Therapy of Renal Diseases and Related Disorders, Second Edition

Therapy of Renal Diseases and Related Disorders, Second Edition

Edited by
Wadi N. Suki
The Methodist Hospital
Baylor College of Medicine
Houston, Texas
and
Shaul G. Massry
Division of Nephrology
University of Southern
California
Los Angeles, California

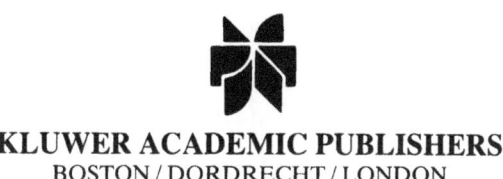

KLUWER ACADEMIC PUBLISHERS
BOSTON / DORDRECHT / LONDON

Distributors for North America:
Kluwer Academic Publishers
101 Philip Drive
Assinippi Park
Norwell, Massachusetts 02061 USA

Distributors for all other countries:
Kluwer Academic Publishers Group
Distribution Centre
Post Office Box 322
3300 AH Dordrecht, THE NETHERLANDS

Library of Congress Cataloging-in-Publication Data
Therapy of renal diseases and related disorders/edited by Wadi N.
  Suki and Shaul G. Massry.—2nd ed.
    p. cm.
  Includes bibliographical references.
  ISBN 0-7923-0676-7
    1. Kidneys—Diseases—Treatment. 2. Urinary organs—
Diseases—Treatment. I. Suki, Wadi N., 1934–
II. Massry, Shaul G.
    [DNLM: 1. Kidney Diseases—therapy. WJ 300 T398]
RC902.T49 1990
616.6′106—dc20
DNLM/DLC
for Library of Congress   90-4136
                                                                   CIP

Copyright © 1991 by Kluwer Academic Publishers
Third Printing 1993
Printed on acid-free paper.

All rights reserved. No part of this publication may be
reproduced, stored in a retrieval system or transmitted in any
form or by any means, mechanical, photocopying, recording, or
otherwise, without the prior written permission of the publisher,
Kluwer Academic Publishers, 101 Philip Drive, Assinippi Park,
Norwell, Massachusetts 02061.

PRINTED IN THE UNITED STATES OF AMERICA.

Contents

Foreword		ix
Preface to the First Edition		xi
Preface to the Second Edition		xiii
Contributors		xv

PART ONE: DISORDERS OF FLUID, ELECTROLYTE, AND ACID-BASE BALANCE

1. Treatment of hypoosmolar and hyperosmolar states STEPHEN BRENNAN AND J. CARLOS AYUS 1
2. Polyuric syndromes WILLIAM P. MULDOWNEY AND MICHAEL H. HUMPHREYS 17
3. Edematous states ARTHUR GREENBERG AND JULES B. PUSCHETT 27
4. Disorders of potassium metabolism JACQUES J. BOURGOIGNIE, JAMES R. OSTER, GUIDO O. PEREZ, AND DOLLIE F. GREEN 45
5. Disorders of calcium metabolism AARON HALABE AND ROGER A.L. SUTTON 91
6. Disorders of magnesium metabolism THOMAS DYCKNER 111
7. Disorders of phosphate metabolism MOSHE LEVI AND JAMES P. KNOCHEL 121
8. Nephrolithiasis and nephrocalcinosis JOAN H. PARKS AND FREDRIC L. COE 139
9. Metabolic alkalosis SANDRA SABATINI AND NEIL A. KURTZMAN 159
10. Metabolic acidosis ROBERT M.A. RICHARDSON AND MITCHELL L. HALPERIN 177
11. Diabetic ketoacidosis HORACIO J. ADROGUÉ, JORGE BARRERO, AND GEORGE M. DOLSON ... 193
12. Renal tubular acidosis FERNANDO SANTOS, GAD KAINER, AND JAMES C.M. CHAN 207
13. Respiratory acid-base disturbances GREGORIO I. CASAR AND R. KEITH WILSON 223
14. Mixed acid-base disorders JOHN T. HARRINGTON AND NICOLAOS E. MADIAS 233
15. Fluid and electrolyte abnormalities in children ADRIAN SPITZER AND RICHARD NEIBERGER 245
16. Fluid and electrolyte disorders in the surgical patient HERVY H. HINER, JR. AND WADI N. SUKI 263
17. Fluid and electrolyte disorders in the thermally injured CHARLES BAXTER 277
18. Acute renal failure DAVID M. GILLUM, JOHN D. CONGER, AND ROBERT J. ANDERSON 285

PART TWO: INTRINSIC PARENCHYMAL DISEASE

A. Glomerular

19. Acute glomerulonephritis and glomerulonephritis in bacterial endocarditis DAVID S. BALDWIN AND JOEL NEUGARTEN 305

20. Nephrotic syndrome GERALD C. GROGGEL AND WAYNE A. BORDER 317
21. Goodpasture's syndrome CURTIS B. WILSON 333
22. Hematuria and IgA nephropathy JOJI OHNO 343

B. Tubulointerstitial

23. Urinary tract infections MARVIN FORLAND 349
24. Vesicoureteral reflux and reflux nephropathy PRISCILLA KINCAID-SMITH 363
25. Genitourinary tuberculosis JAMES E. GOW 387

PART THREE: RENAL INVOLVEMENT IN SYSTEMIC DISEASE

26. Systemic lupus erythematosus SUSAN L. ANDREW AND DAVID P. HUSTON 395
27. Vasculitic diseases of the kidney JAMES E. BALOW AND HOWARD A. AUSTIN III 413
28. Noninflammatory vascular diseases of the kidney GARABED EKNOYAN 425
29. Thrombotic microangiopathy ELLIN LIEBERMAN 443
30. Renal involvement in dysproteinemias DOMINIQUE GANEVAL AND JEAN-PIERRE GRÜNFELD ... 453
31. Hyperuricemic nephropathy EDWARD R. AHRENS AND THOMAS H. STEELE 469
32. Renal disorders in liver disease MURRAY EPSTEIN 477
33. Renal complications of pregnancy JOHN M. DAVISON, ADRIAN I. KATZ, AND MARSHALL D. LINDHEIMER 495
34. Diabetic nephropathy ELI A. FRIEDMAN 533

PART FOUR: HEREDITARY AND CONGENITAL DISEASES

35. Renal cystic disorders JARED J. GRANTHAM, JOANN B. RECKLING, AND SHARON L. SLUSHER 543
36. Renal disorders in sickle hemoglobinemia STEPHANIE LEAR AND ROBERT M. ROSA 573
37. Inherited renal tubular disorders RUSSELL W. CHESNEY 581

PART FIVE: NEOPLASIA

38. Cancers of the kidney and urinary tract PETER T. SCARDINO AND MADELINE CANTINI 593

PART SIX: CHEMICAL AND PHYSICAL INJURIES

39. Toxic nephropathies JOHN F. MAHER 613
40. Acute drug intoxications JAMES F. WINCHESTER 639

PART SEVEN: CHRONIC RENAL FAILURE

A. Medical therapy

41. Prevention of progression of renal insufficiency GIUSEPPE MASCHIO, LAMBERTO OLDRIZZI, AND CARLO RUGIU 649
42. Renal insufficiency EBERHARD F. RITZ 659
43. Anesthesia and surgery in the patient with renal failure DAVID R. BEVAN 669
44. Nutritional management of the uremic patient MARKUS TESCHNER AND AUGUST HEIDLAND 675
45. Cardiovascular complications of uremia and dialysis J. CARLOS AYUS AND R.K. KROTHAPALLI 697
46. Renal osteodystrophy SHAUL G. MASSRY 711
47. Neurologic and psychiatric disorders in renal failure SUHAIL AHMAD AND CHRISTOPHER R. BLAGG 719
48. Hematologic disorders in renal failure K.M. KOCH 733

B. Peritoneal dialysis

49. Acute, intermittent, and cycled peritoneal dialysis JOSE A. DIAZ-BUXO 739
50. Continuous ambulatory peritoneal dialysis ROBERT A. MACTIER AND KARL D. NOLPH 755

C. Hemodialysis

51. Dialysis access surgery GEORGE P. NOON AND H. DAVID SHORT 775
52. Dialyzers, dialysates, and water treatment N.K. MAN AND J.L. FUNCK-BRENTANO 791
53. Membrane biocompatibility ALFRED K. CHEUNG.. 813
54. Dialysis, ultrafiltration, and hemofiltration RAYMOND C. VANHOLDER, NICOLAS H. HOENICH, AND SEVERIN M. RINGOIR 841
55. Use of drugs in uremia and dialysis D. CRAIG BRATER 853

D. Transplantation

56. Donor and recipient selection STUART M. FLECHNER 867
57. Immunosuppression and treatment of rejection YVES F. CH. VANRENTERGHEM.................. 887
58. Tubular and metabolic dysfunction following kidney transplantation J. WINAVER, J. GREEN, AND O. S. BETTER.. 905
59. Renal transplantation in systemic inherited and metabolic disease ELEANOR D. LEDERER AND WADI N. SUKI 921
60. Complications of renal transplantation JOHN A. MURIE AND PETER J. MORRIS 943

PART EIGHT: MISCELLANEOUS

61. The catheter GRANNUM R. SANT AND EDWIN M. MEARES, JR. 955
62. Nonsurgical management of vesicourethral dysfunction J. KEITH LIGHT......................... 969

Index 975

Foreword[1]

"Where are all these kidney patients coming from? A few years ago we had never heard of kidney disease and now you are speaking of patients in the hundreds of thousands and indeed potentially millions." My reply, not meant to be grim, was "From the cemetery, Sir." This is a summary of some Congressional testimony I once gave on behalf of extending kidney disease under Medicare. Where indeed were all the patients with kidney disease in the United States before World War II? They were certainly not under the care of nephrologists! Nephrology was not listed in the questionnaires for any state or the American Medical Association as a subspecialty or even as a special interest. Indeed, even in the late 1960s, when I wrote the American Medical Association editor and asked why nephrology had not been included on a questionnaire to American physicians about their specialty interests, I received a "tongue in check" answer, "What's nephrology?" Indeed, for those of us who bridge back, it is often hard to realize the rapid evolution of our specialty. For uremia, we gave low-protein diets, adequate hydration, attention to fluid and electrolytes, comfort, and prayer. In my first two years at Georgetown, where every death in the hospital was reviewed, my nephrology division made death conference all but a few weeks out of the first two years. In a 1961 book on uremia[2] I wrote:

> The reversibility of uremic coma has received some attention but could use more. In a further effort to discourage pessimism we have therefore placed a capital 'R' following each of the potentially reversible types of renal disease. It is our sincere hope that the number of 'R's will provide a pleasant surprise for the many physicians and medical students who want to think of the uremic syndrome as a terminal state during which little treatment can be instituted except that designed for the comfort of the patient.

This is not to say that the science underlying nephrology was inactive. Quite to the contrary, many cases of fruitful science relating to the kidney area not only existed but flourished and had a profound impact on many young clinicians. Thomas Addis raised to a state of applied perfection the study of the urinary sediment, clinically practical kidney function tests, and the natural history of a number of kidney diseases including glomerulonephritis. William Goldring, Herbert Chasis, Dana Atchley, and others studied the effects of hypertension, endocarditis, and circulatory diseases on the kidney and spawned successive generations of alert clinical investigators, who began to chronicle the natural histories of a wide variety of kidney diseases. Quantitative studies of renal function flourished under a school headed by Homer Smith, and surprisingly precise techniques were developed for studying a whole range of explicit nephron functions. Imagine the joy with the advent of vascular catheterization to be able to apply extraction ratios and the Fick principle in a precise way to an organ such as the kidney by sampling arterial blood, venous blood, and the output of the urine! One had a quantitative handle on the entire function of a vital organ — perhaps for the first time in biologic history. One no longer looked only at the street side of the revolving door; one could find out, for example, that if ammonia did not go into the acid trap of the urine, it indeed might go back into the circulation via the renal vein.

The same story unfolded for a broad range of physiologic substances. In the metabolic school of nephrology, represented perhaps most brilliantly by Professor John Peters at Yale, a host of pioneer investigators applied the methods of quantitative clinical biochemistry to the elements of the blood whose homeostasis was so carefully regulated by the kidney. His deep interest in endocrinology and metabolism pointed our way to appreciate the endocrine role of the kidney in making or releasing a whole array of potent hormones affecting bodily function (e.g., erythropoietin, renin, aldosterone, etc.), and indeed the very survival of the human organism. The role of the kidney in controlling vitamin D metabolism, calcium absorption, parathyroid function, and the complex inter-relationships comprising calcium/phosphorous homeostasis, bone growth, and bone repair were only mistily appreciated and became one of the great metabolic success stories of postwar nephrology and metabolism. Postwar nephrology rushed to the fore and supplied nephrologists with such wonderful tools as the flamephotometer, electro-

---

[1] Revised for the second edition.

[2] Schreiner GE Maher JF: Uremia, Chemistry and Pathogenesis & Treatment. Charles C. Thomas, Springfield, IL, p 24, 1961.

phoresis, microchemistry, immunoassay, sonography, renal biopsy, immunofluorescence, electron microscopy, and unclear magnetic resonance, and permitted a total integration of form, histologic structure, and function. Clinical nephrology became indeed the real fusion of biochemistry, physiology, immunology, renal endocrinology, and the focus of newer imaging techniques.

With this precision in diagnosis, one could realistically hope for rational therapy, and one could be optimistic that some day the correct therapy would be correctly applied to the correct patient with the appropriately diagnosed disease.

With the evolution of such developments, an expert observer could indeed realistically hope that out of the myriad and mushrooming books of nephrology would come one with a message of constructive hope, focusing on the treatment of renal disease. Indeed, Dr. Suki and Dr. Massry have fulfilled that hope with this book, which is appropriately entitled, *The Therapy of Renal Disease and Related Disorders*. They have systematically taken the available scientific information and fused it into a practical text of therapy for the patient. The first section, entitled "Disorders of Fluid, Electrolyte and Acid-Base Balance," covers some of the more challenging general conditions, such as hyperosmolar and hypoosmolar states, polyuria, edema, and acute renal failure. The book then proceeds systematically to disorders of the ions, potassium, calcium, magnesium, phosphate, and the major quartet of acid-base balance, embracing alkalosis and acidosis in its clinically presentable forms. The book proceeds to the intrinsic parenchymal diseases, covering the major areas of glomerular and tubular interstitial disorders and what can be done about them. From there it launches into the vast sea of relationships with systemic diseases such as SLE, vasculitis, hyperuricemia, dysproteinemia, liver disease, pregnancy, and diabetes, among others. Adequate attention is paid to genetic and congenital disorders, including the genetic counseling of families beset by genetically determined disorders. Neoplasia, chemical and physical injuries, and a number of other unusual events are considered with practical insights. Then the book tackles the vast problem of uremia and the newer experience with diet, dialysis, and transplantation.

Uremia is to the nephrologist what the baby is to the pediatrician, for it is the final common pathway of literally hundreds of disease processes that lead to scarring and destruction of nephrons.

We estimate that there are well in excess of 300,000 patients in the world living on the varied methodologies represented by the three basic forms of substituted kidney function — hemodialysis, peritoneal dialysis, and renal transplantation: over 100,000 persons in the United States alone, well over 110,000 in the countries compromising the EDTA Registry, and over 100,000 in the Pacific Rim. If we add on South America, Africa, and the lesser developed nations, the total could well be over 400,000 by the time this book is printed. These 400,000 plus persons and their families, who have intimate, repetitive personal experiences with uremia, serve as living withnesses of the medical progress of nephrology in the past three decades. They are witnesses of the fact that many of today's kidney patients have indeed, literally, "come from the cemetery."

But it is not enough to consider only the techniques of substitution therapy. For with living patients come not only the facets of uremia that are not yet handled by therapy, such as cardiovascular complications, renal osteodystrophy, anemia, disorders of immune surveillance, nutritional problems, etc., but there is also a necessity to know which particular patients fit which particular therapy best, and to choose the optimum time for applying one particular therapy to one particular patient. Indeed, the management of the uremic patients becomes essentially a life plan for that person, and the ills that kidney patients have live on with them, instead of going prematurely with them to the grave.

This is a book that is unique among many books available today. This is a book that presents material positively. This is a book that blends the analytical aspects of diagnosis with the hard realities of scientific and appropriate therapy. This is a book that will be enjoyed by young nephrologists and by physicians with a wide diversity of interests. Most of all, it is a book that will be deeply appreciated by their patients.

George E. Schreiner, M.D.
Distinguished Professor of Medicine
Former Director, Division of Nephrology
Georgetown University School of Medicine

Preface to the First Edition

In the last fifteen years, many books and monographs have been published which deal with different aspects of renal structure and function, and the various renal diseases. The number of published works reflects the explosion of scientific knowledge about the kidney and its diseases. Parallel with this increased knowledge have come major advances in the handling and management of patients suffering from disorders of the kidney. These advances, many of which are life-saving, in large measure have been responsible for the emergence of nephrology as a full-fledged medical specialty.

In spite of the progress made in the therapy of renal diseases and related disorders, there has not been a text devoted fully to this subject. The present text attempts to bring together in one ready reference what is known about renal therapeutics today thereby focusing attention on this vital aspect of nephrology and recording the present state-of-the-art.

The major strides forward in renal therapy shall be clear to the reader of this volume. Areas where advances or breakthroughs are still needed or where solid, objective proof of efficacy is still lacking shall be equally clear. The rapid pace of new research on renal therapy continued during the period that this text was in preparation, and this rapid pace attests to the vitality of nephrology as a discipline. We look forward to the preparation of new editions of this volume reflecting substantive advances which will continue to be made.

It is fitting, in closing, to acknowledge the generosity of each of the contributing authors who have given selflessly of their precious time to prepare their respective chapters, and the forbearance of our publisher, who has waited patiently as the process of assembling and editing this volume proceeded.

Wadi N. Suki
Shaul G. Massry

Preface to the Second Edition

It is said that a static science is a dead science, and to any observer of nephrology it is quite clear that there has been nothing static about this discipline. Even while the first edition was under preparation, newer treatments were being developed, the efficacy of new treatments was being tested, and the results of such trials were being published. It is impossible to capture in a book all the progress that is being made in a particular discipline that is changing rapidly, for to do so would be akin to capturing motion in a still picture. One can convey the impression of motion in a still picture, but it takes a video or a movie to capture motion. And so it is in nephrology, a field in which it should be clear to any one who takes more than a cursory look that major developments and important advances are being made steadily. We were almost prophetic, therefore, when we said in the preface to the first edition:

> The rapid pace of new research on renal therapy continued during the period that this text was in preparation, and this rapid pace attests to the vitality of nephrology as a discipline. We look forward to the preparation of new editions of this volume reflecting substantial advances which will continue to be made.

No sooner had the first edition come out in print than had a process of obsolescence already begun to set in as the wheels of progress kept on turning — hopefully leading us all forward. We were almost prophetic in predicting "the preparation of new editions." So now we come back with a new edition to report on some of the advances that were made since the first edition, and luckily for us all, and above all for our patients, advances have been made and continue to be made as we write these words. We have invited many of the past authors to update their chapters, while several new authors were invited to rewrite chapters on topics previously covered or to write new chapters on topics not previously covered. The task of writing a chapter is an onerous task and, having ourselves written many chapters for many texts, we are keenly aware of the time and effort that goes into the preparation of a chapter. In addition, it is all for very little reward, whether it is in terms of monetary returns to the author or in terms of the academic recognition that the author derives from writing a chapter, as compared with a scientific article in a peer-reviewed journal reporting original scientific research. One can only conclude, therefore, that hundreds of authors undertake the task of writing a chapter propelled not by the motive of profit but by that of the noble commitment to convey to their fellow physicians the latest advances in their respective areas of expertise, with the aim of bettering the health of their patients and of raising the standards of the care they receive. It is fitting then to bear in mind that a text such as this is a tribute to each of the authors who contributed to it, and all of us who shall consult this text, as we tackle the complexities of managing our patients, are in their debt.

Wadi N. Suki
Shaul G. Massry

Contributors

CHAPTER 1

Stephen Brennan, M.D.
Assistant Professor of Medicine
Department of Medicine
Baylor College of Medicine
Houston, Texas 77030

J. Carlos Ayus, M.D.
Professor of Medicine
Department of Medicine
Baylor College of Medicine
Houston, Texas 77030

CHAPTER 2

William P. Muldowney, M.D.
Fellow in Nephrology
San Francisco General Hospital
San Francisco, California 94110

Michael H. Humphreys, M.D.
Chief, Division of Nephrology
San Francisco General Hospital
Associate Professor of Medicine
University of California
San Francisco, California 94110

CHAPTER 3

Arthur Greenberg, M.D.
Associate Professor of Medicine
Renal-Electrolyte Division
University of Pittsburgh School of Medicine
Pittsburgh, Pennsylvania 15261

Jules B. Puschett, M.D.
Professor and Chairman
Department of Medicine
Tulane University School of Medicine
1430 Tulane Avenue
New Orleans, Louisiana 70112-2699

CHAPTER 4

Jacques J. Bourgoignie, M.D.
Professor of Medicine
Chief, Division of Nephrology
University of Miami/Jackson Memorial Medical Center
VA Medical Center
Miami, Florida 33101

James R. Oster, M.D.
Professor of Medicine
University of Miami
VA Medical Center
Miami, Florida 33101

Guido O. Perez, M.D.
Professor of Medicine
University of Miami
VA Medical Center
Miami, Florida 33101

Dollie F. Green, M.D.
Assistant Professor of Clinical Medicine
University of Miami School of Medicine
Miami, Florida 33101

CHAPTER 5

Aaron Halabe, M.D.
Visiting Scientist
Department of Medicine
Vancouver General Hospital
University of British Columbia
Vancouver, B.C., Canada V5Z 1M9

Roger A.L. Sutton, M.D.
Vancouver General Hospital
Laurel Pavillion-3
910 West 10th Avenue
Vancouver, B.C., Canada, V5Z 1M9

CHAPTER 6

Thomas Dyckner
Associate Professor of Medicine
Department of Internal Medicine
Nacka Sjukhus
Nacka, Sweden

CHAPTER 7

Moshe Levi, M.D.
Assistant Professor of Medicine
University of Texas
Southwestern Medical Center
and Chief, Home Dialysis
VA Medical Center
Dallas, Texas 75216

James P. Knochel, M.D.
Professor of Medicine
University of Texas
Southwestern Medical Center
and VA Medical Center
Dallas, Texas 75235-9030

CHAPTER 8

Joan H. Parks, M.B.A.
Nephrology Section
Box 28
University of Chicago
5841 South Maryland Avenue
Chicago, IL 60637

Fredric L. Coe, M.D.
Professor of Medicine
Department of Medicine
Michael Reese Hospital
University of Chicago
Chicago, Illinois 60616

CHAPTER 9

Sandra Sabatini, Ph.D., M.D.
Professor of Medicine
Department of Internal Medicine
and Physiology
Texas Tech University
Health Sciences Center
Lubbock, Texas 79430

Neil A. Kurtzman, M.D.
Professor of Medicine
Chairman, Department of Medicine
Texas Tech University
Health Sciences Center
Lubbock, Texas 79430

CHAPTER 10

Robert M.A. Richardson, M.D.
University of Toronto
Division of Nephrology
Toronto General Hospital
and St. Michael's Hospital
Toronto, Ontario, Canada M5B 1A6

Mitchell L. Halperin, M.D.
Professor of Medicine
University of Toronto
Toronto General Hospital
and St. Michael's Hospital
Toronto, Ontario, Canada M5B 1A6

CHAPTER 11

Horacio J. Adrogué, M.D.
Associate Professor of Medicine
Department of Medicine
Baylor College of Medicine
Houston, Texas 77030

Jorge Barrero, M.D.
Fellow in Nephrology
Department of Medicine
Baylor College of Medicine
Houston, Texas 77030

George M. Dolson, M.D.
Assistant Professor of Medicine
VA Medical Center
Houston, Texas 77030

CHAPTER 12

Fernando Santos, M.D.
Professor of Pediatrics
University of Oviedo
Ministerio de Sanidad y Consumo
Instituto Nacional de la Salud
Hospital "NTRA. STA. de Covadonga"
Oviedo, Asturia
Spain

Gad Kainer, M.B., B.S.. F.R.A.C.P.
Visiting Scholar, Department of Pediatrics
Virginia Commonwealth University's
Medical College of Virginia
Richmond, Virginia 23298

James C.M. Chan, M.D.
Professor and Vice Chairman
Department of Pediatrics
Chairman, Division of Nephrology
Children's Medical Center
Department of Pediatrics
Virginia Commonwealth University's
Medical College of Virginia
Richmond, Virginia 23298

CHAPTER 13

Gregorio I. Casar, M.D.
Instructor in Medicine
Pulmonary Section
Baylor College of Medicine
Houston, Texas 77030

R. Keith Wilson, M.D.
Associate Professor
Department of Medicine
Director of Respiratory Care Services
Baylor College of Medicine
and The Methodist Hospital
Houston, Texas 77030

CHAPTER 14

John T. Harrington, M.D.
Professor of Medicine
Tufts University School of Medicine
and Chief of Medicine
Newton-Wellesley Hospital
Newton, Massachusetts

Nicolaos E. Madias, M.D.
Professor of Medicine
Tufts University School of Medicine
and Chief, Division of Nephrology
New England Medical Center Hospitals
Boston, Massachusetts 02111

CHAPTER 15

Adrian Spitzer, M.D.
Professor of Pediatrics
Director, Division of Nephrology
Albert Einstein College of Medicine
Bronx, New York 10461

Richard Neiberger, M.D., Ph.D.
Assistant Professor
Department of Pediatrics
Albert Einstein College of Medicine
Bronx, New York 10461

CHAPTER 16

Hervy H. Hiner, Jr. M.D.
Assistant Professor of Medicine
Department of Medicine
Baylor College of Medicine
Houston, Texas 77030

Wadi N. Suki, M.D.
Professor of Medicine
Chief, Renal Section
Baylor College of Medicine
Houston, Texas 77030

CHAPTER 17

Charles Baxter, M.D.
Professor of Surgery
Department of Surgery
University of Texas
Health Sciences Center
Dallas, Texas 75235

CHAPTER 18

David M. Gillum, M.D.
Assistant Professor of Medicine
Department of Medicine
Baylor College of Medicine
Houston, Texas 77030

John D. Conger, M.D.
Associate Professor of Medicine
Division of Renal Diseases
VA Medical Center
Denver, Colorado 80220

Robert J. Anderson, M.D.
Professor of Medicine
Chief, Medical Service
University of Colorado
Health Sciences Center
Denver, Colorado 80220

CHAPTER 19

David S. Baldwin, M.D.
New York University Medical Center
Renal Section
New York, N.Y. 10016

Joel Neugarten, M.D.
Montefiore Hospital
111 East 210th Street
Bronx, New York 10467

CHAPTER 20

Gerald C. Groggel, M.D.
Assistant Professor of Medicine
University of Vermont
D305 Given Building
Burlington, Vermont 05405

Wayne A. Border, M.D.
Professor of Medicine
Chief, Division of Nephrology & Hypertension
University of Utah
Health Science Center
Salt Lake City, Utah 84132

xviii *Contributors*

CHAPTER 21

Curtis B. Wilson, M.D.
Professor of Medicine
Department of Immunology
Research Institute of Scripps Clinic
La Jolla, California 92037

CHAPTER 22

Joji Ohno, M.D.
Professor Emeritus
Department of Internal Medicine
Juntendo University School of Medicine
Tokyo, Japan

CHAPTER 23

Marvin Forland, M.D.
Associate Dean for Clinical Affairs
Professor of Medicine
University of Texas
Health Science Center
San Antonio, Texas 78284-7790

CHAPTER 24

Priscilla Kincaid-Smith, M.D.
Professor of Medicine
Department of Medicine
University of Melbourne
Director of Nephrology
The Royal Melbourne Hospital
Parkville, Victoria 3052
Australia

CHAPTER 25

James E. Gow, M.D
Ingerthorpe
Liverpool L23 6 UL
England

CHAPTER 26

Susan L. Andrew
Clinical Immunology Senior Fellow
Department of Medicine
Baylor College of Medicine
Houston, Texas 77030

David P. Huston, M.D.
Associate Professor
Department of Medicine
and Microbiology and Immunology
Baylor College of Medicine
Director, Immunology Service
and Immunotherapy Unit
The Methodist Hospital
Houston, Texas 77030

CHAPTER 27

James E. Balow, M.D.
Clinical Director, NIDDK
Chief, Kidney Disease Section
National Institutes of Health
Bethesda, Maryland 20892

Howard A. Austin III, M.D.
Chief, Nephrology Service, NIDDK
National Institutes of Health
Bethesda, Maryland 20892

CHAPTER 28

Garabed Eknoyan, M.D.
Professor of Medicine
Department of Medicine
Baylor College of Medicine
Houston, Texas 77030

CHAPTER 29

Ellin Lieberman, M.D.
Children's Hospital of Los Angeles
P.O. Box 54700
Los Angeles, California 90054-0700

CHAPTER 30

Dominique Ganeval, M.D.
Department de Nephrologie
Hopital NECKER
Paris, France

Jean-Pierre Grünfeld, M.D.
Professeur of Medicine
Department de Nephrologie
Hopital NECKER
Paris, France

CHAPTER 31

Edward R. Ahrens, M.D.
Fellow in Nephrology
Department of Medicine
University of Wisconsin
Madison, Wisonsin 53706

Thomas H. Steele, M.D.
Professor of Medicine
Department of Medicine
University of Wisconsin
Madison, Wisconsin 53706

CHAPTER 32

Murray Epstein, M.D.
Professor of Medicine
University of Miami
Chief, Renal Section
VA Medical Center
Miami, Florida 33125

CHAPTER 33

John M. Davison, M.D.
Professor of Medicine
and Obstetrics & Gynecology
University of Chicago
Chicago, Illinois 60637

Adrian I. Katz, M.D.
Dept. of Medicine
University of Chicago
5841 S. Maryland
Chicago, Illinois 60637

Marshall D. Lindheimer, M.D.
Dept. of Medicine
University of Chicago
5841 S. Maryland
Chicago, Illinois 60637

CHAPTER 34

Eli A. Friedman, M.D.
Professor of Medicine
Department of Medicine
State University of New York
Health Science Center
Brooklyn, New York

CHAPTER 35

Jared J. Grantham, M.D.
Professor of Medicine
Director, Division of Nephrology
University of Kansas Medical Center
Kansas City, Kansas 66103

Joann B. Reckling, R.N., M.N.
Research Assistant
Division of Nephrology
University of Kansas Medical Center
Kansas City, Kansas 66103

Sharon L. Slusher, R.N.
Nurse Coordinator
University of Kansas Medical Center
Kansas City, Kansas 66103

CHAPTER 36

Stephanie Lear, M.D.
Department of Medicine
Beth Israel Hospital and Harvard Medical School
Boston, Massachusetts 02215

Robert M. Rosa, M.D.
Assistant Professor of Medicine
Harvard Medical School
Associate Director
Clinical Research Center
Beth Israel Hospital
Boston, Massachusetts 02215

CHAPTER 37

Russell W. Chesney, M.D.
Le Bonheur Professor and Chair
Department of Pediatrics
The University of Tennessee, Memphis
848 Adams, Room 306
Memphis, Tennessee 38104

CHAPTER 38

Peter T. Scardino, M.D.
Professor of Urology
Department of Urology
Baylor College of Medicine
Houston, Texas 77030

Madeline Cantini, R.N.
Department of Urology
Baylor College of Medicine
Houston, Texas 77030

CHAPTER 39

John F. Maher, M.D.
Professor of Medicine
Director, Nephrology Division
F. Edward Hebert School of Medicine
Bethesda, Maryland 20814-4799

CHAPTER 40

James F. Winchester, M.D.
Professor of Medicine
Department of Medicine
Division of Nephrology
Georgetown University Medical Center
Washington, D.C. 20007

CHAPTER 41

Giuseppe Maschio, M.D.
Division of Nephrology
Instituti Ospitalieri
Verona, Italy

Lamberto Oldrizzi, M.D.
Assistant Professor of Nephrology
Division of Nephrology
University of Verona
Verona, Italy

Carlo Rugiu, M.D.
Assistant Professor of Nephrology
Division of Nephrology
University of Verona
Verona, Italy

CHAPTER 42

Eberhard F. Ritz, M.D.
Professor of Medicine
Sektion Nephrologie
Klinikum der Universitat Heidelberg
Heidelberg, Germany

CHAPTER 43

David R. Bevan, M.D.
Professor and Chairman
Department of Anesthesia
McGill University
Montreal, Quebec, Canada

CHAPTER 44

Markus Teschner, M.D.
Nephrologische Abteilung
Medizinische Universitatsklinik
Wurzburg, Germany

August Heidland, M.D.
Professor of Medicine
Chief, Nephrologische Abteilung
Medizinische Universitatsklinik
Wurzburg, Germany

CHAPTER 45

J. Carlos Ayus, M.D.
Professor of Medicine
Department of Medicine
Baylor College of Medicine
Houston, Texas 77030

R.K. Krothapalli, M.D.
Clinical Assistant Professor of Medicine
Department of Medicine
University of Alabama
Birmingham, Alabama

CHAPTER 46

Shaul G. Massry, M.D.
Professor of Medicine
Chief, Division of Nephrology
University of Southern California
Los Angeles, California 90033

CHAPTER 47

Suhail Ahmad, M.D.
Associate Professor of Medicine
University of Washington
Medical Director
Scribner Kidney Center
Seattle, Washington 98915

Christopher R. Blagg, M.D. F.R.C.P.
Executive Director
Northwest Kidney Center
Seattle, Washington 98122

CHAPTER 48

K.M. Koch, M.D.
Department of Nephrology
Center of Internal Medicine
Hannover Medical School
Federal Republic of Germany

CHAPTER 49

Jose A. Diaz-Buxo, M.D.
Director, Home Dialysis
Metrolina Kidney Center
Associate Clinical Professor of Medicine
University of North Carolina
Charlotte, North Carolina 28204

CHAPTER 50

Robert A. Mactier, M.D.
Renal Fellow
Division of Nephrology
Department of Medicine
University of Missouri
Columbia, Missouri 65212

Karl D. Nolph, M.D.
Director, Division of Nephrology
Professor of Medicine
Department of Medicine
University of Missouri
VA Hospital and Dalton Research Center
Columbia, Missouri 65212

CHAPTER 51

George P. Noon, M.D.
Professor of Surgery
Department of Surgery
Baylor College of Medicine
Houston, Texas 77030

H. David Short, M.D.
Assistant Professor of Surgery
Department of Surgery
Baylor College of Medicine
Houston, Texas 77030

CHAPTER 52

N.K. Man, M.D.
Department of Nephrologie
Hopital NECKER
Paris, France

J.L. Funck-Brentano, M.D.
Professeur of Medicine
Department of Nephrologie
Hopital NECKER
Paris, France

CHAPTER 53

Alfred K. Cheung, M.D.
Assistant Professor of Medicine
University of Utah School of Medicine
VA Medical Center
Salt Lake City, Utah 84148

CHAPTER 54

Raymond C. Vanholder, M.D.
Nephrology Department
University Hospital
Universitair Ziekenhuis
Ghent, Belgium

Nicolas H. Hoenich, M.D.
Department of Medicine
University of Newcastle-upon-Tyne
Newcastle-upon-Tyne, United Kingdom

Severin M. Ringoir, M.D.
Director, Nephrology Division
Nephrology Department
Universitair Ziekenhuis
Ghent, Belgium

CHAPTER 55

D. Craig Brater, M.D.
Director of Clinical Phamacology
Professor of Medicine
Indiana University School of Medicine
Indianapolis, Indiana 46202

CHAPTER 56

Stuart M. Flechner, M.D.
Associate Professor of Surgery (Urology)
Director, Division of Transplantation
Department of Surgery
Stanford University School of Medicine
Stanford, California 94305

CHAPTER 57

Yves F. Ch. Vanrenterghem, M.D.
Universitaire Ziekenhuizen Leuven
Department of Nephrology
Leuven, Germany

CHAPTER 58

J. Winaver, M.D.
Department of Nephrology
Rambam Medical Center
and Department of Physiology
Faculty of Medicine
Technion, Haifa, Israel

J. Green, M.D.
Department of Nephrology
Rambam Medical Center
and Department of Physiology
Faculty of Medicine
Technion, Haifa, Israel

O.S. Better, M.D.
Department of Nephrology
Rambam Medical Center
and Department of Physiology
Faculty of Medicine
Technion, Haifa, Israel

CHAPTER 59

Eleanor D. Lederer, M.D.
Assistant Professor of Medicine
Department of Medicine
Baylor College of Medicine
Houston, Texas 77030

Wadi N. Suki, M.D.
Professor of Medicine
Chief, Renal Section
Baylor College of Medicine
Houston, Texas 77030

CHAPTER 60

John A. Murie, M.A., M.D., F.R.C.S.
Consultant Surgeon
The Royal Infirmary
Edinburgh, U.K.

Peter J. Morris, M.D.
Nuffield Department of Surgery
University of Oxford
John Radcliffe Hospital
Oxford, England

CHAPTER 61

Grannum R. Sant, M.D.
Associate Professor of Urology
Department of Urology
Tufts University School of Medicine
and New England Medical Center Hospitals
Boston, Massachusetts 02111

Edwin M. Meares, Jr., M.D.
Charles M. Whitney Professor and Chairman
Department of Urology
Tufts University School of Medicine
and New England Medical Center Hospitals
Boston, Massachusetts 02111

CHAPTER 62

J. Keith Light, M.D.
Associate Professor of Urology
Scott Department of Urology
Baylor College of Medicine
Houston, Texas 77030

CHAPTER 1

Treatment of Hypoosmolar and Hyperosmolar States

STEPHEN BRENNAN & J. CARLOS AYUS

INTRODUCTION

Under usual conditions, the osmolarity of the extracellular fluid (ECF) is maintained within an extremely narrow range. When this range is exceeded, the cells of the body are subject to an injurious influx or efflux of water, which preserves the uniform tonicity of all body fluids. Thus, in situations where the osmolarity of body fluids is disturbed, the principal pathophysiology is related to the inability of cells to maintain normal volume (and hence structure and function). Of course, each of the somatic cells of the body has the ability to regulate its own volume; when this regulatory ability is exceeded, symptoms referable to hypoosmolarity or hyperosmolarity appear. Before discussing specific clinical syndromes of deranged plasma tonicity, it is appropriate to review some important aspects of cell volume regulation.

CELL VOLUME REGULATION

Several elements participate in the determination of any cell's volume. Since most mammalian cells are easily distensible, hydrostatic pressure gradients cannot be maintained across cell membranes. Furthermore, there can be no separation of charge across cell membranes; electroneutrality must be maintained. Water is in thermodynamic equilibrium across cell membranes; thus, cell solute content ultimately determines cell volume at any given osmolarity.

Within cells, the solutes can be broadly grouped into two classes. First are those solutes that do not undergo significant transmembrane transport. These include large anionic macromolecules such as proteins, enzymes, and the like. The second group of intracellular solutes are those that are able to undergo substantial movement into or out of cells. Examples of such species would be Na^+, K^+, amino acids, glucose, and other small organic and inorganic molecules. It is the ability of the cell to control the content of these solutes that is the mechanism of cell volume regulation.

The cell content of solutes in the steady state is a classic problem in mass balance. On the one hand, most cells contain a pump, the so-called Na-K-ATPase pump, which actively extrudes Na^+ ions from the cytoplasm while simultaneously accumulating K^+ ions within the cytoplasm. The Na^+/K^+ ratio of this pump is believed to be $3:2$, resulting in the net exit of solute from the cell interior. On the other hand, cell membranes have a finite permeability to many ions, resulting in their leak into or out of cells, as determined by the prevailing electrochemical potential. This pump-leak model has been hypothesized as the mechanism by which regulation of cell volume and ionic composition can occur simultaneously. Minor changes in ionic permeability or pump activity can have profound effects on cell volume.

Several excellent reviews have appeared that cover many aspects of cell volume regulation in great detail (1, 2). It is beyond the scope of this chapter to present these findings in depth. Instead, we propose to discuss only those aspects of cell volume regulation that are most pertinent to clinically significant abnormalities in plasma tonicity. Specifically, we will cover the adaptive response of the brain to derangements in extracellular tonicity. These reactions are summarized in Table 1.

ADAPTATION TO HYPOTONIC ECF

Several in-vitro and in-vitro studies attest to the remarkable ability of neuronal cells to resist swelling when exposed to a hypotonic milieu. Nearly 50 years ago, Yannet was unable to document an increase in brain water content in cats after 24 hours of exposure to ECF hypoosmolarity (3). He did find, however, that brain K^+ content had diminished significantly, and proposed that the loss of this solute prevented the development of brain swelling. Other studies have examined the time course of the adaptive response. Data of Arieff et al. (4) have shown that an 18% decrease in ECF osmolarity (from 297 to 244 mOsm/kg) caused an increase in brain water content of 17% with very little change in cellular Na^+, K^+, or Cl^- contents within the first 2 hours. Other groups have also demonstrated volume regulatory decreases in intracellular electrolytes (5). In other words, brain cells act as nearly ideal osmometers during acute exposure to hypotonic ECF. How-

Table 1. Adaptive response of the brain to altered plasma tonicity

Time course	Hypotonicity	Hypertonicity
Immediate Minutes-hours	Cell swelling ↑ brain water	Cell shrinkage ↓ brain water
Intermediate Hours-days	Loss of ions Na^+, K^+, Cl^-	Gain of ions Na^+, K^+, Cl^-
Long term Days-weeks	Loss of amino acids Taurine, glutamine, glutamate	Gain of solutes ↑ Amino acids ↑ Idiogenic osmoles

ever, over the subsequent 1–3 weeks, despite a continued decline in plasma osmolarity to 215 mOsm/kg, cellular water recovered to within 7% of control values. This was accomplished by loss of cellular osmoles amounting to 229 mOsm/kg dry weight which could be accounted for entirely by loss of Na^+ and K^+ plus their accompanying anions. More recent data (6) suggest that depletion of intracellular amino acids (particularly glutamine, glutamate, and taurine) is an important adaptive response late in the course of experimental hyponatremia. One potential mechanism that probably is involved in brain cell volume regulation is inhibition of Na-H exchange (7).

In-vitro studies of brain tissue slices have been difficult to interpret due to problems maintaining physiologic water and ion contents. Since the retina is an extension of cerebral gray matter, it has been used in some experimental systems that measure neuronal adaptation to hypotonicity. With this technique, acute decreases in ECF osmolarity from 283 to 247 mOsm/kg resulted in a very rapid increase in cell water, with no change in cell Na^+ and K^+ contents, which were maintained over 120 minutes of observation (8). These studies confirm that little adaptive change in the solute content of brain occurs in the first few hours of hypoosmolarity, but an extremely efficient adaptive process can occur thereafter.

Direct comparisons between studies examining adaptation of brain and other tissues (e.g., muscle) to cellular swelling may not be valid in most cases, since many experimental differences (e.g., duration and severity of hypotonicity, the way in which it was induced, analytic methods, etc.) exist. However, studies examining the correlation between cell volume homeostasis in various tissues of the same animal have been performed and in general support the notion that volume regulatory decreases in brain cells are both faster and more complete than in muscle cells (9).

ADAPTATION TO HYPERTONIC ECF

The response of excitable cells to a hyperosmolar external fluid is analogous to the response seen during hypoosmolar fluid challenge. Initially the cells shrink due to osmotic water abstraction, but ultimately the cells nearly regain the water content they had in the control state by virtue of net solute uptake. Several important differences also exist. These are mainly in the types of solutes that accumulate within the cells as well as the mechanisms by which they accumulate.

There is some uptake of electrolytes during adaptation to hyperosmolarity in rat brains (10–12). However, while regulatory decreases in brain cell volume occur largely due to decreases in the cytoplasmic content of monovalent cations, these are not the predominant solutes accumulated within the cytosol during regulatory increases in cell volume. Recent studies have provided good support for the notion that unmeasured organic substances, specifically amino acids (13), account for much of the increase in total brain osmoles. Studies of hypernatremia have shown that over the course of 7 days, the water content of the brain decreases by approximately 10% but ultimately recovers to within 98–99% of control (14). This is accompanied by an increase in brain solute content of 235 mOsm/kg dry weight, from 948 to 1183 mOsm/kg dry weight. Of this increase, inorganic ions (Na^+, K^+, Cl^-) accounted for 40 mOsm/kg, whereas amino acids increased by 126 mM/kg. The remaining 69 mOsm/kg increase in solute content was composed of unknown substances, the so-called idiogenic osmoles. The formation of idiogenic osmoles has also been detected in hyperosmolar states due to hyperglycemia and uremia. It is of interest that idiogenic osmole formation does not occur in hyperosmolar states induced by infusion of mannitol or glycerol (15).

In summary, cells of the brain behave as if they were osmometers when subjected to alterations in the ECF osmolarity. Some adaptation to changes in cell volume occurs over the subsequent hours to days, more completely in the brain than in the other tissues. These adjustments are made by alterations in cell solute content. During hypotonicity, cell swelling is reversed mainly by extrusion of Na^+ and K^+ (with their attendant anions). In hypertonic media, uptake of these inorganic ions is responsible for only a minority of cell volume regulation; the major intracellular solutes are amino acids and "idiogenic osmoles."

HYPOOSMOLAR STATES

In clinical practice, hypoosmolar states are usually suspected when the plasma sodium is found to be low. Before embarking on an aggressive therapeutic regimen, however, it is vital to prove that the plasma osmolarity is indeed low. The presence of hyponatremia usually implies hypoosmolarity as well; nevertheless, actual measured osmolarity may be low, normal, or even elevated in patients with hyponatremia. Several excellent reviews discuss these syndromes of "pseudohyponatremia" in great detail and the interested reader is referred to them for a more in-depth treatment of this subject (16, 17). For the sake of convenience, in this chapter we will use the term *hyponatremia* to mean a state of true hypotonic hyponatremia in which the plasma osmolarity has been proven to be low.

In theory, it is possible that hyponatremia could result from the ingestion of large volumes of solute-free water.

In practice, however, subjects with normal renal function are able to excrete over 20 l of free water daily (18), so pure water intoxication in patients with normal renal function is rare. Conversely, hyponatremia could result from losses of salt that far exceed water losses; however, the hemodynamic consequences of such massive losses would likely bring the patient to medical attention before clinically important hypotonicity developed. The most common settings in which hyponatremia occurs involve a combination of the three factors that contribute to the development of a hypoosmolar state. Thus, a relative excess of free water ingestion, impairment of free water excretion, and losses of salt in excess of water occur together to cause significant hyponatremia. The physiology of normal water excretion will be briefly summarized here. A number of recent reviews provide a more detailed consideration of this topic (16, 19).

The diluting segment of the nephron needs adequate water and solute delivery in order to generate free water. A decrease in solute ingestion (as seen in malnutrition or malabsorption) or in the glomerular filtration rate (GFR), or an increase in proximal tubular reabsorption (or both) may diminish the amount of fluid delivered to the distal nephron and thus limit the renal capacity to excrete water. Furthermore, tubulointerstitial nephropathies or administration of diuretics may depress free water excretion by disturbing the normal structure or function of the diluting segment. Finally, the dilute tubular fluid present in the late portion of the thick ascending limb of Henle's loop must be allowed to traverse the remaining portions of the nephron without substantial water reabsorption taking place. The water permeability of the most distal nephron sites is determined in large part by the amount of circulating antidiuretic hormone, arginine vasopressin (AVP). The role of AVP in the distal nephron is to increase water permeability in responsive segments, thus permitting reabsorption of water generated in the diluting segment. Suppression of AVP synthesis and/or release is required for the elaboration of a maximally dilute urine. In normal circumstances, very small decreases in plasma osmolarity are sufficient to suppress maximally the release of AVP from the posterior pituitary. Although plasma osmolarity is thought to be the predominant regulatory influence on AVP release in healthy adults, experimental and clinical observations have shown that AVP secretion is also modified by nonosmotic pathways. Examples of nonosmotic regulation of AVP include volume depletion, nausea, and pharmacologic agents.

Most reviews of the treatment of hyponatremia attempt to classify patients into groups based on a judgement of whether the total body sodium is increased, decreased, or normal. Although this approach is useful in gaining insight into the pathophysiology of the electrolyte disorder, we have elected to view the problem from a slightly different perspective. In general, the treatment of true hypotonic hyponatremia is based on two factors: its severity and the speed with which it develops. Our discussion of the therapy of hypoosmolarity will therefore aim to separate patients whose hyponatremia developed rapidly (over a matter of a few hours) from those whose course has evolved more gradually (a time frame of days to weeks). This scheme will allow some insight into the pathophysiology of the central nervous system (CNS) dysfunction, which is the hallmark of severe symptomatic hyponatremia, as well as providing the means to understand and avoid the most feared complication of the treatment of hyponatremia, central pontine myelinolysis (CPM).

ACUTE HYPONATREMIA

Although many different factors come into play, it is apparent from a review of the literature that the majority of cases of acute hyponatremia occur in relatively few clinical settings (Table 2). The situations of perioperative hyponatremia, hypotonic states complicating treatment with oxytocin, and hyponatremia due to decompensated psychosis and compulsive water drinking are described below.

As early as 1953, water retention out of proportion to sodium retention was noted in surgical patients, accompanied by decreases in urine output and plasma sodium, and an increase in urine salt excretion (20). The factors responsible for this can be broadly classified into alterations in AVP secretion, changes in intrarenal water handling, excessive fluid administration, and drug effects (Table 3). In surgical patients, it has been found that AVP levels measured by bioassay increase by 5- to 50-fold compared with preoperative values (21). There is a slow decline of AVP levels to control values, which usually occurs by the third postoperative day, but high levels occasionally persist until the fifth postoperative day.

Preoperative patients frequently have nonosmotic stimuli for AVP secretion. These include clinical or subclinical volume depletion, nausea, an edema-forming disorder, pain, and anxiety. When these patients are subjected to the additional surgical stimulus for AVP release, extremely high AVP levels can be attained. Chung et al. (22) found that at least 4.4% of surgical procedures were complicated by hyponatremia and that postoperative patients accounted for 25% of all episodes of hyponatremia in their institution.

Despite abnormalities in AVP metabolism or renal function, hyponatremia will not develop unless excess free water is administered. Only a small minority of surgical patients develop hyponatremia, and symptomatic hypo-

Table 2. Common clinical settings for acute hyponatremia

Perioperative hyponatremia
Psychiatric disturbances
  Psychogenic polydipsia
  Acute psychosis
  Drug effects
Oxytocin administration
  Obstetrical
  GI bleeding
Diuretic induced

Table 3. Factors altering water balance in perioperative patients

Elevated ADH levels
  Preoperative volume depletion
  Nausea
  Surgical stimulation
  Pain
Renal water handling
  Glomerular filtration/ ↑ proximal reabsorption
    Preoperative volume depletion
    Intraoperative blood loss
    Hypotension
  Diluting segment dysfunction
    Water reabsorption
      ADH dependent
      ADH independent
Excessive water ingestion
  Hypotonic intravenous fluids
  Other (irrigant fluids)
Drugs
  Narcotics
  Diuretics
  Antiemetics

natremia is rarer still. It is the failure to recognize the compromised ability of the patient to maintain water balance that most often causes water intoxication to occur. Whereas at least 20 l of fluid can usually be excreted daily without difficulty, Arieff has shown that the administration of as little as 8.8 l of water over 2 days can lead to devastating hyponatremia in postoperative women (23).

Another factor may be operating in men undergoing transurethral resection of the prostate (TURP). If obstruction of even a low grade is present, high hydrostatic pressures may be transmitted to the AVP-responsive segments of the kidney and water reabsorption will be greater at any level of permeability than in the unobstructed state. There also may be unrecognized water intake in patients undergoing TURP. It has been estimated that irrigant fluid can be absorbed at a rate of 20 ml/min or higher (24), depending on such factors as the size and congestion of the prostate, the presence of infection, hydrostatic pressure of the irrigant, and experience of the surgeon (25). Because of the routine use of electrocautery during TURP, electrolyte solutions cannot be used as an irrigating fluid. Instead, mannitol, glycine, or sorbitol are the favored fluids. In a procedure lasting 2 hours, upwards of 2.4 l of these sodium free solution might be absorbed. This is often sufficient to decrease plasma sodium by 15–20 mEq/l and to induce symptoms. In men undergoing TURP, another frequently overlooked cause of altered mental status is acute ammonia toxicity, which results from the metabolism of absorbed glycine (26, 27). Ammonia levels as high as 1000 μM/l have been reported in these subjects (28), even associated with brainstem lesions on magnetic resonance imaging (MRI) scans of the brain.

Oxytocin is a drug that is used commonly to hasten labor and in the treatment of gastrointestinal (GI) hemorrhage. AT relatively low doses (< 20 mU/min) oxytocin has little antidiuretic potency. However, at doses of 50 mU/min or greater, urine flow can be inhibited in a dose-dependant fashion to less than 10% of preinfusion rates (29). In most cases, doses of over 20 mU/min are not employed. Occasionally, infusions of this degree are required in especially difficult labor or to deliver the products of conception after intrauterine fetal death, miscarriage, or elective abortion (30–32). Since water is the usual vehicle for oxytocin delivery, increasing the drug dose will cause a simultaneous increase in antidiuretic activity and hypotonic fluid delivery. If doses of oxytocin in the antidiuretic range need to be employed, it is prudent to increase the concentration of the solution rather than simply to increase the infusion rate.

Psychotic patients with psychogenic polydipsia are also at risk for severe hyponatremia (33). Although many neuroleptic agents are said to stimulate the release of AVP, the number of reports in which this has been well documented is surprisingly small. Water clearance in a hyponatremic psychotic patient was abnormal when he received haloperidol, but not during a drug-free interval (34). A similar result has been reported in a patient receiving thiothixene (35). Chlorpromazine has been reported to cause elevated levels of AVP in psychotic subjects compared with pretreatment values (36). However, most investigators have been unable to reproduce these findings in other patients or normal subjects. Several studies have found that treatment with thiothixene, haloperidol, or chlorpromazine in schizophrenic patients or normal volunteers resulted in no change in free water clearance or AVP levels unless hypotension occurred (37–43). It was postulated that the alpha-adrenergic antagonist effect of these agents caused blood pressure to drop, with a resultant nonosmotic stimulus for AVP release (44). Nicotine has also been implicated in one patient as a cause of abnormal water clearance (45).

AVP release may be excessive in some patients with schizophrenia as an integral part of their psychiatric disturbance (33). A patient has been described with markedly abnormal water clearance during a presentation in a mentally decompensated state, which became normal after the administration of neuroleptic agents (46). Drugs used for the treatment of psychosis have been found to inhibit the release of AVP, which normally occurs in response to the dopaminergic agonist apomorphine (41). This is of particular interest, since the most widely held theory of the pathophysiology of schizophrenia is that the psychosis is caused by excessive dopaminergic activity in the brain. Patients will occasionally present with schizophrenia and water intoxication prior to treatment with antipsychotic drugs, and hyponatremia will improve following their institution (46, 47). AVP levels may also decline in some of these patients (43). The response of plasma AVP levels to water loading can also be instructive in this respect. At least one patient has been described in whom AVP levels bore no relationship to plasma osmolarity (48), and several studies have found evidence for a "reset osmostat," allowing release of AVP at plasma osmolarities at which it

Table 4. Signs and symptoms of hyponatremia

Headache
Nausea/vomiting
Lethargy/weakness
Hallucinations
Bizarre behavior
Urinary/fecal incontinence
Seizures
Extrapyramidal reaction
Fixed dilated pupils
Impaired temperature regulation
Opisthotonus
Bradycardia
Hypoventilation/respiratory depression
Decorticate/decerebrate posturing
Coma

Table 5. Causes of ↑ ADH activity in chronic hyponatremia

Unregulated ADH secretion
  SIADH
Diuretic-induced hyponatremia
  Volume depletion
  Hypotension
  Angiotensin
Edema-forming disorders
  ↓ "effective" blood volume
  Diuretics
Miscellaneous
  Hypothyroidism
  Glucocorticoid deficiency

normally would be completely suppressed (48, 49). Patients who are compulsive water drinkers can also develop hyponatremia at lower levels of water intake. Polydipsic subjects who are receiving psychiatric medications may have increased thirst because of dryness of the mouth (as a cholinergic side effect of the drug) or direct stimulation of the hypothalamic thirst center (33).

The development of symptoms in hyponatremia depends mainly on the rate at which it develops as well as its severity. This is predictable from knowledge of the response of the brain to acute changes in ECF osmolarity, as discussed above. Since the brain is encased within a rigid compartment, very little parenchymal swelling can occur before intracranial pressure increases and CNS symptoms develop. These symptoms are variable (Table 4). On occasion respiratory arrest may be the first indication that hyponatremia has occurred. More common symptoms include nausea and vomiting, agitation, irritability, delirium, weakness, and seizures. Cerebral edema due to hyponatremia can be detected both radiographically (50) and postmortem (51). The mortality of acute symptomatic hyponatremia may be as high as 50% (17).

CHRONIC HYPONATREMIA

There are many entities that are associated with chronic hyponatremia in humans. These have conventionally been divided into groups based on the status of the ECF volume. In a sense, such a classification is artificial because much of the same pathology is at work in all groups. The presence or absence of symptoms is independent of whether the patient is volume expanded, euvolemic, or volume depleted. In brief, all groups have some nonosmotic stimulus for antidiuretic hormone (ADH) release and relatively excessive water intake. We will thus consider the problem of chronic hyponatremia from the perspective of the underlying stimulus for ADH secretion (Table 5).

The syndrome of inappropriate ADH secretion (SIADH) is an entity of many different etiologies, although the most common reasons are disease of the pulmonary and central nervous systems. Hypotonic hyponatremia is present, in addition to urine that is less than maximally dilute (52). In practice, urine osmolarity usually exceeds that of plasma, but that is not required for the diagnosis. A urine osmolarity of 200 mOsm/kg is inappropriately high for a person with a plasma osmolarity of 240 mOsm/kg in whom ADH ought to be suppressed maximally, and urine osmolarity should be less than 100 mOsm/kg. SIADH is essentially a diagnosis of exclusion in which causes for appropriate nonosmotic release of ADH (such as volume depletion, heart failure, and cirrhosis) have been excluded, there is no evidence of endocrine dysfunction (such as hypothyroidism or adrenal insufficiency), which would interfere with normal water handling, and renal function is normal. Ingestion of drugs that increase AVP levels or potentiate its action in the kidney should be ruled out.

Edema-forming disorders (congestive heart failure, cirrhosis with ascites, and the nephrotic syndrome) are also frequently associated with hyponatremia. The ECF-volume status in each of these syndromes is grossly expanded, but there is a great deal of controversy soncerning the status of the much more elusive " effective blood volume." Most researchers agree that in heart failure (CHF) patients, the decrease in cardiac output leads to a decrease in the effective blood volume. The issue is not nearly as clear with respect to ascites and the nephrotic syndrome (NS). In any event, regardless of whether actual blood volume is increased, decreased, or unchanged, the kidneys behave as if they are hypoperfused in the majority of patients with these three disorders. Thus, GFR (while variable) tends to decrease, proximal tubular salt and water reabsorption are increased, and urinary excretion of sodium is very low. This may be magnified by treatment with dietary sodium restriction and diuretic agents, which are commonly employed in these patients. By activation of baroreceptor afferents in the cardiovascular system, liver, or kidneys, AVP release is stimulated. Because of the intrarenal abnormalities just discussed, free water clearance is submaximal and hyponatremia ensues in the face of elevated AVP levels. This can perhaps be conceptualized in a teleologic way by considering that the kidney has as its first priority the maintenance of adequate ECF volume. This defense of volume homeostasis will occur even at the expense of plasma tonicity if possible.

A sizeable number of patients receiving diuretics will ultimately develop hyponatremia. Although this process is frequently mild and asymptomatic, it can be severe and quite acute (53–56). Several processes interact to allow this to occur. When diuretics are being used in the treatment of an edema-forming condition, it may be difficult to separate the effects of the underlying disease from those of the diuretic itself; any additional factors related to the diuretic will be synergistic with the primary pathologic process, in any case. The negative sodium balance induced by the diuretic will represent an additional stimulus for the nonosmotic release of AVP. Agents with a preferential site of action in the cortical diluting segment (such as thiazides) will further impair the ability to excrete a water load. Host factors also predispose to the development of diuretic-induced hyponatremia. These include malnutrition, advanced age, and female gender. In some patients, marked stimulation of thirst is a probable predisposing factor.

The symptoms of chronic hyponatremia are different in several important ways when compared with acute hyponatremia. The most important distinguishing feature between the two is the fact that chronic hyponatremia is much more likely to be an asymptomatic process. Due to the efficiency of cell volume regulation, neuronal swelling is less likely to occur in those patients in whom hyponatremia develops gradually. Therefore, those symptoms that are related to cerebral edema and increased intracranial pressure are much less likely to be early features of the presentation of chronic as opposed to acute hyponatremia. On the other hand, symptoms of neuronal dysfunction due to changes in the transmembrane electrical potential are more likely. These include lethargy, GI complaints, depression of the sensorium, weakness, apathy, and ultimately coma (4). Although no precise correlation exists between the severity of symptoms and the degree of hyponatremia (17), the clinician will probably detect the most severe dysfunction in subjects with plasma sodium less than 120 mEq/l.

The impact of female gender on the development of symptoms related to hypoosmolarity of the plasma is becoming more widely appreciated. Studies performed in rabbits (57) showed a higher mortality during chronic hyponatremia in female rabbits (86%) as compared with male animals (24%). In the same study, the brain content of water, sodium, and potassium were all lower in male rabbits than in females. It has recently been shown that sodium transport is decreased in synaptosomes isolated from the brains of female, but not male, rats with chronic hyponatremia (58). This is presumably due to differences in the availability of AVP and differential responses of AVP to female versus male sex hormones. The importance of hormonal regulation in the brain response to hyponatremia is emphasized in the recent report of a woman treated with clomiphene citrate and human chorionic gonadotropin for infertility. She developed symptomatic hyponatremia following ingestion of a water load in preparation for a pelvic ultrasound (59).

Table 6. Therapy of hyponatremia

MEASURE PLASMA OSMOLALITY

Acute hyponatremia
  Prevention
  Asymptomatic = fluid restriction
  Symptomatic
    Hypertonic saline ± furosemide
    Normal saline
Chronic hyponatremia
  Asymptomatic
    Fluid restriction
    Therapy of underlying disease
  Symptomatic
    Hypertonic saline ± furosemide
    Normal saline
    Therapy of underlying disease
    Lithium
    Demeclocycline
    AVP inhibitors (experimental)

TREATMENT OF HYPOTONIC STATES (TABLE 6)

Acute hyponatremia

When acute hyponatremia occurs, it is important to recognize and treat it promptly. The first symptoms are apt to be quite dramatic (e.g., seizures and/or respiratory arrest) and may indicate a far advanced process for which any therapy is less likely to produce a good outcome. Thus, awareness of the situations in which an unrecognized acute hypotonic state is possible is the first and most important step in management. The most common situation in which this occurs is the postoperative patient. As discussed above, multiple factors conspire against the ability of the kidney to excrete a water load in surgical subjects; thus every postoperative patient should be considered at risk for the development of hyponatremia and appropriate prophylactic measures should be taken. If they are not and respiratory arrest ensues, treatment after the fact is often associated with a very bad outcome, both in terms of mortality and neurologic morbidity. A summary of 23 reports of patients with acute hyponatremia is presented in Table 7. One hundred percent of patients in whom hyponatremia was suspected and treated early (often before the results of serum sodium determinations were available) were neurologically normal after treatment, whereas severe neurologic disability or death occurred in 25 of 76 patients (33%) in whom recognition (and hence treatment) were delayed (23, 25, 29–32, 46, 60–75).

The most important step to be taken in the prevention of postoperative hyponatremia is a careful consideration of the choice of intravenous fluids administered. It is common practice to infuse hypotonic solutions to patients in the perioperative period. This is seldom an ideal choice

Table 7. Effect of delayed recognition on outcome in acute hyponatremia

	Outcome	
	Normal n (%)	Disability or death n (%)
Early Rx	13 (100)	0 (0)
Late Rx	51 (67)	25 (33)

in patients with normal renal function. Unless there is a definite reason to suspect the existence of hypotonic fluid losses, isotonic sodium chloride is preferable. The rate of administration must be supervised carefully in this situation to avoid fluid overload. One could argue that hypotonic fluids are preferable to normal saline in postoperative patients with renal dysfunction, cirrhosis, or CHF, because the risk of fluid overload is substantially higher in patients receiving greater amounts of sodium; on the other hand, these subjects are also at the greatest risk for the development of hyponatremia. If adequate monitoring can be performed, the careful administration of isotonic solutions may be safer than the indiscriminate use of solutions containing free water.

The goals of treatment in acute hyponatremia are to reduce cellular water and to increase ECF sodium concentration only to the degree necessary to render the patient seizure free and alert. This seldom if ever requires that the sodium level be corrected entirely to normal. Under no circumstance should the patient be allowed to develop hypernatremia, and in fact it should be rare that correction to a serum sodium above 130 mEq/l is necessary as the initial treatment. The most frequent therapy employed is hypertonic saline solutions, often in conjunction with a loop-acting diuretic such as furosemide. The combination of fluid and diuretic is a logical attempt to address both the hyponatremia itself and the water overload that it signifies. It is often useful to remember that "isotonic" sodium chloride solutions are in fact hypertonic to the patient with hypoosmolarity and can be employed until the most basic laboratory and clinical investigations have been completed. These should include, at a minimum, a review of prescribed medications, a good neurologic and general physical examination, and serum osmolarity. Loop diuretics have the property of causing a diuresis of water in excess of solute when given acutely, and can thus be used to accelerate water excretion. Care must be taken, however, to exclude underlying ECF volume depletion before potent diuretics are considered.

Chronic hyponatremia

In patients with chronic asymptomatic hyponatremia, aggressive therapy with hypertonic saline is not indicated. This is particularly true if the hyponatremia is mild to moderate in severity (plasma sodium > 120 mEq/l). In patients who are obviously volume depleted, isotonic saline is clearly the fluid of choice. In patients in whom adrenal insufficiency or hypothyroidism have been identified, appropriate endocrine replacement is warranted. If the patient has received any drugs associated with hyponatremia, they should be discontinued if possible. In most cases of asymptomatic hyponatremia, however, none of these factors are present; water restriction is the cornerstone of therapy in those subjects. By and large, if a patient is able to maintain a fluid restriction of approximately 1 l/day, negative water balance will occur and the serum sodium will be corrected. If a greater degree of precision in calculation of the desired fluid restriction is required, a relatively simple calculation can be performed. As a rough guide, the total excreted solutes of a normal subject on a regular diet amounts to approximately 10 mOsm/kg body weight, or about 600–700 mOsm/day in the average 70 kg man. Therefore, the formula:

$$V = [\text{weight (kg)} \cdot 10]/[\text{minimum Uosm}],$$

where [minimum Uosm] is the lowest attainable urine osmolarity, will provide the clinician with the greatest volume of fluid intake (V) that can be associated with negative fluid balance. By way of example, if a patient weighing 60 kg has a minimum Uosm of 450 mOsm/kg H_2O, any fluid intake less than $(60)(10)/(450) = 1.3$ l/day will be associated with a correction of hyponatremia.

Several medical measures have been proposed for the long-term management of chronic hyponatremia. When lithium is used in the treatment of bipolar disorders, some patients develop polyuria, polydipsia, and hypernatremia (76). Lithium has been used to treat a few patients with SIADH with a modest response (77). Its use has not been reported in hyponatremia associated with edema-forming disorders. Toxicity of the kidneys, CNS, heart, and thyroid have all been reported in patients receiving long-term lithium treatment for affective disorders (78–83). Demeclocycline (DMC), a tetracycline antibiotic used in the treatment of acne, was fortuitously discovered to be associated with a nephrogenic diabetes insipidus when administered in doses of 600–1200 mg/day (84, 85). It has been successfully employed by several groups treating patients with SIADH, including subjects unresponsive to lithium (77, 86, 87). However, acute renal failure and renal tubular toxicity have been attributed to DMC in hyponatremic patients with CHF or cirrhosis (88–91). Several other drug regimens have been reported in the treatment of chronic hyponatremia. These include urea administration and inhibitors of AVP such as vasopressinoic acid (92–94). More experience with these agents is required before they can receive broad recommendation. Finally, correction of the functional state of volume depletion that exists in CHF and decompensated cirrhosis is often associated with an improvement of hyponatremia. In cirrhosis this can sometimes be achieved following the placement of a LeVeen shunt (95), and in CHF the use of vasodilators can improve cardiac output and renal perfusion, and ultimately renal water excretion can increase (96).

Rate of correction versus degree of correction

In patients with severe symptomatic hyponatremia, water restriction may not be sufficient to relieve symptoms. Although there is some data to suggest that even very severe chronic hyponatremia in symptomatic patients is best treated by conservative measures (97), the majority of clinical and laboratory experience suggests that the mortality and morbidity (particularly irreversible CNS sequelae) of slow correction by water restriction alone is unacceptable (4, 17, 23, 51, 98, 99). Therefore, more rapid correction of hyponatremia with hypertonic saline is indicated in symptomatic patients. In some patients, simultaneous administration of furosemide is necessary to prevent circulatory overload and acute pulmonary edema.

There has been a lively controversy in the literature regarding the rate at which the hypoosmolarity should be corrected. Some authors argue that the development of a rare neurologic syndrome known as central pontine myelinolysis (CPM) is the result of rapid correction of long-standing hyponatremia, and propose that serum sodium should not rise at a rate greater than 0.5 mEq/l/hr (100, 101). Other investigators point out that CPM seems to develop only when chronically hyponatremic patients are inadvertently made hypernatremic during acute treatment or if the absolute increase in serum sodium exceeds 25 mEq/l in the first 24–48 hours of therapy (98, 102, 103). It is of interest that CPM does not develop as a result of hyponatremia per se or due to the treatment of acute hyponatremia.

These observations can be most easily explained by referring to the nature of cell volume homeostasis described earlier. In acute hyponatremia, neuronal water content is increased and solute content is normal. In this case, treatment with hypertonic fluids causes the extraction of excess water and a prompt return to the baseline state. On the other hand, a patient with chronic hyponatremia has nearly normal brain cell volume but decreased brain cell solute. During rapid correction, cell volume will tend to decrease, and there will be a lag period before the neurons switch from a state of net solute exit to net solute entry. During this vulnerable period, if cell volume change are excessive, neuronal damage can result in the development of CPM. Thus, if the total change in ECF osmolarity is limited, the neurons are not exposed to osmotic stresses outside their regulatory range and CPM is less likely to occur.

There are excellent clinical and experimental data to support this view. If the data of patients with CPM developing after active correction of hyponatremia are carefully examined, it can be found that the vast majority of them underwent correction to normonatremic or hypernatremic levels early in their treatment (104). This is clearly excessive, since symptoms are virtually always relieved with correction to mildly hyponatremic levels. Of patients who were never hypernatremic or normonatremic, the serum sodium increased by more than 25 mEq/l in the first 48 hours of therapy (Figure 1). Preexisting liver disease, structural lesions of the CNS, diuretic use, advanced age, and female gender were predisposing factors in the majority

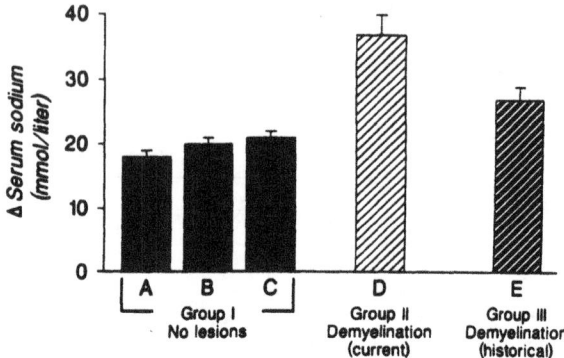

Figure 1. Influence of magnitude of change in serum sodium on the development of demyelinating lesions of the CNS. Patients in group I (no demyelination) had a smaller increment in serum sodium immediately after correction with hypertonic saline (A), 24 hours later (B), and 48 hours later (C) than concurrent patients who developed demyelinating lesions (Group II, D) or historic controls (Group III, E). Reproduced from Ayus JC, et al., Treatment of symptomatic hyponatremia and its relation to brain demage. A prospective study, N Engl J Med 317:1190–1195, 1987, with permission.

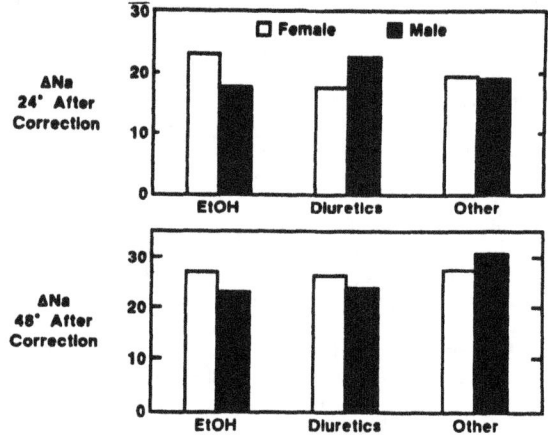

Figure 2. Absolute change in serum sodium concentration 24 and 48 hours after treatment in patients who developed CPM in the setting of alcohol abuse (EtOH), current use of diuretics, or other conditions. Reproduced from Brennan S, et al.: Central pontine myelinolysis and electrolyte disorders. In: *Neurologic Manifestations of Systemic Disorders.* Little Brown, Boston, 1989, in press, with permission.

of patients (Figure 2) (104). An episode of hypoxia or anoxia greatly increases the risk of CPM (102). The major risk factors for the development of CPM are summarized in Table 8. Despite the fear of CPM during the correction of hyponatremia, overall patient survival is improved when the correction is rapid (> 0.7 mEq/l/hr), as compared with slower rates (98) (Figure 3). The mortality of hyponatremia in a recent study was 30%, both in patients treated either by slow infusion of saline or by water restriction (105). Six reports of 108 patients undergoing rapid correction (> 0.6 mEq/l/hr) of severe symptomatic acute or chronic hyponatremia demonstrate the safety and efficacy of this approach (54, 102, 106–111).

Animal experiments have been conducted in order to delineate the relationship between the correction of severe hyponatremia and the development of demyelinating brain lesions. It has been clearly shown that demyelination occurs when severe hyponatremia is corrected to normonatremic or hypernatremic values, even when accomplished relatively slowly by water restriction alone (112). On the other hand, rapid correction to mildly hyponatremic levels did not cause significant brain injury. Another study in rats has shown that untreated severe hyponatremia in rats resulted in significant morbidity and mortality, whereas rapid correction to mildly hyponatremic levels was associated with 100% survival of the animals without any evidence of brain lesions, as long as the absolute change in serum sodium was less than 25 mEq/l (99) (Figure 4). Other studies in the literature have come to similar conclusions. Thus, both animal and human studies clearly demonstrate that early recognition and rapid correction is safe and effective in the treatment of severe symptomatic chronic hyponatremia.

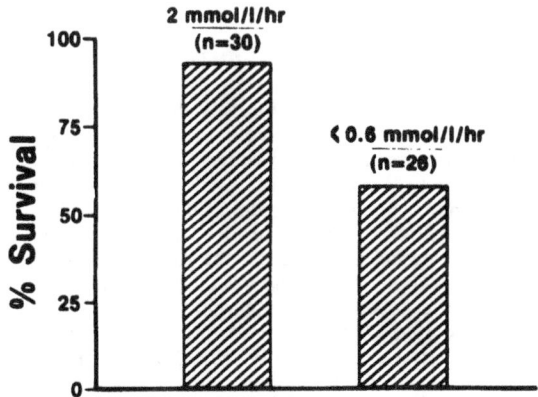

Figure 3. Survival in patients with symptomatic hyponatremia as a function of the rate of correction. During correction of severe symptomatic hyponatremia to mildly hyponatremic levels, patient survival was imporved in subjects who were corrected rapidly (2 mM/l/hr) with hypertonic saline as compared with patients who underwent slow correction (< 0.6 mM/l/hr). Reproduced from Ayus JC, et al.: Changing concepts in the treatment of severe symptomatic hyponatremia: Rapid correction and possible relation to central pontine myelinolysis. Am J Med 79:897–902, 1985, with permission.

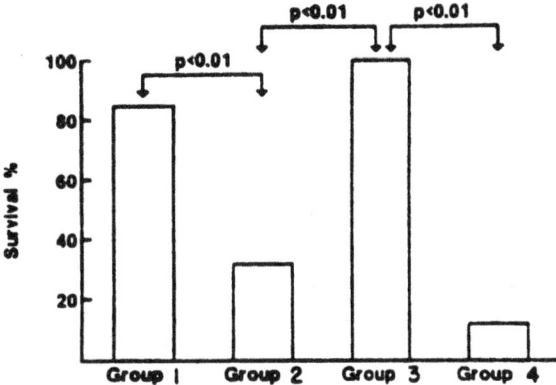

Figure 4. Survival rates in groups of rats with hyponatremia. Group 1: Mild hyponatremia (serum sodium 120–130 mEq/l) with spontaneous correction. Group 2: Severe hypontremia (serum sodium < 120 mEq/l) with spontaneous correction. Group 3: Severe hyponatremia with rapid correction by administration of 855 mM NaCl with an absolute change in serum sodium of < 25 mEq/l in the first 24 hours. Group 4: Severe hyponatremia with rapid correction by administration of 855 mM NaCl with an absolute change in serum sodium of > 25 mEq/l in the first 24 hours. Reproduced from Ayus JC, et al.: Symptomatic hyponatremia in rats: Effect of treatment on mortality and brain lesions. Am J Physiol 257 (Renal Fluid Electrolyte Physiol 26):F18–F22, 1989, with permission.

Table 8. Major risk factors for development of cerebral demyelinating lesions in patients with symptomatic chronic hyponatremia

1. Coexistent hypoxic-anoxic episode (respiratory arrest seizures)
2. Correction of sodium to normo- or hypernatremic levels within the first 48 hours of therapy
3. Absolute change in serum sodium > 25 mM/l within the first 48 hours of therapy
4. Hypernatremia in patients with severe liver disease (even in the absence of prior hyponatremia)
5. Female gender

In summary, acute hyponatremia usually occurs because of a combination of increased ingestion of water, increased excretion of salt, and decreased renal free water clearance. The clinical settings in which it develops include postoperative patients, subjects with psychiatric disturbances, men undergoing TURP, and women treated with oxytocin. The object of treatment is to raise the plasma osmolarity rapidly to the lowest level that is associated with symptomatic improvement followed by a more gradual correction to normal levels. This treatment is required in order to prevent long-term neurologic sequelae. If respiratory arrest or coma develop, the prognosis is usually quite grave, even if hyponatremia is ultimately corrected.

On the other hand, chronic hyponatremia is often asymptomatic and well tolerated. Symptoms of chronic hypoosmolarity are primarily related to changes in transmembrane electrochemical gradients, since cell volume regulation is nearly complete within 1–3 days. The patient with asymptomatic hyponatremia does not require aggressive therapy and is best managed by fluid restriction with or without adjunctive pharmacologic measures. Patients with liver disease, structural lesions of the CNS, a history of diuretic use, advanced age, and female gender are at greatest risk for developing symptomatic hyponatremia. When symptoms are present, rapid treatment is required, using hypertonic saline with a loop diuretic if indicated. The guidelines of treatment are to raise the plasma sodium by no more than 20–25 mEq/l over the first 48 hours; correction beyond mildly hyponatremic levels (130 mEq/l) is not necessary, and correction to hypernatremic levels (> 140 mEq/l) is contraindicated. Failure to adhere to these guidelines can predispose patients to CPM. Rapid treatment of symptomatic hyponatremia improves survival and the neurologic outcome when compared with gradual correction.

HYPEROSMOLAR STATES

Because sodium with its accompanying anions comprises the great majority of osmoles in the plasma, hypertonicity is always present if hypernatremia is present. However, a hyperosmolar state can exist in the absence of hypernatremia if another solute (such as glucose) is present in excessive amounts. The subject of hyperglycemic nonketotic hyperosmolar coma is discussed in detail in another chapter of this book and will not be covered here. We will present features of other hyperosmolar states, particularly those associated with hypernatremia.

The plasma osmolarity should be determined early during the clinical evaluation of hypertonic states. The major solutes that contribute to plasma osmolarity in normal subjects are sodium and potassium, with their accompanying anions, urea, and glucose. An estimate of osmolarity that is useful clinically is obtained from the formula:

$$P_{osm} = ([Na + K] \cdot 2) + BUN \text{ (mg/dl)}/2.8 + glucose \text{ (mg/dl)}/18.$$

Unfortunately, this equation only estimates the true osmolarity; it does not take into account the possible presence of other osmotically active substances, nor does it provide as insight into the contribution a given species makes to the "effective osmolarity." This is particularly true in the case of urea. Urea diffuses throughout the total body water in a fairly short period of time and consequently does not cause fluid shifts between water compartments under ordinary circumstances; it is not an "effective" osmole. Even astronomically high levels of BUN do not cause clinically important abnormalities of water balance, unless they are caused by the rapid administration of exogenous urea.

If one assumes that urinary solute excretion of 10 mOsm/kg body weight take place daily to preserve a steady state, the minimum volume of urine that must be excreted in 24 hours can be estimated from the following formula:

$$V = [\text{weight (kg)} \cdot 10]/[\text{maximum } U_{osm}]$$

where [maximum U_{osm}] is the highest attainable urinary osmolarity. In a normal 70-kg subject with a maximum U_{osm} of 1000 mOsm/kg, this will correspond to 700 ml of urine in 24 hours. If one further assumes that insensible water losses amount to about 500–1000 ml/day, total daily water losses will be close to 1500 ml/day. This figure will obviously increase in persons unable to concentrate their urine maximally or with greater amounts of insensible water loss. Therefore, in addition to an intact urinary concentrating mechanism and appropriate stimulation of AVP, prevention of hypertonicity also depends on the adequate ingestion of water. A major factor in most cases of clinical hypernatremia is impaired thirst or restricted access to water. Hyperosmolarity may also occur because of the acute administration or ingestion of hypertonic fluids (such as hypertonic saline, sodium bicarbonate, glucose, mannitol, or radiographic contrast dyes).

This brief discussion of the pathophysiology of hypernatremia serves to highlight three important points in the evaluation of the patient with hypertonicity. First, the osmolarity of plasma and urine must be determined in order to assess the adequacy of the pituitary-renal water conservation mechanism. Second, urine volume must be measured and carefully compared with fluid intake on order to assess the intactness of the thirst response. Third, all ingested drugs (and infant formulas, if appropriate) must be reviewed and/or examined in order to ensure that the patient has not been exposed to hypertonic solution.

CLINICAL FEATURES OF HYPERTONICITY

The structural CNS lesions of hypernatremia are a direct consequence of adaptive cell-volume regulation. Hypernatremia is associated with an acute decrease in intracranial pressure (113), as neuronal cells shrink due to an egress of water. Some of this fluid finds its way into the vascular tree; the remainder resides in the interstices of the brain, resulting in edema of the extracellular space. Physical separation of the brain from the meninges ensues, damage to the delicate bridging veins occurs, and intracranial hemorrhage (subdural, subarachnoid, or intracerebral) frequently develops (113–118). Thrombosis of the venous sinuses is another characteristic finding. These pathologic observations have been made in patients as well as in experimental models of hyperosmolarity.

By and large, hyperosmolar states are seen at the extremes of age. A study of hypernatremia in childhood revealed that 45 of 50 pediatric patients with plasma sodium values greater than 149 mEq/l were under the age of 18 months (118). Conversely, a study of older patients with plasma sodium levels above 148 mEq/l demonstrated a mean age of 78 years in the study population (119). In both groups, water intake tends to be limited; in the young children, an inability to express thirst and to obtain water for themselves is present, whereas normal thirst is depressed in older patients (119, 120). Other special problems characterize both age groups. In infants, renal water conservation is not yet fully developed, and insensible water losses via the skin and lungs account for at least 50% of daily fluid loss (121). Predisposition to febrile illnesses in general, and diarrheal illnesses in particular, put the very young at high risk for excessive water losses and consequent hypernatremia. Among older patients, dependence upon others for certain aspects of day-to-day living increases with age. Of elderly patients with hypernatremia, only 38% lived independently prior to hospitalization (119). The increasing predisposition to infectious diseases that occurs in the aged will tend to increase insensible water losses. As part of the aging process, many aspects of renal function deteriorate, including urinary concentrating ability (122).

The signs and symptoms of hypernatremia are variable. In experimental hyperosmolarity, findings include nystagmus, myoclonic jerking of the extremities, and ultimately respiratory failure and death (123). The electroencephalogram (EEG) reveals loss of normal fast frequencies and occasional decreases in voltage, but the abnormal limb movements are not associated with EEG discharges (123). The myoclonus in this case is attributable to a direct effect of the hypertonicity on the muscles. In human subjects, preexisting abnormalities of mental status may make it difficult to detect any new neurologic findings. In addition, since hypernatremia frequently occurs in the setting of a coexistent pathologic process, it may be difficult to ascribe any particular symptom or group of symptoms to hypertonicity per se. In infants, male gender predominates (118, 124). There may be alternating periods of lethargy and irritability (125). Tachypnea is frequently present and may be severe. A history compatible with gastroenteritis is frequently obtained and may be the cause of the hypernatremia (126); conversely, neusea and vomiting are often seen, even in the absence of diarrhea, and may be due to the effects of hyperosmolarity on the CNS itself (127). Seizures are commonly present and correlate with the degree of hypernatremia (118, 128). Associated laboratory abnormalities include metabolic acidosis and hyperglycemia (125, 126). The abnormalities in glucose metabolism are important therapeutically and will be addressed further below.

In the elderly some important differences exist (119–129). When considering only patients who were hypernatremic at the time of hospital admission, women were predominant. Although nearly half the hypernatremic patients had a febrile illness, other associated conditions assume more prominence than in infants. These include the postoperative state, diuretic administration, excessive intravenous solute administration (including nutritional supplements), and diabetes mellitus as the leading causes. Depression of the sensorium is frequently present and is highly correlated with the degree of hypernatremia. Altered mental status is also an independent predictor of subsequent mortality at any level of hypernatremia (119).

Hypernatremia is associated with considerable long-term morbidity and mortality, both in children and adults. One study in neonates identified 24 babies with hypernatremia; 17 of these children died, the majority of whom (11 infants) succumbed to intracranial hemorrhage (117). Another series of 114 pediatric patients reported a total incidence of brain damage due to hypernatremia of 14% (130). Most other studies in children report morbidity and mortality figures between these two extremes, with survivors of hypernatremia having a 10–15% likelihood of having permanent neurologic deficits (126). In adults, the figures are similar. The mortality in elderly patients with hypernatremia was found to be 42% in one study, and neurologic morbidity as assessed by changes in the level of care was present in 38% of the survivors (119). One especially noteworthy finding in this series was the fact that mortality was higher in patients with hypernatremia developing in the hospital. The authors attributed this finding to a more complicated clinical setting and delayed recognition of hypertonicity in the hospitalized subjects.

TREATMENT OF HYPEROSMOLAR STATES

The goal of therapy in hypernatremia is the reduction of plasma osmolarity towards normal by the administration of solute-free water or the removal of excess solute or both. Removal of solute is usually accomplished by the administration of diuretics or institution of dialysis (131). When water administration is planned, the major therapeutic questions are the type of fluid to be given and its rate and route of ingestion. Water can be extremely toxic if given injudiciously; such textbook statements as "the euvolemic hypernatremic patient who has sustained pure water losses requires water replacement as a 5% dextrose infusion" (132) necessitate scrutiny before they are casually applied.

In adult patients with hypernatremia, the usual fluid given to supply free water is 5% dextrose in water (D_5W). The free water deficit is calculated as follows:

Deficit (l) = $0.6 \cdot$ weight (kg) $\cdot$ [(current PNa)/140 − 1].

This deficit is subsequently replaced over a period of 36–72 hours, with relatively rapid replacement taking place in the first several hours of therapy. Several assumptions underlie this approach, both stated and unstated. The stated assumptions are that water is in nearly instantaneous equilibrium across all cell membranes, and that overly rapid correction can lead to cell swelling and clinical deterioration. The usually unstated assumption is that the dextrose in D_5W can be rapidly metabolized to CO_2 and is the equivalent of pure water in its clinical effects. This assumption has recently been questioned, and is in fact not literally true (133). Infusion of glucose-containing solutions may lead to a deterioration in CNS function by raising the serum osmolarity.

One liter of D_5W contains 50 g, or 278 mM, of glucose. If glucose is distributed equally throughout the ECF volume (15 l), at a blood glucose concentration of 5 mM

(90 mg/dl) the total glucose content in the human body is 75 mM (13.5 g). Therefore, without metabolism 1 l of D_5W will cause a nearly fourfold increase in glucose concentration and will potentially aggravate the hyperosmolar condition. Additionally, an osmotic diuresis due to glucose will hasten renal water losses and slow correction of the hypertonic state.

It has been estimated that in the normal state the total glucose oxidative capacity of the body is 8–9 g/hr (133). Thus, even if glucose metabolism is completely normal, if D_5W is infused at a rate that exceeds 200 ml/hr (equivalent to 10 g glucose/hr), the blood glucose concentration may increase. Furthermore, the metabolism of glucose is seldom if ever normal in patients with hypernatremia. As noted previously, children with hypertonic states commonly have hyperglycemia, consistent with insulin resistance (125). In fact, glucose intolerance has been documented in a rat model of hypernatremia (134) and as a complication of diabetes insipidus following suprasellar surgery in humans (135). In clinical practice, this may be due to or exacerbated by high levels of catecholamines and/or glucocorticoids in the circulation, related to the stress of an acute illness.

We therefore recommend that solutions containing glucose not be considered as first-line agents in the treatment of hypernatremia. Instead, fluid should be administered as distilled or tap water if possible, obviating any dependence on metabolism to provide solute-free water. Since pure water cannot be delivered parenterally without the risk of hemolysis, we suggest that the GI tract be used whenever feasible. If this approach is not possible, infusion of D_5W should not exceed 200 ml/hr, and the blood glucose concentration must be carefully monitored and aggressively treated if it becomes elevated. The use of oral solutions has been safely applied in children with hypernatremia due to gastroenteritis (136, 137), but to our knowledge only one adult patient with severe symptomatic hypernatremia has been reported in whom oral rehydration with tap water has been effectively accomplished (138).

The optimal rate of correction of hypernatremia is being reexamined. On the one hand, rapid correction may seem urgent because of the marked CNS depression. However, consideration of the mechanisms of cell volume adaptation make this option less attractive. Presumably, in hypertonicity of several days' duration, cell volume has expanded nearly to normal by the active accumulation of electrolytes, amino acids, and idiogenic osmoles. When treatment is begun, plasma osmolarity will begin to decrease, water will enter CNS cells, and brain edema may ensue. It is possible that adaptive decreases in cell volume are delayed in this setting, since it probably takes time for the cells to switch from a state of net solute accumulation to one of net solute loss. One could predict that symptoms reminiscent of acute hypotonicity may be a complication of excessively rapid correction of hypernatremia. This prediction has been borne out both experimentally and clinically. In rabbits made chronically hypernatremic by the administration of hypertonic saline, acute correction of the hyperosmolar state was associated with increases in brain water content that were virtually indentical to those seen in previously normal animals given the same volume of solute-free water (139). Seizures were noted in 55% of the animals during the acute correction of hypernatremia. In humans, rehydration seizures occur when the rate of correction of hypernatremia exceeds 0.5–0.7 mEq/l/hr (136, 137, 139, 140). This complication may be somewhat less likely to occur when hydration is accomplished orally rather than intravenously (141). Studies in rats have shown that correction of severe hypernatremia to middly hypernatremic levels (plasma Na 147–149 mM/l) is accompanied by normalization of neurologic findings within 24 hours, and unremarkable CNS histology at the end of 1 month (142).

In summary, hypernatremia occurs when water ingestion is inadequate to correct for fluid losses in the urine, GI tract, or elsewhere (insensible losses). It occurs most commonly at the extremes of age and is very frequently an iatrogenic problem. The clinical presentation depends on the rate of development and the severity of the hypertonic state, and the presence of symptoms is associated with a poor neurologic outcome. The most common CNS lesion is intracranial hemorrhage.

The ideal treatment of hypernatremia represents a balance between free-water administration and solute (sodium) excretion. Sodium removal can be accomplished with diuretics or dialysis. Infusion of glucose-containing fluids such as D_5W can be associated with a worsening of the hypertonic state and they should not be administered unless solute-free solutions cannot be absorbed via the GI tract. Overzealous correction can be accompanied by rehydration seizures, which are probably due to acute cerebral edema from CNS cellular water uptake. This can be avoided by gradual parenteral treatment if oral replacement is not a viable option.

REFERENCES

1. Siebens AW: Cellular volume control. In: DW Seldin, G Giebisch, eds, *The kidney: Physiology and Pathophysiology*. Raven Press, New York, pp 91–115, 1985.
2. Fishman RA: Cell volume, pumps and neurologic function: Brain's adaptation to osmotic stress. *Res Publ Assoc Nerv Ment Dis* 53:159–171, 1974.
3. Yannet H: Changes in the brain resulting from depletion of extracellular electrolytes. *Am J Physiol* 128:683–689, 1940.
4. Arieff AI, Llach F, Massry SG: Neurological manifestations and morbidity of hyponatremia: Correlation of brain water and electrolytes. *Medicine* (Baltimore) 55:121–129, 1976.
5. Melton JE, Patlak CS, Pettigrew KD, Cserr HF: Volume regulatory loss of Na, Cl, and K from rat brain during acute hyponatremia. *Am J Physiol* 252 (Renal Fluid Electrolyte Physol 21): F661–F669, 1987.
6. Thurston JH, Hauhart RE: Brain amino acids decrease in chronic hyponatremia and rapid correction causes brain dehydration: Possible clinical significance. *Life Sci* 40:2539–2542, 1987.
7. Adler S, Simplaceanu V: Effect of acute hyponatremia on rat brain pH and rat brain buffering. *Am J Physiol* 256 (Renal Fluid Electrolyte Physiol):F113–F119, 1989.

8. Ames A III, Isom JB, Nesbett FB: Effects of osmotic changes on water and electrolytes in nervous tissue. *J Physiol* (London) 117:246–262, 1965.
9. Woodbury DM: Effect of acute hyponatremia on distribution of water and electrolytes in various tissues of the rat. *Am J Physiol* 185:281–286, 1968.
10. Cserr HF, DePasquale M, Patlak CS: Regulation of brain water and electrolytes during acute hyperosmolarity in rats. *Am J Physiol* 253 (Renal Fluid Electrolyte Physiol 22): F522–F529, 1987.
11. Cserr HF, DePasquale M, Patlak CS: Volume regulatory influx of electrolytes from plasma to brain during acute hyperosmolarity. *Am J Physiol* 253 (Renal Fluid Electrolyte Physiol 22):F530–F537, 1987.
12. Pullen RGL, DePasquale M, Cserr HF: Bulk flow of cerebrospinal fluid into brain in response to acute hyperosmolarity. *Am J Physiol* 253 (Renal Fluid Electrolyte Physiol 22):F538–F545, 1987.
13. Baxter CF, Ortiz CL: Amino acids and the maintenance of osmotic equilibrium in brain tissue. *Life Sci* 5:2321–2329, 1966.
14. Arieff AI, Guisado R, Lazarowitz VC: Pathophysiology of hyperosmolar states. In: TE Andreoli, JJ Grantham, FC Rector Jr, eds, *Disturbances in Body Fluid Osmolality*. American Physiological Society, Bethesda, MD pp 227–250, 1977.
15. Guisado R, Arieff AI, Massry SG: Effects of glycerol infusion on brain water and electrolytes. *Am J Physiol* 227:865–872, 1974.
16. Berl T, Anderson RJ, McDonald KM, Schrier RW: Clinical disorders of water metabolism. *Kidney Int* 10:117–132, 1976.
17. Covey CM, Arieff AI: Disorders of sodium and water metabolism and their effects on the central nervous system. In: BM Brenner, JH Stein, eds, *Contemporary Issues in Nephrology. Sodium and Water Homeostasis*, Vol I. Churchill Livingstone, New York, pp 212–241, 1978.
18. Barlow ED, deWardener HE: Compulsive water drinking. *Q J Med* 28:235–258, 1959.
19. Humes HD: Disorders of water metabolism. In: Kokko JP, Tannen RL, eds, *Fluids and Electrolytes*. Saunders, Philadelphia, pp 118–149, 1986.
20. LeQuesne LP, Lewis AAG: Postoperative water and sodium retention. *Lancet* 1:153–158, 1953.
21. Moran WH Jr, Miltenberger FW, Shuayb WA, Zimmerman B: The relationship of antidiuretic hormone to surgical stress. *Surgery* 56:99–108, 1964.
22. Chung HM, Kluge R, Schrier RW, Anderson RJ: Postoperative hyponatremia: A prospective study. *Arch Intern Med* 146:333–336, 1986.
23. Arieff AI: Hyponatremia, convulsions, respiratory arrest, and permanent brain damage after elective surgery in healthy women. *N Engl J Med* 314:1529–1535, 1986.
24. Hagstrom RS: Studies on fluid absorption during transurethral prostatic resection. *J Urol* 73:852–859, 1955.
25. Still JA Jr, Modell JH: Acute water intoxication during transurethral resection of the prostate, using glycine solution for irrigation. *Anesthesiol* 38:98–99, 1973.
26. Roesch RP, Stoelting RK, Lingeman JE, Kahnoski RJ, Backes DJ, Gephardt SA: Ammonia toxicity resulting from glycine absorption during a transurethral resection of the prostate. *Anesthesiol* 58:577–579, 1983.
27. Ryder KW, Olson JF, Kahnoski RJ, Karn RC, Oei TO: Hyperammonemia after transurethral resection of the prostate: A report of two cases. *J Urol* 132:995–997, 1984.
28. Weissman JD, Weissman BM: Pontine myelinolysis and delayed encephalopathy following the rapid correction of acute hyponatremia. *Arch Neurol* 46:926–927, 1989.
29. Whalley PJ, Pritchard JA: Oxytocin and water intoxication. *JAMA* 186:601–603, 1963.
30. Lilien AA: Oxytocin-induced water intoxication. A report of a maternal death. *Obstet Gynecol* 32:171–173, 1968.
31. Gupta DR, Cohen NH: Oxytocin, "salting out", and water intoxication. *JAMA* 220:681–683, 1972.
32. Morgan DB, Kirwan NA, Hancock KW, Robinson D, Howe JG, Ahmad S: Water intoxication and oxytocin infusion. *Br J Obstet Gynecol* 84:6–12, 1977.
33. Raskind M, Barnes RF: Water metabolism in psychiatric disorders. *Semin Nephrol* 4:316–324, 1984.
34. Peck V, Shenkman L: Haloperidol-induced syndrome of inappropriate secretion of antidiuretic hormone. *Clin Pharmacol Ther* 20:442–444, 1979.
35. Ajlouni K, Kern MW, Tures JF: Thiothixene-induced hyponatremia. *Arch Intern Med* 134:1103–1105, 1974.
36. Shah DK, Wig NN, Chaudhury RR: Antidiuretic hormone levels in patients with weight gain after chlorpromazine therapy. *Indian J Med Res* 61:771–776, 1973.
37. Fishman CM: Water intoxication and thioridazine (letter). *Ann Intern Med* 82:852, 1975.
38. Fowler RC, Kronfol ZA, Perry PJ: Water intoxication, psychosis, and inappropriate secretion of antidiuretic hormone. *Arch Gen Psychiatr* 34:1097–1099, 1975.
39. Kosten TR, Camp W: Inappropriate secretion of antidiuretic hormone in a patient receiving piperazine phenothiazines. *Psychosomatics* 21:351–355, 1980.
40. Miller M, Moses AM, Rao KJ: Water intoxication and thioridazine (letter). *Ann Intern Med* 82:852, 1975.
41. Kendler KS, Weitzman RE, Rubin RT: Lack of arginine vasopressin response to central dopamine blockade in normal adults. *J Clin Endocrin Metab* 47:204–207, 1978.
42. Rowe JW, Shelton RL, Helderman H: Influence of the emetic reflex on vasopressin release in man. *Kidney Int* 16:729–735, 1979.
43. Raskind MA, Courtney ND, Backus FI: Antipsychotic drugs and plasma vasopressin. In: *Scientific Proceedings, 135th Annual Meeting, American Psychiatric Association*, Toronto, pp 222–223, 1982.
44. Berl T, Cadnapaphornchai P, Harbottle JA: Mechanism of suppression of vasopressin during alpha-adrenergic stimulation with norepinephrine. *J Clin Invest* 53:219–227, 1974.
45. Rosenbaum JF, Rothman JS, Murray GB: Psychosis and water intoxication. *J Clin Psychiatr* 40:287–291, 1979.
46. Dubovsky SL, Grabson S, Berl T, Schrier RW: Syndrome of inappropriate secretion of antidiuretic hormone with exacerbated psychosis. *Ann Intern Med* 79:551–554, 1973.
47. Brown RP, Kocsis JH, Cohen SK: Delusional depression and inappropriate antidiuretic hormone secretion. *Biol Psychiatr* 18:1059–1063, 1983.
48. Robertson GL: The pathophysiology of ADH secretion. In: G Tolis, ed, *Clinical Neuroendocrinology: A Pathophysiological Approach*. Raven Press, New York, pp 247–260, 1979.
49. Hariprasad MK, Eisinger RP, Nadler IM: Hyponatremia in psychogenic polydipsia. *Arch Intern Med* 140:1639–1642, 1980.
50. Berginer VM, Osimani A, Berginer J, Barmeir E: CT brain scan in acute water intoxication. *J Neurol Neurosurg Psychiatr* 48:841–842, 1985.
51. Lipsmeyer E, Ackerman G: Irreversible brain damage after water intoxication. *JAMA* 196:286–288, 1966.

52. Nolph KD, Schrier RW: Sodium, potassium, and water metabolism in the syndrome if inappropriate antidiuresis. *Annu Rev Med* 31:315–327, 1980.
53. Ayus JC: Diuretic induced hyponatremia. *Arch Int Med* 146:1295–1296, 1986.
54. Ashouri OS: Severe diuretic-induced hyponatremia in the elderly. *Arch Int Med* 146:1355–1357, 1986.
55. Friedman E, Shadel M, Halkin H, Farfel Z: Thiazide induced hyponatremia. Reproducibility by single dose rechallenge and an analysis of pathogenesis. *Ann Intern Med* 110:24–30, 1989.
56. Ashraf N, Locksley R, Arieff AI: Thiazide induced hyponatremia associated with death or neurologic damage in outpatients. *Am J Med* 70:1163–1168, 1981.
57. Ayus JC, Krothapalli RK, Arieff AI: Sexual difference in survival with severe symptomatic hyponatremia (abstract). *Kidney Int* 33:180, 1088.
58. Fraser CL, Kucharczyk J, Arieff AI, Rollin C, Sarnacki P, Norman D: Sex differences result in increased morbidity from hyponatremia in female rats. *Am J Physiol* 256 (Regulatory Integrative Comp Physiol 25):R880–R885, 1989.
59. Scoccia B, Scommegna A: Carbamazepine-induced hyponatremia after transabdominal follicular ultrasound examination. *Fertility Sterility* 50:984–985, 1988.
60. Aasheim GM: Hyponatremia during transurethral surgery. *Can Anaesth Soc J* 20:274–280, 1973.
61. Kirschenbaum MA: Severe mannitol-induced hyponatremia complicating transurethral prostatic resection. *J Urol* 121:687–688, 1979.
62. Sunderrajan S, Bauer JH, Vopat RL, Wanner-Barjenbruch P, Hayes A: Posttransurethral resection hyponatremic syndrome: Case report and review of the literature. *Am J Kidney Dis* 4:80–84, 1984.
63. Bartholemew LG, Scholz DA: Reversible postoperative neurological symptoms. *JAMA* 162:22–26, 1956.
64. Scott JC Jr, Welch JS, Berman IB: Water and sodium depletion in surgical patients. *Obstet Gynecol* 26:168–175, 1965.
65. Zimmerman B, Wangensteen OH: Observations on water intoxication in surgical patients. *Surgery* 31:654–669, 1952.
66. Deutsch G, Goldberg M, Dripps RD: Postoperative hyponatremia with the inappropriate release of antidiuretic hormone. *Anesthesiology* 27:250–256, 1966.
67. Harrison RH III, Boren JS, Robison JR: Dilutional hyponatremic shock: Another concept of the transurethral resection reaction. *J Urol* 75:95–110, 1956.
68. Ting S, Eshaghpour E: Inappropriate secretion of antidiuretic hormone after open heart surgery. *Am J Dis Child* 134:873–874, 1980.
69. Appelt GL, Benson GS, Corriere JN Jr: Transient blindness. Unusual initial symptom of transurethral prostatic resection reaction. *Urology* 13:402–404, 1979.
70. Henderson DJ, Middleton RG: Coma from hyponatremia following transurethral resection of the prostate. *Urology* 15:267–271, 1980.
71. Fusz RE, Lauler DP, Cohen P: Diuretic-induced hyponatremia and sustained antidiuresis. *Am J Med* 33:783–791, 1962.
72. Swanson AG, Iseri OA: Acute encephalopathy due to water intoxication. *N Engl J Med* 258:831–834, 1958.
73. Devereaux MW, McCormick RA: Psychogenic water intoxication: A case report. *Am J Psychiatry* 129:628–630, 1972.
74. Langgard H, Smith WO: Self-induced water intoxication without predisposing illness. *N Engl J Med* 266:378–381, 1962.
75. Raskind M: Psychosis polydipsia and water intoxication. *Arch Gen Psychiatry* 30:112–114, 1974.
76. Singer I, Forrest JN, Jr: Drug induced states of nephrogenic diabetes insipidus. *Kidney Int* 10:82–95, 1976.
77. White MG, Fetner CD: Treatment of the syndrome of inappropriate secretion of antidiuretic hormone. *N Engl J Med* 292:390–392, 1975.
78. Harris CA, Dirks JH: Effect of acute lithium infusion on proximal and distal tubular reabsorption in rat (abstract). *Fed Proc* 32:381A, 1973.
79. Hullin RP, Coley VP, Birch NS, Thomas TH, Morgan DB: Renal function after long-term treatment with lithium. *Br Med J* 1:1457–1459, 1979.
80. Hallgren R, Alm PO, Hellsing K: Renal function in patients on lithium treatment. *Br J Psychiatr* 135:22–27, 1979.
81. Hansen HE, Hestbech J, Sorensen JL, Norgaard K, Heliskov J, Amdisen A: Chronic interstitial nephropathy in patients on long-term lithium treatment. *Q J Med New Series* 68:577–591, 1979.
82. Tangedahl TN, Gau GT: Myocardial irritability associated with lithium carbonate therapy. *N Engl J Med* 287:867–869, 1972.
83. Hurtig HI, Dyson WL: Lithium toxicity enhanced by diuresis. *N Engl J Med* 290:748–749, 1974.
84. Roth H, Becker KL, Shalhoub RJ, Katz S: Nephrotoxicity of demethylchlorotetracycline hydrochloride. *Arch Intern Med* 120:433–435, 1967.
85. Lazar R, Kerman L, Kanter A: Demethylchlorotetracycline hydrochloride and nephrogenic diabetes insipidus. *Cutis* 6:881–883, 1970.
86. Cherrill DA, Stote RM, Birge JR, Singer I: Demeclocycline treatment in the syndrome of inappropriate antidiuretic hormone secretion. *Ann Intern Med* 83:654–656, 1975.
87. deTroyer A: Demeclocycline treatment of syndrome of inappropriate antidiuretic hormone secretion. *JAMA* 237:2723–2726, 1977.
88. Miller PD, Linas SL, Schrier RW: Plasma demeclocycline levels and nephrotoxicity. Correlation in hyponatremic cirhotic patients. *JAMA* 243:2513–2515, 1980.
89. Oster JR, Epstein M, Ulano HB: Deterioration of renal function with demeclocycline administration. *Curr Ther Res* 20:794–800, 1976.
90. Carrilho F, Bosch J, Arroyo V, Mas B, Viver J, Rodes J: Renal failure associated with demeclocycline in cirrhosis. *Ann Intern Med* 87:195–197, 1977.
91. Cox M, Shook A, Singer I: Demeclocycline-induced azotemia, natriuresis, and antikaliuresis in congestive heart failure (abstract). *Clin Res* 27:495A, 1979.
92. Decaux G, Brimioulle S, Genette F, Mockel J: Treatment of the syndrome of inappropriate secretion of antidiuretic hormone by urea. *Am J Med* 69:99–106, 1980.
93. Decaux G, Genette F: Urea for long term treatment of syndrome of inappropriate secretion of antidiuretic hormone. *Br Med J* 283:1081–1083, 1981.
94. Sawyer WH, Pang PKT, Seto J, McEnroe M, Lammek B, Manning M: Vasopressin analogs that antagonize antidiuretic responses by rats to the antidiuretic hormone. *Science* 212:49–58, 1981.
95. Greig PD, Blendis M, Lanyer B, Taylor BR, Colapinto RF: Renal and hemodynamic effects of peritoneovenous shunt. II. Long term effects. Gastroenterology 80:119–125, 1981.
96. Dzau VJ, Colucci WS, Williams GH, Curfman G, Meggs L, Hollenberg NK: Sustained effectiveness of converting enzyme inhibition in patients with severe congestive heart failure. *N Engl J Med* 302:1373–1379, 1980.
97. Sterns RH: Severe symptomatic hyponatremia: Treatment

and outcome. A study of 64 cases. *Ann Intern Med* 107:656–664, 1987.
98. Ayus JC, Krothapalli RK, Arieff AI: Changing concepts in the treatment of severe symptomatic hyponatremia: Rapid correction and possible relation to central pontine myelinolysis. *Am J Med* 79:897–902, 1985.
99. Ayus JC, Krothapalli RK, Armstrong DL, Norton HJ: Symptomatic hyponatremia in rats: Effect of treatment on mortality and brain lesions. *Am J Physiol* 257 (Renal Fluid Electrolyte Physiol 26):F18–F22, 1989.
100. Kleinschmidt-DeMasters BK, Norenberg MD: Rapid correction of hyponatremia causes demyelination: Relation to central pontine myelinolysis. *Science* 211:1068–1070, 1981.
101. Illowsky BP, Laureno R: Encephalopathy and myelinolysis after rapid correction of hyponatremia. *Brain* 110:855–867, 1987.
102. Ayus JC, Krothapalli RK, Arieff AI: Treatment of symptomatic hyponatremia and its relation to brain demage: A prospective study. *N Engl J Med* 317:1190–1195, 1987.
103. Arieff AI: Hyponatremia associated with brain damage. *Adv Intern Med* 32:325–344, 1987.
104. Brennan S, Ayus JC: Central pontine myelinolysis and electrolyte disorders. In: *Neurologic Manifestations of Systemic Disorders*, Little Brown, Boston, 1989, in press.
105. Hochman I, Cabili S, Peer G: Hyponatremia in internal medicine ward patients: Causes, treatment and prognosis. *Isr J Med Sci* 25:73–76, 1989.
106. Cheng JC, Zikos D, Skopicki HA, Peterson DR, Fisher KA: Correction of symptomatic hyponatremia (abstract). *Kidney Int* 33:186, 1988.
107. Decaux G, Unger J, Brimioulle S, Mockel J: Hyponatremia in the syndrome of inappropriate secretion of antidiuretic hormone. Rapid correction with urea, sodium chloride, and water restriction therapy. *JAMA* 247:471–474, 1982.
108. Worthley LIG, Thomas PD: Treatment of hyponatraemic seizures with intravenous 29.2% saline. *Br Med J* 292:168–170, 1986.
109. Hantman D, Rossier B, Zohlman R, Schrier R: Rapid correction of hyponatremia in the syndrome of inappropriate secretion of antidiuretic hormone. *Ann Intern Med* 78:870–875, 1973.
110. Ghanem A: Hyponatraemia and hypo-osmolality (letter). *Lancet* 2:572, 1988.
111. Ayus JC, Olivero JJ, Frommer JP: Rapid correction of severe hyponatremia with intravenous hypertonic saline. *Am J Med* 72:43–48, 1982.
112. Ayus JC, Krothapalli RK, Armstrong DL: Rapid correction of severe hyponatremia in the rat: Histopathological changes in the brain *Am J Physiol* 248 (Renal Fluid Electrolyte Physiol 17):F711–F719, 1985.
113. Luttrell CN, Finberg L, Drawdy LP: Hemmorhagic encephalopathy induced by hypernatremia. II. Experimental observations on hyperosmolarity in cats. *Arch Neurol* 1:153–160, 1959.
114. Finberg L, Kiley J, Luttrell CN: Mass accidental salt poisoning in infancy: A study of a hospital disaster. *JAMA* 184:187–190, 1963.
115. Elton NW, Elton WJ, Nazareno JP: Pathology of acute salt poisoning in infants. *Am J Clin Pathol* 39:252–264, 1963.
116. Luttrell CN, Finberg L: Hemorrhagic encephalopathy induced by hypernatremia. I. Clinical, laboratory, and pathologic observations. *Arch Neurol Psychiatr* 81:424–432, 1959.
117. Simmons MA, Adcock EW III, Bard H, Battaglia FC: Hypernatremia and intracranial hemorrhage in neonates. *N Engl J Med* 291:6–10, 1974.
118. Morris-Jones PH, Houston IB, Evans RC: Prognosis of the neurological complications of acute hypernatremia. *Lancet* 2:1385–1389, 1967.
119. Snyder NA, Feigal DW, Arieff AI: Hypernatremia in elderly patients. A heterogenous, morbid, and iatrogenic entity. *Ann Intern Med* 107:309–319, 1987.
120. Phillips PA, Rolls BJ, Ledingham JGG, Forsling ML, Morton JJ, Crowe MJ, Wollner L: Reduced thirst after water deprivation in healthy elderly men. *N Engl J Med* 311:753–759, 1984.
121. Weil WB, Wallace WM: Hypertonic dehydration in infancy. *Pediatrics* 17:171–181, 1956.
122. Beck N, Byung PY: Effect of aging on urinary concentrating mechanism and vasopressin-dependent cAMP ub rats. *Am J Physiol* 243 (Renal Fluid Electrolyte Physiol 12):F121–F125, 1982.
123. Dodge PR, Sotos JF, Gamstorp I, DeVito D, Levy M, Rabe T: Neurophysiologic disturbances in hypertonic dehydration. *Trans Am Neurol Assoc* 87:33–36, 1962.
124. Hill ID, Mann MD, Bowie MD: Hypernatraemic dehydration: A prospective study in children with diarrhoeal disease. *S Afr Med J* 59:479–481, 1981.
125. Haddow JE, Cohen DL: Understanding and managing hypernatremic dehydration. *Pediatr Clin N Am* 21:435–441, 1974.
126. Hogan GR: Hypernatremia-problems in management. *Pediatr Clin North Am* 23:569–574, 1976.
127. Ross EJ, Christie SBM: Hypernatremia. *Medicine* 48:441–473, 1969.
128. Perkin RM, Levin DL: Common fluid and electrolyte problems in the pediatric intensive care unit. *Pediatr Clin North Am* 27:567–586, 1980.
129. Mahowald J, Himmelstein D: Hypernatremia in the elderly: Relation to infection and mortality. *J Am Geriatr Soc* 29:177–180, 1981.
130. Macaulay D, Watson M: Hypernatraemia in infants as a cause of brain damage. *Arch Dis Child* 42:485–491, 1967.
131. Miller M, Finberg L: Peritoneal dialysis for salt poisoning. *N Engl J Med* 263:1347–1350, 1960.
132. Bichet DG, Levi M, Schrier RW: Polyuria, dehydration, and overhydration. In: Seldin DW, Giebisch G, eds, *The Kidney: Physiology and Pathophysiology*. Raven Press, New York, pp 851–984, 1985.
133. Marsden PA, Halperin ML: Pathophysiological approach to patients presenting with hypernatremia. *Am J Nephrol* 5:229–235, 1985.
134. Nitzan M, Zelmanovsky S: Glucose intolerance in hypernatremic rats. *Diabetes* 17:579–581, 1968.
135. Freidenberg GR, Kosnik EJ, Sotos JF: Hyperglycemic coma after suprasellar surgery. *N Engl J Med* 303:863–865, 1980.
136. Pizarro D, Posada G, Levine ML: Hypernatremic diarrheal dehydration treated with "slow" (12-hour) oral rehydration therapy: A preliminary report. *J Pediatr* 104:316–319, 1984.
137. Blum D, Brasseur D, Kahn A, Brachet E: Safe oral rehydration of hypertonic dehydration. *J Pediatr Gastroenterol Nutr* 5:232–235, 1986.
138. Franco-Saenz R, Wolffing BK, Rivers RJ: Case report: Hypodipsia and hypernatremia in congenital hydrocephalus. *Am J Med Sci* 297:385–386, 1989.
139. Hogan GR, Dodge PR, Gill SR, Master S, Sotos JF: Pathogenesis os seizures occurring during restoration of plasma tonicity to normal in animals previously chronically hypernatremic. *Pediatrics* 43:54–64, 1969.
140. Kahn A, Blum D, Casimir G, Brachet E: Controlled fall in natremia in hypertonic dehydration: Possible avoidance of

rehydration seizures. *Eur J Pediatr* 135:293–296, 1981.
141. Hogan GR, Dodge PR, Gill SR, Pickering LK, Master S: The incidence of seizures after rehydration of hypernatremic rabbits with intravenous of ad libitum oral fluids. *Pediatr Res* 18:340–345, 1983.
142. Ayus JC, Krothapalli R, Spark J, Freiberg M: Severe hypernatremia in rats: Effect of treatment on brain function and histology (abstract). *Kidney Int* 35:214, 1989.

CHAPTER 2

Polyuric Syndromes

WILLIAM P. MULDOWNEY & MICHAEL H. HUMPHREYS

INTRODUCTION

Urine volume normally is closely matched to the dietary intake of water and is largely independent of the intake of solute over the range encountered in normal diets. Water balance in the face of varying intake is achieved by renal regulation of urine volume through the operation of the concentrating and diluting mechanism: Extrarenal fluid losses via the skin and lungs, and in stool, occur, but they are relatively constant and do not contribute to the pathophysiology of polyuric states. Although urine volume is regulated independently of solute excretion in most circumstances, the two are related at the extremes: very low rates of solute excretion may impair the ability to maintain water balance and result in dilutional hyponatremia, while extremely high rates of solute excretion may obligate urinary water excretion and lead to negative water balance and hypernatremia. This circumstance of solute diuresis is one of the polyuric syndromes and will be discussed more fully below.

NORMAL WATER BALANCE

Water balance results from a dynamic interplay between water intake and renal water excretion. The components participating in normal water balance are schematized in Figure 1. Water intake is dictated chiefly by thirst and attendant water-seeking behavior. Two general mechanisms participate in the stimulation of thirst. In one, water loss leads to an increase in body fluid osmolality and consequent *cellular dehydration*: Cells in regions of the central nervous system undergoing this process activate neural pathways; giving rise to the sensation of thirst. Water ingestion corrects the state of cellular dehydration and the sense of thirst subsides. This mechanism accounts for water intake in most day-to-day circumstances. Thirst is also stimulated by *hypovolemia* independent of any increase in body fluid osmolality. The hypovolemia may be real, as from hemorrhage, or sensed, as occurs in congestive heart failure and cirrhosis of the liver. Hypovolemia activates thirst through neural pathways involving high- and low-pressure baroreceptors and through the action of circulating angiotensin II on the CNS, particularly the subfornical organ (1). Thirst, like hunger, is also subject to modulation from higher centers, and water intake may occur because of conditioned behavior rather than dictated by a sense of thirst resulting from cellular dehydration or hypovolemia. The extreme case of this is *psychogenic polydipsia*, another of the polyuric syndromes to be discussed below.

The regulation of renal water excretion is achieved through adjustments in the secretion of vasopressin (ADH) from the neurohypophysis and through the operation of the renal concentrating mechanism (Figure 1). The factors that stimulate ADH secretion are similar to those stimulating thirst. A period of water deprivation leads to negative water balance from continuing renal and extrarenal water losses. Body fluid osmolality rises, and ADH secretion is stimulated through osmoreceptors in the CNS lying close to the supraoptic nucleus. ADH secretion can also be stimulated nonosmotically by hypovolemia and hypotension. The afferent pathways mediating this stimulation are the high-pressure baroreceptors located in the aortic arch and carotid sinus, and the low-pressure baroreceptors in the right and left atria (Figure 1). In addition, it has recently been shown that renal afferent nerves stimulate ADH secretion in the cat (2), although the importance of this mechanism in overall regulation is not yet clear. ADH then promotes water conservation by increasing the water permeability of the renal collecting duct, thereby allowing the excretion of a smaller volume of more concentrated urine. Thus, the same factors involved in stimulating thirst and water intake, on the one hand, also activate increased ADH secretion and water conservation, on the other.

These same pathways also operate to suppress ADH excretion in the face of a dilute body fluid osmolality and/or blood volume expansion. The sensitivity of ADH secretion to small changes in body fluid osmolality is so great that one of the major challenges facing the clinician caring for a polyuric patient is to discriminate excessive water intake, with secondary, appropriate suppression of ADH secretion, from a primary impairment in ADH secretion with a secondary or reactive increase in thirst and water intake. At times the differentiation between two conditions can be extremely difficult, even though the

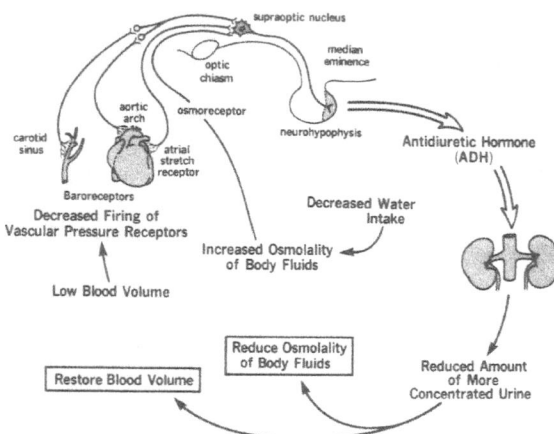

Figure 1. Schematic view of the regulation of water balance. In the face of decreased fluid intake, an increase in body fluid osmolality is sensed by osmoreceptors in the CNS and leads to ADH secretion; hypovolemia, detected by pressure receptors, also triggers ADH release. ADH then acts on the kidneys to conserve water and thereby correct body fluid osmolality and restore blood volume. This system operates in reverse in response to excess water intake or expanded blood volume: ADH is suppressed and dilute urine is excreted. Polyuric syndromes can best be understood in this framework.

underlying mechanisms leading to polyuria are radically different.

The ability of the kidneys to excrete urine that is appropriately dilute or concentrated also depends on several intrarenal factors, in addition to the proper regulation of circulating ADH concentration. First, reabsorption of filtered NaCl in the water-impermeable thick ascending limb of Henle's loop leads to the formation of a dilute tubular fluid in the early distal convoluted tubule; further solute removal in later nephron segments and the absence of an ADH effect leads to the excretion of large volumes of dilute urine. This process of NaCl reabsorption in the thick limb also produces the hypertonic medullary interstitium required for concentration of the urine in the presence of ADH-induced increases in the water permeability of the collecting duct. Recent studies have shown that ADH also stimulates NaCl transport in the medullary thick ascending limb (3), and action that would increase the tonicity of the interstitium, allowing excretion of a more concentrated urine. Thus, interference with function of the thick limb, as results from diuretic administration, will interfere with both the diluting and concentrating abilities. Second, the hypertonicity of the interstitium is maintained by the low rate of medullary blood flow, chiefly through the vasae rectae. Any increase in medullary blood flow accelerates the return of medullary solute to the general circulation and reduces the hypertonicity of the medulla. This washout of the medulla reduces the urinary concentrating ability. Two factors that increase medullary blood flow are osmotic diuresis and protracted water diuresis, circumstances usually associated with polyuria. This must be kept in mind in the interpretation of diagnostic tests discussed below (water deprivation, ADH administration) in the polyuric patient. Some diuretics also increase medullary blood flow. Third, appropriate excretion of free water also depends on optimal delivery of solute (NaCl) out of the proximal tubule to the diluting segment in the thick ascending limb. In states of volume depletion, proximal reabsorption is increased, and distal delivery is correspondingly reduced, so that urine dilution is impaired. Advantage of this fact is taken in the treatment of diabetes insipidus (DI) by producing mild volume depletion with diuretics, thereby limiting solute delivery to the diluting segment and reducing free water excretion. Fourth, excessive rates of solute excretion limit tubular water reabsorption and obligate high urine volumes regardless of the state of hydration of the patient. The resulting osmotic diuresis is a common cause of polyuria. Finally, renal water excretion also depends on an appropriate response of collecting duct epithelium to circulating ADH. Although a full description of the cellular actions of ADH is beyond the scope of this chapter, the elements of this response include binding of the peptide to its receptor, activation of adenylate cyclase and the formation of cyclic adenosine-3,5'-monophosphate, activation of a protein kinase, and phosphorylation of membrane proteins, with an increase in the permeability of the luminal membrane to water. Interference with any of these steps will produce partial or complete nephrogenic DI, as discussed below. Drugs that do this include lithium ion and demeclocycline; indeed, advantage has been taken of this effect of these agents in the treatment of the syndrome of inappropriate ADH secretion (SIADH) (4). ADH also stimulates the production of prostaglandins by renal medullary interstitial cells (5). These prostaglandins antagonize the effect of ADH to increase collecting duct water permeability. Interference with this effect of ADH by inhibition of prostaglandin synthesis with nonsteroidal antiinflammatory agents may potentiate the action of ADH on urine concentration (6).

CLASSIFICATION OF POLYURIC SYNDROMES

Since urine volume normally reflects water intake, a wide range is possible depending on habitual intakes. However, it is customary to regard urine volumes greater than 3 l/24 hr as indicative of polyuria. Defined in this manner, polyuria can be regarded as *appropriate* if the large urine volume is secondary to excessive fluid intake. In this circumstance, all aspects of the diluting mechanism are operating appropriately to maintain water balance. More commonly, polyuria is *inappropriate* due to some limitation on the ability of the kidneys to reabsorb water sufficiently. In such cases, water intake is driven by the sense of thirst; the magnitude of the intake will reflect the magnitude of the defect in renal water reabsorption. It has also become customary to describe polyuric states as *pri-*

Table 1. Classification of polyuric states

I. Primary polyuria — polyuria due to solute-free water loss from absence of ADH or impairment of its action on the renal tubule
   A. Central DI (pituitary, vasopressin-responsive DI)
      1. Idiopathic (familial and nonfamilial forms)
      2. Following head trauma, brain surgery, or hypophysectomy
      3. Resulting from space-occupying lesions: tumors (primary or metastic), granulomas, infiltrative diseases, vascular aneurysms
      4. Following viral or bacterial infections
   B. Nephrogenic DI
      1. Congenital
      2. Acquired
         a. Renal disease
            i. chronic renal failure of any cause
            ii. tubulointerstitial disease, particularly involving the medulla: Sjogren's syndrome, amyloidosis, medullary cystic disease, polycystic kidney disease, sickle cell disease, obstructive uropathy
            iii. transient renal dysfunction: postobstructive diuresis, nonoliguric acute renal failure, diuretic phase of oliguric acute renal failure, nonoliguric prerenal azotemia
         b. Electrolyte abnormalities
            i. hypercalcemia
            ii. hypokalemia
   C. Increased free water intake with appropriate polyuria
      1. Compulsive water drinking (psychogenic polydipsia)
      2. Primary neurogenic polydipsia
      3. Excessive administration of hypotonic intravenous fluids

II. Secondary polyuria — polyuria resulting from obligatory solute excretion (osmotic diuresis) or impairment of solute reabsorption
   A. Osmotic diuresis
      1. Glucose: uncontrolled diabetes or excess intravenous glucose administration
      2. Urea
         a. Endogenous: marked protein catabolism (burns, severe trauma, rhabdomyolysis), some cases of postobstructive diuresis or recovery from oliguric acute renal failure
         b. Exogenous: excessive administration of high-protein tube feedings or parenteral nutrition
      3. Miscellaneous
         a. Mannitol
         b. Glycerol
         c. Angiographic dyes
   B. Impaired solute (NaCl) reabsorption
      1. Diuretics
      2. Nonoliguric acute renal failure
      3. Diuretic phase of oliguric acute renal failure

mary if they result from the suppression or absence of ADH secretion or impairment of its action on the kidneys, and *secondary* if they occur as a consequence of renal abnormalities, even though circulating ADH concentrations would, if measured, be found to be elevated. Accordingly, central DI, nephrogenic DI, and psychogenic polydipsia are examples of primary polyuria, while osmotic diuresis and other disorders of tubular transport are illustrative of secondary polyuric states. Although these distinctions are arbitrary, they nevertheless can be used to provide a useful framework with which to classify the various polyuric syndromes. Table 1 reflects such a classification scheme.

DATA REQUIRED FOR ESTABLISHING PROPER DIAGNOSIS

Once a patient is recognized as being polyuric, data from history, physical examination, and laboratory studies must be used to characterize the basis for the polyuria. The *history* may indicate whether the onset was abrupt or gradual and temporally related to head trauma, prescribed medications, or nutritional or other therapy of concurrent disease. It will also give information about patterns of fluid intake. The *physical examination* is useful for revealing the state of hydration and may provide clues to underlying diseases causing or contributing to the polyuria, e.g., diabetes. Laboratory tests are required in order to assign the disorder to the proper diagnostic category. Serum sodium concentration and osmolality should be routinely measured, as should the blood glucose and urea nitrogen concentrations. Hematocrit and total protein determinations may be useful in gauging the degree of hemoconcentration resulting from negative water balance. Urinary measurements necessary for accurate diagnosis and management include the 24-hour urinary volume as well as urine osmolality, sodium, and, occasionally, urea nitrogen concentrations. in cases of polyuria from suspected glucose osmotic diuresis, some measure of urinary glucose is also necessary. As will be discussed subsequently, urine osmolality will play a key role in proper diagnosis, since it reflects the degree to which the polyuric state is chiefly a solute-free water diuresis or a combination of high solute and water excretion. Urinary specific gravity may provide similar information; however, because the specific gravity is influenced by the nature of the solutes dissolved in the urine, whereas osmolality is a measure of the osmotic activity of all dissolved solutes regardless of their nature, the latter measurement is preferred. Measurement of urine and serum creatinine concentrations in addition to sodium concentrations also permits calculation of fractional sodium excretion [FE_{Na}, $(U/P_{Na} \div U/P_{cr}) \times 100$], useful in evaluating the possibility of solute diuresis in polyuric patients.

It is usually the case that, even with skillful interpretation of data derived from history, physical examination, and the laboratory tests just described, it is not possible to assign patients with certainty to the proper diagnostic category. To do this, it is necessary to evaluate the response to water deprivation and the subsequent administration of exogenous ADH (7). The standardized test is carried out in the inpatient setting where close monitoring will detect symptomatic dehydration and volume depletion at the earliest stages before harmful levels are reached. It is performed over a 12- to 16-hour period, usually overnight for the sake of convenience; the goal is to evaluate the renal response to a rise in plasma osmolality above 295 mOsm/kg H_2O or a decrease in body weight of 3-5%. When these conditions are achieved, a urine osmolality less than 300 mOsm/kg H_2O suggests that the patient's polyuria results from central or nephrogenic DI, while a U_{osm} greater than 300 mOsm/kg H_2O indicates at least partial responsiveness of the urinary concentrating mechanism, as occurs with partial central or nephrogenic DI or psychogenic polydipsia (Table 2).

These interpretations are further refined by evaluating the patient's response to the administration of 5 U of aqueous ADH subcutaneously. Urine is collected over the ensuing 2 hours; an increase in U_{osm} of 50% or greater is observed in patients with complete central DI, and an increase of 15% or greater is characteristic of partial central DI. Patients in whom U_{osm} fails to increase by even 15% after exogenous ADH are polyuric because of nephrogenic DI, whether partial or complete. The rare patient with psychogenic polydipsia may also exhibit no change (< 15% increase) in U_{osm} after ADH administation. The reason for this is that the state of virtually constant water diuresis that these patients undergo washes out the hypertonic medullary interstitium, preventing further urine concentration, even though the cellular actions initiated by ADH are presumably intact. However, such patients will typically have a higher U_{osm} after dehydration than patients with either central or nephrogenic DI (Table 2) (7).

The sequential steps in the diagnostic approach to the polyuric patient are outlined in Figure 2. Since patients with the various forms of DI usually have an intact thirst

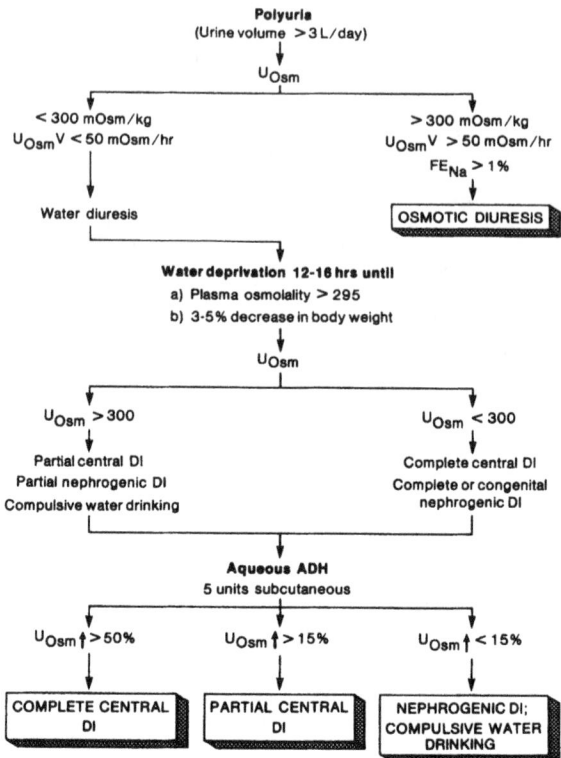

Figure 2. Diagnostic approach to the major polyuric syndromes.

Table 2. Fluid deprivation and exogenous vasopressin test in polyuria

	Number of cases	Mean U_{osm} with dehydration	U_{osm} after vasopressin	% change (n U_{osm})
Normal subjects	9	1067 ± 68.7	978 ± 79.4	−8.9 ± 3.0
Complete pituitary diabetes insipidus	18	168 ± 13	445 ± 52	180 ± 41.4
Partial pituitary diabetes insipidus	12	437.0 ± 33.6	548.6 ± 28.2	28.5 ± 4.7
Compulsive water drinking	7	738.2 ± 52.9	779.8 ± 73.1	5.0 ± 2.2

Source: Date from Miller M, Dalakos T, Moses AM, et al.: Recognition of partial defects in antidiuretic hormone secretion. Ann Intern Med 73:72, 1970. Adapted for *Renal and Electrolyte Disorders*, 2nd ed. R. Schrier, Little Brown & Co, Boston, 1980.

mechanism, the screening laboratory values outlined earlier will be close to normal, provided that free access to water is available. For this reason, the water deprivation protocol is usually necessary. Patients with polyuria from osmotic diuresis are often less able to increase water intake as dehydration develops because of associated CNS disease and will therefore be more likely to have aberranrt laboratory results. In such patients, the measured rate of solute excretion (U_{osm} × urine flow rate) will be greater than 50 mOsm/hr (about 1 mOsm/min or > 1200 mOsm/24 hr), and FE_{Na} > 1% despite dehydration and volume depletion.

PRIMARY POLYURIC SYNDROMES

Central diabetes insipidus

Central (pituitary) DI is classified as *partial* if residual ADH secretion permits elaboration of at least a modestly concentrated urine, or *complete* if urine is persistently hypotonic to plasma. It may be permanent or transient; transient, incomplete forms of central DI are more common following injury to the median eminence of the hypothalamus or the neurohypophysis, while lesions of the

ADH-synthesizing neurons of the supraoptic and paraventricular nuclei are typically more severe and permanent. Central DI occurs from trauma and following neurosurgery in about 25% of cases, and as a result of space-occupying lesions in another 25%. However, about half the cases have no discernible cause (8, 9). Clinically, this form of DI is usually abrupt in onset and is accompanied by urine volumes of 3–10 l per day or more with urine osmolality varying from 50 to 200 mOsm/kg H_2O. Patients suffer from marked nocturia and express a preference for ice water replacement fluids. Hyperosmolality and hypernatremia only develop if the patient has a disordered thirst mechanism or if adequate replacement fluids are not available; this can become a major consideration in the comatose patient, in whom serious hypernatremia can develop in a matter of hours.

Following acute injury to the hypothalamic-neurohypophyseal axis, a patient may exhibit the full-blown picture of DI, with polydipsia, polyuria, and the excretion of large amounts of dilute urine. This is followed in a few days by the "normal interphase," in which urine is concentrated and the urine volume is normal, but during which time an ingested water load is retained and not excreted, indicative of excessive ADH secretion. This excessive ADH occurs as a result of leakage of previously synthesized hormone from damaged neurons. Within a few more days, polyuria and polydipsia recur, and the patient enters the chronic stage of central DI, as no further ADH is available for release into the circulation. This triphasic response requires close attention on the part of the clinician to aviod the development of either hyperosmolality or hypoosmolality.

When DI is present for a long duration, both hydroureter and hydronephrosis can develop, reflecting the high urine output. Bladder volume may become very large, even to the point where nocturia may subside. DI can occur at any age, and both sexes are affected. Because it can be familial, other family members should be questioned about polyuria.

Nephrogenic diabetes insipidus

Nephrogenic DI is also termed *vasopressin-resistant DI* because administration of ADH does not result in elaboration of a more concentrated urine (Figure 2, Table 2). Nephrogenic DI can rarely result from inheritance of an X-linked homozygous gene; it typically presents in infancy with marked dehydration and hypotonic urine (10–12). The basis for vasopressin resistance is not known, although the failure of urinary cAMP excretion to increase in response to ADH administration suggests a defect in hormone action prior to the generation of this nucleotide (13). Nephrogenic DI occurs more commonly as an acquired abnormality resulting from renal disease and from certain drugs. The renal diseases that cause this abnormality have as a common feature primary involvement of the renal medulla, with attendant disruption of the processes involved in the development and maintenance of the hypertonic interstitium and/or the permeability of the collecting duct; GFR is often well preserved. Sjogren's syndrome (14), amyloid involvement of the collecting duct (15), myeloma (16), medullary cystic disease (17), and polycystic kidney disease (17) are some causes of this form of nephrogenic DI. Bilateral partial urinary tract obstruction can also present as a polyuric state with excretion of hypotonic urine, and ADH-resistant polyuria also develops in some cases following relief of urinary tract obstruction, contributing to postobstructive diuresis (18). In obstructive uropathy, it appears that the polyuria results from a decrease in water permeability of the collecting duct resulting from the obstruction. Sickle cell disease also can result in excretion of hypotonic urine, although through a different mechanism: In the oxygen-poor and low-flow environment of the renal medulla, sludging and sickling of red cells occurs, leading to infarction and fibrosis of the interstitium and loss of medullary hypertonicity (19, 20). Loss of maximum concentrating ability occurs in any form of chronic renal insufficiency and is roughly proportional to the deline in GFR; it seldom is sufficient to produce symptomatic polyuria. ADH-resistant hyposthenuria has also been observed in far advanced renal failure (21). However, this is usually not a clinical problem because the low GFR limits the volume of urine. It has also been suggested that a vasopressin-resistant concentrating defect can occur in states of prerenal azotemia, leading to a syndrome of polyuric prerenal failure (22).

A number of drugs can also produce nephrogenic DI (23) (Table 3). The most common of these is lithium, usually in the form of lithium carbonate prescribed for the treatment of manic-depressive illness. Lithium interferes with the ADH-stimulated increase in cAMP generation in the collecting tubule, thereby producing DI; this adverse consequence of the drug can occur even with blood levels in the therapeutic range, but is more common with toxic levels (> 2 mM/l) (23–25). Patients will report increased thirst and water intake in response to the polyuria. Demeclocycline has a similar action but is less commonly prescribed (26). Other agents that can result in nephrogenic DI are listed in Table 3. Two electrolyte disturbances also result in polyuria. Hypercalcemia of any cause impairs urinary concentration by decreasing medullary hypertonicity and leading to medullary nephrocalcinosis (27, 28), and by inhibiting the stimulation of cAMP caused by ADH (29). Chronic hypokalemia also impairs

Table 3. Drugs known to cause nephrogenic diabetes insipidus

Lithium
Demeclocycline
Colchicine
Vinblastine
Methoxyflurane
Amphotericin B
Aminoglycoside antibiotics
Cisplatinum
Dextropropoxyphene

urinary concentration; although the mechanism is not known, it is associated with reduced medullary hypertonicity (30) and is independent of renal prostaglandins (31). Both hypokalemia and hypercalcemia in the rat lead to polydipsia: Rats drink more water than necessary to overcome the concentrating defect (32, 33). This polydipsia then contributes to the polyuria characteristic of these conditions.

Acquired nephrogenic DI in general tends to be milder than complete central DI. Urine volume is typically less than 4–6 l/day, and with maximum dehydration patients can usually achieve a urine hypertonic to plasma, although there is no further response to exogenous ADH (Figure 2, Table 2).

Compulsive water drinking

Compulsive water drinking is also known as psychogenic polydipsia. The basis for polyuria relates solely to excessive water ingestion; the appropriate suppression of ADH secretion then leads to the excretion of the ingested fluid as hypotonic urine. Patients with this entity are usually middle-aged women with a history of psychiatric disorders (34, 35); rarely, structural lesions of the base of the brain and the hypothalamus may produce intense thirst, so-called primary neurogenic polydipsia. Because polyuria in this setting is driven by excessive water intake, plasma osmolality is usually below 280 mOsm/kg H_2O, in distinction to patients with central or nephrogenic DI, in whom plasma osmolality is usually above 285 mOsm/kg H_2O (34). However, sufficient overlap in these numbers usually dictates that the response to the dehydration test be evaluated (Figure 2, Table 2)

SECONDARY POLYURIA

States of secondary polyuria result from tubular abnormalities in reabsorption of filtered solute with obligatory water loss secondary to the transport defect. The situations in which secondary polyuria occurs are listed in Table 1. Chief among them is osmotic diuresis (36), but secondary polyuria can also occur as a result of impaired tubular reabsorption from diuretic administration of from damage in nonliguric acute renal failure or the recovery (diuretic) phase of oliguric acute renal failure. The clinical settings in which secondary polyuria arises are usually straightforward and pose no major diagnostic problem. Functionally, they are characterized by a high rate of solute excretion (often > 50 mOsm/hr), urine osmolality > 300 mOsm/kg H_2O, and FE_{Na} > 1%. In the case of osmotic diuresis, the involved solute is also evident from the clinical setting and can be confirmed by measuring urinary glucose or urea nitrogen; mannitol diuresis must be suspected in patients infused with this agent, and diuresis from angiographic dye infusion can be indicated by a very high urine specifc gravity (> 1.040).

TREATMENT OF POLYURIA

Treatment of polyuria and its consequences is directed at two distinct goals: treatment of the underlying disorder, which usually involves chronic management, and treatment, often emergency, of the complications resulting from the polyuria.

Treatment of primary polyuria

The basic for treatment rests on an accurate diagnosis, and the approach outlined above should be followed to do this.

CENTRAL DIABETES INSIPIDUS (DI)

Since the basic abnormality in central DI is absence of ADH, therapy is primarily directed at hormone replacement. A variety of agents and preparations is available. In acute situations (e.g. postoperatively), a short-acting ADH preparation such as aqueous vasopressin is preferred because of the relatively short half-life (4–6 hours); it can be administered subcutaneously in a dose of 5–10 U. For chronic therapy, a synthetic ADH analog, desamino-D-arginine-vasopressin (desmopressin, DDAVP) has achieved widespread success. This compound has an antidiuretic-to-pressor ratio of approximately 2000:1, compared to a 1:1 ratio for the natural ADH, as well as a longer duration of action (6–24 hours) due to delayed metabolic clearance (37, 38). It is administered intranasally in doses of 10–20 μg every 12–24 hours, with the dosage adjusted according to the response. Absorption by this route of administration may be impaired by nasal congestion, as during upper respiratory infection. This compound is well tolerated and virtually free of major side effects; it also has a low antigenic propensity. A long-acting, intramuscularly administered hormone preparation, vasopressin tannate in oil, is also available; its duration of action is 24–72 hours, and this factor, coupled with the need for IM injections, has limited its utility, particularly since DDAVP has become available. Absorption of this compound is variable unless the mixture is warmed and shaken prior to injection to ensure even dispersion of the hormone in the vehicle. Because of its long duration of action, water intoxication can occur with excessive water ingestion or infusion.

Nonhormonal therapy is also useful in the treatment of central DI, particularly partial lesions. The mainstay of such pharmacologic therapy is chronic diuretic administration; the agents to be recommended are of the thiazide class of diuretics. By producing negative sodium balance, these diuretics decrease GFR modestly and stimulate reabsorption in the proximal tubule. This limits the amount of filtrate delivered distally and thus the volume of free water that can be generated (39). Once established, this effect can be maintained, even without continued diuretic treatment, if salt intake is sufficiently reduced, but it is generally more practical to administer the diuretic chronically. The sulfonylurea hypoglycemic agents chlorpropamide and possibly tolbutamide are also effective, because they enhance residual ADH release and because they augment the renal actions of ADH (40, 41), possibly through inhibition of ADH-stimulated prostaglandin synthesis (42). Nonsteroidal antiinflammatory drugs such as indomethacin, which also inhibit renal prostaglandins, will also decrease urine output in patients with partial central DI (43). The lipid-lowering agent clofibrate and the anticonvulsant carbamazepine have also been shown to be effective in this setting, and carbamazepine may be synergistic with chlorpropamide when both are used together (44, 45). Complications of therapy include hypoglycemia with the sulfonylureas and water intoxication with all agents if water intake is excessive. Clofibrate and carbamazepine have other side effects that limit their usefulness in this setting.

NEPHROGENIC DIABETES INSIPIDUS

Congenital nephrogenic DI is usually severe and mandates careful attention of fluid balance (through measurement of body weight) and uninterrupted access to water for children with this problem. Neither exogenous ADH nor drugs, such as chlorpropamide, that protentiate its action is effective, and diuretic therapy coupled with a restricted sodium intake is required. With this regimen, urine volume can be reduced to 3–4 l/day.

Treatment of acquired nephrogenic DI depends on the basis for the DI. In renal disease, polyuria is usually mild and may not warrant specific treatment. Many of these forms of renal disease may also be associated with sodium wasting and renal tubular acidosis, and attention must be given to these possibilities and to the need for supplementation with sodium chloride or sodium bicarbonate. With bilateral urinary tract obstruction, relief of the obstruction represents the treatment for the polyuria. However, no specific treatment exists for the other renal diseases associated with nephrogenic DI. When the nephrogenic DI results from drug therapy, it is generally true that cessation of the responsible drug will restore the ability to concentrate the urine, although indomethacin has been shown to be effective in this form of DI as well (46, 47). Evidence suggests that lithium may impair urinary concentrating ability for up to a year after it is discontinued (48). In addition, lithium has proven so useful in the management of manic-depressive psychosis that its discontinuation may pose a real therapeutic bind, and some degree of nephrogenic DI may have to be accepted as a consequence of the continued use of this agent. The polyuria resulting from hypercalcemia and hypokalemia also usually resolve when the underlying abnormality responsible for these electrolyte disorders is identified and treated.

COMPULSIVE WATER DRINKING

Treatment of compulsive water drinking is in a sense straightforward, since the components involved in the normal maintenance of water balance (Figure 1) are intact and the polyuria results solely from excessive water intake. Therefore, simple restriction of water ingestion is the only measure required, However, this will need to be accompanied by psychiatric consultation and treatment in nearly all cases. Management of such patients is further complicated by the fact that psychotropic drugs often prescribed to facilitate psychiatric management may themselves have effects on water metabolism, usually to produce hyponatremia and mimic SIADH. If water intake persists at high levels, serious, even life-threatening, hypoosmolality can develop. A similar problem can occur in a patient with compulsive water drinking if the basis for the polyuria is felt erroneously to be central DI rather than compulsive water drinking. Administration of a diuretic to such an individual may also run the risk of producing serious hyponatremia (49).

Treatment of secondary polyuria

Once a polyuric state is recognized as being secondary, the treatment is usually self-evident. The solute responsible for osmotic diuresis should be stopped (mannitol, angiographic dye) or treated (glucose in diabetics). If it results from a urea diuresis, the urea load should be reduced by reducing the amount of nitrogen in enteral or parenteral feedings. If the urea results from marked hypercatabolism from trauma or burns, it may not be possible to alter the rate of solute excretion, and adequate free water must be provided. In all cases of secondary polyuria, hypovolemia must be corrected if present. Since osmotic diuresis results in excretion of a hyponatric urine with respect to plasma, hypernatremia often occurs with or without volume depletion and must be corrected with administration of hypotonic solutions. Polyuria resulting from the diuretic phase of oliguric acute renal failure, or from nonoliguric acute renal failure or postobstructive diuresis, is obligatory and should be managed according to standard principles of fluid therapy. In these settings, particularly postobstructive diuresis, it may become ambiguous whether the polyuria results from the acquired transport defect or merely reflects the appropriate excretion of infused salt and water, i.e., whether the clinician "is chasing his tail." Since most postobstructive diureses are short lasting (< 72 hours), it may be appropriate after this interval to reduce fluid intake to half the volume of urine output in the previous 24 hours (50). If, under careful clinical monitoring, circulatory function is well maintained, replacement therapy can safely be reduced further. If the patient maintains persistent polyuria despite clinically evident volume depletion, then further fluid support is still necessary.

Treatment of complications

Complications of polyuria relate chiefly to the hyperosmolality, which can result from solute-free water loss in DI, and to the attendant hypovolemia. In patients with central or nephrogenic DI, restriction of access to water intake for any reason (usually obtundation or coma) will lead to water loss and progressive hyperosmolality. The hyperosmolality in this setting is reflected precisely by hypernatremia. Any serum sodium concentration above 145 mEq/l should draw the attention of the clinician, and levels above 150 mEq/l demand prompt attention (51). Serious morbidity and mortality occur with levels above 160 mEq/l. In patients with DI, the degree of hypernatremia can be used to estimate the magnitude of the water deficit, since the water loss can be considered to be solute free:

$$\text{Water deficit} = \frac{P_{Na} - 140}{140} \times \text{TBW},$$

where P_{Na} is the measured serum sodium concentration and TBW is total body water. This latter term can be estimated as a fraction of body weight and varies with age and sex, being lower in women than men at any age and reaching a maximum value of 0.6 in young adult men; it is lower in childhood and old age. In hypernatremic DI patients, the figure should be reduced, since water has been preferentially lost from the body. With these thoughts in mind, one can estimate that the water deficit in a 30-year-old man weighing 65 kg with a serum sodium concentration of 168 mEq/l would be

$$\text{Water deficit} = \frac{(168 - 140)}{140} \times 0.55(65) = 7.15 \text{ l}.$$

Treatment of the hypernatremia should be carried out with hypotonic fluids. The *rate* at which fluid is administered should be no faster than to lower the serum sodium concentration by 2 mEq/hr, since more rapid correction may produce or exacerbate CNS side effects, including coma, seizures, and permanent brain damage. In patients in whom hypovolemia is so profound as to compromise the circulation, then resuscitation must be with crystalloid and/or colloid solutions until the circulation is adequately supported.

Patients with secondary polyuria may also be hyperosmolar, but here a more complex effect on serum sodium concentration exists. Solutes such as urea or glycerol freely cross cell membranes and so do not influence the distribution of water between intracellular and extracellular fluid compartments. In such patients, the hyperosmolality does not directly affect the serum sodium concentration, and hypernatremia, when it occurs, results from excretion of urine with a rather low (29–60 mEq/l) sodium concentration under the influence of the osmotic diuresis. On the other hand, hyperglycemia in diabetics, or high mannitol levels, obligates the transfer of water from intracellular to extracellular compartments, since these solutes are effectively confined to the extracellular space. This redistribution of water initially results in hyponatremia, although hyperosmolality exists. Later, osmotic diuresis causes greater water than sodium loss so that hypernatremia develops. Indeed, the presence of a normal or elevated serum sodium concentration in a diabetic patient with hyperosmolar coma is a grave sign, since correction of the hyperosmolality by insulin administration will cause extracellular water to redistribute back into cells, making the hypernatremia even worse unless large amounts of free water are given simultaneously. A general description of these relationships has been provided (52); a rough rule of thumb is to remember that the serum sodium concentration will fall or rise 1.6 mEq/l for every rise or fall in blood glucose concentration of 100 mg/dl (53).

Treatment of hyperosmolality in secondary polyuria is addressed at a) removal of the responsible solute, e.g., insulin treatment of hyperglycemia, cessation of mannitol infusion, reduction of protein intake in tube feedings; b) provision of crystalloid or colloid infusions to support the circulation if symptomatic hypovolemia is present; c) provision of hypotonic fluids to correct any hypernatremia, using the guidelines developed above.

Other complications may result from secondary polyuria, chiefly loss of other electrolytes such as potassium and magnesium. Replacement should be provided, using serum levels to monitor adequacy.

ACKNOWLEDGMENTS

William P. Muldowney is a Fellow in Nephrology at the Division of Nephrology of San Francisco General Hospital. He is supported by a matching fellowship from the National Kidney Foundation and the National Kidney Foundation of Northern California.

REFERENCES

1. Simpson JB, Epstein AN, Camardo JS Jr: Localization of receptors for the dipsogenic action of angiotensin II in the subfornical organ of rats. *J Comp Physiol Psychol* 92:768, 1978.
2. Caverson MM, Ciriello J: Effects of stimulation of afferent renal nerves on plasma levels of vasopressin. *Am J Physiol* 252:R801, 1987.
3. Hall DA, Varney DM: Effect of vasopressin on electrical potential differences and chloride transport in mouse medullary thick ascending limb of Henle. *J Clin Invest* 66:792, 1980.
4. Forrest JN Jr, Cox M, Hong C, et al.: Superiority of demyclocycline over lithium in the treatment of chronic syndrome of inappropriate secretion of antidiuretic hormone. *N Engl J Med* 298:173, 1978.
5. Beck TR, Hassid A, Dunn MJ: The effect of arginine vasopressin and its analogs on the synthesis of prostaglandin E_2 by rat renal medullary interstitial cells in culture. *J Pharmacol Exp Ther* 215:15, 1980.
6. Gross PA, Schrier RW, Anderson RJ: Prostaglandins and water metabolism: A review with emphasis on in vivo studies. *Kidney Int* 19:839, 1981.
7. Miller M, Dalakos T, Moses AM, et al.: Recognition of partial defects in antidiuretic hormone secretion. *Ann Int Med* 73:721, 1970.
8. Moses AM, Notman DD: Diabetes insipidus and syndrome of inappropriate antidiuretic hormone secretion. *Adv Int Med* 27:73, 1982.
9. Coggins CH, Leaf A: Diabetes insipidus. *Am J Med* 42:807, 1967.
10. Robinson MG, Kaplan SA: Inheritance of vasopressin resistant ('nephrogenic') diabetes insipidus. *Am J Dis Child* 99:164, 1960.
11. Silverstein E, Tobian L: Pitressin-resistant diabetes insipidus

with massive hydronephrosis. *Am J Med* 30:819, 1961.
12. Carter RD, Goodman AD: Nephrogenic diabetes insipidus accompanied by massive dilation of the kidneys, ureters and bladder. *J Urol* 89:366, 1963.
13. Fichman MP, Brooker G: Deficient renal cyclic adenosine 3′, 5′-monophosphate production in nephrogenic diabetes insipiduc. *J Clin Endocrinol Metab* 35:35, 1972.
14. Shearn MA, Tu W: Nephrogenic diabetes insipidus and other defects of renal tubular function in Sjogren's syndrome. *Am J Med* 39:312, 1965.
15. Carone FA, Epstein FH: Nephrogenic diabetes insipidus caused by amyloid disease: Evidence in man of role of collecting ducts in concentrating urine. *Am J Med* 29:539, 1960.
16. Smithline N, Kassirer J, Cohen JJ: Light-chain nephropathy, tubular dysfunction and light-chain proteinuria. *N Engl J Med* 294:71, 1976.
17. Holliday MA, Egar TJ, Morris CR, et al.: Vasopress in resistant hyposthenuria in chronic renal disease. *Am J Med* 42:378, 1967.
18. Earley LE: Extreme polyuria in obstructive uropathy: Report of a case of 'water-losing nephritis' in an infant with discussion of polyuria. *N Engl J Med* 255:600, 1956.
19. Levitt MF, Hausser AD, Levy MS, et al.: The renal concentrating defect in sickle cell disease. *Am J Med* 29:611, 1960.
20. Buckalew VM Jr, Someren A: Renal manifestations of sickle cell disease. *Arch Intern Med* 133:660, 1974.
21. Tannen RL, Regal EM, Dunn MJ, et al.: Vasopressin-resistant hyposthenuria in advance chronic renal disease. *N Engl J Med* 280:1135, 1969.
22. Miller PD, Krebs RA, Neal BJ, et al.: Polyuric prerenal failure. *Arch Int Med* 140:907, 1980.
23. Singer I, Forrest JN: Drug-induced states of nephrogenic diabetes insipidus. *Kidney Int* 10:82, 1976.
24. Singer I, Rotenberg D, Puschett JB: Lithium-induced nephrogenic diabetes insipidus: In vivo and in vitro studies. *J Clin Invest* 51:1081, 1972.
25. Myers JB, Morgan TO, Carney SL, et al.: Effects of lithium on the kidney. *Kidney Int.* 18:601, 1980.
26. Singer I, Rotenberg D: Demeclocycline-induced nephrogenic diabetes insipidus. *Ann Intern Med* 79:679, 1973.
27. Mannitius A, Levitin H, Epstein FH: On the mechanism of impairment of renal concentrating ability in hypercalcemia. *J Clin Invest* 39:693, 1960.
28. Zeffren JL, Heinemann HO: Reversible defect in renal concentrating mechanism in patients with hypercalcemia. *Am J Med* 33:54, 1962.
29. Back N, Sigh H, Reed E, et al.: Pathogenic role of cyclic AMP in the impairment of urinary concentrating ability in acute hypercalcemia. *J Clin Invest* 54:1049, 1974.
30. Manitius A, Levitin H, Beck D, et al.: On the mechanism of impairment of renal concentrating ability in potassium deficiencies. *J Clin Invest* 39:684, 1960.
31. Berl T, Aisenbrey GA, Linas SL: Renal concentrating defect in the hypokalemic rat is prostaglandin independent. *Am J Physiol* 238:F37, 1980.
32. Berl T, Linas S, Ainsenbrey G, et al.: On the mechanism of polyuria in potassium depletion. The role of polydipsia. *J Clin Invest* 60:620, 1977.
33. Levi M, Peterson L, Berl T: Mechanism of concentrating defect in hypercalcemia. Role of polydipsia and prostaglandins. *Kidney Int* 23:489, 1983.
34. Barlow ED, De Wardener HE: Compulsive water drinking. *Q J Med* 28:235, 1959.
35. Dubovsky SL, Grabon S, Berl T, et al.: Syndrome of inappropriate secretion of antidiuretic hormone with exacerbated psychosis. *Ann Int Med* 79:551, 1973.
36. Gennari FJ, Kassirer JP: Osmotic diuresis. *N Engl J Med* 291:714, 1974.
37. Kosmas ME: Evaluation of a new antidiuretic agent, desmopressin acetate (DDAVP). *JAMA* 240:1896, 1978.
38. Ziai F, Waller R, Rosenthal IM: Treatment of central diabetes insipidus in adults and children with desmopressin. *Arch Intern Med* 138:1382, 1978.
39. Earley LE, Orloff J: The mechanism of antidiuresis associated with the administration of hydrochlorothiazide to patients with vasopressin-resistant diabetes insipidus. *J Clin Invest* 41:1988, 1962.
40. Moses AM, Numann P, Miller M: Mechanism of chlorpropamide-induced antidiuresis in man. Evidence for release of ADH and enhancement of peripheral action. *Metabolism* 22:59, 1973.
41. Froyshov I, Haugen HN: Chlorpropamide treatment in diabetes insipidus. *Acta Med Scand* 183:397, 1968.
42. Zusman RM, Keiser HR, Handler JS: Inhibition of vasopressin-stimulated prostaglandin E biosynthesis by chlorpropamide in the toad urinary bladder. Mechanism of enhancement of vasopressin-stimulated water flow. *J Clin Invest* 60:1348, 1977.
43. Fichman MP, Speckart P, Zia P, et al.: Antidiuretic response to prostaglandin inhibition in primary and nephrogenic diabetes insipidus. *Clin Res* 23:505A, 1977.
44. Wales JK: Treatment of diabetes insipidus with carbamazepine. *Lancet* 2:948, 1975.
45. Rado JP: Combination of carbamazepine and chlorpropamide in the treatment of 'hyporesponders' pituitary diabetes insipidus. *J Clin Endocrinol Metab* 38:1, 1974.
46. Usberti M, Dechaux M, Guillot M, et al.: Renal prostaglandin E_2 in nephrogenic diabetes insipidus. Effects of inhibition of prostaglandin synthesis by indomethacin. *J Pediat* 97:476, 1980.
47. Delaney V, dePertuz Y, Nixon D, et al.: Indomethacin in streptozocin-induced nephrogenic diabetes insipidus. *Am J Kidney Dis* 9:79, 1987.
48. Bucht G, Wahlin A: Renal concentrating capacity in long-term lithium treatment and after withdrawal of lithium. *Acta Med Scand* 207:309, 1980.
49. Kennedy RM, Earley LE: Profound hyponatremia resulting from a thiazide induced decrease in urinary diluting capacity in a patient with primary polydipsia. *N Engl J Med* 282:1185, 1970.
50. Vaughan ED Jr, Gillenwater JY: Diagnosis, characterization and management of post-obstructive diuresis. *J Urol* 109:286, 1973.
51. Feig PV: Hypernatremic and hypertonic syndromes. *Med Clin North Am* 65:271, 1981.
52. Moran SM, Jamison RL: The variable hyponatremia response to hyperglycemia. *West J Med* 142:49, 1985.
53. Katz MA: Hyperglycemia-induced hyponatremia. Calculation of expected serum sodium depression. *N Engl J Med* 289:843, 1973.

CHAPTER 3

Edematous States

ARTHUR GREENBERG & JULES B. PUSCHETT

INTRODUCTION

Except when edema is due to local phenomena such as obstruction to venous flow from a thrombus or an inflammatory reaction from infection, the final common pathway responsible for edema formation is retention of salt and water by the kidney. Whether responding appropriately to the patient's condition as in hypovolemic shock, or in a counterproductive manner, as in congestive heart failure, the kidney's attempt to preserve body volume results from its perception of a reduction in vascular filling in the arterial circuit. Accordingly, the first consideration in treatment of edema is correction of the underlying disorder, if that can be achieved. When the deranged physiology is irreversible, the mainstays of therapy are a reduction in the salt content of the diet and the administration of diuretic agents. The diuretics currently available share the capability of impairing sodium chloride or bicarbonate reabsorption at one or more sites along the tubular system. They are of three basic types: a) agents, including the thiazide group, that are modestly natriuretic and useful for the treatment of mild to moderate edema: b) high-ceiling diuretics, such as furosemide which are more potent and thus are useful with severe or "resistant" edema: c) special purpose agents, such as spironolactone and triamterene, prescribed not so much for their natriuretic potency, which is small, but because of their ability to reduce potassium secretion. Like any other drug, diuretics cause side effects. In general, the more potent the diuretic, the greater its potential for producing adverse effects and the greater its expected severity.

After a discussion of general concepts, this chapter will discuss the therapy of the important disease states commonly accompanied by edema formation. Although an extensive search of the literature has been performed, the techniques and methods employed and recommended are largely those of the authors. The recommendations presented are firmly grounded in physiologic principles but are based upon empiric observations.

AVAILABLE TREATMENT MODALITIES

As edema results from the abnormal retention of sodium and water, the treatment modalities are self-evident: the reduction of sodium intake by dietary restriction and the augmentation of sodium excretion by diuretic administration. Bedrest may also lead to a diuresis (1). Since only modest reductions in sodium intake and the level of activity are achievable chronically in outpatients, diuretic administration becomes increasingly important as the edema becomes more severe.

The morbidity of abnormal sodium retention is dependent upon both intravascular and interstitial fluid excess. A increase in intravascular volume leads to hypertension and, in patients with preexisting heart disease, to congestive heart failure. Increased interstitial fluid predisposes to skin breakdown and cellulitis. When massive, it leads to a decrease in mobility. In addition to the practical difficulties with clothing and shoes caused by wide fluctuations in weight, edema is uncomfortable. Patients complain of puffiness and bloating. Patient intolerance of the simple cosmetic effects is variable; some, especially adolescents and young adults, tolerate them poorly.

Although the complete resolution of edema should be sought, this goal is not always achievable without severe side effects. Diuretics work by promoting renal excretion of filtered sodium. In cirrhotic and nephrotic patients who are hypoalbuminemic, mobilization of edema fluid from the interstitium into the intravascular space is impaired. Intravascular volume depletion with resultant prerenal azotemia frequently complicates diuresis in such patients and limits the achievable diuresis. In disorders characterized by intravascular fluid accumulation, e.g., congestive heart failure, prerenal azotemia occurs if the diuresis is overvigorous or if previously well-controlled patients on a stable diuretic regimen reduce their sodium intake without a concomitant reduction in the diuretic dosage. As a practical matter, it is often advisable and it may be necessary to settle for less than complete resolution of edema.

Diet therapy

Although the average dietary intake of sodium is quite variable, estimates of sodium consumption in the United States range from 100–300 mEq/day (3–7 g). The sodium contents of various sodium-restricted diets are listed in Table 1. Dietary restriction is of vital importance in the therapy of edema. If sodium intake is reduced, the need for sodium excretion is similarly diminished. It may be

Table 1. Sodium restricted diets

Sodium content		Description
4 g	175 mM	No added salt; suitable for outpatients
2 g	87 mM	Mild restriction; suitable for outpatients; excludes obviously salty foods
1 g	43 mM	Moderate restriction; rarely achievable by outpatients
500 mg	22 mM	Severe restriction
250 mg	11 mM	Rigid restriction; unpalatable

difficult to further augment sodium excretion in patients with extreme sodium avidity due to cirrhosis or nephrotic syndrome or to increased excretion in patients with a markedly decreased glomerular filtration rate (GFR) and decreased filtered sodium loads. By restricting intake, however, the physician may reduce as much as 10-fold the amount of sodium that must be excreted in order to achieve balance or a net diuresis.

Physicians are frequently lax in explaining to patients the rationale behind sodium restriction. Poor compliance results. Counseling of the patient, and more importantly, the family member who prepares the meals, is essential. The help of a dietitian interested in working with patients is key. The nutritionist can interview the patient's family to obtain specific data about eating habits and may make an estimate of sodium intake. Based on the physician's diet prescription, the nutritionist can then make specific suggestions for meals and may emphasize which foods are proscribed. When thoughtfully applied, restrictions need not seriously disrupt other family members, who may replace salt omitted from recipes by adding it to cooked food.

OUTPATIENT MANAGEMENT

Diets readily suitable for outpatients include the no-added-salt and 2 g sodium restriction. These are simple to understand and do not require precise meal planning. The 1 g sodium diet is much more restrictive and difficult to follow. It requires careful planning and a high degree of patient motivation. Although of value, it is infrequently achievable.

INPATIENT DIETS

All patients receiving diuretics to treat edema should be on a sodium restricted diet. If diuretic resistance is suspected, the restriction should be severe, 1000 mg. Although available, the 250 mg or 500 mg diets are unpalatable and are rarely used for the management of edema. Once a suitable diuretic regimen has been established and discharge is anticipated, sodium intake should be liberalized to simulate the outpatient diet that a patient will follow.

It is essential to include both dietary and parenteral sodium in calculations of intake. Note that 1 l of 0.2% saline contains 34 mM (787 mg) of sodium. Carbenicillin contains 5 mM of sodium (125 mg) per gram of drug. Careful efforts at rigorous dietary restriction may be abrogated by the administration of even a single liter of dilute saline solution.

SALT SUBSTITUTES

The commercially available salt substitutes all contain potassium. They are useful in patients with a tendency to become hypokalemic and represent an underutilized and palatable form of potassium replacement. Obviously, they are contraindicated in patients with renal failure. Salt substitutes containing a mixture of potassium and sodium salts are also contraindicated, as there is no rationale for their use.

Bed rest

Patients frequently report that dependent edema worsens during the course of the day and disappears overnight. Most of this change, of course, represents a shift of edema fluid out of dependent areas into interstitial spaces elsewhere. In patients who spend much time at bedrest, edema shifts from the ankles to the sacrum and scrotum or labia.

In addition to these shifts in the location of edema fluid, prolonged bedrest does lead to a net diuresis. With assumption of the supine position, central blood volume increases, as does renal and splanchnic perfusion. Such factors are especially important in patients with edema due to congestive heart failure. Limitation of activity may drop the demand on impaired cardiac reserve below the level of cardiac output that can be supplied by the diseased myocardium. If this is the case, the pathophyiologic events that lead to edema are no longer present and the edema may resolve completely. In patients with moderately advanced renal failure, the mechanism for fluid accumulation is different and bedrest is of little additional value.

Diuretics

Although proper diet selection and careful reduction of sodium administration may reduce the tendency for positive sodium balance, such measures alone are rarely sufficient to effect a diuresis because of the remarkable ability of the kidney to reabsorb filtered sodium. Untreated patients with cirrhosis or nephrotic syndrome are capable of reducing daily urinary sodium excretion to 1 to 2 mM, representing a fractional sodium excretion well below 0.01%. Clearly, sodium restriction alone will not lead to a significant reduction in edema, as each kilogram of edema fluid represents approximately 140 mM of accumulated sodium.

Diuretics act largely by inhibiting renal reabsorption of filtered sodium, although in certain circumstances they may increase the glomerular filtration rate. Functionally and anatomically, the nephron is divided into several sections, including the glomerulus, proximal tubule, de-

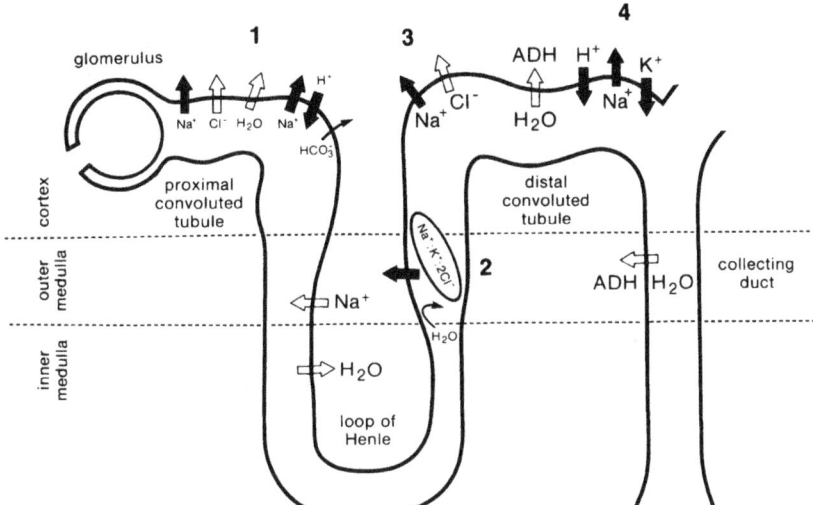

Figure 1. Sites of fluid and electrolyte transport in the nephron. In this schematic depiction of the major sites of fluid and electrolyte transport within the nephron, the solid arrows at each locus represent the actively transported moiety and the open arrows indicate passive reabsorption. The loop of Henle is shown as essentially impermeant to water, whereas in the distal tubule and collecting duct, water reabsorption occurs when vasopression (ADH) is present. Numbers refer to sites of action of diuretics (see text).

Table 2. Sodium reabsorption along the nephron

Site	Filtered sodium reabsorbed (%)
Proximal convoluted tubule	65–70
Loop of Henle	15–20
Distal convoluted tubule	5–10
Late distal tubule and collecting duct	2–3

scending and ascending limbs of the loop of Henle, distal tubule, and collecting duct (Figure 1). As noted in Table 2, the bulk of sodium reabsorption occurs in the proximal tubule, with lesser amounts being reabsorbed more distally. Although proximal reabsorption averages 65% of the filtered load, in extreme cases of sodium avidity it may exceed 90%. It is useful to classify diuretics according to their sites of action (Table 3). A listing of other characteristics of these agents is provided in Table 4.

PROXIMALLY ACTING DIURETICS

Since the bulk of sodium reabsorption occurs in the proximal tubule, it might be expected that proximally acting diuretics would be the most effective in promoting a diuresis. In practice this has not been the case. Most of the available proximally active diuretics work by carbonic anhydrase inhibition (Figure 1, site 1). Bicarbonate and sodium reabsorption are decreased. Although micropuncture studies indicate that benzolamide, one such agent, can increase sodium delivery out of the proximal tubule from 40% to 60%, the net increase in urinary chloride excretion is substantially less (2). This reflects the marked capacity of the distal nephron (in particular, the loop of Henle) to augment solute reabsorption and to largely negate the effect of proximally acting diuretics. At most,

Table 3. Site of action and potency of diuretics

Agent	Primary site	Secondary site	Fractional excretion of sodium (%)
Acetazolamide	Proximal tubule		3–5
Furosemide	Ascending loop of Henle	Proximal tubule[a]	20–25
Ethacrynic acid Bumetanide	Ascending loop of Henle	Proximal tubule	20–25
Thiazides	Distal tubule	Proximal tubule[a]	5–8
Metolazone	Distal tubule	Proximal tubule[b]	5–8
Spironolactone Triamterene Amiloride	Distal tubule and collecting duct		2–3

[a] Proximal action mediated by carbonic anhydrase inhibition.
[b] Proximal action mediated by inhibition of phosphate-linked sodium transport.

carbonic anhydrase inhibitors increase fractional sodium excretion by 3–5%. Even this effect is lost as serum bicarbonate levels fall.

For these reasons, proximally acting agents have not been widely utilized. They may provide some synergistic effect when given with more distally acting agents, as may distally active agents such as chlorothiazide and metolazone, which have modest proximal activity (*vide infra*).

The most frequently used carbonic anhydrase inhibitor is acetazolamide, which may be given as 250 or 500 mg po or I.V. bid. Dichlorphenamide and methazolamide are also available. These agents should not be used in individuals with renal failure, as severe metabolic acidosis may result.

Table 4. Relative potency of diuretic drugs: Onset and duration of action

Class	Usual dose range	Dose frequency per day	Onset after oral dose (hr)	Onset after I.V. dose	Duration of effect oral (or I.V.)	Maximal fractional sodium excretion (percent of filtered load)	Comments
Thiazides/thiazidelike							
Hydrochlorothiazide	50–100 mg	1–2	2	—	6–12 hr	5–8	Thiazides are ineffective in the presence of renal insufficiency.
Chlorthalidone	25–50 mg	1	2	—	48–72 hr	5–8	Long-acting thiazides (e.g., quinethazone & chlorothalidone) produce hypokalemia more predictably than shorter acting agents.
Metolazone	2.5–20 mg	1	1	—	12–24 hr	5–8	This drug is similar in potency to thiazides but, unlike thiazides, it is effective in states of renal insufficiency. Use with loop blockers provides an extremely potent diuretic action in patients with resistant edema.
Carbonic anhydrase inhibitors							
Acetazolamide	250–1000 mg	1–2	1–2	30–60 min	8–12 hr	3–5	Renal effect may become blunted by presence of metabolic acidosis due to the drug or by other clinical situations in which metabolic acidosis is present.
Loop blockers[a]							
Furosemide	20–320 mg	1–2	0.5	5 min	6–8 hr (2–3 hr I.V.)	20–25	Dosage of agents in this group is best determined by titration on an individual basis. These drugs are markedly kaliuretic and are effective in states of renal insufficiency. Frequent and/or high-bolus (I.V.) doses may result in ototoxcity.[b]
Ethacrynic acid	50–250 mg	1–2	0.5	5 min	6–8 hr (2–3 hr I.V.)	20–25	
Bumetanide	0.5–10.0 mg	1–2	0.5	5 min	4–6 hr (2–3 hr I.V.)	20–25	

Table 4. (Cont.)

Class	Usual dose range	Dose frequency per day	Onset after oral dose (hr)	Onset after I.V. dose	Duration of effect oral (or I.V.)	Maximal fractional sodium excretion (percent of filtered load)	Comments
Antikaliuretic agents							
Spironolactone	25–400 mg	1–4	48–72	—	3–4 days after cessation of therapy	2–3	Effect of spironolactone is dependent on presence of aldosterone, and is gradual in onset and reversal.
Triamterene	100–300 mg	1–2	2–4	—	7–9 hr	2–3	These agents act independently of the patient's aldosterone status. They may produce azotemia, hyperkalemia, and/or metabolic acidosis.
Amiloride	5–10 mg	1	2	—	24 hr	2–3	

[a] Equipotent doses of these three drugs are furosemide 40 mg, bumetanide 1 mg, and ethacrynic acid 50 mg. Relative potency of bumetanide may be less in renal insufficiency.
[b] The duration of action of the I.V. form is prolonged in renal insufficiency.
Modified, with permission from Pitts, T.O. In: Appendix to Puschett, J.B., Greenberg, A. (eds): *The Diuretic Manual*. Elsevier, New York, 1985.

DIURETICS ACTING ON THE LOOP OF HENLE: "HIGH-CEILING" DIURETICS

The most potent diuretic agents are those that block solute reabsorption in the ascending limb of the loop of Henle (Figure 1, site 2). Initially thought to be a site of active sodium transport with accompanying passive chloride reabsorption, the thick ascending limb was later reported to be a site of active chloride transport with passive sodium reabsorption. More recent evidence has shown that reabsorption in this segment actually involves the electroneutral cotransport of two chloride ions with a sodium and a potassium ion (3). Although this segment ordinarily accounts for reabsorption of only 15–20% of the filtered load, the more distal segments (distal convoluted tubule and collecting duct; Figure 1, sites 3 and 4) are unable to markedly increase sodium reabsorption as delivery increases. Thus, increased delivery of sodium out of the loop results in a significant increase in urinary sodium excretion. Three agents — furosemide, bumetanide, and ethacrynic acid — are currently available in the United States. For the most part, these drugs act from the luminal surface of the renal tubular cell and are dependent upon filtration and secretion into the tubular lumen for their action. They are weak organic acids whose secretion may be blocked by competition with other drugs, such as probenecid, that compete for secretion by the same pathway (4). In addition to its effect on transport, furosemide may also augment sodium excretion by virtue of its intrarenal hemodynamic effects. These may be partly mediated by the effect of loop diuretics in increasing prostaglandin synthesis. Thus, coadministration with nonsteroidal antiinflammatory agents has been shown to reduce the natriuretic and diuretic effect of the loop blockers (5, 6). The natriuretic effect of these drugs can be related to their urinary excretion rate with a curve that is S shaped. At low excretion rates, there is little natriuretic effect. At middle ranges, natriuresis increases strikingly as the drug excretion rate increases, but at higher drug excretion rates a plateau phase is observed. It should be clear that optimum drug usage will provide for a drug excretion rate near the top of the steep part of this sigmoid curve. If a low dose that falls on the early, flat part of the curve fails to produce a diuresis, repeating that dose is unlikely to effect a diuresis. Thus, the dose of these agents should be progressively increased until an effective dose is established. Then, this dose can be repeated up to four times daily, as needed (7).

Furosemide is available as 20, 40, and 80 mg tablets; ethacrynic acid in 50 mg tablets. Bumetanide is available as 0.5, 1, and 2 mg tablets. Forty milligrams of furosemide is approximately equipotent with 50 mg of ethacrynic acid. In patients with normal renal function, the equipotent dose of bumetanide is 1 mg. However, with renal failure, the dosage equivalency ratio for furosemide and bumetanide is more on the order of 20:1 (8).

Although as much as 500–1000 mg of furosemide have been used, patients who fail to respond to 240–320 mg rarely respond to higher doses. Experimental evidence suggests that the plateau dosage may be as low as 160 mg (9). As the incidence of side effects, including gastrointestinal upset and (usually reversible) ototoxicity increases with the dosage, it is inadvisable to give more than 320 mg at a single dose. Large intravenous doses should be given slowly over 30-45 minutes to minimize ototoxicity.

The side effects of ethacrynic acid appear to be more severe, and permanent deafness has been reported (10). Therefore, the use of this agent should be reserved for patients with known hypersensitivity to furosemide or other sulfonamide derivatives. If given intravenously, it should be used with great caution and only by infusion, not intravenous push. A further reason to use slow infusion rates is that rapid administration leads to local venous irritation with pain and burning.

Ethacrynic acid and furosemide have no synergistic effect. Forty milligrams of furosemide plus 50 mg of ethacrynic acid are no more potent than 80 mg of furosemide. There is no rationale for combination therapy with these two agents. Bumetanide is a nontoxic alternative to ethacrynic acid in patients in whom furosemide is contraindicated. Thus, there is little or no current indication for the use of the most ototoxic of these drugs, ethacrynic acid.

AGENTS ACTING PRIMARILY IN THE DISTAL TUBULE

Thiazides

These agents are of moderate potency and may lead to a 5-8% increase in fractional sodium excretion. Their principal site of action is the distal tubule (Figure 1, site 3), although some modest proximal effects, probably based on carbonic anhydrase inhibition, are demonstrable (11).

Thiazides are safe and inexpensive and are first-line drugs in patients with normal renal function. They have little effect in patients with a GFR less than 30 ml/min (serum creatinine > 2.5-3 mg/dl) and therefore should not be used in patients with azotemia. Most agents have 8- to 12-hour durations of action and may be given twice a day. Chlorthalidone has a longer half-life and may be given once a day. Except for this difference, the action and side effects of the different thiazides are identical; the physician is well advised to gain experience with any one (or two) preparations rather than to use multiple drugs from this group of agents. The therapeutic range of the thiazides is much narrower than that of the high-ceiling agents. While progressively increasing diuresis may be seen as furosemide doses are increased from 20 to 320 mg (a 16-fold increase in dosage), there is little additional benefit of increasing the dose of hydrochlorothiazide beyond 100 mg daily after an initial dose of 25 or 50 mg.

Metolazone

Metolazone, like the thiazides, acts primarily on the distal tubule. Alone, its diuretic effect is also modest. Its potential advantages are that its effects appear to last up to 24 hours or longer, and that it retains efficacy in patients with markedly reduced renal function. In addition, metolazone inhibits phosphate-linked sodium transport in the proximal nephron (12) and as such may have a synergistic effect when used with a loop blocker (*vide infra*). It is available in 2.5, 5, and 10 mg tablets.

Potassium-sparing agents

These agents act by blocking potassium-linked sodium reabsorption in the late distal tubule and collecting duct (Figure 1, site 4). As these sites reabsorb relatively little sodium, these agents increase fractional excretion of sodium by only 2-3% of the filtered load.

Spironolactone is a competitive inhibitor of aldosterone and may be useful in cirrhosis, nephrotic syndrome, and congestive heart failure if secondary hyperaldosteronism is present. Triamterene directly blocks potassium secretion and is useful even when secondary hyperaldosteronism is absent. Amiloride also has a direct effect on distal potassium secretion. The principal use for these agents is to obviate the kaliuresis that may accompany the use of other diuretics. Except in the three states listed above, the natriuretic effect is minor. The use of these agents in patients with renal failure requires extreme caution. Profound hyperkalemia may accompany their administration. This is of potentially great significance in diabetics who are prone to hyporeninemic hypoaldosteronism and lack insulin to defend against hyperkalemia (13). Spironolactone may lead to acidosis in cirrhotics, as acid excretion is also inhibited (14). Spironolactone is available as 25, 50, or 100 mg tablets. The usual dosage is 100-400 mg in divided doses. It is also available in combination tablets containing 25 mg hydrochlorothiazide and 25 mg spironolactone or 50 mg of each.

Triamterene is available as 50 or 100 mg capsules. The dosage ranges from 100 mg on alternate days to 300 mg daily. The usual starting dosage is 100 mg bid. It, too, is available as a combination capsule containing 25 mg hydrochlorothiazide and 50 mg triamterene. Amiloride is available as 5 mg tablets. The starting dosage is 5 mg daily. Up to 20 mg daily may be used, although it is rare to require more than 10 mg. A combination product containing 50 mg hydrochlorothiazide and 5 mg amiloride has been marketed.

SIDE EFFECTS OF DIURETIC THERAPY

For a complete discussion of the idiosyncratic effects of these agents, the reader is referred to the standard pharmacology text (15). The pharmacologic side effects of these agents are primarily disturbances of sodium, fluid, and electrolyte homeostasis. An excessive diuresis, of course, leads to volume depletion with signs of circulatory collapse. This is readily reversed by discontinuation of the diuretic, liberalization of salt intake, and administration of appropriate parenteral fluids, as needed. The more difficult question of subtle decreases in plasma volume associated with diminished renal plasma flow and GFR is discussed below in the sections dealing with separate disease entities.

Hypokalemia and metabolic alkalosis may be corrected by administration of potassium as its chloride salt.

Although some authorities (16) have advocated the routine use of potassium supplementation in hypertensive patients to prevent potassium depletion with possible attendant complications such as a propensity to arrhythmias, worsened hyperglycemia, and hyperuricemia, this indication is controversial. The authors are in general in agreement with the arguments brought forth by opponents of routine supplementation (17, 18). However, in patients with edema and profound secondary hyperaldosteronism that markedly increases the tendency toward potassium loss, some treatment of hypokalemia will likely be necessary. An alternative to potassium supplementation is the use of antikaliuretic diuretics. Because of the grave risks of hyperkalemia, these agents should be used with caution in patients with renal failure or in diabetics. In such patients, efforts to raise serum potassium should be used only after hypokalemia has developed, not prophylactically. Potassium and potassium-sparing diuretics should be used together only in extraordinary circumstances and only with frequent, in-hospital monitoring of potassium levels.

Hyponatremia may result from diuretic therapy if volume depletion serves as a nonosmotic stimulus to ADH release. This may be a particular problem in patients receiving thiazides or metolazone, whose major site of action is in the cortical diluting site (Figure 1, site 3). Hyponatremia has been reported after minimal exposure to these agents (19), appears to be an idiosyncratic reaction, and may have severe consequences (20, 21).

COMBINATION THERAPY IN DIURETIC RESISTANCE

The requirements for successful diuresis are listed in Table 5. Diuretic resistance may occur if one or more of these mechanisms are inoperative. The most frequent cause of diuretic resistance in outpatients is poor compliance. Patients frequently diurese well in hospital where prior outpatient therapy has failed because medication compliance is enforced. In addition, dietary restriction may be more adequately imposed in the hospital. A more subtle cause of diuretic resistance is diminished bioavailability of the drug due to bowel edema and decreased absorption (22, 23). Diminished or delayed absorption of the drug may be obviated by intravenous administration of the agent. As the diuresis proceeds and bowel edema diminishes, an increased amount of the drug may be absorbed, resulting in overdiuresis.

For diuretics to significantly increase sodium excretion, there must be substantial delivery of sodium to the tubular lumen. When GFR is markedly reduced and sodium delivery to the tubular system is negligible, no diuretic will be

Table 5. Requisite conditions for diuretic efficacy

1. Delivery of diuretic to the nephron site at which it acts
2. Delivery of sodium to the site at which the diuretic acts
3. Inhibition of sodium reabsorption by the diuretic
4. Failure of more distal nephron sites to reabsorb the increased sodium load

effective. In some disorders, like congestive heart failure, proximal sodium reabsorption may be markedly increased. As a result, little sodium is delivered to the loop where the more potent diuretics act. As congestive heart failure improves and cardiac output and renal perfusion improve, proximal sodium reabsorption decreases and distally active diuretics may regain their potency.

Actual resistance to diuretic agents may occur with severe renal failure when the drugs are not secreted or filtered into the tubular lumen. Extra-renal metabolism of the drug may play a more important role in its elimination when renal excretion is impaired (24).

Finally, diuretics may be ineffective if sites more distal to the site inhibited by the drug can increase reabsorption, thus blunting the more proximal effects of the agent.

Several of these factors may act in concert, depending upon the clinical situation. In chronic renal failure, although less drug may be secreted into the tubular lumen, the actual response of sodium excretion to furosemide excretion may be supranormal in each remnant nephron. Since the total number of nephrons is decreased, however, the absolute amount of sodium excretion is diminished (25). In contrast, in nephrotic syndrome and heart failure, diminished drug absorption and delivery to the tubule because of edema is accompanied by a decreased sodium excretory response to whatever diuretic reaches the tubule (26, 27).

Diuretic resistance is not necessarily static. As the underlying condition is corrected with the treatment of fluid retention, patients refractory to large doses of the drug

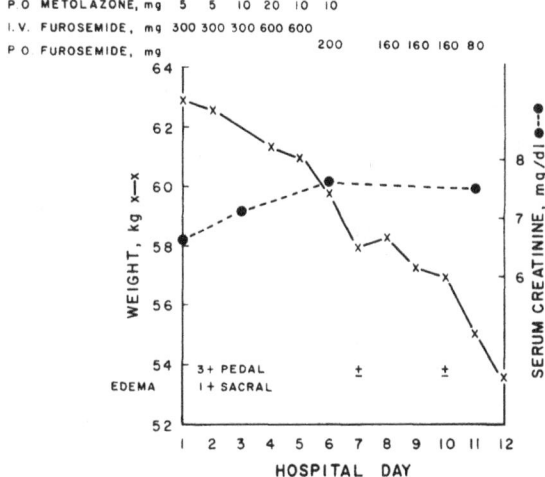

Figure 2. This diabetic patient with chronic renal failure, the nephrotic syndrome, and congestive heart failure developed progressive edema while receiving 160 mg furosemide daily as an outpatient. In hospital on a 2 g sodium restriction, he showed a minimal response to 10 mg oral metolazone and up to 600 mg I.V. furosemide daily. With resolution of congestive heart failure and edema, he responded vigorously to 80 mg furosemide orally.

may later become sensitive to much smaller doses. This may be because of improved bioavailability or because of less renal tubular resistance to the drug (24). As congestive heart failure improves and cardiac output and renal perfusion increase, proximal sodium reabsorption decreases and distally active diuretics may regain their potency. The course of such a recovery of diuretic sensitivity is shown in Figure 2.

In states of diuretic resistance the use of combination therapy may be valuable. In particular, to obviate the problems caused by sequential reabsorption of sodium at different nephron sites, treatment by sequential nephron blockade may be useful. By giving a combination of a proximally acting agent such as acetazolamide and a loop blocker such as furosemide, an effect greater than the diuresis seen with either agent alone may result. Thiazides have also been used to block reabsorption distal to the loop. Metolazone, with distal and proximal effects (the latter not dependent on carbonic anhydrase inhibition), has been used for this purpose. It appears to have a significant effect when given with furosemide (28–30). This agent offers the further advantage of its utility in patients with renal failure. A diuresis not previously obtainable or simplification of a patient's medication regimen may thus be achieved.

TREATMENT OF SPECIFIC CLINICAL CONDITIONS

Congestive heart failure

A rational approach to the treatment of cardiac failure has to include a determination of the severity of the heart failure and the urgency of the required treatment. Patients with pulmonary edema will, of course, require emergency treatment, whereas patients with incipient or slowly progressive congestive heart failure should receive less aggressive therapy. As with other diseases, the least complicated method of treatment is preferred. This may range from as little as dietary sodium restriction or intermittent diuretic therapy to a complicated regimen combining several diuretic drugs, "unloading" agents. and digitalis. A suggested approach is summarized in Table 6 and in the discussion that follows.

MILD CONGESTIVE HEART FAILURE

This disorder is characterized by an elevated venous pressure with right heart failure. GFR is usually well preserved, although there may be a modest impairment in renal blood flow. Transudation of fluid from the venous circulation into the interstitial space occurs with consequent development of detectable edema. The majority of such patients can be managed with dietary sodium restriction and diuretic administration. The latter may be given on a daily basis, on alternate days, or 4–5 times per week. The thiazide diuretics provide generally good results (31). An advantage of intermittent therapy in this setting is that it minimizes side effects. Therapy might be initiated with 50 mg hydrochlorothiazide or an equivalent dosage of another agent. The starting dose can be doubled if the response is inadequate. At the starting dose, hypokalemia is not usually a problem, but, especially at the higher dosage, the serum potassium level should be checked periodically. Thiazides are ineffective when the GFR is less than 30 ml/min (32, 33); when congestive heart failure is complicated by renal insufficiency, other agents should be chosen.

Metolazone is a potential alternative. Compared to the thiazides, this agent has two advantages: a) Its action appears to be more prolonged (up to 48 hours) and b) it is effective even in advanced renal insufficiency. The long duration of effect may be used to advantage by administering 2.5–5.0 mg on alternate days in some patients. Others will require a daily dosage if the response is inadequate. In patients with renal insufficiency, higher doses (up to 20 mg daily) may be required (34–36). Although controversy continues to exist as to whether or not digitalis should be employed at this stage of heart failure (37–39), in our view it is seldom necessary.

MODERATE CONGESTIVE HEART FAILURE

In these patients, renal blood flow is invariably reduced because of a decrease in the effective arterial volume.

Table 6. Therapeutic considerations in congestive heart failure

Severity	Clinical findings	RBF	GFR	Therapy
Mild	None or mild peripheral edema with exertional dyspnea	Normal or slightly decreased	Normal	Thiazides, metolazone
Moderate	Moderate peripheral edema; vascular congestion and/or pleural effusion	Moderately reduced	Moderately reduced	Digitalis, loop blockers, thiazides, or antikaliuretic agents as adjuncts; angiotensin-converting inhibitors as unloading agents once patient stabilized
Severe	Significant peripheral edema; dyspnea at rest; marked pulmonary congestion or edema	Severely reduced	Severely reduced	Combination diuretic therapy: loop blockers with metolazone; angiotensin-converting inhibitors as unloading agents; nitrates short term

Frequently, measurable decrements in GFR also occur. As a consequence of alterations in physical factors within the kidney and variations in humoral function that accompany the severe heart failure, sodium reabsorption in both proximal and distal nephron segments is intense. With more significant impairment of sodium excretion than in mild congestive heart failure, the tendency to positive sodium balance is even greater. Generalized volume overload with worsening peripheral edema, as well as pulmonary vascular congestion occur. Here, digitalis therapy is indicated in conjunction with diuretics. For patients with normal or mildly impaired kidney function (GFR values > 50% of normal), a standard digitalizing dose of 1.0–1.5 mg digoxin followed by 0.25 mg/day is appropriate. With more advanced renal insufficiency, the dose should be adjusted downward to 25–75% of the standard dosage in patients with GFR values in the range of 10–15 ml/min and to 10–25% of the usual dosage when GFR is less than 10 ml/min (40). For patients who are virtually anephric and receiving dialysis, 0.125 mg on alternate days or every third day frequently suffices. Toxicity should be monitored by watching for symptoms and by following the electrocardiogram and serum digoxin level.

Thiazides are rarely of value unless given in combination with other agents. Initial therapy with a more potent agent, one acting to impair sodium reabsorption at the loop of Henle (see Table 6), is more appropriate. For exmple, oral furosemide, beginning at a dosage of 40 mg/day, will often be sufficient, especially when combined with digoxin. If the clinical response is inadequate, the dosage may be increased or an additional agent may be added. As emphasized earlier, if a single dose is inadequate, then a higher dose should be used rather than repeating the ineffective dose more than once per day. Once an effective dosage has been determined, it may be repeated later in the day if the diuresis trails off after several hours and a greater loss of salt and fluid, as reflected by a decrement in the patient's weight, is desired.

An alternative approach is to block sodium chloride reabsorption at more than one site in the nephron. Because of the low cardiac output, effective arterial filling is diminished, even though the venous circuit is full. Renin release will be augmented and secondary hyperaldosteronism will be present. Therefore, administration of an agent acting at the sodium-potassium-hydrogen exchange site in the late distal convoluted tubule and collecting duct (spironolactone, triamterene, or amiloride) may prove useful. The natriuretic effect of these drugs is modest, but they have the additional benefit of reducing potassium excretion and the tendency to hypokalemia. If GFR is not markedly diminished, the combination of a thiazide and a loop blocker may prove helpful. This regimen impairs sodium reabsorption at two adjacent transport sites in the nephron: the thick ascending limb of the loop of Henle and the early distal convoluted tubule (see Figure 1). For example, a patient might receive 50 mg hydrochlorothiazide with 40–120 mg furosemide in the morning. The drugs could be repeated in the afternoon, if necessary.

Such a regimen is likely to be highly kaliuretic. Hypokalemia may be controlled by adding spironolactone or triamterene to complete distal nephron blockade. Alternatively, KCl could be administered. As noted above, giving both the potassium-sparing agents and KCl together is rarely necessary and is fraught with danger.

As noted above, patients with moderate congestive heart failure may have a modest reduction in renal blood flow or changes in its intracortical distribution (31) that result in a mild decrement in GFR. This is manifest as a modest elevation in serum creatinine with a disproportionate rise in blood urea nitrogen. A BUN of 50 mg/dl with creatinine 2.0 mg/dl is a representative example. Here, the usual 10:1 ratio of BUN to creatinine has been disturbed. This so-called prerenal pattern results from the augmentation of distal nephron urea reabsorption that occurs with diminished urine flow. Creatinine is not reabsorbed and the modest increase in serum creatinine concentration reflects the very small fall in GFR that is present. Depending upon the cardiac output, prerenal azotemia may be improved or worsened by diuresis. If the induced reduction of extracellular and plasma volume restores the myocardium to a more favorable position on the Starling curve, cardiac output will increase with an improvement or stabilization of renal hemodynamics. The BUN and creatinine will then remain the same or fall. If, however, cardiac output is unimproved, further diuretic-induced volume contraction will worsen prerenal azotemia. This is especially likely where cardiac output is preload dependent. In some cardiac patients, it may be necessary to accept a compromise between induction of a further reduction of GFR and toleration of some degree of edema. Thus, to keep the patient out of florid pulmonary edema, some stable level of elevated BUN and creatinine may have to be accepted. This occurrence is more likely with severe congestive heart failure, as discussed below. Alternatively, in the patient with moderate congestive heart failure, a small amount of residual edema may provide insurance against the rapid or progressive increment in BUN and creatinine that will result from volume depletion.

SEVERE CONGESTIVE HEART FAILURE

When cardiac output is profoundly reduced, total renal blood flow is markedly compromised and GFR is significantly reduced. With a fall in GFR, the filtered load of sodium falls. Also, as the fall in GFR is proportionately less than the fall in renal blood flow, the filtration fraction (GFR/renal blood flow) is increased. The resulting physical forces, including plasma oncotic pressure and decreased peritubular capillary hydrostatic pressure, strongly enhance the reabsorption of sodium from the tubular lumen. The combined effect of diminished load and augmented proximal fractional reabsorption is to markedly decrease the delivery of sodium out of the proximal tubule. In animal models of congestive heart failure, it has been difficult to demonstrate specific alterations in proximal tubular transport (41, 42). Whether these observations can be extrapolated to humans is problematic; such studies are difficult or impossible to perform in humans. Nonetheless, patients with advanced congestive heart failure behave as though proximal reabsorption were greatly stimulated (31, 43). The augmented reabsorption at this site cannot be much inhibited by the usual diuretic agents, as they lack important proximal activity. A further effect of diminished effective arterial volume or pressure is to stimulate aldosterone secretion. This hormone stimulates distal tubular sodium reabsorption, leading to a further decrement in renal sodium excretion.

The physiologic principles outlined earlier in this chapter suggest the therapeutic maneuvers that are useful in these patients. Besides verifying adequate digitalization, the physician may employ combination diuretic therapy aimed at inhibiting sodium transport at those sites in the nephron where reabsorption is most intense. The most logical approach is to block the transport system sequentially (see section on combination therapy in diuretic resistance). A useful regimen is the combination of metolazone and furosemide (44). Commonly, 5–10 mg of metolazone is accompanied by 40–120 mg of furosemide. These oral dosages may be increased to 20 and 240 mg, respectively. Intravenous diuretics may be successful if large doses of oral drug have failed because of impaired gastrointestinal absorption. It is important when switching from oral to intravenous drug to begin with a lower dose. Rapid intravenous infusion bypasses the delay in gastrointestinal absorption and may cause urinary diuretic excretion to rise rapidly. Small dosages may thus result in a dramatic natriuresis and diuresis. A suggested starting dose is 5–10 mg of oral metolazone, followed an hour later by 40–80 mg of intravenous furosemide. This sequence allows a delay to permit metolazone absorption from the gut and may allow the effects of the two drugs to peak simultaneously. The dosage of both drugs may be increased on a graded schedule. The metolazone need not be repeated for about 24 hours, but the effect of furosemide will have worn off in about 4–6 hours. We do not recommend giving more than 20 mg of metolazone or 240–320 mg of furosemide per 24-hour period.

The potential for further elevation of the BUN and creatinine levels with successful diuretic therapy is even greater in this group than in those patients with moderate degrees of cardiac failure. In addition, these patients are more vulnerable to the development of arrhythmias because of changes in potassium concentration. Volume contraction may further worsen pre-existent hyponatremia. For intractable congestive heart failure, "unloading" agents have been introduced. These may be an effective adjunct to diuretic treatment (45–48). Nitrates and angiotensin-converting enzyme inhibitors appear to have the best long-term effect. Other agents, such as hydralazine and prazosin, have been disappointing. Calcium-channel blockers may be employed, but at least one, nifedipine, has the potential for worsening renal function in patients with coexisting chronic renal insufficiency (49).

In the small group of patients in whom all of the measures described above have been fruitless, dialysis should be considered as a method for fluid removal. Because of the tenuous cardiovascular status of such patients, peritoneal dialysis is often preferred to hemodialysis. In addition, it may be preferable to employ a chronic Tenckhoff catheter rather than acutely placing a trocar-type catheter. The former is preferred for the following reasons: a) The pain and trauma as well as the likelihood of a vagal episode are less with surgical placement. b) Since repeated dialyses are likely, the need for repeated catheter placements is obviated. c) Repeat dialyses with a chronic catheter are easier to manage technically.

When hemodialysis is necessary (for technical or other reasons), it is advisable to keep the blood flow rate low and to keep the length of each procedure as brief as possible, commensurate with the accomplishment of fluid removal and biochemical improvement. A typical dialysis might last for 3 hours with a blood flow of 125–150 ml/min. As an alternative, slow continuation ultrafiltration or chronic arteriovenous hemofiltration may be employed (50). Chronic dialysis therapy should not be commenced without careful reflection on a case-by-case basis. It is necessary to attempt to determine the quality of life that can be achieved. In each instance, the decision to begin, to continue, or to stop dialysis should be a joint one, arrived at after discussion with the patient, family, and referring physician. The cause of death in such patients is invariably a cardiovascular event, reflecting progression of the underlying cardiac disease.

PULMONARY EDEMA

The availability of potent fast-acting loop diuretics radically altered the treatment of this medical emergency (51, 52). In patients with normal renal function, 40–80 mg of furosemide or 1–2 mg of bumetanide should be administered intravenously. In acute pulmonary edema, furosemide may have an important extrarenal vasodilator action that improves cardiac function even before a diuresis occurs (53). The significance of this effect is uncertain. Some studies in patients with chronic congestive heart failure show a vasodilator effect (54); others suggest an early vasoconstrictor effect of the drug (55). Whatever the effect of these small, direct hemodynamic effects, it is clear that a marked symptomatic and objective improvement occurs in association with the diuresis. In patients without pre-existing renal disease, it is rare for loop diuretics to be insufficient. However, additional benefit may be seen when nitrates are used to promote venous pooling and diminish preload until the effect of the diuresis is seen. Inotropic agents such as dobutamine or dopamine may have additional efficacy (46), as may hemofiltration without dialysis (56).

Acute glomerulonephritis

Although edema in this disorder may be massive, it usually presents as subtle periorbital or hand edema, noted by the patient upon arising and disappearing during the course of the day. The sodium retention of acute glomerulonephritis results from the combined effects of diminished GFR and increased fractional reabsorption of sodium (57). Unless patients have nephrotic-range proteinuria, their plasma volume is increased (57) and the ability to mobilize interstitial fluid is unimpaired. They may be treated as aggressively as needed with diuretics, without fear of induction of significant prerenal azotemia.

As volume overload is a significant contributor to hypertension in such patients, hypertension is an indication for vigorous treatment. As renal failure may be present and as titration of the diuretic over a wide range of renal functional changes may become necessary, furosemide or an alternative loop agent is the diuretic of choice. Because of the tendency to hyperkalemia, the potassium-sparing diuretics should be avoided.

Nephrotic syndrome

This disorder is characterized pathogenetically by abnormalities in glomerular basement membrane function that lead to the excretion of more than 3.5 g of urinary protein per day. Eventually, as the loss of protein in the urine outstrips the ability of the liver to produce plasma proteins, hypoalbuminemia develops. While it is clear that plasma colloid osmotic pressure is reduced, thus favoring the transudation of fluid from the intravascular interstitial compartment, this process alone does not adequately explain the edema formation characteristic of this syndrome. Indeed, the pathogenetic sequence remains uncertain because the important physiologic parameters are difficult to study directly in human subjects and because there is a confusion about what measurements should be made. Much has been written about plasma volume in this disorder (57). Patients with nephrotic syndrome may have plasma volumes that are low, normal, or high, yet they all have edema (58, 59). What appears to be most important is not the absolute numerical value of plasma volume, but rather its effect on arterial filling. Even though measured plasma volume may be high, effective perfusion of the arterial circuit is inadequate in patients with the nephrotic syndrome. The final common pathway for edema development is a signal from an as yet unidentified receptor or receptors that results in enhanced renal sodium reabsorption. Whether this is a predominately proximal or distal effect within the kidney is uncertain (60, 61). Neither is it known with certainty whether physical or humoral factors are the primary determinants.

Therapy of the individual disease states that produce nephrotic syndrome is beyond the scope of this chapter but is discussed elsewhere in this book. Nonspecific methods of controlling edema are in order in patients who have not yet responded to more specific treatment or in patients with disorders for which there is no specific treatment.

The most important initial step is restriction of sodium intake, as detailed above in the section on diet therapy. Except in refractory patients, this restriction need not be onerous. For many patients, a no-added-salt regimen suffices.

Diuretic administration is usually indicated. Most patients with normal GFR will respond to the thiazide diuretics. Hydrochlorothiazide and chlorthalidone in a dosage of 50–100 mg daily or an equivalent amount of another benzothiadiazine derivative may be employed. It is generally wiser, however, to initiate treatment with a loop agent, since these high-ceiling agents have a broader therapeutic range. The usual starting dose of furosemide or bumetanide is 40 mg or 1 mg/day, respectively. When patients fail to respond adequately to initial doses, higher doses should be combined with more severe sodium restriction, such as a 2-g sodium intake. It is again important to establish the lowest effective dose by using escalating doses of the agent. Once an effective dose is found, it may be repeated during a given 24-hour period if more aggressive therapy is required. With furosemide, for instance, the usual pattern is to begin with 40 mg and to increase the dose to 80 mg then 160 mg then 240 mg or 320 mg. If an inadequate result occurs, even with these larger doses, an intravenous route should be selected, beginning with a 40 mg dose. Should large doses of intravenous drug prove ineffective, combinations of the loop agent with metolazone may be tried. When the filtered load of bicarbonate is normal, a carbonic anhydrase inhibitor may also be effective. An example of this form of therapy would be the combination of 500 mg acetazolamide and 120 mg furosemide, both given intravenously.

Intravenous hyperoncotic albumin therapy has been used as a means of achieving a diuresis in patients with edema from the nephrotic sydrome. Although efficacious, this agent should be reserved for patients with truly resistant edema. The rationale for its use is that hyperoncotic albumin will increase plasma colloid oncotic pressure. This, in turn, favors mobilization of fluid from the interstitium to the intravascular space. This albumin effect is ephemeral (62). Several other actions of the agent may be potentially more important. First, volume expansion attending albumin administration inhibits proximal tubular transport by a complex series of intrarenal and extrarenal events (63). This will be of special benefit if a loop-active agent is used to provide sequential blockade. Second, albumin has a potentially antinatriuretic effect. To the extent that its infusion raises the oncotic pressure of the peritubular capillary blood, this maneuver tends to favor *reabsorption* rather than excretion of sodium (60). Third, the increase in intravascular volume that accompanies the albumin infusion may elevate GFR, an effect that would favor increased sodium *excretion*. Whether albumin infusion proves effective in inducing a diuresis will depend upon the relative contributions made by each of the renal and extrarenal factors described. An example of this therapeutic approach is to give 240 mg of furosemide intravenously while infusing 12.5–25 g of salt-poor albumin rapidly. The advisibility of this treatment depends, of course, upon the patient's ability to tolerate volume expansion from a cardiovascular standpoint.

As was discussed in the section on congestive heart failure, aggressive diuretic therapy may be detrimental if it reduces intravascular volume acutely and leads to a reduction in renal blood flow and a decrease in GFR. All of the

Acute renal failure

The improved prognosis of nonoliguric acute renal failure (ARF) as compared with the oliguric variety has been stressed (64). Diuretics may play a role in the conversion of oliguric to nonoliguric acute renal failure or in the protection from the development of acute renal failure. In experimental ARF, this effect has not been consistently demonstrable (65, 66). Although some clinical trials have suggested a role for diuretic therapy (10), others have not (67–69). Although it remains unclear whether diuretics actually convert oliguric to nonoliguric acute renal failure or merely indentify those patients with acute renal failure who retain diuretic responsiveness, as a practical matter patients with nonoliguric renal failure are easier to manage. Fluid and sodium overload is less severe and less rigorous dietary restriction is necessary. As potassium excretion parallels urinary volume, hyperkalemia is often less severe in patients with nonoliguric acute renal failure.

Thus, a course of diuretics is indicated in patients with acute renal failure, provided that any volume deficits have already been repleted. In addition, diuretics and sodium restriction are indicated in patients presenting with acute renal failure and edema from excess prior oral sodium intake or sodium administration. It is impossible to predict who will respond to treatment or at what dosage a response will be seen. Treatment should be given with 40 mg furosemide I.V. If no response is seen, 80 mg may be given 2–3 hours later. If there is no response, the dose is doubled to 160 mg and finally to 320 mg. Although these are the customary limiting doses, more recent work has suggested that 160 mg may be an appropriate maximum dosage (9). Bumetanide, in a dosage of 1–10 mg, might be a suitable alternative. As discussed above, there is little value but considerable risk with higher dosages. These large dosages may be employed up to twice daily of a response is seen. If furosemide or bumetanide fail, it is usually because of a diminished GFR. Accordingly, sequential blockade is not of additional value. Thiazides are not useful in this setting at all because of the low GFR. Acetazolamide is typically contraindicated because of accompanying metabolic acidosis. Antikaliuretic agents are contraindicated because of the tendency to hyperkalemia. If they have failed initially, furosemide or bumetanide may be tried later in the course of the patient's illness, but they are usually ineffective in this setting until the spontaneous diuresis that heralds impending recovery has begun.

In the volume-overloaded diuretic refractory patient, sodium restriction is of prime importance. In the severely ill patient with acute renal failure, careful selection of intravenous fluids is necessary. Where fluid must be given with medications or for hyperalimentation, sodium-free fluids should be chosen. When hyponatremia has occurred in the edematous or volume-overloaded patient, the proper treatment is an additional water restriction, rather than a substitution of sodium-containing intravenous fluids. When conflicting requirements or volume overload cannot be managed conservatively, dialysis becomes necessary.

Chronic renal failure

Fractional sodium excretion is increased in patients with chronic renal failure as a part of the adaptive mechanism for the diminished nephron mass (70). Nevertheless, the absolute capacity to excrete sodium is diminished due to the marked decrease in GFR and the filtered sodium load. Sodium intake may readily exceed the maximal excretory capacity. Volume overload then results and leads to edema and hypertension.

Where sodium restriction alone has proven inadequate, diuretics are necessary. Thiazides are of no value in patients with a GFR less than 30 ml/min. If the patient is seen early in his course, thiazides may still be useful. If, however, the diagnosis suggests that azotemia will progress, it is probably best to initiate therapy with furosemide, as it can be progressively titrated as the patient's renal function diminishes.

The treatment of edema in patients with uncomplicated chronic renal failure is straightforward. Salt restriction and progressive doses of furosemide or bumetanide should be used until edema is controlled. Furosemide in a dosage up to 240–320 mg daily is usually adequate to control patients who are not end stage. Failure to control edema with such dosages in the non-nephrotic patient suggests a lack of compliance with diet or medication.

In the patient with chronic renal failure and either congestive heart failure or the nephrotic syndrome or both, control of edema may be more difficult. The most common such patients are diabetics with end-stage renal disease. Patients with amyloidosis or focal glomerulosclerosis might also progress in such a fashion. Because cardiac output may be dependent upon preload, these patients may develop prerenal azotemia superimposed upon their preexisting chronic renal failure if they are too vigorously diuresed. In particular, this occurs because diuretics may decrease plasma volume faster than interstitial fluid can be mobilized, due to the diminished plasma oncotic pressure. In such patients, the physician treads a narrow path between underdiuresis with edema and congestive heart failure, and overdiuresis with diminished cardiac output and worsening renal function. Although edema may be controllable, it is frequently at the cost of diminished renal function. Patient morbidity is usually less with early institution of dialysis.

Although "salt-losing nephropathy" is rare, patients with chronic renal failure are unable to rapidly decrease sodium excretion (71). This characteristic, when encountered, is usually seen in patients with interstitial nephropathy. Such patients are particularly at risk for volume depletion with resultant prerenal azotemia when intercurrent gastrointestinal disease leads to a reduction in sodium intake. Similarly, edematous patients admitted to the hospital may have an overly rapid diuresis if compliance with long-ignored dietary restrictions and the diuretic regimen is restored.

Idiopathic edema

This clinical syndrome occurs exclusively in women and is almost invariably confined to the child-bearing years. It is characterized by recurring bouts of generalized edema. While they may wax and wane, these episodes demonstrate no specific periodicity and, in particular, are unrelated to the menstrual cycle (72). Despite a significant amount of investigative effort, the etiology and pathogenesis of this entity remain obscure. Except when treatment with diuretics has seen initiated, patients do not uniformly demonstrate secondary hyperaldosteronism. Renin levels are not altered in any consistent fashion, despite the observation that the disorder is most pronounced in the upright posture and that a diuresis occurs when the patient is able to remain supine for 24–48 hours (72, 73). Neither abnormalities of water balance, including regulation of the secretion of antidiuretic hormone or the adenylate cyclase system, appear to be causative (72, 73). By exclusion, the disorder is a defect in the normal homeostasic response to upright posture, perhaps related to the sympathetic nervous system or other humoral mechanisms.

The diagnosis is confirmed by having the patient perform twice daily weights, upon arising and in the evening, and by having her record urine output for each 12-hour segment of the day for several days. An intradiem weight gain exceeding 1 kg with a major increase in urinary output during nocturnal recumbency is characteristic. The disorder has a predilection for patients who have other somatic complaints. Emotional lability may be a feature and patients may become panic stricken when large weight gains occur. Two principles of therapy are key. First, constant reassurance and a sympathetic and patient attitude on the part of the physician are essential. Second, the tendency to overmedicate with diuretics should be avoided. For women who are only mildly or moderately symptomatic, postural therapy combined with a mild diuretic taken intermittently is appropriate. During periods of fluid retention, the patient should attempt to remain supine, except to go to the bathroom. The use of diuretics should be restricted to symptomatic periods or on an alternate-day or 5 times per week basis. A suitable schedule would be hydrochlorothiazide 50 mg on alternate days or every day but Wednesday and Sunday. Metolazone, 2.5 mg, may be used on a similar schedule. Only in the most resistent cases should loop-blocking agents be employed. Tachyphylaxis is a regular problem when unlimited or unsupervised diuretic administration is practiced. Spironolactone may be helpful in selected patients, particularly when given with a thiazide. In some patients, support stockings may be beneficial. One additional caution is in order: Patients with this disorder tend toward self-medication and often solicit medications from more than one physician.

Premenstrual syndrome

This condition is characterized by the development of irritability and depression or other behavioral symptoms, headaches, and peripheral edema, beginning about 5–10 days prior to the onset of menses. These symptoms subside as menstruation proceeds. Patients may be aware of tender, swollen, and often painful breasts and abdominal bloating, as well as edema of the extremities; from 1 to 3 kg of weight may be gained. The exact pathophysiology of this disorder is unknown. A relationship to changes in estrogen or progesterone levels has been suggested, but neither this nor a relationship to secondary hyperaldosteronism has been proved (74, 75). Care should be taken not to confuse this disorder with idiopathic edema. Therapy of the edema of premenstrual syndrome is symptomatic. Therapy with 25–50 mg of hydrochlorothiazide for several days prior to the menses is generally effective. Spironolactone may be used as an alternative. Progestational agents and sedatives may be of value in selected patients. As with idiopathic edema, overtreatment of the volume expansion should be avoided.

Toxemia of pregnancy

Preeclampsia is defined as the occurrence of hypertension, edema, and proteinuria after the 20th week of gestation. When accompanied by convulsions, the disorder is termed *eclampsia*. Young primigravidas are most frequently affected but multiparas older than 35, diabetics, and patients with twin pregnancy or hydatidiform mole are also at increased risk.

Most authorities recommend admission to hospital as the initial treatment of preeclampsia. The pathophysiology of this disorder is incompletely understood, but vasospasm appears to play a major role in the hypertension (76). Because plasma volume is decreased compared to normal pregnancy despite the presence of edema, this condition is an exception to the general principle that salt restriction and diuretics should be used to treat edema. Perhaps the only time where it is agreed that diuretics are useful in this condition is when heart failure has resulted from the severe hypertension. Delivery of the fetus, if sufficiently mature, is the preferred treatment of preeclampsia. When there is insufficient fetal maturity or if the mother is too ill for immediate delivery, magnesium sulfate is the mainstay of treatment. Hydralazine is the favored antihypertensive, as treatment with this agent does not appear to decrease uterine blood flow (77).

Cirrhosis, ascites, and hepatorenal syndrome

DEFINITIONS AND PATHOGENESIS

There is substantial debate about the mechanism of edema and ascites formation in hepatic disease. This disorder and its treatment have been extensively reviewed (78–81). Traditionally, the "underfilling" theory implicated a diminished plasma oncotic pressure as the cause of transudation of fluid from the abnormal hepatic vasculature and lymphatics into the abdomen as ascites and from systemic capillaries as edema fluid. Plasma volume was decreased and renal sodium retention occurred secondarily. An important feature of this model, a decrease in plasma volume in such patients, has not been a uniform finding. Subsequent work suggests that abnormal renal sodium retention due to hormonal or physical factors leads to sodium retention, which precedes the ascites and edema formation, and that the latter occur as "overflow" phenomena (82, 83). The relative roles of these two potential mechanisms is unknown. A modest chronic impairment of GFR is common in cirrhosis and its incidence is probably underestimated, since a fall in creatinine production due to muscle wasting may blunt the rise in serum creatinine and mask a fall in clearance (80). Some patients with severe liver failure, however, develop progressive azotemia and oliguria. This functional renal impairment developing in the setting of severe liver disease is termed *hepatorenal syndrome*. In some cases it is preceded by overvigorous attempts at diuresis, but frequently it is spontaneous. Although spontaneous remission has been reported (84), the usual outcome is fatal unless hepatic disease improves or hepatic transplantation is performed. When a diuresis has preceded the development of the hepatorenal syndrome, it may be impossible to distinguish the hepatorenal syndrome from prerenal azotemia. Since all such patients are edematous, the distinction lies in the unmeasurable "effective arterial volume." A series of elegant studies have shown that it is impossible to distinguish clinically between those patients who are hypotensive with low cardiac output and high peripheral vascular resistance (prerenal azotemia) and those who are hypotensive with normal or high cardiac outputs and low peripheral vascular resistance due to presumed arteriovenous shunting (hepatorenal syndrome) (85). The former group may respond to volume repletion.

TREATMENT

Because of the risk of inducing hepatorenal syndrome if it is not already present, and because volume depletion or hypokalemia may worsen hepatic encephalopathy, diuresis in patients with cirrhosis must be deliberate and meticulous. Nearly 20 years ago, it was shown that cirrhotic patients could mobilize only 900 ml of ascitic fluid per day, although edema fluid could be mobilized more rapidly (86). Therefore, it was recommended that no more than 0.5 kg/day weight loss be sought in patients who have ascites alone and that the weight loss of edematous patients be limited to 1 kg/day. A more recent study has confirmed these findings with regard to ascites mobilization, but recommends more rapid diuresis of edema. Provided that azotemia does not supervene, more than 2 kg/day can be removed successfully (87). Although the former recommendations may be too conservative, the latter have not yet gained wide acceptance.

Initially, patients should be placed at bedrest on a 1 g sodium diet. If hyponatremic, their water intake should be restricted as well. Approximately 15% of patients will have a spontaneous diuresis (79). If no weight loss occurs, treatment with a diuretic should be initiated. Athough other drugs have been used as initial agents with success (88, 89), the greatest experience has been with spironolactone, which has been preferred not only because of safety, but perhaps also because of increased efficacy compared with other agents (90). After a starting dosage of 100 mg daily in divided doses, the dosage may be increased over several days to 400 mg daily. Dosages up to 1000 mg daily have been used, and titration of the dose according to the urinary sodium/potassium ratio (a ratio greater than 1 indicating inhibition of aldosterone action) has been recommended (91). If no response is seen to spironolactone, small doses of a second agent should be used. Furosemide or an alternative loop blocker seems a logical choice, although metolazone or thiazide may also be employed. The dosage of the second agent may be progressively increased until an adequate diuresis or azotemia develops.

Some short-term benefit may arise from albumin infusion to increase mobilization of edema fluid just before an intravenous dose of furosemide. This is expensive and has no end point. It should be used only as a temporizing effort in patients in whom improvement in liver function is expected. Ascites reinfusion has been advocated for the same purpose, but has proved to be cumbersome and is associated with troublesome side effects.

Much recent attention has been given to the LeVeen peritoneal-venous shunt and comparable devices that allow for continuous ascites reinfusion. Although initial uncontrolled reports have shown dramatic success with ascites (92) and the hepatorenal syndrome (93, 94), the selection criteria in these studies were not uniform. Furthermore, the procedure is not without risk. Potential complications include venous occlusion, disseminated intravascular coagulation, and variceal bleeding (95). Patients with intraabdominal sepsis, recent esophageal variceal bleeds or bilirubin greater than 8 mg/dl should be excluded (92). The procedure appears to be of value in some patients, but selection criteria should be rigorous (95, 96). A more recent study found no long-term benefit of this procedure (97).

REFERENCES

1. Ring-Larsen H, Henriksen JH, Wilken C, Clausen J, Pals H, Christensen NJ: Diuretic treatment in decompensated cirrhosis and congestive heart failure: Effect of posture. *Br Med J* 292:1351–1353, 1986.
2. Kunau RT: The influence of the carbonic anhydrase inhibitor, benzolamide (CL 11, 366) on the reabsorption of chloride, sodium and bicarbonate in the proximal tubule of the rat. *J Clin Invest* 51:294–306, 1972.
3. Greger R, Schlatter E, Lang F. Evidence for electroneutral sodium co-transport in the cortical thick ascending limb of Henle's loop of rabbit kidney. *Pflügers Arch* 396:308–314, 1983.
4. Leary WP, Reyes AJ: Drug interactions with diuretics: *S Afr Med J* 65:455–461, 1984.
5. Favre L, Glasson PH, Riondel A, Vallotton MB: Interaction of diuretics and non-steroidal anti-inflammatory drugs in man. *Clin Sci* 64:407–415, 1983.
6. Chennavasin P, Seiwell R, Brater DC: Pharmacokinetic-dynamic analysis of the indomethacin-furosemide interaction

in man. *J Pharmacol Exp Ther* 215:77–81, 1980.
7. Brater DC: Resistance to loop diuretics. Why it happens and what to do about it? *Drugs* 30:427–443, 1985.
8. Allison MEM, Lindsay MK, Kennedy AC: Oral bumetanide in chronic renal failure. *Postgrad Med J* 51:47–50, 1975.
9. Brater DC, Anderson SA, Brown-Cartwright D: Response to furosemide in chronic renal insufficiency: Rationale for limited dose. *Clin Pharmacol Ther* 40:134–139, 1986.
10. Kjellstrand CM: Ethacrynic acid in acute tubular necrosis. *Nephron* 9:337–348, 1972
11. Steinmuller SR, Puschett JB: Effects of metolazone in man: Comparison with chlorothiazide. *Kidney Int* 1:169–181, 1972.
12. Puschett JB, Steinmuller SR, Rastegar A, Fernandez P: Metolazone: Mechanism and site of action. In: AF Lant, GM Wilson eds, *Modern Diuretic therapy in the treatment of cardiovascular and Renal disease.* Exerpta Medica, Amsterdam, pp 168–175, 1973.
13. Goldfarb S, Cox M, Singer I, Goldberg M: Acute hyperkalemia induced by hyperglycemia; hormonal mechanisms. *Ann Int Med* 84:426–432, 1976.
14. Gabow PA, Moore S, Schrier RW: Spironolactone-induced hyperchloremic acidosis in cirrhosis. *Ann Int Med* 90:338–340, 1979.
15. Gilman AG, Goodman LS, Rall TW, Murad F (eds): *Goodmen and Gilman's The Pharmacolgical Basis of Therapeutics*, 7th ed. Macmillan New York, 1985.
16. Kaplan NM: Problems with the use of diuretics in the treatment of hypertension. *Am J Nephrol* 6:1–5, 1986.
17. Freis ED: The cardiovascular risks of thiazide diuretics. *Clin Pharmacol Ther* 39:239–244, 1986.
18. Papademetriou V: Diuretics, hypokalemia, and cardiac arrhythmias: A critical analysis. *Am Heart J* 111:1217–1224, 1986.
19. Ashraf N, Lochsky R, Arieff AI: Thiazide-induced hyponatremia assoicated with death or neurologic damage in outpatients. *Am J Med* 70:1163–1168, 1981.
20. Sterns RH, Riggs JE, Schochet SS: Osmotic demyelination syndrome following correction of hyponatremia. *N Engl J Med* 314:1535–1542, 1986
21. Ashouri OS: Severe diuretic-induced hyponatremia in the elderly. A series of eight patients. Arch Intern Med 146:1355–1357, 1986.
22. Odlind BG, Beermann B: Diuretic resistance: Reduced bioavailability and effect of oral furosemid. *Br Med J* 2:1577, 1980.
23. Vasko MR, Brown-Cartwright D, Knochel Jp, Nixon JV, Brater DC: Furosemide absorption altered in decompensated congestive heart failure. *Ann Intern Med* 102:314–318, 1985.
24. Brater DC: Pharmacodynamic and pharmacokinetic considerations in the therapy of patient with resistant edema. In: JB Puschett, A Greenberg, eds, *Diuretics II Chemistry, Pharmacology, and Clinical Applications.* Elsevier, New York, pp 308–314, 1987.
25. Brater DC, Anderson SA, Brown-Cartwright D: Response to furosemide in chronic renal insufficiency: Rationale for limited doses. *Clin Pharmacol Ther* 40:134–139, 1986.
26. Brater DC, Day B, Burdette A, Anderson S: Bumetanide and furosemide in heart failure. *Kidney Int* 26:183–189, 1984.
27. Keller E, Hoppe-Seyler G, Schollmeyer P: Disposition and diuretic effect of furosemide in the nephrotic syndrome. *Clin Pharmacol Ther* 32:442–449, 1982.
28. Gunstone RF, Wing AJ, Shani HGP, Njemo D, Sabuka EMW: Clinical experience with metolazone in fifty-two African patients: Synergy with furosemide. *Postgrad Med J* 47:789–793, 1971.
29. Epstein M, Lepp BA, Hoffman DS, Levinson R: Potentiation of furosemide by metolazone in refractory edema. *Current Ther Res* 21:656–667, 1977.
30. Oster JR, Epstein M, Smoler S: Combined therapy with thiazide-type and loop diuretic agents for resistant sodium retention. *Ann Intern Med* 99:405–406, 1983.
31. Puschett JB: Physiologic basis for the use of new and older diuretics in congestive heart failure. *Cardiovas Med* 2:119–134, 1977.
32. Frazier HS, Yager H: The clinical use of diuretics. *N Engl J Med* 246–248, 1973.
33. Reubi FC, Cottier PT: Effect of reduced glomerular filtration rate on responsiveness to chlorothiazide and mercurial diuretics. *Circulation* 23:200–210, 1961.
34. Dargie HJ, Allison MEM, Kennedy AC, Gray MJB: High dosage metolazone in chronic renal failure. *Br Med J* 4:196–198, 1972.
35. Craswell PW, Ezzat E, kopstein J, Varghese Z, Moorhead JF: Use of metolazone, a new diuretic, in patients with renal disease. *Nephron* 12:63–73, 1973.
36. Paton RR, Kane RE: Long-term diuretic therapy with metolazone of renal failure and nephrotic syndrome. *J Clin Pharm* 17:243–251, 1977
37. Tobin JR: The treatment of congestive heart failure. Digitalis glycosides are still the primary mode of therapy. *Arch Int Med* 138:453–454, 1978.
38. Lemberg L: Digitalis in congestive heart failure. *Arch Intern Med* 138:451–452, 1978.
39. Spector R: Digitalis therapy in heart failure: A rational approach. *J Clin Pharm* 19:692–696, 1979.
40. Bennett WM, Aronoff GR, Morrison G, Golper TA, Pulliam J, Wolfson M, Singer I. Drug prescribing in renal failure: Dosing guidelines for adults. *Am J Kidney Dis* 3:155–193, 1983.
41. Schneider EG, Dresser TP, Lynch RE, Knox FG: Sodium reabsorption by proximal tubule of dogs with experimental heart failure. *Am J Physiol* 220:952–957, 1971
42. Stumpe KO, Reinelt B, Ressel C. Klein H, Kruck F: Urinary sodium excretion and proximal tubule reabsorption in rats with high-output heart failure. *Nephron* 12:261–274, 1974.
43. Bell NH, Schedel HP, Bartter FC: An explanation for abnormal water retention and hypo-osmolality in congestive heart failure. *Am J Med* 36:351–360, 1964.
44. Puschett JB, McCrary RF: Metolazone in the therapy of congestive heart failure. In: RD Scott, ed, *Clinical Cardiology and Diabetes.* Futura, Mt. Kisco, NY, pp 47–55, 1980.
45. Braunwald E: Vasodilator therapy — a physiologic approach to the treatment of heart failure. *N Engl J Med* 297:331–333, 1977.
46. Cohn JN: Vasodilator therapy of congestive heart failure. In: *Advances in Internal Medicine,* Year Book Medical Publishers, Vol. 28. Chicago, pp 293–315, 1980.
47. Sutton FJ: Vasodilator therapy. *Am J Med* 80 (Suppl 2B):54–58, 1986.
48. Dollery CT, Corr L: Drug treatment of heart failure. *Br Heart J* 54:234–242, 1985.
49. Diamond JR, Cheung JY, Fang LST: Nifedipine-induced renal dysfunction. Alterations in renal hemodynamics. *Am J Med* 77:905–909, 1984.
50. Golper TA: Continuous ateriovenous hemofiltration in acute renal failure. *Am J Kidney Dis* 6:373–396, 1985.
51. Diuretics and the treatment of pulmonary edema (editorial). *N Engl J Med* 279:160, 1968.
52. Robin ED, Cross CE, Zelis R: Pulmonary edema. *N Engl J Med* 288:239–245, 292–304, 1973.

53. Dikshit K, Vyden JK, Forester JS, Chatterjie K, Prakash R, Swan HJC: Renal and extra-renal hemodynamic effects of furosemide in congestive heart failure after acute myocardial infarction. *N Eng J Med* 288:1087–1090, 1973.
54. Brater DC, Chennavasin P, Dehmer GJ: Prolonged hemodynamic effect of furosemide in congestive heart failure. *Am Heart J* 108:1031–1032, 1984.
55. Francis GS, Siegel RM, Goldsmith SR, Olivari MT, Levine TB, Cohn JN: Acute vasoconstrictor response to intravenous furosemide in patients with chronic congestive heart failure. *Ann Intern Med* 103:1–6, 1985.
56. Gerhardt RE, Abdulla AM, Mach SJ, Hudson JB: Isolated ultrafiltration in the treatment of fluid overload in cardiogenic shock. *Arch Intern Med* 139:358–359, 1979.
57. Glassock RJ: Sodium homeostasis in acute glomerulonephritis and the nephrotic syndrome. *Contrib Nephrol* 23:181–203, 1980.
58. Mees EJD, Roos JC, Boer P, Yoe OH, Simatupand TA: Observations on edema formation in the nephrotic syndrome in adults with minimal lesions. *Am J Med* 67:378–384, 1979.
59. Meltzer JI, Keim HJ, Laragh JH, Sealey JE, Jan K, Chen S: Nephrotic syndrome: Vasoconstriction and hypervolemic types indicated by renin-sodium profiling. *Ann Intern Med* 91:688–696, 1979.
60. Grausz H, Lieberman R, Earley LE: Effect of plasma albumin on sodium reabsorption in patients with nephrotic syndrome. *Kidney Int* 1:47–54. 1973.
61. Kuroda S, Aynedjian HS, Bank N: A micropuncture study of renal sodium retention in nephrotic syndrome in rats: Evidence for increased resistance to tubular fluid flow. *Kidney Int* 16:561–571, 1979.
62. Davison AM, Lambie AT, Virth AH, Cash JD: Salt-poor albumin in the management of the nephrotic syndrome. *Br Med J* 1:481–484, 1974.
63. Bourgoignie J, Penell JP, Jacob AI: Sodium metabolism and volume regulation. In: HC Gonick, ed, *Current nephrology*, Vol 3. Houghton Mifflin, Boston, pp 1–4, 1979.
64. Anderson RJ, Linas SL, Berns AS, Henrich WL, Muller TR, Gabow PA, Schrier RW: Non-oliguric acute renal failure. *N Engl J Med* 296:1134–1138, 1977.
65. Ufferman RC, Jaenike JR, Freeman RB, Pabico RC: Effects of furosemide on low-dose mercuric chloride acute renal failure in the rat. *Kidney Int* 8:362–367, 1975.
66. Lindner A, Cutler RE, Goodman WG: Synergism of dopamine plus furosemide in preventing acute renal failure in the dog. *Kidney Int* 16:158–160, 1979.
67. Epstein M, Schneider NS, Befeler B: Effect of intrarenal hemodynamics in acute renal failure. *Am J Med* 58:510–515, 1975.
68. Kleinecht D, Ganeval D, Gonzalez-Duque LA, Fermanian J: Furosemide in acute oliguric renal failure, a controlled trial. *Nephron* 17:51–58, 1976.
69. Brown CB, Oggs CS, Cameron JS: High dose furosemide in acute renal fialure: A controlled study. *Clin Nephrol* 15:90–96, 1981.
70. Bricker NS: On the pathogenesis of the uremic state. An exposition of the "trade-off" hypothesis. *N Engl J Med* 286:1093–1099, 1972.
71. Danovitch GM, Bourgoignie J, Bricker NS: Reversibility of the "salt-losing" tendency of chronic renal failure. *N Eng J Med* 296:14–19, 1977.
72. Feldman HA, Jayakumar S, Puschett JB: Idiopathic edema: A review of etiologic concepts and management. *Cardiovasc Med* 3:475–488, 1978.
73. Streeten DHP, Dalakos TG, Souma M, Fellerman H, Clift GV, Schletter FE, Stevenson CT, Speller PJ: Studies of the pathogenesis of idiopathic oedema. The roles of postural changes in plasma volume, plasma renin activity aldosterone secretion rate, and glomerular filtration rate in the retention of sodium and water. *Clin Sci Mol Med* 45:347–373, 1973.
74. Goldsmith L, Weiss G. Puberty, adolescence, and the clinical aspects of normal menstruation. In: N Danforth, JR Scott, PJ DiSaia, CB Hammond, WN Spellacy, eds, *Obstetrics and Gynecology*. JB Lippincott, Philadelphia, 1986.
75. Daly MJ, Winn H, Willson JR: Sexual responses of women, dysmenorrhea, and premenstrual tension. In: JR Willson, ER, Garrington, WJ Ledger, eds, *Obstetrics and Gynecology*. CY Mosby, St. Louis, 1983.
76. Lindheimer MD, Katz AK: The kidney in pregnancy. In: BM Brenner, FC Rector Jr, eds, *The Kidney*, 3rd ed. WB Saunders, Philadelphia, 1986.
77. Wonley RJ: Pregnancy-induced hypertension. In: N Danforth, JR Scott, PJ DiSaia, CB Hammond, WN Spellacy, eds, *Obstetrics and Gynecology*. JB Lippincott, Philadelphia, 1986.
78. Epstein M: Deranged sodium homeostasis in cirrhosis. *Gastroenterology* 76:622–635, 1979.
79. Linas SL, Anderson RJ, Miller PD, Schrier RW: Rational use of diuretics in cirrhosis. In: M Epstein, ed, *The Kidney in Liver Disease*. Elsevier North-Holland, New York, pp 313–323, 1978.
80. Pitts TO, Van Thiel DH: The pathogenesis of renal sodium retention and ascites formation in Laennec's cirrhosis. In: M Galanter, ed, *Recent Developments in Alcoholism*. Plenum, New York, pp 379–440, 1986.
81. Rocco VK, Ware AJ: Cirrhotic ascites. Pathophysiology, diagnosis, and management. *Ann Intern Med* 105:573–585, 1986.
82. Lieberman FL, Denison EK, Reynolds TB: The relationship of plasma volume, portal hypertension, ascites, and renal sodium retention in cirrhosis: The overflow theory of ascites formation. *Ann NY Acad Sci* 170:202–206, 1970.
83. Levy M: Sodium retention and ascites formation in dogs with experimental portal cirrhosis. *Am J Physiol* 233:F572–F585, 1977.
84. Goldstein H, Boyle JD: Spontaneous recovery from the hepatorenal syndrome: Report of four cases. *N Engl J Med* 272:285–288, 1965.
85. Tristani FE, Cohn JN: Systemic and renal hemodynamics in oliguric hepatic failure: Effect of volume expansion. *J Clin Invest* 46:1894–1906, 1967.
86. Shear L, Ching S, Gabuzda GJ: Compartmentalization of ascites and edema in patients with hepatic cirrhosi. *N Eng J Med* 282:1391–1396, 1970.
87. Pockros PJ, Reynolds TB: Rapid diuresis in patients with ascites from chronic liver disease: The importance of peripheral edema. *Gastroenterology* 90:1827–1833, 1986.
88. Hillenbrand P, Sherlock S: Use of metolazone in the treatment of ascites due to liver disease. *Br Med J* 4:266–270, 1971.
89. Moult PJA, Lunzer MR, Trash DB, Sherlock S: Use of bumetanide in the treatment of ascites due to liver disease. *Gut* 15:988–992, 1974.
90. Lang GR, Westenfelder C, Nascimento L, Dhupelia VB, Arruda JAL, Kane RE. Metolazone and spironolactone in cirrhosis and the nephrotic syndrome. *Clin Pharmacol Ther* 21:234–243, 1976.
91. Eggert RC: Spironolactone diuresis in patients with cirrhosis and ascites. *Br Med J* 4:401–403, 1970.
92. Wapnick S, Grosberg S, Kinney M, Azzara V, LeVeen HH:

Renal failure in ascites secondary to hepatic, renal and pancreatic disease. *Arch Surg* 113:581–585, 1978.
93. Fullen WD: Hepatorenal syndrome: Reversal by peritoneovenous shunt. *Surgery* 82:337–341, 1977.
94. Pladson TR, Parish RM: Hepatorenal syndrome. Recovery after peritoneovenous shunt. *Arch Int Med* 137:1248–1249, 1977.
95. Blendis LM, Greig PD, Langer B, Baigrie RS, Ruse J, Taylor BR: The renal and hemodynamic effects of the peritoneovenous shunt for intractable hepatic ascites. *Gastroenterology* 77:250–257, 1979.
96. Epstein M: The LeVeen shunt for ascites and hepatorenal syndrome. *N Engl J Med* 302:628–630, 1980.
97. Linas SL, Schaefer JW, Moore EE, Good JT, Jr, Gransiracusa R: Peritoneovenous shunt in the management of the hepatorenal syndrome. *Kidney Int* 30:736–740, 1986.

CHAPTER 4

Disorders of Potassium Metabolism

JACQUES J. BOURGOIGNIE, JAMES R. OSTER, GUIDO O. PEREZ & DOLLIE F. GREEN

Causes of potassium abnormalities are multiple. They may be observed in a variety of clinical settings from the office to the emergency room, and they confront the endocrinologist, nephrologist, cardiologist, gastroenterologist, as well as the surgeon and the anesthesiologist. Many derangements of potassium homeostasis are confusing and poorly understood. Not infrequently, they are iatrogenically induced. All carry the potential of life-threatening consequences. The importance of recognizing the etiology of changes in potassium homeostasis is critical for appropriate therapeutic intervention. Similarly, an adequate understanding of potassium homeostasis is necessary for preventing or minimizing iatrogenic potential causes of serious hyperkalemia or hypokalemia. For these reasons, a brief overview of normal potassium homeostasis and regulating factors is presented prior to considering specific clinical entities and treatment modalities.

POTASSIUM HOMEOSTASIS

Potassium is the major intracellular cation, and only 2% of total body potassium is extracellcular (Figure 1) (1). Counterregulatory mechanisms operate on multiple organs to maintain potassium homeostasis.

External potassium balance

External potassium balance, or the absence of an appreciable difference between dietary intake and excretion, operates to maintain total body potassium within narrow limits. The typical American diet contains about 1 mEq of potassium/kg body weight per day (2). Ninety percent is normally excreted by the kidneys and less than 10% in the feces, with minimal losses through skin. Thus, changes in potassium input or in potassium excretion by the kidney, gastrointestinal trast, or skin may be expected to alter total body potassium and result in conditions of either potassium accumulation or potassium deficit.

The kidneys are responsible for maintaining external potassium balance because stool potassium losses normally remain relatively constant (3). Potassium is freely filtered across the glomerular capillaries. Most is reabsorbed in the proximal convoluted tubule and in ascending limb of Henle's loop so that the fractional delivery of filtered potassium to the earliest portion of the distal tubule is only 5–10%. Thus, most of the potassium excreted in the urine is secreted by the "late" distal tubule and the cortical collecting duct. The principal cells are thought to effect potassium secretion as the result of transport across the basolateral and luminal membranes. The basolateral membrane is the site of the active uptake of potassium mediated by Na-K-ATPase. The subsequent secretion of potassium across the apical membrane is believed to occur passively because the electrochemical gradient is favourable for diffusion into the lumen and the potassium conductance of the apical membrane is high (4).

Individual factors influencing renal potassium excretion are listed in Table 1. The most important are functional renal mass [estimated as glomerular filtration rate (GFR)], plasma and intracellular potassium concentrations, distal tubular fluid flow rate, tubular availability of anions (chloride and impermeant anions), the acid-base status, and hormonal influences, including mineralocorticoid and glucocorticoid hormones. These factors exert their influences from either the luminal side (flow rate, sodium and anion concentrations, transepithelial potential difference) or from the peritubular side (dietary intake, plasma potassium concentration, the acid-base status, and hormones) (4).

The rate of fluid flow through the distal tubule is an important factor influencing potassium excretion. Increases in luminal flow rate independent of solute excretion, as assessed by continuous microperfusion, facilitate potassium excretion (5).

Changes in the tubular sodium concentrations between 40 and 100 mM do not seem to affect potassium excretion. Nevertheless, luminal sodium concentrations less than 35 mM appear to be limiting for potassium excretion (6). A decrease in transtubular potential difference may then act to impede potassium movement into the lumen. Sodium concentrations of this magnitude are rarely obtained, except under conditions of water diuresis when the tubular fluid sodium concentration may drop to 25–30 mM (7). Infusions of sodium salts whose anions are poorly

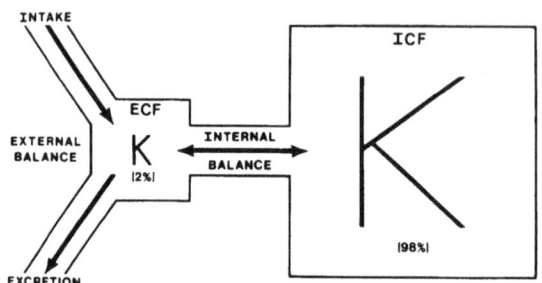

Figure 1. Potassium balance. The content of the small extracellular fluid (ECF) potassium pool is determined both by the difference between intake and excretion (external potassium balance) and by exchange with the much larger potassium pool in the intracellular fluid (ICF) (internal potassium balance). Reprinted with permission from: RH Sterns, et al.: Medicine 60:339–354, 1981 (1).

Table 1. Factors modifying the renal excretion of potassium

Functional renal mass	Acid-base status
Tubular fluid flow rate	Steroid hormones
Distal sodium delivery	Mineralocorticoids
Transepithelial potential difference	Glucocorticoids
Anion availability	Catecholamines
(chloride versus others)	Antidiuretic hormone
Dietary intake	
Plasma potassium concentration	

Table 2. Factors modifying the distribution of potassium between the extracellular and the intracellular space

Acid-base status	Catecholamines
Extracellular fluid tonicity	Beta$_2$-adrenergic system
Insulin	Alpha-adrenergic system
Aldosterone	

reabsorbed (such as sulfate or penicillins) increase potassium excretion. This may be related to increases in tubular flow rate and in the electrical potential difference. The results of recent microperfusion studies suggest, however, that chloride concentrations in the lumen below 10 mM are associated with augmented potassium secretion (8). Although the mechanism of this effect has not been elucidated, it might contribute to the increased potassium excretion in the presence of poorly reabsorbable anions.

The transepithelial potential difference influences the passive movement of potassium from cells to the lumen. Although not an important regulator of potassium excretion under physiologic circumstances, the potential difference may play a role in several pathophysiologic conditions. For example, administration of amiloride, by impeding sodium entry into the cell, leads to hyperpolarization of the apical membrane and reduction of the transepithelial potential. This causes the fall in potassium secretion observed with administration of this agent (9). Decreased transepithelial potential, and thus decreased potassium secretion, has been postulated to be the cause of hyperkalemia in the "chloride shunt" syndrome (10) (vide infra).

An increase in dietary potassium intake results in a greater number of Na-K-ATPase pump units per cell in potassium-secreting epithelia (4). When the extracellular potassium concentration increases, distal potassium secretion is directly stimulated, independently of flow rate and mineralocorticoid activity (11, 12). Alkalosis stimulates urinary potassium losses whereas acute acidosis inhibits distal renal potassium secretion (4). In chronic acidosis, the results are more variable and, in general, potassium excretion is stimulated because of changes in other variables regulating potassium excretion such as mineralocorticoid activity (13). Finally, hormonal agents, especially mineralocorticoids, act from the peritubular side to enhance the rate of potassium secretion. They increase the basolateral membrane area in the collecting ducts, presumably reflecting an increase in Na-K-ATPase pump sites (12). Perfusion of rabbit cortical collecting tubules in vitro has shown that the effects of mineralocorticoids are mediated by a) increased basolateral uptake, b) increased electrochemical gradient, and c) increased potassium conductance of the tubular membrane (14).

The kaliuresis accompanying glucocorticoid (as opposed to mineralocorticoid) administration results from alterations in GFR, sodium, and fluid delivery to the distal nephron, rather than from a direct glucocorticoid receptor-mediated potassium secretory effect (14).

Several other hormones affect potassium excretion (14). Epinephrine decreases urinary potassium excretion. This influence is localized to the cortical collecting tubule and represents a selective beta$_1$ agonistic effect (15). In-vivo microperfusion experiments of the distal convoluted tubule of Brattleboro rats have also delineated a clear effect of antidiuretic hormone to stimulate potassium secretion (7). The physiologic and pathophysiologic significance of these responses to epinephrine and antidiuretic hormone have not been defined.

Internal potassium balance

Besides the mechanisms modulating the external balance of potassium, potassium homeostasis is also greatly influenced by an internal balance system that governs the distribution of potassium between the extracellular and the intracellular spaces (1). Intracellular potassium is quantitatively most abundant in tissues with the largest cell mass: muscles, liver, and red blood cells. Thus, small changes in internal potassium balance or cell breakdown may greatly affect the extracellular (and serum) potassium concentration. In contrast with changes in the external balance, internal redistribution of potassium is not immediately associated with net changes in total body potassium.

The distribution of potassium in and out of the cells is also modulated. Modifying factors are listed in Table 2. The most important appear to be the acid-base status, extracellular tonicity, and hormonal influences, including that of insulin, catecholamines, and aldosterone. The role of these factors will be discussed separately with the specific clinical entities in which their impact in altering potassium homeostasis may be important.

Assessment of total body potassium

As a consequence of the dual balance system for potassium, each of which may affect extracellular potassium concentration independently and often in a counterregulatory fashion, and because total body potassium is not easily quantitated and, therefore, not routinely measured, changes in potassium homeostasis are not readily assessed from measurements of the serum potassium concentration. In contrast, variations in the serum potassium concentration outside the normal narrow range of 3.5–5.0 mEq/l are easily and rapidly recognized in the laboratory. Nevertheless, because the relationship between the serum potassium concentration and total body potassium is not a constant, changes in extracellular potassium do not necessarily mirror changes in total body potassium. Both hypokalemia and hyperkalemia may be associated with a normal total body potassium. Conversely, in certain clinical settings, such as diabetic ketoacidosis, a normal serum potassium is usually indicative of severe potassium depletion. Thus, changes in potassium homeostasis are not always properly assessed from the concentration of serum potassium and may even be overlooked in the absence of clinical symptomatology.

One must distinguish between those disorders wherein total body potassium remains constant, in which changes in serum potassium result from a redistribution of potassium between the extracellular and the intracellular spaces, and those in which changes in serum potassium concentration are associated with concomitant changes in total body potassium (16, 17). In the former, therapy aimed at counterbalancing the internal maldistribution of potassium should theoretically suffice to correct the hyperkalemia or hypokalemia without intervention directed at removing or adding potassium to the body. In contrast, in the latter, overall balance and potassium homeostasis can only be restored by subtraction or addition of potassium.

There are limitations to this concept. Indeed, in many situations of deranged potassium homeostasis, a mixed condition prevails because of counterbalancing or concomitant influences of specific disorders on external and internal potassium balance mechanisms. Even within a single organ such as the kidney, opposite influences on potassium excretion can be recognized. For instance, the influence of the decreased distal fluid delivery prevailing in states of extracellular fluid volume depletion, a condition that favors potassium retention, may be counterbalanced by that of an increase in aldosterone and/or antidiuretic hormone secretion, which stimulate distal tubular potassium secretion (13).

Physiologic effects of potassium

The intracellular distribution of potassium establishes the internal milieu and the resting membrane potential of cells (18). Potassium plays an important role in activating a variety of enzymes and cell functions, and is critical in determining neuromuscular excitability. The latter is not a function of serum potassium concentration alone, but of the ratio between the intracellular and extracellular potassium concentrations. Because intracellular potassium (K_i) is so much higher than extracellular potassium (K_e), and because variations in the extracellular potassium concentration are proportionally greater and develop more rapidly than changes in intracellular potassium, important changes in the ratio K_i/K_e are mainly produced by alterations of K_e. The K_i/K_e ratio is not constant.

The rapidity with which the serum potassium concentration changes critically influences the K_i/K_e ratio and the clinical manifestations of potassium imbalance (19). Thus, in acute hypokalemia, secondary to severe diarrhea or vomiting, K_i/K_e rises, thereby increasing the resting membrane potential to produce hyperpolarization with symptoms of muscle weakness or paralysis. Conversely when acute hyperkalemia develops, as in rhabdomyolysis or in acute renal failure, K_i/K_e decreases, resulting in depolarization and arrhythmias (Figure 2) (20). Such effects are markedly attenuated when the serum potassium concentration changes gradually; in this case, commensurate changes in intracellular potassium minimize changes in K_i/K_e and in the resting membrane potential. Even important changes in the serum potassium concentration

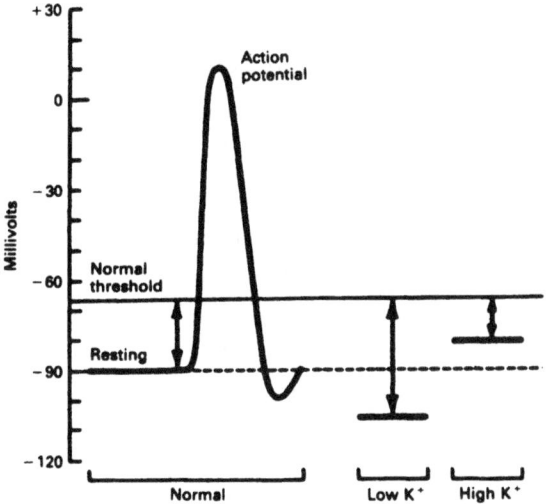

Figure 2. The action potential of skeletal muscles and effect of potassium homeostasis. The solid horizontal line delineates the normal threshold potential of depolarization; the broken line shows the resting potential when potassium homeostasis is normal. In acute hypokalemia, the resting potential is more negative (relative hyperpolarization). This increases the gap between the resting potential and the threshold potential at which an action potential is propagated. In acute hyperkalemia, the resting potential is less negative (relative depolarization) and is closer to the threshold potential. Reprinted with permission from: RS Brown: Kidney Int 30:116–127, 1986 (20).

may not be reflected clinically and may not alert the clinician to the underlying disturbance. The physician, therefore, must have a high degree of suspicion and must assess the etiology and the possible consequences of changes in potassium homeostasis from the clinical setting and from measurements of the serum potassium concentration.

CLINICAL APPROACH TO HYPERKALEMIA AND HYPOKALEMIA

A useful outline to evaluate the etiology of changes in serum potassium is depicted in Figure 3. As indicated above, hyperkalemia or hypokalemia may result from changes in the internal potassium balance or redistribution of potassium between intracellular and extracellular compartments without net changes in total body potassium. They may also stem from external potassium imbalance, which is associated with net changes in total body potassium. The latter may result from an abnormal intake of exogenous potassium and/or from potassium losses or retention at the output level. Changes in output may be of renal or extrarenal origin. Finally, measurements of serum potassium sometimes return from the laboratory with unexpected results. The physician must be aware that factitious changes in serum potassium concentration are possible.

Factitious changes in serum potassium

Table 3 lists causes of factitious or artifactual changes in serum (or plasma) potassium concentration. In these situations, the concentration of circulating potassium is actually normal but is changed during or after the time of blood withdrawal prior to serum (or plasma) analysis in the laboratory. These errors are rare and, generally result in hyperkalemia.

Errors due to the analytical method used for measuring potassium are quite unusual. Potassium measurements by

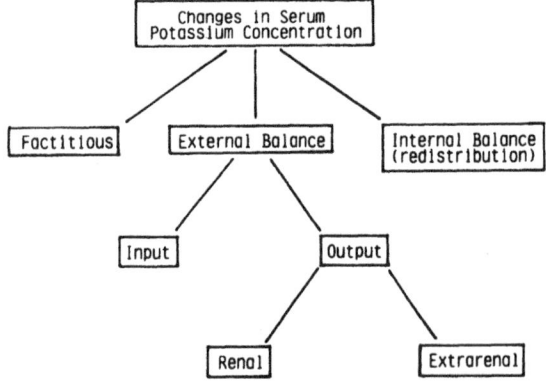

Figure 3. Diagram of mechanisms potentially responsible for changes in serum potassium concentration.

Table 3. Sources of factitious or artifactual changes in serum (or plasma) potassium concentration

Hyperkalemia
- Ischemic blood drawing (fist-clenching)
- Extracorporeal hemolysis
- Delayed separation of serum (or plasma) in the presence of:
  - Thrombocytosis $> 1 \times 10^6/mm^3$
  - Leukocytosis $> 7 \times 10^4/mm^3$
  - Familial defect in red blood cell membrane

Hypokalemia
- Leukemic cells: $3 \times 10^4 - 7.4 \times 10^5/mm^3$

automated chemical analysis, flame photometry, or the potassium-specific electrode are highly reliable.

Artifactual hyperkalemia (or normokalemia masking true hypokalemia) can occur if serum samples are improperly obtained. Since human erythrocytes have a very high potassium concentration (> 120 mEq/l), hemolysis within the collection tube can introduce a major error (21). Thus, aspiration of blood through a small-bore needle into a vacuum tube may, on occasion, produce gross hemolysis. The laboratory technician usually makes a note of obvious hemolysis on the laboratory report.

Another source of spurious hyperkalemia is sustained contraction of the forearm muscles (fist-clenching) during or just prior to withdrawal of blood. In this setting, especially when a tight tourniquet is used, potassium may be translocated from the active and slightly ischemic muscle cells into the blood. This phenomenon may (unpredictably) elevate the serum potassium by as much as 2.7 mEq/l (22, 23).

If clotted or heparinized blood is allowed to stand too long before separation of serum or plasma, potassium may be released by cells and may progressively increase the extracellular potassium concentration. This may occur when blood containing a very large number of platelets ($> 10^6$) or leukocytes ($> 10^5$) clots within the collection tube, releasing potassium into the serum (24, 25). The same phenomenon can occur when normal heparinized blood samples are left for 2–3 hours at room temperature before separation of the cells and plasma. Cold storage of blood samples accelerates this process (26). The laboratory reports hyperkalemia, often to a striking degree, but the true concentration of potassium within the circulation is not elevated.

There is also a rare condition of familial pseudohyperkalemia, in which a defect in the red blood cell membrane results in apparent hyperkalemia when the collection tube remains for some time in a warm environment prior to cell separation (27).

Artifactual hypokalemia has been described in association with a high white blood count in myeloproliferative disorders. If blood from leukemic patients is permitted to stand at room temperature for 2–3 hours, the white blood cells may extract potassium from plasma and spuriously lower the measured value (28).

In these conditions, the patient, of course, has none

of the clinical manifestations of hyperkalemia or hypokalemia, and the electrocardiogram is normal.

Laboratory and diagnostic procedures

A list of initial laboratory and diagnostic procedures that are often helpful in the evaluation of patients with apparent hyperkalemia or hypokalemia is presented in Table 4.

If a physician receives an unexpected report of hyperkalemia or hypokalemia in a patient without any apparent reason, he or she should consider the possibility of some type of artifact. If a repeat determination reveals a similar value, a plasma sample should be obtained while avoiding or minimizing the use of a tourniquet and undue muscular effort. Blood can be aspirated directly into a heparinized syringe, rather than into a vacuum tube, and then gently transferred into a heparin-containing collection tube after removing the needle and stopper. The blood sample should immediately be brought to and processed by the laboratory and the plasma should be quickly separated from the circulating cells. Normally, differences in potassium concentration between serum and plasma should not exceed 0.2–0.3 mEq/l (29). Platelet and white blood cells should also be counted.

An electrocardiogram should be obtained to assess the physiologic significance of the alleged change in serum potassium concentration. If the electrocardiogram indicates hyperkalemia or hypokalemia, or if the laboratory confirms prior results, blood urea nitrogen and serum creatinine concentrations must be measured to assess renal function. The concentrations of other serum electrolytes and the acid-base status should be evaluated to help in the differential diagnosis. A 1–2 ml "spot" urine sample for measuring pH, sodium, potassium, chloride, and creatinine concentrations before therapy is instituted may ultimately prove extremely helpful in the differential diagnosis of the etiology of hypokalemia. In certain situations, special tests to measure renin activity and aldosterone in plasma or to rule out urinary tract obstruction can be rapidly obtained.

Table 4. Initial laboratory and diagnostic procedures often helpful in the evaluation of a patient with hyperkalemia or hypokalemia

A. Electrocardiogram
B. Repeat blood potassium levels using heparinized blood obtained without the use of a tourniquet or fist-clenching
C. Platelet and white blood cell counts
D. Blood urea nitrogen and serum creatinine concentrations to assess renal function
E. Serum sodium, chloride, and bicarbonate concentrations
F. Arterial blood gas values
G. Measurement of urinary pH and concentrations of sodium, potassium, chloride, and creatinine on spot urine sample
H. Plasma aldosterone and renin activity (special situations)
I. Renal ultrasonography (special situations)

HYPERKALEMIA

Hyperkalemia results from increased potassium input, abnormal transcellular distribution, or decreased renal or gastrointestinal excretion. It may represent a most serious electrolyte disturbance because of cardiotoxicity and frequent absence of premonitory clinical manifestations. Thus, the clinician must be aware of the most common disorders predisposing to severe hyperkalemia, such as renal failure, tissue necrosis, and certain medications that impair potassium homeostasis. Understanding the pathophysiologic mechanisms responsible for hyperkalemia helps the physician anticipate and prevent this potentially life-threatening electrolyte disturbance.

As a result of transcellular potassium distribution

Ninety-eight percent of total body potassium is located within the intracellular water. The activity of Na-K-ATPase is the main factor responsible for the maintenance of this gradient. Thus, factors interfering with the activity of this system, such as impaired function of beta$_2$ adrenoceptors, intoxication with cardiac glycosides, and perhaps insulin deficiency, frequently result in hyperkalemia, particularly during potassium administration (30). In addition, shifts of potassium from the intracellular to extracellular space occur with some types of acidemia, exercise, hypertonicity, aldosterone deficiency, in hyperkalemic periodic paralysis, and with medications and tissue damage (Figure 4).

ACIDOSIS

When protons enter cells, potassium moves out into the extracellular space. Changes in serum bicarbonate per se, independent of changes in blood pH, also influence the serum potassium concentration (31, 32). The effect of acidemia on serum potassium concentration depends on the acuteness of onset, whether it is metabolic or respiratory in origin, and, if metabolic, whether caused by mineral or organic acids.

Chronic acidosis is generally associated with increased urinary potassium excretion and therefore does not produce hyperkalemia (13); whereas acute acidemia inhibits distal tubular potassium secretion (33). Respiratory acidosis causes less hyperkalemia, perhaps because of easy passage of CO_2 into cells (thereby causing more similar changes in pH in both compartments). Mineral acids cause marked increases in serum potassium concentration (34). On the other hand, hyperkalemia is frequently absent when the acidosis is induced by organic acids (34). It has been postulated that, because the organic anion penetrates the cell, the potassium ion remains in the intracellular compartment. There is evidence, however, that organic acids stimulate insulin release (35) and that epinephrine release during certain organic acidoses prevents acute increases in serum potassium. In diabetic acidosis, hyperkalemia is frequent at the time of presentation despite the presence of substantial deficits in total body potassium. The etiology of the increase in serum potassium in diabetic

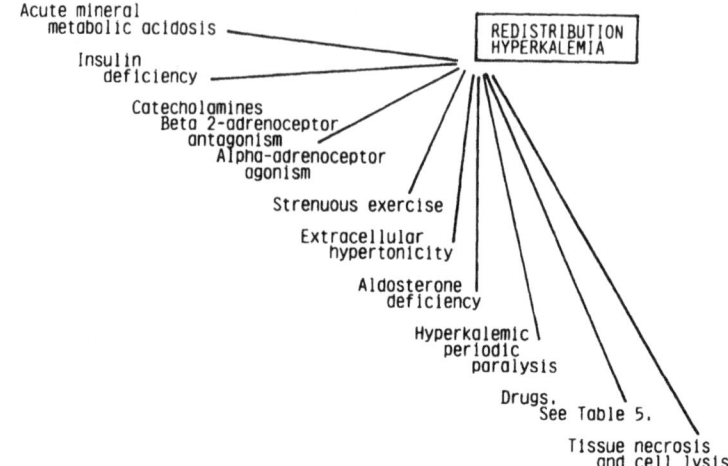

Figure 4. Causes of hyperkalemia as a result of redistribution of potassium between intracellular and extracellular space (no increase in total body potassium).

ketoacidosis is complex and is related in part to factors other than acidemia per se, such as decreased renal function, hyperosmolality, insulin deficiency, and increased catabolism (36).

INSULIN DEFICIENCY

The phenomenon of insulin-stimulated tissue potassium uptake has been carefully evaluated (30, 37–43). In healthy volunteers, utilizing the insulin clamp technique, it has been shown that most of the initial decline in serum potassium concentration associated with increases in plasma insulin as small as 25 µU/ml is accounted for by hepatic uptake. Subsequently, uptake by peripheral tissues is the main factor responsible for the continued decline in serum potassium levels (40). Potassium uptake by forearm muscles is also stimulated by intraarterial infusion of insulin, independent of glucose utilization (41).

The cellular mechanism(s) responsible for the effect of insulin on potassium uptake remains incompletely understood (30). Most investigators have shown that insulin hyperpolarizes muscle and adipose tissue cells, even in the absence of glucose transport. The effect may be due to stimulation of Na-K-ATPase or to changes in the permeability with enhanced potassium influx.

It is unclear, however, if a negative-feedback control loop exists between insulin and potassium. In dogs, infusions of potassium causing increases in serum levels greater than 1.5 mEq/l result in significant increases in plasma insulin (40). Increases of serum potassium concentration smaller than 1.0 mEq/l, however, are associated with little or no changes in peripheral insulin levels (42). To evaluate the possibility that portal (but not peripheral) insulin levels might increase with small increments in serum potassium levels, Martinez et al. (43) recently sampled portal vein blood in dogs given an infusion of potassium chloride designed to result in increments of serum potassium concentration less than 1 mEq/l. Portal insulin levels did not increase, suggesting an insensitive feedback mechanism.

It is well established that basal insulin secretion is needed to maintain potassium tolerance (39). Insulin deficiency may, therefore, contribute to the phenomenon of glucose-induced hyperkalemia. Diabetic subjects may manifest paradoxical hyperkalemia during acute glucose loads (44–46), particularly in patients with hypoaldosteronism and chronic renal failure. The low blood levels of insulin (and aldosterone in some cases) may be insufficient to counteract the hypersomolarity-induced efflux of potassium from cells (vide infra). Therefore, it is important to recognize that hyperglycemia, spontaneous or induced by glucose administration, may be associated with marked hyperkalemia in patients at risk.

After intravenous infusion of glucagon, a transient increase precedes a progressive decrease in the serum potassium concentration (47, 48). The secondary fall is presumably due to the concomitant increase in insulin secretion. Thus, glucagon may have a hyperkalemic effect, but only in insulinopenic subjects.

CATECHOLAMINES

Early studies in experimental animals have shown that the administration of epinephrine produces an initial increase followed by a subsequent decline in the extracellular potassium concentration (49, 50). The transient initial hyperkalemia originates from hepatic release, whereas the subsequent decrease reflects increased tissue uptake. The latter is mediated by stimulation of beta$_2$ adrenoceptors and appears to require activation of adenylate cyclase and the resultant stimulation of Na-K-ATPase.

The important role of the adrenergic nervous system in the regulation of potassium homeostasis in humans has been documented in several recent studies (56–61). Epinphrine enhances, whereas beta-adrenergic blockade impairs, extrarenal disposal of an intravenous potassium load in normal volunteers. Beta-adrenergic blockade also exaggerates the hyperkalemia induced by exercise (56) and further impairs potassium homeostasis in patients with chronic renal failure undergoing maintenance hemodialysis (57). Thus, beta$_2$ adrenergic inhibition may cause hyperkalemia and should be used with caution in patients with disturbed potassium homeostasis. Hyperkalemia is less likely to occur when a selective beta$_1$-adrenergic inhibitor is given (57, 62).

The effects of alpha-adrenergic stimulation on potassium homeostasis have also been evaluated by several investigators (58, 59). Alpha-adrenergic agonists exaggerate the hyperkalemia produced by intravenous administration of potassium in healthy volunteers (59). Conversely, alpha-adrenergic blockade attenuates the increase in serum potassium associated with phenylephrine infusion (59) or with exercise (61).

EXERCISE

During muscle-cell contraction, potassium is released from cells. This local increase in potassium is believed to promote the normal rise in blood flow during exercise, so-called exercise hyperemia (63). Transient increases in serum potassium concentration are seen regularly after modest exercise. In contrast, severe hyperkalemia after exhaustive physical activity may indicate rhabdomyolysis. The release of potassium during exercise is attenuated in physically trained individuals and is enhanced in subjects pretreated with propranolol (56, 61).

EXTRACELLULAR HYPERTONICITY

Hyperkalemia may be caused by hyperosmolality, especially in the setting of hyperglycemia in decompensated diabetes mellitus (64–66). An increase in serum potassium concentration occurs after administration of solutes that remain primarily in the extracellular fluid compartment, thereby producing hypertonicity (e.g., mannitol). The efflux of potassium has been postulated to occur because the diffusion of water out of cells raises the intracellular potassium concentration, thus favoring its outward diffusion. On the other hand, there is no evidence to suggest that extracellular hypotonicity leads to hypokalemia (64).

MINERALOCORTICOIDS

In addition to their effects on the kidney to increase renal potassium excretion, mineralocorticoids have an effect an sweat glands, salivary glands, and the colonic epithelium. It remains controversial, however, whether these agents exert an important effect on potassium uptake by other extrarenal tissues such as muscle or liver. In-vitro studies have yielded conflicting data (67, 68), and mineralocorticoids have been reported to cause both increases and decreases in tissue potassium content. The results of in-vivo studies, however, imply an effect of mineralocorticoids on extrarenal potassium homeostasis (69). Balance studies in adrenalectomized dogs suggest that aldosterone increases the intracellular to extracellular potassium concentration ratio (70). In adrenalectomized rats receiving glucocorticoid replacement, aldosterone substantially improves extrarenal potassium homeostasis; and, when epinephrine is given with aldosterone, the defect in extrarenal potassium metabolism is completely corrected (69, 71). In studies of patients with hyporeninemic hypoaldosteronism, Perez et al. (72) have also demonstrated that in addition to a defect in renal excretion, these patients appear to transfer less potassium from the extracellular to the intracellular compartment. Thus, mineralocorticoids may influence extrarenal potassium homeostasis, although the mechanisms responsible for this effect have not been elucidated.

Glucocorticoid administration results in transient increases in renal potassium excretion. The acute administration of these agents may also cause transient increases in serum potassium concentration (69). Because these changes are associated with a kaliuresis, they must be due to release of potassium from tissues. Glucocorticoids also have an important effect on the gut to increase the fecal potassium content. An effect of chronic glucocorticoid replacement on extrarenal potassium homeostasis has not been clearly demonstrated (69).

HYPERKALEMIC PERIODIC PARALYSIS

This rare, inherited disease, characterized by transient attacks of paralysis and hyperkalemia precipitated by cold exposure, exercise, and potassium loading is transmitted as an autosomal dominant disorder (73). During attacks, there is a shift of potassium from cells to extracellular fluid. Myotonia, particularly of the tongue, is one of the salient characteristics. Attacks can be prevented by a high carbohydrate diet, thiazide diuretics, and acetazolamide, presumably by increasing cellular potassium uptake. Recently, administration of beta$_2$-adrenergic agonists has been shown to ameliorate or prevent the attacks (74).

DRUGS

In addition to hypertonic solutions, beta$_2$-adrenoceptor antagonists, alpha-adrenoceptor agonists, and acute glucocorticoid administration, other agents may lead to hyperkalemia by redistributing potassium extracellularly (Table 5).

Severe intoxication with substances such as digitalis (75) and oleander tea (76), which inhibit Na-K-ATPase, may result in hyperkalemia due to release of potassium from cells. Likewise, administration of cationic amino acids such as arginine hydrochloride may obligate efflux of potassium from cells in order to maintain electrical neutrality. Severe lithium intoxication in experimental animals may be associated with hyperkalemia. Slight increments in plasma potassium levels may be seen in humans during chronic lithium therapy, but frank hyperkalemia is rarely observed (77). Impaired uptake of potas-

Table 5. Drug-induced hyperkalemia

A. *Altered potassium distribution between intracellular and extracellular space*

    Hypertonic solutions
        glucose (with insulin deficiency)
        mannitol
    Catecholamines
        $Beta_2$-adrenoceptor antagonists
        Alpha-adrenoceptor agonists
    Steroids
        Mineralocorticoid deficiency
        Acute glucocorticoid administration
    Digitalis, oleander tea
    Arginine
    Lithium
    Fluoride
    Succinylcholine
    Dantrolene (potentiated by verapamil)
    Agents causing acute tumor lysis
    Drug-induced rhabdomyolysis
    Drug-induced hemolysis

B. *Increased potassium input*

    Potassium supplements (oral or intravenous)
    "Salt substitutes"
    Potassium penicillin
    Transfusion of stored blood
    Collins' solution (post-transplantation)

C. *Decreased potassium output*

    Beta-adrenergic antagonists
    Nonsteroidal antiinflammatory agents
    Angiotensin-converting enzyme inhibitors
        captopril
        enalapril
    Cyclosporin
    Heparin
    Potassium-sparing diuretics
        spironolactone
        triamterene
        amiloride
    Drug-induced renal failure

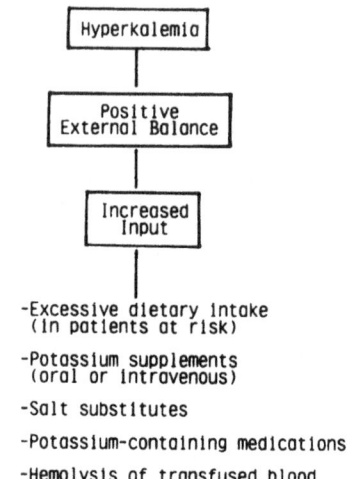

Figure 5. Causes of hyperkalemia as a result of increased total body potassium from increased exogenous potassium input.

sium by cells may be the cause of hyperkalemia in fluoride poisoning (78). The use of depolarizing agents such as succinylcholine during anesthesia may release potassium from cells by increasing the permeability of the muscle membrane. This effect may be exaggerated in damaged or denervated muscle from which massive amounts of potassium may be released. Finally, agents that cause acute tumor lysis, rhabdomyolysis, or hemolysis may induce severe hyperkalemia.

As a result of increased potassium input (Figure 5)

DIET

The normal kidney has a remarkable ability to excrete potassium. Adaptive facilitation of the renal and extrarenal potassium homeostatic mechanisms permits normal subjects to ingest large amounts of potassium safely. A daily potassium intake of 6 mEq/kg body weight can be ingested over 24 hours by normal subjects without increasing serum potassium above 6 mEq/l (79). Up to 640 mEq of potassium chloride have been administered orally daily to patients with acromegaly or myasthenia gravis, and populations subsisting mainly on potatoes apparently suffered no ill effects from a presumed daily intake of 500–1000 mEq of potassium (79).

The phenomenon of potassium adaptation has been evaluated extensively in experimental animals (71, 80–82). Rats fed high-potassium diets survive severe potassium challenges; adrenalectomy prevents this adaptation, suggesting a role for mineralocorticoids. High potassium diets, per se, increase the basolateral membrane area and the Na-K-ATPase density of potassium secretory epithelia. These changes also occur in adrenalectomized animals. Definitive proof for increased tissue potassium uptake during potassium loading is limited, however.

When a single load of potassium of 0.25 mEq/kg body weight is administered acutely by mouth to normal subjects, the maximal increase in plasma potassium concentration averages 0.39 ± 0.1 mEq/l (46). Three hours after the load, serum potassium returns to baseline values. During this interval, two thirds of the load are excreted in the urine. Of the amount retained, half is translocated to the intracellular compartment. Subjects receiving 0.5 mEq of potassium chloride per kg of body weight exhibit a maximal increment in plasma potassium concentration of about 0.8 mEq/l, which occurs 60–90 minutes after administration of the load (72). In the 4 hours following ingestion, approximately half of the load is excreted in the urine. Of the amount retained, approximately one third is translocated intracellularly. Single oral doses of approximately 1 mEq/kg body weight may result in increments of serum potassium exceeding 1 mEq/l, and after doses of

2–2.5 mEq/kg weight, potassium concentrations may reach 6–8 mEq/l (79). This information is important when administrating potassium therapeutically.

In patients with impaired potassium homeostasis such as diabetics (46), or in those with chronic renal failure (72), administration of even small amounts of potassium may result in marked increments in plasma potassium concentration. For example, Perez et al. (83) recently described two patients in whom administration of the usual replacement dose of potassium chloride resulted in life-threatening hyperkalemia. In patients with mild-to-moderate chronic renal failure, the impaired acute potassium tolerance is related primarily to defective renal rather than extrarenal mechanisms (72). As expected, patients with hypoaldosteronism transfer less potassium into cells and have an even greater impairment of renal potassium excretion (72). It should be noted, however, that in spite of impaired acute tolerance, the 24-hour balance for potassium is generally maintained in chronic renal failure through adaptive mechanisms permitting excretion of the daily load (84).

In a study of anuric patients with chronic renal failure on maintenance hemodialysis, Fernandez, Oster, and Perez (85) observed maximal increments in serum potassium concentration of 1.06 ± 0.13 mEq/l after a small oral dose of potassium (0.25 mEq/kg body weight). When expressed as a percentage of the retained load, the amount of potassium translocated into cells was small, suggesting that advanced uremia is associated with impaired extrarenal mechanisms of potassium disposal.

In the absence of both renal and extrarenal homeostatic mechanisms, administered potassium remains in the extracellular compartment. Thus, small amounts of potassium (i.e., approximately 25 mEq) would be expected to result in increments of serum potassium concentration approaching 2 mEq/l (83). Recent studies also demonstrate that regularly dialyzed patients exhibit an impaired kaliopenic response to administration of beta$_2$ adrenoceptor agonists (86).

For obvious reasons, tolerance to intravenous administration of potassium in humans has not been evaluated systematically. Keith et al. (87) described a volunteer who received 950 ml of a 1% solution of potassium chloride intravenously over 91 minutes. The serum concentration of potassium increased from a control value of 4.5 mEq/l to a value of 5.5 mEq/l. Severe pain was noted along the vein in which the infusion was given.

DRUGS

A major cause of hyperkalemia secondary to increased potassium input is the administration of potassium supplements. A large study of the risk of oral potassium supplements was carried out by the Boston Collaborative Drug Surveillance Program (88). Hyperkalemia was documented in 4% of 4900 patients receiving potassium chloride supplements, and there were seven deaths. In a study in hospitalized patients, 27 of 6199 patients died from adverse drug reactions, and five of the deaths could be attributed to potassium chloride supplements (89). Accidental potassium overdose has been observed in patients taking nonprescription potassium supplements, such as potassium citrate to alkalinize the urine or salt substitutes. The latter contain 10–13 mEq of potassium per gram. Potassium-containing medications, such as high doses of penicillin, or transfusion of stored or hemolyzed blood, may lead to hyperkalemia.

As a result of decreased potassium output

RENAL

Numerous pathophysiologic entities lead to hyperkalemia as a result of decreased urinary potassium excretion (Figure 6).

Decreased GFR

In acute oliguric renal failure, hyperkalemia is common once the GFR falls below 15–20 ml/min. This is due not only to the low GFR, decreased distal sodium delivery and flow rate, and tubular damage, but also to the frequently associated increased tissue catabolism. In contrast, hyperkalemia is uncommon in chronic renal failure, unless the GFR falls to less than 10 ml/min or a complication occurs, i.e., the patient develops marked acidosis or hypercatabolism (90–94). In addition, the onset of aldosterone deficiency, the development of tubular dysfunction, or the administration of certain drugs may result in dangerous increases in plasma potassium levels.

Adaptative mechanisms that help maintain potassium balance in patients with advanced chronic renal failure include increased Na-K-ATPase in undamaged distal nephrons, increased fecal potassium excretion, and perhaps hyperaldosteronism. The latter has been difficult to demonstrate, and low, normal, or high aldosterone levels have been reported in patients with chronic renal failure. Nevertheless, in dogs with chronic renal insufficiency, an increase in serum potassium markedly stimulates aldosterone secretion (95). Moreover, the important role of aldosterone in the maintenance of potassium homeostasis in chronic renal disease becomes apparent following administration of aldosterone inhibitors or the development of spontaneous or drug-induced hypoaldosteronism (vide infra). Under these circumstances, patients with only moderate renal insufficiency and GFRs of 50–70 ml/min may manifest life-threatening hyperkalemia.

Hypoaldosteronism

The untreated patient with Addison's disease typically presents with hyperkalemia and hyponatremia (96). Most patients manifest azotemia, and they may exhibit mild-to-moderate hyperchloremic metabolic acidosis. Reversible adrenal insufficiency induced by ketoconazole was recently described (97).

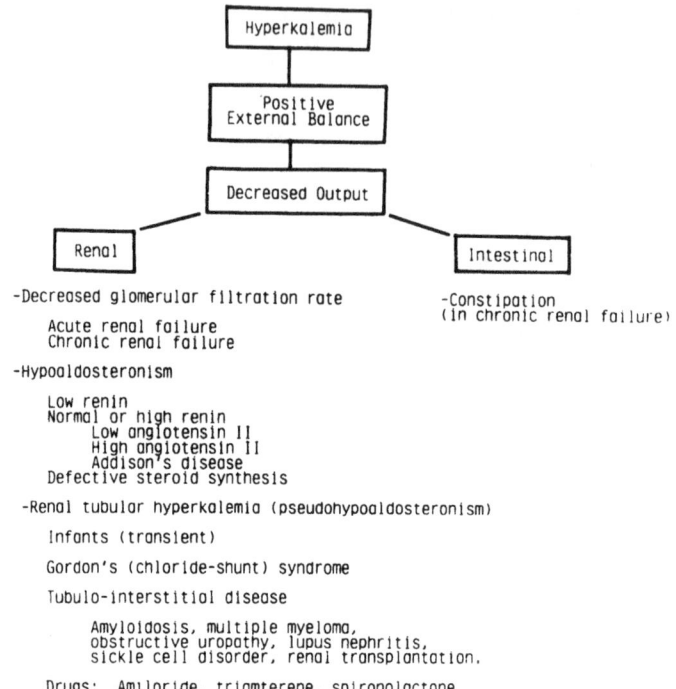

Figure 6. Causes of hyperkalemia as a result of increased total body potassium from decreased potassium output.

Deficiency of enzymes involved in the biosynthetic pathways for mineralocorticoids may result in "salt wasting," hyperkalemia, and acidosis (98, 99). Defects in the early synthetic steps decrease production of all adrenal steroids and are lethal (98). Deficiencies in the intermediate steps are responsible for the various adrenogenital syndromes. The only one of these syndromes that is characterized by mineralocorticoid deficiency is complete 21-hydoxylase deficiency ("salt-losing" form), which is associated with decreased cortisol and aldosterone secretion, as well as an increase in adrenal androgen production (99). A congenital defect in the final steps required for the biosynthesis of aldosterone results in hypoaldosteronism, but normal production of cortisol and adrenal androgen (100).

The syndrome of hyporeninemic hypoaldosteronism (SHH) is by far the most common form of isolated mineralocorticoid deficiency in the adult. Considerable interest in this syndrome has evolved in the last several years, and what was originally thought to be a rarity (100–103) is now recognized frequently. The presence of unexplained persistent hyperkalemia, typically in the range of 5.5–6.5 mEq/l, in disproportion to the decrement of renal function, is the usual diagnostic clue.

Hypoaldosteronism is an acquired defect secondary to insufficient stimulation of the adrenal gland by the renin-angiotensin system. Hypo-, normo-, and hyper-reninemic forms can be recognized. The hyporeninemic variety may be idiopathic or induced by drugs (nonsteroidal anti-inflammatory agents). The normo-reninemic or hyper-reninemic variety associated with decreased circulating levels of angiotensin II results from an endogenous (idiopathic) or drug-induced (captopril, enalapril) inhibition of angiotensin-converting enzyme. When hypoaldosteronism is associated with normal circulating levels of renin and angiotensin II, the abnormality may be of primary adrenal origin (idiopathic, critical illness) or may be drug induced (cyclosporin A, heparin) (102–104) (vide infra).

In most patients, SHH is associated with chronic renal disease, usually of the tubulointerstitial type. At least a third or more of the patients have diabetes mellitus. Most patients exhibit mild-to-moderate chronic renal insufficiency and a normal glucorticoid production and response to ACTH stimulation. The majority of patients are in the fifth to seventh decades of life, and many are hypertensive. As expected from the aldosterone deficit, these patients manifest hyperkalemia and hyperchloremic acidosis. Most patients remain asymptomatic, and hyperkalemia-related electrocadiographic manifestations are uncommon. The natural course of SHH remains unclear.

Interpretation of the precise role of aldosterone deficiency in the causation of hyperkalemia in this syndrome is confounded by the concomitant presence of several other factors that often perturb potassium homeostasis, including diabetes mellitus and chronic renal failure. Likewise, patients with primary adrenocortical insufficiency frequently exhibit decreased GFR, sodium depletion, oliguria, and acidosis, all factors that may influence potassium homeostasis (105).

The role of acidosis in contributing to hyperkalemia in SHH is controversial. Not all hyperkalemic patients with SHH are acidotic (106), and correction of the acidosis does not necessarily reverse the hyperkalemia. Furthermore, as indicated above, the relationship between serum potassium and extracellular pH is exceedingly complex, and hyperkalemia is often not a concomitant of acidemia. Nevertheless, Halperin et al. (107) have suggested that it is precisely with the hyperchloremic type of metabolic acidosis that hyperkalemia is most likely to occur, unless obviated by concomitant urinary or gastrointestinal losses of potassium.

Other factors may be related to the development of hyperkalemia in SHH. Schambelan and Sebastian (102) have reported that the serum potassium of their 22 patients was directly proportional to the 24-hour urinary excretion of potassium, suggesting the importance of dietary intake of potassium in influencing the blood level. In addition, some patients with SHH have a relative tubular resistance to aldosterone (101–103). Such a phenomenon could conceivably relate in part to the presence of renal insufficiency.

Despite these considerations, it seems clear that mineralocorticoid deficiency per se has an important role in the pathogenesis of the hyperkalemia of SHH. Whereas correction of acidosis may not correct the hyperkalemia, administration of mineralocorticoids almost always does (106), together with marked improvement in the low fractional excretion of potassium.

There have been relatively few studies of renal potassium handling in patients with SHH. In the patients of Perez, Oster, and Vaamonde (108), hyperkalemia appeared to be related to a fractional excretion of potassium that was abnormally low for the observed degree of renal insufficiency. Furthermore, potassium excretion was increased only slightly by sodium sulfate, but was substantially improved by desoxycorticosterone.

Various medications have been shown to induce hypoaldosteronism (Table 5). Beta-adrenergic blocking agents are known to decrease plasma renin activity and may secondarily decrease aldosterone production. Nevertheless, hyperkalemia, after administration of these agents, is believed to be due primarily to their extrarenal inhibition of beta$_2$ adrenoceptors (20). Probably the most common cause of drug-induced hypoaldosteronism is the use of nonsteroidal antiinflammatory drugs, which inhibit prostaglandin synthetase and decrease renin release (109–111). The hyperkalemia and the frequently associated decrease in renal function associated with administration of nonsteroidal antiinflammatory agents usually subside after discontinuation of these drugs. Angiotensin-converting enzyme inhibitors, such as captopril or enalapril, decrease the synthesis of angiotensin II and aldosterone, and may cause marked hyperkalemia, especially in patients with reduced renal function (112). The hyperkalemic effect of cyclosporin in renal transplant patients may be related, in part, to inhibition of prostaglandin synthesis (113), but more likely appears to result from a specific blockade of angiotensin II-mediated aldosterone production (114). Heparin administration may cause hyperkalemia, presumably by directly inhibiting aldosterone biosynthesis (115).

Renal tubular defects (tubular hyperkalemia or pseudohypoaldosteronism)

Hyperkalemia attributed to decreased renal potassium excretion resistant to correction by exogenous mineralocorticoids has been described in patients exhibiting normal to moderately reduced GFR (116–123). This finding, referred to as *pseudohypoaldosteronism* (116) or *renal tubular hyperkalemia* (119), has been reported as a transient abnormality in infants, in patients with an unusual condition characterized by hyperkalemia, acidosis, hypertension, and normal GFR (Gordon's syndrome or chloride-shunt syndrome), and in patients with a variety of predominantly tubulointerstitial diseases.

In the pseudohypoaldosteronism of infancy, patients present with failure to thrive, renal sodium wasting, acidosis, and an elevated plasma renin activity and plasma aldosterone concentration (116). No structural abnormality of the kidney has been reported, and recent data suggest a genetic predisposition. The leading hypothesis is that the primary abnormality is a defect in renal sodium handling.

Patients with the chloride-shunt or Gordon's syndrome (117) may show an abnormal increase in distal tubular chloride reabsorption such that the mineralocorticoid-induced, charge-dependent driving force for potassium and hydrogen-ion secretion is attenuated by the voltage-shunting effect of excessive chloride reabsorption. It is believed that the increase in distal sodium chloride reabsorption also causes an expansion of the extracellular fluid volume, hypertension, and hypoaldosteronism. Of interest, a similar defect has been postulated as a contributing pathogenic mechanism in patients receiving drugs that inhibit prostaglandin synthesis.

The third group of patients with renal tubular hyperkalemia includes those with tubulointerstitial renal disease and varying aldosterone levels (118–123). As mentioned above, some patients with SHH may exhibit tubular resistance to replacement doses of mineralocorticoids. It is possible that both abnormalities arise independently as a consequence of structural renal damage. On the other hand, they may be causally related. For example, chronic hyperchloremia and acidosis might conceivably depress renin production, which in turn could lead to hypoaldosteronism.

Hyperkalemia has been reported in patients with renal amyloidosis and in those with multiple myeloma and widespread tubular infiltration (119). In patients with obstructive uropathy, it has been postulated that a failure of distal tubular sodium reabsorption reduces the transtubular potential difference, thus interfering with both potassium and hydrogen-ion secretion (120). In contrast to patients who have hypoaldosteronism, these subjects also may exhibit an inability to acidify the urine during acidosis.

A defect in renal potassium excretion has been described in patients with sickle cell disease (121). The abnormality occurs in patients with HbSS or HbSC disease as well as in those with sickle cell trait (HbAS). Although some patients have been found to have hypoaldosteronism, the defect may originate from damage to the medullary and papillary architecture. A similar defect has been found in patients with systemic lupus erythematosus (122), presumably related to the extensive tubulointerstitial inflammation found in some cases and in patients following renal transplantation (124). Of note, antibodies against the tubular basement membrane have been described in these three nephropathies, and it is tempting to postulate that they are pathogenically associated with the potassium-secreting defect.

Potassium-sparing diuretics, which act on the nephron to reduce potassium excretion, may induce severe hyperkalemia in patients at risk or in patients receiving medications interfering with other regulatory mechanisms of potassium homeostasis. Spironolactone, a competitive antagonist of aldosterone, interferes with the usual mineralocorticoid regulation of potassium transport, resulting in functional hypoaldosteronism. In contrast, amiloride and triamterene indirectly block the secretion of potassium, even in the absence of aldosterone, in late distal and collecting tubular cells (9, 125).

GASTROINTESTINAL

Increased colonic secretion of potassium may help maintain potassium balance in patients with chronic renal failure in whom stool potassium may equal 30% or 40% of the amount of potassium ingested. Therefore, constipation may interfere with this route of potassium disposal and may contribute to the development of hyperkalemia in patients with chronic renal failure.

Clinical consequences of hyperkalemia (Table 6)

CARDIAC EFFECTS

The risk of cardiotoxicity overshadows all other clinical manifestations of hyperkalemia. Characteristic electrocardiographic changes of hyperkalemia begin to appear at serum levels of 5.5–6.5 mEq/l (126). The initial change usually consists of the peaking of T waves in association with a normal or decreased QT interval. As the extracellular potassium concentration rises from 6.5 to 7.5 mEq/l, the QRS complex widens and the PR interval increases. At a serum potassium level exceeding 8 mEq/l, the P wave disappears, there is marked widening of the QRS complex, and a sine wave pattern appears that progresses to ventricular fibrillation or asytole (126). Hyperkalemic cardiotoxicity is increased in patients with preexisting heart disease or abnormalities of cardiac conduction or rhythm.

Experimental studies in Purkinje cells have shown that conduction velocity and membrane excitability decrease at serum potassium concentrations above 7.0 mEq/l (127). The effect is mediated by a reduction in the number of

Table 6. Clinical manifestations of hyperkalemia

A. Cardiovascular effects
   Peaked T waves
   Shortened QT interval
   Widening of QRS complex
   Absent P waves
   "Sine waves"
   Ventricular fibrillation or asystole
B. Neuromuscular effects
   Weakness
   Paresthesias
   Flaccid paralysis
   Respiratory failure
C. Metabolic effects
   Increased aldosterone secretion
   Decreased renin activity
   Increased catecholamines
   Decreased prostaglandins
D. Renal and acid-base effects
   Increased sodium excretion
   Increased distal potassium secretion
   Decreased proximal bicarbonate reabsorption
   Decreased renal ammoniagenesis
   Decreased acid excretion

sodium channels available for activation. The abnormalities are potentiated by hypocalcemia, hypomagnesemia, hyponatremia, and acidosis. It is noteworthy that hyperkalemia does not seem to interfere with cardiac contractility.

NEUROMUSCULAR EFFECTS

The first symptoms of hyperkalemia generally include paresthesias and weakness of the extremities. They may be followed by weakness or flaccid paralysis of the ascending type (128). The weakness may affect the respiratory muscles and may result in respiratory failure. The deep tendon reflexes are intact early but decrease progressively as paralysis ensues. Sensory abnormalities are usually absent.

METABOLIC EFFECTS

Hyperkalemia directly stimulates aldosterone production by the adrenal gland (72). Increments in serum potassium concentration as small as 0.2–0.3 mEq/l may increase plasma aldosterone levels. Hyperkalemia also directly decreases renin secretion (129). The effects of potassium on insulin and glucagon production were already discussed (vide supra). Although hypokalemia or potassium deficiency may increase prostaglandin synthesis and depress catecholamine production, the effects of hyperkalemia on these hormones have not been systematically evaluated (130, 131).

RENAL AND ACID-BASE METABOLISM

One of the main effects of hyperkalemia on the kidney is to alter the set point for bicarbonate reabsorption in the proximal tubule to induce bicarbonaturia (132–134). As previously discussed, hyperkalemia directly promotes increased potassium secretion in the distal nephron. Although the resultant stimulation of aldosterone production would be expected to favor distal hydrogen ion secretion, the associated increase in cell pH would be expected to decrease proton secretion. In addition, acute increases in ambient potassium suppress renal ammoniagenesis, presumably as a result of intracellular alkalosis (135). The net result of hyperkalemia in experimental animals is a decrease in net acid excretion, leading to the development of hyperchloremic metabolic acidosis.

MANAGEMENT OF HYPERKALEMIA

General principles

The management of an individual patient with hyperkalemia depends very much on the circumstances. First, the immediate (acute) therapy may differ considerably from long-term maneuvers; and second, therapy must be influenced greatly by the severity of the hyperkalemia, as reflected both by the serum potassium concentration and the presence of clinical manifestations (vide infra). In most circumstances, hyperkalemia is a rather straightforward management problem. Uncommonly, it constitutes either a true medical emergency, demanding almost instantaneous appropriate action, or a chronic challenge to the clinician's ingenuity.

Acute therapy

The general approach to the acute management of hyperkalemia is outlined in Table 7. The first priority is to determine its severity. This is accomplished not only by knowing the serum concentration of potassium and its expected rate of increase, but more importantly by assessing the presence of life-threatening clinical manifestations, particularly, serious electrocardiographic or other cardiovascular changes, or neuromuscular abnormalities (e.g., weakness, paralysis). Generally, emergent serum levels are in excess of 7.0–7.5 mEq/l, but lower values may prove fatal when the level is rapidly rising. Similarly, a normal electrocardiogram does not necessarily imply the absence of an immediate threat to life.

Levinsky (136) has classified the severity of hyperkalemia in a clinically useful manner. In this schema, minimal hyperkalemia is defined as serum potassium levels less than 6.5 mEq/l with absent or very mild electrocardiographic changes. Moderate hyperkalemia includes serum levels between 6.5 and 8.0 mEq/l or electrocardiographic changes limited to peaking T waves. Finally, severe hyperkalemia indicates a serum potassium concentration greater

Table 7. General approach to the acute management of severe hyperkalemia

A. Determination of severity
  1. Serum [K] and the acuteness and rate of its rise
  2. Clinical manifestations — EKG, cardiovascular, neuromuscular

B. When possible, rapid determination of etiology. Some therapeutic modalities may specifically "counteract" certain pathophysiologic abnormalities (see Table 9).

C. Immediate discontinuation of all sources of potassium intake and agents that perturb potassium homeostasis

D. Reversal of membrane abnormalities
  1. Calcium gluconate or chloride
  2. Hypertonic NaCl (to hyponatremic patients)

E. Redistribution of potassium from the extracellular compartment to the intracellular space
  1. Sodium bicarbonate
  2. Insulin-glucose
  3. Stimulators of beta$_2$ adrenoceptors

F. External removal of potassium
  1. In stools — cation exchange resin (polystyrene sulfonate)
  2. In urine — increase urine flow rate and distal tubular delivery of sodium (loop diuretic)
  3. By dialysis
  4. By exchange transfusion [in neonates (171)]

than 8.0 mEq/l or QRS widening, heart block, or ventricular arrhythmias (136).

When the electrocardiogram is abnormal and the serum potassium exceeds 6.0–6.5 mEq/l, emergency therapy should be initiated. In the presence of a sine-wave pattern, an attempt should be made to reverse the adverse membrane effect by infusing calcium (vide infra). With less severe electrocardiographic changes, immediate therapy is aimed at effecting a shift of potassium from the extracellular to the intracellular compartment. Subsequently, definitive therapy should be geared to remove potassium from the body (vide infra). In contrast, if the serum potassium is less than 6.0 mEq/l, and the electrocardiogram is normal, the patient can usually be managed simply with potassium-restricted diets and discontinuation of medications known to affect potassium homeostasis.

As discussed by Kassirer and Wish (137), there are several general principles that pertain to the treatment of acute hyperkalemia. First, one should look for and correct any associated serious abnormalities, such as hyponatremia or acidosis. Second, the efficacy of therapy must be carefully monitored by serial electrocardiograms and determinations of serum potassium. Third, it is important for the clinician to recognize that the therapy for life-threatening acute hyperkalemia should not be a stepwise application of the various modalities. Rather, this medical emergency often justifies a "shotgun" approach, i.e., simultaneous initiation of an array of procedures designed to: a) counter the membrane effects of hyperkalemia, b) redistribute potassium intracellularly, and c) remove it from the body. Obviously, an important therapeutic factor is the immediate interruption of all sources of potassium input (external and internal) into the extracellular fluid and discontinuation of all medications that individually, or acting in concert, perturb potassium homeostasis. Fourth, the expected rate of increase of serum potassium has to be taken into consideration, since aggressive treatment is indicated when one anticipates marked and sustained increases in serum potassium levels.

Whenever possible, rapid determination of the pathogenic factors relating to the patient's hyperkalemia may be of considerable value in guiding therapy and providing prognosis regarding anticipated difficulties. For example, hyperkalemia related to ill-advised, excessive chronic administration of potassium to a patient with mild renal insufficiency is generaly of short duration, whereas that related to massive rhabdomyolysis with subsequent oligoanuric acute renal failure often proves to be a challenge for many days.

REVERSAL OF MEMBRANE ABNORMALITIES

Calcium salts

The intravenous administration of one of the salts of calcium is indicated for the acute therapy of life-threatening hyperkalemia. Intravenous infusion of calcium carries potential risks, particularly in large, rapidly given doses, or in patients concomitantly receiving digitalis preparations. The use of calcium, therefore, should be employed with caution and reserved for the patient who already had evidence of serious hyperkalemia-induced myocardial dysfunction, e.g., widening of the QRS complex (or other severe electrocardiograpohic changes) or severe neuromuscular manifestations.

Calcium administration acts to reverse the altered relationship between the resting and the threshold potential caused by hyperkalemia; the serum potassium concentrations is unaffected. Specifically, a rise in serum calcium increases the threshold potential and tends to correct hyperkalemia-induced polarization blockade. Although hypocalcemia potentiates the adverse electrical effects of severe hyperkalemia, calcium administration is usually helpful, even in the absence of hypocalcemia. Continuous electrocardiographic monitoring is recommended during the intravenous adminstration of calcium. This serves not only to identify the expected action of the medication, which may appear within 1–3 minutes and last approximately 30–60 minutes (rapid urinary excretion of calcium and tissue uptake obviates a longstanding effect), but as a clue to excessive or too rapid administration reflected in a marked shortening of the Q-T interval. In particular, the intravenous administration of calcium to a patient receiving cardiac glycosides carries a considerable risk and may induce such evidence of digitalis intoxication as multifocal premature ventricular contractions or even ventricular fibrillation.

The usual recommendation is for an infusion of 10–30 ml (one to three 10 ml ampules) of 10% calcium gluconate given undiluted over a 4- to 6-minute period. Alternatively, 5–10 ml may be given over 2–3 minutes. It should be noted that the manufacturer of at least one preparation of calcium gluconate cautions not to exceed a rate of infusion of approximately 1.5 ml/min, but it is not stated if this pertains to the treatment of hyperkalemia (or severe hypocalcemia) (138). In a patient receiving digitalis, administration of calcium must be carried out more cautiously, for example, either by giving a smaller amount or by diluting the medication with 100 ml of 5% dextrose and infusing this slowly over 20–30 minutes.

In the absence of the desired response, dosing with calcium may be repeated after approximately 5–10 minutes. It has been suggested that lack of response to a second dose indicates that further infusion will not be helpful. Some authors suggest that the initial dose of calcium gluconate can be followed or replaced by an intravenous infusion of 30 ml of the 10% solution in a liter of 5% dextrose in water.

Worthley and Phillips (139) have suggested that calcium chloride, rather than calcium gluconate, should be the preferred intravenous form. They believe that the chloride salt is better and more predictably retained, that the resultant elevation of plasma calcium concentration is more predictable, and that it provides a greater inotopic effect (139). The Invenex Laboratories' preparation of $CaCl_2$ USP is a dihydrate ($CaCl_2 \cdot 2 H_2O$) (140). Therefore, the molecular weight is 147 (Ca = 40, 2 Cl = 71, $2 H_2O$ = 36). In 1 g of the salt (10 ml of a 10% solution), the amount of elemental calcium is $(40)(1000)/147$ = 272 mg. The equivalent weight of calcium is 20; therefore, the number of milliequivalents of calcium per gram of $CaCl_2 \cdot 2 H_2O$ = 272/20 = 13.6 mEq. This means that, volume for volume, calcium chloride provides approximately three times more elemental calcium than does calcium gluconate. For example, the Invenex Laboratories' preparation of 10% calcium gluconate (6% of the total calcium is actually provided as calcium D-saccharate) contains 4.65 mEq of calcium per 10 ml ampule (138). It has also been postulated that, milliequivalent for milliequivalent, calcium chloride is less complexed and produces a greater increase in serum ionized calcium than calcium gluconate (139). Despite its apparent frequent use, we are unaware, however, of any specific reports regarding the use of calcium chloride for the treatment of severe hyperkalemia. If calcium chloride is given, smaller doses should be initially employed than with calcium gluconate. For example, one of the manufacturers recommends that the rate of injection (it is not stated if this pertains to the treatment of hyperkalemia) should not exceed 0.5–1.0 ml of 10% $CaCl_2$ per minute (140).

During or following the intravenous administration of calcium, patients may complain of tingling sensations, heat waves, a sense of oppression, and a chalky taste. Rapid injection and/or overdosage may result in vasodilation, hypotension, weakness, lethargy, intractable nausea and vomiting, coma, bradycardia, arrhythmias, syncope, or cardiac arrest. Calcium should be injected through a small needle into a large vein. This decreases the risk of an overly rapid rise in serum calcium or extravasation into the perivenous tissues, which may result in local necrosis. Calcium chloride solutions are irritating to veins and must not be injected subcutaneously or intramuscularly.

Sodium

In hyperkalemic patients with hyponatremia and hypovolemia, a beneficial effect of sodium administration on cardiac and neuromuscular function has been suggested. Presumably, this relates to antagonism of the effects of hyperkalemia on cell membranes. For this purpose, hypertonic sodium bicarbonate, 50–100 ml of either a 7.5% or an 8.4% solution, may be given intravenously over 5–10 minutes. Alternatively, 50–100 mEq of sodium bicarbonate may be added to a liter of 0.9% NaCl and infused at a rate of approximately 250 ml/hr.

REDISTRIBUTION OF POTASSIUM

Sodium bicarbonate

The administration of sodium bicarbonate remains the most effective emergency maneuver to reduce serum potassium concentration rapidly. The mechanism of action involves the intracellular redistributive effect, not only of an increasing pH, but of an increasing serum bicarbonate per se, even when pH remains constant (32). Thus, this form of therapy is usually indicated regardless of the baseline acid-base status. Nevertheless, it is most effective in the acidotic patient, because acidemia may be at least in part responsible for the hyperkalemia. If renal function is adequate sodium bicarbonate administration also facilitates the urinary excretion of potassium.

There are several acceptable ways to administer bicarbonate: a) 50–100 ml (one or two ampules) of either 7.5% or 8.4% sodium bicarbonate (from 45 or 50 mEq, respectively, to from 90 to 100 mEq, respectively) are given intravenously over 5–10 minutes and repeated, if necessary, after 15 minutes; b) 90–150 mEq of sodium bicarbonate can be added to 1000 ml of 5% or 10% dextrose in water, and 500 ml of the resulting solution is infused in 30 minutes (if volume overload is not present), with the rest given during the subsequent 2–3 hours).

In general, the serum potassium-lowering effect of bolus injections of sodium bicarbonate begins after 5–10 minutes (with slow infusion, the onset of action is somewhat delayed).

The duration of action is also variable, but typically is about 2 hours. According to the limited data of Fraley and Adler (31, 32), one should expect a fall in serum potassium of about 0.18 mEq/l per 1.0 mEq rise in bicarbonate when pH increases and of 0.13 mEq/l per 1.0 mEq rise in bicarbonate when pH remains unchanged. In hyperkalemic patients, the decrement in serum potassium subsequent to bicarbonate administration may average 1.3 mEq/l per 0.1 unit pH increase (16).

The principal potential adverse effects of sodium bicarbonate administration are volume overload, hypernatremia, alkalemia, and rapid reduction in ionized serum calcium. Pre-exsiting hypervolemia and/or congestive heart failure is a contraindication to administration of sodium bicarbonate unless it is previously or concomitantly corrected with diuretics. One must remember that each milliliter of an 8.4% solution of sodium bicarbonate contains 1.0 mEq of sodium and 2.0 mOsm of solutes/ml (i.e., a sodium concentration of 1000 mEq/l and an osmolality of 2000 mOsm/kg H_2O). Overly enthusiastic administration of these hypertonic solutions can quickly induce serious hyperosmolality.

Patients with underlying hypocalcemia (as in those with severe chronic renal failure) may develop tetany when given sodium bicarbonate unless an infusion of calcium is given first (or concomitantly, into a different vein). Similarly, a patient with severe hyperkalemia caused by massive rhabdomyolysis with acute renal failure may develop sodium-bicarbonate-induced tetany when his or her acidemia (which "protected" the serum ionized calcium level) is corrected (141).

Insulin-glucose

Provision of insulin-glucose ameliorates hyperkalemia by facilitating the intracellular redistribution of potassium. This is believed to occur by virtue of the action of insulin causing depolarization of cell membranes, and not because of the intracellular transport of glucose per se; that is, it is the insulin that effects the reduction in serum potassium concentration, not the glucose. Glucose is given to obviate the hypoglycemia that would follow administration of insulin alone. Of course, in a patient whose glucose-pancreas axis is intact, infusion of glucose will evoke a sufficient release of endogenous insulin. If glucose is given to a diabetic patient whose insulin release is inadequate, so that hyperglycemia (and hence hyperosmolarity) results, the serum potassium concentration may actually increase, particularly if hypoaldosteronism is also present (46).

For the above mentioned reasons, severely hyperkalemic patients, even if known not to be diabetic, should receive insulin and glucose, rather than glucose alone. Approximately 1 U of insulin is recommended for each 5 g of glucose administered. We suggest mixing the aqueous insulin directly into 10% dextrose (or giving it "IV push" when small volumes of 50% dextrose are used). Obviously, if the patient is hyperglycemic, no glucose should be given initially. There are several convenient methods for administering insulin-glucose: a) 50 ml of 50% dextrose in water (25 g of glucose) together with 5 U insulin given over 2–5 minutes. Continuous infusions of greater than 10% solutions of dextrose produce osmotic damage to the vessel wall unless infused through a central line; b) 500 ml of 10% dextrose, together with 10 U insulin, given over 30–60 minutes (if volume overload is not a problem); and c) 1000 ml of 10% dextrose together with 20 U of insulin, with one third of the solution given in the first 30 minutes and the remainder over the subsequent 2–3 hours. Method a can be repeated, if necessary, or can be followed by either b or c. The latter two techniques lend themselves nicely to the additional maneuver of adding sodium bicarbonate (50–100 mEq/l) to the dextrose solutions.

The major potential adverse effects of insulin-glucose administration are hyperglycemia, hypoglycemia, and volume overload. Obviously, careful surveillance of the patient's volume status and serum glucose level is essential.

EXTERNAL REMOVAL OF POTASSIUM

Cation exchange resins

For many years, one of the mainstays of therapy of hyperkalemia has been the oral or rectal administration of the cation exchange resin sodium polystyrene sulfonate (Kayexalate®, Winthrop–Breon Laboratories). Although not acting with sufficient rapidity to serve as the keystone of emergency management, Kayexalate often provides a crucial adjunctive measure and is often of great value in the chronic management of and prophylaxis against hyperkalemia.

As implied in its generic name, Kayexalate is an ion-exchange resin provided in the sodium phase. The degree of release of sodium in exchange for potassium binding is variable and differs in the in-vitro versus the in-vivo setting, but is believed to average approximately 33%. Thus, the potential load of sodium approximates 1.4 mEq/g (142). Lesser amounts of magnesium and calcium may also be removed. It is believed that the action of Kayexalate occurs predominantly in the colon, the principal site of potassium secretion in the gastrointestinal tract. Presumably, patients with a nonfunctioning or absent colon may not benefit from its administration.

The efficiency of Kayexalate is believed to be greater when the medication is ingested than when it is administrated as an enema. The rectal route is needed in patients whose upper gastrointestinal tract is not intact, in those who are unable to swallow adequately, or when administration via a nasogastric tube is deemed inadvisable. A recent report has documented the possibility of pneumonitis secondary to aspiration of particles of sodium polystyrene sulfonate (143). It is important, therefore, to avoid the oral route of administration in the seriously ill patient predisposed to aspiration and always to position patients appropriately to facilitate safe ingestion.

The dosage of Kayexalate varies with the setting. In general, however, the oral dose for an adult is 15–25 g given one to four times per day mixed in water or in 20% sorbitol syrup (approximately 5 ml per gram of resin). In enema form, the usual dosage is 30–50 g given every 6 hours, well mixed with 100–200 ml of water plus sorbitol or with 20% dextrose (in water). The enemas should be retained for at least 30–60 minutes, if possible (which may require the insertion of a balloon-type rectal catheter), and should be preceded and followed by a cleansing enema. Resin enemas may be given at hourly intervals, if necessary. The effect of Kayexalate begins after approximately 1–2 hours. A single enema may reduce the serum potassium concentration by as much as from 0.5–2.0 mEq/l.

Hourly 30 g Kayexalate enemas may result in potassium removal rates of close to 30 mEq/hr.

In addition to pneumonitis (143), potential adverse effects of sodium polystyrene sulfonate include sodium overload, potassium depletion, gastric irritation, and severe constipation, even to the point of intestinal obstruction or fecal impaction. Kayexalate-induced constipation is treated or prevented by coadministration of the osmotic cathartic sorbitol (10–20 ml of 70% syrup as needed). Not a very palatable product, Kayexalate has even been incorporated into candy (144).

Severe metabolic alkalosis may develop when magnesium/aluminum-hydroxide-type antacids (or similar laxatives) are given together with Kayexalate (145). Although antacids themselves constitute a substantial alkali load (146), they only rarely produce metabolic alkalosis in the patient not otherwise at risk. Probably because the resin obviates formation of insoluble magnesium carbonate, coadministration of resin and "nonabsorbable" alkali imbalances the ratio of the gastrointestinal consumption of HCl and sodium bicarbonate usually obtained when antacids are given alone (145–146). Joint administration of sodium polystyrene sulfonate and antacids also appears to reduce potassium binding (142). Finally, a recently described complication of Kayexalate in sorbitol enemas is of concern. Lillemoe and his associates (147) described five postoperative hyperkalemic uremic patients (four of whom died) who developed ischemic necrosis of the colon in close temporal relation to the use of these enemas. None had preexisting symptoms of colonic ischemia. Furthermore, using a rat model, these investigators demonstrated similar lesions in both uremic and nonuremic animals (invariably in the former group) given enemas containing either sorbitol alone or Kayexalate in sorbitol but not saline or Kayexalate alone (147). As a result of these observations, the authors no longer use Kayexalate in sorbitol enemas in uremic patients during the perioperative period or other times of stress.

Peritoneal dialysis and hemodialysis

Because of the efficacy of the other therapeutic maneuvers, dialysis, particularly in the patient without severe renal failure, is generally considered to be a method of last resort in the management of severely hyperkalemic patients.

Hemodialysis, because of its high flow of dialysate, is more efficient in removing potassium than is peritoneal dialysis. The potassium clearance typically exceeds 100 ml/min (149), and as much as 40–50 mEq of potassium can be removed in the first hour. Obviously, the lower the potassium concentration of the dialysate, the faster the rate of removal. Nevertheless, one should not use a zero-potassium (no potassium) dialysate, since this carries the potential risk of overly rapid or excessive decrements in serum potassium. In the unusually severe case (the traumatized and hypercatabolic patient in danger of developing rapid hyperkalemia), a 1–2 mEq potassium/l dialysate will suffice to control the hyperkalemia. Potassium can be withheld from peritoneal dialysis fluid for the first few exchanges (provided that the patient is not receiving digitalis or similar drugs); after three to six cycles, potassium chloride, 3 mEq/l, is added to the dialysis solution. It is important to remember that either form of dialysis reduces serum potassium concentration, not only by external removal, but by internal redistribution related to increasing blood bicarbonate and pH (and sometimes glucose) levels caused by provision of dialysate buffer (bicarbonate or acetate). The rapid correction of acidosis by dialysis may cause sudden and marked shifts of potassium from the extracellular to the intracellular space that may result in severe or even fatal hypokalemia (148). A low-potassium dialysate should not be used in digitalized patients.

Feig and his associates have increased our understanding of the influence of hemodialysis (using a "no-K bath") on potassium metabolism (149). It should be pointed out, however, that these studies were carried out in patients undergoing chronic maintenance hemodialysis, rather than in patients with severe acute hyperkalemia. Indeed, the mean predialysis plasma potassium was only 4.4 ± 0.9 (SD) mEq/l (149). These investigators made two major observations. First, in contrast to BUN, there was a marked postdialytic rebound of plasma potassium concentration. This was postulated to relate to a rate of extracellular translocation of intracellular potassium that was slower than that of external potassium removal (which averaged 1.2 ± 0.2 mEq/kg for the 3 hours of dialysis). Second, the amount of potassium removal and the magnitude of the decrement in plasma potassium correlated directly with the pretreatment plasma potassium concentration (149). The latter phenomenon could not be explained solely by greater removal, because the change in plasma potassium factored by the amount of potassium removed also correlated with the baseline plasma potassium concentration, i.e., a given rate of potassium removal produced a greater fall in potassium concentration when plasma potassium was high. The authors concluded, therefore, that the state of potassium balance exerts an influence on the volume of distribution of potassium such that the latter appears to be smaller when the plasma potassium concentration is higher (149).

Finally, Sherman and his colleagues (150) have recently shown that approximately 40% of the potassium removed by dialysis is not accounted for by the plasma-dialysate gradient, body weight, or serum carbon dioxide content (i.e., the major factors presumed to influence potassium removal). The investigators postulated that differences in the level of trancellular potassium flux were most likely explanation for the observed variability of potassium removal. For example, the 28% increase (p = 0.16) in potassium removal noted with a glucose-free dialysate might have been related to lower plasma insulin level, which could have facilitated the intracellular to extracellular movement of potassium (150).

As mentioned, peritoneal dialysis removes potassium at a much slower rate than hemodialysis. For example, if 2 L of dialysate containing no potassium are exchanged per hour, and if the patient's serum potassium is 7.0 mEq/l, approximately 14 mEq of potassium could be removed per hour, assuming complete equilibration. In clinical use, the typical rate of removal is between 180 and 240 mEq in 36–48 hours. Nolph et al. (151) compared the potassium-removing efficacy of two different peritoneal dialysis solutions (1.5 vs. 7.0% dextrose, both without potassium). The 7% solution provided a significantly higher potassium clearance, which averaged 25 ml/min (corresponding to a removal rate of approximately 12.5 mEq/hr at a serum potassium of 8.0 mEq/l).

Diuretics

In the absence of renal failure, considerable amounts of potassium may be excreted in the urine. To this end, the patient may be given solutions of sodium chloride and/or sodium bicarbonate intravenously, together with furosemide at initial doses of 40 mg orally or intravenously. When renal insufficiency is present, a larger dose is needed. Loop diuretics will increase the delivery of sodium to the distal nephron and enhance the tubular flow rate at the same site, thereby facilitating potassium excretion. Obviously, the patient's fluid volume and acid-base status must be closely monitored.

Chronic therapy

Prevention of dangerous acute increases in serum potassium concentration is an important component of the chronic management of longstanding hyperkalemia (e.g., in some patients with chronic renal failure). Useful modalities are outlined in Table 8. This sometimes involves therapy for certain well-defined causes of hyperkalemia (Table 9), for example, that associated with hyporeninemic hypoaldosteronism (Table 10) or with Gordon's syndrome (vide infra).

Dietary restriction of potassium is important, particularly avoidance of sudden ingestion of relatively large amounts of potassium. For example, adaptive changes in

Table 8. Modalities useful in the chronic therapy of long-standing hyperkalemia

A. Maneuvers "specific" for certain conditions (see Table 9)

B. Dietary restriction of potassium

C. Limitation or avoidance of the use of, and reduction of dosage of, medications adversely affecting potassium homeostasis; careful monitoring of patients using such medications

D. Prevention and treatment of reductions of GFR and/or oliguria

E. Prevention and treatment of hypovolemia

F. Prevention and treatment of acidemia

G. Prevention and treatment of prolonged constipation in patients with chronic renal failure

H. External removal of potassium (as outlined in Table 7)

Table 9. Examples of therapeutic modalities for the treatment or prevention of hyperkalemia that "specifically" counteract certain pathophysiologic states

A. Thiazide diuretic in familial hyperkalemia (Gordon's syndrome)
B. Furosemide and/or fludrocortisone in hyporeninemic hypoaldosteronism
C. Fludrocortisone (and glucocorticoid) in patients with Addison's disease
D. Albuterol or acetazolamide in hyperkalemic periodic paralysis; stimulators of beta$_2$ adrenoceptors for other conditions, including chronic renal failure
E. Dantrolene to reduce risk of anesthesia-induced malignant hyperthermia syndrome (of note, however, dantrolene itself may cause or contribute to hyperkalemia [165])
F. Debridement of grossly necrotic muscle, drainage of large hematomas

Table 10. Therapy of hyperkalemia in patients with hyporeninemic hypoaldosterism

A. Acute
   Same as emergency therapy for most causes of hyperkalemia
B. Chronic
   1. Avoidance of excessive dietary potassium, particularly large amounts at one time
   2. Avoidance of medications that impair potassium homeostasis (see Table 5); avoidance of hyperglycemia
   3. Furosemide (in the smallest effective dose)
   4. Fludrocortisone (added to regimen if furosemide alone does not suffice)
   5. Sodium polystyrene sulfonate (usually not needed)
   6. Sodium citrate or sodium bicarbonate (usually not needed and may not be helpful in reducing serum potassium)
   7. Trial-and-error manipulation of dietary sodium intake (see text)

chronic renal failure may permit a daily excretion of "normal amounts" of potassium but fail to protect against the threat of an acute load (72, 84). In patients at risk, single, small oral amounts of potassium may produce a marked increase in serum potassium (83). As a rule, one attempts to reduce the daily dietary potassium intake of patients to less than approximately 65 mEq. Since the atomic weight of potassium is 39, 65 mEq corresponds to approximately 2.5 g of elemental potassium (1000/39 = 25.6 mEq/g).

An important mode of preventive therapy is to limit the use of medications that are known to affect potassium homeostasis adversely (152). If such medications are deemed necessary, they should be used in minimal dosage, for as short a time as possible, with careful monitoring of serum potassium. The use of two or more such agents in patients at risk is certainly contraindicated.

Finally, situations that place additional constraints on internal or external homeostatic mechanisms must be obviated or corrected (1). Thus, the potential acute reduction of GFR or a dramatic decrease in urine flow rate, extracellular fluid volume contraction (which limits the distal delivery of sodium and volume), and acidemia must be carefully anticipated, and avoided, if possible.

Management of selected specific conditions

SYNDROME OF HYPORENINEMIC HYPOALDOSTERONISM (SHH)

It has been suggested that the renal acidification defect frequently associated with SHH (Type 4 renal tubular acidosis) is the most common form of renal tubular acidosis (153). Certainly, it is one of the most frequent causes of hyperkalemia in patients with diabetic nephropathy or chronic interstitial nephropathy and mild-to-moderate renal insufficiency (102, 103).

The treatment of acute severe hyperkalemia in patients with SHH is similar to that of the emergency management of life-threatening hyperkalemia of any etiology. Similarly, most of the basic principles of chronic management (Table 8) do not differ (e.g., avoidance of certain medications, excessive potassium intake) importantly from those appropriate for the other states of chronic hyperkalemia. Dietary restriction of potassium is important since the degree of hyperkalemia in SHH appears to be proportional to the level of potassium intake (102). Diabetic patients with hypoaldosteronism appear to be particularly at risk of hyperglycemia-induced hyperkalemia (45, 46, 154, 155). Kayexalate therapy is usually not needed on a long-term basis. Of interest, correction of acidosis with chronic alkali loading does not necessarily have a beneficial effect on serum potassium concentration (108, 156), indicating, as mentioned above, that in some patients, acidemia is not an important cause of the hyperkalemia.

When patients with SHH become sodium depleted, one might anticipate that they incur a substantial risk of worsening hyperkalemia because of a constraint on the delivery of sodium and volume to the distal nephron. Perez et al. (157), however, demonstrated that this need not be the case. After experimentally induced sodium depletion, both plasma renin activity and plasma aldosterone concentration were substantially higher than after a previous period of simple dietary sodium restriction; and, an increase in serum potassium concentration occurred in only 1 of 5 subjects so treated (157). Similarily, Radó et al. (158) observed six patients with "outpatient hyperkalemia" whose increased levels of serum potassium prior to admission appeared to relate to high dietary levels of sodium intake, which in turn resulted in "phsyiological suppression" of plasma renin and aldosterone. In practice, for an individual patient with SHH, one cannot predict the effect of a change in sodium intake; so, if control of his or her hyperkalemia is inadequate, the clinician may attempt cautious upward and downward adjustments on a trial-and-error basis.

The seemingly obvious form of therapy for SHH might appear to be chronic administration of a mineralocorticoid such as fludrocortisone. Despite frequent tubular resistance necessitating pharmacologic doses (0.4–1.0 mg/day), such therapy may be efficacious in reducing the serum potassium concentration (103, 156). Part of the beneficial effect of mineralocorticoid administration has been shown to be on an extrarenal base (103, 156). Nevertheless, it carries the risk of inducing sodium retention with subsequent worsening of congestive heart failure, hypertension, and edema, especially in elderly chronically ill patients (103). Sometimes sodium retention occurs even when potassium excretion is not enhanced. For these reasons, and because of its proven efficacy and safety when properly used, furosemide, in relatively low dosage (e.g., 40–120 mg/day), appears to be the agent of choice for the treatment of SHH (156). Its improvement of potassium homeostasis and acidosis appears to be based both on a renal and an extrarenal effect, since there is not significant correlation between the decrement in serum potassium concentration and the cumulative urinary excretion of potassium (156). For patients who do not repond adequately to furosemide alone, fludrocortisone should be added to the regimen (156). Finally, when giving furosemide, the clinician should watch for the occasional patient who may develop volume contraction and a clinically important exacerbation of azotemia. Nevertheless, in the study of Sebastian, Schambelan, and Sutton (156), furosemide induced decreases in creatinine clearance that were not progressive.

HYPERKALEMIC PERIODIC PARALYSIS

Attacks of this very uncommon and troublesome, but only rarely fatal, condition are reduced in frequency by avoidance of excessive exercise, exposure to cold, and sudden intake of relatively large amounts of potassium (73, 74, 159, 160). Until recently, chronic therapy was based on long-term administration of thiazide diuretics, the carbonic anhydrase inhibitor, acetazolamide (159), or acetazolamide plus fludrocortisone. Preliminary data now suggest the value of an alternative, more attractive method: inhalation (74) or ingestion (73) of the $beta_2$-adrenoceptor stimulator albuterol (called salbutamol in Great Britain), which translocates potassium into cells.

Albuterol inhalation, when employed at the onset of an attack, prevented both the hyperkalemia and the muscle weakness in several patients challenged with exercise or oral potassium chloride (73). Furthermore, 13 of 15 patients who employed this approach chronically were well satisfied with the results. Preliminary data in one patient suggest that a daily dose of one 2 mg albuterol tablet prevents attacks without side effects (74). Some patients may also require continued medication with acetazolamide (73).

Successful administration of albuterol to patients with hyperkalemic periodic paralysis raises the possibility that the use of this or other agonists of $beta_2$ adrenoceptors, such as terbutaline, might be helpful in patients with hyperkalemia of other etiologies in conjunction, or as an alternative, to insulin. At present, the data in this regard are limited and should be considered preliminary. For example, Montoliu et al. (161) have demonstrated recently that the intravenous administration of 0.5 mg albuterol decreased hyperkalemia in a group of dialysis patients with renal failure from 5.5 to 4.4 mEq/l ($p > 0.001$) in 30 minutes; and Vitez (162) has reported favourable results following the intravenous infusion of epinephrine in 2 of 3 patients with hyperkalemia of diverse pathogenesis.

HYPERKALEMIA ASSOCIATED WITH THE MALIGNANT HYPERTHERMIA SYNDROME (MHS)

The MHS occurs primarily in anesthetized patients (particularly those receiving potent inhalation agents or succinylcholine) with preexisting trauma, burns, or neuromuscular disease (163, 164). There is also an important hereditary predisposition. Therapy of this condition is in part preventative, and early recognition is critical. In patients at risk, pretreatment with dantrolene and avoidance of triggering agents and stress is used to reduce the likelihood of the syndrome. The MHS is postulated to result from a sudden rise in the concentration of ionized calcium within the myoplasma. Metabolic processes are markedly accelerated to stimulate production of heat, CO_2, and lactate, and result in depletion of ATP. The latter presumably impairs the activity of Na-K-ATPase, which results in a redistribution of potassium from the intracellular into the extracellular space (163). Dantrolene, a medication related to phenytoin, is believed to act by reducing the release of calcium from muscle sarcoplasmic reticulum. It may be used for both prophylaxis and therapy of the MHS (163). Of note, a patient was recently reported with malignant hyperthermia and coronary artery disease who was treated with verapamil and developed hyperkalemia and myocardial depression when given dantrolene parenterally (165).

RHABDOMYOLYSIS (AND HEMATOMA)-RELATED HYPERKALEMIA

Hyperkalemia caused by massive rhabdomyolysis and the associated acute renal failure may become a difficult management problem. This relates to the potential for release of very large amounts of intracellular potassium into the extracellular fluid in the face of markedly limited urinary excretion. It is probable that the accompanying high-anion-gap-type severe metabolic acidosis may also be contributory (166). To prevent severe hyperkalemia, such patients must be recognized early because they may require daily and prolonged hemodialysis. In addition, if large amounts of necrotic muscle are present, surgical debridement may be mandatory. In analogy, absorption of potassium from very large hematomas (e.g., intraperitoneal, retroperitoneal) may be similarly problematic, and aspiration or drainage of the hematoma may be indicated, depending upon the site and risk of such a procedure.

HYPERKALEMIA ASSOCIATED WITH SEVERE DIGITALIS TOXICITY

Hyperkalemia may complicate digoxin toxicity. As discussed above, severe hyperkalemia, caused by inhibition of Na-K-ATPase, may be a feature of life-threatening toxicity to digitalis, particularly when a massive overdose has occurred (167) or when renal failure exists (168). Preliminary data now indicate the efficacy of administering sheep-derived purified Fab fragments of digoxin-specific antibodies (75). Thus, in a multicenter evaluation in patients resistant to conventional therapy, 11 of whom had hyperkalemia, Smith et al. (75) reported full recovery in 21 patients. Unfortunately, specific details of the serum potassium response to antibody administration were not provided.

GORDON'S SYNDROME (CHLORIDE-SHUNT SYNDROME)

Gordon's syndrome (and closely related disorders) is a rare hereditary disease whose distinguishing feature is hyperkalemia despite a normal GFR (117, 169). The other principal clinical features are hyperchloremic metabolic acidosis, hypertension in adult patients, hypoaldosteronism (relative or absolute), and hyporeninism. Inconsistent characteristics are short stature, intellectual impairment, and muscle weakness (117, 169).

The pathophysiology of this syndrome, which has been called the mirror image of Bartter's syndrome, remains incompletely defined. A reasonable working hypothesis is that deficiency of a chloruretic or natriuretic hormone (atrial natriuretic peptide, natriuretic prostaglandins), or excessive chloride permeability in the distal nephron, results in sodium retention, volume expansion, suppression of the renin-angiotensin-aldosterone axis, and decreased excretion of potassium (117, 169). Increased dietary intake of sodium chloride has been observed in some patients, which may exacerbate the various findings. Therapy for the metabolic features of Gordon's syndrome consists of dietary restriction of sodium chloride and/or the chronic administration of thiazide diuretics (furosemide is said to be less efficacious) (117, 168). The excellent response to these modalities provides support for the abovementioned pathogenic formulation.

HYPERKALEMIA CAUSED BY RENAL TUBULAR DEFECTS

As discussed above, various tubular defects may be associated with renal hyperkalemia. In analogy with renal tubular acidosis, we have grouped these conditions under the rubric *renal tubular hyperkalemia* (119). In patients with these abnormalities, one cannot predict which, if any, agent might facilitate urinary potassium excretion, and the clinician must often rely on a trial-and-error sequential approach using furosemide, acetazolamide plus bicarbonate, thiazide-type diuretics, and mineralocorticoid, and search for and relieve urinary tract obstruction. In a study carried in both patients and experimental animals, Rastogi et al. (170) demonstrated that in hyperkalemic distal renal tubular acidosis, the administration of furosemide may result in an enhancement of urinary potassium excretion, particularly when the diuretic causes an increased excretion of acid.

DRUG-INDUCED HYPERKALEMIA

The danger of the development of drug-induced hyperkalemia in the patient at risk has already been emphasized, especially when more than one drug is used simultaneously (152). Sometimes, therefore, it is not necessary to discontinue all of the potentially culpable agents. Rather, it may suffice to stop some of them and to reduce the dosage of others. Of course, the patient must be closely monitored.

HYPOKALEMIA

Hypokalemia is usually defined as a serum potassium concentration less than 3.5 mEq/l. Hypokalemia, like hyperkalemia, may result from the abnormal transcellular distribution of potassium. In this instance, hypokalemia develops without a deficit in total body potassium. In most situations, however, a decrease in extracellular potassium concentration reflects a potassium deficit from excessive losses and/or decreased intake.

Hypokalemia may be found in more than 20% of hospitalized patients (172–174). It may be a transient event in many instances, with the serum potassium concentration rising back to normal spontaneously without potassium supplements (172). In half of unselected patients with a serum potassium below 2.8 mEq/l, no apparent cause of hypokalemia may be identified (172).

Lawson et al. (173, 174) identified 73 patients with serum potassium below 2.0 mEq/l and 472 with a serum potassium level less than 2.4 mEq/l among 58,167 hospitalized patients, for an overall incidence of severe hypokalemia of almost 1%. Mortality in patients with severe hypokalemia was 30% compared to 8% in age- and sex-matched normokalemic patients. The causes of severe hypokalemia (serum potassium levels below 2.0 mEq/l) involved drugs in one third of the cases, inadequate intake in 26%, gastrointestinal losses in 14%, and renal losses in 12%. Serum potassium was less than 3.0 mEq/l in 5.2%. Drugs, most commonly diuretics, and intravenous fluids accounted for the moderate hypokalemia in 56% of patients.

In the outpatient setting, chronic diuretic therapy of hypertension is the most common cause of hypokalemia. From 10%–30% of hypertensive patients given a daily dose of diuretic will develop hypokalemia. In a recent series of 158 nonedematous hypertensives, all under age 65 and receiving no digitalis or potassium supplements, 29% had a plasma potassium concentration below 3.4 mEq/l after 2 years of treatment (175).

As a result of transcellular potassium distribution

Hypokalemia from redistribution of potassium may be caused by alkalosis, insulin excess, changes in catecholamines, attacks of familial or episodic paralysis, and by drugs (Figure 7).

ALKALOSIS

Both an elevated blood bicarbonate and an elevated pH resulting from a decreased P_{CO_2} may produce hypokalemia

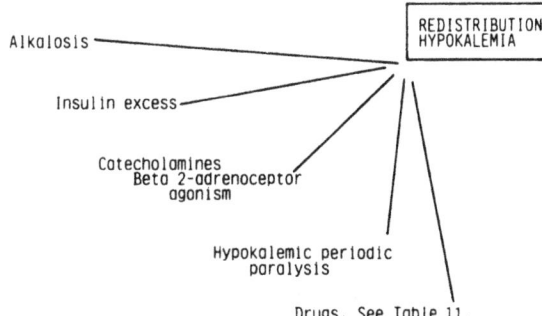

Figure 7. Causes of hypokalemia as a result of redistribution of potassium between intracellular and extracellular space (no decrease in total body potassium).

by translocating extracellular potassium into cells in exchange for hydrogen ions. Teleogically, the movement of protons from cells into the extracellular fluid serves to return the pH of the extracellular fluid to a normal range. The shift of potassium tends to be greater in metabolic alkalosis, wherein plasma bicarbonate is increased, than in respiratory alkalosis, wherein plasma bicarbonate is decreased (16).

Severe hypokalemia has been recorded in association with various forms of bicarbonate administration, including transdermal from absorption of bicarbonate applied in the form of baking soda to treat a diaper rash (176), or from the chronic daily consumption of 2–3/liters of bicarbonated water (Vichy Saint Yorre contains 70 mEq of sodium bicarbonate per liter) for 3–4 years (177). One must remember, however, that patients with metabolic alkalosis are not hypokalemic simply because of redistribution of potassium; rather, the dominant cause is total body potassium depletion production by alkalosis-induced urinary losses of potassium.

INSULIN EXCESS

The effects of insulin on cellular potassium uptake have been discussed. Insulin, with or without glucose, can decrease serum potassium concentration by shifting potassium into cells. Hypokalemia may complicate insulin treatment of diabetic ketoacidosis. This is particularly evident when potassium deficits exist that may have been underestimated or when high doses of insulin are administered (178, 179). Hypokalemia may also develop in patients with an intact pancreas challenged with an acute glucose load. The release of endogenous insulin shifts potassium intracellularly.

CATECHOLAMINES

Beta$_2$-adrenergic and alpha-adrenergic functions modify the transcellular potassium distribution in opposite directions. The former stimulates intracellular potassium uptake (60) whereas the latter opposes it (58).

Disorders of Potassium Metabolism 65

Normally, hypokalemia secondary to excess endogenous beta$_2$-adrenergic activity is rarely encountered, perhaps because of the opposing effects of alpha-adrenergic stimulation on potassium redistribution. As mentioned earlier, beta-adrenergic stimulation protects against dangerous hyperkalemia during vigorous exercise whereas alpha-adrenergic stimulation has an important role in preventing and mitigating postexercise hypokalemia (61).

Clinically, hypokalemia averaging 3.3 mEq/l has been observed in 70% of 73 patients admitted to the hospital with acute severe head injury, a condition known to be associated with high epinephrine levels and hypertension (180, 181). The serum potassium concentration was reduced by about 0.9 mEq/l as compared with values in randomly selected outpatient controls. Increase in plasma epinephrine and modest hypokalemia are also observed in 10–15% of patients with acute myocardial infarction (182–184). Nevertheless, a causal relationship between beta$_2$-adrenergic stimulation and hypokalemia has not been formally established in these situations. Whether hypokalemia after myocardial infarction represents an epiphenomenon related to the extent of the injury or results from an increase in epinephrine associated with stress is currently debated (185).

On the other hand, hypokalemia complicating the exogenous administration of beta$_2$-adrenergic agonists has been reported in the treatment of premature labor and of asthma. Beta$_2$-adrenergic agonists are used intravenously in the treatment of premature labor (186–188). During therapy, serum potassium levels decrease to 2.5–3.0 mEq/l and return to normal values within 30 minutes to 2 hours after discontinuation of the drug. In this setting, administration of beta$_2$-adrenergic blocking agents reverses the hypokalemia.

Beta$_2$-adrenergic agonists are also given with increasing frequency parenterally or by inhalation for the treatment of asthma. A dose-related decrease in serum potassium (about 1 mEq/l) has been described with inhalation of fenoterol (189). This observation suggested that an overdose of beta$_2$-agonists, in conjunction with the increase in epinephrine present during a stressful asthma attack, carried a risk of rapid hypokalemia and might be incriminated in an increasing number of sudden and unexpected deaths observed in young patients with asthma, mostly using inhalational beta$_2$-agonists (189). Concomitant use of theophylline may enhance the hypokalemia (190). These patients exhibit both hyperinsulinemia and elevated plasma catecholamine levels, which may contribute in lowering serum potassium concentration.

HYPOKALEMIC PERIODIC PARALYSIS

Whereas severe hypokalemia from any cause can lead to paralysis, hypokalemic periodic paralysis refers to a rare syndrome, which is either familial with autosomal dominant transmission or occurs sporadically in thyrotoxic patients, especially but not exclusively in those of Oriental extraction. It is characterized by recurrent attacks of flaccid paralysis, which may last up to 24 hours and affect the limbs and trunk. During attacks, there is a shift of extracellular potassium intracellularly (191).

Attacks usually begin in childhood or adolescence; they may occur daily or weekly, or only episodically at several-year intervals. The paralytic episodes are precipitated by rest after vigorous exercise, by high carbohydrate meals, or administration of glucose, glucose plus insulin, epinephrine, or glucagon (16).

During an attack, serum potassium decreases by 1–2 mEq/l, and a serum potassium of 2.0 mEq/l is not unusual. Typically, serum potassium returns toward normal without any specific therapy, concomitant with an improvement in muscle strength. The hypokalemia may be associated with dangerous cardiac arrhythmias (192).

The nature of the cell membrane defect may involve reduced excitability and an increased sodium conductance, which are exacerbated by a reduction of extracellular potassium (193).

DELIRIUM TREMENS

Hypokalemia with a serum potassium concentration less than 3.5 mEq/l occurs in about 50% of patients hospitalized for alcoholic withdrawal (194). The etiology of the hypokalemia in these patients may results from a combination of poor intake, respiratory alkalosis, ketosis, vomiting, diarrhea, and magnesium depletion. In one study, a uniform occurrence of hypokalemia with a mean serum potassium of 2.9 mEq/l has been observed to occur a few hours to 1 day before a crisis of delirium tremens (195). The hypokalemia has been attributed to maldistribution of 160–240 mEq of potassium. The serum potassium concentration normalized spontaneously after a few days. In contrast, delirium tremens did not occur in patients who did not develop hypokalemia (195). This fascinating observation needs confirmation.

DRUGS (TABLE 10)

Several drugs that may induce hypokalemia by redistributing potassium between the extracellular and intracellular space have already been discussed, including bicarbonate, insulin (exogenous and endogenous), and beta$_2$-adrenergic agonists. Barium and chloroquine intoxication and administration of blood, drugs, or fluids in a clinical setting, wherein avid utilization of extracellular potassium exists may also lead to hypokalemia.

Barium poisoning

Ingestion of 1–15 g of soluble barium salts (196, 197) or barium chloride burns (198) may lead to hypokalemia with flaccid paralysis, vomiting, and diarrhea. Hypokalemia may be profound (serum potassium < 2.0 mEq/l) and results from the specific blocking by barium of cellular potassium exit channels (9, 199).

Chloroquine intoxication

Two cases of severe hypokalemia (serum potassium concentration, 1.1 mEq/l) have been reported after acute intoxication with massive doses (10 g) of chloroquine resulting in cardiopulmonary arrest (200). The hypokalemia was protracted and persisted for 22 and 33 hours. Despite administration of large amounts of parenteral potassium, urinary excretion of potassium was minimal, indicating that the hypokalemia resulted from cellular potassium entry. The severe and resistant hypokalemia suggested that chloroquine, rather than treatment of the cardiopulmonary arrest, was responsible for potassium redistribution.

Theophylline overdose

Hypokalemia has been reported as an incidental finding in patients with a theophylline overdose. In a series of 22 patients with self-inflicted theophylline overdose, hypokalemia (serum potassium concentration ranging from 3.4 to 2.2 mEq/l) was observed in all patients (201). The decrease in serum potassium correlated with the concomitant serum theophylline concentrations.

The origin of theophylline-induced hypokalemia may be multifactorial. Theophylline, a phosphodiesterase inhibitor, increases cyclic AMP and Na-K-ATPase activity of the cell membrane, thereby enhancing the intracellular movement of potassium. As mentioned above, theophylline may potentiate the adverse effects of parenteral terbutaline (190). Likely factors also include theophylline-induced increases in plasma catecholamine and insulin, in combination with mild respiratory alkalosis resulting from stimulation of the respiratory center. Theophylline is also a mild diuretic.

An equivalent degree of hypokalemia, with serum potassium levels falling to less than 3.5 mEq/l 25% of the time, has also been reported after consumption of 180–360 mg of caffeine, a dose equivalent to the amount of caffeine contained in two cups of strong coffee (202). Caffeine has pharmacologic properties similar to those of theophylline.

Toluene sniffing

Sniffing of paint or glue may result in severe hypokalemia with a mean serum potassium concentration of 1.7 mEq/l, resulting in quadriparesis, sparing the central and respiratory muscles. The hypokalemia has been attributed to renal tubular acidosis, but it may in part be due to potassium redistribution intracellularly, since it is most often associated with a low urinary potassium concentration (203).

"Utilization" of extracellular potassium

Transfusion of frozen and washed erythrocytes may decrease the serum potassium concentration by 1 mEq/l and may be associated with premature ventricular beats when serum potassium decreases to less than 3 mEq/l. The hypokalemia results from potassium entry into blood cells that were depleted of potassium during the process of freezing and washing (204). This complication does not occur with transfusion of conventionally prepared blood. With the latter, hyperkalemia, rather than hypokalemia, may be observed.

Similarly, when treatment of pernicious anemia is initiated, the production of new blood cells "consumes" potassium, and hypokalemia of dangerous and even fatal proportion may result (205). Since patients with pernicious anemia may have diarrhea, they may have an underlying potassium depletion. Therapy should include the provision of sufficient potassium to replete body stores.

As analogous phenomenon may develop in anabolic states. Hypokalemia below 3.0 mEq/l has been observed in 18% of patients on total parenteral nutrition as a result of potassium redistribution into cells (206). The hypokalemia can be easily prevented by incorporating sufficient amounts of potassium in the parenteral nutrition fluid. For patients with a normal renal function, 90–120 mEq/day is recommended, and for patients in renal failure, 40–50 mEq/day (207).

As a result of decreased potassium input

Hypokalemia may derive from an inadequate intake of potassium (Figure 8). If potassium intake is eliminated, the kidneys adjust by decreasing potassium excretion to about 5–10 mEq/day, but only after several days (208). In the meantime, a deficit of 200–300 mEq may have developed. With stool potassium losses remaining constant at about 10 mEq/day, minimal intake of potassium, therefore, should equal 20–25 mEq daily to avoid a deficit. Higher intakes of potassium per day may be necessary to compensate for intercurrent losses.

A concern is the finding of surveys that certain groups of impoverished people, especially the elderly, consume a diet that may only contain 25 mEq of potassium daily (209–211). Potassium deficits from inadequate intake are easy to envision under these conditions. Thus, the longer the reduced intake, the larger the cumulative potassium depletion. Nevertheless, although reduced potassium intake in the elderly or the alcoholic patient with poor dietary habits may lead to total body potassium depletion, hypokalemia often is only modest.

Eating disorders associated with psychological problems often lead to severe potassium deficits (212). Hypokalemia may be modest, and blood pH may be normal, unless self-induced vomiting and/or use of diuretics or laxatives coexist. Fifty percent of hospitalized patients with anorexia nervosa have a serum potassium concentration of less than 3.5 mEq/l, and serum potassium levels as low as 1.5 mEq/l have been reported (213). Bulimarexia, like anorexia nervosa, affects young women but is ten times more frequent. In a series of 275 bulimic patients, 88% reported self-induced vomiting; 60%, laxative abuse; and 33%, diuretic abuse (214, 215).

Drastic reduction in potassium absorption, as in geophagia, may lead to severe hypokalemia. Some types of clay do not contain potassium and bind potassium in the gut to make it unavailable for absorption (216).

As a result of increased potassium output

Total body potassium depletion from increased potassium loss is the major cause of severe hypokalemia and can develop through losses in sweat (rarely), urine (common), or feces (most common) (Figure 9). Other conditions

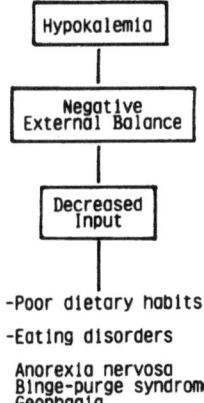

Figure 8. Hypokalemia as a result of decreased total body potassium from decreased intestinal potassium absorption.

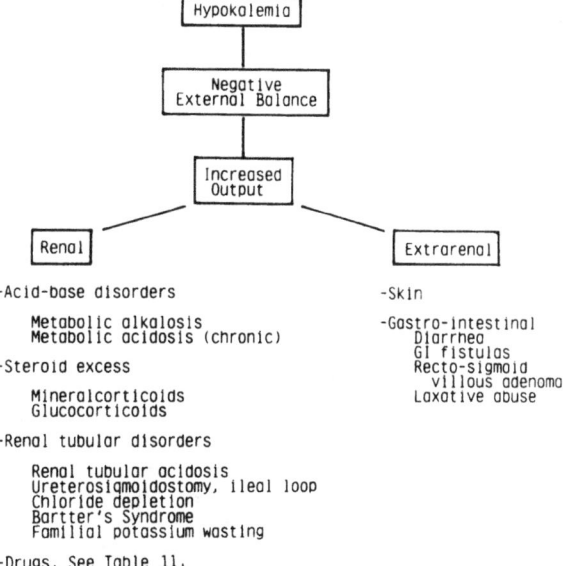

Figure 9. Hypokalemia as a result of decreased total body potassium from increased potassium output.

being equal, losses of potassium are markedly enhanced in all three organs if hyperaldosteronism coexists.

A careful history most often will orient the clinician to the etiology of the hypokalemia. When a specific diagnosis is not readily evident, the use of a flow diagram based on measurements of urinary potassium and acid-base status is often helpful to assist in the differential diagnosis of hypokalemia associated with potassium deficits (217). Two schemes are presented in Figures 10 and 11. In instances of hypokalemia of obscure origin, measurements in blood and urine collected on admission before treatment is started (see Table 4) may be most useful.

EXTRARENAL LOSSES OF POTASSIUM

After 3–5 days of extrarenal potassium losses, urinary potassium excretion values less than 20 mEq in a 24-hour urine collection, less than 20 mEq/g creatinine in a spot urine specimen, or a urinary fractional excretion of potassium (U/P K ÷ U/P creatinine × 100) less than 6% in the presence of adequate amounts of urinary sodium (greater than 100 mEq/day), indicate appropriate renal potassium conservation and suggest that extrarenal losses are responsible for the hypokalemia (217).

Skin losses of potassium

Potassium in sweat averages 9 mEq/l. Losses through skin can exceed 100 mEq/day during vigorous exercise, especially in hot climates. Hypokalemia, however, rarely occurs, and urinary potassium excretion may remain elevated as a consequence of secondary hyperaldosteronism (218). On the other hand, hypokalemia (serum potassium from 1.6–3.4 mEq/l) is the rule in nonexertional heat stroke (218). Prolonged hypothermia may also produce mild hypokalemia by a shift of potassium from the extracellular to the intracellular space (219).

Gastrointestinal losses of potassium

Losses of gastric fluid through vomiting or nasogastric suction are frequently associated with potassium deficits. Nevertheless, in these instances, measurements of urinary potassium indicate that the hypokalemia actually results from renal, rather than extrarenal, losses of potassium. These are secondary to volume depletion with hyperaldosteronism, chloride depletion, metabolic alkalosis, and delivery of large amounts of bicarbonate to the distal nephron. Indeed, gastric fluid contains only 5–10 mEq of potassium per liter. When the loss of hydrochloric acid is minimized in patients receiving nasogastric suction by the administration of H_2-receptor antagonists, hypokalemia does not develop despite continuous gastric aspiration. An interesting aspect of the hypokalemic metabolic alkalosis associated with vomiting is that once the vomiting abates, both the alkalosis and the hypokalemia can be corrected by administering sodium chloride without potassium supplementation (17). This suggests that volume depletion is necessary to maintain the alkalosis, presumably by enhancing tubular reabsorption of bicarbonate. The alkalosis, therefore, maintains the hypokalemia by causing extracellular to intracellular redistribution of potassium and by enhancing urinary potassium losses.

Intestinal potassium losses occur from all types of diarrheas (malabsorptive, secretory, hormonal, infectious, or drug induced [cytosine-arabinoside (20)], from gastrointestinal fistulas, and from villous adenoma of the rectosigmoid colon. A metabolic acidosis from losses of bicarbonate and/or organic anion in stool characterizes secretory diarrhea; whereas, blood pH may be variable in other types. The potassium concentration is less than 10–20 mEq/l in intestinal fluid, except in secretions of villous adenoma, where it may reach 100 mEq/l (221). Nevertheless, large losses of potassium are not unusual in severe diarrhea and may reach several hundred milli-

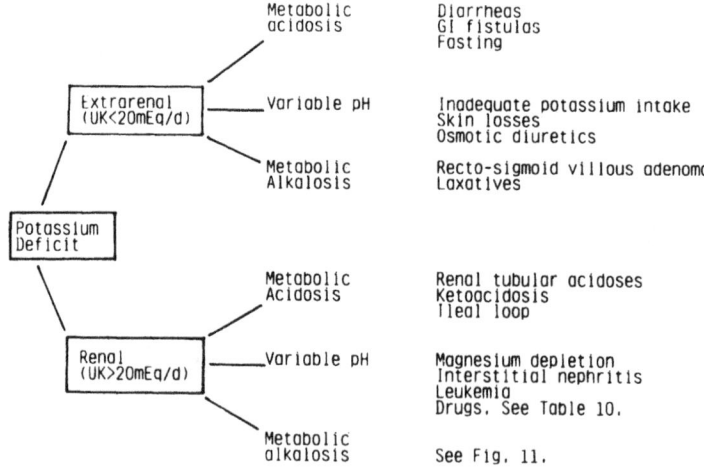

Figure 10. Differential diagnosis of hypokalemia with total body potassium deficit (negative external balance).

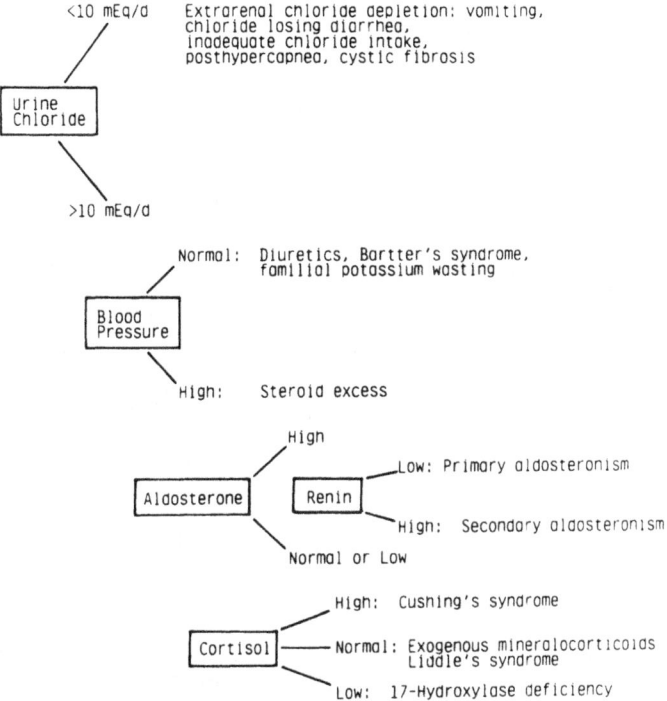

Figure 11. Differential diagnosis of hypokalemia with total body potassium deficit and metabolic alkalosis.

equivalents of potassium per day in cholera. Intestinal losses of potassium are related to the volume of fluid lost, but not as dramatically as the losses of sodium (2).

Chronic laxative abuse is a cause of severe intestinal potassium loss that is often difficult to diagnose, as the patient may not acknowledge such practice (222). The diagnosis may be helped by identifying phenolphthalein in urine and stool, and magnesium in stool (223). Alkalosis is usual. But blood pH may be normal in chronic laxative users, and urinary potassium concentration is unpredictable depending on the severity of the hypokalemia and the status of the extracellular fluid volume (222).

RENAL LOSSES OF POTASSIUM

Substantial urinary losses of potassium (i.e., 40–80 mEq/day) in a hypokalemic patient receiving adequate amounts of dietary sodium indicate that the kidneys fail to conserve potassium appropriately. This may result from tubular defects and/or hormonal or pharmacologic influences. It should be remembered, however, that renal conservation of potassium develops slowly. Therefore, urinary potassium may exceed 20 mEq/l in acute hypokalemia of short duration or in situations wherein a potassium-wasting diuretic was only recently discontinued (less than 1 week).

The acid-base status may help differentiate different forms of renal potassium losses.

Renal losses with metabolic acidosis

Metabolic acidosis is seen in distal (classic, Type I) and in proximal (Type II) renal tubular acidosis. In distal renal tubular acidosis, the potassium wasting reflects the utilization of potassium for cation (sodium/potassium) exchange, since hydrogen ion cannot be secreted maximally; from hyperaldosteronism secondary to chronic metabolic acidosis; and conceivably from a separate tubular defect. In proximal renal tubular acidosis, the inability to reabsorb bicarbonate proximally results in a markedly increased bicarbonate and fluid delivery to the distal potassium secretory sites (224).

Hypokalemic metabolic acidosis with flaccid paralysis may also occur when ureteral urine is diverted into the sigmoid colon or into an ileal loop with outlet obstruction; urinary sodium chloride is absorbed in exchange for potassium and bicarbonate. Serum potassium concentration and the acid-base status are usually normal in patients with an unobstructed ileal bladder.

As already mentioned, potassium deficits are always present in patients with diabetic ketoacidosis. This results from the osmotic diuresis due to glycosuria and from the substantial ketoanionuria. Nevertheless, hypokalemia is usually absent due to the combined effects of plasma hypertonicity, lack of insulin, renal failure, increased catabolism, and possibly the acidosis itself. Therefore, a normal or low extracellular potassium concentration in a patient with diabetic ketoacidosis usually indicates a severe underlying potassium deficit, which can exceed 10 mEq/kg body weight (225, 226).

Renal losses with variable blood pH

Renal losses of potassium associated with a variable pH (depending on the extracellular fluid volume status and the underlying pathophysiology) include polyuric states secondary to tubular injury from hypercalcemia, severe potassium deficit, diuretic phase of acute tubular necrosis, or postobstructive diuresis. Potassium losses can be severe and reach 6–36 mEq/hr in postobstructive diuresis (16). When extracellular fluid volume depletion develops or when the potassium deficit is severe, metabolic alkalosis ensues. In conditions of tubular injury, magnesium is also lost in urine, and magnesium depletion itself may lead to renal potassium wasting and a severe hypokalemia that is refractory to treatment with potassium supplements alone. Renal potassium wasting may occur in patients with acute or chronic leukemia in whom tubular damage (lysozymuria) develops (173, 227) and in patients with interstitial nephritis (rarely) (228).

Renal losses with metabolic alkalosis

The differential diagnosis of potassium deficits and hypokalemia associated with metabolic alkalosis, based on measurements of urinary chloride, blood pressure, plasma aldosterone, renin, and cortisol, is outlined in Figure 11.

Renal potassium losses in patients whose chloride depletion is of extrarenal origin are associated with very low urinary chloride excretion (< 10 mEq/day). In these instances, the metabolic alkalosis and the hypokalemia are typically responsive to the administration of sodium chloride alone unless extremely large potassium deficits exist. When potassium losses are large and exceed 500 mEq, the severe potassium deficit may result in an alkalosis that is associated with urinary chloride losses and that is no longer corrected by sodium chloride (16). Treatment then consists of providing large amounts of potassium chloride supplements to bring the serum potassium concentration above 3.0 mEq/l, to correct the existing acid-base abnormality, and then to evaluate the underlying etiology of the hypokalemia (17).

In contrast, when renal losses of potassium and chloride coexist in metabolic alkalosis, the hypokalemia is not responsive to sodium chloride administration. In this situations, a normal blood pressure may serve to separate tubular losses of potassium due to diuretics, Bartter's syndrome, or familial potassium wasting from conditions of steroid excess (either mineralocorticoids or glucocorticoids) associated with hypokalemia and high blood pressure. Differentiation between the various clinical entities of steroid excess is made by measuring plasma aldosterone and renin activity to separate primary (adrenal adenoma or hyperplasia) and secondary (renovascular hypertension, malignant hypertension, renin-secreting tumor) hyperaldosteronism, and by measuring cortisol and response to ACTH to diagnose primary and secondary Cushing's syndrome (ectopic ACTH-secreting tumors, exogenous glucocorticoid administration) (16).

In hypokalemic hypertensive patients with metabolic alkalosis and normal or low plasma levels of aldosterone and cortisol, an exogenous source of mineralocorticoid must be suspected, as seen in patients given exogenous mineralocorticoids by various routes [parenteral, oral, topical (228), as well as nasal (229)]. The same findings pertain to licorice users (230) or to patients given carbenoxolone for the treatment of gastric ulcer (231). Licorice (some chewing tobaccos and snuff contain licorice), which contains glycyrhizinic acid, and carbenoxolone (a glycyrhitenic acid derivative) potentiate mineralocorticoid activity (232). Liddle's syndrome is a familial syndrome with hypertension that mimics primary aldosteronism but in which excess mineralocorticoid cannot be identified (233). Cortisol production is blocked in 17-hydroxylase deficiency syndromes that are associated with adrenogenital abnormalities (16).

Renal losses due to drugs

A number of drugs may cause hypokalemia as a result of renal potassium losses (Table 11). The acid-base status is variable depending on the underlying associated pathology, but is often normal unless extracellular fluid volume depletion is part of the clinical picture, renal tubular acidosis ensues, or hypokalemia is severe.

CISPLATIN AND ANTIBIOTICS

Diffuse tubular toxicity may develop following the administration of cisplatin, aminoglycosides, amphotericin B, viomycin, polymyxin B, rifampin, or capreomycin (227, 234–239). In these instances, renal losses of magnesium and potassium occur, leading to hypomagnesemia, hypokalemia, and hypocalcemia.

High-dose sodium penicillin and its derivatives (ticarcillin, carbenicillin, ampicillin, nafcillin, amoxicillin, and cephalexin) may induce potassium losses by acting as osmotic and poorly reabsorbed anions in tubular fluid (240).

GOSSYPOL

The use of gossypol, an extract from cotton seed oil used for male contraception in the People's Republic of China, has been associated with hypokalemic paralysis in 1% of more than 8000 volunteers (241). The hypokalemia stems from renal potassium losses, but the tubular mechanism affected by gossypol has not been defined. The incidence of hypokalemia is enhanced by a low dietary potassium intake. In the majority of patients, recovery was prompt following potassium repletion. Nonetheless, in some

Table 11. Drug-induced hypokalemia

A. *Altered potassium distribution between intracellular and extracellular space*

    Bicarbonate (parenteral, oral, transdermal)
    Insulin — glucose (endogenous insulin)
    Beta$_2$-adrenergic agonists (epinephrine, albuterol, terbutaline, ritodrine)
    Barium (soluble salts) intoxication
    Chloroquine intoxication
    Theophylline overdose (caffeine)
    Toluene sniffing*
    Increased "utilization" of extracellular potassium
        Transfusion of frozen-washed erythrocytes
        Treatment of pernicious anemia
        Total parenteral nutrition

B. *Decreased potassium input*

    Some clays adsorb potassium in the gut

C. *Increased potassium output*

    Intestinal
        Laxatives
        Cytosine arabinoside
    Renal
        Antimitotics: cisplatin
        Nephrotoxic antibiotics
            Aminoglycosides, viomycin, capreomycin, polymyxin B, rifampin
            Amphotericin B*
            Penicillins (high dose)
        Gossypol
        L-DOPA
        Diuretics
            Osmotic agents
            Carbonic anhydrase inhibitors
            Loop diuretics
            Thiazides
        Steroids
            Mineralocorticoids
            Glucocorticoids
            Glycyrrhizinic acid (licorice) and its derivative (carbenoxolone)

* May also cause renal tubular acidosis.

patients, episodes of hypokalemia recurred for several months after cessation of gossypol administration.

L-DOPA

A correlation has been described between hypokalemia and hyperaldosteronism in Parkinsonians treated with L-DOPA (242).

DIURETICS

Drugs inhibiting fluid and sodium reabsorption proximally to the "distal" tubular secretory sites of potassium induce urinary potassium losses, potentially leading to hypokalemia. They include osmotic agents (glucose, urea, mannitol, poorly reabsorbed anions) and diuretics, such as carbonic anhydrase inhibitors, loop diuretics, and thiazides (125, 243). The increased potassium secretion results from increased rates of sodium and tubular fluid delivery to the distal nephron. Potassium losses are proportional to the diuretic and natriuretic potency of the drugs and to their duration of action. Other factors enhance the kaliuresis induced by diuretics, principally the extracellular fluid volume status and the level of plasma aldosterone. Thus, potassium losses are increased in sodium-replete individuals with a large urinary output and in patients with hyperaldosteronism. Large urine volumes, metabolic alkalosis, and the simultaneous use of two potassium-wasting diuretics acting at different sites in the renal tubule also increase the incidence and severity of potassium deficits. As the extracellular fluid volume contracts, metabolic alkalosis develops, which may enhance the hypokalemia by shifting potassium intracellularly. Although carbonic anhydrase inhibitors are only mild diuretics, the distal delivery of large amounts of bicarbonate as a result of proximal tubular carbonic anhydrase inhibition may lead to severe urinary potassium losses and metabolic acidosis (125, 243).

In nonedematous patients given diuretics, the serum potassium concentration decreases progressively for the first week to 10 days of treatment and remains stable (244) or eventually improves (245) thereafter. The fall in serum potassium concentration ranges from 0.3–1.2 mEq/l, depending on the dose and type of diuretic used, and levels below 3.0 mEq/l occur in less than 5% of patients (246). Most patients receiving diuretics have a serum potassium between 3.3 and 3.8 mEq/l (246). The incidence of hypokalemia is higher with thiazide derivatives given chronically than with loop diuretics and is greatest with long-acting thiazides such as chlorthalidone (244). The hypokalemia is associated with relatively small changes in total body potassium (< 300 mEq) (246, 147).

Severe hypokalemia is uncommon with long-term diuretic therapy whereas mild hypokalemia may occur in 5–20% of patients given low-dose chronic diuretics. Among 169 hypertensive patients ingesting an unrestricted diet without potassium supplements evaluated by Sandor (175), the serum potassium concentration was below 3.4 mEq/l in 29% and below 3.0 mEq/l in 13% after 2 years of treatment. In a large study of 5000 hypertensive patients, Licht et al. (248) observed a prevalence of serum potassium less than 3.5 mEq/l in 11% of patients given 50 mg of hydrochlorothiazide per day, 8.1% given 25 mg chlorthalidone per day, 2.2% given 25 mg hydrochlorothiazide per day, and 3.1% given 40 mg furosemide per day. Among 1318 patients with congestive heart failure given potassium-wasting diuretics alone without potassium supplements, 78 (or 5.9%) developed hypokalemia with a serum potassium concentration of less than 3.5 mEq/l (174).

Clinical consequences of hypokalemia

There are many serious complications of hypokalemia. Like hyperkalemia, they involve cardiac, muscular, metabolic, and renal abnormalities. A detailed account of the

Table 12. Clinical manifestations of hypokalemia

A. *Cardiovascular effects*

    Depressed ST segments
    Appearance of U waves
    Ventricular ectopic beats
    Ventricular couplets
    Ventricular tachycardia or fibrillation
    Increased risk of digitalis toxicity
    Orthostatic hypotension

B. *Muscular effects*

    Myalgia, weakness, cramps
    Paralysis
    Rhabdomyolysis with myoglobinuria
    Hypodynamic ileus
    Decreased ureteral peristalsis

C. *Metabolic effects*

    Abnormal carbohydrate metabolism
    Reduced muscle glycogen content and synthesis
    Increased glucose intolerance
    Precipitation of overt diabetes mellitus
    Reduced insulin release during hyperglycemia
    Hyperlipidemia
    Increased renin activity
    Decreased aldosterone secretion

D. *Renal and acid-base effects*

    Increased production of ammonia by the kidney
    Decreased protein synthesis
    Negative nitrogen balance
    Growth retardation
    Hepatic encephalopathy or coma
    Metabolic alkalosis
    Nephrogenic diabetes insipidus
    Increased risk of pyelonephritis
    Incomplete syndrome of distal renal tubular acidosis
    Increased urinary excretion of prostaglandin

consequences of hypokalemia has been presented by Knochel (210) (Table 12).

CARDIAC EFFECTS

In cardiac muscle, hypokalemia increases the resting membrane potential, increases the duration of the action potential and of the refractory period, increases automaticity, increases the threshold potential, and decreases conductivity (20). These alterations predispose to the development of arrhythmias, particularly of the reentrant variety. The most common arrhythmias are supraventricular tachyarrhythmias (ectopic atrial tachycardia with block, nonparoxysmal junctional tachycardia), and ventricular tachycardia and fibrillation. More subtle, early electrocardiographic manifestations of hypokalemia, rarely evident at a serum potassium concentration above 3.0 mEq/l, include low-voltage, flattened T waves; depressed ST-T segments; and U waves. T-U fusion may produce pseudo Q-T prolongation. The presentation of unusually peaked precordial U waves may simulate tall T waves of hyperkalemia except for their association with an apparently prolonged Q-T interval, which actually represents a Q-U interval (249).

Hypokalemia predisposes to digitalis intoxication, which, in the presence of mild hypokalemia, may develop at "therapeutic" serum levels of the cardiac glycoside (250).

The risk of arrhythmias are among the most dangerous side effects of hypokalemia. The fact that hypokalemia may also be responsible for reentry phenomena and delayed conduction phenomena that are common to ischemia, hypoxia, and the effects of digitalis therapy perhaps explains why even mild hypokalemia may be arrhythmogenic, particularly in patients experiencing myocardial ischemia, hypoxia, or receiving digitalis (vide infra).

MUSCULAR EFFECTS

Severe potassium deficiency may have important effects on smooth-muscle function, including hypodynamic ileus, impaired pressor responsiveness to catecholamine or angiotensin infusion, and postural hypotension.

Skeletal muscle appears to be the main organ affected in potassium deficiency. Modest potassium deficiency may be associated with a persistent increase in serum creatinine kinase activity and muscle weakness. Severe potassium deficiency, especially when serum potassium falls below 2 mEq/l, may be associated with frank rhabdomyolysis and evident myoglobinuria or paralysis, including respiratory arrest from paralysis of respiratory muscles. Chronic potassium deficiency may favor the development of rhabdomyolysis if an acute event that places heavy metabolic demand on the muscle is superimposed (210).

METABOLIC EFFECTS

Metabolic effects of hypokalemia include glucose intolerance, complications resulting directly from increased renal ammonia production such as protein and nitrogen wasting, and hepatic coma in susceptible patients with advanced liver disease (210). Hypokalemia also suppresses aldosterone and insulin secretion and increases renin secretion.

RENAL AND ACID-BASE EFFECTS

Hypokalemia also has numerous effects on the kidney. In addition to increased ammoniagenesis, hypokalemia may decrease renal blood flow and GFR, predispose to urinary tract infection, impair the renal concentrating ability, alter renal acidification, and maintain metabolic alkalosis (16).

The effects of potassium depletion on prostaglandin production are variable. Increases in urinary prostaglandin excretion have been documented in humans with potassium depletion secondary to vomiting or diuretic administration; potassium depletion, however, associated with primary aldosteronism or DOCA administration to humans does not appear to increase prostaglandin excretion (16). In Bartter's syndrome, prostaglandins appear to play an important role in many of the manifestations of the syndrome.

The systemic effects of hypokalemia appear both maladaptive and adaptive. Whereas the cardiac and muscular complications are clearly deleterious, the hormonal effects of aldosterone and insulin suppression and the renal effects of increased ammonium excretion may be protective by facilitating maintenance of normokalemia through decreased cellular uptake and decreased urinary losses.

CLINICAL SIGNIFICANCE OF MILD HYPOKALEMIA

There is unanimous agreement on the dangers of moderate to severe hypokalemia (serum potassium concentration < 3.0 mEq/l). On the other hand, controversy exists on the incidence and importance of clinical events associated with mild chronic hypokalemia, particularly on the heart, and on the risk/benefit ratio for prevention or therapy of mild hypokalemia developing in nonedematous patients receiving diuretics chronically. The issue relates to the arrhythmogenic potential of mild hypokalemia (serum potassium concentration of 3.0–3.5 mEq/l).

Until recently, mild hypokalemia was believed to be of little clinical importance, except in the digitalized patient. Recent observations, however, have indicated an increased incidence of ventricular arryhythmias in hypertensive patients treated with potassium-wasting diuretics. Therefore, the concern exists that diuretic-induced hypokalemia may result in sudden death. This might explain the relative lack of reduced frequency in fatal cardiac events, as opposed to the uniform decrease in the number of cerebrovascular accidents that has been observed in most multicenter studies on the control of hypertension in which thiazides were part of the study protocol (251–254). In contrast, the recent European Working Party on High Blood Pressure in the Elderly Trial demonstrated that control of hypertension decreases coronary deaths (255). Of interest in this study, a combination of a thiazide diuretic with a potassium-sparing diuretic was used.

The appropriate concern regarding the potential cardiotoxicity of mild hypokalemia secondary to diuretic administration has resulted in a vast and conflicting literature. Until a prospective, randomized, placebo-controlled study of potassium correction for the prevention of arrhythmias is done, neither the effect of treatment nor the rate of complications of such treatment will be known.

The arguments are summarized hereunder. On the one hand:
1. Studies employing ambulatory monitoring of the electrocardiogram indicate that diuretic-induced ventricular ectopy in hypertensive patients may be more common than previously recognized (256–259).
2. Ventricular arrhythmias increase with exercise in patients maintained on thiazides chronically (260).
3. Thiazides have been implicated not only because of their kaliuretic effects, but also because of the loss of magnesium associated with their use (260).
4. The simultaneous administration of potassium and magnesium has prevented the occurrence of exercise-induced arrhythmias (260).
5. Separately, hypokalemia may complicate the course of patients with acute myocardial infarction, possibly as a result of epinephrine release and beta$_2$-adrenergic stimulation (261–265).
6. Patients with mild diuretic-induced hypokalemia may become more hypokalemic if they sustain a stressful event such as an acute myocardial infarction (263).
7. At least seven studies have shown that the prevalence of arrhythmias following myocardial infarction increases as serum potassium concentration falls below 3.5 mEq/l (263) and is inversely related to the level of serum potassium for concentration values from < 3.0 to 4.5 mEq/l (184).
8. The arrhythmias appear related to hypokalemia, rather than to prior diuretic use, since hypokalemic patients not taking diuretics may have an equivalent frequency of ventricular arrhythmias following myocardial infarction (263).

On the other hand
1. Hypokalemia with diuretics develops only in a small number of subjects, about 20% on low-dose diuretics (vide supra).
2. At least five studies have not confirmed an increased incidence of diuretic-induced arrhythmias (266).
3. The arrhythmogenic and hypokalemic potential of other drugs has not always been taken into consideration (265).
4. No fatality from diuretic-induced hypokalemia has been documented (266).
5. The temporal relationship between hypokalemia and ventricular arrhythmias need be demonstrated (266).
6. Administration of potassium alone may not suppress the frequency of diuretic-associated ventricular arrhythmias (258).
7. Only a small proportion of patients (10–15%) develop hypokalemia following myocardial infarction (182–184); and, when hypokalemia occurs, only about one third develop arrhythmias (265) Thus, overall, diuretic-induced hypokalemia accounts only for a small number of instances of ventricular fibrillation postmyocardial infarction (266).
8. On admission of patients with acute myocardial infarction, hypokalemia does not predict an increased occurrence of arrhythmias (268), and survival at 3 months is the same for patients with hypokalemia or with normokalemia who experience ventricular fibrillation after myocardial infarction (265).
9. The risk/benefit ratio may be too expensive in dollars and in complications (gastrointestinal and hyperkalemic) for systematic prevention of diuretic-induced hypokalemia (266, 267, 269, 270). Moreover, potassium administration does not always correct diuretic-induced hypokalemia (269).

The interrelationship between potassium, diuretics, myocardial infarction, and arrhythmias is complex. Thus, whereas lowered serum potassium following myocardial infarction may be documented, other variables, such as age (271), diuretics per se (264), and the presence of underlying mocardial pathology (272–274) may have an influence independent of the serum level of potassium. Hypokalemia also occurs in patients with acute medical conditions other than myocardial infarction and, in many instances, is spontaneously reversible (172). The role of adrenergic stimulation in the etiology of ventricular arrhythmias may be predominant since the same issue of potentially lethal cardiac arrhythmias has been raised in a series of sudden deaths observed in asthmatics inhaling $beta_2$-adrenergic agonists (vide supra). Whether adrenergic stimulation is directly cardiotoxic to the myocardium or indirectly so by changing the local environment is unknown. Whatever the mechanism, the apparent protection and improved long-term survival observed in patients who are maintained on $beta_2$-adrenergic blockers after their first myocardial infarction is interesting in the present context (275, 276).

MANAGEMENT OF HYPOKALEMIA

The correction of hypokalemia may not be straightforward and is influenced by multiple clinical factors. The choices depend on the clinical context. The severity and the acuteness of the hypokalemia, the presence of symptoms, and the existence and the magnitude of concurrent potassium deficits dictate the approach to therapy. The acid-base and the extracellular fluid volume status, the presence of interacting drugs, and the associated underlying disorders also modify therapy importantly.

There are several modalities with which to correct existing hypokalemia or to prevent its potential development. One is to increase potassium intake by administering potassium supplements, either orally or parenterally. Another is to prevent extracellular potassium entry into the intracellular space by administering $beta_2$-adrenergic antagonists or to reverse a maldistribution of potassium between the extracellular and intracellular spaces by correcting an alkalemic condition. A third is to decrease urinary potassium output by using potassium-sparing diuretics to decrease distal tubular potassium secretion, or by inducing hypoaldosteronism with nonsteroidal antiinflammatory drugs or angiotensin-converting enzyme inhibitors. A fourth modality of correcting hypokalemia is to use a combination of the above.

Despite the abovementioned complexities, the treatment of hypokalemia need not be complicated, provided that certain general principles are kept in focus (Table 13).

General principles

1. Hypokalemia per se does not necessarily justify therapy with potassium supplements or potassium-sparing diuretics (137). The etiology of the hypokalemia needs to be recognized. The clinical context, the patient's history and physical examination, and routine laboratory blood and urinary tests outlined in Table 4 will usually orient the physician to the nature (potassium redistribution vs. deficit) and the etiology of a decrease in serum potassium concentration. In hypokalemia resulting from intracellular potassium shifts, potassium replacement may not be necessary or need only be minimal to restore nomokalemia. In contrast, liberal amounts of potassium may be necessary in other circumstances, especially if losses of potassium continue.
2. Associated acid-base abnormalities, particularly metabolic acidosis and alkalosis, and sodium chloride and water deficits must be assessed and recognized. The correction of extracellular fluid volume deficits and/or metabolic alkalosis is the first, and sometimes the only, step necessary to correct hypokalemia. As indicated earlier, once vomiting has abated, the hypokalemic metabolic alkalosis of vomiting or nasogastric aspiration can be fully corrected by extracellular volume repletion with sodium chloride and minimal potassium replacement (17).
3. Normokalemia or hypokalemia in a context of meta-

Table 13. Principles of management of hypokalemia

1. The clinical context dictates the need for therapy of hypokalemia. Hypokalemia per se does not necessarily justify treatment with potassium supplements or potassium-sparing diuretics.
2. Assess the etiology (redistribution vs. deficit) of the hypokalemia.
3. Assess and correct acid-base and extracellular fluid volume abnormalities.
4. Assess the level of renal function.
5. Assess and correct serum tonicity and serum magnesium, if needed.
6. Normokalemia or hypokalemia in a context of metabolic acidosis or serum hypertonicity often indicates potassium deficits.
7. Potassium-sparing diuretics should not be used in patients at risk (patients with decreased renal function or patients receiving other drugs impeding potassium homeostasis).
8. Only resistant hypokalemia justifies the use of two simultaneous treatment modalities of hypokalemia.
9. Assess the potential contribution of medications to hypokalemia and the underlying pathophysiology causative of hypokalemia and correct, whenever possible.
10. Evaluate concurrent medications and/or existing clinical conditions that may aggravate the consequences of hypokalemia.
11. Discontinue treatment of hypokalemia whenever potassium concentration is about 3.5–4.0 mEq/l for fear of "overshoot" hyperkalemia or until a pattern of response is clearly established.
12. Whenever treating hypokalemia, follow the response to treatment by serial measurements of serum potassium concentration and, if indicated, acid-base status.
13. The oral route of potassium replacement, using potassium chloride, is the safest and the preferred modality of treatment. The intravenous route of therapy should be reserved for extreme situations.

bolic acidosis or serum hypertonicity often means severe total body potassium depletion. Correction of the acid-base and electrolyte abnormalities may be difficult. Too rapid alkalinization may exacerbate the hypokalemia, whereas too rapid administration of potassium, without concurrent correction of the acidosis or the hypertonicity, may lead to severe hyperkalemia. In these instances, both abnormalities must be corrected concomitantly (137).
4. The use of potassium-sparing diuretics is potentially dangerous and is usually contraindicated in patients with decreased renal function, and in patients concomitantly receiving other drugs impeding potassium homeostasis (see Table 5). With rare exceptions, their use should be restricted to patients with hypokalemia and intact renal function. They should not be administered concurrently with oral or parenteral potassium supplements; and, when they are used, they should be used cautiously, with serum potassium concentration measured at regular intervals.
5. Only in unusual instances of resistant hypokalemia may it be indicated to use more than one therapeutic modality to correct hypokalemia. Such instances may occur in renal tubular acidosis or Bartter's syndrome. In patients with these conditions, large amounts of potassium supplements may be needed in addition to potassium-sparing diuretics or drugs preventing aldosterone production.
6. Hypokalemia is not a disease per se, but a manifestation of an underlying pathophysiologic condition. The potential contribution of medications to hypokalemia, and the underlying etiology of hypokalemia, should be vigorously pursued and corrected, whenever possible.
7. Concurrent medications and/or clinical conditions must be assessed that may aggravate a given level of hypokalemia and may render severe an otherwise mild form of hypokalemia. This especially applies to patients on digitalis therapy and to patients with organic heart disease (273, 274, 277).
8. When hypokalemia is initially corrected, treatment should be discontinued whenever the serum potassium concentration reaches 3.5–4.0 mEq/l. Indeed, once total body potassium stores are replenished, the relationship between increases in total body potassium and changes in serum potassium concentration is no longer linear; that is, for any given change in total body potassium, changes in serum potassium concentration are much more apparent at serum potassium concentrations above 4 mEq/l than below 3.5 mEq/l (20). "Overshoot" hyperkalemia can easily develop by overtreating hypokalemia, particularly in patients at risk, such as diabetics or patients with chronic renal insufficiency.
9. When correcting hypokalemia, serum potassium concentration and, if indicated, the acid-base status must be closely monitored. This may require several measurements a day in acute instances of combined potassium-acid-base disorders, or merely weekly measurements in instances of uncomplicated mild hypokalemia.

In brief, the clinical context governs the answers to such questions as when to treat, whom to treat, and how to treat hypokalemia.

When to treat?

There is general agreement that severe hypokalemia, defined by a serum potassium concentration less than 2 mEq/l, must be treated. This level of hypokalemia is usually associated with potassium deficits and is treated by administering potassium. Depending upon the clinical circumstances, however, the need for oral versus parenteral potassium supplements may be highly variable. For the patient with paresthesias, muscle weakness, or flaccid paralysis, or the patient with cardiac arrhythmias, parenteral potassium is necessary. One must remember, however, that parenteral potassium is administered directly into the extracellular space, thus modifying the K_i/K_e ratio, and therefore membrane potential, before entering the intracellular space. In contrast, in the nonemergent situation of an asymptomatic patient without cardiac arrhythmia, oral potassium supplementation may suffice to treat even severe hypokalemia.

When moderate hypokalemia exists, with serum potassium concentrations between 2 and 3 mEq/l, the consensus is also to treat. Moderate hypokalemia, however, may not always be associated with potassium deficits, but may simply reflect a translocation of extracellular potassium into the intracellular space. In this instance, intervention aimed at preventing further intracellular entry of potassium from the extracellular space, with administration of only minimal amounts of potassium, may suffice to correct the hypokalemia.

Finally, there is no absolute answer as to when mild hypokalemia, with a serum potassium concentration between 3 and 3.5 mEq/l, must be treated or prevented. The same principles formulated for the treatment or the prevention of mild hypokalemia in nonedematous patients receiving chronic diuretic therapy are applicable to the treatment of mild hypokalemia observed in other clinical circumstances (vide infra).

Whom to treat?

Indications for treatment of hypokalemia and prophylactic management are listed in Table 14. As indicated above, symptomatic and asymptomatic patients with a serum potassium concentration consistently below 3.0 mEq/l should be treated with an aim of maintaining the serum potassium concentration above 3.5 mEq/l. In patients at risk, such as patients receiving digitalis or those with organic heart disease, including left ventricular hypertrophy in hypertensive patients, and patients with any other disorder that is conducive to development of severe hypokalemia, serum potassium should be maintained at 3.5–4.0 mEq/l (273, 274, 277, 278).

Table 14. General indications for prophylactic management and potassium replacement in hypokalemia

Prophylaxis
- Diuretic therapy in the presence of cardiac disease (including left ventricular hypertrophy)
- Digitalized patients at risk of hypokalemia
- Patients with severe liver disease

Replacement
- Moderate-to-severe hypokalemia (serum K^+ <3 mEq/l) without symptoms
- Mild hypokalemia (serum K 3.0–3.5 mEq/l) in the presence of organic heart disease, acute myocardial infarction, acidemia, or signs and symptoms of hypokalemia.

How much to treat?

In the average 70-kg man, total body potassium is approximately 50 mEq/kg. As indicated earlier, changes in serum potassium concentration are a poor index of changes in total body potassium, particularly in the presence of acid-base disturbances.

In the absence of acid-base abnormalities, Sterns et al. (1) reviewed case studies in which decreases in serum potassium concentration and its associated total body potassium changes were simultaneously measured. The study included normal human volunteers undergoing experimental potassium depletion and nonalkalotic hypokalemic patients receiving replacement therapy. A linear relationship was evident between the fall in serum potassium concentration and the reduction in total body potassium. When the serum potassium concentration fell by 1 mEq/l, from 4.0 to 3.0 mEq/l, the body potassium deficit was 200–300 mEq/70-kg body weight. At a serum potassium concentration of 2.5 mEq/l, the potassium deficit was abot 500 mEq; and at 2 mEq/l, the deficit was close to 700 mEq. Thus, in the presence of a normal acid-base status, each decrease in serum potassium concentration of 0.27 mEq/l represents approximately a 100-mEq potassium loss (1).

For any given deficit of potassium, acidemia produces a higher serum potassium concentration, which might lead to underestimation of potassium losses. In contrast, alkalemia lowers the serum potassium concentration and tends to cause an overestimation of potassium deficits. Thus, hyperkalemia in the presence of acidosis may be indicative of severe potassium depletion, since some acidosis shift potassium out of cells. On the other hand, in the face of alkalosis, hypokalemia may not necessarily indicate total body potassium depletion, since potassium tends to shift intracellularly.

How to treat?

ACUTE THERAPY

The level of hypokalemia that demands emergency treatment is highly variable and depends on clinical circumstances. As already indicated, the more acute the hypokalemia develops, the more severe the symptoms will be.

The oral route of administration (liquid or tablet) is the safest and preferred mode of potassium replacement. Oral potassium should be given, preferably as a liquid with or after meals, or as the wax matrix tablet, which must be swallowed and not allowed to dissolve in the mouth. The usual dosage required in hypokalemic states ranges from 40 to 120 mEq per day depending on the clinical situation and the estimated potassium deficit (287). A partial list of current formulations for oral replacement therapy is shown in Table 15.

In treating hypokalemia, regardless of the route of administration, one must closely follow serum potassium concentration, keeping in mind that potassium must traverse the extracellular space before reaching the depleted intracellular compartment. The use of large doses of potassium intravenously is often associated with abrupt increases in serum potassium concentration and profound changes in neuromuscular excitability, even in the face of severe potassium depletion. Nevertheless, the intravenous route is indicated when oral therapy is not feasible or in the case of life-threatening hypokalemia, i.e., paralysis or serious arrhythmias.

When potassium is provided by the intravenous route, the use of peripheral veins is preferred over a central route. Infusions of potassium chloride, potassium acetate, and potassium phosphate must be administered slowly as

Table 15. Commonly used oral potassium preparations

Preparation	Manufacturer	Strength (mEq/15 ml)
Liquids		
Potassium chloride	(various)	10, 15
10%		20
20%		40
Kay Ciel	Berlex	20
Kaon Cl 20%	Adria	40
Klorvess	Sandoz	20
Potassium gluconate		20
		(as potassium gluconate)
Kaon	Adria	45
Tri-K		(potassium acetate, potassium bicarbonate, and potassium citrate)
Powders		
(to 2 oz. water)		(per packet)
K-Lor	Abbot	15
Kay Ciel	Berlex	20
Klyte/Cl	Mead Johnson	25
Tablets and capsules		
Slow K	Ciba	8-wax matrix
Klotrix	Mead Johnson	10-wax matrix
Micro-K Extentabs	Robins	8-controlled release (microencapsulated)

dilute solutions. The standard undiluted potassium chloride solutions contain 2 mEq each of K^+ and Cl^- per ml. The maximum rate at which potassium can be safely given into peripheral veins is usually in the range of 10–20 mEq/hr. Higher rates of infusion may be administered if the clinical status warrants a more rapid correction of the hypokalemia (16). For example, rates higher than 40 mEq/hr have been advocated in certain life-threatening complications such as quadriparesis with respiratory compromise (280, 281). Cardiac monitoring with frequent measuring of serum potassium is mandatory to avoid the known cardiac and neuromuscular effects of hyperkalemia. In most circumstances, 20–40 mEq of potassium are added to each liter of saline or dextrose solution.

One must be aware of the decrement in serum potassium of about 0.2–1.4 mEq/l seen when potassium is administered with glucose solutions. This is presumably secondary to the enhanced insulin secretion stimulated by a glucose load. The results of a recent study comparing administration of potassium in glucose versus mannitol solutions for the treatment of familial hypokalemic periodic paralysis suggest that mannitol solutions may be more effective in both improving potassium levels and correcting the symptoms (280).

Under controlled situations, potassium can also be administered subcutaneously (hypodermoclysis). The concentration, however, should not exceed 10 mEq/l. This archaic method has recently been advocated as an alternative for potassium replacement in the elderly patient with poor venous access (282).

In summary, except in extreme situations, intravenous potassium should be given peripherally in concentrations of 20–40 mEq/l and at rates not greater than 10–20 mEq/hr, preferably in a non-dextrose-containing solution. When fluid restriction is necessary, up to 20 mEq per 100 ml can be given cautiously over 1 hour using a microdrip device. During replacement, frequent monitoring of the clinical status, electrocardiogram, and serum potassium concentration is indicated.

It is critical that, regardless of the type of diluent, the solution be thoroughly mixed to avoid infusing a concentrated solution of potassium, which has been associated with fatal hyperkalemia (283).

In the setting of severe hypokalemia, or in the event that peripheral venous access is unavailable, potassium can be delivered into the femoral vein with the tip of the catheter not in close proximity to the heart (284). The rate of administration should not exceed 60 mEq/hr, as rates exceeding this have been associated with severe cardiac disturbances (285, 286).

CHRONIC THERAPY

Potassium supplementation

Dietary intake. The success of diet in the management of hypokalemia depends on an enthusiastic physician and a compliant patient (279). It is most effective in patients with mild hypokalemia such as the nonedematous hypertensive patient receiving thiazide diuretics with a serum potassium concentration less than 3.5 but greater than 3.0 mEq/l (287).

Although increased consumption of foods rich in potassium may prove feasible in some cases, this approach is not without limitations. The physician must be wary about the excess caloric intake, along with the expense of ingesting foods rich in potassium. For example, to provide an additional 60–80 mEq supplement of potassium, a person must ingest four to six bananas daily (one medium-sized banana = 14 mEq) or drink up to five to seven cups of orange juice daily (half cup = 6.4 mEq). Moreover, potassium in food is not in the form of the chloride salt.

Potassium salts. The specific potassium salt to be used depends on the etiology of the hypokalemia and the acid-base status.

There are several salts of potassium available, the neutral salts, including potassium chloride or potassium phosphate, and the alkaline salts, e.g., potassium bicarbonate or their metabolic precursors, e.g., acetate, citrate, and gluconate, which contain from 4 to 13 mEq of potassium per gram.

Potassium chloride is most frequently used, perhaps because potassium chloride best corrects the hypokalemia associated with hypochloremic metabolic alkalosis secondary to diuretic therapy or to the loss of gastric fluid.

In the presence of hypochloremia, the use of potassium bicarbonate or its precursors is often ineffective (288). The non-chloride-containing salts are usually indicated in clinical situations in which hypokalemia is associated with acidosis, such as secretory diarrhea and renal tubular acidosis.

In the presence of severe metabolic acidosis and severe potassium deficiency, one must follow an aggressive approach. Because the bicarbonate and potassium deficits are not equal, one may have to administer potassium chloride and bicarbonate simultaneously in two different infusions. Potassium should be dissolved in 0.45% sodium chloride and may have to be administered at rates greater than 20–30 mEq/hr in order to correct the potassium deficit. Rapid correction of acidosis without correction of the potassium deficiency may lead to worsening of hypokalemia (137).

Potassium has been formulated into several preparations: liquid form, enteric-coated tablet (no longer on the market), wax matrix formulations, and a more recent form, the microencapsulated preparation (Table 15).

The liquid form, the first to appear on the market, although the least expensive, is quite unpopular because of its unpalatable taste and unpleasant side effects, e.g., nausea, heartburn, and diarrhea, especially in patients with delayed gastric emptying.

The use of enteric-coated preparations is no longer advocated for the treatment of hypokalemia. Enteric-coated tablets dissolve rapidly in the presence of an alkaline pH in the small intestine and present a high local concentration of potassium upon disintegration of the tablet. Their use led to an incidence of gastrointestinal ulceration of 40–50 per 100,000 patient-years and has resulted in several reported deaths (289).

The preparations most often used today are the slow-release formulations, which consist of either sugar-coated (SlowK®, KaON Cl), or film-coated (Klotrix®, K-tab®) tablets, with the potassium salt imbedded in a wax matrix to provide approximately 8–10 mEq per tablet, respectively. These tablets were designed to release potassium ions into the intestinal tract slowly, over a period of hours, to avoid ulcerations.

Although in general the wax matrix formulation is considerably safer than the enteric-coated tablets, the new microencapsulated potassium chloride formulations may be preferable. For example, in 48 healthy volunteers, ingestion of the wax matrix tablets was associated with a high incidence of upper gastrointestinal lesions unaccompanied by symptoms (289). This effect was exacerbated by drugs that decreased gastric emptying. These observations have been confirmed, thus emphasizing the importance of avoiding the wax matrix formulation in clinical conditions associated with delayed gastric emptying, i.e., pyloric stenosis, gastric stasis, and old age.

Although absorption of potassium from the wax matrix is considerably slower than from the liquid preparation, recent bioavailability studies comparing the different formulations during chronic ingestion did not show statistically significant differences among the liquid form, wax matrix, or the microencapsulated preparations, as assessed by the amount of potassium excreted over a 24-hour period (190, 291).

Potassium-sparing diuretics

This form of therapy is usually indicated in those clinical situations wherein prevention of hypokalemia is the goal (292). Recent studies suggest that potassium-sparing diuretics may be more effective than potassium supplements in maintaining a positive potassium balance during diuretic therapy (292, 293). Nevertheless, these agents are not without side effects, the most serious being severe or fatal hyperkalemia (294), which can occur even in patients with a normal GFR (295). They should be used only when the risks of hypokalemia clearly outweigh those of therapy (277) (Table 14).

In general, potassium-sparing diuretics should be used with caution in diabetics and the elderly and are contraindicated in those patients with evidence of renal dysfunction or in those ingesting drugs that further interfere with potassium homeostasis (137, 277, 278).

Spironolactone. Spironolactone acts as a competitive antagonist of aldosterone at the distal tubule. Spironolactone is the most expensive of the potassium-sparing diuretics, and its use is associated with many undesirable side effects, e.g., gynecomastia in men and hirsutism in women. Its use is mainly beneficial in the cirrhotic patient at risk of developing hepatic encephalopathy as a result of hypokalemia and in patients with disease states associated with a mineralocorticoid excess. Dosages depend upon the degree of potassium deficit and the clinical situation. The usual dosage ranges from 50 to 100 mg daily, but dosages as high as 400 mg/day are sometimes justified (16).

Amiloride. Amiloride is a weak diuretic that acts on the luminal membrane of the distal tubule to block sodium reabsorption, is aldosterone independent, and decreases transmembrane potential. It is effective at dosages as low as 5 mg/day, with a maximal response often achieved at 40 mg/day. Dosages exceeding 20 mg/day are usually not recommended (16).

Triamterene. This agent, like amiloride, is aldosterone independent. It is usually combined with a fixed dosage of hydrochlorothiazide (Diazide®, Maxzide®) and is quite popular among clinicians. Like other potassium-sparing diuretics, triamterene should be avoided in patients who are at an increased risk for developing hyperkalemia (16).

Management of selected specific conditions

HYPOKALEMIC PERIODIC PARALYSIS

Carbonic anhydrase inhibitors, such as acetazolamide (250–750 mg/day) or dichlorphenamide are effective in eliminating attacks and in improving interattack weakness, possibly in part by inducing and maintaining a modest metabolic acidosis (297–298). Diazoxide may be useful temporarily (299). Patients should be instructed to avoid vigorous activity as well as high carbohydrate loads to prevent recurrent attacks. Sporadic thyrotoxic hypokalemic paralysis disappears with correction of the thyrotoxicosis. Unlike familial hypokalemia (300), paralytic episodes are improved in the thyrotoxic variety by administration of beta$_2$-adrenergic blockers (301, 302).

BARIUM POISONING

Treatment consists of precipitation of barium in the stomach as insoluble barium sulfate by oral administration of magnesium or sodium sulfate (5–10 g), gastric lavage, support for treatment of respiratory paralysis, and administration of large amounts of potassium parenterally (197). Removal of barium is hastened with saline diuresis and furosemide to increase renal excretion (197). Magnesium sulfate given parenterally may be contraindicated; acute renal failure may have developed from intrarenal precipitation of barium sulfate in a patients intoxicated with barium chloride and given intravenous magnesium sulfate (197).

BARTTER'S SYNDROME

The hallmarks of Bartter's syndrome are hypokalemic alkalosis in association with hyperreninemia, hyperaldosteronism, hyperplasia of the juxtaglomerular apparatus, and a normal blood pressure. These patients exhibit renal potassium and chloride wasting and are resistant to the pressor effects of angiotensin II and norepinephrine (303).

Increased urinary prostaglandin excretion is found in most, but not in all, cases of Bartter's syndrome, indicating that facilitated prostaglandin production represents an epiphenomenon rather than the primary abnormality responsible for the disease (303). Other findings include elevated plasma bradykinin and urinary kallikrein levels; increased urinary excretion of epinephrine and norepinephrine; and a defect in platelet aggregation. Less common associations include hyperuricemia, hypercalcemia, and hypomagnesemia (303); an increase in erythrocyte sodium concentration and an increase in passive sodium permeability of the red blood cell membrane, which is reversible upon correction of hypokalemia (304); a defect in salt reabsorption in the distal tubule (305); contraction of extracellular fluid volume as a result of chloride wasting (306); and decreased rates of urinary calcium excretion (307).

Whether the proximate cause of Bartter's syndrome is a defect in chloride reabsorption at a distal nephron site or a renal potassium-losing abnormality remains unresolved (308, 309).

Familial and congenital forms of renal potassium wasting different from classic Bartter's syndrome have been described in hypokalemic patients with normal plasma renin activity and aldosterone, normal fractional chloride reabsorption, a normal juxtaglomerular apparatus, and evidence of interstitial disease (303, 308) or with hypercalciuria in preterm infants (310). Diuretic or laxative abuse and cystic fibrosis can mimic Bartter's syndrome (311, 312). The hypokalemic alkalosis results from chloride depletion owing to urinary losses in the former, and to high sweat chloride in the latter condition.

The treatment of the hypokalemia of Bartter's syndrome is difficult and includes potassium repletion by administering potassium supplements and decreasing renal potassium wasting with potassium-sparing diuretics and prostaglandin synthetase inhibitors.

Prostaglandin inhibitors, such as indomethacin, correct a number of the manifestations of Bartter's syndrome. Non-steroidal antiinflammatory drugs uniformly decrease plasma renin activity and, to a lesser extent, plasma aldosterone; reverse the diminished pressor response to angiotensin II and norepinephrine; decrease urinary kallikrein excretion; and reverse the defect in platelet aggregation (303). The defect in distal chloride reabsorption and the impaired urinary concentration ability, however, are unresponsive to prostaglandin inhibition (308), and hypokalemia is only partially corrected to a serum potassium concentration of about 3.0 mEq/l (303). Nevertheless, therapy with indomethacin should be tried, as it can be helpful in those patients who can tolerate long-term administration of the drug without gastrointestinal problems. The effects of indomethacin, however, on serum potassium may be transient (313) or minimal (314, 315).

Aldosterone antagonists given alone are of limited value in increasing serum potassium concentration, although their use, in combination with other therapy, may be beneficial in some patients. Long-term use of captopril may also increase serum potassium concentration (316, 317). Amiloride (10–40 mg/day) given alone or concurrent with potassium supplements, prostaglandin synthetase inhibitors, or angiotensin-converting enzyme inhibitors improves serum potassium levels in most patients with Bartter's syndrome (318–320). The combination of propranolol and a potassium-sparing diuretic, or propranolol and indomethacin, has been shown to normalize the serum potassium concentration in some patients (313). Finally, reversal of Bartter's syndrome has been described after renal transplantation in a child with focal and segmental glomerulosclerosis (321).

CHRONIC DIURETIC THERAPY

The issue of diuretic-associated hypokalemia and ventricular ectopy has already been reviewed. The controversy regarding the clinical importance and the need to correct mild hypokalemia is unresolved. No single position is entirely tenable. Whether increased ventricular ectopy is a function of hypokalemia, hypomagnesemia, or both, or of additional yet unknown factors, is uncertain. Convincing evidence that increased ventricular ectopy actually increases mortality in these patients is lacking; and whether potassium repletion prevents cardiac death in this circumstance is entirely unknown.

In patients with acute myocardial infarction, the relationship between hypokalemia and ventricular ectopy is clear, although it may not be one of cause and effect. Hypokalemia may be a marker for high catecholamine levels, which may provoke arrhythmias (277). Nevertheless, the practice of prescribing potassium supplements in this setting is common and should be advocated until some other therapeutic intervention proves superior.

The new more bioavailable preparations of the fixed-dose thiazide/potassium-sparing drug combination have the potential for drug-related adverse effects (322). Nevertheless, in a post-marketing surveillance study of 47,465 patients treated with a fixed-dose combination of hydrochlorothiazide and triamterene, hyperkalemia (defined as a serum potassium concentration exceeding 5.5 mEq/l) was reported in only 0.2% of patients (323). There were no deaths related to hyperkalemia, although several hospitalizations occurred. When hyperkalemia developed, a known contraindication to a potassium-sparing diuretic was usually documented. These included azotemia (serum creatinine $\geq$ 2.5 mg/dL), diabetes mellitus (often with an element of renal insufficiency), and concurrent use of an angiotensin-converting enzyme inhibitor (323).

We believe that prevention and/or correction of mild hypokalemia is not always indicated when chronic therapy with potassium-wasting diuretics is prescribed. Conversely, hypokalemia should be prevented or corrected in specific populations of patients at risk from hypokalemia-induced ventricular arrhythmias. Patients without clinical evidence of organic heart disease do not show an increase in ventricular arrhythmias with mild hypokalemia and need not receive potassium supplements (257, 272). On the other hand, patients who have historical, physical, radiographic, and/or electrocardiographic (including left ventricular hypertrophy) evidence of organic heart disease have shown an increased frequency and severity of ventricular ectopy when treated with diuretics. This risk can be reduced by normalizing the serum potassium concentration despite continuation of diuretics (257, 273, 277). Mild hypokalemia should be prevented and/or corrected to a serum potassium concentration of about 3.5–4.0 mEq/l in these patients (273, 274) and in any patient receiving digitalis preparations. This limit is chosen because the incidence of ventricular tachycardia and ventricular fibrillation decreases sharply when the serum potassium concentration exceeds 3.5 mEq/l in patients with acute myocardial infarction (263). Appropriate replacement of magnesium may need to be provided as well (vide infra).

Prevention or correction of diuretic-induced hypokalemia can also be safely achieved by limiting the dose of diuretic and using the lowest effective dose, restricting sodium intake, and use of at least 60 mEq per day of a potassium supplement. Additional measures may include using a combination of potassium-losing and potassium-sparing diuretics (which also will spare magnesium), addition of an angiotensin-converting enzyme inhibitor or a beta-adrenergic blocking drug, and careful attention to changes in the patient's condition during long-term follow up (274, 324).

EATING DISORDERS

The management of hypokalemia in eating disorders is difficult and may be frustrating because of the low level of patients cooperation. The multifactorial pathogenesis of the hypokalemia often requires a team approach (including psychiatric, dietetic, and social services) of the underlying psychological disorder. Antidepressants may be needed in certain patients. For success, self-motivation is necessary; the patient must make as many decisions as possible. These therapeutic features have been recently emphasized by Lucas (325) and by Oster (212).

MAGNESIUM DEFICIENCY

Magnesium and potassium deficiency often occur concurrently as a result of inadequate intake (total parenteral nutrition, alcoholism), gastrointestinal losses (diarrhea, alcoholism, laxative abuse, malabsorption), or renal losses due to diuretics, antibiotic or cisplatin nephrotoxicity, hyperaldosteronism, postobstructive diuresis, or during the recovery phase of acute tubular necrosis (326). Therefore, in hypokalemic conditions, the serum magnesium concentration should be measured and hypomagnesemia corrected.

The importance of recognizing magnesium deficiency in the etiology of the hypokalemia is that the latter may be refractory to potassium supplementation unless magnesium replacement is also achieved.

Hypomagnesemia (defined by a serum magnesium concentration < 1.25 mEq/l) can be expected in approximately 7–11% of hospitalized patients (exclusive of intensive care unit patients). About 40% of hypokalemic patients may have concurrent low levels of serum magnesium (327, 328).

Both potassium and magnesium depletion have been associated with cardiac arrhythmias, and administration of both potassium and magnesium may be necessary to correct the arrhythmias (260).

Potassium-sparing diuretics appear to reduce renal losses of magnesium. When long-term treatment is considered with diuretics, a combination of hydrochlorothiazide and triamterene has been shown to prevent both hypokalemia and hypomagnesemia (329).

Magnesium deficiency should be prevented, and patients at risk of developing hypomagnesemia because of limited intake and/or increased magnesium losses should be given 10–15 mEq of magnesium daily (330).

Whenever possible, and certainly for mild magnesium depletion, the oral route of replacement is preferable, but may be limited by magnesium-induced diarrhea. Magnesium-containing antacids such as Mylanta®, Maalox®, Riopan®, or Gelusil® contain 7–10 mEq magnesium/5 ml, of which about 6–16% may be absorbed. Thus, a 30 ml qid dose of Maalox TC®, which contains 10 mEq of magnesium per 5 ml, might provide 38 mEq of absorbable magnesium per day (330). Milk of magnesia is a suspension of magnesium oxide containing approximately 3 mEq/ml (330). Magnesium aspartate hydrochloride is also used for oral therapy (331).

When hypomagnesemia is severe and symptomatic, the parenteral route (providing from 30 to 120 mEq/day) may be necessary, providing that renal function is adequate. The standard preparation of magnesium sulfate ($MgSO_4 \cdot 7H_2O$) is usually available in 10% or 50% solutions. One gram of magnesium sulfate provides 98 mg (8.1 mEq) of elemental magnesium (330).

HYPERALDOSTERONISM

The combination of suppressed plasma renin activity (under stimulated conditions) and high aldosterone levels (under conditions of salt loading) represent the best diagnostic indices of primary aldosteronism. Classically, potassium supplements and spironolactone improve the hypokalemia and the hypertension of patients with adenoma, whereas it may not correct the hypertension in patients with bilateral hyperplasia. This distinction, however, is not absolute (308). On the other hand, amiloride may be effective in correcting the hypokalemia in patients with both adrenal adenoma and bilateral hyperplasia (308).

Treatment of hypokalemia in secondary aldosteronism depends on the underlying disease. The syndrome abates after removal of the primary cause such as a renin-secreting tumor, correction of renal artery stenosis in renovascular hypertension, or treatment of malignant hypertension. In instances of nephrotic syndrome or advanced liver disease with ascites, only palliative treatment may be available. In these instances, a combination of therapeutic measures to correct hypokalemia is often necessary. This may include potassium supplementation, administration of potassium-sparing diuretics, correction of potential magnesium deficits, and correction of existing acid-base abnormalities and extracellular fluid volume deficits.

RENAL TUBULAR DISORDERS

Renal tubular acidosis, particularly of the distal variety (Type I), can lead to profound total body potassium deficits as a result of renal potassium losses. In contrast, the hypokalemia associated with proximal renal tubular acidosis is usually mild, unless the patient is treated. The administration of bicarbonate may then lead to severe potassium losses (16). The administration of potassium supplements and potassium-sparing diuretics may be needed to correct the hypokalemia of proximal tubular acidosis because of the large amounts of bicarbonate rejected by the proximal tubule that reach the distal tubule. In these instances, potassium bicarbonate is the replacement salt of choice, but it may be poorly effective in spite of large amounts of supplementation. In distal renal tubular acidosis, doses of 40–80 mEq of potassium per day are sufficient to maintain potassium balance (16).

CISPLATIN AND NEPHROTOXIC ANTIBIOTICS

When cisplatin, large doses of penicillin or penicillin derivatives, or nephrotoxic antibiotics are necessary, a primary concern should be one of prevention of hypokalemia by measuring serum potassium concentration serially and administering potassium supplements if indicated. If hypokalemia develops, the primary treatment is removal of the offending agent. If this is not possible, large amounts of potassium (and sometimes magnesium) supplementation may be necessary, together eventually with potassium-sparing diuretics if renal function is normal. Cisplatin-induced hypokalemia may be prevented by amiloride (332).

INTESTINAL LOSSES OF POTASSIUM

Classically, potassium losses accruing as a result of secretory diarrhea are associated with bicarbonate losses. In these instances, potassium bicarbonate (or an organic anion salt of potassium) replacement is appropriate.

DIALYSIS

Hypokalemia may be a complication of hemodialysis despite the use of a dialysate containing potassium (333). This problem can occur in association with marked predialysis acidosis. With institution of dialysis and rapid correction of the acidosis, a major redistribution of potassium may occur from the extracellular to the intracellular space at a rate exceeding the capacity of potassium transfer across the dialysis membrane to compensate. As a result, severe hypokalemia may develop (148).

Patients taking digoxin have a high rate (39%) of serious arrhythmias during dialysis. Such patients should be dialyzed against a bath containing 3.0–3.5 mEq/l of potassium, and quinidine sulfate (100 mg by mouth, 45 minutes prior to dialysis) should be given to prevent arrhythmia (333).

Hypokalemia has also been observed in 10–19% of patients undergoing acute peritoneal dialysis (334, 335); it is usually moderate and without clinical significance, except in digitalized patients, in whom it may cause severe arrhythmias. Severe hypokalemia may occur with prolonged peritoneal lavage (continuous ambulatory peritoneal dialysis) and may be aggravated by peritonitis, dextrose loading, or correction of acidosis. To correct this problem, 2–4 mEq/l of potassium chloride should be added to dialysis solutions (336).

ACKNOWLEDGMENTS

The authors are grateful to Mrs. Sonia Barton for her skilled secretarial assistance.

REFERENCES

1. Sterns RH, Cox M, Feig PV, Singer I: Internal potassium balance and the control of the plasma potassium concentration. *Medicine* (Baltimore) 60:339–354, 1981.
2. Holbrook JT, Patterson KJ, Bodner JE, Douglas LW: Sodium and potassium intake and balance in adults consuming self-selected diets. *Am J Clin Nutr* 40:786–793, 1984.
3. Fordtran JS: Speculations on the pathogenesis of diarrhea. *Fed Proc* 26:1405–1414, 1967.
4. Field MJ, Berliner RW, Giebisch GH: Regulation of renal potassium metabolism. In: MM Maxwell, CR Kleeman, RG Narins eds, *Clinical Disorders of Fluid and Electrolyte Metabolism*. McGraw-Hill, New York, pp 119–146, 1987.
5. Good DW, Wright FS: Luminal influences on potassium secretion: Sodium concentration and fluid flow rate. *Am J Physiol* 236:F192–F205, 1979.
6. Good DW, Velasquez H, Wright FS: Luminal influences on potassium secretion: Low sodium concentration. *Am J Physiol* 246:F609–F619, 1984.
7. Field MJ, Stanton BA, and Giebisch GH: Influence of ADH on renal potassium handling: A micropuncture and microperfusion study in Brattleboro rats. *Kidney Int* 25:502–511, 1984.
8. Velasquez H, Wright FS, Good DW: Luminal influences on potassium secretion: Chloride replacement with sulfate. *Am J Physiol* 242:F46–F55, 1982.
9. Koeppen BM, Biagi BA, Giebisch GH: Intracellular microelectrode characterization of the rabbit cortical collecting duct. *Am J Physiol* 244:F35–F47, 1983.
10. Schambelan M, Sebastian A, Rector FC Jr: Mineralocorticoid resistant renal hyperkalemia without salt wasting (type II pseudohypoaldosteronism). Role of increased renal chloride reabsorption. *Kidney Int* 19:716–727, 1981.
11. Field MJ, Stanton BA, Giebisch GH: Differential acute effects of aldosterone and dexamethasone and hyperkalemia on distal tubular potassium secretion in the rat kidney. *J Clin Invest* 74:1792–1802, 1984.
12. Stanton B, Pan L, Deetjen H, Guckian V, Giebisch GH: Independent effects of aldosterone and potassium on in-

duction of potassium adaptation in rat kidney. *J Clin Invest* 79:198–206, 1987.
13. Scandling JD, Ornt DB: Mechanism of potassium depletion during chronic metabolic acidosis in the rat. *Am J Physiol* 252:F122–F130, 1987.
14. Field MJ, Giebisch GJ: Hormonal control of potassium excretion. *Kidney Int* 27:279–387, 1985.
15. Katz LD, D'Avella J, DeFronzo RA: Effect of epinephrine on renal potassium excretion in the isolated perfused rat kidney. *Am J Physiol* 247:F331–F338, 1984.
16. Tannen RL: Potassium disorders. In: JP Kokko, RL Tannen, eds, *Fluid and Electrolytes*. WB Saunders, Philadelphia, pp 150–228, 1986.
17. Gabow PA, Peterson LN: Disorders of potassium metabolism. In: RW Schrier, ed, *Renal and Electrolyte Disorders*. Little, Brown, Boston pp 207–249, 1986.
18. Shanes AM: Electrochemical aspects of physiological and pharmacological action in excitable cells: II. The action of potential and excitations. *Pharmacol Rev* 10:165–273, 1958.
19. Saxton CR, Seldin DW: Clinical interpretation of laboratory values. In: JP Kokko, RL Tannen, eds, *Fluids and Electrolytes*. WB Saunders, Philadelphia, pp 3–63, 1986.
20. Brown RS: Nephrology Forum. Extrarenal potassium homeostasis. *Kidney Int* 30:116–127, 1986.
21. Mather A, Mackie NR: Effects of hemolysis on serum electrolyte value. *Clin Chem* 6:223–227, 1960.
22. Skinner SL: A cause of erroneous potassium levels. *Lancet*, 1:478–480, 1961.
23. Romano AT, Young GN Jr: Mild forearm exercise during venipuncture, and its effects on potassium determinations. *Clin Chem* 2:303–304, 1977.
24. Ingram RH Jr, Seki M: Pseudohyperkalemia with thrombocytosis. *N Engl J Med* 267:895–900, 1962.
25. Chumbley LC: Pseudohyperkalemia in acute myelocytic leukemia. *JAMA*, 211:1007–1009, 1970.
26. Wills MR, Fraser ID: Spurious hyperkalemia. *J Clin Pathol* 17:649–650, 1964.
27. Stewart GN, Carrol RJM, Fyffe JA: Familial pseudohyperkalemia: A new syndrome. *Lancet* 2:175–177, 1979.
28. Naparstek Y, Gutman A: Spurious hypokalemia in myeloproliferative disorders. *Am J Med Sci* 288:175–177, 1984.
29. Smith JD, Bia MJ, DeFronzo RA. Clinical disorders of potassium metabolism. In: AI Arieff, RA DeFronzo, eds, *Fluid, Electrolyte and Acid-Base Disorders*. Churchill Livingstone, New York, pp 413–509, 1985.
30. Bia MJ, DeFronzo RA: Extrarenal potassium homeostasis. *Am J Physiol* 240:F257–F268, 1981.
31. Fraley DS, Adler S: Isohydric regulation of plasma potassium by bicarbonate in the rat. *Kidney Int* 9:333–343, 1976.
32. Fraley DS, Adler S: Correction of hyperkalemia by bicarbonate despite constant blood pH. *Kidney Int* 12:354–360, 1977.
33. Malnic G, de Mello-Aires M, Giebisch G: Potassium transport across renal distal tubules during acid-base disturbances. *Am J Physiol* 221:1192–1208, 1971.
34. Perez GO, Oster JR, Vaamonde CA: Serum potassium concentration in acidotic states. *Nephron* 27:233–243, 1981.
35. Adrogué HJ, Chap Z, Ishida T, Field JB: Role of the endocrine pancreas in the kalemic response to acute metabolic acidosis in conscious dogs. *J Clin Invest* 75:798–808, 1985.
36. Adrogué HJ, Lederer ED, Suki WN, Eknoyan G: Determinants of plasma potassium levels in diabetic ketoacidosis. *Medicine* 65:163–172, 1986.
37. Alexander EA, Perrone RD: Regulation of extrarenal potassium metabolism. In: MH Maxwell, CR Kleeman, RG Narins, eds, *Clinical Disorders of Fluid and Electrolyte Metabolism*. McGraw-Hill, New York, pp 105–117, 1987.
38. Santeusano F, Faloona G, Knochel JP, Unger RH: Evidence for a role of endogenous insulin and glucagon in the regulation of potassium homeostasis. *J Lab Clin Med* 81:809–817, 1973.
39. DeFronzo RA, Sherwin RS, Dillingham M, Hendler R, Tamborlane WV, Felig P: Influence of basal insulin and glucagon secretion on potassium and sodium metabolism. *J Clin Invest* 61:472–479, 1978.
40. DeFronzo RA, Felig P, Ferrannini E, Wahren J: Effect of graded doses of insulin on splanchnic and peripheral potassium metabolism in man. *Am J Physiol* 238:E421–E427, 1980.
41. Andres R, Baltzman MA, Cader G, Zierler KL: Effect of insulin on carbohydrate metabolism and on potassium in the forearm of man. *J Clin Invest* 41:108–114, 1962.
42. Cox M, Sterns RH, Singer I: The defense against hyperkalemia: The roles of insulin and aldosterone. *N Engl J Med* 299:525–532, 1978.
43. Martinez R, Rietberg R, Skyler J, Oster JR, Perez GO: Effect of hyperkalemia on insulin secretion. *Experientia*. In press.
44. Goldfarb S, Strunk I, Goldberg M: Paradoxical glucose induced hyperkalemia: Combined aldosterone and insulin deficiencies. *Am J Med* 59:744–750, 1975.
45. Goldfarb S, Cox M, Singer I, Goldberg M: Acute hyperkalemia induced by hyperglycemia: Hormonal mechanisms. *Ann Intern Med* 84:426–432, 1976.
46. Perez GO, Lespier L, Knowles R, Oster JR, Vaamonde CA: Potassium homeostasis in chronic diabetes mellitus. *Arch Intern Med* 137:1018–1022, 1977.
47. Pettit GW, Vick RL, Kastello MD: The contribution of renal and extrarenal mechanisms to hypokalemia induced by glucagon. *Eur J Pharmacol* 41:437–441, 1977.
48. Burton SD, Mandon CE, Ishida T: Dissociation of potassium and glucose efflux in isolated perfused rat liver. *Am J Physiol* 212:261–266, 1967.
49. D'Silva JH: The action of adrenaline on serum potassium. *J Physiol* 82:393–398, 1934.
50. D'Silva JH: The action of adrenaline on serum potassium. *J Physiol* 86:219–228, 1936.
51. DeFronzo RA, Bia M, Birkhead G: The effect of epinephrine on potassium homeostasis. *Kidney Int* 20:83–91, 1981.
52. Rosa RM, Silva P, Young JB, Landsberg K, Brown RS, Rowe JW, Epstein FH: Adrenergic modulation of extrarenal potassium disposal. *N Engl J Med* 302:431–434, 1980.
53. Bia MJ, Tyler K, DeFronzo RA: Regulation of extrarenal potassium homeostasis by adrenal hormones in rats. *Am J Physiol* 242:F641–F644, 1982.
54. Struthers AD, Reid JL: The role of adrenal medullary catecholamines in potassium homeostasis. *Clin Sci* 66:377–382, 1984.
55. Clausen T: Adrenergic control of $Na^+ - K^+$ homeostasis. *Acta Med Scand Suppl* 672:111–115, 1983.
56. Carlsson E, Fellenius E, Lundborg P, Svensson L: Beta-adrenoceptor blockers, plasma potassium, and exercise. *Lancet* 2:424–425, 1978.
57. Arrizabalaga P, Montoliu J, Martinez-Vea A, Andreu L, Lopez Pedret J, Revert L: Increase in serum potassium caused by beta 2-adrenergic blockade in terminal renal failure: Absence of mediation by insulin or aldosterone. *Proc Eur dialysis Transplant Assoc* 20:572–574, 1983.

58. Todd EP, Vick RL: Kalemotrophic effect of epinephrine: Analysis with adrenergic agonists and antagonists. *Am J Physiol* 220:1963–1969, 1971.
59. Williams ME, Rosa RM, Silva P Brown RS, Epstein, FH: Impairment of extrarenal potassium disposal by alpa-adrenergic stimulation. *N Engl J Med* 311:145–149, 1984.
60. Brown MJ, Brown DC, Murphy MD: Hypokalemia from beta 2-receptor stimulation by circulating epinephrine. *N Engl J Med* 309:1414–1419, 1983.
61. Williams ME, Gervino EV, Rosa RM, Landsberg L, Young JB, Silva P, Epstein FH: Catecholamine modulation of rapid potassium shifts during exercise. *N Engl J Med* 312:823–827, 1985.
62. Struthers AD, Reid JL, Whitesmith R, Rodger JC: The effect of cardioselective and nonselective beta-adrenoceptor blockade on the hypokalemic and cardiovascular responses to adrenomedullary hormone in man. *Clin Sci* 65:143–147, 1983.
63. Kjellmer I: The role of K ions in exercise hyperaemia. *Med Exp* (Basel) 5:56–60, 1961.
64. Moreno M, Murphy C, Goldsmith C: Increase in serum potassium resulting from the administration of hypertonic mannitol and other solutions. *J Lab Clin Med* 73:291–294, 1969.
65. Makoff DL, Da Silva JA, Rosenbaum BJ, Levy SE, Maxwell MH: Hypertonic expansion: Acid-base and electrolyte changes. *Am J Physiol* 218:1201–1207, 1970.
66. Makoff DL, Da Silva JA, Rosenbaum BJ: On the mechanism of hyperkalemia due to hyperosmotic expansion with saline or mannitol. *Clin Sci* 41:383–393, 1971.
67. Lim VS, Webster GD: The effect of aldosterone on water and electrolyte composition of incubated rat diaphragms. *Clin Sci* 33:261–270, 1967.
68. Adler S: An extrarenal action of aldosterone on mammalian skeletal muscle. *Am J Physiol* 218:616–621, 1970.
69. DeFronzo RA, Bia M: Extrarenal potassium homeostasis. In: DW Seldin, G Giebisch, eds, *The Kidney: Physiology and Pathophysiology*. Rover Press, New York pp 1179–1206, 1985.
70. Young DB, Jackson TE: Effects of aldosterone on potassium distribution. *Am J Physiol* 243:R526–R-530, 1982.
71. Alexander EA, Levinsky NG: An extrarenal mechanism of potassium adaptation. *J Clin Invest* 47:740–748, 1968.
72. Perez GO, Pelleya R, Oster JR, Kem DC Vaamonde CA: Blunted kaliuresis afrer an acute potassium load in patients with chronic renal failure. *Kidney Int* 24:656–662, 1983.
73. Clausen T, Wang P, Ørskov H, Kristensen O: Hyperkalemic periodic paralysis. Relationships between changes in plasma water, electrolytes, insulin and catecholamines during attacks. *Scand J Clin Lab Invest* 40:211–220, 1980.
74. Wang P, Clausen T: Treatment of attacks in hyperkalemic periodic paralysis by inhalation of salbutamol. *Lancet* 1:221–223, 1976.
75. Smith TW, Butler VP, Haber E, Fozzard H, Marcus FI, Bremmer WF, Schulman IC, Philips A: Treatment of life-threatening digitalis intoxication with digoxin-specific Fab antibody fragments. *N Engl J Med* 307:1357–1362, 1982.
76. Haynes BE, Besser HA, Wightman WD: Oleander tea: Herbal draught of death. *Ann Emerg Med* 14:350–353, 1985.
77. Coggans F: Acute hyperkalemia during lithium treatment of manic illness. *Am J Psych* 137:860–861, 1980.
78. McIvor M, Baltazar R, Beltran J, Mower MM, Wenk R, Lustgarten J, Salmon J: Hyperkalemia and cardiac arrest from fluoride exposure during hemodialysis. *Am J Card* 51:901–902, 1983.
79. Schwartz WB: Potassium and the kidney. *N Engl J Med* 253:601–608, 1955.
80. Adam WR, Dawborn JK: Potassium tolerance in rats. *Aust J Exp Biol Med Sci* 50:757–786, 1972.
81. Fisher KA, Binder HJ, Hayslett JP: Potassium secretion by colonic mucosal cells after potassium adaptation. *Am J Physiol* 231:987–994, 1976.
82. Wright FS, Strieder N, Fowler NB, Giebisch G: Potassium secretion by distal tubule after potassium adaptation. *Am J Physiol* 221:437–448, 1971.
83. Perez GO, Oster JR, Pelleya R, Caralis PV, Kem DC: Hyperkalemia from single small oral doses of potassium chloride. *Nephron* 36:270–271, 1984.
84. Bourgoignie JJ, Kaplan M, Pincus J, Gavellas G, Rabinovitch A: Renal handling of potassium in dogs with chronic renal insufficiency. *Kidney Int* 20:482–490, 1981.
85. Fernandez J, Oster JR, Perez GO: Impaired extrarenal disposal of an acute oral potassium load in patients with end-stage renal disease on chronic hemodialysis. *Mineral Electrolyte Metab* 12:125–129, 1986.
86. Stemmer CL, Perez GO, Oster JR: Impairment of β 2-adrenoceptor stimulated potassium uptake in endstage renal disease. *J Clin Pharmacol* 27:628–631, 1987.
87. Keith NM, Osterberg AE, Burchell HB: Some effects of potassium salts in man. *Ann Intern Med* 16:879–892, 1942.
88. Lawson DH: Adverse reactions to potassium chloride. *Q J Med* 43:433–440, 1974.
89. Shapiro S, Slone D, Lewis GP, Jick H: Fatal drug reactions among medical inpatients. *JAMA* 216:467–472, 1971.
90. Silva P, Brown RS, Epstein FH: Adaptation to potassium. *Kidney Int* 11:466–475, 1977.
91. Kahn T, Kaji DM, Nicolis G, Krakoff LR, Stein RM: Factors related to potassium transport in stable chronic renal disease. *Clin Sci Mol Med* 54:661–666, 1978.
92. Schon DA, Silva P, Hayslett JP: Mechanism of potassium excretion in renal insufficiency. *Am J Physiol* 227:1323–2330, 1974.
93. Schultze RG, Taggart DD, Shapiro H, Pennell JP, Caglar S, Bricker NS: On the adaptation in potassium excretion association with nephron reduction in the dog. *J Clin Invest* 50:1061–1068, 1971.
94. Bourgoignie JJ, Jacob AI, Sallman AL, Pennell JP: Water, electrolyte, and acid-base abnormalities in chronic renal failure. *Semins Nephrol* 1:91–111, 1981.
95. Bourgoignie JJ, Gavellas G, Van Putten V, Berl T: Potassium aldosterone response in dogs with chronic renal insufficiency. *Miner Electrolyte Metab* 11:150–154, 1985.
96. Brown JJ, Fraser R, Lever AF, Robertson JIS, James VHT, McCusker J. Wynn V: Renin, angiotensin, corticosteroids, and electrolyte balance in Addison's disease. *Q J Med* 37:97–118, 1968.
97. Tucker WS, Snell BB, Island DG, Gregg CR: Reversible adrenal insufficiency induced by ketoconazole. *JAMA* 253:2413–2414, 1985.
98. Migeon CJ: Diagnosis and treatment of adrenogenital disorders. In: LJ DeGroot, GF Cahill, L Martini, DH Nelson, WD Odell, JT Potts, E Sternberger, AI Winegrad, eds, *Endocrinology*. Grune & Stratton, New York, pp 1203–1224, 1979.
99. Mulaikal RM, Migeon CJ, Rock JA: Fertility rates in female patients with congenital adrenal hyperplasia due to 21-hydroxylase deficiency. *N Engl J Med* 316:178–182, 1987.
100. Ulick S: Diagnosis and nomenclature of the disorders of the

terminal portion of the aldosterone biosynthetic pathway. *J Clin Endocr Metab* 43:92–96, 1976.
101. Perez G, Siegel L, Schreiner GE: Selective hypoaldosteronism with hyperkalemia. *Ann Intern Med* 76:757–763, 1972.
102. Shambelan M, Sebastian A: Hyporeninemic hypoaldosteronism. *Adv Intern Med* 24:385–405, 1978.
103. DeFronzo RA: Nephrology forum: Hyperkalemia and hyporeninemic hypoaldosteronism. *Kidney Int* 17:118–134, 1980.
104. Findley JW, Adams AH, Raff H: Selective hypoaldosteronism due to endogenous impairment in angiotensin II production. *N Engl J Med* 316:1632–1635, 1987.
105. Perez GO, Oster JR, Vaamonde CA: Renal acidification in patients with mineralocorticoid deficiency. *Nephron* 17:461–473, 1976.
106. Vaamonde CA, Perez GO, Oster JR: Syndrome of aldosterone deficiency. In: J Arruda, N Kurtzman, eds, *Symposium on Disorders of Tubular Transport: Physiological and Clinical Implications. Miner Electrolyte Metab* 5:121–134, 1981.
107. Halperin ML, Bear R, Goldstein MB, Richardson RMA, Robson WLM: Interpretation of the serum potassium concentration in metabolic acidosis. *Clin Invest Med* 2:55–57, 1979.
108. Perez GO, Oster JR, Vaamonde CA: Renal acidosis and renal potassium handling in selective hypoaldosteronism. *Am J Med* 57:809–816, 1974.
109. MacCarthy EP, Frost GW, Strokes GS: Indomethacin-induced hyperkalemia. *Med J Aust* 1:550, 1979.
110. Goldszer R, Coodley EL, Posner MJ, Simons WM, Schwartz AB: Hyperkalemia associated with indomethacin. *Arch Inten Med* 141:802–804, 1981.
111. Nesher G, Zirman A, Hershko C: Hyperkalemia associated with sulindac therapy. *J Rheumatol* 13:1084–1085, 1986.
112. Packer M, Kessler PD, Gottlieb SS: Adverse effects of converting-enzyme inhibition in patients with severe congestive heart failure: Pathophysiology and management. *Postgrad Med J* 62 (Suppl 1):179–182, 1986.
113. Kahan BD: CsA nephrotoxicity. *Transplant and Immunol* 3:1–11, 1987.
114. Stern N, Lusky S, Petrasck D, Jensen G, Eggena P, Lee DBN, Tuck ML: Cyclosporin A-induced hyperreninemic hypoaldosteronism. A model of adrenal resistance to angiotensin II. *Hypertension* 9:III31–III35, 1987.
115. Edes TE, Sunderranjan EV: Heparin-induced hyperkalemia. *Arch Intern Med* 145:1070–1072, 1985.
116. Oberfield SE, Levine LS, Carey RM, Bejar R, New MI: Pseudohypoaldosteronism. Multiple target organ unresponsiveness to mineralocorticoid hormones. *J Clin Endocr Metab* 48:228–234, 1979.
117. Gordon RD: The syndrome of hypertension and hyperkalemia with normal GFR. A unique pathophysiologic mechanism for hypertension. *Clin Exp Pharm Physiol* 13:329–333, 1986.
118. Perez GO, Pelleya R, Oster JR: Renal tubular hyperkalemia. *Am J Nephrol* 2:109–114, 1982.
119. Mehta BR, Cavallo T, Rummers AR, DuBose TD: Hyporeninemic hypoaldosteronism in a patient with multiple mycloma. *Am J Kidney Dis* 4:175–178, 1984.
120. Batlle DC, Arruda JAL, Kurtzman NA: Hyperkalemic distal renal tubular acidosis associated with obstructive uropathy. *N Engl J Med* 304:373–380, 1981.
121. DeFronzo RA, Taufield PA, Black H, McPhedran P, Cooke CR: Impaired renal tubular potassium secretion in sickle cell disease. *Ann Intern Med* 90:310–316, 1979.
122. DeFronzo RA, Cooke CR, Goldberg M, Cox M, Myers, AR, Agus ZS: Impaired renal tubular potassium secretion in systemic lupus erythematosus. *Ann Intern Med* 86:268–271, 1977.
123. Kiley J, Zager P: Hyporeninemic hypoaldosteronism in two patients with systemic lupus erythematosus. *Am J Kidney Dis* 4:39–43, 1984.
124. DeFronzo RA, Goldberg M, Cooke CR: Investigations into the mechanism of hyperkalemia following renal transplantation. *Kidney Int* 11:357–365, 1977.
125. Kokko JP: Site and mechanism of action of diuretics. *Am J Med* 77(5A):11–17, 1984.
126. Dittrich KL, Walls RM: Hyperkalemia: ECG manifestations and clinical considerations. *J Emerg Med* 4:449–455, 1986.
127. Dominguez G, Fozzard HA: Influence of extracellular K^+ concentrations on cable properties and excitability of sheep cardiac Purkinje fibers. *Circ Res* 26:565–574, 1970.
128. Pollen RH, Williams RH: Hyperkalemic neuromyopathy in Addison's disease. *N Engl J Med* 273–278, 1960.
129. Sealey JE, Clark I, Bull MB, Laragh JH: Potassium balance and the control of renin secretion. *J Clin Invest* 49:2119–2127, 1970.
130. Zusman RM, Keiser HR: Regulation of prostaglandin E_2 synthesis by angiotensin II, potassium, osmolality, and dexamethasone. *Kidney Int* 17:277–283, 1980.
131. Landsberg L, Young JB: Fasting, feeding and regulation of the sympathetic nervous system. *N Engl J Med* 298:1295–1301, 1978.
132. Chan YL, Biagi B, Giebisch G: Control mechanisms of bicarbonate transport across the rat proximal convoluted tubule. *Am J Physiol* 242:F532–F543, 1982.
133. Kunau RT Jr, Frick A, Rector FC Jr, Seldin DW: Micropuncture study of the proximal tubular factors responsible for the maintenance of alkalosis during potassium deficiency in the rat. *Clin Sci* 34:223–231, 1968.
134. Levine DZ, Walker T, Nash LA: Effects of KCl infusions on proximal tubular function in normal and potassium depleted rats. *Kidney Int* 4:318–325, 1973.
135. Tannen RL, McGill J: Influence of potassium in renal ammonia production. *Am J Physiol* 231:1178–1184, 1976.
136. Levinsky NG: Management of emergencies VI: Hyperkalemia. *N Engl J Med* 274:1076–1077, 1966.
137. Kassirer JP, Wish JB: Disorders of potassium metabolism. In: WN Suki, SG Massry, eds, *Therapy of Renal Diseases and Related Disorders*. Martinus Njhoff, Boston, pp 63–81, 1984.
138. Calcium Gluconate Injection, USP. Package Insert, Invenex Laboratories, Revision, April, 1984.
139. Worthley LIG, Philips PH: Intravenous calcium salts (letter). *Lancet* 2:149, 1980.
140. Calcium Chloride Injection, USP. Package Insert, Invenex Laboratories, Revision, April, 1983.
141. Knochel JP: Rhabdomyolysis and myoglobinuria. In: WN Suki, G Eknoyan, eds, *The Kidney in Systemic Disease*. John Wiley and Sons, New York, pp 263–284, 1981.
142. Kayexalate brand of sodium polystyrene sulfonate, USP. Package Insert, Winthrop-Beron Laboratories, Revision, January, 1984.
143. Haupt HM, Hutchins GM: Sodium polystyrene pneumonitis. *Arch Intern Med* 142:379–381, 1982.
144. Johnson K, Gardner ME: Kayexalate candy. *Am J Hosp Pharm* 35:1034–1035, 1978.
145. Madias NE, Levey AS: Metabolic alkalosis due to absorption of "nonabsorbable" antacids. *Am J Med* 74:155–158, 1983.

146. Stemmer CL, Oster JR, Vaamonde CA, Perez GO, Rogers AI: Effect of routine doses of antacid on renal acidification. *Lancet* 2:3–6, 1986.
147. Lillemoe KD, Romolo JL, Hamilton SR, Pennington LR, Burdick JE, Williams GM: Intestinal necrosis due to sodium polystyrene (Kayexalate) in sorbitol enemas: Clinical and experimental support for the hypothesis. *Surgery* 101:267–272, 1987.
148. Wiegand CF, Davin TD, Raij L, Kjellstrand CM: Severe hypokalemia induced by hemodialysis. *Arch Intern Med* 141:161–170, 1981.
149. Feig PV, Shook A, Sterns RH: Effect of potassium removal during hemodialysis on the plasma concentration. *Nephron* 27:25–30, 1981.
150. Sherman RA, Hwang ER, Bernholc AS, Eisinger RP: Variability in potassium: Removal by hemodialysis. *Am J Nephrol* 6:284–288, 1986.
151. Brown ST, Ahearn DJ, Nolph KD: Potassium removal with peritoneal dialysis. *Kidney Int* 4:67–69, 1973.
152. Ponce SP, Jennings AE, Madias NE, Harrington JT: Drug-induced hyperkalemia. *Medicine* 64:357–370, 1985.
153. McSherry E: Nephrology forum: Renal tubular acidosis in childhood. *Kidney Int* 20:799–809, 1981.
154. Radó JP, Bános C, Gercsák G, Molnár Z, Pat E, Csabuda M: Glucose-induced hyperkalemia developing in the upright position in captopril-treated hypertensives. *Res Commun Chem Pathol Pharmacol* 38:161–164, 1982.
155. Montoliu J, Revert L: Lethal hyperkalemia associated with severe hyperglycemia in diabetic patients with renal failure. *Am J Kidney Dis* 5:47–48.
156. Sebastian A, Schambelan M, Sutton JM: Amelioration of hyperchloremic acidosis with furosemide therapy in patients with chronic renal insufficiency and type 4 renal tubular acidosis. *Am J Nephrol* 4:287–300, 1984.
157. Perez GO, Lespier LE, Oster JR, Vaamonde CA: Effect of alterations of sodium intake in patients with hyporeninemic hypoaldosteronism. *Nephron* 18:259–265, 1977.
158. Radó JP, Boer P, Dorhout Mees EJ, Simatupang T: "Outpatient hyperkalemia" syndrome in renal and hypertensive patients with suppressed aldosterone production. *J Med* 10:145–157, 1979.
159. Riggs JE, Griggs RC, Moxley III, Lewis ED: Acute effects of acetazolamide in hyperkalemic periodic paralysis. *Neurology* 31:725–729, 1981.
160. Pope HG Jr, Hudson JI, Poskanzer DC, Yurgelum-Todd D: Familial hyperkalemic periodic paralysis and bipolar disorder: A linkage and treatment study. *Biol Psychiat* 19:1449–1459, 1984.
161. Montoliu J, Lens XM, Revert L: Potassium-lowering effect of albuterol for hyperkalemia in renal failure. *Arch Intern Med* 147:713–717, 1987.
162. Vitez TS: Treatment of hyperkalemia with epinephrine. *Anesthesiology* 65:350–351, 1986.
163. Britt BA: Malignant hyperthermia. *Can Anaesth Soc J* 32:666–677, 1985.
164. Ward RJ, Eisele JW, Reay DT, Horton WG: Hemolysis and hyperkalemia complicate malignant hyperpyrexia during anesthetic death. *J Foren Sci* 31:543–545, 1986.
165. Rubin AS, Zablocki AD: Hyperkalemia, verapamil and dantrolene. *Anesthesiology* 66:246–247, 1987.
166. McCarron DA, Elliott WC, Rose JS, Bennet WM: Severe mixed metabolic acidosis secondary to rhabdomyolysis. *Am J Med* 67:905–908, 1979.
167. Smith TW, Wilkerson JT: Suicidal and accidental digoxin ingestion: Report of five cases with serum digoxin level correlations. *Circulation* 44:29–36, 1971.
168. Papadakis MA, Wexman MP, Fraser C, Sedlacek SM: Hyperkalemia complicating digoxin toxicity in a patient with renal failure. *Am J Kidney Dis* 5:64–66, 1985.
169. Gordon RD, Hodsman GP: The syndrome of hypertension and hyperkalaemia without renal failure: Long term correction by thiazide diuretic. *Scot Med J* 31:43–44, 1986.
170. Rastogi S, Bayliss JM, Nascimento L, Arruda JAL: Hyperkalemic renal tubular acidosis: Effect of furosemide in humans and in rats. *Kidney Int* 28:801–807, 1985.
171. Lorch V, Jones FS, Hoersten IR: Treatment of hyperkalemia with exchange transfusion. *Transfusion* 25:390–391, 1985.
172. Morgan DB, Young RM: Acute transient hypokalemia: New interpretation of a common event. *Lancet* 2:751–752, 1982.
173. Lawson DM, Henry DA, Lowe JM, Gray JMB, Morgan HG: Severe hypokalemia in hospitalized patients. *Arch Intern Med* 139:978–980, 1979.
174. Price BJ, Paterson KR, Onyanga-Omara F, Donnelly T, Gray JM, Lawson DH: Record linkage study of hypokalemia in hospitalized patients. *Postgrad Med J* 62:187–191, 1986.
175. Sandor FF, Pickens PT, Crallan J: Variations of plasma potassium concentrations during long-term treatment of hypertension with diuretics without potassium supplements. *Br Med J* 284:711–715, 1982.
176. Gonzalez J, Hogg RJ: Metabolic alkalosis secondary to baking soda treatment of a diaper rash. *Pediatrics* 67:820–822, 1981.
177. Camous JP, Gibelin P, Benoit P, Baudouy M, Varenne A, Morand P: Hypokaliemie avec troubles du rythme graves induite par l'eau de Vichy. *Presse Medicale* 15:2212–2213, 1986.
178. Kreisberg RA: Diabetic ketoacidosis: New concepts and trends in pathogenesis and treatment. *Ann Intern Med* 88:681–695, 1978.
179. Burghen GA, Etteldorf JH, Fisher JN, Kitabchi AQ: Comparison of high-dose and low-dose insulin by continuous intravenous infusion in the treatment of diabetic ketoacidosis in children. *Diabetes Care* 3:15–20, 1980.
180. Robertson CS, Clifton JL, Taylor AA, Grossman RG: Treatment of hypertension associated with head injury. *J Neurosurgery* 59:455–460, 1983.
181. Conci F, Procaccio F, Boselli L: Hypokalemia from beta 2-receptor stimulation by epinephrine (letter), *N Engl J Med* 310:1329, 1984.
182. Dyckner T, Helmers C, Lundman T, Webster PO: Initial serum potassium level in relation to early complications and prognosis in patients with acute myocardial infarction. *Acta Med Scand* 197:207–210, 1975.
183. Nordrehaug JE: Malignant arrhythmias in relation to serum potassium values in patients with an acute myocardial infarction. *Acta Med Scand* 647(5):101–107, 1981.
184. Solomon RJ, Cole AG: Importance of potassium in patients with acute myocardial infarction. *Acta Med Scand* 647(5):87;93, 1981.
185. Whelton PK, Whelton A, Walker WG: Preface. In: *Potassium in Cardiovascular and Renal Medicine*. Marcel Dekker, New York. pp V–VI, 1986.
186. Ingemarsson I, Arulkumaran S, Kottegoda SR: Complications of beta-mimetic therapy in preterm labour. *Aust NZ J Obstet Gynaecol* 25:182–189, 1985.
187. Hendricks SK, Keroes J, Katz M: Electrocardiographic changes associated with ritodrine-induced maternal tachy-

cardia and hypokalemia. *Am J Obstet Gynaecol* 154:921–923, 1986.
188. Moravec MA, Hurlbert BJ: Hypokalemia associated with terbutaline administration in obstetrical patients. *Anesth Analg* 59:917–920, 1980.
189. Haalboom JRE, Deenstra M, Struyvenberg A: Hypokalemia induced by inhalation of fenoterol. *Lancet* 1:1125–1127, 1985.
190. Smith SR, Kendall MJ: Potentiation of the adverse effects of intravenous terbutaline by oral theophylline. *Br J Clin Pharmacol* 21:451–453, 1986.
191. Zierler K: Family periodic paralyses. In: Whelton PK, Whelton A, Walker WG, eds, *Potassium in Cardiovascular and Renal Medicine*. Marcel Dekker, New York, pp 133–142, 1986.
192. Johnson V, Winternitz WW: Hypokalemic periodic paralysis. *South Med J*: 77:1207–1209, 1984.
193. Rüdel·R, Lehmann–Horn F, Ricker K, Küther G: Hypokalemic periodic paralysis: In-vitro investigation of muscle fiber membrane parameters. *Muscle Nerve* 7:110–120, 1984.
194. Blachley J, Knochel JP: Alcohol-induced disturbances in electrolyte and acid-base homeostasis. In: JP Kokko, RL Tannen, eds, *Fluids and Electrolytes*. WB Saunders, Philadelphia, pp 515–547, 1986.
195. Wadstein J, Skude J: Does hypokalemia precede delirium tremens? *Lancet*, 2:549–551.
196. Berning, J: Hypokalemia of barium poisoning (letter). *Lancet*, 1:110, 1975.
197. Wetherill SF, Guarino MJ, Cox RW: Acute renal failure associated with barium chloride poisoning. *Ann Intern Med* 95:187–188, 1981.
198. Stewart DW, Hummel RP: Acute poisoning by a barium chloride burn. *J Trauma* 24:768–70, 1984.
199. Roza O, Berman LB: The pathophysiology of barium: Hypokalemic and cardiovascular effects. *J Pharmacol Exp Ther* 177:433–439, 1971.
200. Lofaso F, Baud FJ, Halna du Fretay X, Bismuth C, Staikowsky F, Sidhom N: Hypokaliemié au cours d'intoxications massives par la chloroquine. *Presse Méd* 16:22–24, 1987.
201. Hall KW, Dobson KE, Dalton JG, Chignone MC Penner SB: Metabolic abnormalities associated with intentional theophylline overdose. *Ann Intern Med* 101:457–462, 1984.
202. Passmore AP, Kondewe GB, Johnston GD: Caffeine and hypokalemia. *Ann Intern Med* 105–468, 1986.
203. Streicher HZ, Gabow PA, Moss AM, Kono D, Kaehny WD: Syndromes of toluene sniffing in adults. *Ann Intern Med* 94:758–762, 1981.
204. Rao TLK, Mathru M, Salem MR, Adel AE: Serum potassium level following transfusion of frozen erythrocytes. *Anesthesiology* 52:170–172, 1980.
205. Hesp R, Chanarin L, Tait CE: Potassium changes in megaloblastic anemia. *Clin Sci Mol Med* 49:77–79, 1975.
206. Weinsier RL, Bacon J, Butterworth CE Jr: Central venous alimentation: A prospective study of the frequency of metabolic abnormalities among medical and surgical patients. *J Parent Extracorp Nutrition* 6:421–425, 1982.
207. Inadomi DW, Kopple JD: Fluid and electrolyte disorders in total parenteral nutrition. In: MM Maxwell, CR Kleeman, RG Narins eds, *Clinicial Disorders of Fluid and Electrolyte Metabolism*. McGraw-Hill, New York pp 945–967, 1987.
208. Squires RD, Huth EJ: Experimental potassium depletion in normal human subjects: I. Relation of ionic intakes to the renal conservation of potassium. *J Clin Invest* 38:1134–1148, 1959.
209. Grim CE, Luft FC, Miller JZ, Meneely JR, Batterbee HD, Hames CG, Dahl LK: Racial differences in blood pressure in Evans County, Georgia. Relationship to sodium and potassium intake and plasma renin activity. *J Chron Dis* 33:87–94, 1980.
210. Knochel JP: Diuretic-induced hypokalemia. *Am J Med* 77(5A):18–27, 1984.
211. Knochel JP: Complications of total parenteral nutrition. *Kidney Int* 27:489–496, 1985.
212. Oster JR: The binge-purge syndrome: A common albeit unappreciated cause of acid-base and fluid-electrolyte disturbances. *South Med J* 80:58–67, 1987.
213. Warren SE, Steinberg GM: Acid-base and electrolyte disturbances in anorexia nervosa. *Am J Psychiat* 136:415–418, 1979.
214. Pope HG Jr, Hudson JI, Yurgelun–Todd D: Anorexia nervosa and bulimia among 300 suburban women shoppers. *Am J Psychiat* 141:292–294, 1984.
215. Mitchell JE, Hatsukami D, Eckert Ed, Pyle RL: Characteristics of 275 patients with bulimia. *Am J Psychiatry* 142:482–485, 1985.
216. Gonzalez JJ, Owens W, Ungaro PC, Werk EE, Wentz PW: Clay ingestion: A rare cause of hypokalemia. *Ann Intern Med* 97:65–66, 1982.
217. Narins RG, Jones ER, Stom MC, Rudnick MR, Bastl CP: Diagnostic strategies in disorders of fluid, electrolyte and acid-base homeostasis. *Am J Med* 72:469–520, 1982.
218. Knochel JP, Reed G: Disorders of heat regulation. In: MH Maxwell, CR Kleeman, RG Narins, eds, *Clinical Disorders of Fluid and Electrolyte Metabolism*. McGraw-Hill, New York, pp 1197–1232, 1987.
219. Koht A, Cane R, Cerullo LJ: Serum potassium levels during prolonged hypothermia. *Intensive Care Med* 9:275–277, 1983.
220. Slavin RE, Dias MA, Saral R: Cytosine arabinoside induced gastrointestinal toxic alterations in sequential chemotherapeutic protocols: A clinical pathologic study of 33 patients. *Cancer* 42:1747–1759, 1978.
221. Davis JE, Scavey PW, Sessions JT Jr: Villous adenomas of the rectum and sigmoid colon with severe electrolyte depletion. *Ann Surg* 155:806–816, 1962.
222. Oster JR, Materson BJ, Rogers AI: Laxative abuse syndrome. *Am J Gastroenterol* 74:451–458, 1980.
223. Krefs GJ, Fortran JS: Diarrhea. In: JS Schleisinger, MH Fortran, eds, *Gastrointestinal Disease*. WB Saunders, Philadelphia, pp 811–829, 1983.
224. Rocher LL, Tannen RL: The clinical spectrum of renal tubular acidosis. *Ann Rev Med* 37:319–331, 1986.
225. Beigelman PM: Potassium in severe diabetic ketoacidosis. *Am J Med* 54:419–420, 1973.
226. Soler NG, Dixon K, Bennett MA, Fitzgerald MG, Malins JM: Potassium balance during treatment of diabetic ketocidosis. *Lancet* 2:665–667, 1972.
227. O'Regan, Carson S, Chesney RW, Drummond KN: Electrolyte and acid-base disturbances in the management of leukemia. *Blood* 49:345–353, 1977.
228. Braden GL, Germain MJ, Fitzgibbons JP: Impaired potassium and magnesium homeostasis in acute tubulointersititial nephritis. *Nephron* 41:273–278, 1985.
229. Montoliu J Botey A, Trilla A, Revert L: Pseudoprimary aldosteronism from the topical application of 9-alpha-fluoroprednisolone to the skin. *Clin Nephrol* 22:262–266, 1984.
230. Gilli M, Cocito D: Hypokalemic myopathy caused by

fluoroprednisolone in a nasal spray. Observations in 2 cases. *Minerva Med* 74:1463–1467, 1983.
231. Cuspidi C, Gelosa M, Moroni E, Sampieri L: Pseudo-Conn's syndrome after habitual ingestion of liquorice. Report on various clinical cases. *Minerva Med* 72:825–830, 1981.
232. Ganguli PC, Mohamed SD: Long-term therapy with carbenoxolone in the prevention of recurrence of gastric ulcer. Natural history and evolution of important side-effects and measures to avoid them. *Scand J Gastroenterology* 65:63–71, 1980.
233. Takeda R, Morimoto S, Uchida K, Nakai T, Miyamoto M, Hashiba T, Yoshimitsu K, Kin KS, Miwa V: Prolonged pseudoaldosteronism induced by glycyrrhizin. *Endocrinol Jpn* 26:541–547, 1979.
234. Wang C, Chan TK, Yeung RT, Coghlan JP, Scoggins BA, Stockigt JR: The effect of triamterene and sodium balance on renin. aldosterone, and erythrocyte sodium transport in Liddle's syndrome, *J Clin Endocrinol Metab* 52:1027–1032, 1981.
235. Keating MJ, Sethi MR, Bodey GP, Samaan NA: Hypocalcemia with hypoparathyroidism and renal tubular dysfunction associated with aminoglycoside therapy. *Cancer* 39:1410–1414, 1977.
236. Zaloga GP, Chernow B, Pock A, Wood B, Zartitsky A, Zucker A: Hypomagnesemia is a common complication of aminoglycoside therapy. *Surg Gynecol Obstet* 158:561–565, 1984.
237. Schwartz JS, Kempa JS, Vasilomanolakis EC, Szidon JP, Coe FL, Jao W: Viomycin-induced electrolyte abnormalities. *Repiration* 40:284–292, 1980.
238. Steiner RW, Omachi AS: A Bartter's-like syndrome from capreomycin, and a similar gentamicin tubulopathy. *Am J Kidney Dis* 7:245–249, 1986.
239. Cheng JT, Kahn T: Potassium wasting and other renal tubular defects with rifampin nephrotoxicity. *Am J Nephrology* 4:379–382, 1984.
240. Brunner FP, Frick PG: Hypokalemia, metabolic alkalosis and hypernatremia to "massive" sodium penicillin therapy. *Br Med J* 4:550–552, 1968.
241. Qian SZ: Gossypol-hypokalaemia interrelationships. *Int J Androl* 8:313–324, 1985.
242. Granerus AK, Jagenurg R, Svanborg A: Kaliuretic effect of L-DOPA treatment in Parkinsonian patients. *Acta Med Scand* 201:291–297, 1977.
243. Dirks JH, Sutton RAL (eds): *Diuretics: Physiology, Pharmacology, and Clinical Use*. WB Saunders, Philadelphia, 1985.
244. Morgan DB, Davidson C: Hypokalemia and diuretics: An analysis of publications. *Br Med J* 2:905–908, 1980.
245. Lemieux G, Beauchemin M, Vinay P, Gougoux A: Hypokalemia during the treatment of arterial hypertension with diuretics. *Can Med Assoc J* 122:905–907, 1980.
246. Kassirer JP, Harrington JT: Diuretics and potassium metabolism. A reassessment of the need, effectiveness and safety of potassium therapy. *Kidney Int* 11:505–515, 1977.
247. Papedemetriou V, Freis ED: In: Whelton PK, Whelton A, Walker WG, eds, *Potassium in Cardiovascular and Renal Medicine*. Marcel Dekker, New York, pp 281–292, 1986.
248. Licht JM, Haley RJ, Pugh B, Lewis SB: Diuretic regimens in essential hypertension: A comparsion of hypokalemic effects, B.P. control and cost. *Arch Intern Med* 143:1694–1699, 1983.
249. Reddy GV, Schamroth L, Schamroth CL: Tall and peaked U-waves in hypokalemia. *Chest* 91:605–67, 1987.

250. Sundam S, Burma DP, Vaish SK: Digoxin toxicity and electrolytes: A correlative study. *Acta Cardiol* (Bruxelles) 38:115–123, 1983.
251. Multiple Risk Factor Intervention Trial Research Group: Multiple risk factor intervention trial: Risk factor changes and mortality results. *JAMA* 248:1465–1477, 1982.
252. Helgeland A: Treatment of mild hypertension: A five year controlled drug trial. The Oslo study. *Am J Med* 69:725–732, 1980.
253. Veterans Administration Cooperative Study Group on Antihypertensive Agents: Effects of treatment on morbidity in hypertension. *JAMA* 213:1143–1152, 1970.
254. Multiple Risk Factor Intervention Trial Research Group: Baseline rest electrocardiographic abnormalities, antihypertensive treatment, and mortality in the Multiple Risk Factor Intervention Trial. *Am J Cardiol* 55:1–15, 1985.
255. Amery A, Birkenhager W, Brixho P, Bulpitt C, Clement D, Deruyttere M, De Schaepdryver A, Dollery C, Fagard R, Forette F, Forte J, Hamdy R, Henry J, Joossens J, Leonetti G, Lund–Johansen P, O'Malley K, Petrie J, Strasser T, Tuomilehto J, Williams B: Mortality and morbidity results from the European Working Party on High Blood Pressure in the Elderly Trial. *Lancet* 1:134–1354, 1985.
256. Holland OB, Nixon JV, Kuhnert L: Diuretic-induced ventricular ectopic activity. *Am J Med* 70:762–768, 1981.
257. Caralis PV, Materson BJ, Perez–Stable E: Potassium and diuretic-induced ventricular arrhythmias in ambulatory hypertensive patients. *Mineral Electrolyte Metab* 10:148–153, 1984.
258. Holland OB: Diuretic-induced ventricular arrhythmias. In: Whelton PK, Whelton A, Walker WG, eds, *Potassium in Cardiovascular and Renal Medicine*. Marcel Dekker, New York, pp 255–260, 1986.
259. Whelton PK: Thiazide-associated cardiac arrhythmias: Experience in the general population. In: Whelton PK, Whelton A, Walker WG, eds, *Potassium in Cardiovascular and Renal Medicine*. Marcel Dekker, New York, pp 269–280, 1986.
260. Hollifield JW: Thiazide diuretics, hypokalemia, and cardiac arrhythmias. *Am J Med* 77(5A):28–32, 1984.
261. Parker M, Gottlieb SS, Blum MA: Immediate and long-term pathophysiologic mechanisms underlying the genesis of sudden cardiac death in patients with congestive heart failure. *Am J Med* 82(3A):4–10, 1987.
262. Cooper WD, Vandenburg MJ: Relationship between initial serum potassium values and cardiac arrhythmias in patients with acute myocardial infarction. In: Whelton PK, Whelton A, Walker WG, eds, *Potassium in Cardiovascular and Renal Medicine*. Marcel Dekker, New York, pp 171–186, 1986.
263. Solomon, RJ: Importance of potassium in the development of arrhythmias during acute myocardial infarction. In: Whelton PK, Whelton A, Walker WG, eds, *Potassium in Cardiovascular and Renal Medicine*. Marcel Dekker, New York, pp 187–192, 1986.
264. Reid JL: Catecholamines and hypokalemia during and after myocardial infarction. In: Whelton PK, Whelton A, Walker WG, eds, *Potassium in Cardiovascular and Renal Medicine*. Marcel Dekker, New York, pp 203–218, 1986.
265. Nordrehaug JE: Association between hypokalemia and cardiac arrhythmias in patients with acute myocardial infarction. In: Whelton PK, Whelton A, Walker WG, eds, *Potassium in Cardiovascular and Renal Medicine*. Marcel Dekker, New York, pp 193–202, 1986.
266. Harrington JT: Are physicians obsessed with the treatment of hypokalemia? In: Whelton PK, Whelton A, Walker WG, eds, *Potassium in Cardiovascular and Renal Medicine*.

Marcel Dekker, New York, pp 479–486, 1986.
267. Harrington JT, Isner JM, Kassirer JP: Our national obsession with potassium. *Am J Med* 73:155–159, 1985.
268. Nordrehaug JE: Hypokalemia, arrythmias, and early prognosis in acute myocardial infarction. *Acta Med Scand* 217:299–306, 1985.
269. Kassirer JD, Harrington JT: Diuretics and potassium metabolism: A reassessment of the need, effectiveness, and safety of potassium therapy. *Kidney Int* 11:105, 1977.
270. Kassirer JP, Harrington JT: Fending off the potassium pushers. *N Engl J Med* 312:785–787, 1985.
271. Flamenbaum W: Diuretic use in the elderly: Potential for diuretic-induced hypokalemia. *Am J Cardiol* 57:38A–43A, 1986.
272. Madias JE, Madias NE, Gavras HP: Nonarrhythmogenicity of diuretic-induced hypokalemia. Its evidence in patients with uncomplicated hypertension. *Arch Intern Med* 144:2171–2176, 1984.
273. Caralis PV, Perez–Stable E: Electrolyte abnormalities and ventricular arrhythmias. *Drugs 31* (Suppl 4):85–100, 1986.
274. Materson BJ, Caralis PV: The continuing controversy over diuretic-associated ventricular ectopy and potassium supplements. In: JB Puschett, A Greenburg, eds, *Diuretics. II: Chemistry, Pharmacology, and Clinical Applications.* Elsevier Science, New York, pp 669–676, 1987.
275. Norwegian Multicenter Study Group: Timolol-induced reduction in mortality and reinfarction in patients surviving acute myocardial infarction. *N Engl J Med* 304:801–807, 1981.
276. Beta-Blocker Heart Attack Trial Research Group: A randomized trial of propranolol in patients with acute myocardial infarction. I. Mortality results. *JAMA* 247:1707–1714, 1982.
277. Tannen RL: Nephrology Forum. Diuretic-induced hypokalemia. *Kidney Int* 28:988–1000, 1985.
278. Stanazek WF, Romankiewicz JA: Current approach to management of potassium deficiency. *Drug Intell Clin Pharm* 19:176–84, 1985.
279. Luce J: Potassium supplementation. *Am J Clin Nutrit* 33:2053–2062, 1980.
280. Griggs RC, Resnick J, Engel WK: Intravenous treatment of hypokalemic periodic paralysis. *Arch Neurol* 40:539–540, 1983.
281. Abramson E, Arky: Diabetic acidosis with initial hypokalemia. *JAMA* 196:401–403, 1966.
282. Schen RJ, Arieli: Administration of potassium by subcutaneous infusion in the elderly patients. *Br Med J* 285:1167–1168, 1982.
283. Bergman N, Vellar I: Potential life threatening variations of drug concentrations in intravenous infusion systems. Potassium chloride, insulin and heparin. *Med J Aust* 2:270–272, 1982.
284. DeFronzo RA, Bia M: Intravenous potassium chloride therapy. *JAMA* 245:2446, 1982.
285. Pullen H, Doig A, Lambie AT: Intensive intravenous potassium replacement therapy. *Lancet* 2:809, 1967.
286. Swales JD: Hypokalemia and the electrocardiogram. *Lancet* 2:1365, 1964.
287. Kosman ME: Management of potassium problems during long term diuretic therapy. *JAMA* 230:743–748, 1974.
288. Schwartz WB, van Ypersele de Strihou C, Kassirer SP: Role of anions in metabolic alkalosis and potassium deficiency. *N Engl J Med* 279:630–639, 1968.
289. McMahon GF, Ryan JR, Akdamar K, Ertan A: Upper gastrointestinal lesions after potassium chloride supplements: A controlled clinical trial. *Lancet* 2:1059–1060, 1982.
290. Skoutakis VA, Acchiardo SR, Wojclechowski N, Carter C, Melikan AP, Cheremos AN: The comparative bioavailability of liquid wax-matrix and the micro-encapsulated preparations of potassium chloride. *J Clin Pharmacol* 25:619–621, 1985.
291. Ben-Ishay D, Engleman K: Bioavailability of potassium from a slow-release tablet. *Clin Pharmacol Therap* 142:250–258, 1973.
292. Morgan TO: Potassium replacement: Supplements or potassium-sparing diuretics? *Practical Therapeutics Drugs* 18:218–25, 1979.
293. Jackson PR, Ramsay LE: Relative potency of spironolactone, triamterence and potassium chloride in thiazide-induced hypokalemia. *Br J Clin Pharmacol* 14:257–263, 1982.
294. Sjoberg WE, Kreisle JE: Hyperkalemia and sudden death during spironolactone (Aldactone) therapy. *Tex State J Med* 58:1022–1024, 1962.
295. Feinfeld DA, Carvounis CP: Fatal hyperkalemia and hyperchloremic acidosis. Association with spironolactone in the absence of renal impairment. *JAMA* 240:1516, 1978.
296. Goulon M, Raphael JC, Simon N: Paralysie périodique familiale avec hypokalémie. Etudes hémodynamiques et métaboliques: Effets favorable de l'acétazolamide. *Rev Neurol (Paris)* 134:655–672, 1978.
297. Dalakas MC, Engel WK: Treatment of "permanent" muscle weakness in familial hypokalemic periodic paralysis. *Muscle Nerve* 6:182–186, 1983.
298. Johnsen T: Effect upon insulin, glucose and potassium concentrations of acetazolamide during attacks of familial periodic hypokalemic paralysis. *Acta Neurol Scand* 56:533–541, 1977.
299. Johnsen T: Trial of the prophylactic effect of diazoxide in the treatment of familial periodic hypokalemia. *Acta Neurol Scand* 56:525–532, 1977.
300. Johnsen T: Treatment of familial periodic hypokalemia with propranolol. *Acta Neurol Scand* 56:613–619, 1977.
301. Yeung RTT, Tse TF: Thyrotoxic periodic paralysis. Effect of propranolol. *Am J Med* 57:584–590. 1974.
302. Conway MJ, Siebel JA, Eaton RP: Thyrotoxicosis and periodic paralysis: Improvement with beta blockade. *Ann Intern Med* 81:332–326, 1974.
303. Tannen RL: Potassium metabolism. In: HC Gonick, eds, *Current Nephrology*, Vol 6. John Wiley and sons, New York, pp 151–186, 1983.
304. Korff JM, Siebens AW, Gill JR: Correction of hypokalemia corrects the abnormalities in erythrocyte sodium transport in Bartter's syndrome. *J Clin Invest* 74:1724–1729, 1984.
305. Uribarri J, Alveranga D, Oh MS, Kukar NK, Carroll HJ: Bartter's syndrome due to a defect in salt reabsorption in the distal convoluted tubule. *Nephron* 40:52–56, 1985.
306. Boer P, Hené RJ, Koomans HA, Nieuwenhuis MG, Geyskens GG, Dorhout Mees EJ: Blood and extracellular fluid volume in patients with Bartter's syndrome. *Arch Intern med* 143:1902–1905, 1983.
307. Rudin A, Sjogren B, Aurell M: Low urinary calcium excretion in Bartter's syndrome. *N Engl J Med* 310:1190, 1984.
308. Tannen RL: Potassium metabolism. In: HC Gonick, eds, *Current Nephrology*, Vol 9. Year Book Medical Publishers, Chicago, pp 359–399, 1986.
309. Garrick R, Ziyadeh FN, Jorkasky D, Goldfarb S: Bartter's syndrome: A unifying hypothesis. *Am J Nephrology* 5:379–384, 1985.
310. Proessmans W, Devlieger H, Van Assche A, Eggermont E, Lÿnen P: Bartter's syndrome in two siblings. Antenatal and

neonatal observation. *Int J Pediat Nephrology* 6:63–70, 1985.
311. Jamison RL, Ross JC, Kempson RL, Sufit CR: Surreptitious diuretic ingestion and pseudo-Bartter's syndrome. *Am J Med* 73:142–147, 1982.
312. Davidson AG, Snodgrass GJA: Cystic fibrosis mimicking Bartter's syndrome. *Acta Paediatr Scand* 72:781–783, 1983.
313. Favre H, Glasson P, Flory ED, Dray F, Vallotton MB: Bartter's syndrome: Recurrence in the course of a treatment inhibiting prostaglandin synthesis. *Schweiz Med Wochenshcr* 109:142–147, 1979.
314. Barbour GL, Day JO: Asymptomatic Bartter's syndrome. *Southern Med J* 71:1341–1344; 1349, 1978.
315. Kornerup HJ, Pedersen EB, Petersen VP: Bartter's syndrome without hyperplasia of the juxtaglomerular apparatus, treated with indomethacin. *Acta Med Scand* 204:235–239, 1978.
316. Hené RJ, Koomans HA, Boer P, Dorhout Mees EJ: Long-term treatment of Bartter's syndrome with captopril. *Br Med J* 285:695, 1982.
317. Hené RJ, Koomans HA, Dorhout Mees EJ, Stolps AVD, Verhoef GEG, Boer P: Correction of hypokalemia in Bartter's syndrome by enalapril. *Am J Kidney Dis* 9:200–205, 1983.
318. Griffing GT, Komanicky P, Aurecchia SA, Sindler BH, Melby JC: Amiloride in Bartter's syndrome. *Clin Pharmacol Ther* 31:713–718, 1982.
319. Griffing GT, Aurecchia SA, Sindler BM, Melby JC: The effect of amiloride on the renin-aldosterone system in primary aldosteronism and Bartter's syndrome. *J Clin Pharmacol* 22:505–512, 1982.
320. Griffing FT, Melby JC: The therapeutic use of a new potassium-sparing diuretic, amiloride, and a converting enzyme inhibitor, MK-421, in preventing hypokalemia associated with primary and secondary hyperaldosteronism. *Clin Exper Hypertension* 5A:779–801, 1983.
321. Blether SL, Van Wyk JJ, Lorentz WB, Jennnette JC: Reversal of Bartter's syndrome by renal transplantation in a child with focal, segmental glomerular sclerosis. *Am J Med Sci* 289:31–36, 1985.
322. Materson BJ: Diuretic-associated hypokalemia. *Arch Intern med* 145:1966–1967, 1985.
323. Hollenberg NK, Bannon JA: The PACT Study: Postmarketing surveillance in 47,465 patients treated with Maxzide (triamterene/hydrochlorothiazide). *Am J Med* 80(4A):30–36, 1986.
324. Robertson JIS: Diuretics, potassium depletion, and the risk of arrhythmias. *Eur Heart J* 5A:25–28, 1984.
325. Lucas AR: "Pigging out." *JAMA* 247:82, 1982.
326. Whang R: Magnesium deficiency: Pathogenesis, prevalence and clinical implication. *Am J Med* 82(3A):24–29, 1987.
327. Whang R, Oei TO, Aikawai JK, Watanabe A, Vannatta J, Fryer A, Markanich M: Predictors of clinical hypomagnesemia. Hypokalemia, hypophosphatemia, hyponatremia, and hypocalcemia. *Arch Intern med* 144:1794–1796, 1984.
328. Boyd JC, Bruns DE, Wills MR: Frequency of hypomagnesemia in hypokalemic states. *Clin Chem* 29:178–179, 1983.
329. Davidov ME, Becker FE, Hollifield JW: Serum magnesium and potassium levels in hypertensive patients after a therapeutic switch from hydrochlorothiazide plus a potassium supplement to Maxzide. *Am J Med* 82(3A):48–51, 1987.
330. Oster JR: Magnesium. *Southern Med J* 78:1111–1120, 1985.
331. Dychner T: Potassium/magnesium depletion: Is your patient at risk of sudden death? *Am J Med* 82(3A):52, 1987.
332. Jureidini KF: Prevention of cis-platinum nephrotoxicity with amiloride hydrochloride. *Second Asian Pacific Congress Nephrology*, p 41, 1983.
333. Morrison J, Michelson EL, Brown S, Morganroth J: Mechanism and prevention of cardiac arrhythmias in chronic hemodialysis patients. *Kidney Int* 17:811–819, 1980.
334. Vaamonde CA, Michael UF, Metzger RA, Carroll KE: Complications of acute peritoneal dialysis. *J Chronic Dis* 28:637–659, 1975.
335. Valk TW, Swartz RD, Hsu CH: Peritoneal dialysis in acute renal failure: Analysis of outcome and complications. *Dial Transpl* 9:48–53, 1980.
336. Spital AH, Sterns RH: Potassium supplementation via the dialysate in continued ambulatory peritoneal dialysis. *Am J Kidney Dis* 6:173–176, 1985.

CHAPTER 5

Disorders of Calcium Metabolism

AARON HALABE & ROGER A.L. SUTTON

GENERAL CONSIDERATIONS

The adult human body contains 1.3 kg of calcium of which 99% is contained in bones and teeth, 1% in cells of soft tissue, and 0.15% in the extracellular fluid (1). The bone calcium is in the form of hydroxyapatite crystals, and the exchange of calcium between bone and extracellular fluid occurs by two mechanisms: bone turnover, which is concerned with replacement and remodeling of bone and involves coupled osteoclastic resorption and osteblastic deposition, and homeostatic equilibration, which is concerned with the regulation of the plasma calcium level (2, 3). The normal total plasma calcium concentration is 4.5–5.1 mEq/l (9–10.2 mg/dl). Of the total calcium 40–43% is bound to plasma protens (mainly albumin), 5–10% is combined with anions such as citrate and phosphate to form nonionized complexes, and the remaining 40–50% is free ionized calcium. Only this last fraction is physiologically active. In addition, a small amount of calcium is also bound to serum globulins.

Factors such as blood pH, serum sodium concentration, and abnormalities of serum proteins can alter the relationship between total and ionized calcium levels. An increase in pH increases the binding of calcium to albumin (4), and in addition a rise in the plasma bicarbonate concentration increases the formation of calcium bicarbonate complexes. The combined effect is a change in ionized calcium of 0.08 mEq/l (0.16 mg/d1) for each 0.1 U change in pH (5, 6). The serum sodium concentration may affect the binding of calcium to albumin, as described by Walser et al. (7). A serum sodium concentration less than 120 mEq/l causes an increase in protein-bound calcium, whereas a sodium concentration greater than 150 mEq/l causes a decrease in the protein-bound calcium. Abnormal serum proteins with increased affinity for calcium occur in certain IgG myeloma patients (8). Furthermore, in severe hypoalbuminemia associated with the nephrotic syndrome, albumin may have an increased affinity for calcium (9). At any given ionized calcium concentration in the plasma, a change in serum proten levels alters the total calcium concentration, as in conditions of hemoconcentration and venous stasis (10) and with changes in posture (11).

CALCIUM HOMEOSTASIS

The concentration of ionized calcium is normally maintained within a narrow range (2–2.5 mEq/l or 4–4.9 mg/dl) through the actions of PTH, vitamin D metabolites, and possible calcitonin in their three target organs: the skeleton, the kidney, and the small intestine (Figure 1). PTH is secreted by the parathyroid glands in response to a fall in the serum ionized calcium level and protects against hypocalcemia by producing the release of skeletal mineral (12, 13) and by direct actions on the kidney to enhance tubular reabsorption of calcium (14–18) and to increase the synthesis of 1,25-dihydroxyvitamin D_3 (calcitriol), which in turn promotes intestinal calcium absorption (19).

Vitamin D derived from the diet or synthesized in the skin is metabolized by the liver to 25-hydroxy vitamin D_3 (calcidiol), the major circulating form of vitamin D. Calcidiol has a half-life of 20–25 days and its synthesis is not tightly regulated. The plasma level reflects the body stores of vitamin D. Calcidiol is further metabolized by the enzyme 25-l-alpha hydroxylase in the kidney to calcitriol, the most active form of vitamin D. This hormone increases the absorption of calcium and phosphate in the gut (20, 21) and, together with PTH, enhances bone resorption (22). The plasma level of this hormone is tightly regulated, and the main stimulators of its production are PTH and a low serum phosphorus level, while hypercalcemia inhibits its production. Patients with renal failure have a decreased activity of the enzyme 25-1-alpha-hydroxylase.

Calcitonin inhibits bone resorption (23, 24) but has no proven role in normal homeostasis or in protecting against hypercalcemia in humans. On a normal dietary calcium intake of 800 mg per day in the adult, the fecal calcium is about 600 mg. Thus, the daily net absorption is about 200 mg (being equal to the urinary calcium in an individual in metabolic balance), and the fractional absorption is about 25% of the intake (Figure 1). The fractional

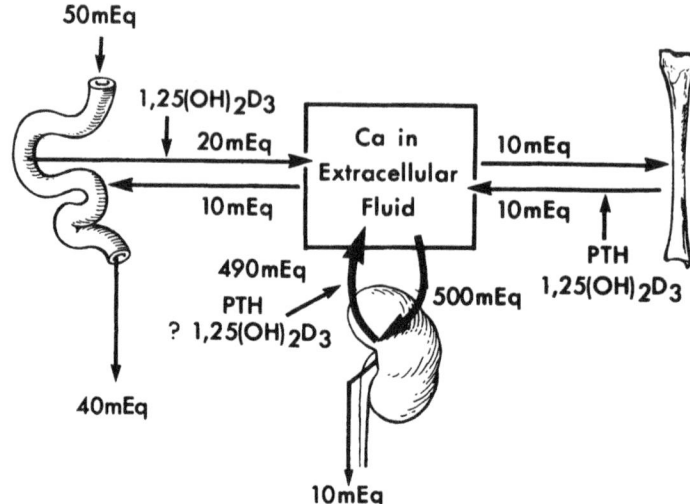

Figure 1. Major sites of calcium exchanges between the extracellular fluid and the bone, kidney, and intestine. Approximate size of fluxes are shown in mEq/day as well as the sites of action of PTH and 1,25-(OH)$_2$D$_3$. Modified from Kanis JA, Journal of Bone Joint Surgery, 64B:542, 1982. First published in BM Brenner, FC Rector, eds, WB Saunders, Philadelphia, 1986. Figure 15–1).

absorption increases with a reduction in intake (25), in part as a result of increased calcitriol production (26).

HYPERCALCEMIA

The diagnosis of hypercalcemia has been increasing in recent years, probably as a result of the use of automated methods for measuring serum calcium. The incidence of hypercalcemia is reported to be in the range of 0.3–5% in the general population (27). Hypercalcemia may be masked in the presence of hypoalbuminemia. If facilities are available, the determination of the ionized calcium level can be used to confirm the presence of true hypercalcemia.

Parfitt (28) has divided hypercalcemia into two pathophysiologic types: equilibrium and disequilibrium hypercalcemia. The first type is exemplified by chronic hyperparathyroidism, in which the plasma calcium concentration is stable, bone resorption may be normal, and the hypercalcemia is not due to a net increase in skeletal calcium release. By contrast, in disequilibrium hypercalcemia as (exemplified by multiple myeloma or metastatic carcinoma), there is a net increase in bone resorption. The plasma calcium level in these cases is unstable and tends to show a progressive rise.

Disequilibrium hypercalcemia can also occur in severe hyperparathyroidism with gross bone resorption, or if renal calcium excretion is reduced due to dehydration or thiazide diuretics. A third variety of hypercalcemia, which may be called *hyperabsorptive hypercalcemia*, shares features of both the equilibrium and disequilibrium types and may be associated with vitamin D intoxication, sarcoidosis, or the milk alkali syndrome. In these conditions there is an increase in intestinal calcium absorption, and tubule calcium reabsorption may be increased as a result of alkalosis, volume depletion, or possibly the direct action of vitamin D.

Causes of hypercalcemia (Table 1)

MALIGNANCY

Malignancy is the commonest cause of hypercalcemia in hospitalized patients. Malignant hypercalcemia has been described in association with many different tumours. It can be divided into three major groups: patients with solid tumors with or without bone metastases and patients with hematologic malignancies.

In patients with solid tumors without bone metastases, the hypercalcemia is due to the production by tumor cells of a circulating mediator of osteolytic bone resorption. This clinical syndrome is known as *humoral hypercalcemia of malignance* (HHM). These patients have abnormalities of renal tubular function resembling those of primary hyperparathyroidism, including increased cyclic AMP production (29), and inhibition of phosphorus reabsorption. These patients generally have low serum calcitriol levels, unlike the normal or high levels of primary hyperparathyroidism. However, patients with humoral hypercalcemia of malignancy do not have renal tubular bicarbonate wasting, as may be found in primary hyperparathyroidism (30), and the presence of hyperchloremic acidosis is more suggestive of hypercalcemia from a parathyroid origin.

The mediators of humoral hypercalcemia of malignancy may include tumor growth factors (TGF) and PTH-like

Table 1. Etiology of hypercalcemia

A. *Common Causes*
   Primary hyperparathyroidism (in outpatients)
   Malignancy (in inpatients)

B. *Infrequent Causes*
   Chronic renal failure (secondary and tertiary hyperparathyroidism)
   Hyperthroidism
   Sarcoidosis
   Recovery phase of acute renal failure
   Immobilization

C. *Rare Causes*
   Familial hypocalciuric hypercalcemia
   Other granulomatous diseases
   Adrenal insufficiency
   Pheochromocytoma
   Islet cell tumors with pancreatic cholera syndrome

D. *Drugs*
   Thiazides
   Vitamin-D intoxication
   Vitamin A
   Lithium

factors (31). The hypercalcemia of breast carcinoma is usually associated with extensive bone destruction. In these patients, an impairment of renal tubular calcium excretion has recently been reported to play a major role in potentiating the hypercalcemia associated with increase osteoclastic bone resorption (32).

Hematologic malignancies are frequently associated with hypercalcemia, particularly multiple myeloma and T-cell lymphoma. About 25% of patients with multiple myeloma develop hypercalcemia. The causes of hypercalcemia include local factors produced by myeloma cells, for example, osteoclastic activating factor (31), but renal mechanisms, including an impaired glomerular filtration rate, may also play an important role. Patients with HTLV Type I-associated lymphoma may have increased calcitriol levels (33). In this disease hypercalcemia is not usually associated with a reduced glomerular filtration rate, suggesting that osteotropic factors or local production of calcitriol may be the cause of the hypercalcemia. Recently it has been shown that a polypeptide with amino acid sequence homologies with PTH has a role in the syndrome of HHM (34, 35). The possibility of the simultaneous occurrence of a parathyroid adenoma and malignancy should be kept in mind (36-40). Singer et al. found that 4.4% of 105 patients with malignancy and hypercalcemia had primary hyperparathyroidism (41).

PRIMARY HYPERPARATHYROIDISM

Primary hyperparathyroidism may be associated with adenoma, hyperplasia, or carcinoma of the parathyroid glands and may be sporadic, familial, or hereditary. The familial form of primary hyperparathyroidism is autosomal dominant, with a high degree of penetrance. It may manifest itself as primary parathyroid hyperplasia alone or as a part of the multiple endocrine neoplasia (MEN) syndromes.

In Type I MEN, primary hyperparathyroidism occurs in 95% of the patients and is associated with pituitary, pancreatic, adrenal, or thyroid adenomas. In Type II MEN, primary hyperparathyroidism is present in 20-30% of the patients who usually present with medullary carcinoma of the thyroid and/or pheochromocytoma. Primary hyperparathyroidism also occurs in association with other systemic diseases such as sarcoidosis (42, 43), cancer (44, 45), meduallry sponge kidney (46, 47), Hashimoto's disease, thyrotoxicosis, and Cushing's syndrome.

Hypercalcemia is the usual biochemical clue in primary hyperparathyroidism, but it is not invariably present. Normocalcemic primary hyperparathyroidism, may occur because the end-organ responsiveness of the skeleton to PTH is blunted, for example, because of coexisting vitamin D deficiency (48-51), magnesium deficiency (52), pancreatitis (53), renal failure, or possibly hypothyroidism (54). Determination of the plasma ionized calcium level may be helpful in identifying some cases of normocalcemic primary hyperparathyroidism (55).

The laboratory findings of hypercalcemia, hypophosphatemia, and a normal or high alkaline phosphatase in the presence of a high PTH and/or elevated urinary cyclic AMP excretion (expressed per unit of GFR) in a patient with or without nephrolithiasis or nephrocalcinosis and a normal or high calcitriol (56, 57) strongly suggest the diagnosis of primary hyperparathyroidism. Preoperative localization of the enlarged glands can be achieved by noninvasive methods such as ultrasound examination of the neck with high resolution (58, 59) or double tracer subtraction scanning of the neck (60). In surgical series of patients with primary hyperparathyroidism, about 80% have an adenoma and about 20% have hyperplasia of all four glands.

The treatment of choice for adenoma is removal by an experienced surgeon, who will usually identify all the other glands (61). Subtotal parathyroidectomy is performed for hyperplasia. Persisting hypercalcemia after unsuccessful surgical exploration necessitates reevaluation and preoperative localization by cervical and thoracic venous sampling for PTH measurement, together with arteriography (62, 63) and computed tomography (64, 65).

FAMILIAL HYPOCALCIURIC HYPERCALCEMIA (FHH)

This entity is inherited as an autosomal dominant (66-68). It is characterized by early onset of hypercalcemia, a tendency to hypermagnesemia, normal serum phosphorus, normal urinary concentrating ability, reduced fractional urinary calcium excretion, and a lack of clinical manifestations such as renal calculi, azotemia, or bone disease. Indices of parathyroid function including PTH level and urinary cyclic AMP excretion indicate that the glands are not suppressed. Parathyroid surgery should not be undertaken, except in patients with severe complications, when total parathyroidectomy should be performed (69).

THIAZIDE DIURETICS

Thiazides are the only diuretic agents that cause hypocalciuria. Under certain circumstances this may contribute to the production of hypercalcemia. In addition, the natriuresis causes extracellular fluid contraction and increased serum levels of protein. Thiazide-induced hypercalcemia is common in patients with primary hyperparathyroidism or increased bone turnover of other causes. Hypercalcemia in response to these agents in normal subjects without underlying disorders of calcium metabolism is partly related to hemoconcentration and elevation of protein-bound calcium (70). Thiazides also have a direct effect on bones and potentiate the skeletal action of PTH. If a patient who is receiving thiazide diuretics develops hypercalcemia, the diuretics should be stopped and an evaluation for an underlying cause of the hypercalcemia, especially primary hyperparathyroidism, should be undertaken.

HYPERVITAMINOSIS D

Vitamin D intoxication is most commonly iatrogenic, occurring in the course of treatment with large doses of vitamin D for hypoparathyroidism (71), vitamin D-resistant rickets, and osteomalacia. In this condition the serum level of calcitriol is normal (72), and the calcidiol level is high. This may account for the long persistence of the intoxication, since the half-life of calcidiol is 10–20 days (73), compared with less than 24 hours for calcitriol.

SARCOIDOSIS AND OTHER GRANULOMATOUS DISORDERS

Hypercalcemia has been noted in 1–20% of patients with sarcoidosis. Hypercalciuria is even more frequent than hypercalcemia. There is intestinal hyperabsorption of calcium, hypersensitivity to sunlight and to exogenous vitamin D, and suppression of PTH. The metabolic abnormality is responsive to glucocorticoids. It is now known that the cause of hypercalcemia in sarcoidosis and some other granulomatous disorders is the unregulated nonrenal production of calcitriol, as in alveolar macrophages, and it is likely that the granulomatous tissue may be the source of the hormone (74–77).

MILK ALKALI SYNDROME

This entity is characterized by hypercalcemia, alkalosis, and renal impairment, and it occurs in acute, subacute, and chronic forms. Currently it is most often related to the ingestion of antacids containing calcium carbonate. This syndrome can be accompanied by nephrocalcinosis and renal insuffuciency. Calcium carbonate alone can produce the syndrome.

OTHER ENDOCRINE CAUSES

In hyperthyroidism, some authors report an incidence of hypercalcemia of 15–20% and even 50% as determined by ionized calcium determinations (79, 81), but severe hypercalcemia is uncommon. The hypercalcemia is caused by direct stimulation of bone resorption by the thyroid hormone (82–84). It may respond to treatment with propranolol. Primary hyperparathyroidism may coexist with hyperthyroidism (85).

Pheochromocytoma may be associated with hypercalcemia, even in the absence of primary hyperparathyroidism (86, 87). The hypercalcemia disappears after removal of the pheochromocytoma. Adrenal insufficiency may be associated with hypercalcemia (87, 88), which is partly attributable to hemoconcentration and an increase in protein-bound calcium. Acromegaly has been reported to be associated with hypercalcemia (90). Patients with acromegaly may have high intestinal calcium absorption (91) and enhanced bone resorption (92), probably due to elevated calcitriol levels (93). Hypercalcemia in patients with acromegaly may also be due to parathyroid hyperplasia as a part of the syndrome of multiple endocrine neoplasia Type I. Islet cell tumors of the pancreas producing the pancreatic cholera syndrome may be associated with hypercalcemia (94).

VITAMIN A INTOXICATION

Hypercalcemia due to vitamin A intoxication is associated with increased bone resorption, modeling defects in the long bones, periosteal calcification, nephrocalcinosis, and renal insufficiency (95). Although vitamin A enhances PTH secretion (96), PTH excess has not been documented in human vitamin A intoxication. Hypercalcemia in this entity responds to glucocorticoid therapy (95).

Signs and symptoms of hypercalcemia

The signs and symptoms of hypercalcemia are listed in Table 2. Symptoms are influenced by the rate of change in the ionized calcium in the ECF or may be caused by the underlying disease in nonparathyroid hypercalcemia.

The hypercalcemic patient can present without symptoms or with anorexia, nausea, vomiting, constipation, polyuria, nocturia, and hypertension. Other symptoms may include emotional lability, depression, neuromuscular weakness, somnolence, confusion, and even coma.

Patients may have signs of gout, pseudogout, or chondrocalcinosis, especially patients with hypercalcemia of parathyroid origin. Soft-tissue calcifications in the cornea may be present in hypercalcemia, especially when accompanied by high serum phosporus levels as in renal failure. Hypertension may be present in acute and chronic hypercalcemia, and may be reversible after correction of the hypercalcemia.

Diagnostic evaluation

The diagnosis of hypercalcemia should be based on at least two determinations of the serum calcium level. In addition, serum phosphorus and protein levels should be determined. The urinary excretion of calcium, phosphorus,

Table 2. Signs and symptoms of hypercalcemia

Renal
  Impaired urinary concentration
  Polyuria
  Nephrocalcinosis and nephrolithiasis
  Acute or chronic renal failure

Gastrointestinal
  Anorexia, nausea, vomiting
  Constipation, pancreatitis, peptic ulcer

Neurologic
  Personality changes
  Psychiatric disturbances
  Disorientation
  Confusion, muscle weakness, myopathy

Cardiac
  Shortening of QT interval
  Vertricular arrhythmias
  Complete heart block
  Hypertension
  Synergistic digitalis effect

Extraskeletal calcification

and cyclic AMP may be helpful in the differential diagnosis of hypercalcemia.

Determination of urinary calcium and the calcium to creatinine clearance ratio are important in identifing the entity of familial hypocalciuric hypercalcemia. Calcium to creatinine clearance ratios below 0.01 are usual in patients with FHH, whereas in primary hyperparathyroidism values are usually greater than 0.01. Serum PTH is not elevated in the majority of cases of FHH and the tendency to mild hypermagnesemia may be another useful clue. Hypercalciuria in the presence of renal failure suggests sarcoidosis (43).

The association of hypercalcemia with lymphadenopathy, an elevated ESR, and slight abnormalities in the liver function in the absence of malignancy should raise the possibility of sarcoidosis. In these cases, serum PTH should be low unless primary hyperparathyroidism coexists. Serum calcitriol levels are increased in hypercalcemic sarcoidosis, and may be normal or increased in primary hyperparathyroidism.

Vitamin D intoxication should be considered as a cause of hypercalcemia in patients with hypercalciuria and a low concentration of PTH. The finding of a high serum calcidiol level confirms the diagnosis. In this situation cessation of vitamin D will lead to reveresal of the hypercalcemia, although this may be slow.

Patients who develop hypercalcemia because of thiazide administration may be identified by a proper drug history. The drug should be stopped and the patient followed, since the possibility of underlying primary hyperparathyroidism exists and the patient should be investigated.

Parathyroid activity is best assessed with one of the newer PTH assays. It can also be estimated by determining the tubular reabsorption of phosphorus (TRP or TMP/GFR), provided renal function is normal. High values of phosphate reabsorption exceeding 85% are incompatible with primary hyperparathyroidism. Lower values may also be found in malignant hypercalcemia. The presence of hyperchloremic acidosis may also be of diagnostic value in differentiating between patients with hyperparathyroidism and those with hypercalcemia from other causes.

Before good PTH assays became available, determination of the urinary cyclic AMP/GFR ratio was useful in making the diagnosis of primary hyperparathyroidism (97). Patients with primary hyperparathyroidism usually have increased or normal serum calcitriol levels. In the presence of renal failure, however, serum levels may actually be low (98, 99).

Suppression tests involving measurements of PTH or urinary cyclic AMP after the infusion of calcium (100), or of urinary cyclic AMP after an oral calcium load (101), may provide useful information. In the past, a steroid suppression test was sometimes employed (102). Most patients with hyperparathyroidism remain hypercalcemic despite oral prednisone or hydrocortisone. Provocation tests including phosphate depletion or thiazide administration have been advocated. High-resolution ultrasound examination of the neck, and double tracer subtraction scaning are noninvasive methods that may be employed for imaging the enlarged parathyroid glands (58–60).

The x-ray findings support the diagnosis of hyperparathyroidism but, in the case of bone changes, rarely present, include subperiosteal bone resorption, erosion of distal phalangeal tufts or distal ends of clavicles, nephrolithiasis (radioopaque), and nephrocalcinosis. A chest x-ray should be performed in every patient with hypercalcemia and may provide evidence suggesting lung cancer, lymphome or sarcoidosis, or parathyroid cyst.

Additional tests such as serum and urine electrophoresis, and thyroid and adrenal function tests may help to reveal the cause of hypercalcemia.

Therapy (Table 3)

The therapy of hypercalcemia depends on the severity and clinical condition of the patient, as well as the underlying cause. Severe (disequilibrium) hypercalcemia requires IV fluids, and other measures such as furosemide, phosphate, calcitonin, or mithramycin, while mid hypercalcemia may not need therapy. We will first review the modalities that are used to treat hypercalcemia and then consider the management of hypercalcemia due to some specific causes.

TREATMENT MODALITIES

Extracellular fluid volume expansion

The acutely ill patient should be admitted to the hospital, where serum electrolytes, calcium, magnesium, and phosphorus, as well as renal function tests, may be closely monitored. Initial treatment is aimed at replacing fluid and electrolyte losses, promoting urinary calcium excretion, and decreasing calcium influx into the extracellular fluid from the bones and intestine. The administration of saline

Table 3. Treatment of hypercalcemia

Therapy	Mechanism of action	Dose	Side effect	Contraindication
Saline	↑ UCaE	IV 2–3/l every 3–4 hrs	Pulmonary edema, hypokalemia	Congestive heart failure, hypertension,
Furosemide	↑ UCaE	IV 100 mg/hr	Volume depletion, hypokalemia, hypomagnesemia	Renal insufficiency
Intravenous phosphate	↑ Ca deposition into bone	1–2 mM/kg every 6–8 hrs	Hypocalemia, soft-tissue calcification, hypotension	Renal insufficiency, hyperphosphatemia
Oral phosphate		1–1.5 g/day in divided doses	Diarrhea, GI upset hypotension, soft-tissue calcif.	Renal insufficiency
Mithramycin	↓ Bone resorption	IV 25 µg/kg	Hemorrhage, hepatotoxicity, thrombocytopenia	Renal insufficiency, bleeding disorder, liver impairment, nausea & vomiting
Calcitonin	↓ Bone resorption	1–5 U/kg IM every 12–24 hr	Nausea, vomiting, allergy, resistance	Thrombotic allergy
Cortisone	↓ Bone resorption	150 mg/24 hr	Hypocalcemia, sodium retention	Steroid excess
Indomethacin or aspirin	PG synthetase inhibitors	50–100 mg/day 2–3 g/day	GI bleeding, impaired renal function, salt retention	Gastric or duodenal bleeding ulcer

(2 l of 0.85% saline over 2–3 hours or 3–6 l/m² of saline per 24 hours) to maintain a urine output of at least of 250 ml/m²/hr will restore the extracellular fluid volume, raise the GFR, and decrease tubular reabsorption of calcium. Caution is required in elderly patients and in those with renal impairment or with cardiovascular disease who are taking digitalis, where rapid changes in body fluid volume or electrolye levels may be dangerous.

Enhanced urinary excretion of calcium

After expanding the extracellular fluid volume, the administration of furosemide (103, 104) or ethacrynic acid will augment the urinary excretion of calcium due to further inhibition of calcium reabsorption in the ascending limb of the loop of Henle. Furosemide should be given after the initial 2 l of saline every 2–4 hours in a dose of 1–3 mg/kg (or ethacrynic acid 20–40 mg every 1–2 hours) in order to maintain urinary flow rates of 250–500 ml/hr. It is important not to give furosemide before extracellular fluid expansion since the natriuresis induced by furosemide can contract the extracellular fluid volume and aggravate the hypercalcemia. In addition, furosemide may augment hypomagnesemia and hypokalemia, increasing the risk of cardiac arrhythmias. Usually 20–40 mEq of KCL and 15–30 mg of magnesium per liter of infused saline are adequate the replenish the losses of these electrolytes. If the urinary output is between 5 and 10 l in 24 hours, urinary calcium excretion may increase to 1–2 g/day, decreasing the serum calcium concentration by 2–4 mg/dl. The use of furosemide with saline permits a greater rate of infusion without the risk of pulmonary edema. Thiazide diuretics should be avoided in hypercalcemia, because a decrease in urinary calcium excretion may result from an enhanced reabsorption in the kidney (104–106).

Careful avoidance of prerenal azotemia is imperative, since dehydration may aggravate the hypercalcemic state. The risk of eighth cranial nerve damage from loop diuretics is greatest in patients with renal failure, in the elderly, and with its concurrent use along with other ototoxic medications. Patients with a low serum phosphorus level should be treated with oral phosphate (in addition to saline) in divided doses totaling 500–1400 mg of elemental phosphorus per day (107).

Inorganic phosphate

The administration of either oral or intravenous inorganic phosphate is effective in reducing serum calcium levels (107, 108) by causing a shift of calcium out of the extracellular fluid into bone (109). Bone resorption is also inhibited (110). This therapy is contraindicated in renal failure and in the presence of serum phosphorus levels above 5 mg/dL. The use of intravenous phosphate may be associated with soft-tissue calcification (111), tetany and convulsions (112), hypocalcemia, acute renal failure, hypotension, and even death if given too rapidly. One gram of elemental phosphorus as the sodium or potassium salt (33 mM) infused with saline over a period of 8–16 hours is a safe and effective dose for the acute control of hypercalcemia. Calcium levels begin to fall within minutes after the infusion is begun (113), but the nadir may not occur until a week after the infusion (114). No more than one such infusion per day and no more than 2 days of consecutive intravenous phosphate infusions should be administered. Oral phosphate therapy is also effective for chronic hypercalcemia (107, 115) (calcium above 12 mg/dL) in patients with hyperparathyroidism in whom surgery has to be delayed, or in those with persistent hypercalcemia after the surgical exploration (116). It has also been used in the chronic treatment of patients with malignant hypercalcemia. It is best given at the end of meals and may not be well tolerated because of diarrhea and gastrointestinal upset. The daily dose is 1–3 g of elemental phosphorus in three divided doses. Multiple myeloma not complicated by renal failure responds particularly well to phsophate (117). Phosphate may increase the efficacy of calcitonin therapy, since the calcitonin may increase the renal clearance of phosphate, thereby attenuating its own effectiveness when used alone. Phosphate should be used cautiously in sarcoidosis or vitamin D intoxication, as these conditions are often accompanied by elevated serum phosphate levels.

Diphosphonates

Diphosphonates are drugs that inhibit bone resorption (118), resulting in a decrease in serum calcium levels and in urinary calcium excretion (119). Because of their P-C-P structure, they are resistant to hydrolysis by natural pyrophosphatases. Some diphosphonates also interfere with osteoblastic activity and bone mineralization, and may cause osteomalacia with long-term use. Dichloromethylene diphosphonate (Cl_2MDP), given orally or parenterally, is effective for hypercalcemia due to myeloma, breast cancer, parathyroid carcinoma, and other malignancies (120–123). Given parenterally it is as effective as mithramycin. Osteomalacia does not appear to be induced by this drug; unlike etidronate disodium (EHDP, Didronel R). Following IV administration of Cl_2MDP, the serum calcium starts to fall within 24 hours, the maximum response occurring after 4 or 5 days. Oral APD usually decreases serum calcium within 72 hours, but it may take longer. APD, like Cl_2MDP, may not cause osteomalacia. APD is reported to be effective for malignant hypercalcemia as well as for Paget's disease (124, 125, 162). Long-term use of EHDP is associated with the development of osteomalacia. Cl_2MDP was withdrawn from clinical use following the occurrence of leukemia in patients taking the drug.

Calcitonin

The administration of calcitonin causes hypocalcemia and hypophosphatemia by inhibiting the bone resorptive capacity of the osteoclast. It also acts on the kidney to decrease the tubular reabsorption of calcium, phosphorus, and sodium. Calcitonin was recently shown to be involved in the regulation of calcitriol, having a direct stimulatory effect on its production in the rat (126). Calcitonin is useful in treating hypercalcemia secondary to malignancy or lymphoproliferative disorders or in patients in whom mithramycin is contraindicated, in cases of primary hyperparathyroidism with hypercalcemic crisis who are undergoing surgery, and in other emergency situations (125). The degree of serum calcium reduction that can be obtained with calcitonin is usually less than with mithramycin or inorganic phosphate (128–130). Its effect may decrease after a few days of therapy, possibly as a result of antibody formation or rebound parathyroid stimulation (131). Calcium escape may be avoided by the addition of steroids or phosphates (117–133). Calcitonin therapy may be especially appropriate for patients with congestive heart failure or uremia, because mithramycin, forced diuresis, and inorganic phosphate produce special problems in these patients. Since the concurrent administration of mithramycin and calcitonin has been reported to produce severe hypocalcemia (133), it is recommended that calcitonin should be discontinued by the third day of mithramycin therapy (133). Calcitonin is available as the human, salmon, and pig hormone. Salmon calcitonin has a greater potency and a longer half-life than the porcine variety (128, 134). Periodic examination of the urine sediment is advisable, since chronic administration has been associated with renal tubular epithelial sloughing (135). The recommended dose is 0.5–4 MRC units/kg intramuscularly every 12 hours to a maximum of 8 MRC units/kg every 6 hours. The serum calcium level starts to decrease within 1–2 hours, with a maximal effect at 8–10 hours. Many patients become normocalcemic within a few hours after the initial therapy. The advantages of calcitonin include its rapid onset of action and safety, especially in patients with renal failure. The side effects may include flushing, nausea, and vomiting, which occurs in 10% of treated patients.

Glucocorticoids

Glucocorticoids may inhibit the activity of both osteoclasts and osteoblasts (136). They may increase renal calcium clearance (137, 138), inhibit prostaglandin activity (139), and have a direct cytotoxic effect on malignant cells (139). In multiple myeloma, glucocorticoids may block the bone-resorbing effect of OAF (140). They are effective in hypercalcemia due to granulomatous disease, vitamin D intoxication, and malignancies such as lymphoma, leukemia, and myeloma. In malignancy they may interfere with the production or action of osteoclast activating factors and prostaglandins, thus inhibiting bone resorption, or they may cause tumor lysis. In sarcoidosis they reduce the intestinal absorption of calcium and may reduce the synthesis of calcitriol by the granulomatous tissue. In vitamin D intoxication, steroids decrease both bone resorption and intestinal calcium absorption. The side effects of glucocorticoids are numerous and well known. They may be more pronounced in patients with malignancies who have a poor nutritional status and are receiving chemotherapy. Steroids, given with calcitonin, can increase its efficacy in lowering the serum calcium in patients with malignancies. The recommended dose of glucocorticoids for the management of hypercalcemia is 40–100 mg/day of prednisone or its equivalent, and most patients respond within 5–10 days [139]. Glucocorticoids should not be used to treat the hypercalcemia of primary hyperparathyroidism, because they are ineffective. On the other hand, they may be used in the suppression test for the differential diagnosis of hypercalcemia.

Mithramycin

This is a potent cytotoxic antibiotic that blocks bone resorption through an inhibition of the DNA-dependent RNA activity in the osteoclast (142–145), and is effective in the management of hypercalcemia of malignancy. It may also prevent vitamin D-related calcium absorption from the gastrointestinal tract (146). The recommended dose is 25 µg/kg intravenously. It may be administered in 50 ml of 5% of dextrose over 3 hours, and it should be avoided in patients with renal or liver disease or in patients with thrombocytopenia. Repeated doses can be given every 3–4 days, but toxicity usually limits the use to 2–3 weeks. Its onset of action is at 6–12 hours, with a peak effect at 48–92 hours, and the duration of action is 2–7 days. The complications of mithramycin when given in large doses include thrombocytopenia due to bone marrow suppression, nephrotoxicity, platelet dysfunction, and hepatocellular necrosis.

Prostaglandin synthetase inhibitors

Prostaglandins may exhibit PTH-like effects that result in calcium mobilization from bone (147–150). Although some cases of malignant hypercalcemia may respond to therapy with prostaglandin synthetase inhibitors such as indomethacin or aspirin, these agents are not recommended for the routine therapy of malignant hypercalcemia. In hypercalcemic patients with malignancy without bone metastasis, a trial with these agents is justified in doses of 50–100 mg/day of indomethacin or 2–4 g/day of aspirin when conventional therapies have not produced adequate control of the hypercalcemia. If no response is apparent in 5–7 days, therapy should be discontinued. Treatment with prostaglandin inhibitors can acutely reduce renal blood flow and cause renal function to decline. Side effects of indomethacin include nausea, vomiting, diarrhea, and gastrointestinal ulceration and bleeding. Severe frontal headache, dizziness, vertigo, mood alteration, asthma, fluid retention, visual and retinal changes, blood dyscrasias, renal failure, and dermatitis have also been reported (151).

Dialysis

Peritoneal dialysis and hemodialysis with calcium-free dialysate (152, 153) are highly effective for acute lowering of the serum calcium, mainly in oliguric hypercalcemic patients or in patients who do not respond to other modalities of treatment. This therapeutic approach is rarely needed, but can be life-saving in addition to other measures, especially in patients with congestive heart failure or renal failure.

TREATMENT OF HYPERCALCEMIA DUE TO SPECIFIC CAUSES

Primary hyperparathyroidism

A minority of patients with primary hyperparathyroidism have severe (disequilibrium) hypercalcemia and require urgent medical therapy with fluids and loop diuretics, phosphate, or calcitonin to bring the hypercalcemia under control before surgery is undertaken, or sometimes before a diagnosis can be made.

The definitive treatment of hypercalcemia in primary hyperparathyroidism is surgical. Specific indications for surgery include:
1. Patients with disequilibrium hypercalcemia regardless of the level of serum calcium
2. Patients with bone diseaes (osteitis fibrosa cystica), active renal stone disease, pancreatitis, active peptic ulcer disease, or neuropsychiatric manifestations
3. Patients with asymptomatic hypercalcemia and serum calcium above 12 mg/dl

Surgery should be undertaken by an experienced parathyroid surgeon, who will usually attempt to identify all four glands, even if the enlarged parathyroid has been localized preoperatively by the new non-invasive methods. The identification and removal of the parathyroid adenoma usually restores normocalcemia. Patients who are known to have multiple endocrine adenomatosis should have a total parathyroidectomy with autotransplantation in a center where it is feasible, or excision of 3 and 3/4 glands in a center where autotransplantation is not available. The importance of identifying FHH is that no treatment is usually required. On rare occasions, with severe hypercalcemia total parathyroidectomy may be indicated.

Primary hyperparathyroidism is now most commonly identified as a result of routine screening in asymptomatic patients. It is, of course, essential to make a definitive diagnosis (PTH assay) in such patients and where appropriate, to exclude other diagnoses such as renal, lung, or breast malignancy (by chest x-ray, abdominal ultrasound, and mammogram). The management of such patients is controversial, but when hypercalcemia is mild (< 12 mg/dl), especially in older patients (> 60 years), surgery is often felt not to be justified. Long term followup for 7–9 years of nonoperated patients showed no difference in mortality, renal function, blood pressure, serum, or urinary calcium between the nonoperated and the operated groups (154–156).

Patients in whom surgery is contraindicated, is refused, or has failed, who are symptomatic and/or have serum calcium levels above 12 mg/dl, can be controlled with oral phosphates (107). Phosphate reduces serum and urinary calcium and shoul be used with caution, since it may potentiate a decline in renal function and promote metastatic calcification. Initial reports of the efficacy of cimetidine

(157) or adrenergic beta blockers (158, 159) in ameliorating hyperparathyroidism have not been confirmed. Dichloromethylene diphosphonate reduces serum calcium and may prove useful, but it is not available for clinical use. Diphosphonates may lower the serum calcium level towards normal by antagonizing the PTH effect on bone in primary hyperparathyroidism (160).

Malignant hypercalcemia

As with primary hyperparathyroidism, patients may present with severe (disequilibrium) hypercalcemia requiring urgent treatment (such as fluids, loop diuretics, diphosphonates, inorganic phosphate, or calcitonin) or may have milder hypercalcemia, initially presenting a diagnostic problem. The definitive treatment is that of the malignancy — either surgery, radiotherapy, or chemotherapy. If treatment of the malignancy is impossible or ineffective in correcting hypercalcemia, many treatment modalities can be effective. Corticosteroids (e.g., prednisone 60–100 mg/day) are usually effective in hemopoietic malignancies (but may take 5–10 days for the full effect) but are less frequently effective in solid tumors with or without metastases. Recently a small comparative study has been reported in malignant hypercalcemia (161), which indicates that no single agent was universally effective, but oral phosphate and mithramycin were the most effective. More recently, IV diphosphonates and gallium nitrate have been shown to be highly effective in malignant hypercalcemia (see Addendum).

Oral phosphate may be useful in the management of malignant hypercalcemia, alone or in combination, for example, with steroids or calcitonin, and is given in a dose of 1–3 g elemental phosphorus per day.

In patients who do not respond to steroids and/or phosphate, the administration of diphosphonates or mithramycin is advised. Mithramycin has a rapid onset action (12 hours), with a peak at 42–92 hours and a long effect. The drug can be repeated every 3–4 days. Although many side effects have been reported (see text), the dose of 25 μg/kg seems is relatively safe. In patients with breast cancer and bone metastases, the administration of this drug in addition to chemotherapy may promote bone healing.

In patients in whom the use of mithramycin is contraindicated, calcitonin may be given. This drug has minimal toxicity and may lower serum calcium by 1–1.5 mEq/l (2–3 mg/dl), but resistance develops, thus rapidly limiting its use. The recommended dose is 4 MRC U/kg salmon calcitonin every 12 hours. The administration of calcitonin in combination with glucocorticosteroids or phosphates may delay the appearance of resistance.

Although the new group of diphosphonates have been reported to be effective in the management of hypercalcemia of malignancy, their use is limited in North America since only EHDP (Didronel R) is avaiable in Canada and the U.S.A.. EHDP is effective in malignant hypercalcemia only when given parenterally. Dichloromethylene diphosphonate (Cl_2MDP) is effective orally or parenterally for hypercalcemia due to myeloma, breast cancer, parathyroid carcinoma, and other malignancies, but is also not available. APD is highly effective orally for malignant hypercalcemia and is available in Europe. Recent studies show a striking reduction in morbidity when given to patients with breast cancer and bone metastases (162).

Other hypercalcemias

Thiazide associated hypercalcemia should be managed by withdrawal of the drug and further investigation. Patients with vitamin D intoxication require vitamin D withdrawal. With calcitriol overdosage, hypercalcemia rapidly reverses (1–2 days), whereas with native vitamin D it may persist for weeks. In the meantime, glucocorticoids (e.g., prednisone 40–60 mg/day) and a low calcium intake will control the hypercalcemia.

Hypercalcemia associated with granulomatous diseases generally responds well to corticosteroids, e.g., prednisone 30–60 mg/day.

The milk alkali syndrome is managed by withdrawal of the oral calcium supplement and institution of alternative antacid regimes such as cimetidine.

Beta-adrenergic blockers are effective in the treatment of hypercalcemic thyrotoxicosis. The intravenous administration of 10 mg/hr of propranolol has been observed to reverse the hypercalcemia of thyrotoxicosis (159). Oral therapy is also effective at doses of 80–100 mg/day, and the response becomes apparent within a week. This therapy is contraindicated in the presence of congestive heart failure or bronchospasm.

OTHER POTENTIAL THERAPIES FOR HYPERCALCEMIA

WR 2721

Ethyl-phosphorothioic acid [WR 2721, S-2-(3-aminopropylamine] is a potent hypocalemic agent that inhibits parathyroid hormone secretion and action both in vivo and in vitro (163). In parathyroidectomized rats, WR 2721 produced hypocalcemia, in part through a reduction in osteoclastic activity (164). In vivo it has been used in hypercalcemia due to carcinoma of the parathyroid (165) and in the treatment of hypercalcemia induced by vitamin D (166).

Chloroquine

This antimalarial drug was first reported to be effective in hypercalcemic sarcoidosis in 1963 (167). Recently, the efficacy of chloroquine in two patients with sarcoidosis has been reported (168), with restoration of the serum levels of calcitriol to normal, but without change in the serum calcidiol, suggesting that this drug may prevent, directly or indirectly, the l-alpha hydroxylation of the calcidiol by the activated macrophage. The use of chloroquine appears promising in those cases where calcitriol production is increased, and it may cause fewer side effects than the steroids. Routine ophthalmologic examinations can allow chloroquine to be prescribed with little risk of retinopathy.

Ketoconazole

Reduction of serum calcitriol levels with ketoconazole has recently been reported (169). This antimycotic drug impairs the synthesis of ergosterol in fungal membranes as a result of interference in the reactions involved in the removal of the 14-alpha-methyl groups of lanosterol, the precursor of ergosterol. Ketoconazole induces blockade of cytochrome P450 dependent enzymes involved in the synthesis of hormones from cholesterol. This drug has recently been administered to nine normal men (169) and shown to decrease the serum levels of calcitriol without any changes in the serum levels of calcidiol, PTH, or serum phosphorus, suggesting a direct inhibitory effect of the drug on the renal l-alpha-hydroxylase enzyme. Direct support for this mechanism is provided by a recent report that ketoconazole is a competitive inhibitor of l-alpha-hydroxylase in the cultured chick kidney cell (170). This drug may prove to be useful in those cases where increased production of calcitriol is the cause of hypercalcemia or severe hypercalciuria, as in sarcoidosis or other granulomatous diseases. However, further studies are required before its use can be recommended.

Cisplatinum

Recently, cisplatinum has been reported to be effective therapy for cancer-associated hypercalcemia in humans (171) and in a mouse experimental model (172).

Diphosphonates and gallium nitrate (see Addendum)

HYPOCALCEMIA

Hypocalcemia is defined as a decrease in the level of ionized calcium in serum. As with hypercalcemia, hypocalcemia may also be artifactual due to a reduction in serum albumin. Hypocalcemia develops when either PTH is deficient, as in hypoparathyroidism, or when an end-organ resistance to PTH exists either as inherited pseudohypoparathyroidism or acquired as in vitamin D deficiency, magnesium deficiency, or hyperphosphatemia (Table 5). Hypocalcemia is less frequent than hypercalcemia as a laboratory finding. Its incidence in the general population is reported to be 0.6% (29).

Clinical manifestations (Table 4)

Hypocalcemia may be asymptomatic, or may present as a medical emergency manifested by seizures, tetany, ventricular arrythmias, or intractable congestive heart failure. The patient often presents with paresthesias of the distal extremities and perioral area, but muscle cramps, carpopedal spasm, laryngeal spasm, tetany, and seizures may also be the presenting features. Subclinical tetany may be revealed by a positive Chvostek or Trousseau sign. These signs may also be present in hypomagnesemic hypocalcemic patients, and a positive Chvostek sign is reported

Table 4. Signs and symptoms of hypocalcemia

Neuromuscular
  Paresthesiae
  Tetany
  Numbness
  Myopathy
  Chvostek's and Trousseau's signs
  Papilledema
  Increased intracranial pressure
  Seizures
Ectodermal
  Alopecia
  Cataracts
  Dermatitis
  Moniliasis, brittle nails
Cardiovascular
  Prolongation of QT interval
  Ventricular arrhythmias
  Congestive heart failure
  Hypotension
Psychiatric
  Dementia
  Psychosis
  Mental retardation
  Affective disorders

Table 5. Causes of hypocalcemia

PTH deficiency
  Primary — idiopathic, congenital and familial
  Secondary — following surgery for thyroid and parathyroid glands, amyloid or iron deposition, metastases
PTH resistance
  Pseudohypoparathyroidism Type I–II
  Hypomagnesemia
Vitamin-D deficiency
  Nutritional rickets and osteomalacia
  Renal failure
  Renal tubular disorders
Vitamin-D resistance
  1,25-$(OH)_2D_3$ resistance (Type II vitamin-D-dependent rickets)
Drugs: Mithramycin, calcitonin, colchicine, IV citrate, furosemide
Calcium binding and sequestration
  Tumor lysis, rhabdomyolisis, acute pancreatitis, phosphate enemas, osteoblastic metastases

to be present in 10% of normal people. Chvostek's sign is elicited by tapping over the facial nerve to produce a facial twitch. Eyelid muscle contraction is said to be pathognomonic of hypocalcemia. Trousseau's sign is elicted by inflating the blood pressure cuff to greater than systolic pressure for 3 minutes, and the test is positive when carpal spasm occurs 1–2 minutes after release. Chronic and moderate hypocalcemia may cause such non specific symptoms as weakness, fatigue, irritability, alteration in memory, and affective disorders. Papilledema (173, 174), bilateral cataracts (175), and calcification of the basal ganglia have been described in both PTH deficiency and PTH resistance (176, 177). Resistance to digitalis therapy has also been reported in hypocalcemia (178).

Causes of hypocalcemia (Table 5)

HYPOPARATHYROIDISM

Surgical hypoparathyroidism may result from thyroid, parathyroid, or radical neck surgery and may be transitory or permanent. Hypoparathyroidism may occur following therapy with ^{131}I (179, 180) and in association with acute pancreatitis (181, 182), metastasis to the parathyroid glands (183), amyloid deposition, and iron deposition in the glands in patients with thalassemia (184). Idiopathic PTH deficiency may be sporadic or familial, and unassociated with other disorders (185). The disease often has its onset in childhood, but may be of adult onset, particularly in the sporadic cases. Hypoparathyroidism may be a manifestation of the autoimmune polyglandular failure syndrome (186, 187) and may be associated with mucocutaneous candidiasis and Addison's disease as well as other autoimmune disorders such as diabetes mellitus, Hashimoto's thyroiditis, alopecia, ovarian dysgenesis, vitiligo, and pernicious anemia.

PSEUDOHYPOPARATHYROIDISM

The clinical syndromes of pseudohypoparathyroidism (PTH resistance) represent states of hypocalcemia resulting from refractoriness to the peripheral actions of PTH and may be accompanied by a multitude of abnormal somatic and mental abnormalities, including short stature, round face, subnormal intelligence, thickset body habitus, brachy dactyly, and subcutaneous calcifications (186, 187). However, patients with biochemical features may lack any of these somatic features. The biochemical abnormality is designated usually as Type I or II (188). In Type I there is renal and skeletal resistance to PTH, and the administration of exogenous PTH does not cause phosphaturia or an increase in urinary cyclic AMP (189, 190). It has been suggested that this resistance is due to a reduction of the N or G protein of the adenylate cyclase system, as has been described in red blood cells, cultured skin fibroblasts, and renal tissue from patients (191, 192). Deficient membrane G unit activity is associated with decreased responsiveness to various polypeptide hormones, including PTH, TSH, glucagon, and gonadotropins. Type II patients have similar features to Type I, but in this variant PTH elicits a normal increase in urinary cyclic AMP without phosphaturia (193, 194). Type I is inherited as an x-linked dominant, whereas the inheritance pattern of Type II is unknown (195). Pseudohypoparathyroid patients are usually hypocalcemic and hyperphosphatemic, and have normal or elevated serum concentrations of PTH (196). There is a failure of l-alpha-hydroxylation of calcidiol in pseudohypoparathyroidism (197).

PTH resistance also occurs in severe magnesium deficiency (in which there is also an impairment of PTH release)

Table 6. Serum vitamin-D level

Condition	25-(OH)D$_3$	1,25-(OH)$_2$D$_3$
Nutritional D deficiency	Low	Normal or low
Malabsorption	Low	Normal or low
Hypoparathyroidism & low pseudohypoparathyroidism	Normal	Low
Anticonvulsant therapy	Low	Normal or low
Chronic renal failure	Normal	Low
Nephrotic syndrome	Normal or low	Normal
Vitamin-D-dependent rickets		
Type I	Normal	Low
Type II	Normal	High
Sex-linked hypophosphatemia	Normal	Normal or low
Oncogenic osteomalacia	Normal	Normal or low

and in chronic renal failure. In both of these circumstances hypocalcemia results from the inability of secreted PTH to restore normal serum calcium levels.

VITAMIN D DEFICIENCY

Vitamin D, together with PTH, is responsible for skeletal calcium mobilization in order to maintain calcium homeostasis. In vitamin D deficiency, this effect of PTH is impaired. Table 6 summarizes the disorders of vitamin D deficiency and resistance, and the associated abnormalities of serum levels of vitamin D metabolites.

Vitamin-D deficiency due to diet or impaired conversion of vitamin D to calcitriol can result in hypocalcemia and a failure of bone to mineralize normally. Profound hypocalcemia is unusual in vitamin D deficiency since secondary hyperparathyroidism occurs. Patients with renal failure have hypocalcemia due to resistance to the action of PTH on bone, attributable in part to calcitriol deficiency. They have decreased intestinal calcium absorption, hypocalciuria, and secondary hyperparathyroidism. The loss of renal mass and the hyperphosphatemia contribute to the decreased calcitriol production in these patients. In the normal neonate at birth PTH is undetectable, and the plasma calcium level exceeds maternal levels (198), but it decreases within the first few days of life. The early onset of neonatal hypocalcemia may be associated with prematurity (199), and maternal hyperparathyroidism or diabetes (200) in both of which the maternal high ionized plasma calcium leads to parathyroid suppression. Late-onset hypocalcemia occurs between days 3 and 21, and is always due to ingestion of a formula with a high phosphate/calcium ratio such as cow's milk (201). Phosphate overload may also lead to hypocalcemia in rhabdomyolysis and in the tumor lysis syndrome, or may be due to excess phosphate ingestion, including phosphate cathartics and sodium phosphate enemas.

Diagnosis of hypocalcemia

Hypocalcemia may be discovered accidentally by a routine calcium determination or because it is clinically suspected.

The history and physical examination may be helpful in providing clues regarding possible surgical hypoparathyroidism or renal failure. The initial laboratory work-up in a hypocalcemic patient should include serum inorganic phosphorus and alkaline phosphatase. Hyperphosphatemia suggests hypoparathryoidism, pseudohypoparathryroidism, renal failure, or occasionally vitamin D deficiency (202) or magnesium depletion (203). Hypophosphatemia can be found in the "hungry bones" syndrome, and in vitamin D deficiency as a result of secondary hyperparathyroidism. The serum alkaline phosphatase level is usually raised in rickets or osteomalacia. When the cause of hypocalcemia is not apparent, a serum magnesium determination should be made, and if it is below 1.0 mEq/l (1.2 mg/dl), the hypocalcemia may be secondary to magnesium depletion. Determination of serum PTH and urinary cyclic AMP is of value in distinguishing between PTH deficiency and PTH resistance (see Table 7). Determination of vitamin D metabolites may also be helpful. Skeletal x-rays for Looser zones and an iliac crest bone biopsy may confirm the diagnosis of osteomalacia in cases where it is suspected. With respect to pseudohypoparathyroidism, the response to PTH administration in terms of its hypercalcemic, phosphaturic, and urinary cAMP effects will permit the differentiation of hypoparathyroidism from pseudohypoparathyroidism Types I and II. The biochemical differential diagnosis of hypocalcemia is summarized in Table 7.

Therapy

MANAGEMENT OF HYPOCALCEMIC EMERGENCIES

Hypocalcemic patients with tetany, carpopedal spasm, ventricular arrhythmias, respiratory failure, refractory congestive heart failure, hypotension, and status epilepticus must be treated as an emergency, even if the underlying cause is not known. An intravenous bolus of 200–300 mg of elemental calcium (10–15 mEq/l) in the form of 10% calcium gluconate (4.5 mEq/l or 93 mg Ca/10 ml) should be given over 2–3 minutes. Those patients with severe or recurrent symptoms should have a continuous infusion of dextrose solution containing an elemental calcium concentration of 15 mg/l (0.75 mEq/l) over 4–6 hours. Patients must be monitored, the total or ionized calcium being checked hourly until the life-threatening symptoms resolve. In patients with refractory hypocalcemia, the possibility of magnesium deficiency should be considered. Most patients with hypocalcemia associated with hypomagnesemia have plasma magnesium levels below 0.8 mEq/l (1.0 mg/dl). Clinical causes of hypomagnesmia include alcoholism, malabsorption, and renal magnesium wasting. Every patient with unexplained hypocalcemia must have a serum magnesium determination. In patients with severe hypomagnesemia, one or two ampoules of a 10% solution of $MgSO_4 \cdot 7H_2O$ (10 ml) should be administered intravenously over a 60-minute period (one ampoule contains 4 mM or 96 mg of magnesium). This may be followed by 2–4 ml of 50% magnesium sulfate solution intramuscularly every 4 hours until the serum magnesium level is normal. Magnesium is contraindicated in patients with renal failure and without clear documentation of magnesium depletion. It must be remembered that patients with hypocalcemia secondary to magnesium depletion may have hypokalemia as well, which should be treated in order to avoid severe arrhythmias.

TREATMENT OF SPECIFIC HYPOCALCEMIC DISORDERS

Hypoparathyroidism and pseudohypoparathyroidism

The long-term treatment of chronic hypocalcemia should be directed to the underlying cause. Hypoparathyroidism

Table 7. Biochemical differential diagnosis of hypocalcemia

Diagnosis	Serum PTH	Serum phosphate	Urinary cAMP	Serum 25-(OH)D	Serum 1,25-(OH)$_2$D
PTH deficiency	D	I	D	N	D
PTH resistance (PHP Type I)	I	I	D	N	D
cAMP resistance (PHP Type II)	I	N-I	I	N	D
25-(OH)D deficiency (nutritional or liver disease) I	I	D	I	D	D-N
1,25-(OH)$_2$D deficiency (renal disease)	I	D	I	N	D
1,25-(OH)$_2$D resistance (Type II vitamin-D-dependent rickets)	I	D	I	N	I

I = increase;
D = decrease.

Table 8. Vitamin-D preparations

Brand name	Ergocalciferol Calciferol	Dihydrotachysterol Hytakerol	b2(OH)D$_3$ One-alpha	1,25-(OH)$_2$D$_3$ Rocaltrol
Strength and form	Cap 50,000 IU 10,000 IU/ml	Cap 0.125 mg 0.25 mg/ml	Cap 0.25, 1.0 µg	Cap 0.25, 0.5 µg
Administration route	PO, IM	PO	PO	PO IV also available
Dose in hypoparathyroidism	25,000–100,000 IU (per day)	0.25–1 mg	0.25–2.0 µg	0.25–1.0 µg
Duration of effects after drug is administered	6–18 weeks	13 weeks	1–3 days	1–5 days

following thyroid or parathyroid surgery causes a fall in the serum calcium level, which may be transitory or permanent, and may result from transient suppression of normal parathyroid glands due to previous hypercalcemia, transient hypoparathyroidism due to surgery, permanent hypoparathyroidism, or rapid remineralization of bones ("hungry bones"). Patients with mild symptoms and a serum calcium level below 8.5 mg/dl can be treated by oral calcium supplementation 1–2 g/day until the transient hypocalcemia is over (usually less than 7–10 days). Several calcium salts are available, and in prescribing them one should take into consideration the content of elemental calcium. The latter constitutes 40% of calcium carbonate, 36% of calcium chloride, 12% of calcium lactate, and 8% of calcium gluconate. Calcium gluconate is generally preferable, being less irritating than calcium chloride. Patients with a serum calcium concentration below 8.5 mg/dl after 10 days of treatment must be considered as having permanent hypoparathyroidism and require additional longterm treatment. A thiazide diuretic such as chlorthalidone (50 mg/day) will produce a small increase in the serum calcium level and may be sufficient in a mild case (204). If these measures fail to restore the plasma calcium level to or near to the normal range, or fail to relieve symptoms, and if hyperphosphatemia is present, vitamin D therapy is indicated (Table 8). Vitamin-D$_2$ (ergocalciferol) is usually required in a dose of 50,000 to 100,000 U/day in severe hypoparathyroidism. When the conversion of vitamin D to calcitriol is impaired, as in PTH deficiency, either the active metabolite, calcitriol, or the synthetic analog, 1-alpha-hydroxy cholecalciferol, is the drug of choice because of the short half-life and the ease of achieving good therapeutic control of serum calcium during the early period of therapy. The only disadvantage of this therapy is the cost. The serum calcium level should be raised to around 8.5 mg/dl, since with further elevations these patients will show marked hypercalciuria due to loss of the hypocalciuric action of PTH. The combination of calcitriol with an oral calcium supplement is particularly liable to cause hypercalciuria; some patients may be better managed without the calcium supplement. An effective dose of l-alpha-vitamin D$_3$ or calcitriol is around 0.5–1.0 µg/day, but some patients may require up to 2 µg/day. The most common side effect of long-term treatment with vitamin D and calcium supplementation is hypercalcemia, which reverses rapidly (usually 1–1½ days for calcitriol or 3–5 weeks for Hytakerol). Nephrocalcinosis, renal insufficiency, and uremia have occurred during chronic management of hypocalcemia with vitamin D. In patients maintained on vitamin D, the serum calcium, phosphorus, and creatinine must be checked at least every 4 months, as dose requirements can change.

Vitamin D deficiency

Hypocalcemia may also result from an alteration of vitamin D metabolism, as in vitamin D deficiency, malabsorption syndromes, postgastrectomy states, hepatobiliary disease, nephrotic syndrome, vitamin D dependency rickets, and end-stage renal disease. In these chronic disorders the goal of therapy is to increase intestinal absorption of calcium using vitamin D sterols, in addition to oral calcium supplementation. In nutritional deficiency where the metabolism and activation of vitamin D is intact, physiologic amounts of D$_2$ (10 µg or 400 U/day) are required. Calcium supplementation is also important in children with rickets to avoid worsening of the hypocalcemia, as bone is rapidly mineralized. In malabsorption states, up to 50,000 U of vitamin D$_2$ or D$_3$ weekly or even daily may be needed. Primary biliary cirrhosis represents the most common hepatic disease associated with the manifestations of vitamin D deficiency. In these patients the levels of calcidiol are often low, and most of the patients have osteoporosis rather than osteomalacia. Therapy with calcitriol (0.5–1.0 µg/day) may be used, but large doses of vitamin D are also effective and less expensive. Patients on anticonvulsants may develop hypocalcemia with or without osteomalacia, and require treatment with vitamin D (205) or with calcitriol (0.2–0.5 µg/day).

Hungry bones syndrome

Patients with the "hungry bones" syndrome have hypocalcemia, hypophosphatemia, and an elevated alkaline phosphatase level of bone origin. This condition may occur after parathyroid surgery in patients with radiographic evidence of osteitis fibrosa (206) and may be severe in patients with chronic renal failure who undergo subtotal parathyroidectomy and have hyperparathyroid bone disease on x-rays. The condition results from the great excess of bone formation over bone resorption and requires prolonged and aggressive treatment with vitamin D and calcium supplements until the bone heals. Calcitriol may be given before surgery in order to increase the serum calcium level to 12 mg/dl and must be continued after surgery in addition to calcium supplements. The recommended dose of calcitriol is 1–2 µg/day but higher doses may be needed. The serum alkaline phosphatase level may be followed as an index of osteoblastic activity and the remineralization process. When the serum alkaline phosphatase level falls to normal, these patients are prone to develop hypercalcemia, and therefore the normalization of the alkaline phosphatase indicates that the doses of vitamin D and calcium should be reduced.

Renal failure

The hypocalcemia of advanced chronic renal failure and/or dialysis patients is best treated with calcitriol or l-alpha-hydroxy vitamin D_3 at a dose of 0.5–2 µg/day.

Vitamin D therapy with any of the available preparations may produce episodes of hypercalcemia. Resistance to treatment is uncommon, but can occur with all metabolites, and has been reversed by cortisone administration, magnesium supplementation, or injections of parathyroid extract (207, 208).

In chronic hypocalcemia the symptoms are not a reliable guide to the success of therapy. Some patients exhibit a marked symptomatic improvement despite depressed serum calcium levels. On the other hand, symptoms can be worsened during respiratory alkalosis, exercise, metabolic alkalosis secondary to vomiting, menstruation, and estrogen administration. For this reason it is essential to educate the hypoparathyroid patient on the signs and symptoms of hypocalcemia. Vitamin D requirements may decrease in hypoparathyroid patients after an episode of vitamin D intoxication and after delivery (postpartum).

REFERENCES

1. Parfitt AM, Kleerekoper M: The divalent ion homeostasis system. Physiology and metabolism of calcium, phosphorus, magnesium and bone. In: MH Maxwell, CR Kleeman, eds, *Clinical Disorders of Fluid & Electrolyte Metabolism.* McGraw–Hill, New York, p269, 1980.
2. Parfitt AM: The actions of parathyroid hormone on bone. 1. *Metabolism* 25:809, 1976.
3. Parfitt AM: The actions of parathyroid hormone on bone. II. *Metabolism* 25:904, 1976.
4. Loken HF, Havell RJ, Gordon GS, Wittinton SL: Ultracentrifugal analysis of protein-bound and free calcium in human serum. *J Biol Chem* 235:3654, 1960.
5. Moore EW: Ionized calcium in normal serum, ultrafiltrates and whole blood determined by ion exchange electrodes. *J Clin Invest* 49:318, 1970.
6. Pedersen KO: The effect of bicarbonate pCO_2 and pH on serum calcium fractions. *Scand J Clin Lab Invest* 27:145, 1970.
7. Walser M, Robinson BH, Duckett JW: The hypercalcemia of adrenal insufficiency. *J Clin Invest* 42:456, 1963.
8. Jaffe JP, Mosher DF: Calcium binding by a myeloma protein. *Am J Med* 67:343, 1979.
9. Lim P, Jacob E, Chio LF, Pwee HS: Serum ionized calcium in nephrotic syndrome. *Q J Med* 179–421, 1973.
10. Berry EM, Gupta MM, Turner SJ, Burns RR: Variations in plasma calcium with changes in plasma specfic gravity, total protein and alburmin. *Br Med J* 4:640, 1973.
11. Husdan H, Rapoport A, Lock S: Influence of posture on the serum concentration of calcium. *Metabolism* 22:787, 1973.
12. Raisz LG: Physiologic and pharmacologic regulation of bone resoprtion. *N Engl J Med* 282:909, 1973.
13. Slatopolsky E, Martin K, Morrissey J, Hruska K: Parathyroid hormone secretion metabolism and biologic actions. *Semin Nephrol* 1:319, 1981.
14. Kleeman CR, Bernstein D, Rockney R, Dowling JT, Maxwell M H: Studies on the renal clearance of diffusible calcium and the role of parathyroid glands on its regulation. *Yale J Biol Med* 34:1, 1961.
15. Widrow SH, Levinsky NG: The effect of parathyroid extract on renal tubular calcium reabsorption in the dog. *J Clin Invest* 41:2151, 1982.
16. Massry SG, Coburn JW, Chapman LW, Kleeman CR: Role of serum calcium, parathyroid hormone and NaCl infusion, on renal calcium and Na clearances. *Am J Physiol* 214:1403, 1968.
17. Shareghi GR, Stoner LC: Calcium transport across segments of the rabbit distal nephron in vitro. *Am J Physiol* 235:F367, 1978.
18. Greger R, Lang F, Oberleithner H: Distal site of calcium reabsorption into the rat nephron. *Pflügers Arch* 374:153, 1978.
19. Favus MJ. Transport of calcium by intestinal mucosa. *Semin Nephrol* 1:306, 1981.
20. Myrtle JF, Norman AW: Vitamin D: A cholecalciferol metabolite highly active in promoting intestinal calcium transport. *Science* 171:79, 1971.
21. Walling MW: Intestinal calcium and phosphate transport. Differential responses to Vitamin D_3 metabolites. *Am J Physiol* 233:E488, 1977.
22. Lee DBN, Brautbar N, Massry SG Renal production and biologic actions of vitamin D metabolites. *Semin Nephrol* 1:335, 1981.
23. Hirsch PE, Munson PL: Thyrocalcitonin.*Physiol Rev* 49:548, 1969.
24. Copp DH: Endocrine regulation of calcium metabolism. *Ann Review Physiol* 32:61, 1970.
25. Nicolayson R: The absorption of calcium as a function of body saturation with calcium. *Acta Physiol Scand* 6:201, 1943.
26. Boyle IT, Gray RW, DeLuca HF: Regulation by calcium of in vivo synthesis of 1,25 hydroxycholecalciferol and 21,25 hydroxycholecalciferol. *Proc Natl Acad Sci USA* 68:2131, 1971.

27. DeCristofaro JB, Tsang, RC: Calcium (review). *Emerg Med Clin North Am* 4(2):207.21, 1986.
28. Parfitt AM: Equilibrium and disequilibrium hypercalcemia. New light on and old concept. *Metab Bone Dis Related* 1:279, 1979.
29. Stewart AF, Horst R, Deftos LJ, Cadman EC, Lang R, Broadus AE: Biochemical evaluation of patients with cancer associated with hypercalcemia. Evidence for humoral and non-humoral groups. *N Engl J Med* 303:1377, 1980.
30. Mundy RG: Pathogenesis of hypercalcemia of malignancy (review). *Clin Endocrinol* (Oxford) 23:705, 1985.
31. Mundy RG, Raisz LG, Cooper RA, Schechter GP, Salmon SE: Evidence for the secretion of an osteoclast stimulating factor in myeloma. *N Engl J Med* 291:1041, 1974.
32. Ralston SH, Fogelman I, Gardiner MD, Boyle IT: Relative contribution of humoral and metastatic factors to the pathogenesis of hypercalcemia in malignancy. *Br Med J* 288:1405, 1984.
33. Breslau NA, McGuire JL, Zerwekh JE, Frenkl EP, Pak CYC: Hypercalcemia associated with increased serum calcitriol levels in 3 patients with lymphoma. *Ann Int Med* 100:1, 1984.
34. Mosley JM, Kubota M, Diefenbach-Jagger H, Wettenhall REH, Kemp BE, Suva LJ, Rodda CP, Ebeling PR, Hudson PJ, Zajac JD, Martin TJ: Parathyroid hormone-related protein purified from a human lung cancer cell line. *Bone Mineral Research Congress* (ASBMR), Abs No. 391, Indianapolis, 1987.
35. Stewart AF, Wu T, Goumas D, Burtis WJ: Amino-terminal sequence of a human HHM-associated adenylate cyclase-stimulating protein contains PTH-like and PTH-unlike domains. *Bone Mineral Research Congress* (ASBMR), Abs No. 392, Indianapolis, 1987.
36. Katz A, Kaplan L, Massry SG, Heller R, Plotkin D, Knight I: Primary hyperparathyroidism in patients with breast carcinoma. *Arch Surg* 101:582, 1970.
37. Kaplan L, Katz AD, Ben Isaac C, Massry SG: Malignant neoplasms and parathyroid adenomas. *Cancer* 28:401, 1971.
38. Far HW, Fahey TJ Jr, Nash AG, Farr CM: Primary hyperparathyroidism in cancer. *Am J Surg* 126:539, 1973.
39. Samaan NA, Hickey RC, Hill CS Jr, Medellin H, Gates R B: Parathyroid tumors. Preoperative localization and association with other tumors. *Cancer* 33:933, 1974.
40. Vichayanrat A, Abramides A, Gardner B, Wallach S, Carter A C: Primary hyperparathyroidism in breast cancer. *Am J Med.* 61:136, 1976.
41. Singer FR, Sharp CF, Rude R K: Pathogenesis of hypercalcemic malignancy. *Miner electrolyte Metab* 2:161, 1979.
42. Robinson RG, Kerwin DM, Tsou E: Parathyroid adenoma with coexistent sarcoid granulomas. Hypercalcemic patient. *Arch Intern Med* 140: 1980.
43. Case records of the Massachusetts General Hospital: Weekly clinicopathological exercises. Case 50-1981. *N Engl J Med* 305:1457, 1981.
44. Farr HW, Fahey TJ Jr, Nash AG, Farr CM: Primary hyperparathyroidism and cancer. *Am J Surg* 126:539, 1973.
45. Heath DA: Hypercalcemia and malignancy. *Ann Clin Biochem* 13:555, 1976.
46. Rao DS, Frame B, Block MA, Parfitt AM: Primary hyperparathyroidism. A cause of hypercalciuria and renal stones in patients with medullary sponge kidney. *JAMA* 237:1353, 1977.
47. Gremillion DH, Kee JW, McIntosh DA: Hyperparathyroidism and medullary sponge kidney. *JAMA* 237:436, 1977.
48. Vaishnava H, Rizvi SNA: Primary hyperparathyroidism associated with nutritional osteomalacia. *Am J Med* 45:640, 1976.
49. Keynes WM, Caird FI: Hypocalcemic primary hyperparathyroidism. *Br Med J* 1:208, 1970.
50. Dent CE, Jones PE, Mullan DP: Masked primary (or tertiary) hyperparathryroidism. *Lancet* 1:1161, 1975.
51. Woodhouse NJY, Doyle FH, Joplin GF: Vitamin D deficiency and primary hyperparathyroidism. *Lancet* 2:282, 1971.
52. Levi J, Massry SG, Coburn JW, Llach F, Kleeman CR: Hypocalcemia in magnesium depleted dogs: Evidence for reduced responsiveness to parathyroid hormone and relative failure of parathyroid gland function. *Metabolism* 23:323, 1974.
53. Cope D, Culver PJ, Mixter CG, Nardi GL: Pancreatitis — a diagnosis clue to hyperparathyroidism. *Ann Surg* 145:857, 1957.
54. Lever EG: Primary hyperparathyroidism masked by hypothyroidism. *Am J Med* 74:144, 1983.
55. Muldowney FP, Freaney R, McMullin JP, Towers RP, Spillane A, O'Connor P, O'Donohoe P, and Moloney M: Serum ionized calcium and parathyroid hormone in renal stone disease. *Q J Med* 45:75, 1976.
56. Pak CYC, Nicar MJ, Peterson R, Zerwekh JE, Snyder W: A lack of unique pathophysiologic background for nephrolithiasis of primary hyperparathyroidism. *J Clin Endocrinol Metab* 53:536, 1981.
57. Broadus AF, Horst RL, Lang R, Littledike ET, Rassmussen H: Circulating 1,25 dihydroxyvitamin D in primary hyperparathyroidism. *N Engl J Med* 302:421, 1980.
58. Edis AJ, Evans TC Jr: High-resolution, real-time ultrasonography in the preoperative location of parathyroid tumors. Pilot study. *N Engl J Med* 301:532, 1979.
59. Brewer WH, Walsh JW, Newsome HH Jr: Impact of sonography on surgery for primary hyperparathyroidism. *Am J Surg* 145:270, 1983.
60. Ferlin G, Borsato N, Camerani M, Conte N, Zotti D: New perspectives in localizing enlarged parathyroids by technetium-thallium subtraction scan. *N Nucl Med* 24:438, 1983.
61. Etiology and treatment of primary hyperparathyroidism (editorial). *Lancet* 1:367, 1983.
62. Brennan MF, Doppman JL, Marx SJ, Spiegel AM, Brown EM, Aurbach GD: Reoperative parathyroid surgery for persistent hyperparathyroidism. *Surgery* 83:669, 1983.
63. Doppman JL, Lawrence E, Mallette MD, Marx SJ, Monchik JM, Broadus A, Spiegel AM, Beazley R, Aurbach GD: *The localization of abnormal mediastinal parathyroid glands. Radiology* 115:31, 1975.
64. Wolverson MK, Sundaram M, Eddelston B, Prendergast J: Diagnosis of parathyroid adenoma by computed tomography for localization of parathyroid adenomas. *J Comput Assist Tomogr* 5:818, 1981.
65. Whitley NO, Bohlman M, Connor TB, McCrea ES, Mason GR, Whitley J E: Computed tomography for localization of parathyroid adenomas. *J Comput Assist Tomogr* 5:812, 1981.
66. Foley TP Jr, Harrison HC, Arnaud CD, Harrison HE: Familial benign hypercalcemia. *J Pediatrics* 81:1060, 1972.
67. Marx SJ, Spiegel AM, Brown EM, Koehler JO, Gardner DG, Brennan MF, Aurbach GD: Divalent cation metabolism. Familial hypocalciuric hypercalcemia versus typical primary hyperparathyroidism. *Am J Med* 65:235, 1978.
68. Marx SJ, Spiegel AM, Brown EM, Windeck R, Gardner DG, Downs RW Jr, Attie M, Aurbach GD: Circulating parathyroid hormone activity: Familial hypocalciuric hypercalcemia versus typical primary hyperparathyroidism. *J Clin*

Endo Metab 47:1190, 1978.
69. Davies M, Klimiuk PS, Adams PH, Lumb GA, Large DM, Anderson DC: Familial hypocalciuric hypercalcemia and acute pancreatitis. *Br Med J* 282:1023, 1981.
70. Stote RM, Smith LH, Wilson DM, Dube WJ, Goldsmith RS, Arnaud CD: Hydrochlorothiazide effects on serum calcium and immunoreactive parathyroid hormone concentrations. Studies in normal subjects. *Ann Intern Med* 77:587, 1972.
71. Hossain M: Vitamin D intoxication during treatment for hypoparathyroidism. *Lancet* 1:1149, 1970.
72. Hughes MR, Baylink D, Jones PG, Haussler MR: Radioligand receptor assay for 25-hydroxyvitamin D_2/D_3, and 1-alpha 25-dihydroxyvitamin D_2/D_3. Application to hypervitaminosis D. *J Clin Invest* 58:61, 1976.
73. Counts SJ, Baylink DJ, Shen FH, Sherrard DJ, Hickman RO: Vitamin D intoxication in an anephric child. *Ann Int Med* 82:196, 1975.
74. Papapoulos SE, Clemens TL, Fraher LJ, Lewin IG, Sandler LM, O'Riordan JLH: 1,25 dihydroxycholecalciferol in the pathogenesis of the hypercalcemia of sarcoidosis. *Lancet* 1:627, 1979.
75. Bell NH, Stern PH, Pantzer E, Sinha TK, DeLuca HF: Evidence that increased circulating l-alpha 25-dihydroxyvitamin D is the probable cause for abnormal calcium metabolism in sarcoidosis. *J Clin Invest* 64:L218, 1979.
76. Barbour GL, Coburn JW, Slatopolsky E, Norman AW, Horst RL: Hypercalcemia in an anephric patient with sarcoidosis: Evidence for extrarenal generation of 1,25-dihydroxyvitamin D. *N Engl J Med* 305:440, 1981.
77. Adams JS, Sharma OP, Singer FR: Metabolism of 25-hydroxyvitamin D_3 by alveolar macrophages in sarcoidosis. *Clin Res* 31:499A, 1983.
78. Baxter JD, Bondy PK: Hypercalcemia of thyrotoxicosis. *Ann Intern Med* 65:429, 1966.
79. Burman KD, Monchik JM, Earll JM, Wartofsky L: Ionized and total serum calcium and parathyroid hormone in hyperthyroidism. *Ann Intern Med* 84:668, 1976.
80. Mosekilde J, Christensen MS: Decreased parathyroid function in hyperthyroidism: Interrelationships between serum parathyroid hormone, calcium-phosphorus metabolism and thyroid function. *Acta Endocrinology* 84:566, 1977.
81. Fritzel D, Malleson A, Marks V: Plasma levels of ionized calcium and magnesium in thyroid disease. *Lancet* 1:1360, 1977.
82. Krane SM, Brownell GL, Stanbury JB, Corrigon H: The effect of thyroid disease on calcium metabolism in man. *J Clin Invest* 35:874, 1956.
83. Adams PH, Jowsey J, Kelly PJ, Riggs BL, Kinney VR, Jones JD: The effects of hyperthyroidism on bone and mineral metabolism in man. *Q J Med* 36:1, 1967.
84. Mundy GR, Shapiro JL, Bandelin JC, Canalis EM, Raisz IG: Direct stimulation of bone resorption by thyroid hormones. *J Clin Invst* 58:529, 1975.
85. Rude RK, Oldham SB, Singer FR, Nicoloff JT: Treatment of thyrotoxic hypercalcemia with propranolol. *N Engl J Med* 294:431, 1976.
86. Finlayson JF, Casey JH: Hypercalcemia and multiple pheochromocytomas. *Ann Intern Med* 82:810, 1975.
87. Heath H, Edis AJ: Pheochromocytoma associated with hypercalcemia and ectopic secretion of calcitonin. *Ann Intern Med* 91;208, 1979.
88. Jorgensen H: Hypercalcemia in adrenocortical insufficiency. *Acta Med Scand* 193:175, 1973.
89. Tuttle SG, Figueroa WG: Hypercalciuria associated with reduction in corticoid therapy after prolonged administration of prednisone and after bilateral adrenalectomy for Cushing's syndrome. *J Clin Invest* 37:937, 1958.
90. Nadarajah A, Hartog M, Redfern B, Thalassinos N, Wright AD, Joplin GE, Fraser TR: Calcium metabolism in acromegaly. *Br Med J* 4:797, 1968.
91. Sjoberg HE: Retention of oral ^{45}calcium in acromegaly. *Horm Metab Res* 1:136, 1969.
92. Riggs BL, Randall RV, Wahner HW, Jowsey J, Kelly PM, Singh M: The nature of the metabolic bone disorder in acromegaly. *J Clin Endocrinol Metab* 34:911, 1972.
93. Eskildsen PC, Lund B, Sorensen OH, Lund BI, Bishop JE, Norman AW: Acromegaly and vitamin D metabolism: Effect of bromocriptine treatment. *J Clin Endocrinol metab* 41:484, 1979.
94. Hirose S, Kobayashi K, Kajikawa K, Sawabu N, Takeuchi J: A case of watery diarrhea, hypokalemia and hypercalcemia associated with nonulcerogenic islet cell tumor of the pancreas. *Am J Gastroenterology* 64:382, 1975.
95. Frame B, Jackson CE, Reynolds WA, Umphrey JE: Hypercalcemia an skeletal effects in chronic hypervitaminosis A. *Ann Int Med* 80:44, 1974.
96. Chertow BS, Williams GA, Norris RM, Baker GR, Hargis GK: Vitamin A stimulation of parathyroid hormone: Interactions with calcium, hydrocortisone, and vitamin E in bovine parathyroid tissues and effects of vitamin A in man. *Eur J Invest* 7:307, 1977.
97. Broadus AE, Mahaffey JE, Bartter FC, Neer RM: Nephrogenous cyclic adenosine monophosphate as a parathyroid function test. *J Clin Invest* 60:771, 1977.
98. Broadus AE, Horst RL, Lang R, Travis, Littledike ET, Rasmussen H: The importance of circulating 1,25 dihydroxy vitamin D, and renal stone formation in primary hyperparathyroidism. *N Eng J Med* 302:421, 1980.
99. Adami S, Milroy EJG, O'Riordan JLH: Primary hyperparathyroidism. In: BEC Nordin, ed, *Metabolic Bone and Stone disease*. Churchill Livingstone, New York, p 112, 1984.
100. Broadus AE, Deftos LJ, Bartter FC: Effects of the intravenous administration of calcium on nephrogenous cyclic AMP. Use a parathyroid suppression test. *J Clin Endocrinol Metab* 46:477, 1978.
101. Broadus AF, Horst RL, Littledike ET, Mahaffey JE, Rasmussen H: Primary hyperparathyroidism with intermittent hypercalcemia: Serial observations and simple diagnosis by means of an oral calcium tolerance test. *Clin Endocrinol* 12:225, 1980.
102. Watson L, Moxham J, Fraser P: Hydrocortisone suppression test and discriminant analysis in different diagnosis of hypercalcemia. *Lancet* 1:1320, 1980.
103. Suki WN, Yium JJ, Von Minden M, Saller-Hebert C, Ecknoyan G, Martinez-Maldonado M: Acute treatment of hypercalcemia with furosemide. *N Engl J Med* 283:836, 1970.
104. Elliott TG, McKenzie WH: Treatment of hypercalcemia. *Drug Intell Clin Pharm* 17:12, 1983.
105. Brickman AS, Massry SG: Changes in serum and urinary calcium during treatment with hydrochlorothiazide. *J Clin Invest* 51:945, 1972.
106. Parfitt AM: The interaction of thiazide diuretics with parathyroid hormone and vitamin D — studies in patients with hypoparathyroidism. *J Clin Invest* 51:1879, 1972.
107. Goldsmith RS, Ingbar SH: Inorganic phosphate treatment of hypercalcemia of diverse etiologies. *N Engl J Med* 274:1, 1966.
108. Herbert LA, Lemann J Jr, Petersen JR, Lennon EJ: Studies

of the mechanism by which phosphate infusion lowers serum calcium concentration. *J Clin Invest* 45:1886, 1966.
109. Massry SG, Mueller E, Silverman AG, Kleeman CR: Inorganic phosphate treatment with hypercalcemia. *Arch Intern Med* 121:307, 1968.
110. Carrol E, Pechet M: Stimulation of bone formation by inorganic phosphate and inhibition of bone resorption by thyrocalcitonin. *J Clin Invest* 46:1043, 1967.
111. Breuer RI, Le Bauer J: Caution in the use of phosphates in the treatment of severe hypercalcemia. *J Clin Endocrinol* 27:695, 1967.
112. Alijouni K, Rosenfeld PS: Treatment of hypercalcemia. *Drug Ther* 4:103, 1974.
113. Lee DBN, Zawada ET, Kleeman CR: The pathophysiology and clinical aspects of hypercalcemic disorders. *Western J Med* 129:278, 1978.
114. Yendt ER: Disorders of calcium, phosphorus, and magnesium metabolism. In: Maxwell MH, Kleeman CR, eds, *Clinical Disorders of Fluid and Electrolyte Metabolism*. McGraw-Hill, New York p 416, 1972.
115. Massry SG, Mueller E, Silverman AG, Kleeman CR: Inorganic phosphate treatment for hypercalcemia. *Arch Intern Med* 121:307, 1968.
116. Coburn JW, Brickman AS, Massry SG: Medical treatment in primary and secondary hyperparathyroidism. *Semin Drug Treatment* 2:117, 1972.
117. Brautbar N, Luboshitzky R: Combined calcitonin and oral phosphate treatment for hypercalcemia in multiple myeloma. *Arch Intern Med* 137:914, 1977.
118. Fleisch H, Felix R: Diphosphonates. *Calif Tissue Int* 27:91, 1979.
119. Shane E, Baquiran DC, Bilezikian J P: Effects of dichloromethylene diphosphonate on serum and urinary calcium in primary hyperparathyroidism. *Ann Intern Med* 95:23, 1981.
120. Breukelen FJM, Bijvoet OLM, Van Oosterom AT: Inhibition of osteolytic bone lesions by (3-amino-l-hydroxypropyliden)-1, l-biphosphonate (A.P.D) *Lancet* 1:803, 1979.
121. Siris ES, Sherman WH, Baquiran DC, Schlatter JP, Osserman EF, Canfield RE: Effects of dichloromethylene diphosphonate on skeletal mobilization of calcium in multiple myeloma. *N Eng J Med* 302:310, 1980.
122. Jacobs TP, Siris ES, Bilezikian JP, Baquiran DC, Shane E, Canfield RE:Hypercalcemia of malignancy: Treatment with intravenous dichloromethylene diphosphonate. *Ann Intern Med* 94:312, 1981.
123. Chapuy MC, Meunier PJ, Alexandre CM, Vignon EP: Effects of disodium dichlormethylene diphosphonate on hypercalcemia produced by bone metatases. *J Clin Invest* 65:1243, 1980.
124. Canfield R, Rosner W, Shinner J, et al.: Diphosphonate therapy of Paget's disease of bone. *J Clin Endocrinol Metab* 44:96, 1977.
125. Frijlink WB, TeVelde J, Bijvoet OLM, Heynen G: Treatment of Paget's disease with (3-amino-l-hyroxypropylidene)-1, l-biphosphonate (A.P.D.) *Lancet* 1:799, 1979.
126. Jaeger P, Williams J, Clemens LT, Hayslett PJ: Evidence that calcitonin stimulates 1,25-dihydroxy production and intestinal absorption of calcium *in vivo*. *J Clin Invest* 78:456, 1986.
127. Silva OL, Becker KL: Salmon calcitonin in the treatment of hypercalcemia. *Arch Intern Med* 132:337, 1973.
128. Habener JF, Singer FR, Deftos LJ, Potts JT: Immunological stability of calcitonin in plasma. *Endocrinology* 90:952, 1972.
129. Singer FR, Aldred JP, Neer RM, Krane SM, Potts JT: An evaluation of antibodies and clinical resistance to salmon calcitonin. *J Clin Invest* 51:2331, 1972.
130. Neer RM, Habener JF, Peacock N, Murray T: Escape from calcitonin (CT) during therapy of hypercalcemia. *Clin Res* 18:676, 1970.
131. Dube WJ, Goldsmith RS, Arnaud SB: Hyperparathyroidism secondary to long term therapy of Paget's disease in bone with calcitonin. In: RV Talmag, PL Munson, eds, *Calcium, Parathyroid Hormone and the Calcitonins. Excerptal Medical*, Amsterdam, p 113, 1972.
132. Au WYW: Calcitonin treatment of hypercalcemia due to parathyroid carcinoma — synergistic effect of prednisone on long-term treatment of hypercalcemia. *Arch Int Med* 135:1594, 1975.
133. Caro JF, Besarab A, Glennon JA: Symptomatic hypocalcemia following combined calcitonin and mithramycin therapy for hypercalcemia due to malignancy. *Cancer Treat Rep* 62:1561, 1978.
134. Deftos LJ, Potts JT: Parathyroid hormone, thyrocalcitonin, vitamin D, bone and mineral metabolism. In: PL Bondy, ed, *Duncan's Disease of Metabolism*. WB Saunders, Philadelphia, p 1225, 1974.
135. Reilly MJ, Kepler JA, Poor DM, Lande NI, Rolf BI, Douglas PM (eds): Am Hosp Form Serv 2:68, 1980.
136. Jee WSS, Roberts WE, Park HZ: Interrelated effects of glucocorticoid and parathyroid hormone upon bone remodelling. In: RV Talmage, PL Munson, eds, *Calcium Parathyroid Hormone and the Calcitonins*. Excerpta Medica, Amsterdam, p 430, 1972.
137. Collins EJ, Garett E, Johnston RL: Effect of adrenal steroids on radiocalcium metabolism in dogs. *Metabolism* 11:716, 1962.
138. Loak H: The action of corticosteroid on the renal reabsorption of calcium. *Acta Endocrinol* 34:60, 1960.
139. Tashian AH, Voelkel EF, McDonough J: Hydrocortisone inhibits prostaglandin production by mouse fibrosarcoma cells. *Nature* 258:739, 1975.
140. Mundy GR, Rick ME, Turcotte R, Kowalski MA: Pathogenesis of hypercalcemia in lymphosarcoma cell leukemia: Role of an osteoclast activating factor-like substance and a mechanism of action for glucocorticoid therapy. *Am J Med* 5:600, 1978.
141. Potts JT: Disorders of the parathyroid gland. In: KJ Isselbacher, RD Adams, E Braunwald, RG Petersdorf, JD Wilson, eds, *Harrison's Principles of Internal Medicine*. McGraw–Hill, p 1838, 1980.
142. Kennedy BJ: New York, Metabolic and toxic effects of mithramycin during tumor therapy. *Am J Med* 49:494, 1970.
143. Singer FR, Neer RM, Murray JM, Keutmann HT, Deftos LJ, Potts JT: Mithramycin treatment of intractable hypercalcemia due to parathryoid carcinoma. *N Engl J Med* 283:634, 1970.
144. Elias EG, Reyn G, Mittelman A: Control of hypercalcemia with mithramycin. *Ann Surg* 175:431, 1972.
145. Smith IE, Powles TJ: Mithramycin for hypercalcemia associated with myeloma and other malignancies. *Br Med J* 1:268, 1975.
146. Parsons V, Baum M: Effect of mithramycin on calcium and hydroxyproline metabolism in patients with malignant disease. *Br Med J* 1:474, 1967.
147. Brereton HD, Halushk PV, Alexander RW, Mason DM, Keiwer HE, DeVita VT Jr: Indomethacin-responsive hypercalceia in a patient with renal-cell adenocarcinoma. *N Eng J Med* 291:83, 1974.
148. Robertson RP, Baylink DJ, Marini JJ, Adkison W: Elevated prostaglandins and suppressed parathyroid hormone asso-

ciated with hypercalcemia and renal cell carcinoma. *J Clin Endocrinol Metab* 41:164, 1975.
149. Brenner DE, Harvey HA, Lipton A, Demers L: A study of prostaglandin E_2, parathormone and response to indomethacin in patients with hypercalcemia of malignancy. *Cancer* 44:556, 1982.
150. Atkins D, Ibbotson KJ, Hillier K, Hunt NH, Hammonds JC, Martin TJ: Secretion of prostaglandins as bone resorbing agents by renal cortical carcinoma in culture. *Br J Cancer* 36:601, 1971.
151. Prescott LF: Anti-inflammatory analgesics and drugs used in rheumatoid arthritis and gout. In: MNG Dukes, ed, *Meyler's Side Effects of Drugs*. American Elsevier, New York, pp 217, 1975.
152. Nolph KD, Stolt M, Maher JF: Calcium free peritoneal dialysis treatment of vitamin D intoxication. *Arch Int Med* 128:809, 1971.
153. Stolz ML, Nolph KD, Maher JF: Factors affecting calcium removal with calcium-free peritoneal dialysis. *J Lab Clin Med* 78:389, 1971.
154. Scholz D, Purnell D: Asymptomatic primary hyperparathyroidism: A 10-year prospective study. *Mayo Clin Proc* 56:473, 1981.
155. Posen S, Clifton–Bligh P, Reeve TS, Wagstaffe C, Wilkinson M: Is parathyroidectomy of benefit in primary hyperparathyroidism? In: B Frame, JT Potts, eds, *Clinical Disorders of Bone and Mineral Metabolism*. Excerpta Medica, Amsterdam, p 154, 1983.
156. Neer R: Natural history of untreated hyperparathyroidism. Presented at Symposium on Clinical Disorders of Bone and Mineral Metabolism. May 1983.
157. Sherwood JK, Ackroyd FW, Garcia M: Effect of cimetidine on circulating parathyroid hormone in primary hyperparathyroidism. *Lancet* 1:616, 1980.
158. Caro JF, Castro JH, Glennon JA: Effect of long-term propranolol administration on parathyroid hormone and calcium concentration in primary hyperparathyroidism. *Ann Int Med* 91:740, 1979.
159. Rude RK, Oldham SB, Singer FR, Nicoloff JT: Treatment of thyrotoxic hypercalcemia with propranolol. *N Eng J Med* 294:431, 1976.
160. Sigurdsson G, Woodhouse NJY, Taylor S, Joplin GF: Stilboestrol diphosphonate in hypercalcemia due to parathryoid carcinoma. *Br Med J* 1:27, 1973.
161. Mundy GR, Wilkinson R, Heath DA: A comparative study of available medical therapy for hypercalcemia malignancy. *Am J Med* 74:421, 1983.
162. Van Holten–Verzamdvoort A, Harinck HIJ, Hermans J, Cleton RJ, Bijvoet OLM: Supportive bisphosphonate treatment reduces morbidity from bone lesions in breast cancer (abstract). *ASBMR*, Bone Mineral Research Congress, Abs No. 390, Indianapolis, 1987.
163. Glover D, Riley L, Carmichael K, et al.: Hypocalcemia and inhibition of parathyroid hormone secretion after administration of WR-2721 (a radioprotective and chemoprotective agent). *N Engl J Med* 309:1137, 1983.
164. Wolf J, Attie M, Fallar M, Goldfarb S: Studies of the hypocalcemic action of WR-2721. *Clin Res* 32:412, 1984.
165. Glover JD, Shaw L, Glick J, Slatopolsky E, Weiler C, Attie M, Goldfarb S: Treatment of hypercalcemia in parathyroid cancer with WR2721, S-2-(3-aminopropylamine) ethylphosphorothoric acid. *Ann Int Med* 103:55, 1985.
166. Weiss J, Wolf J, Slatopolsky E, Fallar M, Attie M, Goldfarb S: Sustained hypocalcemia, inhibition of PTH secretion and correction of Vitamin D induced hypercalcemia with chronic administration of WR-2721 (abstract). *Kidney Int* 27:129(S), 1985.
167. Hunt BJ, Yendt ER: The response of hypercalcemia in sarcoidosis to chloroquine. *Ann Int Med* 59:554, 1963.
168. O'Leary JT, Jones G, Yip A, Lohnes D, Cohanim M, Yendt E: The effects of chloroquine on serum 1,25-dihydroxy vitamin D and calcium metabolism in sarcoidosis. *N Engl J Med* 315:12, 1986.
169. Glass RA, Eil CH: Ketoconazole-induced reduction in serum 1,25-dihydroxy vitamin D. *J Clin Endocrinol Metabolism* 63:766, 1986.
170. Henry HL: Effect of ketoconazole and myconazole on 25-hydroxy D_3 metabolism by cultured chick kidney cells. *J Steroid Biochem* 23:91, 1985.
171. Mishoulam HJ, Lad TE, Khan A, Kukla LJ, Abrahamson EC, McGuire WP, Kukreja SC: Effect of cisplatinum on hypercalcemia of malignancy. *Clin Res* 31:778a, 1983.
172. Kukla LJ, Abrahamson EC, Shevrin DH, Lad TE, Mcguire WP, Kukreja SC: Cisplatinum as treatment for humoral hypercalcemia of malignancy in an athymic mouse model. *Clin Res* 31:739A, 1983.
173. Walsh FB, Murray RG: *Ocular manifestations of disturbances in calcium metabolism*. *Am J Ophth* 36:1657, 1953.
174. Barr DP, MacBride CM, Sanders TE: Tetany with increased intracranial pressure and papilledema. Results from treatment with hydrotachysterol. *Trans Assoc Am Phys* 53:227, 1938.
175. Ireland AW, Hornbrook JW, Neale FC, Posen S: The crystalline lens in chronic surgical hypoparathyroidism. *Arch Int Med* 122:408, 1969.
176. Camp JD: Symmetrical calcification of the cerebral basal ganglia, its roentgeneologic significance in the diagnosis of parathyroid insufficiency. *Radiology* 49:568, 1947.
177. Levine P: Intracranial calcification associated with hypoparathyroidism. *Bull NY Acad Med* 38:632, 1962.
178. Chopra D, Janson P, Sawin CT: Insensitivity to digoxin associated with hypocalcemia. *N Eng J Med* 296:917, 1977.
179. Eipe J, Johnson SA, Kiamko RT, Bronksy D: Hypoparathyroidism following ^{131}I therapy for hyperthyroidism. *Arch Intern Med* 121:270, 1968.
180. Sagel J, Epstein S, Kalk J, Von Mieghen W: Radioactive iodine therapy for thyrotoxicosis at Groote Schuur Hospital over a 6 year period. *Postgrad Med J* 48:308, 1972.
181. Robertson GM, Moore EW, Switz DM, Sizemore GW, Estep HL: Inadequate parathyroid response in acute pancreatitis. *N Engl J Med* 194:512, 1976.
182. Haldiman B, Goldstein DA, Akam M, Massry SG: Renal function and blood levels of divalent ions in acute pancreatitis. A prospective study in 99 patients. *Miner Electrolyte Metab* 3:190, 1980.
183. Horwitz CA, Myers LWP, Foote FW: Secondary malignant tumors of the parathyroid glands. Report of 2 cases with associated hypoparathyroidism. *Am J Med* 52:797, 1972.
184. Brezis M, Shalev O, Leibel B, Berenheim J, Ben Ishay D: Phosphorus retention and hypoparathyroidism associated with transfusion and iron overload in thalassemia. *Miner Electrolyte Metab* 4:57, 1980.
185. Drake TG, Albright F, Bauer W, Castleman B: Chronic idiopathic hypoparathyroidism. Report of 6 cases with autopsy findings. *Ann Intern Med* 12:1751, 1939.
186. Spinner MW, Blizzard RM, Childs B: Clinical and genetic heterogeneity in idiopathic Addison's disease and hypoparathyroidism. *J Clin Endocrinol Metab* 28:795, 1968.
187. Wilson PW, Buckley CE, Eisenbarth GS: Disordered immune function in patients with polyglandular failure. *J*

188. Nusynowitz ML, Frame B, Kolb FO: The spectrum of the hypoparathyroid states. A classification based on physiologic principles. *Medicine (Baltimore)* 55:105, 1976.
189. Klahr S, Slatopolsky E: Urinary phosphate and cyclic AMP in pseudohypoparathyroidism. In: SG Massry, E Ritz, A Rapado, eds, *Homeostasis of Phosphate and Other Minerals.* Plenum, New York, p 173, 1977.
190. Chase LR, Melson GL, Aurbach GD: Pseudohypoparathyroidism: Defective excretion of 3'5'-AMP in response to parathyroid hormone. *J Clin Invest* 48:1832, 1969.
191. Farfel Z, Brickman AS, Kaslow HR, Brothers V, Bourne H: Defect of receptor cyclase coupling protein in pseudohypoparathryoidism. *N Eng J Med* 303:237, 1980.
192. Bourne HR, Kaslow HR, Brickman AS, Farfel Z: Fibroblast defect in pseudohypoparathyroidism Type I. Reduced activity of receptor cyclase coupling protein. *J Clin Endocrinol Metab* 53:636, 1981.
193. Drezner M, Neelon FA, Lebovitz HE: Pseudohypoparathyroidism Type II. A possible defect in the reception of cyclic AMP signal. *N Eng J Med* 289:1056, 1973.
194. Rodriguez HJ, Villareal H, Klahr S, Slatopolsky E: Pseudohypoparathyroidism Type II. Restoration of normal renal responsiveness to parathyroid hormone by calcium administration. *J Clin Endocrinol Metab* 39:693, 1974.
195. Daneman D, Kooh SW, Fraser D: Hypoparathyroidism in childhood. *Clin Endocrinol Metab* 11:211, 1982.
196. Kolb FO, Steinbach HL: Pseudohypoparathyroidism with secondary hyperparathyroidism and osteitis fibrosa. *J Clin Endocrinol* 22:59, 1962.
197. Drezner MK, Neelon FA, Haussler M, McPherson HT, Lebovitz HE: 1,25-dihydroxycholecalciferol deficiency: The probable cause of hypocalcemia and metabolic bone disease in pseudo hypoparathyroidism. *J Clin Endocrinol Metab* 42:621, 1976.
198. Pitkin RM: Calcium metabolism in pregnancy. A review. *Am J Obstet Gynecol* 121:724, 1975.
199. Tsang RC, Light IJ, Sutherland JM, Kleinman LI: Possible pathogenetic factors in neonatal hypocalcemia of prematurity. *J Pediatr* 82:423, 1973.
200. Tsang RC, Chen I-W, Friedman MA, Chen I: Neonatal parathyroid function: Role of gestational age and postnatal age. *J Pediatr* 83:728, 1973.
201. Barltrop D: Neonatal hypocalcemia. *Postgrad J* 51 (Suppl 3): 7, 1975.
202. Rao DS, Parfitt AM, Kleerekoper M, Pumo BS, Mathews M, Frame B: Dissociation of cAMP and phosphaturic response to PTH in human vitamin D deficiency. An acquired disorder simulating pseudohypoparathyroidism. Presented at VII Int. Conference on Calcium Regulating Hormones, Kobe, Japan, 1983.
203. Medalle K, Waterhouse C: A magnesium deficient patient presenting with hypocalcemia and hypophosphatemia. *Ann Intern Med* 79:76, 1973.
204. Porter RH, Cox BA, Heaney D, Hostetter TH, Stinebaugh BJ, Suki W: Treatment of hypoparathyroid patients with chlorthalidone. *N Engl J Med* 298:578, 1978.
205. Peterson P, Gray P, Tolmn KG: Calcium balance in drug-induced osteomalacia: Response to vitamin D. *Clin Pharm Ther* 19:63, 1976.
206. Purnell DC, Scholtz DA, Smith LH, Sizemore GW, Black BM, Goldsmith RS, Arnaud CDP: Treatment of primary hyperparathyroidism. *Am J Med* 56:800, 1974.
207. Parfitt AM: Adult hypoparathyroidism. Treatment with calcifediol. *Arch Int Med* 138:874, 1978.
208. Nagant De Deuxchaisnes C: Hyperparathyroidism. In: LV Avioli, SM Krane, eds, *Metabolic Bone Disease*, Vol 2. Academic Press, New York, 1978.

ADDENDUM

This addendum summarizes some recent important advances which have occurred relating to the diagnosis and treatment of disorders of calcium metabolism.

The parathyroid hormone related protein (PTHRP) that is now believed to mediate most humoral hypercalcemia of malignancy was isolated in 1986, its complementary cDNA has been cloned, and the gene mapped and isolated (209). Assays for circulating PTHRP have been developed and the results reported (210–212). Although the assay is not yet widely available, it is expected to be a valuable tool in diagnosing humoral hypercalcemia of malignancy in which PTH assays give normal or low results. With respect to PTH assays, earlier assays did not reliably separate primary hyperparathyroidism from normal or from hypercalcemia of malignancy. However, the development of double antibody assays for "intact" PTH by several groups (213–215) and their commercial introduction has greatly enhanced the usefulness of PTH assays in making these distinctions, and has rendered many of the other diagnostic tests obsolete.

A recent study has gone a long way towards explaining why overt bone disease (osteitis fibrosa cystica) is an increasingly rare presentation of primary hyperparathyroidism especially in North America. In a study from Paris (216) the patients with primary hyperparathyroidism and osteitis fibrosa cystica tended to be older, had lower glomerular filtration rates and lower 25 (OH)D_3 and calcitriol levels than patients with renal calculi. Bone disease appeared to result from the lower calcitriol levels and the associated lower intestinal calcium absorption.

With respect to the treatment of hypercalcemic disorders, the management of asymptomatic primary hyperparathyroidism has recently been reviewed by Potts (217) who points out that the relationship between osteoporosis and primary hyperparathyroidism is still incompletely understood, and there may be geographical differences; for example vertebral fractures may be commoner in this disease in Europe than in North America. Further work is required before firm recommendations can be made as to which patients should be followed without surgical treatment. The treatment of cancer associated hypercalcemia significantly improves morbidity but has little effect on mortality (218). With respect to the intravenous diphosphonates (or bisphosphonates, as this group of drugs is increasingly called), the use of intravenous aminohydroxypropylidene diphosphonate (APD) in Europe, where it is available (it is not yet released in the U.S.A. and Canada) have shown it to be remarkably effective in malignant hypercalcemia (219). In a randomized study comparing APD, mithramycin and a corticosteroid/

calcitonin regime, APD corrected the hypercalcemia better than the other treatments (220). Intravenous EHDP (etidronate disodium) has also been shown to be very effective therapy for this disorder (221).

Gallium nitrate, originally used as a chemotherapeutic agent, has recently been shown to be effective therapy for cancer related hypercalcemia when given as an IV infusion (222). In randomized studies it has been shown to be more effective than either calcitonin (222) or IV etidronate (223).

Finally, regarding the treatment of hypocalcemic disorders, Yamamoto et al. (224) have recently shown that the dose of calcitriol required to achieve nomocalcemia in pseudohypoparathyroidism is somewhat lower than in hypoparathyroidism, presumably because of the presence of normal PTH levels in the former condition. For the same reason hypercalciuria is less marked during calcitriol therapy in pseudohypoparathyroidism than in hypoparathyroidism.

REFERENCES

209. Bilezikian JP: Parathyroid hormone related peptide in sickness and in health. *N Engl J Med* 322:1151–1153, 1990.
210. Budayr AA, Nissenson RA, Kline RF, et al.: Increased serum levels of a parathyroid hormone-like peptide in malignancy associated with hypercalcemia. *Ann Intern Med* 111:807–812, 1989.
211. Henderson JE, Shustic C, Kramer R, et al.: Circulating concentrations of parathyroid hormone-like peptide in malignancy and hyperparathyroidism. *J Bone Min Res* 5:105–113, 1990.
212. Burtis WJ, Brady BS, Orloff JJ, et al.: Immunochemical characterization of circulating parathyroid hormone-related protein in patients with humoral hypercalcemia of cancer. *N Engl J Med* 322:1106–1112, 1990.
213. Lindall AW, Elting J, Ells J, Rouse BA: Estimation of biologically activate intact parathyroid hormone in normal and hyperparathyroid sera by sequential N-terminal immunoextraction and mid region radioimmunoassay. *J Clin Endocrinol Metab* 57:1007, 1983.
214. Nussbaum SR, Zahradink RJ, Lavinge JR, et al.: Highly sensitive two site immunoradiometric assay of parathyrin and its clinical utility in evaluating patients with hypercalcemia. *Clin Chem* 8:1364–1367, 1987.
215. Blind, E, Schmidt-Gayk H, Scharla S, et al.: Two-site assay of intact parathyroid hormone in the investigation of primary hyperparathyroidism and other disorders of calcium metabolism compared with a midregion assay. *J Clin Endocrinol Metab* 67:353–360, 1988.
216. Patron P, Gardin J-P, Paillard M: Renal mass and reserve of vitamin D: determinants in primary hyperparathyroidism. *Kidney Int* 31:1174–1180, 1987.
217. Potts JT Jr: Management of asymptomatic hyperparathyroidism. *J Clin Endocrinol Metab* 70:1489–1493, 1980.
218. Ralston SH, Gallacher SJ, Patel U, et al.: Cancer associated hypercalcemia, morbidity and mortality. Clinical experience in 126 patients. *Ann Intern Med* 112:499–504, 1990.
219. Harinck HIJ, Bijvoet OLM, Plantingh AST, et al.: Role of bone and kidney in tumour induce hypercalcemia and its treatment with bisphosphonate and sodium chloride. *Am J Med* 82:1133–1142, 1987.
220. Ralston SH, Dryburgh FJ, Cowan RA, et al.: Comparision of aminohydroxypropylidene diphosphonate, mithramycin and corticosteroids/calcitonin in treatment of cancer associated hypercalcemia. *Lancet* 2:907–910, 1985.
221. Etridronate disodium: A new therapy for hypercalcemia of malignancy. *Am J Med* 82 (2A):1–78, 1987.
222. Warrell RP Jr, Israel R, Frisone M, et al.: Gallium nitrate for acute treatment of cancer related hypercalcemia: a randomized double blind comparison with calcitonin. *Ann Intern Med* 108:669–674, 1988.
223. Warrell RP Jr, Murphy WK, Schulman P, O'Dwyer PJ: Gallium nitrate vs. etridronate for acute treatment of cancer related hypercalcemia randomized double blind study. *J Bone Min Res* 5:S271, 1990.
224. Yamamoto M, Takuwa Y, Masuko S, Ogata E: Effects of endogenous and exogenous parathyroid hormone on tubular reabsorption of calcium in pseudohypoparathyroidism. *J Clin Endocrinol Metab* 66:618–625, 1988.

CHAPTER 6

Disorders of Magnesium Metabolism

THOMAS DYCKNER

INTRODUCTION

Magnesium is one of the most abundant intracellular ions in plants and animals. Magnesium is the second most common divalent metal ion in the oceans and the third most common on land. In the precambrian sea, where life is thought to have developed, magnesium held a dominant position. Therefore, it is not surprising that cells have tried to maintain their original environment. In the *milieu interieur*, magnesium is of great importance for many biologic actions, and the ion is essential for growth and life. Even the most primitive energy-producing reactions, such as anaerobic glycolysis, need magnesium as an essential activator in several enzymatic steps.

In the medical profession a frequently encountered misconception is that magnesium is a trace element. The reason for this misconception probably resides in earlier difficulties in obtaining accurate and reproducible determinations of magnesium in plasma, and nowadays in the lack of correlation between plasma and total body magnesium.

Next to potassium, magnesium (atomic weight 24.32) is the most abundant intracellular cation in the human body. The amount of magnesium in the body is approximately 22–28 g, corresponding to about 1000 mM (2000 mEq). More than half of this amount (about 60%) is to be found in bone, where most of it is firmly bound. However, a tiny fraction is adsorbed to the surface of the apatite crystals and is more easily exchangeable.

The remainder is divided between muscles (about 20%) and other soft tissues. The amount and distribution of magnesium in the body is illustrated in Figure 1. It has been demonstrated by several investigators that skeletal muscle magnesium is readily available in deficiency situations. Using radiolabeled magnesium, investigators have found one magnesium pool that can be equilibrated fairly quickly, which consists mainly of extracellular magnesium. There is a second magnesium pool that turns over at about half the rate of the first pool. The second pool mainly consists of intracellular magnesium. Most of the body magnesium, however, is in a pool with a very slow turnover rate, which is mainly skeletal magnesium. About 30% of bone magnesium is exchangeable in vitro, but in vivo only 1% is exchangeable within 24 hours and 5% is exchangeable within a week.

Skeletal muscle is quantitatively the most important tissue, containing about 80% of the total magnesium of the active cell mass. However, only about 5–10% of this is present as free ions in the cytosol. Somewhat less than 0.5% of body magnesium is present in plasma. The plasma magnesium level is remarkably constant. About 30% of plasma magnesium is protein bound, and most of the remaining fraction is in a free ionized form and is filtered through the kidneys. Magnesium is mainly an intracellular ion, and the magnesium concentration in the cell is usually calculated to be 12.5–17 mM/kg of intracellular water. In practice, however, most of the intracellular magnesium is bound to different complexes (e.g., energy-rich phosphate compounds), and the free ionized intracellular magnesium concentration is considerably much lower.

FUNCTIONS OF MAGNESIUM

Magnesium is an essential cofactor for many different enzyme systems (about 300). It is of great importance for splitting reactions and for the transfer of phosphate groups. Thus it is indispensible for the metabolism of adenosine triphosphate (ATP). ATP is involved in the utilization of glucose; the synthesis of fat, protein, nucleic acids, and coenzyme systems; muscle contraction; and some energy-demanding membrane transport systems. Hence, it is understandable that magnesium deficiency may present in many different ways. In plants magnesium plays the same role in the chlorophyll molecule as iron does in the hemoglobin molecule in the animal world.

DAILY REQUIREMENTS AND DIETARY CONTENT

Since the diagnosis of a magnesium deficiency is complicated, difficulties have arisen in establishing the daily magnesium requirement. Most authorities in the field consider an adequate intake to be around 15 mM/day and proportionately more fore children and pregnant women. The supply of magnesium in the diet has decreased during

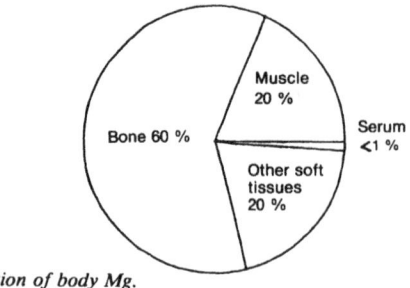

Figure 1. Distribution of body magnesium.

the last decades, mostly due to the increase in industrial processing and refining of our food. Calculations of magnesium content in the western diet have been estimated to between 6 and 12 mM/day, which evidently does not provide an excess.

Abundant amounts of magnesium are found in meat and other animal food products. However, in the case of a low magnesium intake, the simultaneous presence of calcium, phosphate, and protein in the diet have a negative influence on the intestinal absorption of magnesium. Some vegetables, crude rice, cereals, cocoa, nuts, and shellfish contain a form of magnesium that is more easily absorbed. Table 1 shows the magnesium concentration of some foodstuffs.

ABSORPTION

Magnesium is mainly absorbed from the small intestine, chiefly the jejunum, as demonstrated by ^{28}Mg tracer studies, with a maximum blood level at 2 and 8 hours following ingestion. The colon may also play an important role in the absorption of magnesium under certain circumstances. This has been demonstrated in some case reports of hypermagnesemia after giving magnesium-containing solutions by enema. Results from some investigations also indicate a possible compensatory increase in the absorption of magnesium from the colon during diseases of the small intestine, e.g., inflammatory processes that interfere with magnesium absorption in the small intestine.

Normally 30% of total ingested magnesium is absorbed, but there are wide variations due to other components in food. Absorption also depends on the absolute amount of magnesium in food and the magnesium status of the body. With a very low dietary intake (1 mM/day), 75% was absorbed, while a high intake (25 mM/day) resulted in a decrease of the absorption to 24% in one study. In magnesium deficiency the absorption will be increased by increased parathyroid hormone release. However, calcium absorption is favored, which complicates the outcome. Endogenous fecal magnesium excretion is normally low, 1–2%, as determined in trials using intravenous ^{28}Mg.

INTERACTIONS WITH HORMONES AND VITAMINS

A highly complicated and not yet fully understood system of interactions exists between magnesium and various hormones, but there is no evidence of a specific magnesium-regulating hormone. The effects of some hormones on magnesium metabolism are shown in Table 2.

Parathyroid hormone

A mild magnesium deficiency results in an increased release of parathyroid hormone (PTH), whilst a severe deficiency leads to a decrease. In cases of severe magnesium depletion, it has been demonstrated that there is a decreased peripheral sensitivity to exogenously administered PTH. Large doses of PTH in humans increase both the intestinal absorption and the renal reabsorption of magnesium, while small doses seem to have no effect. The situation is complicated by simultaneous changes in the metabolism of calcium and phosphates. Under normal circumstances, PTH does not appear to be essential for the regulation of magnesium balance, which is also true for calcitonin.

Thyroid hormones

In hyperthyroidism, a lowering of serum magnesium is often observed, and the reverse has been demonstrated in

Table 1. Magnesium concentration in some foods

Mg	µg/g fresh weight	mg/100 kcal
Cabbage	166–321	63.8–229.3
Beans	241–1697	49.2–92.8
Crude rice	1477	40.9
Cereals	1032	23.9–42.2
Meat	209–402	7.4–14.7
Fish	207–532	30.4–68.2
Shellfish	154–530	30.8–41.7
Cocoa	4289	94.9
Nuts	1583–3175	26.3–49.3

Table 2. Influence of some hormones on magnesium metabolism

	S-Mg	i.c./e.c.	Excretion	Absorption
Thyroid hormone	−	+	+	(−)
Insulin	−	+	0	0
Adrenal steroids	−	−	+	(−)
Estrogen	−	+	0	?
Catecholamines	+/−	−	?	?
PTH	(−)	(−)	−	+

i.c. = intracellular; e.c. = extracellular

hypothyroidism. Thyroid hormones have been reported to increase the renal excretion of magnesium and to increase the transport of magnesium from the extracellular to the intracellular compartment. The gastrointestinal absorption of magnesium is probably reduced, perhaps due to the fact that thyroid hormone increases vitamin D metabolism.

Insulin

In uncontrolled diabetes mellitus, magnesium is lost from the intracellular compartment, which leads to a temporarily enhanced serum magnesium concentration. However, the urinary excretion of magnesium is raised, resulting in a lowering of the serum magnesium level. Insulin causes a shift of magnesium from the extracellular to the intracellular compartment, resulting in a lowering of serum magnesium, but urinary magnesium does not increase and the gastrointestinal absorption of the ion seems to be unchanged. Hypomagnesemia results in an increase of insulin secretion, while a decrease is seen at high magnesium levels. Administration of glucagon leads to a lowering of the serum magnesium concentration.

Corticoids

An excess of glucocorticoids and/or mineralocorticoids may result in hypomagnesemia, mainly due to a large increase in the excretion of magnesium. With a chronic excess of these hormones, a cellular magnesium depletion may develop. The magnesiuretic effect of aldosterone is secondary to the extracellular volume expansion and to the larger filtered load of sodium, both of which lead to a decreased reabsorption of magnesium. Magnesium depletion, in turn, has been shown to increase aldosterone release, which may result in a vicious circle.

Estrogen

In the studies reported thus far, estrogen appears to cause a slight reduction of the serum magnesium concentration and to increase the uptake of magnesium in soft tissues and bone. The urinary output is not influenced.

Catecholamines

There is a complex relationship between magnesium and catecholamines. Depending on the study design and the time lag between administration and sampling, catecholamines have been reported to both increase and decrease serum magnesium concentration and to reduce tissue magnesium levels. Catecholamines will cause lipolysis with a sizable increase of free fatty acids, which in turn can chelate magnesium. Magnesium and calcium have reciprocal effects on the storage and release of catecholamines from the adrenal medulla with calcium stimulating and magnesium inhibiting the release of catecholamines.

Vitamin D

The effect of vitamin D on magnesium metabolism is difficult to evaluate, since the clinical picture is complicated by simultaneous changes in calcium and phosphate metabolism. Low doses of vitamin D increase the gastrointestinal absorption of magnesium, and physiologic doses may retain a positive magnesium balance. Vitamin D increases the transport of magnesium from the extracellular to the intracellular space.

Thiamine (B_1)

Magnesium and thiamine are in some aspects dependent on each other. In states of magnesium deficiency, the body does not appear to be able to utilize administered thiamine and symptoms of a deficiency may develop. Administration of thiamine in magnesium depletion accentuates the symptoms attributable to magnesium deficiency.

Pyridoxine (B_6)

Vitamin B_6 increases the transport of magnesium into the cells. Like the administration of thiamine, vitamin B_6 aggravates the symptoms of any simultaneous magnesium deficit.

RENAL EXCRETION OF MAGNESIUM — REGULATION OF BODY MAGNESIUM CONTENT AND SERUM MAGNESIUM CONCENTRATION

The ionized fraction of magnesium in serum (about 70%) is filtered in the glomeruli (Figure 2). In health the kidneys are the main organs responsible for the regulation of magnesium metabolism. This role involves both the regulation of the body magnesium content and the control of the serum magnesium concentration. These roles may sometimes give rise to conflicting situations.

The urinary excretion of magnesium is largely dependent on the net absorption of magnesium and the external balance of the ion. To conserve the body magnesium content, the kidneys have to match urinary excretion to net absorption. Simultaneously there is a need to regulate serum magnesium concentration by supplying an adequate amount of magnesium to the extracellular fluid by the process of tubular reabsorption. The situation may be illustrated by the following formula:

Net absorption − ext. balance = Mg_p × GFR − tubular reabsorption.

In the steady state, the result of a change in the renal handling of magnesium is a change in the plasma magnesium concentration or in some other function of the body's magnesium content, but not a change in the rate of urinary excretion of magnesium. Such a change can only be accomplished by a change in load.

The reabsorption of magnesium follows a Tm/GFR

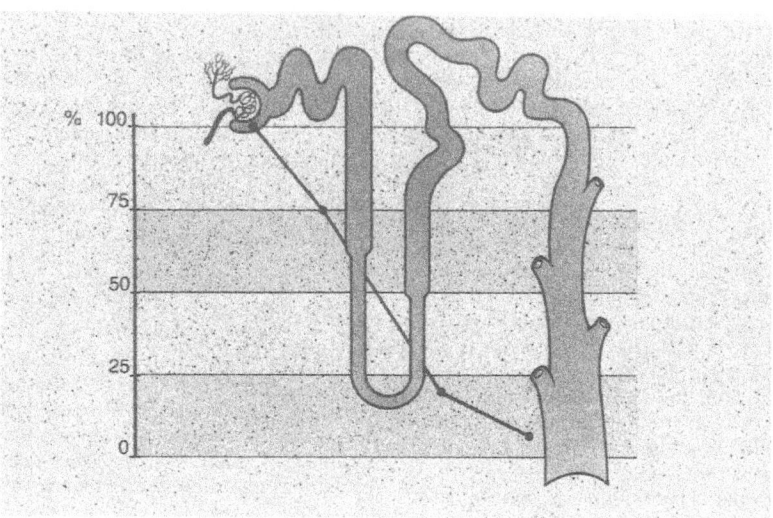

Figure 2. Reabsorption of magnesium throughout the nephron.

model, with a lower limit of about 0.6 mM/l and a less well-defined upper limit of about 1.00–1.50 mM/l. This means that a comparatively small increase in the serum magnesium concentration will result in an increased urinary output of the ion. Active secretion of magnesium in humans has not been demonstrated.

There is no indication of any important extrarenal mechanisms for control of the serum magnesium concentration. Therefore, the serum levels of magnesium are entirely dependent on load/GFR and tubular reabsorption of magnesium according to the formula:

$$Mg_p = \frac{Mg_u}{GFR} \quad \frac{Tm_{Mg}}{GFR}.$$

On a daily basis, tubular reabsorption supplies about 110 mM magnesium to the extracellular fluid, accounting for 90% of the serum magnesium concentration in the fasting state. Load per GFR makes a significant contribution only when the GFR is reduced, but does not become dominant until the GFR falls below 10 ml/min. Impaired tubular reabsorption will result in unchanged urinary excretion and a fall in the serum magnesium concentration in the steady-state condition. According to the Tm/GFR model, a fall in serum magnesium concentration will automatically lead to a reduction of the urinary excretion of magnesium.

The excretion of magnesium varies during the day, with a maximum in the late morning and the lowest excretion in the late evening. Many factors influence the urinary excretion of magnesium (Figure 3). The proximal reabsorption of magnesium is approximately 30–45% of the filtered load and is dependent upon sodium reabsorption. Inhibition of sodium transport due to an increase in the extracellular volume is accompanied by a parallel change in magnesium reabsorption. Generally the change in magnesium clearance is about twice the change in sodium clearance.

Supplying extra calcium or magnesium results in an inhibition of the tubular reabsorption of magnesium. In the latter case, the main effect appears to be caused by a rise in the magnesium concentration on the contraluminal side of the membrane, while an increase in magnesium within the tubular lumen leads to an increase in magnesium reabsorption. Reabsorption in the distal tubules and collecting ducts occurs against an electrochemical gradient by an active, probably magnesium-specific, transport mechanism. There is probably an additional mechanism that is jointly used by calcium and magnesium. Increasing the concentration of either ion decreases the reabsorption of the other and increases its excretion.

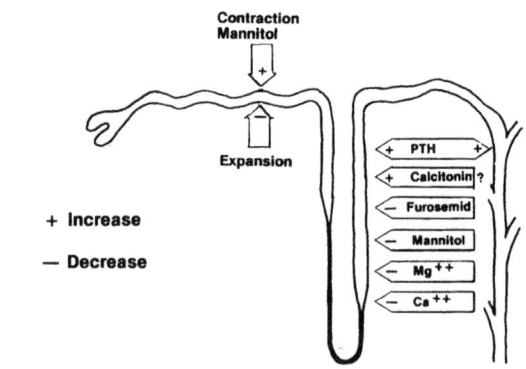

Figure 3. Factors influencing renal handling of magnesium ion.

Parathyroid hormone influences magnesium reabsorption in that high doses increase reabsorption, while low doses have no effect in humans. Aldosterone excess has a negative influence on magnesium metabolism. This is most likely an indirect effect, due to chronic volume expansion and an influence on the renal handling of sodium, leading to increased urinary excretion of magnesium.

CAUSES OF MAGNESIUM DEFICIENCY

Magnesium deficiency is not uncommon. Some factors and diseases leading to a magnesium deficiency are presented in Table 3. Deficiency may arise through reduced intake, reduced absorption, or excessive excretion. On a worldwide basis, malnutrition is one of the most common causes of magnesium deficiency, but even in the Western world, a low intake may be a problem. Through industrial processing the magnesium content of our food has decreased substantially and, to say the least, a normal diet does not contain an excess of magnesium. Elderly people, in particular, who often have an inadequate intake of nutrients, vitamins, and calories and who also may have impaired gastrointestinal absorption, are at risk for developing magnesium deficiency. In the active phase of Crohn's disease, the risk of a magnesium deficiency is noticeable, and following large intestinal resections the risk is obvious.

A primary loss of cellular magnesium will lead to a

Table 3. Some causes of magnesium deficiency

Reduced intake
  Protein calorie malnutrition
  Starvation
  Prolonged I.V. therapy without magnesium supplementation
  Inadequate dietary habits

Intestinal malabsorption
  Malabsorption syndromes, e.g., sprue, pancreatic insufficiency, Mb Crohn
  Resection of small intestine

Loss of body fluids
  Long-term gastric drainage
  Chronic abuse of laxatives
  Intestinal and biliary fistulae
  Prolonged diarrhea

Increased excretion
  1. Decreased Tm/GFR for magnesium (extrinsic)
     Diuretic therapy, notably loop diuretics
     Primary and secondary aldosteronism
     Hyperthyroidism
     ADH excess
     Hyperparathyroidism
     Hypercalcemia
     Chronic alcohol ingestion
  2. Decreased Tm/GFR for magnesium (intrinsic)
     Aminoglycoside nephropathy
     Tubulointerstitial nephropathy
     Bartter's syndrome
     Renal tubular acidosis

secondary negative external balance of the ion, while a primary negative balance will result in secondary losses of magnesium from the cellular compartment. A reduction of net intestinal absorption or of Tm/GFR will lead to a state of chronic hypomagnesemia.

Excessive excretion of magnesiuim may occur as a more or less transient phenomenon in certain stuations or on a more chronic basis. A decreased Tm/GFR for magnesium can be produced either by an influence from extrinsic factors or by a deranged intrinsic situation in the kidneys.

A very common reason for an increased urinary loss of magnesium is the widespread use of conventional diuretics. An increase in urinary losses of magnesium by 25–300% has been observed in several studies. The magnitude of the loss is dependent on the type of diuretic used, the dose, the dosage interval, and the duration of therapy. When ordinary doses of commonly used diuretics were given, the increase in the urinary loss of magnesium remained between 25% and 50%. Low muscle magnesium levels are often seen after a few years of treatment with diuretics, particularly in patients who have other concomitant factors leading to a deficiency, e.g., inadequate dietary habits, reduced gastrointestinal absorption, alcoholism, or aldosteronism. In a study of 597 patients with congestive heart failure and/or arterial hypertension who were on long-term therapy with conventional diuretics, about 40% of the patients presented subnormal muscle magnesium values. This situation could be normalized by combining conventional diuretics with amiloride, spironolactone, or triamterene. Among the diuretics, the loop blockers give rise to the largest magnesium losses from the body. This is not surprising, since magnesium is mainly reabsorbed in the ascending limb of the loop of Henle. The use of thiazides is accompanied by lesser magnesium losses in the urine, since only about 5% of the magnesium filtered is reabsorbed in the distal convoluted tubule. However, other factors may take precedence, e.g., the secondary aldosteronism induced by thiazides, changes of extracellular fluid volume, and changes of sodium load.

The most common cause of the intrinsic decreases of Tm/GFR for magnesium probably is chronic pyelonephritis. In chronic renal failure, there is a reduction of sodium reabsorption due to the need to excrete more sodium per nephron. This reduction of sodium reabsorption is accompanied by a lowered magnesium reabsorption, which will protect the body from a dangerous hypermagnesemia. In the exaggerated form of salt-losing nephropathy, a patient may lose large amounts of sodium and magnesium, which will have to be replaced by oral or parenteral therapy.

About 20% of patients with Bartter's syndrome exhibit hypomagnesemia. Most of these patients probably have a type III Bartter's syndrome, with a localized defect in sodium-chloride transport in the thick ascending limb of the loop of Henle. Amiloride, spironolactone, and triamterene have been tried in some of these patients without any positive effects on serum magnesium levels. However, parenteral magnesium therapy has proved to be effective.

The use of nephrotoxic substances, such as cisplatin,

cyclosporine, capreomycin, carbenicillin, amphotericin B, and gentamycin, may lead to a Bartter's-like syndrome by reducing the tubular reabsorption of magnesium. About half the patients on 70 mg cisplatin/m^2 body surface every 2 weeks will develop hypomagnesemia. The nephrotoxicity may be reduced by adequate hydration of the patient or by simultaneous parenteral thiosulphate administration. Magnesium supplements should be given.

SYMPTOMATOLOGY IN MAGNESIUM DEFICIENCY

With regard to the extensive physiologic role of magnesium in different enzyme systems, it is understandable that the symptomatology of a magnesium deficiency may be both diversified and difficult to explain. A thorough knowledge of the different symptoms that may occur and of the most common factors and disease entities leading to a deficiency will of course make the diagnosis easier. Symptoms of a deficiency principally occur in the nervous system, skeletal muscles, gastrointestinal tract, and cardiovascular system. Symptoms associated with the central nervous system often begin with apathy, depression, difficulty in remembering, and reduced ability to concentrate. In more severe deficiency, confusion or even hallucinations and paranoia ideas may be present.

Neuromuscular symptoms are often prominent in serious deficiency, and patients may present with tremor and muscle twitching. Muscular weakness is common and is probably related to a secondary potassium deficiency. Tremor and fasciculation of the skeletal muscles, numbness, tingling, and cramps may occur, even in mild deficiency states. There is sometimes a positive Chvostek sign. Athetoid movements, ataxia, nystagmus, and tetany have been observed in more severe deficiency.

Gastrointestinal symptoms are common and consist of anorexia, loss of appetite, and indigestion. General abdominal pain, diarrhea, or constipation may occur.

In the cardiovascular system symptoms mainly consist of an increased tendency to paroxysmal supraventricular tachycardias, ventricular ectopic beats, ventricular tachycardia, or even fibrillation.

Many of the symptoms of magnesium deficiency are probably caused by a secondary intracellular potassium depletion. The pathophysiologic mechanisms for the intracellular potassium depletion and the refractoriness to potassium repletion in a magnesium deficiency remain unclear. The maintenance of a high intracellular potassium concentration is dependent on an adequate function of Na-K-ATPase, which in turn uses magnesium as an essential cofactor. Thus, in a magnesium-deficiency situation, a high intracellular potassium concentration cannot be maintained. This mechanism has been demonstrated in vitro but not in vivo. Another mechanism has been demonstrated in vivo, the requirement for magnesium to inhibit the outward migration of potassium from the cell. Whatever the mechanism, there are several studies clearly showing that the intracellular potassium concentration cannot be corrected with potassium alone when there is a concomitant magnesium depletion. Magnesium supplementation alone, however, will correct both the intracellular potassium and magnesium concentrations.

DIAGNOSIS OF MAGNESIUM DEFICIENCY

Unfortunately, there is no single laboratory test to disclose a magnesim deficiency. The fact that serum magnesium shows no correlation to skeletal muscle magnesium is generally accepted. Most authorities in the field consider skeletal muscle magnesium a fairly good indicator of the body's magnesium status. However, serum magnesium is not without value. In a clinical context, the serum magnesium should be determined when there are symptoms consistent with a magnesium deficiency and/or in conditions that may lead to a deficiency. Serum magnesium should therefore be determined in long-term diuretic treatment, especially when there is a tendency to arrhythmias. Simultaneous digitalis therapy makes it even more mandatory to check the serum magnesium concentration. Digitalis intoxication can be aggravated by magnesium deficiency.

Low serum magnesium levels may indicate a magnesium deficiency, but have also been observed in situations of acute stress, such as acute myocardial infarction, surgery, alcohol abstinence, etc. Under these circumstances, low serum magnesium levels are not necessarily an expression of magnesium deficiency. It is to be emphasized, however, that a normal or even a high serum magnesium level does not exclude the existence of a magnesium depletion. For this reason, it is necessary to judge the serum magnesium level together with any symptoms present, but above all, to consider the factors that might lead to a magnesium deficiency. In serious protein disturbances, the serum albumin value should be taken into account, since 30% of magnesium in the serum is protein bound.

Analysis of magnesium in the urine may be of some clinical value. When assessing magnesium in the urine it should be observed that the urinary magnesium excretion depends on the diet. On normal diets, 3–6 mM/day is excreted. A value below 1 mM/day may be a clue to a magnesium deficiency. In clinical practice, urinary magnesium excretion following parenteral administration of magnesium may be used to improve the diagnostic value of magnesium analyses in urine. Many different loading tests have been designed.

In our own practice, when using a loading test, we give 30 mM magnesium sulphate in 500 ml 5% gluose I.V. over 12 hours to an adult. A 24 hour urine specimen is collected from the beginning of the infusion. Note that this test must not be used in patients with renal insufficiency, disturbances of cardiac conduction, or advanced respiratory insufficiency! The infusion is usually accompanied by a moderate fall in blood pressure due to the vasodilatory effect of magnesium. Subjectively the patient may experience tiredness or hot flushes, and often a slight erythematous reaction is observed. In the case of a magnesium deficiency, more than 50% of the administered magnesium is retained. A retention of less than 20–30% indicates that a magnesium deficiency is most unlikely.

GUIDELINES FOR THERAPY

It is evident that the diagnosis of a magnesium deficiency and the estimation of its severity is not very straightforward. Figure 4 represents an attempt to facilitate this assessment and also to suggest some guidelines for therapy. In the presence of pronounced symptoms coupled with low serum magnesium levels, the diagnosis is not difficult. Since in cases of a magnesium deficiency of a moderate or mild degree the symptoms are often vague and not easily recognized, the figure was produced using serum magnesium as the starting point and combining this with common etiologic factors.

In patients with pronounced symptoms and factors capable of producing a magnesium deficit (positive history), intravenous magnesium is given immediately and the urinary magnesium excretion is monitored. It is recommended that the same quantity of magnesium as given in the magnesium loading test (MLT) be administered over the same time period. This makes it possible to confirm the existence of a magnesium deficiency. Magnesium in urine is also assessed during the continuation of therapy to ascertain when the deficiency has been compensated, i.e., when more than 80% of the administered dose is excreted. In severe magnesium depletion, therapy will often have to be continued for 2–3 weeks.

In this context, it should be stressed that magnesium should not be administered at a rate exceeding 30 mM/12 hr to prevent the development of excessively high serum levels. This should be avoided for two reasons: to avoid toxic effects and to eliminate the possibility of exceeding the Tm for magnesium, resulting in the loss of inadvertently large amounts of magnesium in the urine and rendering the interpretation of the loading test impossible. In patients with pronounced symptoms without known factors leading to a deficiency, it is important to perform a loading test for confirmation of the diagnosis. When serum magnesium is low, one should always test for a deficiency by determining the urinary magnesium excretion, and when values are low, it is necessary to perform a diagnostic loading test. However, when the patient presents with slight symptoms and a positive history, oral substitution may be started without any preceding loading tests.

When the loading test indicates a deficiency in patients with symptoms and/or a positive history, oral substitution therapy is suggested. When the history is negative and there are no symptoms, observation is advocated. When the serum magnesium concentration is normal, only the combination of slight symptoms and a positive history gives cause for further investigation. A low serum calcium concentration together with a low serum magnesium level may indicate a serious magnesium depletion, especially

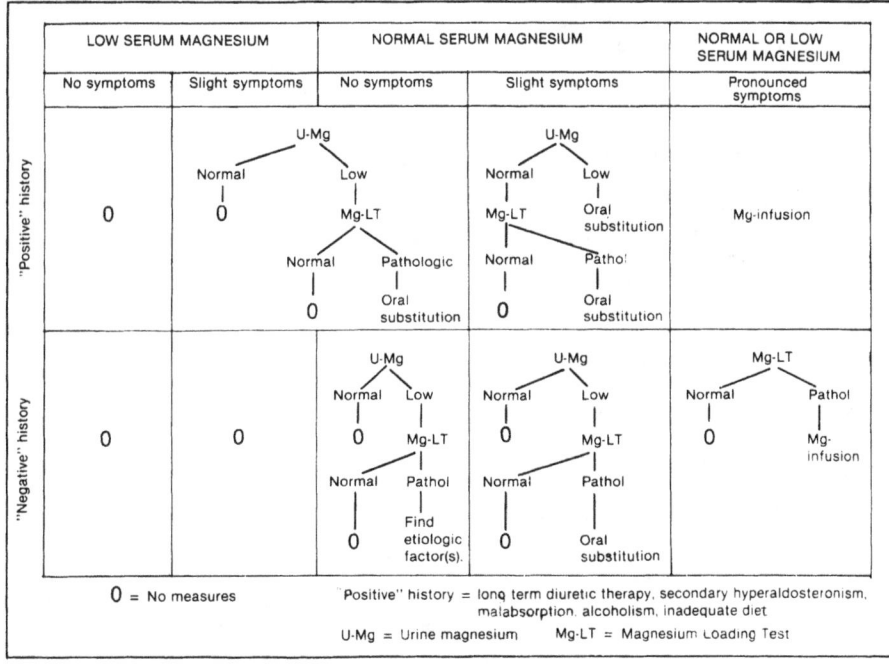

Figure 4. Guidelines for diagnosis and therapy in suspected magnesium deficiency.

when the serum calcium is resistant to calcium administration. A pronounced magnesium depletion will result in a decreased release of PTH from the parathyroid glands and a decreased peripheral response to PTH. This is in contrast to the effect of a slight magnesium deficit, which leads to increased PTH secretion.

With reference to oral magnesium therapy, a suitable daily dose is about 15 mM magnesium, corresponding to the normal daily intake. Magnesium can be administered as chloride, sulphate, oxide, etc. The chloride form is hygroscopic and is therefore most suitably prepared as a solution. It is desirable, of course, to avoid the development of a magnesium deficiency. In long-term diuretic therapy, which is one of the main etiologic factors behind magnesium deficiency in the Western world, potassium-sparing diuretics offer a possibility for treatment. In this situation amiloride, spironolactone, and triamterene have all proved to effectively preserve the intracellular levels of both potassium and magnesium.

CONTRAINDICATIONS FOR PARENTERAL MAGNESIUM ADMINISTRATION

Renal insufficiency (> 200 μM/l s-creatinine) is a contraindication against parenteral magnesium administration, since the body is unable to excrete a large excess of the ion. Administration necessitates careful observation of the patient and close laboratory controls of the serum magnesium concentration. Due to the depressing effect of magnesium on impulse formation and conductivity, bifascicular blocks and advanced AV blocks are contraindications for parenteral magnesium administration. Advanced respiratory insufficiency is another contraindication, since magnesium administration may lead to depressed ventilation and a tendency towards accumulating carbon dioxide.

SYMPTOMS OF MAGNESIUM OVERDOSAGE

In cases of magnesium overdosage, the deep tendon reflexes will first diminish and finally disappear. This is generally accepted to be the first symptom and appears at a serum magnesium concentration of about 2.5 mM/l. At concentrations between 5 and 8 mM/l, respiratory paralysis may appear, and at levels between 8 and 12 mM/l, cardiac arrest in diastole is seen. Cardiac arrest may respond favorably to pacemaker treatment. Intravenous administration of calcium is the generally accepted antidote. In severe intoxication with magnesium, hemodialysis may be contemplated. When the contraindications for parenteral magnesium administration are observed and the recommended dosage is used, a serum magnesium level of more than 2.5 mM/l is extremely rare.

MAGNESIUM AND RENAL STONE DISEASE

Changes of magnesium metabolism may play an important role for the development of renal calcium oxalate stones. Low urinary excretion of magnesium, as seen in magnesium deficiency, decreases the solubility of oxalate, and thus calcium oxalate stones can easily be formed. Several investigations have shown the possibility of a considerable reduction in the occurrence of stones by the administration of magnesium, which will change the calcium/magnesium ratio in urine. An effective treatment consists of 500 mg magnesium hydroxide bid. Treatment with thiazides has also been used with similar results. This mode of treatment induces changes in the calcium/magnesium ratio in urine in the same direction as does magnesium therapy, but in this case by reducing calcium excretion.

HYPERMAGNESEMIA

The most common situation where hypermagnesemia is encountered is in patients with a reduced renal function. However, this hypermagnesemia is usually rather mild, with values around 1.1–1.5 mM/l, and constitutes no immediate threat to the patient. Treatment is generally not needed.

Table 4 lists some of the possible causes of hypermagnesemia. When the GFR and Tm/GFR for magnesium are normal, about a fivefold increase in the magnesium load is required to produce an elevated serum magnesium level. The contribution of magnesium load to serum concentration increases with a reduced GFR, but does not dominate until the GFR has fallen to about 10 ml/min. The tubular reabsorption of magnesium may be increased when there is a contraction of the extracellular fluid volume, as in adrenal insufficiency.

In both hyperparathyroidism and hypothyroidism, an increased tubular reabsorption of magnesium is seen, although in the former case the outcome is complicated by simultaneous changes in calcium metabolism. Endogenously produced hypermagnesemia is related to cell catabolism, but seldom if ever reaches dangerous levels when it is an isolated occurrence.

Magnesium-containing antacids and laxatives are the most common exogenous causes of increased serum magnesium levels. Patients with renal failure and con-

Table 4. Some causes of hypermagnesemia

Increased magnesium load
  1. Endogenous
      Cell catabolism
      Diabetic ketoacidosis
  2. Exogenous
      Magnesium-containing antacids
      Magnesium-containing laxatives
      Magnesium-containing enemas
      Parenteral magnesium therapy

Decreased GFR

Increased Tm/GFR for magnesium
  Mineralocorticoid deficiency
  Hypothyroidism

---

comitant vitamin D treatment are particularly at risk for developing a dangerous hypermagnesemia. Absorption of magnesium from the colon as a result of the administration of magnesium-containing enemas has been described with serum values reaching 8 mM/l. In many countries magnesium is used for the treatment of eclampsia, aiming at a serum magnesium level of between 3 and 4 mM/l. Not infrequently, however, a doubling of these values is attained.

Symptomatic hypermagnesemia is usually accompanied by lethargy, respiratory depression, absent deep tendon reflexes, dilated pupils, hypotension, bradycardia, nausea, and vomiting. Symptoms may be worsened by concomitant hypocalcemia, hyperphosphatemia, and hyperkalemia.

THERAPEUTIC GUIDELINES FOR HYPERMAGNESEMIA

In the majority of cases, hypermagnesemia is mild, and as long as the deep tendon reflexes are still present, no treatment is needed, except cessation of magnesium-containing antacids, laxatives, etc. When severe symptoms are encountered, such as respiratory depression or cardiac dysrhythmias, the administration of 5 mM calcium I.V. is advocated, apart from respiratory support and cardiac monitoring. When the hypermagnesemia presents a threat to the patient's life, hemodialysis is the treatment of choice and usually results in the attainment of safe serum magnesium levels within a couple of hours. When serum magnesium level are above 5 mM/l and the patient has reduced renal function, hemodialysis should be used.

REFERENCES

1. Wacker WEC, Parisi AF: *Magnesium metabolism.* N Engl J Med 278:658–663, 712–717, 772–776.
2. Rude RK, Singer FR: *Magnesium deficiency and excess.* Ann Rev Med 32:245–259, 1981.
3. Gums JG: *Clinical significance of magnesium: A review.* Drug Intell Clin Pharm 21:240–246, 1987.
4. Massry SG: *Role of hormonal and non-hormonal factors in the control of renal handling of magnesium.* Mag Bull 3:277–280, 1981.
5. Cronin RE, Knochel JP: *Magnesium deficiency.* Adv Int Med 28:509–533, 1983.
6. Reyes AJ, Leary WP: *Diuretics and magnesium.* Mag Bull 3:87–99, 1984.
7. Dyckner T, Wester PO: *Clinical significance of diuretic-induced magnesium loss.* Pract Cardiol 10(6):1–4, 1984.

CHAPTER 7

Disorders Of Phosphate Metabolism

MOSHE LEVI & JAMES P. KNOCHEL

INTRODUCTION

A 70-kg adult contains about 700 g of phosphorus. Eighty-five percent of this quantity is in bone, 14% in soft tissues, and the remainder is equally distributed between the teeth, blood, and extravascular fluids. The extracellular fluid pool of phosphorus is only about 600 mg.

In extracellular fluid, phosphorus is present predominately in the inorganic form. In serum, phosphorus exists mainly as $H_2PO_4^{-1}$ and HPO_4^{-2}, their ratio depending upon pH. At 37°C and the ionic strength of plasma, the pKa for phosphorus is 6.8. Using the Henderson–Hasselbach equation, the ratio of HPO_4^{-2}/HPO_4^{-1} under these conditions is about 4:1. Less than 15% of phosphorus is protein bound. The bulk of the intracellular phosphorus is composed of organic compounds, such as sugar phosphate. Only a small fraction of the cytosolic phosphorus is inorganic. Phosphorus is an integral and critical part of all body cells. Key intracellular organic-phosphorus-containing compounds include adenosine triphosphate (ATP), cyclic adenosine monophosphate (cAMP), guanine adenosine monophosphate (cGMP), and nicotine adenosine dinucleotide (NAD). 2,3-disphosphoglycerate (2,3-DPG) is found only in erythrocytes. Other important phosphorus compounds include phospholipids, phosphoproteins, and nucleic acids. Although the concentration of inorganic phosphorus in the cell is very low, it is very important, since it provides the source of phosphorus for synthesis of ATP and it also regulates key intracellular enzymes, including hexokinase, phosphofructokinase, glutaminase, 25-OH-cholecalciferol 1-hydroxylase, and 5′nucleotidase.

REGULATION OF PHOSPHORUS HOMEOSTASIS

The plasma phosphorus level is regulated by absorptive and secretory fluxes in the intestine, the kidney, and the bone, as schematically shown in Figure 1. Although highly variable, a normal adult consumes approximately 20 mg phosphorus/kg body weight/day. In addition, 3 mg phosphorus/kg body weight/day is added to the gastrointestinal tract from digestive juice secretion. Under steady-state conditions, i.e., phosphorus balance, 7 mg/kg body weight/day is excreted in the stool, and 16 mg/kg body weight/day is absorbed by the gastrointestinal tract, resulting in net absorption of 13 mg/kg body weight/day.

INTESTINAL ABSORPTION OF PHOSPHORUS

Most phosphorus is absorbed in the duodenum and jejunum, with minimal absorption occurring in the ileum (1–3). The movement of phosphorus from the intestinal lumen to the blood requires a) transport across the luminal brush border membrane, b) transport through the cytoplasm, and c) transport across the basolateral plasma membrane. The transport of phosphorus across the luminal brush border membrane occurs as a result of a) passive diffusion of phosphorus and b) active transport of phosphorus via the sodium-phosphate cotransport system, which is regulated by 1,25-dihydroxyvitamin D_3 (1–4). With an increasing concentration of phosphorus in the diet, intestinal absorption occurs predominately by passive diffusion of phosphorus across the luminal brush border membrane. On the other hand, with reduced phosphate intake, the intestinal absorption of phosphorus occurs predominately by the active transport mechanism. After a prolonged period of low dietary phosphorus intake, the resultant hypophosphatemia stimulates renal synthesis of $1,25(OH)_2D_3$ from $25(OH)D_3$. The increased levels of circulating $1,25(OH)_2D_3$ then stimulate the sodium-phosphorus cotransporter in the luminal brush border membrane (1–4).

Less is known about the transport of phosphorus through the cytoplasm and across the basolateral membrane; the available evidence indicates that the exit of phosphorus across the basolateral membrane represents a mode of passive transport down its electrochemical gradient (1–4).

RENAL REABSORPTION OF PHOSPHORUS

Ninety to 95% of the inorganic phosphorus in serum is ultrafilterable at the level of the glomerulus. At physiologic levels of serum phosphorus (2.8–4.8 mg/dl in adults),

PHOSPHORUS METABOLISM

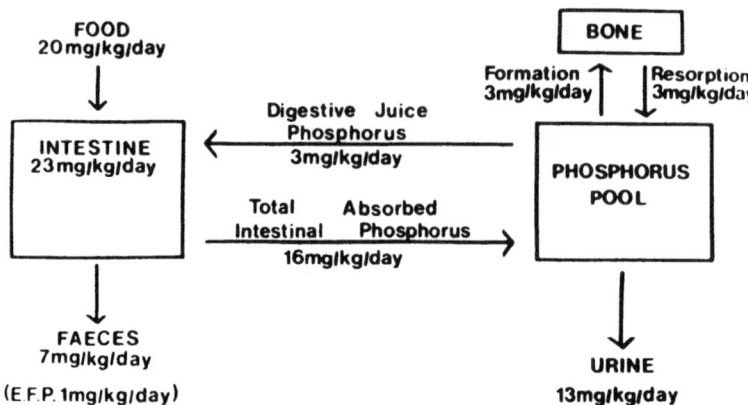

Figure 1. Schema of P metabolism for the normal human adult on an averge P intake patient who is in zero P balance. From: Nordin BEC (ed): *Calcium, Phosphate and Magnesium Metabolism.* Churchill Livingstone, New York, 1976.

approximately 7 g of phosphorus are filtered per day by the kidney (3.8 mg/dl × 180 l/day = 6.84 g/day). Under normal physiologic conditions, 80–90% is reabsorbed by the proximal tubule (the proximal convoluted and the proximal straight tubule) (1–12). However, there is also a significant amount of filtered phosphorus that is reabsorbed in the distal segments of the nephron, including in the distal convoluted tubule, the cortical collecting tubule, and also, to a minor extent, in the inner medullary collecting tubule (Figure 2) (1–12). In addition to the internephron heterogeneity in phosphorus reabsorption, recent evidence also indicates an intranephron heterogeneity. Micropuncture studies in the rat indicate that the deep nephrons have a higher transport maximum for phosphorus than the superficial nephrons, and the deep or juxtamedullary nephrons may have a key regulatory role in phosphorus homeostasis (7).

The majority of the reabsorption and the regulation of phosphorus metabolism takes place in the proximal tubule of the kidney. In recent years the application of in-vitro transport techniques to the study of renal physiology have advanced our understanding of the regulation of phosphorus transport. The transport of phosphorus across the tubular epithelium takes place against its electrochemical gradient and requires the presence of sodium in the luminal fluids. Phosphorus reabsorption by the proximal tubule occurs according to the scheme shown in Figure 3. The cotransport system for sodium and phosphate is located in the apical or luminal brush border membrane. The electrochemical gradient for sodium supplies the energy for the intracellular accumulation of phosphorus. The exit of phosphorus across the basolateral membrane is downhill (passive) and occurs via a sodium-independent pathway. Thus, transcelluar transport of phosphorus is secondary active, ultimately energized by the Na = K = ATPase pump in the basolateral membrane, and is mediated by a sodium-phosphorus cotransport system in the luminal brush border membrane and a sodium-independent mechanism in the basolateral membrane.

Reabsorption of phosphorus in the proximal tubule is affected by many factors, such as diet, hormones, meta-

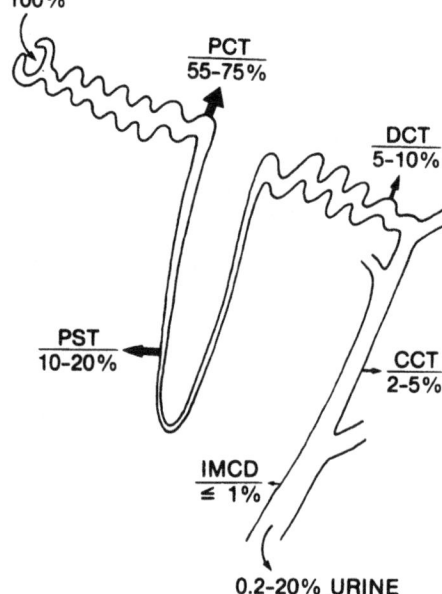

Figure 2. Segmental PO_4 reabsorption as percent of filtered load. PCT = proximal convoluted tubule; PST = proximal straight tubule; DCT = distal convoluted tubule) CCT = cortical collecting tubule; IMCD = inner medullary collecting duct. From: Lau K: Phosphate disorders. In: Kokko JP, Tannen RL, eds, *Fluids and Electrolytes.* WB Saunders, Philadelphia, pp 398–471, 1986.

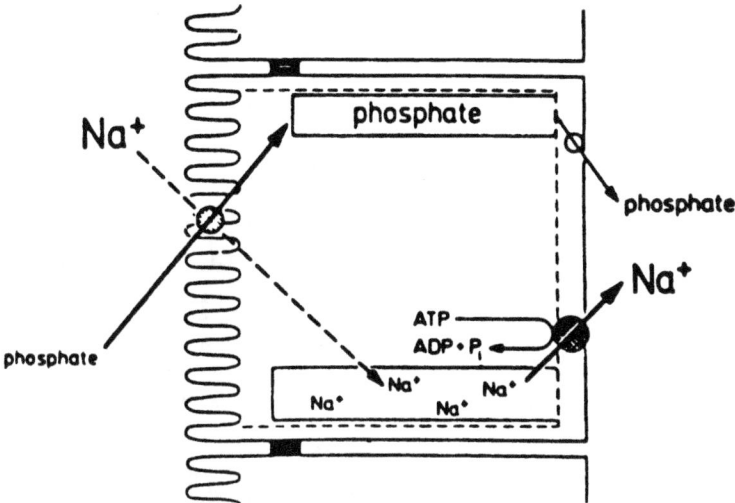

Figure 3. Active transport of inorganic phosphate (Pi) in renal proximal tubule. Apical membrane (brush border) contains a Na-Pi contransport system energized by the transmembrane electrochemical gradient for Na and Pi. Basolateral membrane contains a Na-independent transport system for Pi as well as the Na pump. From: Murer, Malstrom 1987. How renal phosphate transport is regulated. *NIPS* 2:45–48, 1987.

bolism, and plasma ion levels (Table 1). All of these factors alter the transport rate of the sodium-phosphorus cotransport system, suggesting that the luminal brush border membrane entry step is the rate-limiting process and the site for regulation.

HYPOPHOSPHATEMIA

Definition

Hypophosphatemia is defined as an abnormally low concentration of inorganic phosphorus in serum or plasma. It often indicates phosphorus deficiency. However, hypophosphatemia may also occur under a variety of circumstances in which total body phosphorus stores are normal (3, 13–15). Moderate hypophosphatemia may be defined as a serum phosphorus concentration between 2.5 and 1.0 mg/dl; it is common, yet it is not usually associated with signs and symptoms of phosphate deficiency. Severe hypophosphatemia is defined as serum phosphorus levels below 1.0 mg/dl, and patients with severe hypophosphatemia usually display signs and symptoms that require therapy. Phosphorus deficiency is defined as an abnormally low content of total body phosphorus, reflected by a low phosphorus to nitrogen ratio by tissue analysis. Phosphorus deficiency may exist in the absence of hypophosphatemia.

Incidence

In two independent studies the prevalence of moderate hypophosphatemia, defined as serum phosphorus levels less than 2.5 mg/dl, has been found to be 2% of hospital admissions (16–19). The prevalence of severe hypophosphatemia, defined as serum phosphorus levels less than 1.0 mg/dl, has been found to be 0.1–0.25% of consecutively hospitalized patients (16–19).

Causes of hypophosphatemia

As discussed earlier, more than 99% of the total body phosphorus is found in soft tissues and bone, and only

Table 1. Pharmacologic and metabolic factors that regulate renal proximal tubule phosphate transport

Increased transport
  Dietary phosphate deprivation
  Parathyroidectomy
  Vitamin 1,25-$(OH)_2D_3$
  Luminal calcium
  Thyroid hormone
  Insulin
  Growth hormone

Decreased transport
  Dietary phosphate excess
  Parathyroid hormone
  Hypercalcemia
  Extracellular fluid volume expansion
  Proximally acting diuretics
  Luminal glucose
  Acute respiratory acidosis
  Metabolic acidosis
  Metabolic alkalosis
  Glucocorticoids
  Calcitonin
  Aging

Table 2. Causes of hypophosphatemia: Redistribution

Respiratory alkalosis
  Sepsis
  Heat stroke
  Hepatic coma
  Salicylate poisoning
  Gout

Recovery from hypothermia

Hormonal effects
  Insulin
  Glucagon
  Epinephrine
  Adrogens

Nutrient effects
  Glucose
  Fructose
  Glycerol
  Lactate
  Amino acids
  Xylitol

Acute leukemia and lymphoma

Table 3. Causes of hypophosphatemia: Decreased gastrointestinal absorption

Decreased dietary intake

Decreased intestinal absorption
  Vitamin-D deficiency
  Malabsorption
  Steatorrhea
  Secretory diarrhea
  Vomiting
  Phosphate-binding antacids

Intrinsic disorders of intestinal phosphate absorption
  Familial hypophosphatemic rickets
  Aging

---

approximately 0.6% of the total body phosphorus is in the blood and extravascular fluids. Therefore, rapid removal of phosphorus from the blood due to transcellular shift, as occurs in acute hyperventilation and nutrient infusion (Table 2), can result in acute and marked decreases in serum phosphorus concentration. On the other hand, chronic and gradual phosphorus losses caused by impaired intestinal absorption or renal reabsorption (Tables 3 and 4) do not necessarily result in a significant decrease in serum phosphorus concentration, as the large intracellular phosphorus stores can easily compensate for these losses and maintain the serum phosphorus concentration within a normal range. In clinical situations, moderate hypophosphatemia usually results from one or a combination of the following factors: a) redistribution of phosphorus from the extracellular to the intracellular space (Table 2), b) decreased gastrointestinal absorption of phosphorus (Table 3), or c) decreased renal tubular reabsorption of phosphorus (Table 4).

Sometimes some of these factors, especially when they occur in combination, may result in severe hypophosphatemia and may require the immediate attention of the clinician (Table 5). Some of these causes of severe hypophosphatemia will be discussed briefly, as they are the most common causes of hospital-acquired hypophosphatemia.

Respiratory alkalosis

Several clinical conditions, such as fever, sepsis, alcohol withdrawal, salicylate poisoning, central nervous system disorders, and some hypoxic pulmonary diseases, induce hyperventilation, which results in respiratory alkalosis. In addition to the decrease in extracellular fluid (ECF) p_{CO_2} and the increase in ECF pH, there is a similar decrease in intracellular p_{CO_2} and an increase in intracellular pH. The glycolytic pathway, and specifically phosphofructokinase, a key rate-limiting enzyme for glycolysis, is stimulated during intracellular alkalosis (20). This increases formation of sugar phosphates and, in turn, induces intracellular entry of phosphorus, resulting in hypophosphatemia. Urinary phosphorus excretion during acute respiratory alkalosis is minimal, thus confirming the notion that the hypophosphatemia is the result of redistribution of ECF phosphorus (21–23). When acute respiratory alkalosis

---

Table 4. Causes of hypophosphatemia: decreased renal tubular reabsorption

Hyperparathyroidism
  Tubular disorders
  Fanconi syndrome
  Familial hypophosphatemic rickets
  Hypophosphatemia associated with tumors
  Vitamin-D-deficient rickets
  Vitamin-D-dependent rickets

Primary or genetically transmitted idiopathic hypercalciuria

Secondary or acquired tubular disorders
  Diuretic phase of acute tubular necrosis
  Postobstructive diuresis
  Postrenal transplantation
  Glycosuria
  Volume expansion
  Diuretics
  Acid-base abnormalities
  Glucocorticoids

Table 5. Causes of severe hypophosphatemia

Respiratory alkalosis
Hyperalimentation
Dietary deficiency and phosphate-binding antacids
Chronic alcoholism and alcohol withdrawal
Recovery from diabetic ketoacidosis
Nutritional recovery syndrome
Severe thermal burns
Renal transplantation

significant role in promoting intracellular shifts of extracellular phosphorus. When this phenomenon occurs in previously healthy subjects or animals, the resultant hypophosphatemia is mild and transient, as the phosphorylated intracellular compounds release the phosphorus, which is then used for other intracellular metabolic pathways. Hyperalimentation, however, is usually utilized to treat patients with malnutrition, increased catabolism, cachexia, or severe burns. Total phosphorus stores in these patients is often marginal, and as hyperalimentation induces tissue regeneration and repair, phosphorus is incorporated into the new cells. These patients, therefore, can develop progressively severe and persistent hypophosphatemia (24–27). The recognition of this fact has resulted in the inclusion of phosphorus in hyperalimentation formulae and elimination of this potentially important cause of severe phosphatemia.

Phosphate-binding antacids

Most of the antacids nowadays contain aluminum hydroxide or aluminum carbonate and magnesium hydroxide or magnesium carbonate. Both aluminum and magnesium ions complex with phosphorus in the gastrointestinal tract, resulting in decreased phosphorus absorption. In addition, other agents commonly used to treat peptic ulcer disease, including Tums®, that contain calcium carbonate and sucralfate also bind phosphorus and also result in reduced phosphorus absorption. Although the kidney is able to adapt to decreased gastrointestinal phosphorus absorption by reabsorbing most of the filtered phosphorus, because of ongoing obligatory gastrointestinal secretion of phosphorus

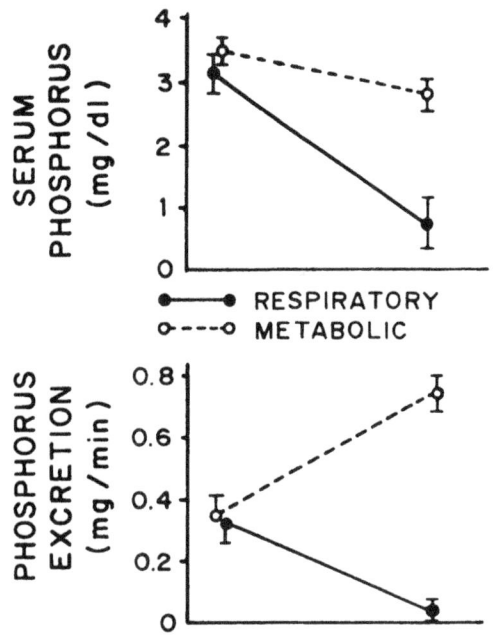

Figure 4. Respiratory alkalosis may depress serum phosphorus concentration markedly in normal subjects and cause virtual disappearance of phosphorus from urine. Serum phosphorus falls only slightly with the same degree of alkalosis produced by infusion of $NaHCO_3$ and is associated with an increase in phosphaturia. From: Mosteller ME, Tuttle EP: Effect of alkalosis on plasma and urinary excretion of in organic phosphate in man. J Clin Invest 43:138–151, 1964.

occurs in a previously healthy subject, the resultant hypophosphatemia is usually quite mild and transient. However, voluntary forced hyperventilation in healthy volunteers has been observed to reduce serum phosphorus to levels as low as 0.3 mg/dl (Figure 4). Similarly, if acute respiratory alkalosis occurs in the setting of previous phosphorus depletion, such as in chronically ill and malnourished patients, then the resultant hypophosphatemia can be quite severe and persistent. This is especially true if the same chronically ill and malnourished patients are also receiving hyperalimentation, as the two have additive effects (Figure 5).

Hyperalimentation

Infusion of glucose, fructose, and other metabolizable nutrients requiring phosphorylation during the glycolytic cycle induces intracellular entry of phosphorus and causes hypophosphatemia. Indeed, when given to healthy animals, infusion of glucose is associated with increases in muscle-cell total phosphorus, adenosine triphosphate, and glucose-6-phosphate (23). Infusion of certain amino acids also causes a similar response. Since both glucose and amino acids induce insulin release, insulin may play a

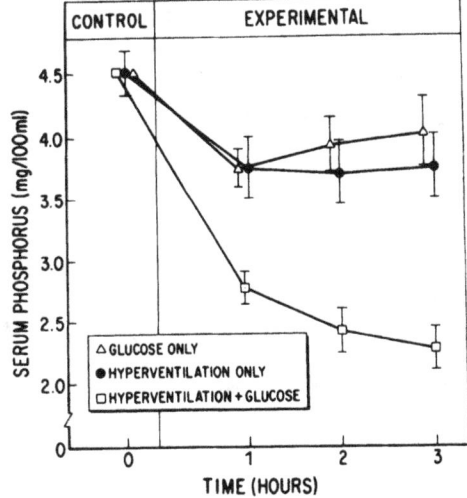

Figure 5. Development of severe hypophosphatemia during hyperventilation. From: Brautbar N, et al.: On the mechanism of hypophosphatemia during acute hyperventilation: Evidence for increased muscle glycolysis. Miner Electrolyte Metab 9:45–50, 1983.

in digestive juices, a negative phosphorus balance can gradually develop. Antacid-induced hypophosphatemia may, therefore, become an important factor when it occurs in patients with hyperventilation who are receiving hyperalimentation, or in patients with uncontrolled diabetes mellitus and chronic alcoholism, as will be discussed next.

Chronic alcoholism and alcohol withdrawal

The chronic alcoholic patient has several reasons for phosphorus depletion, not necessarily accompanied by hypophosphatemia, i.e., reduction in serum phosphorus concentration (Table 6). Most of the chronic alcoholics have decreased gastrointestinal absorption of phosphorus because of their poor intake of food, antacid ingestion for symptoms of gastritis, and sometimes abnormally low $1,25(OH)_2D_3$ levels. In addition, they may also have increased urinary excretion of phosphorus because of direct effects of alcohol, magnesium deficiency, and sometimes use of diuretics in patients with cirrhosis and ascites, all of which result in decreased renal tubular reabsorption of phosphorus (28–34). These factors are compounded in the alcoholic patient who presents to the hospital either with alcohol withdrawal or alcoholic ketoacidosis. In experimental chronic alcoholic intoxication, there occurs a major reduction of muscle phosphorus content despite abundant dietary phosphorus and the lack of hypophosphatemia (30).

Typically, the serum phosphorus concentration is normal on admission to the hospital, although sometimes it may be low or even high. However, the serum phosphorus concentration almost always falls rapidly during the first few hospital days (Figure 6).

In the patient with alcohol withdrawal (delirium tremens), the hyperventilation resulting in respiratory alkalosis and the administration of intravenous fluids containing dextrose cause redistribution of phosphorus to the intracellular compartment. In addition, the use of ant-

Table 6. Causes of hypophosphatemia in the alcoholic patient

Redistribution
  Respiratory alkalosis
  Intravenous hydration with dextrose-containing solutions

Decreased gastrointestinal absorption
  Poor intake of food
  Reduced absorption due to the use of antacids, diarrhea, and vomiting
  Impaired $1,25\text{-}(OH)_2D_3$ metabolism
  Calcitonin secretion
  Nasogastric suction

Decreased renal absorption
  Metabolic acidosis
  Magnesium deficiency
  Increased ethanol levels
  $1,25\text{-}(OH)_2D_3$ metabolism
  Increased calcitonin secretion
  Diuretic administration

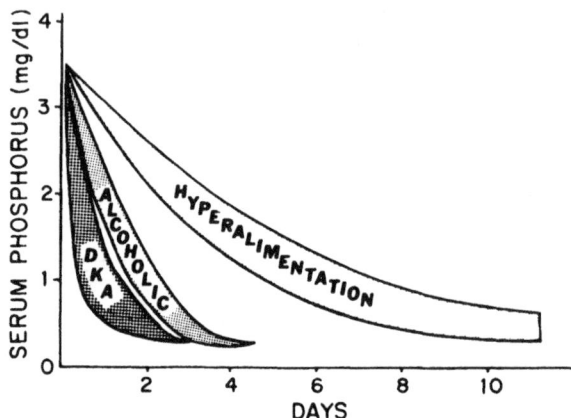

Figure 6. Approximate time when severe hypophosphatemia appears during treatment for diabetic ketacidosis (DKA), alcoholic withdrawal, and hyperalimentation. From: Knohel JP: Hypophosphatemia. In: Massry SG, Glassock RJ, eds, *Textbook of Nephrology*. Williams and Wilkins, Baltimore, pp 3.94–3.99, 1983.

acids causes a decrease in the gastrointestinal absorption of phosphorus, altogether resulting in severe hypophosphatemia.

In the patient with alcoholic ketoacidosis, the nausea and vomiting and the use of antacids and nasogastric suction cause a further decrease in gastrointestinal absorption of phosphorus. The ketoacids also cause a decrease in renal tubular reabsorption of phosphorus.

Diabetic ketoacidosis

In the diabetic patient with ketoacidosis, the resultant glycosuria, ketonuria, osmotic diuresis, and ketoacidosis all decrease renal tubular reabsorption of phosphorus. The presence of nausea and vomiting also result in decreased intake of food and phosphorus. In addition, insulin-dependent diabetic with a long history of poorly controlled diabetes may also have abnormal vitamin $1,25(OH)_2D_3$ metabolism, which causes impairment in gastrointestinal and renal tubular transport of phosphorus. Experimentally, acute metabolic acidosis sharply reduces synthesis of $1,25(OH)_2D_3$.

When the patient with diabetic ketoacidosis first presents to the hospital, the serum phosphorus concentration is usually increased or normal (36), however, once insulin therapy is started, hypophosphatemia may occur within 12–48 hours, as insulin causes a shift of phosphorus from the extracellular fluid to the intracellular compartment. The hypophosphatemia occurs at a time when the initially increased urinary phosphorus excretion becames markedly reduced.

The great majority of patients with diabetic ketoacidosis who have been ill for a short period of time are not seriously phosphorus deficient. Characteristically, these patients have had vomiting for a few days at most and simply have not had sufficient time to become frankly depleted. On the other hand, some patients show severe hypophosphatemia when first admitted to the hospital despite coexistent volume depletion and metabolic acidosis, factors that usually cause elevations of serum phosphorus. The usual setting in this latter group of patients is characterized by a long prodrome, lasting a week or more, of marked polyuria, polydipsia, and the absence of vomiting. The lack of vomiting permits a greater fluid intake, a larger urine volume, and a greater opportunity to become profoundly phosphorus depleted. Most of these patients are young, Type I diabetics. Serum potassium concentrations also tend to be low in this group despite acidosis. In such patients hypophosphatemia becomes very severe during the subsequent hospital course and could be associated with severe morbidity.

Nutritional recovery syndrome

The nutritional recovery of refeeding syndrome represents a constellation of findings, consisting of heart failure and a variety of electrolyte derangements observed during treatment of patients with severe protein calorie malnutrition or starvation. In contrast to hyperalimentation, hypophosphatemia may occur during administration of calories in normal quantities (26).

This syndrome can be reproduced in experimental animals and is commonly seen during overzealous feeding of patients who have lost marked quantities of weight as a result of food fadism or anorexia nervosa. On the basis of clinical descriptions, such patients present with many of the complications observed in starved prisoners after World War II. In addition to hypophosphatemia provoked by nutrients, most of these patients show other serious disturbances such as hypokalemia, hypomagnesemia, and severe glucose intolerance. The observation that feeding with small quantities of skim milk rather than pure carbohydrates caused less morbidity is very likely ascribable to the reduced calories and the higher phosphorus and potassium contents of skim milk.

Severe thermal burns

Patients with severe third-degree burns whose kidney function remains intact often become hypophosphatemic 2–10 days after the injury. Hypophosphatemia may become very severe. According to most observers, as serum phosphorus declines, phosphorus excretion into the urine usually falls to very low levels. Most patients with burns hyperventilate, and consequently respiratory alkalosis may be responsible for the hypophosphatemia. On the other hand, it has been suggested that additional factors, including renal tubular injury, volume expansion as a result of fluid administration, mobilization of retained salt and water from injured tissue, and the resulting diuresis, could also be responsible for the declining serum phosphorus levels.

In a series of 33 patients with severe thermal burns, the lowest values of serum phosphorus occurred in seven patients who died (41). Simultaneous reduction of urinary phosphorus excretion indicated that the depletion of phosphorus was mainly the result of extrarenal mechanisms. However, since fractional excretion of phosphorus still increased, renal losses may also have contributed to the hypophosphatemia. An interesting finding was that these patients showed marked increases in serum calcitonin and catecholamine levels, which may have played a role in the hypophosphatemia (41).

Hypophosphatemia in burns has potentially important connotations, because it can be implicated as a contributing factor in burn-wound sepsis, because of the effects of hypophosphatemia on white cell function, which will be discussed later.

Renal transplantation

Hypophosphatemia is very commonly seen in patients following successful renal transplantation and is of concern because it may play a role in the pathogenesis of severe osteomalacia in some of these patients (42–55). The causes of the hypophosphatemia are multifactorial. In the immediate post-transplantation period, intravascular volume expansion and osmotic diuresis cause marked phosphaturia. The hypophosphatemia in the ensuing several days after a successful renal transplantation may result from a combination of factors: a) administration of glucocorticoids, which inhibit renal phosphorus transport and may also inhibit gastrointestinal absorption of phosphorus; b) ingestion of antacids such as aluminum/magnesium carbonate, which complex with gut phosphorus and inhibit its absorption; c) persistently elevated parathyroid hormone levels, especially in patients with previously severe secondary hyperparathyroidism; and d) an intrinsic renal tubular defect for phosphorus reabsorption that is independent of all other hormonal/metabolic factors and may become further exacerbated during periods of rejection. Sometimes the hypophosphatemia can be severe and may require phosphate replacement therapy. Of note, $1,25(OH)_2D_3$ levels are within the normal range in most of these patients, however, some patients with severe hypophosphatemia following renal transplantation may benefit from short periods of $1,25(OH)_2D_3$ therapy to enhance gastrointestinal and renal tubular phosphorus transport.

Clinical consequences of severe hypophosphatemia

When severe hyposphatemia is associated with phosphorus deficiency, it can result in multiorgan dysfunction (56–62) (Table 7). In some tissues, the cellular effects of phosphorus deficiency are caused by its effects on 2,3-diphosphoglycerate (2,3-DPG), adenosine nucleotides including adenosine triphosphate (ATP), and, in others, secondary electrical disturbances in excitatory tissue. 2,3-DPG levels are decreased in the red blood cells, which causes an increase in the affinity of hemoglobin for oxygen. This results in impaired oxygen delivery to the organs or

Table 7. Consequences of severe hypophosphatemia

Cardiopulmonary
  Decreased cardiac output, cardiac arrhythmia, hypotension
  Decreased vital capacity, impaired diaphragmatic contractility, hypoxia

Neurologic
  Anorexia, irritability, confusion, dysarthria, seizures, coma

Musculoskeletal
  Muscle weakness, decreased transmembrane resting potential, rhabdomyolysis
  Bone pain, psuedofractures, rickets, or osteomalacia

Hematologic
  Impaired function of erythrocytes, platelets, and leukocytes

Endocrine/metabolic
  Hyperinsulinemia, insulin, resistance, decreased glucose metabolism
  Decreased PTH levels, increased 1,25-$(OH)_2D_3$ levels

Renal
  Decreased GFR, decreased T_m for bicarbonate, decreased titratable acid excretion, hypercalciuria, hypermagnesemia

tissue hypoxia. There is also a decrease in the tissue content of ATP and, therefore, a decrease in the availability of energy-rich phosphate compounds for cell function. Reduced cellular phosphorus concentration also stimulates the irreversible deamination of adenosine monophosphate (AMP), which depletes intracellular adenosine nucleotide stores and further impairs the cell's ability to generate ATP. Finally, in phosphorus-deficient alkalosis and in dogs with experimental phosphorus deficiency, the resting transmembrane electrical potential difference across muscle cells is abnormally low and may be the cause of the profound weakness experienced by phosphorus-deficient patients (30, 57).

An especially important hypophosphatemic syndrome is that seen in seriously ill patients managed for prolonged periods of time with intravenous fluids. Typically, a patient is in an intensive care unit setting, may be postoperative, and has been intubated. The patient cannot be extubated at the expected time or, if extubated, develops progressive weakness and progressive respiratory failure characterized by impairment of diaphragm function, hypercarbia, hypoxia and respiratory acidosis (59–61). Neurologic events may also occur and may include ascending paralysis resembling the Guillain–Barre syndrome, mental confusion, and seizure activity. In these cases, the serum phosphorus concentration usually falls to values less than 1.0 mg/dl. Correction of hypophosphatemia quickly improves diaphragm function and cures the respiratory failure. Neurologic dysfunction, however, improves more slowly (57).

TREATMENT OF HYPOPHOSPHATEMIA

The major question in the evaluation of a patient with hypophosphatemia is whether the low serum phosphorus concentration is indicative of a true phosphorus deficiency syndrome (Table 7). It is reemphasized that less than 0.05% of total body phosphorus is present in the extracellular fluid pool; accordingly, hypophosphatemia does not necessarily denote phosphorus deficiency, since it may represent no more than an intracellular shift. For example, in a previously healthy subject, acute hyperventilation, which induces an acute and transient shift of extracellular fluid phosphorus to the intracellular space, can cause a similar degree of hypophosphatemia to that observed after prolonged nausea and vomiting in a chronic alcoholic patient with alcoholic ketoacidosis. The hypophosphatemia in the previously healthy subject with acute hyperventilation, however, is associated with normal body phosphorus stores and does not require treatment, whereas the same degree of hypophosphatemia in the alcoholic patient most likely represents phosphorus deficiency and requires phosphate replacement therapy.

Since most of the clinical consequences of hypophosphatemia are caused by decreased levels and impaired synthesis of 2,3-DPG in erythrocytes, and ATP in all cells including erythrocytes, the measurement of erythrocyte 2,3-DPG and ATP levels would be most helpful in determining whether the decrease in serum phosphorus concentration is associated with a decrease in cellular phosphorus. However, until such measurements become routine in the clinical chemistry laboratory, the clinician has to resort to less perfect, yet quite adequate, means of assessing the patient with hypophosphatemia.

In most cases of hypophosphatemia, a careful history, physical examination, review of the medications and intravenous fluid therapy, and laboratory data, including arterial pH and blood gases, urinary phosphorus, and creatinine for calculation of fractional excretion of phosphorus, can help establish the cause of the hypophosphatemia and determine whether the patient needs phosphate replacement therapy.

In patients with moderate hypophosphatemia (1.0–2.5 mg/dl), if there is no history of previous renal or gastrointestinal losses, and if there is no evidence of the expected consequences of phosphorus depletion, then there is no need for phosphate replacement. This is especially the case if the hypophosphatemia is causes by hyperventilation or nutrient administration, which result in a transient shift of phosphorus from extracellular to intracellular sites. In most of these cases, the identification and treatment of the primary cause usually results in restoration of the blood phosphorus concentration to normal. On the other hand, if the hypophosphatemia occurs in patients who are suspected of having previous renal and gastrointestinal phosphorus losses, who have evidence of malnutrition or increased catabolism, and also, most importantly, if there is evidence of the phosphorus depletion syndrome, then careful replacement of the phosphorus deficiency is indicated.

Patients with severe and sustained hypophosphatemia (< 1.0 mg/dl) usually have depletion of total body phosphorus stores and may require replacement therapy to normalize plasma phosphorus concentration and tissue 2,3-DPG and ATP levels (Figure 7). An important ex-

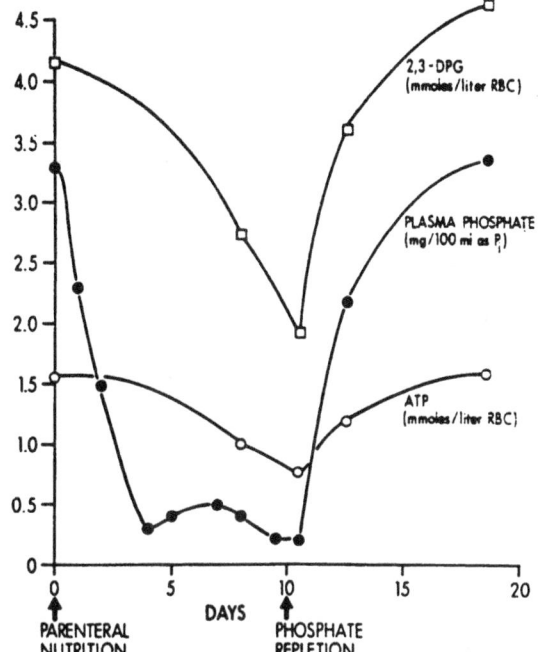

Figure 7. Plasma phosphate, red cell adenosine triphosphate (ATP) and 2,3-diphosphoglycerate (DPG) during parenteral nutrition and phosphate repletion in vivo. From: Lichtman MA, et al.: Reduced red cell glycolysis, 2,3-diphosphoglycerate and adenosine triphosphate concentration, and increased hemoglobin-oxygen affinity caused by hypophosphatemia. Ann Intern Med 74:562–568, 1971.

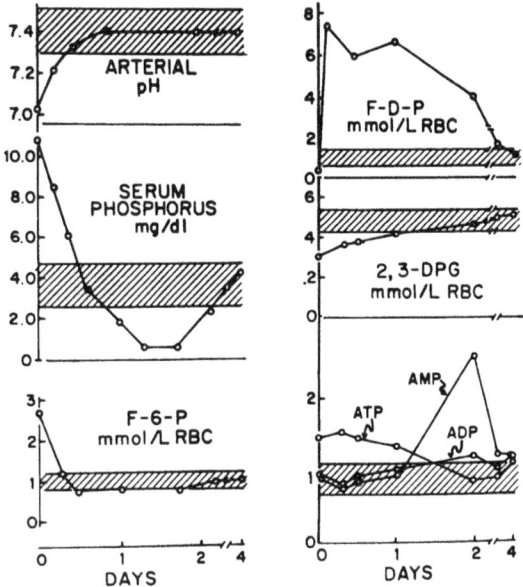

Figure 8. Biochemical data on a patient with diabetic ketoacidosis. A 45-year-old man with glucose 583 mg/dl, pH 7.06, pCO$_2$ 12.6 mmHg, HCO$_3$ 3.3, and ketosis. Abbreviations for red cell components: F-6-P = fructos-6-phosphate; F-D-P = fructose diphosphate; 2,3-DPG = 2,3-diphosphoglycerate; ATP = adenosine triphosphate; AMP = adenosine monophosphate; ADP = adneosine diphosphate. From: Kono N, et al.: Alteration of glycolytic intermediary metabolism in erythrocytes during diabetic ketoacidosis and its recovery phase. Diabetes 30:346–353, 1981.

ception is the common patient with diabetic ketoacidosis whose serum phosphorus is often normal or elevated when first measured, but falls to levels approaching 1.0 mg/dl or less following insulin and fluids. In diabetic ketoacidosis, 2,3-DPG levels are usually lower than normal and, because of its predictable effects on hemoglobin oxygen affinity, it was long believed that it caused tissue hypoxemia and that it played a major role in the pathogenesis of diabetic coma. Phosphate replacement therpay was advocated to enhance recovery of 2,3-DPG levels (63, 64). Recent controlled studies, however, have not shown any statistical difference between recovery of erythrocyte 2,3-DPG levels, glucose utilization rates, or the clinical course of recovery from diabetic ketoacidosis in patients who were randomly assigned to conventional treatment alone or combined with phosphate infusions (65, 66). Therefore, treatment with insulin and fluids, which corrects the acidosis in DKA, results in improvement of the erythrocyte 2,3-DPG levels in spite of the persistent hypophosphatemia (67) (Figure 8). Figure 9 summarizes and compares the effects of hypophosphatemia on red blood cell glycolytic products and adenine nucleotides in patients receiving total parenteral nutrition (25) and in patients during the treatment of diabetic ketoacidosis (67).

Routine phosphate replacement therapy is therefore not necessary in most patients with DKA. It should only be reserved for the occasional patient with severe and persistent hypophosphatemia. As described earlier in this chapter in the discussion dealing with pathogenesis, one should be alert for the typically young, new-onset, Type I diabetic who has been developing diabetic ketoacidosis for many days or weeks before he or she is admitted to a hospital. In these cases, the presence of severe hypophosphatemia before treatment has been initiated, despite coexistent metabolic acidosis, indicates a severe phosphorus deficiency that demands treatment.

In most patients with other causes of severe hypophosphatemia, phosphorus replacement may be delayed if the under-lying causes, such as phosphorus-binding antacids, alcohol, diuretics, and osmotic diuresis due to uncontrolled diabetes, can be identified and treated and/or discontinued. However, in spite of these measures, if the hypophosphatemia persists, and especially if the patient is symptomatic, then phosphorus therapy should be initiated.

If the patient is able to tolerate oral intake, the safest and most efficient mode of therapy is the administration of skim or low-fat (0.5% fat) milk, which contains approximately 0.9 mg phosphorus/ml. Milk is also a rich source

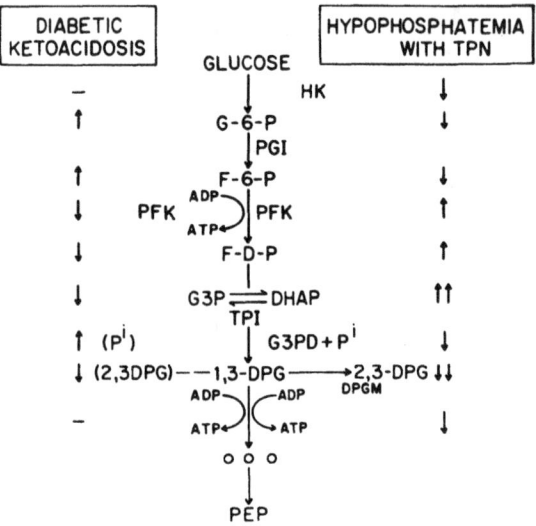

Figure 9. Arrows indicate deviations of red blood cell metabolite concentrations from normal in patients with hypophosphatemia during treatment of DKA and in those with hypophosphatemia induced by total parenteral hyperalimentation (TPN). From: Travis SF, et al.: Alterations of red-cell glycolytic intermediates and oxygen transport as a consequence of hypophosphatemia in patients receiving intravenous hyperalimentation. Engl J Med 285:763–768, 1971.

Table 8. Commonly available phosphorus-containing preparations

	Phosphorus	Sodium	Potassium
Oral preparations	(mg)	(mEq)	(mEq)
K-Phos neutral tablets (Beach)	250/tab	12/tab	2/tab
K-Phos tablets (Beach)	114/tab		3.65/tab
Neutra-Phos-K capsules (Willen Drug Co.)	250/cap		14/cap
Neutra-Phos capsules (Willen Drug Co.)	250/cap	7/cap	7/cap
Fleet Phospho Soda (C.D. Fleet Co.)	149/ml	6/ml	
Parenteral preparations	(mg/ml)	(mEq/ml)	(mEq/ml)
Hyper-Phos-K (Davies, Rose–Hoyt)	67		3.3
In-Phos (Davies, Rose–Hoyt)	25	1.6	0.2
Sodium phosphate (Abbott)	93	4	
Potassium phosphate (Abbott)	93		4

of calcium, potassium, magnesium, and protein, and its use is ideal in malnourished patients. A typical patient with severe hypophosphatemia would require between four and eight cartons of milk (8 oz of milk per carton) per day, as each 8 oz contains approximately 235 mg of elemental phosphorus and the average patient requires 1000–2000 mg phosphorus per day to have body stores repleted within 7–10 days.

If the patient is unable to tolerate milk, then they can be given any of the oral preparations listed in Table 8. The intravenous administration of phosphorus is usually reserved for patients with severe hypophosphatemia who cannot take milk or tablets, or who are overtly symptomatic and have evidence of erythrocyte, platelet, and leukocyte dysfunction; cardiomyopathy; respiratory muscle weakness; or altered mental status as a result of the severe hypophosphatemia (Table 7). Since we do not have adequate means to determine the degree of intracellular phosphorus depletion, we also do not have a satisfactory means to determine the amount of phosphorus that needs to be replaced. An earlier study suggested 2.5–5.0 mg elemental phosphorus/kg body weight be administered intravenously every 6 hours to replete phosphorus in patients with severe hypophosphatemia (68), although the efficacy of this therapy was not validated. A more recent study adminstered 9 mM phosphorus in 0.5 N saline intravenously as a continuous infusion over 12 hours, which corresponds to approximately 2 mg/kg body weight every 6 hours (69). Mean serum phosphorus concentration increased from baseline value of 0.81 mg/dl to 1.27 mg/dl in 12 hours, to 1.67 mg/dl in 24 hours, 2.07 mg/dl in 36 hours, and 2.80 mg/dl in 48 hours (Figure 10). Once a serum phosphorus concentration of 2.0–2.5 mg/dl is achieved, it would be most safe to switch to oral replacement therapy.

An important factor that should also be considered in the treatment of patients with hypoposphatemia is that most of these patients may also have low serum magnesium levels. Of note, phosphorus deficiency may result in increased urinary magnesium excretion, and magnesium

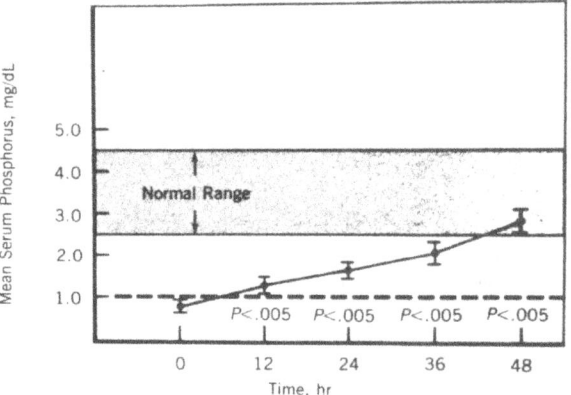

Figure 10. Mean serum phosphorus response to 9 mM of phosphorus given intravenously every 12 hours as a continuous infusion in ten severely hypophosphatemic patients. From: Vannatta JB, et al.: Efficacy of intravenous phosphorus therapy in the severely hypophosphatemic patient. Arch Intern Med 141:885–887, 1981.

deficiency may also result in increased urinary phosphorus excretion. Therefore, in selected patients, the hypomagnesemia, if present, may need to be corrected for the successful correction of the hypophosphatemia. In this regard, milk is also a good source for magnesium as each 8 oz of milk contains 34 mg of this element.

SIDE EFFECTS AND COMPLICATIONS OF TREATMENT OF HYPOPHOSPHATEMIA

The major side effects of phosphorus replacement therapy are diarrhea, especially with oral preparations; and hyperphosphatemia, hypocalcemia, and hyperkalemia if potassium phosphate salts are employed; metabolic acidosis; and volume excess, especially with intravenous preparations (Table 9).

The diarrhea is a dose-related phenomenon, and it can be generally avoided if phosphorus tablets are given in divided doses and if the total dose is limited to four tablets a day.

The hyperphosphatemia is a direct consequence of excessive phosphorus adminstration. Since the intracellular phosphorus depletion cannot be correctly estimated, and since the initial serum concentration response to intravenous phosphorus replacment does not indicate the degree of depletion, and also does not predict the serum concentration response to further therapy, one has to carefully monitor the serum phosphorus concentration every 12 hours during intravenous replacement therapy. One of the consequences of hyperphosphatemia is that it causes hypocalcemia can result in metastatic calcification and hypotension, and can impair renal function. Pulmonary vascular calcification with hypoxia due to a diffusion block may be a fatal complication.

Hyperkalemia may occur in patients with decreased renal function and oliguria, since most of the phosphorus preparations contain potassium. Therefore, serum potassium should be closely monitored during phosphorus administration.

Finally, some of the phosphorus preparations including oral phosphosoda (pH 4.8), acid sodium phosphate (pH 4.9), intravenous sodium phosphate (pH 5.7), and potassium phosphate (pH 6.6) are acidic, and when adminstered in large doses may result in metabolic acidosis.

HYPERPHOSPHATEMIA

Definition

Hyperphosphatemia is defined as a serum phosphorus concentration exceeding 5 mg/dl in adults, although a serum phosphorus concentration up to 6 mg/dl may be considered physiologic in children and adolescents. Hyperphosphatemia usually indicates total body phosphorus excess, however, it may also occur under circumstances in which total body phosphorus stores are normal, as in situations associated with acute redistribution of phosphorus from intracellular to extracellular fluid.

Table 9. Complications related to treatment of hyperphosphatemia

---
Hyperphosphatemia
Hypocalcemia
Hyperkalemia (potassium phosphate)
Metabolic acidosis
Volume expansion (sodium phosphate)
Diarrhea (oral phosphate)

Causes of hyperphosphatemia

Hyperphosphatemia can result from a) redistribution of phosphorus from intracellular compartments to extracellular fluid, b) increased gastrointestinal intake and absorption, or intravenous administration of phosphorus, and c) reduced renal phosphorus excretion, either because of decreased glomerular filtration or increased tubular reabsorption of phosphorus.

RENAL CAUSES OF HYPERPHOSPHATEMIA (TABLE 10)

One of the most common causes of hyperphosphatemia is decreased urinary excretion of phosphorus as a result of reduced GFR associated with chronic or acute renal failure. In chronic and progressive renal failure, phosphorus homeostatsis is maintained by a stepwise increase in phosphorus excretion per functioning nephron. As renal insufficiency progresses and the number of functioning nephrons decreases, however, phosphorus homeostasis can no longer be maintained and hyperphosphatemia develops. Hyperphosphatemia is also very common in acute renal failure, especially in acute renal failure resulting from rhabdomyolysis and tumor lysis syndrome.

Table 10. Causes of hyperphosphatemia

Decreased renal excretion of phosphorus
  Decrease in glomerular filtration rate
    Chronic renal failure
    Acute renal failure
  Increase in tubular reabsorption of phosphorus
    Hypoparathyroidism
    Pseuodhypoparathyroidism Type I and II
    Tumoral calcinosis
    Pseudoxanthoma elasticum
    Hyperthyroidism
    Glucocorticoid deficiency
    Biphosphonate therapy
Increased gastrointestinal absorption of phosphorus
  Ingestion and/or administration of phosphorus laxatives and enemas
  Pharmacologic therapy with vitamin-D metabolites
  Clinical disorders associated with increased vitamin-D levels

Increased renal tubular reabsorption of filtered phosphate can also result in hyperphosphatemia. Parathyroid hormone is an important regulator of tubular reabsorption of phosphorus, and the absence of parathyroid hormone, as in surgical or traumatic hypoparathyroidism, and the tubular resistance to parathyroid hormone, as in pseudohypoparathyroidism Type I and Type II, result in hyperphosphatemia due to the increase in the tubular transport maximum for phosphorus. Hyperphosphatemia is also reported with primary or genetic disorders such as the syndrome of familial tumoral calcinosis and pseudoxanthoma elasticum, in which there is an increase in the tubular transport maximum for phosphorus (70, 71). In tumoral calcinosis and pseudoxanthoma elasticum, abnormal vitamin D metabolism may also play an important pathogenic role, as $1,25(OH)_2D_3$ levels are either normal or increased and can thus result in hyperphosphatemia by causing both increased gatrointestinal absorption and renal tubular reabsorption of phosphorus. Hyperphosphatemia can also occur in acromegaly, hypothyroidism, and glucocorticoid deficiency after surgical correction of hypercortisolism in patients with Cushing's syndrome (72). Finally, biphosphonates which are used in the treatment of Paget's disease of bone (73), surgically untreatable hyperparathyroidism, and hypercalcemia of malignancy associated with metastatic bone disease, can also result in hyperphosphatemia, in part due to enhanced renal tubular reabsorption of phosphate.

GASTROINTESTINAL CAUSES OF HYPERPOSPHATEMIA (TABLE 10)

Hyperphosphatemia can result from an increased oral intake of phosphorus tablets or laxatives and vitamin D therapy, which would result in increased intestinal absorption of phosphorus. Another common cause of hyperphosphatemia is sodium phosphate enemas, which in individuals with renal insufficiency can result in very high levels of hyperphosphatemia and subsequent death. A recent study has shown that phosphorus is certainly absorbed by the colon, and therefore that phosphate enemas should be prescribed with great caution, especially in children and in patients with renal insufficiency (74).

PHARMACOLOGIC CAUSES OF HYPERPHOSPHATEMIA (TABLE 10)

Hyperphosphatemia may result from increased intravenous phosphorus administration during the treatment of hyposphosphatemia or in patients receiving total parenteral nutrition (TPN) (75).

HYPERPHOSPHATEMIA RESULTING FROM REDISTRIBUTION (TABLE 11)

A common cause of hyperphosphatemia is acute respiratory acidosis, which results in redistribution of phosphorus from intracellular pools to the extracellular fluid. Acute metabolic acidosis is also associated with hyperphosphatemia and may be partially responsible for the hyperphos-

Table 11. Causes of hyperphosphatemia

Redistribution of intracellular phosphorus
  Acute respiratory acidosis
  Acute metabolic acidosis

Increased release of intracellular phosphorus
  Burkitt's lymphoma
  Lymphoblastic lymphoma
  Acute lymphoblastic leukemia
  Metastatic small-cell bronchogenic carcinoma
  Metastatic breast adenocarcinoma
  Rhabdomyolysis
  Thyrotoxicosis
  Autoimmune hemolytic anemia

phatemia seen in patients with diabetic ketoacidosis prior to insulin therapy (36) and the hyperphosphatemia in patients with chronic renal failure (76, 77).

HYPERPHOSPHATEMIA RESULTING FROM INCREASED RELEASE OF INTRACELLULAR PHOSPHORUS (TABLE 11)

Hyperphosphatemia resulting from increased entry into the extracellular fluid is most dramatically seen in patients with acute renal failure associated with the crush syndrome or in the acute tumor lysis syndrome. In the latter, marked hyperphosphatemia, hyperkalemia, and hyperuricemia appear shortly after chemotherapy. It is especially apt to follow such treatment for lymphomas, including lymphoblastic lymphoma, Burkitt's lymphoma, and acute lymphoblastic leukemia. This syndrome sometimes happens, even in the absence of chemotherapy, in conditions associated with high cell turnover (78), and the syndrome has also been reported as a complication of chemotherapy of extensive small-cell bronchogenic carcinoma, metastatic breast adenocarcinoma, and during radiotherapy of metastatic medulloblastoma.

In patients with severe rhabdomyolysis due to trauma, extensive tissue destruction secondary to infarction or infection, and especially in intestinal necrosis associated with lactic acidosis, hyperphosphatemia of a pronounced degree may serve as an indication for surgical debridement or removal of the affected tissue. Each of these conditions is generally associated with severe volume depletion and renal failure.

Clinical consequences of hyperphosphatemia (Table 12)

One of the most striking clinical consequences of hyperphosphatemia is related to the reciprocal fall in the serum calcium concentration, which occurs in all cases of hyperphosphatemia, with the exception of tumoral calcinosis, pseudoxanthoma elasticum, and thyrotoxicosis, where serum calcium levels are normal because of the associated increase in $1,25(OH)_2D_3$ levels and the increase in gastrointestinal calcium absorption. In all the other cases, hyperphosphatemia produces hypocalcemia by several mechanisms, including decreased synthesis of

Table 12. Clinical consequences of severe hyperphosphatemia

Hypocalcemia
  Impaired myocardial contractility
  Conduction abnormalities
  Decreased systemic vascular tone
  Hypotension
  Increased neuromuscular excitability

Ectopic calcification
  Vascular
  Soft tissue
  Skeletal muscle
  Cardiac muscle
  Periarticular space

Table 13. Treatment of hyperphosphatemia

Acute hyperphosphatemia
  Increased renal excretion of phosphorus
    Intravenous volume expansion
    Bicarbonate
    Carbonic anhydrase inhibitors
  Shift into intracellular stores
    Glucose-insulin
    Removal from extracellular fluid

Chronic hyperphosphatemia
  Dietary phosphorus restriction
  Decreased gastrointestinal absorption
  Aluminum salts
    Alternagel
    Amphogel
    Basagel
    Alu caps
    Alu tabs
  Magnesium salts
    Magnesium carbonate
    Magnesium hydroxide
  Calcium salts
    Calcium carbonate
    Calcium citrate
  Sucralfate

Disorders of Phosphate Metabolism

$1,25(OH)_2D_3$, decreased absorption of calcium from the gastrointestinal tract, and precipitation of calcium. The hypocalcemia can result in impaired myocardial contractility, conduction abnormalities, decreased systemic vascular reactivity, hypotension, and increased neuromuscular excitability, including tetany, seizure activity, and convulsions.

Another serious side effect of hyperphosphatemia is the high incidence of ectopic calcification, which is caused by the precipitation of Ca-Pi in the form of hydroxyapatite crystals. The factors that control Ca-Pi precipitations include the Ca-Pi concentration product, local pH, circulating levels of PTH, and, most importantly, prior cell injury. Thus, if the calcium phosphorus product rises above 60, especially in the presence of an alkaline pH, a metastatic calcification is likely. This explains the common occurrence of metastatic calcification in patients with Burnet's (milk alkali) syndrome. High levels of PTH also favor ectopic calcification. The ectopic calcification can occur in virtually every organ system, including the heart, lung, brain, muscle, eye, skin, and the periarticular space of the large joints. Vascular calcification can also occur, resulting in necrosis and gangrene of the upper and lower extremities. Finally, it should be noted that there can be ectopic calcification of the kidney as well, resulting in worsening of renal function, which would only further aggregate the hyperphosphatemia (79).

Treatment of hyperphosphatemia (Table 13)

The treatment of hyperphosphatemia depends on the cause, whether it is acute or chronic, and whether renal function is intact. The major treatment modalities include inhibition of gastrointestinal absorption and/or enhancement of urinary excretion of phosphorus.

In acute hyperphosphatemic disorders that are mainly caused by rhabdomyolysis, tumor lysis syndrome, and similar conditions that are associated with an increased entrance of phosphorus from intracellular stores to extracellular fluid, administration of phosphate enemas and laxatives, or administration of phosphorus-containing intravenous fluids and total parenteral nutrition, if renal function is adequate the goal is to induce phosphaturia. This can be most optimally achieved by extracellular fluid volume expansion with intravenous saline, and also by administration of sodium bicarbonate and acetazolamide, a carbonic anhydrase inhibitor. Each of these modalities reduces tubular reabsorption of filtered phosphorus and results in increased urinary excretion of phosphorus. In the treatment of hyperphosphatemia associated with rhabdomyolysis and tumor lysis syndrome, this form of therapy may also be helpful toward prevention of acute tubular necrosis and hyperkalemia. Allopurinol, a xanthine oxidase inhibitor, is also administered to prevent the hyperuremicia that accompanies the hyperkalemia and hyperphosphatemia accociated with the tumor lysis syndrome.

In acute hyperphosphatemic disorders associated with impaired renal function, additional treatment modalities include administration of intravenous insulin and glucose, and hemodialysis or peritoneal dialysis. Insulin and glucose administration cause a shift of extracellular fluid phosphorus to the intracellular space, however, the effects are only transient. Dialysis is an effective mode of therapy for sustained removal of extracellular fluid phosphorus in these conditions. Peritoneal dialysis may be the preferred mode of dialysis, because the frequent exchanges, every 1 or 2 hours, utilized in acute peritoneal dialysis allow for the continuous removal of extracellular fluid phosphorus. Continuous arteriovenous hemodialysis (CAVHD), a recently introduced mode of dialytic therapy, may also be quite suitable in the treatment of patients with severe and sustained hyperphosphatemia.

In chronic hyperphosphatemic disorders associated with renal insufficiency, or enhanced gastrointestinal absorption caused by increased vitamin D levels, the goal is to inhibit gastrointestinal absorption of phosphorus. Since dietary phosphorus restriction to the degree that is required to satisfactorily reduce the serum phosphorus concentration is impractical, the major mode of therapy is the use of certain phosphorus-binding salts, including aluminum, calcium, and magnesium salts.

Side effects and complications of treatment of hyperphosphatemia (Table 14)

Aluminum hydroxide and aluminum carbonate gel and capsules, which are commerically available as Alternagel®, Basaljel®, and Amphogel®, or Alu-Tab® and Alu-Cap®, have been the traditional form of therapy very effectively used in the control of hyperphosphatemia. The major side effects of the aluminum gels are severe constipation and, in the very compliant patient, hypophosphatemia with phosphate depletion, resulting in osteomalacia (80). In addition, recently it has clearly become evident that aluminum in these compounds can be absorbed from the gastrointestinal tract, result in aluminum accumulation in several organs, and can cause chronic anemia, disabling osteomalacia, myopathy, and often fatal encephalopathy (81–84). The present-day strategy is, therefore, to use phosphate-binding salts other than aluminum gels. Magnesium salts are effective phosphate binders, however, since magnesium if also absorbed from the gastrointestinal tract and can result in neuromuscular toxicity, its use is limited in patients with chronic renal failure (85, 86). At the present time the most commonly used phosphate-binding salts are the calcium salts, including calcium carbonate and calcium citrate (87–96). The calcium salts are at least as effective as aluminum gels in binding dietary phosphorus and controlling hyperphosphatemia. They also have the potential advantage that the increase in gastrointestinal calcium absorption may normalize the calcium deficiency that occurs in patients with chronic renal failure. One major side effect, however, is that the increase in gastrointestinal calcium absorption can result in hypercalcemia and can increase the risk of metastatic calcification. Active research is underway to develop and test new nonsoluble and nonabsorbable aluminum compounds and calcium-charged polymers, which are effective phosphate binders, but potentially lack the side effects associated with aluminum, magnesium, and calcium salts (97–99).

ACKNOWLEDGMENTS

The authors would like to thank Ms. Ginny Mitchell for excellent secretarial assistance and the Dallas Veterans Administration Medical Center Medical Media Department for the illustrations.

REFERENCES

1. Lau K: Phosphate disorders. In: JP Kokko, RL Tanner, eds, *Fluids and Electrolytes*. WB Saunders, Philadelphia, pp 398–471, 1986.
2. Lee DB, Kurokawa K: Physiology of phosphorus metabolism. In: MH Maxwell, CR Kleeman, RG Narins, eds, *Clinical Disorders of Fluid and Electrolyte Metabolism*, 4th ed. McGraw-Hill, New York, pp 245–295, 1987.
3. Slatopolsky E, Klahr S: Disorders of phosphorus, calcium and magnesium metabolism. 1988. In: RW Schrier, CW Gottschalk, ed., *Diseases of the Kidney*, 4th ed. Little, Brown, Boston, pp 2865–2920, 1988.
4. Quamme GA, Shapiro RJ: Membrane controls of epithelial phosphate transport. *Can J Physiol Parmacol* 65:275–286, 1987.
5. Bonjour JP, Caverzasio J: Phosphate transport in the kidney. *Rev Physiol Biochem Pharmacol* 100:161–214, 1984.
6. Mizgala CL, Quamme GA: Renal handling of phosphate. *Physiological Rev* 65:431–466, 1985.
7. Knox FG, Hamarati A: Renal regulation of phosphate excretion. In: DW Seldin, G Giebisch, eds, *The Kidney: Physiology and Pathophysiology*. Raven Press, New York, pp 1381–1396, 1985.
8. Gmaj P, Murer H: Cellular mechanisms of inorganic phosphate transport in kidney. *Physiol Rev* 66:376–370, 1986.
9. Hammerman MR: Phosphate transport across renal proximal tubular cell membranes. *Am J Physiol* 251:F385–F398, 1986.
10. Kempson SA, Dousa TP: Current concepts of regulation of phosphate transport in renal proximal tubules. *Biochem Pharmacol* 35:721–726, 1986.
11. Sacktor B, Kinsella JL: Hormonal effects on sodium cotransport systems. *Ann NY Acad Sci* 456:438–444, 1986.
12. Murer H, Malstrom K: How renal phosphate transport is regulated. *NIPS* 2:45–48, 1987.
13. Knochel JP: Deranged phosphorus metabolism. In: DW Seldin, G Giebisch, eds, *The Kidney: Physiology and Pathophysiology*. Raven Press, New York, pp 1397–1416, 1985.
14. Knochel JP, Jacobson HR: Renal handling of phosphorus, clinical hypophosphatemia, and phosphorus deficiency. In: BM Brenner, FC Rector Jr eds, *The Kidney,* 3rd ed. WB Saunders, *Philadelphia* pp 619–662, 1986.
15. Brautbar N, Kleeman CR: Hypophosphatemia and hyperphosphatemia: Clinical and pathophysiologic aspects. In: MH Maxwell, CR Kleeman, RG Narins, eds, *Clinical Disorders of Fluid and Electrolyte Metabolism*, 4th ed. McGraw-Hill,

Table 14. Complications related to treatment of hyperphosphatemia

General
  Hypophosphatemia

Specific
  Aluminum salts
    Constipation
    Aluminum toxicity
      Anemia
      Osteomalacia
      Encephalopathy
  Magnesium salts
    Diarrhea
    Magnesium toxicity
      Neuromuscular
      Hypotension
  Calcium salts
    Calcium toxicity
    Ectopic calcification

New York, pp 789–830, 1987.
16. Betro MG, Pain RW: Hypophosphataemia and hyperphosphataemia in a hospital population. *Br Med J* 1:273–276, 1972.
17. Juan D, Elrazak MA: Hypophosphatemia in hospitalized patients. *JAMA* 242:163–164, 1979.
18. Larsson L, Rebel K, Sorbo B: Severe hypophosphatemia — A hospital survey. *Acta Med Scand* 214:221–223, 1983.
19. King AL, Sica DA, Miller G, Pierpaoli S: Severe hypophosphatemia in a general hospital population. *Southern Med J* 80:831–835, 1987.
20. Trivedi B, Sanforth WH. Effect of pH on the kinetics of frog muscle phosphofructokinase. *J Biol Chem* 211:4110–4114, 1966.
21. Mostellar ME, Tutle EP. Effect of alkalosis on plasma and urinary excretion of inorganic phosphate in man. *J Clin Invest* 43:138–151, 1964.
22. Hoppe A, Metler M, Berndt TJ, Knox FG, Angielski S: Effect of respiratory alkalosis on renal phosphate excretion. *Am J Physiol* 241 (Renal Fluid Electrolyte Physiol 12):F471–F475, 1982.
23. Brautbar N, Leibovici H, Massry SG: On the mechanism of hypophosphatemia during acute hyperventilation: Evidence for increased muscle glycolysis. *Min Elect Metab* 9:45–50, 1983.
24. Lichtman MA, Miller DR, Cohen J, Waterhouse C: Reduced red cell glycolysis, 2, 3-diphosphoglycerate and adenosine triphosphate concentration, and increased hemoglobin-oxygen affinity caused by hypophosphatemia. *Ann Intern Med* 740:562–568, 1971.
25. Travis SF, Sugerman HJ, Ruberg FL, Dudrick SJ, Delivoria-Papadopoulos M, Miller LD, Oski FA: Alterations of red-cell glycolytic intermediates and oxygen transport as a consequence of hypophosphatemia in patients receiving intravenous hyperalimentation. *Engl J Med* 285:763–768, 1971.
26. Silvis SE, DiBartolomeo AG, Aaker HM: Hypophosphatemia and neurological changes secondary to oral caloric intake. A variant of hyperalimentation syndrome. *Am J Gastroenterol* 73:215–222, 1980.
27. Weinsier RL, Krumdieck CL: Death resulting from overzealous total parenteral nutrition: The refeeding syndrome revisited. *Am J Clin Nutrition* 34:393–399, 1980.
28. Kalbfleisch JM, Lindeman RD, Ginn HE, Smith WO: Effects of ethanol administration on urinary excretion of magnesium and other electrolytes in alcoholic and normal subjects. *J Clin Invest* 42:1471–1475, 1963.
29. Stein JH, Smith WO, Ginn HE: Hypophosphatemia in acute alcoholism. *Am J Med Sci* 252:78–83, 1966.
30. Blachley JD, Ferguson ER, Carter NW, Knochel JP: Chronic alcohol ingestion induces phosphorus deficiency and myopathy in the dog. *Trans Assoc Am Physic* 93:110–122, 1980.
31. Knochel JP: Hypophosphatemia in the alcoholic. *Arch Intern Med* 140:613–615, 1980.
32. Ryback RS, Eckardt MJ, Paulter CP: Clinical relationships between serum phosphorus and other blood chemistry values in alcoholics. *Arc Intern Med* 140:673–677, 1980.
33. Adler AJ, Gudis S, Berlyne GM: Reduced renal phosphate threshold concentration in alcoholic cirrhosis. *Min Electrolyte Metab* 10:63–66, 1984.
34. De Marchi S, Cecchin E, Grimaldi F: Reduced renal phosphate threshold concentration in chronic alcoholics: One component of a more complex tubule dysfunction? *Min Electrolyte Metab* 12:147–148, 1986.
35. Schafer RM, Teschner M, Heidland A: Alterations of water, electrolyte and acid-base homeostasis in the alcoholic. *Mineral Electrolyte Metab* 13:1–6, 1987.
36. Kebler R, McDonald FD, Cadnapaphornchai P: Dynamic changes in serum phosphorus levels in diabetic ketoacidosis. *Am J Med* 79:571–576, 1985.
37. Levy LA: Severe hypophosphatemia as a complication of the treatment of hypothermia. *Arch Intern Med* 140:128–129, 1980.
38. Zamkoff KW, Kirshner JJ: Marked hypophosphatemia associated with acute myelomonocytic leukemia. Indirect evidence of phosphorus uptake by leukemic cells. *Arch Intern Med* 140:1523–1524, 1980.
39. Matzner Y, Prococimer M, Polliack A, Rubinger D, Popovtzer MM: Hypophosphatemia in a patient with lymphoma in leukemic phase. *Arch Intern Med* 141:805–806, 1981.
40. Aderka D, Shoenfeld Y, Santo M, Berliner S, Shaklai M, Weinberger A, Pinkhas J: Life-threatening hypophosphatemia in a patient with acute myelogenous leukemia. *Acta Haemat* 64:117–119, 1980.
41. Lenquist S, Lindell B, Nordstrom H, Sjoberg HE: Hypophosphatemia in severe burns. *Acta Chir Scand* 145:1–6, 1979.
42. Moorhead JF, Ahmed KY, Varghese Z, Willis MR, Baillod RA, Tatler GLV: Hypophosphataemic osteomalacia after cadaveric renal transplantation. *Lancet* 20:694–697, 1974.
43. Ward HN, Pabico RC, McKenna BA, Freeman RB: The renal handling of phosphate by renal transplant patients: Correlation with serum parathyroid hormone (SPTH), cyclic 3′,5′-adenosine monophosphate (cAMP) urinary excretion, and allograft function. *Adv Exp Med Biol* 81:173–181, 1977.
44. Nielsen HE, Christensen MS, Melsen F, Torring S: Bone disease, hypophosphatemia and hyperpharathyroidism after renal transplantation. *Adv Exp Med Biol* 81:603–610, 1977.
45. Farrington K, Varghese Z, Newman SP, Affmi KY, Fernando ON, Moorhead JF: Dissociation of absorptions of calcium and phosphate after successful cadaveric renal transplantation. *Br Med J* 1:712–714, 1979.
46. Nielsen HE, Melsen F, Christiensen MS: Spontaneous fractures following renal transplantation. Clinical and biochemical aspects, bone mineral content and bone morphometry. *Min Elect Metab* 2:323–330, 1979.
47. Walker GS, Peacock M, Marshall DH, Giles GR, Davison AM: Factors influencing the intestinal absorption of calcium and phosphorus following renal transplantation. *Nephron* 26:225–229, 1986.
48. Kovarik J, Graf H, Stummvoll HK, Wolf A, Pinggera WF: Tubular phosphate handling after successful kidney transplantation. *Klin Wochenschr* 58:863–869, 1980.
49. Friedman A, Chesney R: Fanconi's syndrome in renal transplantation. *Am J Nephrol* 1:45–47, 1981.
50. Rosenbaum RW, Hruska KA, Korkor A, Anderson C, Slatopolsky E: Decreased phosphate reabsorption after renal transplantation: Evidence for a mechanism independent of calcium and parathyroid hormone. *Kidney Int* 19:568–578, 1981.
51. Lucas PA, Brown RC, Bloodworth L, Woodhead JS: Vitamin D_3 metabolites in hypercalcemic adults after kidney transplantation. *Proc EDTA* 20:213–219, 1983.
52. Bonomini V, Feletti C, Di Felice A, Buscaroli A: Bone remodelling after renal transplantation. *Adv Exp Med Biol* 178:207–216, 1984.
53. Sakhaee K, Brinker K, Helderman JH, Bengfort JL, Nicar MJ, Hull AR, Pak CYC: Disturbances in mineral metabolism after successful renal transplantation. *Min Elect Metab* 11:167–172, 1985.
54. Felsenfeld AJ, Gutman RA, Drezner M, Llach F: Hypophosphatemia in long-term renal transplant recipients: Effects on

bone histology and 1,25-dihydroxycholecalciferol. *Min Elect Metab* 12:333–341, 1986.
55. Parfit AM, Kleerekoper M, Cruz C. Reduced phosphate reabsorption urelated to parathyroid hormone after renal transplantation: Implications for the pathogenesis of hyperparathyroidism in chronic renal fallure. *Min Elect Metab* 12:356–362, 1986.
56. Stoff JS: Phosphate homeostasis and hypophosphatemia. *Am J Med* 72:489–495, 1982.
57. Knochel JP: Neuromuscular manifestations of electrolyte disorders *Am J Med* 72:521–535, 1982.
58. Venditti FJ, Marotta C, Panezai FR. Olderwurtel HA, Regan TJ: Hypophosphatemia and cardiac arrhythmias. *Min Elect Metab* 13:19–25, 1987.
59. Aubier M, Murciano D, Lecocguic Y, Vires N, Jacquens Y, Squara P, Pariente R: Effect of hypophosphatemia on diaphragmatic contractility in patients with acute respiratory failure. *N Engl J Med* 313:420–424, 1985.
60. Rie MA: Hypophosphatemia and diaphragmatic contractility. *N Engl J Med* 314:519–520, 1986.
61. Hasselstrom L, Wimberley PD, Nielsen VG: Hypophosphatemia and acute respiratory failure in a diabetic patient. *Intensive Care Med* 12:429–431, 1986.
62. Lumlertgul D, Harris DCH, Burke TJ, Schrier RW: Detrimental effect of hypophosphatemia on the severity and progression of ischemic acute renal failure. *Min Elect Metab* 12:204–209, 1986.
63. Kanter Y, Gerson JR, Bessman AN: 2,3-diphosphoglycerate, nucleotide phosphate, and organic and inorganic phosphate levels during the early phases of diabetic ketoacidosis. *Diabetes* 26:429–433, 1977.
64. Keller U, Berger W: Prevention of hypophosphatemia by phosphate infusion during treatment of diabetic ketoacidosis and hyperosmolar coma. *Diabetes* 87–95, 1979.
65. Wilson HK, Keuer SP, Lea AS, Boyd AE, Eknoyan G: Phosphate therapy in diabetic ketoacidosis. *Arch Intern Med* 142:517–520, 1982.
66. Fisher JN, Kitabchi AE: A randomized study of phosphate therapy in the treatment of diabetic ketoacidosis. *J Clin Endocrinol metab* 57:177–180, 1983.
67. Kono N, Kuwajima M, Tarui S: Alteration of glycolytic intermediary metabolism in erythrocytes during diabetic ketoacidosis and its recovery phase. *Diabetes* 30:346–353, 1981.
68. Lentz RD, Brown DM, Kjellstrand CM: Treatment of severe hypophosphatemia. *Ann Intern Med* 89:941–944, 1978.
69. Vannatta JB, Whang R, Papper S: Efficacy of intravenous phosphorus therapy in the severely hypophosphatemic patient. *Arch Intern Med* 141:885–887, 1981.
70. Mallette LE, Mechanick JI: Heritable syndrome of pseudoxanthoma elasticum with abnormal phosphorus and vitamin D metabolism. *Am J Med* 83:1157–1162, 1987.
71. Weisinger JR, Mogollon A, Lander R, Bellorin-Font E, Riera R, Abadi I, Paz-Martinez R: Massive cerebral calcifications associated with increased renal phosphate reabsorption. *Arch Intern Med* 146:473–477, 1986.
72. Takuwa Y, Yamamoto M, Matsumoto T, Hata K, Ogata E: Hyperphosphatemia after surgical correction of hypercortosolism in patients with Cushing's syndrome. *Min Elect Metab* 12:119–124, 1986.
73. Challa A, Norrwall AA, Bevington A, Russell RGG: Cellular phosphate metabolism in patients receiving biophosphonate therapy. *Bone* 7:255–259, 1986.
74. Martin RR, Lisehora GR, Braxton M, Barcia PJ: Fatal poisoning from sodium phosphate enema. *JAMA* 257:2190–2192, 1987.
75. Suzuki NT: Hyperphosphatemia in nondialyzed TPN patients. *J Parenter Enter Nutrition* 11:512, 1987.
76. Barsotti G, Lazzeri M, Cristofano C, Cerri M, Lupetti S, Giovannetti S: The role of metabolic acidosis in causing uremic hyperphosphatemia. *Min Elect Metab* 12:103–106, 1986.
77. De Marchi S, Cecchin E: More on the role of metabolic acidosis in causing uremic hyperphosphatemia. *Min Elect Metab* 13:67–68, 1987.
78. Stark ME, Dyer MCD, Coonley CJ: Fatal acute tumor lysis syndrome with metastatic breast carcinoma. *Cancer* 60:762–764, 1987.
79. Lumlertgul D, Burke TJ, Gillum DM, Alfrey AC, Harris DC, Hammond WS, Schrier RW: Phosphate depletion arrests progression of chronic renal failure independent of protein intake. *Kidney Int* 29:658–666, 1986.
80. Delmez JA, Fallon MD, Harter HR, Hruska KA, Slatopolsky E, Teitelbaum SL: Does strict phosphorus control precipitate renal osteomalacia? *J Clin Endocrinol Metab* 62:747–752, 1986.
81. Slatopolsky E: The interaction of parathyroid hormone and alumimum in renal osteodystrophy. *Kidney Int* 31:842–854, 1987.
82. Burnatowska-Hledin MA, Doyle TM, Eadie MJ, Mayor GH: 1,25-dihydroxyvitamin D_3 increases serum and tissue accumulation of aluminum in rats. *J Lab Clin Med* 108:96–102, 1986.
83. Slanina P, Frech W, Ekstrom L-G, Loof L, Slorach S, Cedergren A: Dietary citric acid enhances absorption of aluminum in antacids. *Clin Chem* 32:539–541, 1986.
84. Weberg R, Berstad A: Gastrointestinal absorption of aluminum from single doses of aluminum containing antacids in man. *Eur J Clin Invest* 16:428–432, 1986.
85. O'Donovan R, Hammer M, Baldwin D, Moniz C, Parsons V: Substitution of aluminum salts by magnesium salts in control of dialysis hyperphosphatemia. *Lancet* 19:880–882, 1986.
86. Jennings AE, Bodvarsson M, Galicka-Piskorsha G, Difendorf AS, Simon GM, Levey AS: Use of magnesium hydroxide and low magnesium dialysate does not permit reduction of aluminum hydroxide during continuous ambulatory peritoneal dialysis. *Am J Kid Dis* 8:192–195, 1986.
87. Ramirez JA, Emmett M, White MG, Fathi N, Santa Ana CA, Morawski SG, Fordtran JS: The absorption of dietary phosphorus and calcium in hemodialysis patients. *Kidney Internat* 30:753–759, 1986.
88. Fournier A, Moriniere P, Sebert JL, Dkhissi H, Atik A, Leflon P, Renaud H, Gueris J, Gregoire I, Idrissi A, Garabedian M: Calcium carbonate, an aluminum-free agent for control of hyperphosphatemia, hypocalcemia, and hyperparathyroidism in uremia. *Kidney Int* 29:S114–S119, 19 .
89. Taber TE, Hegmen TF, York S: Calcium carbonate as a phosphate binder in hemodialysis patients. *Trans Am Soc Artif Intern Organs* 32:127–129, 1986.
90. Salusky IB, Coburn JW, Foley J, Nelson P, Fine RN: Effects of oral calcium carbonate on control of serum phosphorus and changes in plasma aluminum levels after discontinuation of aluminum-containing gels in children receiving dialysis. *J Pediat* 5:767–770, 1986.
91. Alon U, Davidai G, Bentur L, Berant M, Better OS: Oral calcium carbonate as phosphate-binder in patients and children with chronic renal failure. *Min Elect Metab* 12:320–325, 1986.
92. Herez G, Kraut JA, Andress DA, Howard N, Roberts C, Shinaberger JH, Sherrard DJ, Coburn JW: Use of calcium

carbonate as a phosphate binder in dialysis patients. *Min Elect Metab* 12:314–319, 1986.
93. Andreoll SP, Dunson JW, Bergstein JM: Calcium carbonate is an effective phosphorus binder in children with chronic renal failure. *Am J Kid Dis* 3:206–210, 1987.
94. Stein HD, Yudis M, Sirota RA: Calcium carbonate as a phosphate binder. *N Engl J Med* 316:109–110, 1987.
95. Almirall J, Campistol JM, Torras A, Revert L: calcium carbonate as phosphate binder in dialysis. *Lancet* 10:799–800, 1987.
96. Cushner HM, Copley JB, Lindberg JS, Foulks CJ: Calcium citrate, a nonaluminum-containing phosphate-binding agent for treatment of CRF. *Kidney Int* 33:95–99, 1988.
97. Schneider HW, Kulbe KD, Weber H, Streicher E: In vitro and in vivo studies with a non-aluminum phosphate-binding compound. *Kidney Int* 29 (Suppl 18):S120–S123, 1986.
98. Larson EA, Ash SR, White JL, Hem Sl: Phosphate binding gels: Balancing phosphate absorption and aluminum toxicity. *Kidney Int* 29:1131–1135, 1986.
99. Vucelic B, Hadzic N, Gragas J, Puretic Z: Changes in serum phosphorus, calcium and alkaline phosphatase due to sucralfate. *Int J Clin Pharm Therapy Toxicol* 24:93–96, 1988.

CHAPTER 8

Nephrolithiasis and Nephrocalcinosis

JOAN H. PARKS & FREDRIC L. COE

INTRODUCTION

From time to time, in most people, the urine separates into a solid and liquid phase. Unlike birds, which regularly produce a semisolid urine, all mammals have renal tubules and urinary collecting systems whose lumens are narrow and easily obstructed. As long as the solid phase in urine consists of very tiny particles, 0.1 to 10 microns in diameter, phase separation is asymptomatic. Larger particles can block tubule lumens or may adhere to papillary surfaces. Once anchored, a particle can then grow, until its dimensions become similar in magnitude to those of the urinary tract, i.e., millimeters to centimeters in diameter. Then, it can cause clinical disease.

Nature of stone disease

Essentially, the main thing a stone can do is cause obstruction. When it enters a ureter, it may suddenly block urine flow, or causes spasm, which has the same functional consequence. Severe pain occurs, usually called *renal colic*. Colic begins suddenly (1), often as a mild ache or scratchy sensation in one flank, and then worsens over 30 minutes or so to reach a plateau of maximum severity (2). It then remains constant, until the stone moves through the ureter or until analgesic medication is used. Renal colic is described as an aching or tearing sensation; nausea, vomiting, and diarrhea are common. Moving about is less uncomfortable than lying still, probably because it is distracting. Stones in the upper ureter cause mainly flank pain; as they move downward, the pain radiates anteriorly and downward over the abdomen, into the pelvis, the groin, and ultimately into the ipsalateral vulva or testicle. Stones at the ureterovesicle junction can cause dysuria, frequency, urgency, and nocturia, and mimic acute cystitis. Stones can obstruct an infundibulum drawing a group of calyces, or the ureteropelvic junction. Pain often comes in spells, when the stones occlude like a ball valve, and disappears suddenly as it rolls away from the orifice it has been blocking. Some stones gradually occlude the ureteropelvic junction or an infundibulum, producing no symptoms despite severe hydronephrosis.

Given their simple nature, stones can produce only a narrow range of disease. Mostly, they cause great pain, which patients dread. Colic episodes frequently require hospitalization and result in a loss of working days. Obstruction may require cystoscopy or even ureteral or renal surgery, which have their own complications, Obstruction, and especially cystoscopy, can predispose to urinary infection, a common complication of stones. Finally, stones can cause hematuria, which is worrisome but is the least important of these morbid effects.

Types of stones

There are calcium, uric acid, cystine, and struvite stones (3); other types — ammonium acid urate, xanthine (4) and triampterine — are known but are rare. The most common stones are composed of calcium (Table 1). Calcium stones contain calcium oxalate, pure or admixed with calcium phosphate, occasionally calcium phosphate alone, and not rarely, calcium oxalate mixed with uric acid (5). Calcium oxalate in stones is crystalline, either the monohydrate or dihydrate form. There is no clinical significance to one or the other. Uric acid stones are composed of the undissociated, protonated form of uric acid. Cystine stones are made of the insoluble amino acid. Struvite is the triple salt of magnesium, ammonium, and phosphate, and forms only as a result of infection with bacteria that possess the enzyme urease. The four types of stones have different natural histories because they usually grow to different sizes; each is detailed separately in the following sections. When radiopaque stones collect in the kidneys in large numbers, the term *nephrocalcinosis* is used descriptively.

Table 1. Classification of types of stones in 1256 patients

	Number	%
Calcium oxalate	801	64
Calcium + uric acid	108	9
Uric acid	26	2
Cystine	8	1
Struvite	72	6
Unknown	213	17
Total	1256	

People at risk

Nephrocalcinosis also has a special and separate meaning. Hypercalcemia, especially when accompanied by elevated serum phosphorus levels, can cause deposits of calcium phosphate in the renal parenchyma, particularly along tubular basement membranes (6). The result is one form of tubulointerstitial nephropathy. Hyperoxaluric states can also do this (7), as calcium oxalate crystals form in tubule lumens and the renal interstitium. Hypercalcemic or hyperoxaluric state may cause papillary stones, as well as cortical deposits. Diffuse parenchymal calcification may be, but is usually not, visible by x-ray; unlike stones, it causes chronic renal damage and renal failure. Radiographically visible calcifications frequently occur in papillary necrosis (8) and tuberculosis (9, 10). Papillary necrosis from any cause results in calyceal calcifications in the areas of tissue injury.

Because it comes in many forms, nephrocalcinosis is usually modified by adjectives. Papillary nephrocalcinosis implies stones or calcification in areas of papillary injury or anatomic distortion, as in medullary sponge kidney (11). Patchy cortical nephrocalcinosis usually implies prior tissue injury or hypercalcemia. The two together suggest hyperoxaluria, combined hypercalcemia, and hypercalciuria, or a process that has damaged papillae and cortex, such as severe infection.

Stones usually begin in adult life and tend to recur. Cystine stones, however, frequently begin in childhood. Calcium stones affect men four times more often than women; uric acid stones are also usually formed by men. The two sexes produce cystine stones equally. Struvite stones occur mainly in women. Affluence and a sedentary life are said to predispose to calcium stones (12), but the reason for the association is not known. Gout is strongly associated with uric acid stones (13), but not with mixed calcium-uric acid stones. Struvite stones usually seem to follow chronic relapsing urinary infection, but there are many cases where no such history is present.

Altogether, it is easy to derive useful generalizations about who gets each type of stone, but there are enough exceptions that each must be viewed as, at best, a broad guideline. A man with struvite stones is not a rare patient, and women with common calcium stones are frequently seen.

Problems of management

Because they cause mainly obstruction, the consequences of stones are managed usually by urologic surgeons, not by the physicians for whom this book is intended. The role of the physician in management is mainly supportive and, of course, diagnostic in that the problem is often first recognized by the nonsurgeon. Nevertheless, we should all be well informed, even as observers.

COLIC

The pain of acute ureteric obstruction by a stone is unendurable and requires analgesic medication. Morphine or another drug is indicated. Abdominal radiographs will usually disclose calcium, cystine, or struvite stones, which are radiopaque; uric acid stones are radiolucent. Intravenous pyelography is needed to assess the degree of urinary obstruction and to detect radiolucent stones. Hospitalization is required if the pain persists with analgesic agents or if there is severe obstruction.

OBSTRUCTION

Assuming an intact contralateral kidney, there is no immediate urgency with regard to an obstructing stone; one can wait for days as it passes. A single abdominal radiograph will document the movement of the stone. If an obstructing stone is stationary or if hydronephrosis is very severe, it must be removed. Cystoscopy is usual. A stone "basket" may be used to move the stone if it is in the lower one-half of the ureter. If an easier measure does not work, one requires ureterolithotomy. Even if surgery is eventually needed, a lower lying stone is desirable; it can be removed using a small incision in the abdomen, whereas for higher stones the surgery requires a subcentral incision and dissection that disturbs the perinephric space.

Certain problems are emergencies, or at least require urgent surgery. Anuria occurs with obstruction of both kidneys or a solitary functioning kidney. Infection can complicate obstruction, and produce sepsis and terrible renal injury. The renal pelvis can leak, allowing urine to enter the perinephric space. Such leaks seal spontaneously once the stone has been removed, but require that stone removal proceed as soon as possible.

INFECTION

Urinary infection usually occurs with stones because of the need for cystoscopy and surgery. Apart from the emergency of infection above an obstructed ureter, management is conventional. A special case is struvite stone, which always arises from infection with bacteria that possess urease. These bacteria, usually *Proteus* species, cannot be eradicated once a stone is present; the goal is palliative reduction of their number (see Struvite Stones).

CHRONIC PAIN

Stones in the kidney, especially, can cause chronic, intermittent pain as they obstruct infundibulae or the ureteropelvic junction. Less often, low ureteric stones at the ureterovesicle junction cause chronic discomfort, mainly dysuria and frequency. Large stones in the kidney that chronically obstruct may cause more damage, but not as much pain as small stones. There is no effective treatment for stone pain, except dissolution or removal of the stones. The main problem is to differentiate it from musculoskeletal pain, which is common in patients with stones who have had many episodes of muscle spasm because of colic. The main characteristic of stone pain is sudden cessation as stones move away from an orifice and sudden recurrence. Often the severe pain will end abruptly, leaving

Table 2. Metabolic and clinical disorders in 915 calcium stone-formers

	No. of patients	%
Idiopathic hypercalciuria	234	26
Hyperuricosuria	132	14
Hypercalciuria & hyperuricosuria	120	13
Primary hyperparathyroidism	59	6
Renal tubular acidosis	8	1
Enteric hyperoxaluria	47	5
Primary hyperoxaluria	3	0.3
Medullary sponge kidney	109	12
Sarcoidosis	7	1
Cushings, Paget's	11	1
No disorder found	185	20
Total	915	

Used with permission from Parks JH, Coe FL: Stone disease in idiopathic hypercalciuria. In: FL Coe, ed, *Hypercalciuric States*. Grune and Stratton, New York, in press.

only residual soreness. When pain encroaches enough upon the quality of life to warrant surgery, the stones should be removed. If they are uric acid or cystine stones, dissolution is possible, though it may take months.

CALCIUM STONES

There are many ways to classify the causes of common stones. We prefer to separate the large group, who have hypercalciuria, hyperuricosuria, or no known disorders, from the small group, whose stones arise from serious systemic disorders. For the former, treatment decisions are based upon the seriousness of the stone disease itself, whereas the latter may require treatment even when the stones are themselves trivial. Our experience (Table 2) illustrates the relative frequencies of these two groups and their subgroups.

Hypercalciuria, hyperuricosuria, or no disorder

NATURAL HISTORY OF STONES

Because of its size, this group of patients has lent itself to the analysis of the natural history of stones and much is known about it. The onset of stones is greatest roughly at the end of adolescence (Figure 1), in the early part of the third decade. Patients who have recurrent stones tend to form them at a rate of about one every 2–3 years (Table 3). The main morbidity, hospitalization, cystoscopy, infec-

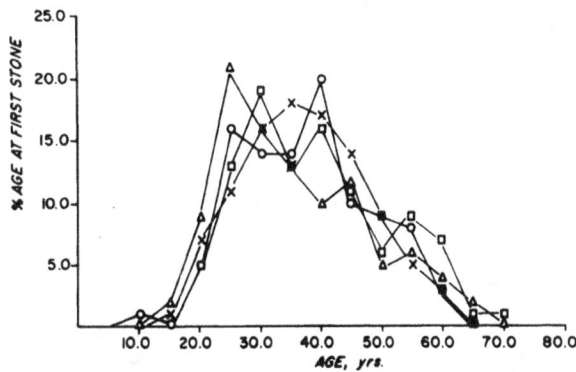

Figure 1. Distribution of age at first stone by metabolic subgroup in patients with calcium stone. Triangle indicates idiopathic hypercalciuria; circle, hyperuricosuria; x, hypercalciuria and hyperuricosuria; square, neither disorder. The percentage of all stones formed by patients in each of the four subgroups is shown for each 5-year age interval. Used with permission.

Table 3. History of stone disease in patients with recurrent calcium nephrolithiasis

	IH	HU	BO	NE	ALL
No. patients	228	108	114	160	610
Percentage of men	68.0	91.0	81.0	82.0	78.0
Age at first stone	33.0	35.2	34.6	36.2	34.6
Pretreatment interval/pt	9.0	7.5	10.1	8.8	8.9
Pretreatment interval/pt yrs	2053	806	1154	1415	5428
Mean interval between stones	2.65	2.84	2.34	2.85	2.68
Interval first to second	4.43	3.83	4.26	4.19	4.23
Interval last stone to entry	1.13	0.92	0.80	1.00	1.06
Total number stones	1929	723	1046	1269	4967
Recurrent stones/100 pt yrs	82.8	76.3	80.7	78.4	80.3
Treatment interval/pt	2.94	3.19	2.68	2.41	2.80
Treatment interval/pt yrs	670	344	306	386	1706
New stones formed	55	28	50	109	242
New stones/100 pt yrs	8.21	8.13	16.35	28.23	14.19
Percentage of pts/no relapse	89.0	88.9	87.7	89.1	88.6

Used with permission from Parks JH, Coe FL: Stone disease in idiopathic hypercalciuria. In: FL Coe, ed, *Hypercalciuric States*. Grune and Stratton, New York, in press.

tion, and surgery rate is easily predicted per 100 stones for a large population (Table 4), though any one individual is quite unpredictable.

There is a common fallacy that stone disease wanes with time (14). We have shown (15), however, that the interval between successive stones does not increase, and may even narrow. Our current series is much larger than our original one and continues to show stable or falling intervals. Since the interval between successive stones does not increase, one cannot say that the disease will tend to improve in any given case, unless some treatment is used.

Patients who have formed only one stone by the time they see a physician also pose special problems. One tends to believe that their disease is not serious and that the single stone, being an isolated event, may not be sufficient reason for detailed work-up and treatment. There are few studies of this problem. In two prospective studies, most people (11, 16) who had formed one stone ultimately formed another (Table 5). Given this fact, we suspect that a solitary stone deserves investigation.

At the other pole of the disease are patients who form large numbers of stones, at least ten. We have called this *accelerated nephrolithiasis* (17). Such patients have the same metabolic disorders as other common stone formers and respond to treatment in a similar way. Why they form as many stones as they do is not known.

IDIOPATHIC HYPERCALCIURIA

This is the most common disorder found in patients with stones. Nearly one-half of calcium stone-formers have it, compared with 5% of people in general. It has been suspected of causing stones ever since it was first described, and contemporary evidence linking it directly to stone production is very strong indeed. The diagnosis requires un-

Table 4. Recurrence of stones with time in solitary stone-formers

Duration of follow-up (yr)	Blacklock[a]		Williams[b]	
	Patients	Percent with recurrence	Patients	Percent with recurrence
1			399	14
2	440	38		
3	337	43		
4	270	48	345	42
5	216	50		
6	188	52		
7	157	56		
8	112	64		
9	85	67	231	61
10–14			158	80
15–19			47	92
20–24			24	98
>25			10	100

[a] Adapted from Blacklock NJ: (12).
[b] Recalculated from Williams RE (16).
Used with permission from Coe (3).

Table 5. Morbidity caused by stone disease in the pretreatment interval and the treatment interval

	IH	HU	BO	NE	ALL
Pretreatment					
Morbidity per 100 patient years					
Cystoscopies	16.66	15.64	15.42	11.59	14.92
Hospitalizations	26.54	29.29	24.78	20.08	24.89
Infections	6.43	2.73	4.25	6.86	5.53
Surgeries	7.55	6.58	6.58	5.23	6.61
Morbidity per 100 stones					
Cystoscopies	16.80	17.43	17.02	12.92	16.31
Hospitalizations	28.25	32.64	27.34	22.38	27.20
Infections	6.84	3.04	4.68	7.64	6.04
Surgeries	8.04	7.33	7.27	5.83	7.23
Treatment					
Morbidity per 100 patient years					
Cystoscopies	2.84	3.77	2.94	2.33	2.93
Hospitalizations	8.06	6.68	5.56	7.51	7.21
Infections	3.58	1.45	1.96	0	2.05
Surgeries	3.43	3.19	1.64	1.29	2.58

Used with permission from Parks JH, Coe FL: Stone disease in idiopathic hypercalciuria. In: Coe FL, ed, *Hypercalciuric States*. Grune and Stratton, New York, in press.

explained hypercalciuria and normocalcemia. The usual upper limits of normal for 24-hour urine calcium are 300 mg (men), 250 mg (women), or 4 mg/kg (either sex).

Etiology

Hypercalciuria is an inherited trait. Our own study of nine families (18) (Figure 2) suggests an autosomal dominant inheritance. Other studies have confirmed ours (19, 20). As expected, hypercalciuria can be detected among children at the same rate as in adults (21). Hypercalciuria also occurs spontaneously among normal laboratory rats (22). Rather than a disease, hypercalciuria, like tallness, may well be a trait conditioned by genetic variability, of interest to physicians only because it seems to enhance the risk of calcium stone production.

Pathogenesis

Virtually all patients with hypercalciuria absorb dietary calcium at a higher rate than normal people do, and their renal tubules reabsorb filtered calcium less perfectly (23). One way this could occur would be a primary increase in intestinal calcium absorption, due either to a disorder of the intestinal epithelial cells or an increase in the serum $1,25(OH)_2D_3$ level. There is good evidence that serum $1,25(OH)_2D_3$ levels are higher than normal in hypercalciuria (24), but calcium hyperabsorption seems to occur in some patients whose $1,25(OH)_2D_3$ levels are normal (25). Calcium hyperabsorption could reduce renal calcium reabsorption by causing post prandial suppression of PTH secretion (Figure 3). PTH stimulates overall tubule calcium reabsorption (26). An alternative model (Figure 3) is a primary defect of renal tubule calcium reabsorption, which

Nephrolithiasis and Nephrocalcinosis   143

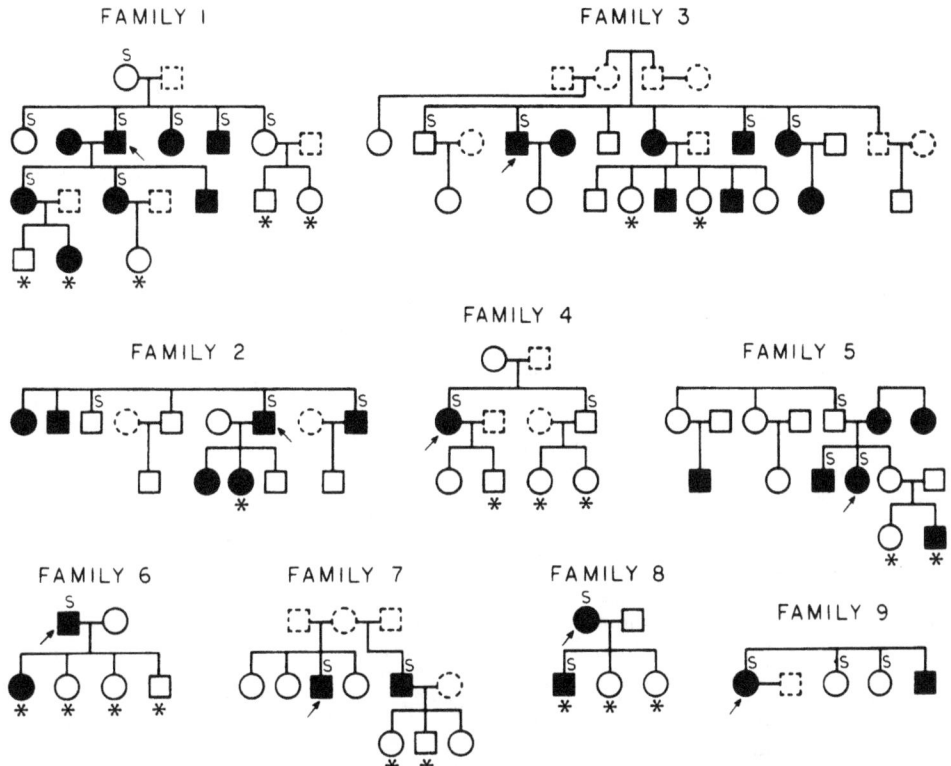

Figure 2. Family pedigrees of nine probands with idiopathic hypercalciuria. Hypercalciuric individuals are shown by dark shading. Stone disease is indicated by S. Children, defined as males or females below the age of 20 years, are indicated by *. Marginal hypercalciuria was present in four siblings, one each in families 1, 2, 3, and 5; in the mother of proband 4; two aunts and one niece in family 5; and one nephew in family 3. Altogether, hypercalciuria occurred in 11 of 24 siblings and 7 of 16 offspring of the probands. The arrows indicate probands. Interrupted symbols indicate relatives not studied; they are given for the sake of pedigree accuracy. Use with permission from Coe FL et al. (18).

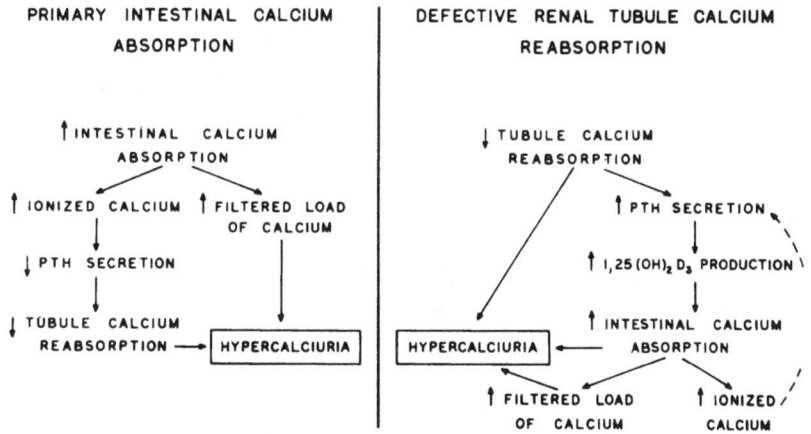

Figure 3. Proposed pathogenesis for two alternative models of idiopathic hypercalciuria. Left panel: Primary intestinal overabsorption. Right panel: Primary defective tubule calcium reabsorption. Dotted line indicates mechanisms tending to restore PTH secretion toward normal. Used with permission from Coe FL and Favus MJ: Disorders of renal stone formation. In: Brenner BM, Rector FC Jr, (eds), The Kidney, and ed. WB Saunders Philadelphia, Chapter 37, 1981.

could lead to intestinal hyperabsorption by producing secondary hyperparathyroidism (27). A third alternative is that neither model is correct and that patients have a dual defect. Renal tubule cells produce $1,25(OH)_2D_3$ and reabsorb calcium. If there were a cellular defect that reduced calcium reabsorption and, at the same time or because of the reabsorptive defect, disturbed the regulation of $1,25(OH)_2D_3$ production, each model could be mimicked, depending upon the relative prominence of the transport and regulatory defects.

The exact pathogenesis of hypercalciuria, if known in a given case, could influence treatment. Thiazide diuretic agents reduce urine calcium excretion (28), probably by stimulating distal-tubule calcium reabsorption (29). However, they may not be ideal for patients with pure intestinal hyperabsorption who could, theoretically, retain calcium that might deposit in soft tissues. A low-calcium diet or a drug like cellulose phosphate that reduces intestinal calcium absorption (30) would be ideal for pure hyperabsorption, but unsafe if renal tubular calcium reabsorption were defective.

Unfortunately, it is difficult to tell the two types of hypercalciuria apart. Normal values of serum PTH and urine cyclic AMP, though expected in absorptive hypercalciuria, were observed in 20 patients of Sutton et al. (31) who had fasting hypercalciuria, a trait that is most compatible with a renal tubule defect. Furthermore, values of fasting urine calcium, urine cyclic AMP, and serum PTH all are distributed continuously in patients with hypercalciuria (32), so that the detection of patients who cannot tolerate a prolonged low-calcium diet must be based upon the potentially arbitrary subdivision of a continuous distribution. Nevertheless, all evidence points to either the separate existence of two forms of hypercalciuria or a single type that includes elements of both a tubule reabsorptive defect and either disordered $1,25(OH)_2D_3$ regulation or excessive intestinal calcium transport; undoubtedly, a better understanding of the pathogenesis will improve the safety of long-term treatment.

Pathogenesis of stones

Hypercalciuria appears to favor the formation of a solid phase by increasing the supersaturation of urine. Urine is supersaturated with respect to a given solid phase if crystals of that phase will grow in the urine. Once growth ceases, the urine is at the equilibrium solubility product for the phase. We (33) measured supersaturation with respect to calcium oxalate monohydrate by measuring the calcium-oxalate product in urine before and after incubation of the urine with seed crystals of calcium oxalate monohydrate at 37°C for 48 hours. The ratio of the concentration products before and after incubation (CPR, or concentration product ratio) is a good index of supersaturation. Patients with hypercalciuria (Figure 4) had a greater statistical tendency to higher than normal CPR values than did other stone-formers. This tendency could easily enhance risk of stone formation.

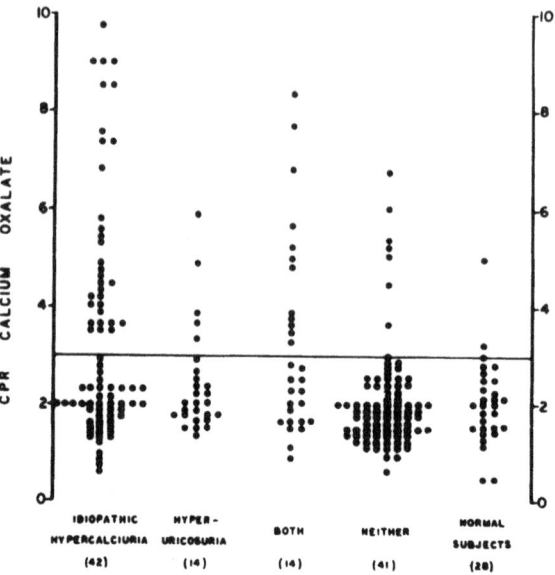

Figure 4. Values of the calcium oxalate concentration ratio (CPR) in 24-hour urine collections from 111 calcium stone-formers and 28 normal subjects. Each point represents a single urine sample. The number of patients in each category is shown in parentheses. One normal subject who had urine CPR values of 3.2 and 5.2 was studied twice. The rest contributed one urine value each to the figure. Forty patients elaborated at least one urine sample with CPR above 3:22 with hypercalciuria, 3 with hyperuricosuria, 9 with both, and 6 with neither. Used with permission from Weber DV et al. (33).

Low-calcium diet

Some of the best data were obtained in the course of a prospective trial of orthophosphate treatment (34). Forty-six patients with calcium stones were treated with only a low-calcium diet and water (Table 6). New stone production fell to 52% of pretreatment and remained low for up to 6 years. In contrast, acid phosphate with the diet prevented the fall in new stone production (Table 6). When the acid phosphate was discontinued, the stone production rate fell to the level seen with diet alone. Unfortunately the patients represented a mixture of normocalciuria and hypercalciuria; nevertheless, they suggest that diet alone has some effect.

Thiazide diuretic agents

Our own data, prospective but not controlled, illustrate the extreme effects of thiazide (see Table 3). The same responses have been documented by Yendt and Cohanim (35), Pak et al. (36), and Maschio et al. (37). The probable mechanism is a reduction of calcium oxalate supersaturation. By lowering urine calcium, thiazide reduces super-

Table 6. Effects of low calcium diet and oral phosphate on stone recurrence

Treatment	Patient years	Stones/100 pt yrs	Stones formed	Stones predicted using rate from		
				BT	T	Placebo + diet
Before treatment (BT)						
(A) Phosphate + diet (25)	183	67	123	—	—	123
(B) Placebo (20)	120	78	94			
(C) Diet (26)	123	57	70			
(B) + (C) (46)	243	67	164			
Treatment						
(A) Phosphate + diet	77	54	42	51.6	—	25.4[a]
(B) Placebo	60	33	20	46.8[a]	—	—
(C) Diet	71	32	23	40.4[a]	—	—
(B) + (C)	131	33	43	86.2[a]	—	—
Follow-up						
(A) Phosphate + diet	86	24	21	57.6[a]	46.4[a]	23.2
(B) Placebo	57	26	15	44.7[a]	18.8	—
(C) Diet	73	27	20	41.6[a]	23.3	
(B) + (C)	130	27	35	87.1[a]	42.9	

Adapted with permission from Ettinger (34). Table 1. Number of patients is in parentheses. "Before treatment" data (BT) were prior to entry into the program; thereafter, all patients received a low-calcium diet during the treatment period (T) and follow-up years. During "treatment" years only, 25 patients received oral phosphate; the other received placebo or diet alone.
[a] Differs significantly from the number observed (p < .001) by the Chi-square method.

saturation (33) (Figure 5), and the reduction appears to persist over many months.

Diet versus thiazide

Clearly thiazide is more effective, but side effects of allergic drug reactions (rare) (Table 7) and hypokalemia, postural giddiness, and impotence detract from their use. In general, thiazide produces hypocalciuria at one third to one half of the full dose, so the latter three complications are not frequent or severe. On the other hand, a low-calcium diet poses a serious risk if used for years in people

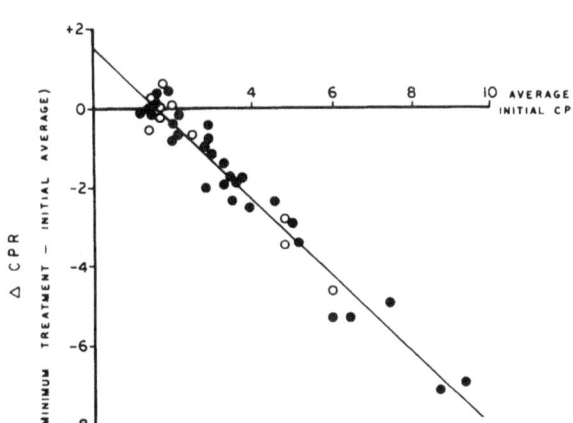

Figure 5. Relation between the maximum fall in the concentration product ratio (CPR) produced by thiazide treatment (y axis) and the magnitude of the average initial 24-hour urine CPR value (x axis) for 30 patients who were hypercalciuric (closed circles) and ten who were not (open circles). The maximum fall in CPR was very closely correlated with the average pretreatment CPR derived from the two pretreatment urine collections (r = 0.95). Their linear regression, shown by the diagonal line, has a slope of 0.97 and a y intercept of $1.60 \times 10^{-6}\,m^2$. Used with permission from Weber DV et al. (33).

Table 7. Drug complications of thiazide

Total number of patients	482
Total patient years on thiazide	1522.86
Patients who discontinued because of side effects	13
Rash	2
Impotence	2
Abdominal pain[a]	2
Photosensitivity	2
Ventricular fibrillation[b]	1
Hypotensive episode	1
Headaches	1
"Weak"	1
Rising alkaline phosphatase	1
Incidence of side effects/pt year	0.0085

[a] After each dose of thiazide.
[b] In a patient who simultaneously lost weight on a liquid diet.

146 Therapy of Renal Diseases and Related Disorders

who cannot conserve calcium normally. We recommend thiazide, at least now, for those people whose clinical stone disease warrants treatment. If thiazide cannot be used or is not acceptable to a patient, a low-calcium diet can be considered if evidence points to normal renal calcium conservation. Minimum criteria should be normal serum PTH, fasting urine cyclic AMP, and calcium (38).

Follow-up, outcome, and prognosis

After 8 weeks of treatment, the urine calcium must be measured. The urine calcium should be below the upper limits of normal. If thiazide is used, the urine sodium should be measured and kept below 200 mEq/24 hr; this reduces potassium wasting and improves the hypocalciuric response to thiazide. Abdominal radiograph should be obtained near the start of treatment to assess the number of stones in the kidneys, and a new one should be obtained yearly. Successful treatment is the formation of no new stones; preexistent stones may pass or require removal, but that must not be viewed as treatment failure. In general, most patients remain stone free. Treatment is long term.

HYPERURICOSURIA

Daily uric acid excretion rates above 800 mg (men) or 750 mg (women) are more frequent in patients with calcium stones than in normal people (39), and a reduction of uricosuria is associated with a marked fall in stone production (40).

Pathogenesis

Dietary purine excess was a common cause in our patients (Figure 6), but occasional patients excreted uric acid at a high rate, even during a low-purine diet and must, therefore, have had a primary state of endogenous uric acid overproduction. If our ten studies are a reasonable guide to what occurs in whole populations, diet could be the main form of treatment. The particular dietary cause of hyperuricosuria that we observed was an excess of meat, fish, and poultry, used in place of bread and grains (Figure 7).

Pathogenesis of stones

Hyperuricosuria raises the supersaturation of urine, mainly with respect to undissociated uric acid (see Table 8). Sodium hydrogen urate supersaturation is not increased by spontaneous hyperuricosuria, whereas it is when hyperurico-

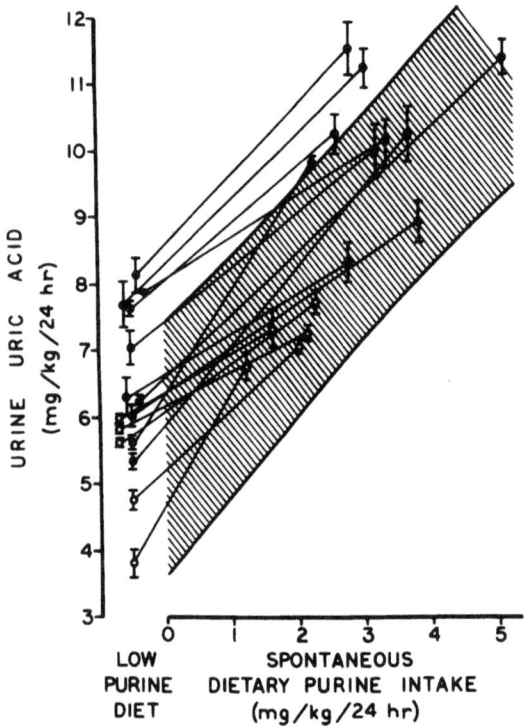

Figure 6. Relation between urine urate excretion and purine intake in patients and normal subjects on ambient and low purine diets. Used with permission from Coe FL, Kavalich AG: Hypercalciuria and hyperuricosuria in patients with calcium nephrolithiasis. N Engl J Med 291:1344–1350, 1974.

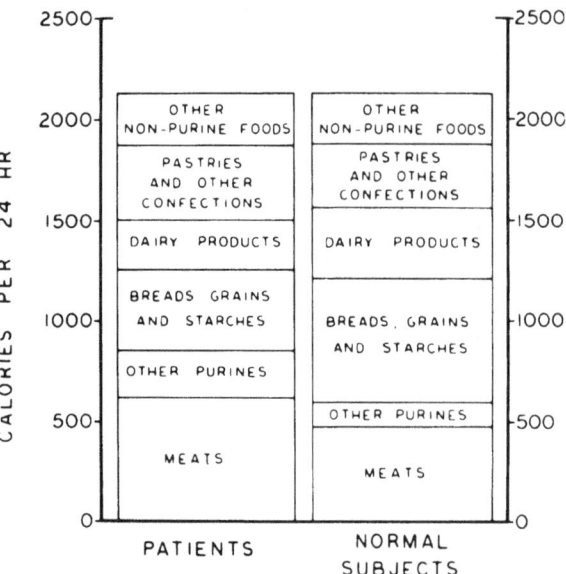

Figure 7. Diets of patients and normal subjects. Calories consumed in each of six broad food categories are similar for the two groups, except for meats and other high-purine foods, and for breads, grains, and starches, which differ markedly. Used with permission from Coe FL, Moran E, Kavalich AG: The contribution of dietary purine overconsumption to hyperuricosuria in calcium oxalate stone formers. J Chron Dis 29:793–800, 1976.

Table 8. Summary of urinary uric acid saturation measurements[a]

24-hour urine values	Metabolic group				
	Normal (n = 20)	IH (n = 20)	HU (n = 12)	Both (n = 14)	Neither (n = 17)
No. of samples	24	69	36	42	51
Total uric acid, mg/l	503 ± 32	421 ± 23	575 ± 28	616 ± 27[g]	462 ± 32
Urine volume, ml	1268 ± 65	1717 ± 133[h,j]	1501 ± 79[f]	1397 ± 70	1387 ± 90
Urine pH	6.22	5.92	5.62[g]	5.74[g]	5.67[h]
Undissociated uric acid,[b] mg/l	57 ± 8[j]	84 ± 11	155 ± 21[h]	150 ± 16[i]	128 ± 18[g]
CPR, monosodium urate	2.8 ± 0.03[c]	2.2 ± 0.2	2.7 ± 0.2	3.1 ± 0.2	2.2 ± 0.2
Initial [Na] · [urate],[c] m² × 10⁻⁵	37 ± 4	27 ± 3	35 ± 4	42 ± 3[j]	29 ± 3
Final [Na] · [urate],[d] m² × 10⁻⁵	13.2 ± 0.7	11.0 ± 0.5	12.0 ± 0.6	12.9 ± 0.5	13.2 ± 1.0
Sodium concentration, mEq/l	131 ± 8[j]	118 ± 7	130 ± 7	149 ± 7[k]	132 ± 7[j]

[a] All values, except for the numbers of samples and the numbers of people in each metabolic group (in parentheses), are the means ± SEM. Abbreviations used are IH = idiopathic hypercalciuria; HU = hyperuricosuria; CPR = concentration product ratio; [Na] = sodium concentration (mEq/l); [urate] = urate = urate concentration (mM/l).
[b] The mean equilibrium value, determined in 26 urine samples of pH below 5.6, after 48 hours of incubation with crystals of uric acid, was 905 mg/l.
[c] Before incubation with crystals of sodium hydrogen urate.
[d] After 48 hours of incubation with crystals of sodium hydrogen urate.
[e] Based upon the study of the 16 of the 20 normal subjects who had CPR measurements.
[f] $p < 0.05$, compared with control.
[g] $p < 0.02$, compared with control.
[h] $p < 0.01$, compared with control.
[i] $p < 0.001$, compared with control.
[j] $p < 0.05$, men vs. women.
[k] $p < 0.02$, men vs. women.
Used with permission from Coe et al. (41).

suria is induced under controlled conditions (41), because a high-meat diet lowers urine pH. In other words, spontaneous hyperuricosuria favors the formation of uric acid crystals in urine.

Uric acid crystals have lattice dimensions that resemble closely those of calcium oxalate monohydrate (Table 9). Computer analysis of the topography of surface changes of the two crystals shows a very good matching (42). This means that calcium and oxalate ions could attach themselves to the surface of uric acid crystals and begin to grow into a crystal of calcium oxalate, as they could on a surface of calcium oxalate itself.

Such a phenomenon could facilitate calcium stone production, because there is an energy barrier that must otherwise be overcome to produce calcium oxalate in urine. As calcium-oxalate supersaturation increases in a solution with little solid phase, calcium and oxalate ions in solution will collide at a higher frequency. At sufficient supersaturation, usually 10–12 times above the solubility limit in urine. collisions become so frequent that ion clusters of a sufficient size to be stable begin to form. Size is critical because the electrostatic forces that hold ions together increase with the total mass, whereas the escaping tendency of an ion from a cluster back into solution is related to the surface of the cluster. Homogeneous nucleation, the process of de-novo creation of calcium oxalate nuclei, therefore requires extreme supersaturation. By contrast, the growth of calcium oxalate crystals occurs at all levels of supersaturation, however slight. Therefore, heterogeneous nuclei of uric acid, by providing a preformed surface, could permit the formation of calcium oxalate in urine, even if urine supersaturation never exceeded the normal range of one to three times the solubility limit.

An alternative view is that crystals of uric acid or sodium hydrogen urate could adsorb and remove from solution normally occurring, protective inhibitors of crystallization. Such inhibitors, macromolecules, are responsible for the fact that homogeneous nucleation of calcium oxalate occurs at CPR values of 10–12 in urine and at only 8 in buffer (43), and that calcium oxalate crystal growth is greatly reduced by even dialyzed urine (44). We have been

Table 9. Geometrical correspondence between naturally occurring faces of uric acid and calcium oxalate crystals

	Face	Dimensions (Å)
Uric acid	100	6.21 × 7.40
Uric acid · 2H$_2$O	100	6.35 × 7.40
CaOx · H$_2$O[a]	001	6.28 × 14.57
CaOx · 2H$_2$O[b]	101	12.30 × 7.34
NaH urate · H$_2$O	100	3.567 × 8.693
	010	9.097 × 3.567

[a] Whewellite or calcium oxalate monohydrate.
[b] Weddellite or calcium oxalate dihydrate.
Used with permission from Coe (88).

unable to show any reduction of urinary crystal growth inhibition by hyperuricosuria (Figure 8). Others have (45). The differences probably are because uric acid crystals are favored by the spontaneous hyperuricosuria we study, whereas induced hyperuricosuria at a fixed urine pH near 6 favors sodium hydrogen urate crystal formation. Urate crystals appear to adsorb acidic macromolecules (46), whereas uric acid crystals may not.

Diet

Correction of dietary purine intake to achieve a normal level should reverse hyperuricosuria and raise urine pH in most patients, and is therefore the ideal approach. Unfortunately, we have had difficulty achieving a chronic reduction of intake and have not acquired a large body of long-term treatment data. Most patients resist change because they believe that an isocaloric exchange of breads, grains, and starches for meat will cause weight gain or will be less enjoyable.

Allopurinol

Because of this reluctance, we have a large experience with allopurinol. Given at a low dose of 100 mg twice daily, allopurinol will lower uric acid excretion to normal in virtually all patients. New stone production is greatly reduced. Smith et al. (47) have done a placebo-controlled trial of allopurinol in patients with calcium stones and mild hyperuricosuria (see Table 10); the drug was greatly-superior to placebo.

Diet versus drug

Certainly, diet is preferable if it can be used and should be offered in every case. If refused or if follow-up urine values show an inadequate fall in uric acid excretion, allopurinol is indicated. Sometimes people will modify their diets over several years of allopurinol treatment, so that the drug can be discontinued.

Complications

In our experience (Table 11), we have never encountered a dangerous complication of allopurinol. In four patients, a skin rash developed; one patient showed an increase in alkaline phosphatase that led to discontinuation of the drug; two patients developed cataracts, which were once thought to be a complication of allopurinol, and the drug was stopped; one patient discontinued the drug because of gastrointestinal distress. This is a total incidence of eight drug reactions in 1000.49 patient years of therapy.

Allopurinol and thiazide

By chance, patients can have hypercalciuria and hyperuricosuria, and require dual treatment. The results of treatment are excellent (see Table 3).

NO METABOLIC DISORDER

This group may exist mainly because of the arbitrary nature of the diagnostic criteria that we all use to define hypercalciuria and hyperuricosuria. The upper limits of normal are defined by the upper 5% of values encountered among people who are normal in that they have not formed stones. Such criteria may underestimate the risk of stones conferred by values of urine calcium of uric acid that are nevertheless not uncommon in normal people, just as blood pressure levels in many people who have had a stroke or heart attack are only moderately above the mean pressure among people who have not (48). However, in the absence of correct data to evaluate this notion, every clinician must expect to encounter people in whom no obvious metabolic disorder exists. We have reasoned that, since they cannot tolerate normal values of urine calcium and oxalate without forming stones, lower than normal values may be needed to protect them.

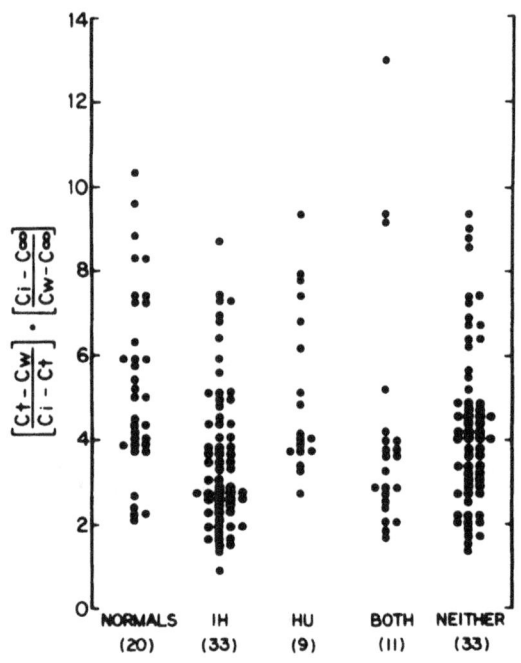

Figure 8. Inhibitor levels in each metabolic class. Numbers of subjects in parentheses. Used with permission from Coe FL, Margolis HC, Deutsch LH, Strauss AL: Urinary macromolecular crystal growth inhibitors in calcium nephrolithiasis. Miner Electrol Metab 3:268–275, 1980.

Diet

The Ettinger data (see Table 6) show a fall in stone production with diet (34). The effect is modest but the risk of treatment is low. This may be a sufficient approach for

Table 10. Effects of allopurinol on new stone production by recurrent calcium oxalate stone-formers with serum urate levels greater than 6 mg/100 ml[a]

Year of follow-up	Allopurinol-treated patients — New stones			Placebo-treated patients — New stones			χ^{2c}	p
	Yes	No	All[b]	Yes	No	All		
0.5	21	28	49	30	13	43	6.57	< 0.01
1	11	27	38	24	3	27	20.70	< 0.001
2	10	20	30	19	1	20	16.84	< 0.001
3	6	17	23	12	1	13	14.54	< 0.001
4	4	15	19	11	1	12	14.73	< 0.001
5	2	10	12	4	1	5	5.97	< 0.02

[a] Adapted from Smith (49). The numbers are patients who have or have not formed new stones at each follow-up interval.
[b] Includes patients remaining in the study; some were lost due to failure of treatment compliance, personal decisions to leave the study, or drug intolerance. Patients entered the study at different times and therefore had varying lengths of total follow-up.
[c] Calculated χ^2 for placebo- vs. allopurinol-treated patients; p values are for one degree of freedom.
Used with permission from Coe (3).

Table 11. Drug complications of allopurinol

Total number of patients	246
Total patient years on allopurinol	1000.49
Patients who discontinued because of side effects	8
Rash	4
Liver enzyme changes	1
Cataract	2
Abdominal pain[a]	1
Incidence of side effects/pt yr	0.008

[a] After each dose of allopurinol.

patients with uncomplicated stone disease of modest clinical significance.

Thiazide

We (Table 3) have observed a strong effect of thiazide. The treatment reduced new stone formation; 89% of patients were free of stones at 2.41 years of follow-up. Thiazide probably is the best treatment for patients who have had severe stone disease.

MEDULLARY SPONGE KIDNEY

This is an inherited disorder in which the distal ends of the terminal collecting ducts are dilated (49). On intravenous pyelogram, this "tubular extaria" causes rays of thin lines of contrast material to extend upward from the calyces into the renal papillae. Small stones form in the collecting ducts, leading to papillary nephrocalcinosis (50). Hypercalciuria is frequent in medullary sponge kidney (MSK) and has been viewed as a possible consequence of the tubule defect (11). Cases of primary hyperparathyroidism and MSK have been described in which renal hypercalciuria has been thought to lead to secondary parathyroid stimulation and, ultimately, an adenoma (51). Patients with MSK are said to be at abnormal risk of urinary infection.

Our observations contradict these ideas. We observed 111 cases of MSK among 1224 calcium stone-forming patients. Of these, two had hyperparathyroidism, a fraction equal to that of the whole series. A higher proportion of MSK patients than other stone-formers were women (Figure 9), and women with stones are hypercalciuric more frequently than men; this sex difference is what caused hypercalciuria to be unduly associated with MSK. When the sexes are compared separately, MSK and hypercalciuria are not associated (Figure 9). The same is true of infection; women have more than men, with or without MSK.

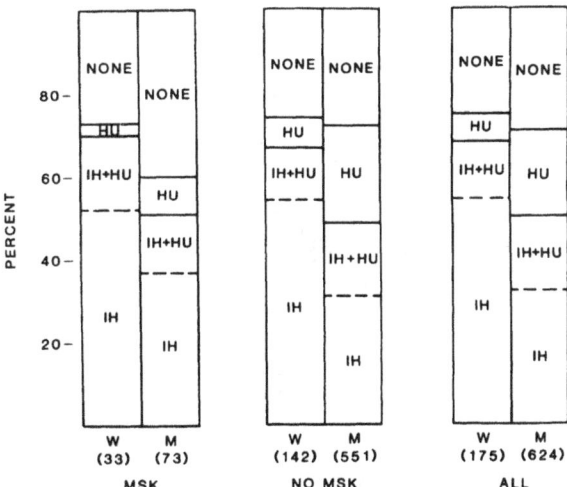

Figure 9. Percent of women (w) and men (m) calcium stone-formers with and without medullary sponge kidney (MSK). IH-idiopathic hypercalciuria; HU-hyperuricosuria. Used with permission from Parks JH, Coe FL, Strauss AL: Calcium nephrolithiasis in women.

The only really unusual characteristic of MSK is a high rate of stone production. Even so, the morbidity per stone was low, so the clinical severity of stone disease was not remarkably worse than usual.

Primary hyperparathyroidism

PATHOGENESIS OF STONES

Primary hyperparathyroidism results from either hyperplasia of several parathyroid glands or a single adenoma (52). Disease results from overproduction of parathyroid hormone (PTH). PTH causes the release of bone mineral (53). It stimulates the renal cell 1-α-25 (OH)D$_3$ hydroxylase to increase the production of 1-α-25 (OH)$_2$D$_3$ (1,25 D$_3$), which increases calcium absorption by the small intestine (51) and colon (52). It reduces renal tubule phosphorus reabsorption, causing hypophosphatemia, which may also stimulate 1,25 D$_3$ production, and increases renal tubule calcium reabsorption (54). The combination of increased intestinal calcium absorption and bone dissolution causes hypercalciuria, just as a high meat intake can cause hyperuricosuria; the increased tubule calcium reabsorption, however, permits the kidney to increase calcium excretion only at the expense of an increased filtered load of calcium, in other words, only when hypercalciuria occurs can the urine excretion rate match calcium entry into the plasma.

Stones occur mainly because of hypercalciuria. Urine supersaturation with respect to calcium oxalate and calcium phosphate are both increased (55). In our experience (56) with 56 cases, calcium oxalate stones were the most common.

CLINICAL CHARACTERISTICS

The diagnosis is based upon finding unexplained hypercalcemia. Among 1132 patients, we observed persistent hypercalcemia in 66 and all had primary hyperparathyroidism, except ten who had unexplained intermittent hypercalcemia (7), and a few others with hyperthyroidism, medica meatosum, sarcoidosis, and multiple myeloma (one each). The entire list of disorders that one should exclude is sarcoidosis, vitamin D intoxication, malignant tumor, Paget's disease, hyperthyroidism, and familial hypocalciuric hypercalcemia; the last, however, is not a cause of stones.

We found that hypercalcemia was often mild, despite severe hypercalciuria (Figure 10) in patients with stones. If slight hypercalcemia were overlooked, a diagnosis of idiopathic hypercalciuria would result. These results emphasize the importance of even slight hypercalcemia in patients with renal stones. They also illustrate how easy it is to find cases of "normocalcemic" primary hyperparathyroidism by overestimating the upper limit of normal for serum calcium.

Stone disease in our patients was not very different from that in idiopathic hypercalciuria (Table 12). Stones occurred at the same rate in patients with severe hypercalcemia as in the majority with very mild hypercalcemia. After parathyroidectomy, stones occurred in only one patient, who was still hypercalciuric. Hyperchloremic metabolic acidosis, azotemia, and hypertension were very rare.

TREATMENT

There are few alternatives to surgical parathyroidectomy. Since the abnormal glands result from benign neoplasia,

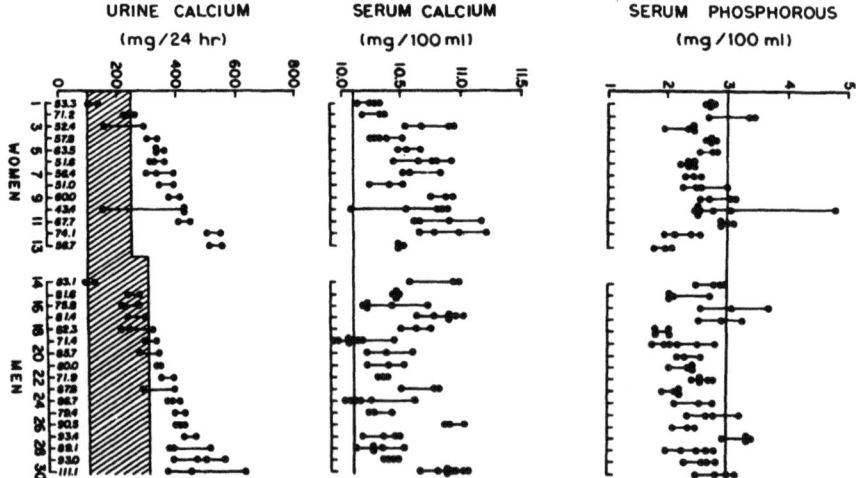

Figure 10. Selected characteristics of 30 patients with primary hyperparathyroidism and mild hypercalcemia. All values are shown for each patient. Body weight (kg) is shown above each number. The usual normal limits for calcium excretion (cross-hatched), upper limit for serum calcium (10.1 mg/dl), and lower limit for serum phosphorus (horizontal lines) are used.

Table 12. Morbidity in 48 patients with proven hyperparathyroidism

Morbid event	Mean serum calcium level < 11 mg/dl		Mean serum calcium level > 11 mg/dl[a]	
	Women (13)	Men (17)	Women (10)	Men (8)
Total stones before surgery	32	58	31	14
Pt yrs from first stone to treatment	66	121	46	13
Recurrent stones/patient[b]	29	34	46	47
Recurrent stones/100 pt years	1.46	2.41	2.87	1.0
Hospitalizations/100 stones	62	52	39	64
Cystoscopies/100 stones	12	10	16	14
Surgical procedures/100 stones	28[c]	17	19	36
Patient years since treatment	23	32	14	15
Stones formed since treatment	0[d]	0	0	1[e]
Azotemia[f]	0	1	2	0
Hypertension	0	2	1	0

[a] Five patients (four women) were hyperchloremic (> 108 mm/l), compared with none of the 30 patients with mild hypercalcemia (χ^2 = 8.3, p < .001); venous carbon dioxide content was low (< 24 mm/l) in two of these, both women.
[b] Calculation omits the first stone for each patient.
[c] The excess of surgical procedures among women is not significant (χ^2 = 2.44, p = NS).
[d] Combined predicted new stones (patient years since treatment times pretreatment stone-formation rate) for men (6.67) and women (10.88) = 17.6. This differs significantly from the total new stones formed (none; χ^2 = 17.6; p < .001).
[e] Predicted new stones for men and women, 13.3 (χ^2 = 11.4, p < .001); the single, new-stone occurred in the patient who remained hypercalciuric after curative parathyroidectomy. The method for predicting new stones is as in previous footnote.
[f] Serum creatinine level above 1.2 mg/dl (men), 1.0 mg/dl (women).
Used with permission from Parks et al. (56).

their removal is curative. A single enlarged gland is simply removed. If two or more are large, treatment requires removal of three or three and a half glands. Probably a better approach is to remove all cervical parathyroid tissue and transplant part of one gland to the forearm, preserving the rest by freezer banking (57). If the forearm tissue regrows or is too ample, more can be removed under local anesthesia, whereas a second neck exploration would otherwise result.

A rare patient cannot or will not be treated surgically. Medical treatment for them is very unsatisfactory. Oral phosphate has been used (58). A single recent study describes an oral disphosphonate as reducing urine calcium. The effects on stone formation are not established.

Hyperoxaluria

Urine oxalate concentration affects urine supersaturation with respect to calcium oxalate more than calcium concentration does, so hyperoxaluric state above 45 mg oxalate/24 hr easily cause calcium oxalate stones. Most hyperoxaluria is of enteric origin; rare patients have primary oxalate overproduction as a hereditary trait.

ENTERIC HYPEROXALURIA

Oxalate (COOH-COOH) is common in plants, and is present in almost all diets. It can be absorbed all along the intestine (60), but the exact mechanisms of transport are not yet known. Hyperoxaluria can occur when dietary oxalate is very high, or because of excessive oxalate absorption.

Dietary hyperoxaluria

Some foods (Table 13) are very high in oxalate, and excessive use can cause hyperoxaluria. This condition is diagnosed by history and is confirmed by reversal of hyperoxaluria upon a change in diet. Ascorbic acid can raise oxalate production and lead to hyperoxaluria. The magnitude of dietary hyperoxaluria is usually 50–60 g/24 hr, and it is below that from other causes.

Ileal resection or bypass

When the colon is intact and functioning, loss of ileum because of resection or bypass procedures that exclude ileum from the intestinal stream causes hyperoxaluria. The excessive oxalate is absorbed in the colon. One reason may be that fat malabsorption fosters chelation in the lumen of dietary calcium by unabsorbed lipids, so that the free ionic oxalate concentration can increase (61). Another is that bile salts and fatty acids may increase the permeability of colon mucosa to oxalate.

Hyperoxaluria from resection or bypass can be severe, up to 150–200 mg/day. Stones are very frequent, but the oxalate may also produce renal damage. In part, renal damage may reflect tubule plugging with masses of calcium oxalate crystals. It may also involve interstitial deposits of crystals that cause a tubulointerstitial nephropathy. These interstitial deposits may arise as calcium and oxalate are

Table 13. Foods with high oxalate content (0.1% or over)

Asparagus
Beets
Beet tops
Black tea
Brussel sprouts
Chenopodium
Chocolate
Cocoa
Dill
Dried figs
Gelatin (includes jello)
Ground pepper
Lambs quarters (vegetable)
Lime peel
Nuts, including peanuts
Ovaltine
Parsley
Poke (vegetable)
Poppy seeds
Purslane (vegetable)
Rhubarb
Sorrel
Soybeans
Spinach
Swiss chard (vegetable)
Unripe bananas
Wheatgerm

reabsorbed, together, from the tubule fluid or because plasma oxalate levels are increased by excessive intestinal oxalate absorption. The tubulointerstitial nephropathy can produce acute (62) or chronic (63) renal failure.

Treatment depends upon the cause. Bypass procedures should be reversed if hyperoxaluria is present. If reversal is impossible, or ileal resection is the basis for hyperoxaluria, medical treatment can be effective. A low-fat diet lessens oxaluria (64), perhaps because less fatty acids enter the colon lumen to bind calcium (65) or to increase colonic mucosal permeability (66). High calcium intake, of 1–4 g calcium daily, may lower oxalate absorption (67). The oral resin, cholestyramine, is very effective, as it chelates oxalate as well as bile salts (7). Cholestyramine is difficult to use because it may worsen diarrhea or cause abdominal pain in patients with bowel disease, and it chelates vitamin K so that prothrombin time may increase and bleeding may occur, as well as drugs such as digitalis glycosides. For these reasons, a low-fat diet and oral calcium are preferable first-line treatments.

Other disorders of the urine are frequent and should be treated. Urine volume may be low because of extrarenal (enteric) water losses; increased fluids, taken as small volumes of water at frequent intervals during the day, can increase urine flow. Enteric bicarbonate losses lower urine pH, raising the risk of uric acid crystallization, and urine citrate may be reduced because of the modest systemic acid load (68). Supplemental alkali is helpful. It can be given as the sodium or potassium salt of citric acid, depending upon the need for potassium replacement.

OVERPRODUCTION OF OXALATE

Primary hyperoxaluria

One will encounter only a rare example of hereditary hyperoxaluria, due to overproduction; we have observed three cases in 10 years, among 1285 patients with stones. Urine oxalate excretion is 100–300 mg/24 hr, and stones may begin even in childhood (69). There are two types: Type I is due to a deficiency of 2-oxoglutarate:glyoxylate carboligase; most patients have it. Type II is very rare and is the deficiency of D-glyceric dehydrogenase; l-glyceric aciduria accompanies oxaluria. Primary hyperoxaluria usually causes not only severe stone disease, but also chronic renal failure (7). The diagnosis is easily missed once renal failure is serious, an oxalate excretion falls to nearly normal. There is no ideal treatment. High-dose pyridoxine, 200–400 mg/day, may reduce oxalate excretion. The diet should be free of oxalate. Magnesium, as the oxide (450 mg/day) or hydroxide (210 mg/day), will increase urine magnesium and help to complex oxalate. Oral, inorganic neutral phosphate, 2 g/day, also seems to reduce stone formation (7).

Ascorbic acid

In some patients, very large amounts of ascorbic acid may increase oxalate production and excretion (70). Diagnosis is by history and treatment is straightforward.

Other hyperoxaluric states

Pyridoxine deficiency causes hyperoxaluria in animals (71); no human counterpart has been described. Ethylene glycol and the anesthetizing agent methoxyflurane both can cause hyperoxaluria from oxalate overproduction. Acute oxalate tubulointerstitial nephropathy occurs, but does not cause stone disease.

Renal tubular acidosis

Recurrent stones are a clinical problem only in hereditary (type I) distal renal tubular acidosis; the other varieties are not stone-forming conditions. The pathogenesis of renal tubular acidosis is detailed elsewhere in this book. We focus here upon the mechanism of stone production and treatment.

PATHOGENESIS OF STONES

The three components that lead to stones are alkaline urine, hypercalciuria, and low urine citrate level, and the stones are composed of calcium phosphate. In an alkaline urine, more phosphate exists in the form of PO_4^{3-} than at lower pH values, and the solubility for calcium phosphate salts is easily exceeded. Urine citrate normally complexes calcium and reduces supersaturation; the low citrate level in renal tubular acidosis raises free urine calcium ion concentration, as does hypercalciuria, thus forming stones.

Mechanism of hypercalciuria

Chronic metabolic acidosis, produced by subnormal renal acid excretion, causes hypercalciuria (72). The acidosis reduces fractional calcium absorption by the renal tubule (73). In normal people, intestinal calcium absorption may increase (74), but the net balance of calcium becomes negative as urine losses overbalance the net intestinal absorption. In balance studies, calcium balance in renal tubular acidosis is less positive than normal and frequently is negative (75). How acidosis reduces renal tubule calcium reabsorption is unknown. In the single micropuncture study available, the main site of reduced reabsorption appeared to be the cortical or medullary collecting tubules (76).

Reason for low urine citrate

Renal cells increase their oxidation rate for citric acid during metabolic acidosis (77). The result is less citrate in the urine. This cell response may arise at the mitochondrial level, as renal cortical cell mitochrondria increase their citrate oxidation rate when bathed in an acid medium.

NATURAL HISTORY AND TREATMENT OF STONES

Stones are very frequent in this disease. We observed 96 stones/100 patient years at risk in six patients (78) and very high recurrence rates among the other 12 patients who we found described in previous reports. Nephrocalcinosis is common. The volume of stones retained in the kidney or passed is very large compared with usual calcium oxalate stones. A main reason for the large amounts of stones is that both calcium and phosphate are present in urine at high concentrations (2–5 mM/l) compared with oxalate (100–50 μM/l), so that a considerable mass of crystals can accumulate.

Treatment with 2–4 mEq/kg body weight/day of alkali seems to be very effective. We observed a great reduction of stone formation and found a similar reduction in cases published by others. Alkali lowers urine calcium and increases urine citrate, removing 2 of the 3 factors favoring stones. The form of alkali is not important. Sodium bicarbonate tablet (two 10-grain tablets provide 14.5 mEq of base) and Shohl's solution (1 ml provides 1 mEq of base as citrate) are both inexpensive and practical.

Other causes of calcium stones

Calcium stones can occur in all of the hypercalciuric states. In particular, they occur in sarcoidosis, vitamin D excess, Cushing's syndrome, hyperparathyroidism, immobilization, and Paget's disease (3). Malignant tumors frequently cause hypercalciuria, but not stones. Perhaps the lack of stones reflects the relatively short duration of hypercalciuria. Each of the hypercalciuric states that causes stone is diagnosed by renal clinical means; they all require treatment, both because of stones and because of their general systemic effects.

URIC ACID STONES

Pathogenesis of stones

Uric acid stones are composed of uric acid itself, not one of its salts. One proton of uric acid is readily dissociable in normal urine (pK = 5.38), which has a pH near 6 (3). Urate, the product of the dissociation, forms salts with sodium, potassium, and ammonium (79) that can crystallize, but they rarely do in urine, even though normal urine is frequently as metastably supersaturated with respect to some of them, especially sodium hydrogen urate, as it is with respect to undissociated uric acid itself (80). Why the salts almost never form crystals in urine is not clear, but since undissociated uric acid forms the only important crystal found in uric acid stones, the entire discussion that follows will concern it, and we will refer to *undissociated uric acid* simply as *uric acid*. *Total urate* will mean uric acid and the dissociated acid.

Urine uric acid concentration (U) must be related to total urate excretion (T), urine volume (V), and urine pH by:

$$U = T \div [V \cdot X (1 + \Sigma)],$$

where Σ is 10 raised to the exponent (pH − pK) and pK for uric acid is 5.31. The equation derives simply from the acid-base dissociation equation and the fact that T must equal the sum of U and dissociated uric acid. When urine pH is equal to 5.31, Σ is 1 and U will be o.5 (T ÷ V); as pH falls, (1 + Σ) converges as 1 and U is closely approximated by (T ÷ V). In actual practice, urine pH is the main factor that can regulate whether uric acid will crystallize, because normal values for T are 400–800 mg/24 hr and urine volume is usually 1–2 l, whereas the solubility of uric acid is only 96 ± 2 mg/l. In other words, values for T ÷ V are 200–800 mg/l, but at normal values of urine pH, around 6–6.2, (1 + Σ) is large enough that U does not greatly exceed its solubility constant (41). Even so, hyperuricosuria and low urine flow rates can contribute to uric acid crystallization.

All forms of uric acid lithiasis are caused by these three factors. In the most common, spontaneous disease or stones associated with gout, low urine pH is the main factor; hyperuricosuria is usually a minor problem. Intestinal diseases, including inflammatory ileocolitis, ileostomy, and small bowel bypass, reduce urine flow as well as pH by causing extrarenal losses of water and bicarbonate. Very severe hyperuricosuric states, such as Lesch-Nyhan syndrome (79), some malignant neoplasms, and tumor-lysis sydrome (79), can cause uric acid stones, even without low urine pH. Whatever the underlying conditions may be, therapy always is based upon identifying the contributions of urine pH, urine volume, and total waste excretion to uric acid supersaturation, and making whatever changes are needed to bring the uric acid concentration below 96 mg/l.

To do this, we need a convenient nomogram, such as Figure 11 provides. In this case, U is shown as a function of (pH) for various values of (T ÷ V). The data for a given patient can be viewed on this figure, and one can estimate the changes in pH of (T ÷ V) needed to reduce U to below its solubility limit.

Clinical stones disease

Uric acid lithiasis is clinically more varied than its calcium counterpart. Stones may be small and discrete and, in passing, produce typical and individual bouts of colic, hematuria, and obstruction. They may silently grow to large proportions, filling the pelvis and calyces of a kidney, and are especially easy to assess because they are radiolucent. Uric acid may also form a crystalline sludge, which causes transient pain or hematuria, but passes as gravel or as a dispersed sand that escapes detection. The gravel may be red, because uric acid crystals absorb a red pigment, uricine (80), from urine. The native crystals are actually white. Finally, masses of crystals may plug the ureter entirely, causing anuria or unilateral obstruction. Such massive plugging may be painless.

Treatment

URINE PH

How far urine pH must rise can be estimated from Figure 11, but as a rule there is little advantage to raising pH above 6.5. For chronic treatment, oral citrate in the form of Shohl's solution or an equivalent is best. The usual starting doses are 1–2 mEq/kg/day of base. Alkalis must be given at least four times daily, the last dose being given at bedtime. Urine pH should be measured at intervals during the day as well as in the 24-hour urine, and the timing of treatment should be adjusted to achieve even control. If the pH falls overnight, as judged by the pH of the first voided morning urine, 250 mg acetozolamde may be added at bedtime.

Massive ureteral obstruction by uric acid requires special treatment. If there is urine flow, bicarbonate should be given intravenously, 6–8 mg/kg/day, along with acetozolamide, 250 mg, to achieve a maximally alkaline urine. This can rapidly dissolve the crystals. Given anuria, patency of the urinary tract must be achieved by retrograde ureteral catheterization; then use of alkali will be effective.

HYPERURICOSURIA

Unless it is very elevated, total urate excretion requires no individual treatment. If T exceeds 1000 mg/24 hr, however, a reduction can be useful in lowering U; the exact benefit in a given case can be estimated from Figure 11. If hyperuricosuria is due to excessive purine intake, as judged by history, the diet should be altered. In general, a purine excess is rarely present unless the dietary intake

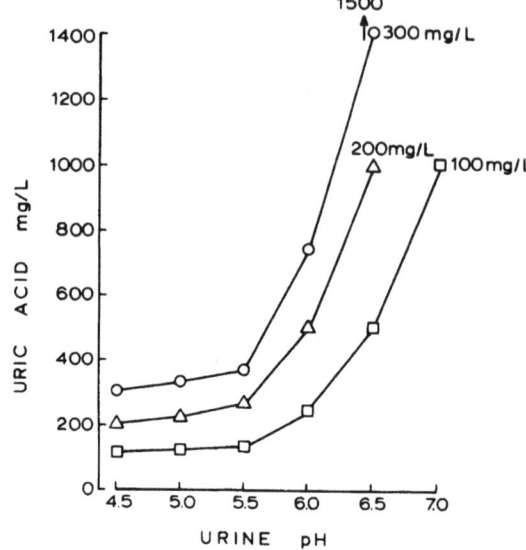

Figure 11. A nomogram for estimating the extent of urine saturation with respect to uric acid. Used with permission from Coe FL et al. (3).

of meat, fish, and poultry exceeds $\frac{3}{4}$ lb daily. When the diet cannot be altered, or when hyperuricosuria appears to be due to endogenous overproduction, allopurinol can be used. A reasonable starting dose is 100 mg twice daily. The treatment of massive hyperuricosuria due to tumor lysis or to Lesch-Nyhan syndrome always requires allopurinol, usually at a dose of 300–400 mg daily. One should emphasize that the treatment of hyperuricosuria is an adjunct to the increase of urine pH; uric acid stones are rarely due to hyperuricosuria and can usually be prevented by raising the urine pH.

INCREASED URINE VOLUME

The goal of treatment is to provide a reasonable volume, 1.5–2 l daily; this is sufficient to prevent uric acid stones if the urine pH is raised above 6. Usually, urine volume is not a major problem in pathogenesis or treatment. It is a problem, however, in patients with ileostomy, intestinal bypass, or inflammatory bowl disease, and these patients may be intolerant of a large fluid intake. For them, one may do best by recommending frequent, small amounts of water throughout the day.

Calcium-uric acid stones

About 10% of any large stone-forming group will manufacture either uric acid and calcium stones or mixed stones containing both crystals. The reason they do so is that their urine is excessively supersaturated with both calcium oxalate and uric acid (Figure 12). Treatment must be

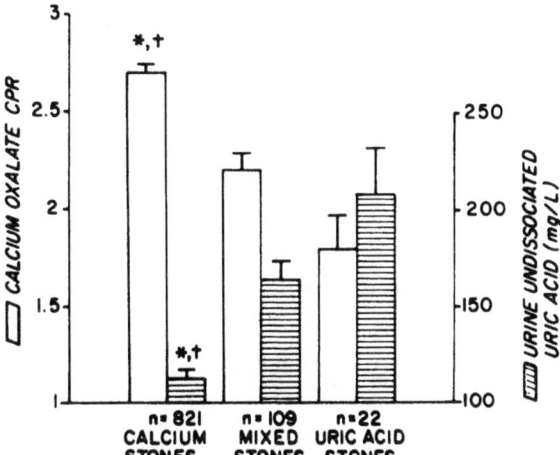

Figure 12. Calcium oxalate and undissociated uric acid supersaturation in stone-forming patients. Values for CPR (open bars) of above 1 indicate supersaturation (see text). The solubility of undissociated uric acid (hatched bars) in urine is 96 ± 3 mg/l (16), so supersaturation can be calculated by dividing the concentrations by 96. This figure presents all available measurements in patients with pure calcium, mixed calcium-uric acid, and pure uric acid stones. For CPR, there were values from 431, 56, and 9 patients for calcium, mixed, and uric-acid formers, respectively; corresponding numbers of patients providing undissociated uric acid values were 811, 106, and 22. All values are means ± SEM. Used with permission from Millman S, Strauss AL, Coe FL: Pathogenesis and clinical course of mixed calcium-uric acid nephrolithiasis.

directed against both types of stones; when this is done, the results of treatment are equal to those for either pure calcium or uric acid stone disease.

Dissolution of stones

Uric acid stones can, in practice, be dissolved simply by a sustained reduction of uric acid supersaturation. This is in contrast to calcium oxalate stones, in which dissolution is not usually practical. For this reason, large uric acid stones need not always be approached surgically. During dissolution, large stones may fragment, preceding typical attacks of renal colic.

CYSTINURIA

Cystinuria is an inherited disease in which dibasic amino-acid transport is reduced in both the renal tubule and in intestinal mucosal cells (81). The only known clinical consequence of the transport disorder is that cystine, which is insoluble, crystallizes in the urine to form stones. The stones themselves produce the usual problems of episodic colic attacks and may grow large enough to fill the renal pelvis, as uric acid stones frequently do. They are radiopaque because of the sulfur in cystine, but less so by far than the usual calcium stones. Cystinuria frequently produces stones during childhood.

The diagnosis of cystinuria requires either documented passage of a cystine stone or excretion of cystine in clinically significant amounts. Heterozygotes for cystinuria, who usually have an incomplete transport defect (82), may excrete as much as 80–150 mg/24 hr of cystine. Since urine can dissolve 300 mg/l, this virtually never results in stones. Homozygous cystinuria usually leads to the excretion of above 300 mg of cystine daily. The nitroprusside screening test, which is easily performed (83), detects both heterozygous and homozygous cystinuria; it is useful for excluding the disease, but by itself is not sufficient for the diagnosis of clinically significant cystinuria.

The goal of treatment is to reduce the urine cystine concentration to below 300 mg/l, and a high fluid intake is the best approach to initiating treatment. The volume of urine required can be estimated only from an accurate measurement of daily cystine excretion. Water must be ingested at regular intervals throughout the day and also at night, as cystine excretion is constant. In general, patients must awaken to empty their bladder at least once nightly.

Cystine, being an acid, is more soluble as urine pH increases, but the effects of pH begin only above 7. Supplemental alkali, as sodium bicarbonate or sodium citrate, 2–4 mEq/kg/24 hr, can be given in four divided doses daily to raise the urine pH. The effects of alkali are minor compared with water, so this represents adjunctive treatment, to be used if water alone is not sufficient in the volumes that a particular patient is willing to ingest.

D-penicillamine is effective, but should always be reserved for patients whose stone disease persists despite water and alkali. Allergic reactions to D-penicillamine, which include skin rash, fever, and even the nephrotic syndrome, occur eventually in over half of the patients and prevent further use of the agent. This drug acts by forcing a soluble complex with cysteine and will prevent stones in those patients who can use it.

STRUVITE STONES

The triple salt, magnesium-ammonium phosphate, or struvite, occurs in human stones only because of infection of the urinary tract with bacteria that possess the enzyme urease. *Proteus*, *Klebsiella*, *Pseudomonas*, and *Aerobacter* species are usually the cause; *E. coli* never possess the enzymes (84). Urease decomposes urea to ammonia, which hydrolyzes by taking up a proton from water to form ammonium ions and in the process greatly increases the pH of the urine. In alkaline urine, phosphate readily lowers its protons to form PO_4^{3-}, which crystallizes with NH_4^+ and Mg^{2+} to form struvite. An alkaline urine with a high ammonium concentration is never produced by the kidney, because renal excretion of ammonium depends upon an acid pH in tubular fluid, so struvite stones cannot be formed without infection.

Clinically, struvite stones differ from the rest in that staghorn calculi are usual, whereas the passage of small stones is uncommon. On the other hand, struvite stones frequently occur because of infection caused by urologic instrumentation or surgery in patients who have had repeated episodes of calcium stones due to metabolic causes, so there is often a history of passing small stones. Even though calcium stones are a frequent antecedent, and such stones occur in men more often than women, struvite stones occur mostly in women. This illustrates the greater vulnerability of women to persistent urinary infection.

Diagnosis is best made by documenting struvite stones by crystallographic analysis. It is suspected from the radiographic appearance of the stones, which are large, branched, and variably radiodense from place to place. Urine culture may not reveal the organisms, but culture of the stones themselves virtually always does (85).

The problem of treating a patient who has a large struvite stone in one or both kidneys includes the timing of surgery and the selection of antimicrobial agents. Surgery should be considered if there is significant intrarenal obstruction manifested by dilated calyces, recurrent systemic infection — as opposed to simple chronic bacteriuria (which is frequently present), or significant pain. Some patients, perhaps because of infection that is otherwise silent, lose weight or are fatigued, and improve with surgery. Naturally, serious ureteropelvic obstruction requires surgical treatment.

Antimicrobial agents vary depending upon the setting. If stones are present, one can hope only to reduce colony counts, and therefore the rate of stone growth (86); chronic penicillin is usually reasonable for this purpose. After stone removal, one can hope to eradicate the infection using bacterocidal drugs chosen on the basis of culture. The newest agent, acetohydroxamic acid (87), inhibits bacterial urease; however, it is still experimental and is not generally available.

The outcome of treatment is disappointing. Stone removal is followed by recurrence in over half of patients by 5 years (87). Frequently, retained fragments are found immediately after surgery. After several recurrences, the affected kidney usually must be removed, because recurrent symptomatic stones cannot be tolerated, yet perinephric scarring makes pyelolithotomy impractical. The frequency of recurrence and difficulties of subsequent surgery make the decision about surgery difficult, in that one should wait until there is a clear need, yet not so long that renal damage is severe or the quality of a patient's life has been excessively compromised. There is no substitute in this situation for clinical judgement.

Because treatment is unsatisfactory, prevention is especially important. Infection with a urease-possessing bacteria is serious in anyone, but particularly in a stone-forming patient who may have stones in the kidneys that can become infected and be a nidus for a large struvite stone. Such infections should be cured before retained infected stones occur by using a full course of a bacterocidal agent, even if hospitalization is required. Follow-up, with repeated treatment if necessary, is essential.

REFERENCES

1. Coe FL: Renal colic and flank pain. In SG Massry, RJ Glassock eds, *Textbook of Nephrology*. Elsevier, New York, 1980.
2. Bretland PM: *Acute Ureteric Obstruction*. Appleton-Century-Crofts, London, 1972.
3. Coe FL: *Nephrolithiasis: Pathogenesis and Treatment*. Year Book Medical, Chicago, 1978.
4. Greene ML, Fujimoto WY, Seegmiller JE: Urinary xanthine stone: A rare complication of allopurinol therapy. *N Engl J Med* 280:426, 1969.
5. Coe FL: Calcium-uric acid nephrolithiasis. *Arch Intern Med* 138:1090, 1978.
6. Schneider AF, Reaven EP, Reaven GA: A comparison of renal calcification produced by parathyroid extract or calcium gluconate. *Endocrinology* 67:733–743, 1960.
7. Smith LH Jr: Enteric hyperoxaluria and other hyperoxaluria states. In: FL Coe, BM Brenner, JM Stein, eds, *Nephrolithiasis*. Churchill-Livingstone, New York, 1980.
8. Hare WSC, Poynter JD: The radiology of renal papillary necrosis as seen in analgesic nephropathy. *Clin Radiol* 25:423–428, 1974.
9. Roylance J, Penry, JB, Rhys-Davies E, Roberts M: The radiology of tuberculosis of the urinary tract. *Clin Radiol* 21:163–172, 1970.
10. Friedenberg RM: Tuberculosis of the genito urinary system. *Semin Roentgenol* 6:310–318, 1971.
11. Yendt ER, Jarzylo S, Finnis WA, et al.: Medullary sponge kidney (tubular ectasia) in calcium urolithiasis. Presented at the Fourth International Symposium on Urolithiasis Research, *Williamsburg, Va*, June 22–26, 1980.
12. Blacklock NJ: The pattern of urolithiasis in the Royal Navy. In: A Hodgkinson, BEC Nordin, eds, *Renal Stone Research Symposium*, JA Churchill, London, pp 33–47, 1968.
13. Yu TF, Gutman AB: Uric acid nephrolithiasis in gout: Predisposing factors. *Ann Intern Med* 67:1133, 1967.
14. Marshall V, White RH, Chaput de Saintonge M, et al.: The natural history of renal and ureteric calculi. *Br J Urol* 47:112–124, 1975.
15. Coe FL, Keck J, Norton E: The natural history of calcium urolithiasis. *JAMA* 238:1519–1523, 1977.
16. Williams RE: Long-term survey of 538 patients with upper urinary stone. *Br J Urol* 35:416–437, 1963.
17. Coe FL, Parks JH, Strauss A: Accelerated nephrolithiasis. *JAMA* 244:809–810, 1980.
18. Coe FL, Parks JH, Moore E: Familial idiopathic hypercalciuria. *N Engl J Med* 300:337–340, 1979.
19. Hamed IA, Czerwinski AW, Coats B, Kaufman C, Altmiller DH: Familial absorptive hypercalciuria and renal tubular acidosis. *Am J Med* 300:337, 1979.
20. Meches K, Szelid ZS: Autosomal dominant inheritance of hypercalciuria. *Eur J Pediatr* 133:239–242, 1980.
21. Moore E, Coe FL, McMann B, Favus M: Idiopathic hypercalciuria in children: Prevalence and metabolic characteristics. *J Pediatr* 92:906–910, 1978.
22. Favus MJ, Coe FL: Evidence for spontaneous hypercalciuria in the rat. *Miner Electrolyte Metab* 2:150–154, 1979.
23. Peacock M, Nordin BEC: Tubular reabsorption of calcium in normal and hypercalciuric subjects. *J Clin Pathol* 21:353, 1968.
24. Shen FH, Baylink DJ, Nielsen RL, Sherrard DJ, Ivey JL, Haussler MR: Increased serum 1,25 dihydroxyvitamin D in idiopathic hypercalciuria. *J Lab Clin Med* 90:955, 1977.
25. Haussler MR, Baylink DJ, Hughes MR, Brumbough PF,

Wergedal JF, Shen FH, Nielsen RL, Counts SJ, Bursac KM, McCain TA: The assay of 1,25-dihydroxyvitamin D_3: Physiologic and pathologic modulation of circulating hormone levels. *Clin Endocrinol* 5:151s, 1976.
26. Goldberg M, Azuz ZS, Goldfarb S: Renal handling of phosphate, calcium and magnesium. In: BM Brenner, FC Rector Jr, eds, *The Kidney*, vol. 1. WB Saunders, Philadelphia, pp 344-390, 1976.
27. Pak CYC, Galosy RA: Fasting urinary calcium and adenosine 3',5'-monophosphate: A discriminant analysis for the identification of renal and absorptive hypercalciuria. *J Clin Endocrinol Metab* 48:260, 1979.
28. Quamme GA, Wong NLM, Sutton RAL, Dirks JH: Interrelationship of chlorothiazide and parathyroid hormone: A micropuncture study. *Am J Physiol* 229:200, 1975.
29. Costanzo LS, Windhager EE: Calcium and sodium transport by the distal convoluted tubule of the rat. *Am J Physiol* 235: F492, 1978.
30. Pak CYC, Delea CS, Bartter FC: Successful treatment of recurrent nephrolithiasis (calcium stones) with cellulose phosphate. *N Engl J Med* 190:175, 1974.
31. Sutton RAL, Walker VR: Responses to hydrochlorothiazide and acetazolamide in patients with calcium stones: Evidence suggesting a defect in renal tubular function. *N Engl J Med* 302:709-713, 1980.
32. Coe FL, Favus MJ, Crockett T, Strauss AL, Parks JH, Porat A, Sen P, Gantt CL, Sherwood LM: Effects of low-calcium diet on urine calcium excretion, parathyroid function and serum 1,25(OH)$_2$D$_3$ level in patients with idiopathic hypercalciuria and normal subjects. *Am J Med*, 1982.
33. Weber DV, Coe FL, Parks JH, Dun MSL, Tembe V: Urinary saturation measurements in calcium nephrolithiasis. *Ann Intern Med* 90:180, 1979.
34. Ettinger B: Recurrence of nephrolithiasis: A six-year prospective study. *Am J Med* 67:245, 1979.
35. Yendt ET, Cohanim M: Prevention of calcium stones with thiazides. *Kidney Int* 13:397, 1978.
36. Pak CYC, Peters P, Hurt G, Kadesky M, Fine M, et al.: Is selective therapy of recurrent nephrolithiasis possible? *Am J Med* 71:615-622, 1981.
37. Maschio G, Tessitore N, D'Angelo A, Fabris A, Pagano F, et al.: Prevention of calcium nephrolithiasis with low dose thiazide, amiloride and allopurinol. *Am J Med* 71:623-626, 1981.
38. Pak CYC, Kaplan R, Bone H, Townsend J, Waters O: A simple test for the diagnosis of absorptive, resorptive and renal hypercalciuria. *N Engl J Med* 292:497-500, 1975.
39. Gutman AB: Uric acid nephrolithiasis. *Am J Med* 45:756, 1968.
40. Coe FL: Hyperuricosuric calcium oxalate nephrolithiasis. *Kidney Int* 13:418, 1978.
41. Coe FL, Strauss AL, Tembe V, Dun SL: Uric acid saturation in calcium nephrolithiasis. *Kidney Int* 17:662-668, 1980.
42. Mandel NS, Mandel GS: Epitaxis between stone forming crystals at the atomic level. In: FL Coe, BM Brenner, JH Stein, eds, *Contemporary Issues in Nephrology: Nephrolithiasis*. Churchill Livingstone, New York, 1980.
43. Pak CYC, Holt K: Nucleation and growth of brushite and calcium oxalate in urine of stone formers. *Metabolism* 25: 665-673, 1976.
44. Ito H, Coe FL: Acidic peptide and polyribonucleotide crystal growth inhibitors in human urine. *Am J Physiol* 233:F455, 1978.
45. Robertson WG, Knowles F, Peacock M: Urinary acid mucopolysaccharide inhibitors of calcium oxalate crystallization. In R Fleisch, WG Robertson, LH Smith, W Vahlensieck, eds, *Urolithiasis Research*. Plenum Press, London, 19
46. Pak CYC, Barella PE, Holt K, et al.: Effect of oral purine load and allopurinol on the crystallization of calcium salts in the urine of patients with hyperuricosuric calcium urolithiasis. *Am J Med* 65:593, 1978.
47. Smith MJV: Placebo vs. allopurinol for renal calculi. *J Urol* 117:690, 1977.
48. Freis ED: Age, race, sex and other indices of risk in hypertension. *Am J Med* 55:275-280, 1973.
49. Kuiper JJ: Medullary sponge kidney. In: KD Gardner Jr, ed, *Cystic Diseases of the Kidney*. John Wiley, New York, 1976.
50. Coe FL: The clinical and laboratory assessment of the patient with renal disease. In: BM Brenner, FC Rector Jr, eds, *The Kidney*, Vol 2. WB Saunders, Philadelphia, pp 765-805, 1976.
51. Stella FJ, Massry SG, Kleeman CR: Medullary sponge kidney associated with parathyroid adenoma. *Nephron* 10:322-336, 1973.
52. Golden A and Canary JJ: The parathyroid gland. In: JMB Bloodworth Jr, ed, *Endocrine Pathology*. Williams and Wilkins Baltimore, p 181, 1968.
53. Parfitt AM: PTH and osteoblasts, the relationship between bone turnover and bone loss, and the state of the bones in primary hyperparathyroidism. *Metabolism* 25:1033-1061, 1976.
54. Agus ZS, Chiu PJS, Goldberg, M: Regulation of urinary calcium excretion in the rat. *Am J Physiol* 232:F454-460, 1977.
55. Favus MJ, Kathpalia SC, Coe FL, Mond A: Calcium active transport by rat descending colon: Response to dietary calcium restriction and 1,25(OH)$_2$D$_3$. *Am J Physiol* 238:675-678, 1980.
56. Parks JH, Coe FL, Favus MJ: Hyperparathyroidism in nephrolithiasis. *Arch Intern Med* 140:1479-1481, 1981.
57. Coe FL, Favus MJ, Kathpalia SC, Jao W, Sherwood LM: Calcium and phosphorus disorders of malignant origin. In: R Reisselbach, ed, *Cancer and the Kidney*. WB Saunders, Philadelphia, 1981.
58. Broadus AE, Horst RL, Lang R, Rasmussen IH: Distinct pathophysiologic subgroups in primary hyperparathyroidism: Role of serum 1,25(OH)$_2$D$_2$ and response to phosphorus therapy. *Clin Res* 27:363A, 1979.
59. Binder HJ: Intestinal oxalate absorption. *Gastroenterology* 67:441, 1974.
60. Hofmann AF, Thomas PJ, Smith LH, McCall JT: Pathogenesis of secondary hyperoxaluria in patients with ileal resection and diarrhea. *Gastroenterology* 58:960, 1970.
61. Vainder M and Kelly J: Renal tubular dysfunction secondary to jejunoileal bypass. *JAMA* 235:1257, 1976.
62. Cryer PE, Garber AJ, Hoffstein P, Lucas XX, Wise L: Renal failure after small intestinal bypass for obesity. *Arch Intern Med* 135:1610, 1975.
63. Anderson K, Jagenburg R: Fat reduced diet in the treatment of hyperoxaluria in patients with ileopathy. *Gut* 15:360, 1974.
64. Dobbins JW, Binder HJ: Effects of bile salts and fatty acids on the colonic absorption of oxalate. *Gastroenterology* 70: 1896, 1976.
65. Chadwick VS, Phillips JF, Hofmann AF: Measurements of intestinal permeability using low molecular weight polyethylene glycols (PEG 400). *Gastroenterology* 73:247, 1977.
66. Hofman AF, Poley JR: Role of bile acid malabsorption in pathogenesis of diarrhea and steatorrhea in patients with ileal resection: I. Response to cholestyramine or replacement of dietary long chain triglycerides by medium chain triglyceride.

Gastroenterology 62:918, 1972.
67. Elliot JS, Soles WP: Excretion of calcium and citric acid in patients with small bowel disease. *J Urol* 111:810, 1974.
68. Williams HE, Smith LH Jr: Primary hyperoxaluria. In: JP Stanbury, B Wyngaarden, DS Fredrikson, eds, *The Metabolic Basis of Inherited Disease*. McGraw-Hill, New York, p 196, 1972.
69. Hockaday TDR, Clayton JE, Frederick Ew, Smith LH Jr: Primary hyperoxaluria. *Medicine* 43:315, 1964.
70. Hagler L, Herman RH: Oxalate metabolism. *Am J Clin Nutr* 26:758, 882, 1006, 1242, 1973.
71. Gershoff SN, Faragella FF: Endogenous oxalate synthesis and glycine, serine, deoxypridoxine interrelationships in vitamin B_6-deficient rats. *J Biol Chem* 234:2391, 1959.
72. Coe FL, Firpo JJ Jr: Evidence for mild reversible hypoerparathyroidism in distal renal tubular acidosis. *Arch Intern Med* 135:1485–1488, 1975.
73. Lemann J Jr, Litzow JR, Lennon EJ: Studies of the mechanism by which chronic metabolic acidosis augments urinary calcium excretion in man. *J Clin Invest* 46:1318, 1967.
74. Lemann J Jr, Litzow JR, Lennon EJ: The effect of chronic acid loads in normal man: Further evidence for the participation of bone mineral in the defense against chronic metabolic acidosis. *J Clin Invest* 45:1608, 1966.
75. Greenberg AJ, McNamara H, McCrory WW: Metabolic balance studies in primary renal tubular acidosis: Effects of acidosis on external calcium and phosphorus balances. *J Pediatr* 69:610, 1966.
76. Sutton RAL, Wong NLM, Dirks JH: Effects of metabolic acidosis and alkalosis on sodium and calcium transport in the dog kidney. *Kidney Int* 15:520–533, 1979.
77. Simpson DP: Regulation of renal citrate metabolism by bicarbonate ion and pH: Observations in tissue slices and mitochondria. *J Clin Invest* 46:225, 1967.
78. Coe FL, Parks JH: Stone disease in hereditary renal tubular acidosis. *Ann Intern Med* 93:60–61, 1980.
79. Holmes EW Jr: Uric acid nephrolithiasis. In: FL Coe, BM Brenner, JH Stein, eds, *Contemporary Issues in Nephrology: Nephrolithiasis*, Vol 5, Churchill Livingstone, New York, 1980.
80. Pinto B, Rocha E, Ruiz-Marcellan FJ: Isolation and characterization of uricine from uric acid stones. *Kidney Int* 10:437, 1976.
81. Crawhall JC, Purkiss P, Watts RWE, Young EP: The excretion of amino acids by cystinuric patients and their relatives. *Ann Human Genet* 33:149, 1969.
82. Resnick MJ, Goodman HO, Boyce WH: Heterozygous cystinuria and calcium oxalate urolithiasis. *J Urol* 122:52, 1979.
83. Hambraeus L: Comparative studies of the value of two cyanide-nitroprusside methods in the diagnosis of cystinuria. *Scand J Lab Clin Invest* 15:657, 1963.
84. Chute R, Suby HI: Prevalence and importance of urea-splitting bacterial infections of the urinary tract in the formation of calculi. *J Urol* 44:590, 1943.
85. Griffith DB, Bruce RR, Fishbein WN: Infection (urease)-induced stones. In: FL Coe, BM Brenner, JH Stein, eds, *Nephrolithiasis*, Vol 5, Churchill Livingstone, New York, 1980.
86. Griffith DB: Struvite stones. *Kidney Int* 13:372, 1975.
87. Griffith DB, Gibson JR, Clinton CW, Musher DM: Acetohydroxamic acid: Clinial studies of a urease inhibitor in patients with staghorn renal calculi. *J Urol* 119:9, 1978.

CHAPTER 9

Metabolic Alkalosis

SANDRA SABATINI & NEIL A. KURTZMAN

INTRODUCTION

Metabolic alkalosis is a primary pathophysiologic event characterized by a gain of bicarbonate or a loss of nonvolatile acid from extracellular fluid. More simply put, it is a primary increase in plasma bicarbonate concentration (normal plasma HCO_3 = 24 mEq/l). Like all acid-base disturbances, metabolic alkalosis commonly complicates the course of patients with preexisting disorders. An understanding of its pathophysiology makes the diagnosis and management of metabolic alkalosis a relatively simple process.

In this chapter we discuss the basic mechanisms of hydrogen ion secretion and bicarbonate reabsorption by the kidney; a summary of the factors modulating these processes in the proximal tubule and the distal nephron are then considered. The generation and maintenance of metabolic alkalosis are reviewed; this is followed by a summary of the specific pathophysiologic states associated with this acid-base disorder. Finally, we conclude with a discussion of therapy.

RENAL SECRETION OF HYDROGEN

Reabsorption of bicarbonate (bicarbonate reclamation)

Most available evidence suggests that bicarbonate reabsorption in the proximal tubule is mediated by a sodium/hydrogen antiporter localized in the brush border membrane (1–6). Recent evidence, however, now documents the presence of a proton-translocating ATPase (H^+-ATPase), although its physiologic role is as yet unknown (6–10). The proximal tubule probably does not reabsorb bicarbonate as such, although speculation concerning this mechanism persists in the literature.

The salient features of bicarbonate reabsorption in the proximal tubule are shown in Figure 1. The hydrogen ion probably results from the dissociation of carbonic acid ($H_2CO_3 \rightleftharpoons H^+ + HCO_3$), which has been formed by the hydration of carbon dioxide and water, the end products of intermediary metabolism ($CO_2 + H_2O \rightleftharpoons H_2CO_3$).* The proton is then secreted into the tubular lumen in exchange for sodium, maintaining electrical neutrality, where it reacts with the filtered bicarbonate to form carbonic acid. Carbonic acid, in turn, dissociates to carbon dioxide and water. Carbonic anhydrase, an enzyme found on the luminal surface of proximal tubular cells (11, 12), catalyzes the dissociation to CO_2 and H_2O. Carbon dioxide diffuses into the renal proximal tubular cell, beginning the cycle again. There is some evidence that carbonic acid may enter the cell directly (13, 14). The bicarbonate formed secondary to proton secretion is passively returned to the blood, either by neutral chloride exchange or by conductive bicarbonate-facilitated diffusion (1).

The source of energy for proton secretion by the proximal tubule appears to be the sodium-potassium ATPase (Na-K-ATPase), an enzyme found in abundance on the basolateral surface of proximal tubular cells (10, 15–17).

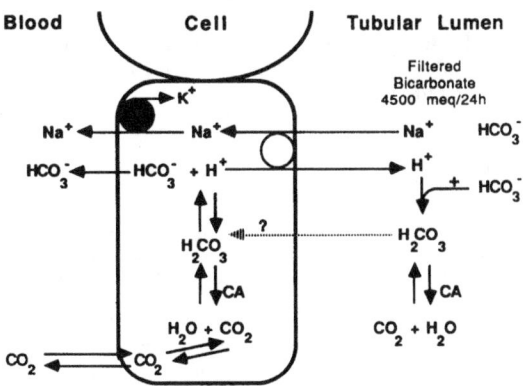

Figure 1. Hydrogen ion secretion by the proximal tubule. Na/H antiporter (○) accounts for ≃85% of proximal tubule acidification. Not shown is electrogenic hydrogen ion secretion (H-ATPase), probably localized at the tubular lumen. CA = carbonic anhydrase; dark circle (●) = active transport.

---

*Alternatively: $H_2O \rightarrow H^+ + OH^-$, and $OH^- + CO_2 \rightarrow HCO_3^-$.

The enzyme generates the electrochemical gradient for luminal sodium entry by maintaining a low intracellular sodium ($\simeq 12$ mEq/l). Basolateral sodium exit, mediated by Na-K-ATPase activity, thus supplies the energy for luminal Na/H exchange (secondary active transport). Electrogenic proton secretion (H^+-ATPase), to the extent that it occurs in the proximal tubule, depends upon intracellular ATP and in some species also depends upon chloride (8).

The proximal tubule generates a small, lumen positive voltage ($\simeq +3$ mV). It is a "leaky" epithelium with a low electrical resistance. The proximal tubule generates a relatively small pH gradient; the pH at the end of the proximal tubule is only about 6.8 (the glomerular ultrafiltrate pH is 7.4). Because of these properties, this segment of the nephron is a high capacitance system capable of reabsorbing about 90% of all the bicarbonate present in the ultrafiltrate, $\simeq 4500$ mEq HCO_3/day. Bicarbonate reabsorption by the proximal tubule (i.e., Na/H exchange) is affected by many factors (see Table 1) each of which are discussed in the subsequent section.

Factors affecting bicarbonate reabsorption

EXTRACELLULAR VOLUME

The state of the extracellular volume is one of the major factors controlling bicarbonate reabsorption (18, 19). When extracellular volume is expanded, proximal sodium reabsorption falls, presumably as a consequence of decreased activity in the Na/H antiporter. Bicarbonate reabsorption thus decreases secondarily. Conversely, when the extracellular volume is contracted, sodium reabsorption is enhanced, as is that of bicarbonate. Bicarbonate reabsorption in the normal human is essentially complete until the plasma level reaches a value of $\simeq 26$ mEq/l (the bicarbonate T_m) (20, 21). In volume-contracted subjects, however, no T_m is seen and this observation required modification of the T_m concept. As now used, HCO_3 T_m defines the maximal rate of bicarbonate reabsorption observed under the particular set of circumstances in which it is measured, not the maximal rate possible. For example, HCO_3 T_m is higher in normal subjects than it is in volume-expanded subjects.

Chloride deficiency stimulates bicarbonate reabsorption

Table 1. Factors influencing bicarbonate reabsorption

Increased HCO_3 reabsorption	Decreased HCO_3 reabsorption
Volume contraction	Volume expansion
Potassium depletion	Potassium excess
Hypercapnia ($\uparrow$ arterial p_{CO_2})	Hypocapnia ($\downarrow$ arterial p_{CO_2})
Glucose	—
Hypoparathyroidism	Hyperparathyroidism
Hypercalcemia	Hypocalcemia
—	Phosphate depletion
Vitamin D	Vitamin-D deficiency
—	Acetazolamide

(22, 23). Since chloride depletion almost invariably means salt depletion, and consequently contraction of the extracellular volume, it is likely that chloride depletion enhances bicarbonate reabsorption through contraction of the extracellular volume. There is no evidence that chloride per se affects the Na/H antiporter, but it does appear to alter H^+-ATPase activity in some species (8).

GLOMERULAR FILTRATION RATE AND THE FILTERED LOAD OF BICARBONATE

The classic studies of Pitts and colleagues (20, 21) first demonstrated that bicarbonate reabsorption varied in proportion with changes in glomerular filtration rate. They also noted that at low levels of filtered load, bicarbonate reabsorption by the kidney was complete and no bicarbonate appeared in the urine. When the plasma bicarbonate reached 26–28 mEq/l, however, there was no further increase in the bicarbonate reabsorptive rate and bicarbonate began to appear in the urine. While they called this the tubular maximum (T_m) for bicarbonate, it was not a true T_m, because it had to be expressed as reabsorption per GFR, rather than reabsorption per unit time.

More recently several investigators have argued that the filtered load of bicarbonate is a major determinant of bicarbonate reabsorption. Using clearance techniques, Langberg et al. (24) demonstrated that in dogs, bicarbonate reabsorption is a function both of the filtered bicarbonate and arterial pH and that there was no evidence for special effects of the plasma bicarbonate, p_{CO_2}, or glomerular filtration rate. Using micropuncture techniques, Cogan et al. (25) demonstrated a tight relationship in the superficial proximal tubule between bicarbonate reabsorption and the filtered load in both normal and acidotic rats. Extracellular volume expansion did not inhibit proximal bicarbonate reabsorption independent of filtered load. Substantiating these findings is the study by Berry and Cogan (26) in which isolated perfused proximal tubules from rabbits, subjected to in vitro volume expansion (induced by changing luminal protein concentration), showed no change in bicarbonate reabsorption while salt transport was significantly reduced. This observation is in sharp contrast to the earlier in vivo work of Cohen (27) demonstrating that there was a correction of the metabolic alkalosis during volume expansion when the glomerular filtration rate (and hence, the filtered load of bicarbonate) was maintained constant by aortic constriction. The differences in these contrasting data await elucidation.

The resolution of these conflicting studies has major application to our understanding of the forces that maintain clinical metabolic alkalosis. If the filtered load of bicarbonate is the main determinant of its excretory rate, then subjects with persistent metabolic alkalosis must have a decline in the filtered load of bicarbonate, which can only result from a decrease in the glomerular filtration rate, since the plasma bicarbonate concentration is high. Correction of metabolic alkalosis would therefore be seen as the result of maneuvers that increase the filtered load of bicarbonate, resulting in increased urinary excretion of bicarbonate. If the study of Cohen (27) bears more keenly on clinical metabolic alkalosis, then attention to factors other than the filtered load should be more important in its maintenance (e.g., changes in volume, potassium homeostasis, etc).

PLASMA p_{CO_2}, BLOOD pH, AND CELL pH

An acute fall in p_{CO_2} depresses proximal bicarbonate reabsorption, and conversely a rise in plasma p_{CO_2} enhances bicarbonate reabsorption (28). The mechanism for this effect may be due to an alteration of intracellular pH, a change in renal hemodynamics, or both.

To examine the first issue, Langberg and coworkers (24) found that the effect of altering p_{CO_2} on bicarbonate reabsorption correlated better with a change in extracellular pH than with the change in arterial p_{CO_2}. When the p_{CO_2} was changed in proportion to the plasma bicarbonate concentration (such that the arterial pH remained constant), bicarbonate reabsorption did not change as compared to control. On the other hand, when arterial pH was allowed to change, bicarbonate reabsorption was increased when pH fell and decreased when it rose (24). This study concluded that extracellular pH was a major determinant of proximal bicarbonate reabsorption. Another explanation, however, is possible, and that is that changes of the extracellular pH merely reflect changes in the cell pH, and it is the cell pH that is the critical determinant of changes in bicarbonate reabsorption. Changing pH by altering the plasma p_{CO_2} results in a rapid change of the cell pH (as opposed to changing the extracellular bicarbonate concentration) owing to the easy diffusibility of carbon dioxide across cell membranes. For example, an increase in p_{CO_2} decreases cell pH; this decrease would enhance bicarbonate reabsorption by stimulating the Na/H antiporter of the brush border membrane.

The hemodynamic effect of alterations in p_{CO_2} is well known (28). An acute fall in the p_{CO_2} causes renal vasodilation and a fall in glomerular filtration rate, and bicarbonate reabsorption rises markedly. If one prevents the fall in glomerular filtration rate by infusion of vasopressors, the effect of hypercapnia on bicarbonate reabsorption is of much less magnitude.

In summary, the effects of alterations in plasma p_{CO_2} are probably mediated via two mechanisms. The first, and probably most important, is mediated by an alteration of extracellular pH, which in turn changes cell pH. The second is modulted by an alteration of renal hemodynamics, which subsequently changes bicarbonate reabsorption, either through a tubular effect or by a change in filtered load.

CARBONIC ANHYDRASE

The enzyme, carbonic anhydrase, plays a major role in the renal transport of bicarbonate (29). Its importance is easily demonstrable by observing the effect of administering enzyme inhibitors, acetazolamide or benzolamide.

Infusion of acetazolamide results in a prompt bicarbonate diuresis. Under such conditions, about 30% of the filtered bicarbonate appears in the urine (30-32). If one measures bicarbonate transport in the superficial proximal tubule, however, different results are observed. In this nephron segment, infusion of inhibitors of carbonic anhydrase activity decreases bicarbonate transport by a magnitude of 70-100% (29, 30). In other words, whole kidney bicarbonate reabsorption is affected to a much lesser degree than is superficial proximal tubule bicarbonate transport. This indicates that there is a major carbonic-anhydrase-independent pathway for bicarbonate reabsorption. It also indicates that the site in the nephron where this process takes place is not the superficial proximal tubule. The site of major carbonic-anhydrase-independent bicarbonate reabsorption may be the deeper proximal tubules, which are inaccessible to micropuncture assessment, the more distal segments of the nephron, or both. Bicarbonate transport occurs in the medullary thick ascending limb (medullary and cortical) and the collecting duct (32-34). In the deeper structures, there is a gradient for bicarbonate from lumen to blood, and as such passive bicarbonate transport probably occurs (32). The thick ascending limb and the collecting duct are capable of electrogenic proton secretion. In the papillary collecting duct, H-ATPase activity increases in response to chronic bicarbonate loading, as evidenced by substantial H-ATPase activity (35).

Another interesting difference between in vivo and in vitro studies is the effect of amiloride on carbonic-anhydrase-independent bicarbonate reabsorption. In vitro studies in collecting tubule (36) and turtle bladder (37, 38) show an almost complete inhibition of either total CO_2 transport or hydrogen ion secretion by acetazolamide. Animals treated with acetazolamide excrete only about 30% of the filtered bicarbonate in the urine (32, 33), and amiloride administration superimposed on acetazolamide induces an additional increase in bicarbonate excretion of approximately 10% (33). Amiloride acts mainly in the cortical collecting tubule, suggesting strongly that there is substantial carbonic-anhydrase-independent bicarbonate reabsorption in this nephron segment. Such was demonstrated by Frommer et al. (32) in the rat, thus the apparent discrepancy between the in vivo clearance studies and the in-vitro studies is now clear.

Finally, if distal nephron acidification is to a large extent dependent upon the presence of carbonic anhydrase activity, then one would predict that the infusion of acetazolamide (or a similar drug) would decrease the rate of distal urinary acidification. When acetazolamide is infused to animals under a variety of experimental conditions, it does not decrease the urine-blood p_{CO_2} gradient (a marker of distal acidification), suggesting that, in vivo, distal acidification is not inhibited by blocking carbonic anhydrase activity (39). This is in sharp contradistinction to the effect of amiloride, which consistently lowers the urine-blood p_{CO^2} gradient (40). Taken further, these results suggest that there is a large component of distal urinary acidification that is independent of carbonic anhydrase activity. In vitro, at least, even carbonic-anhydrase-independent acidification, albeit small in absolute terms, is affected by voltage (38).

POTASSIUM

It has been known for many years that bicarbonate reabsorption by the kidney is inversely proportional to the level of body potassium stores (41). In other words, bicarbonate reabsorption is depressed in potassium-loaded animals and is increased in potassium-depleted animals. The demonstration that hypokalemic metabolic alkalosis could be corrected by the administration of sodium chloride alone casts doubt on the role of potassium as a regulator of bicarbonate reabsorption (22), however, it was subsequently demonstrated that potassium exerts a regulatory role over bicarbonate reabsorption, which is independent of any effect attributable to volume.

Kurtzman et al. (42) studied bicarbonate reabsorption in three groups of dogs: one with potassium depletion (induced by a potassium-free diet and desoxycorticosterone), a second with hyperkalemia, and a third normal group. Bicarbonate reabsorption fell in all three groups following volume expansion with isotonic saline (Figure 2). The higher the fractional chloride excretion, the lower the bicarbonate reabsorption. At any given level of fractional chloride excretion, bicarbonate reabsorption was higher in potassium-depleted animals than in normal animals; bicarbonate reabsorption was higher in normal animals than in those that were potassium loaded. When salt excretion was very low, and by inference volume was markedly contracted, there was no difference in bicarbonate reabsorption among the three groups (Figure 2). These authors concluded that volume expansion depressed bicarbonate reabsorption in potassium-loaded, normal, and potassium-depleted animals, but that, independent of volume, the state of body potassium stores affected bicarbonate reabsorption. It also became clear that volume contraction, a major stimulus to increase bicarbonate reabsorption, could completely overcome the depressive effect of potassium loading on bicarbonate reabsorption. A micropuncture study by Kunau et al. (43) and a microperfusion by Chan et al. (44) demonstrated a direct effect of hypokalemia on the capacity of the proximal tubule to reabsorb bicarbonate. It is likely that the effects of potassium on hydrogen ion secreton are mediated by changes in cell pH such that potassium deficiency causes a decrease in cell pH, subsequently increasing bicarbonate reabsorption.

GLUCOSE

Patients returning to a normal diet after prolonged fasting commonly develop metabolic alkalosis (45). Glucose loading elevates bicarbonate reabsorption in these patients. Glucose infusion has been shown to enhance bicarbonate reabsorption in normal dogs (46). This seems to be a direct effect of glucose, since insulin administration does not raise bicarbonate reabsorption. It has also been shown in humans that glucose loading enhances acid excretion, a function of the distal nephron (47). The mechanism for this is not known.

PARATHYROID HORMONE (PTH), CALCIUM, PHOSPHATE, AND VITAMIN D.

Administration of pharmacologic doses of PTH to dogs and to humans leads to an increase in bicarbonate excretion (48, 49). The effect of PTH on bicarbonate reabsorption is of small magnitude, despite the high doses used in these studies, and appears to be related to decreased Na/H antiporter activity of the proximal tubule (50). Animals with thyroparathyroidectomy have increased Na/H exchange activity (50). The hormone also indirectly affects distal nephron acidification; chronic administration of PTH (1–34) to humans increases net acid excretion because of increased distal phosphate delivery (51, 52).

Acute hypercalcemia enhances bicarbonate reabsorption in normal dogs (48). This effect of hypercalcemia is seen in thyroparathyroidectomized animals, suggesting that calcium per se, independent of PTH, has an effect on hydrogen ion secretion.

Chronic phosphate depletion leads to a decrease in bicarbonate reabsorption (53), apparently by decreasing the intracellular hydrogen ion concentration, and thus increasing the cell pH. Siegfried et al. (54) have shown that vitamin D enhances bicarbonate reabsorption. Whether this effect is mediated through calcium is not yet known.

ALDOSTERONE

The mineralocorticoid, aldosterone, plays no role in proximal bicarbonate reabsorption (55–57). Microchemical and autoradiographic techniques by Farman et al. (58, 59) have demonstrated that there is no binding of ^{3}H-

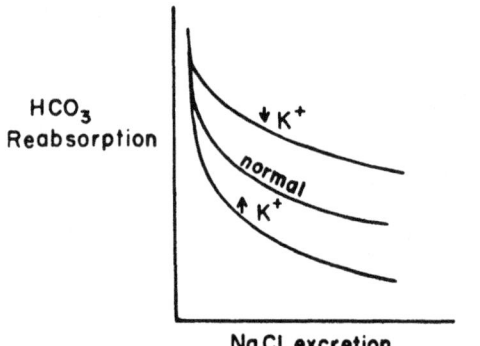

Figure 2. Effect of potassium depletion and hyperkalemia on proximal bicarbonate reabsorption. When volume is normal (i.e., high NaCl excretion), hypokalemia increases HCO_3 reabsorption and vice versa, as compared to control. When volume is contracted (i.e., low NaCl excretion), no effect of potassium is observed in HCO_3 reabsorption, indicating that volume is an overriding stimulus affecting proximal HCO_3 reabsorption. Adapted from: Kurtzman et al., Metabolism 22:481, 1973.

aldosterone to proximal convoluted tubules of the rabbit. Rather, specific binding occurred in the distal nephron (cortical collecting tubule). Aldosterone excess enhances acid secretion and results in metabolic alkalosis; aldosterone deficiency is associated with metabolic acidosis (60, 61). This effect of aldosterone on acid secretion is a consequence of an effect of the hormone on the distal nephron to stimulate electrogenic proton secretion (62, 63). Whether this occurs solely in the cortical collecting tubule or in other segments of the distal nephron (medullary thick ascending limb and papillary collecting duct) is not yet known.

In summary, as shown in Table 1, the following factors seem to be important regulators of bicarbonate reabsorption: Extracelluar volume expansion depresses bicarbonate reabsorption, whereas extracellular volume contraction enhances it; high plasma p_{CO_2} increases and low plasma p_{CO_2} decreases bicarbonate reabsorption; and hyperkalemia depresses bicarbonate reabsorption and hypokalemia increases it. PTH and phosphate depletion depress bicarbonate reabsorption; acute hypercalcemia and vitamin D enhance bicarbonate reabsorption. Glucose loading enhances bicarbonate reabsorption, whereas acetazolamide administration decreases it. Aldosterone has no effect on proximal bicarbonate reabsorption, but it is necessary for efficient distal urinary acidification.

Renal acid excretion (bicarbonate regeneration)

Despite the high efficiency of the proximal tubule in reabsorbing bicarbonate (i.e., bicarbonate reclamation), progressive acidemia would result if there were not a second mechanism whereby the kidney replenishes the extracellular bicarbonate used to neutralize endogenous acids (i.e., bicarbonate regeneration). Shown in Figure 3 is the schema for hydrogen ion secretion by the distal nephron, the site believed responsible for bicarbonate regeneration. The factors controlling distal urinary acidification differ from those controlling bicarbonate reabsorption in the proximal tubule.

As a consequence of dietary intake and intermediary metabolism, there is a daily production rate of endogenous acid of 1–1.5 mEq/kg body weight. These hydrogen ions result from the metabolism of sulfoproteins and phosphoproteins, as well as from the incomplete oxidation of fats and carbohydrates. The acids produced daily are immediately neutralized by the buffers present in the extracellular fluid, resulting in the consumption of bicarbonate. The distal nephron regenerates the consumed bicarbonate such that 70–100 mEq/day of acid is excreted. As a consequence of normal distal urinary acidification, acid-base homeostasis is maintained and the acid balance is zero (i.e., intake equals output).

Net acid excretion = (Urinary titratable acid excretion + NH_4^+ excretion) − urinary HCO_3 excretion.

Under normal conditions virtually no bicarbonate appears in the urine, as it is completely reabsorbed, mainly by the proximal tubule, hence the main components of renal acid

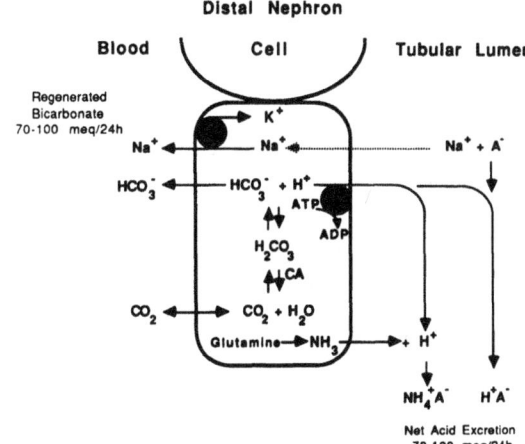

Figure 3. Hydrogen ion secretion by the distal nephron. Electrogenic hydrogen ion secretion (H-ATPase) accounts for virtually all acidification in the distal nephron, although Na/H antiporter activity is found in papillary collecting duct cells in culture. CA = carbonic anhydrase; dark circle (•) = active transport.

excretion are titratable acid and ammonium. If the distal nephron excretes excess acid, additional bicarbonate is regenerated on a milliequivalent for milliequivalent basis and metabolic alkalosis will result.

TITRATABLE ACID EXCRETION

Titratable acid refers to the hydrogen ions present in the urine in the form of weak acid anions. The pK of the buffer pair, the amount of the buffer present, and the urine pH determines the amount of titratable acid excreted daily.

pK of the buffer pair. The most abundant buffer present in urine is phosphate (pK = 6.8), followed by creatinine (pK = 5.0) and urate (pK = 5.33). According to the Henderson–Hasselbalch equation,

$$pH = pK + \log \frac{A}{HA},$$

where A is the conjugate base and HA is the weak acid. From this equation, the pH equals the pK when the concentration of A equals that of HA (i.e., the log of 1 = 0). This means that when the pH equals the pK, 50% of the buffer is present in the nonionized form. As pH is increased, more of the buffer will exist in the nonionized form (and vice versa). An ideal buffer has a pK between the blood pH ($\simeq 7.4$) and final urine pH, as it can then accept both hydrogen and hydroxyl ions. The phosphate buffer pair (pK = 6.8) has a ratio of 1:1 (Na_2HPO_4:NaH_2PO_4) at a urine pH of 6.8. At a pH of 7.4 (blood) the ratio is 4:1. If 1000 μM of phosphate are filtered at the glomerulus daily, 800 μM will be in the monohydrogen form (Na_2HPO_4) and can accept 300 μM hydrogen as pH falls from 7.4 to 6.8 (at pH 6.8, 500 μM each is present as the monohydrogen and the dihydrogen form of phoshate). At a urine pH of 5.5, most of the phosphate exists as dihydrogen phosphate (NaH_2PO_4) and the other weak acids such as creatinine, urate, and other organic acids assume more importance.

Amount of urinary buffer

The amount of buffer present in the urine directly determines the amount of titratable acid excreted. Phosphate is the most abundant buffer present in the urine. On a normal diet its concentration is relatively constant, consequently the bulk of titratable acid is phosphate.

Urine pH

The urine pH is the final determinant of titratable acid excretion. The lower the urine pH, the greater the amount of titratable acid, limited of course by the restrictions described above (i.e., pK, buffer concentrations).

AMMONIUM EXCRETION

Ammonia (NH_3) is a weak base that is thought to be freely diffusible across cell membranes. In the renal cell, NH_3 is formed from glutamine and, depending upon the nephron segment, primarily results from the activity of the phosphate-dependent glutaminase (distal nephron) or phosphate-independent glutaminase enzymes (proximal tubule).

Because of the pK of the $NH_3:NH_4^+$ buffer pair (pK 9.4), intracellular NH_3 synthesized ionizes in the tubular lumen, where it accepts a proton and remains trapped. Urine pH is a major determinant influencing NH_4^+ excretion; the relationship is an inverse one in that NH_4^+ excretion increases as urine pH falls. The acute changes in ammonium excretion are simply related to changes in NH_3 distribution, not synthesis; more NH_3 diffuses into the tubular lumen than diffuses into the peritubular blood. If urine pH is increased acutely (with HCO_3 or acetazolamide), urinary NH_4^+ will dissociate and NH_3 diffuses into the peritubular blood. Recent experiments suggest the NH_4^+ may be secreted as such across some membranes (64, 65). If this is true, our present concepts regarding ammonium excretion require modification.

Potassium depletion stimulates NH_3 production in vivo and in vitro, presumably by stimulating glutamine uptake by the renal tubular cell (66, 67). Potassium deprivation of 1-week duration stimulates titratable acid excretion in the isolated perfused rat kidney (68).

ROLE OF DISTAL SODIUM DELIVERY, BUFFER CONTENT, ALDOSTERONE, AND BLOOD pH ON NET ACID EXCRETION

Distal sodium delivery

The state of sodium reabsorption by the distal nephron has a major impact on net acidification. This effect is the result of the negative potential difference generated by the active transport of sodium in the distal nephron. The generation of a lumen negative potential difference accelerates the rate of proton transport, even though hydrogen ion secretion occurs in the absence of sodium transport. Thus, factors that interfere with sodium reabsorption, and therefore with the generation of a lumen negative potential difference, can markedly reduce the overall rate of distal acidification (46, 69). The influence of sodium transport on acidification is clearly illustrated by the effect of the diuretic agent, amiloride. In the turtle bladder this drug reduces proton secretion only in the open-circuited condition (46); that is to say, amiloride exerts an effect on acidification only when there is a lumen negative potential difference, which it reduces to zero. If the potential difference is restored to control values in the continued presence of amiloride, acidification returns to control values. This component of acidification reduced by amiloride is, therefore, the "voltage-dependent" component. In intact animals, amiloride inhibits distal urinary acidification, presumably through its effect on the luminal potential difference. The voltage-dependent component of acidification may, under a variety of normal and abnormal circumstances, be the critical modulator of net acidification.

Any event that reduces distal sodium transport, all other things being equal, results in a reduction in distal acidification. Such a reduction in distal sodium transport could result from an intrinsic abnormality in the tubule's capacity to transport sodium, from a decreased availability of sodium for transport as the consequence of decreased distal delivery of the cation, or because of aldosterone deficiency. An example of the role of decreased distal delivery is the decreased capacity to acidify the urine seen in patients with severe liver disease. At one time it was postulated that patients with cirrhosis had an intrinsic defect in distal acidification similar to that observed in patients with distal renal tubular acidosis. This defect was tentatively ascribed to the hypergammaglobulinemia commonly observed in patients with profound hepatic damage. The impaired capacity to acidify the urine that is commonly observed in patients with cirrhosis is, at least in part, the result of the impaired distal delivery of sodium; increasing distal sodium delivery (either with a diuretic or infusion of sodium sulfate) results in a relatively normal acidification response. Assessment of distal acidification in this clinical setting is further clouded by the ubiquitous finding of respiratory alkalosis in patients with cirrhosis, a disturbance that also inhibits distal acidification (71, 72).

Clinical examples of overt acid retention secondary to impaired distal acidification as a result of a reduction in the voltage-dependent component of acidification are the acidoses seen in some patients with obstructive uropathy (73) and hemoglobin-S (74).

Since the generation of lumen negative potential favors the secretion of potassium as well as protons, a defect in sodium transport should be reflected by diminished potassium excretion and hyperkalemia, as well as a reduction of acidification. Thus, full expression of a defect in the generation of a lumen negative voltage secondary to defective sodium transport would be a tendency to sodium wastage (which might be seen only following dietary sodium restriction), a reduced capacity to excrete potassium, hyperkalemia, reduced acid excretion, and metabolic acidosis (75).

Another mechanism that might retard the development of a lumen negative voltage is accelerated chloride transport (76). If the permeability of the distal nephron to chloride is increased, then sodium will be reabsorbed in an electrically silent fashion. This type of abnormality would likewise be reflected by hyperkalemia and metabolic acidosis, but would be associated with a tendency to sodium retention rather than sodium wastage. The ensuing volume expansion resulting from increased salt reabsorption should lead to the development of hypertension in such an afflicted patient.

Consider the reverse, i.e., an increase in the negativity of the luminal potential difference. Under conditions where sodium absorption is increased or chloride is decreased, the lumen would become more electrically negative. Hydrogen and potassium excretion would increase and hypokalemic metabolic alkalosis should ensue. Infusion of Na_2SO_4 makes the tubule lumen more negative and markedly stimulates hydrogen and potassium secretion. In some reports there is an attendant metabolic alkalosis as well. The clinical states that may be associated with this mechanism are discussed in the section on pathophysiologic states associated with metabolic alkalosis.

Buffer content

Under ordinary circumstances, a large fraction of acid excreted in the urine is in the form of titratable acid, the remainder being ammonium. Since most of titratable acid is phosphate, a reduction in the filtered load of phosphate (as may be seen with phosphate depletion) or an acceleration of proximal phosphate reabsorption would result in decreased delivery of phosphate to the distal nephron. This, in turn, would be reflected by a decrease in titratable acid formation and a brief period of acid retention. Such a mechanism in and of itself should not cause metabolic acidosis, because as soon as a small degree of acid was retained, ammoniagenesis would be stimulated and acid excretion returned to an appropriate level as a consequence of increased ammonium excretion.

Prolonged phosphate depletion results in a defect in acidification that cannot be attributed totally to the absence of phosphate as a urinary buffer. Not only does phosphate deprivation impair proximal acidification (52), but evidence from animals strongly suggests that distal acidification is also reduced (77). The overall impact of phosphate deprivation on acid-base regulation is somewhat mitigated by the fact that phosphate depletion stimulates the extrarenal buffering capacity (65). This enhancement of buffering tends to prevent a major reduction in extracellular pH secondary to the reduction in acid excretion.

The other main urinary buffer is ammonia. Under conditions of increased acid delivery to the circulation, the renal response is to excrete the extra acid in the form of ammonium. In addition to acidemia, there are a number of other factors that regulate the kidney's ability to enhance ammoniagensis and, thus, increase ammonium excretion. Aldosterone likely participates in the regulation of ammoniagenesis (79, 80). Increased levels of aldosterone enhance ammoniagenesis, while the reverse is seen in the absence of the steroid. A similar effect of potassium on ammoniagenesis has also been observed. Hyperkalemia inhibits ammonia production while hypokalemia stimulates it (67, 81–83). The relative contributions of aldosterone and potassium are difficult to dissect because aldosterone deficiency is usually associated with hyperkalemia, and both conditions suppress ammonia production (75, 80). Similarly, aldosterone excess is usually associated with hypokalemia, both of which stimulate ammonia production.

Aldosterone

In general, aldosternone excess favors acid excretion while aldosterone deficiency reduces it. There are a number of mechanisms whereby aldosterone may modulate distal acidification. The hormone is not required to generate large pH gradients between the blood and urine. This can be demonstrated both in vitro and in vivo. In the turtle bladder, the addition of aldosterone results in an increase in proton conductance, but not in a proton motive force (84). In the dog, the rat, and the human, an aldosterone deficiency is associated with acid retention, but with an intact ability to lower urine pH during acidemia (75, 80, 85).

Aldosterone may modulate distal acidification through its effect on sodium transport. By enhancing sodium reabsorption and increasing the negativity of the tubular lumen, the voltage-dependent component of acidification would be enhanced. This effect on the proton pump appears to be direct. Furthermore, if aldosterone deficiency results in salt wastage and volume contraction, then distal sodium delivery may be reduced. Aldosterone also, as mentioned above, modulates ammoniagenesis. Since aldosterone is a major potassium-regulating hormone, its effect on potassium may also modulate ammoniagenesis and urinary acid excretion. Finally, if volume is contracted as a consequence of aldosterone deficiency, renal blood flow, and thus glutamine delivery, might be reduced, with a subsequent reduction in ammoniagenesis.

In and of itself, aldosterone probably plays a relatively small role in regulating overall acid excretion. Otherwise, normal humans rendered mineralocorticoid deficient retain acid, but only for a short period of time and only in an amount sufficient to lower the serum bicarbonate concentration less than 2 mEq/l (86). This situation, however, likely does not apply to patients in whom an aldosterone deficiency is associated with a reduced glomerular filtration rate (80). Under these conditions, aldosterone may be critical for maintenance of acid-base homeostasis.

Blood pH

As blood pH falls, the normal kidney excretes a urine with a pH less than 5.5. This occurs as early as 2 hours after the development of acidemia. The immediate response to acidemia is to increase urinary titratable acid by increasing urinary phosphate excretion. Once the urinary buffers are titrated, the kidney increases ammoniagenesis, such that ammonium excretion, under conditions of chronic acidemia, will rise fivefold to tenfold (87).

Extrarenal buffering

While the kidney is the primary organ responsible for the maintenance of normal acid-base homeostasis, it is apparent that extrarenal mechanisms could account for a small rise in plasma bicarbonate as well. Fraley and Adler (88) studied the extrarenal effects of PTH on the handling of an acid load in both dog and rats, and it is clear from their data that the extrarenal effects of parathyroid hormone are opposite to the renal effects. In their experiments, the animals were first acutely nephrectomized and then received a constant acid infusion. Animals that had been previously thyroparathyroidectomized (TPTX) were unable to buffer the acid load and had a lower arterial pH and plasma bicarbonate than did controls or TPTX animals receiving PTH. Changes in skeletal muscle pH were insufficient to account for the buffering that occurred following PTH infusion.

We further examined this issue using the same model in several groups of rats (78, 89). Animals with secondary hyperparathyroidism, induced by four-fifths renal infarction (chronic renal failure) or 24-hour bilateral ureteral obstruction (acute renal failure), were able to buffer a constant acid infusion better than were similar groups of animals that had previous TPTX (78). If bone resorption was prevented by prior administration of diphosphonates, the mortality rate was higher than in nontreated animals. Chronic phosphate depletion, a syndrome accompanied by a low parathyroid hormone levels in humans, was associated with enhanced extrarenal buffering. Thyrocalcitonin to intact, but not TPTX, rats was associated with a decrease in extrarenal buffering. By contrast, chronic vitamin-D administration was found to increase the buffering capacity as compared to control (89).

These results suggest that states of parthyroid hormone excess (either primary or secondary) are important to enhanced extrarenal buffering. The source of alkali released into the extracellular space is likely to be from bone. The effects of phosphate depletion and vitamin D in increasing extrarenal buffering are independent of parathyroid hormone and are likely to represent direct effects on bone metabolism.

More recently, several balance studies have demonstrated that chronic administration of either parathyroid hormone or vitamin D results in a sustained increase in plasma bicarbonate concentration, which, as stated, is probably from bone. Since the increased bicarbonate is not excreted by the kidney, the induction of hypercalcemia following these two hormones likely has an effect on the kidney of increasing overall bicarbonate reabsorption. That this effect is due to parathyroid hormone and vitamin D rather than the coexisting hypercalcemia was demonstrated by the observation that when hypercalcemia was induced as the consequence of prolonged administration of calcium salts, the reverse effect was observed; that is to say, the plasma bicarbonate concentration decreased (90, 91).

In summary, acid excretion by the kidney takes place by two mechanisms. In the proximal tubule, bicarbonate reclamation occurs as a consequence of Na/H exchange. Many factors contribute to the control of bicarbonate reabsorption and these are outlined in Table 1. Acid excretion also occurs by the formation of titratable acid and ammonium (bicarbonate regeneration), primarily a function of the distal nephron. The urine pH affects the formation of both titratable acid and ammonium, whereas the amount of buffer filtered affects only titratable acid formation. Aldosterone is the major hormone affecting distal urinary acidification. The plasma bicarbonate concentration may also be modified by changes in extrarenal buffering. Many agents affect extrarenal buffering in addition to their known effects on the kidney. These factors, taken together, regulate the metabolic component in acid-base homeostasis under both normal and pathologic conditions.

GENERATION OF METABOLIC ALKALOSIS

Metabolic alkalosis must be considered in two phases: the generation of new bicarbonate, and the maintenance of a high plasma bicarbonate concentration, the latter being accomplished by increased tubular reabsorption. In order to generate metabolic alkalosis, one must have a gain of base or a loss of acid (Table 2). The gain of base may result from the administration of alkaline solutions, and the loss of acid may be by the gastrointestinal tract or the kidney.

The body produces about 60–100 mEq of acid daily as the consequence of normal metabolism. The kidney is thus required to excrete 60–100 mEq of acid daily. For each milliequivalent of acid excreted in the urine, 1 mEq of new bicarbonate will be generated and added to the blood, maintaining normal acid-base homeostasis. In order for the kidney to generate metabolic alkalosis, the net acid excretion must increase, at least transiently, resulting in the addition of excess amounts of bicarbonate to the blood. Depletion of hydrochloric acid from the stomach as the consequence of vomiting or nasogastric suction leaves behind large quantities of bicarbonate in the blood.

If new bicarbonate is added to the blood (regardless of the mechanism), it does not necessarily follow that metabolic alkalosis will ensue. The new bicarbonate may be excreted by the kidney, thus preventing metabolic alkalosis. It is clear that in order for sustained metabolic alkalosis to be present, the excess bicarbonate generated or administered must not be excreted, i.e., the high bicarbonate present in the filtrate must be reclaimed by the kidney

Table 2. The generation and maintenance of metabolic alkalosis

Generation	Maintenance	Example
I. *Loss of acid from extracellular space*		
A. Loss of gastric fluid (HCl)	↓ EAV	Vomiting
B. Loss of acid into urine: increased distal Na delivery in presence of hyperaldosteronism	K depletion + aldosterone excess ↓ EAV + K depletion (contributing factor)	Primary aldosteronism Diuretic administration
C. Loss of acid into cells: K deficiency		K deficiency
D. Loss of acid into stool	K deficiency + EAV ↓	Congenital chloride-losing diarrhea
II. *Excessive HCO_3 loads*		
A. Absolute		
Oral or parenteral loads of HCO_3 or alkalinization salts	↓ EAV, oral or IV administration K deficiency	$NaHCO_3$ administration, milk alkali syndrome
Metabolic conversion of the salts of organic acids to HCO_3, (e.g., ketones, lactate)	↓ EAV, K deficiency, oral or IV administration	Lactate, acetate, or citrate administration
B. Relative		
Alkaline loads in renal failure	Renal failure	Alkali administration to patients with renal failure
III. *Posthypercapnic states*	↓ EAV	Correction of chronic hypercapnia in presence of low-salt diet

EAV = effective arterial volume; adapted from Seldin and Rector (116).

in order to maintain the metabolic alkalosis. An increase in bicarbonate reabsorptive capacity that is unaccompanied by the gain of bicarbonate or the loss of acid cannot generate metabolic alkalosis.

The kidney can generate metabolic alkalosis if there is an increased capacity of the distal nephron to secrete hydrogen ion at a time when there is adequate distal sodium delivery. Aldosterone excess increases both sodium and chloride reabsorption in the distal nephron and enhances potassium and sodium secretion. The retained salt results in extracellular volume expansion, which in turn depresses proximal reabsorption, increasing distal sodium delivery. Patients with an aldosterone excess commonly have metabolic alkalosis. This type of metabolic alkalosis is almost invariably accompanied by hypokalemia. The data of Kurtzman et al. (55) suggest that both hyperaldosteronism and hypokalemia are required for the kidney to generate metabolic alkalosis. Dogs were potassium depleted by the administration of the potassium exchange resin, Kayexalate®, and deoxycorticosterone acetate (DOCA). Their diet contained both sodium chloride and sodium bicarbonate. After a few days all the animals developed metabolic alkalosis. When the DOCA was discontinued, the metabolic alkalosis rapidly corrected without correction of the hypokalemia. When DOCA was again restarted in these same potassium-depleted animals, metabolic alkalosis recurred, but only if the dosage of DOCA was very high. Once the metabolic alkalosis returned, sodium bicarbonate was removed from the diet and replaced with equal amounts of potassium bicarbonate. This resulted in the correction of both the potassium depletion and the metabolic alkalosis, even though excessive amounts of DOCA were still being administered. In this animal model of primary aldosteronism, both the generation and maintenance of metabolic alkalosis were dependent on the simultaneous presence of potassium depletion and aldosterone excess. Either factor alone was unable to generate (or maintain) metabolic alkalosis. Thus, the generation (and the maintenance) of metabolic alkalosis in patients with primary mineralocorticoid excess is likely to be the consequence of accelerated distal hydrogen ion secretion, which is driven by both steroid excess and potassium depletion.

FACTORS THAT MAINTAIN METABOLIC ALKALOSIS

As shown in Table 3, there are a number of factors that play a role in the maintenance of metabolic alkalosis (18,92). In perhaps all patients with metabolic alkalosis, the glomerular filtration rate in decreased. This reduction prevents the increase in bicarbonate from being filtered at the glomerulus. Thus, although the plasma bicarbonate concentration is elevated, the signal is not recognized by the kidney and bicarbonate excretion is not increased. There may be an additional effect of volume contraction to stimulate tubular bicarbonate absorption independent of filtered load. Atrial natriuretic hormone corrects metabolic alkalosis, presumably by its effect of increasing the glomerular filtration rate (93).

Hypokalemia perpetuates metabolic alkalosis by decreasing the filtered load of bicarbonate. This is thought to be due to the reduction in the glomerular filtration rate because of increased renal vascular resistance (94, 95). Tubular reabsorption of bicarbonate is likely to be directly stimulated by potassium depletion and is most likely to be the result of intracellular acidosis (44).

A role for hypochloremia seems likely in the maintenance of metabolic alkalosis. Hypochloremia stimulates renin release, resulting in a decrease in the glomerular filtration rate (96, 97). The effect of low chloride is inde-

Table 3. Factors that maintain metabolic alkalosis by decreasing urinary bicarbonate excretion

Factor	Proposed mechanism
Decreased glomerular filtration rate	Increases fractional HCO_3 reabsorption, preventing the elevated plasma HCO_3 concentration from exceeding T_m
Volume contraction	Stimulates proximal tubular HCO_3 reabsorption
Hypokalemia	Decreases glomerular filtration rate and increases proximal tubular HCO_3 reabsorption
Hypochloremia*	Increases renin, decreases glomerular filtration rate, and decreases distal chloride delivery ($\uparrow H^+$ secretion by the medullary collecting tubule
Passive backflux of HCO_3	Favorable concentration gradients for passive movement from proximal tubular lumen to blood
Aldosterone	Increases Na-dependent H^+ secretion in cortical collecting tubule and Na-independent H^+ secretion in medullary collecting tubule

*Animal models are associated with hypokalemia, thus the precise role of chloride is not clearly understood.

pendent of volume contraction and aldosterone. The resultant decrease in the glomerular filtration rate decreases the filtered bicarbonate, which in turn decreases urinary bicarbonate excretion. Furthermore, there may be a role for chloride in the more terminal portions of the nephron. If sodium-independent hydrogen ion secretion is favored by a low urine chloride concentration in the medullary collecting tubule, then chloride depletion may further accelerate acid secretion and serve to maintain an elevated bicarbonate concentration. A decrease in distal chloride delivery would decrease the Cl/HCO_3 antiporter, thus maintaining the high bicarbonate concentration (98–100). In this regard, chloride dependency of the H^+-ATPase enzyme has been shown in vitro in mammalian kidney (8). If these results can be translated to the intact kidney, chloride depletion should decrease acid secretion, not increase it, as suggested above.

There may also be a role for passive bicarbonate backflux in the maintenance of metabolic alkalosis (101). At the glomerulus there is an increase in the bicarbonate concentration at the proximal tubule during metabolic alkalosis as compared to normal, all other things being equal. Thus, the increase in salt and water reabsorption that occurs in subjects with metabolic alkalosis, combined with the decrease in hydrogen ion secretion, will result in an increase in the bicarbonate concentration of the urine as it traverses the proximal tubule. This may exceed the blood concentration, resulting in a gradient for bicarbonate transport from the lumen to blood. In micropuncture study in rats following bicarbonate loading, Cogan and Liu (102) did not observe gradients high enough to result in significant backflux, although such may occur in other models of metabolic alkalosis.

Finally, aldosterone increases acidification in the collecting tubule. In the cortical segment this is probably secondary to the steroid-induced stimulation of sodium transport, while in the medullary collecting duct the effect is probably on proton secretion per se (62, 63, 103).

PATHOPHYSIOLOGIC STATES ASSOCIATED WITH METABOLIC ALKALOSIS

Gastric alkalosis

With vomiting or gastric drainage, profound metabolic alkalosis may occur as each milliequivalent of acid (HCl) lost from the stomach represents 1 mEq of bicarbonate added to the extracellular fluid. Profound hypokalemia and volume contraction also occurs in gastric alkalosis. These result from mechanisms other than the loss of sodium and potassium in vomitus or drainage per se as there is little sodium and potassium present in gastric juice (Table 4).

The sequence of events is outlined in Figure 4 and is as follows: The loss of hydrochloric acid results in a rise in plasma bicarbonate with little change in sodium or potassium. When the plasma bicarbonate exceeds the reabsorptive capacity of the proximal tubule, bicarbonate appears in the urine. This bicarbonate is delivered to the distal nephron as sodium bicarbonate, where some of the sodium is exchanged for potassium. Thus, as shown in Table 5, the early phase of gastric alkalosis is associated with a high urine pH, and with high sodium and potassium excretion. Urine chloride is low owing to its loss in gastric juice. Overall, this represents the loss of salt and water, with a resultant contraction of the effective arterial volume: The sodium is lost in the urine, the chloride is lost in the vomitus, and water is lost in both. With the contraction of the effective arterial volume, proximal bicarbonate reabsorption by the kidney increases and the generated metabolic alkalosis is thus maintained. As this occurs, decreased amounts of bicarbonate and sodium are delivered to the distal nephron. Because of the volume contraction, aldosterone is stimulated. Urine sodium excretion falls and potassium excretion increases; because of the decrease in distal bicarbonate delivery, the urine pH falls

Table 4. Composition of gastric juice

	Concentration	
	Mean	Range
Sodium (mEq/l)	20	10–30
Potassium (mEq/l)	10	5–40
Chloride (mEq/l)	120	80–170
Hydrogen (nEq/l)	90	65–150
Volume (ml/24 hr)	1000	400–5000

Metabolic Alkalosis   169

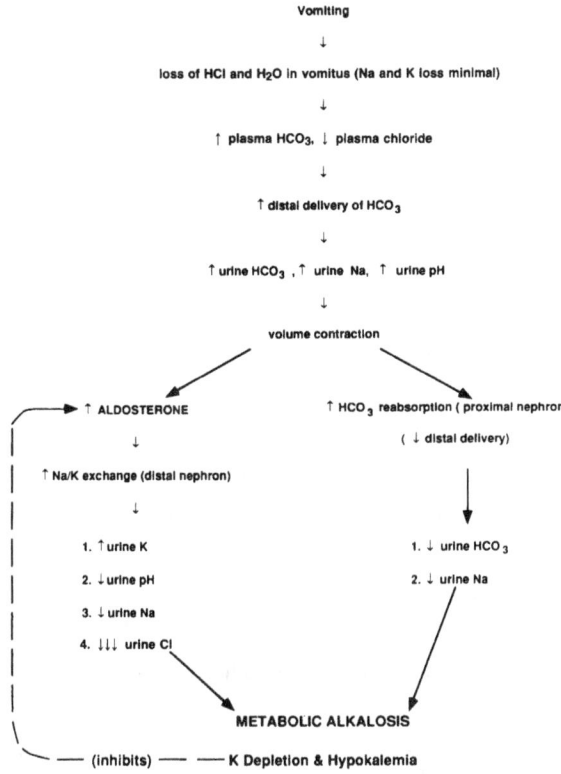

Figure 4. Schema for the pathogenesis of gastric alkalosis.

as bicarbonate disappears from the urine (Table 4, late phase).

With the development of potassium depletion, aldosterone secretion now falls; however, proximal bicarbonate reabsorption remains high, both because of volume contraction and hypokalemia. While aldosterone levels are found to be in the "normal range," when corrected for the hypokalemia present a profound state of secondary hyperaldosteronism exists. Note that both early and late in gastric alkalosis, urine chloride is the *only* accurate marker of the state of volume; it is always low. Use of the urine sodium alone may yield incorrect information as regards effective arterial volume, as it is high early in gastric alkalosis and low only late in the disorder (Table 5).

Therapy is directed towards correction of the salt, potassium, and water deficits. In patients without severe cardiac, hepatic, or renal disease, the urine chloride is used to assess adequate replacement. A urine chloride concentration greater than 40 mEq/l usually indicates that sufficient salt has been administered.

Mineralocorticoid excess

Many clinical conditions are associated with mineralocorticoid excess and metabolic alkalosis. These may be associated with hyperreninemic states or with hyporeninemia. Examples of each are given in Table 6. The metabolic alkalosis in these conditions occurs in the following way:
1. Increased sodium reabsorption by the distal nephron with enhanced potassium excretion
2. Expansion of extracellular volume with depression of proximal sodium reabsorption
3. Increased distal delivery of sodium with enhanced acid and potassium excretion.

Metabolic alkalosis ensues because acid excretion is enhanced by two separate mechanisms: potassium depletion, which increases acid secretion in the presence of aldosterone, and the secondary aldosteronism itself. If volume expansion is prevented by giving a very low sodium diet to a mineralocorticoid-treated animal, metabolic alkalosis does not occur (104). With a low-sodium diet, proximal reabsorption is increased and very little sodium reaches the distal nephron, thus preventing the sodium for hydrogen exchange.

In the presence of mineralocorticoid and adequate dietary NaCl, distal acidification is increased and the metabolic alkalosis is both generated and maintained by this effect. Potassium depletion and volume expansion counterbalance one another, and a change in proximal bicarbonate reabsorption plays little role in maintaining this form of metabolic alkalosis.

Accelerated hypertension is a state in which there is renal underperfusion, high renin, and increased aldosterone. A mild metabolic alkalosis may be seen, although usually only hypokalemia is noted. Renin-producing tumors include hemangiopericytomas (juxtaglomerular apparatus hyperplasia), Wilm's tumors, renal hamartomas, and occasionally lung malignancies. Unilateral renal artery stenosis or stenosis to a solitary kidney (as may be seen in the transplanted kidney) increases renin. Secondary hyperaldosteronism results and, as a consequence of accelerated potassium and hydrogen ion secretion, causes metabolic alkalosis.

The patient with primary aldosteronism clinically may have unilateral adrenal adenoma, bilateral adrenal hyperplasia, or, rarely, adrenal carcinoma. These disorders are the second most common cause of secondary hypertension (1–2%). Surgical resection of the adenoma usually results in complete correction of the abnormalities although ≃15% may still have hypertension. Adrenal carcinoma is usually associated with increased desoxycorticosterone and may be coincident with increased glucocorticoid production as well. The etiology of the increased aldosterone is unknown in patients with bilateral adrenal hyperplasia

Table 5. Urinary electrolytes in gastric alkalosis

	Na	K	Cl	HCO$_3$	pH
	mEq/l				
Early phase	↑	↑	↓	↑	↑
Late phase	↓	↑	↓	↓	↓

Table 6. Clinical states associated with metabolic alkalosis

Syndrome	Mineralocorticoid production	Renin	Volume	Hypertension	Hypokalemia
Unilateral RAS	↑	↑	↑	+	±
Accelerated hypertension	↑	↑	↑	+	±
Hemangiopericytoma	↑	↑	↑	+	±
Primary aldosteronism	↑	↓	↑	+	+
Adrenogenital syndromes (11- and 17-β-hydroxylase deficiency)	↑ (DOC)	↓	↑	+	+
Licorice	↓	↓	↑	+	+
Liddle's syndrome	↓	↓	↑	+	+
Vomiting	↑	↑	↓	−	+
Diuretics	↑	↑	↓	±*	+
Bartter's syndrome	↑	↑	↓	−	+
Congenital chloride-losing diarrhea	↑	↑	↓	−	−
Posthypercapnic alkalosis	↑	↑	↓	−	±

RAS = renal artery stenosis; DOC = desoxycorticosterone.
*Hypertension may be the underlying reason why diuretics were initially prescribed, and BP may not be below normal.

and the disorder is heterogeneous in nature. A subset of patients responds to exogenous aldosterone, another subset responds to dexamethasone, and a third does not respond to either. Clearly, much basic work must be done to unravel the cellular defects in each of these subgroups before we can make a rational approach to therapy.

The adrenogenital syndromes causing metabolic alkalosis are the 11- and 17-β-hydroxylase deficiencies (105). The defects result in high levels of desoxycorticosterone due to high ACTH levels resulting from the glucocorticoid synthesis. In 11-hydroxylase deficiency there is excess androgen synthesis, resulting in precocious puberty in males and virilization in females. With 17-β-hydroxylase deficiency, both androgen and estrogen synthesis is blocked and both sexes develop primarily female characteristics. Upon entering puberty no secondary sex characteristics develop. Both defects are associated with metabolic alkalosis, hypokalemia, and hypertension. Glucocorticoids are needed to reduce the female virilization in 11-hydroxylase deficiency and sex hormones are required in 17-β-hydroxylase deficiency for development of secondary sex characteristics.

Liddle's syndrome was described to characterize a group of patients with hypertension and metabolic alkalosis who behaved as though they had mineralocorticoid excess, but none could be found (106). The defect is probably one in which the distal nephron sodium reabsorption is enhanced. The abnormalities can be reversed with amiloride or triamterene. This illustrates the voltage-dependent acidification that we described in vitro.

Licorice ingestion (natural licorice) results in hypokalemic metabolic alkalosis. Aldosterone and renin are low, but a component of licorice, glycyrrhizic acid, has aldosteronelike actions. The compound is also present in some chewing tobaccos and in the United States, is the more common. Carbenoxolone, a new agent used in Europe to treat peptic ulcer disease is similar to glycyrrhizic acid, and one of its limitations is the development of hypertension and hypokalemic metabolic alkalosis.

"Contraction" alkalosis (diuretic administration)

Administration of thiazides, ethacrynic acid, and furosemide is commonly associated with metabolic alkalosis. It has been suggested that ethacrynic acid and furosemide, which have their diuretic site of action in the loop of Henle, may induce metabolic alkalosis without loss of acid (107). This alkalosis has been called contraction alkalosis and is thought to be due to enhanced excretion of sodium and chloride without proportional loss of bicarbonate (bicarbonate reabsorption in the loop of Henle is small in magnitude). It should be pointed out, however, that adrenalectomized dogs treated with maintenance doses of dexamethasone and DOCA and with furosemide failed to develop metabolic alkalosis. When the dogs were volume contracted at a time when large amounts of DOCA were given, metabolic alkalosis developed (60). The generation of this type of metabolic alkalosis is due to enhanced acid excretion brought on by potassium depletion and secondary hyperaldosteronism. Once generated, diuretic – induced metabolic alkalosis is maintained by volume contraction and potassium depletion.

Contraction per se seems a simplistic explanation for this type of metabolic alkalosis. It seems likely that excess renal acid excretion must occur for it to develop. Excess acid excretion could occur if increased lumen negativity resulted because of decreased chloride permeability in the collecting duct.

Bartter's syndrome

Bartter's syndrome is typically associated with metabolic alkalosis. It has been suggested that this syndrome represents a form of salt wastage due to the defective reabsorption of sodium chloride in the loop of Henle (108, 109). This salt wastage leads to a contracted plasma volume, which stimulates renin and aldosterone production. Potassium reabsorption also seems to be impaired, since adrenalectomy does not correct the severe hypokalemia found in these patients. The generation of metabolic alkalosis seems to result from severe potassium depletion and mineralocorticoid excess in the presence of increased distal delivery of sodium; enhanced proximal reabsorption secondary to a contracted plasma volume maintains the alkalosis.

Congenital chloride-losing diarrhea

Patients with this rare disease have hyperchloremia, a high stool chloride concentration, and absence of chloride in the urine (110, 111). The stool chloride concentration is higher than the sum of the sodium and potassium concentration. This is in contrast to all other diarrheal states, in which the sum of the sodium and potassium concentration in the stool is higher than the chloride concentration. These patients have a defect in chloride-bicarbonate transport in the ileum. They are unable to transport chloride against an electrochemical gradient; this defect results in a loss of chloride and acid in the stool, which in turn causes metabolic alkalosis. Distal proton secretion may also be impaired as the H^+-ATPase depends on chloride.

Posthypercapnic metabolic alkalosis

Chronic hypercapnia enhances acid and chloride excretion. At the same time, it stimulates proximal bicarbonate reabsorption, maintaining an increased concentration of plasma bicarbonate. Following the return of the p_{CO_2} to normal, there usually is retention of chloride and excretion of bicarbonate in the urine. If patients with hypercapnia are on a low-salt diet or are treated with diuretics so that volume is contracted, proximal reabsorption will be enhanced and bicarbonate reabsorption will remain elevated following the return of the p_{CO_2} to normal, resulting in posthypercapnic metabolic alkalosis.

Correction of this type of metabolic alkalosis usually can be accomplished by salt administration. This syndrome may result if the "effective" arterial volume is contracted for any reason, such as congestive heart failure. In this latter instance, successful treatment of the heart failure is required to correct the alkalosis; salt administration here is contraindicated.

Postfasting metabolic alkalosis

It has been well established that fasting patients returning to a normal diet with a high glucose content may develop metabolic alkalosis. Bicarbonate reabsorption measured in these patients correlates with the sodium balance (45). Bicarbonate reabsorption is low in the first week of fasting when the sodium balance is negative, but high in the second and third weeks when the sodium balance becomes positive. Glucose administration leads to a further increase in bicarbonate reabsorption and worsens the metabolic alkalosis. The matinenance of this type of metabolic alkalosis seems to be caused by contracted extracellular volume and the enhancing effect of glucose on bicarbonate reabsorption. The mechanism responsible for the generation of this type of metabolic alkalosis is not clear at the present time, though it may be secondary to increased acid excretion.

Hypercalcemia and hypoparathyroidism

A few cases of metabolic alkalosis have been reported in association with hypoparathyroidism; hypercalcemia is more commonly associated with metabolic alkalosis. It is likely that parathyroid hormone depresses bicarbonate reabsorption and its absence enhances it (48, 49). Hypercalcemia increases bicarbonate reabsorption by suppressing parathyroid hormone secretion and by a direct effect on renal hydrogen ion secretion. Although these observations explain the maintenance of metabolic alkalosis in these conditions, they leave unsolved the question of how metabolic alkalosis is generated. Parathyroid hormone has been shown to have an inhibitory effect on acid excretion, and theoretically this lack of parathyroid hormone could lead to enhanced acid excretion (51).

The generation of metabolic alkalosis secondary to hypercalcemia has been attributed to a greater availability of the buffering capacity of the skeleton secondary either to bone destruction or increased bone turnover. As mentioned previously, recent work suggests that parathyroid hormone has a direct effect on skeleton, which mobilizes buffer into the extracellular compartment (78, 89). Thus patients with hypercalcemia and hyperparathyroidism may develop metabolic alkalosis as a consequence of enhanced transfer of buffer from bone to the circulation.

Excessive bicarbonate loads

Administration of sodium bicarbonate in doses up to 140 g/day for periods extending to 3 weeks produces metabolic alkalosis, with the plasma bicarbonate ranging between 33 and 36 mEq/l. A linear relationship was noted between the doses of sodium bicarbonate administered and the rise in serum bicarbonate. If volume contraction or potassium depletion does not develop, the metabolic alkalosis will correct as soon as bicarbonate administration ceases, because of the kidney's intrinsic capacity to excrete enormous amounts of bicarbonate. In renal failure, however, a smaller dose of sodium bicarbonate may produce metabolic alkalosis because of the limited capacity of the severely diseased kidney to excrete a sodium load.

Respiratory compensation

Metabolic alkalosis may lead to compensatory hypoventilation and consequent CO_2 retention. Uncomplicated metabolic alkalosis is not always associated with alveolar hypoventilation. The magnitude of the hypoventilation in metabolic alkalosis is not great; the p_{CO_2} is usually not higher than 55 mmHg. This is in contrast with metabolic acidosis, where a reduction in plasma bicarbonate is always associated with a marked reduction in p_{CO_2}.

EFFECTS OF METABOLIC ALKALOSIS

Metabolic alkalosis affects the central nervous system in a variety of ways. Cerebral blood flow decreases, although not to the extent seen with respiratory alkalosis. Lethargy and confusion occurs, and if the alkalemia is severe, coma and seizures may result. Metabolic alkalosis decreases the respiratory center, decreasing the drive for ventilation; it also blunts the respiratory response to p_{CO_2}. While alveolar hypoventilation is usually not a problem in normal individuals, it may be a substantial problem in the patient with chronic pulmonary disease. In acute metabolic alkalosis, oxygen affinity increases (Bohr effect) for all tissues, worsening the already compromised cerebral hypoxia. With chronic alkalosis, erythrocyte 2, 3-diphosphoglycerate levels increase, tending to overcome the Bohr effect.

Neuromuscular irritability occurs in metabolic alkalosis and is manifested by muscle twitching, spasm, and tetany. A positive Chvostek's and Trousseau's sign are usually easily elicited and are thought to be related to the decreased ionizable calcium universally seen with alkalemia (metabolic and respiratory). High blood pH increases the protein binding of calcium, thus reducing the ionized calcium in the extracellular fluid. This is exacerbated by the hypomagnesemia seen in virtually all patients with metabolic alkalosis. Additionally, intracellular calcium may be decreased, although whether the mechanisms are purely the result of a chemical interaction or are in part hormonal is not known. An alkaline pH decreases aldosterone release in response to angiotensin II in perfused bovine adrenal glands, and the response to norepinephrine is reduced in the isolated turtle heart when perfused at pH 8 (112, 113). The mechanisms for at least part of these findings is likely to be related to an altered cytosolic calcium.

The effects of metabolic alkalosis on cardiac function in humans is not well understood. A small positive inotropic effect probably occurs in acute metabolic alkalosis, but this is also associated with a decrease in peripheral vascular resistance. In vitro the inotropic response to norepinephrine is reduced with high (and low) pH. Electrocardiographic changes reported with metabolic alkalosis include Q-T prolongation, U waves, and atrial and ventricular arrhythmias. The arrhythmias are more severe in patients on digitalis and may be the result of the hypokalemia.

Hypomagnesemia and hypokalemia frequently coexist with metabolic alkalosis (114, 115). Both of these cations are predominately intracellular, and with chronic alkalosis the low plasma values usually are reflected by low tissue levels. Hypokalemia is associated with abnormalities in the electrical properties of the heart and muscle; there is a decrease in muscle blood flow due to vasoconstriction, and abnormal responses to a variety of hormones and drugs occur. Hypokalemia causes a concentrating defect in the kidney. Hypomagnesemia worsens the kaliuresis, thus metabolic alkalosis may be associated with profound deficiencies of these important intracellular cations. The effect of magnesium deficiency is less well understood, but the ion is an ubiquitous part of all intracellular and membrane-bound ATPases. Na-K-ATPase (as well as Ca-ATPase and H^+-ATPase) depends upon magnesium and, if cellular levels fall, a variety of abnormal transport processes could result. Defects in the membrane potential alone would alter the function of excitable tissues (i.e., heart, skeletal muscle, and nerves) and nonexcitable tissues as well. The requirement of the Na-K-ATPase for magnesium has a K_m of 0.8–1.2 mM; under normal conditions the intracellular free magnesium concentration varies from 0.2 to 3.0 mM, with the highest concentration being found in heart. Magnesium may effect non-ATP-dependent transporters as well. Magnesium increases the activity of calcium-stimulated K channels; its absence presumably does the reverse. In many studies, magnesium depletion increases the tissue calcium concentration, an ion important as a "second messenger" in a variety of hormonal and nonhormonally mediated events.

THERAPY OF METABOLIC ALKALOSIS

Once the pathophysiology of the type of metabolic alkalosis is delineated, the treatment is simple. If volume contraction is the underlying mechanism, it should be restored to normal. Potassium and magnesium deficits should be corrected. If primary mineralcorticoid excess is present, it may be antagonized with spironolactone (200–400 mg/day) prior to definitive therapy.

Acid administration, carbonic anhydrase inhibition, and hemodialysis using an acid bath are techniques that may be used on rare occasions to treat metabolic alkalosis. In the patient with posthypercapnic metabolic alkalosis, pulmonary disease, and lethargy, 250 mg acetazolamide should result in a prompt bicarbonate diuresis if the volume status is normal. Often, however, this is precisely the patient who may have contraction of "effective" arterial volume due to congestive heart failure, and in such a circumstance the effect of this proximally acting diuretic may be blunted.

Infusion of a dilute soluton of hydrochloric acid (NH_4Cl or arginine hydroclroide) into a large central vein may be accomplished over an 18- to 24-hour period if the volume administered will not compromise cardiovascular function. NH_4Cl is absolutely contraindicated in the patient with hepatic failure, as it increases blood ammonia levels and may precipitate hepatic encephalopathy. Arginine and NH_4Cl will worsen the azotemia in patients with renal insufficiency, and arginine alone causes large shifts of potassium out of cells, regardless of any existing acid-base abnormalities. In the potassium-depleted patient, as virtually all of these patients are, small potassium shifts may lead to life-threatening cardiac arrhythmias, respiratory paralysis, and death.

If hydrochloric acid infusion is indicated, the concentration prepared by the pharmacy is 100–200 mEq/l. To calculate the amount needed, an initial estimate assumes that the acid is distributed only in the extracellular space (i.e., 20% body weight). This underestimates the amount, as the true space is approximately 50% of body weight. Careful titration of the blood with frequent measurements of pH and p_{CO_2} is mandatory. In the patient with renal failure or in a patient in whom the fluid status is precarious, dialysis against a high-chloride/low-bicarbonate bath may be indicated. While peritoneal dialysis or hemodialysis may be performed, hemodialysis probably allows the more precise regulation of fluids. Again, careful attention to blood pH and p_{CO_2} is necessary.

The therapeutic modalities just described (i.e., acid infusion or dialysis and carbonic anhydrase inhibitors) have very specific and limited indications, and may be very hazardous when improperly applied. Their use should be reserved for the physician who is expert in the management of renal disease in general and acid-base disturbances in particular.

ACKNOWLEDGMENTS

This work was supported in part by grants from the National Institutes of Health, #RO1-DK-36119 and RO1-DK-36199. Dr. Sabatini is the recipient of a Research Career Development Award, #K04-DK01527.

The excellent typographical and editorial assistance of Ms. Sondra Rogers is greatly appreciated.

REFERENCES

1. Alpern RJ, Warnock DG, Rector FC: Renal acidification mechanisms. In: BM Brenner, FC Rector Jr, eds, *The Kidney*, 3rd ed. WB Saunders, Philadelphia, p 206, 1986.
2. Sabatini S, Kurtzman NA: Overall renal regulation. In: DW Seldon, G Giebisch, eds, *Regulation of Acid-Base Balance*. Raven Press, New York, in press, 1988.
3. Chan YL, Giebisch G: The relationship between sodium and bicarbonate ion transport in the rat proximal convoluted tubule. *Am J Physiol* 240:F222, 1981.
4. Bichara M, Paillard M, Leirel F, Gardin JP: Hydrogen ion transport and acidification in rat proximal convoluted tubules: Na/H exchange. *Am J Physiol* 238:F445, 1980.
5. Akiba T, Rocco VK, Warnock DG: Parallel adaptation of rabbit renal cortical Na/H antiporter and Na/HCO$_3$ cotransporter in metabolic acidosis and alkalosis. *J Clin Invest* 80:308, 1987.
6. Kurtz I: Apical Na/H antiporter and glycolysis dependent H-ATPase regulate intracellular pH in rabbit S$_3$ proximal tubule. *J Clin Invest* 80:928–935, 1987.
7. Sabatini S, Kurtzman NA: Proton ATPase activity along the rat nephron. *Clin Res* 35:663A, 1987.
8. Ait-Mohammed AK, Marsay S, Barlet C, Khadouriz C, Doucet A: Characterization of N-ethylmaleimide-sensitive proton pump in rat kidney. *J Biol Chem* 261:12526, 1986.
9. Sabolic I, Burchard R: Characteristics of the proton pump in rat renal cortical endocytic vesicles. *Am J Physiol* 250:F818, 1986.
10. Kinne-Saffran E, Kinne R: Proton pump activity and Mg-ATPase activity in rat kidney cortex brush border membranes: Effect of proton "ATPase" inhibitors. *Pflügers Arch* 407:180, 1986.
11. Wistrand PJ, Kinne R: Carbonic anhydrase activity of isolated brush-border and basal-lateral membranes of renal tubular cells. *Pflügers Arch* 370:121, 1977.
12. Lönnerholm G, Ridderstrale Y: Intracellular distribution of carbonic anhydrase in the rat kidney. *Kidney Int* 17:162, 1980.
13. Malnic G, de Mello-Aires M: Kinetics of bicarbonate reabsorption in proximal tubule of the rat. *Am J Physiol* 220:1759, 1971.
14. Costa-Silva VL, Campiglia SS, de Mello-Aires M, Giebisch G: Role of luminal buffers in renal tubuar acidification. *J Mem Biol* 63:13, 1981.
15. Skou JC: Enzymatic basis for active transport of Na$^+$ and K$^+$ across cell membranes. *Physiol Rev* 45:596, 1965.
16. Glynn IM, Karlish SJD: The sodium pump. *Ann Rev Physiol* 37:13, 1975.
17. Kinne R, Schmitz JE, Kinne-Saffran E: The localization of the Na$^+$-K$^+$ ATPase in the cells of the rat kidney cortex. *Pflügers Arch* 329:191, 1971.
18. Sabatini S, Kurtzman NA: The maintenance of metabolic alkalosis: Factors which decrease bicarbonate excretion. *Kidney Int* 25:357, 1984.
19. Kurtzman NA: Regulation of renal bicarbonate reabsorption by extracellular volume. *J Clin Invest* 49:586, 1970.
20. Pitts RF, Lotspeich WD: Bicarbonate and the renal regulation of acid-base balance. *Am J Physiol* 147:138, 1946.
21. Pitts RF, Ayer JL, Schiess WA: The renal regulation of acid-base balance in man. III. The reabsorption and excretion of bicarbonate. *J Clin Invest* 28:35, 1949.
22. Kassirer JP, Schwartz WB: The response of normal man to selective depletion of hydrochloric acid. Factors in the genesis of persistent gastric alkalosis. *Am J Med* 40:10, 1966.
23. Schwartz WB, Van Ypersele de Striou C, Kassiere JP: Role of anions in metabolic alkalosis and potassium deficiency. *N Engl J Med* 279:630, 1968.
24. Langberg H, Mathisen O, Holdaas H, Kiil F: Filtered bicarbonate and plasma pH as determinants of renal bicarbonate reabsorption. *Kidney Int* 20:780, 1981.
25. Cogan MG, Maddox DAL. Lucci MS, Rector FC Jr: Control of proximal bicarbonate reabsorption in normal and acidotic rats. *J Clin Invest* 64:1168, 1979.
26. Berry CA, Cogan MA: Influence of peritubular protein on solute absorption in the rabbit proximal tubule. *J Clin Invest* 68:506, 1981.
27. Cohen JJ: Selective Cl retention in repair of metabolic alkalosis without increasing filtered load. *Am J Physiol* 218:165, 1970.
28. Kurtzman NA: Relationship of extracellular volume and CO$_2$ tension to renal bicarbonate reabsorption. *Am J Physiol* 219:1299, 1970.
29. Maren TH: Current status of membrane bound carbonic anhydrase. *Ann NY Acad Sci* 341:246, 1980.
30. Cogan MG, Maddox DA, Warnock DG, Lin ET, Rector FC: Effect of acetazolamide on bicarbonate reabsorption in the proximal tubule of the rat. *Am J Physiol* 237:F447, 1979.
31. Lucci MS, Warnock DG, Rector FC Jr: Carbonic anhydrase-dependent bicarbonate reabsorption in the rat proximal tubule. *Am J Physiol* 236:F58, 1979.
32. Frommer JP, Laski ME, Wesson DE, Kurtzman NA: Internephron heterogeneity for carbonic anhydrase-independent bicarbonate reabsorption in the rat. *J Clin Invest* 73:1034, 1984.

33. Cruz–Soto M, Frommer JP, Itsarayoungyuen K, Batlle DC, Arruda JAL, Kurtzman NA: Carbonic anhydrase-independent bicarbonate reabsorption in rats with chronic papillary necrosis. *Min Elect Metab* 10:319, 1984.
34. Laski ME, Kurtzman NA: Characterization of acidification in the cortical and medullary collecting tubule of the rabbit. *J Clin Invest* 72:2050, 1983.
35. Sabatini S, Kurtzman NA: The profile of H-ATPase activity in rat nephron after chronic metabolic aicdosis. *Clin Res* 36:46, 1988.
36. McKinney TD, Burg MB: Bicarbonate absorption by rabbit cortical collecting tubules in vitro. *Am J Physiol* 234(2):141, 1978.
37. Schwartz JH, Rosen S, Steinmetz PR: Carbonic anhydrase function and the epithelial organization of H^+ secretion in turtle urinary bladder. *J Clin Invest* 51:2653, 1972.
38. Sabatini S, Kurtzman NA: Evidence for voltage regulation of carbonic anhydrase independent acidification in the turtle bladder. *Min Elect Metab* 11:277, 1985.
39. Rubinstein H, Batlle DC, Roseman MK, Sehy JT, Arruda JAL, Kurtzman NA: Urinary p_{CO_2} during carbonic anhydrase inhibition *Min Elect Metab* 5:49, 1981.
40. Arruda JAL, Subbarayudu K, Dytko G, Mola R, Kurtzman NA: Voltage dependent distal acidification defect induced by amiloride. *J Lab Clin Med* 95:407, 1980.
41. Fuller GR, MacLeod MB, Pitts RF: Influence of administration of potassium salts on the renal tubular reabsorption of bicarbonate. *Am J Physiol* 182:111, 1955.
42. Kurtzman NA, White MG, Rogers PW: The effect of potassium and extracellular volume on renal bicarbonate reabsorption. *Metabolism* 22:481, 1973.
43. Kunau RT, Frick A, Rector FC, Seldin DW: Micropuncture study of the proximal tubular factors responsible for the maintenance of metabolic alkalosis during potassium deficiency in the rat. *Clin Sci* 34:223, 1968.
44. Chan YL, Biagi B, Giebisch G: Control mechanisms of bicarbonate transport across rat proximal convoluted tubule. *Am J Physiol* 242:F532, 1982.
45. Steinbaugh B, Schloeder FX: Glucose-induced alkalosis in fasting subjects. *J Clin Invest* 51:1326, 1972.
46. Suki WN, Herbert CS, Steinbaugh B, Martinez–Maldonado M, Eknoyan G: Effects of glucose on bicarbonate reabsorption in the dog kidney. *J Clin Invest* 54:1, 1974.
47. Garrett ES, Nahmias C: The effect of glucose on the urinary excretion of sodium and hydrogen ion in man. *Clin Sci Mol Biol* 47:589, 1974.
48. Crumb CK, Martinez–Maldonado M, Eknoyan G, Suki WN: Effects of volume expansion, purified parathyroid extract and calcium on renal bicarbonate absorption in the dog. *J Clin Invest* 54:1287, 1974.
49. Karlinsky ML, Sager DS, Kurtzman NA, Pillay VKG: Effect of parathormone and cyclic adenosine monophosphate on renal bicarbonate reabsorption. *Am J Physiol* 227:1226, 1974.
51. Hulter HN, Peterson JC: Acid-base homeostasis during chronic PTH excess in humans. *Kidney Int* 28:187, 1985.
52. Hulter HN: Effects and interrelationships of PTH, Ca, vitamin D, and Pi in acid-base homeostasis. *Am J Physiol* 248:F739, 1985.
53. Gold LS, Massry SG, Arieff AI, Coburn JW: Renal bicarbonate wasting during phosphate depletion. *J Clin Invest* 52:2556, 1973.
54. Siegfried D, Kumar R, Arruda JAL, Kurtzman NA: Influence of vitamin D on bicarbonate reabsorption. In: Massry SG, Ritz E, eds, *Phosphate Metabolism*. Plenum Press, New York, p 395, 1978.
55. Kurtzman NA, White MG, Rogers PW: Aldosterone deficiency and renal bicarbonate reabsorption. *J Lab Clin Med* 77:931, 1971.
56. Lynche RE, Schneider ES, Willis LR, Knox FS: Absence of mineralocorticoid-dependent sodium reabsorption in dog proximal tubule. *Am J Physiol* 223:40, 1972.
57. Muryama Y, Suki A, Tadoro M, Sakai F: Microperfusion of Henle's loop in the kidney of the adrenalectomized rat. *J Pharm Pharmacol* 18:518, 1968.
58. Farman N, Vandewalle A, Bonvalet JP: Aldosterone binding in isolated tubules. Biochemical determination in proximal and distal parts of the rabbit nephron. *Am J Physiol* 242:F63, 1982.
59. Farman N, Vandewalle A, Bonvalet JP: An autoradiographic study of concentration dependency in the rabbit nephron. *Am J Physiol* 242:F69, 1982.
60. Kurtzman NA, White MG, Rogers PW: Pathophysiology of metabolic alkalosis. *Arch Intern Med* 131:702, 1973.
61. Batlle DC, Kurtzman NA: Acid-base physiology and pathophysiology. *Contemp Nephrol* 3:191, 1985.
62. Mujais SK: Effects of aldosterone on rat collecting tubule N-ethylmaleimide-sensitive adenosine triphosphatase. *J Lab Clin Med* 109:34, 1987.
63. Stone DK, Seldin DW, Kokko JP, Jacobson HR: Mineralocorticoid modulation of rabbit medullary collecting duct acidification. *J Clin Invest* 72:77, 1983.
64. Kurtzman NA: Ammonia secretion and urinary acidification. *Semin Nephrol* 2:1, 1982.
65. Arruda JAL, Dytko G, Withers L: Ammonia transport by the turtle urinary bladder. *Am J Physiol* 246:F569, 1984.
66. Tannen RL: The effect of uncomplicated potassium depletion on urine acidification. *J Clin Invest* 49:813, 1970.
67. Sastrasinh S, Tannen RL: Effect of potassium on renal NH_3 production. *Am J Physiol* 244:F383, 1983.
68. Kornandakieti C, Tannen RL: Hydrogen ion secretion by the distal nephron in the rat: Effect of potassium. *J Lab Clin Med* 104:293, 1984.
69. Batlle DC, Sehy JT, Roseman MK, Arruda JAL, Kurtzman NA: Clinical and pathophysiological spectrum of acquired distal renal tubular acidosis. *Kidney Int* 20:389, 1981.
70. Better OS, Goldschmidz, Chaimowitz D, Alroy GG: Defect in urinary acidification in cirrhosis: The role of excessive tubular reabsorption of sodium in its etiology. *Arch Intern Med* 130:77, 1972.
71. Giammarco RA, Goldstein MB, Halperin ML, Stinebaugh BJ: The effect of hyperventilation on distal nephron hydrogen ion secretion. *J Clin Invest* 58:77, 1976.
72. Batlle DC, Schlueter W, Gutterman C, Kurtzman NA: Assessment of collecting tubule hydrogen ion secretion in acute respiratory alkalsis using the urinary p_{CO_2}. *Pflugers Arch* 411:692, 1988.
73. Batlle DC, Arruda JAL, Kurtzman NA: Hyperkalemic distal renal tubular acidosis associated with obstructive uropathy. *N Engl J Med* 304:373, 1981.
74. Batlle DC, Itsarayoungyuen K, Arruda JAL, Kurtzman NA: Hyperkalemic hyperchloremic metabolic acidosis in sickle cell hemoglobinopathies. *Am J Med* 72:188, 1982.
75. Batlle DC, Kurtzman NA: Distal renal tubular acidosis: Pathogenesis and classification. *Am J Kidney Dis* 1:328, 1982.
76. Schambelan M, Sebastian A, Rector FC Jr: Mineralocorticoid-resistant renal hyperkalemia without salt wasting (type II pseudohypoaldosteronism): Role of increased renal chloride reabsorption. *Kidney Int* 19:716, 1981.

77. Arruda JAL, Julka NK, Rubenstein H, Sabatini S, Kurtzman NA: Distal acidification defect induced by phosphate deprivation. *Metabolism* 29:826, 1980.
78. Arruda JAL, Julka NK, Rubinstein H, Cruz-Soto M, Sabatini S, Batlle DC, Kurtzman NA: Parathyroid hormone and extrarenal acid-base buffering. *Am J Physiol* 239:533, 1980.
79. Hulter HN, Ilnicki L, Harbottle J, Sebastian A: Impaired renal H^+ secretion and ammonia production in mineralocorticoid-deficient glucocorticoid-replete dogs. *Am J Physiol* 232:F136, 1977.
80. Batlle DC: Hyperkalemic hyperchloremic metabolic acidosis associated with selective aldosterone deficiency and distal renal tubular acidosis. *Semin Nephrol* 1:260, 1981.
81. Tannen RL: Relationship of renal ammonia production and potassium homeostasis. *Kidney Int* 11:453, 1977.
82. Tannen RL, McGill J: The influence of potassium on renal ammonia production. *Am J Physiol* 231:1178, 1976.
83. Tannen RL, Kunin SA: Effect of potassium on ammoniagenesis by renal mitochondria. *Am J Physiol* 231:44, 1976.
84. Al-Awqati Q, Norby LH, Mueller A, Steinmetz PR: Characteristics of stimulation of H^+ transport by aldosterone in turtle urinary bladder. *J Clin Invest* 58:351, 1976.
85. DiTella PJ, Sodhi B, McCreary J, Arruda JAL, Kurtzman NA: Mechanism of the metabolic acidosis of selective mineralocorticoid deficiency. *Kidney Int* 14:466, 1978.
86. Sebastian A, Sutton JM, Hulter HN: Effect of mineralocorticoid replacement therapy on renal acid-base homeostasis in adrenalectomized patients. *Kidney Int* 18:762, 1981.
87. Vinay P, Allignet E, Pichette C, Watford M, Lemieux G, Gougoux A: Changes in renal metabolite profile and ammoniagenesis during acute and chronic metabolic acidosis in dog and rat. *Kidney Int* 17:312, 1980.
88. Fraley DS, Adler S: An extrarenal role for parathyroid hormone in the disposal of acute acid loads in rats and dogs. *J Clin Invest* 63:985, 1979.
89. Arruda JAL, Alla V, Rubinstein H, Cruz-Soto M, Sabatini S, Batlle D, Kurtzman NA: Metabolic and hormonal factors influencing extrarenal buffering of an acute acid load. *Min Elect Metab* 8:36, 1982.
90. Hulter H, Sebastian A, Toto RD, Bonner EL, Ilnicki LP: Renal and systemic acid-base effects of chronic hypercalcemia-producing agents: Calcitriol, PTH and intravenous calcium. *Kidney Int* 21:445, 1982.
91. Mitinick P, Greenburg A, Coffman T, Kelepauris E, Wolf CT, Gadfare S: Effects of two models of hypercalcemia on renal acid base metabolism. *Kidney Int* 21:613, 1982.
92. Jacobson HR, Seldin DW: On the generation, maintenance and correction of metabolic alkalosis. *Am J Physiol* 245:F425, 1983.
93. Cogan MG: Atrial natriuretic factor ameliorates chronic metabolic alkalosis by increasing glomerular filtration. *Science* 229:1405, 1985.
94. Linas SL, Dickmain D: Mechanism of the decreased renal blood flow in the potassium-depleted conscious rat. *Kidney Int* 21:757, 1982.
95. Cogan MG, Liu FY: Metabolic alkalosis in the rat: Evidence that reduced glomerular filtration rather than enhanced tubular bicarbonate reabsorption is responsible for maintaining the alkalotic state. *J Clin Invest* 7:1141, 1983.
96. Abboud HE, Luke RG, Galla JH, Kotchen TA: Stimulation of renin by acute selective chloride depletion. *Circ Res* 44:815, 1979.
97. Kotchen TC, Guthrie GP, Boucher LD, Lorenz JN, Oh CE: Disassociation between plasma renin and plasma aldosterone induced by dietary glycine hydrochloride. *Am J Physiol* 254:E187, 1988.
98. Galla JL, Bonduris DN, Dumbald SL, Luke RG: Segmental chloride and fluid handling during corrections of chloride-depletion alkalosis in the rat. *J Clin Invest* 73:96, 1984.
99. Galla JH, Luke RG: Effect of chloride and extracellular fluid volume on bicarbonate reabsorption along the nephron in metabolic alkalosis in the rat: A reassessment of the classical hypothesis of the maintenance of metabolic alkalosis. *J Clin Invest* 80:41, 1987.
100. Craig DM, Galla JH, Bonduris DN, Luke RG: Importance of the kidney in the correction of chloride-depletion alkalosis in the rat. *Am J Physiol* 250:F54, 1986.
101. Alpern R, Cogan M, Rector FC: Effect of luminal bicarbonate concentration on proximal acidification in the rat. *Am J Physiol* 243:F53, 1982.
102. Cogan MG, Liu FY: Metabolic alkalosis in the rat. *J Clin Invest* 71:1124, 1983.
103. Stokes JB, Ingram MJ, Williams AD, Ingram D: Heterogeneity of the rabbit collecting tubule: Localization of mineralocorticoid hormone action to the cortical portion. *Kidney Int* 20:340, 1981.
104. Seldin DW, Welt LG, Cort JH: The role of sodium salts and adrenal steroids in the production of hypokalemic alkalosis. *Yale J Biol Med* 29:229, 1956.
105. Bondy PK: Disorders of the adrenal cortex. In: JD Wilson, DW Foster, eds, *Textbook of Endocrinology*, 7th ed. WB Saunders, Philadelphia, p 816, 1985.
106. Liddle GW, Bledsoe T, Coppage WS: A familial renal disorder simulating primary aldosteronism but with negligible aldosterone secretion. *Trans Assoc Am Phys* 76:188, 1963.
107. Cannon PJ, Heineman HO, Alber MS, Laragh JL, Winters RW: 'Contraction' alkalosis after diuresis of edematous patients with ethacrynic acid. *Ann Intern Med* 62:979, 1965.
108. Kurtzman NA, Gutierrez LF: The pathophysiology of Bartter's syndrome. *JAMA* 234:758, 1975.
109. Gill JR, Bartter FC: Evidence for a prostaglandin independent defect in chloride reabsorption in the loop of Henle as a proximal cause of Bartter's syndrome. *Am J Med* 65:766, 1978.
110. Carrow DC: Congenital alkalosis with diarrhea. *J Ped* 26:519, 1945.
111. Evansen TM, Stanbury SW: Congenital chloridorrhea or so-called congenital alkalosis with diarrhea. *Gut* 6:29, 1965.
112. Carrel JE, Landry AS, Elliot ME, Goodfriend D: Effect of pH on adrenal angiotensin receptors and responses. *J Lab Clin Med* 108:23, 1986.
113. Sabatini S, Barboriak JJ, Hardman HF: Utilitzation of glucose in the anaerobically perfused turtle heart. *J Pharmacol Exp Ther* 155:395, 1967.
114. See Chapter 4, this edition.
115. See Chapter 6. this edition
116. Seldin Dw, Rector FC: The generation and maintenance of metabolic alkalosis. *Kidney Int* 1:306, 1972.

CHAPTER 10

Metabolic Acidosis

ROBERT M.A. RICHARDSON & MITCHELL L. HALPERIN

INTRODUCTION

Of all the acid-basic disorders, metabolic acidosis is the one most likely to be associated with serious morbidity or even death. Examples are the lactic acidosis of shock states and servere acidosis associated with methanol or ethylene glycol poisoning; these require urgent therapy to prevent a fatal outcome. On the other hand, metabolic acidosis may be mild, chronic, and of little immediate clinical consequence. Examples include certain types of renal tubular acidosis (RTA) or chronic diarrhea.

The therapy for metabolic acidosis will be determined in part by the severity of the acidosis and the rapidity of its development. A number of other factors must be be considered with respect to therapy, including the potassium status, the degree of respiratory compensation, the potential for rapid reversal of the acidosis, and specific treatment directed at the underlying cause. While some broad generalizations with regard to alkali therapy may be made, the use of alkali and other treatment modalities are best discussed with reference to each specific disorder. In this chapter, we shall briefly review the pathogenesis of and the diagnostic approach to metabolic acidosis, provide some general principles of treatment, and then discuss individual disorders separately.

METABOLIC ACIDOSIS: PATHOGENESIS AND DIAGNOSTIC APPROACH

Metabolic acidosis is caused by acid gain or sodium bicarbonate loss. Both result in a rise in Blood [H^+] (a fall in pH), and a fall in the plasma bicarbonate concentration. The causes are listed in Table 1. Since metabolic acidosis is not a specific diagnosis, the underlying cause must be accurately determined in order to provide optimal therapy.

Acid overproduction from endogenous sources (lactic, ketoacidosis), intoxications (methanol, ethylene glycol, or salicylate), or failure to generate "new" bicarbonate in the kidney because of renal failure will all cause metabolic acidosis in association with an increased plasma anion gap. In contrast, renal or gastrointestinal sodium bicarbonate loss and failure of renal new bicarbonate generation with a normal or near normal glomerular filtration rate (GFR) will all cause metabolic acidosis with a normal plasma anion gap. Therefore calculation of the plasma anion gap is the most important step to determine the pathogenesis of metabolic acidosis (1–3) (Figure 1).

The plasma anion gap has therapeutic as well as diagnostic implications. An elevated plasma anion gap may indicate the presence of an organic anion, which can be metabolized to produce bicarbonate. An example is β-hydroxybutyrate in ketoacidosis (Equation 1). Furthermore, the magnitude of the elevation of the plasma anion gap in that situation can provide a semiquantitative estimate of how much bicarbonate will be generated with treatment of the underlying disorder. These aspects will be discussed in more detail later.

The initial diagnostic pathway for determining the cause

Table 1. Etiology of metabolic acidosis

1. *With an increased plasma anion gap*
   a. *Endogenous acid overproduction*
      Lactic acidosis (hypoxia)
      Ketoacidosis (insulin lack)
      D-lactic acidosis (altered gut flora and/or transit time)
   b. *Exogenous intoxications*
      Methyl alcohol (methanol)
      Ethylene glycol
      Salicylate
      Paraldehyde
   c. *Failure of renal new bicarbonate generation (very low GFR)*
      Renal failure (low GFR)
2. *With a normal plasma anion gap*
   a. *Gastrointestinal bicarbonate loss*
      Diarrhea, ileus, fistula drainage, T-tube drainage, villous adenoma, ileal conduit
   b. *Urine bicarbonate loss*
      Proximal renal tubular acidosis
      Carbonic anhydrase inhibitors
   c. *Failure of renal new bicarbonate generation (GFR not very low)*
      Low distal H^+ secretion
      Low NH_3 availability
         Hyperkalemia
         Medullary interstitial disease
   d. *Acid production with urinary organic anion loss (see Figure 6)*

178 Therapy of Renal Diseases and Related Disorders

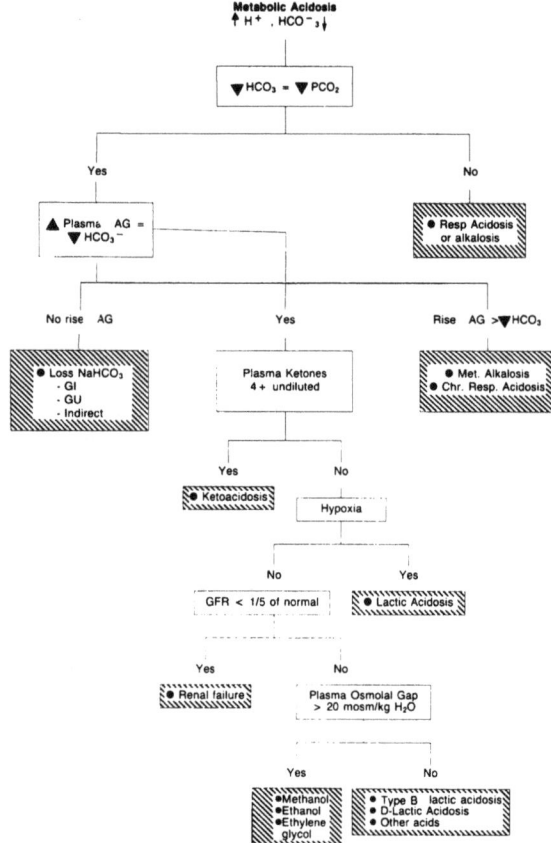

Figure 1. Approach to patients with metabolic acidosis. Metabolic acidosis is present when there is a rise in plasma [H$^+$] and a fall in bicarbonate concentration. The degree is respiratory response is first assessed by comparing the fall in P$_{CO_2}$ from 40 mmHg to the fall in [HCO$_3^-$] from 25 mM; these falls should be almost equal. The basis of the acidosis (acid addition vs. NaHCO$_3$ loss) is then determined by comparing the rise in the plasma anion gap to the fall in the plasma [HCO$_3^-$]; more detailed flow sheets appear in Figures 2–4. Solid triangles represent change from normal values. Reprinted with permisssion from the authors: Halperin ML, Goldstein MB: *Fluid, Electrolyte, and Acid-Base Emergencies.* WB Saunders, Philadelphia, 1988.

of metabolic acidosis is shown in Figure 1. If the plasma anion gap is increased, and the cause for this elevation is unclear from clinical examination and routine laboratory investigation, the plasma osmolal gap (7) should be determined by the following formula:

Plasma osmolal gap = Measured osmolality
– [(2X plasma [Na])
+ blood glucose (mg/dl)/18
+ BUN (mg/dl)/2.8].

If SI units are used,

Plasma osmolal gap = Measured osmolality
– [(2X plasma [Na])
+ blood glucose (mM) and urea (mM)].

A plasma osmolal gap of more than 20 mOsm/kg H$_2$O indicates the presence of a significant quantity of an unmeasured solute such as ethanol, methanol, or ethylene glycol, which could be confirmed with specific assays. A value less than 10 mOsm/kg H$_2$O would fit with lactic acidosis, ketoacidosis, renal failure, or salicylate intoxication. Measurement of plasma salicylate, glucose, ketones, creatinine, and lactate would assist in the diagnosis, depending on the clinical context (see Figure 2 for approach to wide anion gap types of metabolic acidosis).

If the plasma anion gap is normal, the diagnosis is metabolic acidosis of the sodium bicarbonate loss type (Figure 3). Its etiology can be ascertained by measuring urinary bicarbonate and ammonium excretion rates (4). Urine ammonium should be high if the cause of the acidosis is gastrointestinal bicarbonate loss or previous renal bicarbonate loss, and not high if the metabolic acidosis is of renal origin. Details of the interpretation of the urine "net charge" as an index of urine ammonium excretion rate are given in Goldstein et al. (5) and Appendix 1. The finding of a low urine ammonium then leads to the diagnosis of *RTA* and a second category (Figure 4) in which renal acidification disorders are identified. A third category for the plasma anion gap is called a *hybrid* (Figure 5). In this case the plasma anion gap is elevated, but the increase in the plasma anion gap above normal is significantly less than the fall in the plasma bicarbonate concentration from normal. In this setting, the urine "net charge" is used to estimate urine ammonium excretion, and therefore the renal contribution to acidosis could be misleading, because one possible explanation for this hybrid is ketoacidosis with loss of the anion (primarily β-hydroxybutyrate) in the

Table 2. Rationale and modes of therapy in metabolic acidosis

A. *Questions concerning NaHCO$_3$ therapy in metabolic acidosis*
1. What is the rate of H$^+$ production?
2. Can this augmented rate of H$^+$ production be diminished?
3. How severe is the metabolic acidosis?
4. Is the respiratory response adequate?
5. Can the patient make bicarbonate quickly?
6. What is the plasma potassium concentration?

B. *Modes of therapy*
1. Stop H$^+$ production
    Oxygen delivery for type A lactic acidosis, insulin for DKA, ethanol for methanol, or ethylene glycol intoxication
2. High leverage to change blood [H$^+$]
    Ventilation if P$_{CO_2}$ too high
    Reexpand circulating volume if this is the cause for tissue hypoxia
3. Ensure patient does not get worse
    Specific measures (see #1)
    Can buy time during very severe acidosis by giving sodium bicarbonate
    Replace bicarbonate deficit especially if:
        Sodium bicarbonate loss caused the acidosis
        Low NH$_4^+$ excretion
    Additional role of bicarbonate
        excrete ASA$^-$ anion in alkaline urine

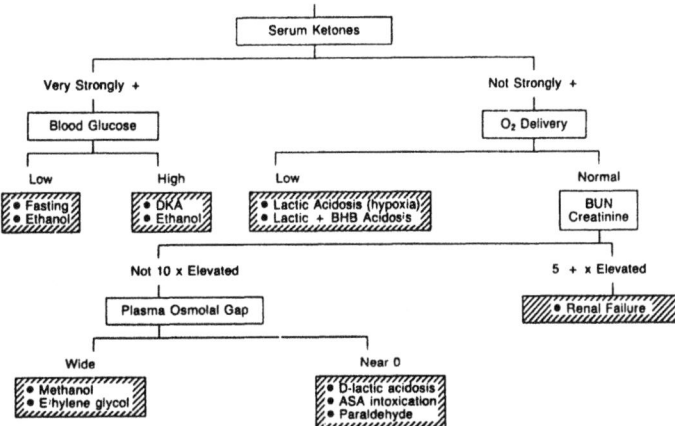

Figure 2. Approach to the patient with metabolic acidosis and a wide plasma anion gap. Parameters to assess are shown in the open boxes and diagnostic categories are shown in the hatched boxes. For more discussion, see text and references 1–3. BHB = B-hydroxybutyrate, DKA = diabetic ketoacidosis, ASA = acetosalicylate. Reprinted with permission from the authors: Halperin ML, Goldstein WB: *Fluid, electrolyte, and Acid-Base Emergencies.* WB Saunders, Philadelphia, 1988.

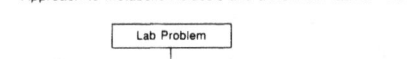

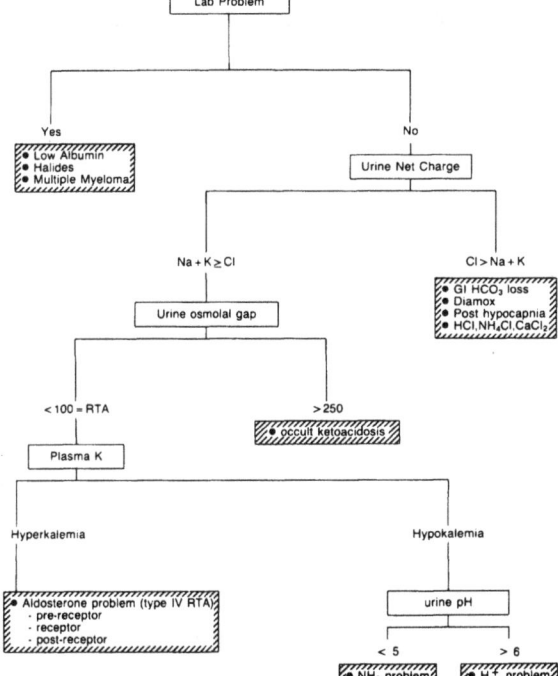

Figure 3. Approach to patients with metabolic acidosis and a normal plasma anion gap. For details, see legend to Figure 2 and the text. The urine net charge is discussed in Appendix 1 and the urine osmolal gap in Appendix 2. The approach to renal tubular acidosis is shown in Figure 4. Reprinted with permission from the authors: Halperin ML, Goldstein MB: *Fluid, Electrolyte, and Acid-Base Emergencies.* WB Saunders, Philadelphia, 1988.

urine, reducing the plasma anion gap (Figure 6). The urine ammonium excretion is usually high in this setting, and it can be assessed using the urine osmolal gap [for details see Halperin et al. (6) and Appendix 2].

THERAPY OF METABOLIC ACIDOSIS — GENERAL CONSIDERATIONS (TABLE 2)

Once the cause of the metabolic acidosis is determined, rational therapy can be instituted. The question of whether to give alkali therapy, and how much to give, is certainly important, but other measures to prevent or correct the acidosis can be even more important. In this section, the general principles that govern the treatment of metabolic acidosis will be discussed, including those that apply to exogenous bicarbonate administration. Thus, before discussing alkali treatment, several questions will be considered:

Can H^+ production be stopped?

Consider two patients with severe metabolic acidosis (pH 7.05, plasma $[HCO_3^-]$ 8 mM); one has diabetic ketoacidosis (DKA), the other has severe diarrhea from an ileostomy. Although H^+ production in the patient with DKA is high (may be 100 mmol/hr), it can be arrested with insulin. In contrast, the rate of H^+ production (or $NaHCO_3$ loss) in the patient with diarrhea is likely to be lower, but may not be readily reduced (Table 3). Therefore, alkali therapy might be more urgent in the patient with diarrhea than in the patient with DKA.

In methanol and ethylene glycol poisoning, ongoing H^+ production can be diminished with ethanol administration, which slows metabolism of the toxins to their acid endproducts. In renal failure or RTA, in contrast to all the above

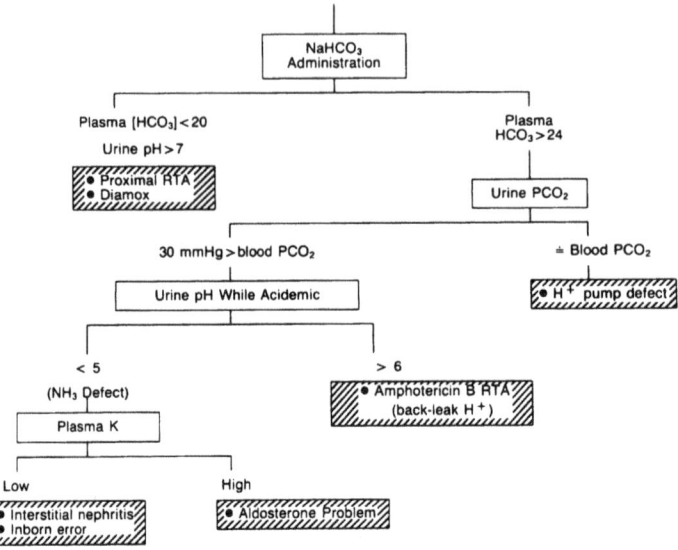

Figure 4. Approach to patients with renal tubular acidosis. For details, see legend to Figure 2. First proximal RTA is ruled out by determining whether bicarbonaturia occurs during acidemia. At this time, examining the urine P_{CO_2} helps identify patients with a defect in distal nephron H^+ secretion (27). While acidemic, patients with distal RTA have a low rate of NH_4^+ excretion (a positive "net charge" in urine electrolytes) (5); those whose urine pH is 5 or less have low NH_3, most commonly due either to hyperkalemia or interstitial renal disease. Reprinted with permission of the authors: Halperin ML, Goldstein MB: *Fluid, Electrolyte, and Acid-Base Emergencies.* WB Saunders, Philadelphia, 1988.

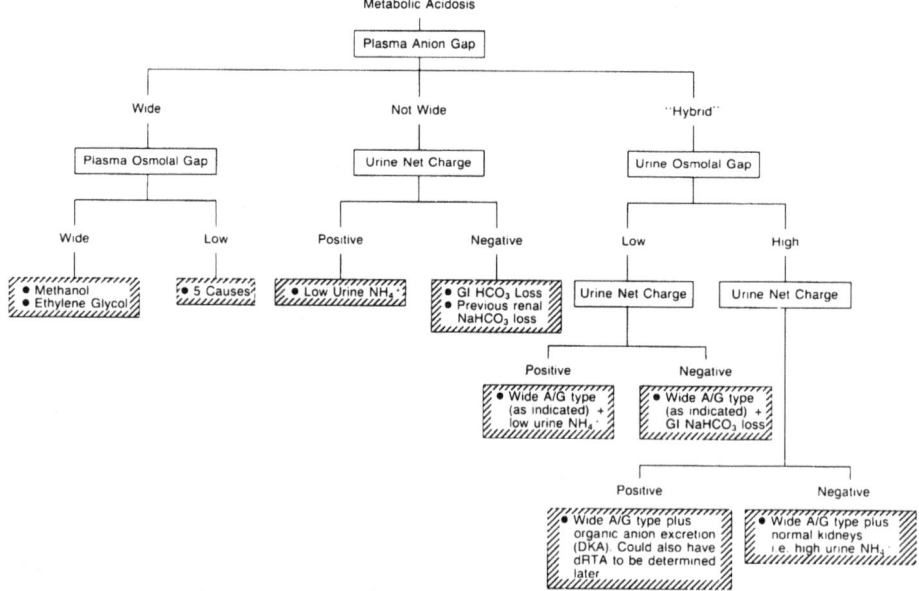

Figure 5. General approach to patients with metabolic acidosis. For details, see legend to Figure 2 and the text. The basis of this approach is to relate the decline in the plasma bicarbonate concentration to the rise in the plasma anion gap. Three main categories of metabolic acidosis could result, simple wide anion gap type (Figure 2), normal anion gap type (Figure 3), and a "hybrid" mixture of these types (i.e., the rise in the plasma anion gap is less than the fall in the plasma bicarbonate concentration). Reprinted with permission of the authors: Halperin ML, Goldstein MB: *Fluid, Electrolyte, and Acid-Base Emergencies.* WB Saunders, 1988.

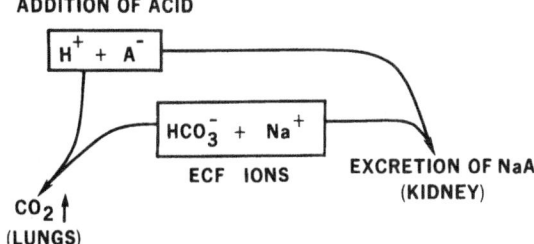

Figure 6. Loss of sodium bicarbonate from the ECF during ketoacidosis. The production of β-hydroxybutyric acid ($H^+ + A^-$) yields metabolic acidosis when $H^+ + A^-$ are retained or A^- without H^+ (or NH_4^+) are excreted. However, the plasma anion gap will not be elevated if the β-hydroxybutyrate anion is excreted in the urine with sodium. Metabolic acidosis persists because the H^+ that are produced are not removed by metabolism of β-hydroxybutyrate to neutral end products (equation 1) and the excretion of β-hydroxybutyrate is not accompanied by the excretion of ammonium. Reprinted with permission from the authors: Halperin ML, Goldstein MB: *Fluid, Electrolyte, and Acid-Base Emergencies.* WB Saunders, Philadelphia, 1988.

examples, the H^+ production rate is only close to 3 mmol/hr (Table 3) and reducing the rate of H^+ production is not important therapeutically.

Is there an organic anion available for metabolism to bicarbonate?

Consider two patients with severe metabolic acidosis (pH 7.05, plasma $[HCO_3^-]$ 8 mM, anion gap 30 mEq/l); one has DKA, the other has methanol poisoning. In the patient with DKA, approximately 18 mM of organic anion (largely β-hydroxybutyrate and acetoacetate) are available for metabolism to neutral end products such as CO_2 and H_2O, thus generating bicarbonate

$$\begin{matrix} CH_3 \\ CHOH \\ CH_2 \\ COO^- \end{matrix} + 4.5O_2 \rightarrow 3CO_2 + 3H_2O + HCO_3^-. \qquad (1)$$

Table 3. Approximate rates of H^+ production during metabolic acidosis. All rates are expressed as mmol H^+/hr. The body can only buffer up to 1000 mmol of retained H^+.

Type of Acidosis	Mechanism	Rate (mmol/hr)
1. RTA or renal failure	Normal H^+ production, but low NH_4^+ excretion	3
2. Diarrhea	$NaHCO_3$ loss	4–20
3. Methanol intoxication	Synthesis of formic acid	40
4. Diabetic ketoacidosis	Synthesis of B-HB due to insulin lack	60
5. D-lactic acidosis	Abnormal gut flora	?
6. L-lactic acidosis	Low O_2 (must involve the liver)	3600 if 100% anoxia

Thus, exogenous bicarbonate therapy might not be necessary or even advisable, providing that an adequate amount of insulin is given. In contrast, the organic anions accumulating in methanol intoxication (formate, lactate) either cannot be metabolized further (formate) or will not be metabolized until the toxic end products of methanol metabolism are removed (lactate). Therefore, exogenous bicarbonate might have to be given to the patient with methanol intoxication.

Is respiratory compensation appropriate?

In metabolic acidosis, the blood P_{CO_2} falls due to hyperventilation mediated by peripheral and central chemoreceptors. The fall in P_{CO_2} from normal is usually 1.0 – 1.3 mm Hg for each 1 mM fall in plasma bicarbonate concentration from normal (25 mM). Thus in patients with metabolic acidosis, the observed P_{CO_2} should be compared with the expected value; if the P_{CO_2} is *higher* than expected, respiratory acidosis is present and the cause should be determined (Figure 1). For example, a higher than expected P_{CO_2} in a comatose patient with methanol intoxication may signal incipient respiratory failure from CNS depression, an obstructed upper airway, or aspiration pneumonia, each requiring specific intervention. It is therapeutically important to identify respiratory acidosis, since the superimposed respiratory disorder can markedly worsen the degree of acidemia (Table 4, example B). In such instances, correcting the cause of the respiratory problem or institution of intubation and assisted ventilation may allow rapid improvement in the degree of acidemia.

What is the plasma potassium concentration?

Metabolic acidosis may be associated with normal, low, or high plasma potassium values, depending on the balance of exogenous potassium administration, renal potassium excretion, gastrointestinal potassium loss, and shifts of potassium across the cell membrane. Clearly exogenous bicarbonate administration is beneficial in hyperkalemic states. It is unlikely to cause immediate problems if the plasma potassium concentration is normal; however, if

Table 4. Impact of small changes in $[HCO_3^-]$ or PCO_2 on the acid-base status of the patient with a plasma $[HCO_3^-]$ of 5 mM

	$[H^+]$ (nM)	pH	P_{CO_2} (mm Hg)	$[HCO_3^-]$ (mM)
A. Stable metabolic acidosis	92	7.04	19	5
B. Small reduction in hyperventilation	144	6.86	30	5
C. Small fall in plasma $[HCO_3^-]$	152	6.82	19	3

Note that the small fall in plasma bicarbonate concentration in C or a slight increase in P_{CO_2} in B converts a modest acidemia into a severe one.

hypokalemia is present, bicarbonate therapy may have to be postponed until severe hypokalemia can be ameliorated. Examples are patients with diarrhea and potassium loss, distal hydrogen ion secretory disorders (classical distal RTA), and some patients with diabetic ketoacidosis. These patients may present with severe acidosis, but if the plasma potassium is, for example, 2.0 mM or less, the administration of bicarbonate without potassium could cause life-threatening hypokalemia, resulting in cardiac arrhythmia or respiratory arrest.

Is the acidosis very severe?

Bicarbonate therapy is indicated in severe metabolic acidosis (vide infra) but how is *severe* defined? In fact, this definition is arbitrary. While it is clear that when blood pH falls to less than 6.90, death or permanent neurological damage may result, it is not clear whether the acidemia itself or the underlying disorder (shock, methanol poisoning, etc.) have caused irreversible cell damage. Certainly many patients with diabetic ketoacidosis or lactic acidosis due to seizures have had blood pH values less than 6.90 and have had complete recovery with no apparent sequellae. On the other hand, there is some evidence that moderate acidemia (pH < 7.20) can impair cardiac contractility and diminish the cardiac response to catecholamines. Hence, we would recommend that when either the blood pH is less than 7.0 or the plasma bicarbonate concentration is less than 8 mM, therapy with sodium bicarbonate is advisable. Why either a low pH or a low bicarbonate concentration should be criteria for therapy is illustrated in the following three examples:

Consider a patient who has these plasma values: pH 7.04, P_{CO_2} 19 mmHg, HCO_3^- 5 mM. This patient has severe metabolic acidosis with normal respiratory compensation. Although the pH fall is not life threatening at present, a small further reduction of plasma bicarbonate concentration to 3 mM without a further fall in P_{CO_2} would result in a pH of 6.82 (Table 4, example C). Similarly, if the patient could not continue to hyperventilate and the P_{CO_2} rose to 30 mmHg, the blood pH would fall to 6.86 (Table 4, example B). Therefore in this setting, alkali therapy should be given to get the patient out of danger until definitive therapy can be acheived.

Consider a second patient who has the following plasma values: pH 6.96, P_{CO_2} 45 mmHg, HCO_3^- 10 mM. In this case, the plasma HCO_3 concentration is not reduced to a level that would threaten the patient's life, but the patient has a coexisting respiratory acidosis. The pH of less than 7.00 indentifies this patient as being at high risk, and the patient should be ventilated. Since the P_{CO_2} might rise further, correction of the cause of the respiratory acidosis (which may require intubation and assisted ventilation) is indicated.

Consider a third patient who has the following plasma values: pH 7.22, P_{CO_2} 15 mmHg, HCO_3^- 6 mM. In this case the pH is not life threatening but this is because the P_{CO_2} is so low. Since the plasma bicarbonate concentration is less than 8 mM, alkali could be given to raise the plasma bicarbonate level to a safer level as continued acid production or a diminished degree of hyperventilation could lead to a marked fall in blood pH.

When is ventilation therapy required?

When the P_{CO_2} is too high for the degree of acidosis, ventilation therapy offers the quickest and quantitatively most valuable way to raise the plasma pH. It is important to recognize that the administration of sodium bicarbonate in an acidemic patient is a CO_2-producing process, and if the patient is being ventilated the P_{CO_2} will rise if alveolar ventilation is not increased.

When is bicarbonate therapy advisable?

The indications for bicarbonate therapy are summarized in Table 2. Having asked the questions, How fast are hydrogen ions being produced? Can the rate of H^+ production be diminished?, and Can the patient make bicarbonate?, the following guidelines can be used:
1. Plasma bicarbonate concentration less than 8 mM or pH less than 7.0
2. Problems with hyperventilation if there is a delay instituting assisted ventilation (i.e., moderate metabolic acidosis with respiratory acidosis)
3. Moderate metabolic acidosis where there is no organic anion that can be metabolized to yield bicarbonate (see equation 1, i.e., normal plasma anion gap type of acidosis, certain intoxications), especially if there is a kidney disease that results in a low rate of NH_4^- excretion
4. For metabolic acidosis of only moderate severity (i.e., plasma bicarbonate concentration close to 10 mM, pH close to 7.10), the indications for bicarbonate therapy are less clear and the clinician must use his or her judgement based on the factors discussed above.

CALCULATION OF THE QUANTITY OF BICARBONATE TO ADMINISTER

When calculating the amount of sodium bicarbonate to administer, one should assume a volume of distribution of 50% of total body weight. This is to account for 60% of the H^+ load that was buffered in the ICF. The initial bicarbonate therapy should aim at removing the patient from immediate danger, i.e., raising the plasma bicarbonate concentration to 10–12 mM. The rapidity with which the sodium bicarbonate is given will be determined by the severity of the acidemia, the cardiac status of the patient, and the potassium status. For example, a 70 kg patient who has a plasma bicarbonate concentration of 4 mM will require at least 245 mM of bicarbonate to raise the plasma bicarbonate concentration to 11 mM (11 − 4 or 7 mM × 50% of body weight or 35l = 245 mM). If the patient is free of heart disease, and is hyperkalemic and not hypernatremic, he or she can receive 50–100 mM of sodium bicarbonate in the hypertonic form, with perhaps the remainder as an isotonic infusion (3 amps = 132 mM of bicarbonate in 1 l of water). This calculation assumes that there is no ongoing H^+ production. This is essentially true in metabolic acidosis due to renal disease, but may grossly the underestimate bicarbonate requirements in lactic acidosis or methanol intoxication where the rate of H^+ generation is high (Table 3). Blood gases should be determined frequently to judge the adequacy of treatment (use a venous source unless you need to know the PO_2).

With very low plasma bicarbonate concentrations, the volume of distribution of bicarbonate exceeds 50% of total body weight owing to a higher proportion of intracellular fluid H^+ buffering.

The tonicity of the sodium bicarbonate administered should be determined by the patient's tonicity; if the patient is hypertonic (e.g., diabetic ketoacidosis) do not give hypertonic sodium bicarbonate.

THERAPEUTIC OPTIONS IN PATIENTS WITH METABOLIC ACIDOSIS, RENAL FAILURE, AND ECF VOLUME EXPANSION

Gastric HCO_3^- generation

The stomach generally generates 150 mM of bicarbonate daily, and this can be mobilized as a therapeutic tool in challenging patients. One can insert a nasogastric tube, stimulate gastric acid secretion with pentagastrin (provided the patient has not received histamine-receptor blockers and is not achlorhydric), and remove even greater amounts of HCl. One must ensure that the nasogastric tube is well situated to remove most of the acid. The periodic installation of antacids down the tube will help to prevent complications secondary to excess acid secretion. Should sufficient sodium be removed via this route, it will diminish the danger of administration of some sodium bicarbonate intravenously.

Phlebotomy and dialysis

If the patient with severe metabolic acidosis is in frank pulmonary edema, in addition to the usual therapeutic maneuvers (diuretics, oxygen, morphine, digitalis), one should do a phlebotomy early to allow the administration of sodium bicarbonate, as acidemia may also impair cardiac function. The phlebotomized blood should be centrifuged and the cells returned to the patient. If the patient has renal failure, early dialysis with a bicarbonate bath should be planned.

Ventilation

One should consider ventilating patients with an elevated P_{CO_2} early to lower their P_{CO_2} to an appropriate degree for their acidemia (fall in plasma bicarbonate concentration from 25 mM should equal the fall in P_{CO_2} from 40 mmHg). One can influence the acid-base state much faster by lowering the P_{CO_2} than by the administration of bicarbonate. In patients with pulmonary edema, ventilation will also be beneficial for the pulmonary edema if the patient can tolerate the positive end-expiratory pressure.

TREATMENT OF SPECIFIC CAUSES OF METABOLIC ACIDOSIS

Ketoacidosis

The pathogenesis, diagnosis, and treatment of diabetic ketoacidosis (DKA) is discussed in Chapter 00. Therefore we shall just provide an outline in Table 5 for the differential diagnosis but will not discuss therapy.

Lactic acidosis

Lactic acidosis may be classified into two major categories: Type A, in which lactic acid production is increased and its removal is impaired because of tissue hypoxia; Type B, in which hepatic lactate removal is impaired for reasons other than hypoxia (Table 6). Type A is much more common than Type B. Both, but particularly Type A, are associated with a very high mortality rate (for review, see 8–11).

Type A lactic acidosis is difficult to treat for a number of reasons. Lactate and H^+ production rates may be extremely rapid (up to 3600 mmol/hr in total body anoxia, Table 3), so that life-threatening acidemia occurs within minutes. It is often very difficult to reduce the rate of H^+ production because of the nature and severity of the underlying process (cardiogenic shock, gram-negative sepsis, etc.). Finally, the massive amounts of sodium bicarbonate that would be required to titrate ongoing acid production can cause severe ECF volume expansion (pulmonary edema) and hypernatremia; furthermore, the increase in blood pH resulting from bicarbonate therapy may actually increase lactate and H^+ production rates by stimulating glycolysis (12), adding to the sodium bicarbonate load required.

TYPE A LACTIC ACIDOSIS

The only treatment of type A lactic acidosis that can be successful is reducing the rate of H^+ production. The most important measures lead to an increase in arterial perfusion to tissues, especially the liver, which is the primary site of lactate removal. Raising arterial pressure may be a simple matter of expanding the intravascular volume with saline or colloid, but it may require measures to increase myocardial function, such as inotropic agents or afterload reduction. In the setting of cardiogenic shock, more aggressive measures such as an intraaortic balloon pump or even cardiac surgery may be necessary. Obviously, oxygen therapy to correct hypoxemia, transfusion of red cells to correct severe anemia, surgical resection of ischemic tissue, and antibiotic treatment of sepsis are all indicated in certain circumstances.

Table 5. Etological classification of ketoacidosis

Cause	Special features	Treatment
1. *Insulin deficiency with normal B cells*		
a. Hypoglycemia Fasting	Never find plasma/[HCO$_3$] < 18 mM or AG > 19 mEq/l; plasma [glucose] not < 3 mM	Glucose cures it quickly
Liver problem, e.g., glycogen storage disease, Type I or a defect in glugoneogenesis (GNG)	Hypoglycemia can be marked Plasma [HCO$_3$] can be < 18 mM If defect in GNG, may also have lactic acidosis	Glucose eliminates ketoacidosis Special therapy for underlying disease
b. Inhibition of insulin release High α-adrenergics Ethanol with vomiting yeilding marked ECF volume contraction	Pernicious vomiting, almost in shock Ketoacidosis may be severe Mixed acid-base disorders Blood [glucose] may be low, normal, or high	NaCl to restore ECF volume KCl to replace K deficit B vitamins Phosphate Glucose only if hypoglycemic
2. β-*cell destruction* (diabetes mellitus)	Severe hyperglycemia Severe ketoacidosis ECF volume very low K depletion with hyperkalemia Look for underlying disease and treat it	Insulin NaCl, KCl Threat of hypokalemia in 2 hours Glucose needed in 6 hours
3. *Other causes*		
a. Excessive lipolysis Postexercise	High FFA mobilization continues but oxidation rate slows	No real danger, no special treatment
Salicylate overdose	Activates tissue lipase Hyperventilation CNS toxicity K depletion	Remove ASA by promoting excretion + GI lavage; dialysis may be necessary

If the above measures do not immediately reverse the acidosis, bicarbonate therapy may be necessary to "buy time" for the other measures to begin to reduce H$^+$ production [see Appendix 3 and Narins and Cohen (13) for a more detailed discussion]. The guidelines for bicarbonate therapy are the same as are given above under General Considerations. Bicarbonate should be given to raise plasma bicarbonate to 10–12 mM. With normal respiratory compensation (P$_{CO_2}$ close to 25 mmHg), blood pH will be at a reasonably "safe" level (7.15–7.25). Although there is some evidence that at blood pH values less than 7.20, myocardial depresssion occurs; this is controversial (13). Certainly there is little advantage in raising blood pH much above 7.20, and indeed this may stimulate glycolysis (12) and therefore H$^+$ and lactate production.

The major problems associated with massive sodium bicarbonate therapy in lactic acidosis are ECF volume expansion and hypertonicity. Hypertonicity may be minimized by giving at least some of the bicarbonate isotonically – for example, adding 2–3 ampules of sodium bicarbonate (88–132 mM) to 1 l sterile water (glucose should not be present in this solution which is discussed in detail later). One can try to treat the problem of ECF volume expansion with a loop diuretic, but these are ineffective when the kidneys are underperfused; alternatively, hemodialyisis against a bicarbonate bath can provide a large net bicarbonate load and not a large sodium gain. Note that dialysis does not treat the cause of the lactic acidosis; it merely allows more vigorous bicarbonate therapy. Peritoneal dialysis with lactate buffer would be inappropriate, because the rate of metabolism of this dialyzable lactate to generate new bicarbonate will be grossly impaired and peritoneal dialysis may be ineffective in a shock state because of poor splanchnic perfusion.

The other measure that can lead to endogenous bicarbonate formation is the use of the activator of pyruvate dehydrogenase, dichloroacetate (14). Recall that this effect requires oxygen consumption and is of limited value in these patients unless it helps restore oxygen delivery by improving myocardial function (there is some evidence that this occurs).

TYPE B LACTIC ACIDOSIS

There is not the same urgency here as the rate of H$^+$ accumulation is much lower than in Type A lactic acidosis.

Lactic acidosis due to thiamine deficiency

This form of lactic acidosis is entirely preventable by giving thiamine. The clinical setting where it is most prevalent is in the alcoholic or in areas where nutritional intake is inadequate. The major danger is not the acidosis but rather the CNS lesion that is caused by local glycolysis that is accelerated by reversal of alcoholic ketoacidosis with glucose therapy.

Table 6. Classification of lactic acidosis

I. *Reduced oxygen delivery vs. demand (Type A)*
  A. Low blood oxygen content
     Low arterial P_{O_2} (O_2-poor air or lung problem)
     Hemoglobin problem (severe anemia, altered hemoglobin)
  B. Decreased tissue perfusion
     Local arterial obstruction
     Loss of arterial blood volume (hemorrhage, venous pooling as in septic shock)
     Cardiac disease
  C. High tissue demand for oxygen
     Severe exercise
     Uncouplers of oxidative phosphorylaxion
     Hypermetabolism (fever, thyrotoxicosis)
     Very large tumor burden
  D. Inhibited tissue oxygen utilization
     Cyanide and other drugs that inhibit oxidative phosphorylation

II. *Reduced lactate removal without hypoxia (Type B)*
  A. Liver disease (extensive)
     Infiltration with tumor cells
     Damage (e.g., cirrhosis)
  B. Interference with normal liver metabolism (Figure 7)
     1. Increased NADH production (ethanol)
     2. Decreased NADH oxidation (cyanide)
     3. Increased pyruvate production (e.g., very large tumor burden)
     4. decreased pyruvate metabolism (e.g., drugs such as phenformin; inborn errors of metabolism such as pyruvate dehydrogenase deficiency or gluconeogenic enzyme defects; nutritional problems such as thiamine deficiency)

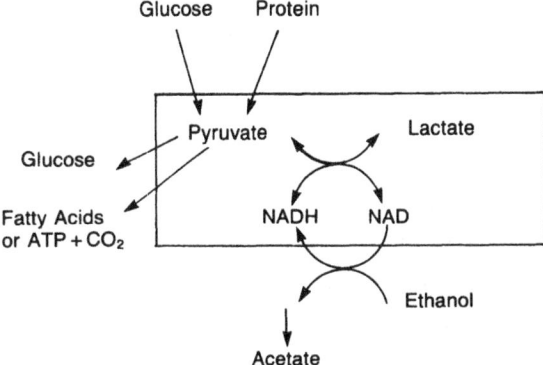

Figure 7. Etiology of lactic acidosis: Role of ethanol. Lactate can be made via only one reaction, which is catalyzed by the near-equilibrium enzyme lactate dehydrogenase (enclosed in the rectangle). In this reaction, NADH is converted to NAD. Lactate will accumulate if the concentration of its precursors, pyruvate and/or NADH, increase. Pyruvate is formed from glucose or protein and is removed in gluconeogenesis or via flux through pyruvate dehydrogenase (dichloroacetate activates this enzyme and flux will increase if oxygen is available). Ethanol oxidation produces NADH in the liver; this causes pyruvate conversion to lactate, lactic acidosis, and lower rates of glyuconeogenesis. However, lactic acidosis should be mild because ethanol oxidation can only occur in the liver.

Ethanol-induced lactic acidosis

The cause of lactic acidosis is hepatic ethanol metabolism that generates NADH, leading to diversion of pyruvate to lactate (Figure 7). Thus ethanol must be being metabolized at the time this diagnosis is made. Furthermore, since all other tissues can oxidize the lactate produced, the degree of lactic acidosis is always mild if this is the sole cause. No specific treatment is required.

Drug-induced lactic acidosis (Table 7)

The drugs in question accumulate if their intake is high or if excretion is low (especially with prerenal failure in the case of phenformin). Although the degree of lactic acidosis may be severe, the chances of survival are good. The measures required are neutralizing the H^+ excess with sodium bicarbonate, reducing H^+ production with insulin, accelerating lactate metabolism (dichloroacetate), and eliminating the drug by renal excretion or dialysis (phenformin).

Lactic acidosis due to tumors

There are three major subgroups to consider:
1. Tumor infiltration into the liver that compromises the normal hepatic lactate clearance.
2. The release of metabolites from necrotic tumor masses, which leads to inhibition of hepatic gluconeogenesis (e.g., a product of the amino acid tryptophan that can inhibit phosphenolpyruvate carboxykinase, a key gluconeogenic enzyme).
3. It is possible that an exceedingly large tumor burden an synthesize so much lactic acid, given its biochemistry, that it would exceed the capacity of even a normal liver to remove it (greater than 100 mmol/hr).

Obviously, all three mechanisms may operate to produce this type of lactic acidosis. In addition, should hypoxia or hypotension supervene, the lactic acidosis will be greatly aggravated.

Treatment must be directed at the primary causes and, as expected, the prognosis will generally reflect the behavior of the tumor and the liver pathology.

POTENTIAL DISADVANTAGES OF NaHCO₃ THERAPY IN CHRONIC (TYPE B) LACTIC ACIDOSIS

The lactic acid production rate declines as the $[H^+]$ rises (12). Therefore the administration of sodium bicarbonate, by diminishing the $[H^+]$, will increase glucose conversion to lactic acid. This may have two important clinical implications:
1. If the source of glucose is the lean body mass (gluconeogenesis), considerable muscle mass may be lost as a result of sodium bicarbonate therapy(15, 16).
2. If 150 mmol of $NaHCO_3$ are given in 1 l of 5% glucose

Table 7. Drugs associated with lactic acidosis

Biguanides
Streptozotocin
Salicylate
Isoniazid
Alcohols
    Ethanol, methanol, ethylene glycol
Sugars
    Fructose, sorbitol, xylitol

(− 300 mmol of glucose), − 600 mmol of H^+ and lactate$^-$ (2 lactate + 2 H^+ from each glucose) could be produced from the glucose, whereas only 150 mmol of bicarbonate were provided.

SUMMARY

Recall that lactic acidosis represents a heterogeneous group of diseases. Hence there is no specific therapy for lactic acidosis. The specific cause must be identified and treated if possible. Sodium bicarbonate merely "buys a little time" before the cause is reversed. Finally, dichloroacetate will accelerate lactic acid oxidation; however, it requires oxygen delivery to be effective.

Salicylate intoxication

The most common acid-base disturbance associated with salicylate intoxication is respiratory alkalosis due to central respiratory stimulation. Metabolic acidosis may complicate the picture, however, especially in children. Because even toxic salicylate levels are usually considerably less than 10 mM (140 mg/dl), the elevation of the plasma anion gap in salicylate-associated metabolic acidosis is due to the accumulation of not only salicylate, but also β-hydroxybutyrate, sometimes lactate, and other unidentified organic anions. Acidemia is usually mild because of coexisting respiratory alkalosis.

The diagnosis of salicylate intoxication may be suspected in a patient with a known history of salicylate ingestion (which may be therapeutic, accidental, or suicidal) who has a wide plasma anion gap type of metabolic acidosis, respiratory alkalosis, and possibly other symptoms such as tinnitus. Suspicion will be increased by finding unexplained ketosis (salicylate activates tissue lipase) and hypouricemia (high-dose salicylate is uricosuric). It is confirmed by the absence of a plasma osmolal gap and the detection of salicylate in the blood. Other clues are the presence of hypokalemia, urine sodium plus potassium being much higher than the urine chloride concentration in acid urine, and finally unexpected clinical findings, such as the adult respiratory distress syndrome.

Treatment of salicylate intoxication is aimed at increasing urine salicylate excretion and preventing cell (especially brain) accumulation of salicylates. Salicylate is a weak organic acid that is transported across cells and renal epithelia, primarily in the undissociated form (Figure 8). Therefore, alkalinizing the urine reduces salicylate reab-

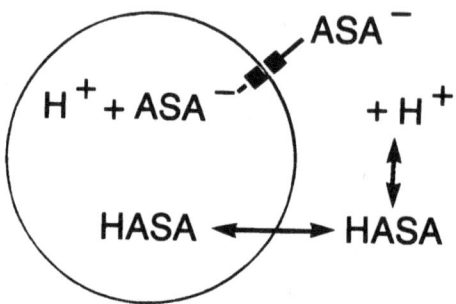

Figure 8. Importance of nonionic diffusion during salicylate intoxication. The circle represents a cell membrane or the luminal membrane of a kidney tubule. In nonionic diffusion, the weak acid (HASA), but not is conjugate base (ASA$^-$ anion), crosses cell membranes quickly enough. Hence, the HASA concentration is equal on both sides of the membrane but the ASA$^-$ anion will be trapped in alkaline urine or in a more alkaline ECF (vs. the ICF [H^+]). Reprinted with permission from the authors: Halperin ML, Goldstein MB: *Fluid, Electrolyte, and Acid-Base Emergencies.* WB Saunders, Philadelphia, 1988.

sorption by the kidney and markedly enhances its excretion; similarly, alkalinizing the ECF tends to prevent salicylate accumulation in cells, therefore acidemia should be avoided.

Alkalinizing the urine can be achieved with sodium bicarbonate administration. The major risk of this therapy is excessive elevation of blood pH because of coexistent respiratory alkalosis. One approach is to add 1 ampule (44 mmol) sodium bicarbonate to each liter of one-half normal saline and infuse at 300–500 ml/hr to achieve a forced alkaline diuresis. If the blood pH exceeds 7.55 as a result of this therapy, acetazolamide (500 mg) should be given to promote bicarbonate excretion. Be careful to avoid inducing metabolic acidosis, as this will increase the toxicity of salicylates (Figure 8).

The major complication of forced alkaline diuresis therapy is sodium and water retention, which could be managed with administration of a loop diuretic. It has been suggested that alkalinization of the urine alone with sodium bicarbonate (without large volumes of saline) may be just as effective in promoting salicylate excretion and may avoid problems with fluid retention (17).

In severe intoxications complicated by the adult respiratory distress syndrome, cardiovascular instability, etc., hemodialysis is the treatment of choice, although, if it is not available, peritoneal dialysis may be used.

Methanol intoxication

Methanol is an inexpensive and widely available intoxicant that is used as a solvent (xerox fluid), an antifreeze, and a fuel. Ingestion either as a suicide attempt or unwittingly as an ethanol substitute can result in severe metabolic acidosis, blindness, and death (18, 19). Methanol itself causes an intoxication similar to that induced by ethanol. Its serious toxicity derives from the fact that it is metabolized by hepatic alcohol dehydrogenase to formaldehyde and subsequently to formic acid. These end products are respondsible for the neurotoxicity (particularly the optic nerve) and severe metabolic acidosis. One ounce (30 ml) of methanol can yield 1000 mmol of formic acid. Because the affinity of methanol for alcohol dehydrogenase is much less than that of ethanol (100-fold higher K_m), methanol blood levels decline much more slowly and, of greater importance, the toxic products of methanol metabolism accumulate slowly so that clinical manifestations of methanol poisoning may appear 24–48 hours after ingestion.

The clues to suspect the diagnosis are: a history of ingestion (sometimes difficult to elicit); symptoms of altered vision, abdominal symptoms such as nausea or pain, and the presence of a wide plasma osmolal gap: later, the diagnosis is confirmed by finding a high blood methanol level. Above all, a high degree of suspicion is required. Physical examination may be normal, show varying degrees of a reduced level of consciousness and there may be retinal edema. Of note, the normal circulating volume helps distinguish this type of acidosis from DKA, alcoholic ketoacidosis, and most patients with Type A lactic acidosis.

TREATMENT OF METHANOL POISONING

The toxicity of methanol and the associated severe acidemia are both related to the metabolism of methanol to formaldehyde and the organic acid formic acid catalyzed initially by hepatic alcohol dehydrogenase. As methanol itself is relatively nontoxic, the approach to therapy is to retard its metabolism by competing for the availability of *alcohol dehydrogenase* and then to remove the methanol and toxic metabolites by dialysis. Since alcohol dehydrogenase also catalyzes the metabolism of ethanol, and as its affinity for ethanol is far greater than for methanol, the provision of ethanol is the most effective way to lower the rate of methanol metabolism.

Chronic drinkers may have higher levels of alcohol dehydrogenase and therefore the chronic alcoholic could be more threatened by methanol intoxication (by both acidemia and toxicity). However, if an alcoholic who has also been drinking ethanol, and then is exposed to methanol, is more protected than his or her colleagues who have not coincidentally ingested ethanol. For the same reason (higher alcohol dehydrogenase levels), the chronic drinker will require a higher rate of ethanol administration to maintain therapeutic levels of ethanol.

There are three major components of therapy:
1. Establishment and maintenance of adequate ethanol levels to prevent methanol metabolism
2. Correction of life-threatening acidemia
3. Removal of methanol.

Ethanol Therapy

1. Establish therapeutic blood levels of ethanol of 100 mg/dl (22 mM) by giving 0.6 g of ethanol/kg body weight I.V. or orally (about 4 oz whiskey orally in a 70-kg man).
2. Maintain this blood ethanol level for the duration of intoxication. In chronic drinkers, give 0.15 g/kg/hr and in nondrinkers give 0.07 g/kg/hr, which can be given orally or I.V. (about 1–2 oz whiskey PO/hr in a 70-kg man).

Correction of acidemia

The indications for bicarbonate administration are given in the section on General Considerations.

Removal of methanol

Methanol is best removed by hemodialysis, but if unavailable peritoneal dialysis will remove some methanol (18). Blood ethanol levels can be maintained by adding ethanol to the dialysate. Hemodialysis is best performed using two separate access lines, which allows higher blood flow rates and lower recirculation; a dialysis membrane with a high urea clearance; and a bicarbonate bath to help correct for the acidosis. Since patients may require dialysis for prolonged periods (more than 12 hours) a dialysis machine with ultrafiltration control is preferred to limit unwanted changes in ECF volume.

Blood levels of ethanol should be monitored during therapy, and the rate of ethanol infusion should be adjusted accordingly to account for differences in rates of absorption, metabolism, and removal.

Ethylene glycol intoxication

Because ethylene glycol is readily available (automobile antifreeze), relatively inexpensive, and not unpleasant to the taste, it may be ingested as an intoxicant. It causes fulminant metabolic acidosis, severe central nervous system toxicity, and acute tubular necrosis. As with methanol, the products of ethylene glycol metabolism cause the toxicity. Ethylene glycol is also metabolized by hepatic alcohol dehydrogenase to a number of end products, including glyoxalic, glycolic, and oxalic acids. Following the initial toxicity associated with profound metabolic acidosis and CNS manifestations (confusion, coma, seizures), patients may develop congestive heart failure and respiratory failure. Those who survive usually have acute tubular necrosis, which is generally of the oliguric form (20, 21).

Ethylene glycol intoxication should always be suspected in patients with metabolic acidosis and an increased plasma anion gap, especially if the patient appears intoxicated and denies ethanol intake or if the odor of ethanol is not evident. The index of suspicion can be increased greatly by finding oxalate crystals in the urine. As with methanol, a wide plasma osmolol gap is helpful in the absence of ethanol. The diagnosis is confirmed by detecting ethylene glycol in the blood.

THERAPY

The principles of therapy of ethylene glycol intoxication are identical to those for methanol. The additional complication of acute tubular necrosis may limit the quantity of sodium bicarbonate that may be given, as it is generally of the oliguric variety. Therefore, acute pulmonary edema may become a feature of therapy for ethylene glycol intoxication. The use of nasogastric suction and pentagastrin stimulation of gastric acid secretion may ameliorate both the acidemia and the pulmonary edema while dialysis is being arranged. Because of the acute renal failure, early dialysis is critical. As with methanol, hemodialysis is the preferred method to remove ethylene glycol and its metabolites; however, if it is not available, peritoneal dialysis should be carried out. As with methanol, ethanol should be given as a loading dose followed by a maintenance dose, and ethanol should be added to the dialysate. Ethanol levels should be maintained at about 100 mg/dl (22 mM) until all the ethylene glycol has been removed.

Organic acid load from the GI tract (D-lactic acidosis)

Certain bacteria in the GI tract may convert carbohydrate (cellulose) into organic acids. The two factors that make this possible are slow GI transit (blind loops, obstruction) and change of the normal flora (usually with antibiotic therapy). The most prevalent organic acid is D-lactic acid (22). Since humans metabolize this isomer somewhat more slowly than L-lactate (23), and production rates can be very rapid, life-threatening acidosis can be produced.

There are three additional points that should be noted with respect to D-lactic acidosis:
1. The usual laboratory test for lactate is specific for the L-lactate isomer. Hence the laboratory report for "lactate" will not be elevated.
2. GI bacteria produce D-lactate, amines, and other compounds, which may cause clinical symptoms related to CNS dysfunction (personality changes, gait changes, confusion, etc.).
3. Some of the D-lactate will be lost in the urine if the GFR is not too low (23). Hence the degree of rise in the plasma anion gap may not be as high as expected for the fall in the plasma bicarbonate concentration later in the course of this disorder.

Threatment will be directed at the gastrointestinal problem and at ensuring that the patients do not die of severe metabolic acidosis (give sodium bicarbonate if necessary).

Renal acidoses (see Chapter 12 for more details)

As described in Table 1, renal disorders may cause metabolic acidosis with either a normal or increased anion gap. Whether the anion gap is elevated or not depends primarily on the GFR, i.e., with a low GFR a number of anions, including phosphate, sulphate, and others, may be retained, raising the plasma anion gap. The plasma anion gap does not usually exceed 22 mEq/l or about 10 mEq/l above normal. Be sure to examine the plasma albumin level, as this is the most important constituent of the normal plasma anion gap and hypoalbuminemia is not an uncommon feature in this patient group.

LOSS OF SODIUM BICARBONATE IN THE URINE

The mechanism for the acidosis in proximal renal tubular acidosis is primarily the loss of bicarbonate in the urine (despite acidosis, the rate of NH_4^+ excretion is lower than in other forms of metabolic acidosis). Bicarbonate loss is usually due to reduced reclaiming or recycling of filtered bicarbonate in the proximal tubule and may be identified by finding an alkaline urine pH (> 7.0) when the plasma bicarbonate concentration is low. This disorder may be due to drug administration (carbonic anhydrase inhibitors such as acetazolamide) or to a tubular disorder, in which case the condition is called *proximal RTA*.

Proximal RTA is characterized by a steady state (urine acid excretion equals dietary acid production) but at a lowered plasma bicarbonate concentration. This lowered plasma bicarbonate concentration is sometimes called the *threshold for bicarbonate excretion*. When plasma bicarbonate falls below the threshold, net acid excretion exceeds the net acid production from the diet. When the plasma bicarbonate rises above the threshold (such as after eating when gastric H^+ secretion is stimulated), bicarbonaturia will occur. The most important points about proximal RTA therapeutically are that the acidosis is usually mild and that complications due to the acidosis are minor. These facts alone argue against alkali therapy. In addition, if exogenous sodium bicarbonate is given, as the plasma bicarbonate concentration rises temporarily bicarbonate excretion will rise proportionately. Massive amounts of bicarbonate may be required to normalize the plasma bicarbonate concentration and this effect is transient. In addition, the large increase in delivery of sodium and bicarbonate to the cortical collecting duct may augment potassium secretion, resulting in hypokalemia. Therefore, since acidemia is usually mild, asymptomatic, and difficult or dangerous to treat, sodium bicarbonate treatment should not be attempted in the adult.

REDUCED AMMONIUM EXCRETION

The kidney normally maintains acid-base balance by excreting sufficient ammonium to balance acid generation from dietary protein. The principal mechanism for H^+ excretion is as ammonium (1). Ammonium excretion should increase in metabolic acidosis and depends on the rate of ammonium synthesis in the cortex of the kidney, transfer of ammonium to the outer medulla where it dissociates to NH_3, and trapping of NH_3 in the collecting duct as ammonium by secretion of H^+ by the collecting duct. Reduced ammonium excretion can result from a) low NH_3 availability, b) reduced collecting duct H^+ secretion, or c) a combination of both. Therapy of the three most common clinical examples of these disorders will be discussed:

Renal failure

As GFR falls, ammonium synthesis by the renal cortex falls, reducing NH_3 availability. Metabolic acidosis is therefore typical of advanced renal failure, although the degree of acidosis is variable. It is rarely fulminant, and urgent bicarbonate therapy is seldom necessary. The metabolic acidosis may contribute to fatigue and anorexia, however, and the chronic acidosis may in part be buffered in bone, contributing to the bone loss seen in uremia. Therefore it is probably reasonable to give oral sodium bicarbonate to these patients to maintain the plasma bicarbonate close to 20-25 mM. With the onset of dialysis therapy, the acid-base balance is maintained by bicarbonate or bicarbonate precursor (acetate, lactate) addition from the dialysis fluid.

Distal RTA (classical RTA)

This disorder is primarily due to reduced H^+ secretion by the collecting duct, resulting in reduced trapping of NH_3 as ammonium (4). It is often complicated by disorders of calcium homeostasis (osteopenia, growth retardation, calcium stones, nephrocalcinosis), hypokalemia, and progressive renal failure (see Chapter 12 for details). In this disorder, if any of the above complications are present, sodium bicarbonate (or equivalent alkali given as the potassium salt) should be given to normalize the plasma bicarbonate concentration. This therapy has been shown to prevent most of the complications listed above. How much alkali is required? Since the daily normal acid load from the diet is usually about 70 mmol/day, in the complete absence of urine H^+ excretion a maximum of 70 mmol of alkali (5–6 g sodium bicarbonate/day) would be required to maintain acid-base homeostasis once the bicarbonate deficit has been replaced. Since urine net acid excretion is usually reduced but not absent, considerably less bicarbonate is usually required. Supplemental potassium is often required as well.

Distal RTA may occasionally present with severe hypokalemia ($K^+ < 2$ mM), producing symptoms of muscle weakness or even paralysis. Metabolic acidosis may also be moderately severe, but administration of alkali alone could cause respiratory arrest by causing movement of potassium into cells and worsening the hypokalemia. In this instance, potassium bicarbonate should be given first; larger amounts may be given by an oral or by a nasogastric tube than intravenously; be sure the patient can absorb this potassium, i.e., bowel sounds are present. Glucose-containing solutions should be avoided, since they may stimulate insulin release, which may also cause a potassium shift into the cells. The addition of potassium, sparing diuretics such as amiloride will reduce the ongoing urine potassium loss and facilitate correction of the hypokalemia. Sodium bicarbonate administration may have to be delayed until the plasma potassium value is above 3.0 mM.

RTA with hyperkalemia

Reduced ammonium excretion is commonly associated with hyperkalemia; several mechanisms may be involved in the pathogenesis of the disorder. Hypoaldosteronism may be present, causing reduced urine potassium loss and hyperkalemia. This leads to reduced ammonium excretion, primarily because hyperkalemia inhibits ammoniagenesis (there is also diminished aldosterone-stimulated collecting duct H^+ secretion). Another mechanism for the disorder is tubulointerstitial disease affecting the cortical collecting duct, making it less responsive to aldosterone.

Therapy depends on the pathogenesis and on the patient's ECF volume. In patients with hypoaldosteronism due to adrenal disease, ECF volume and blood pressure are usually reduced and aldosterone replacment with 0.05–0.1 mg fludrocortisone per day plus saline administration is the usual treatment of choice. Glucocorticoid deficiency, if present, should also be corrected.

Patients with secondary hypoaldosteronism (hyporeninemic hypoaldosteronism) are frequently ECF volume expanded and hypertensive. An example is patients with non-insulin-dependent diabetes mellitus with nephropathy. In these patients, fludrocortisone may aggravate sodium retention. Additional therapeutic alternatives would include diuretics such as furosemide to increase urine potassium and sodium excretion, or potassium exchange resins such as Kayexalate to increase fecal potassium loss. Correction of hyperkalemia by either mechanism will improve ammonium excretion.

Patients with primary tubular dysfunction (for example, obstructive nephropathy) who do not respond to mineralocorticoid may be treated with oral sodium bicarbonate. This will correct the acidosis, and also the hyperkalemia, by causing a shift of potassium into cells and by increasing renal potassium excretion due to increased distal sodium and/or volume delivery. Alternatively, if patients with primary tubular dysfunction are ECF volume expanded or hypertensive, diuretic therapy may be helpful. As in patients with classical distal RTA, only modest amounts of bicarbonate are required to maintain near-normal plasma bicarbonate concentrations (usually 25–50 mmol/day).

APPENDIX 1: INTERPRETATION OF URINE "NET CHARGE"

The kidney maintains acid-base balance by performing two functions: reabsorbing (reclaiming) filtered bicarbonate and generating new bicarbonate by excreting "net acid." Net acid is excreted as ammonium and $H_2PO_4^-$, and the amount is equal to aicd produced from the diet during steady state. The principal renal adaptation to metabolic acidosis is an increase in ammonium excretion; therefore, knowing the urine ammonium content would be very useful in differentiating renal from nonrenal causes of the normal anion gap type of metabolic acidosis. In those due to nonrenal causes, urine ammonium excretion should be high (much greater than 80 mmol/day); for those in which there is a renal cause of metabolic acidosis, ammonium excretion will be low (less than 40 mmol/day). Since measurement of urine ammonium is not a routine laboratory determination, a convenient method to estimate urine ammonium is to use the urine anion gap or "urine net charge" (5).

Since the sum of urine cations equals the sum of urine anions, an increase in urine ammonium must be balanced by an increase in urine anion excretion, usually chloride. Therefore, as the urine ammonium content increases, the urine net charge, (calculated as urine [sodium] + [potassium] − [chloride]) becomes progressively negative. The relationship between urine ammonium and urine net charge can be described by the equation (5):

$$\text{urine NH}_4^+ = -0.8 \text{ (urine net charge)} + 82.$$

The simplest method of using this correlation is that a positive urine net charge in the presence of metabolic acidosis indicates inappropriately low urine ammonium excretion (i.e., in a 24-hour urine that has less than 80 mmol of NH_4^+). However, if the urine net charge is negative, urine ammonium excretion is greater than 80 mmol/day, and therefore there must be a nonrenal source of the acidosis.

The urine net charge should not be used as an index of ammonium excretion under the following circumstances: alkaline urine (pH > 7.0) because of a high urine bicarbonate concentration; therapy with large doses of penicillin; and excretion of large quantities of other anions such as β-hydroxybutyrate or salicylates. These potential pitfalls can be circumvented using the urine osmolal gap (see Appendix 2 for details). Furthermore, this test should not be used for precise determinations of urine ammonium but rather for an estimate of the renal response to metabolic acidosis for diagnostic purposes.

APPENDIX 2: THE URINE OSMOLAL GAP

The urine net charge or anion gap (5) will detect urine NH_4^+ when it is excreted as NH_4Cl. This is the usual case; however, in ketoacidosis, the urine may contain NH_4^+ β-hydroxybutyrate. This will not be detected by the urine net charge. With a high index of suspicion and measurements of urine osmolality, sodium, potassium, chloride, glucose, and urea, the urine osmolal gap can be calculated (7). It is usually less than 100 mOsm/kg H_2O. Excretion of NH_4^+ plus β-hydroxybutyrate can be implied if the measured urine osmolality is 200 mOsm/kg H_2O greater than the urine osmolality calculated from the above constituents (equation 2).

$$\text{Urine osmolal gap} = \text{measured osmolality} - [\text{Glucose (mM)} + \text{urea (mM)} + \text{Na} + \text{K} + \text{Cl}] \quad (2)$$

or

$$\text{urine NH}_4^+ = \frac{2(\text{urine [Na] + [K]}) + \text{urine glucose (mM)} + \text{urine urea (mM)}}{2}.$$

APPENDIX 3: SHOULD $NaHCO_3$ BE GIVEN TO A PATIENT WITH TYPE A LACTIC ACIDOSIS?

The answer to this question would certainly have been yes a decade ago; however, there is a degree of uncertainty now because of the work of Arieff and collagues (24, 25). We shall address this question at a much more fundamental level and try to provide a rationale for the variety of clinical circumstances associated with lactic acid accumulation.

First, recognizing that lactic acidosis represents many diseases, one cannot have a general treatment that will be valid in all cases. For example, lactic acidosis occurs with exercise, shock, hepatic insufficiency, etc.; treatments do differ in each case. Therefore, sodium bicarbonate is not a specific treatment; rather, it is a temporary measure that has benefits and risks.

We think that the clinician must answer three questions before deciding whether sodium bicarbonate should be given. The questions are:

1. *Why are excessive quantities of lactic acid accumulating?* The rationale for this question is that you must decide if the rate of H^+ production will be decreased spontaneously or with specific therapy. If the role of H^+ production is likely to be reduced with specific therapy, sodium bicarbonate probably will not be needed (e.g., exercise- or convulsion-induced lactic acidosis).
2. *How quickly will lactic acid be produced?* The rationale for this question is illustrated in the following example: During total anoxia 60 mmol of lactic acid are produced each minute (Table 3). Given a total buffer capacity of close to 1000 mmol (11), the patient will die in just a few minutes unless the H^+ production rate is diminished. Since sodium bicarbonate cannot be infused at this rate (and the sodium load would also be lethal), sodium bicarbonate is of little benefit. Even if only the liver were hypoxic, the infusion of sodium bicarbonate will only "buy a little time." Therefore, the only rational treatment is to reverse tissue hypoxia. In the case of hepatic insufficiency, unless the compromised liver function can be reversed, sodium bicarbonate treatment will be of very little value.
3. *How severe is the acidosis?* As discussed in the section on general principles of sodium bicarbonate therapy, sodium bicarbonate will have greater therapeutic leverage during severe acidosis. Furthermore, ventilation therapy will be appropriate if the P_{CO_2} is higher than anticipated, given the degree of metabolic acidosis (Table 4).

One other point can be made: The experimental models that were designed to evaluate sodium bicarbonate therapy do not resemble clinical Type A lactic acidosis. For example, a dog breathing air with a low oxygen content has low oxygen delivery to tissues. However, cardiac output in these animals is markedly increased, and small changes in cardiac output will cause large changes in lactic acidosis. Thus if the sodium bicarbonate given decreased cardiac output by a small amount (or increased tissue oxygen demand), this would lead to worsening lactic acidosis. In contrast, Type A lactic acidosis due to shock is usually accompanied by a very low cardiac output; in this setting, sodium bicarbonate might have a very different effect on cardiac output and hence lactic acid production rate. Given this uncertainty, we feel that strong statements concerning possible benefits or risks of $NaHCO_3$ are not warranted (see also 13 and 26).

In summary, sodium bicarbonate is not a specific therapy for lactic acidosis. Whereas it may cause a greater degree of harm in certain situations in animal models, it may buy a little time in patients with severe lactic acidosis and thereby permit the clinician to reverse the cause of lactic acid accumulation. No impact on survival can be expected unless the cause of the lactic acid overproduction is reversed.

REFERENCES

1. Emmet ME, Narins RG: Clinical use of the anion gap. *Medicine* 56:38, 1977.
2. Oh MS, Carroll HJ: The anion gap. *N Engl, J Med* 297:814–817, 1977.
3. Gabow PA: Disorders associated with an altered anion gap. *Kidney Int* 27:472–483, 1984.
4. Halperin ML, Goldstein MB, Richardson RMA., Stinebaugh BJ: Distal renal tubular acidosis syndromes: A pathophysiological approach. *Am J Nephrol* 5:1–8, 1985.
5. Goldstein MB, Bear RA, Richardson RMA, Marsden PA, Halperin ML: The urine anion gap: A clinically useful index of ammonium excretion. *Am J Med Sci* 29:198–202, 1986.
6. Halperin ML, Margolis BL, Robinsion LA, Halperin RM, West ML, Bear RA: The urine osmolar gap: Clue to estimate urine ammonium in "hybrid" types of metabolic acidosis. *Clin Invest Med* 11:198–202, 1988.
7. Glasser L, Sternglanz PD, Combie J, Robinson A: Serum osmolality and its applicability to drug overdose. *Am J Clin Pathol* 60:695–699, 1973.
8. Cohen RD, Woods HF: Lactic acidosis revisited. *Diabetes* 32:181–191, 1983.
9. Park R, Arieff AI: Lactic acidosis: Current concepts. *Clin Endocr Metab* 12:339–359, 1983.
10. Madias NE: Lactic acidosis. *Kidney Int* 29:752–774, 1986.
11. Halperin ML, Fields ALA: Lactic acidosis – emphasis on the carbon precursors and buffering of the acid load. *Am J Med Sci* 289:154–159, 1985.
12. Halperin ML, Connors HP, Relman AS, Karnovsky ML: Factors that control the effect of pH on glycolysis in leukocytes. *J Biol Chem* 244:384–390, 1969.
13. Narins RG, Cohen JJ: Bicarbonate therapy for organic acidosis: The case for its continued use. *Ann Int Med* 106:615–618, 1987.
14. Stacpoole PW, Harman EM, Curry SH, Baumgartner TG, Misbin RI: Treatment of lactic acidosis with dichloroacetate. *N Engl J Med* 309:390–396, 1983.
15. Fields ALA, Wolman SL, Halperin M L: Chronic lactic acidosis in a patient with cancer: Therapy and metabolic consequences. *Cancer* 47:2026–2029, 1981.
16. Fraley DS, Adler S, Bruns FJ, Zett B: Stimulation of lactate production by administration of bicarbonate in a patient with a solid neoplasma and lactic acidosis. *N Engl J Med* 303:1100–1102, 1980.
17. Prescott LF, Balali-Mood M, Critchley JAJH, Johnstone AF, Proudfoot AT: Diuresis or urinary alkalinization for salicylate poisoning? *Br Med J* 285:1383–1386, 1982.
18. Gonda A, Gault H, Churchill D, Hollomby D: Hemodialysis for methanol intoxication. *Am J Med* 64:749–757, 1978.
19. McCoy HG, Cipolle RJ, Ehlers SM, Sawchuk RJ, Zaske DE: Severe methanol poisoning. *Am J Med* 67:804–807, 1979.
20. Parry ME, Wallach R: Ethylene glycol poisoning. *Am J Med* 67:804–807, 1979.
21. Peterson CD, Collins AJ, Bullock ML, Keane WF: Ethylene glycol poisoning. *N Engl J Med* 304:21–23, 1981.
22. Oh MS, Phelps KR, Traube M, Barbosa-Saldivar JL, Boxhill C, Carroll HJ: D–lactic acidosis in man with short–bowel syndrome. *N Engl J Med* 301:249–252, 1979.
23. Oh MS, Uribarri J, Alveranga D, Lazar I, Bazilinski N, Carroll HJ: Metabolic utilization and renal handling of D-lactate in men. *Metabolism* 34:621–625, 1985.
24. Arieff AI, Leach W, Park R, Lazarowitz VC: Systemic effects of $NaHCO_3$ in experimental lactic acidosis in dogs. *Am J Physiol* 242:F586–F591, 1982.
25. Graf H, Leach W, Arieff A I: Metabolic effects of sodium bicarbonate in hypoxic lactic acidosis in dogs. *Am J Physiol* 249:F630–F635, 1985.
26. Stacpoole PW: Lactic acidosis: The case against bicarbonate therapy. *Ann Int Med* 105:276–279, 1986.
27. Halperin ML, Goldstein MB, Haig A, Johnson MD, Stinebaugh BJ: Studies on the pathogenesis of type I (distal) renal tubular acidosis as revealed by the urinary P_{CO_2} tensions. *J Clin Invest* 53:669–677, 1974.

CHAPTER 11

Diabetic Ketoacidosis

HORACIO J. ADROGUÉ, JORGE BARRERO & GEORGE M. DOLSON

INTRODUCTION

The term *diabetes* (a siphon, in Greek) was coined by Aretaeus the Cappadocian during the second century AD as a description of the polyuria that accompanies this disease. He graphically described the illness as "a melting down of the flesh and limbs into urine," associated with an unquenchable thirst, nausea, and vomiting, and rapid death (1). Even before Aretaeus, Egyptian physicians writing in the Papyrus Ebers described polyuria that, in retrospect, may have been the osmotic diuresis of diabetes mellitus. Thomas Willis (1621–1675), namesake of the Circle of Willis, noted the sweet taste of the urine and attributed the increasing incidence of diabetes in England to "good fellowship and gusling down chiefly of unallayed wine." Matthew Dobson during the later half of the eighteenth century published a case report of a young man with diabetes and performed experiments on the urine, finding both protein and sugar. He observed the patient's serum and noted that it was also sweet and rather opaque. A prominent physician, Adolph Kussmaul, recognized that the hyperpnea of diabetic patients in coma was neither due to a primary lung disease not associated with lack of oxygen; the respiratory pattern of these patients now bears his name. Several years later (1889, 1890), Oskar Minkowsky induced diabetes mellitus in dogs by removal of the pancreas (2). During this century our understanding of the pathogenesis of diabetes mellitus and, as a consequence, the management of the disease has grown substantially due to contributions by researchers studying the clinical and basic biochemical aspects of the illness.

PATHOPHYSIOLOGY

Humans are able to utilize energy from carbohydrates, fats, or proteins, and energy-rich foods consumed during times of plenty can be stored as the complex carbohydrate glycogen, or as the energy-dense triacylglycerals. The biochemical systems that regulate these processes rely on the availability of insulin, which represents one of the most prominent regulators of tissue metabolism (3–6).

Complex carbohydrates are broken down into simple sugars and absorbed by the GI tract, with glucose being the predominant sugar. Glucose is taken into cells and can be metabolized to pyruvate by anerobic glycolysis, generating two moles of ATP from each mole of glucose. The maximum ATP yield can be realized, however, only if pyruvate can be metabolized all the way to carbon dioxide and water through the citric acid cycle and the cytochrome oxidase chain. Should the cell's energy stores be replete, glucose is not oxidized but rather is converted to glycogen, a complex polysaccharide that acts as a compact storage form for carbohydrate. Glycogen synthesis occurs primarily in the liver and muscle, and is stimulated when insulin is present. If serum glucose, and thus insulin levels are decreased as, for example during fasting, glycogen is broken down into glucose. Alternatively, lactate, which is generated during anaerobic glycolysis, can be converted into pyruvate and ultimately into glucose in the liver and renal cortex. Amino acids and glycerol can also be converted into glucose in the liver, as described below.

Protein can be utilized as either a structural component in cell growth or as an energy substrate. Reductions in serum insulin (as after an overnight fast) enhance protein breakdown and mobilization of amino acids. In the liver and renal cortex, these amino acids are converted into pyruvate or oxaloacetate and enter the gluconeogenic pathway. The final product of this pathway, glucose, is then returned to the circulation and is used to support energy metabolism by other tissues, notably muscle and brain. Thus, from an energy utilization point of view, protein may be transformed into and subsequently used as glucose.

Fatty acids in the form of triacylglycerals are the primary energy storage metabolite in humans, since they are anhydrous and contain approximately twice the energy per gram of carbohydrates. These lipids are stored in the fat cells of adipose tissue. When insulin levels are low and epinephrine, norepinephrine, glucagon, and cortisol are relatively elevated, the stored triacylglyceral is hydrated, forming glycerol and free fatty acids, which are released into the circulation. In the liver, glycerol is converted into pyruvate and ultimately into glucose. The free fatty acids can be used by many cells as an energy substrate. After uptake by the cell, fatty acids are transported to the mitochondria, where they are converted into acetyl Co A and enter the citric acid cycle, where ultimately they are broken down into carbon dioxide and water by the cytochrome oxidase chain, generating ATP. If free fatty acids are in great excess with respect to the availability of glucose for tissue oxidation, the surplus fatty acids are converted into acetoacetic acid. Acetoacetic acid is in equilibrium with β-hydroxybutyric acid and acetone, with final concentrations of β-hyproxybutyric acid being three times those of acetoacetic acid. These ketone bodies circulate in the blood and are the preferential energy sources for myocardium and the renal cortex, and during prolonged fasting they can be used by the central nervous system as well. Thus fatty acids, glycerol, and ketoacids are versatile and are widely used metabolic substrates that reach maximum serum levels during periods of fasting when glucose levels would be expected to be low.

In summary, the interaction of the various energy pathways provides adaptability by allowing a variety of metabolic fuels to be used. The balance between the various metabolic pathways is in large part maintained by insulin. Thus the key to understanding the pathophysiology of diabetes mellitus lies with the understanding of insulin's role in regulating normal human metabolism.

Insulin physiology

The insulin molecule contains 51 amino acids and has a molecular weight of 5800. It is composed of A and B chains, which are linked by disulfide bridges. Insulin is synthesized by beta cells in the pancreatic islets of Langerhans as a prohormone, then is released in its active circulating form. Native insulin has a circulatory half-life of 4–5 minutes and is primarily degraded by the liver.

Glucose is the most potent stimulus for insulin secretion. The mechanism by which glucose triggers insulin secretion is not entirely known but appears to be mediated, at least in part, either through glucoreceptors or as a result of changes in cellular levels of metabolic products of glucose metabolism within islet cells (5). Regardless, cell cAMP and cytosolic calcium levels rise in pancreatic beta cells after they are exposed to glucose, leading to insulin release. Insulin release is biphasic and consists of an initial rapid burst, which reaches a peak within 2 minutes and rapidly declines, followed by a more prolonged release commencing 5–10 minutes after stimulation and lasting approximately 1 hour. Overall, the rapid response of the beta cells to glucose provides a basic mechanism for tight regulation of the serum glucose, which normally varies by no more than 30–40 mg/100 ml over 24 hours.

There are other factors controlling insulin release besides glucose (5, 6). Amino acids stimulate insulin release, possibly through the action of gastrointestinal secretagogues. Of all the secretagogues, there is the most evidence for a role of gastric inhibitory polypeptide, which enhances the effects of glucose on insulin release. Neurogenic factors also play an important role in the control of insulin release. The alpha-adrenergic effects of catecholamines, especially epinephrine and norepinephrine, result in inhibition of glucose-mediated insulin release, whereas beta-adrenergic effects (i.e., isoproterenol) amplify the glucose-induced insulin release. Both of the above actions are mediated through changes of cell cAMP levels. The parasympathetic nervous system also acts on the pancreas and stimulates glucose-mediated insulin secretion through the vagus nerve. Thus, control of insulin secretion is accomplished through an intricate system that integrates controlling signals at several levels.

Insulin ultimately leads to enhanced glucose utilization and storage by acting on the liver, muscles, and adipose tissue. These tissues represent the primary targets for insulin action. In the adipocyte, insulin inhibits lipolysis, thus decreasing the transfer of fatty acids and glycerol to the liver; in the hepatocyte, insulin enhances esterification rather than oxidation of free fatty acids; and in peripheral tissues, insulin stimulates the oxidation of ketones. The action of insulin on these tissues is mediated by an effect at the cell membrane, where it binds to a receptor that in turn either triggers the generation of one or more second messengers or, alternatively, is followed by the internalization of the insulin molecule. The net result of insulin action in the liver is to decrease glycogenolysis, gluconeogenesis, and ketogenesis, and to stimulate glycogen and fatty acid synthesis. Insulin affects muscles, resulting in enhanced glucose and amino acid uptake and the promotion of protein and glycogen synthesis. In addition, in adipose tissue glycerol and fatty acid synthesis is stimulated. Thus, insulin serves to stockpile ingested nutrients as energy-rich compounds in the liver, muscle, and adipose tissue.

Effects of insulin deficiency

The development of diabetic ketoacidosis (DKA) involves a series of closely interrelated derangements of energy metabolism and of body fluid volume and composition, the fundamental nature of which has not been completely unraveled (5, 7). A synopsis of the most prominent metabolic alterations present in diabetic ketoacidosis is depicted in Figure 1. The role of an enhanced level of the counterregulatory hormones in the disturbed metabolism that is characteristic of DKA is presented in Figure 2. The composite clinical picture in full-blown DKA on admission includes hyperglycemia with hyperosmolality, metabolic acidosis due to the accumulation of ketoacids, extracellular and intracellular fluid (ECF and ICF, respectively) volume depletion, and varying degrees of electrolyte deficiency, particularly of potassium and phosphate (8, 9). Since proper correction of the alterations in volume status, acid-base, and electrolyte composition is critical for survival, a clear understanding of the pathogenesis of these derangements is essential for the adequate management of DKA (10).

Hyperglycemia and serum electrolytes

Insulin deficiency, either absolute or relative, results in hyperglycemia because of an impairment in glucose utilization by most tissues and the excessive hepatic

Diabetic Ketoacidosis

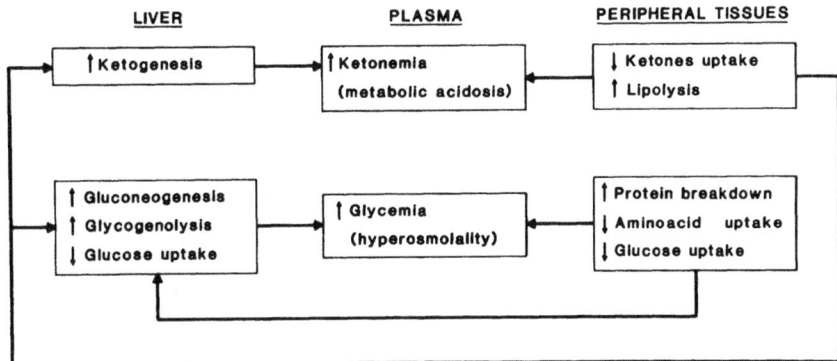

Figure 1. Cardinal alterations in DKA.

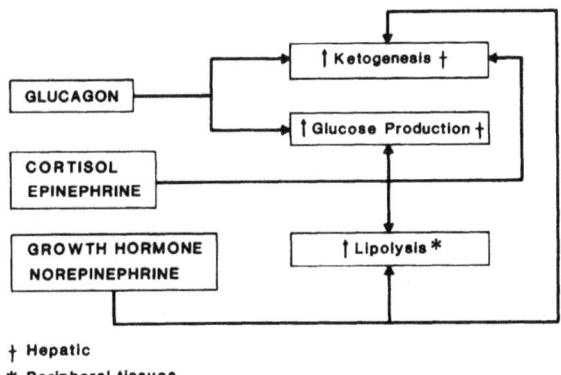

† Hepatic
* Peripheral tissues

Figure 2. Counterregulatory hormones in DKA.

production of glucose. The increase in effective osmotic pressure of the ECF consequent to the elevated glucose level causes a shift of water out of cells, most prominently from skeletal muscle. The resulting expansion of the ECF compartment is brief due to simultaneous renal and extrarenal losses of fluids. The increased filtered load of glucose, due to hyperglycemia, exceeds the renal tubular reabsorptive capacity, resulting in massive glycosuria, which is a hallmark of DKA. During the osmotic diuresis caused by the glycosuria, 75–150 ml/kg of water and 4–10 mEq/kg of sodium and chloride are lost in the urine (Table 1). Urinary water losses are disproportionately greater than the accompanying electrolyte losses, an event that should elevate the serum sodium and chloride levels. However, other factors also act to modify the serum concentration of sodium and chloride. First, the osmotic shift of water from cells into the vascular space dilutes the serum sodium (11). Further, the migration of sodium to the ICF compartment in the replacement of potassium losses decreases the serum sodium. Chloride, however, may be less depressed than sodium because urinary losses of sodium (as ketone salts) are significantly greater than losses of chloride. Alternatively, because of chloride losses secondary to vomiting, depression of serum chloride may be enhanced. Differences in the magnitude of these phenomena from one patient to another accounts for the variability in plasma composition observed on presentation. Table 2 reviews the admitting laboratory values of patients admitted with the diagnosis of DKA. Note that usually serum sodium and chloride are depressed. Elevations in the serum sodium suggest a profound water depletion, which may be seen in severely decompensated patients.

Prerenal azotemia due to volume depletion is a classic finding in DKA and is usually reversible, but occasionally it may progress to acute tubular necrosis (12, 13). Typically, the levels of urea nitrogen, creatinine, total proteins, uric acid, hematocrit, and hemoglobin are all elevated on admission, a reflection of ECF volume contraction, but they decrease significantly when water and electrolyte deficits are corrected. Thus, as a consequence of the severe hypertonic volume depletion and major metabolic derangements, deterioration in mental status, renal function, and cardiovascular function may all occur.

Acid-base changes

Insulin by its triple action on adipose, hepatic, and peripheral tissues is currently considered to be the major regulator of both production and utilization of ketones

Table 1. DKA: Water and electrolyte deficits (per kg body weight)

Water	70–150 ml
Sodium	4–10 mEq
Chloride	5–7 mEq
Potassium	3–10 mEq
Phosphorus	0–2 mEq
Magnesium	0.2–1 mEq

Table 2. Laboratory abnormalities on admission for DKA

Glucose	350–750 mg/dl			Values below 200 mg/dl ("euglycemic DKA") may be seen especially in alcoholics or pregnant isulin-dependent diabetics Values above 1000 mg/dl may be seen, especially in severe volume contraction leading to renal failure with loss of glycosuria (HHS may develop concomitantly). Concentration not related to severity of DKA
Blood ketones	Postive in undiluted plasma			The nitroprusside reagent (Ketostix, Acetest) does not react with β-hydroxybutyrate; color reaction is mostly (> 80%) due to acetoacetate
Bicarbonate	< 15 mM			Always reduced in DKA that is uncomplicated with metabolic alkalosis or respiratory acidosis
pH	< 7.30			Always reduced in DKA that is uncomplicated with metabolic alkalosis
	Low	Normal	High*	
Sodium	67%	26%	7%	Body stores are depleted; concentration dependent on blood glucose and relative water loss
Chloride	33%	45%	22%	
Potassium	18%	43%	39%	Body stores are depleted
Magnesium	7%	25%	68%	
Phosphate	11%	18%	71%	Decreases with insulin therapy and volume repletion
Calcium	28%	68%	40%	
BUN, creatinine	High			Since creatinine may be spuriously elevated (crossreaction with acetoacetate), BUN may better reflect renal function
WBC count	Usually high			Is not indicative of infection; is associated with lymphopenia and eosinopenia
Hb, Hct, total protein	Frequently increased			Due to intravascular volume depletion
SGOT, SGPT, LDH, CPK	high (20–65%)			Partially due to interference of acetoacetate in colorimetric methods Elevated CPK may be related to phosphate depletion and possible rhabdomyolysis
Amylase	Often increased			Isoenzyme evaluation reveals that origin is: pancreas (50%), salivary glands (36%), mixed (14%) of cases

From Kreisberg (7).

(5–7). Thus, insulin deficiency initiates a sequence of metabolic events that results in hyperketonemia due to both overproduction and decreased utilization of ketones (Figure 1). Ketogenesis is further stimulated by glucagon, which causes an increase in substrate supply and stimulates the oxidation of fatty acids in the liver. Other counterregulatory hormones involved in the metabolic derangement of DKA are catecholamines and cortisol (Figure 2). Further, the resulting acidosis may increase tissue resistance to the effects of exogenous insulin (14, 15). The net effect of the complex hormonal imbalance that results is stimulation of gluconeogenesis, ketogenesis, and lipolysis, and depression of glycolysis and glycogenesis.

During the development of DKA, ketoacids released into the ECF are titrated by bicarbonate and other body buffers. This buffering process results in an increase of plasma unmeasured anions and accounts for the classical acid-base pattern of metabolic acidosis associated with an increased anion gap (AG) (3, 16, 17). This latter term refers to those plasma anions, other than chloride and bicarbonate, that balance the positive charges of sodium and potassium:

$$AG = (Na^+ + K^+) - (Cl^- + HCO_3).$$

In uncomplicated DKA, the increment in AG above its normal value should be approximately equal to the decrement in plasma bicarbonate. Thus, the ratio of excess AG to that of bicarbonate deficit should be about 1:

$$(\text{Excess AG})/(\text{bicarbonate deficit}) = 1.0,$$

where excess AG (mEq/l) equals measured AG minus normal AG, and bicarbonate deficit (mEq/l) equals normal plasma bicarbonate minus measured plasma bicarbonate.

However, patients are often admitted with DKA and have a metabolic acidosis with an excess AG/bicarbonate deficit that is quite different than 1 (9, 16, 18). To understand these different acid-base and electrolyte patterns in DKA, the factors known to alter the stoichiometric relationship between the increment in AG and the decrement in serum bicarbonate must be evaluated (19). A decrement of the numerator or an increment of the denominator will decrease the magnitude of the ratio, whereas changes in the opposite direction will increase the value. The mechanisms that can alter this ratio are summarized in Table 3. It should be recognized that patients with DKA may have a concomitant alteration in acid-base status, resulting in a normal blood pH or even presenting with an alkalemic state (20).

Until recently, the role of the kidney as a major factor in the pathogenesis of the variable acid-base and electrolyte

Table 3. Ratio of excess plasma anion gap (AG) over bicarbonate deficit in DKA[1-3]

Increase above unity	Decrease below unity
Findings on admission	
1. Severe ECF volume deficit	1. Mild ECF volume deficit
2. Major impairment of renal function	2. Minor impairment of renal function
3. Higher values of Hct, Hb, serum proteins, BUN, creatinine, uric acid	3. Lower values of Hct, Hb, serum serum proteins, BUN, creainine, uric acid
Cause (before and after admission)	
1. Vomiting	1. Renal excretion of sodium salts of ketones
2. Exogenous bicarbonate therapy	2. Chloride-containing infusions
3. Renal acid excretion	3. Hypocapnia-induced suppression of HCO_3 reabsorption
4. Hyperproteinemia	
5. Tissue titration (Na^+/H^+ exchange)	4. RTA

[1] $AG = (Na^+ + K^+) - (Cl^- + HCO_3^-)$.
[2] Excess AG (mEq/l) equals measured AG minus normal AG, and bicarbonate deficit (mEq/l) equals normal plasma bicarbonate minus measured plasma bicarbonate.
[3] Expected value is 1.0 since the bicarbonate deficit is the result of its titration by ketoacids.

pattern in DKA was unrecognized (16, 19). It was demonstrated that on admission for DKA, some patients had pure AG acidosis, others had pure hyperchloremic acidosis, and the rest had a combination of both disturbances. However, when the data was analyzed as a group, the results obtained were consistent with the classic patten of AG acidosis in all the patients (16). The overall level of renal function on admission was found to be the major determinant of the type of metabolic acidosis. Laboratory data indicative of the status of the ECF volume were compared in patients who on admission had mainly "AG acidosis" to those of patients who had mainly "hyperchloremic acidosis." It was observed that the mean values of BUN, serum creatinine, plasma proteins, uric acid, and hematocrit and hemoglobin were all lower in patients with "hyperchloremic acidosis" than in those with "AG acidosis." These results indicate that the severity of the ECF volume deficit is greater in patients presenting with AG acidosis as compared to those with hyperchloremic acidosis. These findings were taken to mean that patients with DKA who develop significant volume depletion, as a result of osmotic diuresis and vomiting, will present with the classic AG type of metabolic acidosis because of a reduced excretion of ketone salts consequent to volume depletion. Conversely, patients with DKA who are able to maintain salt and water intake, thus preventing the development of volume depletion, will present with variable degrees of hyperchloremic acidosis, due to the urinary excretion of ketone salts and a concomitant retention of chloride. Strong support for this hypothesis was obtained from a group of balance studies, which demonstrated that the retention of chloride in excess of sodium, associated with urinary excretion of ketones of a magnitude comparable to that of retained chloride, fully explained the development of hyperchloremic acidosis in the early period after admission (16). A similar mechanism could account for the development of hyperchloremic acidosis prior to admission.

Considering that in DKA the patient is unable to properly metabolize ketoacids, whether these compounds are retained in the ECF or are lost in the urine as sodium and/or potassium salts, theoretically should not have any major effect on the severity the acid-base disorder. The data gathered confirmed this prediction because no difference in the severity of the hypobicarbonatemia was found between the two forms of metabolic acidosis at the time of admission (16). One may wonder why hyperchloremic acidosis is repeatedly recognized only in the recovery phase of DKA but not at the time of admission. Since the accepted treatment of DKA involves the administration of rather large amounts of saline infusions, most patients develop obvious hyperchloremic acidosis in the early period after admission. By contrast, the magnitude of the hyperchloremic acidosis before admission is smaller, making its recognition less likely. Furthermore, unless the ratio of excess anion gap to that of bicarbonate deficit is evaluated in each patient on admission for DKA, a large number of patients having only a component of hyperchloremic acidosis will go unrecognized. In addition, most studies that have evaluated the relationship between the excess AG and the bicarbonate deficit on admission simply compared the mean values of both parameters, so that individual variations in the excess AG/bicarbonate deficit ratio were, by necessity, hidden.

The hyperchloremic acidosis observed in DKA is usually brief, and it is considered to have no adverse clinical consequence. Since the development of this variety of acidosis results from the renal loss of bicarbonate precursors (ketone salts other than ammonium) accompanied by the retention of chloride, these patients should theoretically have a slower rate of recovery from the acid-base disturbance. Indeed, prospective studies have demonstrated that patients admitted with a greater component of hyperchloremic acidosis had, at any given time after admission, a smaller increment in their plasma bicarbonate above their admission levels (16). It appears that the more rapid recovery from metabolic acidosis in patients with DKA presenting with AG acidosis is consequent to the equimolar conversion of the retained ketone salts to bicarbonate after insulin administration. It might then be postulated that in patients with severe renal insufficiency who develop DKA, the underlying reduction in renal function will assure the retention of bicarbonate precursors; thus the acid-base disturbance will be rapidly reversed once insulin is provided. Whereas, to our knowledge, data in support of such a notion are not currently available, in the few instances we have had the opportunity to observe severe DKA in subjects with reduced renal function, the recovery from the acid-base disturbance was notably fast.

Potassium

The development of diabetic ketoacidosis (DKA) is usually accompanied by varying degrees of total body potassium depletion, which results from multiple causes, including massive kaliuresis, decrease intake, and frequent vomiting (3, 17). Yet plasma potassium levels are rarely low at the time of hospitalization, ranging in most instances from normal to high levels, and occasionally attaining dangerously elevated values (3, 4). This paradoxical relationship has been classically attributed to the concomitant changes in blood acidity that would effect a shift in potassium out of the cells in exchange for hydrogen ions moving intracellularly (21).

Several of the metabolic derangements observed in patients presenting with DKA are known to alter potassium metabolism and may contribute to the development of hyperkalemia. Endogenous ketoacidemia and hyperglycemia correlate with increased plasma potassium concentration on admission for patients with diabetic ketoacidosis (22). However, exogenous ketoacidemia and hyperglycemia in the otherwise normal experimental animal fails to increase plasma potassium levels (23, 24), so it would seem that the insulin deficit per se is the major cause of the hyperkalemia that develops in diabetic ketoacidosis (22).

Serum pH and bicarbonate levels are known to alter plasma potassium levels (21). While several studies have indicated that the changes in plasma potassium concentration observed during acute acid-base disorders are consequent to the attendant changes in plasma pH, others have shown that a low plasma bicarbonate concentration, under isohydric conditions, may induce hyperkalemia (25, 26). Increased effective serum osmolality is another abnormality characteristic of DKA that may affect serum potassium, since extracellular hypertonicity resulting from infusion of saline, mannitol, or glucose has been shown to result in the translocation of potassium-rich cell water to the extracellular compartment (27). Hyperglycemia of either endogenous or exogenous origin unaccompanied by ketoacidosis has been repeatedly shown to result in hyperkalemia in insulin-deficient diabetics, especially when hypoaldosteronism is also present (24).

Glucagon may also play a role in the hyperkalemia of DKA. This hormone may cause an increased potassium output from the liver, an effect that is usually transient because of the counter regulatory enhancement of insulin secretion. However, in the presence of an impaired insulin secretion, as in patients with DKA, increments in plasma glucagon levels may result in uncontrolled hyperkalemia (28).

An additional mechanism that may be involved in the deranged potassium homeostasis observed in DKA is the sympathetic system. Potassium tolerance has been found to be markedly impaired in chemically sympathectomized animals, but is improved in animals given a simultaneous infusion of epinephrine (29). The effects of the adrenergic agents on the internal potassium balance are mediated by their effect on the plasma levels of insulin and glucagon, and by a direct cellular effect. Therefore, any physiologic condition or pharmacologic maneuver that stimulates an alpha-adrenergic response or blocks the beta-adrenergic system could result in hyperkalemia, particularly during states of increased potassium load. It is then possible that during diabetic ketoacidosis there may be a suboptimal epinephrine response or altered peripheral sympathetic activity, resulting in potassium movement from the intracellular to the extracellular space, as well as an impairment in cellular entry of potassium.

In summary, acidemia with a decrease in serum bicarbonate, elevation of plasma anion gap, plasma hyperosmolality, glucagon, and sympathetic nervous system dysfunction induce a kalemic response that results from an insulin deficiency (22). Overall, insulin deficiency is probably the major protagonist of the complex hormonal disarray that is responsible for the hyperkalemia. Insulin has been shown to exert an effect on the transcellular shifts of potassium and on the physiologic control of the plasma level of this electrolyte (30, 31). An impairment in the extrarenal disposal of a potassium load has been well defined during insulin deficiency. This hormone is known to enhance the uptake of potassium in the liver, muscles, and adipose tissue. The insulin-induced cellular potassium uptake is only partially dependent on glucose entry into cells, and other glucose-independent mechanisms have been implicated (32, 33).

Phosphate

Serum phosphate levels fluctuate widely in patients with DKA, even though overall phosphate depletion has occurred. Several studies have demonstrated elevated serum phosphate levels in patients with DKA upon initial examination (4, 34). With insulin and fluid therapy, the phosphate concentration drops to normal or low levels. In a recent study, the initial serum phosphate level was found to correlate positively with the serum effective osmolality, glucose, and anion gap (34). This suggests that in the absence of insulin and in the presence of elevated glucose, serum osmolality, and metabolic acidosis, phosphate is shifted from cells into the interstitial and vascular spaces. Further, the osmotic diuresis of hyperglycemia leads to decreased renal reabsorption of phosphate, accounting for the depletion of total body phosphate with time. Then, with appropriate therapy, phosphate is shifted back into cells, rapidly lowering the serum levels. Early research suggested that the relative phosphate depletion of DKA is harmful, as phosphate replacement seemed to improve mortality. A more recent study, however, was unable to document that phosphate replacement makes any difference in the course of treated DKA (35). Thus it is difficult to make unequivocal recommendations regarding replacement therapy. The actual consequences of these shifts are not known.

Alterations in mental status

The differential diagnosis of an alteration in mental status in a diabetic is broad and includes primary central nervous

Table 4. DKA: Differential diagnosis

Toxic encephalopathy (ethanol, methanol, ethylene glycol, opium and narcotics, salicylates)
Trauma (head)
metabolic encephalopathy (hypoglycemia, uremia, hyperosmolar nonketotic coma)
Meningitis
Cerebrovascular accident/brainstem hemorrhage
Gastroenteritis
Pneumonia

system diseases, drug or ethanol intoxication, uremia, hypoglycemia, and hyperglycemia (Table 4). This differential should be considered in any diabetic with an alteration in mental status. During the past 30 years, a subset of comatose patients with hyperglycemia but without severe acidosis have been described (36–39). Typically, these nonketotic hyperglycemic patients in coma are older, have adult-onset or Type-II diabetes mellitus, and appear to have sufficient insulin to suppress fatty acid mobilization and subsequent ketone generation, but insufficient insulin to prevent hyperglycemia (40). The hyperglycemia and associated hyperosmolality appears to be the primary factor responsible for the alteration in mental status. It is hypothesized that the elevation in serum and CSF osmolality causes brain shrinking and leads to the alteration in mental status. With appropriate therapy, the hypertonicity resolves, the CNS returns to its normal size, and the patients recover.

Alternatively, patients in DKA may be admitted with a relatively normal mental status and become unconscious within the first 12 hours of therapy (41), even while serum glucose and ketoacidosis are improving. These patients are typically (but not exclusively) children or young adults, and have a higher mortality than would be expected (42). Often, the deaths of these patients are unexpected, as they do not have the underlying vascular, cardiac, and renal abnormalities found in older diabetics. At autopsy, these patients appear to have cerebral edema (42). The pathogenesis of this condition has been investigated by several authors but remains poorly understood (43–46). Osmotic disequilibrium between brain cells and the CSF is often cited. Comparison of blood and spinal fluid upon admission of decompensated diabetics revealed a lower CSF glucose, relatively normal pH and ketones, but a markedly elevated CSF osmolality (47). With time, brain cells develop an increase in their osmolality to match that of the CSF and thus defend themselves against shrinkage. A sudden decrease in CSF osmolality with volume loading or a fall in blood sugar will then cause brain swelling. The effects of rapid crystalloid volume loading in diabetics with DKA has been studied, and some degree of brain swelling or increase in CSF pressure was found (41, 48, 49). Clinically, patients in DKA with hyponatremia who receive insulin and more than 4 l of fluid per square meter within 24 hours may have an increased risk of developing cerebral edema (49). Alterations in CSF pH (47, 50) and oxygen tension (51) after intravenous bicarbonate therapy may also play a part. After bicarbonate therapy the CSF pH may decrease acutely, since carbon dioxide but not bicarbonate can rapidly cross the blood-brain barrier. Also, oxygen tension in the CNS was found to decrease, possibly due to acute shifts in the hemoglobin-oxygen dissociation curve with changes in pH; brain swelling may be secondary to either of these two factors as well (49). We must emphasize that the above proposed mechanisms are only hypotheses and the pathogenesis of cerebral edema under these conditions is not definitively known. Still, it seems prudent to avoid excessively aggressive volume replacement, sudden changes in the patient's serum sodium, or excessive use of bicarbonate. Fortunately, the development of clinically apparent cerebral edema associated with the therapy of DKA is not common. But, the fact that it occurs in young otherwise healthy patients pinpoints the importance of careful observation of all patients receiving therapy for DKA for the earliest signs of mental deterioration.

CLINICAL CONSIDERATIONS

The initiating events leading to the development of DKA are listed in Table 5. Not infrequently, DKA is precipitated by a seemingly trivial illness, including dietary indiscretions or overindulgence in ethanol. In addition, DKA may be the presenting manifestation in patients with undiagnosed diabetes (52).

The patient's historical and physical findings are in large part explainable by the underlying pathophysiology of the disease (Table 6). Patients may complain of polyuria, polydipsia, progressive weakness, and weight loss, all due to the osmotic diuresis of hyperglycemia. Abdominal pain, anorexia, nausea, and vomiting also occur frequently, and may constitute the patient's chief complaint. Indeed, these abdominal symptoms may be so severe as to require consideration of surgery for an abdominal catastrophe, only to fortunately have the abdominal pain resolve with treatment of the DKA. Changes in the patient's mental

Table 5. DKA: initiating events

1. Omission/reduction of insulin dose
2. Acute illness/infection
    Pneumonia
    Pyelonephritis
    Septicemia
    Mucormycosis
3. Emotional/other stress
4. Myocardial infarction, cerebrovascular accident
5. Intraabdominal catastrophes, pancreatitis
6. Pregnancy
7. Undiagnosed diabetes
8. Undetermined
9. Initiating events features
    Stress hormone release
    Insulin deficit
    Fasting, salt and water depletion

Table 6. DKA: symptoms and signs

- Anorexia, nausea, vomiting
- Abdominal pain, "acute abdomen"
- polyuria, polydipsia, volume depletion
- Headache, lethargy, stupor, coma
- Weakness, hypotonia
- Dyspnea, hyperpnea (Kussmaul type), acetone breath
- uncoordinated ocular movements; fixed dilated pupils

status over hours or days are also frequently reported and correlate with the degree of serum hypertonicity due to hyperglycemia. Other illnesses that should be included in the differential diagnosis are listed in Table 4. On physical examination, patients may be normotensive in spite of their volume losses, but they generally are tachycardic and exhibit orthostatic hypotension. The patient's temperature may be slightly elevated. If the patient is very acidotic, Kussmaul respirations will be noted, and the breath will smell of acetone, resembling the odor of Juicy Fruit™ gum. Abdominal tenderness, sometimes with spasm and rebound, is commonly seen. Abnormal mental status with altered deep tendon reflexes and neck rigidity may all be due to DKA, but other CNS disease processes will have to be considered (Table 4). Coma in the patient in DKA may be secondary to the metabolic derangements in the patient's acid-base status or serum electrolytes or, alternatively, may result from hypertonicity, stroke, CNS bleeding, anoxia after cardio-pulmonary arrest, or infection. Thus, the diagnosis of DKA can be made in a patient wih a compatible history and physical who has a metabolic acidosis, ketonemia, and hyperglycemia. The various labora-

Table 7. Initial assessment of DKA

Bedside evaluation
H & P
1. Make diagnosis promptly
2. Rule out hypoglycemia
3. Establish initiating event
4. Obtain body weight

Blood and urine testing: Confirm diagnosis by finding heavy glycosuria and ketonuria and by a strongly positive serum Acetest reaction (at least in undiluted serum)

Chest x-ray

Clinical laboratory
Blood
1. Glucose (repeat every 1–2 hours)
2. pH, PCO_2, and electrolytes (repeat every 2–4 hrs)
3. BUN, creatinine, osmolality
4. CBC
5. Cultures

Urine
1. Glucose
2. Ketones
3. Cultures

tory abnormalities found on admission in DKA are listed in Table 2.

The initial assessment of DKA involves both bedside evaluation and gathering of data from the clinical laboratory (53–55). The major aspects of this initial evaluation are summarized in Table 7.

The successful treatment of diabetic ketoacidosis depends on early diagnosis, aggressive treatment, the recognition of underlying diseases that may have predisposed the patient to DKA, and personal followup by the patient's physician (55–58). Considering that infection may be the precipitating factor of DKA as well as an important complication, maximal efforts should be made to search for the possible sites of infection and the identification of the causative microorganisms. The basic therapeutic goals and requirements for the successful management of a patient with DKA are listed in Table 8. Diabetic ketoacidosis is a medical emergency and should be treated as such. There are two conditions that carry a high risk of death, the comatose or severely obtunded patient and those in shock. These patients require the specialized care that is summarized in Table 9. Mortality from diabetic ketoacido-

Table 8. DKA: Basic therapeutic goals and requirements

Goals
1. Repletion of intravascular volume and maintenance of an adequate circulation
2. Reversal with insulin of the altered intermediary metabolism
3. Correction of electrolyte and acid-base imbalance
4. Correction of initiating event

Requirements
1. Competent, responsible physician continuously available
2. 24-hour availability of laboratory facilities
3. Equipment and drugs for handling medical emergencies, including those specific for DKA (regular insulin, normal and half-normal saline, 5% glucose in water, $NaHCO_3$, KCL and K-phosphate solutions)
4. Completion of flow sheet with hourly evaluation of vital signs, mental condition, urine tests, serum chemistries, insulin intake, fluid administration (IV, oral), urine output, electrolyte intake, and other medication

Table 9. Emergency therapy in DKA (possible)

Comatose, severely obtunded
- Admit to ICU
- Rule out hypoglycemia (if doubts administer 50 ml of 50% glucose)
- Give O_2, consider endotracheal intubation
- Stomach distension or vomiting: temporary tracheal intubation followed by nasogastric tube with continuous suction (to prevent pulmonary aspiration)

Shock
- Admit to ICU
- Monitor arterial blood pressure, central venous pressure, urine output
- Administer plasma volume expanders (plasminate, serum albumin, LMW dextran, 0.9% saline)

sis has steadily declined since the 1930s, from a high of greater than 40% to currently reported values of less than 5% (55, 59). This decline is due not only to improvements in medical technology, but also to the widespread appreciation of the seriousness and consequences of DKA.

Fluid therapy (Tables 10 and 11)

Upon admission, the patient with DKA should immediately undergo an assessment of vascular volume and cardiovascular function. Hyperglycemia leads to both cellular and extracellular volume depletion. An average 70 kg man may loose 5–7 l of water before being admitted to the hospital. Overall, during the first 24 hours, the patient requires fluids sufficient to provide both replacement of volume deficit and ongoing losses including nasogastric, other gastrointestinal, and insensible losses. Typically this requires infusing 6–10 l or more within the first 24 hours (60). Fluid challenges of this magnitude require that the patient receive careful monitoring for signs of pulmonary edema. Central venous or pulmonary artery catheterization may be required to correctly monitor vascular volume in some patients. Although efforts should be made to avoid bladder catheterization in patients with DKA in order to prevent the initiation or exacerbation of a urinary

Table 10. Differential distribution of standard solutions for intravenous use

Solution	% of volume infused		
	Intravascular	Interstitial	Intracellular
Plasminate 5% albumin	100	0	0
"Normal saline" (0.9% NaCl)	25	75	0
"Half-normal saline" (0.45% NaCl)	17	53	30
5% dextrose in water	10	30	60

Table 11. Fluid therapy in DKA[1]

Shock present (see Table 9)
- Kind
  - a. Plasminate, albumin, 5% albumin
  - b. 0.9% NaCl if the above not available
  - c. NaHCO$_3$,[4] 1–2 ampules (44–88 mEq) to be added per liter of IV infusion[2] when
    blood pH < 7.00 or T$_{CO_2}$ < 5 mM
    Discontinue NaHCO$_3$ in IV infusion when T$_{CO_2}$ > 8–10 mM
- Rate
  - a. 10 ml/kg/hr; if response is inadequate double infusion rate
  - b. Change kind and rate of infusion when shock is corrected to those indicated initially when shock is absent

Shock absent
- Kind
  - a. Normal saline — 0.9% NaCl — (initially) since 1) corrects ECF volume depletion as an ideal solution; 2) prevents a too rapid decrease of ECF osmolality; 3) decreases the risk of cellular swelling (i.e., brain) in comparison with hypotonic solution (0.45% NaCl)
  - b. Half-normal saline — 0.45% NaCl-plus 1 ampule (44 mEq) NaHCO$_3$ per liter when
    blood pH < 7.00 or T$_{CO_2}$ < 5 mM
    Discontinue NaHCO$_3$ in IV infusion when T$_{CO_2}$ > 8–10 mM
- Rate
  - a. Initial 2 hr 400 ml/hr, MILD (5% BW) depletion
    700 ml/hr, MODERATE (10% BW) depletion
    1000 ml/hr, SEVERE (15% BW) depletion
  - b. After 2 hr Decrease initial rate to half unless hemodynamic instability persists
    Change to 0.45% NaCl only if 1) hypernatremia develops, and
    2) signs of cerebral edema are absent (i.e., worsening of mental status, papilledema
    Start 5% dextrose in water[3] when blood glucose decreases to 250 mg/dl with the addition of 0.45% or 0.9% NaCl in the solution if significant ECF volume deficit, hyponatremia or cerebral edema are present
    Monitor urine output hourly (should be at least 30–60 ml/hr) and adjust if necessary, rate of infusion
  - c. After 4 hr of no vomiting or gastric suction start with clear liquids orally (up to 100–200 ml/hr if tolerated) and reduce according rate of IV fluids
  - d. After 8–12 hr from start of clear liquids, begin solid foods

[1] Repairs salt and water deficit and the altered hemodynamic status and renal function; in addition decreases level of counterregulatory hormones and enhances glucosuria.
[2] Bicarbonate should not be given by IV bolus unless hyperkalemia is present because of risk of lethal hypokalemia
[3] IV solutions without (or with low) electrolyte content repair free water deficit.
[4] See Table of Bicarbonate Replacement Therapy for further details. Initial rate includes maintenance needs (~100 ml/hr) plus replenishment of the depleted status of body fluids over a 12-hr period; best estimate of the severity of volume depletion is "weight loss" minus "tissue loss" of 1 lb/day of fasting before admission.

tract infection, a catheter may be inserted if the patient is stuporous or urine output cannot be monitored.

The first consideration in planning fluid therapy in DKA is to stabilize the patient hemodynamically by means of albumin-containing solutions if he or she is in shock (see Tables 9–11 for details). Thereafter, normal saline (0.9% NaCl) should be infused (61–64). Although the estimated water and salt losses in patients with DKA demonstrate the hypotonic nature of overall fluid deficit, other considerations (61–65) mandate the use of normal saline instead of half-normal saline during the initial several hours of treatment with only few exceptions that are outlined in Table 11.

Potassium and phosphate (Table 12)

Recall that the typical patient with DKA has a potassium deficit of about 6 mEq/kg at the time of admission, yet the initial serum potassium will often be normal or elevated. However, with insulin and bicarbonate therapy, the serum potassium level rapidly drops as potassium shifts intracellularly. Thus, potassium supplementation is required (55–58). Specifically, after the initial fluid challenge has restored the urinary output and if serum potassium is below 3.5 mEq/l, an IV infusion of 10–20 mEq/h is started and continued until the DKA is controlled and the serum potassium is 4.0–5.0 mEq/l. Serum potassium should be checked periodically during the infusion, and the potassium infusion rate should be adjusted as needed.

Phosphate deficit may also occur, but the benefit of giving phosphate as part of the routine therapy of DKA is disputed. The initial elevated serum phosphate levels fall with therapy and patients may become hypophosphate-mic. In one study, a total of 45 mM of phosphate was given and found to prevent post-treatment hypophosphatemia. However, this dose did not change the overall outcome of therapy, so the efficacy of treatment remained an open question (35). Although plasma phosphate may decrease to levels that are known to be associated with serious complications (i.e., respiratory failure, hemolysis, and impaired skeletal muscle and heart function), phosphate depletion in DKA is evident as a chemical abnormality that is usually not associated with clinical manifestations (66). Since phosphate administration may impose special risks (i.e., hypocalcemia, hypomagnesemia), it is not recommended (66, 67) in the usual therapy of DKA (Table 12).

Bicarbonate (Tables 13 and 14)

Historically, clinicians have felt that expedient correction of the metabolic acidosis was beneficial to the patient in DKA. Accordingly, bicarbonate was often given within the first few hours of treatment. However, bicarbonate administration should theoretically be unnecessary because ketones, when finally metabolized to CO_2 and H_2O, regenerate bicarbonate. Indeed, in DKA the early administration of bicarbonate may actually be harmful, leading to a worsening of the CNS acidosis and hypokalemia, and causing metabolic alkalosis after the DKA has resolved. The advantages and disadvantages of bicarbonate replacement therapy in DKA are summarized in Table 13. It is immediately apparent that the controversy in terms of the usefulness and indications of bicarbonate administration is based on differences in the appreciation of risks and benefits by different workers (68, 69). Table 14 summa-

Table 12. Potassium supplementation (KCl)[1] in the therapy of DKA

Should *not be* added to the initial 2 l of IV infusion to avoid hyperkalemia since
    a. Urinary output is initially unknown
    b. Initial $[K^+]_p$ is most frequently normal or high

Should *be* added[2] to the third liter of IV infusion and subsequently if
    a. Urinary output is adequate (should be at least 30–60 ml/hr) and
    b. $[K^+]_p < 5.0$ mEq/l
Rate of IV K^+ supplementation:
    a. 20–30 mEq/hr if $[K^+]_p < 4.0$ mEq/l
    b. 10–20 mEq/hr if $[K^+]_p > 4.0$ mEq/l
Concentration of K^+ in IV infusions:
    a. 20 mEq/l when IV supplementation is started and subsequently if $[K^+]_p < 4.0$ mEq/l, and IV infusion rate is 1 l/hr or higher
    b. 40 mEq/l (maximum) if $[K^+]_p < 4.0$ mEq/l and IV infusion rate is < 1 l/hr
Monitoring of K^+ supplementation is accomplished by:
    a. $[K^+]_p$ every 2–4 hrs during the initial 12–24 hrs of therapy
    b. ECG every 30–60 min during the initial 4–6 hrs (i.e., only lead II)

Exception to the above rules on K^+ supplementation: Add K^+ to the initial 2 liters of IV fluids if
    a. Initial $[K^+]_p < 4.0$ mEq/l and
    b. Adequate diuresis is secured

---

[1] Since phosphate replacement therapy is of unproven clinical signficancy and potentially dangerous (i.e., hypocalcemia, hypomagnesemia) potassium phosphate *should not* be infused unless serum phosphate < 0.5 mg/dl; then 10 mM potassium phosphate may be added to IV infusion.
[2] Decreased $[K^+]_p$ during therapy is multifactorial: a) insulin-mediated cellular uptake of K^+, b) dilution due to volume repletion by IV fluids, c) correction of metabolic acidosis, d) urinary K^+ losses.

Table 13. Bicarbonate replacement therapy in DKA* (Part I)

Advantages
1. May improve hemodynamic status if shock persists after volume repletion and significant metabolic acidosis is present
2. Increases myocardial contractility and enhances the cardiac and vascular responses to catecholamines; these mechanisms are involved in the positive hemodynamic effects
3. Helps correction of hyperkalemia, especially in the oligoanuric patient
4. May prevent a rapid fall in CSF osmolality and therefore may decrease the risk of cerebral edema
5. May improve cell metabolism and function (including CNS) that were depressed by severe acidosis
6. May improve the acidosis-induced glucose intolerance and insulin resistance

Disadvantages
1. May precipitate hypokalemia or worsen it, leading to cardiac arrhythmias (especially in digitalized patients) and/or dysfunction of respiratory muscles (respiratory failure)
2. May produce pulmonary edema and hypoxemia due to ECF volume expansion
3. May reduce cerebral blood flow (pH effect) and O_2 delivery to the brain
4. May worsen hypophosphatemia due to cellular uptake of phosphate and depress O_2 delivery from RBC (increased affinity of Hb for O_2) to tissues
5. May produce hypernatremia and increased serum osmolality
6. May further decrease CSF pH, leading to worsening of CNS function
7. May produce overshoot (rebound) alkalosis once conversion of ketone salts to bicarbonate takes place
8. May aggravate lactic acidosis if present
9. May predispose to tetany resulting from hypocalcemia plus alkalosis

*Bicarbonate should not be used in the standard treatment of DKA.

rizes our recommendations in terms of goals, indications, and dose estimation in bicarbonate therapy (69, 70). Yet, some studies found that administration did nothing to improve the recovery of patients with DKA who presented with arterial pH of 6.9–7.19 (71, 72). It should be recognized that in the presence of severe hypobicarbonatemia (i.e., $TCO_2 < 5$ mM), relatively small increments in CO_2 tension or in plasma organic acids may profoundly decrease blood pH to dangerously low levels (69, 73, 74). After weighing the arguments for and against the use of bicarbonate, it appears that the careful administration of bicarbonate to severely acidotic patients, especially those with hyperchloremic metabolic acidosis, to support their arterial pH at 7.1 or 7.2 and serum bicarbonate at approximately 10 is more beneficial than harmful.

Insulin therapy (Table 15)

Insulin is central to the regulation of ketone production and glucose utilization, thus adequate plasma insulin levels must be present if DKA is to be reversed (75, 76). The plasma insulin level that is required for one-half maximal oxidation of glucose in normal humans has been found to be about 5 µM/ml. In a 70 kg man, an IV injection of 7 U of regular insulin achieves peak plasma levels of approximately 1000 µM/ml, a clearly supraphysiologic level. In the years immediately following the discovery of insulin, DKA was treated with insulin doses of about 180 U over 12 hours, given IM. Then, in the 1940s diabetologists increased the doses of insulin based on several studies that suggested that pharmacologic doses of insulin improved patient survival. At the time, however, other studies disputed the need for such large doses of insulin. In the end, though, the use of high-dose insulin became the accepted practice. Then, in the early 1970s, several well-designed clinical trials documented the efficacy of low-dose insulin, which was satisfactorily confirmed thereafter (77–79). Currently, in patients with DKA the accepted practice is to give regular insulin as a low dose of a continuous IV infusion or IM at small intervals.

Table 14. Bicarbonate replacement therapy in DKA[1] (Part II)

Indications
1. Severe acidemia resulting from a decreased T_{CO_2} (pH < 7.00, $T_{CO_2} < 5$ mM), independently of the concomitant hemodynamic status
2. Significant metabolic acidosis (pH < 7.15, $T_{CO_2} < 10$ mM), that
   is associated with shock unresponsive to correction of volume depletion
   persists or has worsened after several hours of therapy
   is of the hyperchloremic variety ($\Delta AG/\Delta T_{CO_2} < 20\%$) instead of the usual high anion gap acidosis
   is associated with worsening of mental status and CNS depression
3. Severe hyperkalemia ($[K^+]_p > 7$ mEq/l)

Goals and dose estimation
1. If $T_{CO_2} < 5$ mM (indication 1), it should be increased to 8–10 mM only
2. If $T_{CO_2} < 10$ mM (indication 2), it should be increased to 13–15 mM
3. Dose estimation: (desired plasma T_{CO_2}-current plasma T_{CO_2}) × kg (BW) × 0.5[2]
4. Calculated bicarbonate dose may be added[2] to IV infusion (1–2 ampules 44–88 mEq $NaHCO_3$ per liter) or given by IV bolus (50% of estimated dose immediately, and the rest within 2–4 hrs provided that hypokalemia is not present or is simultaneously treated and evidence of pulmonary edema is not found)
5. Monitor blood acid-base status every 30–60 min (for 2–4 hr) after initiation of bicarbonate therapy to adjust dose to patient's needs

[1] Bicarbonate should not be used in the standard treatment of DKA.
[2] Derives from the "apparent space of distribution" of bicarbonate (retained HCO_3 mEq/kg/Δ $HCO_3^-_p$ from preinfusion) that is approximately 50% body weight (0.5) in normals, but increases in hypobicarbonatemic states; thus this formula underestimates bicarbonate requirements.

Table 15. DKA: Outline of insulin therapy[1,2]

A. *Continuous infusion (IV)*
  1. Set up piggy-back (50–200 ml) into IV line with regular insulin in normal saline (1 U/ml) after pre-flush of IV tubing (10–20 ml) to allow insulin adherence to plastic
  2. Give initial IV bolus of 0.2 U per kg of actual body weight, followed by
  3. Continuous IV drip of 0.1 U per kg of actual body weight per hour
  4. Double rate of infusion if blood glucose does not decrease in a 2-hour interval (expected drop is 40–80 mg/dl per hour or 10% of initial value)
  5. Give a dose (10–30 U) of regular insulin subcutaneously (SC) when blood glucose decreases to 300 mg/dl and continue with SC insulin injection every 4 hrs with sliding scale (i.e., 5 U if below 150 mg/dl, 10 U if 150–200 mg/dl, 15 U if 200–250 mg/dl, 20 U if 250–300 mg/dl)
  6. Stop insulin infusion when blood glucose decreases to 250 mg/dl and start 5% dextrose in water
  7. Insulin NPH or lente may be given when subcutaneous regimen is started (see 5)

B. *Intramuscular injection (IM) (deltoid muscle)*
  1. Give initial loading dose of 20 U regular insulin followed by 10 U at 1- to 2-hour intervals; IM route should not be used if hypotension is present
  2. Double insulin dose if blood sugar does not decrease in a 2-hour interval (expected drop is 40–80 mg/dl per hour or 10% of initial value)
  3. Start 5% dextrose in water and double time interval of insulin dose to be given SC instead of IM, when blood sugar decreases to 250 mg/dl; at this time insulin NPH or lente may be given SC
  4. Start use of sliding scale (see 5 above) for insulin dose when blood glucose decreases to 250 mg/dl

[1] The half-life of regular insulin administered IV is 4–5 min, IM is 2 hours, and SC is 4 hours.
[2] correction of hyperglycemia (below 300 mg/dl) and ketosis usually occur in 4–6 hours and 12–24 hours, respectively.

Typically an initial IV bolus of 10 U of regular insulin is given and an IV drip of 0.1 U/kg/hr is started. Serum glucose will fall at approximately 10% per hour. As the glucose approaches 250, D5 should be included in the IV fluids and the blood glucose should be followed closely. Recall that the basic problem in DKA is that cells are starved for glucose, and treatment requires that adequate glucose be provided for use by the cells. Hence both adequate glucose and insulin levels must be provided. The IV insulin rate is decreased to 1 or 2 U per hour so that the patient's blood glucose level remains between 100 and 200. Subcutaneous insulin (regular or long acting) is started when the patient can take PO nourishment and ketosis has stopped. Occasionally patients in DKA will exhibit marked insulin resistance (15). Should the blood glucose level not decrease at an insulin dose of 0.1 U/kg/hr, double or triple that dose may be needed. Care must be taken to decrease the dose as the patient's blood sugar approaches 250 or 300.

Table 16. Complications of DKA

1. Severe shock
   Volume depletion and hypovolemia
   Myocardial infarction
   Overwhelming sepsis
2. Cerebrovascular thrombosis, disseminated intravascular coagulation
3. Pulmonary edema, cardiogenic and noncardiogenic
4. Cerebral edema (potentially irreversible and fatal)
5. Hypokalemia and hyperkalemia
6. Acute tubular necrosis (renal failure)

Complications (Table 16)

A number of life-threatening complications may develop in the course of DKA in spite of adequate medical care (80, 81). Shock of cardiac origin or resulting from sepsis or volume depletion, and cerebral thrombosis/edema are among the most prominent complications (3, 82). Cerebral edema leading to death or responsible for chronic sequelae (83) is fortunately rare, yet milder forms may be regularly found with the standard treatment of DKA (49). The etiology remains undefined, since it is not consistently associated with bicarbonate therapy, hyponatremia and/hyposmolality, plasma glucose levels, or excessive hypotonic fluid replacement (46).

ACKNOWLEDGMENTS

We are indebted to Debby S. Verrett for skillful assistance in preparing the manuscript.

REFERENCES

1. Major RH: *Classic Description of Disease.* Charles C. Thomas, Springfield, II, pp 234–237, 1945.
2. Mering J, Minkowski O: Diabetes mellitus after extirpation of the pancreas. *Arch F Exper Path U Pharmakol* 375:26, 1889–1890.
3. Felig P: Diabetic ketoacidosis. *N Engl J Med* 290:1360–1363, 1974.
4. Kreisberg RA: Diabetic ketoacidosis: New concepts and trends in pathogenesis and treatment. *Ann Int Med* 88:681–695, 1978.
5. Karam JH, Salber PR, Forsham PH: Pancreatic hormones and diabetes mellitus In: FS Greenspan, PH Forsham, eds, *Basic and Clinical Endocrinology.* Lange Medical Publications, East Norwalk, CT, pp 523–574, 1986.
6. Skillman TG: Diabetes mellitus. In: EL Mazzaferri, ed, *Endocrinology.* Medical Examination Publishing, New York, pp 595–665, 1986.
7. Kreisberg RA: Diabetic ketoacidosis, alcoholic ketosis, lactic acidosis, and hyporeninemic hypoaldosteronism. In: M Ellenberg, H Rifkin, eds, *Diabetes Mellitus.* Medical Examination Publishing, New York, pp 621–653, 1983.
8. Felts PW: Ketoacidosis. *Med Clin North Am* 67:831–843, 1983.

9. Oster JR, Epstein M: Acid-base aspects of ketoacidosis. *Am J Nephrol* 4:137–151, 1984.
10. Keller U: Diabetic ketoacidosis: Current views on pathogenesis and treatment. *Diabetologia* 29:71–77, 1986.
11. Roscoe JM, Halperin ML, Rolleston FS, Goldstein MB: Hyperglycemia-induced hyponatremia: Metabolic considerations in calculation of serum sodium depression. *Can Med Assoc J* 112:452–453, 1975.
12. Trever RW, Cluff LE: The problem of increasing azotemia during management of diabetic acidosis. *Am J Med* 24:368–375, 1958.
13. Linton AL, Kennedy AC: Diabetic ketosis complicated by acute renal failure. *Postgrad Med J* 39:364–366, 1963.
14. Whittaker J, Cuthbert C, Hammond VA, Alberti KGMM: The effects of metabolic acidosis in vivo on insulin binding to isolated rat adipocytes. *Metabolism* 31:553–557, 1982.
15. Pedersen O, Beck-Nielsen H: Insulin resistance and insulin-dependent diabetes mellitus. Diabetes Care 10:516–523, 1987.
16. Adrogue HJ, Wilson H, Boyd AE III, Suki WN, Eknoyan G: Plasma acid-base patterns in diabetic ketoacidosis. *N Engl J Med* 307:1603–1610, 1982.
17. Kleeman CR, Narins RG: Diabetic acidosis and coma. In: Maxwell MH, Kleeman CR, eds, *Clinical Disorders of Fluid and Electrolyte Metabolism*. McGraw-Hill, New York, pp 1339–1377, 1980.
18. Gamblin GT, Ashburn RW, Kemp DG, Beuttel SC: Diabetic ketoacidosis presenting with a normal anion gap. *Am J Med* 80:758–760, 1986.
19. Adrogue HJ, Eknoyan G, Suki WN: Diabetic ketoacidosis: Role of the kidney in the acid-base homeostasis re-evaluated. *Kidney Int* 25:591–598, 1984.
20. Cronin JW, Kroop SF, Diamond J, Rolla AR: Alkalemia in diabetic ketoacidosis. *Am J Med* 77:192–194, 1984.
21. Adrogue HJ, Madias NE: Changes in plasma potassium concentration during acute acid-base disturbances. *Am J Med* 71:456–467, 1981.
22. Adrogue HJ, Lederer ED, Suki WN, Eknoyan G: Determinants of plasma potassium levels in diabetic ketoacidosis. *Medicine* 65:163–172, 1986.
23. Adrogue HJ, Chap Z, Ishida T, Field JB: Role of the endocrine pancreas in the kalemic response to acute metabolic acidosis in conscious dogs. *J Clin Invest* 75:798–808, 1985.
24. Goldfarb S, Cox M, Singer I, Goldberg M: Acute hyperkalemia induced by hyperglycemia: Hormonal mechanisms. *Ann Int Med* 84:426–432, 1976.
25. Fraley DS, Adler S: Isohydric regulation of plasma potassium by bicarbonate in the rat. *Kidney Int.* 9:333–343, 1976.
26. Fraley DS, Adler S: Correction of hyperkalemia by bicarbonate despite constant blood pH. *Kidney Int* 12:354–360, 1977.
27. Makoff DL, DaSilva JA, Rosenbaum BJ, Levy SE, Maxwell MH: Hypertonic expansion: Acid-base and electrolyte changes. *Am J Physiol* 218:1201–1207, 1970.
28. Massara F, Martelli S, Cagliero E, Camanni F, Molinatti GM: Influence of glucagon on plasma levels of potassium in man. *Diabetologia* 19:414–417, 1980.
29. Silva P, Spokes K: Sympathetic system in potassium homeostasis. *Am J Physiol* 241:F151–F155, 1981.
30. Cox M, Sterns RH, Singer I: The defense against hyperkalemia: The roles of insulin and aldosterone. *N Engl J Med* 299:525–532, 1978.
31. DeFronzo RA, Sherwin RS, Dillingham M, Hendler R, Tamborlane WV, Felig P: Influence of basal insulin and glucagon secretion on potassium and sodium metabolism. *J Clin Invest* 61:472–479, 1978.
32. Clausen T, Kohn PG: The effect of insulin on the transport of sodium and potassium in rat soleus muscle. *J Physiol (Lond)* 265:18–42, 1977.
33. Moore RD, Rabovsky JL: Mechanism of insulin action on resting membrane potential of frog skeletal muscle. *Am J Physiol* 236:C249–C254, 1979.
34. Kebler R, McDonald FD, Cadnapaphornchai P: Dynamic changes in serum phosphorus levels in diabetic ketoacidosis. *Am J Med* 79:571–576, 1985.
35. Wilson HK, Keuer SP, Lea AS, Boyd AE, III, Eknoyan G: Phosphate therapy in diabetic ketoacidosis. *Arch Int Med* 142:517–520, 1982.
36. Danowski TS, Nabarro JDN: Hyperosmolar and other types of nonketoacidotic coma in diabetes. *Diabetes* 14:162–165, 1965.
37. Jackson WPU, Forman R: Hyperosmolar nonketotic diabetic coma. *Diabetes* 15:714-721, 1966.
38. Johnson RD, Conn JW, Dykman CJ, Pek S, Starr JI: Mechanisms and management of hyperosmolar coma without ketoacidosis in the diabetic. *Diabetes* 18:111–116, 1969.
39. Arieff AI, Carroll HJ: Nonketotic hyperosmolar coma with hyperglycemia: Clinical features, pathophysiology, renal function, acid-base balance, plasma-cerebrospinal fluid equilibria and the effects of therapy in 37 cases. *Medicine* 51:73–94, 1972.
40. Matz R: Coma in the nonketotic diabetic. In: M Ellenberg, H Rifkin, eds, *Diabetes Mellitus*. Medical Examination Publishing, New York, pp 655–666, 1983.
41. Clements RS, Morrison AD, Blumenthal SA, Winegrad AI: Increased cerebrospinal-fluid pressure during treatment of diabetic ketosis. *Lancet* 2:671–675, 1971.
42. Young E, Bradley RF: Cerebral edema with irreversible coma in severe diabetic ketoacidosis. *N Engl J Med* 276:665–669, 1967.
43. Arieff AI, Kleeman CR: Studies on mechanisms of cerebral edema in diabetic comas. *J Clin Invest* 52:571–583, 1973.
44. Arieff AI, Kleeman CR: Cerebral edema in diabetic comas. II. Effects of hyperosmolality, hyperglycemia and insulin in diabetic rabbits. *J Clin Endocrinol Metab* 38:1057–1067, 1974.
45. Guisado R, Arieff AI: Neurologic manifestations of diabetic comas: Correlation with biochemical alterations in the brain. *Metabolism* 24:665–679, 1975.
46. Winegrad AI, Kern EFO, Simmons DA: Cerebral edema in diabetic ketoacidosis. *N Engl J Med* 312:1184–1185, 1985.
47. Ohman JL, Marliss EB, Aoki TT, Munichoodappa CS, Khanna VV, Kozak GP: The cerebrospinal fluid in diabetic ketoacidosis. *N Eng J Med* 284:283–290, 1971.
48. Fein IA, Rackow EC, Sprung CL, Grodman R: Relation of colloid osmotic pressure to arterial hypoxemia and cerebral edema during crystalloid volume loading of patients with diabetic ketoacidosis. *Ann Int Med* 96:570–575, 1982.
49. Krane EJ, Rockoff MA, Wallman JK, Wolfsdorf JI: Subclinical brain swelling in children during treatment of diabetic ketoacidosis. *N Engl J Med* 312:1147–1151, 1985.
50. Assal JP, Aoki TT, Manzano FM, Kozak GP: Metabolic effects of sodium bicarbonate in the management of diabetic ketoacidosis. *Diabetes* 23:405–411, 1974.
51. Bureau MA, Begin R, Berthiaume Y, Shapcott D, Khowry K, Gagnon N: Cerebral hypoxia from bicarbonate infusion in diabetic acidosis. *J Pediatrics* 96:968–973, 1980.
52. Matz R: Uncontrolled diabetes mellitus: Diabetic ketoacidosis and hyperosmolar coma. In: M Bergman, ed, *Princi-*

ples of Diabetes Management. Medical Examination Publishing, New York, pp 109–121, 1987.
53. Beigelman PM, Martin HE, Miller LV, Grant WJ: Severe diabetic ketoacidosis. *JAMA* 210:1082–1086, 1969.
54. Taylor AL: Diabetic ketoacidosis. *Postgrad Med* 68:161–173, 1980.
55. Vignati L, Asmal AC, Black WL, Brink SJ, Hare JW: Coma in diabetes. In: *Joslin's Diabetes Mellitus.* Lea and Febiger, Philadelphia, pp 526–552, 1985.
56. Davidson MB: Diabetic ketoacidosis and hyperosmolar nonketotic coma. In: MB Davidson, ed, *Diabetes Mellitus: Diagnosis and Treatment.* Wiley Medical, New York, pp 193–241, 1981.
57. Kitabchi AE, Matteri R, Murphy MB: Optimal insulin delivery in diabetic ketoacidosis (DKA) and hyperglycemic hyperosmolar nonketotic coma (HHNC). *Diabetes Care* 5:(Suppl 1):78–87, 1982.
58. Beigelman PM: Severe diabetic ketoacidosis. In: PM Beigelman, D Kumar, eds, *Diabetes Mellitus for the Houseofficer.* Williams & Wilkins, Baltimore, pp 23–36, 1986.
59. Ellemann K, Soerensen JN, Pedersen L, Edsberg B, Andersen OO: Epidemiology and treatment of diabetic ketoacidosis in a community population. *Diabetes Care* 7:528–532, 1984.
60. Johnson DG: Diabetic ketoacidosis. In: R Bressler, DG Johnson DG, eds, *Management of Diabetes Mellitus.* John Wright PSG, Boston, pp 153–174, 1982.
61. Kandel G, Aberman A: Selected developments in the understanding of diabetic ketoacidosis. *Can Med Assoc J* 128:392–397, 1983.
62. Brown RH, Rossini AA, Callaway CW, Cahill GF: Caveat on fluid replacement in hyperglycemic, hyperosmolar, nonketotic coma. *Diabetes Care* 1:305–307, 1978.
63. Fulop M: The treatment of severely uncontrolled diabetes mellitus. *Adv Int Med* 29:327–356, 1984.
64. Khardori R, Soler NG: Hyperosmolar hyperglycemic nonketotic syndrome. *Am J Med* 77:899–904, 1984.
65. Gundersen HJG, Christensen NJ: Intravenous insulin causing loss of intravascular water and albumin and increased adrenergic nervous activity in diabetics. *Diabetes* 26:551–557, 1977.
66. Foster DW, McGarry JD: The metabolic derangements and treatment of diabetic ketoacidosis. *N Engl J Med* 309:159–169, 1983.
67. Nattrass M, Hale PJ: Clinical aspects of diabetes ketoacidosis. In: M Nattrass, JV Santiago JV, eds, Churchill Livingstone, Edinburgh, pp 231–238, 1984.
68. Levine SN, Loewenstein JE: Treatment of diabetic ketoacidosis. *Arch Int Med* 141:713–715, 1981.
69. Narins RG, Arieff AI: Alkali therapy of metabolic acidosis due to organic acids. *AKF Nephrol Lett* 2:13–22, 1985.
70. Adrogue HJ, Brensilver J, Cohen JJ, Madias NE: Influence of steady-state alterations in acid-base equilibrium on the fate of administered bicarbonate in the dog. *J Clin Invest* 71:867–883, 1983.
71. Lever E, Jaspan JB: Sodium bicarbonate therapy in severe diabetic ketoacidosis. *Am J Med* 75:263–268, 1983.
72. Morris LR, Murphy MB, Kitabchi AE: Bicarbonate therapy in severe diabetic ketoacidosis. *Ann Int Med* 105:836–840, 1986.
73. Madias NE, Adrogue HJ: Influence of chronic metabolic acid-base disorders on the acute CO_2 titration curve. *J Appl Physiol* 55:1187–1195, 1983.
74. Madias NE, Bossert WH, Adrogue HJ: Ventilatory response to chronic metabolic acidosis and alkalosis in the dog. *J Appl Physiol* 56:1640–1646, 1984.
75. Kitabchi AE, Young R, Sacks H, Morris L: Diabetic ketoacidosis: Reappraisal of therapeutic approach. *Ann Rev Med* 30:339–357, 1979.
76. Kozak GP, Rolla AR: Diabetic comas. In: GP Kozak, ed, *Clinical Diabetes Mellitus,* WB Saunders, Philadelphia, pp 109–145, 1982.
77. Fisher JN, Shahshahani MN, Kitabchi AE: Diabetic ketoacidosis: Low-dose insulin therapy by various routes. *N Engl J Med* 297:238–241, 1977.
78. Pfeifer MA, Samols E, Wolter CF, Winkler CF: Low-dose versus high-dose insulin therapy for diabetic ketoacidosis. *Southern Med J* 72:149–154, 1979.
79. Carroll P, Matz R: Uncontrolled diabetes mellitus in adults: Experience in treating diabetic ketoacidosis and hyperosmolar nonketotic coma with low-dose insulin and a uniform treatment regimen. *Diabetes Care* 6:579–585, 1983.
80. Maccario M, Messis CP: Cerebral edema complicating treated non-ketotic hyperglycemia. *Lancet* 2:352–353, 1969.
81. Beigelman PM: Severe diabetic ketoacidosis (diabetic coma). *Diabetes* 20:490–500, 1971.
82. Halmos PB, Nelson JK, Lowry RD: Hyperosmolar nonketoacidotic coma in diabetes. *Lancet* 2:675–679, 1966.
83. Keller RJ, Wolfsdorf JI: Isolated growth hormone deficiency after cerebal edema complicating diabetic ketoacidosis. *N Engl J Med* 316:857–859, 1987.

CHAPTER 12

Renal Tubular Acidosis

FERNANDO SANTOS, GAD KAINER & JAMES C.M. CHAN

ROLE OF THE KIDNEY IN HYDROGEN ION REGULATION

The kidney's role in the prevention of acidosis is to excrete hydrogen ions in the form of titratable acid and ammonium, and to reabsorb bicarbonate present in the glomerular filtrate or formed during the process of urinary acidification in the distal tubule.

The main site of bicarbonate reabsorption is the proximal renal tubule. Approximately 80–90% of the 4500 mM of bicarbonate filtered by the glomerulus each day is reabsorbed by the kidney in normal adults. The remainder is almost totally reabsorbed by the distal renal tubule. The efficiency of the infant kidney is 60–70% reabsorption in the proximal tubule, from a smaller filtered bicarbonate load of 2500 mM/day. A proportionately smaller fraction is reabsorbed by the distal renal tubule (1–4). Infants have a lower renal threshold for bicarbonate that persists until at least during the first year of life (3–5).

Micropuncture studies have shown that sodium ion reabsorption is accompanied by hydrogen ion secretion (6). Carbonic acid is formed from the union of bicarbonate with the hydrogen ion, which, under the enzymatic influence of carbonic anhydrase in the proximal tubule luminal membrane, is hydrolyzed to CO_2 and H_2O. Carbon dioxide diffuses readily from the basolateral membrane of the proximal tubule cells to enter the extracellular bicarbonate pool. The overall rate of bicarbonate reabsorption in the proximal tubule is a transport maximum mechanism, but reabsorption is also directly proportional to the rate of sodium reabsorption and is also under the influence of carbonic anhydrase, extracellular CO_2 tension, parathyroid hormone, potassium concentration, and extracellular fluid volume (6).

In the distal tubule, secreted hydrogen ions combine with filtered phosphate, which has not been reabsorbed, and other nonvolatile buffers, e.g., citrate and creatinine, to form titratable acids. Ammonia, produced by the action of glutaminase on glutamine in the distal tubular cells, combines with hydrogen ions to produce ammonium. Net urinary acid excretion is the difference between titratable acid and ammonium minus any residual bicarbonate (6–9).

In the hydrated patient with normal plasma bicarbonate concentrations, the finding of urinary bicarbonate excretion in excess of 15% of the filtered load in adults and 25% in infants would point to the presence of a proximal tubular defect in bicarbonate reabsorption (3, 8).

It is important to note that, in infants, plasma bicarbonate is usually 4–5 mM/l lower than adult concentrations of 24 mM/l. The difference is made up by chloride ions. The venous plasma bicarbonate concentration is higher than the arterial concentration by several mM/l due to the higher CO_2 from tissue metabolism.

CONCEPT AND CLASSIFICATION

Renal tubular acidosis (RTA) is a disorder resulting from a defect in proximal bicarbonate reabsorption and/or distal hydrogen ion secretion. RTA is characterized by a biochemical picture of hyperchloremic metabolic acidosis with a normal or moderately reduced glomerular filtration rate. The anion gap is characteristically normal (1) (Table 1).

Common clinical features of RTA in children include failure to thrive and recurrent episodes of vomiting and dehydration (2–4). In addition, clinical signs related to underlying diseases and specific manifestations of the different forms of RTA (rickets, hyperkalemia, nephrocalcinosis) can also be found.

Table 1. Metabolic acidosis with normal anion gap

Renal tubular acidosis
Early uremic acidosis
Dilutional acidosis
Acid loads
Bicarbonate losses
  Diarrhea
  Ureterosigmoidostomy
  Intestinal fistulas
  Drugs
    Calcium chloride
    Magnesium sulfate
    Cholestyramine

Several types of RTA are usually described (3, 5). Type I RTA results from inadequate elimination of hydrogen ions in the distal nephron. Type II RTA is characterized by massive bicarbonaturia secondary to defective proximal bicarbonate reabsorption. Type IV RTA is characterized by hyperkalemia and defective ammonium excretion resulting from aldosterone deficiency or tubular resistance to aldosterone actions. Type I RTA associated with severe bicarbonate wasting was once described as Type III RTA (6). It is a hybrid form of RTA combining permanent distal acidification derangement with a transient defect of proximal bicarbonate reabsorption. Type III RTA is currently considered to be a variant of Type I RTA, exclusively found in infants and children, rather than being a distinct entity in itself (3).

DIAGNOSTIC APPROACH

Identification of patients with RTA and their characterization by the different types of RTA require the use of various specific tests.

Urine pH and net acid excretion measurements during spontaneous or induced systemic acidosis

The kidney contributes to maintenance of acid-base homeostasis by means of two principal mechanisms: reabsorption of filtered bicarbonate and fixed acid excretion, which is coupled with regeneration of bicarbonate utilized in the buffering process of these nonvolatile acids.

About 85% of filtered bicarbonate is reabsorbed within the proximal tubule. The remaining 15% of filtered bicarbonate is reabsorbed in the distal nephron segments. Complete reabsorption of filtered bicarbonate results in a decrease of urine pH to approximately 6. In the healthy individual, urine pH can be lowered one or two additional units within the distalmost portions of the nephron. This ability to lower urine pH to a range of 4.3–4.5 is unique to the distal tubule and collecting ducts, and it is accomplished by active hydrogen ion secretion (5, 7, 8).

The bulk of hydrogen ion secreted in the distal nephron is buffered by the two major urinary buffers: ammonia and phosphate. Ammonia combines with hydrogen ions and is excreted as ammonium. Disodium monohydrogen phosphate combines with secreted hydrogen ions to form monosodium dihydrogen phosphate, which is excreted as titratable acid. The term *titratable acid* refers to the amount of alkali needed to titrate an acid urine back to a pH of 7.4 (5).

The sum of titratable acid and ammonium minus bicarbonate constitutes the net acid excretion. Under normal conditions, the total daily net acid excretion equals the total endogenous acid production from diet and intermediary metabolism (9, 10). As shown by Chan (11), the rate of endogenous acid production (mEq/kg body weight/day) is higher in children than in adults (Figure 1). In general terms, it is estimated that healthy adults generate 1–2 mEq of endogenous acid/kg/day (5, 9), whereas this amount is approximately 2–3 mEq/kg/day in infants and children.

According to the previous discussion, evaluation of urine pH and net acid excretion should constitute one of the first steps in the study of patients suspected of having RTA. The urine pH should be measured from freshly voided urine. If the net acid excretion cannot simultaneously be measured, urine should be frozen at $-22°C$, which preserves reproducible and stable values up to 12 months of storage (12).

Challenged by metabolic acidosis (Figure 2), normal

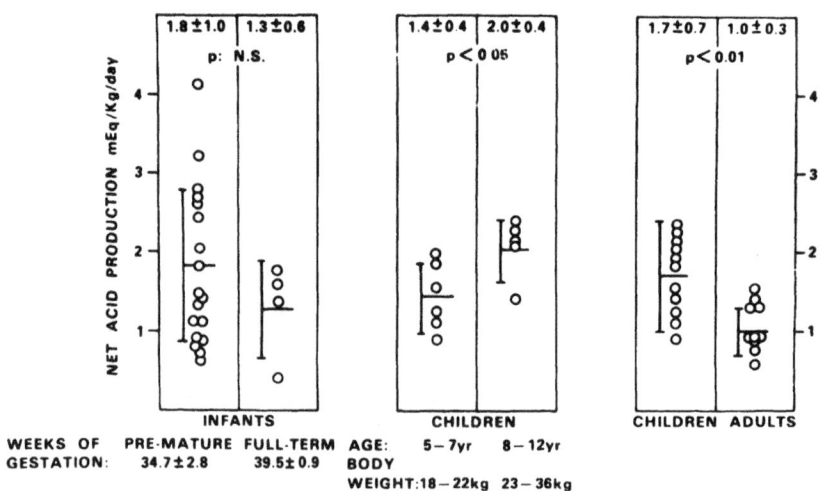

Figure 1. Rate of endogenous acid production in different age groups. Replotted from data of Chan (11).

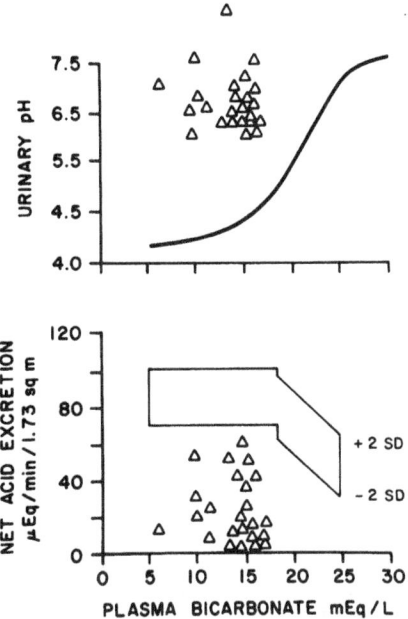

Figure 2. Response of net acid excretion and urinary pH to metabolic acidosis in children with primary Type I RTA as compared with normal values of control population. Reprinted from reference 14 with permission of S. Karger AG, Basel.

subjects are able to lower the urine pH below 5 and to increase the net acid excretion up to 70–100 μEq/min/1.73 m² body surface area (3, 13, 14). In patients with RTA, minimum urine pH and maximum net acid excretion can usually be assessed in the face of spontaneous metabolic acidosis. Moderate acidosis (serum bicarbonate < 16 or 17 mEq/l) is sufficient to evaluate urinary acidification, and it is not necessary to induce severe systemic acidosis (15, 16). It should be noted that special attention must be paid to patients with proximal RTA because they are able to achieve a normal minimum urinary pH only when the serum bicarbonate concentrations fall below the renal bicarbonate threshold. Only with these low concentrations of serum bicarbonate can the filtered bicarbonate be completely reabsorbed, with the cessation of bicarbonate wasting.

In patients with mild acidosis (serum bicarbonate concentration > 17 mEq/l) should acid loading tests be performed. Ammonium chloride at a single dose of 75–100 mEq/m² body surface area, orally administered over 1 hour in gelatin-coated capsules, is a potent acidifying agent (17, 18). In order to achieve a maximal stimulus of ammonium excretion, ammonium chloride can also be given at a dose of 0.1 g/kg body weight daily for 3–5 days (19). Arginine hydrochloride (100–150 mEq H⁺/m² body surface area infused intravenously) (20) and calcium chloride (2 mEq/kg orally) (21) have been used as alternative acidifying agents.

Assessment of the fractional excretion of bicarbonate in the face of normal plasma bicarbonate concentrations

Calculation of bicarbonate wasting at normal plasma concentrations of bicarbonate is a useful procedure to establish the differential diagnosis among the various types of RTA. Bicarbonaturia can easily be estimated by calculating the fractional excretion of bicarbonate that is equal to the ratio:

$$\frac{\text{Urine bicarbonate (mEq/l)} \times \text{plasma creatinine (mg/dl)}}{\text{Plasma bicarbonate (mEq/l)} \times \text{urine creatinine (mg/dl)}} \times 100.$$

In patients with RTA, achieving normal concentrations of plasma bicarbonate (22–24 mEq/l) requires the administration of adequate amounts of alkali. The oral sodium bicarbonate load (2–3 mEq/kg body weight) is usually enough in patients with the types of RTA in which the urinary loss of bicarbonate is small. By contrast, in patients with considerable bicarbonate wasting, intravenous administration of bicarbonate infusions may be needed. During alkali supplementation, special care should be taken to minimize extracellular volume expansion (22, 23).

Assessment of urinary P_{CO_2} in alkaline urine

Theoretically, reduced distal elimination of hydrogen ions could result from: a) impaired hydrogen ion secretion b) back-leak of either carbonic acid or secreted hydrogen ions, and c) distal secretion of bicarbonate. Experimental and clinical findings do not support this last possibility. In turn, impairment in hydrogen ion secretion could result from: a) an intrinsic defect in the proton pump b) inability of the tubular cell to secrete hydrogen ions against an unfavorable chemical (tubular lumen pH lower than blood pH) or electrical (abnormal luminal positive difference) gradient, and c) lack of available sodium in the tubular fluid to be exchanged with hydrogen ions (15, 24–27).

Measurement of urinary P_{CO_2} in highly alkaline urine, induced by bicarbonate loading, allows assessment of the hydrogen secretory capacity of the distal nephron in the face of a favorable chemical gradient (urine pH > blood pH) (28–31). Secreted hydrogen ions enter the tubular lumen and combine with bicarbonate anions to form carbonic acid, which dehydrates slowly into CO_2 and H_2O, since carbonic anhydrase is absent in the luminal side of the distal nephron cells. Delayed dehydration of carbonic acid takes place in the medullary collecting duct and lower urinary tract, where the medullary trapping of P_{CO_2} and the disadvantageous surface to volume relationship limit CO_2 diffusion out of the urine. Thus, the urinary CO_2 content rises, and measurement of P_{CO_2} in alkaline urine can be used as a reliable index of distal hydrogen ion secretion — provided a high urinary bicarbonate concentration, which can react with secreted hydrogen ions, is simultaneously present (25, 32). Under these conditions, normal individuals are capable of increasing urine P_{CO_2} above 70 mmHg and achieving a P_{CO_2} difference between urine and blood 25–30 mmHg (26).

Assessment of urine minus blood P_{CO_2} gradient during neutral sodium phosphate load

Normally, neutral sodium phosphate administration results in a significant rise in urine P_{CO_2} of at least 25 mmHg above blood P_{CO_2}, when the urine pH is about 6.8 (pK of phosphate buffer system) and the urinary phosphate concentration is greater than 20 mM/L (33). Under these conditions, phosphate represents a potent stimulus for proton secretion and, additionally, it reacts with the hydrogen ions secreted into the tubular lumen to form acid phosphate, which is much less diffusible than carbonic acid. The further reaction of acid phosphate with bicarbonate to form carbonic acid and subsequently CO_2 takes place in the distalmost segments of the nephron and lower urinary tract, where back diffusion of CO_2 is limited, giving rise to increased urinary CO_2 content (34).

Thus, theoretically at least, neutral phosphate administration should revert both the acidification defect secondary to acid back-leak and that resulting from a reduced rate of distal hydrogen ion secretion.

Assessment of urine pH following sodium sulfate infusion

In normal individuals in which a state of sodium avidity has been induced, sodium sulfate brings about a fall of urine pH below 5.5 and a kaliuretic response (15, 33, 36). Sodium sulfate infusion increases distal delivery of sodium because sulfate is a poorly reabsorbable anion. Sodium is reabsorbed and the sulfate anion remains in the tubular fluid, which increases the luminal negative potential difference. Consequently, potassium and proton secretions are stimulated. In addition, high lumen electronegativity restricts back-diffusion of secreted acid.

As shown by Batlle et al. (33), sodium sulfate infusion (500 ml solution of 4% sodium sulfate over a period of 45–60 minutes) induced a fall of urine pH as well as significant increases of sodium, potassium, and net acid excretion in normal subjects given 1 mg of oral fludrocortisone over the 12 hours preceding the test. Similar findings were reported by Rodriguez–Soriano et al. (37) in control children receiving 0.2 mM sodium sulfate at an initial intravenous dose of 5 ml/kg body weight × 0.3 followed by infusion of 0.75 ml/min/1.73 m² body surface area for 90 minutes, after oral administration of 0.1 mg of fludrocortisone the day before the test

It is reasonable to hypothesize that patients with RTA, in whom impairment of hydrogen ion secretion results from either the inability to overcome an unfavorable electrical gradient, low distal sodium delivery, or acid back-leak, can respond normally to sodium sulfate testing, provided that the capacity of the tubular cells to both secrete hydrogen ions and reabsorb sodium is preserved.

Assessment of urine pH after furosemide administration

In normal subjects, furosemide administration (1–2 mg/kg body weight) induces a marked decrease of urine pH in association with a significant increase of net acid excretion. This effect is maximum 2–3 hours after furosemide administration (38–40).

Furosemide increases sodium distal delivery and inhibits chloride reabsorption. Thus, furosemide stimulates urinary acidification by a mechanism similar to that of sodium sulfate, since it provides a large amount of sodium available to be exchanged with hydrogen ions and, at the same time, enhances the electronegativity of the tubular lumen by depressing chloride reabsorption.

Accordingly, patients with RTA should show concordant responses to both furosemide and sodium sulfate tests.

Patients with Type IV RTA, in whom hyperkalemia could be worsened by acid loading, may be investigated using furosemide to stimulate urinary acidification (39).

Table 2. Etiological spectrum of Type I RTA

A. Isolated primary defect
B. Secondary defects
  1. Tubulo-interstitial renal disorders
      Obstructive uropathy
      Medullary sponge kidney
      Renal transplantation
      Nephrocalcinosis induced by metabolic and endocrine disorders
        vitamin-D intoxication
        hyperparathyroidism
        idiopathic hypercalciuria
        Wilson's disease
        hyperthyroidism
  2. Genetically transmitted systemic diseases
      Ehlers–Danlos syndrome
      Marfan's syndrome
      Osteopetrosis with associated nerve deafness
      Sickle cell anemia
      Elliptocytosis
      Carbonic anhydrase deficiency
      Hereditary fructose intolerance
      Fabry's disease
  3. Autoimmune diseases
      Sjogren's syndrome
      Hypergammaglobulinemic disorders
      Systemic lupus erythematosus
      Chronic active hepatitis
      Thyroiditis
  4. Toxin or drug induced
      Amphotericin B
      Lithium
      Analgesics
      Cyclamate
      Toluene
  5. Hyponatriuric states
      Nephrotic syndrome
      Hepatic cirrhosis

TYPE I RTA (DISTAL RTA)

The distinctive feature of distal RTA is the inability of the distal nephron to maximally lower urine pH in spite of simultaneous systemic metabolic acidosis.

The etiology of distal RTA is listed in Table 2. As shown in this table, Type I RTA is a syndrome caused by a heterogeneous group of disorders. In some of these disorders, the underlying mechanism potentially responsible for the defective urinary acidification has been identified. Table 3 attempts to present a diagnostic approach useful to distinguish among the different pathophysiologic mechanisms causing Type I RTA (15, 16, 25, 26, 31, 33, 41–47). It should be noted that some of the mechanisms and responses shown in the table still need additional clinical or experimental clarifications, but they are proposed on the basis of theoretical considerations. It is also of interest that Batlle et al. (48) reported a small number of adult patients who had a normal capacity to maximally lower urine pH in metabolic acidosis conditions and inability to normally increase the urine minus blood P_{CO_2} gradient. According to their hypothesis (48), these patients had a decrease in the rate of distal hydrogen ion secretion that could only be determined during bicarbonate loading. In their view, assessment of P_{CO_2} in highly alkaline urine may represent the most sensitive test to investigate distal acidification.

Whereas the acquired forms of distal RTA are frequently observed in adult individuals, most children with Type I RTA have the primary or idiopathic form. It may occur sporadically or be transmitted as an autosomal dominant trait (49).

Failure to thrive is the most common presenting symptom in children having primary Type I RTA (14). Vomiting and diarrhea, polyuria-polydipsia, poor feeding, and recurrent episodes of dehydration are also frequent clinical manifestations (2, 3, 14, 50). These symptoms usually appear in infancy or early childhood (3, 14).

Biochemically, primary distal RTA, like other types of RTA, is characterized by a sustained metabolic acidosis with hyperchloremia and a normal anion gap (1, 51).

Diagnosis of Type I RTA should be established by using the specific tests described here: Urine pH is higher than 5.5 in the face of systemic metabolic acidosis. Simultaneously, net acid excretion is less than 70 µEq/min/ 1.73 m² body surface area (Figure 2).

Fractional excretion of bicarbonate is below 5% once normal plasma concentrations of bicarbonate have been achieved (Figure 3). However, it should be noted that a proximal leak of bicarbonate is frequently associated with a distal defect in infants with Type I RTA (22, 52, 53). Thus, in these small patients, values of fractional excretion of bicarbonate higher than 5% are usually found (Type III RTA). Proximal impairment is transient and, as children are growing, the exaggerated loss of bicarbonate disappears, and a typical pattern of pure distal RTA becomes manifest (50). Associated signs of generalized proximal tubular dysfunction (glycosuria, hyperaminoaciduria) are characteristically absent.

In patients with primary Type I RTA in whom the mechanism for the distal acidification defect could be studied, no response to the different tests administered to stimulate hydrogen ion secretion has been observed (15, 37). Urinary P_{CO_2} is inappropriately low, both in alkaline urine and after phosphate load (Figure 4). In turn, inability to decrease urine pH below 5.5 cannot be reversed with either sodium sulfate infusion or furosemide administration (Table 3). These findings are entirely consistent with an intrinsic derangement of the proton pump as the

Table 3. Proposed pathophysiologic mechanisms causing distal RTA

Hypothetic mechanism	Alkaline urine (U–B P_{CO_2})	Phosphate administration (U–B P_{CO_2})	Sulfate infusion U_{pH}	U_k	Furosemide test U_{pH}	Clinical experimental example
I. Impaired H⁺ secretion						
A. Proton pump failure	Low	Low	>5.5	Normal or high	>5.5	Primary defect, nerve deafness
B. Inability to overcome an adverse gradient						
1. Chemical	Normal	Normal-low	>5.5	Normal	>5.5	No evidence
2. Electrical (voltage defect)						
a. Severe blockade of distal Na reabsorption	Low	Low	>5.5	Low	>5.5	Obstructive uropathy, amiloride
b. Reversible impairment of Na reabsorption	Low	Normal	<5.5	Normal	<5.5	Sickle cell anemia, lithium
c. Lack of Na available to be exchanged with H⁺	Normal	Normal	<5.5	Normal	<5.5	Nephrotic syndrome
II. Back diffusion of acid						
A. Hydrogen ion	Normal	Normal	<5.5	Normal	<5.5	Amphotericin B
B. Carbonic acid	Low	Normal	<5.5	Normal	<5.5	No evidence

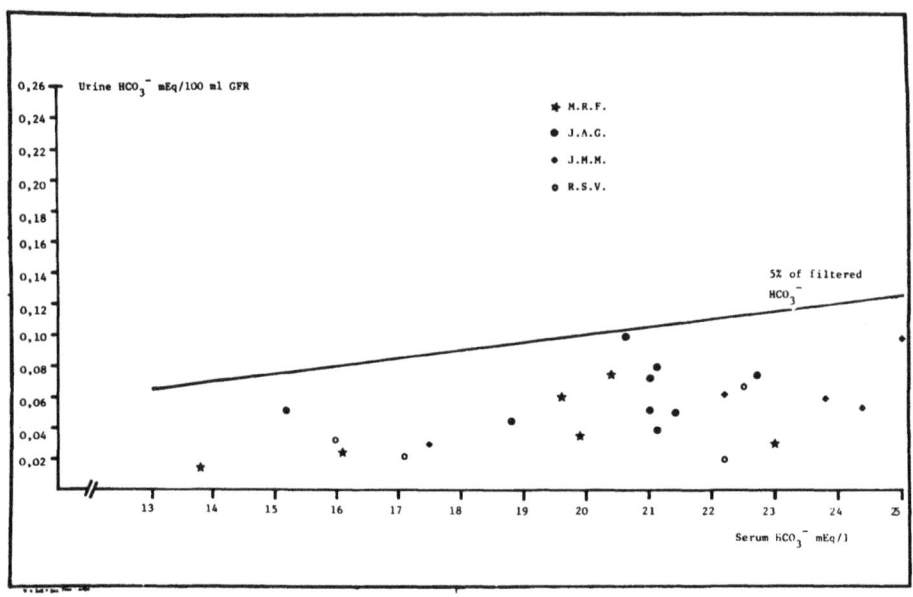

Figure 3. Fractional excretion of bicarbonate in four patients with distal RTA. Note bicarbonaturia lower than 5% of filtered bicarbonate at normal serum bicarbonate concentrations.

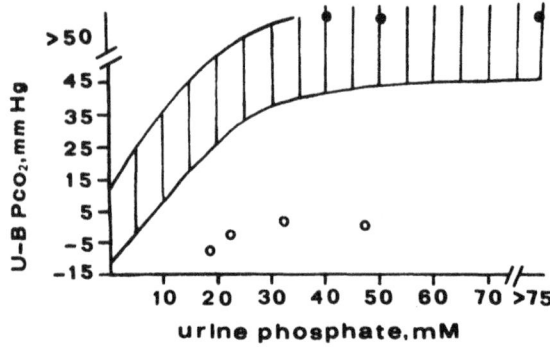

Figure 4. Low urine to blood P_{CO_2} gradient (U-B P_{CO_2}) in four patients with Type I RTA (○) after phosphate loading.

mechanism causing impaired distal acidification in this varient of Type I RTA.

It has been generally assumed (49, 54) that hypokalemia, associated with excessive hyperaldosteronism-dependent renal potassium wasting (55), is a typical feature of classic Type I RTA. However, the pattern of serum potassium concentration in children with primary distal RTA is not uniform, and low, normal, and high values of serum potassium can be found (14). Likewise, a hyperkalemic form of voltage-dependent distal RTA has been reported (44) in some adult individuals with obstructive uropathy.

Hypocitraturia and hypercalciuria are characteristic biochemical findings in patients with distal RTA. Hypocitraturia is believed to be due to enhanced proximal tubular reabsorption of filtered citrate resulting from an acidosis-induced low intracellular concentration of citrate in the tubular epithelium (56). Norman et al. (57) measured urinary excretion of citrate in members of three families with familial distal RTA. Their results support the concept that hypocitraturia may constitute a useful marker to identify otherwise asymptomatic individuals with mild or incomplete forms of Type I RTA.

Hypercalciuria is frequently found in patients with primary Type I RTA. It has been classically proposed that the hypercalciuria of distal RTA is most likely due to bone dissolution secondary to the body's attempt to buffer the retained acid with bone calcium salts (56, 59). However, convincing evidence supporting this hypothesis is lacking. Normal vitamin D-parathyroid hormone metabolism (60) without radiologic evidence of bone abnormality (59) are usually found in individuals with distal RTA. At present, the exact mechanism underlying hypercalciuria secondary to Type I RTA still remains to be elucidated.

Renal calcifications resulting from hypercalciuria and hypocitraturia are commonly present in patients with distal RTA (59) (Figure 5). Nephrocalcinosis and/or nephrolithiasis have been radiologically demonstrable in 63% of 43 patients having distal RTA, nephrocalcinosis representing most of these cases (59). The incidence of nephrocalcinosis could be even higher through the generalized use of renal ultrasound exploration, a method reported to be more sensitive than abdominal radiographs for detecting

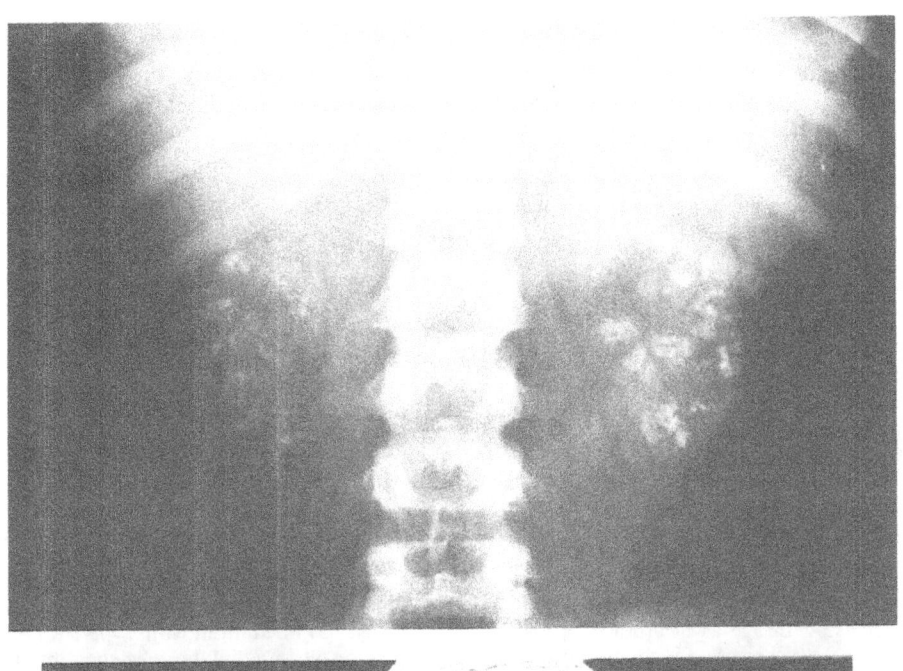
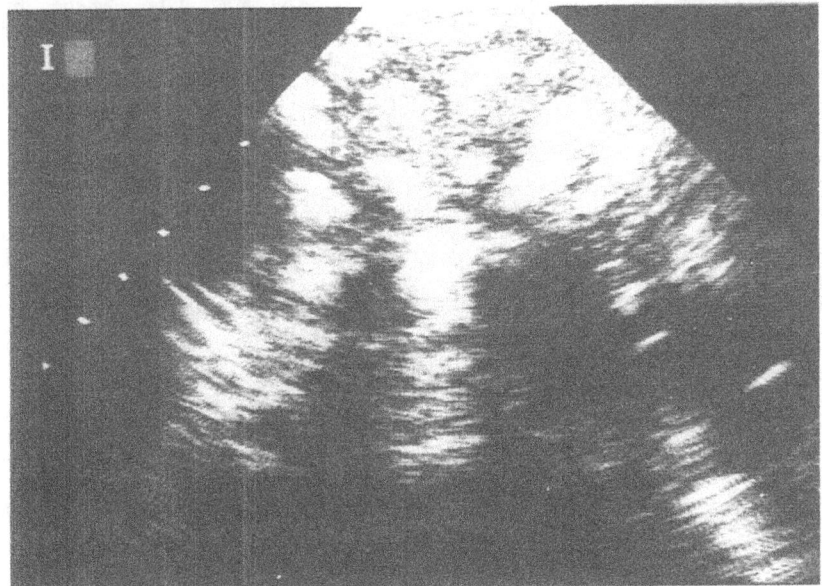

Figure 5. Distal RTA-related nephrocalcinosis demonstrable by abdominal radiographs (A) and ultrasonography (B).

renal parenchymal calcifications (61). However, it should be taken into account that nephrocalcinosis may be the cause, rather than the consequence, of the acidification defect in some patients with secondary forms of distal RTA.

Nephrocalcinosis along with hypokalemia may account in large part for the decreased tubular concentrating ability and secondary polyuria of many patients with Type I RTA (8).

A large number of descriptions of RTA (4, 5, 54)

include the presence of bone abnormalities within the radiographic features of distal RTA. From the study of Brenner et al. (59) in which radiographic findings in a large group of patients with RTA were evaluated, such a statement can no longer be supported. Brenner et al. (59) clearly showed that skeletal abnormalities such as rickets or osteopenia are radiographically absent in nonazotemic subjects with Type I RTA.

The treatment of primary Type I RTA should be directed at the correction of systemic acidosis in order to improve the growth rate of pediatric patients; to reduce the risk of nephrocalcinosis or, at least, halt its progression; to maintain a normal glomerular filtration rate; and to reverse serum potassium abnormalities.

Correction of metabolic acidosis requires daily alkali supplementation. The dose of alkali should be calculated on the basis of estimated endogenous production of nonvolatile acid (approximately 1 mEq/kg body weight/day in adults and 2–3 mEq/kg body weight/day in children) and the magnitude of bicarbonaturia. Thus, whereas adults need about 1 or 2 mEq/kg/day alkali supplementation, most children require higher doses, above 2 or 3 mEq of base/kg/day (2, 14, 51). Particularly high doses of alkali are needed in infants with Type I RTA and associated proximal wasting of bicarbonate. In these patients, alkali requirements decrease with age as bicarbonate proximal leak disappears (50). In either case, it should be emphasized that the alkali dosage must be determined in each patient as a result of the amount of base required to achieve normal plasma bicarbonate concentrations (22–24 mEq/l). Lower doses of alkali will not result in the desirable therapeutic effect and higher doses will produce expansion of extracellular fluid volume and, subsequently, additional urinary loss of bicarbonate.

Various preparations for alkali therapy are commercially available (Table 4). Sodium bicarbonate and Shohl's solution are the preparations most frequently used in the treatment of patients with distal RTA. Sodium bicarbonate, because of intragastric CO_2 production, may produce abdominal bloating and belching. Shohl's solution is a combination of sodium citrate and citric acid (98 and 140 g/l, respectively). The citric acid is converted to CO_2 + H_2O, while the citrate is converted to bicarbonate anion. Shohl's solution diluted with chilled ginger ale or fruit juice is often preferable and more palatable than sodium bicarbonate (5).

Although sporadic cases of transient distal RTA have been reported (62), it should be pointed out that, as a rule, primary Type I RTA is a permanent disorder. Therefore, alkali therapy must be continued for life to avert the recurrence of clinical and biochemical anomalies, although, especially in children, periodic adjustments of alkali dosage may be needed (50).

As shown in Figure 6, sustained correction of metabolic acidosis brings about a significant improvement in the growth rate in such a way that normal height can be attained, provided sufficient amounts of alkali are administered to maintain normal plasma bicarbonate concentrations (14, 63).

The exact mechanism by which chronic metabolic acidosis impairs growth remains to be determined. It is known that acidosis interferes with human growth hormone release and affects collagen metabolism (3). Furthermore, elevated urinary excretion of sulfate has been demonstrated (64, 65) in children with Type I RTA. Such sulfate loss may result in a sulfate deficiency that contributes to growth failure in affected children. Likewise, calcium balance improves following acidosis correction (65, 66). However, in contrast to adult subjects, children with distal RTA show a positive calcium balance under metabolic acidosis conditions; poor growth secondary to suboptimal calcium balance cannot be ruled out (65).

Prevention of nephrocalcinosis constitutes a critical aim in the treatment of distal RTA. In addition to clinical manifestations related to interstitial damage, massive renal parenchymal calcifications cause deterioration of the glomerular filtration rate (8). As shown by McSherry (3), Santos and Chan (14), the appearance of nephrocalci-

Table 4. Commercial preparation for alkali supplementation

Drug	How supplied	Dosage equivalent
Bicitra	Solution: 5 ml = 500 mg sodium citrate 300 mg citric acid	1 ml = 1 mEq base
Calcium carbonate	Tablet: 420, 650 mg Powder: 1000 mg per ½ teaspoon	1 g = 22.3 mEq base
Polycitra	Solution: 5 ml = 550 mg potassium citrate 500 mg sodium citrate 334 mg citric acid	1 ml = 2 mEq base
Polycitra-K	Solution: 5 ml = 1100 mg potassium citrate 334 mg citric acid	1 ml = 2 mEq base
Sodium bicarbonate	Tablet: 325, 650 mg Solution: 1 ml = 1 mEq	325 mg = 4 mEq base 1 ml = 1 mEq base
Shohl's solution	Solution: 1000 ml = 140 g citric acid 90 g hydrated crystalline sodium citrate	1 ml = 1 mEq base

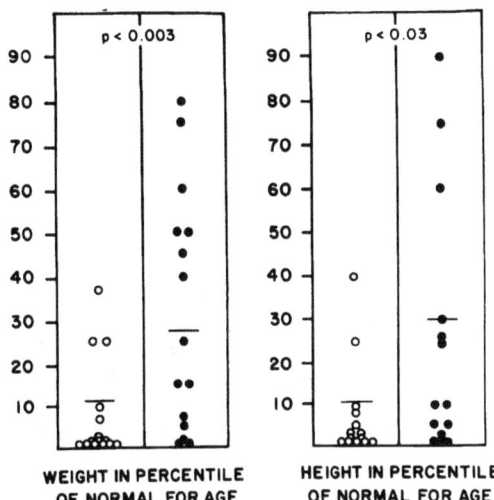

Figure 6. Significant improvement in the growth rate of children with primary distal RTA after 12 months of alkaline therapy. Weight and height at the moment of diagnosis (open circles) and after treatment (solid circles) are presented. Reprinted from Santos and Chan (14) with permission of S. Karger AG, Basel.

nosis, as well as the impairment of glomerular filtration rate, can be prevented in children with primary distal RTA who have been adequately treated since infancy and early childhood. It is also known that, once established, nephrocalcinosis does not revert, even though appropriate alkali supplementation is initiated (67). Unfortunately, nephrocalcinosis can be present at the moment of diagnosis, even in infants (46, 50).

As mentioned above, hypercalciuria and hypocitraturia are the most important factors known to be involved in the pathogenesis of renal calcium deposition in patients with Type I RTA. The correction of acidosis with alkali therapy usually restores normal citrate excretion (57). The hypercalciuric effect of metabolic acidosis has long been recognized. Studies in normal subjects (68) have indicated that chronic metabolic acidosis gives rise to hypercalciuria by decreasing renal tubular calcium reabsorption through a direct action on intracellular metabolism. Rodriguez-Soriano et al. (50) have demonstrated an inverse relationship between urinary excretion of calcium and plasma bicarbonate concentration in five children with primary distal RTA. Such a correlation between the magnitude of calciuria and the degree of acidosis has not been confirmed in other studies, including those involving pediatric patients (14). Moreover, hypercalciuria is not invariably present in acidotic individuals with Type I RTA (14, 60, 67). Hypercalciuria, if present, may persist in spite of correction of acidosis in some patients (4, 14). In addition, sodium intake related to alkali administration may also play a significant role in the magnitude of urine calcium excretion. Accordingly, the response of calciuria to alkali therapy is not uniform in all patients with primary distal RTA.

Serum potassium disturbances tend to normalize following sustained correction of metabolic acidosis (3, 14). In patients with hypokalemia at the moment of diagnosis, the renal wasting of potassium is usually ameliorated with alkali treatment (69–71). This effect is attributed to the alkali-induced reexpansion of the extracellular space and the subsequent removal of the stimulus for renin and aldosterone secretions. Therefore, potassium supplements are not usually required in the long-term treatment of patients with primary distal RTA.

In summary, primary distal RTA has a good prognosis provided early diagnosis is established and adequate alkaline treatment is implemented.

Table 5. Etiologic spectrum of Type II renal tubular acidosis

Primary
Sporadic or transient infantile
Idiopathic or genetic

Secondary
Decreased carbonic anhydrase enzyme activity
  Genetically determined
  Drug Related: Acetazolamide
               Sulfanilamide
               Mafenide acetate
               Outdated tetracyclines
               6-mercaptopurine
Toxin induced
  Heavy metals: Lead
                Mercury
                Cadmium
Gentically transmitted
  Cystinosis
  Tyrosinosis
  Galactosemia
  Fructose intolerance
  Glycogen storage disease Type I
  Metchromatic leukodystrophy
  Leigh's syndrome
  Lowe's syndrome
  Wilson's disease
  Pyruvate carboxylase deficiency
Renal diseases
  Nephrotic syndrome
  Renal vein thrombosis
  Post renal transplantation
  Medullary cystic disease
  Amyloidosis
  Sjogren's syndrome
  Multiple myeloma
Disordered calcium metabolism
  Secondary hyperparathyroidism and chronic hypocalcemia
  Vitamin-D deficiency
  Vitamin-D dependency
Miscellaneous conditions
  Congenital heart disease
  Malignancy
  Osteopetrosis

TYPE II RTA (PROXIMAL RTA)

Proximal renal tubular acidosis (Type II RTA) is due to the reduced capacity of the proximal tubule to reabsorb bicarbonate, resulting in bicarbonate wasting (5).

Primary Type II RTA (Table 5) is a sporadic and transient disorder with a predominantly male incidence (72). But familial forms, transmitted by autosomal dominant and recessive inheritance, with both sexes equally affected, have been described (72). An isolated bicarbonate reabsorption defect is usually transient (2); however, persistence into adult life has been described (72, 73).

Secondary Type II RTA can be due to many etiologic factors (Table 5), characterized by failure of the proximal tubule to reabsorb 75–80% of filtered bicarbonate. The presence of a low renal threshold for bicarbonate results in >15% of the filtered bicarbonate appearing in the urine when the patient's serum bicarbonate is normalized with alkali therapy (2, 74–78). Osteodystrophy in patients with pure bicarbonate-losing disease is not prevalent, but is a constant feature if accompanied by hyperphosphaturia (5).

Other defects in proximal renal tubular function, such as reabsorption of a range of small molecular weight substances that are filtered by the glomerulus and are normally absorbed by the proximal convoluted tubule by energy-consuming active transport, may also be present. Such disorders are described under the broad category of Fanconi syndrome (6, 78–80).

The clinical features at the time of presentation vary with the cause of the Type II acidosis. One of the most striking features is the small stature. Growth failure in these children is universal. Osteodystrophy and rickets are often advanced at the time of diagnosis. It should be noted that secondary Type II RTA may occur in patients with dietary vitamin D deficiency.

The child may be polyuric, polydipsic, and nocturic, and is generally miserable and irritable. Appetite is poor and may not improve with treatment of acidosis and electrolyte imbalance in patients with Fanconi syndrome. The patient comes with a history of failure to thrive, vomiting and diarrhea or constipation, and may even present in a state of shock.

In some children with primary proximal bicarbonaturia, the condition is transient or self-limiting; these children do not have the usual clinical finding of rickets, but do follow the pattern of growth failure. In general, the urinary calculi or nephrocalcinosis encountered in distal tubular acidosis (RTA Type I) are not seen in proximal RTA, probably because of the chelating effect of urinary citrate, which is decreased in distal RTA but is excreted in large amounts in proximal RTA (5, 81).

Whilst patients with Type II RTA usually present in childhood, adult patients may be diagnosed late or may acquire the disorder in a secondary form. Disorders with diverse etiologies ranging from mercury poisoning, inherited syndromes such as osteopetrosis and metachromatic leukodystrophy, ureterosigmoid anastomosis, and acquired idiopathic nephrotic syndrome with glomerulosclerosis have been implicated in proximal tubular dysfunction. Sprue or gastrointestinal malabsorption leading to a severe nutritional deficiency of vitamin D and an increased requirement for calcium and phosphate is more commonly implicated (82–86).

Substances commonly appearing in abnormally large amounts in the urine of patients with Type II RTA include bicarbonate (may be normal when serum bicarbonate is very low), phosphate, amino acids, glucose, lysozyme, immunoglobulin, uric acid, and citrate.

Some primary autosomal recessive disorders associated with secondary Type II RTA are cystinosis, fructose intolerance, galactosemia, and tyrosinemia.

Regardless of the factors that cause the original clinical and biochemical manifestation of Type II RTA, the main biochemical determinants of therapy, after elimination of treatable causes, are still such factors as loss of bicarbonate in large amount, loss of phosphate in moderate amounts, or loss of potassium and sodium ions.

Patients with Type II RTA and those with Fanconi syndromes often require a large amount of alkali and potassium replacement, as well as supplementation with calcium, phosphate, and vitamin D metabolites. The dose must be titrated to each individual patient's needs. The amounts of alkali therapy is 5–15 mEq/kg/day, with about half the amount being in the form of potassium salts to offset the increasing loss of this ion in the urine as a consequence of alkali treatment. It is worthwhile to try to keep the patient's extracellular volume slightly depleted, as expansion of the extracellular space promotes phosphaturia and bicarbonaturia. In some cases the use of hydrochlorothiazide in doses of 1.5–2.0 mg/kg/day has been recommended in two divided doses. The effect of diuretic-induced hypovolemic alkalosis enhances proximal tubular phosphate reabsorption and hypocalciuria. Monitoring serum potassium is essential due to the kaliuretic effect of this diuretic (3, 13, 87).

TYPE IV RENAL TUBULAR ACIDOSIS

Type IV RTA is the most commonly diagnosed form of RTA (3) and is characterized by potassium retention (2, 51, 74, 77, 88). This hyperkalemia is not caused by reduction in the glomerular filtration rate (3, 51). Hyperkalemic metabolic acidosis may be identified at times in patients with reduced glomerular filtration rates due to obstructive uropathy (44). Type IV renal tubular acidosis must be included in the differential diagnosis of any patient presenting with hyperchloremic metabolic acidosis with elevated urinary pH and reduced potassium excretion. It should be emphasized that, under conditions of systemic acidosis, an acid urine pH may be encountered (3, 5, 88, 89, 90).

The basic defect in Type IV RTA is best understood as a reduction in aldosterone levels or reduced responsiveness by the distal tubule to the actions of aldosterone (3, 74, 91, 92).

The transport of sodium, potassium, and hydrogen ions in the distal tubules and collecting ducts is influenced by aldosterone. Sodium reabsorption is enhanced by aldosterone and potassium, and hydrogen ion excretions are increased. In the medullary collecting ducts, aldosterone stimulates hydrogen ion secretion independently of sodium reabsorption (93–95). Thus lack of aldosterone results in a salt-wasting state, with retention of potassium and hydrogen, which lead to the hyperchloremic metabolic acidosis associated with hyperkalemia and hyponatremia.

RTA Type IV subtype 1

This includes primary aldosterone deficiency, as in Addison's disease; congenital adrenal hyperplasia; and isolated hypoaldosteronism (96). The most common autosomally inherited defect in congenital adrenal hyperplasia is 21-hydroxylase deficiency, accounting for approximately 90% of the cases. Deficiency in 18-hydroxylase and 18-dehydrogenase enzymes, responsible for the final steps in aldosterone production, may present with the pure-salt-losing Type IV RTA and without the other manifestations of adrenal hyperplasia (96, 97). As expected, the serum and urinary aldosterone concentrations are reduced, and the plasma renin activity is markedly elevated. As a result of salt wasting, patients often present with reduced intravascular volume, hypotension, and shock (98–100).

Type IV, subtype 1 RTA is treated by supplementation with physiologic doses of mineralocorticosteroids and increased salt intake. Plasma renin activity should be monitored regularly as one of the most useful parameters of sufficient replacement therapy (74). With replacement of physiologic doses of mineralocorticosteroids, normalization of urine acidification and body fluid pH maintenance is achieved (89).

RTA Type IV, subtype 2

Type IV RTA, subtype 2 is more common in adult patients than children. It presents with hyperchloremic, hyperkalemic acidosis with alkaline urine pH and usually a concomitant reduction in the glomerular filtration rate. Plasma renin activity, and serum and urinary aldosterone concentrations are low. Many diseases causing chronic interstitial and vascular changes with reduction in renal parenchyma have been implicated.

Type IV RTA, subtype 2 is encountered secondary to diabetes mellitus, chronic pyelonephritis, interstitial nephritis, obstructive uropathy, nephrosclerosis, and hyperuricemia (gout).

Salt wasting is not encountered, possibly because there is sufficient aldosterone present, together with the reduction in the glomerular filtration rate due to chronic interstitial nephritis from the above primary disease. Not surprisingly, these patients respond to mineralocorticosteroids, but there is tubular resistance to their effect and supranormal doses are usually needed. Potassium restriction promotes increased ammonia production and net acid excretion. The use of furosemide in conjunction with mineralocorticosteroids provides greater therapeutic benefit by enhancing potassium excretion together with increased distal tubular hydrogen secretion (3, 73, 74, 101–103).

Type IV RTA, subtype 3

This type of renal tubular acidosis is found most commonly in adolescents, but children and adults can be affected. Most cases are sporadic, but familial involvement has been described (104). It is characterized by excessive chloride reabsorption by the distal tubule, leading to hypervolemia, hypertension, reduced plasma renin activity, and secondary hypoaldosteronism (90, 105, 106). The hyperkalemic acidosis is corrected by administration of thiazide diuretics or by salt restriction (3, 51). The glomerular filtration rate is usually normal. Affected children may present with short stature. Unlike Type IV RTA, subtype 2, treatment with mineralocorticosteroids is contraindicated, as it can aggravate the hypertension and does not increase potassium excretion (107).

Type IV RTA, subtype 4

This form of tubular acidosis is due to pseudohypoaldosteronism. The primary condition occurs most frequently in infants, in whom the genetically determined maturation defect of tubular aldosterone sensitivity usually resolves by the second year of life (108, 109), but more commonly it is secondary to obstructive uropathy and is found in the post-operative phase after relief of the obstruction (110). Infants with duodenal atresia and Type IV RTA have been described, as well as neonates with renal vein thrombosis presenting with hyperkalemia and pseudohypoaldosteronism (111). Adult patients with chronic tubulointerstitial nephritis and patients following renal transplantation also present with secondary forms of Type IV RTA (112). Replacement of salt loss and administration of sodium bicarbonate in large amounts is often necessary (3, 74, 107).

Type IV RTA, subtype 5

This type of tubular acidosis is the result of an incomplete, though ultimately reversible, distal tubular insensitivity to two of the three actions of aldosterone. The sodium reabsorption effect of aldosterone is intact, but there is inability of aldosterone to modulate hydrogen and potassium ion excretion. Patients are, therefore, affected with hyperkalemic metabolic acidosis with reduced renal excretion of hydrogen and potassium, but with normal urinary and serum sodium concentration, and the blood pressure is normal. This type of RTA has also been observed in infants with severe unilateral neonatal renal disease (3, 74, 113, 114).

The condition is characterized by hyperchloremic, hyperkalemic acidosis with an intact ability to acidify urine when serum bicarbonate concentrations are brought to normal, but low net acid excretion persists. The blood pressure, aldosterone, and renin concentrations are normal. There is no salt wasting. The glomerular filtration rates are normal. Urinary citrate excretion is elevated in children with Type IV RTA, subtype 5, and the urinary calcium excretion is normal, which account for the lack of nephrocalcinosis in untreated patients (3).

Failure to thrive, with short stature in untreated children, may be reversed with alkali treatment, the dose being dependent on the degree of bicarbonate loss. Alkali therapy (sodium bicarbonate) should not include potassium-containing salts. To achieve sustained correction of acidosis and to maintain the serum bicarbonate concentrations of 21–23 mEq/l, treatment with 4–20 mEq NaHCO$_3$/body kg/per day is needed. Catch-up growth and ultimately normal stature can be anticipated in those in whom the diagnosis is made early and appropriate treatments are instituted. Followup over 5–7 years has shown that alkali treatment is no longer necessary. In view of these observations, it has been hypothesized that the reason for this disorder is tubular immaturity with reduced numbers of aldosterone receptors secondary to the short distal tubules characteristic of infants. With maturation of the receptors, the syndrome disappears (3, 74, 115).

SUMMARY

The understanding of the physiology and pathophysiology of the renal tubule has been advanced considerably over the past three decades with the advent of micropuncture techniques for studying renal tubular function. Clinical observations and careful evaluation of laboratory results, together with research aimed at understanding the functional deficits in patients with the various subtypes of renal tubular acidosis, have led to a more cogent approach to the investigation and management of patients with hyperchloremic metabolic acidosis.

ACKNOWLEDGMENT

The authors would like to thank Virginia Murrell for secretarial assistance.

REFERENCES

1. Oh MS, Carroll HJ: The anion gap. *N Engl J Med* 297:814–817, 1977.
2. Nash MA, Torrado AD, Greifer I, Spitzer A, Edelmann CM Jr: Renal tubular acidosis in infants and children. *J Pediatr* 80:738–748, 1972.
3. McSherry E: Renal tubular acidosis in childhood. *Kidney Int* 20:799–809, 1981.
4. Donckerwolcke RA: Diagnosis and treatment of renal tubular disorders in children. *Pediatr Clin North Am* 29:895–906, 1982.
5. Chan JCM: Renal tubular acidosis. *J Pediatr* 102:327–340, 1983.
6. Morris RC Jr: Renal tubular acidosis. Mechanisms, classification and implications. *N Engl J Med* 281:1405–1413, 1969.
7. Chan JCM: Fluid-electrolyte and acid-base disorders in children. *Curr Probl Pediatr* 11:1–55, 1981.
8. Chan JCM: Acid-base disorders and the kidney. *Adv Pediatr* 30:401–471, 1983.
9. Relman AS, Lennon EJ, Lemann J Jr: Endogenous production of fixed acid and measurements of the net balance of acid in normal subjects. *J Clin Invest* 40:1621–1630, 1961.
10. Lennon EJ, Lemann J Jr, Litzow JR: The effects of diet and stool composition on the net external acid balance of normal subjects. *J Clin Invest* 45:1601–1607, 1966.
11. Chan JCM: Hydrogen ion production secondary to metabolism of sulfur-amino acids organic acids. *Nutr Metab* 22:288–294, 1978.
12. Chan JCM: The rapid determination of urinary titratable acid and ammonium and evaluation of freezing as a method of preservation. *Clin Biochem* 5:94–98, 1972.
13. Chan JCM: Nutrition and acid-base metabolism. *Fed Proc* 40:2423–2428, 1981.
14. Santos F, Chan JCM: Renal tubular acidosis in children. Diagnosis, treatment, and prognosis. *Am J Nephrol* 6:289–295, 1986.
15. Batlle D, Kurtzman NA: Distal renal tubular acidosis: Pathogenesis and classification. *Am J Kidney Dis* 1:328–344, 1982.
16. Kurtzman NA: Acquired distal renal tubular acidosis. *Kidney Int* 24:807–819, 1983.
17. Wrong O, Davis HEF: The excretion of acid in renal diseases. *Q J Med* 28:259–313, 1959.
18. Chan JCM, Alon U: Tubular disorders of acid-base and phosphate metabolism. *Nephron* 40:257–279, 1985.
19. Arruda JAL, Kurtzman NA: Metabolic acidosis and alkalosis. *Clin Nephrol* 7:201–215, 1977.
20. Loney LC, Norling LL, Robson AM: The use of arginine hydrochloride infusion to assess urinary acidification. *J Pediatr* 100:95–98, 1982.
21. Oster JR, Hotchkiss JL, Carbon M, Farmer M, Vaamonde CA: A short duration renal acidification test using calcium chloride. *Nephron* 14:281–285, 1975.
22. Rodriguez-Soriano J, Vallo A, Garcia-Fuentes M: Distal renal tubular acidosis in infancy: A bicarbonate wasting state. *J Pediatr* 86:524–532, 1975.
23. Hutcheon RA, Kaplan BS, Drummond KN: Distal renal tubular acidosis in children with chronic hydronephrosis. *J Pediatr* 89:372–376, 1976.
24. Sebastian A, Morris RC Jr: Renal tubular acidosis. *Clin Nephrol* 7:216–230, 1977.
25. Stinebaugh BJ, Schloeder FX, Tam SC, Goldstein ME, Halperin ML: Pathogenesis of distal renal tubular acidosis. *Kidney Int* 19:1–7, 1981.
26. Halperin ML, Goldstein MB, Richardson RMA, Stinebaugh BJ: Distal renal tubular acidosis syndromes: A pathophysiological approach. *Am J Nephrol* 5:1–8, 1985.
27. Batlle DC, von Riotte A, Schlueter W: Urinary sodium in the evaluation of hyperchloremic metabolic acidosis. *N Engl J Med* 316:140–144, 1987.
28. Halperin ML, Goldstein MB, Haig A, Johnson MD, Stinebaugh BJ: Studies on the pathogenesis of type I (distal) renal tubular acidosis as revealed by the urinary P_{CO_2} tension. *J Clin Invest* 53:669–677, 1974.
29. Arruda JAL, Nascimiento L, Kumar SK, Kurtzman NA: Factors influencing the formation of urinary carbon dioxide tension. *Kidney Int* 11:307–317, 1977.
30. Stinebaugh BJ, Esquenazi R, Schloeder FX, Suki WN,

Goldstein MB, Halperin ML: Control of the urine-blood P_{CO_2} gradient in alkaline urine. *Kidney Int* 17:31–39, 1980.
31. DuBose TD Jr: Hydrogen ion secretion by the collecting duct as a determinant of the urine to blood P_{CO_2} gradient in alkaline urine. *J Clin Invest* 69:145–156, 1982.
32. Donckerwolcke RA, Valk C, van Wijngaarden–Penterman MJG, van Stekelenburg GJ: The diagnostic value of the urine to blood carbon dioxide tension gradient for the assessment of distal tubular hydrogen secretion in pediatric patients with renal tubular disorders. *Clin Nephrol* 19:254–258, 1983.
33. Batlle DC, Sehy JT, Roseman MK, Arruda JAL, Kurtzman NA: Clinical and pathophysiologic spectrum of acquired distal renal tubular acidosis. *Kidney Int* 20:389–396, 1981.
34. Stinebaugh BJ, Schloeder FX, Gharafry E, Suki WN, Goldstein MB, Halperin ML: Mechanism by which neutral phosphate infusion elevates urine P_{CO_2}. *J Lab Clin Med* 89:946–958, 1977.
35. Schwartz WB, Jenson RL, Relman AS: Acidification of the urine and increased ammonia excretion without change in acid-base equilibrium: Sodium reabsorption as a stimulus to the acidifying process. *J Clin Invest* 34:673–680, 1955.
36. Seldin DW, Coleman AJ, Carter N, Rector FC Jr: The effect of Na_2SO_4 on urinary acidification in chronic renal disease. *J Lab Clin Med* 69:893–903, 1967.
37. Rodriguez–Soriano J, Vallo A, Castillo G, Oliveros R: Pathophysiology of primary distal renal tubular acidosis. *Int J Pediatr Nephrol* 6:71–78, 1985.
38. Rastogi SP, Crawford C, Wheeler R, Flanigan W, Arruda JAL: Effect of furosemide on urinary acidification in distal renal tubular acidosis. *J Lab Clin Med* 104:271–282, 1984.
39. Stine KC, Linshaw MA: Use of furosemide in the evaluation of renal tubular acidosis. *J Pediatr* 107:559–562, 1985.
40. Batlle DC: Segmental characterization of defects in collecting tubule acidification. *Kidney Int* 30:546–554, 1986.
41. Rodriguez–Soriano J, Vallo A, Castillo G, Oliveros R: Defect in urinary acidification in nephrotic syndrome and its correction by furosemide. *Nephron* 32:308–313, 1983.
42. Hulter HN, Ilnicki LP, Licht JH, Sebastian A: On the mechanism of diminished urinary carbon dioxide tension caused by amiloride. *Kidney Int* 21:8–13, 1982.
43. Batlle D, Itsarayoungyuen K, Arruda JAL, Kurtzman NA: Hyperkalemic hyperchloremic metabolic acidosis in sickle cell hemoglobinopathies. *Am J Med* 72:188–192, 1982.
44. Batlle DC, Arruda JAL, Kurtzman NA: Hyperkalemic distal renal tubular acidosis associated with obstructive uropathy. *N Engl J Med* 304:373–380, 1981.
45. Harrington JT, Hulter HN, Cohen JJ, Madias NE: Mineralocorticoid-stimulated renal acidification: The critical role of dietary sodium. *Kidney Int* 30:43–48, 1986.
46. Peces R, Santos F, Ortego F, Fernandez–Vega F, Malaga S, Alvarez–Grande J: Pathophysiologic mechanism of distal renal tubular acidosis with nerve deafness. *Nephron*, in press.
47. Batlle D, Gaviria M, Grupp M, Arrude JAL, Wynn J, Kurtzman NA: Distal nephron function in patients receiving chronic lithium therapy. *Kidney Int* 21:477–485, 1982.
48. Batlle D, Grupp M, Gaviria M, Kurtzman NA: Distal renal tubular acidosis with intact capacity to lower urinary pH. *Am J Med* 72:751–758, 1982.
49. Seldin DW, Wilson JD: Renal tubular acidosis. In: JB Stambury, *The Metabolic Basis of Inherited Disease*. McGraw-Hill, New York, pp 1618–1633, 1980.
50. Rodriguez–Soriano J, Vallo A, Castillo G, Oliveros R: Natural history of primary distal renal tubular acidosis treated since infancy. *J Pediatr* 101:669–676, 1982.
51. Cogan MG, Rector FC Jr: Acid-base disorders. In: BM Brenner, FC Rector Jr, *The Kidney*. WB Saunders, Philadelphia, pp 457–517, 1986.
52. McSherry E, Sebastian A, Morris RC Jr: Renal tubular acidosis in infants: The several kinds, including bicarbonate-wasting, classic renal tubular acidosis. *J Clin Invest* 51:499–514, 1972.
53. Sebastian A, McSherry E, Morris RC Jr: Impaired renal conservation of sodium and chloride during sustained correction of systemic acidosis in patients with type 1, classic renal tubular acidosis. *J Clin Invest* 58:454–469, 1976.
54. Toto RD: Metabolic acid-base disorders. In: JP Kokko, RL Tannen, *Fluids and Electrolytes*. WB Saunders, Philadelphia, pp 229–304, 1986.
55. Sebastian A, McSherry E, Morris RC Jr: Renal potassium wasting in renal tubular acidosis. *J Clin Invest* 50:667–678, 1971.
56. Narins RG, Goldberg M. Renal tubular acidosis: Pathophysiology, diagnosis and treatment. *Disease-a-Month* 23:1–68, 1977.
57. Norman ME, Feldman NI, Cohn RM, Roth KS, McCurdy DK: Urinary citrate excretion in the diagnosis of distal renal tubular acidosis. *J Pediatr* 92:394–400, 1978.
58. Lemann JJ Jr, Litzow JR, Lemmon EJ: The effects of chronic acid loads in normal man: Further evidence for the participation of bone mineral in the defense against chronic metabolic acidosis. *J Clin Invest* 45:1608–1614, 1966.
59. Brenner RJ, Spring DB, Sebastian A, McSherry EM, Genant HK, Palubinskas AJ, Morris RC Jr: Incidence of radiographically evident bone disease, nephrocalcinosis, and nephrolithiasis in various types of renal tubular acidosis. *N Engl J Med* 307:217–221, 1982.
60. Chesney RW, Kaplan BS, Phelps M, DeLuca HF: Renal tubular acidosis does not alter circulating values of calcitriol. *J Pediatr* 104:51–55, 1984.
61. Alon U, Brewer WH, Chan JCM: Nephrocalcinosis: Detection by ultrasonography. *Rediatrics* 71:970–973, 1983.
62. Leumann EP, Steinmann B: Persistent and transient distal renal tubular acidosis with bicarbonate wasting. *Pediatr Res* 9:767–773, 1975.
63. McSherry E, Morris RC Jr: Attainment and maintenance of normal stature with alkali therapy in infants and children with classic renal tubular acidosis. *J Clin Invest* 61:509–527, 1978.
64. Chan JCM: Urinary sulfate excretion in children with classic renal tubular acidosis. *Nutr Metab* 22:257–261, 1978.
65. Chan JCM: Calcium and hydrogen ion metabolism in children with classic (type I, distal) renal tubular acidosis. *Ann Nutr Metab* 25:65–78, 1981.
67. Wrong OM, Feest TG: The natural history of distal renal tubular acidosis. *Contr Nephrol* 21:137–144, 1980.
68. Lemann J Jr, Litzow JR, Lennon EJ: Studies of the mechanism by which chronic metabolic acidosis augments urinary calcium excretion in man. *J Clin Invest* 46:1318–1328, 1967.
69. Chan JCM: Acid-base, calcium, potassium and aldosterone metabolism in renal tubular acidosis. *Nephron* 23:152–158, 1979.
70. Hruska KA, Ban D, Avioli LV: Renal tubular acidosis. *Arch Intern Med* 142:1909–1913, 1982.
71. Sebastian A, Hulter HN, Kurtz I, Maher T, Schambelan M: Disorders of distal nephron function. *Am J Med* 72:289–307, 1982.
72. Brenes LG, Brenes JN, Hernandez MM: Familial proximal renal tubular acidosis. A distinct clinical entity. *Am J Med* 63:244–252, 1977.

73. Winsnes A, Monn E, Stokke O, Feyling T: Congenital persistent proximal type renal tubular acidosis in two brothers. *Acta Paediatr Scand* 68:861–868, 1979.
74. Roth KS, Buckalew VM Jr, Chan JCM: Renal tubular disorders. In: HC Gonick, ed, *Current Nephrology, Vol 8. Year Book Medical Publishers, Chicago*, pp 87–137, 1985.
75. Kossoy AF, Weir MR: Renal tubular acidosis in infancy: A clinical approach to diagnosis and treatment. *South Med J* 79:1256–1258, 1986.
76. Rodriquez-Soriano J, Boichis H, Edelmann CM Jr: Bicarbonate reabsorption and hydrogen ion excretion in children with renal tubular acidosis. *J Pediatr* 71:802–813, 1967.
77. Rector FC Jr, Martin GC: The renal acidosis. *Hosp Practice* 99–111, 1980.
78. Rodriguez-Soriano J, Edelmann CM Jr: Renal tubular acidosis. *Ann Rev Med* 20:363–382, 1969.
79. Roth K, Foreman JW, Segal S: The Fanconi syndrome and mechanism of tubular transport dysfunction. *Kidney Int* 20:705–716, 1981.
80. Sebastian A, McSherry E, Morris RC Jr: On the mechanism of renal potassium wasting in renal tubular acidosis associated with the Fanconi syndrome (Type 2 RTA). *J Clin Invest* 50:231–243, 1971.
81. Norman ME, Cohn RM, McCurdy DK: Urinary citrate excretion in the diagnosis of distal renal tubular acidosis. *J Pediatr* 92:394–400, 1978.
82. Bourke E, Delaney VB, Mosawi M, Reavey P, Weston M: Renal tubular acidosis and osteopetrosis in siblings. *Nephron* 28:268–272, 1981.
83. McConnell JB, Murison J, Stewart WK: The role of the colon in the pathogenesis of hyperchloraemic acidosis in ureterosigmoid anastomosis. *Clin Science* 57:305–312, 1979.
84. Husband P, McKellar WJD: Infantile renal tubular acidosis due to mercury poisoning. *Arch Dis Child* 45:264–268, 1970.
85. Rodriguez Soriano J, Rivera JM, Vallo A, Prats-Vinas JM, Castillo G: Proximal renal tubular acidosis in metachromatic leukodystrophy. *Helv Pediat Acta* 33:45–52, 1978.
86. McVicar M, Exeni R, Susin M: Nephrotic syndrome and multiple tubular defects in children: An early sign of focal segmental glomerulosclerosis. *J Pediatr* 97:918–922, 1980.
87. Knox FG, Osswald H, Marchand GR, Spielman WS, Haas JA, Brendt TJ, Youngberg SP: Phosphate transport along the nephron. *Am J Physiol* 233:F261–268, 1977.
88. Arruda JAL, Kurtzmann NA: Mechanism and classification of deranged distal urinary acidification. *Am J Physiol* 239:515–523, 1980.
89. Morris RC Jr: Renal tubular acidosis. *N Engl J Med* 304:418–420, 1981.
90. Licht JH, Amundson D, Hsueh WA, Lombardo JV: Familiar hyperkalemic acidosis. *Q J Med* 54:161–176, 1985.
91. Morris RC Jr, Sebastian A, McSherry E: Renal acidosis. *Kidney Int* 1:322–340, 1972.
92. Sebastian A, Schambelan M, Lindefeld S, Morris RC Jr: Amelioration of metabolic acidosis with fludrocortisone therapy in hyporeninemic hypoaldosteronism. *N Engl J Med* 297:576–583, 1977.
93. Malnic G, Klose RM, Giebisch G: Micropuncture study of distal tubular potassium and sodium transport in rat nephron *Am J Physiol* 211:529–547, 1966.
94. McKinney TD, Burg MG: Bicarbonate secretion by rabbit cortical collecting tubules in vitro. *J Clin Invest* 61:1421–1427, 1978.
95. Stone DK, Seldin DW, Kokko JP, Jacobson HR: Anion dependence of medullary collecting duct acidification. A sodium independent effect. *J Clin Invest* 72:77–83, 1983.
96. Oetliker OH, Zurbrugg RP: Renal tubular acidosis in salt losing syndrome of congenital adrenal hyperplasia (CAH). *J Clin Endoc Metab* 31:447–450, 1970.
97. Ulick S: Diagnosis and nomenclature of the disorders of the terminal portion of the aldosterone biosynthetic pathway. *J Clin Endoc Metab* 43:92–96, 1976.
98. Cleveland WW, Green OC, Wilkins L: Deaths in congenital adrenal hyperplasia. *Pediatrics* 29:3–17, 1962.
99. Posner JB, Jacobs DR: Isolated analdosteronism I. Clinical entity, with manifestations of persistent hyperkalemia, periodic paralysis, salt losing tendency and acidosis. *Metabolism* 13:513–521, 1964.
100. Posner JB, Jacobs DR: Isolated analdosteronism II. The nature of the adrenocortical enzymatic defect, and the influence of diet and various agents on electrolyte balance. *Metabolism* 13:522–531, 1964.
101. Rastogi S, Bayliss JM, Nascimento L, Arruda JAL: Hyperkalemic renal tubular acidosis: Effect of furosemide in humans and in rats. *Kidney Int* 28:801–807, 1985.
102. Ashouri OS: Hyperkalemic distal renal tubular acidosis and selective aldosterone deficiency; combination in a patient with lead nephropathy. *Arch Intern Med* 145:1306–1307, 1985.
103. Oh MS, Carroll HJ, Clemmons JE, Vagnucci AH, Levison SP, Whang SM: A mechanism for hyporeninemic hypoaldosteronism in chronic renal disease. *Metabolism* 23:1157–1166, 1974.
104. Brautbar N, Levi J, Rosler A, Leitesdorf E, Djaldeti M, Epstein M, Kleeman CR: Familial hyperkalemia, hypertension, and hyporeninemia with normal aldosterone levels. A tubular defect of potassium handling. *Arch Intern Med* 138:607–610, 1978.
105. Spitzer A, Edelmann CM, Goldberg LD, Hanneman PH: Short stature, hyperkalemia and acidosis: A defect in renal transport of potassium. *Kidney Int* 3:251–257, 1973.
106. Schambelan M, Sebastian A, Rector FC Jr: Mineralocorticoid resistant renal hyperkalemia without salt wasting (type II pseudohypoaldosteronism): Role of increased chloride reabsorption. *Kidney Int* 19:716–727, 1981.
107. Emmett M, Seldin DW: Clinical syndromes of metabolic acidosis and metabolic alkalosis. In GW Seldin, G Giebisch, eds, *The Kidney: Physiology and Pathophysiology.* Raven Press New York, pp 1567–1639, 1985.
108. Schambelan M, Sebastian A, Hutler HN: Mineralocorticoid excess and deficiency syndromes. In: Brenner, Stein, *Acid-Base and Potassium Homeostasis* Churchill Livingstone, New York, pp 232–268, 1978.
109. Dillon MJ, Leonard JV, Buckler JM, Ogilvie D, Liyylstone D, Honour JW, Shackleton CHL: Pseudohypoaldosteronism. *Arch Dis Child* 55:427–434, 1980.
110. Rodriguez Soriano J, Vallo A, Oliveros R, Castillo G: Transient pseudohypoaldosteronism secondary to obstructive uropathy in infancy. *J Pediatri* 103:375–380, 1983.
111. Duffee J, Kodroff MB, Chan JCM: Discussion. In: Glassock, Dehydration, renal vein thrombosis and hyperkalemic renal tubular acidosis in a newborn. *Am J Nephrol* 3:232–239, 1983.
112. Rado JP, Szende L, Szucs L: Hyperkalemia unresponsive to massive doses of aldosterone and renal tubular acidosis in a patient with chronic interstitial nephritis: Clinical and experimental studies. *J Med* 7:481–510, 1976.
113. Alon U, Kodroff MB, Broecker BH, Kirkpatrick BV, Chan JCM: Renal tubular acidosis type 4 in neonatal unilateral kidney diseases. *J Pediatr* 104:855–860, 1984.

114. Brown JJ, Frase R, Lever AF, Robertson JIF, James VHT, McCusker J, Wynn V: Renin, angiotensin, corticosteroids, and electrolyte balance in Addison's disease. *Q J Med* 37:97–118, 1968.

115. McSherry E, Portale A, Gates J. Non-azotemic, non-hyporeninenmic type 4 renal tubular acidosis (RTA) observed in early childhood (abstract). *Kidney Int* 14:769, 1978.

CHAPTER 13

Respiratory Acid-base Disturbances

GREGORIO I. CASAR & R. KEITH WILSON

INTRODUCTION

The hydrogen ion concentration of plasma at any moment is a function of the ratio between the partial pressure of carbon dioxide and the bicarbonate concentration. Therefore, the only way a change in plasma acidity can occur is through a change in the partial pressure of carbon dioxide (P_{CO_2}) or bicarbonate concentration. Primary changes in the P_{CO_2} are the hallmark of respiratory acid-base disturbances. When P_{CO_2} is above normal the disorder is called *respiratory acidosis* and when below normal is denoted as *respiratory alkalosis*. Under normal conditions these disturbances give rise to physiologic responses that lead to changes in the plasma bicarbonate concentration; primary hypocapnia is followed by a secondary decrease in bicarbonate, whereas primary hypercapnia is followed by a secondary rise in plasma bicarbonate (H_{CO_3}). Thus, the degree to which plasma acidity is altered in response to primary changes in the partial pressure of CO_2 is a reflection not only of the initiating change, but also of the secondary change in the plasma bicarbonate concentration (1–4).

From the preceding overview, it is clear that the respiratory acid-base status is closely linked to the balance between CO_2 production and CO_2 excretion. Under basal conditions, a normal adult generates approximately 20,000 mM (400 l) of CO_2 daily. This figure sharply contrasts with the daily production of fixed acid (50–80 mM). From these numbers it becomes readily apparent why it only requires a few minutes of dysfunction in the excretion of CO_2 before we see dramatic changes in CO_2 and pH. Aside from providing fresh oxygen, the lungs are in charge of removing CO_2 from venous blood by a finely integrated mechanism that involves the central nervous system the respiratory cage, and the balance between ventilation and perfusion (Figure 1). It requires approximately 5 l of air per minute to keep a remarkably constant partial pressure of CO_2. The CO_2 is produced in the mitochondria as a result of oxidative phosphorylation, however intracellular P_{CO_2} is not identical for all cells. It is lower in tissues with low metabolic activity and high perfusion (i.e., skin) and highest in tissues with high metabolic activity for their perfusion (i.e., myocardium). Therefore the mixed P_{CO_2} is the integrated mean of the body as a whole. There is a continuous gradient of P_{CO_2} from the mitochondria through the cytoplasm, the venous blood, the alveolar gas, and ambient air. Most of the CO_2 entering the circulation is converted to nongaseous form for transport by mechanisms that depend on certain properties of hemoglobin. However, diffusion is the traditional driving force that is responsible for the steady flow of CO_2 from tissues to the blood and from the blood to the alveolar spaces (5–8).

The rate of CO_2 elimination by the lungs is equal to the product of alveolar ventilation (V_A) and alveolar CO_2 concentration. Because the concentration of CO_2 in the alveolar gas is proportional to the partial pressure of CO_2 in the alveolar space ($pACO_2$), the following relationship may be written:

$$CO_2 \text{ excretion} = V_A \times pACO_2. \tag{1}$$

Diffusion equilibrium for CO_2 across the alveolar capillary wall is achieved extremely rapidly, thus $pACO_2$ and P_{CO_2} are virtually identical. Furthermore, in the steady state the rate of CO_2 excretion is equivalent to the rate of CO_2 production:

$$P_{CO_2} = \frac{CO_2 \text{ production}}{V_A} K. \tag{2}$$

Consequently, P_{CO_2} is an excellent index of the adequacy of VA. Before going any further, it is important to emphasize the concepts of alveolar ventilation and effective alveolar PO_2. Minute ventilation (VE) refers to the amount of air being exhaled in 1 minute and is calculated as a product of tidal volume (VT) x the respiratory rate (F):

$$VE = VT \times F. \tag{3}$$

However, the amount of fresh air reaching the alveoli (VA) equals VE minus dead space (VD). Therefore,

$$VA = VE - VD \times F. \tag{4}$$

Effective alveolar PO_2 refers to the dependency of alveolar PO_2 on the inspired fraction of oxygen (FIO_2), barometric pressure, partial pressure of CO_2, and respiratory quotient RQ, according to the alveolar gas equation:

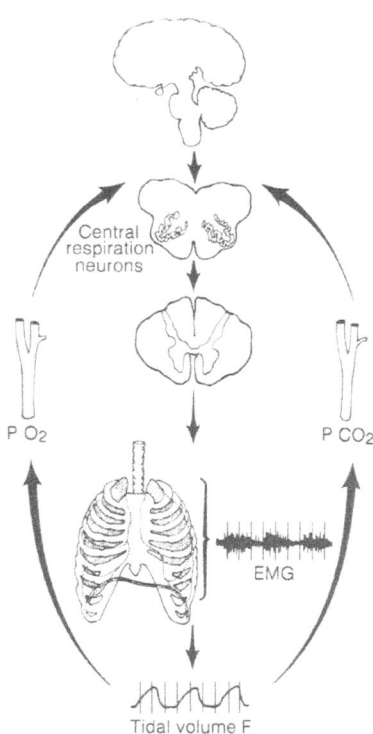

Figure 1. The respiratory system. Including the central controller, the efferents, the ventilatory pump (respiratory muscles and rib cage), major airways, lungs, and efferents. Disruption at any level could result in alveolar hypoventilation (see text).

$$pAO_2 = FIO_2 \times (BP - 47) - \frac{P_{CO_2}}{RQ}. \qquad (5)$$

From the above equation it is readily apparent that increments in the partial pressure of carbon dioxide will displace oxygen from the alveoli, causing hypoxemia. It is important to appreciate that the hypoxemia related to carbon dioxide retention can be overcome by increasing the fraction of inspired oxygen or by increasing the pressure. However, the hypercapnia can only be relieved by increasing the alveolar ventilation (9–11).

ACUTE RESPIRATORY ACIDOSIS

Respiratory acidosis refers to the acid-base disorder resulting from a primary increment in the partial pressure of carbon dioxide. Acute respiratory acidosis is said to be present when the partial pressure of carbon dioxide is higher than 45 mmHg in a person with a previously normal P_{CO_2}. The physiologic consequences of an acute rise in P_{CO_2} are twofold, on the one hand, a rapid fall in pH, and on the other, a decline in the effective alveolar PO_2 as a result of displacement of alveolar oxygen by carbon dioxide with subsequent hypoxemia. Acidosis and hypoxemia interact in a dreadfully synergistic way in all aspects of cellular metabolism, and the lack of their prompt reversal leads to irreversible cellular damage (19).

Clinical instances of acute respiratory acidosis are generally sorted into two major groups according to whether the lungs are normal or abnormal (Table 1). The cardinal feature of both groups is an abnormally high P_{CO_2}. Invariably a drop in arterial PO_2 accompanies the hypercapnia. In patients with normal lungs, either the drive from respiratory neurons is at fault or the chest bellows is operating ineffectively. In contrast, in the patient with abnormal lungs, the abnormal blood gas levels result from widespread imbalances between alveolar ventilation and perfusion. The distinction between these two groups is based on the premise that in patients with normal lungs the fall in arterial PO_2 corresponds torr by torr to the rise of arterial P_{CO_2}. In other words, the alveolar arterial gradient for oxygen is normal (10–13).

Patients with renal disease are at risk for the development of acute respiratory acidosis. Several reasons account for this propensity. The clearance for most drugs is decreased, making these patients susceptible to prolonged respiratory depression secondary to narcotics and/or benzodiazepines (14). The elimination of aminoglycosides is markedly impaired and the well-known capacity of these agents to block neuromuscular transmission is enhanced. Indeed, respiratory arrest may occur following intraperitoneal installation of these antibiotics (15). On the other hand, it is not uncommon for the renal patient to be hypoalbuminemic, with a consequent decreased binding ability. Finally, also common in renal patients is caloric and protein malnutrition. It is now clearly established that malnutrition has an important detrimental effect on the working capacity of the diaphragm, and respiratory muscle fatigue occurs at lower working loads (16, 17).

Severe acute respiratory acidosis (pH < 7.10, P_{CO_2} > 80 and PO_2 < 50) is a life-threatening situation in which endotracheal intubation and artificial ventilation should

Table 1. Causes of acute respiratory acidosis

Acute alveolar hypoventilation with normal lungs
  Central respiratory depression
    Sedatives and/or narcotic overdose
    General anesthesia
    Brainstem infarction
    Metabolic alkalosis
  Neuromuscular defects
    Tetanus, botulism
    Drugs (depolarizing or nondepolarizing muscle relaxants, aminoglycosides)
    Myasthenia gravis crisis
    Myxedema coma
  Mechanical abnormalities of the major airway and/or thoracic cage
    Upper airway obstruction
    Flail chest
    Pneumothorax
    Hemothorax

be promptly instituted (18, 19). If the situation is less critical and no immediate respiratory support is required, some diagnostic and therapeutic maneuvers should be attempted, aimed at correcting the primary pathologic process. The use of naloxone is warranted if an overdose of narcotics is suspected. Clearing the airway and removing any foreign objects is a first-order intervention. Providing an artificial oral airway to assure that a backward displacement of the tongue is not obstructing the hypopharynx can be life saving. Placement of a chest tube in the presence of pneumothorax or massive pleural effusion is appropriate. Neostigmine may be given in cases of myasthenia gravis. Treatment of pulmonary edema or the treatment of bronchospasm in patients with asthma will usually improve ventilation, and epinephrine may be helpful in anaphylactic reactions.

In the patient with acute respiratory acidosis, emphasis should be placed on the immediate correction of hypoxemia and acidosis, since the hypercapnia per se is not associated with major toxic effects.

CHRONIC RESPIRATORY ACIDOSIS

Chronic hypercapnia is a commonly encountered acid-base disorder. As in the case of acute respiratory acidosis,

Table 2. Causes of chronic respiratory acidosis

Chronic alveolar hypoventilation with normal lungs

Central respiratory depression
    Primary alveolar hypoventilation (Ondine curse)
    Obesity hypoventilation syndrome
    Bulbar poliomyelitis
    Encephalitis
Neuromuscular disorders
    Guillain-Barre syndrome
    Bilateral cervical cordotomy
    Bilateral diaphragmatic paralysis
    Muscular dystrophy
    Amyotrophic lateral sclerosis
    Multiple sclerosis
    Polymyositis
    Mitochondrial myopathy
    Hypokalemic myopathy
    Familial hypokalemic or hyperkalemic periodic paralysis
Thoracic cage mechanical abnormalities
    Kyphoscoliosis
    Scleroderma
    Ankylosing spondylitis
    Tracheal stenosis

Chronic alveolar hypoventilation with abnormal lungs

Chronic obstructive airway disease
    Chronic bronchitis
    Emphysema
    Cystic fibrosis
    Bronchiectasis
End-stage restrictive lung disease

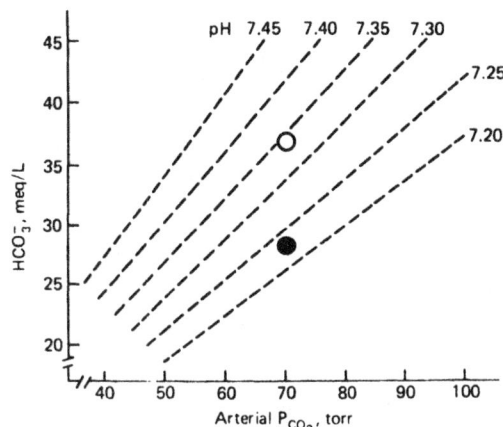

Figure 2. Schematic representation of acute versus chronic hypercapnia. For the same level of arterial P_{CO_2}, patients with chronic hypercapnia (open circles) have a much milder acidosis. After Sandham (33).

it can be observed in patients with normal lungs, but is far more common in patients with chronic lung disease (Table 2). During chronic hypercapnia, the plasma bicarbonate concentration increases as a consequence of renal adaptive responses, producing an acceleration of the rate of sodium-hydrogen exchange along the nephron (20), in contrast with acute respiratory acidosis, in which body buffering accounts for virtually all the increments in plasma bicarbonate. During chronic hypercapnia, the rate of net acid excretion leads to a negative hydrogen-ion balance and the generation of new bicarbonate ions. This newly generated bicarbonate is conserved by the augmented rate of bicarbonate reabsorption (22) (Figure 2). As bicarbonate stores are being augmented, chloride stores are correspondingly depleted as a result of the enhanced urinary chloride excretion associated with an increased excretion of ammonia (21). The factors that motivate the renal response to chronic CO_2 retention are not clear. There is some evidence to suggest that they may be directly mediated through an elevated partial pressure of CO_2 in the kidneys (23).

The treatment of chronic respiratory acidosis is difficult and oftentimes unsuccessful, due to the fact that the underlying condition commonly is far advanced and irreversible. However, it is important to invest time and effort in trying to revert as many factors as possible to optimize the alveolar ventilation and ventilation perfusion relationships. In the rare patient with pure central apnea, the use of progesterone, protriptyline, aminophylline, and, recently, almitrene may be followed by marked improvement (24–27). In patients with obstructive sleep apnea, commonly associated with marked obesity, a weight-reduction regimen, if attained, is usually followed by improvement (28). When this fails, the use of nasal continuous positive airway pressure (CPAP), genioglossus nerve stimulation, and, as a last resort, temporary or permanent tracheostomy sometimes normalizes the arterial blood gases (29, 30). In a recent report, uremic patients with obstructive sleep apnea and severely altered sleep patterns showed marked objective and subjective improvement after hemodyalysis (31). Some patients with idiopathic bilateral diaphragmatic paralysis with intact phrenic nerves are treated with diaphragmatic pacing (32, 33). Patients with the obesity hypoventilation syndrome have a component of obstruction and an increased central threshold for CO_2, and weight reduction and respiratory stimulants sometimes are very effective (34). In patients with chronic obstructive pulmonary disease, optimizing pulmonary toilet, the use of inhaled and oral bronchodilators, the management of secretions, the treatment of infections, the use of diuretics, and sometimes the use of corticosteroids are usually followed by improvement (35–37).

ACUTE RESPIRATORY ACIDOSIS PLUS CHRONIC RESPIRATORY ACIDOSIS

In patients with chronic respiratory acidosis, a new steady state emerges when the augmented filtered load of bicarbonate is precisely balanced by the accelerated rate of bicarbonate reabsorption. Net acid excretion returns to the level required to offset the daily endogenous acid production. Not infrequently this delicate balance is disrupted as a result of respiratory infections, increased bronchospasm, overuse of respiratory depressants, fluid overload, and/or congestive heart failure. As a result, further acidosis, hypoxemia, and hypercarbia develop. Again, as in the case of acute respiratory acidosis when the condition is extreme, immediate intubation should be performed. In less extreme cases, treatment of the underlying precipitating etiology should be attempted.

How much oxygen should be administered to this group of patients? The answer is simple: enough to attain a safe hemoglobin saturation. The debate continues amongst respiratory physiologists and clinicians as to whether there is a group of patients who are "sensitive" to oxygen, in whom the central respiratory neurons are driven by hypoxia, and once this stimulus is removed the patient will cease to breathe (38). If indeed this group of patients exists, it is the overwhelming minority. Recent evidence suggests that the mechanism for the progressive hypoxia is much more complex, involving not only central drive, but also ventilation perfusion relationships and lysis of pulmonary hypoxic vasoconstriction (39). During acute exacerbations of respiratory acidosis, oxygen should be administered rationally, but one must never incur the error of withholding a secure oxygen saturation.

The management of an intubated patient with far advanced lung disease is complex. Complications frequently occur, and the weaning process may be prolonged. However, the outlook for these patients has changed dramatically, with a reported mortality of 20% as compared with 80% in older series (40).

RESPIRATORY ACIDOSIS AND METABOLIC ACIDOSIS

An acid-base disturbance due to combined respiratory acidosis and metabolic acidosis has been repeatedly described in patients undergoing general anesthesia associated with inadequate ventilation. The observed "base deficit" has been attributed to the production of fixed acids secondary to hypoventilation. A striking feature of the acid-base disturbance was the disappearance of the metabolic acidosis without alkali therapy as soon as proper ventilation was secured. The nature of this obscure acid-base disorder has been clarified and represents a "pseudo-metabolic acidosis" associated with acute hypercapnia (41, 42).

In order to properly understand the pathophysiology of the disturbance, we should first clarify some basic concepts. It is frequently but erroneously concluded that the increment in plasma bicarbonate concentration during hypercapnia is just the result of the renal response to a primary increment in CO_2 tension. However, humans or animals without any kidney function, or simply a blood sample under in-vitro conditions, will develop hyperbicarbonatemia during acute hypercapnia. This reaction is explained as follows: Hydration of carbon dioxide results in the formation of carbonic acid, which subsequently dissociates into a hydrogen ion and a bicarbonate ion. The hydrogen ion is, to some extent, bound by the nonbicarbonate buffers, thus the reaction is further sustained, resulting in an increment in plasma bicarbonate. This reaction,

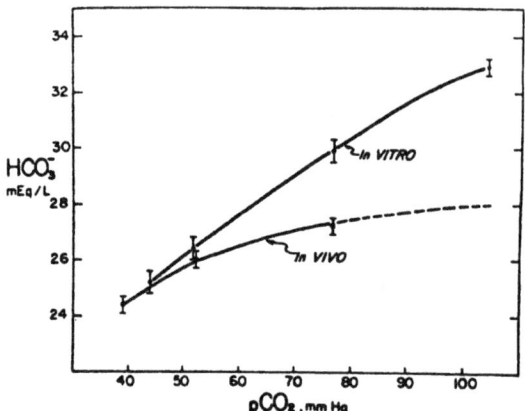

Figure 3. Comparison of the effects of in-vivo and in-vitro equilibration with carbon dioxide on the levels on plasma bicarbonate. The lower curve represents the in-vivo response and was drawn by inspection through the average bicarbonate. The dotted extension is a calculated extrapolation. The upper curve was drawn through the average bicarbonate concentration during in-vitro titration of blood from normal volunteers. From Brackett (3) with permission.

$$CO_2 + H_2O = H_2CO_3 = H_{CO_3} + H^+$$
$$H_{CO_3} + H^+ + Buf^- + X^+ = Buf\,H^+ + H_{CO_3} + X^+\star,$$

is best known as the *interaction reaction* of body buffers and is responsible for the rise in plasma bicarbonate during acute hypercapnia. It is of most interest to compare the in-vivo and in-vitro carbon dioxide titration curves of whole blood, as shown in Figure 3. It can be seen that the rise in plasma bicarbonate for a given change in P_{CO_2} is significantly greater under in-vitro conditions.

Furthermore, whereas the buffer base and base excess remain unchanged during the hypercapnia under in-vitro conditions, both parameters progressively decrease under in-vivo conditions, in proportion to the increment in carbon dioxide tension. In in-vitro conditions the newly formed bicarbonate fully remains in the compartment where it was generated. However, for each millimole of new bicarbonate, one millimole of nonbicarbonate buffer has bound equal amounts of hydrogen ions, losing temporarily its buffer capacity. Hence it is obvious that under in-vitro conditions, buffer base and base excess remain unaltered during acute hypercapnia. Under in-vivo conditions the effects are quite different: Acute hypercapnia acting upon the intravascular and cellular compartments, rich in nonbicarbonate buffers, results in the production of significant quantities of new bicarbonate, increasing the concentration of bicarbonate in these compartments. Carbon dioxide, a rapidly diffusible gas, increases its tension to a similar degree in the interstitial fluid, which, as opposed to the intravascular and intracellular fluid, is practically devoid of nonbicarbonate in the interstitial compartment. Therefore, the concentration of this ion initially remains unchanged. The concentration gradient for bicarbonate created thereby among the body fluid compartments leads to the migration of bicarbonate thereby among the body fluid compartments leads to the migration of bicarbonate from the intravascular, and possibly from the intracellular, to the interstitial compartment. Thus, the small rise in plasma bicarbonate during acute hypercapnia under in-vivo as compared with in-vitro conditions, as well as the base deficit observed in vivo, are the result of the previously described transitory loss of bicarbonate from the blood to the interstitial fluid. When acute hypercapnia disappears, the opposite sequence of events takes place, and bicarbonate ions move back from the interstitial to the intravascular compartment, and hence the base deficit disappears. The phenomenon of false metabolic acidosis that accompanies acute hypercapnia is thus the result of compartmental redistribution of bicarbonate. Figure 4 depicts the magnitude of this phenomenon in the adult as compared with the newborn. Whereas in the adult an acute rise in P_{CO_2} up to 100 mmHg results in a base deficit of about 6.7 mEq/l, in the newborn the effect is even greater, the base deficit reaching approximately 10.3 mEq/l. The greater effect in the newborn is due to a stronger buffering capacity within the intravascular compartment (blood volume, 100 ml/kg as compared with 70 ml/kg in the adult; Hb, 18 g% as compared with 15 g%), as well as the bigger

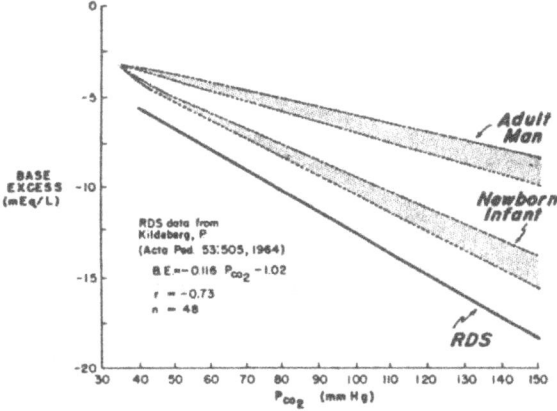

Figure 4. Effects of acute hypercapnia on blood base excess under in-vivo conditions. Predicted CO_2 equilibration curves in adult man and newborn infant, and data obtained from infants in respiratory distress syndrome (RDS). From Suki (3) with permission.

extracellular fluid volume (400–450 ml/kg as compared with 230–270 ml/kg in the adult). If, for example, a newborn develops severe respiratory depression, with Pa_{CO_2} up to 100 mmHg resulting from the administration of narcotics to the child during labor, it is expected to see a base deficit of 10 mEq/l, which does not represent a true metabolic acidosis and will disappear with the correction of the hypoventilation.

On the other hand, respiratory acidosis associated with real — as opposed to pseudo — metabolic acidosis represents a major acid-base emergency. Neither component needs to be markedly abnormal for plasma acidity to be severely deranged. The combination of respiratory acidosis and metabolic acidosis is commonly seen in patients during cardiopulmonary arrest in chronic obstructive pulmonary disease complicated by septic shock, in severe renal failiure complicated by respiratory failure in fulminating pulmonary edema, and in poisoning with various drugs and toxic agents.

Arterial pH below 7.10, either of respiratory or metabolic origin, is very poorly tolerated (43). Thus, immediate means to correct the process are indicated by the use of intravenous bicarbonate and/or mechanical ventilation, depending upon the degree of derangement of each component. Patients presenting with respiratory acidosis and metabolic acidosis should be given sodium bicarbonate, in addition to the previously mentioned measures, to improve oxygenation and alveolar ventilation. The aim of therapy is to bring back blood pH to a safer value. An approximation of immediate bicarbonate requirements may be obtained by multiplying the desired increment in plasma bicarbonate by 50% of body weight in kilograms, which represents the apparent space of distribution of bicarbonate under normal conditions. Since the space of distribution of bicarbonate increases with severe acidosis, this formula will underestimate the bicarbonate requirements. It should be pointed out that correction of tissue hypoxia may regenerate bicarbonate from lactate, thus significantly decreasing the requirement of exogenous bicarbonate. A similar situation is found in most cases of metabolic acidosis due to an increased anion gap, when the underlying disorder is corrected.

The use of sodium bicarbonate during cardiopulmonary resuscitation and to treat severe organic acidosis has been questioned (61, 62). However, the burden of proof remains squarely with those decrying its use as adjunctive therapy in patients whose immediate survival is threatened by severe acidemia (63).

Alkali administration also represents the emergency treatment for hyperkalemia. Acidemia is associated with potassium release from the intracellular compartment and elevation in the plasma potassium concentration. The quantitative aspects of this phenomenon in the case of metabolic acidosis are as follows: a decrease in plasma pH of 0.1 unit leads to an increase in the plasma potassium concentration of about 0.6 mEq/l (46, 47). This pattern seems to be correct in the case of metabolic acidosis due to infusion of mineral acids. In sharp contrast, acute organic-acid acidosis is not associated with a significant change in the plasma potassium concentration (24). Experimental infusion of organic acid fails to produce a significant plasma potassium response (41–43). In addition, spontaneous recovery from grand-mal seizure-induced lactic acidosis in humans was not accompanied by hyperkalemia (44). However, if high levels of plasma potassium are present n a patient with respiratory acidosis plus metabolic acidosis, bicarbonate should be administered, and it will result in depression of the plasma potassium level. In patients with renal failure and severe hyperkalemia, ion-exchange resins should also be administered. If the patient has significant volume expansion, heart failure, or renal failure, and significant amounts of alkali are required to correct the acidemia, dialysis with sodium bicarbonate may be the best therapeutic alternative.

RESPIRATORY ALKALOSIS

Respiratory alkalosis is the acid-base disturbance initiated by a reduction in the carbon dioxide tension. Increased alveolar ventilation is the only process that can result in a period of negative carbon dioxide balance and hence in a reduction in carbon dioxide tension (Table 3).

As in respiratory acidosis, the changes in serum bicarbonate induced by acute respiratory alkalosis are rapid and are largely independent of renal action. With chronicity, renal compensation is responsible for lowering serum bicarbonate, causing pH to approach normality. In acute respiratory alkalosis, the fall in bicarbonate is not great enough to prevent the P_{CO_2}/H_{CO_3} ratio from falling and the pH, therefore, increases. The fall in the hydrogen ion concentration is proportional to the fall in P_{CO_2}. The situation in acute respiratory alkalosis exactly mirrors that seen in acute respiratory acidosis. In both settings the change in hydrogen ion approximates 80% of the change in P_{CO_2}.

Chronic suppression of renal acid excretion will eventually cause bicarbonate to decrease even further, and arterial pH approximates normal. Respiratory alkalosis appears to be unique among the simple acid-base disturbances in the body's ability to compensate pH to normal (8).

A serious condition initially associated with an apparently benign respiratory alkalosis is sepsis. The mechanism by which early sepsis induces alveolar hyperventilation is unclear, but has been attributed to subclinical pulmonary edema with irritation of the stretch receptors, a direct effect of endotoxin on the central nervous system, and/or alteration in cellular metabolism secondary to endotoxin or other products. The initial respiratory alkalosis is sometimes followed by progressive hypoxemia and the development of fulminant noncardiogenic pulmonary edema, oftentimes referred to as *adult respiratory distress syndrome* (ARDS) (50–53).

In large series, the mortality for ARDS ranges between 50% and 75% (53). By far the most important prognostic factor is the number of systems and/or organs failing. When only the lungs are affected by the underlying process, survival approaches 60%. When four or more systems are involved, mortality is almost 100% (54, 59). Prompt intervention and intensive support are paramount in the management of the syndrome. The pulmonary capillary wedge pressure (PCWP) should be kept at the lowest range that is compatible with adequate tissue perfusion. However, it is important to keep in mind several factors: The optimal cardiac output for septic patients with ARDS is not known. It has been demonstrated that in septic patients an abnormal dependency

Table 3. Causes of alveolar hyperventilation

Anxiety
Central nervous systems disorders (CVA, tumor, meningitis, encephalitis)
Drugs (salicylates, overdose of analeptics, cocaine, nicotine, xanthines, dinitrophenol)
Hormones (progesterone, T3, T4)
Catecholamines
Fever
Hyperthyroidism
Endotoxemia
Pregnancy
Metabolic acidosis
Liver failure
Delirium tremens
Pulmonary edema
Pulmonary embolism
Pulmonary fibrosis
High altitudes
Hypoxemia
Hypotension
Anemia
Mechanical overventilation

between oxygen delivery and oxygen consumption operats, and the higher the delivery, and thus the higher the consumption, the better the prognosis (54, 55). In the septic patient who is mechanically ventilated with positive end-expiratory pressure (PEEP), the pulmonary capillary wedge pressure does not reflect the left ventricular end-diastolic volume and could be misleading (51–53). For these reasons, keeping the PCWP on the "low side" could be dangerous. Our management strategy in these patients is to: a) Try to revert and/or treat the underlying process and b) keep adequate perfusion and oxygenation by the use of vasopressors and/or fluids, even at the cost of higher PCWP.

The controversy between the use of crystalloids or colloids in the management of ARDS continues. It has been argued theoretically that even though albumin gives an immediate improvement in hemodynamics, eventually the administered albumin will leak into the lungs and drag additional water with it. However, there is no evidence that exogenous (administered) albumin (or any other substance) is handled differently than the same endogenously produced substance. In the critically ill patient, it seems reasonable to correct a low plasma albumin concentration and plasma oncotic pressure ($< 20\,mmHg$) with appropriate amounts of 25% albumin (58, 59). Finally, some studies have demonstrated an impressive improvement in the survival of septic patients with refractory ARDS by the use of hemofiltration. Beneficial effects are attributed to removal by the procedure of middle-size molecules that may be playing an important pathophysiologic role in septic patients (60).

METABOLIC ALKALOSIS AND RESPIRATORY ALKALOSIS

The additive effects of coexisting metabolic and respiratory alkalosis on pH may result in severe alkalemia. The superimposition of one disorder upon the other precludes any attempt at compensation for either primary disorder. Thus, normal metabolic compensation, which lowers serum bicarbonate, thereby acting to return pH toward normal in respiratory alkalosis, is prevented by the associated primary metabolic alkalosis. Similarly, the hypoventilation and increased P_{CO_2} that is elicited by an act to lower pH in metabolic alkalosis is prevented by the attendent primary alkalosis.

Cardiac output has been shown to fall, while total vascular resistance increases during marked alkalosis (64). Cardiac arrhythmias may result and may remain refractory to all therapies until the pH is lower (65). Alkalosis-induced arrhythmias are more common if the patient is digitlized or severely potassium and/or magnesium depleted. Respiratory alkalosis is a potent cerebral vasoconstrictor, and metabolic alkalosis has similar but less potent effects (66). Alkalemia also shifts the hemoglobin dissociation curve to the left, thereby increasing the affinity of hemoglobin for oxygen, which in turns tends to reduce tissue oxygenation (67). Together, these effects combine to produce cerebral hypoxia and may result in confusion, seizures, and coma. The cerebral effects of respiratory alkalosis and hypoxemia are additive. All these factors may contribute to the markedly increased mortality of patients with severe alkalosis (68). This mixed respiratory and metabolic disorder is most commonly found in the intensive care unit setting, where a multiplicity of medical problems occur. The respiratory component arises from excessive mechanical ventilation, hypoxemia, sepsis, liver disease, and pain. The metabolic component results from vomiting, nasogastric suction, massive blood transfusions, the use of lactated Ringer's solution, and high-dose antacid therapy.

The presence of severe alkalosis represents a medical emergency and should be treated immediately. When the primary etiology is not amenable to prompt reversal, hydrochloric acid or amonium chloride intravenously, or acetazolamide should be administered. When the patient is mechanically ventilated, hypoventilation with sedation should be instituted.

RESPIRATORY ACIDOSIS AND METABOLIC ALKALOSIS

More than half of the patients with chronic respiratory acidosis have an associated metabolic alkalosis. Respiratory acidosis induces a compensatory metabolic response that increases the bicarbonate concentration. When acute or chronic respiratory acidosis is associated with an inappropriately elevated bicarbonate concentration, mixed respiratory acidosis and metabolic alkalosis may be diagnosed.

Patients with chronic obstructive pulmonary disease and respiratory acidosis are often subjected to salt restriction, diuretics, and occasionally glucocorticoids, which makes them prone to the development of metabolic alkalosis. Renal bicarbonate production and renal bicarbonate reabsorption are increased in this setting, providing mechanisms for both generating and maintaining metabolic alkalosis. The elevated pH will diminish respiratory drive and may therefore worsen the pulmonary disorder (69, 70).

Metabolic alkalosis is often accompanied by potassium depletion, which can in turn produce muscle weakness. Hypokalemic myopathy generally begins in the proximal muscles in the lower extremities, but may progress to involve all skeletal muscles. When respiratory muscles are affected, hypoventilation will result (71).

Occasionally, patients with severe metabolic alkalosis are found to have marked hypercarbia and are said to exhibit "supersensitive" respiratory compensation for metabolic alkalosis. When studied following reversal of the acid-base disturbance, these patients have normal respiratory control mechanisms. However, since many of these patients also have severe hypokalemia, it is likely that in some instances the marked hypercarbia was really due to hypokalemic-induced respiratory muscle fatigue and respiratory acidosis. Also, several studies have demonstrated that in patients with acute respiratory acidosis and metabolic alkalosis, treatment with either acetazolamide or ammonium chloride reversed the metabolic alkalosis and markedly improved the hypoventilation. Therefore, in the treatment of these mixed acid-base disturbances, particular attention should be paid to the repletion of chloride, potassium, intravascular volume, and occasionally to the use of acetazolamide and acidifying salts.

REFERENCES

1. Maxwell M, Kleeman C: Clinical Disorders of Fluid and Electrolyte Metabolism, 3rd ed. *McGraw Hill*, pp 184–232, 1980.
2. Cohen JJ, Madias NE: Respiratory acidosis and alkalosis. In: DW Seldin, G Giebish, eds, The Kidney, Physiology and Pathophysiology. Raven Press, New York, 1985.
3. Brackett NC Jr, Wingo CF, Muren O, Solano JT: *Acid-base response to chronic hypercapnia in man.* N Engl J Med 280:124–130, 1969.
4. Madias NE, Androgue HJ, Horowitz GL, Cohen JJ, Schwartz WB: A redefinition of acid base equilibrium in man: CO_2 as a key determinant of normal plasma bicarbonate concentration. *Kidney Int* 10:612, 1969.
5. Rose BD: *Clinical Physiology of Acid-Base and Electrolyte Disorders.* McGraw Hill, New York, 1977.
6. Androgue HJ, Suki WN: Respiratory acid base disorders. In: *Therapy of Renal Diseases.* WN Suki, ed, Martinus Nijhoff, Boston, 1984.
7. Rahn H: Gas transport from the external environment to the cell. In: AVS Rueck, Porter R, eds, *Development of the Lung.* Boston, Little Brown, 1967.
8. Narins RG, Emmet M: Simple and mixed acid-base disorders. A practical approach. *Medicine (Baltimore)* 59:161–187, 1980.
9. Fishman A: *Pulmonary Diseases and Disorders.* McGraw Hill, New York, pp 417–444, 1980.
10. Murray JF: *The Normal Lung*, 2nd ed. WB Saunders Philadelphia pp 211–233, 1986.
11. Fraser R, Pare P: *Diagnosis and Diseases of the Chest.* WB Saunders, Philadelphia, pp 106–116, 1977.
12. Madias NE, Cohen JJ: Respiratory acidosis, In: JJ Cohen, JP Kassirer, eds, *Acid-Base.* Little, Brown, Boston, pp 307–348, 19–.
13. Whitelaw WA: The respiratory pump. In: CA Guenter, MH Welch, eds, *Pulmonary Medicine*, 2nd ed JB Lippincott, Philadelphia, 1982.
14. Goodman A, Goodman L, Gilman A: *The Pharmacological Basis of Therapeutics.* McMillan New York 6th ed, pp 1671–1373, 19–.
15. Rosalo EF, Oram-Smith: Peritoneal lavage treatment in experimental peritonitis. *Ann Surg* 175:384, 1972.
16. Arora NS, Rochester DF: Effect of body weight and muscularity on human diaphragm muscle mass, thickness and area: *J App Physiol* 52:64–70, 1980.
17. Arora NS, Rochester DF: Respiratory muscle strength and maximal voluntary ventilation in undernourished patients. *Am Rev Resp Dis* 126:5–8, 1982.
18. Shibel EM, Moser KM (Eds): Respiratory Emergency. Saint Louis, CV Mosby, 1977.
19. Downing SE, Mitchell JH, Wallace AG: Cardiovascular responses to ischemia, hypoxia and hypercapnia of the central nervous system. *Am J Physiol* 204:881–887, 1963.
20. Van Ypersele de Strihou C, Gulyassy PF, Schwartz WB: Effects of chronic hypercapnia on electrolyte and acid-base equilibrium. III. Characteristics of the adaptive and recovery process as evaluated by provision of alkali. *J Clin Invest* 41:2246–2253, 1972.
21. Polak A, Haynie GD, Hays RM, Schwartz WB: Effects of chronic hypercapnia on electrolyte and acid-base equilibrium. I. Adaptation. *J Clin Invest* 40:1223–1237, 1961.
22. Dulfano MJ, and Ikishawa S: Quantitative acid-base relationships in chronic pulmonary patients during the stable state. *Am Rev Resp Dis* 93:251–256, 1966.
23. Schwartz WB Cohen JJ: The nature of the renal response to chronic disorders of acid-base equilibrium. *Am J Med* 64:417–428, 1978.
24. Giradoux J: Ondine, a Romantic Fantasy in Three Acts. English version by M. Valency. New York, French, 1956, Act 3, 1, 179.
25. Guilleminault C, Dement WC: *Sleep Apnea Syndromes.* Alan R. Liss, New York, 1978.
26. Mellins RB, Balfour HH Jr, Turino GM, Winters RW: Failure of automatic control of ventilation (Ondine's curse). *Medicine* 49:487–504, 1976.
27. Sutton FD Jr, Szillich CW, Creagh CE, Pierson DJ, Weil JV: Progesterone for outpatient treatment of Pickwickian syndrome. *Ann Intern Med* 83:476–479, 1975.
28. Kronenberg RS, Gabel RA, Severinghaus JW: Normal chemoreceptor function in obesity before and after ileal bypass surgery to force weight reduction. *Am J Med* 59:349–353, 1975.
29. Tenney SM, Ou LC: Hypoxic ventilatory response of cats at high altitude: An interpretation of "blunting." *Resp Physiol* 32:185–199, 1977.
30. Glenn WWL, Gee JBL, Cole DR, Farmer WC, Shaw RK, Beckman CB: Combined central alveolar hypoventilation and upper airway obstruction. Treatment by tracheostomy and diaphragm pacing. *Am J Med* 64:50–60, 1978.
31. Fein AM, Niederman MS: Reversal of sleep apnea in uremia by dialysis. Arch Intern Med 147:1355–1356, 1987.
32. Farmer WC, Glenn WWL, Gee JBL: Alveolar hypoventilation syndrome. Studies of ventilatory control in patients selected for diaphragm pacing. *Am J Med* 64:39–49, 1978.
33. Sandham JD, Shaw DT, Guenter CA: Acute supine respiratory failure due to bilateral diaphragmatic paralysis. *Chest* 72:96–98, 1977.
34. Ingram RH, Bishop BJ: Ventilatory response to carbon dioxide after removal of chronic upper airway obstruction. *Am Rev Resp Dis* 102:645–647, 1970.
35. Guilleminault C, Eldridge FL, Tilkian A, Simmons FB, Dement WC: Sleep apnea syndrome due to upper airway obstruction. *Arch Intern Med* 137:296–300, 1977.
36. Menashe VD, Farrehi C, Miller M: Hypoventilation and cor pulmonale due to chronic upper airway obstruction. *J Pediatr* 67:198–203, 1965.
37. Phillipson EA: Regulation of breathing during sleep. *Am Rev Resp Dis* 115:217–224, 1977.
38. Bone RC, Pierce AK, Johnson RL: Controlled oxygen administration in acute respiratory failure in chronic obstructive pulmonary disease. *Am Rev Resp Dis* 108:232–240, 1973.
39. Anthonisen NR: Hypoxemia and O_2 therapy. *Am Rev Resp Dis* 126:729–733, 1982.
40. Aubier M, Murciano D, Milic-Emili J: Effects of the administration of O_2 on ventilation and blood gases in patients with chronic obstructive pulmonary disease during

acute respiratory failure. *Am Rev Resp Dis* 122:747–754, 1980.
41. Shaw LA, Messer AC: The transfer of bicarbonate between the blood and tissues caused by alterations of the carbon dioxide concentration in the lungs. *Am J Physiol* 100:122–136, 1932.
42. Winters RW: Studies of acid-base disturbances. *Pediatrics* 39:700–712, 1967.
43. Kassirer JP: Serious acid-base disorders. *N Engl J Med* 291:773–776, 1974.
44. Ostrea EM Jr, Odell GB: The influence of bicarbonate administration on blood pH in a "closed system": Clinical implications. *J Pediatr* 80:671–680, 1972.
45. Dell RB, Winters RW: Acid base effects of hypertonic sodium bicarbonate solutions: A commentary. *J Pediatr* 80:681–682, 1972.
46. Scribner BH, Burnell JM: Interpretation of the serum potassium concentration. *Metabolism* 5:468–479, 1956.
47. Gabow P: Disorders of potassium metabolism. In: RW, Schrier ed, Renal and Electrolyte Disorders. Little Brown, Boston, pp 143–165, 1976.
48. Van Ypersele de Strihou C: Potassium homeostasis in renal failure. *Kidney Int* 11:491–504, 1977.
49. Blair E: Hypocapnia, and gram-negative bacteremic Shock. *Am J Surg* 119:433–439, 1970.
50. Simmons DH, Nicoloff J, Guzo LB: Hyperventilation and respiratory alkalosis as signs of gram-negative bacteremia. *JAMA* 174:2196, 1960.
51. Kaplan AI Sahn SA, Petty TL: Incidence and outcome of the respiratory distress syndrome in gram-negative Sepsis. *Arch Intern Med* 139:867, 1979.
52. Petty TL: Indicators of risk, course, and prognosis in adult respiratory distress syndrome. *Am Rev Resp Dis* 132:471, 1985.
53. Fowler AA, Hamman RR, Zenbe GO: Adult respiratory distress syndrome, Prognosis After Onset. *Am Rev Resp Dis* 133:472–478, 1985.
54. Bland RD, Shoemaker WL, Abraham E: Hemodynamic and oxygen transport patterns in surviving and non-surviving postoperative patients. *Crit Care Med* 13:85, 1985.
55. Sibbald WJ, Calvin J, Driedger A: Right and left ventricular preload and diastolic ventricular compliance — Implications for therapy in critically ill patients. In: *Critical Care State of the Art*. Fullerton, CA, Society of Critical Care Medicine, 1982.
56. Alderman EL, Glanz SA: Acute hemodynamic interventions shift the diastolic presure volume curve in men. *Circulation* 54:622–671, 1976.
57. Calvin JE, Driedger AA, Sibbald WJ: Does the pulmonary capillary wedge pressure predict left ventricular preload in critically ill patients? *Crit Care Med* 9:437–443, 1981.
58. Hrupt MT, Rackow EL: Colloidosmotic pressure and fluid resuscitation with hetastarch. Albumin, and saline solution. *Crit Care Med* 1982; 10, 159, 1982.
59. Hankeln, K., Randel, C., "Comparison of Hydroxyethyl Starch and, Lactated Ringer's Solution on Hemodynamics and Oxygen Transport on Critically III Patients in Prospective Crossover Studies, *Crit Care Med* 17:133–135, 1989.
60. Barzilay E Lev A, Lesmies C: Continous hemofiltration as an adjunt therapy for acute system organ failure (AOSE), *Rev Esp Anestesiol Reanim* 34:459, 1987.
61. Stalpodt PW: Lactic acidosis: The case against bicarbanate therapy. *Ann Intern Med* 105:276–279, 1986.
62. Graf H, Leach W, Arieff: Evidence of detrimental effect of bicarbonate therapy in hypoxic lactic Acidosis. *Science* 227:754–756, 1985.
63. Narins R, Cohen JJ: Bicarbonate therapy for organic acidosis: The case for its continuous use. *Ann Internal Med* 106:615–618, 1987.
64. Mitchell JH, Wildenthal K, Johnson RL: The effects of acid-base disturbances on cardiovascular and pulmonary function. *Kidney Int* 1:375, 1972.
65. Ayres SM, Grace WJ: Inappropriate ventilation and hypoxemia as causes of cardiac arrhythmias. *Am J Med* 46:495–505, 1969.
66. Betz E, Heuser D: Cerebral cortical blood flow during changes of acid-base equilibrium of the brain. *J Appl Physiol* 23:726, 1976.
67. Finch CA, Lenfant C: Oxygen transport in man. *N Engl J Med* 286:407, 1972.
68. Wilson RF, Gibson D, Percinel AK, Ali MA, Baker G, Leblanc LP, Lucas C: Severe alkalosis in critically ill surgical patients. *Arch Surg* 105:197, 1972.
69. Bear R, Goldstein M, Phillipson E, Hammeke M, Feldman R: Effects of metabolic alkalosis on respiratory function in patients with chronic obstructive pulmonary disease. *Can Med Assoc J* 117:900, 1977.
70. McCurdy DK: Mixed metabolic and respiratory acid-base disturbances; diagnosis and treatment. In: RM, Rogers, ed, *Respiratory Intensive Care*. Springfield, IL, Charles C. Thomas, pp 107–129, 1986.
71. Schwartz WB, Van Ypersele De Stihou C, Kassirer JP: Role of anions in metabolic alkalosis and potassium deficiency. *N Engl J Med* 279:630–639, 1968.

CHAPTER 14

Mixed Acid-Base Disorders

JOHN T. HARRINGTON & NICOLAOS E. MADIAS

INTRODUCTION

Virtually all recent discussions of the diagnosis and management of mixed acid-base disturbances have focused exclusively on the acid-base disorders per se and have relegated the patient and the clinical setting to a subordinate position. In the 1980s several excellent reviews utilizing primarily a laboratory approach have appeared (1–3). In this laboratory-dominated approach, the acid-base data first are examined to determine whether they are consistent with any of the simple acid-base disorders; if the acid-base data do not fit, and assuming that they reflect a steady state, one can confidently conclude that a mixed acid-base disturbance is present (4). For instance, in a patient with a plasma bicarbonate concentration of 8 mEq/l, the finding of a Pa_{CO_2} level substantially greater than the value anticipated for simple metabolic acidosis establishes the presence of a concomitant element of respiratory acidosis and thus the presence of a mixed acid-base disorder.

In this chapter, prior to turning to a discussion of the major clinical settings in which mixed acid-base disorders are common, we will define quantitatively the anticipated adaptive responses to the four simple acid-base disorders, discuss an overall graphic presentation of these cardinal disorders (the template), and then review the major mixed acid-base disorders, using the very same template as a guide. We believe that mixed acid-base disturbances are best categorized into four major groups: a) coexistence of a metabolic and a respiratory acid-base disturbance, b) coexistence of two respiratory acid-base disorders, c) coexistence of two metabolic acid-base disturbances, d) coexistence of three or more of the cardinal acid-base disorders.

Given this introductory, background information, we will then focus on the clinical situations in which mixed acid-base disturbances most commonly occur. In our experience, these clinical situations are limited and include: a) cardiac arrest, b) sepsis, c) drug intoxications (especially alcohol, salicylates, and sedatives), and d) organ failure (especially renal, hepatic, and pulmonary failure). Following our analysis of the mixed acid-base disturbances seen in these four clinical settings (and their treatment), we will discuss briefly mixed acid-base disturbances seen in a variety of other situations. We believe that this patient-centered approach allows the physician not only to more readily diagnose mixed acid-base disturbances, but, more importantly, to *anticipate* them. Bia and Thier have stated in fact that "mixed acid-base disturbances are most commonly predictable on the basis of the clinical setting and physical examination: laboratory data serve mainly to confirm the clinical impression" (1). This anticipatory approach also provides the physician with the potential to prevent the development of these complex disorders, many of which are associated with a high mortality rate.

LABORATORY APPROACH TO ACID-BASE DISORDERS

Extensive clinical and laboratory investigations over the past 25 years have yielded considerable information regarding the expected adaptive response to each of the four simple acid-base disturbances. Detailed discussions of relevant data regarding adaptation to each simple acid-base disturbance can be found elsewhere in this book and in Cohen et al. (3). Here we will briefly review the quantitative relationships for the mean whole-body adaptive responses for the simple acid-base disturbances (Table 1) (4). Computerized diagnostic systems, based on these quantitative relationships, are being developed to aid in the rapid diagnosis of mixed acid-base disorders (5).

Metabolic acidosis

Metabolic acidosis, defined as a primary decrease in plasma bicarbonate concentration, is accompanied by a decrement in Pa_{CO_2} that is proportional to the decrement in bicarbonate concentration. Nearly a dozen studies have explored the $\Delta Pa_{CO_2}/\Delta [HCO_3^-]$ relationship in *steady-state* metabolic acidosis; in general, it takes about 12 hours for such a steady state to be reached. In careful studies carried out in normal subjects given NH_4Cl for several days and in stable patients with chronic uremic acidosis, Lennon and Lemann demonstrated that, on average, the

Table 1. Mean whole-body response equations for primary acid-base disorders

Disorder	Equation
Metabolic acidosis	$\Delta Pa_{CO_2} \cong 1.2\Delta[HCO_3^-]$
Metabolic alkalosis	$\Delta Pa_{CO_2} \cong 0.7\Delta[HCO_3^-]$
Respiratory acidosis	
Acute	$\Delta[HCO_3^-] \cong 0.1\Delta Pa_{CO_2}$
	$\Delta[H^+] \cong 0.75\Delta Pa_{CO_2}$
Chronic	$\Delta[HCO_3^-] \cong 0.3\Delta Pa_{CO_2}$
	$\Delta[H^+] \cong 0.3\Delta Pa_{CO_2}$
Respiratory alkalosis	
Acute	$\Delta[HCO_3^-] \cong 0.2\Delta Pa_{CO_2}$
	$\Delta[H^+] \cong 0.75\Delta Pa_{CO_2}$
Chronic	$\Delta[HCO_3^-] \cong 0.5\Delta Pa_{CO_2}$
	$\Delta[H^+] \cong 0.5\Delta Pa_{CO_2}$

Pa_{CO_2} fell by 1.1 mmHg for each 1 mEq/l decline in plasma bicarbonate concentration (6). Several other studies have corroborated the quantitative findings of these two groups of investigators. Alpert and his colleagues (7) showed that the adequacy of the respiratory response for steady-state metabolic acidosis could be determined using the following formula:

$$Pa_{CO_2} = 1.54 [HCO_3^-] + 8.36 \pm 1.1.$$

On average, the empirically derived relationship states that for every 1 mEq/l fall in bicarbonate concentration, there is a 1.1–1.4 mmHg fall in Pa_{CO_2} (8).

Metabolic alkalosis

In contrast to the well-defined ventilatory response in metabolic acidosis, the quantitative aspects of the $\Delta Pa_{CO_2}/\Delta [HCO_3^-]$ relationship in steady-state metabolic alkalosis are less well defined (9, 10). Nevertheless, available experimental and clinical data do allow one to state that the Pa_{CO_2} probably rises by $\cong 0.7$ mmHg for each 1 mEq/l rise in the plasma bicarbonate concentration. The validity of this quantitative relationship is strongest for patients in whom the plasma bicarbonate concentration is less than 40 mEq/l. Limited data do suggest, however, that the relationship holds for patients with plasma bicarbonate concentrations between 40 and 75 mEq/l as well. In fact, this straight-line relationship between ΔPa_{CO_2} and $\Delta[HCO_3^-]$, with no apparent plateau, can rarely result in the generation of overt (ventilator-dependent) respiratory failure (9).

Respiratory acidosis

In both respiratory acidosis and respiratory alkalosis, the alteration in bicarbonate concentration that ensues as a consequence of the primary alteration in Pa_{CO_2} is time-dependent. Thus, in both respiratory acidosis and respiratory alkalosis, we must consider the anticipated adaptive response in plasma bicarbonate concentration for both *acute* and *chronic* situations. The acute steady state is established instantaneously. Mechanisms are then activated that result in generating the chronic steady state over the next 3 days. For respiratory acidosis, defined as a primary increase in Pa_{CO_2}, the acute phase (though evolving) operationally encompasses approximately the first 1–3 days of hypercapnia; full expression of the adaptive response for respiratory acidosis develops, as noted, within 72 hours or so of a given increment in Pa_{CO_2}.

Respiratory acidosis thus has different anticipated responses in plasma bicarbonate concentration, depending on the time elapsed from the onset of hypercapnia. In *acute* respiratory acidosis, Brackett, Cohen, and Schwartz demonstrated that increasing degrees of hypercapnia are associated with a curvilinear rise in plasma bicarbonate concentration, the successive increments diminishing in magnitude at successively higher levels of Pa_{CO_2} (11). The increment in plasma bicarbonate concentration during acute hypercapnia stems virtually exclusively from titration of nonbicarbonate body buffers, and there is little increase in renal acid excretion. Consequently, little change in plasma bicarbonate concentration ensues. Thus, plasma bicarbonate rises by no more than 3–4 mEq/l, even when Pa_{CO_2} is increased acutely to 80–90 mmHg. In acute respiratory acidosis, therefore, the plasma bicarbonate concentration does not rise to greater than 30 mEq/l or so. This quantitative relationship can be best approximated by a 0.1 mEq/l rise in plasma bicarbonate for each 1 mmHg acute increment in Pa_{CO_2} (12, 13).

By contrast, the relationship between plasma hydrogen ion concentration and Pa_{CO2} is strikingly linear over a range of Pa_{CO_2} extending from normal to 90 mmHg. The average rise in plasma hydrogen ion concentration amounts to approximately 0.75 nEq/l for each 1 mmHg acute rise in Pa_{CO_2} (11).

In *chronic* respiratory acidosis, a substantial transient increase in renal acid excretion (which exceeds endogenous acid production) generates a sizable increase in the plasma bicarbonate concentration. Detailed animal observations revealed that in chronic hypercapnia the relationship between the plasma bicarbonate concentration and Pa_{CO_2} is curvilinear, successive increments in bicarbonate concentration diminishing somewhat in magnitude at progressively higher levels of Pa_{CO_2}. Yet, over the range of Pa_{CO_2} values between 40 and 90 mmHg, which encompasses most values encountered clinically, this curvilinear relationship is closely approximated by a straight line with a slope of 0.3. Over this range, therefore, each 1 mmHg chronic increment in Pa_{CO_2} is associated, on average, with an approximate 0.3 mEq/l increment in the steady-state plasma bicarbonate concentration. The corresponding relationship between the plasma hydrogen ion concentration and Pa_{CO_2} is strikingly linear (as in acute respiratory acidosis), hydrogen ion concentration rising on average by 0.3 nEq/l for each 1 mmHg chronic elevation in Pa_{CO_2} (12–15).

Respiratory alkalosis

Respiratory alkalosis, defined as a primary decrease in Pa_{CO_2}, also has a time-dependent response in the plasma bicarbonate concentration. In acute respiratory alkalosis, the plasma bicarbonate concentration falls only modestly and is usually not lower than 18–20 mEq/l (16). This fall is accounted for principally by the alkaline titration of the nonbicarbonate buffers of the body. The acute, secondary change in the plasma bicarbonate concentration is substantially greater in magnitude than that observed during acute hypercapnia of comparable degree, falling by approximately 0.2. mEq/l for each 1 mmHg acute decrease in Pa_{CO_2}. Thus, a reduction in plasma bicarbonate of 3–4 mEq/l occurs within minutes after Pa_{CO_2} is lowered to 20–25 mmHg. The resulting change in plasma hydrogen ion concentration, however, is strikingly similar numerically to that observed during acute hypercapnia. On average, the plasma hydrogen ion concentration decreases by approximately 0.75 nEq/l for each 1 mmHg acute reduction in Pa_{CO_2}, hr. Over the next several days of sustained hypocapnia, the plasma bicarbonate concentration falls further due to a suppression of renal net acid excretion. Approximately 2–3 days are required after the onset of a given decrement in Pa_{CO_2} before the plasma bicarbonate concentration ceases to fall and a new steady state of acid-base equilibrium supervenes. Studies in experimental animals and humans indicate that each 1 mmHg chronic decrement in Pa_{CO_2} is associated with a fall in the plasma bicarbonate concentration averaging 0.5 mEq/l (13, 17, 18). Evidence suggests that this response is not influenced by the prevailing level of plasma bicarbonate concentration at the onset of hypercapnia. Consequently, the impact of the secondary change in the plasma bicarbonate concentration on the plasma hydrogen ion concentration is critically dependent on the level of the plasma bicarbonate concentration prior to adaptation to hypocapnia (18). In the dog, where the normal level of the plasma bicarbonate concentration is approximately 21 mEq/l, the constant $\Delta[HCO_3^-]/\Delta Pa_{CO_2}$ relationship of 0.5 results in a relatively flat slope for $\Delta[H+]/\Delta Pa_{CO_2}$ of about 0.17 nEq/l (19). In humans, with a normal plasma bicarbonate concentration on the order of 24–25 mEq/l, the same $\Delta[HCO_3^-]/\Delta Pa_{CO_2}$ relationship is translated into a much steeper $\Delta[H^+]/\Delta Pa_{CO_2}$ slope of about 0.5 (13, 18).

ACID-BASE TEMPLATE

Figure 1 shows the full range of anticipated responses (so-called 95% confidence bands) for each of the major acid-base disorders just discussed, as defined by the available empiric observations.

The plasma bicarbonate concentration is plotted on the horizontal axis and Pa_{CO_2} on the vertical axis. The hydrogen ion concentration and pH are plotted in a fan-shaped fashion in the interior of the graph. Acute and chronic respiratory acidosis are plotted in that area of the template displaying elevated Pa_{CO_2} values. Metabolic alkalosis is plotted in the area of the template displaying elevated plasma bicarbonate concentrations. Metabolic acidosis and both acute and chronic respiratory alkalosis are plotted in the lower left-hand portion of the template, both meta-

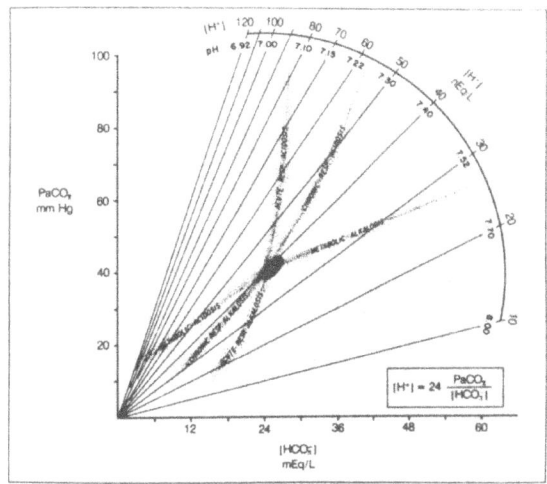

Figure 1. Acid-base template. Ninety-five percent confidence bands for the simple acid-base disorders are represented by the stippled areas. These areas were empirically derived, using the equations in Table 1. From Harrington et al. (4); used with permission of Little, Brown and Company. See text for full discussion of its use.

bolic acidosis and respiratory alkalosis being characterized by hypocapnia and hypobicarbonatemia. The shaded areas roughly outline the 95% confidence bands for the Pa_{CO_2}-bicarbonate relationships for these simple acid-base disorders. The equations used in the preceding discussion have been used to define these confidence bands. It must be emphasized that the relationship between the plasma bicarbonate concentration and Pa_{CO_2} for each of the simple acid-base disorders are derived from empiric data obtained under steady-state conditions. A certain time interval is required for each secondary adaptive response to reach completion or to be eradicated once the initiating, primary disturbance has been corrected. Thus, a mixed acid-base disturbance may be incorrectly diagnosed when only a simple disturbance is present, because insufficient time has elapsed for the secondary response to develop or to resolve.

On the other hand, assuming a steady state is present, a valid set of acid-base data that falls outside any of these confidence bands definitively indicates that a mixed acid-base disorder is present. One, however, should not fall into the trap of assuming that a set of acid-base data that does fall within one of the confidence bands provides conclusive proof that that acid-base disorder is present. Acid-base data falling within the expected range of a simple acid-base disorder are consistent with, but not diagnostic of, the particular disorder. This situation results because the range of physiologic responses for any simple disturbance is wide enough to permit the superimposition of another disturbance without necessarily shifting the acid-base data outside the anticipated boundaries for a simple disorder. Moreover, the simultaneous presence of several acid-base disorders may result in a set of acid-base data that is consistent with a single acid-base disorder. Triple acid-base disorders can result in acid-base data that fall within a single confidence band. For instance, consider a patient with chronic respiratory acidosis (Pa_{CO_2} of 60 mmHg and a plasma bicarbonate concentration of 32 mEq/l) who developed an acute decrement in Pa_{CO_2} (e.g., from intubation) to a level of 44 mmHg, resulting in a plasma bicarbonate concentration of 30 mEq/l. Although, the data would then fit within the metabolic alkalosis confidence band, the patient's acid-base status actually reflects a mixed respiratory acid-base disorder. Thus, the confidence bands should best be utilized as indicating that a given set of acid-base data that fall within a band is *consistent* with, rather than *diagnostic* of, a given acid-base disorder (4).

MIXED ACID-BASE DISORDERS

Mixed metabolic and respiratory acid-base disorders

A variety of mixed acid-base disorders is subsumed under this heading. By definition, such an overall disorder exists whenever there are primary alterations in *both* determinants of plasma acidity, i.e., the plasma bicarbonate concentration (metabolic component) and the Pa_{CO_2} (respiratory component). When the directional change in bicarbonate and Pa_{CO_2} are in opposition, the change in pH will be maximal and vice versa. For instance, with an increase in Pa_{CO_2} (respiratory acidosis) and a decrease in plasma [HCO_3^-] (metabolic acidosis), severe acidemia results. Conversely, with an increase in both Pa_{CO_2} (respiratory acidosis) and in plasma [HCO_2^-] (metabolic alkalosis), there may be little or no change in the blood pH.

The acid-base data of patients with mixed *metabolic and respiratory* acidosis usually reside between the metabolic acidosis and the acute respiratory acidosis bands in the left upper section of the template. Occasionally, however, the data may even track into the area adjacent to the chronic respiratory acidosis band. Throughout this broad area, severe acidemia is found, a direct result of the combination of the simultaneous hypercapnia and hypobicarbonatemia.

The acid-base data of most patients with mixed metabolic and respiratory alkalsosis are found in the broad area occupying the right lower section of the template, directly opposite the region just discussed. Analogous to combined metabolic and respiratory acidosis, the acid-base data in patients with combined metabolic and respiratory alkalosis can approach the chronic respiratory alkalosis band. The most severe instances of alkalemia correspond to this area, a result of the combination of concomitant hypocapnia and hyperbicarbonatemia.

Patients with mixed *metabolic alkalosis and respiratory acidosis* usually have acid-base data that reside between those two bands in the right upper section of the template. This common mixed acid-base disturbance also can result in data that reside near the band of acute respiratory acidosis. The fact that the changes in Pa_{CO_2} and bicarbonate are directionally the same (both increased and therefore offsetting each other's effect on plasma acidity), results in the observation that the pH typically is little changed from normal.

Patients with mixed *metabolic acidosis and respiratory alkalosis* can have data that reside anywhere between the band for metabolic acidosis and that for acute respiratory alkalosis. Similar to mixed metabolic alkalosis and respiratory acidosis, the changes in Pa_{CO_2} and bicarbonate concentration are directionally the same (both decreased in this instance), and hence, again the blood pH is normal or nearly normal. When the independent changes in Pa_{CO_2} and [HCO_3^-] are such that the acid-base coordinates rest between the bands for acute and chronic respiratory alkalosis, a detailed history, and especially knowledge of the clinical setting, are required to distinguish possible mixed metabolic acidosis and respiratory alkalosis from mixed respiratory (acute and chronic) alkalosis.

Mixed respiratory acid-base disturbances

The notion of mixed respiratory acid-base disturbances at first glance appears to be a contradiction in terms. One obviously cannot have simultaneously an elevated (respiratory acidosis) and a depressed (respiratory alkalosis) Pa_{CO_2}. A mixed respiratory disturbance instead refers to the combination of the time-defined phases of acute and chronic respiratory acidosis or alkalosis. For instance, in patients with obstructive lung disease and persistent chronic respiratory acidosis, a superimposed element of acute hypercapnia frequently results from chest infection. In contrast to the relative frequency of mixed acid-base disorders in chronic respiratory acidosis, chronic respiratory alkalosis is less often associated with other acid-base disorders. Such patients, however, can develop a second stimulus to ventilation, resulting in the combination of acute and chronic respiratory alkalosis. For instance, patients with central hyperventilation from a brain tumor can develop a septic complication, resulting in acute hypocapnia superimposed on whatever level of chronic hypocapnia had prevailed. Finally, one frequently does see patients with chronic respiratory acidosis in whom ventilatory support is required. If there is an inordinate reduction in the Pa_{CO_2} to a frankly hypocapnic range, the patient will be left with a still elevated plasma bicarbonate concentration (the original adaptive response to chronic hypercapnia will be somewhat lessened because of an acute buffering effect) and concomitant acute hypocapnia; such an occurrence will markedly shift the patient's pH to the alkaline range.

Elucidation of the nature of such complex acid-base disorders usually requires detailed knowledge of the patient's history and clinical course as well as the use of ancillary laboratory data; mere reliance on the template or any other acid-base road map will be often unrewarding.

Mixed metabolic acid-base disturbances

The acid-base template is of little use in diagnosing the presence of a mixed metabolic acidosis and alkalosis or of mixed metabolic acidoses (e.g., the patient with diabetic ketoacidosis and concomitant lactic acidosis). Full and detailed knowledge of the clinical history, previous acid-base status, and ancillary data [particularly valuable is the pattern and composition of the plasma unmeasured anions (20)] and, most importantly, the clinical setting, are required to unravel such complex metabolic disturbances. Finally, triple acid-base disorders (e.g., the patient with chronic respiratory acidosis who develops hypocapnia subsequent to intubation for ventilatory failure and concomitantly develops lactic acidosis from associated pulmonary sepsis) also must be diagnosed by the history, ancillary data, and, most importantly, the clinical setting.

CLINICAL SETTINGS COMMONLY ASSOCIATED WITH MIXED ACID-BASE DISORDERS

Cardiac arrest

On *a priori* grounds, it is self-evident that cessation of cardiac and pulmonary functions in the nonresuscitated patient leads to lactic acidosis because of tissue hypoxia (21) and acute respiratory acidosis secondary to retention of endogenously produced carbon dioxide (12). In the setting of closed-chest cardiac massage, the situation is, however, more dynamic and complex. Fortunately, good quantitative clinical data are available. Chazan and his colleagues closely analyzed the mixed metabolic and respiratory acidosis of treated cardiac arrest (22). Twenty-two patients were studied and an element of metabolic acidosis was present in almost all patients. Moreover, in a substantial percentage, the metabolic acidosis was compounded by the simultaneous presence of hypercapnia. For the sake of simplicity, these 22 patients with mixed metabolic and respiratory acidosis were subdivided by the authors into eight patients with predominantly metabolic acidosis, ten patients with predominantly respiratory acidosis, and four patients whose classification was uncertain. In those with predominant metabolic acidosis, plasma bicarbonate ranged between 6 and 16 mEq/l, whereas in those ten patients labeled as primarily respiratory acidosis, plasma bicarbonate levels ranged from 16 to 24 mEq/l. The Pa_{CO_2} was lower (17–36 mmHg) in the patients with predominant metabolic acidosis and elevated (62–93 mmHg) in those with predominant respiratory acidosis. Accordingly, the arterial pH was 7.15–7.35 in 5 of the 8 predominant metabolic acidosis patients, but was strikingly lower, 6.86–7.09, in 8 of the 10 patients with severe hypercapnia in addition to hypobicarbonatemia.

Most of the patients with predominant metabolic acidosis had myocardial infarction, although a comparable number of patients with predominant respiratory acidosis also had myocardial infarctions. It was striking that 8 of the 11 patients with substantial hypercapnia and acute respiratory acidosis had major pulmonary problems, including pulmonary edema, aspiration, pneumothorax, and pulmonary hypertension. More than 20 years ago, the astute authors pointed out the ineffectiveness of alkali therapy in those cardiac-arrest patients with predominant respiratory acidosis and the need for careful attention to ventilator therapy, particularly in patients with preexisting pulmonary problems. Further, the authors were prescient in recognizing that the progression of the acidosis in cardiac arrest victims treated with closed-chest message was quite variable. They strongly recommended that alkali therapy should not be based on any static prescription, based on duration from the arrest or the weight of the patient, but rather should be based on serial observations of pH, Pa_{CO_2}, and plasma bicarbonate concentration. Long before other authors had commented on the substantial risks of excess alkali therapy in this setting (e.g., hypernatremia, volume overload, subsequent metabolic alkalosis), these authors recommended the use of only small amounts of sodium bicarbonate and close attention to the details of vigorous passive hyperventilation. The most recent suggestions and recommendations from the American Heart Association's task force on advanced cardiac life support (23), in fact, are broadly consistent with the recommendations of Chazan at al. from some 20 years earlier.

Recently, Weil and his colleagues have pointed out the substantial differences in P_{CO_2} between arterial and mixed venous blood during cardiopulmonary resuscitation (CPR). In 16 patients (who had arterial and pulmonary catheters in place prior to cardiac arrest), arterial blood pH and P_{CO_2} averaged 7.41 and 32 mmHg, respectively, during CPR versus 7.15 and 74 mmHg in mixed venous blood (24). If mixed venous blood more closely reflects the myocardial tissue acid-base status, these data strongly suggest the importance of hypercapnia (respiratory acidosis) as a major contributor to tissue acidemia (especially cardiac), again emphasizing the critical role of adequate ventilation in CPR.

Our own practice is consistent both with that of the American Heart Association's task force and the report of Chazan and his colleagues. Effective external cardiac compression, yielding adequate cardiac output and tissue oxygenation, will hold lactic acidosis in abeyance until cardiac function stabilizes. Effective ventilation can prevent the development of respiratory acidosis in patients whose acid-base values were normal prior to arrest. In patients who have metabolic acidosis or respiratory acidosis prior to the cardiac arrest, however, a more vigorous approach is required. For instance, if the patient is known to have severe metabolic acidosis (plasma bicarbonate < 10–12 mEq/l) prior to the cardiac arrest, more vigorous use of sodium bicarbonate in this setting is not only suggested, but is mandatory. Sufficient bicarbonate should be given to keep the whole blood pH above 7.15 and the plasma bicarbonate concentration above 15 mEq/l or so. Usually one can calculate the amount of bicarbonate required by assuming that administered H_{CO_3} is distributed through an *apparent* space of distribution that is approximately twice the calculated extracellular fluid volume (ECF is ≅ 20% total body weight; thus one needs to multiply total body weight by 40% in order to calculate the apparent space of distribution of bicarbonate). For example, in an 80-kg individual whose plasma [HCO_3^-] is 10 mEq/l, and in whom the goal of therapy is a bicarbonate concentration of 15 mEq/l, the desired increment of 5 mEq/l is multiplied by the 32 l apparent space of distribution (0.4 × 80 kg = 32 l). Thus, 32 × 5, or 160 mEq, of bicarbonate are required. In patients with profound acidosis (plasma [HCO_3^-] < 5 mEq/l), however, the *apparent* space of distribution approaches 100% of body weight (25). The theoretical risk of stimulating lactic acidosis by administering alkali (e.g., as in certain patients with solid tumors) probably does not occur in these patients (21). Given the beneficial effects of alkali therapy in reversing the depressent cardiovascular effects of severe acidemia, we, as well as others, believe judicious alkali therapy is appropriate in this setting (21, 26).

Just as aggressive alkali therapy may be required in the patient with metabolic acidosis prior to cardiac arrest, so the patient with a P_{CO_2} greater than 60 mmHg prior to arrest needs aggressive respiratory therapy and probably intubation to restore effective gas exchange. In the intensive care unit setting, where arrests are more likely to occur, it is mandatory that the physician in charge of the resuscitation team know the most recent acid-base data available *prior* to the cardiac arrest, as well as at frequent intervals throughout the resuscitative effort. The dynamic interaction of a preexisting acid-base disorder with a new acid-base abnormality caused by a catastrophe such as a cardiac arrest is not sufficiently appreciated. Mixed acid-base disturbances are not static "pigeon-holes" into which one can easily fit a patient. Rather the variety of factors that independently affect Pa_{CO_2} and plasma bicarbonate concentration demand analysis on an ongoing basis, especially in the patient undergoing cardiopulmonary resuscitation.

Sepsis

Bacterial sepsis can be associated with several acid-base disturbances, but the interplay of two acid-base disturbances usually predominates. This mixed disorder is composed of lactic acidosis, secondary to shock (8, 12) and respiratory alkalosis as a consequence of sepsis-induced hyperventilation (19, 27, 28). From an acid-base perspective, the lactic acidosis of septic shock appears no different from that of hemodynamic shock, but detailed modern studies are lacking. Elements of both metabolic (lactic) acidosis and respiratory alkalosis are seen in many patients. If a single acid-base disturbance is present, however, it is more likely to be respiratory alkalosis. Several quantitative studies of the acid-base disorders seen in septic patients are available. For instance, Winslow and his colleagues studies 50 patients with bacteremic shock; the Pa_{CO_2} was 30 mmHg or less in 19 of the 30 patients in whom the Pa_{CO_2} was measured (28). Strikingly, 18 of these 19 patients with bacteremic shock *and* a Pa_{CO_2} less than 30 mmHg died. These observations by Winslow and his colleagues are in concert with those by Mazzara, Ayres, and Grace, who, in addition, showed that the death rate in respiratory alkalosis correlated strongly with its severity, rising to near 90% in patients with Pa_{CO_2} levels of 15 mmHg or less (29). Blair studied 30 selected patients with so-called refractory bacteremic shock (27). Twenty-one of the thirty patients had decreased Pa_{CO_2} and in 17, the Pa_{CO_2} was reduced in association with an alkaline blood pH, thus definitively indicating the presence of respiratory alkalosis. In this study pH, Pa_{CO_2}, and bicarbonate were not correlated with outcome, whereas the degree of lactic acid accumulation was (see below). Simmons and his colleagues (30) studied 11 patients with gram-negative bacteremia (proven in six and presumptive in five), but without shock in order to find a clinical sign of the presence of bacteremia. All 11 patients had elevated arterial pH values and depressed Pa_{CO_2} levels; visible hyperventilation was noted in 8 of the 11 patients. Fever, salicylates, cirrhosis, and cerebral lesions were eliminated as the cause of the respiratory alkalosis. Simmons and his colleagues in this seminal paper on the close relationship between sepsis and respiratory alkalosis noted that most of the patients originally were misdiagnosed as simply having pneumonitis.

Hyperventilation in a septic patient thus can be, and is frequently, due to respiratory alkalosis alone. If lactic acidosis ensues, secondary hyperventilation (from the acidemia) will occur and acid-base data are required to determine the nature of the hyperventilation. As stated above, the lactic acidosis of bacteremic sepsis has been much less studied than the respiratory alkalosis. However, it is evident that lactic acidosis will develop whenever there is a substantial degree of tissue hypoxia. In the study by Blair referred to earlier (27), plasma lactate averaged 6.2 mM/l in those patients who died and only 2.8 mM/l in the survivors. Although it was at one time argued that respiratory alkalosis itself leads to progressive lactic acidosis, those early observations have not been documented. Observations by Arbus and his colleagues demonstrated that, even with severe hypocapnia, lactate levels are usually not elevated (16).

The plasma bicarbonate concentration falls in both metabolic acidosis and respiratory alkalosis, the mix of which is seen in septic patients. In this setting, it is thus even more important than usual to know the time course of the respiratory alkalosis in order to determine the reason for the decline in the plasma bicarbonate concentration. In acute respiratory alkalosis, there is little change in the plasma bicarbonate concentration, whereas with sustained hypocapnia, the plasma bicarbonate concentration falls progressively because of a reduction in renal acid excretion (19). In patients with chronic respiratory alkalosis, approximately 50–60% of the fall in the plasma bicarbonate concentration that occurs is offset by an increase in the plasma chloride concentration (due to sodium loss and slight volume contraction), and the remaining 40–50% is offset by an increase in the concentration of unmeasured anions *other* than lactate. Given this slight but definite increase in the anion gap in chronic respiratory alkalosis, and the decline in the plasma bicarbonate concentration in both respiratory alkalosis and metabolic acidosis, one must directly measure lactate levels (and not infer them from a depressed plasma bicarbonate concentration and an elevated anion gap) in order to definitively state that a patient with bacteremic sepsis has both metabolic (lactic) acidosis and respiratory alkalosis.

Therapy of the mixed acid-base disturbance of bacteremic sepsis, whether gram positive or gram negative, centers predominantly on prompt, appropriate antibiotic therapy and vigorous volume repletion. Mortality is clearly related to the speed with which appropriate antibotic therapy is instituted. Even the resolution of the acid-base abnormalities is dependent on therapy of the underlying disease, rather than on therapy directed at acid-base abnormalities per se. Usually no therapy is required for the hypocapnia and respiratory alkalosis, whereas vigorous volume repletion (as well as antibiotics) is indicated in the patient with bacteremic shock. We administer 250–300 cc of normal saline every 15–20 minutes until the blood pressure rises (or central venous pressure rises inordinately). Bacteremic shock has long been known to be characterized by a greatly reduced peripheral vascular resistance and an increased, but inadequate, cardiac output. In our opinion, alkali therapy is rarely needed in these individuals and should be given only in the minority of patients with profound lactic acidosis as a transient measure. Efforts should be directed at raising blood pressure and tissue perfusion, thereby reducing the production of lactic acid. However, if the blood pH falls to less than 7.15, the adverse cardiac consequences of acidema per se argue for its judicious use here, as well as in the patients with lactic acidosis of cardiac arrest (21, 26).

Just as in the cardiac arrest patient, septic shock can occur in patients with a preexisting acid-base disorder. If septic shock is superimposed on a patient with pulmonary failure and preexisting hypercapnia, a triple acid-base disorder can ensue, composed of variable elements of shock-induced lactic acidosis (causing a fall in plasma bicarbonate and a rise in the anion gap), chronic respiratory acidosis (and its attendent, adaptive rise in the plasma bicarbonate concentration), and a new, sepsis-induced respiratory alkalosis (the superimposed fall in Pa_{CO_2}). Analysis of such a complex acid-base disorder requires detailed knowledge of the patient's clinical course and serial acid-base measurements.

Drug intoxications

ALCOHOL

Even in the era of the AIDS epidemic, alcohol abuse remains one of the major public health problems currently afflicting this country and the rest of the world. Given the high use and abuse of alcohol, and its profound metabolic consequences, it is not surprising that alcohol is one of the major causes of mixed acid-base disturbances. In fact, in our own experience, alcohol is the single most common cause of triple acid-base disturbances. The classic triple acid-base disturbance of the alcoholic is composed of metabolic alkalosis (from vomiting), lactic acidosis (from severe volume depletion, hypotension, and alcohol per se), and acute respiratory alkalosis (from sepsis, hypotension, hepatic failure, and the anxiety of the withdrawal syndrome). Much more commonly than this triple acid-base disturbance, however, alcoholic patients suffer from a combination of two acid-base disorders, mixed metabolic acidosis and metabolic alkalosis. The resultant pH can be either frankly acidemic (31) or alkalemic (32). The vomiting frequently seen in alcoholics gives rise to loss of hydrogen ion from the body and produces hypericarbonatemia. If the same alcoholic is unfortunate enough to suffer from concomitant alcohol-induced acidosis, the elevated plasma bicarbonate level, in effect, is back-titrated to normal, or even to below-normal values. The acid-base laboratory clue to the diagnosis of mixed metabolic acidosis and the metabolic alkalosis of alcoholism is the finding of an anion gap that is elevated to a greater degree than that calculated from the observed alteration in the plasma bicarbonate concentration. The anion gap should be calculated whenever an acid-base disorder is suspected, but it is absolutely essential to the diagnosis of mixed metabolic acidosis and alkalosis. Often, the plasma bicarbonate concentration may be perfectly normal, but the finding of an elevated anion gap in the range of 25–30 mEq/l points to the presence of a "hidden" metabolic alkalosis masked by the simultaneous presence of alcohol-induced acidosis.

Halperin and his colleagues have reviewed their experience with metabolic acidosis in the alcoholic and have demonstrated conclusively that it is a mixed metabolic acidosis (31). The authors carefully examined 13 episodes of acidosis in ten patients with alcoholic acidosis. In 9 of the 13 episodes, the patients were also markedly volume contracted. Plasma sodium and potassium concentrations were normal and the plasma glucose ranged from 28 to 235 mg/dl, averaging 134 ± 22 mg/dl. The mean blood pH was 7.29 and the mean bicarbonate concentration was 13 mEq/l; the mean anion gap was elevated at 34 mEq/l. Lactate levels averaged 7 mEq/l, comparable to those noted in previous studies (32, 33). The mean β-hydroxybutyrate level was 2 mEq/l, substantially less than that reported in previous studies (32–34), while acetate levels were minimally elevated at 2 mEq/l. As stressed by these investigators (31), the severity of alcoholic ketoacidosis (β-hydroxybutyric acidosis) is enhanced if patients are both starved and metabolizing alcohol. In all 13 episodes reported, protracted vomiting had led to cessation of alcohol intake prior to admission. It seems likely, therefore, that cessation of alcohol intake in these patients contributed to the lower β-hydroxybutyrate level than that previously noted. Clearly, however, in the individual alcoholic patient with mixed metabolic acidosis, the decline in plasma bicarbonate results from additive effects of lactic acidosis, β-hydroxybutyric acidosis, and acetic acidosis.

Treatment of alcoholic acidosis requires attention to all of the patient's medical problems (35). In regard to the fluid and electrolyte problems per se, prompt correction of volume depletion (with normal saline) demands priority. Most patients also are potassium depleted, despite normokalemia at admission, and require potassium repletion, either as potassim chloride or perhaps as potassium phosphate [given the likelihood that these patients are often phosphate depleted as well (36)]. We administer 30–40 mEq/l and 80–120 mEq/day for the first 2 days or so of hospitalization. There is little need for exogenous insulin in these patients, but sufficient glucose (as D5NS) must be administered to prevent hypoglycememia (35). Many of these patients have no hepatic glycogen stores because of little oral intake (other than alcohol) in the several days before appearing in the hospital emergency room. With restitution of extracellular fluid volume and provision of glucose, rapid recovery from alcohol-induced acidosis occurs, so that most patients have virtually normal electrolytes within 24 hours after admission. Indeed, in the study by Halperin and his coleagues, the plasma bicarbonate concentration, which was 13 mEq/l on admission, had risen to 21 mEq/l within just 5–6 hours after admission, and without exogenous alkali therapy (31).

In the alcoholic patient with a triple acid-base disturbance (i.e., metabolic alkalosis from vomiting, alcohol-induced lactic acidosis, and sepsis-induced acute respiratory alkalosis), considerable attention must be focused at the outset of therapy on the reason for, and the treatment of, sepsis. Concomitantly, volume depletion must be rapidly corrected (see section on sepsis). In any alcoholic patient in whom the P_{CO_2} is substantially reduced, one needs to look for evidence of hepatic insufficiency (a common cause of respiratory alkalosis) and evidence of other drug ingestion (e.g., salicylates). Rarely, alcoholics also suffer from a mixed metabolic acidosis because of simultaneous ingestion of ethyl alcohol and either methyl alcohol or ethylene glycol (8). Toxicologic analysis of blood and urine, as well as a detailed history, usually leads to this diagnosis. Finally, alcoholics frequently develop severe alkalemia secondary to a mixed respiratory alkalosis and metabolic alkalosis (from protracted vomiting). Use of H_2 blockers to reduce further gastric-acid loss is indicated, as well as standard therapy of gastric alkalosis, i.e., correction of the chloride, sodium, and potassium deficits (9). We administer 150–250 cc/hr of normal saline (with 40 mEq/l of potassium) until the volume depletion and alkalosis are corrected.

SALICYLATES

Just as with alcohol, acute and chronic salicylate intoxication remain important public health problems. The ubiquity of the use of aspirin in American society and its persistent usage in suicide attempts make knowledge of its acid-base effects mandatory. Salicylates affect the acid-base balance clinically by at least two independent mechanisms: a) salicylates increase endogenous acid production and b) they increase alveolar ventilation. In regard to the increase in endogenous acid production, it is striking that children under the age of 4 years are at much greater risk than older children or adults for metabolic acidosis from salicylate intoxication. The anion gap is increased in the salicylate-induced metabolic acidosis of infancy and early childhood, but the relative role of the various organic acids has not yet been totally deciphered. The plasma salicylate levels are rarely greater than 3–5mM/l, however, even when the anion gap is substantially greater.

In regard to the effect of salicylates on P_{CO_2}, the increase in alveolar ventilation clinically almost always overrides the pathophysiologic effect of salicylate on uncoupling oxidative phosphorylation, which increases carbon dioxide production. The increased alveolar ventilation is a direct effect of salicylates on the CNS respiratory center. Given the lesser likelihood of developing metabolic acidosis in adults, salicylates can produce pure respiratory alkalosis in adults, but mixed respiratory alkalosis and metabolic acidosis is seen frequently. In one study, more than 50% of adults had a mixed respiratory alkalosis and an anion-gap-type metabolic acidosis (37). Indeed, in the absence of other causes of this mixed acid-base disorder, the finding of mixed metabolic acidosis and respiratory alkalosis should suggest salicylate intoxication (8). In one series, nearly 30% of patients were not diagnosed until 72 hours after admission to the hospital (37). In contrast to the low mortality rate of patients with known overdosage, the mortality rate was 25% in those in whom the diagnosis was overlooked for the first 3 days of hospitalization. In children under the age of 4, the final acid-base equilibrium is determined by the cumulative effects of salicylates on P_{CO_2} (producing respiratory alkalosis) and the effect of salicylates in increasing endogenous acid production (producing metabolic acidosis). As pointed out by Gabow, the degree to which the anion gap is elevated can be helpful in identifying the cause of unexplained metabolic acidosis (20). Patients with salicylate-induced metabolic acidosis commonly have anion gaps of 17–19 mEq/l. Levels substantially higher than that, even in the patient with known salicylate intoxication, should suggest either concomitant lactic acidosis or ingestion of another toxin such as ethylene glycol or methanol (20).

Treatment of mixed respiratory alkalosis and metabolic acidosis of salicylate intoxication centers on elimination of salicylates from the body. Treatment with alkali has the potential advantage of directly treating the acidosis and, by causing an alkaline diuresis, facilitating the excretion of salicylates (8). Given the likelihood that hypocapnia will persist after recovery from acidosis, treatment with alkali poses both theoretical and real problems, but only if excess alkali is given. In one study of 50 patients treated with IV D5 ½ (or ¼) normal saline (supplemented with sodium bicarbonate and potassium chloride), on average, approximately 5 l of fluid, 200 mEq of sodium bicarbonate, and 125 mEq of potassium chloride were given with overall good results. However, substantial alkalemia (pH > 7.55) did occur in 15 patients, hypokalemia (< 3.2 mEq/l) occurred in 15 patients, and pulmonary edema was seen in three elderly patients, emphasizing the risks inherent in a regimen deliberately designed to produce an alkaline diuresis (37). Close patient monitoring, both clinically and biochemically, is thus required in these patients to achieve the desired good effect (prompt reduction in plasma salicylate level) without causing significant adverse effects.

SEDATIVE OVERDOSE

Overdosage with sedatives, including opiates and barbiturates, in the past has resulted in a high frequency of depression of the respiratory center and acute respiratory acidosis in patients attempting suicide. The more widespread use of benzodiazepines rather than barbiturates has reduced the incidence of barbiturate-associated respiratory acidosis, but combined overdosage (usually as suicide attempts or suicide gestures) of several central psychoactive agents still do frequently result in respiratory depression and respiratory acidosis. Overdose of a variety of narcotic agents (e.g., heroine, methadone, morphine, etc.) also can lead to noncardiogenic pulmonary edema, thereby worsening the hypercapnia and accompanying hypoxemia. Patients with sedative-induced respiratory acidosis are at risk of developing a mixed acid-base disturbance for two major reasons. First, the frequent accompaniment of hemodynamic instability and overt hemodynamic shock makes lactic acidosis a common superimposed problem. Secondly, in a patient who attempts suicide by taking multiple medications, vomiting frequently occurs prior to coming into the hospital or gastric lavage with drainage of gastric contents is induced in hospital emergency rooms [in an appropriate attempt to remove the offending agent(s)]; both of these scenarios can lead to metabolic alkalosis. The more dangerous of these complicating acid-base disturbances is obviously lactic acidosis. In a patient with hypercapnia, even a mild fall in the plasma bicarbonate concentration quickly leads to lethal levels of acidemia. Treatment of such patients demands careful attention to their ventilatory status and prompt intubation to manage both hypercapnia and hypoxemia. Volume restitution should be carried out vigorously in the emergency room, using 250–300 ml of normal saline every 15 minutes until adequate blood pressure and tissue perfusion are obtained. Alkali should be reserved for those patients whose pH falls to less than 7.15; it is clearly a temporal measure while intubation is being carried out. Intubation and subsequent mechanical ventilation will rapidly reduce Pa_{CO_2} and thus will rapidly raise blood pH. In the patient who has noncardiogenic pulmonary edema from drug overdose, mechanical ventilation with positive pressure breathing is mandatory and sodium bicarbonate is contraindicated in this setting.

Organ Failure

RENAL FAILURE

Patients with profound renal insufficiency have difficulty in excreting their daily endogenous acid load. As a consequence, there is a gradual fall in the plasma bicarbonate concentration. Early in the course of chronic renal failure, the slight decline in the plasma bicarbonate concentration is offset by a rise in the chloride concentration. Thus a hyperchloremic metabolic acidosis is characteristic of early renal insufficiency (8, 38). As renal function further deteriorates, sulfate, phosphate, and various organic anions are retained, leading to a rise in the anion gap that parallels the further decline in the plasma bicarbonate concentration. In the steady state, the acid-base data in these patients thus are characterized by a mild-to-moderate depression of the plasma bicarbonate concentration, a mild-to-moderate reduction in pH, and an appropriate reduction of Pa_{CO_2} (38). Patients with advanced renal failure often develop superimposed illnesses and thus a variety of mixed acid-base disturbances. The patient with preexisting metabolic acidosis who develops respiratory insufficiency for any reason is in particular danger of severe acidosis because of the combined metabolic and respiratory acidosis. Prior to any needed surgical procedures, azotemic patients should be well dialyzed to bring their plasma bicarbonate concentration to > 20 mEq/l.

Two other acid-base disturbances are frequently superimposed on uremic acidosis, metabolic alkalosis and respiratory alkalosis. In the first instance, the plasma bicarbonate concentration can rise to normal or even above normal, depending on the magnitude of the alkali added or the gastric acid lost. The uremic patient chronically is more at risk from metabolic alkalosis than are normals because of an absolute reduction in the ability to excrete administered bicarbonate because of the profound decline in the glomerular filtration rate. In one study, 3 mEq/kg of oral $NaHCO_3$ in salt-restricted uremic patients raised the mean plasma bicarbonate concentration from 19 to 30 mEq/l in just 4 days (39).

While uremic patients can develop metabolic alkalosis for any of the usual reasons, it is most often due to vomiting and the loss of acid gastric juice. Interestingly, they also are at risk of developing superimposed metabolic alkalosis for reasons unique to the uremic patient; it has been well demonstrated that the administration of either neutral phosphate or cation-exchange resins will make usually nonreasonable antacids (e.g., aluminum hydroxide, magnesium hydroxide) absorbable (40). Phosphate and the cation-exchange resins bind magnesium and aluminum, making them unavailable for the formation of insoluble carbonate salts, thereby allowing absorption of the so-called non-absorbable alkali (in turn, producing a rise in the plasma bicarbonate concentration). In one uremic patient so treated, the bicarbonate concentration rose to 44 mEq/l and seizures resulted from the severe alkalosis (41). Usually, no acute treatment is required for this acid-base disturbance per se because its magnitude is modest. Attention should be directed at the cause and treatment of the metabolic alkalosis. In the rare patient with severe hyperbicarbonatemia, dialysis against a low-bicarbonate dialysate is indicated.

The second disturbance, respiratory alkalosis, may be difficult to detect because the uremic patient typically has a low plasma bicarbonate concentration and a depressed

Pa_{CO_2} (as the adaptive response of metabolic acidosis). Thus, the possibility of respiratory alkalosis (often due to sepsis because of the frail condition of many of these patients) should be considered in any uremic individual in whom the respiratory rate rises, coupled within evidence of hemodynamic instability. These patients need to be rigorously evaluated both from an acid-base and from an infectious disease standpoint.

RESPIRATORY FAILURE

Patients with chronic obstructive pulmonary disease (COPD) and CO_2 retention, as well as patients with acute obstructive disease (e.g., status asthmaticus), obviously have respiratory acidosis as their initial acid-base disturbance. Such patients need to be carefully monitored for alterations in the metabolic component of the acid-base equation because they are at particular danger of hypoxia-induced lactic acidosis. Indeed, acute respiratory acidosis and lactic acidosis comprise one of the more common mixed acid-base disturbances. In such a setting, the rapid decline in plasma bicarbonate concentration that would ensue (if lactic acidosis occurred), when coupled with the prevailing hypercapnia, can rapidly lead to severe and lethal acidemia (4).

In addition to lactic acidosis, patients with elevated Pa_{CO_2} values are frequently sick enough to have concomitant vomiting and metabolic alkalosis. Diuretics frequently are used in the patient with cor pulmonale, thus often resulting in the common mixed disturbance of respiratory acidosis and metabolic alkalosis. Metabolic alkalosis can be perpetuated during resolution of the hypercapnia in these patients (or indeed even in patients in whom the rise in plasma bicarbonate was appropriate for the rise in Pa_{CO_2}) by rigid salt restriction, thus resulting in the entity of posthypercapnic metabolic alkalosis. Treatment with potassium chloride (40–80 mEq/day), or rarely oral NH_4Cl, 1–3 g ($\cong$ 8 mEq of hydrogen ion/g) qid with meals to lessen the chance of gastric irritation is indicated. NH_4Cl should not be given to patients with severe hepatic or renal insufficiency. Lastly, COPD patients can develop such severe respiratory insufficiency that intubation and mechanical ventilation is required. In this setting, the patient's whole blood pH can suddenly swing wildly from severe acidemia to severe alkalemia, due to combined hypocapnia and a persistently elevated plasma bicarbonate concentration. Careful attention to the depth and rate of ventilatory support must be observed in order to prevent severe alkalemia. Alkalemia is particularly a problem in the patient with preexisting metabolic alkalosis and obviously much less of a problem in the patient with preexisting acidosis.

HEPATIC FAILURE

It has been known for many years that patients with hepatic insufficiency are prone to a variety of mixed acid-base disturbances (42). Even in those individuals who have not ingested alcohol as the cause of hepatic insufficiency, mixed-acid base disturbances are common. The most common simple acid-base abnormality is chronic respiratory alkalosis; the etiology remains unclear, but the concentration of ammonia best correlates with the severity of hypocapnia (19). Frequently superimposed on the respiratory alkalosis is metabolic alkalosis, due either to vomiting or to the administration of diuretics. This combined alkalemia can result in pH values above 7.7 (43), causing a metabolic enephalopathy or seizures. One cannot raise the P_{CO_2} in such patients, hence efforts must be directed at lowering the bicarbonate concentration by administration of sufficient chloride, usually as KCl, but if necessary NH_4Cl, as just described in the section on respiratory failure. Given the severity of their liver disease, patients with hepatic failure are also at risk for concomitant lactic acidosis, due either to their original disease, to hemodynamic instability, or to gram-negative sepsis. At one time it was thought that the lactate accumulation seen in patients with hepatic failure and respiratory alkalosis was an appropriate adaptive response, accounting in part for the fall in plasma bicarbonate in respiratory alkalosis. It is now clear that such is not the case and that the rise in lactate levels is due to superimposed lactic acidosis (19). Finally, these patients who frequently have gastrointestinal bleeding are subjected to gastric drainage, which in turn can lead to the loss of acid gastric juice, and thus metabolic alkalosis. The frequent use of H_2 blockers has made this less of a problem than in the past, but it is still a common clinical problem.

REFERENCES

1. Bia M, Thier SO: Mixed acid-base disturbances: A clinical approach. *Med Clin North Am* 65:347–361, 1981.
2. Narins RG, Emmett M: Simple and mixed acid-base disorders: A practical approach. *Medicine* 59:161–187, 1980.
3. Cohen JJ, Kassirer JP, Gennari FJ, Harrington JT, Madias NE, eds, *Acid-Base*. Little, Brown, Boston, 1982.
4. Harrington JT, Cohen JJ, Kassirer JP: Mixed acid-base disturbances. In: Cohen JJ, JP Kassirer, FJ Gennari, JT Harrington, NE Madias, eds, *Acid-Base*. Little, Brown, Boston, 1982.
5. Schreck DM, Zacharias D, Grunau CFV: Diagnosis of complex acid-base disturbances: Physician performance versus the microcomputer. *Ann Emerg Med* 15:164–170, 1986.
6. Lennon EJ, Lemann J Jr: Defense of hydrogen ion concentration in chronic metabolic acidosis. A new evaluation of an old approach. *Ann Int Med* 65:265–274, 1965.
7. Albert S, Dell RB, Winters RW: Quantitative displacement of acid-base equilibrium in metabolic acidosis. *Ann Int Med* 66:312–322, 1964.
8. Harrington JT, Cohen JJ: Metabolic acidosis. In: JJ Cohen, JP Kassirer, FJ Gennari, Harrington JT, Madias NE, eds, *Acid-Base*. Little, Brown, Boston, 1982.
9. Harrington JT, Kassirer JP: Metabolic alkalosis. In: JJ Cohen, JP Kassirer, FJ Gennari, JT Harrington, NE Madias, eds, *Acid-Base*. Little, Brown, Boston, 1982.

10. Harrington JT: Nephrology Forum: Metabolic alkalosis. *Kidney Int* 26:88–97, 1984.
11. Brackett NC Jr, Cohen JJ, Schwartz WB: Carbon dioxide titration curve of normal man. Effect of increasing degrees of acute hypercapnia on acid-base equilibrium. *N Engl J Med* 272:6–12, 1965.
12. Madias NE, Cohen JJ: Respiratory acidosis. In: JJ Cohen, JP Kassirer, FJ Gennari, JT Harrington, Madias NE, eds, *Acid-Base*. Little, Brown, 1982.
13. Gennari FJ: Respiratory acidosis and alkalosis. In: MH Maxwell, CR Kleeman, RG Narins, eds, *Clinical Disorders of Fluid and Electrolyte Metabolism*. McGraw–Hill, New York, 1987.
14. Madias NE, Wolf CJ, Cohen JJ: Regulation of acid-base equilibrium in chronic hypercapnia. *Kidney Int* 27:538–543, 1985.
15. Brackett NC Jr, Wingo CF, Muren O, Solano JT: Acid-base response to chronic hypercapnia in man. *N Engl J Med* 280:124–130, 1969.
16. Arbus GS, Hebert LA, Levesque PR, Etsten BE, Schwartz WB: Characterization and clinical application of the "significance band" for acute respiratory alkalosis. *N Eng J Med* 280:117–123, 1969.
17. Cohen JJ, Madias NE, Wolf CJ, Schwartz WB: Regulation of acid-base equilibrium in chronic hypocapnia. Evidence that the response of the kidney is not geared to the defense of extracellular [H^+]. *J Clin Invest* 57:1483–1489, 1976.
18. Madias NE, Schwartz WB, Cohen JJ: The maladaptive renal response to secondary hypocapnia during chronic HCl acidosis in the dog. *J Clin Invest* 60:1393–1401, 1977.
19. Gennari FJ, Kassirer JP: Respiratory alkalosis. In: JJ Cohen, JP Kassirer, FJ Gennari, JT Harrington, NE Madias, eds, *Acid-Base*. Little, Brown, Boston, 1982.
20. Gabow PA: Nephrology Forum: Disorders associated with an altered anion gap. *Kidney Int* 27:472–483, 1985.
21. Madias NE: Nephrology Forum: Lactic acidosis. *Kidney Int* 29:752–774, 1986.
22. Chazan JA, Stenson R, Kurland GS: The acidosis of cardiac arrest. *N Engl J Med* 278:360–364, 1968.
23. Standards and guidelines for cardiopulmonary resuscitation (CPR) and emergency cardiac care (ECC). *JAMA* 255:2905–2932, 1986.
24. Weil MH, Rackow EC, Trevino R, Grundler W, Falk JL, Griffel MI: Difference in acid-base state between venous and arterial blood during cardiopulmonary resuscitation. *N Engl J Med* 315:153–156, 1986.
25. Garella S, Dana CL, Chazan JA: Severity of metabolic acidosis as a determinant of bicarbonate requirements. *N Engl J Med* 289:121–126, 1973.
26. Narins RG, Cohen JJ: Bicarbonate therapy for organic acidosis: The case for its continued use. *Ann Int Med* 106:615–618, 1987.
27. Blair E: Acid-base balance in bacteremic shock. *Arch Intern Med* 127:731–739, 1971.
28. Winslow EJ, Loeb HS, Rahimtoola SH, Kamath S, Tunnar RM: Hemodynamic studies and results of therapy in 50 patients with bacteremic shock. *Am J Med* 54:421–432, 1973.
29. Mazzara JT, Ayres SM, Grace WJ: Extreme hypocapnia in the critically ill patient. *Am J Med* 56:450–456, 1974.
30. Simmons DH, Nicoloff J, Guze LB: Hyperventilation and respiratory alkalosis as signs of gram-negative bacteremia. *JAMA* 174:2196–2199, 1960.
31. Halperin ML, Hammeke M, Josse RG, Jungas RL: Metabolic acidosis in the alcoholic: A pathophysiologic approach. *Metabolism* 32:308–315, 1983.
32. Fulop M, Hoberman HD: Alcoholic ketosis. *Diabetes* 24:785–790, 1975.
33. Levy LJ, Duga J, Girgis M, Gordon EE: Ketoacidosis associated with alcoholism in nondiabetic subjects. *Ann Int Med* 78:213–219, 1973.
34. Cooperman MT, Davidoff F, Spark R, Pallotta J: Clinical studies of alcoholic ketoacidosis. *Diabetes* 23:433–439, 1974.
35. Cahill GF Jr: Nephrology Forum: Ketosis, *Kidney Int* 20:416–425, 1981.
36. Ritz E: Nephrology Forum: Acute hypophophatemia. *Kidney Int* 22:84–94, 1982.
37. Anderson RJ, Potts DE, Gabow PA, Rumack BH, Schrier RW: Unrecognized adult salicylate intoxication. *Ann Int Med* 85:745–748, 1976.
38. Widmer B, Gerhardt RE, Harrington JT, Cohen JJ: Serum electrolyte and acid-base composition: The influence of graded degrees of chronic renal failure. *Arch Intern Med* 139:1099–1102, 1979.
39. Husted FC, Nolph KD, Maher JF: $NaHCO_3$ and NaCl tolerance in chronic renal failure. *J Clin Invest* 56:414–419, 1975.
40. Madias NE, Levey AS: Metabolic alkalosis due to absorption of "nonreabsorbable" antacids. *Am J Med* 74:155–158, 1983.
41. Ziessman HA: Alkalosis and seizure due to a cation-exchange resin and magnesium hydroxide. *South Med J* 69:497–499, 1976.
42. Zieve L: Pathogenesis of hepatic coma. *Arch Intern Med* 118:211–223, 1966.
43. Cohen JJ, Kassirer JP: Illustrative cases. In: JJ Cohen, JP Kassirer, FJ Gennari, JT Harrington, NE Madias, eds, *Acid-Base*. Little, Brown, Boston, Chapter 15 (patient 21), 1982.

CHAPTER 15

Fluid and Electrolyte Abnormalities in Children

ADRIAN SPITZER & RICHARD NEIBERGER

INTRODUCTION

A physician caring for children is faced with the challenge of evaluating and treating fluid and electrolyte disturbances in patients that range from a 900-g premature infant with dehydration from evaporative water loss secondary to phototherapy to a 100-kg high-school football tackle with dehydration sustained during practice in the hot summer months. The mechanism of dehydration is similar; the goal of therapy is similar; however, the quantities of water and electrolytes necessary to correct the imbalance are dramatically different, even when expressed per unit of body weight.

The incidence of fluid and electrolyte disturbances is higher in infants and children than in adults, and their effects are compounded by a number of characteristics that make fluid and electrolyte balance precarious. These are: a) a high ratio of body surface area to body weight b) a high basal metabolic rate, c) a rapid turnover of body fluids, d) a high body water content, and e) immaturity of discrete renal functions.

The ratio of body surface area (BSA) to body weight (BW) ranges from $0.043\,m^2/kg$ BW in a term newborn to $0.025\,m^2/kg$ BW in the average 70 kg adult. The relatively high BSA/BW ratio prevailing in the infant and the young child promotes conductive and convective water losses. The basal calorie requirement is about 55 kcal/kg/24 hours in infancy as compared to 25–30 kcal/kg/24 hours at maturity. Dissipation of the relatively large amount of energy generated by metabolic processes and the excretion of the metabolic waste products requires large amounts of water.

Differences in body composition between children and adults

The percent of BW comprised of water decreases with age (Figure 1). Total body water (TBW) represents ~80% of BW at birth, ~70% at 6 months, and ~60% at 1 year of age. The intracellular fluid represents only ~30% of BW at birth and increases to 45% by 3 years. The extracellular water volume, on the other hand, decreases from 45% of BW at birth to 30% at 6 months and to 25% at 1 year.

Subsequently, TBW and intracellular water increase while extracellular water decreases until around the age of 4 years, when values similar to those encountered in adults are reached: TBW at 65–70%, extracellular water at 20–25%, and intracellular water at 45–50% of BW.

The composition of intracellular fluid is thought to be similar in infants and adults, although no direct measurements have been made using modern methods of investigation (e.g., ion-specific electrodes, neutron activation, NMR). The composition of extracellular fluid differs from that in adults in two notable aspects. First, in the newborn, serum potassium is higher (4.5–6.5 mEq/l) than in the adult (3.5–5.5 mEq/l). Second, serum bicarbonate is lower in the newborn (18–22 mEq/l in full-term babies and 14–18 mEq/l in premature infants) than in the adult (22–26 mEq/l). Both serum potassium and serum bicarbonate concentrations reach adult values by 6 months of age.

Differences in renal function between children and adults

GLOMERULAR FILTRATION RATE

Filtration of fluid through the glomerular capillary begins in the fetus during the first trimester of gestation. Functional kidneys are not essential to fetal development, as demonstrated by the fact that bilateral renal agenesis is not associated with phenotypic abnormalities; however, urine contributes to the formation of amniotic fluid, which protects the fetus against mechanical injuries and is necessary for the development of the lung. The 25-fold increase in the absolute rate of glomerular filtration that occurs during maturation (Tables 1 and 2) is due predominantly to changes in the glomerular capillary surface area and, to a lesser degree, to increases in the glomerular filtration pressure. There is little if any change in the permeability characteristics of the glomerular capillary membrane.

URINE CONCENTRATION AND DILUTION

Following 12–14 hours of water deprivation, neonates are unable to concentrate their urine above 600–700 mOsm/kg H_2O. The limited concentrating ability is due both to morphologic and functional factors. Among the former is

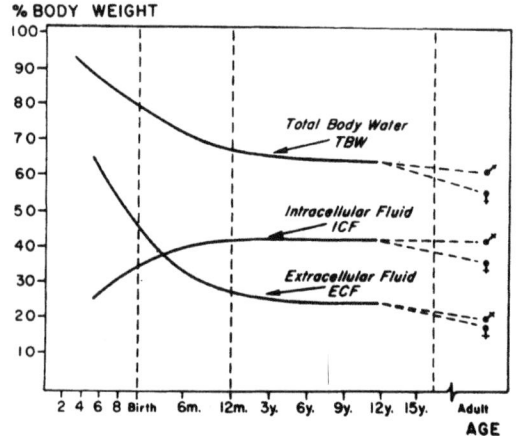

Figure 1. Total body water, intracellular fluid, and extracellular fluid as a function of age. From Winters RW (4).

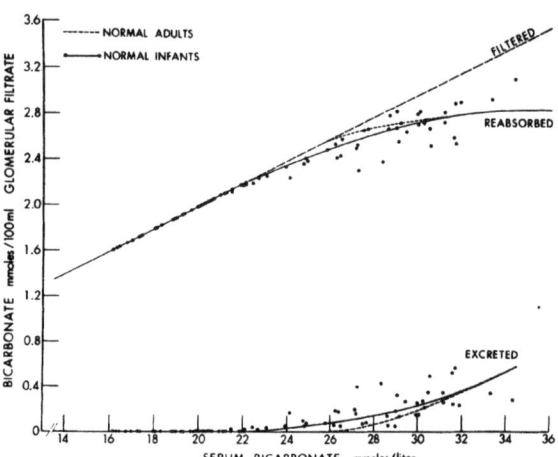

Figure 2. Filtered, reabsorbed and excreted bicarbonate in infants and adults. Note the lower threshold in infants. From Edelmann CM (7).

Table 1. Glomerular filtration rates (ml/min/1.73 m^2) in premature infants

Gestational age Weeks	Postnatal age 1	2–8	>8
25–28	11.0 ± 5.4	15.5 ± 6.2	47.4 ± 21.5
29–34	15.3 ± 5.6	28.7 ± 13.8	54.4

From Schwartz GJ (5).

Table 2. Glomerular filtration rates (ml/min/1.73 m^2) in full-term infants and children

Age	GFR
2–8 days	39 (17–60)*
4–28 days	47 (26–68)
37–95 days	58 (30–86)
1–6 months	77 (39–114)
6–12 months	103 (49–157)
12–19 months	127 (62–191)
2–12 years	127 (89–165)

* Mean (range)
From Goldsmith DI (8).

Table 3. Hydrogen ion excretion in children

Age (years)	<1	1–15
Urine pH	<5.0	<5.5
Titratable acid	62	52
(μEq/min/1.73 m^2)	(43–111)	(33–71)
Ammonium	57	73
(μEq/min/1.73 m^2)	(42–79)	(46–100)

From Edelmann CM, et al. (7).

REABSORPTION OF BICARBONATE AND EXCRETION OF HYDROGEN IONS

As already indicated (Figure 2), newborns and infants maintain a lower serum bicarbonate concentration than adults due to a lower renal threshold for bicarbonate (18–22 mEq/l). In addition, the ability to acidify the urine is limited, due mainly to low excretion of urinary buffers, while hydrogen ion production per kilogram body weight is twofold greater in the infant than in the adult (Table 3).

DISORDERS OF WATER VOLUME

The volume and osmolality of the extracellular fluid are tightly regulated by processes modulating the intake, absorption, and excretion of NaCl and water. Often, fluid and electrolyte disturbances are classified in terms of osmolality (hypertonic, isotoic, and hypotonic). Except for a few circumstances (Table 4), serum tonicity is determined by the concentration of sodium (Table 5). In clinical practice, disorders of sodium and water are so closely related that the two are approached simultaneously. However, for didactic purposes it is important to address first

the shortness of the loops of Henle; among the latter are the relative inability to reabsorb NaCl in excess of water in the ascending limb of Henle's loop and, possibly, the hyporesponsiveness of the collecting duct to vasopressin. Adult levels of urine concentration are attained by 6–12 months of age.

Newborns are able to lower urinary osmolality to 40–50 mOsm/kg H$_2$O. However, the low GFR limits their ability to excrete a water load as expeditiously as adults.

Table 4. Osmotically active substances potentially present in the blood of infants or children

Glucose	Alcohols
Mannitol	Ethylene glycol
X-ray contrast material	Glycine
Urea	

Table 5. Frequency of various types of dehydration among infants and children

Type	Plasma Na (mEq/l)	Frequency
Isotonic	130–150	60%
Hypotonic	< 130	15%
Hypertonic	> 150	25%

Table 6. Causes of hypovolemia in infants and children

Skin losses
  High ambient temperature
  Fever
Respiratory losses
  Sustained hyperventilation
  Salicylate intoxication
Gastrointestinal losses
  Vomiting
  Diarrhea
  Enteric drainage
Urinary losses
  Diabetes mellitus
  Concentrating defects
  Diabetes insipidus
  Mineralocorticoid deficiency
Diuretic therapy

the issues related to fluid volume and then those concerning fluid composition.

Hypovolemia

Dehydration is by far the most common disturbance encountered in children. The gastrointestinal tract, kidneys, lungs, and skin are the four pathways by which water and electrolytes are lost from the body. The major causes of hypovolemia in infants and children are listed on Table 6. In moderate diarrhea (8–12 stools per 24 hours), an infant loses about 35 ml water/kg BW per 24 hours; in severe cases (12–20 stools per 24 hours) loss can approach 75 ml/kg per 24 hours. The amount of total fluid lost with vomiting or diarrhea may be as high as 6 liters per day in a 10-year-old, 30 kg child. Renal losses may also reach several liters per day in conditions such as diabetes mellitus, diabetes insipidus, or obstructive nephropathy. Respiratory water loss may amount to 1–2 liters per day in large children with severe tachypnea. Sweat loss can go up to 800 ml per day in infants and up to 4 liters per day in a 10-year-old, 30 kg child. Losses of this magnitude quickly produce dehydration if not replaced. The rate of sweating varies with the body temperature and is controlled in part by the autonomic nervous system.

The first aim of the diagnostic process is to establish the severity of dehydration (Table 7). Important elements of history are: age, mechanism of dehydration (e.g., vomiting vs. diarrhea, etc.), nature of the primary disease (renal, cardiac, or respiratory), and estimation of the amount of fluid intake, and of urinary and gastrointestinal losses during the past few days. The physical examination allows one to assess: weight (assume an acute weight loss to represent water), sensorium (increasing stupor with worsening dehydration), skin turgor (decreases with increasing degrees of dehydration), humidity of mucous membranes, resistance of the anterior fontanel and of the eyeballs, and respiratory and heart rates. Among laboratory data of help are: the serum creatinine and urea concentrations (a rise is due mainly to a fall in GFR rather than to the loss of water per se) and the specific gravity or osmolality of the urine (in dehydrated patients with normal kidneys, the urine should be maximally concentrated).

An increase in heart rate, associated with a decrease in blood pressure and with stupor, is indicative of shock. An intravenous line should be placed immediately and an

Table 7. Guide to estimating water deficits

Degree of dehydration	Weight loss (%)	Sensorium	Skin turgor	Mucous membranes	Anterior fontanel	Eyeballs	Respiratory rate	Heart rate	Blood pressure	Urine volume
Mild	3–5	Normal	Normal or decreased	Usually normal	Normal	Normal	Normal	Normal	Normal	Normal
Moderate	6–10	Lethargic	Decreased	Slightly dry	Depressed	Slightly sunken	Increased	Increased	Normal	Decreased
Severe	11–15	Semicomatose	Decreased	Dry	Sunken	Sunken	Increased	Increased	Normal or decreased	Decreased
Extreme	15	Comatose	Markedly decreased	Very dry	Clearly visible, no pulsations	"Hollow-eyed"	Increased	Increased	Decreased	Markedly decreased

From Finbeg L (9).

isotonic solution such as plasma, 5% albumin, Ringer's lactate, or normal saline should be administered in an amount of 20 cc/kg BW over a 15-minute period. This treatment should be repeated until a normal pulse and blood pressure are reestablished. Then, or in patients with lesser degrees of dehydration at the outset, fluid requirements should be calculated on the basis of a) estimated deficits, b) maintenance needs, and c) replacement of continuing abnormal losses. The sum of a, b, and c is equal to the total amount of fluid necessary for treatment. This estimate is based on several assumptions and may have to be modified at short intervals.

An accurately measured acute change in body weight is the single best indicator of the magnitude of the water deficit. Unfortunately, this is rarely available and the degree of dehydration has to be estimated from the physical findings (Table 7). Dehydration is frequently classified as mild (5%), moderate (10%), and severe (15%). The percentage refers to the decrease in body weight. The deficit should be replaced during the first 24 hours of therapy, with one-half the amount being given over the first 8 hours and the other half during the ensuing 16 hours.

Maintenance fluid requirements consist of the amounts of water lost by a normal individual of appropriate size through the skin, lungs, kidneys, and gut. These can be computed on the basis of metabolic rate, body surface area, or weight. Calculating water requirements on the basis of caloric expenditure is somewhat cumbersome, while estimation on the basis of body weight is rather inaccurate. We prefer to estimate maintenance fluid requirements on the basis of body surface area, allowing 1400–1600 ml H_2O per m^2. The average body surface area (BSA) of a 3 kg newborn is $0.2 m^2$; of a 10 kg-infant (about 1 year), $0.5 m^2$; of a 30 kg child (about 10 yrs of age), $1.0 m^2$; of a 60 kg individual, $1.5 m^2$; and of an average 70 kg adult, $1.73 m^2$. While this approach is satisfactory, it should not be forgotten that maintenance requirements reflect the amounts of water utilized for temperature regulation (insensible water loss), solute homeostasis (urinary loss), and elimination of solid waste (gastrointestinal loss). Each of these components may change with the conditions prevailing during treatment. For example, insensible water loss may decrease to zero when the infant is placed in an atmosphere saturated with water, as is the case in an incubator, or it may increase when the ambient temperature is high.

Continuing abnormal losses can be estimated or in many cases measured directly. They occur through normal routes (skin, kidney, intestine) or through abnormal routes (fistula, drainage). Increases in water expenditure associated with increases in the metabolic rate are present in fever, hyperthyroidism, and salicylism. The water allowance for increases in body temperature is about 7% of the amount of maintenance fluid for each degree above 38°C. Other hypermetabolic states (burns, heat stroke, respiratory infection) many increase water losses by as much as 75%. On the other hand, hypometabolic states (hypothyroidism or cooling) decrease water needs by 10–25%. In conditions characterized by the inability to concentrate the urine, such as renal dysplasia, diabetes insipidus, or hypokalemia, the excretion of a given solute load may obligate a large volume of water. A similar phenomenon occurs in diabetes mellitus, prompted by the presence of high concentrations of glucose in the glomerular filtrate (osmotic diuresis).

Hypervolemia

Volume expansion is consequent to retention of salt and water (Table 8). A sudden increase in weight is probably the single most reliable indicator of fluid retention. For edema to become apparent, the TBW must be expanded by at least 5% (500 ml for a 1-year-old, 10 kg infant or 1500 ml for a 10-year-old, 30 kg child).

In addition to edema, hypervolemia may be associated with ascites, increased respiratory rate, orthopnea, paroxysmal nocturnal dyspnea, and pulmonary edema. In the absence of these signs, the diagnosis of volume expansion is difficult to make. It should be suspected in patients with excess mineralocorticoid activity, inappropriate antidiuretic hormone secretion, and renal failure. Volume excess is best treated by therapy designed to affect the cause (e.g., inotropic drugs in congestive heart failure). In some cases (e.g., hypervolemia of acute glomerulonephritis), fluid restriction in excess of fluid output may be adequate. When this is not sufficient, or as adjunct therapy, diuretics should be considered. In children who have sufficient residual renal function, a daily or twice daily dose of hydrochlorothiazide (2 mg/kg BW per 24 hours PO) or furosemide (1–6 mg/kg BW per 24 hours PO) can be used. If hypokalemia develops, supplemental potassium (1–2 mEq/kg BW per 24 hours PO) should be added to the treatment.

Serious management problems are posed by fluid overload complicating acute renal failure. Children with this complication may require dialysis (hemodialysis or peritoneal) or continuous arteriovenous hemofiltration to achieve fluid removal. If the normal body weight of the child is known, therapy should be designed to return fluid volume to normal (assuming that each milliliter of fluid removed is equivalent to 1 g of body weight).

Also difficult to manage are children with low serum albumin (0.8–1.2 g/dl) secondary to nephrotic syndrome or liver failure. Often these patients accumulate several liters of fluid and respond poorly to treatment with diuretics, in part because enhanced reabsorption of fluid in the proximal tubule results in decreased delivery of salt and water to the distal segments of the nephron, where most of

Table 8. Common causes of water retention in children

Nephrotic syndrome	Heart failure
Protein-losing enteropathy	Renal failure
Cirrhosis	Inappropriate antidiuretic
Malnutrition	hormone secretion

the diuretics act. In such patients, we recommend treatment with a 25% solution of albumin (0.5–1.0 g/kg BW) administered intravenously over 30–60 minutes and furosemide (1–2 mg/kg BW) given by the same route during the last 15 minutes of the albumin infusion. This treatment often produces a brisk diuresis that lasts for 1–2 hours. If necessary, this regimen can be repeated every 8 hours for 1–3 days. The most serious complications of overaggressive fluid removal are related to intravascular volume depletion and circulatory collapse. Permanent loss of renal function has also been reported following prolonged administration of albumin solution. For this reason, we limit the use of albumin/furosemide therapy to hypoalbuminemic children who have congestive heart failure, pulmonary edema, scrotal edema preventing ambulation, or tissue breakdown and do not extend the treatment beyond 3 days.

DISTURBANCES IN BODY FLUID COMPOSITION

Disturbances in fluid composition should be evaluated in a manner similar to those in volume, starting with estimation of the electrolyte deficit and proceeding through maintenance requirements and ongoing losses.

The deficits of sodium and bicarbonate can be calculated from the following formula:

$$(C_d - C_a) \times (\text{vol. distr.} \times BW) = \text{amount required (mEq)},$$

where C_d = concentration desired (mEq/l), C_a = actual concentration (mEq/l), vol. distr. = apparent volume of distribution, and BW = body weight (kg).

The apparent volume of distribution is the volume of body fluid that the electrolyte appears to be dissolved in. It is a virtual volume that does not reflect a specific anatomic structure. For example, in a premature infant in whom extracellular water is 60% of body weight, the volume of distribution for sodium is 0.7, whereas in an adult in whom the extracellular water is 40% of body weight, the apparent volume of distribution for sodium is 0.6. The same values can be used for the apparent volume of distribution of bicarbonate. Alternatively, one can use the amounts of electrolytes derived empirically by Winters (4) for infants with moderate-to-severe degrees of dehydration (Table 9).

The amounts of electrolytes required for maintenance are (mEq/m² BSA per 24 hours): sodium 35–50, potassium 30–40, bicarbonate 10–15, and magnesium 2–4.

The composition of the extrarenal abnormal losses varies with the source (Table 10). As a rule of thumb, losses through the gastrointestinal route can be considered to be half isotonic. Renal losses can be measured in the majority of patients.

Hyponatremia

The most common causes of hyponatremia are vomiting and/or diarrhea followed by replacement of fluid losses with solutions containing little or no sodium. Other reasons that need to be considered are (Table 11): factitious (hyperglycemia, hyperlipidemia, etc.), primary salt loss (salt-losing enteropathy or nephropathy), inappropriate ADH secretion, mineralocorticoid deficiency, cirrhosis of the liver, and congestive heart failure. With the aid of the history, a physical examination, and measurements of electrolytes in serum and urine, it should be possible to identify the mechanism of hyponatremia. Therapy can then be directed at decreasing water intake, increasing water output, or increasing salt intake to bring the serum sodium into the normal range.

In patients with very low serum sodium (100–120 mEq/l) with or without seizures, the serum sodium should be brought rapidly to 125–130 mEq/l. This can be accomplished by giving intravenously a hypertonic sodium chloride solution (3%) over 5–10 minutes. Full correction of the

Table 10. Composition of extrarenal abnormal losses

Fluid	Na⁺	K⁺	Cl⁻	Protein g%
		—mEq/l—		
Gastric	20–80	5–20	100–150	–
Pancreatic	120–140	5–15	90–120	–
Small intestine	100–140	5–15	90–130	–
Bile	120–140	5–15	80–120	–
Ileostomy	45–135	3–15	20–115	–
Diarrheal	10–90	10–80	10–110	–
Sweat				
Normal	10–30	3–10	10–35	–
Cystic fibrosis	50–130	5–25	50–110	–
Burns	140	5	110	3–5

From Winters RW (4).

Table 9. Probable values of water and electrolyte deficits for moderate to severe dehydration in infants

Type of dehydration	Range of plasma [Na⁺] (mEq/l)	Water (ml/kg)	Na⁺ (mEq/kg)	K⁺ (mEq/kg)	Cl⁻ + HCO₃⁻ (mEq/kg)
Isotonic	130–150	100–150	7–11	7–11	14–22
Hypertonic	>150	120–170	2–5	2–5	4–10
Hypotonic	<130	40–80	10–14	10–14	20–28

From Winters RW (4).

Table 11. Differential diagnosis of hyponatremic states

Disorder	Serum osmolality	Urine concentration[a]	Urine sodium[b]	Weight change	Edema	Other
Vomiting, diarrhea	Low	High	< 10 mEq/l	Decrease	No	Dehydration
Hyperglycemia	Normal or high	Variable	Variable	Variable	No	Glucosuria, ketoacidosis
Hyperlipidemia	Normal	Variable	Variable	Variable	No	
Salt-losing nephropathy	Low	High	> 20 mEq/l	Decrease	No	Evidence of renal disease
SIADHS	Low	High	> 20 mEq/l	Increase	No	CNS, pulmonary disease; drugs
Mineralocorticoid deficiency	Low	High	> 20 mEq/l	Decrease	No	Hyperkalemia
Congestive heart failure	Low	High	< 10 mEq/l	Increase	Yes	Evidence of heart disease
Nephrotic syndrome	Low	High	< 10 mEq/l	Increase	Yes	Proteinuria, hypoalbuminemia
Cirrhosis	Low	High	< 10 mEq/l	Increase	Yes	Evidence of liver disease
Acute and chronic renal failure	Low	High	> 20 mEq/l	Increase	Sometimes	Azotemia, oliguria, evidence of renal disease
Diuretic excess	Low	High	> 20 mEq/l	Decrease	No	History of diuretic administration
Chloride loss or deprivation,[c] cystic fibrosis with excess sweating	Low	High	< 10 mEq/l	Decrease	No	Metabolic alkalosis, hypokalemia

[a] In the presence of serum hypoosmolarity, any degree of urine concentration is inappropriate, even when the urine might otherwise be considered dilute. In the conditions listed, the urine osmolality might be considered high, even when it is less than that of plasma.
[b] The lower sodium levels do not apply in patients who are receiving diuretics.
[c] Examples include chloride diarrhea, low chloride formulas.
Note: SIADHS = syndrome of inappropriate ADH secretion. From Gauthier (29).

sodium deficit can be then achieved in 24–48 hours.

Some investigators claim that increase in serum sodium concentration in excess of 0.5 mEq/l per hour may result in pontine demyelination. No evidence supporting this assertion comes from studies done in children.

SYNDROME OF INAPPROPRIATE SECRETION OF ANTIDIURETIC HORMONE

This syndrome, characterized by relatively high sodium excretion in the presence of hyponatremia, is associated with many disease states: meningitis, brain tumors, perinatal asphyxia, head trauma, cystic fibrosis, asthma, pneumonia, tuberculosis, lung tumors, hypothyroidism, and drugs, to mention only a few. The symptoms are generally absent until the serum sodium falls below 120 mEq/l. Then the patient may exhibit anorexia, nausea, vomiting, irritability, confusion, stupor, and convulsions.

The treatment of choice for inappropriate ADH secretion is water restriction until the serum sodium returns to normal. If the serum sodium is below 120 mEq/l when the patient is first evaluated, we recommend to rapidly increase the serum sodium to 125–130 mEq/l to prevent the symptoms of water intoxication. Two drugs that interfere with the renal action of ADH have been used to treat ADH excess. Demeclocycline (1.0–1.2 g per 24 hours) was demonstrated to be effective in adults and in the few children over the age of 9 years in whom it has been used. Tetracyclines are not recommended for children under 8 years because they can produce staining of the definitive teeth. Lithium was also used in adults but not in children.

Hypernatremia

Hypernatremia is defined as a concentration of sodium in serum exceeding 150 mEq/l. In children hypernatremia is mainly produced by: a) administration of replacement solutions containing sodium chloride in concentrations higher than those in the fluids lost and b) addition of salt instead of sugar to baby formula. Mild degrees of hypernatremia can also occur in patients who are unable to form a concentrated urine (e.g., reset hypothalamic osmostat, central and nephrogenic diabetes insipidus).

The aim of the treatment is to return the serum sodium gradually to the normal range. The correction should be slow. As hypertonicity develops, water moves out of brain cells. This acts as a stimulus for the production of idiogenic osmoles (primarily taurine and sorbitol) that prevent further cell shrinkage. Once this adaptation occurs, an acute reduction in plasma osmolality causes cerebral edema, which may lead to seizures and death. Some authors suggest that serum sodium may be corrected by as much as 2 mEq/l per hour. Others, particularly pediatricians, recommend a more cautious approach, aiming for a decrease in serum sodium of 0.5–1 mEq/l per hour. There are no studies comparing the outcomes of these two methods. The sodium content of the solution used for correction of hypernatremia may vary with the conditions, as long as the rate of fall in the serum sodium concentration is not exceeded. In most cases of hypernatremic dehydration, the sodium deficit is relatively small. Correction can be achieved within 48 hours by using a solution of 5% dextrose in water containing 25–75 mEq/l of sodium as chloride or bicarbonate. In severe hypernatremia (serum sodium > 200 mEq/l) peritoneal dialysis may be effective (12). Whenever possible, appropriate steps should also be taken to correct the cause of hypernatremia.

EXAMPLE

The principles of diagnosis and treatment described herein can best be summarized by applying them to a specific case. Let us consider a 12-month-old infant who presented at the emergency room because of vomiting and diarrhea. The mother recounted that the baby was in good health until 2 days before, when he became anorexic, developed a slight fever (37.8°C rectally), vomiting, and diarrhea. She estimated that the child vomited five to six times and passed about ten watery stools per 24 hours. He retained only the tea the mother gave him in small quantities.

The child was born at term with a weight of 3.4 kg and, according to the mother, grew and developed well. She did not know his weight prior to the current illness.

Physical examination revealed an alert but cranky child, in a good state of nutrition. His skin and bucal mucosa were dry, the anterior fontanel was slightly depressed, the turgor was diminished, but the extremities were pink and warm. The heart rate was 110/min, regular, and the BP was 80/50 mmHg. The initial measurement of serum electrolytes revealed (mEq/l): sodium 125, potassium 4.5, chloride 100, and bicarbonate 15.

The clinical and laboratory findings led to the diagnosis of hyponatremic dehydration with metabolic acidosis. The degree of dehydration was estimated to be about 10%. Considering an ideal weight of 10 kg for age, the fluid deficit was estimated to be 1000 ml. The maintenance fluid requirements, based on a surface area of $0.5 m^2$, were 750 ml. The ongoing abnormal losses were estimated to be 300 ml per 24 hours. Thus, the total amount of fluid required for the first 24 hours was 2 liters.

The electrolyte deficits represented the sum of the electrolytes lost with the 1 liters of fluid and those calculated by the formula presented earlier. They were found to amount to 210 mEq of sodium and 45 mEq of bicarbonate. The potassium deficit was too small to justify immediate correction. Maintenance electrolytes were estimated at 20 mEq of sodium, 20 mEq of potassium, and 10 mEq of bicarbonate per 24-hours. The abnormal gastrointestinal losses were estimated to be 10 mEq each of sodium and potassium over a 24-hour period. Chloride was given in an amount equal to that of the cations. Thus, the electrolyte solution required for the treatment of this infant contained (in mEq/l): Na^+, 105; K^+, 15; HCO_3^-, 22.5; Cl^-, 97.5; roughly similar to a ⅔ normal Ringer's solution.

As is the custom, half of the entire amount (in this case 1 liter) was administered during the first 8 hours (~2 cc/min) and the remaining half (1 liter) was infused during the ensuing 16 hours (~1 cc/min).

It should be rather obvious that the calculations are based on a number of assumptions that may or may not be correct. It is, for instance, very likely that the potassium losses were underestimated in this infant due to the acidosis that, by shifting K^+ from the cells in the ECF, has maintained serum K^+ concentration within the normal range. Consequently, the condition of the patient and the serum electrolyte concentrations should be checked at intervals that vary with the severity of the fluid and electrolyte disturbance, but *not* to exceed 6–8 hours. Adjustments in the rate of administration or in the composition of the fluid should be made as necessary. Valuable indicators of the adequacy of therapy are the rate of urine excretion and the urine osmolality. A urine volume of ≥ 2 ml/kg per hour and a urine osmolality of 400–600 mOsm/l usually reflect appropriate therapy.

ORAL REHYDRATION

Orally administered solutions of salt and water were successfully used for the treatment of diarrhea by D.C. Darrow in the late 1940s and early 1950s. The physiologic basis of this treatment remained, however, unknown until the 1960s, when it became apparent that the sodium-glucose cotransport system present in the intestine obligates water absorption, even during diarrheal illness.

The benefits of oral rehydration therapy include: low cost (five to ten dollars per day vs. several hundreds of dollars per day of hospitalization for IV therapy), simplicity of administration, and safety. Complications including hypernatremia, periorbital edema, hypokalemia, and hyponatremia have been reported, but their relationship to therapy was not always clear. Babies with mild degrees of dehydration (10% or less) secondary to diarrheal disease are particularly suited for this form of therapy. The replacement solution, given during the first 2–3 hours of therapy, should contain 74–90 mEq/l of sodium and should be administered in amounts of 40–50 ml/kg BW to infants with < 5% dehydration and up to 100 ml/kg BW to infants with 5–10% dehydration. The maintenance solution should contain 50 mEq/l of sodium given at a rate of 50 ml/kg BW per 24 hours. There are a number of commercially available preparations that fulfill these requirements (Table 12). Vomiting may be a contraindication for

Table 12. Commercially available oral rehydration solutions

Product	Na^+	K^+	Cl^-	Base	Glucose (g/l)
	—mEq/l—				
Rehydration					
WHO oral rehydration salts	90*	20	80	30 (citrate)	20
Pedialyte-RS (Ross)	75	20	65	30 (citrate)	25
Maintenance/prevention					
Infalyte (Pennwalt)	50	20	40	30 (bicarb)	20
Lytren (Mead Johnson)	50	25	45	30 (citrate)	20
Pedialyte (Ross)	45	20	35	30 (citrate)	25
Resol (Wyeth)	50	20	50	34 (citrate)	20

* Concentrations when diluted (one package to 1 liter water).

oral rehydration, although some babies will stop vomiting when given small but frequent (10 ml every 30 minutes) feedings of rehydration solution or other clear liquids (ginger ale, apple juice, etc.).

In areas of the world where diarrheal illness is a leading cause of infant mortality and medical care is scarce, oral fluid and electrolyte therapy has also been used to treat children with more severe forms of dehydration (> 10%). In our country such children should be hospitalized and subjected to standard intravenous therapy.

DISORDERS OF POTASSIUM BALANCE

Hypokalemia

Hypokalemia may be due to: a) a shift of potassium from the serum into cells, b) inadequate intake or c) an abnormal loss of potassium, either through the kidneys or the gastrointestinal tract (Table 13). When extrarenal potassium losses are associated with hypovolemia, stimulation of the renin-angiotensin-aldosterone system often potentiates hypokalemia by increasing the urinary excretion of potassium.

Symptoms of hypokalemia, unlikely until serum potassium falls below 2.5 mEq/l, are generally related to effects on smooth and skeletal muscles. They include weakness, paralysis, and intestinal ileus. Occasionally, polyuria secondary to decreased concentrating capacity may be the initial complaint. In other cases, neurologic disturbances such as lethargy, confusion, and tetany may cause the patient to seek medical help.

Many of the causes of hypokalemia, such as inadequate

Table 13. Causes of hypokalemia in children

I. Shift of potassium into cells
   A. Alkalosis (metabolic, respiratory)
   B. Hypokalemic periodic paralysis
   C. Insulin administration
II. Inadequate potassium intake
III. Abnormal potassium loss
   A. Extrarenal
      1. Gastrointestinal
         a. vomiting
         b. diarrhea
         c. ureterosigmoidostomy
         d. laxative abuse
      2. Skin
         a. excessive sweating
         b. burns
   B. Renal
      1. Diuretics
      2. Diabetic ketoacidosis
      3. Excess mineralocortocoid activity
      4. Bartter syndrome
      5. Renal tubular acidosis
      6. Miscellaneous (Liddle syndrome, magnesium deficiency, amphotericin B)

intake (potassium salts are so abundant in most foods that an infant or child would have to have a very unusual diet to develop hypokalemia on the basis of diet alone), chronic use of diuretic drugs, laxative abuse, uretero-sigmoidostomy, and antibiotic usage can be identified by history. Chronic self-induced vomiting combined with laxative and diuretic abuse has been identified as the cause of severe hypokalemia in several adolescents who used this method for weight-reduction purposes. In the absence of skin, gastrointestinal, or renal potassium losses, hypokalemia is due to redistribution of potassium, usually consequent to systemic alkalosis that drives potassium into the cells. This syndrome requires no potassium supplementation, but rather treatment directed at the cause.

Of special concern is the insulin-dependent diabetic child with ketoacidosis who may lose potassium through the kidneys due to osmotic diuresis while maintaining a normal serum potassium concentration due to shifting of potassium from the cells as a consequence of acidosis. In such a patient, rapid rehydration associated with normalization of acidosis and hyperglycemia may produce rapid potassium uptake by cells and may result in marked hypokalemia. Calculation of water, sodium chloride, and bicarbonate replacement for the child with diabetic ketoacidosis should be approached as previously described. Once it is apparent that renal failure is not present, potassium (30–40 mEq/l) must be added to the infusion fluids. During the first 24 hours of therapy it is often helpful to give half of the potassium with phosphate, as phosphate depletion is almost always present and it may contribute to urinary potassium losses. Once the serum glucose is ≤300 mg/dl, glucose should be added to the infusion fluid. By the second day, the patient can usually be returned to oral intake, which should be rich in sodium chloride, potassium, inorganic phosphate, and water. Frequent monitoring of electrolytes and glucose is necessary until the fluid and electrolyte balance are restored.

The primary cause of hypokalemia secondary to renal loss is often difficult to establish. Narins et al. (11) have proposed an approach that we have found to be quite helpful (Figure 3). Patients are first separated into two groups on the basis of blood pressure. Hypertensive patients with low urinary potassium are likely to have a disorder of the renin-angiotensin-aldosterone system or a defect in the synthesis of mineralocorticoid hormones. Patients with normal blood pressure are first divided into two groups based on the amount of bicarbonate in the blood. Those with a low serum bicarbonate concentration are likely to have renal tubular acidosis. The patients with high serum bicarbonate are subdivided further according to the amount of chloride in the urine. The presence of a low urinary chloride is indicative of extrarenal potassium losses, whereas a high urine chloride points towards a heterogeneous group of conditions that require specific work-up for identification.

In renin-mediated hypertension with hypokalemia secondary to a tumor, removal of the tumor generally solves the problem. Renal artery stenosis may be corrected by angioplasty. Alternatively, the hypertension can

Urine K⁺ loss >0.5 meq/kg per 24 hrs. in euvolemic patient on normal sodium diet

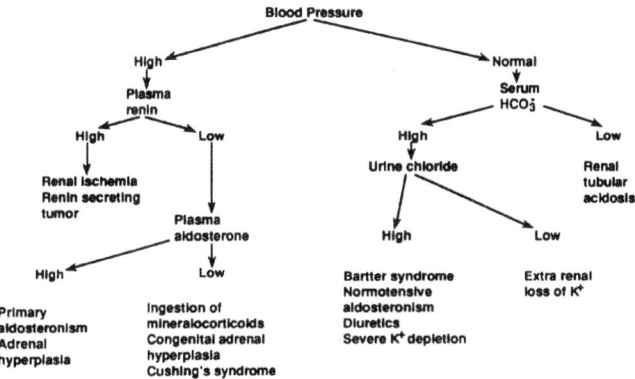

Figure 3. Evaluation of renal potassium loss. (Adapted from Narins et al. (11)].

be treated with captopril (1–6 mg/kg BW per 24 hours PO).

Both adrenal adenoma and adrenocortical hyperplasia are rare in children. Treatment consists of surgical removal of adrenal tissue or supplemental potassium intake and administration of spironolactone (1–3 mg/kg BW per 24 hours PO). If potassium wasting is caused by ingestion of mineralocorticoids or mineralocorticoidlike substances, the offending substance should be stopped.

In patients with normal blood pressure, elevated serum bicarbonate, and low urine chloride, extrarenal potassium loss should be suspected. Causes include persistent vomiting, nasogastric drainage, enteric fistula, etc. The treatment requires a combination of decreasing output, if possible, and increasing potassium intake.

In patients with normal blood pressure, elevated serum bicarbonate, and elevated urine chloride, conditions involving renal potassium wasting (Bartter syndrome, normotensive aldosteronism, diuretic use, renal tubular acidosis, and severe potassium depletion) should be considered. Each of these conditions responds at least partially to potassium supplementation. Some patients with Bartter syndrome have responded to treatment with nonsteroidal antiinflammatory drugs (indomethacin, 2–5 mg/kg BW per 24 hours or ibuprofen, 25 mg/kg BW per 24 hours, given PO), combined with potassium supplementation (2–10 mEq/kg BW per 24 hours).

The two most common diuretics used in children are furosemide and hydrochlorothiazide. Both produce kaliuresis and thus they may produce potassium depletion. This can be corrected by stopping the diuretic, reducing the dose, or increasing K⁺ intake by 2–3 mEq/kg BW per 24 hours, repeating the measurement of serum K⁺ several days later, and adjusting intake as necessary. Finally, a potassium-sparing agent such as spironolactone (1–3 mg/kg/BW per 24 hours) may be added.

In most patients with Type II RTA (proximal renal tubular acidosis), potassium supplementation is not necessary. In Type I RTA (distal renal tubular acidosis), it may be necessary to administer about half the alkali dose (bicarbonate or citrate) as a potassium salt. For instance, if 6 mEq/kg BW per 24 hours of bicarbonate are necessary to prevent acidosis, 3 mEq/kg BW per 24 hours can be given as sodium citrate and the remaining 3 mEq/kg BW per 24 hours as potassium citrate.

The magnitude of the total body potassium loss cannot be estimated accurately from the serum potassium concentration. A 1 mEq/l decrease in serum potassium probably reflects a 5–10% decrease in total body potassium as potassium moves from cells to extracellular fluid to compensate for chronic potassium loss. In patients with potassium depletion, potassium should be supplemented at two to three times the maintenance level (4–6 mEq/kg per 24 hours) until serum concentration is restored to normal.

Hyperkalemia

In children, disorders of potassium metabolism producing hyperkalemia are more common and are more likely to be life threatening than those resulting in hypokalemia. It is good practice to perform an electrocardiogram whenever serum potassium is found to exceed 6 mEq/l. The earliest manifestation of hyperkalemia seen on the ECG is an increase in the amplitude of T waves. Later, widening of the QRS complex occurs and the P waves become wide and flattened. Ectopic rhythms may also appear. Elevation of serum potassium is generally caused by one or more of the following: a) movement of potassium from the intracellular into the extracellular fluid compartment, b) increased potassium input, and c) decreased potassium excretion (Figure 4, Table 14).

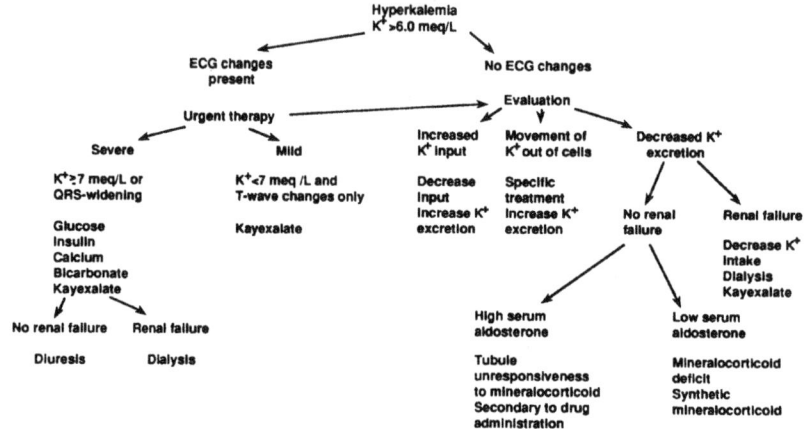

Figure 4. Guide to the treatment of hyperkalemia.

Table 14. Causes of hyperkalemia in children

I. Shift of potassium
   A. Acidosis
   B. Arginine infusion
   C. Digoxin intoxication
   D. Insulin deficiency
   E. Exercise and beta blocker
   F. Familial periodic hyperkalemic paralysis
   G. Insulin deficiency
   H. Succinylcholine
II. Increased potassium input
   A. Endogenous
      1. Major tissue destruction
         a. intravascular hemolysis
         b. tumorlysis
         c. burns
         d. rhabdomyolisis
   B. Exogenous
      1. Transfusion of stored blood
      2. Hemolysis
      3. Administration of potassium-containing medicinals
III. Decreased potassium excretion
   A. Renal failure
   B. Impaired distal tubular potassium secretion with normal mineralocorticoid secretion (Spitzer–Weinstein syndrome, pseudohypoaldosteronism, sickle cell disease, renal allografts)
   C. Mineralocorticoid deficiency (hypoaldosteronism, hyporeninemia, enzymatic defect in mineralocorticoid synthesis, Addison disease)
   D. Drugs (Captopril, Aldactone®)

The shift of potassium out of the cells is a common phenomenon but is rarely a cause of serious complications. The diagnosis can be made by identifying the presence of acidosis and by excluding increased input or decreased excretion of potassium. The treatment must be directed at the specific cause, e.g., correction of acidemia or insulin replacement in insulin-dependent diabetes mellitus.

If hyperkalemia is due to high potassium intake in the presence of normal renal function, the therapeutic measures should consist of decreasing potassium intake and promoting kaliuresis by increasing urine flow and alkalinizing the urine. Urine flow can be increased by administering a solution of 5% dextrose in water, 20 ml/kg BW over 20 minutes, and then continuing the infusion at two to three times the maintenance rate. Furosemide may be administered intravenously, 1–2 mg/kg BW every 4 hours. Alkalinization of the urine may be achieved by giving $NaHCO_3^-$, one dose of 2 mEq/kg BW, and then continuing with 1–2 mEq/kg BW per hour. During vigorous diuresis potassium excretion can be expected to exceed 0.05 mEq/kg BW per hour.

The ability of the human to excrete potassium is primarily a function of the mineralocorticoid-sensitive segment of the renal distal tubule. Mineralocorticoid deficiency may be secondary to abnormal production, or secretion, or to altered biologic activity of the ACTH or aldosterone. A similar clinical picture can be produced by unresponsiveness of the renal tubule to aldosterone. The patient with primary mineralocorticoid deficiency should be given synthetic mineralocorticoids (9-alpha-flurocortisone, 0.05–0.1 mg per 24 hours) or, in a case of emergency, DOCA (1 mg IM). In hyporeninemic hypoaldosteronism, therapy may not be necessary. If sodium chloride wasting is extreme, synthetic mineralocorticoid may be used as above. Infants with pseudohypoaldosteronism (end-organ unresponsiveness), transient or permanent, should receive salt supplementation (whatever is required to normalize serum sodium). In individuals in whom hyperkalemia is suspected to be drug induced, the causative agent should be stopped and replaced by another with a lesser hyperkalemic effect. An example would be replacing a beta blocker with a calcium-channel blocker in a patient with hypertension (22). When decreased renal potassium excretion occurs because of renal failure, potassium intake should be restricted to 1–2 mEq/kg BW per 24 hours.

The most difficult therapeutic problems associated with hyperkalemia occur in children who have increased intake and decreased excretion, such as a leukemic patient undergoing induction therapy who develops sepsis, requires transfusion of blood products, becomes hypotensive, and develops acute renal failure. A child with serum potassium exceeding 6 mEq/l and ECG changes consistent with hyperkalemia needs immediate attention. Treatment measures should be aimed at reversing the depolarizing effect of elevated extracellular potassium, enhancing the transfer of extracellular potassium into the cells, and removing excess potassium. These measures should be instituted simultaneously (Figure 4).

Calcium gluconate 0.5–1.0 ml/kg BW of a 10% solution given IV over 5–10 minutes under ECG monitoring is generally effective in decreasing the depolarization produced by elevated serum potassium. If one dose of calcium gluconate does not produce improvement in the ECG, a second dose should be administered. The effect of calcium gluconate lasts for 30–60 minutes, until calcium is taken up by cells.

Alkalization of the extracellular fluid with sodium bicarbonate (1–2 mEq/kg BW given IV over 5–10 minutes) promotes cellular uptake of potassium. The effect can be expected to last 1–4 hours. Calcium and bicarbonate should not be mixed in the same container because they will precipitate as calcium carbonate.

Insulin-dependent glucose uptake, exhibited by liver and muscle cells, enhances cellular potassium uptake and thus decreases serum potassium. This can be accomplished by infusing 0.5–1.0 g/kg BW of glucose over 15–20 minutes. In newborns, the dose of glucose should not exceed 400 mg/kg BW. The effect lasts for 4–6 hours. Some physicians recommend the addition of 1–2 U of insulin for each 3 g of glucose infused; others claim that in individuals with normal islet cell function, addition of insulin is not necessary.

The final step in the treatment of hyperkalemia is removal of the excess potassium from the body. There are several ways to achieve this goal. One is by increasing urinary potassium excretion (described before). Another is by administering a sodium-exchange resin such as polystyrene sulfonate (Kayexalate R). The dose for children is 0.5–1.0 g/kg BW given either orally (in 3–4 ml water per gram resin) or mixed with a 70% solution of sorbitol as an enema to be retained for 15–30 minutes. This regimen can be repeated every 2–3 hours, as necessary. If the above measures are not effective, attention should be directed towards the existence of a large source of potassium (rhabdomyolisis) or renal failure. In individuals with renal failure and hyperkalemia, dialysis is the treatment of choice. Up to 50 mEq of potassium can be removed in 1 hour of hemodialysis. Peritoneal dialysis can remove 10–30 mEq of potassium per 24 hours, with hourly exchanges and no potassium in the dialysate.

DISORDERS OF CALCIUM BALANCE

Hypercalcemia

The total calcium level measured in serum consists of three fractions: ionized calcium, protein-bound calcium, and calcium bound to small molecules (e.g., phosphate). It is the ionized calcium that is the physiologically important component. Hypercalcemia can be defined as a total serum calcium >11 mg/dl in the presence of normal albumin and globin concentrations or a serum concentration of ionized calcium of >6 mg/dl. Whenever possible, therapeutic decisions regarding disturbances in calcium homeostasis should be based on measurements of ionized calcium.

Signs and symptoms of hypercalcemia are generally nonspecific and include nausea, vomiting, abdominal discomfort, constipation, confusion, hallucinations, impaired memory, weakness, twitching, easy fatigability, polyuria, polydipsia, renal colic, and hypertension.

Hypercalcemia results from increased calcium absorption from the gut, decreased renal excretion, or increased bone resorption. There are no reports indicating the incidence of hypercalcemia and the distribution of primary causes in infants and children, but ectopic production of PTH secondary to breast or lung cancer, or bone invasion by malignancy or chronic granulomatous diseases, are very rare in children. The most common causes of hypercalcemia in the pediatric population are listed in Table 15.

Table 15. Causes of hypercalcemia in infants and children

Infants
Iatrogenic
Hyperparathyroidism
Williams syndrome
Milk alkali syndrome
Children
Hypercalcemic hypocalciuria
Hyperthyroidism
Granulomatous diseases (sarcoid)
Primary hyperparathyroidism
Secondary hyperparathyroidism
Immobilization
Vitamin-D or vitamin-A intoxication
Excessive calcium intake
Adrenal insufficiency
Malignancy

Iatrogenic hypercalcemia is commonly encountered in infants expected to develop hypocalcemia who are treated preventively with large amounts of calcium. In most cases, correction of hypercalcemia can be achieved by decreasing or discontinuing calcium administration.

Hyperparathyroidism is rare in infants. In addition, infants may be less sensitive than adults to the renal phosphaturic effect of PTH. Neonates of untreated hypoparathyroid mothers have high PTH levels because of chronic intrauterine exposure to hypocalcemia. This form of hyperparathyroidism usually resolves without treatment. In another form of hyperparathyroidism (autosomal recessive parathyroid hyperplasia), the infants have marked hypercalcemia associated with bone changes and elevated PTH. The treatment of choice is subtotal parathyroidectomy.

Williams' syndrome and its variants are thought to be produced by hyper-responsiveness to vitamin D. These infants are generally stigmatized (elfin facies, retarded physical and mental development, and cardiac abnormalities). Treatment consists of a diet low in calcium and low in vitamin D.

Older children and adolescents have the potential to develop any of the forms of hypercalcemia seen in adults; however, the majority of children with hypercalcemia fall into one of the following groups:

IMMOBILIZATION SECONDARY TO CASTING OF FRACTURES OR MAJOR BURNS

This form of hypercalcemia responds to saline diuresis (three to four times the maintenance requirement) and furosemide 1–2 mg/kg BW bid. Large amounts of calcium are excreted in urine, but a positive calcium balance is reestablished as soon as the child becomes ambulatory.

VITAMIN D OR VITAMIN A INTOXICATION

Often stopping the vitamin intake is all that is required. If life-threatening hypercalcemia is present, refer to the section on management of severe hypercalcemia.

SECONDARY HYPERPARATHYROIDISM

Frequently, secondary hyperparathyroidism is present in children with chronic renal failure, even when vigorous attempts have been made to control it by using phosphate binders, calcium, and vitamin D supplementation. Following renal transplantation, serum calcium may rise and serum phosphate may remain low. Calcium and phosphate concentrations usually return to normal within 1–3 weeks, without therapy. Occasionally, parathyroidectomy is required.

If serum calcium is >11 mg/dl or if the patient is symptomatic, methods to lower serum calcium should be used. Infusion of a normal solution of saline (200–300 ml/kg BW per 24 hours) or administration of furosemide (1 mg/kg BW q 6 hours) promotes a dramatic and often sufficient increase in urinary calcium excretion. Prednisone (2 mg/kg BW per 24 hours) or hydrocortisone (10 mg/kg BW per 24 hours) have been reported to lower serum calcium but require several days to take effect. We have administered salmon calcitonin 4–10 IU/kg BW IV or IM to several children with severe hypercalcemia (12–15 mg/dl) and found it to have an immediate effect on lowering serum calcium. In severe hypercalcemia associated with renal failure, dialysis should be considered.

Hypocalcemia

Hypocalcemia is much more common among children than hypercalcemia. It may be defined as a total serum calcium of < 7 mg/dl in the presence of normal serum albumin and serum phosphate concentrations, or as an ionized calcium < 2.5 mg/dl.

Clinical manifestations of hypocalcemia fall within four categories: a) neurologic, including tetany, positive Chvostek and Trousseau signs, muscle spasms and cramps, weakness, and seizures; b) respiratory, including apnea, bronchospasm, and laryngeal spasm; c) cardiovascular, including heart failure and hypotension; and d) psychiatric, including anxiety, dementia, depression, irritability, and psychosis.

The concentration of calcium in serum is modulated mainly by PTH and vitamin D. The following abnormalities in parathyroid function may result in hypocalcemia: a) deficient production or release of PTH; b) end-organ insensitivity to PTH; and c) secretion of an immunologically reactive but biologically inactive PTH molecule.

Among the patients who fall into the first category, it is important to identify those who have hypoparathyroidism due to an autoimmune process because of the risk of other autoimmune endocrine abnormalities, particularly Addison disease. Patients with end-organ insensitivity may be separated from those in which the disease is due to biologically inactive PTH on the basis of the lack of renal responsiveness to exogenous PTH. Unfortunately, PTH is not available in the United States.

If the presentation is acute and symptomatic, administration of calcium IV is indicated. Otherwise, patients with hypoparathyroidism (all forms) can be treated effectively with calcium and vitamin D administered orally. Any one of many calcium preparations can be given in amounts that provide approximately 50 mg of elemental calcium per kg BW per day, divided into three or four doses. The maximum dose is about 1 g of elemental calcium per day. Vitamin D is given in dosages of 50–125 μg per day.

There are several primary mechanisms that account for vitamin D abnormalities conducive to hypocalcemia: a) deficient intake b) decreased absorption c) decreased hydroxylation d) increased elimination and e) end-organ resistance to vitamin D.

Deficient intake combined with low sunlight exposure was once a common cause of rickets and hypocalcemia among the children of the United States. At present, cow's milk and infant formula are enriched with vitamin D, and breast-fed babies are supplemented with vitamin D. Consequently, vitamin D-deficient rickets is rarely seen in this country. The recommended daily dose of vitamin D is 10 μg. Inadequate vitamin D intake should be suspected on the basis of history. On physical examination, one shoule look for bowed legs, muscle weakness, enlarged costochondral junctions, and craniotabes. Radiographs may reveal alterations of the long bones, with widening of the wrists and knees. Laboratory evaluation may include measurements of circulating 25-$(OH)D_3$, 1,25-$(OH)_2D_3$, PTH, serum Ca, P, Mg, alkaline phosphatase, and total Co_2. Treatment consists of ensuring adequate calcium and phosphorus in the diet and vitamin D supplementation in doses of 2000–5000 IU daily for 1–2 months (100 IU = 2.5 μg).

Decreased absorption of vitamin D occurs in individuals with fat malabsorption or short gut syndromes. It is a rare cause of hypocalcemia in children. The diagnosis may be suspected on the basis of history. Laboratory evaluation is similar to that described for vitamin D deficiency. These patients should be advised to decrease fat intake and to supplement their vitamin D and calcium intake. If oral supplementation does not produce satisfactory results, an IM preparation of vitamin D (i.e., ergocalciferol) should be considered. Measurement of vitamin D derivatives in serum may be used as a gauge of body vitamin D stores.

Decreased hydroxylation of vitamin D is most common in children with liver disease or renal failure. These patients respond to administration of 1,25-$(OH)_2D_3$. Dosages of 0.015–0.05 μg/kg BW per 24 hours up to a maximum of 2.0 μg per 24 hours are recommended.

If vitamin D elimination is increased due to stimulation of liver metabolism by drugs (such as phenobarbital or phenytoin), additional vitamin D is necessary. Measurement of vitamin D derivatives in serum may serve as a guide for supplementation.

Vitamin D resistance is a very unusual cause of hypocalcemia and rickets in children of the United States. Some of these patients will respond to very large doses of vitamin D and calcium supplementation or to 1,25-$(OH)_2D_3$.

Calcium deficiency alone is a rare cause of hypocalcemia in children. It may be suspected in children with malabsorption syndromes and very unusual diets, and in teenage nursing mothers. Concomitant vitamin D deficiency should be ruled out. Treatment consists of calcium supplementation. The recommended daily dietary elemental calcium intake is 360 mg for a term infant in the first 6 months of life, 540 mg in the second 6 months, 800 mg between the ages of 1 and 10 years, and 1200 mg between the ages of 12 and 18 years. If calcium deficiency is present, supplementation to increase daily calcium by 50–100% should resolve the problem.

Several cases were reported of infants given large oral doses of phosphate or phosphate-containing enemas who developed dramatic hyperphosphatemia and hypocalcemia. Some of these children have died. Treatment should be directed towards decreasing absorption of phosphate from the gut by giving a large dose of a phosphate binder (aluminum hydroxide, 20 mg/kg BW PO) and increasing phosphate removal by hemodialysis.

Drugs contribute to hypocalcemia, either by increasing elimination or by binding calcium. In most cases, the drug (furosemide, aminoglycoside antibiotics, cisplatinum, amphotericin B, digitalis, insulin, citrate) cannot be discontinued, and calcium replacement or supplementation is necessary.

Children wih acute or chronic renal failure develop hypocalcemia through the same mechanisms as those described in adults. Children with acute renal failure may require supplemental calcium (IV or PO) pending the return of renal function. Children with chronic renal failure can be given calcium carbonate (25 mg/kg BW per 24 hours PO), both as a calcium supplement and as a phosphate binder. In addition, they should receive 1,25-$(OH)_2D_3$, 0.015–0.05 μg/kg BW per 24 hours.

It is often helpful to separate hypocalcemia into that occurring in the perinatal period and that occuring later on in life (Table 16). However, there is no firm dividing line as some conditions causing hypocalcemia may occur at all ages.

HYPOCALCEMIA OF INFANCY

Early-onset perinatal hypocalcemia develops within the first 72 hours after birth, usually in sick infants (asphyxia, sepsis). The serum calcium concentration in the fetus is dependent primarily on the active transport of calcium by the placenta. At birth, the calcium stores are low and the ability to mobilize calcium from these stores is tenuous at best. Consequently, a stressful situation can result in hypocalcemia. When symptoms of hypocalcemia are present, 2 ml/kg BW of a 10% solution of calcium gluconate (200 mg calcium per kg BW) should be infused over 5–20 minutes. In the absence of symptoms, hypocalcemia can be treated with a 10% solution of calcium gluconate 5 ml

Table 16. Causes of hypocalcemia in children

I. Perinatal
  A. Early onset
  B. Late onset
  C. Congenital disorders
  D. Metabolic disorders
  E. Drug induced
  F. Maternal disorders
II. Infants and children
  A. Critical illness
  B. Abnormalities of PTH
    1. Decreased secretion
    2. Decreased end-organ responsivity
    3. Secretion of abnormal PTH molecule
  C. Abnormalities of vitamin D
    1. Deficient intake or absorption
    2. Decreased hydroxylation or increased elimination
    3. End-organ resistance
  D. Calcium deficiency
  E. Hyperphosphatemia
  F. Drugs
  G. Renal failure

(500 mg)/kg BW per 24 hours IV given slowly under cardiac monitoring. Once serum calcium returns to normal, calcium infusion should be reduced to 200 mg/kg BW per 24 hours.

Another form of early-onset hypocalcemia is secondary to inadequately treated maternal hyperparathyroidism. The elevated level of maternal parathyroid hormone causes hypercalcemia, which inhibits the parathyroid glands of the fetus. Once separated from the mother, the baby develops hypocalcemia. This diturbance responds to oral calcium supplementation (50–75 mg/kg BW of elemental calcium per 24 hours) and resolves within 1–2 weeks.

Late-onset perinatal hypocalcemia generally develops 6–8 days following birth and is due to hyperphosphatemia. It was much more common when large numbers of infants were fed cow's milk, which has a high phosphate content.

Much of the transfer of calcium from the mother to the fetus occurs during the last trimester of pregnancy. Infants born 1–2 months early have low calcium stores and may develop hypocalcemic rickets. Supplementation with calcium (200–250 mg/kg BW of elemental calcium per 24 hours), phosphate (80–150 mg/kg BW per 24 hours), and vitamin D provides adequate mineral for bone formation.

There are two congenital disorders associated with neonatal hypoparathyroidism and hypocalcemia: the DiGeorge syndrome and idiopathic hypoparathyroidism. Both are very rare. The DiGeorge syndrome is characterized by agenesis of the thymus and parathyroid glands. Most of these children die of infection. Oral calcium supplementation results in adequate serum calcium levels. Treatment with PTH would be appropriate, but the hormone is not available in the United States. Transplantation of parathyroid tissue should be curative of hypoparathyroidism.

Transient idiopathic hypoparathyroidism is usually a benign, self-limited disorder of infancy characterized by persistent hypocalcemia and hyperphosphatemia. It requires treatment with calcium and a vitamin D metabolite for as long as 1 year. There have also been reports of sex-linked and sporadic forms of hypoparathyroidism. These patients can be usually managed with calcium supplementation; only seldom is vitamin D necessary. Congenital hypoparathyroidism caused by the absence of the parathyroid glands can be distinguished from transient neonatal hypoparathyroidism on the basis of undetectable PTH levels in the patients with the former condition.

Hypocalcemia may be found in abnormalities of lipid metabolism, acid-base disturbances, and hypomagnesemia. When possible, correction of the primary cause will restore calcium levels to normal. If correction of the cause is not possible, calcium supplementation should be implemented.

Drugs such as diuretics, aminoglycosides, cisplatinum, amphotericin B, digitalis, insulin, and citrate may reduce serum calcium by one or more of the following mechanisms: increased renal excretion, increased cellular uptake, and direct binding of calcium.

Abnormalities of calcium metabolism in the mother (hypoparathyroidism, vitamin D deficiency) may affect

Table 17. Causes of hypocalcemia among children in the intensive care unit

Hypoparathyroidism	Pancreatitis
Hyper-hypomagnesemia	Chelating drugs
Vitamin-D deficiency	Hungry-bone syndrome
Hyperphosphatemia	Toxic shock syndrome
Sepsis	Fat embolism

From Zaloga GP (25).

calcium homeostasis in offspring. The disorders generally respond to calcium replacement until the calcium regulatory mechanisms develop.

HYPOCALCEMIA OF CHILDHOOD

Hypocalcemia is often encountered during critical illness. It may occur in half or more of the children admitted to pediatric intensive care units. The disturbance is generally multifactorial (Table 17).

If the serum ionized calcium is low and the patient is symptomatic, we recommend administration of 1–2 ml/kg BW of a 10% solution of calcium gluconate (100–200 mg calcium/kg BW), given IV at a rate not to exceed 1 ml/min, under careful monitoring of the heart rate. Once the serum ionized calcium exceeds 2.5 mg/dl, continuous infusion of 100–200 mg/kg BW per 24 hours (up to 6 g per 24 hours) is generally adequate to maintain serum calcium within the normal range. In case of severe hypocalcemia, we have used up to 500 mg/kg BW per 24 hours of a 10% solution of calcium gluconate without complications. When the child improves and oral alimentation is resumed, hypocalcemia resolves.

DISORDERS OF ACID-BASE BALANCE

In utero, the placenta performs the role of removing hydrogen ions and maintaining the serum bicarbonate concentration of the fetus within the normal range. In the term infant at birth, the pH is 7.25 (7.11–7.36) and the Pa_{CO_2} is 51 (37–79) mmHg. One hour after birth, the newborn is in a state of metabolic acidosis, the pH is 7.30 (7.2–7.48) and the Pa_{CO_2} is 34 mmHg. This resolves within a few hours after birth.

Metabolic acidosis

Conditions producing acidemia are more common than those producing alkalemia. Metabolic acidosis is characterized by a low serum bicarbonate concentration and a low pH.

A flow diagram (Figure 5), adapted from the work of Narins et al. (19), is useful in evaluating primary disturbances in hydrogen and bicarbonate ions concentrations. These authors divide patients with metabolic acidosis in

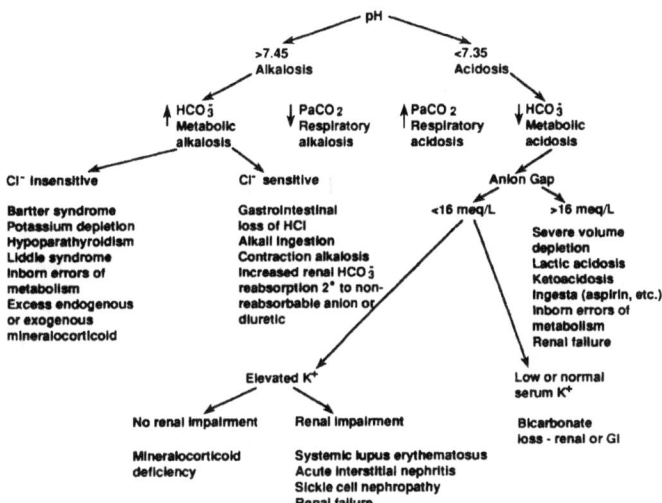

Figure 5. Evaluation of acid-base disturbances. [Adapted from Narins et al (11)].

two categories according to the magnitude of the difference (gap) between the anions (Cl^- + HCO_3^-) and the cations (Na^+ + K^+) present in plasma.

METABOLIC ACIDOSIS WITH LARGE ANION GAP

If the anion gap is > 16 mEq/l, the conditions to be considered are: a) severe volume depletion, b) lactic acidosis, c) ketoacidosis, d) ingestion of toxic substances, and e) renal failure.

Severe volume depletion can be secondary to vomiting, diarrhea, and hemorrhage. It can generally be suspected on the basis of the history and physical examination. Evaluation and treatment are as described in the previous section on hypovolemia. Lactic acidosis occurs in conditions characterized by poor tissue oxygenation, or it can be secondary to drugs, toxins, and liver impairment. Treatment should be directed at alleviating the primary cause (i.e., improving tissue oxygenation in shock). Patients with mild lactic acidosis require no additional treatment; those with more severe forms (pH < 7.20, HCO_3^- < 12 mEq/l) should receive an infusion of bicarbonate to elevate serum bicarbonate concentration into the 15–18 mEq/l range.

Ketoacidosis is fairly common among diabetic children. If the child is also volume depleted, lactic acid may also contribute to acidemia. Diabetic ketoacidosis can be suspected on the basis of the history and should be confirmed by laboratory evaluation of blood glucose and acetone. Treatment includes fluid, electrolyte, and insulin administration. Infusion of bicarbonate should be reserved for patients with pH < 7.2 and HCO_3^- < 12 mEq/l. The goal of therapy is to raise and then to maintain serum HCO_3^- in the 15–18 mEq/l range until physiologic mechanisms can come into play and afford full correction. Toddlers and adolescents are most likely to ingest toxic materials. Many toxic materials may produce profound metabolic acidosis with a large anion gap (salicylic acid, antifreeze fluid, etc.). It is always helpful to consider the possibility of ingestion and, when suspected, to perform blood or urine screening. Supportive care (maintenance of patent airways and normal blood pressure, replacement of fluid and electrolyte deficits) receive highest priority. If the nature of the ingestum can be determined, a toxicology book may be consulted for specific treatment. In most areas, rapid information can be obtained from the local poison control center (dial P-O-I-S-O-N-S).

Acute or chronic renal failure may or may not be associated with an ion gap acidosis. Treatment depends on the pathogenesis of renal failure but, in general, bicarbonate replacement to maintain the serum HCO_3^- in the 20–24 mEq/l range, is indicated.

Inborn errors of metabolism associated with acidemia are very rare. They should be considered in the young infant who is failing to thrive and in whom severe acidosis with an anion gap is present. Conditions presenting with such a picture include: maple-syrup urine disease, propionic acidemia, methylmalonic acidemia, multiple carboxylase deficiency, 3-ketothiolase deficiency, isovaleric acidemia, glutaric aciduria, and lactic acidemia. When first seen, such infants usually require supportive care (i.e., fluid replacement for persistent vomiting, bicarbonate to correct acidosis, glucose to correct hypoglycemia). The specific diagnosis must be made through specialized testing (measurement of amino acids, fibroblast cultures, etc). The care of infants with these conditions is best coordinated through a tertiary center that is experienced in disturbances of metabolism. In the future, treatment of these conditions through genetic engineering may become possible.

METABOLIC ACIDOSIS WITH NORMAL ANION GAP

If the child has acidosis and the anion gap is normal (< 16 mEq/l), it is often helpful to examine the serum potassium (Figure 5). If the serum potassium is normal or low, the most common conditions are those producing bicarbonate loss via the gastrointestinal tract (e.g., diarrhea, drainage) or kidney (e.g., diuretics, renal tubular acidosis). Therapy in these instances must be directed to the cause and, if necessary, should be accompanied by bicarbonate supplementation.

If the serum potassium is elevated, renal impairment needs to be considered. If moderate renal impairment is present, consideration should be given to systemic lupus erythematosus, sickle cell nephropathy, interstitial nephritis, or renal failure. If renal impairment is not present, then one should consider the possibility of mineralocorticoid deficiency or ingestion or administration of acidifying agents containing chloride (e.g., NH_4Cl). The diagnosis and the treatment of these conditions is similar in children and adults.

Metabolic alkalosis

Conditions characterized by volume contraction associated with alkalemia and elevated serum bicarbonate concentration are named by some "chloride-sensitive" forms of metabolic alkalosis. They are due to: a) increased loss of HCl, as in pyloric stenosis of the newborn, the most common of this group; b) ingestion of alkali, which should be considered in an otherwise well child who suddenly develops metabolic alkalosis; and c) increased renal bicarbonate reabsorption secondary to administration of a non-reabsorbable anion (antibiotics, diuretics).

Treatment of pyloric stenosis consists of supportive measures (n.p.o., repair of fluid and electrolyte abnormalities through the intravenous route) and surgical removal of stenosis. Administration of an isotonic solution of sodium chloride (20 ml/kg BW over 20 minutes) produces temporary correction of hyperbicarbonatemia and alkalemia. In children who continue to be alkalotic and do not belong to any of the above categories ("chloride insensitive"), the following should be considered: Bartter syndrome, potassium depletion, hypoparathyroidism, excess mineralocorticoid activity (i.e., primary, secondary to hyperreninemia, ingestion of mineralocorticoid or mineralocortocoidlike agents). These conditions are all very rare in children. Treatment is as described for adults.

Respiratory acidosis

Respiratory acidosis results from primary disturbances in ventilation that increase the arterial Pa_{CO_2}. In normal conditions the amount of carbon dioxide exhaled is equal to the amount of CO_2 produced. If there is a pathologic condition that causes hypoventilation and carbon dioxide retention, the total body production of carbon dioxide exceeds excretion, resulting in acidemia. Conditions producing respiratory acidosis include airway obstruction, central nervous system depression, neuromuscular diseases, injuries to the chest wall, and primary lung diseases (e.g., meconium aspiration, asthma, pneumonia, etc.).

Respiratory alkalosis

Respiratory alkalosis results from primary disturbances that cause hyperventilation. Hyperventilation decreases Pa_{CO_2} and shifts the equilibrium of the bicarbonate-carbonic acid system towards alkalosis. Conditions producing respiratory alkalosis include central nervous system injury, drugs such as salicylic acid, liver failure, and anxiety.

Both respiratory acidosis and alkalosis are best treated by specific therapy directed at the underlying mechanism.

DISORDERS OF MAGNESIUM METABOLISM

Magnesium is incorporated into the structure of bones and teeth. In addition, it promotes activation of enzymes involved in carbohydrate metabolism and in muscle and nerve excitability. It is a major intracellular cation.

Magnesium metabolism is not under direct hormonal control (in contrast to calcium). The serum concentration reflects the balance between intestinal absorption and renal excretion. Normally, 20% of the serum magnesium is bound to albumin. About 90% of the filtered magnesium is reabsorbed by the renal tubule.

Hypomagnesemia

Hypomagnesemia (< 1.5 mEq/l) is seen in neonatal tetany, chronic diarrhea, certain types of chronic renal disease, diuretic therapy, hyperparathyroidism, primary hyperaldosteronism, and diabetic acidosis. Symptoms include disorientation, muscle twitching, tremor, corpopedal spasm, and convulsions. Treatment consists of giving magnesium 1–2 mEq/kg BW per 24 hours PO in three or four divided doses. In long-term parenteral fluid therapy, magnesium deficiency can be avoided by providing magnesium 2–4 mEq/m^2 BSA per 24 hours.

Hypermagnesemia

Hypermagnesemia occurs in Addison disease, in acute renal failure, and after prolonged antihypertensive therapy. Drowsiness, respiratory failure, and coma may occur at levels greater than 10 mEq/l. Calcium gluconate at a dose of 500 mg/m^2 BSA IV over 3 hours reverses the symptoms.

FLUID MANAGEMENT OF BURNS

The major pathophysiologic disturbances in the patient with extensive burns are vasodilation and increased capillary permeability, resulting in the loss of fluid and electrolytes. The amount of fluid required for therapy

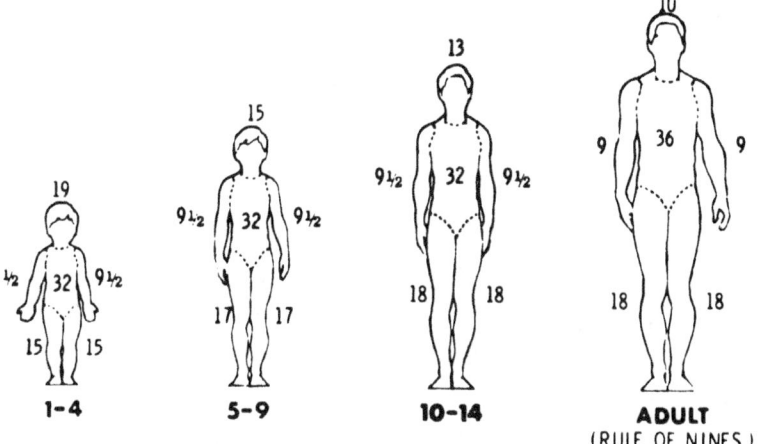

Figure 6. Diagram indicating the body proportions at various ages. The rule of nines frequently used to estimate burn surface in adults does not accurately reflect burn surface in younger individuals. Numbers adjacent to figures indicate percent body surface. Numbers under figures indicate age. From Lund CL and Brower WC (31).

depends on the extent and the degree of the burn. Initially, an isotonic solution (blood, plasma, saline, or Ringer's) should be administered at a rate of 20 ml/kg BW per hour while estimating the area of body surface burned. In children, a relatively larger proportion of the body surface is represented by the head and neck, whereas the lower extremities comprise a relatively smaller proportion than in the adult (Figure 6).

Once an estimate of the burned surface is made, the patient should be given 1600 ml/m^2 of fluid per 24 hours for maintenance, plus 5000 ml/m^2 BSA burned per 24 hours for ongoing losses. Fluid received during the evaluation period should not be deducted from the requirements for the initial 24-hour period.

What the composition of the fluid should be is somewhat controversial. The main objectives are to maintain the blood oncotic pressure, to correct metabolic acidosis, and to provide adequate calories. These goals can be achieved by administering lactated Ringer's with 5% dextrose and 12.5 g albumin per liter. For infants less than 1 year, the concentration of sodium chloride should be decreased to half. Potassium should not be added initially to the intravenous fluids, because a large amount of intracellular potassium is released from injured cells. In addition, acidosis and renal failure may contribute to hyperkalemia. About one half of the total amount of fluid is given during the first 8 hours, the balance during the subsequent 16 hours. Patients with severe burns often develop renal damage and acute anuria. This may be prevented by adding mannitol 0.5–1.0 g (2–4 ml of a 25% solution) per kg of BW to the initial IV solution. The treatment can be repeated as necessary to ensure adequate urine flow. During the second 24 hours, the amount of colloid and electrolyte needed is about half that of the initial day, while the total fluid requirement may remain about the same. The program must be modified according to the general condition of the patient, the degree of hypovolemia, and the functional capacity of the kidney. Though vigorous therapy is required to support the circulation, urine output and body weight must be monitored to avoid a volume overload and cardiac failure.

REFERENCES

1. Spitzer A: The developing kidney and the process of growth. In: DW Seldin G, Giebisch, eds, *The Kidney: Physiology and Pathophysiology*. Raven Press, New York, pp 1979–2015, 1985.
2. Forbes GB: *Human Body Composition, Growth, Aging, Nutrition and Activity*. Springer-Verlag, New York, 1987.
3. Spitzer A: The role of the kidney in sodium homeostasis during development. *Kidney Int* 21:539–545, 1982.
4. Winters RW: *The Body Fluids in Pediatrics*. Little, Brown, Boston, 1973.
5. Schwartz GJ, Brion LP, Spitzer A: The use of plasma creatinine concentration for estimating glomerular filtration rate in infants, children and adolescents. *Pediatr Clin No Am* 34(3):571–590, 1987.
6. Guignard JP, John EG: Renal function in the tiny premature infant. *Clin Perinatol* 13:377–397, 1986.
7. Edelmann CM, et al.: Reabsorption and excretion of bicarbonate in infants and adults. *J Clin Invest* 46:1309–1315, 1967.
8. Goldsmith DI: Clinical and laboratory evaluation of renal function, In: CM Edelmann, ed, *Pediatric Kidney Disease*. Little, Brown, Boston, pp 213–223, 1978.
9. Finberg L: Water and electrolyte physiology. In: AM Rudolph, JIE Hoffman, eds, *Pediatrics*. Appleton and Lange, Norwalk, CT, pp 194–201, 1987.
10. Nash MA: Water and solute homeostasis. In: CM Edelmann, ed, *Pediatric Kidney Disease*. Little, Brown, Boston, pp 290–305, 1978.

11. Narins RG, Jones ER, Strom MC, Rudnick MR, Bastl CP: Diagnostic strategies in disorders of fluid, electrolyte and acid-base homeostasis. *Am J Med* 72:496–519, 1982.
12. Robson AM: The pathophysiology of body fluids. In: RE Behrman, VC Vaughan, eds, *Nelson Textbook of Pediatrics*. WB Saunders, Philadelphia, pp 172–207, 1987.
13. Gruskin AB, Baluarte HJ, Prebis JW, Polinsky MS, Morgenstern BZ, Perlman SA: Serum sodium abnormalities in children. *Pediatr Clin No Am* 29:907–932, 1982.
14. Finch MH, Younoszai KM: Oral rehydration therapy. *South Med J* 80:609–613, 1987.
15. Listernick R, Zieserl E, Davis AT; Outpatient oral rehydration in the United States. *Am J Dis Child* 140:211–215, 1986.
16. Tamer AM, Friedman LB, Maxwell SRW, Cynamon HA, Perez HN, Cleveland WW: Oral rehydration of infants in a large urban U.S. medical center. *J Pediatr* 107:14–19, 1985.
17. Pizarro D, Castillo B, Posada G, Lizano C, Mata L: Efficacy comparison of oral rehydration solutions containing either 90 or 75 millimoles of sodium per liter. *Pediatrics* 79:190–195, 1987.
18. Linshaw ME: Potassium homeostasis and hypokalemia. *Pediatr Clin No Am* 34(3):649–682, 1987.
19. Narins RG, Jones ER, Strom MC, Rudnick MR, Bastl CP: Diagnostic strategies in disorders of fluid, electrolyte and acid-base homeostasis. *Am J Med* 72:503–508, 1982.
20. Kaplan NM: Our appropriate concern about hypokalemia. *Am J Med* 77:1–4, 1984.
21. Bia MJ, DeFronzo RA: Extrarenal potassium homeostasis. *Am J Physiol* 241:F257–F262, 1981.
22. Carlsson E, Fellenius E, Lundborg P, Svensson L: Beta-adrenoceptor blockers, plasma potassium and exercise. *Lancet* 2:424–426, 1978.
23. Root AW: Calcium, phosphate and magnesium disorders In: AR Colon, M Ziai, eds, *Pediatric Pathophysiology*. Little, Brown, Boston, pp 97–125, 1985.
24. Kruse K: Endocrine control and disturbances of calcium and phosphate metabolism in children. *Eur J Pediatr* 146:346–353, 1987.
25. Zaloga GP, Chernow B: Hypocalcemia in critical illness. *JAMA* 256:1924–1929, 1987.
26. Singer FR, Bethune JE, Massry SG: Hypercalcemia and hypocalcemia. *Clin Nephrol* 7:154–162, 1977.
27. Campbell D, Fleischman AR: Perinatal calcium and phosphorous metabolism. *Rev Perinat Med* 5:95–150, 1986.
28. Tsang R, Noginchi A, Steichern JJ: Pediatric parathyroid disorders. *Pediatr Clin No Am* 26:223–249, 1979.
29. Gauthier B, Edelmann C, Barnett H: *Nephrology and Urology for the Pediatrician*. Little, Brown, Boston, pp 49–61, 1982.
30. Donckerwolcke RA: Diagnosis and treatment of renal tubular disorders in children. *Pediatr Clin No Am* 29:895–906, 1982.
31. Lund CL, Brower WC: The estimation of areas of burn. *Surg Gynecol Obstet* 79:352–359, 1944.

CHAPTER 16

Fluid and Electrolyte Disorders in the Surgical Patient

HERVY H. HINER, JR & WADI N. SUKI

INTRODUCTION

The number of surgical procedures that are done each year now totals in the tens of millions (1). As medical science continues to advance, new surgical procedures are being developed, older procedures are becoming more intricate, and the number of the so-called high-risk patients receiving surgery is increasing. These high-risk patients include individuals with preexisting renal and cardiac abnormalities. Consequently, the chances of witnessing renal, fluid, and electrolyte derangements in surgical patients are increased. Despite their increased incidence, these abnormalities can still be effectively managed without a significant increase in morbidity and mortality. Management is made simpler if particular fluid and electrolyte disturbances can be anticipated.

Oliguria, in association with sodium and water retention, was noted in surgical patients as early as 1905 (2). Since then there have been numerous attempts to explain this occurrence by demonstrating decreased renal blood flow (3), increased mineralocorticoid activity (4, 5), or increased levels of ADH (6, 7). Before discussing volume disturbances, a discussion of what normally occurs in the surgical patient is in order.

CONSEQUENCES OF SURGERY

Renal function

It has been well established that a number of anesthetic agents, including halothane, diethyl ether, thiopentone, and fentanyl, reduce the renal blood flow and glomerular filtration rate (GFR) (8–10). Significant decreases in both cortical and medullary renal blood flow have been demonstrated during halothane anesthesia in dogs that were not given large amounts of Ringer's solution during the procedure. A decrease in renal blood flow increases sodium and water absorption in the proximal and distal tubules as a result of changes in glomerulotubular balance, physical forces, and renin secretion (11, 12).

The glomerular filtration rate falls during anesthesia, but rapidly returns to normal following the operation (13, 14). This transient reduction in GFR could reduce the amount of sodium and water excreted as a result of reduced filtration and disturbed glomerulotubular balance.

Mineralocorticoid activity

In 1950 HT Johnson et al. concluded from observations on the concentrations of Na^+ and K^+ in perspiration that there is "increased activity of salt active adrenal steroids in the post-operative period" (15). Shortly afterwards, increased excretion of potassium in the urine again suggested increased mineralocorticoid activity (16). Later, aldosterone was found to be increased in both the urine (4) and blood (17, 18). There is a transient rise in plasma aldosterone on the day of the procedure. The percent increment in plasma aldosterone varies from 200% to 600% depending on the volume status of the patient. There is a sharp reduction in the plasma values after the first post-operative day, with aldosterone levels returning to baseline in a 4- to 5-day period. The increase in aldosterone does not appear to be associated with increased ACTH secretion or serum potassium (18–20). The aldosterone values can be markedly reduced with saline administration, with relatively modest increments in plasma aldosterone levels, which return to baseline after a 1-day period (17). Plasma renin activity is also increased from the time of the procedure to approximately the fifth postoperative day. Surgical patients are usually in positive sodium balance through the fourth postoperative day. However, the blood volume of these individuals is reduced for at least 3 days following surgery. This suggests that diminished intravascular volume may result in stimulation of the renin-angiotensin system, which would then lead to increased aldosterone production. These findings are even more pronounced in patients subjected to cardiopulmonary bypass (18). A positive sodium balance in the presence of diminished blood volume implies that sodium is retained within the extravascular space.

The reasons for the decrement in the circulating blood volume have not been determined. Decreased intravascular oncotic pressure, increased vascular permeability, and altered cellular permeability with intracellular retention of Na^+ and water have been considering (18). Considering that sodium and water retention may occur in adrenalectomized individuals, factors other than adrenal hormones must play a role (21).

ADH

In 1953, Le Quonse observed that the oliguria noted frequently after surgery did not occur in patients with diabetes insipidus (5). Shortly afterwards, elevated levels of bioassayable vasopressin (AVP) were demonstrated in the urine and plasma of postoperative patients (4, 22–25). Because of this, and the frequent occurrence of hyponatremia in the presence of oliguria, inappropriate secretion of AVP was assumed to be at least a partial cause of oliguria and water retention (5). Potential factors responsible for the release of AVP from the posterior pituitary gland during anesthesia and surgery are numerous (11, 26–31) (Table 1). Despite the multitude of possible factors, there is no confirmation of how these various factors interrelate in causing increased secretion of ADH. There appear to be distinct peaks of AVP plasma levels in most patients, with an immediate rise of AVP levels at the time of incision and an even higher elevation of AVP levels immediately after surgery (7, 27). Maximum AVP plasma levels may be more than 20 times greater than the normal levels required to cause maximum antidiuresis under normal conditions (29). In the presence of the elevated AVP levels there is slight to moderate reduction of plasma osmolality 6–30 mOsm/kg, median 19 mOsm/kg, with the maximum urinary concentration ranging from 665 to 941 mOsm/kg.

The degree to which the urine volume varies with AVP secretion is not always consistent and may at times be dependent on the solute load (6, 29). It has also been demonstrated that the maximum urine osmolality that can be produced with exogenous AVP administration is reduced in the perioperative period in comparison with preoperative or late postoperative values (32). This has been attriuted to a decrease flow of solute into the renal medulla. Even with maximum permeability of the renal collecting duct, the reduced medullary tonicity limits the increment of urinary osmolality to a value no higher than the tonicity of the renal medulla (29, 32).

Table 1. Potential causes of increased release of AVP during surgery and anesthesia

---
Stress
Pain
Incision of the skin
Abdominal compression
Visceral traction
Changes in serum osmolality
Hemorrhage
Positive pressure breathing
Hypoxia
Hypercapnia
Adrenergic stimulation
Vagal stimulation

Following surgery the plasma levels of AVP return to normal within 24 hours in many cases, but may be elevated for several days in others (24).

Decreasing renal blood flow, and increased aldosterone and AVP secretion, all probably contribute to sodium and water retention in the perioperative period. Other factors that may contribute to sodium and water retention include surgical trauma of surrounding tissue, and of vasculature and cavity linings, in addition to the increased intracellular sodium and water (33–36). Fortunately, this period of sodium and water retention lasts only 3–4 days and is usually followed by a modest diuresis in the uncomplicated surgical patient.

VOLUME DISORDERS

Volume depletion

Combined deficits of sodium and water occur most commonly in surgical patients (36). The potential causes of volume deficits in the surgical patient are numerous (Table 2). Frequently the presence of volume depletion can easily be established and corrected. Unfortunately, there will be occasions when the volume deficits will be less obvious. In such situations it is still very important to document and correct the deficits to avoid possible hypotension during induction of anesthesia and during the surgical procedure, and to reduce the chance of cardiac, cerebral, or renal

Table 2. Causes of intravascular volume depletion in the surgical patient

---
Vascular
Hemorrhage
Sequestration of intravascular fluid
   Crush injuries
   Soft-tissue trauma
   Hypoalbuminemia
   Intestinal obstruction
   Pancreatitis
   Peritonitis

Gastrointestinal
Decreased oral intake
Vomiting
Nasogastric suctioning
Diarrhea
Enterocutaneous fistulas/drains

Dermal
Increased body temperature
Burns
Open wounds/large avulsions

Renal
Diuretics
Chronic renal insufficiency
Nonoliguric acute renal failure
Tubulointerstitial disease
Postobstructive nephropathy
Adrenal insufficiency

---

ischemia. This is of particular importance in the elderly and in other patients with cardiovascular abnormalities.

Before correcting the volume deficit in a surgical candidate, its presence first must be established in a rational manner. This is done by making use of all available information starting with the history. Volume deficits develop because of an inadequate intake, excessive fluid loss, or a combination of these two factors. Therefore, questions within the history must address whether the patient's fluid intake has been limited. If the intake has been limited, the duration of this limitation must be determined. Likewise, questions within the history should pertain to the possibility of excessive fluid loss. If a history of excessive fluid loss is obtained, the duration of this abnormality also must be determined. Once one determines that the potential of a volume deficit exists, one must then establish its severity. This can be done to some extent by questioning (i.e., are any postural symptoms present?).

If the presence and severity of a volume deficit has been established by the history, the physical examination and other laboratory data can be utilized for further confirmation (Table 3). However, if there is some doubt, the physical examination and other laboratory data may assist in determining the presence of a volume deficit. The physician must always be aware that physical and laboratory parameters are not always specific, and there are always exceptions in interpreting physical, laboratory, and even hemodynamic data. Therefore, the physician must closely scrutinize all data in those individuals with questionable volume deficits, particularly those surgical candidates with severe preexisting renal, pulmonary, or cardiac disease.

Volume overload

Extracellular fluid excess is a less common problem in the routine surgical candidate. This entity develops because of excessive intake, inadequate fluid excretion, or a combination of the two factors. Due to the kidneys' ability to excrete large amounts of sodium and water in the normal individual, the majority of cases of intravascular volume excess will occur in individuals with a limited ability to excrete fluid. This would include mostly individuals with renal insufficiency, congestive heart failure, and patients with mineralocorticoid excess (7).

INTRAOPERATIVE FLUID MANAGEMENT

During surgery, basic fluid loss must be replaced. As simple as this may seem, the problem arises in determining the amount of fluid that is lost or sequestered from the intravascular space. Insensible water losses from perspiration in a normal individual have been estimated to be approximately 0.5 ml/kg BW/hr. Water loss by perspiration can increase considerably during the surgical procedure and can vary between 0.5 and 0.65 ml/kg BW/hr (38–42). This variability is due to a number of factors, including the patient's body temperature, the temperature and humidity of the operating room, the humidity of the anesthetic gas mixtures, the type of surgical procedure, and the size of the surgical wound. Because all of these factors vary independently, water loss is difficult to estimate (38). However, it is said that an adult loses approximately 100–150 ml water per hour during an abdominal operation of moderate length (34, 39, 40).

Exudation of fluid and protein into the field of operation is another source of volume loss. The volume of fluid loss is difficult to quantitate. The amount of fluid loss can increase markedly in patients with major soft-tissue injuries, inflammatory intestinal diseases, and in surgical patients with intestinal obstruction (38). For example, an individual with intestinal fluid obstruction may sequester as much as 6 l of fluid within the intestinal lumen (1). Fluid and protein loss can even be further compounded if surgical trauma is severe and the procedure is of long duration (38). The additional plasma loss from exudation of fluid into the peritoneal cavity in an abdominal operation of moderate duration has been estimated to be approximately 100–200 ml plasma per hour, excluding the amount that is lost directly from bleeding (34). A similar amount of plasma loss also occurs during thoracic surgical procedures (43). Despite these estimations, the amount of plasma loss that occurs in each case must be individualized.

During periods of severe shock or major trauma, displacement of fluid from the extracellular space into the intracellular space may also occur (44, 45). This assumed displacement of water and electrolytes from the extracellular to the intracellular space is accompanied by a fall in the cell membrane potential upon deterioration of the microcirculation. In the elective surgical patient without shock, fluid displacement does not occur (45, 46). An increase in water content of skeletal muscles has been noted during surgery; however, this retention probably occurs in the extracellular space (45, 47, 48). The water content may increase up to 5% during elective surgery (45, 47–49).

Table 3. Potential laboratory abnormalities exhibited in volume depletion

Serum
Hemoconcentration
  ↑ Hematocrit
  ↑ Albumin
  ↑ Ca^{2+}
Increased [HCO_3^-]
Hypokalemia
  (Hyperkalemia may exist if a non-anion gap metabolic acidosis is present)
Increased uric acid
  (In the absence of renal insufficiency or gout)
BUN/creatinine ratio > 20

Urine
↑ Specific gravity
↑ Osmolality
↓ [Na^+] (< 20 mEq/l)
↓ [Cl^-] (< 20 mEq/l)
↓ Fractional excretion of Na^+ (< 1%)

Table 4. Estimation of maintenance operative fluid replacement

Type of surgery	Extent	Fluid replacement
Neurosurgical	Moderate	150–200 ml/hr
Skeletomuscular	Moderate	150–200 ml/hr
Abdominal	Moderate	250–300 ml/hr
Thoracic		450–550 ml/hr
Thoracoabdominal		450–550 ml/hr
Example: Moderate surgery		
Basal perspiration		35 ml/hr
Extra perspiration from wound		25 ml/hr
Estimated urine output		50 ml/hr
Estimate exudation		25 ml/hr
Total		135 ml/hr
Example: Extensive surgery		
Basal perspiration		30 ml/hr
Extra perspiration from wound		125 ml/hr
Urine		40 ml/hr
Estimated exudation in wound		150 ml/hr
Fluid displacement to the extracellular space (5% of extracellular volume in 4 hours)		160 ml/hr
Total		505 ml/hr

Under typical situations fluid may be replaced with a 5% dextrose solution of Ringer's lactate or 5% dextrose solution of one-half normal saline. Blood losses are replaced separately.
Adapted from Thoren L (38).

In determining the amount of fluid that should be replaced during the procedure, the physican must visualize the amount of fluid loss that is occurring. This would include measurement of the output or urine and drains, an estimate of insensible fluid losses from perspiration and exudation, and the amount of sequestered fluid (Table 4).

Plasma and protein replacement

There is usually no need for plasma infusion until plasma loss from bleeding or transudation exceeds 50% of the patient's original blood volume. This is because of the increase in the acute phase proteins occurring within 6–12 hours following operative trauma (50–52). If the serum protein level or colloid osmotic pressure within the intravascular space is allowed to decrease to a point below that in the interstitial space, efflux of fluid from the capillary space into the interstitium would occur. A critical colloid osmotic pressure of 20 mmHg was originally derived from the calculations of Wiederheilm, who also suggested that a decrease of the colloid osmotic pressure by 10 mmHg would be associated with a fluid retention of 5000 ml in the average 70-kg patient (53). If facilities for direct measurement of the colloid osmotic pressure are not available, it can be estimated from the total serum protein within a standard deviation of +3 mmHg by the simple formula:

Colloid oncotic pressure in mmHg = (TSP in g/dl × 4) − 0.8

Thus, a colloid osmotic pressure (COP) of 20 mmHg would be equivalent to having a total serum protein concentration of 5 g/dl (52).

Because approximately 75% of Ringer's lactate or normal saline moves into the interstitial space when given intravenously, four times the amount of calculated blood loss must be given to totally replenish the intravascular space. This could lead to marked edema, which is predominantly located in the skin, subcutaneous tissue, and muscle. Thus, colloids should be administered with crystalloids if blood loss or transfusion requirements exceed 50% of the patient's original blood volume (38).

There have also been attempts to resuscitate patients with moderate blood volume deficits with hypertonic crystalloids. Patients receiving these solutions required a third less volume than individuals that received resuscitation with Ringer's lacatate. Limiting factors for the administration of hypertonic sodium lactate solutions include hypernatremia, hyperosmolality, hypochloremia, and hypokalemia (54). Despite these limitations, investigators have noted improved cardiac function and lowered vascular resistance (55–58). Also, animals in shock receiving hypertonic solutions have been shown to have a better

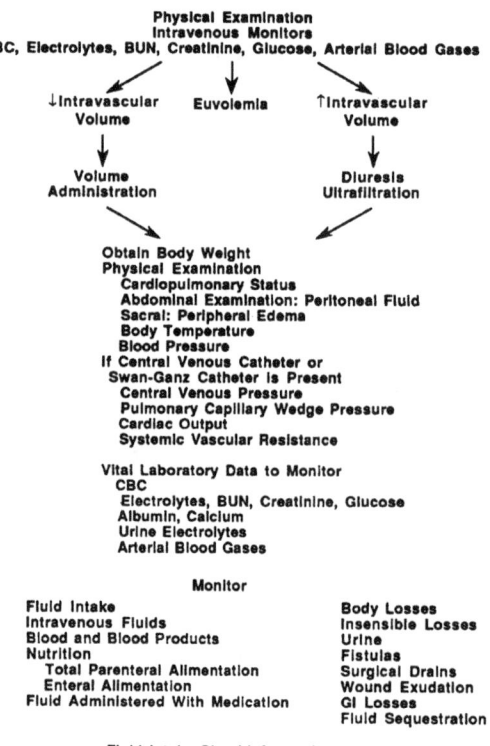

Figure 1. Fluid management during the postoperative period.

survival than animals resuscitated with either Ringer's lactate or normal saline (58–60). Further investigation must be done before hypertonic saline solutions can be used as an established method of blood volume resuscitation in the intraoperative patient.

FLUID MANAGEMENT IN THE POSTOPERATIVE PERIOD

In many patients postoperative fluid management is the most critical period of fluid management in the surgical patient. Fortunately, the majority of elective surgical patients have no major fluid abnormalities postoperatively. This may not be the case in many patients with renal or cardiac abnormalities, hemodynamic instability, or other major medical problems. However, even the most complex cases can be handled easily if approached in an organized manner and monitored closely (Figure 1). The initial step is to determine the patient's fluid balance and the intravascular volume status at the end of the operative procedure. Critically ill patients who have cardiac dysfunction, pulmonary diseases with high pulmonary artery pressure, renal insufficiency, or excessive sequestration of body fluids may temporarily require placement of a Swan–Ganz catheter for optimum fluid management. Fluid losses, including insensible loss and fluid intake, must be monitored closely. Adjustments in fluid administration may have to be made several times per day in complicated surgical cases.

ELECTROLYTE ABNORMALITIES IN THE PERIOPERATIVE PERIOD

Electrolyte disturbances during the perioperative period may lead to serious dysfunction of all major organ systems. If these disturbances are severe enough they may even lead to the death of the surgical patient. In this section, we will discuss the various abnormalities of sodium, potassium, calcium, magnesium, and phosphorus, and also the management of these abnormalities.

Sodium

Sodium is the major cation of extracellular fluid. Sodium and its accompanying anions account for roughly 90% of the osmolality of this compartment. It is also the quantity of this ion in the extracellular fluid compartment that determines an individual's volume status. The serum sodium concentration per se is not an indicator of the quantity of sodium within the body, but only an indicator of the amount of sodium in 1 l of solution. The amount of extracellular fluid volume is an indicator of the total amount of exchangeable sodium within the body.

HYPONATREMIA

Hyponatremia is loosely defined as a serum sodium concentration of less than 130 mEq/l. Hyponatremia may occur in the presence of volume contraction, volume expansion, or euvolemia (Figure 2). Hyponatremia in the presence of volume contraction is an indication of sodium loss in excess of water loss. The loss may be either from renal or nonrenal sources. The presence of excess renal loss of sodium may be determined by demonstrating excess sodium loss in the urine. A urinary sodium concentration of greater than 20 mEq/l in the presence of volume contraction reflects excessive renal sodium wasting by the kidneys. Possible causative factors would be diuretics, sodium-losing nephropathies, mineralocorticoid deficiency, osmotic diuresis, and bicarbonaturia (61, 62). Hyponatremia resulting from diuretics excess is common and is most often due to the thiazides. Diuretics may cause hyponatremia by one of several mechanisms, including increased antidiuretic hormone release (63), having a direct effect on the diluting segments of the nephron (64), and potassium depletion (65).

Urine sodium concentration less than 20 mEq/l in the presence of volume contraction indicates that the renal tubular function is intact and the source of sodium loss must have been extrarenal. Examples include gastrointestinal losses such as vomiting and diarrhea, and those related to sequestration of fluid (i.e., burns, peritonitis, pancreatitis, and intestinal obstruction) (37).

Hyponatremia in the presence of volume expansion depicts an increase in the total body sodium content with an even greater increase in total body water. These patients usually have edema and clinical findings indicative of volume excess. Causes of hyponatremia in this setting include nephrosis, cirrhosis, cardiac failure, and acute and chronic renal failure (Figure 2). Hyponatremia in the presence of euvolemia reflects a normal total body sodium content in the presence of excess total body water. Possible causes include states associated with increased ADH release, antidiuretic drugs, hypothyroidism, hypokalemia, glucocorticoid deficiency, psychosis, and chronic disease (26, 37, 61).

The central nervous system is the organ system affected most by hyponatremia. Symptoms may be nonexistent or include confusion, coma, and convulsion. Symptoms depend on the severity of hyponatremia and the rapidity in which the derangement developed. Symptoms usually do not occur unless the serum sodium is less than 120 mEq/l. The management of hyponatremia is dependent on several factors, including the volume status, the rapidity in which hyponatremia develops, and the presence of symptoms (66, 67).

In addition to being aware of the different causes of hyponatremia, the physician should also be aware of pseudohyponatremia. When this situation exists the serum sodium is not a true indicator of total body water content. Pseudohyponatremia may be found in the presence of hyperglycemia, hyperproteinemia, hypertriglyceridemia, and in the presence of increased blood glycine and mannitol (37).

HYPERNATREMIA

Hypernatremia exists when there is a deficit of total body free water (Figure 3). Like hyponatremia, hypernatremia

268 *Therapy of Renal Diseases and Related Disorders*

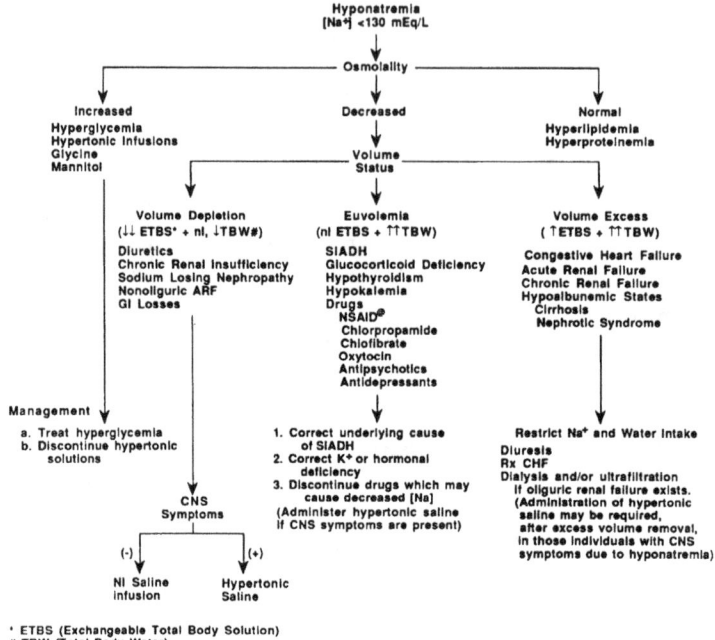

Figure 2. Diagnosis and management of hyponatremia during surgery.

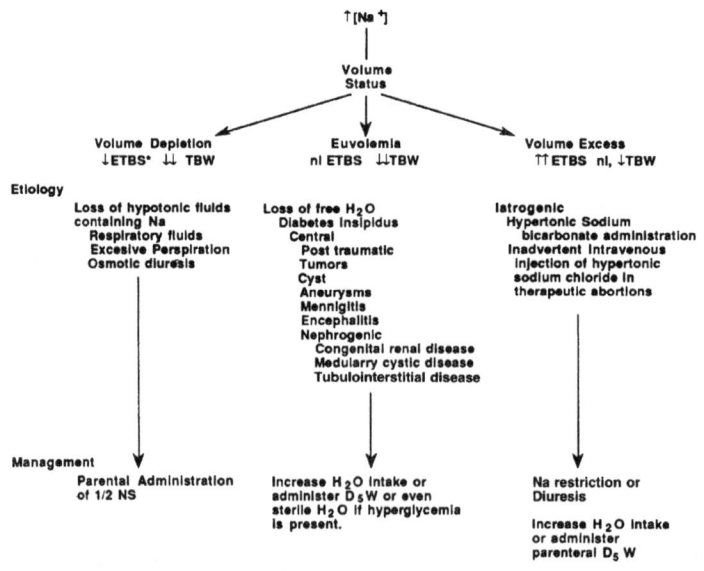

Figure 3. An approach to hypernatremia.

may exist in the presence of volume contraction, volume expansion, and euvolemia. Hypernatremia in the presence of volume contraction reflects a total body water deficit in excess of a total body sodium deficit. This is due to loss of hypotonic fluids from the body. Major sources of hypotonic fluid loss include excessive insensible fluid loss from sweating or hyperventilation, and increased water loss associated with osmotic diuresis (Figure 3). Hypernatremia occurring in the face of volume expansion indicates excess sodium retention in the presence of total body water depletion. Causative factors are most often iatrogenic and include the excessive administration of hypertonic solutions of sodium and excessive replacement of hypotonic fluid loss with isotonic saline solution (Figure 3). Hypernatremia in the presence of euvolemia usually reflects a total body water deficit in the face of a normal total body sodium content. This frequently occurs as a result of a deficiency of ADH release or a loss of ADH function within the kidney (37).

Also, as in hyponatremia, clinical signs reflecting hypernatremia generally involve the central nervous system. Hypernatremia that develops acutely causes cellular dehydration and vascular traction, resulting in intracerebral hemorrhage, thrombosis, confusion, coma, and seizures. When hypernatremia is chronic, central nervous system findings are not as frequent, because of the production of idiogenic osmoles that act as intracellular solutes that counteract neuronal dehydration (68). Management of hypernatremia is dependent on the etiology and volume status of the individual (Figure 3).

Potassium

Each liter of intracellular water contains approximately 150 mEq of potassium, and each liter of extracellular fluid contains approximately 4.5 mEq. The sodium-potassium pumps located within the cellular membrane maintain this gradient between the intracellular fluid and extracellular fluid compartments, thus preventing fatal hyperkalemia (37, 69, 70). Even though the serum potassium concentration is used to assess total body potassium stores, 98% of the total body potassium is actually located intracellularly (69).

HYPOKALEMIA

Hypokalemia may develop in the presence of normal or depleted potassium stores. Hypokalemia occurring in the presence of normal potassium stores reflects translocation of potassium from the extracellular space into the intracellular space. This may be caused by a variety of hormones, drugs, and metabolic disturbances (37, 69–74) (Figure 4).

Hypokalemia that results from potassium depletion occurs secondary to renal losses of potassium or extrarenal losses of potassium. There are numerous causes of both renal and extrarenal losses of potassium (Figure 4). Even though renal conservation of potassium is not as efficient as sodium conservation, renal excretion of potassium may be reduced to less than 20 mEq/day in depleted states by normal functioning kidneys. Therefore, the urinary excre-

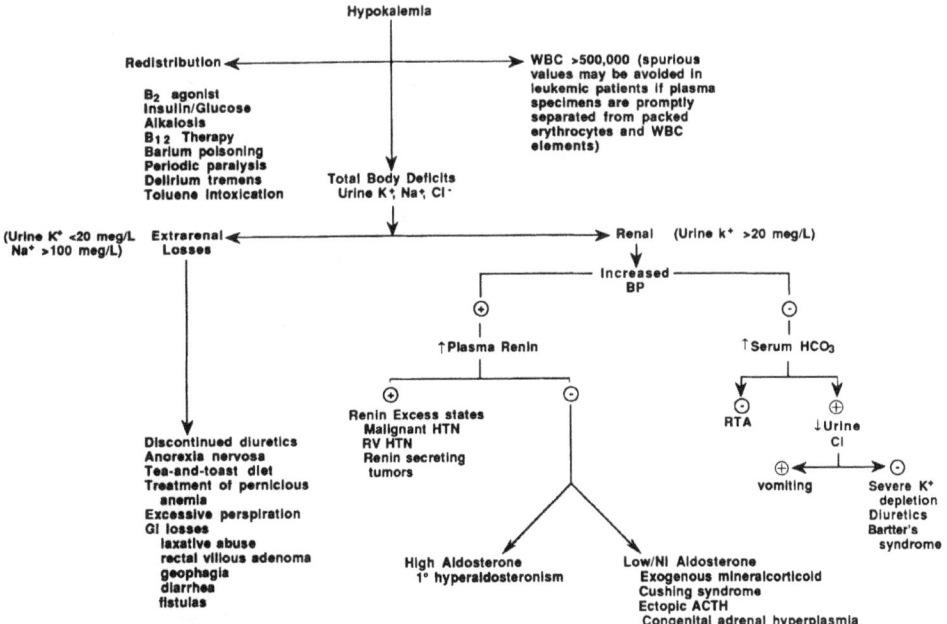

Figure 4. An approach to hypokalemia.

tion of potassium may be used to help differentiate the cause of potassium depletion. To appropriately interpret the urinary excretion of potassium, the patient must be taking a substantial amount of sodium (at least 100 mEq/day).

The clinical manifestations of hypokalemia are numerous, with the most important being neuromuscular and cardiac abnormalities. Practically every major organ system is affected if hypokalemia is severe (Table 5). In patients with potassium depletion, the clinical problems associated with hypokalemia will be more prominent if acute intracellular translocation of potassium occurs (62, 75, 76). Hypokalemia has been stated to be present if serum potassium is 3 mEq/l or less. Recent studies have indicated that moderate chronic hypokalemia (K^+ = 2.6 –3.4 mEq/l) is not associated with an increased incidence of intraoperative arrhythmias (77), however, this may not be the case in an individual receiving digitalis therapy or in one who has a prior history of cardiac arrhythmias (62). Treatment of hypokalemia focuses on replacement. The amount of potassium that is administered depends on whether hypokalemia results from intracellular translocation or whether the patient has acute or chronic potassium depletion. An individual who has a chronic reduction of serum potassium of 1.0 mEq/l may have a total body potassium deficit of 600 mEq (76). Oral potassium supplementation should be sufficient in those patients with mild-to-moderate hypokalemia. Intravenous potassium supplementation should be utilized in severe cases of hypokalemia. In such situations the serum potassium and electrocardiogram should be monitored closely (78).

HYPERKALEMIA

Hyperkalemia may result from either total body potassium excess or redistribution of potassium from the intracellular space to the extracellular space. Spurious hyperkalemia or pseudohyperkalemia is a laboratory artifact that develops from leukocytosis ($5 \times 10^5/mm^3$), thrombocytosis ($7.5 \times 10^5/mm^3$), test tube hemolysis, or ischemic blood drawing. Potassium is released from white blood cells and platelets when blood clots. When marked leukocytosis or thrombocytosis exists, the elevation of serum potassium will be substantial. Because this is a laboratory artifact, no direct harm comes to the patient. These disorders may be distinguished by comparing serum and plasma potassium levels from the same blood sample (37).

As noted earlier, potassium is the major intracellular cation, with less than 2% of the total body potassium contained within the extracellular space. Fatal hyperkalemia may develop if as little as 1.5% of the intracellular potassium is redistributed to the extracellular space. The major causes of redistribution hyperkalemia include mineral acidosis, tissue necrosis, hemolysis, hyperglycemia, periodic paralysis, and drugs (Table 6) (37).

Increased total body potassium may result from excessive potassium intake, limited potassium excretion, or from a combination of the two. Excessive administration of potassium as a sole cause of hyperkalemia is uncommon and is most often iatrogenic when it does occur. Excessive administration of potassium more commonly leads to hyperkalemia in the presence of renal or endocrine ab-

Table 5. Clinical symptoms of hypokalemia

Neuromuscular
Gastrointestinal
    Constipation
    Ileus
Musculoskeletal
    Weakness
    Cramps
    Tetany
    Paralysis
    Rhabdomyolysis
Cardiac
    Digitalis intoxication
    Electrocardiographic changes
    Ventricular ectopy
Renal
    Polyuria/polydipsia
    Metabolic alkalosis
Endocrine
    Carbohydrate intolerance

Table 6. Causes of hyperkalemia

Laboratory artifact
Spurious
    Ischemic venipuncture   Infectious mononucleosis
    Hemolysis   Leukocytosis (WBC > 500,000)
        Thrombocytosis
Normal total body potassium
Redistribution
    B_2 antagonist   Mineral acidosis
    Hyperglycemia   Arginine HCl
    Succinylcholine   Digitalis intoxication
    Fluoride intoxication   Barium poisoning
    Tissue necrosis   Tumor lysis
    Rhabdomyolysis   Periodic paralysis
    Postparathyroidectomy (in the hemodialysis patient)
Excess total body potassium
Increased intake
    Iatrogenic excess K^+ Suicidal attempts with oral K^+
    administration
Decreased renal excretion (GFR < 20 cc/min)
Distal (Type IV) RTA
    Tubulointerstitial disease   Diabetic nephropathy
    Post-transplantation   Obstructive nephropathy
        Lupus nephropathy
Mineralocorticoid defects
    Addison's disease
Drugs
    Angiotensin-converting   Beta blockers
      enzyme inhibitors   Methyldopa
    Nonsteroidal   Cyclosporin
      antiinflammatory   Heparin
      drugs
        Potassium-sparing diuretic
Decreased renal perfusion states
    Severe volume depletion in the elderly or in individuals with marked congestive heart failure

normalities that limit the excretion of potassium. The abnormalities that limit potassium excretion generally fall into one of three categories: limited potassium excretion resulting from severe renal insufficiency, syndromes that result in diminished mineralocorticoid activity, and conditions that limit potassium and hydrogen secretion by the distal tubules (37, 78).

Hyperkalemia may impair myocardial contractility, decrease cardiac conduction and automaticity, and cause hypoventilation (62). These abnormalities are more severe if hyperkalemia develops rapidly. A safe upper limit for the serum potassium concentration has not been defined, but a concentration of 5.5 mEq/l has been considered acceptable. Intraoperative succinylcholine, potassium-containing intravenous solutions, and hypoventilation should, therefore, be avoided if the serum potassium concentration is greater than 5.5 mEq/l.

The management of hyperkalemia is dependent on its severity and the presence of electrocardiographic abnormalities. Calcium salts should be used to aid in the correction of diminished myocardial contractility, heart block, ventricular fibrillation, or other electrocardiographic abnormalities caused by hyperkalemia. If heart block is severe or if asystole exists, a temporary pacemaker may be required. Despite the beneficial effects calcium has on the heart in the setting of hyperkalemia, the serum potassium is not reduced. The serum potassium may be reduced by redistributing the potassium intracellularly with the use of glucose-insulin and/or sodium bicarbonate. Potassium may then be removed from the body with potassium exchange resins or dialysis (79).

Calcium

Calcium is the fifth most abundant inorganic element of the body and is the principal component of the human skeleton. Calcium plays a vital role in neuromuscular function, blood coagulation, membrane function, and multiple enzyme reactions (80). The control of blood calcium is dependent on exquisitely sensitive homeostatic mechanisms involving parathyroid hormone and analogues of vitamin D, and their action on bone, intestine, and the kidney (80). The normal total serum calcium concentration is 8.5–10.5 mg/100 ml, and the normal serum ionized concentration is 4.25–5.25 mg/dl. Fifty percent of the serum calcium is bound to plasma protein, 5% is bound to other anions, and the remaining 45% is ionized and free. It is the ionized fraction that is physiologically active.

HYPOCALCEMIA

Hypoalbuminemia is probably the most common cause of decreased total serum calcium. Because each g/dl of albumin binds approximately 0.8 mg/dl of calcium, the product of 0.8 and the decrement of serum albumin yields the component of hypocalcemia caused by protein depletion. In this setting the physiologically active ionized fraction is not altered.

True hypocalcemia results from decreased bone resorption, decreased intestinal absorption, and calcium sequestration. Decreased bone resorption may be seen in the surgical patient who has renal failure, hypomagnesemia, and also in patients following parathyroidectomy or thyroidectomy. The decreased bone resorption in these individuals is due to either a deficiency of parathyroid hormone or parathyroid hormone resistance. PTH deficiency is most often noted following parathyroid or thyroid surgery. Hypocalcemia following parathyroidectomy usually recovers after a variable period of time, depending on the extent of the surgery and the amount of demineralization of bone prior to surgery. Serum calcium levels may drastically drop immediately following surgery as a result of decreased PTH and the increased uptake of calcium by "hungry bones." The degree of hypoparathyroidism may be estimated 5 days postparathyroidectomy. Serum calcium levels of less than 6 mg/dl at this point suggest permanent hypoparathyroidism. A persistently low PTH level following surgery is also another indicator of hypoparathyroidism (81).

Decreased intestinal absorption of calcium in the surgical patient will most often be secondary to decreased levels of vitamin D and its analogues. Vitamin D malabsorption may be noted in individuals with short bowel syndromes. Calcifediol (25-OH vitamin D) deficiency may occur in individuals with severe liver disease or in those who are taking anticonvulsants. Individuals with renal insufficiency will have decreased calcitriol [$1,25$-$(OH)_2$ vitamin D]. Sequestration of calcium by the formation of calcium soaps in areas of fat necrosis may be noted in individuals with acute pancreatitis. Hyperphosphatemia caused by phosphate ingestion, phosphate enemas, or rhabdomyolysis may lead to severe hypocalcemia because of the precipitation of calcium-phosphate complexes (80, 81).

The clinical presentation of hypocalcemia depends both on its degree and duration. Clinical manifestation of hypocalcemia primarily involves the neuromuscular and cardiovascular systems. The individual exhibiting neuromuscular abnormalities may have hyperactive deep reflexes, positive Chvostek's and Trousseau's signs, muscle cramps, increased irritability, and even seizures. These clinical findings may be further potentiated in the presence of respiratory alkalosis or hypomagnesemia. Acute and chronic hypocalcemia may disturb cardiac function. Acute hypocalcemia may cause hypotension, congestive heart failure, and even ventricular fibrillation. The classic electrocardiographic findings include prolongation of the QT interval, which causes lengthening of the ST segment.

Treatment of hypocalcemia depends on the severity of the abnormality. Mild hypocalcemia may be treated with oral calcium supplements. However, in individuals with severe acute hypocalcemia, intravenous calcium therapy is indicated. One to two ampules of calcium gluconate (10 ml of a 10% solution) should be initially administered over 5 minutes each. This should be followed by a slow infusion of calcium gluconate (1 mg/ml of 5% dextrose in water at 75–100 ml/hr). Patients taking a digitalis preparation should undergo ECG monitoring to avoid digitalis toxicity (80).

HYPERCALCEMIA

The disorders associated with hypercalcemia are numerous (Table 7). The predominant cause of hypercalcemia is hyperparathyroidism, which is estimated to be present in 55% of patients of all ages with hypercalcemia. However, when only older age groups are considered, malignancy may predominate as a cause of hypercalcemia (80).

The clinical manifestations of hypercalcemia are numerous and variable. The severity of the manifestations is dependent on the rate of development of hypercalcemia. Most of the neuropsychiatric/neuromuscular, cardiovascular, and many of the gastrointestinal abnormalities (nausea, vomiting, and anorexia) are noted more often with acute elevations of calcium. Individuals with prolonged elevations may have vascular calcifications, nephrocalcinosis, nephrolithiasis, constipation, duodenal ulcers, weight loss, and skeletal and dermatologic abnormalities.

Diagnostic evaluation should first include a thorough history and physical examination to elicit a history that suggests an associated disorder (i.e., malignancy, renal failure, hyperthyroidism, drugs, etc.). The initial laboratory data should include determinations of serum calcium, phosphorus, alkaline phosphatase, albumin, and total protein. Hypophosphatemia and a chloride: phosphate ratio of greater than 33 is supporting evidence for hyperparathyroidism (81). An elevated alkaline phosphatase in conjunction with a negative roentgenographic evaluation for osteitis fibrosa would suggest malignancy. Radioimmunoassays of PTH may also be obtained to further establish the presence of hyperparathyroidism. The urinary cyclic AMP/creatinine ratio may also be helpful in differentiating various causes of hypercalcemia. The evaluation of hypercalcemia should also include appropriate radiographs.

Treatment of hypercalcemia is dependent on the underlying cause of hypercalcemia and its severity. If hypercalcemia is mild it may be corrected by treating the underlying disease plus the use of oral phosphates, if renal insufficiency is not present. Hypercalcemia of greater severity may require parenteral isotonic saline administration and loop diuretics. Refractory cases of severe hypercalcemia may require calcitonin, cortisone, mithramycin, diphosphonates, and even intravenous sodium EDTA for severely symptomatic individuals with impending cardiac arrest. Hypercalcemia in patients with oliguric renal failure or congestive heart failure may also be corrected by hemodialysis with a low-calcium dialysate (82).

Table 7. Causes of hypercalcemia

I. *Hypercalcemia with inappropriate PTH secretion*
   Primary hyperparathyroidism
     Sporadic
     Hereditary
       Multiple endocrine neoplasia I and II
       Isolated adult hereditary hyperparathyroidism
       Familial hypocalciuric hypercalcemia
   Tertiary hyperparathyroidism
     Malabsorption
     Chronic renal failure
     Post-renal transplant hypercalcemia
   Lithium-associated hyperparathyroidism
   Acute renal failure
   Nonparathyroid malignancies producing PTH
II. *Excessive production of 1,25-dihydroxyvitamin D*
   Granulomatous disorders (sarcoid, tuberculosis, berylliosis, histoplasmosis, coccidiomycosis)
   Lymphomas
   Hypophosphatemia
III. *Excessive skeletal mobilization of calcium*
   Neoplastic production of prostaglandin
   Neoplastic production of osteoclast activating factor
   Humoral hypercalcemia of malignancy
   Direct osteolysis by neoplasm
   Thyrotoxicosis
   Immobilization
IV. *Excessive intestinal absorption of calcium*
   Vitamin D toxicity
   Milk-alkali syndrome
V. *Defective renal excretion*
   Extracellular volume depletion
   Thiazide diuretics
   Milk-alkali syndrome

Magnesium

Magnesium is predominantly an intracellular cation and participates in many membrane enzymatic functions. The serum magnesium concentration is maintained in a range of 1.4–2.0 mEq/l. Approximately 20–35% of plasma magnesium is bound to protein, with the remainder present in a diffusible form that is predominantly ionized magnesium (83, 85). The serum magnesium concentration is the result of a balance between gastrointestinal absorption, soft-tissue deposition, bone deposition/mobilization, and renal reabsorption and excretion (37, 84).

HYPOMAGNESEMIA

Excessive Mg^{2+} losses in the urine and the gastrointestinal tract, bone sequestration, and prolonged dietary restriction may lead to hypomagnesemia (Table 8). In addition to the above, approximately 25–35% of individuals with acute pancreatitis may also develop severe hypomagnesemia. These individuals are believed to develop hypomagnesemia as a result of Mg^{2+} soap formation in areas of fat necrosis around the inflamed pancreas. Many individuals with acute pancreatitis may also have chronic alcoholism. Chronic alcoholism may lead to hypomagnesemia by one of several mechanisms, including starvation and increased intestinal and urinary loss. Chronic alcoholism will be the most common associated problem in the hypomagnesemic surgical patient. Hypomagnesemia may also become evident following surgical correction of hyperparathyroidism in patients with osteitis fibrosis (37). Hypomagnesemia as a result of renal losses may be differentiated from other

Table 8. Hypomagnesemia

Extrarenal causes of hypomagnesemia (< 1–2 mEq/day)
Gastrointestinal losses
    Malabsorption
    Diarrhea
    Alcoholism
    Laxative abuse
Increased bone uptake
    Postparathyroidectomy (hungry bone syndrome)
Decreased intake
    Hyperalimentation
    Starvation

Renal causes of hypomagnesemia (urinary Mg 3–5 mEq/day)
Hyperaldosteronism
SIADH
Diabetic ketoacidosis
Recovery phase of ATN
Aminoglycoside nephrotoxicity
Cisplatinum nephropathy
Loop diuretics
Post-renal obstruction
Phosphate depletion
Hypercalcemia
Alcoholism
Cyclosporin

causes by quantitating 24-hour urine magnesium. Individuals with nonrenal causes of hypomagnesemia should be able to lower their 24-hour urinary excretion to less than 1–2 mEq/day.

Clinical manifestations of hypomagnesemia are mainly neuromuscular and behavioral abnormalities that are very similar to those that are found in hypocalcemia. In addition to this, frank hypocalcemia may be caused by hypomagnesemia. Hypomagnesemia may inhibit the secretion of PTH from the parathyroid gland and may also impair the skeletal response to PTH. Electrocardiographic changes may also occur and include prolongation of the QT interval, decreased amplitude of the T waves, and shortening of the ST segment.

Severe hypomagnesemia may be associated with deficits of 1–2 mEq/kg of body weight. Parenteral magnesium sulfate is usually available as $MgSO_4 \cdot 7 H_2O$. The molecular weight of dehydrated $MgSO_4$ is 246.5 and each gram of salt contains 8.12 mEq of Mg^{2+}; 50 mEq of Mg^{2+} may be given intravenously over 4–6 hours. Intravenous administration should not exceed 100 mEq in a 12-hour period. As an alternative, intravenous administration of $MgSO_4$ may also be given every 2–4 hours in a dose of 16 mEq on the first day of therapy. Magnesium replacement will have to be markedly reduced in patients with renal insufficiency. Careful monitoring of magnesium levels and reflexes is necessary to avoid Mg^{2+} toxicity. The heart rate, respiration, blood pressure, and electrocardiogram will also have to be monitored in patients with renal insufficiency or in those receiving parenteral replacement. Following the repletion of the Mg^{2+} deficit, Mg^{2+} balance may be maintained with the administration of as little as 4 mEq of Mg^{2+} per day. In patients receiving gastric suction, or in those receiving prolonged intravenous fluid therapy, as much as 10–15 mEq of Mg^{2+} per day may be required to maintain adequate Mg^{2+} stores (84, 85).

HYPERMAGNESEMIA

Hypermagnesemia is rarely seen in the perioperative period, particularly in patients with a GFR that exceeds 30 ml/min. But, it may occur in patients with renal insufficiency who are taking Mg^{2+}-containing antacids or laxatives. Hypermagnesemia can also be seen in patients with massive trauma, burns, and in the parturient during treatment of eclampsia (1, 37).

The clinical manifestations of hypermagnesemia are mainly neuromuscular and cardiovascular. Loss of deep tendon reflexes usually occurs when plasma levels exceed 6 mEq/l. Marked sedation, coma, respiratory paralysis, hypotension, and cardiac conduction abnormalities may occur when plasma levels exceed 10 mEq/l (85). The electrocardiographic changes are similar to those found in hyperkalemia, i.e., peaked T waves, widened QRS complex, and depressed ST segments.

Management of hypermagnesemia is dependent on the severity. Intravenous calcium salts may be administered to immediately reduce the toxic effects of hypermagnesemia if the patient is symptomatic. The administration of parenteral saline solution followed by the use of loop diuretics increases the renal excretion of magnesium in those individuals who have adequate renal function. Hemodialysis or peritoneal dialysis will have to be utilized to remove magnesium from the body in those individuals with inadequate renal function (86).

Phosphorus

The human body contains 320 mM of phosphorus/kg body weight (9.9 gm/kg body weight) (37). Eighty percent of the total body phosphorus is contained in bone, 9% in skeletal muscle, and the remainder is located in the viscera and extracellular fluid. Phosphate homeostasis is dependent on gastrointestinal absorption and secretion, renal tubular reabsorption, and transcellular distribution. The maintenance of appropriate phosphate homeostasis is necessary because of the major role that phosphorus plays in intermediary metabolism (37).

Routine measurements of serum phosphorus in clinical laboratories have revealed that hypophosphatemia is a common problem among hospitalized patients (87). The occurrence of hypophosphatemia may be even more frequent in surgical patients (88). The causes of hypophosphatemia are numerous, but usually fall into three categories, which include: decreased dietary intake and intestinal absorption, intracellular shifts, and increased urinary excretion. Despite the great number of causes of hypophosphatemia, the number of entities that may lead to severe hypophosphatemia (phosphorus 1.5 mg/dl) is limited (Table 9) (87, 88). Severe hypophosphatemia is most prevalent in patients in the surgical intensive care units and on the general surgical wards. Several factors could potentially lead to severe hypophosphatemia in the surgical

Table 9. Causes of severe hypophosphatemia

Chronic alcoholism and alcohol withdrawal
Dietary deficiency and phosphate-binding antacids
Severe thermal burns
Sepsis
Recovery from diabetic ketoacidosis
Hyperalimentation
Nutritional recovery syndrome
Respiratory alkalosis
Therapeutic hyperthermia
Renal transplantation

patient and include chronic alcoholism, intravenous glucose administration, hyperalimentation without adequate phosphorus supplementation, sepsis, and respiratory alkalosis. In a recent study the most common cause of hypophosphatemia in surgical patients was intravenous glucose administration, followed by sepsis (88). In the individuals with hypophosphatemia related to sepsis, all but one individual had gram-negative sepsis (88). Sepsis may result in hypophosphatemia by possibly two mechanisms: The first is respiratory alkalosis and the second is a direct effect that the endotoxins may have in reducing serum phosphorus (88–90).

Clinical manifestations of hypophosphatemia are usually not apparent until the serum phosphorus concentration falls below 1 mg/100 ml. Clinical manifestations include deranged myocardial performance (91), precipitation of acute respiratory failure (92, 93), hemolytic anemia (94, 95), myopathy (96), depressed leukocyte function (97), thrombocytopenia (97, 98), seizures, and coma (96, 99). Treatment consists of oral phosphate replacement and, for those unable to take oral therapy, 20 mEq of KH_2PO_4 may be given for every 100 kcal supplied by parenteral nutrition (1).

HYPERPHOSPHATEMIA

Hyperphosphatemia is most frequently seen in the presence of renal insufficiency, but may also be seen in severe trauma and crush injuries, lactic acidosis, tissue ischemia, and hemolysis (87, 96). The consequences of hyperphosphatemia include depression of serum calcium and the predisposition to metastatic calcification of soft tissue. Hyperphosaphatemia may be treated with phosphate-binding antacids and dialysis in those patients with severe renal insufficiency.

CONCLUSION

In this chapter we have discussed the volume changes that occur in the uncomplicated surgical patient and also those fluid and electrolyte abnormalities that may occur during the preoperative, operative, and post-operative period. It was our intent to present this information in a format that will lead to the early recognition of fluid and electrolyte abnormalities so that the management of these disturbances will be more efficient.

REFERENCES

1. Altman M, Suki WN: Preoperative fluid management of the surgical patient. In MH Maxwell, CR Kleeman, RG Narins, eds, *Clinical Disorders of Fluid and Electrolyte Metabolism.* McGraw-Hill, New York, pp 897–916, 1987.
2. Pringle H, Maunsell CB, Pringle S: Clinical effects of ether anaesthesia on renal activity. *B Med J* 11:542–543, 1905.
3. Hardy JD: Role of adrenal cortex in postoperative retention of salt and water. *Ann Surg* 132:189–197, 1950.
4. Llaurado JG, Woodruff MF: Postoperative transient aldosteronism. *Surgery* 42:313–322, 1957.
5. Le Quesne LP, Lewis AAG: Postoperative water and sodium retention. *Lancet* 1:153–158, 1953.
6. Dudley HF, Boling EA, Le Quesne LP, et al: Studies on antidiuresis in surgery: Effects of anesthesia, surgery and posterior pituitary antidiuretic hormone on water metabolism in man. *Ann Surg* 140:354–365, 1954.
7. Haas M, Glick SM: Radioimmunoassayable plasma vasopressin associated with surgery. *Arch Surg* 113:579–600, 1978.
8. Miyazaki M, Muranishi Y, Yokonos S: Anesthesia and renal function. *Jpn J Anesth* 26:497, 1977.
9. Deutsch S, Bastron RD, Peirce EG, et al.: The effects of anesthesia with thiopentone, nitrous oxide, narcotics and neuromuscular blocking drugs on renal function in normal man. *B J Anaesth* 41:807–815, 1969.
10. Gorman HM, Graythorne MWB: The effects of a new neuroleptic-analgesic agent (Innovar) on renal function in man. *Acta Anaesth Scand* 24 (Suppl):111–118, 1966.
11. Arendhorst WJ, Navar LG: Renal circulation and glomerular hemodynamics. In: RW Schrier, CW Gottschalk, eds, *Diseases of the Kidney.* Boston, Little, Brown, pp 65–117, 1988.
12. Anderson RJ, Schrier RW: Renal sodium excretion, edematous disorders, and diuretic use. In: RW Schrier, *Renal and Electrolyte Disorders.* Boston, Little, Brown, pp 79–95, 1986.
13. Habif DV, Papper EM, Fitzpatrick HF, et al.: The renal and hepatic blood flow, glomerular filtration rate and urinary output of electrolytes during cyclopropane, ether, and thiopental anesthesia, operation and the immediate postoperative period. *Surgery* 30:241–255, 1951.
14. Ariel IM, Miller F: The effects of abdominal surgery upon renal clearance. *Surgery* 28:716–728, 1950.
15. Johnson HT, Conn JW, Iob V, et al.: Postoperative salt retention and its relation to increased adrenal cortical function. *Ann Surg* 132:374–385, 1950.
16. Moore FD, Ball MR: Facts and corollaries. In FD Moore, MR Ball, eds., *The Metabolic Response to Surgery.* Springfield, Charles C. Thomas, pp 126–137, 1952.
17. Cochrane JPS: The aldosterone response to surgery and the relationship of this response to postoperative sodium retention. *Br J Surg* 65:744–747. 1978.
18. Barta E, Kuzela L, Tordova E, et al.: The blood volume and the renin-angiotensin-aldosterone system following open-heart surgery. *Resuscitation* 8:137–146, 1980.
19. Hume DM, Bell CC, Barterr F: Direct measurement of adrenal secretion during operative trauma and convalescence. *Surgery* 52:174–187, 1962.
20. Le Quesne LP, Cochrane JPS, Fieldman WR: Fluid and electrolyte disturbances after trauma: The role of adrenocortical and pituitary hormones. *Br Med Bull* 41:212–217, 1985.
21. Forrest APM, Brown DAP, Morris SA, et al.: Metabolic

response to surgery in totally adrenalectomized women. *JR Coll Surg Edinb* 3:33–35, 1957.
22. Cline TN, Cole JW, Holden WD: Demonstration of an anti-diuretic substance in the urine of post-operative patients. *Surg Gynecol Obstet* 96:674–676, 1953.
23. Eisen VD, Lewis AAG: Antidiuretic activity of human urine after surgical operation. *Lancet* 2:361–364, 1954.
24. Moran WH, Miltenberger FW, Shuayb WA, et al.: The relationship of antidiuretic hormone secretion to surgical stress. *Surgery* 56:99–107, 1964.
25. Deutsch S, Goldberg M, Dripps RD: Post-operative hyponatremia with the inappropriate release of antidiuretic hormone. *Anesthesiology* 27:250–256, 1966.
26. Schrier R, Berl T: Nonosmolar factors affecting the release and action of vasopressin. *N Engl J Med* 292:81–88; 141–143, 1975.
27. Moran WH, Zimmerman B: Mechanisms of antidiuretic hormone (ADH) control of importance to the surgical patient. *Surgery* 62:639–644, 1967.
28. Strauss MB, *Body Water in Man. The Acquisition and Maintenance of the Body Fluids*. Little, Brown, Boston, 1975.
29. Fieldman NR, Forsling ML, Le Quesne LP: The effect of vasopressin on solute and water excretion during and after surgical operations. *Ann Surg* 201:383–390, 1985.
31. Ishihara H, Ishida T, Oyama T, et al.: Effects of general anesthesia and surgery on renal function and plasma ADH levels. *Can Anaesth Soc J* 25:312–318. 1978.
32. Gullick HD, Raisz LG: Changes in renal concentrating ability associated with major surgical procedures. *N Engl J Med* 262:1309–1314, 1960.
33. Stillstrom A, Person E, Vinnars E: Postoperative water and electrolyte changes in skeletal muscle: A clinical study with three different intravenous infusions. *Acta Anaesth Scand* 31:284–288, 1987.
34. Kragelund E: Loss of fluid and blood to the peritoneal cavity during abdominal surgery. *Surgery* 69:284–287, 1971.
35. Jarnum S: Plasma protein exudation in the peritoneal cavity during laparotomy. A comparative study in partial gastrectomy and protein-losing enteropathy. *Gastroenterology* 41:107–118, 1961.
36. Shires GT, Williams J, Brown F: Acute change in extracellular fluids associated with major surgical procedures. *Ann Surg* 154:803–810, 1961.
37. Narins RG, Jones ER, Stom MC, et al.: Diagnostic strategies in disorders of fluid, electrolyte, and acid-base homeostasis. *Am J Med* 72:496–520, 1982.
38. Thoren L, Wiklund L: Intraoperative fluid therapy. *World J Surg* 7:581–589, 1983.
39. Baumber CD, Clark RG: Insensible water loss in surgical patients. *Br J Surg* 61:53–56, 1974.
40. Virtue RW, LeVine DS, Aikawa JK: Fluid shifts during the surgical period. RISA and S35 determinations following glucose, saline or lactate infusion. *Ann Surg* 163:523–528, 1966.
41. Coller FA, Maddock WG: Dehydration attendant on surgical operations. *JAMA* 99:875–880, 1932.
42. Lamke LO, Nilsson GE: Water loss by evaporation from abdominal cavity during surgery. *Acta Chir Scand* 143:279–284, 1977.
43. Wranne B: Cardiovascular function after pulmonary surgery. Anesthesia in thoracic surgery. *Int Anaesthesiol Clin* 10:27–39, 1932.
44. Shires GT: Principle and management of hemorrhagic shock, In: GT Shires ed, *Care of the Trauma Patient*. McGraw-Hill, pp 3–51, 1979.
45. Michelsen CB, Askanazi J, Gump FE, et al.: Changes in metabolism and muscle composition associated with total hip replacement. *J Trauma* 19:29–32, 1979.
46. Elwyn DH, Bryan-Brown CW, Shoemaker DC: Nutritional aspects of body water dislocation in postoperative and depleted patients. *Ann Surg* 182:7, 1975.
47. Stjernstrom H, Jorfeldt L, Wiklund L: Influence of abdominal surgical trauma upon some energy metabolites in the quadriceps muscle in man. *Clin Physiol* 1:305–311, 1981.
48. Smith PC, Frank HA, Skillman JJ: Albumin deposition in human lung, skin and skeletal muscle during surgery. *Surg Forum* 26:91–93, 1975.
49. Shires GT: Alterations in cellular membrane function during hemorrhagic shock in primates. *Ann Surg* 176:288–295, 1972.
50. Hogman CF, Andreen M, Rosen I, et al.: Buffy coat poor red cells for improved haemotherapy. Experience with a new storage medium. *Lancet* 1(8319):269–271.
51. Kindmark CO: Sequential changes in plasma proteins in various acute diseases. In: R Bianchi, G Mariani, AS McFarlane, eds, *Plasma Protein Turnover*. The Macmillan Press, London, 1976.
52. Lundsgaard-Hansen P: Component therapy of surgical hemorrhage: Red cell concentrates, colloids and crystalloids. In: JA, Collins, P Lundsgaard-Hansen, eds, *Surgical Hemotherapy*. Bibl Haematol 46:147–169.
53. Wiederhielm CA: Dynamics of transcapillary fluid exchanges. *J Gen Physiol* 52:29, 1968.
54. Shackford SR, Fortlage DA, Peters RM, et al.: Serum osmolar and electrolyte changes associated with large infusions of hypertonic sodium lactate for intravascular volume expansion of patients undergoing aortic reconstruction. *Surg Gyn Obstet* 164:127–136, 1987.
55. Nerlich M, Gunther R, Demling RH: Resuscitation from a hemorrhagic shock with hypertonic saline or lactated Ringer's effect on the pulmonary and systemic microcirculation. *Circ Shock* 10:179–188, 1983.
56. Nakayama S, Sibley L, Gunther RA, et al.: Small-volume resuscitation with hypertonic saline (12,400 mOsm/liter) during hemorrhagic shock. *Circ Shock* 13:149–159, 1984.
57. Gazitua S, Scott JB, Chou CC, et al.: Effect of osmolarity on canine vascular resistance. *Am J Physiol* 217:1216–1223, 1969.
58. Velasco IT, Pontieri V, Silva RE, et al.: Hyperosmotic NaCl and severe hemorrhagic shock. *Am J Physiol* 239:664–674, 1980.
59. Brooks, DK, Williams WG, Manley RW, et al.: Osmolar and electrolyte changes in hemorrhagic shock. *Lancet* 1:521–527, 1963.
60. Monafo WM, Blanhe T, Dietz F: Effectiveness of hypertonic saline solutions in the treatment of murine hemorrhagic shock. *Surg Forum* 20:21–23, 1969.
61. Robertson GL, Berl T: Water metabolism. In: BM Brenner, FC Rector, eds, *The Kidney*. WB Saunders, Philadelphia, pp 408–418, 1986.
62. Stoops CG: Fluid and electrolyte disturbances in the perioperative period. *Indiana Medicine* 80:13–19, 1987.
63. Dunn FL, Brenna TJ, Nelson AE, Robertson GL: The role of blood osmolality and volume in regulating vasopressin secretion in the rat. *J Clin Invest* 52:3212–3219, 1973.
64. Suki WN, Rector FC, Seldin DW: The site of action of furosemide and other sulfonamide diuretics in the dog. *J Clin Invest* 44:1458–1469, 1965.
65. Berl T: Water metabolism in potassium depletion. *Miner Electrolyte Metab* 4:209–215, 1980.
66. Ayus JC, Olivero JJ, Frommer JP: Rapid correction of severe hyponatremia with intravenous hypertonic saline solution.

Am J Med 72:43–48, 1982.
67. Sterns RH: Severe symptomatic hyponatremia: Treatment and outcome. A study of 64 patients. *Ann Int Med* 107:656–664, 1987.
68. Humes DH: Disorders of water metabolism. In: JP Kokko, RL Tannen, eds, *Fluids and Electrolytes.* WB Saunders, Philadelphia, pp 118–149, 1986.
69. Sterns RH, Cox M, Peter UF: Internal potassium balance and control of the plasma potassium concentration. *Medicine* 60:339–354, 1981.
70. Bia MJ, DeFronzo RA: Extrarenal potassium homeostasis. *Am J Physiol* 240 (Renal, Fluid, Electrolyte Physiol 9):F257–F268, 19 .
71. Zieler KL: Effect of insulin on potassium efflux from rat muscle in the presence and absence of glucose. *Am J Physiol* 198:1066–1071, 1960.
72. Vick RL, Todd EP, Leudke DW: Epinephrine induced hypokalemia — relation to liver and skeletal muscle. *J Pharm Exp Ther* 139–141, 19 .
73. Lawson DH, Murray RM, Parker JLW: Early mortality in the megaloblastic anemia. *QJ Med* 1972; XLI (New Series):1–14, 1972.
74. Diengott D, Roza O, Levy N, Muammar S: Hypokalemia in barium poisoning. *Lancet* 11:343–345, 1964.
75. Rose RD: Potassium homeostasis. In: JE Jeffers, M La Barbera, HC De Leo, eds, *Clinical Physiology of Acid-Base and Electrolyte Disorders.* McGraw-Hill, New York, pp 211–224, 1977.
76. Knochel JP: Etiologies and management of potassium deficiency. *Hosp Prac* 22:153–162, 1987.
77. Vitez TS, Soper LE, Wong KC, et al.: Chronic hypokalemia and intraoperative dysrhythmias. *Anesthesiology* 63:130–133, 1985.
78. Batlle DC, Arruda JL, Kurtzman NA: Hyperkalemic distal renal tubular acidosis associated with obstructive uropathy. *N Engl J Med* 304:373–380, 1981.
79. Tannen RL: Potassium Disorders. In: JP Kokko, RL Tannen, eds, *Differential Diagnosis and Management of Fluid, Electrolyte, and Acid-Base Disorders,* WB Saunders, Philadelphia, pp 197–198, 1986.
80. Hughes MR, Suki WN: Hypocalcemia and hypercalcemia. In: WN Suki, SG Massry, eds, *Therapy of Renal Diseases and Related Disorders.* Martinus Nijhoff, Boston, pp 83–99, 1984.
81. Jaun D: Hypokalemia: Differential diagnosis and mechanisms. *Arch Int Med* 139:1166–1171, 1979.
82. Strauch BS, Ball MF: Hemodialysis in the treatment of severe hypercalcemia. *JAMA* 235:1347–1348, 1976.
83. Massry SG: Hypomagnesemia and hypermagnesemia. In: SG Massry, ed, *Textbook of Nephrology.* Williams & Wilkins, Baltimore, pp 3.82–3.85, 1983.
84. Sutton RL, Dirk JH: Calcium and magnesium: Renal handling and disorders of metabolism. In: BM Brenner, FC Rector, eds, *The Kidney.* WB Saunders, Philadelphia, pp 593–598, 1986.
85. Gums JG: Clinical significance of magnesium: A review. *Drug Intell Clini Pharm* 21:240–246, 1987.
86. Ferdinandus J, Pederson JA, Whang R: Hypermagnesemia as a cause of refractory hypotension, respiratory depression, and coma. *Arch Int Med* 141:669–670, 1981.
87. Knochel JP, Jacobson HR: Renal handling of phosphorus, clinical hypophosphatemia and phosphorus deficiency. In: BM Brenner, FC Rector, eds, *The Kidney.* WB Saunders, Philadelphia, pp 638–653, 1986.
88. Halevy J, Bulvik S: Severe hypophosphatemia in hospitalized patients. *Arch Int Med* 148:153–155, 1988.
89. Riedler GF, Scheitlin WA: Hypophosphatemia in septicemia. Higher incidence in gram-negative than in gram-positive infection. *Br Med J* 1:753–756, 1962.
90. Schoenfeld Y, Hager S, Berliner S, et al.: Hypophosphatemia as a diagnostic aid in sepsis. *NY State J Med* 82:163–165, 1982.
91. O'Connor LR, Wheeler WS, Bethune JE: Effect of hypophosphatemia on myocardial performance in man. *N Engl J Med* 297:901–903, 1977.
92. Newman JH, Neff TA, Ziporin P: Acute respiratory failure assoicated with hypophosphatemia. *N Engl J Med* 296:1101–1103, 1977.
93. Aubier M, Murciano D, Lecocevic Y, et al.: Effect of hypophosphatemia on diaphragmatic contractility in patients with acute respiratory failure. *N Engl J Med* 313:420–424, 1985.
94. Knochel JP: The pathophysiology and clinical characteristics of severe hypophosphatemia. *Arch Int Med* 137:203–220, 1977.
95. Klock JC, Williams HE, Mentzer WC: Hemolytic anemia and somatic cell dysfunction in severe hypophosphatemia. *Arch Int Med* 134:360–364, 1974.
96. Lau K: Phosphate disorders. In: JP Kokko, RL Tannen, eds, *Fluids and Electrolytes.* WB Saunders, Philadelphia, pp 398–458, 1986.
97. Craddock PR, Yanata Y, Van Santen L, et al.: Acquired phagocyte dysfunction: A complication of the hypophosphatemia of parenteral alimentation. *N Engl J Med* 290:1403–1407, 1974.
98. Yamata Y, Hebbel RP, Silvis S, et al.: Blood cell abnormalities complicating the hypophosphatemia of hyperalimentation: Erythrocyte and platelets ATP deficiency associated with hemolytic anemia and bleeding in hyperalimented dogs. *J Lab Clin Med* 84:623, 1974.
99. Rosen R, Leach W, Arieff A: Central nervous system dysfunction and hypophosphatemia (abstract). *Kidney Int* 12:460, 1977.

CHAPTER 17

Fluid and Electrolyte Disorders in the Thermally Injured

CHARLES BAXTER

INTRODUCTION

Thermal burns present challenging problems of fluid and electrolyte management. Initially, large volumes of isotonic solutions are required to treat and/or prevent *burn shock*. Postresuscitation management of intravascular and extravascular fluid volumes, increased water requirements, and the management of minor ions (calcium, magnesium, potassium, phosphates, etc.) require a workable understanding of the basic pathophysiology of the burn injury, the complex interaction with treatment regimens, and the differences interposed by age and concomitant disease. Approximately one third of all burn injuries (or one million patients per year) require knowledge of one or more facets of the fluid and electrolyte physiology.

The clinical course of burn injury is characterized by an initial *shock phase* produced by rapid loss of large quantities of extracellular fluid into the injured areas and a lesser loss caused by the intracellular movement of sodium and water into normal tissue cells. Adequate, prompt restoration of fluid volume deficits unveils a hyperdynamic circulatory state that results from severe hypermetabolism.

Insensible water losses through burned skin are increased fourfold to tenfold above normal, while renal handling of water is impaired by high and sustained secretion of antidiuretic hormone. The continuing adrenocortical response results in excretion of large quantities of potassium. Magnesium, calcium, zinc, and copper are either lost through the wound or are utilized in wound repair. Sustained accelerated erythrocyte destruction combined with the blood losses incurred with treatment requires frequent transfusions to maintain the red cell mass. The initial metabolic acidosis during burn shock is rapidly replaced by a respiratory alkalosis, which becomes a mixed alkalosis if potassium depletion goes unattended. Sepsis almost always complicates fluid and electrolyte management, usually between the second and fifth weeks after burn injury. These and other less frequent problems complicate the reaction to therapeutic agents, both topical and systemic pharmacologic therapy.

These abnormalities are divided into those encountered in the resuscitation phase, the immediate postresuscitation period, and the later postburn course, where medical and surgical therapies alter fluid and electrolyte metabolism. Each section emphasizes the common or usual diagnostic and therapeutic considerations, noting the common exceptions encountered in different age groups, burn sizes, and the effect of different therapies.

THE IMMEDIATE POSTBURN PERIOD — BURN SHOCK

Isotonic fluid volume losses begin immediately after injury at an extremely rapid rate. The amount of fluid required for resuscitation was quantitated in 1968 by measuring the extracellular fluid volume deficits (S^{35}) and plasma volumes in primates and after the restoration of these functional extracellular fluid volumes in humans (4, 5). These studies established that the total requirement for sodium averaged 0.52 mEq/kg body weight (BW)/% burn. Translating this quantity of Na^+ into isotonic volume replacement with balanced salt solution (lactated Ringers), a burned patient should receive between 3.8 ml and 4.2 ml of lactated Ringers/kg BW/% total body surface area (TBSA) in the first 24 hours after injury (4). Over one half of this quantity is lost within the first 8 hours after injury, requiring more rapid administration during that interval of resuscitation (Figure 1).

Significant plasma volume deficits accompany the total fluid loss but are unreplaceable in the early postburn period because capillary permeability is so increased that protein molecules ranging from 60,000 to 340,000 daltons pass as freely as sodium ions from the intravascular to extravascular space. This results in a dispropriate decrease in the circulating plasma volume, which cannot be restored by plasma expanders (colloid solutions) until capillary permeability is restored. By 24 hours postburn capillary permeability is restored. By 24 hours postburn capillary permeability has recovered sufficiently to permit rapid restoration of the plasma volume. This is best done with fresh or shelf-stored plasma, requiring 0.5 ml/% burn/kg, administered in the interval between 24 and 36 hours (Figure 1). In very massive burns, the restoration of capillary integrity may be somewhat slower, and additional volumes of plasma may be necessary between 32 and 40 hours following injury. Plasma substitutes are not recommended since they may further impair immunologic

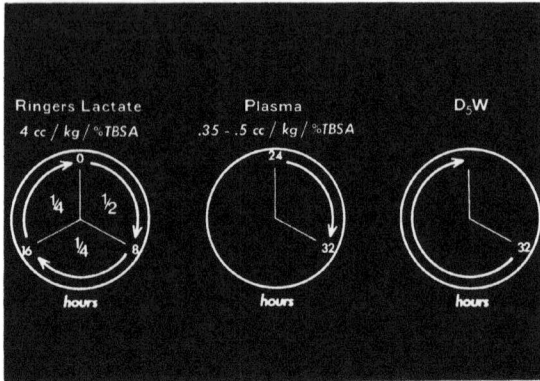

Figure 1. Guideline for fluid resuscitation of burn shock.

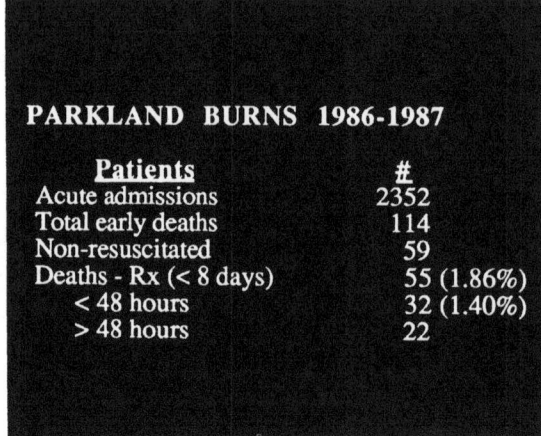

Figure 2. Mortality 1982–1987.

incompetence (28, 31). Water requirements for the first 24 hours are adequately met by the "free" H_2O of lactated Ringers solution. Since the Na^+ concentration is 130 mEq/1, 80 cc of "free" H_2O is given with each liter.

These guidelines to the quantity of isotonic fluid and the rate of its administration are adjusted in accord with the clinical response. The adequacy of resuscitation is monitored principally by urine output. The goal is a flow rate of 50 ml/hr for young adults, 30 ml/hr for the elderly, and 0.5–1 cc/kg/hr for children. Equally important is a clear sensorium.

The best criterion for monitoring resuscitation is restoration of the cardiac output. Invasive catheterization should be avoided unless the course of resuscitation is expected to be difficult or progresses unsatisfactorily.

Restoration of the cardiac output is complete by 8–10 hours in burns below 40% TBSA, but larger burns require 18–24 hours before they are normalized. The blood pressure and pulse are elevated by circulating vasoactive materials released from the burn wound and, therefore, are not indicative of the status of resuscitation. Likewise, hematocrit and hemoglobin remain elevated because of the rapid capillary leak and, therefore, cannot be used as an index of resuscitation until 36-hour postburn injury. Early correction of the metabolic acidosis indicates that adequate organ flow and normal capillary refill times are suggestive of adequate peripheral flow (29). The early mortality (i.e., within < 7 days) is less than 2% (Figure 2). The failures are in massive burns of all ages and less severe burns in the elderly. To attain these results, modification of these routine burn resuscitation guidelines and/or additional therapeutic measures are indicated with concomitant injury or preexisting disease, by age, and by the extent of the burn.

Problems in young and middle-aged adults

Burns above 65% TBSA in these age groups require additional therapies in approximately 20% of the cases. Most often, either a hypoadrenal response or a persistently low cardiac output (myocardial depression) limits the response, while an early *vasoconstrictor shock* state does not relent with fluid replacement alone.

The normal adrenocortical stimulation fails to occur in 20% of patients with massive injury (24) (Figure 3). These

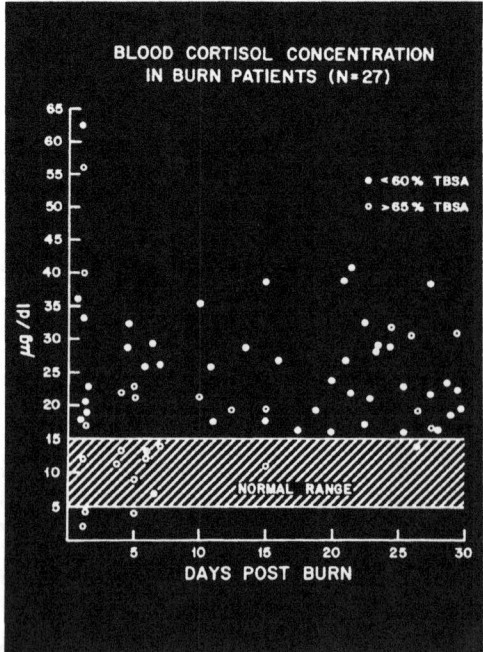

Figure 3. Adeno cortical response showing lack of initial adrenal stimulation patients with > 65% TBSA.

patients react typically as Addisonians, requiring almost twice the normal calculated fluid volume replacements for resuscitation unless it is recognized. Hydrocortisone (100 mg) given every 8 hours returns the volume requirements toward normal. This *adrenal failure* is a temporary state that self-corrects by the third to the fifth day postburn.

Less often, the massively injured, usually greater than 80% TBSA burns, fail to improve their lower cardiac outputs despite increasing the rate of fluid administration to 50–70% above the recommended amounts. Pulmonary edema and right-sided heart failure supervene, while signs and symptoms of shock persist. Depressed myocardial contractility and compliance, demonstrable in both animal (Figure 4) and human studies, underlie the inability of the myocardium to respond (1, 2). Therapeutically, plasmapheresis is often beneficial, whereas all pharmacologic therapies fail. The underlying cause is as yet undetermined, although, it is currently thought to be related to oxygen-radical mediated peroxidation of cell membranes (3, 26).

The third, and rare, cause of resuscitation failure is unrelenting *vasoconstrictor shock*. These patients exhibit large urinary volume flows and persistant systemic signs of shock. Cautious treatment with rapidly reversible vasodilators (25) and increasing the rate of fluid administration alleviates this condition within 12 hours.

Concomitant injury

Inhalation, soft-tissue and/or solid organ injury are common simultaneous injuries that all increase fluid volumes. Damage to the middle and lower airway produces inflammatory edema and later increases in permeability of the pulmonary capillaries. Inhalation injury is characterized by an obstructive ventilatory defect superimposed on the restrictive ventilatory defect found without airway damage (8, 32, 33). The fluid loss from direct parenchymal damage in the lung requires additional fluids, often up to between one third and one half more than in patients without inhalation injury. Evidence of smoke inhalation is determined by a history of an injury in a closed space, damaged mucus membranes in the mouth and hypopharynx, and progressive arterial desaturation. These signs identify this additional fluid-requiring injury.

Mechanical injuries that frequently accompany burns (10% of cases) each have their own fluid requirements, which must be taken into account in the total fluid volume requirements. Injury to visceral organs requires blood replacement. Soft-tissue injury requires principally ECF volume replacement plus replacement of the blood lost.

Pediatric patients

Burns above 25% in children may require larger quantities of lactated Ringers is the first 24 hours because the body surface area to body weight ratio is higher in children. The average amount required is 4.8–5.3 cc/kg/% burn. Calculation on this basis is simpler than attempting to estimate the body surface area in square meters. In children, albumin or plasma administration may be effective earlier (between 12 and 18 hours) postinjury (7). More importantly, burns between 10% and 20% TBSA often have water requirements that are equal to or greater than the amount of calculated volume replacement. Combining the isotonic resuscitation fluid with 5% dextrose and water produces a hypotonic solution, which, when administered as rapidly as is necessary to resuscitate

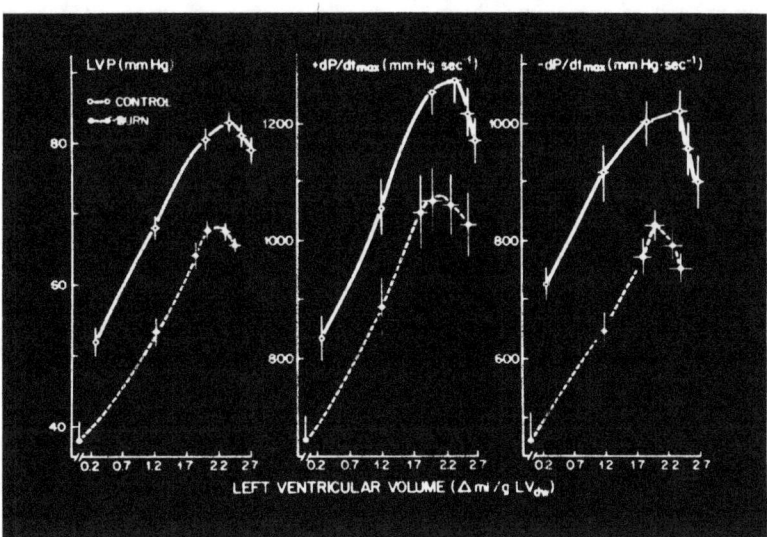

Figure 4. Decreased myocardial contractility and compliance at 24 hours post burn in a 45% third-degree burns in a guinea pig.

the burn injury, often may result in cerebral edema with ensuing convulsions and/or respiratory arrest. The complication is preventable by giving the isotonic resuscitation fluid first, followed by the slow administration of water, either orally or intravenously.

During resuscitation, glucose (2½%) should be added to all fluids administered to children; otherwise, severe hypoglycemia is encountered in over 20% of children below 5 years of age. Hyperoncotic solutions should be avoided (13).

Elderly patients

The heart is most often the limiting factor to successful resuscitation. All major burns are accompanied by a decreased contractility and impaired compliance (17). In the aged, these defects are sufficiently severe in the senescent heart that the cardiac output cannot be restored (17). The resultant underperfusion of vital organs rapidly produces multiple organ failures. The fluid volume requirements are the same as for younger patients, but the impaired heart cannot pump as effectively. Central venous catheter monitoring of the rate of fluid administration is indicated in these individuals. Coronary artery dilation with nitroglycerin will often improve the cardiac output and should be employed initially. If nitroglycerin fails, the balloon counter-pulsation will be effective in improving cardiac output and in preventing myocardial infarction. Myocardial infarction is the most common cause of death in the elderly.

LATER POSTBURN PERIOD

Fluid and electrolyte problems related to wound therapy, sepsis, and/or surgery may be superimposed upon the existing volume, concentration, and compositional changes. Routinely, blood transfusions are necessary every second or third day to replace the continuing red blood cell destruction (14, 19, 20).

Local therapy of the burn wound most often utilizes topical antibacterial creams or ointments, which are removed by debridement in water-filled hydrotherapy tanks. The burn wound (both second and third degree) is a good dialyzing surface. The short contact period of less than 1 hour a day may result in significant absorption of water and chemical (water-soluble antiseptics) employed in hydrotherapy. Simultaneously, cations and anions are lost into the hypotonic hydrotherapy water.

The most common clinical problems arise from absorption of H_2O through the wound. Progressive hyponatremia is frequently noted, particularly if daily water administration is not curtailed to allow for this phenomenon. In small children ($<$ 5 years of age), the rate of water absorption may be sufficiently rapid to produce acute water intoxication, with ensuing convulsions and respiratory arrest. All children with burns over 20% (and lesser burns in infants) should be bathed in an isotonic solution in order to avoid this complication. In all patients, but

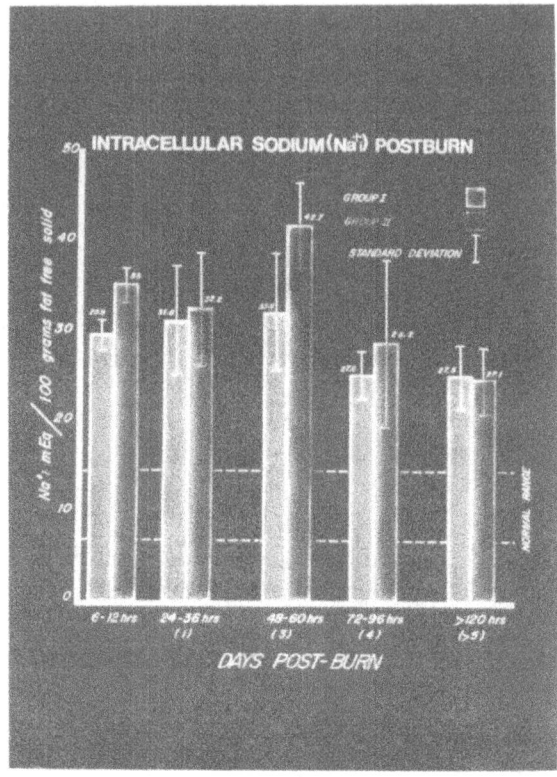

Figure 5. Sustained elevation of intracellular Na^+ concentration in patients with burns of $<$ 40% TBSA (Group 1) and over 40% TBSA) (Group II).

particularly in large burns and in the elderly, daily tanking results in an insidious sodium loss and subsequent shrinking of the extracellular fluid volume. These patients develop signs of moderate ECF volume deficit: loss of interest in their surroundings, lethargy, weakness, and, most importantly, weight loss exceeding more than one-quarter pound per day. Failure to recognize this insidious volume depletion syndrome most often results in pulmonary emboli; pulsation circulatory assist will ensure an adequate circulatory response to administered fluids.

Resuscitation with hypertonic salt solution has been reported to be successful in this setting (21). A solution of 240 mEq Na/l supplies the sodium needs and lessens the water requirements by one third or more. Data does not support an increased survival, but the treatment is sometimes dramatically successful.

Preexisting diseases

Diabetes and alcoholism are special problems. In diabetics, the hyperglycemic response to burn injury may produce hyperosmolar coma, or at least a falsely high urine volume obscuring the use of the urine as an index of adequate resuscitation. Patients with severe peripheral arteriosclerotic vascular disease lack the ability to constrict in the face of plasma volume deficits and shock may be persistent. In these individuals, earlier administration of plasma will restore the circulation, but at the expense of more extensive fluid requirements and pulmonary edema.

The severe alcoholic or cirrhotic patient may require additional volume due to the rapid accumulation of ascites or may not respond due to the myocardial lesion of the disease. The alcoholic patient with a large burn has the highest rate of resuscitation failure.

Electrical burns

High-voltage electrical burns usually involve tissue damage to deeper tissues, especially muscle. Myoglobinuria is always present. The extent of deep-tissue damage is difficult to quantitate initially, and fluid volume requirements vary accordingly. No guidelines are reliable. The best approach is very rapid administration of balanced salt solution (R/L) until the urine output is normalized. Then add mannitol (25–50 g) to each additional 1000 ml to maintain a urine volume of 100–200 ml/hr until the myoglobin has been cleared (6).

IMMEDIATE POSTRESUSCITATION PERIOD

After plasma volume repletion (36 hours postburn), the clinical picture hemodynamically is characterized by a mild tachycardia and systolic hypertension with a normal blood volume and elevated cardiac output (Figure 3). These signs may be misintepreted as a fluid volume overload, because there is obvious edema in all the burn wounds and adjacent normal tissue, the hematocrit is usually lower than normal, and diuresis is beginning. The hyperdynamic circulatory state is a result of the increased oxygen demands of hypermetabolism (30) and the progressive anemia caused by the shortened half-life of the erythrocytes (19, 29).

The actual functional fluid volume status of individual patients is difficult to evaluate. Burn edema is slow to be mobilized because excessive intravascular clotting obstructs venules and lymphatics (34). In addition, sodium is sequestered intracellularly in the cells of solid organs (skeletal muscle, liver, etc.) for at least 10 days (Figure 5). Since sodium, both in the burn wound and that sequestered intracellularly, is not available as functional extracellular fluid, thus the return of the body weight to the preburn level is not an accurate indication of the sodium mass. The severe hypermetabolism that results in rapid weight loss is not quantifiable. Thus, the measurement of body weight decreases does not reflect the functional ECF or intravascular volumes.

The management of water requirements is also difficult. The insensible water loss through burned skin is 4–12 times greater than through normal skin. The actual amount of insensible water loss through the burned area varies in individual patients and depending on whether the wounds are treated open or closed. Also, renal handling of water excretion is impaired by the continued elevated levels of antidiuretic hormone (22). Frequent determination of serum sodium is the only reliable guide to direct the amount of "free" water required. Normal serum osmolarity cannot be assumed. Although serum sodium concentrations can be maintained within a normal range by close attention to water losses and gains, significant increases in osmolarity can occur from a combination of mild hyperglycemia and the toxic level of free fatty acids (14). The total increase in serum osmolarity from these two sources is seldom of clinical importance, but they become significant when the absorption of osmotically active ions, such as polyethylene glycols from topically applied antibacterial agents, becomes a contributing factor.

Compositional abnormalities are also complicated. As previously stated, large amounts of potassium are necessary to maintain normal serum values, and even maintenance of serum concentrations cannot correct the intracellular potassium deficits accompanying the high intracellular sodium concentrations. Urinary potassium excretion continues to be excessive, ranging from a low of 100 mEq/l to a high of > 200 mEq/l under the influence of a continued elevated secretion of ADH and glucocorticoids. A low serum calcium level reflects a decrease in bound calcium (low albumin) and a modest decrease in ionized calcium (presumably due to intracellular movement of the ion). Magnesium depletion requires an additional 8–12 mEq/day to prevent low serum levels.

Chemicals added to the tanking H_2O are also absorbed. Antiseptics, such as Betadine® or Clorox® are often added to hydrotherapy water. Aqueous solutions of Betadine can be absorbed in sufficient quantity that the poly-povidone-iodine (PVP) results in a hyperosmolar state characterized by lethergy, fever, dry mucus membrances, hypertension, oliguria, and, in the most fulminant cases, convulsions. The absorption of hypochlorites may produce a mild acidosis and anemia.

Topical antibiotics and chemotherapeutic agents may also produce fluid and electrolyte problems. The 1% silver sulfadiazine (Silvadene®) topical cream, routinely used in treating burn wounds, has not been a problem. Up to 10% of the sulfadiazine is absorbed, but it rarely reaches even therapeutic levels. Other topicals are employed for special purposes, each having been associated with problems. Aminoglycosides, particularly neomycin, has been responsible for permanent hearing loss (nerve deafness), and prolonged administration may produce acute renal failure. The polyethylene glycols contained in most topical ointments may produce a hyperosmolar syndrome, not unlike that of Betadine in tank water. Sulfamylon® (mafenide acetate) produces a respiratory alkalosis by a direct effect on the respiratory center and produces a superimposed metabolic acidosis by its carbonic anhydrase inhibitor effect. Silver nitrates (½%) applied with wet dressing leaches electrolytes, particularly divalent cations. In addition, the absorbed nitrites cause methemoglobinemia.

Sepsis is almost synonymous with major burns. Colonization of burn wounds begin shortly after injury. While topical antibacterial therapy usually prevents invasive sepsis, the toxic products of bacteria are constantly being absorbed. If invasive sepsis occurs (usually 10^5 organisms/g of burned tissue), the clinical picture of the progressive stages of septic shock soon appears. Sepsis also occurs from the prolonged use of indwelling vascular catheters, urinary catheters, and frequently with pulmonary infections. The accompanying vasodilation requires ECF volume expansion to fill the enlarged vascular tree. The sudden need for volume expansion is usually the first clear-cut sign of invasive sepsis. Simultaneous appropriate antibiotic therapy with hemodynamic and respiratory monitoring may control the sepsis. If not controlled, deterioration in the clinical course is marked by lack of response to additional intravascular or extrascular volume expansion.

Transient bacteremia also follows debridement procedures but is usually self-limited. However, with surgical debridement of large surface areas, the postoperative bacteremia is much more severe.

Early surgical excisions of burn wounds is now widely practiced and is gaining in popularity for most deep dermal and third-degree wounds. Tangential excision of the burn wounds down to a freely bleeding base is the most often performed procedure. Deeper wounds require excision to the investing muscle fascia. When large surface areas (between 10% and 25% TBSA) are excised, a complex postoperative picture is frequently present. In addition to the seeding of bacteria by the operative procedure, blood loss may be excessive and may be difficult to replace completely during the procedure. Approximately 200–250 ml of blood are lost per % TBSA excised. In addition, hypothermia of some degree inevitably results despite warming procedures during the operation. The loss of body heat during operation through open wounds is very rapid in the cold environment of the surgical suite. This complex picture of vasodilatation from the bacterial seeding is difficult to separate from that due to the massive blood loss. Hypothermia, in addition, produces vasoconstriction, which as the patient rewarms requires additional volume expansion.

Throughout the treatment course of burn injury, intravenous alimentation is frequently employed to meet the increased caloric and protein needs of severely catabolized patients. While the patients are subject to all of the known complications of hyperalimentation, the most frequent syndrome observed is hyperosmolar nonketotic coma. This results from persistant attempts to furnish the total caloric needs (2–2½ times normal) with intravenous glucose administration. The osmotic diuresis results in extracellular fluid volume depletion. This complication is predictable if the rate of administration exceeds the capacity of the liver to metabolize glucose (5.5–6.0 mg glucose/kg body wt/min). This abnormality is best treated with 0.45% saline and control of hyperglycemia with insulin.

REFERENCES

1. Adams R, Baxter CR, Parker J: Contractile function of heart muscle from burned guinea pigs. *Circ Shock* 9:63–73, 1982.
2. Adams HR, Baxter CR, Izenberg SD: Decreased contractility and compliance of the left ventricle as complications of thermal injury. *Am Heart J* 108(6):1477–1487, 1984.
3. Alexander F, Mathi M, Teoh KHT, Huval WV, Lelcuk S, Valeri CR, Shepro D, Hechtman HB: Arachidonic acid metabolites mediate early burn edema. *J Trauma* 24(8):709–712, 1984.
4. Baxter CR, Shires GT: Physiological response to crystalloid resuscitation of severe burns. *Ann NY Acad Sci* 150(3):874, 1968.
5. Baxter CR: Fluid volume and electrolyte changes of the early postburn period. *Clin Plastic Surg* 1(4):693–709, 1974.
6. Baxter CR: Present concepts in the management of major electrical injury. *Surg Clin North Am* 50:1041, 1970.
7. Carvajal HF, Linares HA: Effect of burn depth upon oedema formation and albumin extravasation in rats. *Burns* 7:79–83, 1979.
8. Cook WA, Baxter CR, Ferrell JM Jr: Pulmonary circulation after dermal burns. *Vascular Surg* 2(1):1968.
9. Crenshaw CA, Baxter CR, Frenkel EP, Shires GT: Blood viscosity changes in acute burns. *Surg Forum* : – , 1966.
10. Curreri PW, Hicks JE, Illner H, Shires GT, Baxter CR: Inhibition of active sodium transport in erythrocytes from burned patients: Effect of dietary intake. *Surgical Forum* 24:46, 1973.
11. Dobke M, Roberts C, Pearson G, Germany B, Heck E, Baxter CR: A quantitative measurement of complement (C_3) activation in severely burned patients. *J Burn Care Rehab* 5(2):152–7, 1984.
12. Dobke MK, Hayes EC, Baxter CR: Leukotrienes LTB_4 in thermally injured patients' plasma and burn blister fluid. *J Burn Care Rehab* 8(3):189–191, 19 .
13. Goodwin CW, Long JW, Mason AD Jr, Pruitt BA Jr: Paradoxical effect of hyperoncotic albumin in acutely burned children. *J Trauma* 21(1):63–65, 1981.
14. Harris R, Frenkel R, Cottam G, Baxter CR: Lipid mobilization and metabolism after thermal trauma. *J Trauma* 22(3):194–198, 1982.
15. Harris RL, Cottam GL, Baxter CR: The pathogenesis of abnormal erythrocyte morphology in burns. *J Trauma* 21:13–21, 1981.
16. Hilton JG: Effects of alterations of polyunsaturated fatty acid metabolism upon plasma volume loss induced by thermal injury. *J Trauma* 20(8):663–668, 1980.
17. Horton JW, Baxter CR, White DJ: The effects of aging on the cardiac contractile response to unresuscitated thermal injury. *J Burn Care Rehab* 9(1):41–51, 1988.
18. Kefalides NA, Arana JA, Bazan A, Velarde N, Rosenthal SM: Evaluation of antibiotic prophylaxis and gamma-globulin, plasma albumin and saline solution therapy in severe burns. *Ann Surgery* 159(4):496–506, 1964.
19. Loebl EC, Marvin JA, Curreri PW, Baxter CR: Erythrocyte survival following thermal injury. *J Surg Res* 16(2):20, 1974.
20. Loebl EC, Baxter CR, Curreri PW: The mechanism of erythrocyte destruction in the early postburn period. *Ann Surgery* 178(6):681, 1973.
21. Monafo WW: The treatment of burn shock by the intravenous and oral administration of hypertonic lactated saline solution. *J Trauma* 10(7):575–586, 1970.
22. Morgan RJ, Martyn JAJ, Philbin DM, Coggins CH, Burke JF: Water metabolism and antidiuretic hormone (ADH) response following thermal injury. *J Trauma* 20(6):468–472, 1980.
23. Moylan JA Jr, Reckler JM, Mason AD: Resuscitation with hypertonic lactate saline in thermal injury. *Am J Surg* 125:580–584, 1973.

24. Parker CR Jr, Baxter CR: Divergence in adrenal steroid secretory pattern after thermal injury in adult humans. *J Trauma* 5(6):508–510, 1985.
25. Pruitt BA Jr, Mason AD Jr, Moncrief JA: Hemodynamic changes in the early postburn patient: The influence of fluid administration and of a vasodilator (hydralazine). *J Trauma* 11(1):36–46, 1971.
26. Sasaki J, Cottam G, Baxter CR: Lipid peroxidation following thermal injury. *J Burn Care Rehab* 4(4):251–254, 1983.
27. Scheulen JJ, Munster AM: The Parkland formula in patients with burns and inhalation injury. *J Trauma* 22(10):869–871, 1982.
28. Schildt B, Bouveng R, Sollenberg M: Plasma substitute induced impairment of the reticuloendothelial system function. *Acta Chir Scand* 141:7–13, 1975.
29. Sharar SR, Heimbach DM, Green M, Winn RK, Hildebrandt J: Effects of body surface thermal injury on apparent renal and cutaneous blood flow in goats. *J Burn Care Rehab* 9(1):26–30, 1988.
30. Turner WW Jr, Ireton CS, Hunt JL, Baxter CR: Predicting energy expenditures in burned patients. *J Trauma* 25:11–16, 1985.
31. Watson JS, Walker CC, Sanders R: A comparison between dried plasma and plasma protein fraction in the resuscitation of burn patients. *Burns* 3:108–111.
32. Whitener DR, Miller L, Robertson KJ, Baxter CR, Pierce AK: The pulmonary effects of crystalloid fluid replacement in thermal injury. *J Thoracic Surg,* 1980.
33. Whitener D, Whitener L, Robertson K, Baxter CR, Pierce AK: Pulmonary function measurements in patients with thermal injury and smoke inhalation. *Am Rev Respiratory Dis* 122:731–739, 1980.
34. Wilterdink MD, Curreri PW, Baxter CR: Characterization of elevated fibrin split products following thermal injury. *Ann Surgery* 181(2):157, 1975.

CHAPTER 18

Acute Renal Failure

DAVID M. GILLUM, JOHN D. CONGER & ROBERT J. ANDERSON

INTRODUCTION

Acute renal failure (ARF) is broadly defined as an abrupt decrease in renal function sufficient to result in retention of nitrogenous waste in the body. Thus, the hallmark of ARF is rising plasma concentrations of urea nitrogen and creatinine. It is important to note that ARF can occur in the setting of well-maintained urine output as well as oligonanuria. In fact, urine output of 1–2 l/day is the most common form of ARF encountered in contemporary medical practice (1).

Recent studies demonstrate that ARF occurs in 2–5% of all patients admitted to general medical-surgical hospitals (2, 3). The incidence of ARF increases to 10–30% in selected clinical settings such as admission to an intensive care unit, following aminoglycoside administration, and in patients with septic shock (1–12). Despite significant advances in the clinical care of patients with ARF contemporary mortality rates remain high, ranging from 20% to 80% (1–12). Recent controlled studies indicate that ARF developing in hospitalized patients increases mortality by sixfold (3). The high frequency of occurrence and substantial mortality rate demand a thorough understanding of the causes, diagnostic approach, treatment, and prevention of ARF.

ETIOLOGY OF ARF

Abrupt and progressive renal failure is the final common pathway of several disparate extrarenal and renal disorders. Renal excretion of nitrogenous waste begins with ultrafiltration of blood, processing of the ultrafiltrate by the renal tubules, and excretion of the formed urine by the ureter, bladder, and urethra. Based on this overview, it is helpful to classify ARF as due to decreased renal blood flow (prerenal), obstruction to urine flow (postrenal), or a sudden renal parenchymal insult (renal).

Several recent studies indicate that prerenal forms of ARF are common, comprising 40–60% of all cases of ARF (2, 3). The process of formation of an ultrafiltrate of plasma at the glomerular capillary is regulated by Starling forces. Glomerular capillary hydrostatic pressure usually exceeds the hydrostatic pressure within Bowman's capsule and the colloid oncotic pressure within the glomerular capillary, resulting in formation of an ultrafiltrate. When renal perfusion pressure or renal blood flow are reduced to levels that substantially lower the glomerular filtration rate, then prerenal azotemia occurs. The tubular system maximally reabsorbs sodium and water at reduced renal perfusion and glomerular filtration rates as a mechanism to preserve the extracellular fluid volume. Since the predominant mechanism of removal of nitrogenous wastes is via glomerular filtration, and urea reabsorption is increased at reduced tubular flow rates, acute azotemia can occur as a consequence of decreased renal perfusion. From a clinical perspective, prerenal azotemia usually occurs as a result of hypovolemia, septic shock, or marked cardiac failure. Common clinical settings of hypovolemia are listed in Table 1 and include gastrointestinal hemorrhage, severe diarrhea, loss of large volumes of urine from osmotic diuresis (glycosuria) or diuretic agents, and sequestration of extracellular fluid, as occurs in pancreatitis and muscle crush injuries. Not only is prerenal azotemia the most common cause of an abrupt deterioration of renal function, but it is also reversible with appropriate therapy. This is particularly important since prolonged prerenal azotemia may lead to ischemic acute tubular necrosis and consequent high morbidity and mortality rates.

Postrenal forms of ARF are less commonly encountered but are usually amenable to therapy. Obstruction to urine flow as a cause of ARF will be found in 2–4% of all unselected patients with ARF. However, in the elderly, extrarenal obstruction to urine flow will be found in 5–10% of patients with ARF (12). Mechanistically, extrarenal obstruction is more complex than simple obstruction to flow and involves reactive vasoconstriction as well. If obstruction is complete, there is a rapid increase in intratubular pressures that reduce the net hydraulic driving force for glomerular ultrafiltration (13); however, because of the compliance properties of the intrarenal and extrarenal urinary tubules, tubular pressures decline to steady-state levels that are less than the peak pressures measured after acute obstruction. The level of tubular pressures alone under these conditions is not sufficiently elevated to

Table 1. Clinical disorders associated with prerenal azotemia

Volume depletion
  Hemorrhage
  Gastrointestinal losses
  Third space
    Pancreatitis
    Burns
    Peritonitis
    Traumatized tissue
  Diuretic abuse
Cardiac dysfunction
  Congestive heart failure
  Myocardial infarction
  Pericardial tamponade
  Acute pulmonary embolism
Peripheral vasodilation
  Bacteremia
  Antihypertensive medications
Renal vasoconstriction
  Anesthesia
  Surgical operation
  Hepatorenal syndrome
Bilateral renal vascular obstruction
  Embolism
  Thrombosis

Table 2. Clinical disorders associated with postrenal azotemia

Bilateral obstruction of ureters
  Extralumenal
    Tumor: cervix, prostate, endometriosis
    Periureteral fibrosis
    Accidental ureteral ligation during pelvic operation
  Intralumenal
    Sulfonamide and uric acid crystals
    Blood clots
    Pyogenic debris
    Stones
    Edema
    Papillary necrosis
Bladder outlet obstruction
  Prostatic hypertrophy
  Bladder carcinoma
  Bladder infection
  Functional: neuropathy or ganglionic blocking agents
Urethral obstruction

account for the lack of glomerular filtration. Yarger et al. (14) have found that there is renal vasoconstriction in response to ureteral obstruction. The vasoconstriction appears to be mediated by thromboxanes. The vasoconstrictive response to ureteral obstruction reduces the glomerular capillary hydraulic pressure. Thus, reduced glomerular filtration with extrarenal obstruction is the result of both tubular and vascular pressure factors.

In Table 2 are given the conditions that cause postrenal azotemia. It is diagnostically helpful to consider two categories of obstructive uropathy, intrarenal and extrarenal. Intrarenal obstruction to urine flow occurs when tubules are occluded by either crystals (uric acid, methotrexate, calcium oxalate, acyclovir) or by precipitation of protein (multiple myeloma). These forms of ARF often respond to therapy, which includes reduction in the crystal/protein load as well as maintenance of high rates of flow of dilute urine.

Traditionally, postrenal forms of ARF have focused on extrarenal obstruction. In males, bladder neck blockage from prostatic disease is the most common form of extrarenal obstructive uropathy. Obstruction of the upper urinary tract is a less common cause of renal failure, since it requires simultaneous obstruction of both ureters or unilateral ureteric obstruction with either absence of, or severe disease in, the contralateral kidney. Causes of upper urinary tract obstruction include pelvic cancer in females, prostate cancer in males, retroperitoneal fibrosis, and bilateral ureteric occlusion (ligature, stones, clots, pus, papillary tissue).

Once prerenal and postrenal causes of ARF have been considered, the focus of attention should shift to the kidney. When considering renal causes of ARF, it is helpful to think of the major anatomic compartments of the kidney, which include blood vessels, glomeruli, interstitium, and tubules. An abrupt decrease or cessation of the blood supply to the kidney, as occurs in renal embolic, thrombotic, and mechanical occlusion of the renal arteries, can lead to ARF (15–17). A variety of disease processes affecting small renal blood vessels, including malignant hypertension, scleroderma, hemolytic-uremic syndrome, thrombotic thrombocytopenic purpura, and vasculitis, can also result in ARF. An acute inflammatory process involving either the glomerulus or the renal interstititum often produces a clinical spectrum of ARF (1, 18–20). Acute renal vascular, glomerular, and interstitial disorders comprise 1–10% of all patients developing ARF (1, 19).

While disorders of renal vasculature, glomeruli, and interstitium can all produce a clinical picture of ARF, the most common renal cause of acute renal failure has often been termed *acute tubular necrosis*. This is an often-used clinical description, but it is not an entirely appropriate pathologic term.

The primary factors predisposing to acute tubular necrosis are threefold: renal ischemia resulting from prolonged prerenal azotemia (21), nephrotoxins (1–5, 19, 20, 22, 23), and pigmenturia (24). Recent studies indicate that the majority of patients with the clinical syndrome of acute tubular necrosis have more than one of these predisposing factors (3,5).

Renal ischemia is likely to be the most common final pathway of the clinical entity of acute tubular necrosis. A wide variation in the magnitude and duration of renal hypoperfusion has been reported to precede the development of acute renal failure. Ischemia-induced ARF can be either oliguric or nonoliguric in nature and can follow a variety of diverse clinical courses (21, 25, 26). Common contemporary clinical settings of ischemic acute tubular necrosis include burns, abdominal aortic aneurysm surgery

Table 3. Specific etiologies of acute renal failure

Hemodynamic
  Systemic disorders
    Major trauma
    Massive hemorrhage
    Septic shock
    Transfusion reactions
    Pregnancy: postpartum hemorrhage
    Postoperative, particularly cardiac, aortic, and biliary
      surgery
    Medical: pancreatitis, gastroenteritis
  Major blood vessel disease
    Renal artery thrombosis, embolism, or stenosis
    Bilateral renal vein thrombosis
  Diseases of glomeruli and small blood vessels
    Acute post-streptococcal glomerulonephritis
    Systemic lupus erythematosus
    Polyarteritis nodosa
    Schonlein–Henoch purpura
    Subacute bacterial endocarditis
    Serum sickness
    Goodpasture's syndrome
    Malignant hypertension
    Hemolytic-uremic syndrome
    Drug-related vasculitis
    Pregnancy: abruptio placentae, abortion with or without
      gram-negative sepsis: postpartum renal failure
    Rapidly progressive glomerulonephritis, unknown etiology
Nephrotoxins
  Nonsteroidal antiinflammatory agents
  Heavy metals: mercury, arsenic, lead, bismuth, uranium,
    cadmium
  Carbon tetrachloride
  Other organic solvents
  X-ray contrast media
  Pesticides
  Fungicides
  Antibiotics: aminoglycosides, penicillins, tetracyclines,
    amphotericin
  Other drugs and chemical agents: diphenylhydantoin,
    phenylbutazone

and other postoperative states, and gram-negative bacteremia (3, 5).

Nephrotoxins account for 15–25% of all cases of ARF (1–5). Commonly encountered nephrotoxins include nonsteroidal antiinflammatory agents, animoglycoside antimicrobial drugs, radiocontrast material, cyclosporin, amphotericin B, and cisplatin (1–5, 22, 23, 79–29). An additional wide variety of pharmacologic agents are potential nephrotoxins (Table 3).

Another factor predisposing to the clinical entity of acute tubular necrosis is pigmenturia. Both hemoglobinuria and myoglobinuria can result in ARF (24). In the majority of cases, volume depletion coexists with pigmenturia.

CLINICAL AND LABORATORY FEATURES

Specific clinical disorders resulting in prerenal azotemia are listed in Table 1. The most common setting for a reduction in renal perfusion is hypovolemia. A good history will often uncover evidence of excessive fluid loss with inadequate replacement. A physical exam may reveal evidence of fluid loss, hemorrhage, ascites, trauma, or burn injury. Other signs of extracellular fluid volume depletion, such as decreased skin turgor, dry mucous membranes, hypotension, and tachycardia with orthostatic changes in blood pressure and pulse, are often present. In nonhemorrhagic fluid loss the hematocrit may be elevated.

Heart failure with reduced cardiac output produces prerenal azotemia by a mechanism similar to hypovolemia in that renal perfusion and blood flow are reduced. However, the patient will exhibit the systemic clinical parameters of heart failure rather than hypovolemia. Both peripheral vasodilation and vasoconstriction can reduce renal perfusion and produce prerenal azotemia. Assessment for drug exposure, septicemia, hepatic failure, hypotension, and altered skin perfusion all suggest changes in vascular resistance that may cause prerenal azotemia.

The patient's history may provide clues to the presence of postrenal azotemia. Urethral obstruction is suggested by a history of urethritis, hesitancy, urgency, or decreased force of the urine stream. Similar symptoms may be found with prostatic urethral constriction. Genital, prostate, and abdominal examinations may localize the obstruction and detect bladder distention. Determination of residual urine after voiding and cystoscopy will suggest the site and significance of the obstruction. Not only anatomic, but also functional disorders of the bladder may lead to obstruction and postrenal azotemia. Autonomic insufficiency, as in diabetes, spinal cord lesions, and anticholinergic therapy, may cause urinary retention. Determination of residual urine volume will usually confirm the abnormality. Unless there is a single kidney or there is preexisting renal failure, obstruction above the bladder requires that both ureteropelvic systems be involved in order to produce azotemia. Obstruction of the ureters or pelves of the kidneys is due to intraureteral or extraureteral causes. If the obstruction is acute there is usually flank pain and often hematuria. A kidneys-ureters-bladder x-ray (KUB) is useful to determine renal size and, because 85% of renal calculi are radiopaque, may be useful in detecting stones.

Analgesic abuse, sickle cell disease, diabetes mellitus, and acute pyelonephritis are potential causes of papillary necrosis. Gross bleeding from the upper urinary tract may result in ureteral clots. Sulfonamides and chemotherapy for malignancy can cause intraureteral crystal formation. Extraureteral compression is usually the result of tumors, fibrosis, trauma, or inadvertent surgical ligation. While the evidence suggesting obstruction is generally strong on a clinical assessment, ultrasound examination of the renal pelves and proximal ureters is the currently accepted method of diagnosing upper urinary tract obstruction. Intravenous pyelography, while an excellent diagnostic tool for localization, either cannot give good contrast detail because of poor renal function or, in many instances, is discouraged because of nephrotoxicity. Retrograde pyelography is not currently used as a routine procedure for obstruction because of technical difficulty and potential sepsis. However, there can be instances where this technique is still required to diagnose obstruction.

Intrinsic acute renal failure

While intrinsic acute renal failure is largely a diagnosis of exclusion, there are a number of positive clinical features that support its existence. Historically, there is evidence of a hemodynamic insult or exposure to a nephrotoxic substance. Not only must exogenous agents such as antibiotics, nonsteroidal antiinflammaotry drugs, hydrocarbons, glycols, and radiocontrast media be considered, but endogenously induced nephrotoxic disorders such as hyperuricemia, rhabdomyolysis, hemolysis, and hypercalcemia should also be considered. Ischemic injury from hypotension or marked renal vasoconstriction, while usually historically obvious, may occasionally be subtle, as in anesthesia induction or septicemia. Physical examination generally reveals normovolemia or fluid overload, and normal or elevated blood pressure. Other physical findings related to specific etiologies may be present. Trauma, muscle swelling, and tenderness may suggest rhabdomyolysis. Respiratory difficulty may indicate ingestion of hydrocarbons or glycols. Central nervous system dysfunction or coma may also suggest hydrocarbons, glycols, pesticides, or heavy metals. Systemic vasculitis may be accompanied by petechiae or other skin eruptions.

Laboratory features

Laboratory assessment in the acutely uremic patient may be critical in the differential diagnosis, and in determining the severity of the metabolic complications. While it is obvious that blood urea nitrogen (BUN) and serum creatinine (S_{cr}) will both be elevated in acute renal failure, the ratio may be helpful in distinguishing prerenal azotemia from intrinsic acute renal failure. In prerenal azotemia there is a relatively greater fraction of filtered urea reabsorbed than creatinine. As a consequence, the normal ratio of BUN/S_{cr} is elevated. In intrinsic acute renal failure, the dysfunctional tubular system does not increase the fractional reabsorption of urea; therefore, the BUN/S_{cr} ratio remains at approximately 10. Other plasma measurements in acute azotemia states may be diagnostically helpful.

Hepatic enzymes may be elevated in hydrocarbon-induced acute renal failure and in acute interstitial nephritis. Serum hemoglobin and myoglobin levels will be elevated in severe hemolytic states and rhabdomyolysis. Serum creatinine phosphokinase also will be elevated in rhabdomyolysis.

Of greater importance in the differential diagnosis of acute renal failure is the urine volume and composition. Characteristically, azotemic patients are oliguric (< 400 ml/24 hr). However, a significant percent of patients have urine volumes that are above the oliguric range. The greater urine output, however, is a consequence of defective water reabsorption in the distal nephron and does not permit the appropriate excretion of retained nitrogen wastes, which is dependent upon the glomerular filtration rate. In general, high-output acute renal failure does have a somewhat better preserved glomerular filtration rate and has a better prognosis. Anuria is the complete absence of urine and is rare in acute renal failure. More frequently, anuria is associated with obstruction or renal artery thrombosis. The chemical composition of the urine is generally the most reliable laboratory test in establishing the diagnosis of intrinsic renal failure and in distinguishing it from prerenal azotemia. As outlined above, the tubular system is intact in prerenal azotemia but, because of ischemia or nephrotoxicity, is damaged in intrinsic acute renal failure. As a consequence, the urine composition reflects maximal sodium and water conservation in prerenal azotemia, while the capacity of the tubular system to conserve sodium and water is impaired in intrinsic acute renal failure. Table 4 shows the urine composition in acute prerenal azotemia, oliguric and nonoliguric renal failure, and obstructive uropathy (30). These data indicate that while prerenal azotemia can be distinguished from intrinsic acute renal failure and obstructive uropathy, the latter two disorders cannot be separated by the parameters of urine composition shown. However, it is usually more difficult to differentiate between prerenal azotemia and intrinsic acute renal failure, which underscores the diagnostic importance of the urinary indices. The 95% confidence limits for diagnostic urinary indices in prerenal azotemia and intrinsic oliguric acute renal failure are shown in Table 5. Of these values, the renal failure index, which is the urine sodium divided by the urine/plasma creatinine ratio, and the fractional excretion of sodium are the most sensitive

Table 4. Urinary diagnostic indices*

	Prerenal azotemia	Acute oliguric renal failure	Acute nonoliguric renal failure	Acute obstructive uropathy	Acute glomerulonephritis
Urine osmolality, mOsm/kg H$_2$O	518 ± 35	369 ± 20	343 ± 17	393 ± 39	385 ± 61
Urine sodium, mEq/l	18 ± 3	68 ± 5	50 ± 5	68 ± 10	22 ± 6
Urine/plasma urea nitrogen	18 ± 7	3 ± 0.5	7 ± 1	8 ± 4	11 ± 4
Urine/plasma creatinine	45 ± 6	17 ± 2	17 ± 2	16 ± 4	43 ± 7
Renal failure index	0.6 ± 0.1	10 ± 2	4 ± 0.6	8 ± 3	0.4 ± 7
Fractional excretion of filtered sodium	0.4 ± 0.1	7 ± 1.4	3 ± 0.5	6 ± 2	0.6 ± 0.2

Reprinted with permission from Miller et al. (30).
* Values are expressed as mean ± SE.

Table 5. Summary of urinary indices in oliguric renal failure

	Prerenal	Oliguric acute renal failure
Urine osmolality, mOsm/kg H$_2$O	>500	<350
Urine sodium, mEq/l	<20	>40
Urine/plasma urea nitrogen	>8	<3
Urine/plasma creatinine	>40	<20
Renal failure index	<1	>1
Fractional excretion of filtered sodium	<1	>1

Reprinted with permission from Miller et al. (30).

discriminators. However, a combination of indices is useful in ensuring the accuracy of the diagnosis. There are two situations that may obscure the usefulness of urinary chemical composition. Patients who are prerenal may have inappropriately high urinary sodium in the presence of diuretics, preexisting chronic renal failure, or acute metabolic alkalosis. In metabolic alkalosis sodium is lost in the urine with bicarbonate; however, a urine chloride concentration of < 20 mEq/l is consistent with prerenal azotemia, since its enhanced reabsorption is not altered by the elevated tubular bicarbonate (31). The urine sediment is an additional useful assessment in the diagnosis of acute renal failure. An active sediment with tubular epithelial cells, cellular debris, and pigmented granular "renal failure" casts supports the diagnosis of acute renal failure. Microscopic hematuria, a small number of white blood cells and 1$^+$-2$^+$ protein by dipstick are also frequently found. However, the absence of an abnormal sediment does not exclude the presence of intrinsic acute renal failure. Red blood cell casts and quantitative proteinuria > 2.5 g/24 hr indicate the presence of an acute glomerular disorder and are not compatible with acute renal failure. A normal sediment is most often found in prerenal azotemia and postrenal azotemia; however, hematuria may be found with the latter disorder, particularly if the obstructive etiology is a malignancy or an irritant to the urinary tract mucosa. The presence of crystals in the urine, such as uric acid, oxalate with ethylene glycol and methoxyflurane toxicity, and sulfa crystals, may provide an etiologic clue in acute renal failure. Finally, pigmented urine suggests the presence of hemoglobinuria or myoglobinuria.

PATHOPHYSIOLOGY

The pathogenetic mechanisms of acute renal failure have been investigated extensively over several years. There continues to be a lack of consensus concerning the critical factors and events that lead to a reduction in the glomerular filtration rate. Nearly all pathogenetic theories can be reduced to three: hemodynamic abnormalities, tubular fluid back-leak, and tubular obstruction.

Several observations have provided indirect support that vascular events are causally related to functional deterioration in acute renal failure. Three possible hemodynamic changes have been proposed to account for glomerular filtration failure: persistent afferent arteriolar constriction, efferent arteriolar dilatation, and decreased glomerular capillary permeability.

Morphologic data have suggested decreased blood flow particularly in the outer cortex in acute renal failure (32–34). Inert gas washout studies in experimental animals and humans have demonstrated decreased cortical blood flow in acute renal failure (35–38). In uranyl nitrate and norepinephrine acute renal failure in rats, preferential decreases in the outer cortical blood flow have also been shown with radioactive microspheres (39, 40). However, the decreases in cortical blood flow could not account totally for the declines in the glomerular filtration rates. These observations suggest at least a partial role for persistent afferent arteriolar constriction in the pathogenesis of acute renal failure. A number of experimental studies have suggested that the renin-angiotensin system is involved in the maintenance of afferent arteriolar constriction. Juxtaglomerular hypertrophy has been demonstrated in acute renal failure patients (41). Plasma renin is elevated, at least in the early phase of the disease (42, 43). Chronic saline loading in experimental animals attenuates acute renal failure when given prior to induction (44, 45). Conversely, states of volume depletion predispose to both experimental and clinical acute renal failure. Angiotensin inhibition increases the outer cortical blood flow in an experimental acute renal failure model. On the other hand, there are a number of observations that would argue against a significant role for persistent afferent arteriolar constriction. In humans, post-transplant acute renal failure is characterized by a nearly normal renal blood flow pattern. In both ischemic and nephrotoxic disease models, renal blood flow, as determined by electromagnetic flow probe or radioactive microspheres, approaches normal and could not account for the glomerular filtration rate reduction (46). The importance of the renin-angiotensin system in the pathogenesis of acute renal failure has been questioned, since immunization against renin (47), angiotensin antagonists (48), converting-enzyme inhibition (48), and acute saline loading (39) do not protect against experimental acute renal failure.

Efferent arteriolar dilatation was considered a potential mechanism of the glomerular filtration rate reduction based on studies that simultaneously measured intrarenal blood flow, glomerular filtration, and sodium transportation in acute renal failure patients (49). Radioactive sodium and EDTA were infused into the renal artery with an indicator dye. The calculated renal blood flow and glomerular filtration rate were compatible with efferent arteriolar dilatation. Efferent arteriolar dilatation, in turn, was thought to reduce the glomerular capillary hydraulic pressure and thereby to reduce the glomerular filtration rate. However, the findings of this study could have been explained as well by tubular obstruction. There is no direct evidence to support efferent arteriolar dilatation as a pathogenetic process in experimental acute renal failure.

Decreased glomerular permeability has been suggested by a number of experimental models to be a pathogenetic factor in acute renal failure. In a norepinephrine model of acute renal failure, indirect evidence of a reduction in glomerular permeability was found (50). Within models of both uranyl nitrate and mercuric chloride acute renal failure in which direct glomerular dynamics were measured, decreases in the glomerular ultrafiltration coefficient could account for only a fraction of the total glomerular filtration reduction. Therefore, a change in the glomerular permeability is probably only a minor pathogenetic mechanism in acute renal failure.

Tubular fluid backleak

The possibility that tubular fluid backleak was a factor in the pathogenesis of acute renal failure was suggested by the findings of Richards in 1929 (26). He demonstrated that phenolsulfonphthalein, a normally non-reabsorbable marker, leaked from the tubules of mercuric-chloride-poisoned frogs. The presumed mechanism whereby tubular backleak reduces the glomerular filtration rate is as follows: Ultrafiltration from the glomerular capillary loops proceeds according to the net driving pressure for filtration. However, the plasma ultrafiltrate leaks from the tubular system because of ischemic or nephrotoxic injury to proximal tubular cells. The ultrafiltrate is driven into the peritubular capillaries by the postglomerular colloid osmotic pressure. The net effect is that there is absent or marked decrease in the glomerular filtration rate as measured from the excreted urine, depending on the severity of tubular injury. A number of acute renal failure models studied by micropuncture have suggested a loss of lissamine green or inulin from the tubular lumen (52, 54, 55). Since inulin is normally a nonreabsorbable marker, the lack of complete inulin recovery indicates that molecules of at least 5000 MW can back-diffuse through the wall of the tubules. Venkatachalam and colleagues (56, 57) have given anatomical support to the backleak hypothesis by demonstrating disruption of the late proximal tubule and permeability to both inulin and horseradish peroxidase (MW 40,000) in a model of ischemic acute renal failure. The findings of a recent human ischemic acute renal failure study that examined renal hemodynamics indirectly and measured the clearance of dextran of varying molecular weights was compatible with a tubular backleak mechanism (58). There are, however, other micropuncture studies that have not confirmed the backleak hypothesis. In a norepinephrine ischemic acute renal failure model, recovery of radioactive inulin between the early proximal and mid-distal tubule was nearly complete (40).

Tubular obstruction

Like tubular fluid backleak, intratubular obstruction has been proposed as a pathogenetic factor in acute renal failure for several decades. Morphologic studies showed tubular dilatation and necrosis, loss of the cell brush border, and the deposition of the cellular debris in tubular lumens (59–62). The physiologic significance of these findings was later examined using micropuncture methods. Intratubular pressures have been measured in both ischemic and nephrotoxic acute renal failure models. Experimental renal artery clamp (63) and norepinephrine acute renal failure (64) have been found to have intratubular pressures three to four times normal. The magnitude of pressure increase was greatest in the early phase of norepinephrine acute renal failure. In nephrotoxic acute renal failure models such as mercuric chloride (52), uranyl nitrate (51), and glycerol (34), intratubular pressures have not been uniformly increased and more frequently approach normal. It has been argued that the findings of tubular luminal debris and elevated tubular pressures does not prove that obstruction plays an important pathogenetic role (65, 66). However, the magnitude of intratubular pressure elevation in ischemic models (64), the observation that microperfusion at pressures equal to physiologic glomerular hydraulic pressures does not dislodge casts (67), and the normalization of the single-nephron glomerular filtration rate in nehrons with elevated intratubular pressures when the increased pressure is released (64) would all support a definitive role for tubular obstruction in acute renal failure pathogenesis. Experiments in norepinephrine acute renal failure have demonstrated that tubular obstruction is not the only factor in ischemic renal failure. While obstruction appeared to be the major factor in the first 2 days after disease induction, a primary reduction in nephron filtration secondary to vasoconstriction of the afferent vasculature was a factor from 2 to 7 days (64).

The cumulative data indicate that tubular obstruction is an important pathogenetic mechanism, particularly in ischemic acute renal failure. Even in ischemia-induced disease, however, it is unlikely that obstruction is a singular mechanism, but is combined with vascular and, possibly, backleak factors.

Mechanism of cell ischemia in acute renal failure

In hemodynamically induced acute renal failure, the common underlying factor in tubular fluid backleak, tubular obstruction, and, possibly, vascular pathogenetic mechanisms is ischemic cellular injury. Recently, intense interest has focused on the events of cellular ischemia. Much of the investigative effort has been directed at understanding the ischemic changes of renal tubular cells. Increases in cellular calcium and the generation of toxic O_2 metabolites are two of the factors that are related to ischemic injury.

Both in-vivo and in-vitro experiments have demonstrated that alterations in calcium homeostasis can convert a reversible form of cell injury to an irreversible lesion (74). Immediately following a short-term anoxia, cytosolic free calcium is shown to increase from 40 to 60 nM. In other experiments in which isolated proximal tubules were subjected to varying degrees of anoxia, nonlethally injured tubules showed an increase in cell calcium that is partly reversible following reoxygenation (69, 70). These data strongly suggest that changes in calcium (Ca) metabolism precede cell death. Two mechanisms — redistribution of intracellular Ca and disturbances in the transcellular Ca flux — appear to play important roles in setting cytosolic Ca levels following ischemia. Evidence for redistribution comes from studies of isolated perfused cardiac septum subjected to high-flow hypoxia (71). Resting tension was not affected by hypoxia initially. However, within 5 minutes resting tension increased without a concomitant rise in the total cell Ca. Since resting tension is a function of sarcoplasmic Ca content and resting tension increased without a simultaneous rise in total cell Ca, the implication is that there was a shift of Ca from the cytosol to the sarcoplasm. Evidence for a Ca efflux and influx changes to alter total cell and cytosolic free Ca comes in part from a recent study demonstrating that Ca uptake by a suspension of proximal tubules is increased following 30 minutes of anoxia (72). This increase is the result of an increase in the size of both exchangeable cellular Ca pools (glycocalyx and intracellular). Other studies in LLC-MK2 cells have demonstrated that as cytosolic free Ca increases and ATP decreases during anoxia, Ca efflux increased 2.5 times (73). Thus, it does not seem that the increased cytosolic free Ca results from a decreased ability of the cells to actively extrude Ca. Recent studies in cultures of individual nephron segments have been able to demonstrate the deleterious effects of extracellular Ca on the recovery of cells from an anoxic insult (74). Following anoxia, cells incubated in Ca-free media for 2 hours thereafter showed a 46% viability at 48 hours compared to 100% cell death in an incubated Ca-containing medium. The mechanistic role of cell Ca in ischemic cell injury, therefore, appears to be related to the consequences of increased intracellular Ca. Ca is present in the extracellular fluid at concentrations on the order of 10^{-3} M, while cytosolic content is in the range of 10^{-7} M (75). An increase in the normally low permeability of the plasma membrane or failure of transport mechanisms to remove cytosolic Ca leads to cellular Ca overload. Intracellular Ca overload causes detrimental effects, since several cellular processes depend on cytosolic levels of cell Ca. The deleterious effects of Ca overload on mitochondrial function have been well established (76-80). By competing with oxidative phosphorylation, mitochondrial Ca uptake in effect uncouples this process and limits ATP production. Ca produces permeability alterations in the inner mitochondrial membrane by activating membrane phospholipase; Ca has also been shown to precipitate in mitochondrial matrix. Several current investigations are being performed to examine changes in cell membrane permeability, endoplasmic reticulum function, and cellular transport processes as a consequence of increases in cytosolic Ca.

Ischemic renal injury results in a decrease in intracellular ATP and an increase in ATP degradation products including hypoxanthine. The accumulation of hypoxanthine during renal ischemia generates highly reactive oxygen free radicals, since the enzymatic conversion of hypoxanthine to xanthine by xanthine oxidase generates superoxide radical (O_2^-) as a reduction product of molecular oxygen (81). Superoxide radical and its reduction products, hydrogen peroxide (H_2O_2) and hydroxyl radical (OH), can produce cellular injury through lipid peroxidation of mitochondrial, lysosomal, and plasma membranes, which can alter both membrane structure and function (81). Endogenous scavengers protect against oxygen free radical damage under normal physiologic circumstances. Superoxide dismutase rapidly removes O_2^-. Catalase and glutathione peroxidase inactivate H_2O_2. Other scavengers eliminate OH. Under conditions of ischemia, supplies of oxygen radical scavengers may be depleted, and toxic oxygen metabolites may cause cellular injury after reflow of blood and reoxygenation of cells. While oxygen free radicals are difficult to demonstrate biochemically, their effects can be detected by measuring lipid peroxides. The content of malondialdehyde was increased after 60 minutes of renal ischemia and 15 minutes of reflow (82). Furthermore, xanthine oxidase inhibitors, superoxide dismutase, and dimethylthiourea — scavengers of oxygen radicals — protect the kidney from ischemic insult (82-84).

PREVENTION OF ACUTE TUBULAR NECROSIS

Prevention of acute renal failure is the optimal management goal. Unfortunately, it is often difficult to prevent a complicating disorder in the setting of severe illness. In the majority of acute renal failure cases, patients are already seriously ill from surgery, trauma, sepsis, or cardiovascular disorders that are causally related to the acute renal failure. It is these underlying conditions that are often difficult to manage, and as a consequence acute renal failure is difficult to prevent. Nonetheless, some prophylactic approaches appear to decrease the likelihood of acute renal failure.

Several animal studies have shown that volume expansion prior to induction of mercuric or glycerol acute renal failure can prevent or attenuate the decline in the glomerular filtration rate (44, 45, 85, 86). While there are no systematic studies showing that volume expansion prior to exposure to a setting in which acute renal failure is likely to develop have been performed, volume depletion, on the other hand, has been shown to be a risk factor for radiocontrast and aminoglycoside-induced nephropathy (87). Experimental studies in dogs have shown that antecedent treatment with mannitol (88), furosemide (89), or prostaglandins (90) can attenuate ischemic acute renal failure. Mannitol has been shown by some investigators to attenuate the decline in renal function associated with radiocontrast infusion and cardiovascular surgery (91, 92).

Alkalinization of the urine may be of value in disorders in which tubular fluid pH is a factor in pathogenesis. Humphrey et al. (93) demonstrated that sodium bicarbonate infusion may prevent acute renal failure in patients with rhabdomyolysis and myoglobinuria. Sodium bicarbonate diuresis may prevent acute urate nephropathy in patients with malignancy undergoing chemotherapy (94).

Treatment that interferes with the metabolism of nephrotoxins has been useful in acute urate nephropathy and methanol intoxication. Allopurinol will prevent the conversion of xanthine and hypoxanthine to uric acid. Ethanol infusion has been used successfully to prevent the conversion of methanol to formic acid (95).

Acute renal failure secondary to hypercalcemia is a preventable disorder. Volume expansion, furosemide, prednisone, calcitonin, mithramycin, and sodium EDTA all have defined roles in the management of hypercalcemia.

Drug choice, dosage, and frequency of administration can be of critical importance in the prevention of acute renal failure. This is particularly true in elderly patients and in those with preexisting renal disease. Nonsteroidal antiinflammatory drugs are of particular concern in patients with congestive heart failure (96), lupus nephritis (97), nephrotic syndrome (98), and cirrhosis with ascites (99). Sulfa drugs are more likely to cause tubular crystallization in patients who are volume depleted. Finally, although aminoglycosides are frequently used in seriously ill septic patients, their therapeutic range is relatively narrow. The two major errors in aminoglycoside therapy are failure to adjust dosages to creatinine clearance and lean body mass (100–102). While maintaining plasma trough levels at subtoxic levels does not ensure protection from nephrotoxicity, the incidence is markedly reduced.

MANAGEMENT OF PRERENAL AZOTEMIA

Once hypoperfusion of the kidneys is diagnosed by means of the criteria described, then specific therapy to restore perfusion may be initiated. In the patient with marked prerenal azotemia and circulatory instability due to loss of extracellular fluid (e.g., diarrhea, enteric fistula, diuresis), rapid expansion of the intravascular space with 0.9% saline or Ringer's lactate is indicated. In the adult patient, the rate of fluid administration is gauged according to the patient's age, underlying cardiovascular disease, and the urgency of the fluid requirement (i.e., hypotensive patients may require vigorous fluid resuscitation). Patients with hypovolemic shock are best managed with a CVP or Swan–Ganz catheter in place to monitor the hemodynamic response to fluid administration. In the presence of shock, frequent boluses of 100–200 ml up to 1–2 l total fluid may be given the first hour. Thereafter, a rate of infusion is chosen to replace ongoing losses and the remaining fluid deficit in a safe manner. As a general guideline for the average-size adult patient, a rate of 200–250 ml/hr should not be exceeded. Colloid solutions (albumin, plasma, dextran, and hydroxyethyl starch) also have application in volume-depleted states, but controversy continues over the superiority of crystalloids versus colloids for resuscitation in shock states (103). Colloids are most useful in states associated with a low colloid osmotic pressure. Use of dextrans and hydroxyethyl starch may be complicated by hypersensitivity reactions, acute renal failure, and hemorrhagic complications, although hydroxyethyl starch is reported to have a lower risk of hypersensitivity reactions (104). Less acute cases of prerenal azotemia (i.e., excessive diuretic use, salt-wasting nephropathy) may not require parenteral fluid administration and will respond to discontinuing the offending agent and increasing dietary salt consumption. If the diagnosis of prerenal azotemia is correct and has not progressed to ATN, then the response to parenteral volume repletion is gratifyingly prompt. BUN and serum creatinine begin falling and return to baseline values within as little as 24–48 hours if the full deficit is restored. If the patient's weight prior to the acute volume loss is known, then the aim of fluid replacement is to return to the previous weight. When a weight is not available, the physician makes an estimate of Na^+ and fluid losses and administers fluid to restore blood pressure, to establish urine flow in excess of 30 ml/hr, and to avoid volume overload and pulmonary edema, which is of special concern in the elderly and in others with cardiovascular compromise. Avoidance of these complications of volume replacement demands frequent reassessment of the patient with attention to the presence of rales, jugular venous distension, a third heart sound, edema, and daily weights.

Prerenal azotemia resulting from poor cardiac function is more difficult to treat. Impairment of renal sodium excretion is present with only mild cardiac dysfunction, and as cardiac deterioration progresses renal hypoperfusion may result in azotemia (105). Measures to improve cardiac function may also restore renal perfusion, and include the use of diuretics to decrease preload, inotropic agents such as digoxin and dobutamine to improve intrinsic cardiac function, and the use of vasodilators such as hydralazine and captopril to decrease afterload.

MANAGEMENT OF THE PATIENT WITH ACUTE RENAL FAILURE (NONDIALYTIC MANAGEMENT)

Conservative, nondialytic management of acute renal failure is appropriate for those patients in the early phase (oliguric or nonoliguric) with none of the metabolic or medical complications. In general, conservative measures consist of in-hospital observation with close attention to blood pressure, volume status, neurologic function, and evidence of hemorrhagic or infectious complications. Blood should be drawn at least once daily to monitor the serum electrolytes (Na^+, K^+, Cl^-, CO_2), BUN, creatinine, Ca^{2+}, PO_4, and a complete blood count. In the patient with hyperkalemia, more frequent monitoring of the serum K^+ will be required. Measures to avoid infection are vitally important and include scrupulous avoidance of intravenous or urinary catheters if at all possible. The use of prophylactic antibiotics will be considered in more detail, but in general it is not an advisable practice.

Nutritional management of the patient not on dialysis is designed to slow the accumulation of nitrogenous wastes as well as phosphorus, magnesium, potassium, and fluid. Nutritional recommendations include 0.5 g/kg/day of protein with high biologic value or essential amino acids up to a maximum of 40 g/day. In the patient who is not septic or is severely catabolic, this degree of protein restriction supplemented with adequate calories will blunt the rate of rise of BUN, delaying or even precluding the need for dialysis. Total potassium intake must also be restricted, and for the average-size adult between 20 and 40 mEq/day is permitted. Sodium is restricted to prevent volume overload, and for the patient with no overt signs of volume overload, sodium restriction of 87 mEq/24 hr is permissible. Fluid intake in the same patient must be limited to an amount that replaces insensible losses and urinary losses. Given a patient without increased insensible losses (febrile, hyperventilating) 500 ml of fluid plus an amount equal to urinary losses may be allowed. Fluid intake in excess of this amount will lead to hyponatremia.

Hemodialysis for the patient with acute renal failure

Conditions that mandate initiation of dialytic therapy include refractory hyperkalemia, acidosis, volume overload, encephalopathy, pericarditis, and hemorrhage. Although these complications are satisfactorily managed with dialysis, the overall survival of patients with ARF requiring dialysis remains disappointing. Prior to the advent of clinical hemodialysis, mortality from acute renal failure was exceedingly high. The mortality in battle casualties with ARF during World War II was in excess of 90%. By the time of the Korean conflict, dialysis was available, and the mortality of trauma-induced ARF fell to 68% (106). A similar statistic was reported from the Vietnam war, and since that time, despite improvements in dialysis technology, antibiotics, and general medical care, the mortality of the more severe forms of acute renal failure has remained the same (107). The reasons for this disappointing plateau in the mortality figure are not readily apparent, but the claim has been made that the patient with ARF today is more severely ill than cases of ARF in the early years of dialysis. Modern medical technology sustains many more patients with multiple-organ failure, and those patients often have renal involvement requiring dialysis. It has been suggested that in many instances the extrarenal disease is ultimately fatal and that well-managed ARF is not the proximate cause of death in many cases of multiple-organ failure. Firm data to support this contention has not, to the authors' knowledge, been gathered.

Improvement in mortality with the use of intensive dialysis has been described in case reports (108–110). A retrospective evaluation of early and intensive dialysis in ARF reported by Kleinknecht et al. in 1972 compared survival rates of 279 patients not managed with early, intensive dialysis to the survival of 221 patients who were (111). Patients in the first group were managed prior to 1968 and mean BUN predialysis reached 164 mg/dl; after 1968, patients were dialyzed at a mean BUN of 93 mg/dl. The overall mortality was 42% in the group managed prior to 1968, but only 27% in the group managed with early intensive dialysis. Other retrospective studies support a similar reduction in mortality for the intensively dialyzed groups (112, 113). In 1975 Conger reported a prospective study of intensive hemodialysis for the treatment of ARF in Vietnam War caualties (107). Eighteen patients were enrolled in the study and were paired according to the severity of injury. In the intensively dialyzed group, the mean predialysis serum creatinine was maintained at 5 mg/dl, and in the non-intensive dialysis group, the mean predialysis creatinine was 10 mg/dl. Survival was improved and complications were fewer in the intensively dialyzed group. To correct the deficiencies of this study (small numbers, no assessment of nutritional status or antibiotic levels), Conger and others initiated a similar study at the University of Colorado Health Sciences Center Hospital, including 34 patients with ARF of medical and surgical etiologies in whom nutritional status and antibiotic levels were carefully assessed (114). The principal conclusion of the study is that intensive hemodialysis applied to a general population with ARF does not enhance survival. Obviously, this remark does not apply to those patients with clear indications for intensive dialysis such as refractory hyperkalemia, volume overload, severe acidosis, or other complications of ARF that respond to dialysis. Further, it is self evident that a separation in BUN and creatinine for the intensively and non-intensively dialyzed groups must exist beyond which an improvement in the intensively dialyzed population can be demonstrated. Based on this study, a recommendation can be made for maintaining predialysis BUN near 100 mg/dl, and predialysis creatinine at 9.0 mg/dl, a practice that seems well entrenched in clinical nephrology already.

Nutrition in acute renal failure

No clear consensus has been reached regarding the overall importance of nutrition during ARF, and less agreement exists concerning the respective roles of carbohydrates, fats, and protein in the form of essential and nonessential amino acids. While it is apparent that the patient with a prolonged, severe illness who is unable to eat must have nutritional support, conclusive proof that nutritional therapy has an important impact on the course of ARF has not been forthcoming.

In 1967, Berlyne reported that a diet for patients with ARF consisting of 2200 calories, 16 g of high-quality protein, and 500 ml of fluid resulted in improved nutrition, but no clear enhancement of survival was demonstrated (115). The GI route of administration is preferred, but in the intensive care setting intravenous hyperalimentation is often required. Furthermore, little data is available about the effect of enteral nutrition on the course of ARF. Abel and colleagues reported a study in 1973 comparing infusion of 50% glucose only with infusion of 50% glucose and a mixture of essential amino acids (EAAs), and concluded that survival of ARF was improved in patients treated with EAAs (116). This observation has been confirmed by at least one other investigator and has been disputed by several others (117, 118). Freund examined mortality in ARF patients receiving only intravenous glucose or 50% glucose with a mixture of EAAs and nonessential amino acids, and found a higher mortality in the group receiving amino acids (118). Feinstein compared mortality in a prospective double-blind trial of hypertonic glucose + 21 g/day EAAs or 21 g EAAs + 21 g nonessential amino acids per day and found no difference in survival or recovery of renal function between the groups (119). Despite the conflicting evidence about the efficacy of aggressive nutrition in ARF, it has become the standard of practice to institute intensive hyperalimentation early in the course of ARF. Nitrogen balance is improved and survival is not affected adversely, making it a reasonable approach. The resulting accumulation of fluid and the products of protein breakdown often mandate earlier institution of dialysis and ultrafiltration.

Energy requirements for the patient with ARF are difficult to gauge, and some authors suggest using large amounts of calories to minimize protein breakdown. Between 35 and 50 Cal/kg/day is recommended, with the higher energy intakes being reserved for those who are more severely ill (120). It has been suggested that 80% of the caloric requirement be supplied as carbohydrates and 20% as fat (120, 122). The fat is a more efficient source of calories and is necessary to prevent the fatty acid deficiency syndrome. Provision of 5–10% of daily caloric requirements as fat is usually sufficient. Alternatively, administration of two to three 500 ml bottles of a 10% fat emulsion per week will also satisfy the requirements for fatty acids. Hypertonic (50–70%) dextrose is the usual carbohydrate source and is administered at these concentrations to limit fluid intake in the oliguric or anuric patient. The daily protein requirement for the patient with ARF depends upon the frequency of dialysis, as well as any underlying catabolic illnesses. Patients with chronic renal insufficiency undergoing dialysis treatment require 1 g/kg/day of protein (121), and this allowance must be increased for the ARF patient in accordance wth the variables discussed. For patients in need of nitrogen restriction, commercially available solutions of essential amino acids (6.5%) may be administered. Patients receiving frequent dialysis and not under a strict nitrogen limitation may be given an 8.5% amino acid solution that contains approximately 7.15 g of nitrogen. Electrolytes are added to the solution as necessary. In Table 6 are listed the TPN solutions in use at our hospital. Vitamins (B_1, B_2, niacin, B_6, biotin, pantothenic acid, choline) and trace elements (Mn, Zn, Cu, Cr) are added to one bottle daily. Vitamin K (10 mg) is administered twice weekly.

PRACTICAL CONSIDERATIONS IN PARENTERAL HYPERALIMENTATION

The central venous catheter for TPN should be placed by well-qualified personnel, and once secured and its position confirmed by x-ray, it should be scrupulously protected from any use other than alimentation. The initial rate of fluid administration should not exceed 50 ml/hr, and blood glucose must be monitored frequently. In the days that follow, the rate of fluid administration is increased to achieve recommended calorie and protein intakes. Plasma electrolytes must be monitored daily, particularly if the initial solution is electrolyte free. Hypokalemia, hypophosphatemia, and hypomagnesemia are common complications of TPN, and if the renal formula is chosen as the initial solution, K^+, Mg^{2+}, and PO_4^{2-} supplementation will become necessary. Calcium supplementation will also be necessary, along with vitamins and trace elements. During the first weeks of parenteral nutrition, plasma electrolytes, glucose, and BUN are checked at least daily, and plasma calcium, phosphorus, and magnesium are checked two to three times per week. Plasma transaminases are checked several times weekly and total protein, cholesterol, and triglycerides are monitored weekly, initially.

Supplementation with branched-chain amino acids and ketoanalogs of amino acids

Evidence has been presented that infusion of branched-chain amino acids (BCAAs) into septic or postsurgical patients may improve nitrogen balance (122–124). The mechanism for this effect is not understood at present, and the role for BCAA in nutritional support for the patient

Table 6. Solutions for parenteral nutrition

Central formula (with electrolytes)		Renal formula		Central formula (without electrolytes)	
Dextrose 50%	500 ml	Dextrose 70%	500 ml	Dextrose 50%	500 ml
Amino acid 8.5% (essential and non-essential)	500 ml	Amino acid 6.5% (essential only)	230 ml	Amino acid 8.5% (essential and non-essential)	500 ml
Acetate	67.5 mEq	Acetate	15.0 mEq	Acetate	36.5 mEq
Chloride	35.0 mEq	Chloride	7.75 mEq	Chloride	7.0 mEq
Total kcal	1020	Total kcal	1255	Total kcal	1020
Protein	42.5 g	Protein	16.25 g	Protein	42.5 g
Nitrogen	7.1 g	Nitrogen	2.5 g	Nitrogen	7.1 g
Osmolarity	1847	Osmolarity	1940	Osmolarity	1751
Magnesium	5.0 mEq				
Phosphate	15.0 mM				
Potassium	30 mEq				
Sodium	35.0 mEq				

with ARF remains to be defined. Likewise, investigations in animals have demonstrated that the amino acid leucine and its ketoanalog and ketoisocaproate exert a protein-sparing effect. Leucine promotes protein synthesis, while the ketoanalog, alpha ketoisocaproate, prevents protein degradation (125). In humans, infusion of alpha ketoisocaproate into starving, obese subjects exerts a nitrogen-sparing effect (126), but there is a dearth of studies examining the effects of ketoanalogs in the setting of ARF. At the present time a firm recommendation cannot be made for the use of ketoanalogs of amino acids or BCAAs in ARF.

Continuous arteriovenous hemofiltration and other modalities for treatment of ARF

Continuous arteriovenous hemofiltration (CAVH) has now been applied to large numbers of patients with ARF and in certain situations holds distinct advantages over hemodialysis. The procedure involves use of an artifical kidney (Amicon, Hospal) with a high ultrafiltration coefficient, and access to the circulation is achieved with a large-bore catheter in the femoral artery and one in the femoral vein. Because of potential complications of femoral artery catheters, some centers strongly prefer to use Scribner shunts for vascular access. The catheters are in turn connected to the CAVH kidney and the patient's blood pressure supports ultrafiltration without the use of a blood pump. The ultrafiltrate is replaced with intravenous fluid at a high rate and anticoagulation is required (127).

Solutes appear in the ultrafiltrate at concentrations identical to those in plasma water, the exception being those solutes with significant protein binding or large molecular weights (127). The Gibbs–Donnan effect on small solute and electrolyte transfer across the membrane is negligible, and sieving coefficients are close to 1.0. CAVH is not an efficient means of rapid removal of K^+, as the following calculation illustrates.

With 12 l of ultrafiltrate over a 24-hour period, and a plasma K^+ of 4.0 mEq/l, only 4.0 mEq/l × 12 l or 48 mEq K^+ will be removed. However, because of the efficient fluid removal of CAVH, the physician may lower serum K^+ by using intravenous $NaHCO_3$ and glucose with insulin infusions, or alternatively a diffusive dialysis using the CAVH access lines may be accomplished to lower serum K^+.

The solutions for replacement of the ultrafiltrate may be infused into a peripheral vein or may be infused into the CAVH blood lines entering (predilution) or leaving (postdilution) the kidney (128). In theory some advantage is derived from the predilution method in that solute clearance may be increased because of solute diffusion out of RBCs down concentration gradients, and a lower oncotic pressure in the kidney may increase the ultrafiltration rate (UFR). Further, less anticoagulation may be required with the predilution mode. At least one study has confirmed that predilution does enhance urea clearance and UFR (128). The solution most commonly used to replace ultrafiltrate is normal saline (0.9%) with Ca^{2+} and Mg^{2+}

Table 7. Bicarbonate replacement fluid for CAVH (Port, Ann Arbor)

Ingredients of fluid
1 l 0.9% saline + 7.5 ml 10% $CaCl_2$ (10 mEq)
1 l 0.9% saline + 1.6 ml 50% $MgSO_4$ (6 mEq)
1 l 0.9% saline
1 l D_5W + 3 amps $NaHCO_3$ (150 mEq)

Total volume of fluid
4.16 l containing:
Na^+	147 mEq/l
Cl^-	115 mEq/l
HCO_3^-	36 mEq/l
K^+	0 mEq/l
Ca^{2+}	2.4 mEq/l
Mg^{2+}	1.4 mEq/l
Dextrose	1200 mg/dl

Reprinted with permission from Golper TA (127).

additives, and lactate or acetate as a buffering anion. Under conditions in which lactate or acetate infusion is undesirable (i.e., lactic acidosis, hypotension), bicarbonate may be substituted as the anion. A HCO_3^--containing replacement fluid devised by Port is described in Table 7.

For administration of this fluid, a multipronged manifold of the kind used in CCPD is attached to the bags of solution. The manifold in turn connects to intravenous tubing through a high-volume I Med pump (I Med Corp, San Diego, CA) and then to the patient via a peripheral vein or into the kidney circuits (127).

APPLICATIONS OF CAVH

CAVH is ideally suited for the patient with ARF who is hemodynamically unstable (e.g., post cardiac or aneurysm surgery, septic shock), but requires fluid removal and aggressive nutritional support. Paganini has reported his experience with CAVH in severely ill patients with ARF and finds that it is better tolerated than hemodialysis (129). During hemodialysis major contributors to hypotension are the rapid changes in serum osmolality (which results in decreased mobilization of fluid from the cellular compartments) and an associated autonomic dysfunction, neither of which complicate CAVH (130, 131), or pure ultrafiltration. Several investigators have noted that patients who become hypotensive during dialysis do not become hypotensive during pure ultrafiltration, with fluid removal equal to that during dialysis (132). These observations apply as well to CAVH. The early institution of CAVH with removal of large volumes of fluid permits more aggressive TPN, which is especially important in the catabolic patient who may require upwards of 5 l of hyperalimentation fluid daily. Nevertheless, mortality in patients treated with CAVH is high, in large part because the procedure is applied to a subset of critically ill patients with ARF. The suggestion has been made, however, that CAVH may result in improvement of survival over that afforded by conventional dialysis because of improved nutrition (133).

COMPLICATIONS OF CAVH

Prominent among complications of CAVH are those related to vascular access. Because of the proximity of the groin to the perineal area, indwelling catheters placed in this region may be complicated by infection and sepsis more often than catheters at other sites. Long-term catheterization of the femoral artery has been reported to carry a 23% incidence of sepsis, and in several controlled studies of long-term catheterization of the radial and axillary arteries, the incidence of sepsis is not lower (134–138) Hence, catheterization of femoral vessels may not predispose to higher infection rates than catheterization at other sites, especially if proper catheter care is employed (139). Other problems include thrombosis and aneurysm formation at the site of cannulation as well as hemorrhage. Hemorrhage at sites other than the access site may result from the heparinization required. This problem may be circumvented by the use of regional heparinization or lower doses of heparin. For the patient with a coagulopathy resulting from liver disease or other causes, and in patients with thrombocytopenia, anticoagulation may not be necessary.

DRUG REMOVAL BY CAVH

Available information about drug removal in CAVH has recently been summarized by Golper et al. (140). The factor that limits drug permeability across CAVH membranes is the extent of protein binding. Most drugs are relatively small solutes, and size does not limit diffusion across the membranes. With knowledge of a drug's protein binding, sieving coefficient, and the ultrafiltration rate, its removal can be readily computed. For clinical purposes, removal of a drug may be determined by measuring its concentration in the ultrafiltrate and multiplying by the ultrafiltration rate (127).

HEMODIAFILTRATION (CAVHD) AND SCUF

Hemodiafiltration or continuous arteriovenous hemodialysis (CAVHD) and slow continuous ultrafiltration (SCUF) are two modifications to the technique of CAVH that have recently been described (140–143). Hemodiafiltration involves the use of the CAVH procedure with the addition of a diffusive dialysis. This is accomplished by passing a standard peritoneal dialysis solution through the dialysate compartment countercurrent to the blood flow. Gravity alone may be used to pull the dialysate through the kidney, or a pump may be used and the rate adjusted to as high as 500 ml/min. Accurate measurement of the ultrafiltrate becomes difficult with such high flow rates, and an adequate drainage mechanism must be available to handle the large volumes of fluid. Use of such high dialysate flow rates with this technique is ordinarily not practical, but use of dialysate flow rates on the order of 20 ml/min permits accurate measurement of the ultrafiltrate (hence more accurate fluid replacement) and may proceed on a continuous basis. Small molecule clearances are greater with CAVHD than CAVH, and in general the diffusive clearance is equal to the dialysate inflow for rates up to 30 ml/min if the blood flow is > 75 ml/min (140).

SCUF was described by Paganini et al. in 1980 and is a modification of CAVH that is used for removal of excessive fluid in the patient unresponsive to diuretics (143). The technique has been applied to patients with and without acute renal failure. The volume of replacement fluid is considerably smaller than CAVH, and this technique is not suitable for the management of uremia. The rate of ultrafiltration may be controlled by raising the level of the drainage bag, or, alternatively, the fluid line exiting the kidney may be placed in an infusion pump, allowing for precise adjustment of the ultrafiltration rate. Otherwise, SCUF is identical to CAVH.

PERITONEAL DIALYSIS IN ACUTE RENAL FAILURE

There is abundant literature regarding the use of peritoneal dialysis for the treatment of ARF, and in general the mortality figures are similar to those for hemodialysis treatment. In a review of 13 series of patients with ARF treated with peritoneal dialysis (plus a report of their own), Firmat and Zucchini found an average mortality rate of 51%, with a range from 17% to 75% (144). The leading causes of death in these series were sepsis and shock (149–157).

Although peritoneal dialysis is a less efficient means of dialysis, there are certain circumstances that favor its use for ARF. Certain patients are at a greater risk from hemodialysis-induced hypotension, including those with established shock, severe congestive heart failure, recent myocardial infarction, coronary artery disease, and cerebrovascular disease. Patients at risk for bleeding may also be candidates for peritoneal dialysis, because anticoagulation is not required. Often, peritoneal dialysis in this setting is better tolerated. Small children with ARF are often best managed with peritoneal dialysis, principally due to problems in achieving vascular access and their relatively low blood volumes. The adult with none of the aforementioned problems may be successfully managed with peritoneal dialysis if marked catabolism and other complications of renal failure responsive to a more efficient dialysis (i.e., hyperkalemia) are not present. Potassium removal by the peritoneal route is slow, and even at a serum K^+ of 7.0 mEq/l the rate of removal is 12 mEq/hr or less (158). Hourly Kayexelate® enemas (30 g) will remove approximately 30 mEq of K^+/hr and are therefore more efficient than peritoneal dialysis. For the patient with uncontrolled hyperkalemia, hemodialysis is the treatment of choice. Other metabolic complications more amenable to hemodialysis include severe lactic acidosis and hypercalcemia. Peritoneal dialysis effects a relatively slow removal of lactic acid, and absorption of buffer from dialysate is also relatively slow. Some reports have suggested that acetate or bicarbonate are better buffer anions than lactate when peritoneal dialysis must be used in a patient with lactic acidosis (158–161).

The patient with ARF who is markedly catabolic (i.e.,

post trauma, surgery, sepsis) and requires aggressive nutritional support is not a good candidate for peritoneal dialysis.

COMPLICATIONS OF ACUTE RENAL FAILURE

Bleeding

Uremia may impair hemostasis significantly and aggravate any underlying condition that may cause bleeding (e.g., peptic ulcer disease). Abnormalities of hemostasis in uremia result from defects in platelet function, but the intrinsic and extrinsic clotting pathways are usually intact.

Biochemical abnormalities associated with uremia that may result in platelet dysfunction include reductions in platelet ADP and serotonin levels, elevation of cyclic AMP, and reduced generation of thromboxane (162–165). An abnormality of cyclooxygenase in uremic platelets has also been reported (162). Furthermore, there is evidence that the von Willebrand factor component of the coagulation factor VIII (FVIII:VWF) is abnormal. With increasing sophistication in the management of ARF, bleeding problems are less frequent, but still pose some difficult dilemmas.

In the early years of ARF, gastrointestinal hemorrhage resulting from gastric stress ulceration was the second most common cause of death, but, with recognition of the importance of maintaining a more alkaline gastric pH by the use of H_2 receptor antagonists (cimetidine, ranitidine) and liberal antacids, many centers are reporting a dramatic decline in GI bleeding (166, 167). Recent advances in the therapy of bleeding in uremic patients include the use of DDAVP and cryoprecipitate (168, 169). The mechanism of action of cryoprecipitate has not been established, but it does result in increased plasma levels of VWF:VIII. DDAVP results in the release of VWF:VIII multimers from vascular endothelium, which in turn enhances the function of uremic platelets. Several studies report improvement in bleeding times of uremic patients treated with DDAVP. The dose of DDAVP is 0.3 µg/kg in 50 ml of physiologic saline infused over 30 minutes. At least one anecdotal report has claimed improvement of bleeding time with intranasal DDAVP (170). The effect of DDAVP and cryoprecipitate lasts but a few hours, and cryoprecipitate is complicated by its potential for transmission of blood-borne diseases such as AIDS and hepatitis. A recent study reported the use of conjugated estrogens (0.6 mg/kg × 5 days) for uremic bleeding (171). Abnormal bleeding times were corrected, with the earliest effect beginning at 6 hours after administration and peaking between 5 and 7 days. The effect lasted for up to 14 days, and levels of circulating VWF were unaffected. This may prove to be an effective therapy for uremic bleeding in the future.

When hemodialysis is necessary in the patient with hemorrhagic complications, the use of heparin to prevent clotting in the dialyzer is inadvisable. This admonition applies not only to the patient with demonstrated bleeding, but also to the patient who may be at greater risk for bleeding (post surgery, pericarditis). Alternatives to the routine use of heparin include so-called tight heparinization, employing smaller loading and maintenance doses with less prolongation of the clotting time. Citrate anticoagulation has been used successfully in patients at risk for bleeding, but the procedure is cumbersome, requiring a calcium-free dialysate, citrate infusion into the arterial side of the circuit, and maintenance of constant calcium infusion into the venous side of the circuit (172). The method is effective, reduces bleeding complications, and has a low incidence of adverse side effects. A study in 1961 reported significant problems with hypernatremia and acidemia, which were dependent on the rate of infusion of citrate (173). A recent report by Wiegmann et al, examining citrate anticoagulation in a chronic dialysis population demonstrated mild hypernatremia (worse immediately post dialysis) and a high predialysis bicarbonate compared with the heparin-treated group. In general, however, citrate was well tolerated in this group, and the authors assert that the method is a simple one (174). Metabolic alkalosis may complicate citrate anticoagulation when dialysis with high blood flows is performed. This results from a significant citrate infusion into the patient.

Dialysis without the use of anticoagulation is possible if high blood flows across (> 250 ml/min) the dialyzer can be maintained and the kidney is rinsed every 30 minutes or so with 100 cc of saline. In our institution this has proved to be a highly successful alternative to heparin and citrate anticoagulation in the high-risk patient. Some of the success may be attributable to the use of more biocompatible dialysis membranes (cellulose acetate). Because of the success of this method, we have abandoned the use of citrate anticoagulation. A recent report describes a prospective evaluation of hemodialysis without anticoagulation. Out of 262 treatment sessions in 49 patients at increased risk of bleeding, 239 (91%) were successfully completed. There was a relatively low incidence of dialyzer clotting, and no episodes of accelerated bleeding were reported (175). Prostacyclin, which blocks platelet activation and aggregation, has been used as an anticoagulant during hemodialysis. However, prostacyclin may cause symptomatic hypotension, making it unsuitable for use in unstable patients as well as home patients, and it cannot be used without close monitoring and physician attendance.

Infection

Infection is a common problem in the patient with ARF and remains a leading cause of death. There is a high incidence of pulmonary, urinary tract, and wound infection, and septicemia is a common occurrence with an incidence of 51–89% in several large series (176–179). Intraabdominal sepsis is a particularly important determinant of survival, as illustrated by the extremely high mortality in a series of ARF precipitated or complicated by intraabdominal infection (176–182). In the septic patient without an obvious source, intraabdominal sepsis must be vigorously excluded. Abdominal imaging procedures of value include CAT scanning and ultrasound, with the CAT scan the better of the two. Gallium scanning and scanning for indium-labeled white blood cells may be useful, but are hampered by the delay in the results. The importance of reexploration of a suspicious abdomen is emphasized in the aforementioned series. The lowest mortality was reported by Milligan, who operated on 40 of 76 patients once, on 25 twice, and 5 patients underwent three reoperations (183). In the series of Kornhall, 30% of the patients had undiagnosed intraabdominal problems at postmortem, many of which were treatable. Among the potentially treatable problems were abscesses, perforations, and bleeding (184).

The reasons for the increased susceptibility to infection in uremia include malnutrition, poor wound healing, and an overall depression of immune function (185). The use of prophylactic antibiotics in the setting of ARF was examined by Zech et al., who found that the frequency of infection was increased by this practice and is therefore not advisable (186).

Hyperkalemia

Hyperkalemia is a potentially lethal complication of ARF, but one that is eminently treatable. Serum K^+ is followed closely in ARF so that hyperkalemia can be identified early and treated. The signs and symptoms of hyperkalemia are confined largely to the cardiovascular and neuromuscular systems. A rapidly ascending muscular weakness leading to flaccid quadriplegia, but with preservation of cranial nerve function, is occasionally seen with extremely high K^+ (usually > 8.5 mEq/l) (187). Paresthesias have been described and vibratory as well as position sense may be impaired. Respiratory muscle paralysis has also been reported and the muscles of phonation are involved on occasion.

The cardiovascular effects of hyperkalemia are first manifested in electrocardiographic changes. A serum K^+ below 7 mEq/l may result in no changes in the heart, but changes are uniformly present above a K^+ of 8 mEq/l (188). Hyperkalemic changes on electrocardiogram progress from peaking of T waves to prolongation of the PR interval, followed by disappearance of the P waves, and finally, with extreme elevations of the serum K^+, prolongation of the QRS complex and ventricular flutter or fibrillation. Despite its effects on cardiac conduction, hyperkalemia does not seem to affect contractility.

Temporary measures to lower serum K^+, by effecting an internal redistribution include the intravenous administration of $NaHCO_3$, glucose with insulin, and calcium chloride or calcium gluconate. $NaHCO_3$ is generally given as one ampule (50 mEq Na^+) over 5 minutes and may be repeated after 10–15 minutes if the EKG abnormalities persist. Glucose may be administered as one ampule of D_{50} (25 g glucose) along with 5–10 U of regular insulin IV. Calcium is employed to antagonize the cardiac and neuromuscular toxicity of hyperkalemia; 5–10 ml of a 10% solution of calcium gluconate may be injected IV over a 2-minute period (preferably with ECG monitoring). The dose may be repeated after 5 minutes if the ECG findings persist, but further dosing is often ineffective. For the patient receiving digitalis preparations, calcium must be given with extreme caution because of the potential for inducing digitalis toxic arrhythmias. All of the above measures are temporary only, and definitive treatment of hyperkalemia requires its removal from the body using cation exchange resins or dialysis. One such resin is Kayexelate®, which can be given orally or rectally. The recommended oral dose is 20–50 g dissolved in 100–200 ml of a 20% sorbitol solution as often as every 4 hours and given in up to four to five doses per day. The sorbitol is necessary because of the constipating effect of Kayexelate. If oral administration is impossible, 50 g Kayexelate may be given as a retention enema and should be held for 30–60 minutes. As a rule, for each 1 g of Kayexelate 1 mEq K^+ is bound in exchange for 1 mEq Na^+. This Na^+ load may result in volume overload in some patients. Hyperkalemia unresponsive to these conservative measures mandates hemodialysis. Dialysis against a bath without potassium effects a rapid lowering of serum K^+.

Divalent ions

Disturbances in the metabolism of calcium, phosphorus, and magnesium are common in ARF. Hyperphosphatemia with levels greater than 5 mg/dl is an almost universal accompaniment of oliguric ARF, and in cases of severe tissue breakdown the phosphorus may be as high as 20 mg/dl (187). Control of hyperphosphatemia is achieved by oral administration of aluminum hydroxide gels.

Hypocalcemia develops early in the course of ARF and is related to several factors: a) in the presence of hyperphosphatemia, calcium phosphate deposition may occur in the soft tissues (e.g., rhabdomyolysis); b) skeletal resistance to the calcemic action of PTH; and c) reduced levels of $1,25-(OH)_2D_3$ and $25-(OH)D_3$ (190–193).

In the setting of ARF, hypocalcemia is generally not symptomatic, which in part reflects systemic acidosis. Treatment with bicarbonate may precipate symptomatic hypocalcemia in this setting by further lowering the ionized calcium. Hypercalcemia has been reported to complicate the recovery phase of ARF due to rhabdomyolysis and appears to be the result of mobilization of calcium precipated in damaged muscle (191).

Hypermagnesemia may result during the course of ARF from treatment with magnesium-containing antacids or laxatives. These agents should, therefore, not be given to patients with ARF. Certain causes of nephrotoxic ARF (aminoglycosides, cisplatinum) may cause renal Mg^{2+} wasting and hypomagnesemia, and in this instance exogenous Mg^{2+} will be required.

REFERENCES

1. Dixon BS, Anderson RJ: Non-oliguric acute renal failure. *Am J Kidney Dis* 6:71–80, 1985.
2. Hou SH, Bushinsky DA, Wish JB, Cohen JJ, Harrington JT: Hospital-acquired renal insufficiency: A prospective

study. *Am J Med* 74:243–248, 1983.
3. Shusterman N, Strom BL, Murrary TG, Morrison G, West SL, Maislin G: Risk factors and outcome of hospital-acquired acute renal failure. *Am J Med* 83:65–71, 1987.
4. Frankel MC, Weinstein AM, Stenzel KH: Prognostic patterns in acute renal failure. *Clin Exp Dialysis Apheresis* 7:145–167, 1983.
5. Rasmussen HH, Ibels LS: Acute renal failure. Multivariate analysis of causes and risk factors. *Am J Med* 73:211–218, 1982.
6. Bullock ML, Umen AJ, Finkelstein M, Keane WF: The assessment of risk factors in 462 patients with acute renal failure. *Am J Kidney Dis* 5:97–103, 1985.
7. Rasmussen HH, Pitt EG, Ibels LS, McNeil DR: Prediction of outcome in acute renal failure by discriminant analysis of clinical variables. *Arch Int Med* 145:2015–2018, 1985.
8. Cameron JS: Acute renal failure — the continuing challenge. *Q J Med* 59: 337–343, 1986.
9. Wheeler DC, Feehally J, Walls J: High risk acute renal failure. *Q J Med* 61:977–984, 1986.
10. Abreo K, Maorthy AV, Osborne M: Changing patterns and outcome of acute renal failure requiring hemodialysis. *Arch Int Med* 146:1338–1341, 1986.
11. Corwin HL, Teplick RS, Schreiber MJ, Fany LS, Bonventre JV, Coggins CH: Prediction of outcome in acute renal failure. *Am J Nephrol* 7:8–12, 1987.
12. McInnes EG, Levy DW, Chaudhuri MD, Bhan GL: Renal failure in the elderly. *Q J Med* 64:583–588, 1987.
13. Dal Canton A, Corradi A, Stanziale R, Maruccio G, Migone L: Glomerular hemodynamics before and after release of 24-hour bilateral ureteral obstruction. *Kidney Int* 17:491–496, 1980.
14. Yarger WE, Schocken DD, Harris RH: Obstructive nephropathy in the rat: Possible roles for the reninangiotensin system, prostaglandins and thromboxanes in postobstructive renal function. *J Clin Invest* 65:400–412, 1980.
15. Hessman RK, Johnson SF, Coburn JW, Kaufman JJ: Renal artery embolism. *Ann Int Med* 89:477–482, 1978.
16. Textor SC, Novick AC, Tarazi RC, Klimas V, Vidt DG, Pohl M: Critical renal perfusion pressure for renal function in patients with bilateral atherosclerotic renal vascular disease. *Ann Int Med* 102:308–314, 1985.
17. Myers BD, Mitler DC, Mehigan JT, Olcott C, Golbetz H, Robertson CR, Derby G, Spencer R, Friedman S: Nature of the renal injury following total renal ischemia in man. *J Clin Invest* 73:329–341, 1984.
18. McPhaul JJ: Acute glomerular disease presenting as acute renal failure. *Semin Nephrol* 1:21–26, 1981.
19. Hinton AL, Clark WF, Drudger AA: Acute interstitial nephritis due to drugs. *Ann Int Med* 93:735–741, 1980.
20. Pusy CD, Saltissi B, Bloodworth L: Drug-associated acute interstitial nephritis: Clinical and pathological features and the response to high dose steroid therapy. *Q J Med* 52:194–211, 1983.
21. Myers BD, Moran SM: Hemodynamically mediated acute renal failure. *N Engl J Med* 314:97–105, 1986.
22. Corwin HL, Bonventre JV: Renal insufficiency associated with non-steroidal anti-inflammatory agents. *Am J Kidney Dis* 4:147–152, 1984.
23. Kleinknecht D, Handais P, Goldfarb B: Analgesic and nonsteroidal anti-inflammatory drug-associated acute renal failure: A prospective collaborative study. *Clin Nephrol* 25: 275–281, 1986.
24. Gabow PA, Kaehny WD, Kelleher SP: The spectrum of rhabdomyolysis. *Medicine* 61:141–152, 1982.
25. Moran SM, Myers BD: Pathophysiology of protracted acute renal failure in man. *J Clin Invest* 76:1440–1448, 1985.
26. Moran SM, Myers BD: Course of acute renal failure studied by a model of creatinine kinetics. *Kidney Int* 27:928–937, 1985.
27. Matzke GR, Lucarotti RL, Shapiro HS: Controlled comparison of gentamicin and tobramycin nephrotoxicity. *Am J Nephrol* 3:11–17, 1983.
28. Blachley JD, Hill JB: Renal and electrolyte disturbances associated with cisplatin. *Ann Intern Med* 95:628–632, 1981.
29. D'Elia J, Gleason RE, Alday M: Nephrotoxicity from angiographic contrast material. *Am J Med* 72:719–725, 1982.
30. Miller TR, et al.: Urinary diagnostic indices in acute renal failure: A prospective study. *Ann Intern Med* 89:47, 1978.
31. Anderson RJ, Gabow PA, Gross PA: Urinary chloride concentration in acute renal failure. *Miner Electrolyte Metab* 10:92–97, 1984.
32. Cirksena WJ, et al.: Pathogenetic studies in model of pigment nephropathy in the rat. In: U Gessler, K Schroder, Weidinger, eds, *Pathogenesis and Clinical Findings with Renal Failure*. Thieme, Stuttgart, p 105, 1971.
33. Finckh ES, Jeremy D, Whyte HM: Structural renal damage and its relation to clinical features in acute oliguric renal failure. *Q J Med* 31:429, 1962.
34. Oken DE, Arce ML, Wilson DR: Glycerol-induced hemoglobinuric acute renal failure in the rat: I. Micropuncture study of the development of oliguria. *J Clin Invest* 45:724, 1966.
35. Ayer G, et al.: Intrarenal hemodynamics in glycerol-induced myohemoglobinuric acute renal failure in the rat. *Circ Res* 29:128, 1971.
36. Chedru MF, Baethke R, Oken DE: Renal cortical blood flow and glomerular filtration in myohemoglobinuric acute renal failure. *Kidney Int* 1:232, 1972.
37. Hollenberg NK, Adams DF, Oken DE, et al.: Acute renal failure due to nephrotoxins: Renal hemodynamic and angiographic studies in man. *N Engl J Med* 282:1329, 1970.
38. Hollenberg NK, Epstein J, Rosen SM, et al.: Acute oliguric renal failure in man: Evidence for preferential renal cortical ischemia. *Medicine* (Baltimore) 47:455, 1968.
39. Flamenbaum W: Pathophysiology of acute renal failure. *Arch Intern Med* 131:911, 1973.
40. Conger JD, et al.: The effect of acetylcholine on the early phase of reversible norepinephrine-induced acute renal failure. *Kidney Int* 19:399, 1981.
41. Goormaghtigh N: Vascular and circulatory changes in renal cortex in anuric crush syndrome. *Proc Soc Exp Biol Med* 59:303, 1945.
42. Brown JJ, et al.: Renin and acute renal failure: Studies in man. *Br Med J* 1:253, 1970.
43. Kokot F, Kuska J: Plasma renin activity in acute renal insufficiency. *Nephron* 6:115, 1969.
44. DiBona GF, McDonald FD, Flamenbaum W, et al.: Maintenance of renal function in salt-loaded rats despite severe tubular necrosis induced by $HgCl_2$. *Nephron* 8:205, 1971.
45. McDonald FD, et al.: The prevention of acute renal failure in the rat by long-term saline loading: A possible role of renin-angiotensin axis. *So Exp Biol Med* 131:610, 1969.
46. Conger JD, Schrier RW: Renal hemodynamics in acute renal failure. *Ann Rev. Physiol* 42:603–614, 1980.
47. Powell-Jackson JD, Brown JJ, Lever AF, et al.: Protection against acute renal failure in rats by passive immunization against angiotensin II. *Lancet* 1:774, 1972.
48. Baranowski RL, O'Conner GJ, Kurtzman NA: The effect of

1-sarcosine, 8-leucyl angiotensin II on the pressor effect of infused angiotensin II. *Arch Int Pharmacodyn Ther* 209:75, 1974.
49. Reubi R, Grossweiler N, Gurtler R: The renal blood flow in acute renal failure. In: S Shaldon, GC Cooke, eds, *Acute Renal Failure*. Davis, Philadelphia, p 25, 1964.
50. Cox JW, et al.: Studies on the mechanism of oliguria in a model of unilateral acute renal failure. *J Clin Invest* 53:1546, 1974.
51. Blantz RC: The mechanism of acute renal failure after uranyl nitrate. *J Clin Invest* 55:621, 1975.
52. Conger JD, Falk SA: Glomerular and tubular dynamics in mercuric chloride-induced renal failure. *J Lab Clin Med* 107:281–289, 1986.
53. Richards AN: Direct observations of change in function of the renal tubule caused by certain poisons. *Trans Am Assoc Physic* 44:64, 1929.
54. Bank N, Mutz BF, Aynedjian HS: The role of "leakage" of tubular fluid in anuria due to mercury poisoning. *J Clin Invest* 46:695, 1967.
55. Steinhausen M, Eisenbach GM, Helmstadter V: Concentration of lissamine green in proximal tubules of antidiuretic- and mercury-poisoned rats and the permeability of these tubules. *Pflügers Arch* 311:1, 1969.
56. Donohoe JF, et al.: Tubular leakage and obstruction after renal ischemia: Structural-functional correlations. *Kidney Int* 13:208, 1978.
57. Venkatachalam MA, Bernard DB, Donohoe DF, et al.: Ischemic damage and repair in the rat proximal tubule: Differences among the S_1, S_2, S_3 segments. *Kidney Int* 14:31, 1978.
58. Myers BD, Chui F, Hilberman M, Michaels A: Transtubular leakage of glomerular filtrate in human acute renal failure. *Am J Physiol* F319–F325, 1979.
59. Baker SI, Dodds EC: Obstruction of the renal tubules during excretion of hemoglobin. *Br J Exp Pathol* 6:247, 1925.
60. Mason AD Jr, Teschan PE, Muirhead EE: Studies in acute renal failure. III. Renal histologic alterations in acute renal failure in the rat. *J Surg Res* 3:450, 1963.
61. Meroney WH, Rubini ME: Kidney function during acute tubular necrosis: Clinical studies and a theory. *Metabolism* 8:1, 1959.
62. Schrier RW, Cronin RE: Acute renal failure. In: CH Coggins, NB Cummings, eds, *Fogarty International Center Monograph on Prevention of Kidney and Urinary Tract Disease*. US Government Printing Office, Washington, DC, 1978.
63. Tanner GA, Sophasan S: Kidney pressure after temporary renal artery occlusion. *Am J Physiol* 230:1173, 1976.
64. Conger JD, Robinette JB, Kelleher SP: Nephron heterogeneity in ischemic acute renal failure. *Kidney Int* 26:422–429, 1984.
65. Jaenike RJ: Micropuncture study of methemoglobin-induced acute renal failure in the rat. *J Lab Clin Med* 73:459, 1969.
66. Ruiz-Guinazu A, Coelho JB, Pat RA: A methemoglobin-induced acute renal failure in the rat: In vivo observation, histology and micropuncture measurements of intratubular and postglomerular vascular pressures. *Nephron* 4:257, 1967.
67. Burke TJ, Cronin RE, Duchin KL, Peterson LN, Schrier RW: Ischemia and tubule obstruction during acute renal failure in dogs: Mannitol in protection. *Am J Physiol* 238 (Renal Fluid Electrolyte Physiol 7):F305–F314, 1980.
68. Farber JL: The role of calcium in cell death. *Life Sci* 29:1289, 1981.
69. Hunt, D, Humes HD, Weinberg JM: Alterations of cell cation homeostasis during ischemic injury to isolated rabbit tubules (abstract). *Kidney Int* 25:231, 1984.
70. Weinberg JM, Humes HD, Hunt D: Anoxic injury to the renal tubule (abstract). *Kidney Int* 27:106, 1985.
71. Naylor WG, Poole-Wilson PA, Williams A: Hypoxia and calcium. *J Mol Cell Cardiol* 11:683, 1979.
72. Schieppati A, Van Putten V, Burke T, Schrier R: Anoxia increases calcium influx in rat nephron segments (abstract). *Kidney Int* 27:237, 1985.
73. Freudenrich CC, Snowdowne KW, Borle AB: The effect of anoxia on cytosolic free calcium in kidney cells (abstract). *Fed Proc* 43:769, 1984.
74. Wilson P, Schrier RW: Nephron segment and calcium as determinants of anoxic cell death in primary renal cell cultures. *Kidney Int* 29:1172–1179, 1986.
75. Bonventre JV: Cell response to ischemia. In: K Solez, A Whelton, ed, *Acute Renal Failure: Clinical and Morphological Correlations*. Marcel Dekker, New York, 1984.
76. Carafoli E, et al.: A study of Ca ion metabolism in kidney mitochondria during acute uranium intoxication. *Lab Inv* 25:516–527, 1971.
77. Borle A, Clark I: Effects of phosphate induced hyperparathyroidism and parathyroidectomy on rat kidney calcium in vivo. *Am J Physiol* 241:E136, 1981.
78. Lehninger A, et al.: Transport and accumulation of calcium in mitochondria. *Ann NY Acad Sci* 307:160–178, 1978.
79. Mergner WJ, et al.: Studies on the pathogenesis of ischemic cell injury. *Virchows Arch B [Cell Pathol]* 26:17–26, 1977.
80. Arnold PE, Lumlertgul D, Burke TJ, Schrier RW: In vitro versus in vivo mitochondrial calcium loading in ischemic acute renal failure. *Am J Physiol* 248 (Renal Fluid Electrolyte Physiol 17):F845–F850, 1985.
81. Ardaillou R: Reactive oxygen species: Production and role in the kidney. *Am J Physiol* 251 (Renal Fluid Electrolyte Physiol 20):F765–F776, 1986.
82. Paller MS, Hoidal JR, Ferris TF: Oxygen free radicals in ischemic acute renal failure in the rat. *J Clin Invest* 74:1156–1164, 1984.
83. Hansson R, Gustafsson R, Jonsson O, Lundstam S, Pettersson T, Schersten T, Waldenstrom J: Effect of xanthine oxidase inhibition on renal circulation after ischemia. *Transplant Proc* 14:51–58, 1982.
84. Hansson R, Jonsson O, Lundstam S, Pettersson S, Schersten T, Waldenstrom J: Effects of free radical scavengers on renal circulation after ischaemia in the rabbit. *Clin Sci* 65:605–610, 1983.
85. Teschan PE, Lawson NL: Studies in acute renal failure. *Nephron* 3:1, 1966.
86. Thiel G, Wilson DR, Arce ML, et al.: Glycerol-induced hemoglobinuric acute renal failure in the rat: II. The experimental model, predisposing factors, and pathophysiologic features. *Nephron* 4:276, 1967.
87. Schrier RW, Conger JD: Acute renal failure: Pathogenesis, diagnosis, and management. In: RW Schrier, ed, *Renal and Electrolyte Disorders*, 3rd ed. Boston: Little, Brown, pp 423–460, 1986.
88. Cronin RE, et al.: Pathogenic mechanism in early norepinephrine-induced acute renal failure. Functional and histological correlates of protection. *Kidney Int* 14:115, 1978.
89. de Torrente A, et al.: Effects of furosemide and acetylcholine in norepinephrine-induced acute renal failure. *Am J Physiol* 235:F131, 1978.
90. Mauk RH, Patak RV, Fadem SZ, Lifschitz MD, Stein JH:

Studies on the effect of prostaglandin E administration in a nephrotoxic and a vasoconstrictor model of acute renal failure. *Kidney Int* 12:122, 1977.
91. Old CW, Duarte CM, Seidlecki LM, et al.: Effects of mannitol in the prevention of radiocontrast acute renal failure in patients with pre-existing chronic renal failure. *Proc Am Soc Nephrol* 14:31A, 1981.
92. Powers SR, Bora A, Hostnik W, et al.: Prevention of postoperative acute renal failure with mannitol in 100 cases. *Surgery* 55:15–23, 1965.
93. Judson F, Eneas MD, Schoenfeld PY, Humphreys MH: The effect of infusion of mannitol-sodium bicarbonate on the clinical course of myoglobinuria. *Arch Intern Med* 139:801–805, 1979.
94. Klinenberg JR, Bluestone R, Schlosstein L, Waisman J, Whitehouse MW: Urate deposition disease. How is it regulated and how can it be modified? *Ann Intern Med* 78:99–111, 1973.
95. McMartin KE, et al.: Methanol poisoning in human subjects: Role for formic acid accumulation in the metabolic acidosis. *Am J Med* 68:414, 1980.
96. Blackshear JL, Davidman M, Stillman T: Identification of risk for renal insufficiency from nonsteroidal anti-inflammatory drugs. *Arch Intern Med* 143:1130, 1983.
97. Kimberly RP, et al.: Reduction of renal function by newer nonsteroidal anti-inflammatory drugs. *Am J Med* 64:804, 1978.
98. Arisz L, et al.: The effect of indomethacin on proteinuria and kidney function in the nephrotic syndrome. *Acta Med Scand* 199:121, 1976.
99. Zipser RD, et al.: Prostaglandins: Modulators of renal function and pressor resistance in chronic liver disease. *J Clin Endocrinol Metab* 48:895, 1979.
100. Reymann MT, Bradac JA, Coggs CG, Dismukes WE: Correlation of aminoglycoside dosages with serum concentrations during therapy of serious gram-negative bacillary disease. *Antimicrob Agents Chemother* 16:353–361, 1979.
101. Moore RD, Smith CR, Lipsky JJ, Mellits ED, Lietman PS: Risk factors for nephrotoxicity in patients treated with aminoglycosides. *Ann Intern Med* 100:352–357, 1984.
102. Sawyers CL, Moore RD, Lerner SA, Smith CR: A model for predicting nephrotoxicity in patients treated with aminoglycosides. *J Infect Dis* 153:1062, 1986.
103. Billhardt RA, Rosenbush SW: Cardiogenic and hypovolemic shock. *Med Clin North Am* 70:853–876, 1986.
104. Karlson KE, Garzon AA, Shaftan GW, Chu CJ: Increased blood loss associated with administration of certain plasma expanders: Dextran 75, dextran 40, and hydroxyethyl starch. *Surgery* 62: 670, 1967.
105. Dzau VJ: Renal and circulatory mechanisms in congestive heart failure. *Kidney Int* 31:1402–1415, 1987.
106. Teschan PE, Baxter CR, O'Brien TF, et al.: Prophylactic hemodialysis in the treatment of acute renal failure. *Ann Int Med* 59:992, 1960.
107. Conger JD: A controlled evaluation of prophylactic dialysis in posttraumatic acute renal failure. *J Trauma* 15:1056, 1975.
108. Silva H, Pomery J, Rae AI, Rosen SM, Shaldon S: Daily haemodialysis in "hypercatabolic" acute renal failure. *Br Med J* 2:407, 1964.
109. Walsh A, O'Dwyer WF, Woodcock JA, Doyle G, Barry AP: Earlier dialysis in renal failure. *Br J Urol* 33:43, 1961.
110. Parsons FM, Hobson SM, Blagg CR, McCracken BH: Optimum time for dialysis in acute reversible renal failure. Description and value of an improved dialyzer with large surface area. *Lancet* 1:129, 1961.
111. Kleinknecht D, Jungers P, Chanard J, Barband C, Ganeval D: Uremic and non-uremic complications in acute renal failure: Evaluation of early and frequent dialysis on prognosis. *Kidney Int*:190, 1972.
112. Easterling RE, Forland M: A five year experience with prophylactic dialysis for acute renal failure. *Trans Am Soc Artif Int Organs* 10:200, 1964.
113. Fischer RP, Griffin WO Jr, Clark DS: Early dialysis in the treatment of acute renal failure. *Surg Gynecol Obstet* 123:1019, 1966.
114. Gillum DM, Dixon BS, Yanover MJ, et al.: The role of intensive dialysis in acute renal failure. *Clin Nephrol* 25:249–255, 1986.
115. Berlyne GM, Bazzard FJ, Booth EM: The dietary treatment of acute renal failure. *Q J Med* 36:59–83, 1967.
116. Abel RM, Beck CH, Abbott WM, Ryan JA, Barnett OG, Fischer JE: Improved survival from acute renal failure after treatment with intravenous essential L-amino acids and glucose. *N Engl J Med* 288:695, 1973.
117. Baek SM, Makaboli GG, Bryan-Brown CW: The influence of parenteral nutrition on the course of acute renal failure. *Surg Gynecol Obstet* 141:405–408, 1975.
118. Freund H, Harmian S, Fischer JE: Comparative studies of parenteral nutrition in renal failure using essential and nonessential amino acid containing solutions. *Surg Gynecol Obstet* 151:652–656, 1980.
119. Feinstein EI, Blumenkrantz MJ, Healy M, et al.: Clinical and metabolic responses to parenteral nutrition in acute renal failure. *Medicine* 6:124, 1981.
120. Kopple JD: Acute renal failure: Conservative, non-dialytic management. In: RJ Glassock, ed, *Current Therapy in Nephrology and Hypertension, 1984–1985.* CV Mosby, St. Louis, pp 236–242, 1984.
121. Borah MF, Schoenfeld PY, Gotch FA, et al.: Nitrogen balance during intermittent dialysis therapy of uremia. *Kidney Int* 14:491, 1978.
122. Wesson DE, Mitch WE, Wilmore W: Nutritional considerations in the treatment of acute renal failure. In: BM Brenner, JM Lazarus, eds, *Acute Renal Failure.* WB Saunders, Philadelphia, pp 618–642, 1983.
123. Blackburn GL, Desai SP, Keenan RA, et al.: Clinical use of branched chain amino acid enriched solution in the stressed and injured patients. In: M Walser, JR Williamson, eds, *Metabolism and Clinical Implications of Branched Chain Amino and Ketoacids,* Vol 18. Elsevier/North Holland, pp 521–526, 1981.
124. Freund HR, Lapidot A, Fischer JE: The use of branched chain amino acids in the injured septic patient. In: M Walser, JR Williamson, eds, *Metabolism and Clinical Implications of Branched Chain Amino and Ketoacids,* Vol 18. Elsevier/North Holland, pp 527–532, 1981.
125. Goldberg AL, Tischler ME: Regulatory effects of leucine on carbohydrate and protein metabolism. In: M Walser, JR Williamson, eds, *Metabolism and Clinical Implications of Branched Chain Amino and Ketoacids,* Vol 18. Elsevier/North Holland pp 205–216, 1981.
126. Mitch WE, Walser M, Sapir DG: Nitrogen sparing induced by leucine compared with that induced by its ketoanalogue alpha ketoisocaproate, in fasting obese man. *J Clin Invest* 67:553, 1981.
127. Golper TA: Continuous arteriovenous hemofiltration in acute renal failure. *Am J Kidney Dis* 6:373–386, 1985.
128. Kaplan AA: Predilution versus postdilution for continuous arteriovenous hemofiltration. *Trans Am Soc Artif Intern*

Organs 31:1985.
129. Paganini EP, O'Hara P, Nakamoto S: Slow continuous ultrafiltration in hemodialysis resistant oliguric acute renal failure patients. *Trans Am Soc Artif Intern Organs* 30:173–177, 1984.
130. Henrich WL, Woodard TD, Blachley JD, et al.: Role of osmolality in blood pressure stability after dialysis and ultrafiltration. *Kidney Int* 18:480–488, 1980.
131. Swartz RD, Somermeyer MG, Hsu CH: Preservation of plasma volume during hemodialysis depends on dialysate osmolality. *Am J Nephrol* 2:189–194, 1982.
132. Bergstrom J, Asaba H, Furst P, et al.: Dialysis, ultrafiltration and blood pressure. *Proc Eur Dial Transpl Assoc* 13:293–305, 1976.
133. Bartlett RH, Mault JR, Dechert RE, Palmer J, Swartz RD, Port FK: Continuous arteriovenous hemofiltration: Improved survival in surgical acute renal failure? *Surgery* 100:400–408, 1986.
134. Thomas F, Burke JP, Parker J, Orme JT, Gardner RM, Clemmer TP, Hill GA, MacFarlane P: The risk of infection related to radial vs. femoral sites for arterial catheterization. *Crit Care Med* 11:807, 1983.
135. Russell JA, Joel M, Hudson RJ, Mangano DT, Schlobohm RM: Prospective evaluation of radial and femoral artery catheterization sites in critically ill adults. *Crit Care Med* 11:936, 1983.
136. Gurman GM, Kriemerman S: Cannulation of big arteries in critically ill patients. *Crit Care Med* 13:217, 1985.
137. Soderstrom CA, Wasserman DH, Dunham CM, Caplan ES, Cowley RA: Superiority of the femoral artery for monitoring: A prospective study. *Am J Surg* 144:309, 1982.
138. Puri VK, Carlson RW, Bander JJ, Weil MH: Complications of vascular catheterization in the critically ill. A prospective study. *Crit Care Med* 8:495, 1980.
139. Olbricht CJ: Vascular access for CAVH *Proceedings of the Third International Symposium on Acute Continuous Renal Replacement Therapy.* pp 23–26, 1987.
140. Golper TA, Wedel SK, Kaplan AA, et al.: Drug removal during continuous arteriovenous hemofiltration: Theory and clinical observations. *Int J Artif Organs* 8:307, 1985.
141. Geronemus R, Schneider N: Continuous arteriovenous hemodialysis (abstract). *Blood Purif* 2:209, 1984.
142. Ing TS, Purandare VV, Daugirdas JT, et al.: Slow continuous hemodialysis. *Int J Artif Organs* 7:53, 1984.
143. Paganini EP, Nakamoto S: Continuous slow ultrafiltration in oliguric renal failure. *Trans Am Soc Artif Int Organs* 26:201, 1980.
144. Firmat J, Zucchini A: Peritoneal dialysis in acute renal failure. In: Trevino–Becerra A, Boen FS, eds, *Today's Art of Peritoneal Dialysis*. Vol 17, Contributions to Nephrology. S Karger, Basel, p 33, 1979.
145. Alarconon Zurita A, Torre Carballada MA, Sanchez Casajus A, et al.: Complicaciones de la dialisis peritoneal. *Revta Clin Esp* 137:315, 1975.
146. Aye MM, Kulatilake AK, Shackman R: Peritoneal dialysis in surgery. In: DN Kerr, et al., eds, *Proceedings of the European Dialysis Transplant Association*, Vol 2. Excerpta Medica, Amsterdam, p 49, 1965.
147. Barry KG, Schwartz FD, Hano JE, et al.: Peritoneal dialysis: Current applications and recent developments. In: *Proceedings of the Third International congress on Nephrology*. Karger, Basel p 288, 1966.
148. Cameron JS, Ogg C, Trounce JR: Peritoneal dialysis in hypercatabolic acute renal failure. *Lancet* 1:1188, 1967.
149. Derot M, Legrain M, Jacobs C: Indications respectives du rein artificiel et de la dialyse peritoneale dans le traitement de l'insuffisance renale aigue (a propos 537 observations). In: DN Kerr, et al. eds, *Proceedings of the European Dialysis Transplant Association*, Vol 2. Excerpta Medica, Amsterdam, p 44, 1965.
150. Odel HM, Ferris DO, Power MH: Peritoneal lavage as an effective means of extrarenal excretion. *Am J Med* 9:63, 1950.
151. Orofino L, Lampreabe I, Muniz R, et al.: Supervivencia del fracaso renal agudo (FRA) sometido a dialisis. Revision de 82 pacientes. *Revta Clin Esp* 141:155, 1976.
152. Rentero R, Vidaur F, Naranjo P, et al.: Nuestra experiencia en 191 casos de insuficiencia renal aguda. *Revta Clin Esp* 140:243, 1976.
153. Stott RB, Ogg CS, Cameron JS, Bewick M: Why the persistently high mortality in acute renal failure? *Lancet* 2:75, 1972.
154. Tzamaloukas AH, Garella S, Chazan JA: Peritoneal dialysis for acute renal failure after major abdominal surgery. *Arch Surg (London)* 106:639, 1973.
155. Vaamonde CA, Michael UF, Metzger RA, Carroll KE: Complications of acute peritoneal dialysis. *J Chron Dis* 28:637, 1975.
156. Vitacco M, Medilaharzu RY, Caletti MG: Dialisis peritoneal en pediatria. Editorial Ergon, Buenos Aires, 1975.
157. Upadhyaya K, Barwick K, Fishaut M, et al.: The importance of non-renal involvement in hemolytic-uremic syndrome. *Pediatrics* 65(1):115, 1979.
158. Brown ST, Ahearn DJ, Nolph KD: Potassium removal with peritoneal dialysis. *Kidney Int* 4:67, 1973.
159. Dixon SR, McKean WI, Pryor JE, Irvine ROH: Changes in acid base balance during peritoneal dialysis with fluid containing lactate ions. *Clin Sci* 39:51, 1970.
160. Hayat JC: Treatment of lactic acidosis in the diabetic patient by peritoneal dialysis using sodium acetate. A report of cases. *Diabetologia* 10:485, 1974.
161. Sheppard JM, Lawrence JR, Oon RCS, et al.: Lactic acidosis recovery associated with use of peritoneal dialysis. *Aust N Z J Med* 4:389, 1972.
162. Anagnostou A, Kurtzman NA: Hematological consequences of renal failure. In: BM Brenner, FC Rector eds, *The Kidney* WB Saunders, Philadelphia, pp 1631–1656, 1986.
163. Hamet P, Stouder DA, Ginn E, et al.: Studies on the elevated extracellular concentration of cyclic AMP in uremic men. *J Clin Invest* 56:339, 1975.
164. Remuzzi G, Marchesi D, Livio M, Schieppati A, Mecca G, Donati MD, de Gaetano G: Prostaglandins, plasma factors, and hemostasis in uremia. In: G Remuzzi, G Mecca, G de Gaetano, eds, *Hemostasis, Prostaglandin and Renal Disease*. Raven Press, New York, p 273, 1980.
165. Howard MA, Whitworth JA, Hendrix LE, Thomas CB, Firkin BG: Abnormal factor VIII in chronic renal failure. *Med J Aust* 1:148, 1979.
166. Kleinknecht D, Jungers P, Channard J, Barbanel C, Ganeval D, Rondon–Nucete M: Factors influencing immediate prognosis in acute renal failure, with special references to prophylactic hemodialysis. *Adv Nephrol* 1:207, 1971.
167. Kerr DNS: Acute renal failure. In: DAK Black, NF Jones eds, *Renal Disease*. Blackwell Oxford, p 437, 19
168. Janson PA, Jubeliner SJ, Weinstein MS, Peykin D. Treatment of bleeding tendency in uremia with cryoprecipitate. *N Engl J Med* 303:1318, 1980.
169. Mannucci PM, Remuzzi G, Pusiwerei F, et al.: Deamino-8-arginine vasopressin shortens the bleeding time in uremia. *N Engl J Med* 308:8, 1983.

170. Shapiro MD, Kelleher SP: Intransasal deamino-8-D-arginine vasopressin shortens the bleeding time in uremia. *Am J Nephrol* 4:260, 1984.
171. Livio M, Mannucci PM, Vigano G, et al.: Conjugated estrogens for the management of bleeding associated with renal failure. *N Engl J Med* 315:731, 1986.
172. Pinnick RV, Wiegmann TB, Diederich DA: Regional citrate anticoagulation for hemodialysis in the patient at high risk for bleeding. *N Engl J Med* 308:258–261, 1983.
173. Morita Y, Johnson RW, Dorn RE, et al.: Regional anticoagulation during hemodialysis using citrate. *Am J Med Sci* 242:32–42, 1961.
174. Wiegmann TB, MacDougall ML, Diederich DA; Long-term comparisons of citrate and heparin as anti-coagulants for hemodialysis. *Am J Kidney Dis* 9:430–435, 1987.
175. Schwab SJ, Onorato JJ, Sharar LR, Dennis PA: Hemodialysis without anticoagulation. *Am J Med* 83:405, 1987.
176. Cameron JS: Acute renal failure in the intensive care unit today. *Intens Care Med* 12:64–70, 1986.
177. Finn WF: Recovery from acute renal failure. In: BM Brenner, JM Lazarus, eds, *Acute Renal Failure*. WB Saunders, Philadelphia, pp 753–774, 1983.
178. Corwin HL, Bonventre JV: Acute renal failure. Med Clin North Am 70:1037, 1986.
179. Routh GS, Briggs JD, Mone JG, Ledingham JMH: Survival from acute renal failure with and without multiple organ dysfunction. *Postgrad Med J* 56:244, 1980.
180. Moyer C, Cena AF, Chenier R, et al.: Multiple systems failure II. Death predictors in the trauma septic state. The most critical determinants. *J Trauma* 81: 862, 1981.
181. Fry DE, Garrison RN, Heitsch RC, Calhoun K, Polk HC, Jr: Determinants of death in patients with intra-abdominal abscess. *Surgery* 88:517, 1980.
182. Pine RW, Wertz MJ, Lennard ES, Dellinger EP, Carnico CJ, Minshers BH: Determinants of organ malfunction or death in patients with intra-abdominal sepsis. A discriminant analysis. *Arch Surg* 118:242, 1983.
183. Milligan SL, Luft FC, McMurray SD, Kleit SA: Intra-abdominal infection and acute renal failure. *Arch Surg* 113:467, 1978.
184. Kornhall S. Acute renal failure in surgical disease with special regard to neglected complications. *Acta Chir Scan Supp* 419:7, 1971.
185. Dobbelstein H: Immune system in uremia. *Nephron* 17:409, 1976.
186. Zech P, Bouletreau R, Moskovtchenko JF, Beruard M, Favre–Bulle S, Blanc-Brunat N, Traeger J. Infection in acute renal failure. In: J Hamburger, J Crosnier, MH Maxwell, eds, *Advances in Nephrology*, Vol 1. Year Book Medical Publishers, Chicago, 1971.
187. Emanuel M, Metcalf RG; Quadriplegia in hyperkalemia. *J Maine Med Assoc* 157:134, 1966.
188. Epstein FH: Signs and symptoms of electrolyte disorders. In: MH Maxwell, CR Kleeman, eds, *Clinical Disorders of Fluid and Electrolyte Metabolism*. McGraw–Hill, New York, 1980.
189. Massry SG, Arieff AI, Coburn JW, Palmieri G, Kleeman CR: Divalent ion metabolism in patients with acute renal failure. Studies on the mechanism of hypocalcemia. *Kidney Int* 5:437, 1974.
190. Grossman HH, Lange H: Hypercalcemia in acute renal failure. *Annals Intern Med* 69:1332, 1969.
191. deTorrente A, Berl T, Cohn PD, Kawamoto E, Hertz P, Schrier RW: Hypercalcemia of acute renal failure: Clinical significance and pathogenesis. *Am J Med* 61:119, 1976.
192. Llach F, Felsenfeld AJ, Haussler MR: The pathophysiology of altered calcium metabolism in rhabdomyolysis-induced acute renal failure. Interactions of parathyroid hormone, 25-hydroxycholecalciferol and 1,25 dihydroxycholecalciferol. *N Engl J Med* 305:117–123, 1981.
193. Pietrek J, Kokot F, Kuska J: Serum 25-hydroxyvitamin D and parathyroid hormone in patients with acute renal failure. *Kidney Int* 13:178, 1978.

CHAPTER 19

Acute Glomerulonephritis and Glomerulonephritis in Bacterial Endocarditis

DAVID S. BALDWIN & JOEL NEUGARTEN

ACUTE GLOMERULONEPHRITIS

Introduction

The term *acute glomerulonephritis syndrome* refers to the clinical signs and symptoms that are typically observed in association with postinfectious diffuse endocapillary proliferation within glomeruli. The full-blown syndrome consists of the abrupt appearance of salt and water retention, edema, reduced urine output, circulatory congestion, hypertension, hematuria, proteinuria, and decreased filtration rate. All these manifestations do not necessarily occur in each instance of post-infectious glomerulonephritis. Urinary abnormalities, decreased filtration rate, and fluid retention are practically invariable. When these clinical features were thought to occur uniquely in association with diffuse proliferation of mesangial and endothelial cells, polymorphonuclear inflammatory cell reaction, and occasional extracapillary proliferation, which followed infection, the simple term *acute nephritis* was classically applied. As it became apparent, however, that many of these same clinical manifestations could at times characterize the onset of Berger's IgA nephropathy, Henoch–Schonlein purpura, mixed essential cryoglobulinemia, Guillain–Barre–Strohl syndrome, systemic lupus erythematosis, idiopathic mesangiocapillary glomerulonephritis, and systemic vasculitis, the appellation *acute glomerulonephritis syndrome* appeared to be more appropriate (1–3). The following discussion deals primary with the pathophysiology, clinical manifestations, and therapy of the syndrome as it occurs in post-infectious glomerulonephritis.

The course of the acute glomerulonephritis syndrome depends, naturally, on the underlying glomerular disease. In the case of post-infectious acute nephritis, a self-limiting immune complex disease, the large majority of patients experience a spontaneous increase in filtration rate with diuresis and resolution of circulatory congestion, edema, and hypertension within a week of onset, followed ultimately by full recovery of renal function. The acute stage rarely persists longer than several weeks (1, 4, 5). No known therapeutic maneuver will influence the course of the renal lesion or promote histologic healing (4). Therapy is predominantly supportive and is directed toward prevention and management of potentially lethal complications of hypertensive encephalopathy, uremia, hyperkalemia, and pulmonary edema, Over recent years there has been a sharp decline in the mortality from 5–10% to less 1% due to the advent of dialysis, potent diuretics, and antihypertensive agents (5–7). The majority of deaths occur in the elderly, possibly related to the greater incidence in this group of underlying cardiovascular disease (8). Prolonged oligoanuria and irreversible renal failure usually occur when widespread extracapillary proliferation accompanies the endocapillary lesion (7).

Pathophysiology

RENAL INSUFFICIENCY

A reduced glomerular filtration rate (GFR) is probably universal in acute glomerulonephritis; oligoanuric renal failure is infrequent (9). Spontaneous improvement in renal function occurs in the majority, azotemia resolving with the onset of diuresis (9). Extensive clinical and physiologic investigations of the acute phase of glomerulonephritis have been performed by Earle et al. (10). Renal plasma flow (RPF) was unchanged in 50% of patients studied. In the remainder, RPF was only mildly depressed and was associated with a more marked decline in GFR, such that the filtration fraction consistently fell (9). When the clearance of paraaminohippuric acid is corrected for any reduction in its extraction, RPF is found to be normal or elevated in most patients (11). When acute glomerulonephritis is associated with antecedent congestive heart failure or hypertension, the filtration fraction may occasionally be normal (9). The functional tubular capacity is reduced, as evidenced by reductions in maximum reabsorptive and excretory capacities for glucose and paraaminohippurate and in the extraction of the latter (12–14).

SALT AND WATER RETENTION

Fluid retention is universal in patients with acute nephritis and may be manifest by edema, circulatory congestion, or hypertension. Despite early reports of a high protein content in edema fluid, suggesting a possible increase in capillary permeability, Warren and Stead (15) subsequently demonstrated that the fluid is transudative in nature. Heavy glomerular proteninuria with depression in plasma oncotic pressure (nephrotic edema) generally does not play a major role, nor does depressed cardiac function, as will be discussed subsequently. Thus, salt and water retention in acute glomerulonephritis is of primary renal origin and is not attributable to abnormal capillary permeability, hypoproteinemia, or myocardial dysfunction (7, 16), though the latter two may play a contributory role in some patients.

Clinical investigations have not demonstrated a correlation between the magnitude of depression in GFR and the degree of salt and water retention; in fact, massive salt and water retention may occur with only a minor fall in GFR (10, 17). Further, the onset of diuresis is not consistently associated with a rise in GFR (10). A hypothesis has been set forth to explain the occurrence of salt and water retention with what might appear to be an insignificant reduction in GFR (1, 18). It proposes that the decrease in urinary sodium excretion and resultant extracellular fluid volume expansion that follow a reduction in GFR may lead to hemodynamic alterations that restore GFR at the expense of an expanded extracellular volume. In this context, as healing occurs a diuresis may ensue with little detectable increase in GFR.

In light of clinical observations and experimental data obtained in animal models of glomerulonephritis, the following sequence may be postulated to explain the occurrence of marked salt and water retention (19). Reduction in GFR associated with decreased delivery of filtrate may be considered the primary pathogenic mechanism. The fall in GFR may not be apparent in all instances due to compensatory hemodynamic alterations that are themselves dependent, in part, on salt and water retention and extracellular volume expansion. Absolute proximal reabsorption is reduced in concert with the decline in GFR, reflecting alterations in peritubular capillary Starling forces. The extent of salt and water retention must then be related to increased fractional reabsorption in distal segments as a consequence of the fall in GFR and reduced delivery of filtrate. The role of hormonal and neural factors in the pathogenesis of this tubular response remains unclear.

HYPERTENSION

The majority of patients with acute glomerulonephritis manifest hypertension (9). The duration of hypertension is usually short, and the elevation in blood pressure is only modest. Blood pressures that are within the range of normal, especially in children, may nevertheless be elevated when compared to their premorbid level or in retrospect (1). Hypertension develops early in the course and subsides with the onset of spontaneous diuresis (1, 9). Hypertensive encephalopathy occurred in up to 10% of hospitalized patients as reported in the older literature (20). The frequency of this complication has decreased markedly with the advent of potent diuretics and antihypertensive agents (20). In general, cerebral symptomatology correlates with the level of blood pressure; however, encephalopathy may occur with only a moderate elevation in blood pressure (9). Cerebral manifestations include restlessness, decreased level of consciousness, seizures, visual disturbances, aphasia, and paresis (9, 20–22). Overt encephalopathy may be heralded by headache, nausea, or vomiting (23). Though retinal hemorrhages may occur, papilledema is rare, even in patients with full-blown encephalopathy (2, 4, 9, 16, 20, 23). Lumbar puncture may reveal elevated spinal fluid pressure and protein concentration (9). Nonspecific electroencephalographic changes are associated with hypertensive encephalopathy; however, similar changes may occur in the absence of encephalopathy and do not correlate with clinical symptoms or the level of blood pressure. A reduction in blood pressure usually leads to resolution of cerebral symptoms without residual abnormalities (20).

The etiology of hypertension in acute glomerulonephritis is primarily related to salt and water retention, which results in increased cardiac output. Rodriguez–Iturbe et al. (24), Powell (25), and Shahabuddin et al. (26) have studied the renin-angiotensin system in patients with mild-to-moderate hypertension. The severity of hypertension and suppression of plasma renin activity correlated with the degree of fluid retention. Normalization of these parameters occurred with spontaneous diuresis (24, 25). In addition, the percent decrease in blood pressure during diuresis correlated with the percent decrease in weight (24). It was concluded that the renin-angiotensin-aldosterone axis was appropriately suppressed in response to volume expansion and was not involved in sustaining hypertension. Circulating vasoconstrictor substances could not be demonstrated by bioassay (27, 28).

The data supporting a role for neurogenic or hormonal factors in the pathogenesis of hypertension are less convincing. Despite the fact that the aldosterone secretory rate and plasma renin activity are normal or depressed, it has been suggested that they may be inappropriately high for the degree of salt and water retention (1, 16, 22, 24, 25, 29). Extracellular volume expansion may result in increased sensitivity to angiotensin II, raising the possibility that angiotensin-induced vasoconstriction may contribute to hypertension, even in the absence of elevated plasma renin activity (27). The latter was found to increase to elevated levels after the onset of diuresis by Birkenhager et al, (29). They suggested that inadequate suppression of plasma renin by volume expansion contributed to the maintenance of hypertension through increased total peripheral resistance. Furthermore, it has been stated that drug-induced diuresis may not be completely effective in reducing the blood pressure of those with severe hypertension, suggesting that factors other than volume may play some role (22, 30).

CIRCULATORY CONGESTION

Symptoms of circulatory congestion, manifested by dyspnea, orthopnea, cardiomegaly, and pulmonary congestion, are reported in 16–75% of patients (4, 9, 31, 32). The incidence is higher among adults, especially in the elderly, presumably due to underlying cardiovascular disease (9, 33, 34). The pathogenesis of circulatory congestion in acute glomerulonephritis was disputed prior to extensive investigation by Eichna and others (35, 36). In 1948, Gore and Saphir (37) described focal serous myocarditis, characterized by edematous infiltration of the myocardium, in 10% of fatal cases of acute glomerulonephritis. They suggested that a generalized capillary defect with extravasation of plasma proteins may give rise to myocarditis and contribute to the frequent occurrence of cardiac insufficiency and electrocardiographic abnormalities in these patients. Despite these observations, most studies have not demonstrated abnormalities of cardiac histology in patients dying with circulatory congestion (9, 31, 38). Other early investigators attributed circulatory congestion and cardiomegaly to the deleterious effects of hypertension on the heart (9). However, circulatory congestion does not correlate with the level of hypertension and may antedate its onset (9, 31, 32, 39, 40). A sudden marked rise in blood pressure may play a contributory role in the development of myocardial dysfunction in some cases; however, in the majority the modest level and short duration of hypertension is insufficient to precipitate cardiac decompensation and cannot explain the frequent occurrence of cardiomegaly and circulatory congestion (1, 37).

Eichna (12, 35, 36) attributed circulatory congestion to primary salt and water retention. He found that cardiac output was normal or increased, and circulation time and the arteriovenous oxygen difference was normal or decreased, indicating adequate cardiac performance. Elevated blood volume correlates with circulatory congestion, which subsides with the onset of spontaneous diuresis (4, 9). The increase in blood volume is due solely to an increase in plasma volume (7, 40–42). Administration of digitalis to patients with acute glomerulonephritis does not reduce the elevated venous or right ventricular end-diastolic pressures, increase the cardiac output, or initiate a salt and water diuresis, as in patients with underlying myocardial dysfunction and congestive heart failure (4, 12, 16, 35). In a minority of patients with antecedent myocardial disease, primary salt and water retention may precipitate cardiac decompensation, which is then manifested by an elevated circulation time and arteriovenous oxygen difference and decreased cardiac output, which improve after the administration of digitalis. Noncardiac circulatory congestion similar to that observed in acute nephritis may be produced in normal individuals with rapid intravenous administration of salt and water, or prolonged administration of ACTH or corticosteroids, and may occur in patients with renal failure and fluid overload (7, 36). Recent studies have confirmed the work of Eichna et al. (43–48).

Electrocardiographic abnormalities have been reported in 20–100% of patients (31, 33, 38). It has been suggested that these may be related to electrolyte disturbances, hypertension, fluid retention, or myocarditis. No correlation exists, however, between electrocardiographic changes and the level of blood pressure, circulatory congestion, serum creatinine, circulation time, or clinical symptoms (31, 33, 38, 47). Clinical improvement with resolution of cardiomegaly, hypertension, and circulatory congestion often antedates the return of the electrocardiogram to normal (33, 49). Sinus bradycardia or sinus tachycardia may be observed (33, 38, 50, 51). Characteristic are flattening or inversion of the T waves in one or more leads (49, 50). Less frequently observed are left-axis deviation (31); prolongation of the PR, QRS, or QT intervals (20, 49, 50); large upright T waves in lead III (49); or a decrease in the R-wave amplitude (46). Electrocardiographic manifestations of left ventricular hypertrophy occur only rarely with the onset of hypertension and cardiomegaly in acute nephritis (4).

ANEMIA

A normochromic anemia of moderate severity is often observed in acute glomerulonephritis (1). Among ten nephritic patients studied by Eisenberg (41), the hemoglobin concentration was reduced in proportion to the degree of plasma volume expansion and was normalized with the onset of diuresis. The erythrocyte mass remains constant, defining the anemia as dilutional in origin (25, 40, 41). The rapid development of more severe anemia occurs in patients with renal failure and a prolonged acute phase. In these individuals shortened peripheral erythrocyte survival and decreased erythropoesis, as observed in other forms of acute renal failure, may contribute significantly to the anemia (1, 22).

Prevention

Prevention of acute glomerulonephritis that occurs after streptococcal pharyngitis or pyoderma has been attempted systematically by several investigators (52–57). Rammelkamp and Stetson (53, 54, 56) administered either placebo, penicillin, or gamma globulin to patients with epidemic type 12 streptococcal pharyngitis. They reported that penicillin therapy decreased the incidence of acute glomerulonephritis from 11% to 4.5%. Later administration of penicillin to patients in the placebo group was not effective in decreasing the incidence of acute glomerulonephritis. These data were later reevaluated by Kassirer and Schwartz (7), who applied chi square testing and found no statistical difference among the various groups. The incidence of acute glomerulonephritis following scarlet fever, reported to be 1–2%, is not reduced by penicillin therapy, even if administered within 24 hours of the first manifestations of pharyngitis (55). Many other studies document that the occurrence of acute glomerulonephritis following streptococcal pharyngitis or pyoderma is not altered despite prompt institution of antibiotic therapy and eradication of the responsible organism (52, 58–60). Further, antibiotic administration does not influence the course of the disease and will not promote healing or alter the ultimate prognosis (4, 20, 52, 58–60).

Although clinical symptoms related to streptococcal pharyngitis have generally remitted by the time the patient presents with acute glomerulonephritis, streptococci may nevertheless be recovered from the pharynx of these who have not received antibiotic therapy (4). Penicillin should be administered when positive pharyngeal or skin cultures are found in order to prevent suppurative complications and the further spread of nephritogenic streptococci in the population (1, 4, 20, 52, 57–61). Pharyngeal cultures should be obtained from family members and other close contacts and penicillin should be administered when these are positive. In patients who are not allergic to penicillin, a single intramuscular dose of benzathine penicillin G is more effective than oral penicillin in eradicating pharyngeal streptococci (20, 52, 62). Routine screening of close contacts may detect subclinical cases of glomerulonephritis (22). No rationale exists to support the use of penicillin during the early convalescent period or for prolonged chemoprophylaxis in view of the development of type-specific immunity and the unlikelihood of reinfection with nephritogenic streptococci.

Therapeutic approaches

Appropriate management of the patient with acute glomerulonephritis is based on an appreciation of the pathophysiologic basis of its various manifestations. The disease is characteristically a self-limited disorder (58). The vast majority of patients experience a spontaneous diuresis accompanied by remission of circulatory congestion, edema, and hypertension within a week, followed by gradual resolution of urinary abnormalities during succeeding weeks or months. Prolonged oliguria or anuria, exceeding 1 week's duration, is observed in only 5–10% of patients (1, 4, 5, 61). No therapeutic maneuver is know that will influence the severity of renal dysfunction or promote histologic healing (1, 4, 9, 63, 64). Therapy is predominantly supportive and directed toward prevention and management of the potentially lethal complications of uremia, hyperkalemia, hypertensive encephalopathy, and pulmonary edema (4).

DIETARY

Restriction of sodium and fluid intake during acute glomerulonephritis is necessary to alleviate edema and circulatory congestion. Prolonged oliguric acute renal failure may necessitate restriction of dietary potassium and protein as well. Based on studies in humans, several investigators have concluded that manipulation of dietary protein content during the acute phase has no consistent influence on clinical symptoms, the duration of proteinuria and sediment abnormalities, or the rate of healing (65–68). Naeras (67) alternated periods of high- and low-protein feedings, while Mortensen (68) fed diets high or low in protein content to alternate patients. No consistent deleterious effect of high protein intake on the acute course was observed.

PHYSICAL ACTIVITY

Assumption of the upright posture in acute glomerulonephritis has been shown to decrease GFR, RPF, urinary output, and sodium excretion, and to increase hematuria and proteinuria (11). Early authorities recommended enforcement of prolonged bed rest, ranging up to 12 months if proteinuria and sediment abnormalities persisted (4, 6, 20, 22). Subsequent observations have failed to demonstrate a beneficial effect of prolonged bed rest on the clinical course (4, 69, 70). Akerren (69) divided nephritic children into two groups, which differed only in the length of enforced bed rest. The duration of sediment abnormalities and clinical symptoms were not adversely influenced by early ambulation. All patients were free of sequela at the 2-year followup. Bed rest is indicated during the acute phase until edema, gross hematuria, hypertension, and circulatory congestion begin to remit (4, 22). Persistent mild hematuria, or proteinuria, or a minor exacerbation of sediment abnormalities, with ambulation do not represent a contraindication to progressive ambulation and the gradual resumption of normal activities (4, 20, 64).

IMMUNOSUPPRESSIVE THERAPY

Scattered reports ascribe a beneficial effect from the use of corticosteroids in the treatment of acute glomerulonephritis (20, 61, 71–74). However, it is difficult to evaluate the influence of any therapeutic regimen in this disorder, since spontaneous recovery is the rule (1, 20, 63). Even patients with prolonged oliguria, usually with extensive crescent formation, have been reported on rare occasions to undergo spontaneous diuresis (4, 7, 75). Leonard et al. (61), Thorn et al. (76, 77), and Burnett et al. (78) evaluated the effect of ACTH and cortisone administration and concluded that these agents did not favorably influence the course. In fact, edema and hypertension may be exacerbated by corticosteroid therapy (20, 76). Thus, there is no convincing evidence to suggest that corticosteroids favorably alter the natural course of acute glomerulonephritis. These agents have not been shown to accelerate the rate of morphologic healing; cause resolution of azotemia, proteinuria, or hematuria; or decrease the incidence of chronicity (1, 4, 7, 9, 20, 61, 63, 76–78). More recently, anticoagulants in association with corticosteroids and cytotoxic agents have been administered to patients with oliguric crescentic glomerulonephritis of postinfectious origin (79–81). Although this experience is limited, a beneficial effect has been suggested. However, these data must be interpreted cautiously in view of the small number of reported cases without controls and the known occasional occurrence of spontaneous recovery from acute poststreptococcal glomerulonephritis despite the presence of prolonged oliguria and crecents (4, 61, 75). Our own experience utilizing corticosteroids, cytotoxic agents, anticoagulants, and plasmapheresis in the management of patients with oliguric crescentic acute poststreptococcal glomerulonephritis has not demonstrated a favorable influence on the course.

THERAPY OF FLUID RETENTION

Restriction of dietary sodium and fluid intake during the acute phase is necessary in view of primary renal salt and water retention. The role of diuretic administration in the management of fluid retention in acute glomerulonephritis has been investigated by several authors (30, 83, 84). Benzothiadiazide diuretics and their derivatives, with the exception of metalozone, are ineffective in patients with severe impairment of renal function (1). Furthermore, spironolactone and triameterene should not be employed because of the threat of hyperkalemia (1). Furosemide has been shown to be safe and effective in inducing a diuresis in patients with filtration rates as low as 10 ml/min; however, high doses may be required (30, 85, 86). Repetto et al. (30) administered intravenous furosemide to children with acute glomerulonephritis and succeeded in initiating a diuresis with resultant resolution of circulatory congestion and encephalopathy. Significant changes in inulin clearance or in renal hemodynamic parameters were not observed acutely, despite a 23% reduction in retained body water. Though total body water was reduced, the plasma volume was unchanged. Retan and Dillon (83) administered either oral furosemide or placebo to children with acute poststreptococcal glomerulonephritis and edema or hypertension. The average dose of furosemide required to achieve satisfactory diuresis was 5.6 mg/kg/day. Diuretic therapy shortened the duration of edema and hypertension and lessened the need for parenteral antihypertensive agents. Ethacrynic acid, when administered to edematous nephritic children, was associated with diuresis and a reduction in blood pressure (84). Despite the value of potent diuretics in the management of circulatory congestion and massive edema, routine administration of diuretics to those with mild salt and water retention may offer no demonstrable therapeutic benefit, as spontaneous diuresis will occur within 1 week of onset in most cases.

THERAPY OF HYPERTENSION

The majority of patients with acute glomerulonephritis manifest hypertension (9). The duration of hypertension is usually short, and the elevation of blood pressure is rarely severe. Mild elevations in arterial pressure require no treatment; however, marked arterial hypertension and impending or overt encephalopathy are indications for antihypertensive therapy (4, 9, 20, 22, 64). No evidence exists to suggest that this mild hypertension has any deleterious effect (20).

Diuresis induced with furosemide may be effective in the management of mild hypertension; however, several authors have suggested that furosemide-induced diuresis is ineffective in controlling severe hypertension (20, 30, 87). Administration of potent diuretics will, nevertheless, reduce the amount of other antihypertensive agents required to control severe hypertension (22). Peripherally acting vasodilators are the preferred agents (1, 58). Sodium nitroprusside acts directly on vascular smooth muscle to produce dilatation of arteriolar and venous vascular beds and reduction of preload as well as afterload. While total peripheral resistance and arterial pressure are reduced, the effect on cardiac output is variable. Since sodium nitroprusside is metabolized to thiocyanate, and the major route of excretion of thiocyanate is renal, monitoring serum thiocyanate levels during prolonged therapy of azotemic patients is necessary. Gordillo–Paniagua et al. (88) demonstrated the safety and efficacy of sodium nitroprusside in the management of hypertension in children with acute glomerulonephritis. Blood pressure was controlled and encephalopathy resolved without deterioration of renal function. Several investigators have demonstrated the safety and efficacy of diazoxide, a potent peripheral arteriolar vasodilating agent (22, 87, 89). Kohaut et al. (87) administered intravenous diazoxide and furosemide to patients with moderate-to-severe hypertension and achieved a rapid reduction of blood pressure and resolution of encephalopathy. The majority required repeated doses; nevertheless, no serious adverse reactions occurred and azotemia was not exacerbated. Approximately 30% of an administered dose of diazoxide is normally excreted unchanged in the urine; thus, renal failure leads to prolongation of the plasma half-life. On average, 41 hours elapsed before repeat administration of diazoxide was required in the study cited (9). Accumulation of diazoxide may occur after repeated doses in patients with renal function impairment, and hyperglycemia with ketoacidosis may rarely be observed (89). Due to protein binding of diazoxide in excess of 90%, a reduction in dose may be required in the patient with heavy proteinuria and hypoalbuminemia (22). Further, the degree of protein binding is reduced in uremia. Diazoxide is known to cause marked sodium and water retention, which would theoretically limit its utility in acute nephritis. However, neither diuretic insensitivity nor exacerbation of edema was observed by Kohaut et al. (87).

Hydralazine, another direct peripheral vasodilator, has also been shown to be effective in the management of hypertension in acute glomerulonephritis (90, 91). McCrory and Rapoport (90) and Etteldorf et al. (91) treated children with intramuscular hydralazine and achieved a therapeutic reduction in blood pressure in the majority. Transient hemodynamic disturbances lacking clinical consequence occurred in association with the reduction in blood pressure. GFR, filtration fraction, and urinary flow rate were transiently decreased, and renal plasma flow rate (RPF) was variably influenced. Reduction of blood pressure with lesser doses of hydralazine, in association with parenteral reserpine, did not significantly change GFR or RPF, since renal vascular resistance fell (92). Since the renin-angiotensin axis does not appear to play a major role in the pathogenesis of hypertension in acute glomerulonephtiris, propranolol would not be expected to have an important role in its management; however, beta-blocking agents may potentiate the antihypertensive action of peripheral vasodilators by preventing reflex tachycardia. These agents, however, may have adverse hemodynamic sequelae in patients with intrinsic myocardial dysfunction (1). Though not extensively studied, other peripheral vasodilating agents such as prazosin and minoxidil and calcium channel blockers may prove to be efficacious (1, 64).

THERAPY OF RENAL INSUFFICIENCY

Some impairment of renal function is characteristic of acute glomerulonephritis, but severe oligoanuric renal failure is infrequent (50, 93). Prolonged oliguria or anuria is observed in only 5–10% of patients with poststreptococcal glomerulonephritis (61). Management of such patients entails restriction of fluid and dietary sodium, protein, and potassium. Hemodialysis or peritoneal dialysis may become necessary to control circulatory congestion, hyperkalemia, or uremia until spontaneous diuresis ensues. Not infrequently, diuresis fails to occur in such patients, and irreversible renal failure results. The histologic counterpart of this latter course is extensive extracapillary as well as endocapillary proliferation. Performance of a renal biopsy in patients with prolonged oliguria serves to exclude diseases other then diffuse proliferative glomerulonephritis, which may be responsible for acute renal failure.

Despite the frequency of elevated serum potassium levels during the course of acute glomerulonephritis, severe hyperkalemia is uncommon (10, 42, 94). The emergency management of severe hyperkalemia normally includes administration of intravenous dextrose and insulin, calcium, and sodium bicarbonate (95). Sodium polystyrene sulfonate and sorbitol, administered orally or by enema, are employed to promote gastrointestinal potassium excretion (95). In the patient with acute glomerulonephritis, administration of sodium bicarbonate or sodium polystyrene sulfonate may aggravate fluid retention and circulatory congestion. Dialysis may be necessary for the correction of hyperkalemia in those with oligoanuric renal failure.

Prognosis

Despite apparent clinical recovery in the large majority of patients with acute glomerulonephritis, our long-term observations in sporadic cases that required hospitalization suggest a substantial incidence of irreversible renal damage in both adults and children (96). Our followup studies have demonstrated persistent minimal proteinuria and hypertension, and mildly impaired renal function in the majority of patients years after the acute episode (96). Proteinuria or hypertension is present in greater than one third of those examined 3 years or more from the onset. Renal function is reduced in more than one half, occasionally associated with normal urinalyses and blood pressure. In some patients, proteinuria reappears or increases, and hypertension first appears years after subsidence of the acute episode. In addition, exaggerated natriuresis after saline loading, which is not abolished by prior sodium restriction, has been demonstrated years later (97). In the majority, renal biopsies demonstrate partial or complete sclerosis of some glomeruli. Glomerular sclerosis may first appear long after proliferation has subsided, suggesting that clinical and morphologic abnormalities are not merely the end result of the damage inflicted during the acute stage. Terminal uremia developed in 7% of patients within 6 months of onset but very rarely during the following years. Though not invariable, clinical pathologic studies have demonstrated a clear correlation between the severity at onset and the development of chronicity. A large number of mild cases of glomerulonephritis are usually detected during routine surveillance in the course of an epidemic, while sporadic cases tend to be recognized only as a consequence of their severity. This may explain the better prognosis in patients who develop acute poststreptococcal glomerulonephritis during an epidemic. The more favorable prognosis in children, as reported by others, was also evident in our studies, perhaps attributable to the occurrence of milder initial episodes in the young. In addition, when glomerulonephritis follows streptococcal pharyngitis, it may become chronic more frequently than when it follows pyoderma (98). A favorable prognosis has been reported by Travis et al. (5) in children 3–10 years after sporadic glomerulonephritis following upper respiratory or cutaneous infections; by Nissenson et al. (98) in children and adults 7–12 years after predominantly symptomatic, epidemic pyoderma-related nephritis; and by Perlman et al. (99) in children with epidemic pyoderma-related nephritis. Nissenson et al. (100) failed to demonstrate exaggerated natriuresis after saline loading in their patients. In contrast, Garcia et al. (101) found abnormalities in renal function or urinary sediment in 20% of patients 11–12 years after epidemic, pharyngitis-related nephritis. When adults alone were considered, 55% manifested renal abnormalities. Despite the controversy that exists concerning the incidence of chronicity after acute poststreptococcal glomerulonephritis, it is agreed that the ultimate prognosis cannot be favorably influenced by any therapeutic measures undertaken initially.

GLOMERULONEPHRITIS IN BACTERIAL ENDOCARDITIS

Introduction

Glomerulonephritis occurring during the course of bacterial endocarditis was originally recognized as a clinicopathologic entity at the turn of the century. Since its initial description, the natural history of this form of glomerulonephritis has been dramatically influenced by the advent of antibiotic therapy and the changing epidemiology of infective endocarditis.

The occurrence of focal glomerular disease in bacterial endocarditis was first described by Löhlein in 1908 (102). Shortly thereafter Baehr, and later Bell, described both diffuse as well as focal glomerulonephritis at necropsy in acute and subacute endocarditis (103, 104). Because the early focal segmental lesions are necrotic, contain eosinophilic material resembling thrombi, and frequently coexist with infarcts, early investigators proposed that these were the consequence of embolization from vegetations (102, 105). An immune pathogenesis gained favor with the awareness that glomerular disease in patients with right-sided bacterial endocarditis could not be explained on an embolic basis (106–110). The occurrence of diffuse glomerulonephritis, the deposition of immunoglobulin diffusely, and the frequent depression of serum complement levels further supported an immunologic mechanism. This was corroborated by the demonstration ultrastructurally of electron-dense deposits in glomeruli and was further supported by the finding of specific antibody in kidney eluates and by the demonstration of bacterial antigen in the deposits. Direct or indirect immunofluorescence microscopy has identified bacterial antigen in glomerlar deposits accompanying bacterial endocarditis due to *Staphylococcus aureus* and hemolytic *streptococcus* (111–113). Eluates of kidneys obtained at autopsy from patients with enterococcal endocarditis and glomerulonephritis have been shown to contain antibody reactive with bacteria cultured from antemortem blood (114, 115). It is not certain if the deposits form locally by the binding of antibody to glomerular-bound antigen or result from the deposition of circulating complexes.

Clinical features

Renal dysfunction may be the presenting manifestation of basterial endocarditis, at times prompting a diagnosis of primary renal disease when the blood culture results are negative (116). In the preantibiotic era, uremia contributed to the death of 5–10% of patients. This figure fell to 3–4% with the advent of antibiotic therapy (117). In the 1952 series of Spain and King (118), no uremic deaths were observed in 25 penicillin-treated patients with fatal subacute bacterial endocarditis; 9 uremic deaths occurred in 52 untreated patients. Modern experience with uremia is discussed in following sections.

FOCAL GLOMERULONEPHRITIS

The clinical manifestations of focal glomerulonephritis are usually mild. Microscopic hematuria, pyuria, or minimal proteinuria may be observed; heavy proteinuria and hypertension are rare. Renal functional impairment is generally absent or mild. Renal manifestations resolve with control of infection. Infrequently, when focal and segmental glomerular involvement is severe and extensive, renal insufficiency or uremia may supervene (119). Focal glomerulonephritis may occur in the absence of clinical renal involvement (120). Morel–Marogar et al. (120) studied renal biopsies after treatment in eight patients with *S. viridans* subacute bacterial endocarditis who had no clinical evidence of renal disease and found healed or active focal glomerulonephritis in all.

DIFFUSE GLOMERULONEPHRITIS

Our recent experience with diffuse glomerulonephritis in fatal bacterial endocarditis, as observed at a large metropolitan hospital, forms the basis for the following description of the clinical features (119, 121). Renal functional impairment is common, ranging from mild to severe enough to require dialytic support. The duration of antecedent symptoms does not appear to correlate with the level of renal insufficiency on presentation. In the majority, serum creatinine levels reach their peak on the initiation of therapy or during the early days of treatment. With effective antibiotic therapy, recovery of renal function, normalization of serum complement levels, and remission of the other clinical features of glomerulonephritis occur regularly in those with mild or moderate renal functional impairment. Recovery of renal function is less frequent and a fatal outcome is more common in patients who present with renal failure. Since failure of antibiotic therapy to control infection is more frequent in patients with initial uremia than in those with mild renal failure, it may be inferred that the presence of renal failure hinders the efficacy of antibiotic therapy. Alternatively, other factors interfering with a bacterial cure could be responsible for continuing nephritis. In any case, it appears that persistent infective endocarditis engenders severe and unremitting glomerulonephritis. Despite these observations, advanced renal failure may yet remit on occasion when eradication of the infection is possible.

Microscopic hematuria and proteinuria are universal in diffuse glomerulonephritis (121). Gross hematuria may also occur and may result from renal infarction or drug-induced interstitial nephritis. It is generally believed that the nephrotic syndrome is a rare feature of diffuse glomerulonephritis as it occurs in bacterial endocarditis (122); however, it has been noted in 14% of histologically confirmed cases (119). This figure probably overestimates the true incidence of nephrotic syndrome in that heavy proteinuria is likely to be an indication for renal biopsy. Hypertension is rare, contrasting with its frequent occurrence in other forms of acute post infectious endocapillary glomerulonephritis (123). In the few hypertensive patients who have been reported, antecedent essential hypertension generally could not be excluded (119). Because of the difficulty in differentiating cardiac, nephrotic, and "nephritic" edema in patients with endocarditis and glomerulonephritis, the occurrence of primary renal sodium retention and noncardiac circulatory congestion cannot be determined with certainty.

Hypocomplementemia in the course of infective endocarditis frequently accompanies glomerulonephritis but is neither invariable nor specific for renal involvement (107, 108, 112, 124). The level of serum complement is depressed prior to antibiotic therapy in 90% of patients with diffuse, and in 60% of those with focal, glomerulonephritis in subacute bacterial endocarditis (119). In acute bacterial endocarditis with diffuse glomerulonephritis, the level of serum complement is depressed in about 70% of patients; data in patients with focal glomerulonephritis are insufficient (119). The majority of hypocomplementemic patients demonstrate activation of the classical complement pathway (125–127). A high incidence of alternative pathway activation has been described, however, in patients with S. aureus endocarditis and glomerulonephritis (127). The degree of complement depression correlates directly with the severity of renal impairment (127). The serum complement level becomes normal with successful antibiotic therapy and recovery of renal function. Failure to control infection and continuing renal failure is associated with persistent hypocomplementemia (16).

Therapy and prognosis

With the control of infection by antibiotic therapy, urinary abnormalities will normalize in most patients within several days to weeks (119). Occasionally, microscopic hematuria or proteinuria may persist for months to years after bacteriologic cure (121). Renal insufficiency of mild-to-moderate severity also resolves promptly with successful antibiotic therapy; infrequently, transient worsening of renal function may occur prior to recovery. Despite the usual fatal outcome in patients who present with uremia, even severe renal failure may resolve with successful antibiotic therapy, sometimes with continued improvement during weeks or months. Serial renal biopsies reveal almost complete histologic resolution of glomerulonephritis in association with clinical recovery (125). Residua may include expansion of the mesangium or infrequent hyalinized glomeruli. Rarely, renal failure requiring dialysis may persist despite bacteriologic cure. This might be observed more frequently were in not for the high mortality in those who develop uremia.

Several recent reports have suggested that supplementation of antibiotic therapy with plasmapheresis and corticosteroids may promote recovery of renal function in patients with renal failure due to combined endocapillary- and extracapillary proliferative glomerulonephritis (128, 129). However, it is not possible to dissociate the influence of these additional therapeutic modalities from that of antibiotic therapy alone in uncontrolled studies.

Among those cured of endocarditis, later deaths due to progressive renal failure have occasionally been reported (119). The true incidence of chronic renal disease following bacterial endocarditis is not known but appears to be low. In several patients, extensive residual glomerular changes have been observed long after bacteriologic cure (119). Savin et al. (110) reported persistent renal insufficiency, nephrotic syndrome, and sediment abnormalities after a bacteriologic cure of S. aureus endocarditis. Our own studies demonstrate that glomerulonephritis acquired during the course of endocarditis may on occasion prove to be irreversible after a bacteriologic cure and can be followed by persistent renal insufficiency or sediment abnormalities (119, 121). As may be inferred from the preceeding discussion, the course of glomerulonephritis generally closely parallels that of the underlying infective endocarditis. The therapy is directed at eradication of the infection with appropriate antibiotics. Once endocarditis is successfully treated, the eventual complete clinical healing of glomerulonephritis can be anticipated in most cases.

REFERENCES

1. Glassock RJ: Clinical aspects of acute, rapidly progressive and chronic glomerulonephritis. In: LE Earley, CW Gottschalk, eds, *Diseases of the Kidney*, Vol 1. Little, Brown, Boston, pp 691–764, 1963.
2. Glassock RJ, Bennett CM: The glomerulopathies. In: BM Brenner, FC Rector Jr, eds, *The Kidney*, Vol 2. WB Saunders, Philadelphia, pp 1351–1492, 1976.
3. De Wardener HE: *The Kidney*. Churchill Livingstone, Edinburgh, pp 211–215, 1958.
4. Kassirer JP: The treatment of acute poststreptococcal glomerulonephritis. *Kidney* 4:1–6, 1971.
5. Travis LB, Dodge WF, Beathard GA, Spargo BH, Lorentz WB, Caravajal HF, Berger M: Acute glomerulonephritis in children. *Clin Nephrol* 1:169–181, 1973.
6. Lieberman E: Critical analysis of treatment of acute glomerulonephritis exclusive of immunosuppressive drugs. In: J Metcoff, ed, *Acute glomerulonephritis*. Little, Brown, Boston, pp 367–389, 1967.
7. Kassirer JP, Schwartz WB: Acute glomerulonephritis. *N Engl J Med* 265:686–692; 736–741, 1961.
8. Nesson HR, Robbins SL: Glomerulonephritis in older age groups. *Arch Intern Med* 105:23–32, 1960.
9. Nissenson Ar, Baraff LJ, Fine RN, Knutson DW: Poststreptococcal acute glomerulonephritis: Fact and controversy. *Ann Intern Med* 91:76–86, 1979.
10. Earle DP, Farber SJ, Alexander JD, Pelligrino ED: Renal function and electrolyte metabolism in acute glomerulonephritis. *J Clin Invest* 30:421–433, 1951.
11. Bradley SE, Bradley GP, Tyson CJ, Curry JJ, Blake WD: Renal function in renal disease. *Am J Med* 9:766–798, 1950.
12. Farber SJ: Physiologic aspects of glomerulonephritis. *J Chron Dis* 5:87–107, 1957.
13. Watt MF, Howe JS, Parrish AE: Renal tubular changes in acute glomerulonephritis. *Arch Intern Med* 103:690–695, 1959.
14. Earle DP, Segal D: Natural history of glomerulonephritis. *J Chron Dis* 5:3–13, 1957.
15. Warren JV, Stead EA Jr: Protein content of edema fluid in patients with acute glomerulonephritis. *Am J Med Sci* 208:618–622, 1944.
16. Fordham CC, Welt LG: The cardiovascular manifestations of acute glomerulonephritis: Physiologic basis for treatment. *Prog Cardiovasc Dis* 3:382–394, 1961.
17. Blantz RC, Hostetter TM, Brenner BM: Functional adaptations of the kidney to immunological injury. In: CB Wilson, BM Brenner, JH Stein, eds, *Immunologic Mechanisms of Renal Disease. Contemporary Issues in Nephrology*, Vol 3. Churchill Livingstone, New York, pp 122–143, 1978.
18. Glassock RJ, Bennett CM: Glomerular hemodynamics and permselectivity in experimental glomerular disease. In: P Kincaid-Smith, AJF d'Apice, RC Atkins, eds. *Progress in Glomerulonephritis. Perspectives in Nephrology and Hypertension*. John Wiley, New York, pp 159–172, 1979.
19. Neugarten J, Baldwin DS: The acute glomerulonephritis syndrome. In: WN Suki, SG Massry, eds, *Therapy of Renal Diseases and Related Disorders*. Martinus Nijhoff, Boston, pp 183–193, 1984.
20. Strauss MB, Welt LG: Clinical aspects of acute poststrepto-

coccal glomerulonephritis. In: MB Strauss, LG Welt, eds, *Diseases of the Kidney*, Vol 1. Little, Brown, Boston, pp 419–462, 1963.
21. Hughes JG, Hill FS, Davis BC: Electroencephalographic findings in acute nephritis. *J Pediatr* 36:451–459, 1950.
22. Travis LB: Acute postinfectious glomerulonephritis. In: CM Edelmann, ed, *Pediatric Kidney Disease*, Vol 2. Little, Brown, Boston, pp 611–631, 1978.
23. Bord J: Acute glomerulonephritis. *Am J Med* 7:317–335, 1949.
24. Rodriguez-Iturbe B, Baggio B, Colina-Chourio J, Favaro S, Garcia R, Sussana F, Castillo L, Borsatti A: Studies on the renin-aldosterone system in the acute nephritic syndrome. *Kidney Int* 19:445–453, 1981.
25. Powell HR, Rotenberg E, Williams AL, McCredie DA: Plasma renin activity in acute poststreptococcal glomerulonephritis and the haemolytic uraemic syndrome. *Arch Dis Child* 49:802–807, 1974.
26. Shahabuddin SH, Nor MM, Abdullah AM, Mosdeen F: Plasma renin activity and hypertension in acute glomerulonephritis. *Austr NZ J Med* 9:250–253, 1979.
27. Goorno WE, Kaplan NM: Renal pressor material in various hypertensive diseases. *Ann Intern Med* 63:745–751, 1965.
28. Gunnells JC: Circulating vasoconstrictor material in hypertension. *Circulation* 30 (Suppl III):90–91, 1964.
29. Birkenhager WH, Schalekamp MADH, Schlenkamp-Kuyken MPA, Kolsters G, Krauss XH: Interrelations between arterial pressure, fluid-volumes and plasma-renin concentration in the course of acute glomerulonephritis. *Lancet* 1:1086–1087, 1970.
30. Repetto HA, Lewy JE, Brauado JL, Metcoff J: The renal functional response to furosemide in children with acute glomerulonephritis. *J Pediatr* 80:660–666, 1972.
31. LaDue JS: The role of congestive heart failure in the production of the edema of acute glomerulonephritis. *Ann Intern Med* 20:405–422, 1944.
32. Dean JVB: Relation of cardiac enlargement to hypertension in acute and chronic glomerulonephritis. *Am J Med* 1:161–167, 1946.
33. Murphy TR, Murphy FD: The heart in acut glomerulonephritis. *Ann Intern Med* 41:510–532, 1954.
34. Sapir DG, Yardley JH, Walker WG: Acute glomerulonephritis in older patient. *Johns Hopkins Med J* 123:145–152, 1968.
35. Eichna L: Circulatory congestion and heart failure. *Circulation* 22:864–886, 1960.
36. Eichna LW, Farber SJ, Berger AR, Rader B, Smith WW, Albert RE: Non-cardiac circulatory congestion simulating congestive heart failure. *Trans Assoc Am Phys* 67:72–85, 1954.
37. Gore I, Saphir O: Myocarditis associated with acute and subacute glomerulonephritis. *Am Heart J* 36:390–402, 1948.
38. LaDue JS, Ashman R: Electrocardiographic changes in acute glomerulonephritis. *Am Heart J* 31:685–701, 1946.
39. Peters JP: Edema of acute nephritis. *Am J Med* 14:448–458, 1953.
40. Fleisher DS, Voci G, Garfunkel J, Purugganen H, Kirkpatrick J, Wells, C, McElfresh AE: Hemodynamic findings in acute glomerulonephritis. *J Pediatr* 69:1054–1062, 1966.
41. Eisenberg S: Blood volume in patients with acute glomerulonephritis as determined by redioactive chromium tagged red cells. *Am J Med* 27:241–245, 1959.
42. Dodge WF, Travis LB, Haggard ME, Harris LC, Bryan GT, Daeschner CW Jr: Studies of physiology during the early stage of acute glomerulonephritis in children. In: J Metcoff, ed, *Acute Glomerulonephritis*. Little, Brown, Boston, pp 319–338, 1967.
43. Binak K, Simaci N, Ucak D, Harmanci N: Circulatory changes in acute glomerulonephritis at rest and during exercise. *Br Heart J* 37:833–839, 1975.
44. Davies CE: Heart failure in acute nephritis. *Q J Med* 20:163–171, 1951.
45. DeFazio V, Christensen RC, Regan TJ, Baer LJ, Morita Y, Hellems HK: Circulatory changes in acute glomerulonephritis. *Circulation* 20:190–200, 1959.
46. Vardi P, Markiewicz W, Levy J, Adler O, Riss E, Benderley A: The heart in acute glomerulonephritis: An echocardiographic study. *Pediatrics* 63:782–787, 1979.
47. Guz A, Noble NIM, Trenchard D, Garnett ES, Clarkson EM, McDonald SJ, de Wardener HE: The significance of a raised central venous pressure during sodium and water retention. *Clin Sci* 30:295–303, 1966.
48. Earle DP, Taggart JV, Shannon JA: Glomerulonephritis: A survey of the functional organization of the kidney in various stages of diffuse glomerulonephritis. *J Clin Invest* 23:119–137, 1944.
49. Williams RD: Electrocardiographic changes in acute hemorrhagic nephritis. *Johns Hopkins Med J* 65:434–444, 1939.
50. Master AM, Jaffe HL, Dack S: The heart in acute nephritis. *Arch Intern Med* 60:1016–1027, 1937.
51. Rubin MI, Rappaport M: *Am J Dis Child* 55:244–272, 1938.
52. Freedman P, Meister HP, Lee HJ, Smith EC, Co BS, Nidus BD: The renal response to streptococcal infection. *Medicine* 49:433–463, 1970.
53. Stetson CA, Rammelkamp CH Jr, Krause RM, Kohen RJ, Perry WD: Epidemic aute nephritis: Studies on etiology, natural history and prevention. *Medicine* 34:431–450, 1955.
54. Rammelkamp CH Jr: Prevention of acute nephritis. *Ann Intern Med* 43:511–517, 1955.
55. Weinstein L, Bachrach L, Boyer NH: Observations on the development of renal failure and glomerulonephritis in cases of scarlet fever treated with penicillin. *N Engl J Med* 242:1002–1010, 1950.
56. Rammelkamp CH Jr, Stetson CA, Krause RM, Perry WD, Kohn RJ: Epidemic nephritis. *Trans Assoc Am Physic* 67:276–282, 1954.
57. Dillon HC Jr: Streptococcal skin infections and acute glomerulonephritis. *Postgrad Med J* 46:641–652, 1970.
58. Glassock RJ: Clinical features of immunologic glomerular disease. In: CB Wilson, BM Brenner, JH Stein, eds, *Immunologic Mechanisms of Renal Disease. Contemporary Issues in Nephrology*, Vol 3. Churchill Livingston, New York, pp 255–322, 1978.
59. Weinstein L, Le Frock J: Does antimicrobial therapy of streptococcal pharyngitis or pyoderma alter the risk of glomerulonephritis? *Infec Dis* 124:229–231, 1971.
60. Lascyh EE, Frankel V, Vardy PA, Bergner-Rabinowitz S, Olfek, I, Rabinowitz K: Epidemic glomerulonephritis in Israel. *J Infect Dis* 124:141–147.
61. Leonard CD, Nagle RB, Striker GE, Cutler RF, Scribner BH: Acute glomerulonephritis with prolonged oliguria. An analysis of 29 cases. *Ann Intern Med* 73:703–711, 1970.
62. Breese BB, Disney FA, Talpey WB: Penicillin in streptococcal infection. *Am J Dis Chld* 110:125–130, 1965.
63. Dreow HA: Managment of acute glomerulonephritis. *N Engl J Med* 249:144–153, 1953.
64. De Wardener HE: Treatment of acute glomerulonephritis. *Am Heart J* 98:523–525, 1979.
65. Rudebeck J: Clinical and prognostic aspects of acute glomerulonephritis. *Acta Med Scand* 173(Suppl):1–184, 1946.
66. Illingworth RS, Philpott MG, Rendle-Short J: Controlled

investigation of the effect of diet on acute nephritis. *Arch Dis Child* 29:551–555, 1954.
67. Naeras A: Studies on urinary sediment. III. Effect of high protein diet upon the course of nephritis with special reference to the urinary sediment. *Acta Med Scand* 95:359–382, 1938.
68. Mortensen V: Treatment of acute glomerulonephritis with high protein diet. *Acta Med Scand* 129:321–331, 1947.
69. Akerren Y, Lindgren M: Investigation concerning early rising in acute haemorrhagic nephritis. *Acta Med Scand* 151:419–423, 1955.
70. McCrory WW, Fleisher DS, Sohn WB: Effects of early ambulation on the course of nephritis in children. *Pediatrics* 24:395–399, 1959.
71. Iseri LT, Mader IJ: The effect of ACTH on acute glomerulonephritis. *J Lab Clin Med* 42:821, 1953.
72. Danowski TS, Matees FM: Therapy of acute and chronic glomerulonephritis. *J Chron Dis* 5:122–137, 1957.
73. Farnsworth EB: Acute and subacute glomerulonephritis modified by adrenocorticotropin. *Proc Soc Exp Biol Med* 74:57–59, 1950.
74. Nakamoto S, Dunea G, Kolff WJ, McCormack LJ: Treatment of oliguric glomerulonephritis with dialysis and steroids. *Ann Intern Med* 63:359–368, 1965.
75. Harrison CV, Loughridge LW, Milne MD: Acute oliguric renal failure in acute glomerulonephritis and polyarteritis nodosa. *Q J Med* 33:39–55, 1964.
76. Thorn GW, Merril JP, Smith S, Roche M, Frawley TF: Clinical studies with ACTH and cortisone in renal disease. *Arch Intern Med* 86:319–354, 1950.
77. Thorn GW, Fosham PH, Frawley TF, Hill SR, Roche M, Staehelin D, Wilson DL: The clinical usefulness of ACTH and cortisone. *N Engl J Med* 242:865–872, 1950.
78. Burnett Ch, Greer MA, Burrows BA, Sisson JH, Relman AS, Weinstein LA, Colburn CG: The effects of cortisone on the course of acute glomerulonephritis. *N Engl J Med* 243:1028–1032, 1950.
79. Kincaid–Smith P, Saker BM, Fairley KF: Anticoagulants in irreversible acute renal failure. *Lancet* 2:1360–1363, 1968.
80. Gill DG, Turner DR, Chantler C, Cameron JS: The progression of acute proliferative poststreptoccocal glomerulonephritis to severe epithelial crescent formation. *Clin Nephrol* 8:449–452, 1977.
81. Kincaid–Smith P: Severe acute oliguric renal failure in glomerular and vascular disease. In: *The Kidney: A Clinicopathologic Study*. Blackwell, Oxford, pp 259–275, 1975.
82. Neugarten J, Baldwin DS: The acute glomerulonephritis syndrome. In: WN Suki, SG Massry, eds. *Therapy of Renal Diseases and Related Disorders*. Martinus Nijhoff, Boston, pp 183–193, 1984.
83. Retan JW, Dillon HC: Furosemide in the treatment of acute poststreptococcal glomerulonephritis. *South Med J* 62: 157–160, 1969.
84. James JA: Ethacrynic acid in edematous states in children. *J Pediatr* 71:881–886, 1967.
85. Muth RG: Diuretic properties of furosemide in renal disease. *ANN Intern Med* 69:249–261, 1968.
86. Pruitt AW, Boles A: A diuretic effect of furosemide in acute glomerulonephritis. *J Pediatr* 89:306–309, 1979.
87. Kohaut JC, Wilson CJ, Hill LL: Intravenous diazoxide in acute poststreptococcal glomerulonephritis. *J Pediatr* 87: 795–798, 1975.
88. Gordillo–Paniagua G, Valasquez–Jones L, Martini R, Valdez–Bolanos E: Sodium Nitroprusside treatment of severe arterial hypertension in children. *J Pediatr* 87:799–802, 1975.
89. McLaine PN, Drummond KN: Intravenous diazoxide for severe hypertension in children. *J Pediatr* 79:829–832, 1971.
90. McCrory WW, Rapoport M: Effects of hydrazinophthalazine on blood pressure and renal function in children with acute nephritis. *Pediatrics* 12:29–37, 1953.
91. Etteldorf JN, Smith JD, Tharp CP, Tuttle AH: Hydralazine in nephritic and normal children with renal hemodynamic studies. *Am J Dis Child* 89:451–462, 1955.
92. Etteldorf JM, Smith JD, Johnson C: The effect of reserpine and its combination with hydralazine on blood pressure and renal hemodynamics during the hypertensive phase of acute nephritis in children. *J Pediatr* 48:129–139, 1956.
93. Maddox DA, Bennett CM, Deen WM, Glassock RJ: Determinants of glomerular filtration in experimental glomerulonephritis in the rat: Structural and functional observations. *Kidney Int* 5:356–364, 1975.
94. Earle D: Physiologic abnormalities in acute glomerulonephritis. In: J Metcoff, ed, *Acute Glomerulonerphritis*. Little, Brown, Boston, pp 301–317, 1967.
95. Kunis CL, Lowenstein J: The emergency treatment of hyperkalemia. *Med Clin North Am* 65:165–176, 1981.
96. Baldwin DS, Gluck MC, Schacht RG, Gallo G: The long-term course of poststreptococcal glomerulonephritis. *Ann Intern Med* 80:342–358, 1974.
97. Schacht RG, Steele JM Jr, Lowenstein J, Baldwin DS: Failure of sodium restriction to abolish exaggerated natriuresis in poststreptococcal glomerulonephritis. *Nephron* 18:333–341, 1977.
98. Nissenson AR, Mayon–White R, Potter EV, Mayon–White V, Abidh S, Poon–King T, Earle DP: Continued absence of clinical renal disease seven to 12 years after poststreptococcal acute glomeruloneohritis in Trinidad. *Am J Med* 67:255–262, 1979.
99. Perlman LV, Herdman RC, Kleinman H, Vernier RL: Poststreptococcal glomerulonephritis. A ten-year follow-up of an epidemic. *JAMA* 194:63–70, 1965.
100. Nissenson AR, Mayon–White R, Potter EV, Poon–King T, Earle DP: Effect of sodium loading on sodium excretion in patients recovered from poststreptococcal glomerulonephritis. *Cardiovasc Med* 2:779–783, 1977.
101. Garcia R, Rubio L, Rodriguez–Iturbe B: Long-term prognosis of epidemic poststreptococcal glomerulonephritis in Maracaibo: Follow-up studies 11–12 years after the acute episode. *Clin Nephrol* 15:291–298, 1981.
102. Löhlein M: Ueber hamorrhagische nierenaffektionen bei chronischer ulzeroser endokarditia (embolische nicteiterige herd-nephritis). *Med Klin* 6:375–379, 1910.
103. Baehr G: Glomerular lesions of subacute bacterial endocarditis. *J Exp Med* 15:330–347, 1912.
104. Bell ET: Glomerular lesions associated with endocarditis. *Am J Pathol* 8:639–662, 1932.
105. Baehr G, Lande H: Glomerulonephritis as a complication of subacute streptococcus endocarditis. *JAMA* 75:789–790, 1920.
106. Bain RG, Edwards JE, Scheifley CH, Geraci JE: Right-sides bacterial endocarditis and endarteritis. *Am J Med* 24:98–110, 1958.
107. Sherry S: Staphylococcal sepsis and acute renal failure. *Am J Med* 28:430–442, 1960.
108. Glancy DL, Marcus FI, Cuadra M, Ewy GA, Roberts WC: Isolated organic tricuspid valvular regurgitation. *Am J Med* 46:989–996, 1969.
109. Halpern M, Trubek M: Necrotizing arterities and subacute glomerulonephritis in gonococcic endocarditis. *Arch Pathol* 15:35–50, 1933.
110. Savin V, Siegel L, Schreiner GE: Nephropathy in heroin

addicts with Staphylococcal septicemia. In: P Kincaid-Smith, TH Mathew, EL Becker, eds, *Glomerulonephritis, Morphology, Natural History and Treatment*. John Wiley and Sons, New York, pp 397–408, 1973.
111. Yum M, Wheat LJ, Maxwell D, Edwards JL: Immunofluorescent localization of *Staphylococcus aureus* antigen in acute bacterial endocarditis nephritis. *Am J Clin Pathol* 79:832–835, 1978.
112. Pertschuk LP, Woda BA, Vuletin JC, Brigati DJ, Soriano CB, Nicastri AD: Glomerulonephritis due to *Staphylococcus aureus* antigen. Am J Clin Pathol 65:301–307, 1976.
113. Perz GO, Rothfield N, Williams RC Jr: Immune-complex nephritis in bacterial endocarditis. *Arch Intern Med* 136:334–336, 1976.
114. Levy RL, Hong R: The immune nature of subacute bacterial endocarditis nephritis. *Am J Med* 54:645–652, 1973.
115. Iida H, Mizumura Y, Uraoka T, Takata M, Sugimoto T, Miwa A, Yamagishi T: Membranous glomerulonephritis associated with enterococcal endocarditis. *Nephron* 40:88–90, 1985.
116. Lerner IL, Weinstein L: Infective endocarditis in the antibotic era. *N Engl J Med* 274:199–206; 259–266; 302–321, 1966.
117. Gorlin R, Favour CB, Emery FJ: Long-term follow-up study of penicillin-treated subacute bacterial endocarditis. *N Engl J Med* 242:995–1001, 1950.
118. Spain DM, King DW: The effect of penicillin on the renal lesion of subacute bacterial endocarditis. *Ann Intern Med* 36:1086–1089, 1952.
119. Neugarten J, Baldwin DS: Glomerulonephritis in bacterial endocarditis. *Am J Med* 77:297–304, 1986.
120. Morel–Maroger L, Sraer JD, Herreman G, Godeau P: Kidney in subacute endocarditis. Pathological and immunofluorescent findings. *Arch Pathol* 94:205–213, 1972.
121. Neugarten J, Gallo GR, Baldwin DS: Glomerulonephritisi in bacterial endocarditis. *Am J Kidney Dis* 5:371–379, 1984.
122. Glassock RJ: Clinical aspects of acute, rapidly progressive and chronic glomerulonephritis. In: Earley LE, Gotschalk CW, eds, *Diseases of the Kidney*, Vol 1. Little, Brown, Boston, pp 691–793, 1963.
123. Neugarten J, Baldwin DS: The acute glomerulonephritis syndrome. In: WN Suki, SG Massry, eds, *Therapy of Renal Diseases and Related Disorders*. Martinus Nijhoff, Boston, pp 183–193, 1984.
124. Pelletier LL Jr, Petersdorf RG: Infective endocarditis: A review of 125 cases from the University of Washington Hospitals. 1962–72. Medicine (Baltimore) 56:287–313, 1977.
125. Beaufils M, Gilbert C, Morel–Maroger L, Sraer JK, Kanfer A, Meyrier A, Kourelsky O, Vanchon F, Richet G: Glomerulonephritis in severe bacterial infections with and without endocarditis. In: J Hamburger, J Crosnier, MH Maxwell, eds, *Advances in Nephrology*, Vol 7. Year Book Medical, Chicago, pp 217–234, 1977.
126. Kauffmann RH, Thompson J, Valentijn RM, Daha MR, Van Es LA: The clinical implications and the pathogenetic significance of circulating immune complexes in infective endocarditis. *Am J Med* 71:17–25, 1981.
127. O'Connor DT, Weisman MH, Fierer J: Activation of the alternate complement pathway in *Staph. aureus* infective endocarditis and its relationship to thrombocytopenia, coagulation abnormalities, and acute glomerulonephritis. Clin Exp Immunol 34:179–187, 1978.
128. McKenzie PF, Taylor AE, Woodroffe AJ, Seymour AE, Chan YL, Clarkson AR: Plasmapheresis in glomerulonephritis. *Clin Nephrol* 12:97–108, 1979.
129. Rovzar MA, Logan JL, Ogden DA, Graham AR: Immunosuppressive therapy and plasmapheresis in rapidly progressive glomerulonephritis associated with bacterial endocarditis. *Am J Kidney Dis* 7:428–433, 1986.

CHAPTER 20

Nephrotic Syndrome

GERALD C. GROGGEL & WAYNE A. BORDER

DEFINITION

The nephrotic syndrome may be defined as the presence of heavy proteinuria and hypoalbuminemia in association with varying degrees of edema, lipiduria, and hyperlipidemia. One of the earliest clinical pathologic correlations made in nephrology was a description of a group of patients with heavy proteinuria whose kidneys upon examination showed lipid accumulation within the renal tubule as the only abnormality. The renal lesion was called *lipoid nephrosis* and the patients were said to suffer from *nephrosis*. In distinction, other patients with proteinuria had distinctly abnormal glomeruli, showing changes both in proliferation and inflammation. These patients were said to have *nephritis* and often went on to renal failure. It soon became apparent, however, that many patients with abnormal glomeruli or nephritis showed heavy proteinuria and edema that was indistinguishable from that found in patients with lipoid nephrosis. Therefore the term *nephrotic syndrome* was coined to describe the presence of a constellation of findings that was common to certain patients suffering from either lipoid nephrosis or glomerulonephritis. Today it is clear that the nephrotic syndrome is a direct manifestation of injury to the glomerular capillary wall and that such an injury can occur in any form of glomerulopathy. Thus a wide variety of glomerular lesions may be encountered in patients with the nephrotic syndrome.

In another approach Schreiner has arbitrarily defined protein excretion > 3.5 g/24 hr/1.73 m^2 as being nephrotic-range proteinuria (1). Although there is validity in this definition, certain patients can develop the nephrotic syndrome even though they excrete < 3.5 g of protein per 24 hours. Since one cannot place an absolute value on "nephrotic"-range proteinuria, it is more reasonable to use the definition of Earley and Forland, who have stated that the nephrotic syndrome is produced when proteinuria leads to hypoalbuminemia (2). Thus it is the hypoalbuminemia that is the hallmark of the nephrotic syndrome. This definition takes into account the varying capacity of different individuals to adapt to proteinuria by increasing protein synthesis and is consistent with the clinical observation that the degree of proteinuria does not necessarily predict the severity of the nephrotic syndrome.

The major value in the clinical use of the term, *nephrotic syndrome*, is the emphasis that it places on the systemic complications that arise from this syndrome of proteinuria and secondary hypoalbuminemia. The term provides no insight into the etiology and/or pathogenesis of the glomerulonephritis as it was originally thought to do. Nevertheless, it is useful to say that a patient suffers from the *nephrotic syndrome*, since this allows the physician to anticipate a predictable group of complications to which the patient will be susceptible.

PATHOPHYSIOLOGY

The pathophysiology of the nephrotic syndrome begins at the glomerular capillary wall (3). The glomerular capillary wall acts as a barrier to exclude proteins from entering the urinary space by discriminating according to both the molecular size and electrical charge (4, 5). At neutral physiologic pH, the glomerular wall behaves as a graded sieve for molecules bearing little or no electrical charge. Thus such molecules pass the glomerular filter as readily as water and ions when the average molecular radius is less than about 17 Å and are nearly completely excluded from the glomerular filtrate above a radius of about 44 Å. The fractional clearance of neutral molecules, having a molecular radius of 36 Å (the size of albumin in solution), is about 10% of the prevailing glomerular filtration rate. Although the fractional glomerular clearance of albumin has never been directly measured in humans, it is presumed to be much less than 10%, and probably closer to 0.01% (6). This discrepancy is best explained by the fact that albumin is a polyanion at physiologic pH and is thus retarded in its transglomerular passage by electrostatic repulsion via the interactions with the anionic molecules of the capillary wall, particularly heparan sulfate proteoglycan and sialic acid (5). The glomerular capillary wall possess fixed negative (anionic) charges that are located on the endothelial cell surface, throughout the glomerular basement membrane and on the epithelial cell coat. Within the glomerular basement membrane, these anionic sites are composed primarily of heparan sulfate proteoglycan and impose a strong negative charge on the glomerular capillary wall that allows it to electrostatically repel negatively charged plasma proteins (5). Plasma proteins in general are negatively charged, especially albumin, except for some immunoglobulin molecules that are positively charged (cationic). When similar fractional clearance studies are conducted using charged modified anionic or cationic dextran molecules, one can see the clear effect of electrical charge (4). Negatively charged molecules have reduced clearance relative to neutral molecules of the same molecular size. On the other hand, positively charged molecules have an increased clearance relative to neutral molecules of the same size. The size barrier is maintained by the function of the glomerular basement membrane as a coarse gel.

Proteinuria can now be seen to occur by one of two mechanisms (4). Due to injury the size of pores of the glomerular basement membrane can be increased such that there is loss of the size selectivity. A second possibility is the loss of the electrical barrier, which would now allow negatively charged proteins to gain access to the urinary space. In some diseases it is possible that both size and charge abnormalities occur simultaneously and lead to proteinuria. It is also possible that loss of the charge barrier may lead to alterations in the structure of the basement membrane, resulting in the loss of size selectivity as well. Recent studies have shown that the normal glomerular ultrafiltrate contains only trace amounts of albumin, making it impossible for decreased tubular reaborption alone to lead to heavy albuminuria (6). On the other hand, proteins smaller than albumin are freely filtered, and for these proteins, such as light chains or $beta_2$ microglobulin, the proximal tubular reabsorption represents a major site of catabolism. In the presence of tubulointerstitial injury, therefore, these low molecular weight filtered proteins can enter the urine and sometimes accumulate in quantities of 1.0–2.0 g or even greater than 3.5 g. This type of proteinuria is called *tubular proteinuria* and is distinguished from glomerular proteinuria in that it contains little albumin relative to low molecular weight proteins. The overproduction of low molecular weight paraproteins, such as occurs with light chains and multiple myeloma, can occasionally lead to a pseudonephrotic syndrome. In these patients, several grams of light chains can be excreted in the urine, however, hypoalbuminemia and edema do not follow.

Recent studies have also shown that the collection of a 24-hour urine sample is not necessary to quantitate the 24-hour urine protein excretion. Ginsberg et al. have shown that a single voided urine sample can be used to quantitate proteinuria (7). They demonstrated an excellent correlation between 24-hour protein excretion and the protein/creatinine ratio in a single urine sample expressed as milligrams of protein per milligrams of creatinine. In the presence of stable renal function, a protein/creatinine ratio of more than 3.5 corresponded to a protein excretion of 3.5 g per 24 hours.

The sequence of physiologic events leading from proteinuria to the full clinical picture of the nephrotic syndrome is reasonably clear. Once proteinuria results in hypoalbuminemia there is a reduction in the plasma oncotic force. This leads to an unbalancing of Starling's forces in the peripheral capillaries and movement of plasma water into the interstitial space as edema (8). With the reduction of intravascular volume, the hypothetical intrathoracic carotid and intracranial arterial sensors will detect decreased "effective" arterial blood volume and will activate the physical and hormonal mechanisms favoring secondary renal retention of salt and water. Although the intravascular volume is returned toward normal, it is at the expense of ever-increasing edema formation.

Recent studies have also suggested a primary disturbance of renal salt and water excretion in some forms of nephrotic syndrome, since the total plasma volume and "effective" arterial volume may actually be increased in some patients with heavy proteinuria, hypoalbuminemia, and edema (9). These patients often have structural glomerular lesions and suppressed plasma renin levels (10). Experimental work has shown that it is intrarenal factors acting on the distal tubule that enhance renal salt retention (11).

In addition to albumin, other important plasma proteins are lost in the urine as well. Historically, when the proteinuria was confined to the loss of albumin, the proteinuria was said to be selective and when larger proteins such as immunoglobulins and fibrinogen, were present, the proteinuria was said to be nonselective (12). Although an interesting concept, the measurement of protein selectivity has not provided great clinical usefulness. The loss of other plasma proteins, as well as albumin, predisposes to some of the well-recognized complications of the nephrotic syndrome. The continued loss of albumin often leads to a negative nitrogen balance and to a reduction in the lean body mass, but this can often be masked by the associated edema formation. The enhanced renal excretion and increased fractional catabolism of IgG may lead to serious hypogammaglobulinemia. Factors of the alternative pathway of complement, particularly factor B, may be lost in the urine, contributing to defective bacterial opsonization. The loss of transport proteins can lead to true or apparent endocrine deficiency syndromes. This particularly occurs with the loss of thyroglobulin and a reduction in T_4 and thyroxin-binding globulins, giving the apparent picture of hypothyroidism in patients with the nephrotic syndrome. Recently it has been recognized that the loss of the vitamin-D transport protein, vitamin-D binding globulin, leads to defective intestinal calcium transport, hypocalcemia, hypocalciuria, and the subsequent stimulation of parathyroid activity (13, 14). Such hyperparathyroidism and acquired hypovitaminosis D could lead to accelerated bone loss and osteomalacia, and/or osteitis fibrosis cystica, which ordinarily would not occur until there was advanced renal failure. The hypoalbuminemia could also lead to important pharmacologic consequences, since many drugs circulate in an albumin-bound form. Thus, in the nephrotic state high levels of free drug may result, leading to toxicity. The nephrotic syndrome is often described as a *hypercoaguable state* because of both increases and decreases in various clotting factors (15). This term is vague and its exact physiologic significance is unclear. Nevertheless patients with the nephrotic syndrome do suffer from an increased incidence of thromboembolic events (16). A variety of trace metals and their binding proteins are also lost in the urine of nephrotic subjects. Thus iron, zinc, and copper deficiencies may develop and lead to clinical manifestations. Lastly, lipid metabolism is greatly altered in the nephrotic syndrome, leading to elevated plasma levels of VLDL and LDL lipoproteins and reduced levels of HDL (17). These abnormalities can result in a tendency for accelerated atherogenesis. All of these biochemical disturbances must be considered in dealing with the general problem of the nephrotic syndrome as distinct from the specific management of individual lesions, as will be discussed below.

ETIOLOGY AND PATHOLOGIC CLASSIFICATION

Causes of the nephrotic syndrome can be divided into those that are secondary to a systemic illness with kidney involvement and those causes that are related directly to the kidney or are idiopathic. There is nearly an endless list of allergens, microorganisms, drugs, toxins, tumors, and systemic metabolic and hereditary diseases that have been associated with the nephrotic syndrome in individual patients. The most common of these are diabetes mellitus and systemic lupus erythematosus.

A useful approach is to catagorize the clinicopathologic diagnosis in 100 consecutive adult patients presenting with the nephrotic syndrome in general and also a hypothetical list of 100 consecutive patients with the idiopathic nephrotic syndrome. Such hypothetical lists are shown in Tables 1 and 2.

Table 1. The clinicopathologic diagnosis in 100 adult patients presenting with the nephrotic syndrome

Diabetic nephropathy	35
Lupus nephritis	20
Membranous nephropathy	20
Minimal change disease	8
Glomerulosclerosis	5
Mesangial proliferative nephritis	5
Membranoproliferative nephritis	3
Amyloidosis	1
Acute post-infectious glomerulonephritis	1
Rapidly progressive crescentic glomerulonephritis	2

Table 2. Clinicopathologic diagnosis in 100 adult patient with idiopathic nephrotic syndrome

Minimal change disease	15
Mesangial proliferative nephritis	10
Focal sclerosis	15
Membranous nephropathy	50
Membranoproliferative nephritis	5
Others	5

Looking at these lists, one immediately recognizes that they contain nearly all the described forms of human glomerulopathies. For each of these entities, there is an underlying body of basic knowledge, often derived from experimental animals that provides a basis for the understanding of the pathogenesis of the renal lesion. One can apply this information to an individual patient and thus have a more workable approach to the clinical management of the patient with the nephrotic syndrome. As a single entity, diabetic nephropathy is the most frequent cause of the nephrotic syndrome in adults, followed by lupus nephritis. The most common cause of the idiopathic nephrotic syndrome is membranous nephropathy in adults. Other common causes of the idiopathic nephrotic syndrome include minimal change disease, focal segmental glomerulosclerosis, mesangial proliferative nephritis, and membranoproliferative glomerulonephritis. Hypertensive nephrosclerosis is common due to the large number of patients who suffer from hypertension, but only a very small percentage of these patients actually develop the nephrotic syndrome. Although commonly mentioned as a cause of the nephrotic syndrome, amyloidosis is less frequent than one might expect from its prominence in the medical literature. The nephrotic syndrome may occasionally occur as a feature of either acute post-infectious glomerulonephritis or rapidly progressive crescent glomerulonephritis, but this is unusual. Other features of these entities are often more prominent, such as acute onset of renal failure and/or the progression to end-stage renal disease. The presence of proteinuria leading to hypoalbuminemia in these patients has lead to the confusing use of the terms *nephritic* and *nephrotic* to indicate the simultaneous presence of nephrotic syndrome and renal failure. It is preferable to directly state the pathophysiologic abnormality in each patient rather than to resort to the use of clinical terms that lack precision.

GENERAL MANAGEMENT OF THE NEPHROTIC SYNDROME AND ITS COMPLICATIONS

Edema

Edema formation in the nephrotic syndrome correlates reasonably well with the degree of hypoalbuminemia. Based upon a variety of studies in experimental animals, it is generally agreed that hypoalbuminemia leads to a reduction in intravascular volume by allowing water to cross the vessel wall into the interstitial space (8). This intravascular reduction leads to the stimulation of the renin-angiotensin-aldosterone system and other antinatriuretic factors that lead to a positive sodium balance (10). Despite common agreement that such a pathophysiologic sequence occurs, measurements of the intravascular volume in patients with an established nephrotic syndrome have shown a variety of alterations. Thus, plasma volume may be reduced, normal, or even increased (9). Such findings are not inconsistent with the pathogenesis just described in that such measurements may lack the sensitivity to detect small decrements in the intravascular volume or patients may have been studied at a time when the intravascular volume was returned to a normal state; they do suggest that, in addition to secondary renal sodium retention, some renal diseases may induce a primary form of sodium retention, leading to expansion of plasma volume despite hypoalbuminemia. Investigation of the renin-angiotensin system in patients with the nephrotic syndrome has in general shown two groups of patients (10). In one group there is evidence of volume contraction with high plasma renin and aldosterone levels, and a tendency to show clinical signs of orthostatic hypotension and vasoconstriction. In a second group of patients, often with some degree of a depressed glomerular filtration rate, renin and aldosterone seem to be suppressed due to hypervolemia. There is an increased incidence of hypertension in these patients and the nephrotic syndrome is usually resistant to steroid therapy. In the former group of patients, minimal change disease was the most frequent finding, whereas the latter group suffered from a variety of membranous and/or proliferative disorders.

The most important treatment for the edema of the nephrotic syndrome is to attempt to treat the underlying cause of the nephrotic syndrome and thus to reduce the proteinuria. Unfortunately in many cases this is not always possible. Thus in order to decrease edema formation in these patients, it is necessary to produce a negative sodium balance. This can be accomplished by the cautious use of dietary sodium restriction plus a diuretic (18). Since a decreased intravascular volume and symptoms of orthostatic hypotension are seen frequently, one must be careful in the induction of a negative sodium balance to prevent the development of prerenal azotemia and worsening orthostatic hypotension. One usually begins by reducing dietary sodium to 2 g (5 g sodium chloride), which is essentially a no added-salt diet. In the absence of important renal failure, potassium-containing salt substitutes can be prescribed. In the presence of normal renal function, a thiazide diuretic would be the first choice for inducing naturiesis. Use of the loop diuretics such as furosemide in this setting may predispose to extensive volume depletion. A useful adjunct to salt restriction and diuretic therapy is an attempt to mobilize the interstitial fluids by having the patient lie down for a period of time or simply elevate the feet. Experimentally one can induce a natriuresis by immersion to the chin in carefully temperature-controlled water, but this technique has been confined to research use (19). Hypokalemia may occur in some patients receiving potent diuretics and the use of potassium supplementation or a potassium-sparing diuretic such as amiloride may be advisable. It is extremely important to follow the daily weight in patients with the nephrotic syndrome in order to not induce too rapid a volume reduction. Other complications of severe edema in the nephrotic syndrome can be precipitation of acute renal failure secondary to reduced renal perfusion with the development of acute tubular necrosis (20). Several series of nephrotic patients who developed acute renal failure, probably as a result of prolonged or critical renal hypoperfusion, have been reported. Another cause of acute renal failure in the nephrotic syndrome can be due to interstitial renal edema, which leads to collapse of the renal tubules and increased hydrostatic pressure in the proximal tubules and Bowman's space (21). Because renal blood flow can be so tenuous in the nephrotic syndrome, these patients are particularly prone to drug-induced causes of acute renal failure, particularly due to the prostaglandin inhibitors. Infusions of albumin, in general, do not provide a sustained benefit, since the albumin is rapidly lost in the urine. This therapy should only be used in the setting of vascular collapse and hypotension.

Hypoproteinemia

Hypoalbuminemia in the nephrotic syndrome is due to the urinary loss of albumin and to the increased fractional catabolism of albumin in these patients (22). This increased fractional catabolism comes about largely because of the tubular reabsorption of albumin in the kidney and the catabolism of the albumin in the proximal tubule (23). Thus, the amount of albumin in the urine markedly underestimates the total renal loss of albumin. In the past, because of the concern for the development of negative nitrogen balance, these patients were often placed on a high-protein diet. But recent work has shown that in nephrotic patients a high-protein diet (1.6 g/kg) often leads to not only increased albumin synthesis, but also increased albuminuria (24). The overall net effect was a lowering of the serum albumin concentration. While the use of a low-protein diet (0.8 g/kg) led to decreased protein synthesis, but also decreased urinary albumin, and the overall net effect was an increase in serum albumin concentration (24). Thus while long-term studies addressing this issue remain to be performed, it is not appropriate to recommend a high-protein diet to nephrotic patients. As mentioned, the infusion of albumin for purposes of restoring intravascular volume is an expensive procedure that is justified only as emergency treatment (25).

The loss of thyroid-binding globulin in the nephrotic syndrome commonly leads to a low serum total T_4 level (26). However, measurements of free T_4 and thyroid stimulating hormone are normal. So though chemically the patients can appear to be hypothyroid, clinically they are in a euthyroid state (27). This discrepancy is due to the low level of protein-bound thyroxin with a normal level of free T_4 available for tissue metabolism. It is thus not recommended to treat these patients for hypothyroidism.

Hypocalcemia that is out of proportion to the hypoalbuminemia has been described in patients with the nephrotic syndrome. Low levels of 25-hydroxycholecalciferol have been reported, and the level is related to the degree of proteinuria (14). Vitamin D and its metabolites circulate in the plasma bound to vitamin-D binding globulin, which is lost in the urine in the nephrotic syndrome. This is probably the explanation for the development of vitamin-D deficiency. Recently, low serum levels of 1,25-dihydroxycholecalciferol have been reported in the nephrotic syndrome as well (28). The impact of this hypocalcemia is secondary stimulation of parathyroid hormone activity and the induction of hyperparathyroidism, which can lead to significant bone disease. Thus, premature renal osteodystrophy may occur before there is azotemia. Current studies are evaluating the clinical usefulness of supplementing these patients with oral vitamin-D preparations (13).

Hyperlipidemia

Hyperlipidemia has long been recognized as a complication of the nephrotic syndrome. There is a general correlation between the elevation of cholesterol and phosphoslipids, and the degree of proteinuria and hypoalbuminemia. In a recent study of 20 nephrotic patients, 70% were found to have an elevated cholesterol and 85% had a decreased ratio of HDL cholesterol to total cholesterol (17). In the liver there is a relation between the synthetic pathway for albumin and that for lipoproteins (29). Studies in experimental animals with the nephrotic syndrome have shown that there is a general increase in the hepatic synthesis of VLDL, LDL, and HDL (30, 31). The elevation of VLDL, which is rich in triglycerides, is what gives rise to the lactescence of serum seen in severe cases of the nephrotic syndrome. The pathogenesis of the hyperlipidemia of the nephrotic syndrome appears to be due to increased hepatic synthesis of lipoproteins and decreased clearance of lipoproteins from the circulation (32). The increased hepatic lipoprotein synthesis has been felt to be secondary to the increased albumin synthesis, and the increased hepatic albumin synthesis is probably secondary to the decrease in plasma oncotic pressure. However, a recent study has shown that the serum cholesterol in the nephrotic syndrome is dependent only upon the renal clearance of albumin and is completely independent of the rate of albumin synthesis (33). Thus the renal loss of macromolecules appears to play a key role in the hypercholesterolemia of the nephrotic syndrome. Clearance of lipoproteins from the circulation is diminished in the nephrotic syndrome because of reduced lipoprotein lipase enzyme activity and reduced lectothin acyltransferase enzyme activity. The hypoalbuminemia also causes decreased removal of free fatty acids, which leads to decreased lipoprotein lipase activity. Hypoalbuminemia also decreases removal of lysolecthin, which causes decreased LCLT activity. The accumulation of VLDL in the nephrotic syndrome is thought to be due to an inhibition of its conversion to LDL, probably due to the reduction in lipoprotein lipase activity. HDL lipoprotein levels may be reduced in severe proteinuria secondary to losses into the urine (34).

Lipiduria is an expected consequence of the increase in glomerular wall permeability and is not related to the hyperlipidemia (35). Once in the tubule, lipoproteins can form casts, which are seen in the urine sediment; the incorporation of lipoprotein droplets within tubular cells gives rise to oval fat bodies which are proximal renal tubular cells seen to be loaded with lipid droplets that are shed into the urinary tract. Cross polarization shows the characteristic Maltese cross present in the lipid droplets and is an interesting clinical finding.

There is a great deal of controversy over whether the hyperlipidemia of the nephrotic syndrome predisposes to premature coronary heart disease (36, 37). Clearly the hyperlipidemia correlates with the proteinuria. Thus only patients with persistent proteinuria will have sustained elevations of serum lipids and will be at risk for premature coronary heart disease. Most studies investigating the incidence of coronary heart disease in the setting of the nephrotic syndrome have not taken into account the persistence of the proteinuria. Also HDL cholesterol appears to be variably affected in the nephrotic syndrome. However, it would appear that nephrotic patients with long-standing persistent proteinuria and reduced HDL cholesterol are adults followed with the nephrotic syndrome, compared to a control population, no differences in the prevalence of angina, intermittent claudication, or myocardial infarction was found (38). The authors concluded that the early reports showing a greatly increased incidence of ischemic heart disease in unselected patients with the nephrotic syndrome was not a universal finding; but, unfortunately, many of the patients in this series had minimal change disease in which the proteinuria was only intermittently present. The exact magnitude of the risks associated with the hyperlipidemia in the nephrotic syndrome is unknown but is clearly elevated compared to the normal rate for cardiovascular disease.

Given that one should want to reduce the hyperlipidemia to decrease the risks of coronary heart disease, the results of using drugs have not been convincing. In most of the older studies, clofibrate has been employed but has had a high degree of complications, particularly severe muscle necrosis secondary to the increased concentrations of the drug related to the underlying hypoalbuminemia (39). Recent work has shown that gemfibrozil is well tolerated in nephrotic patients and has a beneficial effect on cholesterol and triglycerides (40). In a recent short-term study, the HMG CO-A reductase inhibitor, lovastatin, was well tolerated and was effective for improving the hyperlipidemia of the nephrotic syndrome (41). There is also experimental evidence suggesting that hyperlipidemia may play a role in the progression of chronic renal failure (42). In the rat 5/6 nephrectomy model, the lipid-lowering agent, clofibric acid, was effective in maintaining the glomerular filtration rate and preventing focal glomerulosclerosis (43). Thus this may be another reason for attempting to control the hyperlipidemia of the nephrotic syndrome.

In summary, the best general recommendations are that nephrotic patients remain on a low cholesterol diet and that they maintain their ideal body weight with a reasonable amount of daily exercise. If this is not effective in lowering the hyperlipidemia and they remain persistently proteinuric with a decreased HDL lipoprotein fraction, they should probably be treated with one of the newer lipid-lowering agents. However, one must keep in mind that these patients will be at risk for increased side effects from these drugs.

Thrombotic complications

Several studies have shown a high incidence of renal vein thrombosis in patients with the nephrotic syndrome, usually due to underlying membranous nephropathy. In a review of 151 nephrotic patients, 33 were shown by angiography to have renal vein thrombosis and of these 20 had membranous nephropathy (16). In 27 consecutive patients with membranous nephropathy and the nephrotic syndrome, 13 were found to have renal vein thrombosis at angiography and one further patient developed renal vein thrombosis diagnosed at autopsy (44).

Two forms of renal vein thrombosis are recognized (16). In the acute form there is the sudden onset of flank pain often associated with costovertebral angle tenderness and macroscopic hematuria. This occurs in the setting of severe volume depletion, heat stroke, or major trauma. The second form occurs in patients with nephrotic syndrome where the renal vein thrombosis appears in a clinically silent manner without changes in edema, protein excretion, or the production of renal failure. However, patients have been described where increased proteinuria and worsening of the nephrotic syndrome, along with deterioration of renal function, has been associated with the development of renal vein thrombosis, although it is clear that such findings are not present in the majority of cases. In a review of 31 cases of renal vein thrombosis, 28 of the patients were found to have an underlying renal disorder, with the nephrotic syndrome being the most common complication (45). It is clear that the development of renal vein thrombosis should be considered as a complication of the nephrotic syndrome (46). This is based upon the inability to produce the nephrotic syndrome experimentally by ligation of the renal veins or to produce primary glomerulonephritis by the same technique.

The manner in which the nephrotic syndrome predisposes to renal vein thrombosis is unclear. In general the nephrotic syndrome is associated with increased levels of plasma fibrinogen, factors V and VII, and plasminogen (15, 47, 48). The elevation of these factors probably does not lead to hypercoagulation. There are three mechanisms for controlling the coagulation cascade (49). These include antithrombin III, which is a heparin cofactor that acts to neutralize thrombin and activated factors IX, X, XI, and XII; protein C, which neutralizes activated factors XIII and V; and lastly plasminogen activator, which converts plasminogen to plasmin leading to fibrinolysis. In the nephrotic syndrome there have been reported decreased levels of antithrombin III (50, 51). It is thought that antithrombin III is lost in the urine in states of altered glomerular permeability, but there does continue to be controversy over whether antithrombin III is actually reduced in this disorder. There are also decreased levels of factors IX and XII in the nephrotic syndrome. The loss of antithrombin III could lead to a state of hypercoaguability. The hypoalbuminemia has been shown to correlate with the decreased levels of antithrombin III (51). Both protein C and plasminogen activitor appear to be normal in the nephrotic syndrome (52).

Platelet abnormalities, particularly an increase in platelet aggregability and adhesiveness, have been found in the nephrotic syndrome, and these could lead to the initiation of coagulation (48, 53). These changes in platelet function are felt to be secondary to hypoalbuminemia. Albumin is thought to prevent arachidonic acid release by platelets and thus to prevent its metabolism to platelet-aggregating substances.

It is difficult to make a solid clinical recommendation for the management of hypercoaguability in the nephrotic syndrome since so few studies have been done. All patients with the nephrotic syndrome should not undergo renal angiography since this procedure is associated with serious risks (44). Rather, only those patients with evidence of thromboembolic disease or clinical evidence for renal vein thrombosis, such as sudden deterioration in renal function or worsening of the proteinuria, should be studied. All patients with documented renal vein thrombosis should be treated with anticoagulation, since there is a significant incidence of thromboembolic complications (15). Recently thrombolytic therapy with either streptokinase or urokinase has been shown to be very effective therapy, with lysis of the clot demonstrated by angiography (54, 55). Patients should continue to be treated with anticoagulant therapy for as long as they remain nephrotic. New evidence of thrombosis following discontinuation of therapy have been documented. Presently prophylactic anticoagulation is not recommended, since the complications of anticoagulation therapy are considerable. Prophylaxis should be reserved for the nephrotic patient who becomes at high risk for thrombosis, such as during a period of immobilization.

Infectious complications

Hypogammaglobulinemia is found in the nephrotic syndrome and is thought to result from the loss of immunoglobulins into the urine and also due to increased catabolism of immunoglobulins. In one study of 73 nephrotic children, IgG levels were reduced to 20% of normal (56). In general, serum complement components are not lost in the urine and are not low in the nephrotic syndrome, except in those forms of glomerulonephritis associated with consumption of complement. Factor B, a component of the alternative complement pathway, has been shown to be reduced in the nephrotic syndrome (57). These changes in serum immunoglobulin levels, as well as the protein calorie malnutrition frequently present in the nephrotic syndrome and the use of steroids and immunosuppressive agents to treat the nephrotic syndrome, act together to produce an immune-compromised state. Thus nephrotic syndrome patients are at increased susceptibility for infections, particularly bacterial infections of the lungs and peritoneum. Any infection in the patient with nephrotic syndrome should be taken seriously and treated aggressively with antibiotic therapy. In addition, these patients should have routine immunizations, particularly pneumococcal vaccine and influenza vaccine. There is no evidence that such immunizations are harmful to the underlying glomerular disease, except in minimal change disease, where relapses may be temporarily associated with such immunization.

TREATMENT OF SPECIFIC GLOMERULOPATHIES CAUSING THE IDIOPATHIC NEPHROTIC SYNDROME

Initial clinical evaluation

The physician should emphasize several points in the clinical evaluation of new patients presenting with the nephrotic syndrome (Table 3). In taking the history one should pay particular attention to the presence of diabetes mellitus in the patient's family or any other systemic disorders associated with renal disease. The patient's exposure to drugs and toxins as well occupational history should be carefully examined. It is important to ascertain whether the patient's symptoms are due to the nephrotic syndrome alone, or whether there are other findings suggesting an underlying disease such as diabetes mellitus, malignancy, vasculitis, or lupus erythematosus. The presence of an underlying disorder can often be masked by the presence of the nephrotic syndrome, and unless care is taken this may be overlooked.

The laboratory examination should begin with a standard blood count and urinalysis. At least two separate 24-hour urine collections should be obtained for measurement of total protein and creatinine. The adequacy of the 24-hour urine collection can be determined from the total creatinine excretion, which should be 15–20 mg/kg in females and 20–25 mg/kg in males. If 24-hour urine collections are unable to be obtained, the protein excretion can be accurately estimated from a spot urine collection measurement of both protein concentration and creatinine concentration, with the results expressed as milligrams of protein/milligrams of creatinine (7). The ratio of 1 mg protein/1 mg creatinine corresponds to approximately 1 g/24 hours. Routine chemistry tests should include creatinine (for calculation of creatinine clearance), BUN, albumin, total protein, calcium, phosphorus, cholesterol, triglycerides, HDL cholesterol, and electrolytes. Serologic tests should include antinuclear antibody, C_3 and C_4 components of complement, and hepatitis B surface antigen. A urinary protein immunoelectrophoresis can be performed in order to be certain that the major protein is albumin and to detect the rare patient with a monoclonal gammopathy excreting large quantities of light chain in the urine. Finally, the evaluation should include a standard chest film and electrocardiogram. In the presence of normal renal function, an intravenous pyelogram should be performed to establish that the patient's renal anatomy and kidney size are normal. If there is diminished renal function, renal ultrasonography is preferred.

Once patients with secondary forms of the nephrotic syndrome are eliminated, the clinical abnormalities of patients with idiopathic nephrotic patients are common to all patients and therefore lack diagnostic specificity for the various forms of primary glomerular lesions. Urinalysis will usually show small numbers of leukocytes and/or oval fat bodies in the majority of patients. In addition, 20–50% of patients in each diagnostic category can have microscopic hematuria. Red blood cell casts, although suggestive of glomerulonephritis, are generally uncommon in idiopathic nephrotic syndrome, except in patients with membranoproliferative and mesangial proliferative glomerulonephritis. Because of the absence of distinguishing clinical features, a more accurate diagnostic test is needed. Percutaneous renal biopsy is a low-risk procedure that has a high diagnostic specificity for determining the specific cause of the idiopathic nephrotic syndrome. For this reason, in adult patients with the idiopathic nephrotic syndrome, renal biopsy is mandatory in order to provide the physician with information to allow for counseling the patients in terms of prognosis, planning of therapy, and also for determining the chances of recurrence of this disease in a transplanted kidney should it be necessary in the future.

The glomerulopathies producing the idiopathic nephrotic syndrome are classified according to the findings on light, immunofluorescence, and electron microscopy. Each of these techniques provides separate information concerning the distribution and nature of the lesions as well as clues to the underlying immunopathogenesis. The three techniques should not be viewed as redundant, and if they are unavailable locally the physician performing the biopsy should forward the tissue to another location where all can be performed. It is important for the renal biopsy to be evaluated by someone with experience in renal pathology. If the biopsy cannot be examined in a appropriate way by an experienced pathologist, the patient should be referred to a medical center where such services are available.

Classification of glomerulopathies

Glomerulopathies causing the idiopathic nephrotic syndrome are entities by nature of the combination of clinical and pathologic findings in each case. Due in large part to the availability of renal biopsy, patients are now said to

Table 3. Initial evaluation of patients with the nephrotic syndrome

History:	Search for evidence of a systemic disease such as diabetes mellitus, familial renal disease, exposure to drugs, chemicals, toxins
Physical:	Evidence of a systemic disease, e.g., diabetes mellitus, systemic lupus, vasculitis, etc.
Laboratory:	Complete blood count, two 24-hour urine collections for protein and creatinine, serum creatinine, BUN, electrolytes, calcium, phosphate, albumin, total protein, cholesterol, triglycerides, HDL cholesterol, urinary protein electrophoresis; anti-nuclear antibody, C_3 and C_4 complement; Hepatitis B antigen; chest x-ray, electrocardiogram

suffer not from the nephrotic syndrome but from minimal change disease, focal glomerulosclerosis, mesangial proliferative glomerulonephritis, membranous nephropathy, or membranoproliferative glomerulonephritis. Depending on the age of the patient and certain selection factors such as referral to a medical center, one can estimate the contribution of each of these entities to a population of adult patients with idiopathic nephrotic syndrome. Such an estimate is shown in Table 2.

MINIMAL CHANGE DISEASE (MCD)

The term *minimal change* is taken literally from the microscopic findings that are remarkable for the paucity of abnormal findings. The changes usually consist of a very mild diffuse increase in the amount of mesangial matrix (58). Although glomeruli with global sclerosis can be seen in normal individuals as well as in patients with minimal change disease, the presence of segmental sclerosis would indicate another diagnosis. Tubular interstitial areas are most often normal. The immunofluorescent studies should be negative in patients with true minimal change disease. Correspondingly, no electron-dense deposits are noted by ultrastructural examination, with the only abnormality being effacement of the epithelial foot processes. It is important to emphasize that light microscopy alone is inadequate to diagnose minimal change disease or any other glomerulopathies causing the idiopathic nephrotic syndrome (59). Many cases of steroid unresponsiveness in minimal change disease probably represent incorrect diagnoses that are based upon light microscopic examination alone.

The cause of minimal change disease remains unknown (60). Many tantalizing observations have been made, but to date they remain unproven or unconfirmed. Theoretically minimal change disease could be caused by some factor that alters glomerular capillary wall permeability and is produced by steroid responsive cells such as T lymphocytes (61). Unfortunately, to date no such factor has been identified. Recent work has shown that there is a defect in the charge-selective barrier of the basement membrane in patients with the minimal change nephrotic syndrome (62). It has also been shown that there is generalized loss of membrane negative charge occurring in steroid responsive nephrotic syndrome, particularly in red blood cells and platelets, and that this is probably due to neutralization rather than to the absence of anionic groups (63). Thus an abnormality in T-cell function may lead to changes in the charge of membranes, particularly the glomerular capillary wall, leading to increased permeability.

The natural history of minimal change disease has been much better described in children than in adults due to its higher prevalence in the young (64). It is characterized by a prompt and complete response to corticosteroids in both children and adults. Today the survival at 5 years is 95% or greater. In a child less than age 10 who presents with the absence of hematuria, hypertension, or azotemia, and who has selective proteinuria and a normal C_3 level, the likelihood of the presence of minimal change disease is so great that renal biopsy need not be performed (64). Approximately 95% of such patients will respond to steroid treatment. In older children and adults who present in this manner, or have hematuria, azotemia, hypertension, or a low C_3, renal biopsy is recommended. Glucocorticoids, particularly prednisone, are now uniformly accepted for the treatment of minimal change disease in both children and adults. The mechanism of their effect is unknown but they are likely to work by interfering with cellular immune responses. It has been estimated that without prednisone therapy, about 25% of patients will undergo a spontaneous remission. With the administration of prednisone at 1 mg/kg (usually 60–80 mg/day) for adults, 85% of patients will become protein free within 3–4 weeks, an additional 8% within 8 weeks, and an additional 5% within 12 weeks (64). Thus over 95% of patients will have a complete remission of proteinuria within 12 weeks of prednisone therapy (65, 66). There is now general agreement that daily prednisone therapy is superior to intermittent therapy, however, there is controversy as to whether daily therapy is superior to alternate-day therapy. In adults it is common to begin patients with 120 mg of prednisone/1.73 m^2/day given on alternate days, and it is thought that this leads to a response equal to that of an administration of daily prednisone. In contrast, many pediatric nephrologists prefer to initiate therapy with daily prednisone and after remission has occurred to switch to alternate-day prednisone (67).

After remission of proteinuria, 15–20% of patients will apparently be cured and have no further problems. The remainder of patients eventually relapse, the majority doing so within the first year (68). About half of the patients who relapse will have multiple relapses within a 1-year period. After successful treatment with prednisone, 30–40% of patients will redevelop proteinuria as the prednisone is being tapered, or within 2 weeks of discontinuation of prednisone. These patients are often said to be steroid dependent. After several relapses with retreatment with prednisone, up to 10–50% of patients may fail to demonstrate a response to further prednisone therapy and are labeled *steroid resistant* or *late nonresponders* (66, 69).

In patients who have become steroid resistant, have multiple relapses, or who show serious side effects to steroid therapy, various regimens of cytotoxic drugs have been tried (64). The alkylating agents, cyclophosphamide and chlorambucil, have been used successfully in these patients. Both drugs have been shown to decrease the frequency of relapses or to extend the time until the next relapse occurs. Cyclophosphamide is used in doses of 2–3 mg/kg/day and chlorambucil in doses of 0.1 mg/kg/day, in addition to steroids. A recently described regimen combined prednisone at 1.5–2.0 mg/kg/day with chlorambucil at < 0.3 mg/kg/day for 5–15 weeks (70). After proteinuria disappeared, the prednisone was switched to an alternate-day regimen. Using this form of treatment, 84% of patients remained in remission at 3 years and 78% at 5 years. Recently it has been shown that the benefits of cyclophosphamide or chlorambucil in decreasing relapse rates are limited to those patients who do not display a steroid-dependent behavior (71). Side effects of both drugs include leukopenia, bone marrow suppression, infection, alopecia, vomiting, possible tumor induction, and sterility. In addition, cyclophosphamide is known to cause chemical cystitis, and about 6% of children taking chlorambucil have been reported to have focal seizures.

Of the reported side effects, sterility has been one that has received a great deal of attention (72). Males seem to be at greater risk than females, and the duration of therapy may be equally important as the total dose in producing sterility. At present, cumulative total doses of chlorambucil under 8 mg/kg (73) and cyclophosphamide under 300 mg/kg are thought to be relatively safe from any permanent effects of sterility (74, 75). With these doses the oncogenic risk is also thought to be small. Again, the use of cytotoxic therapy should be reserved for patients with frequent but not steroid-dependent relapses who have also developed unacceptable steroid side effects (76). A recent report has shown that a short course of methylprednisolone pulses followed by low-dose oral prednisone is about as effective as a regimen of high-dose oral steroids but does improve the ratio of risk to benefit associated with treatment of the minimal change nephrotic syndrome (77). Side effects related to treatment were significantly fewer in the group given methylprednisolone than in the control group.

MESANGIAL PROLIFERATIVE GLOMERULONEPHRITIS

Mesangial proliferative glomerulonephritides are glomerular lesions that are characterized primarily by increased cellularity in the mesangial region in patients without well-defined systemic illnesses. This includes a heterogeneous group of disorders that have been primarily defined by immunofluorescent findings (78). The mesangial proliferative glomerulonephritides are defined by proliferation of both mesangial cells as well as the mesangial matrix. Usually each mesangial lobule will contain four to six nuclei, while the peripheral capillary walls will appear normal. Mesangial proliferative glomerulonephritis has long been associated with the nephrotic syndrome in both adult and pediatric patients. There is, however, controversy over whether mesangial proliferative glomerulonephritis is a distinct entity separate from minimal change disease and focal segmental glomerulosclerosis (79). Several reports have appeared recently that indicate it is reasonable to place mesangial proliferative glomerlonephritis between minimal change disease and focal sclerosis in a histologic hierarchy (80). Controversy continues over whether mesangial proliferation infers a worse prognosis than normal light microscopy. Using light microscopy alone, the International Study of Kidney Disease in Childhood found a clear correlation between a poor response to prednisone therapy and the degree of mesangial proliferation (81). Other separate reports, usually involving small numbers of patients, found no difference in the response rate to standard prednisone treatment between patients with only minimal changes and those with mild mesangial proliferation (82).

By immunofluorescence microscopy patients with mesangial proliferative changes can have mesangial deposits of IgA, IgM, and/or C_3. In fact, primary mesangial proliferative glomerulonephritis can be divided into IgA neohropathy (Berger's disease), IgM nephropathy, minimal change disease, or glomerulonephritis with C_3 deposits only (78). But it is the IgM nephropathy that is most commonly associated with the nephrotic syndrome and will be discussed here. In 1978 two groups of patients were reported who had predominant findings of IgM mesangial deposits as well as C_3 deposits (79, 83). Based on these observations, the term *IgM mesangial nephropathy* was coined (79). The ages of these patients ranged from 4 years through 60 years, with a slight male predominance. The majority of the patients were in their second or third decade of life. The clinical presentations of mesangial proliferative glomerulonephritis can be that of a) microscopic hematuria alone, b) microscopic hematuria and asymptomatic proteinuria, or c) microscopic hematuria and the nephrotic syndrome. There is little correlation between the clinical findings and the histologic severity, except in patients with azotemia, who often showed marked mesangial proliferation and lesions, suggesting a focal segmental sclerosing process. In general, the prognosis of patients without the nephrotic syndrome is good, because to date there is little evidence that they develop renal failure. Of the group with the nephrotic syndrome, perhaps 30% will develop mild azotemia, but there are few documented cases of progression to end-stage renal disease. Both hypertension and renal failure are thus uncommon.

By light microscopy the mesangial changes range from mild to severe. In patients with the most mild changes, it would be easy to diagnosis minimal changes disease if only light microscopy were used. In other patients, the degree of mesangial proliferation clearly exceeded the limits usually accepted for the minimal change category. Although immunofluorescence demonstrated IgM deposits in the mesangium in all patients, electron microscopy revealed dense deposits in the mesangium in approximately one third of the patients. Such a disparity between immunofluorescence and electron microscopy has been widely recognized and is likely to be due to the greater sensitivity of immunofluorescence compared to electron microscopy (84). Patients with mesangial proliferative glomerulonephritis who have hematuria alone or hematuria and non-nephrotic proteinuria should be reassured and given general medical treatment for hypertension or other conditions, but should not be treated for the glomerular disease. The reason for this is that the prognosis is favorable without treatment and there is no evidence that any form of treatment is effective. Patients with the nephrotic syndrome with or without azotemia should be considered for treatment. Treatment of mesangial proliferative glomerulonephritis is similar to that of minimal change disease.

The first drug of choice is prednisone in either daily or

alternate-day dosing. Patients should be treated to the point of a remission of the nephrotic syndrome or up to 8 weeks. With this treatment, approximately 50% of the patients can be expected to respond with complete remission of the nephrotic syndrome. However, the majority of patients will relapse as soon as the steroid dose is tapered and therefore would be considered steroid dependent. In a small percentage of patients there will be no resoponse to prednisone. Thus this response to prednisone clearly suggests that these patients do not have minimal change disease, since the expected response rate should be about 95%. If prednisone is ineffective or if the patient has become resistant, cyclophosphamide at a dose of 2 mg/kg can be administered for 8 weeks. It can be given alone or with a low-to-moderate dose of prednisone. There is no evidence that adding prednisone to the cyclophosphamide improves the outcome. The cyclophosphamide does not need to be tapered after the 8-week course.

In a study of 68 pediatric patients, 32% of the patients with positive immunofluorescence were not responsive to prednisone therapy, compared to 2% of patients who had no deposits detected by immunofluorescence (85). It seems likely that the presence of IgM mesangial deposits should be considered as a marker that indicates the possibility of a poor response to prednisone. In a small number of patients, a second renal biopsy has been performed and about 25% of these patients have evidence of focal changes of segmental proliferation or sclerosis. It is possible that IgM deposits may predispose to focal sclerosis by some unique biologic property of IgM. This hypothesis has been suggested in the literature but direct proof of it is lacking. Presently most nephrologists would agree that IgM mesangial proliferative glomerulonephritis is an entity separate from minimal change disease and focal glomerulosclerosis, with a prognosis that lies somewhere between those two entities.

In summary, it is important to recognize the presence of IgM mesangial deposits as a hallmark in patients who will have a less favorable response to standard treatment with prednisone for the nephrotic syndrome than patients with similar histologic findings who do not have the positive immunofluorescence. This is true whether the histologic findings are called minimal change disease or mesangial proliferative glomerulonephritis.

FOCAL AND SEGMENTAL GLOMERULOSCLEROSIS

Focal and segmental glomerulosclerosis or focal sclerosis is responsible for about 10–15% of adult patients with idiopathic nephrotic sundrome and smaller numbers for children, depending on the age. The etiology and pathogenesis of focal sclerosis is unclear. The majority of investigators have found little evidence that focal sclerosis represents an advanced stage of minimal change disease in which the initial lesion has undergone an evolution into the more serious histologic category (86). It is clear that if immunofluorescence is not used as part of the diagnostic criteria of minimal change disease, this entity can be easily confused with focal glomerulosclerosis. If focal sclerosis represented simply an advanced form of minimal change disease, then one would expect the nephrotic syndrome to have been present longer in presenting patients in whom the initial biopsy showed focal sclerosis compared to those in whom the biopsy showed minimal change disease. The evidence indicates that the duration of the nephrotic syndrome is similar in both groups of patients (59). Furthermore, in patients who have come to autopsy with minimal change disease, careful examination of the kidney has not revealed evidence of focal sclerosis. Since focal sclerosis may be missed by a sampling error in the biopsy, it is easy to understand how a patient who is nonresponsive to prednisone therapy and who undergoes a second renal biopsy may then be found to have focal sclerosis.

In addition to idiopathic focal sclerosis, it is now clear that a number of other processes can lead to similar histologic changes. These include a few cases of post-streptococcal glomerulonephritis, heroin-associated glomerulopathy, AIDS nephropathy (87), reflux nephropathy, obstructive nephropathy, analgesic nephropathy, in a setting of renal agenesis, and in many experimental models of renal disease (88). Although some authors have used this nonspecific quality of focal sclerosis as evidence against the diagnostic usefulness of this term, it would seem that this approach denies clear evidence that certain patients presenting with new-onset nephrotic syndrome will have focal sclerosis as the only glomerular lesion. These patients whose disease is termed *idiopathic focal glomerulosclerosis* do consitute a distinct clinical group, making it valuable to continue to use this term.

A few prospective controlled trials of therapy in focal sclerosis have been carried out, and the majority of the clinical information concerning treatment is based upon case reports or uncontrolled studies. In general, the nephrotic syndrome due to focal sclerosis seems to be resistant to both prednisone and cytotoxic therapy. A large retrospective series from France found that only about 20% of patients with focal sclerosis responded to prednisone therapy with a complete or partial remission of proteinuria (89). In a recent review of 46 adults with idiopathic focal segmental glomerulosclerosis, 29 of the patients had nephrotic proteinuria at the time of presentation and 13 had renal insufficiency at presentation (90). A response to therapy was observed in 50% of the patients, but only 16 of the patients were treated. The authors did find that nephrotic patients who responded to therapy had a better course than nonresponders or patients who were not treated. Seventeen percent of their patients progressed to end-stage renal disease. Overall the experience in the United States has indicated that about 25% of patients may respond to treatment. However, it is unclear whether this response rate is any different than the spontaneous remission rate. There is no evidence that other forms of aggressive therapy, such as intravenous methylprednisolone or plasma exchange, have any application in patients with focal sclerosis. It would seem reasonable to begin a 4-week course of prednisone in patients with focal sclerosis who are nephrotic. If there is a response, the steroids can be tapered and switched over to alternate-day therapy. If there is no response, the steroids should be discontinued. Cytotoxic agents have only proved useful in those patients who are steroid dependent or in those who are responsive to steroids but frequently relapse.

Recently there have been some preliminary reports on the use of cyclosporine in the treatment of steroid-resistant idiopathic nephrotic syndrome, particularly focal glomerulosclerosis (91–93). In general, a response in terms of a reduction of proteinuria has been achieved with cyclosporine but this reponse is cyclosporine dependent. Cyclosporine nephrotoxicity was also seen in this setting (92). Cyclosporine does not appear to have any lasting effect on the pathogenesis of focal sclerosis, and presently we cannot recommend its use in the setting of idiopathic nephrotic syndrome. Further studies remain to be performed.

In summary, focal sclerosis remains one of the most resistant lesions causing the idiopathic nephrotic syndrome, and to date there is no evidence that any form of therapy directed at the renal lesion is effective. It is therefore recommended that these patients have their nephrotic syndrome managed by medical treatment alone or be given a brief trial of glucocorticoids if no contraindications are present. One must also be aware of the high incidence of reoccurrence of this lesion in renal allografts.

MEMBRANOPROLIFERATIVE GLOMERULONEPHRITIS (MPGN)

In both children and adults, membranoproliferative glomerulonephritis is the least common form of glomerulopathy that causes the idiopathic nephrotic syndrome, but the prognosis is worse in this disorder than in any of the other causes of the idiopathic nephrotic syndrome. The terminology describing this entity is somewhat confusing. In the United States the term *membranoproliferative glomerulonephritis* has been used, but in France the term *mesangioproliferative glomerulonephritis* is used, and in the United Kingdom *mesangiocapillary glomerulonephritis* is used. The term *membranoproliferative glomerulonephritis* is meant to describe both the abnormalities of the glomerular basement membrane as well as the associated proliferation of mesangium that is found. In general, membranoproliferative glomerulonephritis can be divided into two types, which are distinguished by the location of the electron-dense deposits (94). In Type I MPGN, electron-dense deposits are noted throughout the mesangium and within the subendothelial space. By immunofluorescence there is associated deposition of immunoglobulin and complement. In Type II, electron-dense deposits are noted within the lamina densa of the glomerular basement membrane in an unusual pattern of nodular and fusiform configuration. By immunofluorescence immune deposits can be sparse, whereas there is heavy staining for complement, particularly C_3. Nephritic factor is a substance that was isolated from the serum of patients with MPGN and was subsequently shown to activate complement in serum from normal individuals (95). This nephritic factor is an immunoglobulin that is directed against the C_3 convertase of the alternative pathway and that stabilizes this convertase against degradation by the normal control proteins of the alternative complement pathway (96). Thus the convertase continues to degrade C_3 and contributes to the hypocomplementemia commonly found in MPGN. The role of nephritic factor in the pathogenesis of MPGN remains unclarified (97).

In a large series of both adults and children with MPGN, 50% of the patients presented with the nephrotic syndrome (98). About 90% had hematuria and approximately one third were hypertensive. Importantly, MPGN is the only cause of the idiopathic nephrotic syndrome that is associated with hypocomplementemia. Complement levels should always be measured in all patients with the nephrotic syndrome prior to a renal biopsy. The prognosis of MPGN is poor, with frequent progression to renal failure. In one large series, only 7% of the patients underwent a remission, while after 20 years it is predicted that 90% of patients will have renal failure (98).

The efficacy of various forms of treatment of MPGN remains controversial. In children the use of moderate-dose, alternate-day prednisone for 1–2 years has been reported to slow the progression of the renal lesion, but no control group has been used (99, 100). In a similar use of prednisone in a randomized control study conducted by the International Study of Kidney Disease in Children, there has been some preliminary evidence of benefit in halting progression (101). In this study a percentage of the patients developed hypertension, and this then accelerated the course of the renal failure. In patients who do not develop hypertension, such steroid therapy appears to be of benefit. In adults there has been no corresponding evidence that prednisone therapy is beneficial. In a recent controlled trial of a combination of cyclophosphamide, coumadin, and dipyridamole for 18 months, no benefits of therapy on proteinuria or progression of renal disease were seen (102). Recently two reports of the use of platelet inhibitor therapy in MPGN have been shown to be beneficial (103, 104). Forty patients with Type I MPGN were treated with dipyridamole and aspirin for 1 year in a double-blind, controlled study (103). Renal function was stabilized in the treated group compared to the placebo. In a second prospective trial, warfarin and dipyridamole were used for 1 year (104). Treatment appeared to stabilize renal function when compared to controls. Urinary protein excretion was also decreased with treatment, but bleeding was a complication in this study. Thus it would appear that antiplatelet therapy has a beneficial effect on the progression of the renal disease in this disorder. Presently therapy with asprin and dipyridamole can be recommended for these patinets.

MEMBRANOUS NEPHROPATHY

In adults membranous nephropathy is the single most common cause of the idiopathic nephrotic syndrome. It has been described in patients from age 5 through age 80, but it is a much less frequent finding in children (105). The term *membranous* is meant to indicate the abnormality in the glomerular basement membrane that occurs in the absence of cellular proliferation. It is known that this abnormality is due to the formation of immune deposits on the subepithelial side of the basement membrane and a subsequent reaction of the basement membrane with the formation of spikes that extend between immune deposits and eventually enclose and engulf them. There is much experimental evidence that indicates that the immune deposits form in this disorder by in-situ immune complex formation and not due to deposition of circulating immune complexes (106). In Heymann nephritis, an experimental model of membranous nephropathy induced in the rat by immunization with renal tubular antigen, it is now clear that an antibody forms that reacts directly with an antigen located in the subepithelial space (107). Recently a second mechanism for the in-situ formation of immune deposits in membranous nephropathy has been described in which a cationic antigen bound directly to the anionic sites of the glomerular basement membrane, initiating immune deposit formation (108).

The vast majority of patients with membranous nephropathy present with the nephrotic syndrome or occasionally with asymptomatic proteinuria (105). Hematuria occurs in about 50% of the patients, but hypertension and azotemia at the time of presentation are distinctly unusual. The natural history of membranous nephropathy is variable and difficult to predict in individual patients. About 50% of the patients will have persistent proteinuria with slowly progressive loss of renal function, resulting eventually in renal failure. About 25% of patients will have a spontaneous remission and 25% will have persistent proteinuria, but with stable renal function. Children appear to have a much better prognosis than adults and women may have less severe disease than men (109).

The efficacy of steroids and immunosuppressive agents in membranous nephropathy remains controversial (110). The results of uncontrolled trials of prednisone therapy in membranous nephropathy are contradictory. Many reports have found no response to prednisone therapy, whereas others have reported an improvement. Only one large prospective control study has been reported (111). The collaborative study of adult idiopathic nephrotic syndrome compared oral prednisone therapy with placebo in a double-blind fashion. Treated patients received an 8-week course of high-dose, alternate-day prednisone or placebo, and the prednisone was then tapered over a 6- to 8-week period and withdrawn. Initially, treated patients had more complete remissions and partial remissions than the untreated controls, but this difference was not significant at greater than 4 months. An unexpected finding, after followup of 2 years, was that the treated group had more stable renal function with, only 2 of 34 treated patients having a doubling in serum creatinine, while the control group had 11 of 38 patients who had a doubling in serum creatinine. In general, the decline of renal function was 10% per year in the placebo group, compared to 2% in the prednisone-treated group.

Although reservations have been expressed about the validity of the study because of the poor course of the control group, most nephrologists would now recommend that all patients with idiopathic membranous nephropathy in whom there is no contraindication to glucocorticoid therapy be treated with an 8-week course of alternate-day prednisone at a dose of approximately 2 mg/kg. The steroids are then tapered over 4–6 weeks and discontinued. Whether patients with secondary forms of membranous nephropathy such as that due to malignancy, systemic lupus erythematosus, or other disorders should be treated is unknown at this time.

Several control trials of cytotoxic agents have failed to demonstrate any significant benefit. However, recently a well-controlled study of 81 adults with idiopathic membranous nephropathy was reported in which patients were randomly assigned to symptomatic treatment or to a 6-month course of methylprednisolone and prednisone alternating with chlorambucil every other month for a total of 6 months (112). The treated group had a significantly greater number of sustained remissions as well as preservation of renal function, whereas the control group had progression of their renal disease.

If patients relapse after having a response to steroid therapy, they can be retreated by the same protocol. In patients with membranous nephropathy who do not have the nephrotic syndrome, the prognosis is good in that renal failure is unusual and these patients probably do not need to be treated. The side effects of the 8-week course of alternate-day steroids is minimal, and thus it is recommended that all patients with membranous nephropathy and the nephrotic syndrome should be treated. Other forms of therapy for membranous nephropathy, such as long-term administration of high-dose daily prednisone cannot be recommended because of the high incidence of serious side effects. The use of chronic low-dose daily prednisone has been advocated by one study, but this treatment has not been confirmed (113). A recent report has indicated that cyclophosphamide is beneficial in reversing the decline in renal function in patients with membranous nephropathy (114).

REFERENCES

1. Schreiner GE: The nephrotic syndrome. In: MB Strauss, LG Welt, eds, *Diseases of the Kidney*, Vol 1. Little, Brown, Boston, p 503, 1971.
2. Earley LE, Forland M: Nephrotic syndrome. In: LE Earley, C Gottschalk, eds, *Diseases of the Kidney*. Little, Brown, Boston, p 765, 1979.
3. Brenner BM, Hostetter TH, Humes HD: Molecular basis of proteinuria of glomerular origin. *N Engl J Med* 298:826–833, 1978.
4. Rennke HG, Olson JL, Venkatachalam MA: Glomerular filtration of macromolecules: Normal mechanisms and the pathogenesis of proteinuria. In: GM Berlyne, S Giovanetti, D Thomas, eds, *Contributions to Nephrology*, Vol 24. Karger, Basel, p 30, 1981.
5. Kanwar YS: Biophysiology of glomerular filtration and proteinuria. *Lab Invest* 51:7–21, 1984.
6. Eisenbach GM, Van Liew JB, Boylan JW: Effect of

angiotensin on the filtration of protein in the rat kidney: A micropuncture study. *Kidney Int* 8:80–87, 1975.
7. Ginsberg JM, Chang BS, Matarese RA, Garella S: Use of single voided urine samples to estimate quantitative proteinuria. *N Engl J Med* 309:1543–1546, 1983.
8. Anderson RJ, Schrier RW: Renal sodium excretion, edematous disorders, and diuretic use. In: RW Schrier, ed, *Renal and Electrolyte Disorders*, 3rd ed. Little, Brown, Boston, p 79, 1986.
9. Dorhout MEJ, Roos JC, Boer P, Yoe OH, Simatuppang TA: Observations on edema formation in the nephrotic syndrome in adults with minimal lesions. *Am J Med* 67:378–384, 1979.
10. Meltzer JI, Keim HJ, Laragh JH, Sealey JE, Jan K, Chien S: Nephrotic syndrome: Vasoconstriction and hypervolemic types indicated by renin-sodium profiling. *Ann Intern Med* 91:688–696, 1979.
11. Ichikawa I, Rennke HG, Hoyer JR, Badr KF, Schor N, Troy JL, Lechene CP, Brenner BM: Role for intrarenal mechanisms in the impaired salt excretion of experimental nephrotic syndrome. *J Clin Invest* 71:91–103, 1983.
12. Joachim GR, Cameron JS, Schwartz M, Becker EL: Selectivity of protein excretion in patients with the nephrotic syndrome. *J Clin Invest* 43:2332–2341, 1964.
13. Haldemann B, Healy M, Gelliffe R, Goldstein DA, Pattabhiraman R, Massry SG: Effect of an oral dose of 25-hydroxyvitamin D3 on its blood levels in patients with nephrotic syndrome. *J Clin Endocrinol Metab* 50:470–474, 1980.
14. Sato KA, Gray RW, Lemann J Jr: Urinary excretion of 25-hydroxyvitamin D in health and the nephrotic syndrome. *J Lab Clin Med* 99:325–330, 1982.
15. Llach F: Hypercoagulability, renal vein thrombosis, and other thrombotic complications of nephrotic syndrome. *Kidney Int* 28:429–439, 1985.
16. Llach F, Papper S, Massry SG: The clinical spectrum of renal vein thrombosis: Acute and chronic. *Am J Med* 69:819–827, 1980.
17. Appel GB, Blum CB, Chien S, Kunis CL, Appel AS: The hyperlipidemia of the nephrotic syndrome. Relation to plasma albumin concentration, oncotic pressure and viscosity. *N Engl J Med* 312:1544–1548, 1985.
18. Rose BD: Clinical use of diuretics. In: BM Brenner, JH Stein, eds, *Body Fluid Homeostasis*. Churchill Livingstone, New York, p 409, 1987.
19. Krishna GG, Donovitch GM: Effects of water immersion on renal function in the nephrotic syndrome. *Kidney Int* 21:395–401, 1982.
20. Esparza AR, Kahn SI, Garella S, Abuelo JG: Spectrum of acute renal failure in nephrotic syndrome with minimal (or minor) glomerular lesions. Role of hemodynamic factors. *Lab Invest* 45:510–521, 1981.
21. Lowenstein J, Schacht RG, Baldwin DS: Renal failure in minimal change nephrotic syndrome. *Am J Med* 70:227–233, 1981.
22. Landwehr DM, Carvalho JS, Oken DE: Micropuncture studies of the filtration and absorption of albumin by nephrotic rats. *Kidney Int* 11:9–16, 1977.
23. Cortney MA, Sawin LL, Weiss DD: Renal tubular protein absorption in the rat. *J Clin Invest* 49:1–12, 1970.
24. Kaysen GA, Gamberetoglio J, Jimenz I, Jones H, Hutchinson F: Effect of dietary protein intake on albumin homeostasis in nephrotic patients. *Kidney Int* 29:572–577, 1986.
25. Lewis RT: Albumin: Role and discriminative use in surgery. *Can J Surg* 23:322–328, 1980.

26. Gavin LA, McMahon FA, Castle JN: Alterations in serum thyroid hormones and thyroxine-binding globulin in patients with nephrosis. *J Clin Endocrinol Metab* 46:125–137, 1978.
27. Afrasiabi MA, Vaziri ND, Gwinup G, Mays M, Barton CH, Ness RL, Valenta LJ, Thyroid function studies in the nephrotic syndrome. *Ann Intern Med* 90:335–341, 1979.
28. Goldstein DA, Haldimann B, Sherman D, Norman AW, Massry SG: Vitamin D metabolites and calcium metabolism in patients with nephrotic syndrome and normal renal function. *J Clin Endocrinol Metab* 52:116–121, 1981.
29. Marsh JB, Sparks CE: Hepatic secretion of lipoproteins in the rat and the effect of experimental nephrosis. *J Clin Invest* 64:1229–1237, 1979.
30. Gherardi E, Messori M, Rozzi R, Colandra S: Experimental nephrotic syndrome in the rat induced by puromycin aminonucleoside: Hepatic synthesis of lipoproteins and apolipoproteins. *Lipids* 15:858–863, 1980.
31. Gherardi E, Vecchia L, Colandra S: Experimental nephrotic syndrome in the rat induced by puromycin aminonucleoside. Plasma and urine lipoproteins. *Exp Mol Pathol* 32:128–142, 1980.
32. Bernard DB: Metabolic abnormalities in nephrotic syndrome: Pathophysiology and complication. In: BM Brenner, JH Stein, eds, *Contemporary Issues in Nephrology, Vol 9. Nephrotic Syndrome*. Churchill Livingstone, New York, p 85. 1982.
33. Kaysen GA, Gambertoglio J, Felts J, Hutchison F: Albumin synthesis, albuminuria and hyperlipemia in nephrotic patients. *Kidney Int* 31:1368–1376, 1987.
34. Oetliker OH, Mordasini R, Lutschg J, Riesen W: Lipoprotein Metabolism in nephrotic syndrome in childhood. *Pediat Res* 14:64–66, 1980.
35. Junest D, Wallner J, Karl HJ: Correlation of total cholesterol and protein in urine in patients with the nephrotic syndrome. *Klin Wochenschr* 58:1215–1216, 1980.
36. Mallick NP, Short CD: The nephrotic syndrome and ischaemic heart disease. *Nephron* 27:54–57, 1981.
37. Wass V, Cameron JS: Cardiovascular disease and the nephrotic syndrome: The other side of the coin. *Nephron* 27:58–61, 1981.
38. Wass VJ, Jarrett D, Chilvers C, Cameron JS: Does the nephrotic syndrome increase the risk of cardiovascular disease? *Lancet* 2:664–667, 1979.
39. Bridgman JF, Rossen SM, Thorp JM: Complications during clofibrate treatment of nephrotic syndrome hyperlipoproteinemia. *Lancet* 2:506–508, 1972.
40. Groggel GC, Cheung AK, Ellis-Benigni K, Wilson DE: Treatment of nephrotic hyperlipoproteinemia with gemfibrozil. *Kidney Int* 36:266–271, 1989.
41. Golper TA, Illingworth DR, Morris CD, Bennett WM: Lovastatin in the treatment of multifactorial hyperlipidemia associated with proteinuria. *Am J Kid Dis* 13:312–320, 1989.
42. Moorhead JF, Chan MK, El-Nahas M, Varghese Z: Lipid nephrotoxicity in chronic progressive glomerular and tubulo-interstitial disease. *Lancet* 2:1309–1311, 1982.
43. Kasiske BL, O'Donnell MP, Garvis WJ, Keane WF: Pharmacologic treatment of hyperlipidemia reduces glomerular injury in rat 5/6 nephrectomy model of chronic renal failure. *Circulation Res* 62:367–374, 1988.
44. Wagoner RD, Stanson AW, Holley KE, Winter CS: Renal vein thrombosis in idiopathic membranous glomerulopathy and nephrotic syndrome: Incidence and significance. *Kidney Int* 23:368–374, 1983.
45. Clark RA, Wyatt GM, Colley DP, Renal vein thrombosis:

An underdiagnosed complication of multiple renal abnormalities. *Radiology* 132:43–50, 1979.
46. Schrier RW, Gardenswartz MH: Renal vein thrombosis. *Postgrad Med* 67:83–93, 1980.
47. Vaziri ND: Nephrotic syndrome and coagulation and fibrinolytic abnormalities. *Am J Nephrol* 3:1–6, 1983.
48. Panicucci F, Sagripanti A, Vispi M, Pinori E, Lecchini L, Larsotti G, Giovannetti S: Comprehensive study of haemostasis in nephrotic syndrome. *Nephron* 33:9–13, 1983.
49. Rosenberg RD, Bauer KA: New insights into hypercoagulable states. *Hosp Prac* 21:131–147, 1986.
50. Vaziri ND, Paule P, Toohey J, Hung E, Shahriar A, Darwish R, Pahl M: Acquired deficiency and urinary excretion of antithrombin III in nephrotic syndrome. *Arch Intern Med* 144:1802–1803, 1984.
51. Kauffmann RH, Veltkamp JJ, Van Tilbrug NH, Leendert AVE: Acquired antithrombin III deficiency and thrombosis in the nephrotic syndrome. *Am J Med* 65:607–613, 1978.
52. Soff GA, Sica DA, Marlar RA, Evans HJ, Qureshi GD: Protein C in nephrotic syndrome: Use of a new enzyme-linked immunoadsorbent assay for protein C antigen. *Amer J Hematol* 22:43–49, 1986.
53. Remuzzi G, Marchesi D, Mecca G, de Gaetano G, Silver M: Platelet hypersensitivity in the nephrotic syndrome. *Proc Eur Dial Transplant Assoc* 16:481–494, 1979.
54. Rowe JM, Rasmussen RL, Mader SL, Dimarco PL, Cockett AT, Marder VJ: Successful thrombolytic therapy in two patients with renal vein thrombosis. *Am J Med* 77:1111–1114, 1984.
55. Burrow CR, Walker WG, Bell WR, Gatewood OB: Streptokinase salvage of renal function after renal vein thrombosis. *Ann Intern Med* 100:237–238, 1984.
56. Giangiacomo J, Cleary TG, Cole BR, Hoffslen P, Robson AM: Serum immunoglobulins in the nephrotic syndrome. A possible cause of minimal-change nephrotic syndrome. *N Engl J Med* 293:8–12, 1975.
57. McLean RH, Forsgren A, Bjorksten B, Kim Y, Quie PG, Michael AF: Decreased serum factor B concentration associated with decreased opsonization of *Escherichia coli* in the idiopathic nephrotic syndrome. *Pediat Res* 11:910–916, 1977.
58. Churg J, Habib R, White RHR: Pathology of the nephrotic syndrome in children. A report for the International Study of Kidney Diseases in Children. *Lancet* 1:1299–1302, 1970.
59. Jao W, Pollak VE, Norris H, Lewy P, Pirani CL: Lipoid nephrosis. An approach to the clinicopathologic analysis and dismemberment of idiopathic nephrotic syndrome with minimal glomerular changes. *Medicine* 52:445–468, 1973.
60. Mallick NP: The pathogenesis of minimal change nephropathy. *Clin Nephrol* 7:87–94, 1977.
61. Shalhoub RJ: Pathogenesis of lipoid nephrosis: A disorder of T-cell function. *Lancet* 2:556–558, 1974.
62. Carrie BJ, Salyer WR, Myers BD: Minimal change nephropathy: An electrochemical disorder of the glomerular membrane. *Am J Med* 70:262–268, 1981.
63. Levin M, Smith C, Walters MDS, Gascoine P, Barratt TM: Steroid-responsive nephrotic syndrome: A generalized disorder of membrane negative charge. *Lancet* 1:239–242, 1985.
64. Grupe WE: Relapsing nephrotic syndrome in childhood. *Kidney Int* 16:75–85, 1979.
65. International Study of Kidney Disease in Children: The primary nephrotic syndrome in children. Identification of patients with minimal change nephrotic syndrome from initial response to prednisone. A report of the International Study of Kidney Disease in Children. *J Pediatr* 98:561–564, 1981.
66. International Study of Kidney Disease in Children: Nephrotic syndrome in children: Prediction of histopathology from clinical and laboratory characteristics at time of diagnosis. *Kidney Int* 13:159–165, 1978.
67. International Study of Kidney Disease in Children: Nephrotic syndrome in children. A randomized trial comparing two prednisone regimens in steroid-responsive patients who ralapse early. Report of the International Study of Kidney Disease in Children. *J Pediatr* 95:239–243, 1979.
68. Makker SP, Heymann W: The idiopathic nephrotic syndrome of childhood: A clinical re-evalution of 145 cases. *Am J Dis Child* 127:830–845, 1974.
69. Siegel NJ. Goldberg B, Krassner LS, Hayslett JP: Long term followup of children with steroid responsive nephrotic syndrome. *J Pediatr* 81:251–258, 1972.
70. Williams SA, Makker SP, Inglefinger JR, Grupe WE: Long term evaluation of chlorambucil plus prednisone in the idiopathic nephrotic syndrome of childhood. *N Engl J Med* 302:929–933, 1980.
71. Effect of cytotoxic drugs in frequently relapsing nephrotic syndrome with and without steroid dependence. Arbeitsgemeinschaft für padiatrische nehrologie. *N Engl J Med* 306:451–454, 1982.
72. Lewis EJ: Cholrambucil for childhood nephrosis: A word of caution. *N Engl J Med* 302:963–964, 1980.
73. Collis L, Nieto V, Vila A, Rende J: Chlorambucil treatment in minimal lesion nephrotic syndrome: A reappraisal of its gonadal toxicity. *J Pediatr* 97:653–656, 1980.
74. Hsu AC, Folami AO, Bain J, Ranco CP: Gonadal function in males treated with cyclophosphamide for nephrotic syndrome. *Fertil Steril* 31:173–177, 1979.
75. Trompeter RS, Evans PR, Barratt TM: Gonadal function in boys with steroid-responsive nephrotic syndrome treated with cyclophosphamide for short periods. *Lancet* 1:1177–1179, 1981.
76. Cameron JS: Immunosuppressive agents in the treatment of the nephrotic syndrome and glomerulonephritis in children. *Pediatrician* 8:364–377, 1979.
77. Imbasciati E, Gusmano R, Edefonti A, Zucchelli P, Pozzi C, Grassi C, Della Volpe M, Perfumo F, Petrone P, Picca M, Appiani AC, Pasquali S, Ponticcilli C: Controlled trial of methylprednisolone pulses and low dose oral prednisone for the minimal change nephrotic syndrome. *Br Med J* 291:1305–1308, 1985.
78. Cohen AH, Border WA: Mesangial proliferative glomerulonephritis. *Semin Nephrol* 2: 228–240, 1982.
79. Cohen AH, Border WA, Glassock RJ: Nephrotic syndrome with glomerular mesangial IgM deposits. *Lab Invest* 38:610–619, 1978.
80. Murphy WM, Jukkola AF, Roy S: Nephrotic syndrome with mesangial cell proliferation in children — A distinct entity? *Am J Clin Pathol* 72:42–47, 1979.
81. International Study of Kidney Disease in Children: The primary nephrotic syndrome in children: Clinical significance of histopathologic variants of minimal change and of diffuse mesangial hypercellularity. A Report of the International Study of Kidney Disease in Children. *Kidney Int* 21:39, 1982.
82. Rashid H, Ezedum S, Morley AR, Kerr DN: Nephrotic syndrome with slight proliferative changes in the glomeruli: Response to prednisone. *Br Med J* 2:347–350, 1980.
83. Bhasin HK, Abuelo JG, Nayok R, Esparza AR: Mesangial proliferative glomerulonephritis. *Lab Invest* 39:21–29, 1978.

84. Sterzel RB, Ehrich JHH, Lucia H, Thompson D, Kashgarian M: Mesangial disposal of glomerular immune deposits in acute malarial glomerulonephritis of rats. *Lab Invest* 46:209–214, 1981.
85. Allen WR, Travis LB, Cavallo T, Branhaul BH, Cunningham RJ: Immune deposits and mesangial hypercellularity in minimal change nephrotic syndrome: Clinical relevance. *J Pediatr* 100:188–191, 1982.
86. Cameron JS: The problem of focal segmental glomerulosclerosis. In: P Kincaid–Smith, AJF d'Apice, RC Atkins, eds, *Progress in Glomerulonephritis*. John Wiley & Sons, New York, pp 209–230, 1979.
87. Rao TKS, Filipone EJ, Nicastri AD, Landsman SH, Frank E, Chen CK, Friedman EA: Associated focal and segmental glomerulosclerosis in the acquired immunodeficiency syndrome. *N Engl J Med* 310:669–673, 1984.
88. Goldszer RC, Sweet J, Cotran RS: Focal segmental glomerulosclerosis. *Ann Rev Med* 35:429–449, 1984.
89. Habib R: Focal glomerular sclerosis. *Kidney Int* 4:355–366, 1973.
90. Korbet SM, Schwartz MM, Lewis EJ: The prognosis of focal segmental glomerular sclerosis of adulthood. *Medicine* 65:304–311, 1986.
91. Meyrier A, Simon P, Perret G, Condamin–Meyrier M–C: Remission of idiopathic nephrotic syndrome after treatment with cyclosporine A. *Br Med J* 292:699–792, 1986.
92. Capodicasa G, DeSanto NG, Nuzzi F, Giordano C: Cyclosporin A in childhood — A 14 month experience. *Int J Ped Naphrol* 7:69–72, 1986.
93. Rao TKS, Friedman EA: Prospective trial of cyclosporine (CyA) in refractory nephrotic syndrome in adults: Preliminary findings. *Kidney Int* 31:214, 1987.
94. Habib R, Loriat C, Gubler M-C, Levy M: Morphology and serum complement levels in membranoproliferative glomerulonephritis. *Adv Nephrol* 4:109–138, 1974.
95. Spitzer RE, Vallota EH, Forrestal J: Serum C_3 lytic system in patients with glomerulonephritis. *Science* 164:436–438, 1969.
96. Amos N, Sissons JGP, Peters DK: Binding of nephritis factor by anti-IgG and protein A. *Pathol Biol* (Paris) 25:390–396, 1977.
97. Peters DK: Complement and membranoproliferative glomerulonephritis. In: P Kincaid–Smith, AJF d'Apice, RC Atkins, eds, *Progress in Glomerulonephritis*. John Wiley & Sons, Now York, pp 77–87, 1979.
98. Cameron JS, Turner DR, Heaton J, Williams DG, Ogg CS, Chantler C, Haycock GB, Hicks J: Idiopathic mesangiocapillary glomerulonephritis. Comparison of types I and II in children and adults and long-term prognosis. *Am J Med* 74:175–192, 1983.
99. McEnery PT, McAdams AJ, West CD: Membranoproliferative glomerulonephritis: Improved survival with alternate day prednisone therapy. *Clin Nephrol* 13:117–124, 1980.
100. McEnery PT, McAdams AJ, West CD: The effect of prednisone in a high-dose, alternate-day regimen on the natural history of idiopathic membranoproliferative glomerulonephritis. *Medicine* 64:401–424, 1986.
101. International Study of Kidney Disease in Children: Alternate day steroid therapy in membranoproliferative glomerulonephritis: A randomized controlled clinical trial. A report of the International Study of Kidney Disease in Children. *Kidney Int* 21:150, 1982.
102. Cattran DC, Cardella CJ, Roscoe JM, et al.: Results of controlled drug trial in membranoproliferative glomerulonephritis. *Kidney Int* 27:436–441, 1985.
103. Donadio JV, Anderson CF, Mitchell JC, Holley KE, Ilstrup DM, Fuster V, Chesebro JH: Membranoproliferative glomerulonephritis. A prospective clinical trial of platelet-inhibotor therapy. *N Engl J Med* 310:1421–1426, 1984.
104. Zimmerman SW, Moorthy AV, Dreher WH, Friedman A, Varanasi U: Prospective trial of warfarin and dipyridamole in patients with membranoproliferative glomerulonephritis. *Am J Med* 75:920–927, 1983.
105. Noel LH, Zabetti M, Droz D, Barbanel C: Long term prognosis in idiopathic membranous glomerulonephritis. *Am J Med* 66:82–90, 1979.
106. Couser WG, Salant DJ: In situ immune complex formation and glomerular injury. *Kidney Int* 17:1–13, 1980.
107. Couser WG, Steinmuller DR, Stilmant MM, Slant DJ, Lowenstein LM: Experimental glomerulonephritis in the isolated perfused rat kidney. *J Clin Invest* 62:1275–1287, 1978.
108. Border WA, Ward HJ, Kamil ES, Cohen AH: Induction of membranous nephropathy in rabbits by administration of an exogenous cationic antigen. *J Clin Invest* 69:451–461, 1982.
109. Hopper J, Trew PA, Biava CG: Membranous nephropathy: Its relative benignity in women. *Nephron* 29:18–24, 1981.
110. Cameron JS: Membranous nephropathy: The treatment dilemma. *Am J Kidney Dis* 1:371–375, 1982.
111. Collaborative study of the adult idiopathic nephrotic syndrome: A controlled study of short-term prednisone treatment in adults with membranous nephropathy. *N Engl J Med* 301:1301–1306, 1979.
112. Ponticelli C, Zucchelli P, Passerini P, et al.: A randomized trial of methylprednisolone and chlorambucil in idiopathic membranous nephropathy. *N Engl J Med* 320:8–13, 1989.
113. Bolton WK, Atuk NO, Sturgill BC, Westervelt FB: Therapy of the idiopathic nephrotic syndrome with alternate day steroids. *Am J Med* 62:60–70, 1977.
114. West ML, Jindal KK, Bear RA, Goldstein MB: A controlled trial of cyclophosphamide in patients with membranous glomerulonephritis. *Kidney Int* 32:579–584, 1987.

CHAPTER 21

Goodpasture's Syndrome

CURTIS B. WILSON

INTRODUCTION

Beginning with studies at the turn of the century using crude anti-kidney antisera, anti-glomerular basement membrane (GBM) antibody disease has become the clearest example of antibody-induced glomerular injury (1). In animal studies, it can be clearly shown that glomerular injury produced by anti-GBM antibodies is dose dependent and that temporal features of glomerular binding affect the extent of the inflammatory response and, in turn, the degree of injury induced. The experimental anti-GBM antibody model has been used widely to demonstrate the roles of inflammatory mediators. These mediators include humoral factors such as the complement proteins (both early- and late-acting components) and cellular elements including polymorphonuclear (PMN) leukocytes, monocytes/macrophages, and the enzymatic, oxidative, and other iflammatory elements contained therein (1–3).

The role of anti-GBM antibodies in human glomerulonephritis was clearly shown by Lerner, Glassock, and Dixon in 1967 (4) when these antibodies, which were recovered from the circulation or were eluted from the kidneys of affected individuals, were used successfully to transfer glomerular injury to nonhuman primates. These investigators provided additional evidence of the nephritogenic importance of the antibodies using the observation of inadvertent transfer of anti-GBM antibody-induced injury to a renal transplant, which was placed in an affected individual at a time that anti-GBM antibodies remained in the circulation.

GOODPASTURE'S SYNDROME

The clinical presentation of pulmonary hemorrhage and glomerulonephritis, often rapidly progressive, has come to be termed *Goodpasture's syndrome*. In its classic form, Goodpasture's syndrome is produced by anti-GBM antibodies reactive with antigen(s) present in GBM, alveolar basement membrane (ABM), and occasionally other basement membranes (1, 5). The antibody reaction conforms with the distribution of the reactive basement membrane antigen, which is continuous throughout the basement membrane, exhibiting a characteristic linear pattern of antibody fixation when tissue is studied by immunoflourescence (6). A number of clinical problems, including systemic lupus erythematosus, Wegener's granulomatosis, and other vasculitides, to name a few (Table 1), can present with clinical pictures at least initially indistinguishable from that produced with anti-GBM antibodies (7–9). The overlapping clinical presentations demonstrate the need for an etiologic and immunopathogenic definition in defining the disease process.

Understanding the immunopathogenesis is important since the therapy and outcome vary among different conditions, producing pulmonary hemorrhage and glomerular injury (Goodpasture's syndrome). Rapid diagnosis and the earliest possible institution of appropriate therapy may have considerable impact on the success of treatmet. Immunopathologic study of kidney or lung biopsies and serum assays are available to detect anti-GBM antibodies, There is interest in the recent findings of circulating antibodies that are reactive with cytoplasmic antigens in polymorphonuclear leukocytes (PMN), which are reported in high frequency in patients with Wegener's granulomatosis and, to a lesser extent, in other forms of vasculitis (10).

Table 1. Some conditions presenting with combined renal and pulmonary involvement

Anti-GBM/ABM antibody disease
Systemic lupus erythematosus
Other collagen vascular disorders including progressive systemic sclerosis
Polyarteritis nodosa
Wegener's granulomatosis
Other vasculitides
Mixed essential cryoglobulinemia
Lymphoid granulomatosis
Churg–Strauss syndrome
Hypersensitivity angiitis
Henoch–Schonlein purpura
D-penicillamine and other toxic reactions
Undefined etiology

The reactive antigens in the PMN are multiple, with anti-29 KD antigen, anti-alkaline phosphatase, and anti-myeloperoxidase antibodies reported from different laboratories (11, 12). A portion of patients with anti-GBM antibodies have been found to have anti-PMN reactivity as well (13), and it is suggested that the anti-PMN antibodies may relate to the histologic pattern of disease expression. The pathogenic importance of this newly detected antibody remains to be determined.

SPECTRUM OF ANTI-GBM AND OTHER ANTI-BASEMENT MEMBRANE ANTIBODY-INDUCED DISEASES

This chapter will focus on anti-GBM antibody-induced Goodpasture's syndrome and other clinical manifestations of anti-basement membrane antibody production. Anti-basement membrane antibodies are being observed in an increaseing number of renal and extrarenal diseases (Table 2). In addition to reactions with GBM and ABM, tubular basement membranes (TBM), choroid plexus basement membranes, and perhaps intestinal or skin basement membranes may be targets. Anti-GBM antibodies may also complicate renal transplantation through recurrence of the original immune reaction or de-novo induction of the antibody, in some instances due to basement membrane differences between the host and the transplanted organ (14). Anti-TBM antibody reactions often accompany anti-GBM antibodies. In addition, anti-TBM antibodies may occur as an isolated event, sometimes complicating immune complex forms of glomerular disease or occurring after renal transplantation. This selective TBM antigen system in humans is shared by certain rat strains and is different from the combined GBM/TBM antigen reaction observed in human anti-GBM antibody disease, a nephritogenic antigen system that is also found in rats and other experimental animals.

CLINICAL PRESENTATION AND FINDINGS

The demographics of the clinical presentation of anti-basement membrane antibody disease have changed from our 1973 series (1, 5, 15) with, at present, nearly equal distribution of combined kidney and lung involvement (Goodpasture's syndrome) and kidney involvement only. Very unusually (1–2% of patients), the lung may be the only site of clinical abnormality, even though antibody binding to the GBM can be identified when kidney biopsy material is studied. A bimodal age distribution is found with ages varying from under 5 to over 80. Young adults, particularly males aged 15–35, most commonly present with combined lung and kidney involvement. A second peak of disease occurs beginning at age 50–55, in which females with involvement confined predominately to the kidney are more common. In our experience, the Caucasian race accounts for over 90% of cases, even in military populations where patient selection should not be a factor. There is an unusually high frequency of HLA-DR2 and perhaps other genetic markers (HLA-B7) (16), suggesting that either a unique antibody predisposition or antigen expression may be involved in disease genesis.

Occasionally toxic exposures, including hydrocarbon solvents and fuels, and rarely such diverse events as influenza infections or underlying renal injury, have been temporally associated with disease onset. However, the events responsible for induction of the usually transient anti-GBM antibody response in humans remain poorly understood. Antibiotic administration has been related to anti-TBM antibody production. Of interest, mercuric chloride injection is capable of inducing a brief anti-GBM antibody response in rats, and the rat antibody is cross-reactive with immunopurified human GBM antigen in our human anti-GBM antibody radioimmunoassay. The rat anti-GBM antibodies appear to be part of a polyclonal antibody response induced by the chemical compound and, as part of such a response, may be similar to the occasional reports of anti-GBM antibody in patients with systemic lupus erythematosus. Antigens capable of experimentally inducing anti-GBM antibodies are present in normal human and animal urine; however, it is unknown if self-immunization can occur from this antigen source. Lymhoid stroma contains sufficient antigen to induce anti-GBM antibodies in conjunction with production of anti-lymphocyte sera, and anti-GBM antibody-related glomerular disease has been detected in patients treated for Hodgkin's disease.

Patients frequently (30–50%) report an antecedent flulike illness prior to the onset of pulmonary or glomerulonephritic symptomatology. About 5% have arthritic complaints, with a somewhat higher percentage having arthralgias. The actual onset of disease may be pulmonary, renal, or both. Hemoptysis usually triggers rapid medical attention. When the onset is nephritic, hematuria/protein-

Table 2. Anti-basement membrane antibody diseases

GBM and/or ABM antigens
  Goodpasture's syndrome (combined glomerulonephritis and pulmonary hemorrhage)
  Glomerulonephritis alone, often severe and rapidly progressive; occasionally the glomerulonephritis may be mild and remitting
  Clinical symptoms confined to the lung presenting as idiopathic pulmonary hemosiderosis
  Recurrent or de-novo glomerulonephritis after renal transplantation
TBM antigens
  Tubulointerstitial nephritis — complicating anit-GBM antibody disease, complicating presumed immune complex forms of glomerulonephritis, occasionally seen with drug-induced tubulointerstitial nephritis and rarely occurring as a primary disease
  Recurrent or de-novo tubulointerstitial nephritis after renal transplantation
??Other basement membrane antigens
  Choroid plexus, intestine, skin, etc.

uria that may go undetected until the clinical features related to impending renal failure prompt a physician visit. The renal and pulmonary symptoms may be separated by several months. The nephrotic syndrome is unusal, probably related to the rapidity with which renal failure frequently develops; however, the nephrotic syndrome can be a presentation in the disease, and its presence should not cause the physician to overlook the diagnosis of anti-GBM antibody disease. Hypertension is found in one third or so of affected individuals when first observed. Anemia is present in most patients and is frequently severe. Hypocomplementemia is present in less than one fifth of patients and is usually mild. Abnormalities in liver function studies, including elevated serum glutamic-oxaloacetic transaminase and bilirubin, are present in less than 25% of patients. An occasional patient has been observed with neurologic symptomatology, including dementia or convulsions, which could possibly be related to antibody binding to choroid plexus basement membrane with subsequent disturbance in production or composition of cerebrospinal fluid. The contribution of such postulated injury has been difficult to confirm in the setting of chronic renal failure with its attendant potential for neurologic problems.

The outcome of patients relates, in a general way, to the level of anti-GBM antibody present and is also influenced by the type of clinical presentation and the sex and age of the patient. Younger men presenting with Goodpasture's syndrome have the best expectancy in terms of retention of adequate renal function. Young female patients with Goodpasture's presentations or young males and females having involvement confined to the kidney more often progress to renal failure. The outcome with retention of adequate renal failure is also not as good in older age groups, particularly in those patients presenting with combined pulmonary and lung symptomatology.

From a morphologic viewpoint, the degree of renal involvement varies from focal, sometimes rather mild, proliferative changes to severe crescentic and necrotizing glomerulonephritis, with virtual obliteration of the majority of glomeruli. Crescents in some glomeruli have been found to contain multinucleated giant cells. Tubulointerstitial changes are also observed and are more frequent in patients with combined GBM/TBM reactivity in their antibodies compared to those patients with antibody reactivity restricted to the GBM alone (17). Electron microscopic studies of the affected renal tissue usually reveal a GBM that is free of electron-dense deposits, except in rare patients who may present with what appears to be a combined anti-GBM and immune complex picture. Clinical and pathologic evidence of vasculitis is uncommon. Histologic findings in the lung are usually confined to evidence of intraalveolar hemorrhage.

PULMONARY INVOLVEMENT

The pulmonary involvement in patients with anti-GBM antibody disease is frequently severe and life threatening. It can occur at any time during the course of anti-GBM antibody production and does not correlate well with the absolute level of anti-GBM antibody present. Severe pulmonary hemorrhage, usually associated with hemoptysis, is also suggested by worsening anemia, often bilateral hilar infiltrates on chest x-ray, blood gas abnormalities, and abnormal carbon monoxide studies. The episodes of hemorrhage can require emergent medical management, including intubation and ventilation support. The exact pathogenesis of the pulmonary involvement remains unclear and is difficult to study since lung tissue is not frequently or easily sampled. Transbronchial lung biopsies have been inconsistent in demonstrating the presence of anti-basement membrane antibody binding to the ABM (18–19). When present, the finding is of diagnostic usefulness; however, a negative study does not exclude the binding of antibody to other areas in the lung not sampled. Some recent experimental observations suggest that pulmonary fixation of antibody may not be a constant feature of the disease, as contrasted with fixation in the glomerulus through the fenestrated glomerular endothelium. Studies have demonstrated that experimental anti-GBM antibodies capable of binding to sections of lung will not bind when administered in vivo unless the lung has been previously injured, as during experimental oxygen toxicity studies (20, 21) or, recently in our laboratory, following minute amounts of unleaded gasoline placed into the trachea (22). In the latter studies, we found that the linear fixation of antibody to the ABM was confined to focal areas. It seems a likely possibility that lung binding of the anti-basement membrane antibody and associated, often short-lived, even though severe, episodes of pulmonary hemorrhage may be triggered by events that alter the normal relationship of the vascular compartment with the normally sequestered ABM antigens. This suggestion would correlate with the clinical observations of episodic pulmonary hemorrhage induced in patients with anti-GBM antibody following infectious episodes, physiologic disturbances, or perhaps made manifest by toxic exposures such as cigarette smoking or hydrocarbon fuel exposure (9, 23–27). Management of episodes of pulmonary hemorrhage should include identification and removal of possible stimuli.

DIAGNOSIS

The presence of anti-GBM antibody in tissue is sought using immunohistochemical techniques (Table 3). Most commonly, immunofluorescence studies are used to demonstrate linear deposits of immunoglobulin (predominantly IgG, only occasionally IgA or IgM) in a smooth, continuous pattern along GBM and ABM (1, 5, 6). The specificity of the immunoglobulin deposits is suggested by the absence of albumin or other control serum proteins. The glomerular immunoglobulin deposits are accompanied by complement in one half to two thirds of patients. As histologic damage of the kidney progresses, the architecture of the GBM becomes altered so that perfectly

Table 3. Diagnosis of anti-GBM antibody disease

Kidney or lung biopsy
  Immunofluorescence or immunohistochemical evidence of immunoglobulin deposits conforming to the distribution of the basement membrane
    Usually IgG, infrequently IgA, IgM
    C3 in one half to two thirds
    Fibrin deposits in areas of crescent formation
    Absence of albumin or other proteins not associated with immune reactions
  Elution of antibody from tissues to confirm specificity
    Acidic, basic, chaotropic buffers to remove antibody bound in washed tissue homogenate
    Recovery and concentration of antibody (mean about 35 µg of antibody per gram of tissue)
    Test reactivity of antibody by indirect immunofluoresence or more sensitive radioimmunoassay or ELISA
Detection of circulating anti-GBM antibody
  Indirect immunofluoresence using normal human kidney sections as a target (relatively insensitive, but quite specific)
  Radioimmunoassays or ELISA techniques (specificity and sensitivity of assay chosen must be known)
  Concentration of circulating antibody by perfusion through a human or nonhuman primate kidney (study tissue as described above)
Other measures
  Transfer of disease to nonhuman primate using serum or eluates
  T-cell sensitization assays (specificity unclear)

linear deposits cannot be found in all glomerular loops (Figure 1). The deposits that remain conform to the remaining remnants of basement membrane present. Usually, if sufficient glomeruli are present in the biopsy, some less-damaged glomeruli will retain a more characteristic linear appearance. The glomerular immunoglobulin and complement deposits are often accompanied by striking fibrin deposition in areas of crescent formation. The GBM deposits of immunoglobulin are accompanied by TBM deposits in about 70% of patients. The TBM deposits may be focal, involving the circumference of TBM of only a small portion of tubules or more diffuse, involving the TBM of almost all tubules in the cortex. Anti-basement membrane antibody binding can be sought in other organs as well, including the choroid plexus.

Immunofluorescence studies of linear immunoglobulin deposits need to be confirmed since nonspecific linear immunoglobulin deposits may occur. Such linear background staining is commonly observed in kidneys obtained at autopsy, kidneys that have been perfused in preparation for transplantation, and kidneys from patients with diabetes mellitus. Occasionally, kidney biopsies from other unrelated conditions can have quite bright nonspecific linear background staining. The nonspecific immunoglobulin deposits are usually accompanied by linear albumin deposits that help to define their nonspecific nature. Because of this background problem, it is risky to make the diagnosis of anti-GBM disease based on immunofluorescence findings alone. The presence of anti-GBM antibody suggested by immunohistochemical study should be confirmed by elution of antibody from renal tissue with specificity testing and/or detection of circulating anti-GBM antibody. Elution of needle biopsy tissue may provide sufficient antibody for study with sensitive radioimmunoassay confirmation.

For detection of circulating anti-GBM antibody, the indirect immunofluorescence technique is quite specific when positive; however, the technique is less sensitive than radioimmunoassay and ELISA techniques currently available (Table 3) (28–31). Indirect immunofluorescence also appears to be influenced by the particular tissue target in use, suggesting that some genetic variations in expression of reactive basement membrane antigens may occur. Human kidney sections used as a substrate for the indirect immunofluorescence method are more reliable than nonhuman species, which must rely on crossreactivity.

Over the past 15 or so years, radioimmunoassays and, more recently, ELISA techniques developed in research laboratories have been found useful in detecting anti-GBM antibody in patients. Unfortunately, the assays are not standardized among the laboratories performing them and, in addition, the assays may not be available in a timely manner without special effort by the patient's physician. Since hospital laboratories may send anti-GBM assays rather randomly to outside laboratories, the attending physician should be aware of where samples from his patients are being studied and what the specificity and sensitivity of the particular assay employed is. Correct and rapid diagnosis is important since successful therapy appears to hinge on initiation of therapeutic regimens before irreversible renal injury has occurred.

The fluid-phase anti-GBM antibody radioimmunoassay developed in our laboratory in the early 1970s utilizes an immunopurified human GBM antigen (1, 28, 29) and has been used to detect and follow several hundred patients with anti-GBM antibody disease. The assay has had an excellent correlation with immunofluorescence and elution studies performed in our laboratory. When serum is available early in the course of disease, antibody is detected in almost all patients. Antibody levels may fall rapidly in some patients, so that if the timing of sampling is delayed relative to the onset of disease, circulating antibody may be missed. After antibody is no longer detectable in the serum, it may still be detected bound in the kidney, where its half-life appears to be measured in months. The almost universal decline in antibody in serial followup studies suggests that antibody levels may have been higher prior to the first sample studied. In spite of this, there is a reasonable correlation with the severity of the disease and the level of antibody in the first sample submitted. The average duration of antibody production is about 12–15 months, which may be hastened by the aggressive therapies currently in use. A few patients persist in producing antibody, often at low levels, for up to 4–5 years after the original diagnosis. Limited serial studies suggest that bilateral nephrectomy may also hasten antibody disappearance.

The antigens present in our antigen mixture and reactive

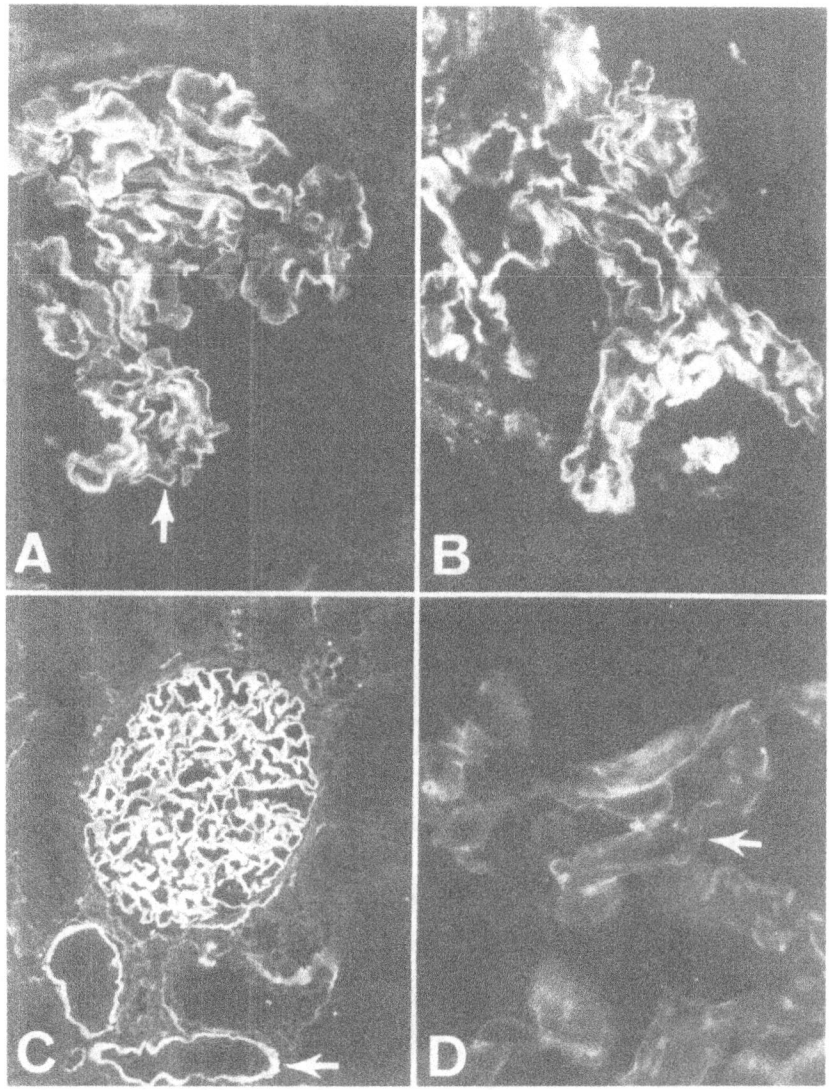

Figure 1. *A*: Nearly continuous linear IgG deposits (arrow) are seen along the GBM of a glomerulus from a patient with anti-GBM antibody-induced glomerulonephritis. The glomerulus is somewhat distorted by the presence of a crescent on the right. *B*: Another glomerulus from the patient depicted in A showing further disruption of glomerular architecture with areas of residual linear staining and other areas containing disrupted and fragmented immune deposits. *C*: Indirect immunofluorescence using a normal human kidney section and an anti-GBM antibody that contains reactivity with the TBM (arrow) of a minority population of tubules. *D*: Indirect immunofluorescence using normal human lung, showing binding of anti-basement membrane antibody (arrow) to the ABM.

with human anti-GBM antibodies are predominantly in the 27-28 kD and 54-56 kD size range using gel electrophoresis of immune precipitates formed with human anti-GBM antibody (32). Studies in several laboratories suggest that the NCl domain of Type IV collagen, an area resistant to collagenase digestion, is the site of the reactive antigen (33-35). This terminal area of the Type IV collagen has a monomer and dimer structure of the size range noted above. This area of the molecule serves for interaction with an adjacent molecule, which, when joined to four additional Type IV collagen molecules by the opposite end of the molecule, designated the 7S region, leads to a meshwork of collagen fibers within the GBM (36, 37). Current studies to determine the Type IV collagen alpha chain origin and subunit structure of the antigenic monomer suggest that a new, incompletely defined Type IV collagen alpha chain may be the possible antigen source (38). Work also proceeds at defining the peptide structure of the reactive antigen site, a finding that, when available, may lead to better detection and possibly immunospecific therapeutic approaches to disease management (39).

The complexity of pathogenic antigens in GBM, which includes, in addition to Type IV collagen, such other components as laminin and heparan sulfate-proteoglycan, remains to be defined. Passive models using antibodies reactive with these isolated components have not had involvement as severe as that produced by more crude extracts of GBM (40–43). Antibodies reactive with these components have been described in Chagas' disease and in poststreptococcal glomerulonephritis (44–46). Patients with IgA nephropathy have been reported to have antibodies reactive with collagenase-sensitive antigens thought to reside in the Type IV collagen alpha chains (47). The immunopathologic significance of these antibody reactions remain to be defined.

The subunit of the NCl felt to be the reactive site of the human anti-GBM antibody appears to be involved in the classic autoimmune anti-GBM antibody model of sheep originally described by Steblay (48, 49). The NCl of the murine Englebreth–Holm–Swarm tumor has also been reported to induce antibody binding to GBM and ABM in C57B1 mice (50). It remains unclear how many antigenic determinants may be involved in the human anti-GBM antibody disease. Two-dimensional gel electrophoresis suggests limited heterogeneity among reactive antigens (51). Subtle difference in antigen reactivity can be observed between patients with combined pulmonary and kidney involvement as compared to those with kidney involvement alone. Studies in our laboratory, for example, have shown that patients with lung involvement more frequently react with ABM by indirect immunofluorescence than do counterparts with similar anti-GMB antibody titers (measured by radioimmunoassay) who lack lung involvement (1).

Questions regarding the tertiary configuration of the epitope and its accessibility to circulating antibody, already suggested to be important in pulmonary injury (see above), may also contribute to accessibility of antigen within the kidney. For example, TBM antigens are not normally accessible to antibody in vivo or in vitro in certain rat strains. The reactivity can be recovered after enzymatic treatment of the basement membrane (52). In hereditary nephritis (Alport's syndrome), certain kindreds lack detectable GBM antigens by indirect immunofluorescence staining (14, 53–55). Recent studies using either enzyme treatment of fetal kidney to expose GBM antigens or acid-urea altered skin to study GBM antigen presence in hereditary nephritis suggest that GBM antigen accessibility in humans may vary as well (56–58). Quantitative variation in the accessibility and content of nephritogenic GBM antigens among basement membranes of different individuals remains to be defined.

Table 4. Management of anti-GBM antibody disease

Rapid and early diagnosis
  Suspicion based on history, clinical features, course, environmental exposures, kidney or lung pathologic studies, etc.
  Kidney and lung biopsy — immunofluoresence/elution detection of anti-GBM antibodies
  Detection of circulating anti-GBM antibodies
Assessment of prognositic variables
  Age, sex, clinical course, degree of renal failure, presence of hemoptysis, level of anti-GBM antibody, renal morphology, and degree of potential reversibility
Treatment to stabilize or recover renal function and/or manage pulmonary hemorrhage
  Theoretical objective is to rapidly lower levels of circulating anti-GBM antibodies and to blunt their effects
    Regimens of immunosuppression coupled with plasma exchange can increase rate of anti-GBM antibody disappearance and show promise in uncontrolled studies
  Benefits must be weighed versus risks
  Monitor anti-GBM antibody levels
  Minimize exposure to immunosuppressive agents
Control of episodic pulmonary hemorrhage
  High-dose parenteral ("pulse therapy") or oral corticosteroids often control episodes of hemorrhage
  Ventilatory support may be required
  Eliminate recognized predisposing factors
  Immunosuppresive regimens with plasma exchange may be beneficial
  Effect, if any, of bilateral nephrectomy unclear

MANAGEMENT

Rapid and accurate diagnosis is essential in the approach to patients with clinical presentations of anti-GBM antibody-induced Goodpasture's syndrome or rapidly progressive glomerulonephritis, as well as less common presentations of otherwise unexplained asymptomatic proteinuria/hematuria, nephrotic syndrome, or idiopathic pulmonary hemosiderosis (Table 4). Diagnosis is based on a combination of immunofluorescence and/or elution study of renal (or lung) biopsy material and confirmation of the presence of anti-GBM antibodies with serum assays. In addition to helping establish an etiologic diagnosis, kidney biopsy studies give some indication of the acuteness and severity of the inflammatory histologic change in the glomeruli, which very often includes crescentic changes that may be quite extensive. The character of the crescentive infiltrate and the degree of irreversible scarring that has already occurred are elements to be considered in forming a treatment plan. This information, combined with an assessment of the clinical course, can be used to establish some idea of the expected outcome, which must be weighed against the risks of the aggressive immunosuppressive and plasma exchange regimens currently felt to be of benefit in the management of patients with anti-GBM antibody-associated Goodpasture's syndrome or glomerulonephritis alone. It should go without saying that the expectations for an individual who develops clinical symptomatology slowly and who maintains renal function near a normal level with relatively mild histologic involvement on kidney biopsy will have a better prognosis than an individual with rapid onset of renal failure over a few days with extensive loss of glomeruli and severe crescentic involvemet of those glomeruli that remain when biopsied. A portion of the former type of patient may not progress, even without treatment, whereas many of the latter type of patient lack sufficient residual kidney substance to regain function, even with the most extensive treatment program. The diversity of clinical severity and the related propensity for progression make critical evaluation of therapeutic approaches difficult. Very large number of patients would need to be available to set up sufficiently well-matched subgroups to study the best immunosuppressive and/or plasma exchange protocols in a critical fashion. Based on historic controls, the current aggressive therapies appear to have significant benefit, making it hard to justify trials that include an untreated control group.

The clinican must then use as much historic, clinical, and laboratory data as he can gather to plan the therapeutic approach for each patient. Age, sex, and clinical presentation are factors. The level of circulating anti-GBM antibody, the clinical activity of the process judged on history, changing serum creatinine values, urinary sediment findings, and the type and intensity of morphologic change (in particular, the percentage and type of crescents) within the kidney are also important elements for an informed decision regarding treatment for the renal involvement. Since the disease can progress very rapidly and the outcome correlates with the degree of damage present at onset of therapy, delays in starting therapy need to be minimized. When pulmonary hemorrhage is also a feature of the clinical picture, its frequency and intensity, as monitored by degree of anemia, chest x-ray findings, and amounts of hemoptysis, require additional consideration. Since, as noted above, infection (particularly pulmonary infections) may actually precipitate episodes of pulmonary hemorrhage, particular care must be taken in immunosuppressive programs to guard against falling into a cycle of increasing immunodepression and infection complicating ventilatory support therapies.

The Hammersmith group originated the combined immunosuppression and plasma exchange management program for patients with anti-GBM antibody disease and have recently reviewed their results (15, 59). This study was comprised of a mail survey group (mortality 25%) and a group treated at the Hammersmith (mortality 16%). Of 30 patients receiving the full treatment (Table 5), all but one was free of antibody within 8 weeks. In the combined groups, 21 of 27 patients with normal or moderate renal failure (serum creatinine < 6.0 mg/dl) improved renal function or retained adequate renal function to avoid dialysis. In contrast, only 1 of 12 patients with serum creatinine > 6.0 mg/dl had an improvement in renal function.

Table 5. Immunosuppresive and plasma exchange protocols

Savage et al., 1986 (15)
  Prednisolone 60/mg/day, which is gradually reduced
  Cyclophosphamide 3 mg/kg/day for 8 weeks or less if antibody gone (white blood cell count > 3500/mm^3 and no infection)
  Patients < 55 years also receive azathioprine 1 mg/kg/day
  At least 14 daily 4-L plasma exchanges with plasma protein replacement
Johnson et al., 1985 (19)
  Prednisone 2 mg/kg/day for 1 week, reduced to 1 mg/kg/day for 3 weeks, then taper to alternate-day dosage for 3 months
  Cyclophosphamide 2 mg/kg/day for 3 months then 1 mg/kg/day less if glomerular filtration rate < 10 ml/min (white blood cell count maintained > 4000/mm^3, platelet count > 100,000/mm^3)
  Methylprednisolone 1 g daily for 1–3 days for either severe pulmonary hemorrhage or fulminant renal failure (increase in serum creatinine > 1.0 mg/dl/day)
  Four-liter plasma exchanges every 3 days with frozen plasma replacement until circulating anti-GBM antibody < 5% binding by radioimmunoassay or no recovery of renal function after 30 days on dialysis
Walker et al., 1985 (60)
  Prednisolone 0.5–1.5 mg/kg/day
  Cyclophosphamide 1–2 mg/kg/day
  Antiplatelet therapy (sulphinpyrazone 400–800 mg/day, dipyridamole 100–400 mg/day)
  Four-liter plasma exchange daily for 3–5 days, then on alternate days, decreasing related to outcome.

Johnson et al. (19) randomized the addition of plasma exchange therapy in a group of patients with anti-GBM antibody disease who were receiving a standard immunosuppressive regimen (Table 5). The plasma exchange was less frequent than in the Hammersmith study. Addition of plasma exchange hastened the disappearance of circulating anti-GBM antibody. The outcome of the groups was related more to the severity of renal involvement (serum creatinine and percentage of crescents) at the onset of management than the added use of plasma exchange. Of interest, a patient with 50% crescents in the non-plasma exchange group progressed to dialysis, in contrast to a patient in the plasma exchange group with 70% crescents who did not require dialysis.

Walker et al. (60) have also reported a series treated with a more varied immunosuppressive and plasma exchange protocol with the addition of antiplatelet agents (Table 5). Of their patients, 73% had improvement in renal function (at least 30% reduction in serum creatinine) and 41% had long-term recoveries of renal function. Five patients with anuria showed no improvement in renal function; however, of six patients with severe oliguria or dialysis, 30% had long-term recovery of renal function (serum creatinine < 3.0 mg/dl for 24–44 months). The latter observation makes it more difficult to decide when to withold therapy based entirely on clinical severity when first seen and points out the need for full consideration of the multiple prognostic factors listed above.

The long-term outlook of patients and the duration of therapy remains unclear. Exacerbation of anti-GBM antibody responses is uncommon and therapy is generally tapered as soon as the clinical picture warrants. Renal failure may develop after initial favorable results and the disappearance of circulating anti-GBM antibody, suggesting that consideration be given to including such items as protein restriction and blood pressure control to preserve residual function, which may be compromised by progressive sclerosis.

TRANSPLANTATION

As can be seen from the foregoing, many patients with anti-GBM antibody disease lose renal function and come under consideration for renal transplantation. Recurrent disease, based either on transplantation while nephritogenic levels of anti-GBM antibody remain in the circulation or by reexacerbation of the anti-GBM antibody response, is a concern for transplantation management.

The commonly accepted practice is to delay transplantation until circulating antibody has disappeared (1). The decline in antibody can be hastened by the therapeutic approaches outlined in the previous section. Limited evidence also suggests that bilateral nephrectomy may have a similar effect, although this is seldom done today. It appears that once antibody production has diminished to undetectable levels, reappearance of sufficient antibody to cause clinical probelms is uncommon in the well-immunosuppressed transplant recipient. The contribution of immunosuppression is suggested by the example of an identical twin transplantation studied in our laboratory (61). The nonimmunosuppressed recipient of the isograft rapidly redeveloped circulating anti-GMB antibody, which had been absent 2 years before transplantation. Clinical evidence of a recurrence was noted and was blunted by institution of immunosuppression. The clinician must then weigh the risks and problems inherent in long-term dialysis versus the risk of recurrent disease. The occasional transplant prior to complete disappearance of antibody (62) suggests that perhaps a "safe" level of antibody could be determined; however, most patients can wait until antibody production is no longer detectable.

The final problem in transplantation comes when GBM antigens present in the transplant can lead to immunization of the recipient who may lack these antigens, such as in the case of some kindreds of hereditary nephritis (Alport's syndrome) (14). Such immunization can lead to sufficient anti-GBM antibody to result in severe glomerulonephritis in the transplant with loss of function. Care should be taken to classify patients with suspected hereditary nephritis in terms of their GBM antigenic makeup. This can be done best by special study of renal biopsy material. A recent report suggests that denatured skin biopsies can also be used for this purpose (58), which, if successful, will allow more complete family screening. The finding of a similar antigenic defect in hereditary nephrititis in Samoyed dogs (63) should serve as model that may be of help in studying the potential for induction of anti-GBM antibodies by introduction of new GBM antigens via transplantation. This dog model may also provide a means of determining if immunospecific immune modulation could be used for management of this subgroup of individuals with hereditary nephritis who require renal transplantation.

ACKNOWLEDGMENTS

This is publication No. 5267-IMM from the Department of Immunology, Research Institute of Scripps Clinic, La Jolla, California, USA. This work was supported in part by United States Public Health Service Grants DK-20043, DK32353, and AG-04342; and Biomedical Research Support Grant RRO-5514.

REFERENCES

1. Wilson CB, Dixon FJ: The renal response to immunological injury. In: BM Brenner, FC Rector Jr, eds, *The Kidney*, 3rd ed. WB Saunders, Philadelphia, pp 800–889, 1986.
2. Cybulsky AV, Quigg RJ, Salant DJ: Role of the complement membrane attack complex in glomerular injury. In: BM Brenner, JH Stein, eds, CB Wilson, guest ed, *Contemporary Issues in Nephrology*. Churchill-Livingstone, New York, 1988, pp 57–86.
3. Johnson RJ, Klebanoff SJ, Couser WG: Oxidants in glomerular injury. In: BM Brenner, JH Stein, eds, CB Wilson, guest ed, *Contemporary Issues in Nephrology*. Churchill–Livingstone, New York, 1988, pp 87–110.
4. Lerner RA, Glassock RJ, Dixon FJ: The role of antiglomerular basement membrane antibody in the pathogenesis of human glomerulonephritis. *J Exp Med* 126:989–1004, 1967.
5. Wilson CB, Dixon FJ: Anti-glomerular basement membrane antibody-induced glomerulonephritis. *Kidney Int* 3:74–89, 1973.
6. Wilson CB, Dixon FJ: Diagnosis of immunopathologic renal disease. (editorial) *Kidney Int* 5:389–401, 1974.
7. Leatherman JW, Sibley RK, Davies SF: Diffuse intrapulmonary hemorrhage and glomerulonephritis unrelated to antiglomerular basement membrane antibody. *Am J Med* 72:401–410, 1982.
8. Boyce NW, Holdsworth SR: Pulmonary manifestations of the clinical syndrome of acute glomerulonephritis and lung hemorrhage. *Am J Kidney Dis* 8:31–36, 1986.
9. Wilson CB: Immunologic diseases of the lung and kidney (Goodpasture's syndrome). In: AP Fishman, ed, *Pulmonary Diseases and Disorders*, 2nd ed. McGraw-Hill New York, 1988.
10. van der Woude FJ, Rasmussen N, Lobatto S, Wiik A, Permin H, van Es LA, van der Giessen M, van der Hem GK, The TH: Autoantibodies against neutrophils and monocytes: Tool for diagnosis and marker of disease activity in Wegener's granulomatosis. *Lancet* 1:425–429, 1985.
11. Lockwood CM, Bakes D, Jones S, Whitaker KB, Moss DW, Savage CO: Association of alkaline phosphatase with an autoantigen recognized by circulating anti-neutrophil antibodies in systemic vasculitis. *Lancet* 1:716–720, 1987.
12. Falk RJ, Terrell R, Jennette JC: Anti-granulocyte cytoplas-

mic autoantibody (AGCA) specific for myeloperoxidase (MPO) in vasculitis related and idiopathic necrotizing and crescentic glomerulonephritis (abstract) *Kidney Int* 33:313, 1988.
13. Lockwood CM, Jayne DR, Marshall P, Jones S, Savage COS: A prospective study of the incidence of anti-GBM and anti-neutrophil cytoplasm antibodies in patients with rapidly progressive nephritis (abstract). *Kidney Int* 33:329, 1988.
14. McCoy RC, Johnson HK, Stone WJ, Wilson CB: Absence of nephritogenic GBM antigen(s) in some patients with hereditary nephritis. *Kidney Int* 21:642–652, 1982.
15. Savage COS, Pusey CD, Bowman C, Rees AJ, Lockwood CM: Antiglomerular basement membrane antibody mediated disease in the British Isles 1980–4. *Br Med J* 292:301–304, 1986.
16. Rees AJ, Peters K, Amos N, Welsh KI, Batchelor JR: The influence of HLA-linked genes on the severity of anti-GBM antibody-mediated nephritis. *Kidney Int* 26:444–450, 1984.
17. Andres G, Brentjens J, Kohli R, Anthone R, Anthone S, Baliah T, Montes M, Mookerjee BK, Prezyna A, Sepulveda M, Venuto R, Elwood C: Histology of human tubulointerstitial nephritis associated with antibodies to renal basement membranes. *Kidney Int* 13:480–491, 1978.
18. Beechler CR, Enquist RW, Hunt KK, Ward GW, Knieser MR: Immunofluorescence of transbronchial biopsies in Goodpasture's syndrome. *Am Rev Respir Dis* 121:869–872, 1980.
19. Johnson JP, Moore J, Jr, Austin HA, III, Balow JE, Antonovych TT, Wilson CB: Therapy of anti-glomerular basement membrane antibody disease: Analysis of prognostic significance of clinical, pathologic and treatment factors. *Medicine* 64:219–277.21, 1985.
20. Jennings L, Roholt OA, Pressman D, Blau M, Andres GA, Brentjens JR: Experimental anti-alveolar basement membrane antibody-mediated pneumonitis. I. The role of increased permeability of the alveolar capillary wall induced by oxygen. *J Immunol* 127:129–134, 1981.
21. Downie GH, Roholt, OA, Jennings L, Blau M, Brentjens JR, Andres GA: Experimental anti-alveolar membrane antibody-mediated pneumonitis. II. Role of endothelial damage and repair, induction of autologous phase, and kinetics of antibody deposition in Lewis rats. *J Immunol* 129:2647–2652, 1982.
22. Yamamoto T, Wilson CB: Binding of anti-basement membrane antibody to alveolar basement membrane after intratracheal gasoline instillation in rabbits. *Am J Pathol* 126:497–505, 1987.
23. Beirne GJ, Wagnild JP, Zimmerman SW, Macken PD, Burkholder PM: Idiopathic crescentic glomerulonephritis. *Medicine* 56:349–381, 1977.
24. Rees AJ, Lockwood CM, Peters DK: Enhanced allergic tissue injury in Goodpasture's syndrome by intercurrent bacterial infection. *Br Med J* 2:723–726, 1977.
25. Donaghy M, Rees AJ: Cigarette smoking and lung haemorrhage in glomerulonephritis caused by autoantibodies to glomerular basement membrane. *Lancet* 2:1390–1393, 1983.
26. Leaker B, Walker RG, Becker GJ, Kincaid-Smith P: Cigarette smoking and lung hemorrhage in anti-glomerular-basement-membrane nephritis. *Lancet* 2:1039, 1984.
27. Wilson CB: Drug- and toxin-induced nephritides: Antikidney antibody and immune complex mediation. In: G Porter, ed, *Nephrotoxic Mechanisms of Drugs and Environmental Toxins*. Plenum, New York, pp 383–392, 1982.
28. Wilson CB, Marquardt H, Dixon FJ: Radioimmunoassay (RIA) for circulating antiglomerular basement membrane (GBM) antibodies. *Kidney Int* 6:114a, 1974.
29. Wilson CB: Radioimmunoassay for anti-glomerular basement membrane antibodies. In: NR Rose, H Friedman, eds, *Manual of Clinical Immunology*, 2nd ed. American Society for Microbiology, Washington DC, pp 886–894, 1980.
30. Fish AJ, Kleppel M, Jeraj K, Michael AF: Enzyme immunoassay of anti-glomerular basement membrane antibodies. *J Lab Clin Med* 105:700–705, 1985.
31. Bowman C, Lockwood CM: Clinical application of a radioimmunoassay for auto-antibodies to glomerular basement membrane. *J Clin Lab Immunol* 17:197–202, 1985.
32. Wilson CB, Holdsworth SR: Anti-glomerular basement membrane (GBM) antibody-induced disease. In: W Zurukzoglu, M Papadimitriou, M Pyrpasopoulos, M Sion, C Zamboulis, eds, *Proceedings of the 8th International Congress of Nephrology*. S Karger, Basel, pp 910–916, 1981.
33. Wieslander J, Barr JF, Butkowski RJ, Edwards SJ, Bygren P, Heinegard D, Hudson BG: Goodpasture antigen of the glomerular basement membrane: Localization of noncoloagenous regions of type IV collagen. *Proc Natl Acad Sci USA* 81:3838–3842, 1984.
34. Kefalides NA, Ohno N, Wilson CB: Antigenic components of bovine lens capsule that cross-react serum from Goodpasture's syndrome. *Fed Proc* 43:779, 1984.
35. Wieslander J, Heinegard D: The involvement of Type IV collagen in Goodpasture's syndrome. *Ann NY Acad Sci* 460:363–374, 1985.
36. Butkowski RJ, Wieslander J, Wisdom BJ, Barr JR, Noelken ME, Hudson BG: Properties of the globular domain of Type IV collagen and its relationship to the Goodpastures antigen. *J Biol Chem* 260:3739–3747, 1985.
37. Timpl R: Recent advances in the biochemistry of glomerular basement membrane. *Kidney Int* 30:293–298, 1986.
38. Butkowski RJ, Langeveld JPM, Wieslander J, Hamilton J, Hudson BG: Localization of the Goodpasture epitope to a novel chain of basement membrane collagen (abstract). *Proceedings of the Xth International Congress of Nephrology*, London, 1987.
39. Kefalides NA, Abrams WR, Ohno N, Wilson CB, Rosenbloom J: Indentification of antigenic determinants in the NC-1 domain of Type IV collagen reactive with Goodpasture sera (abstract) *FASEB J* 2:A629, 1988.
40. Yaar M, Foidart JM, Brown KS, Rennard SI, Martin GR, Liotta L: The Goodpasture-like syndrome in mice induced by intravenous injections of an-Type IV collagen and anti-laminin antibody. *Am J Pathol* 107:79–91, 1982.
41. Makino H, Gibbons JT, Reddy MK, Kanwar YS: Nephritogenicity of antibodies to proteoglycans of the glomerular basement membrane-I. *J Clin Invest* 77:142–156, 1986.
42. Miettinen A, Stow JL, Mentone S, Farquhar MG: Antibodies to basement membrane heparan sulfate proteoglycans bind to the laminae rarae of the glomerular basement membrane (GBM) and induce subepithelial GBM thickening. *J Exp Med* 163:1064–1084, 1986.
43. Feintzeig ID, Abrahamson DR, Cybulsky AV, Dittmer JE, Salant DJ: Nephritogenic potential of sheep antibodies against glomerular basement membrane laminin in the rat. *Lab Invest* 54:531–541, 1986.
44. Szarfman A, Terranova VP, Rennard SI, Foidart JM, De Fatima M, Scheinman JI, Martin GR: Antibodies to laminin in Chagas' disease. *J Exp Med* 155:1161–1171, 1982.
45. Fillit H, Damle SP, Gregory JD, Volin C, Poon-King T, Zabriskie J: Sera from patients with poststreptococcal glomerulonephritis contain antibodies to glomerular heparan sulfate proteoglycan. *J Exp Med* 161:277–289, 1985.
46. Kefalides NA, Pegg MT, Ohno N, Poon-King T, Zabriskie J, Fillit H: Antibodies to basement membrane collagen and to

laminin are present in sera from patients with poststreptococcal glomerulonephritis. *J Exp Med* 163:588–602, 1986.
47. Cederholm B, Wieslander J, Bygren P, Heinegard D: Patients with IgA nephropathy have circulating anti-basement membrane antibodies reacting with structures common to collagen I, II, and IV. *Proc Natl Acad Sci USA* 83:6151–6155, 1986.
48. Steblay RW: Glomerulonephritis induced in sheep by injection of heterologous glomerular basement membrane in Freund's complete adjuvant. *J Exp Med* 116:253–271, 1962.
49. Bygren P, Wieslander J, Heinegard D: Glomerulonephritis induced in sheep by immunization with human glomerular basement membrane. *Kidney Int* 31:25–31, 1987.
50. Wick G, Von der Mark J, Doetrocj H, Timpl R: Globular domain of basement membrane collagen induces autoimmune pulmonary lesions in mice resembling human Goodpasture disease. *Lab Invest* 55:308–317, 1986.
51. Yoshioka K, Kleppel M, Fish AJ: Analysis of nephritogenic antigens in human glomerular basement membrane by two-dimensional gel electrophoresis. *J Immunol* 134:3831–3837, 1985.
52. Zanetti M, Wilson CB: Characterization of anti-tubular basement membrane antibodies in rats. *J Immunol* 130:2173–2179, 1983.
53. Jeraj K, Kim Y, Vernier RL, Fish AJ, Michael AF: Absence of Goodpasture's antigen in male patients with familial nephritis. *Am J Kidney Dis* 6:626–629, 1983.
54. Savage COS, Pusey CD, Kershaw MJ, Cashman SJ, Harrison P, Hartley B, Turner DR, Cameron JS, Evans DJ, Lockwood CM: The Goodpasture antigen in Alport's syndrome: Studies with a monoclonal antibody. *Kidney Int* 30:107–112, 1986.
55. Savage COS, Reed A, Kershaw M, Pincott J, Pusey CD, Dillon MJ, Barratt TM, Lockwood CM: Use of a monoclonal antibody in differential diagnosis of children with haematuria and hereditary nephritis. *Lancet* 1:1459–1461, 1986.
56. Jeraj K, Fish AJ, Yoshioka K, Michael AF: Development and heterogeneity of antigens in the immature nephron: Reactivity with human anti-glomerular basement membrane autoantibodies. *Am J Pathol* 117:180–183, 1984.
57. Yoshioka K, Michael AF, Velosa J, Fish AJ: Detection of hidden nephritogenic antigen determinants in human renal and nonrenal basement membranes. *Am J Pathol* 121:156–165, 1985.
58. Kashtan C, Fish AJ, Kleppel M, Yoshioka K, Michael AF: Nephritogenic antigen determinants in epidermal and renal basement membranes of kindreds with Alport-type familial nephritis. *J Clin Invest* 78:1035–1044, 1986.
59. Lockwood CM, Boulton-Jones JM, Lowenthal RM, Simpson IJ, Peters DK, Wilson CB: Recovery from Goodpasture's syndrome after immunosuppressive treatment and plasmapheresis. *Br Med J* 2:252–254, 1975.
60. Walker RG, Scheinkestel C, Becker GJ, Owen JE, Dowling JP, Kincaid-Smith P: Clinical and morphologic aspects of the management of crescentic anti-glomerular basement membrane antibody (anti-GBM) nephritis/Goodpasture's syndrome. *Q J Med* 54:75–89, 1985.
61. Almkuist RD, Buckalew VM, Hirszel P, Maher JF, James PM, Wilson CB: Recurrence of anti-glomerular basement membrane antibody mediated glomerulonephritis in an isograft. *Clin Immunol Immunopathol* 18:54–60, 1981.
62. Cove-Smith JR, McLeod AA, Blamey RW, Knapp MS, Reeves WG, Wilson CB: Transplantation, immunosuppression and plasmapheresis in Goodpasture's syndrome. *Clin Nephrol* 9:126–128, 1978.
63. Jansen B, Thorner PS, Singh A, Patterson JM, Lumsden JH, Valli VE, Baumal R, Basrur PK: Hereditary nephritis in Samoyed dogs. *Am J Pathol* 116:175–178, 1984.

CHAPTER 22

Hematuria and IgA Nephropathy

JOJI OHNO

INTRODUCTION

Distorted erythrocytes in the urine or dysmorphic erythrocyturia and erythrocyte casts with no clot formation are characteristic features of renal parenchymal hematuria, often seen in glomerulonephritis and infrequently in interstitial nephritis. In addition to these features, the presence of proteinuria that exceeds the amounts estimated from local bleeding, such as in pelvic or ureteral stone, bladder tumor, is also an evidence of glomerular hematuria. Glomerular hematuria is almost universally observed in both primary and secondary glomerulonephritides.

The mechanism of the glomerular hematuria includes thinning and tiny breaks of the glomerular capillary basement membrane caused by inflammatory and, rarely, hereditary changes. The most common cause of glomerular hematuria in clinical medicine is of course acute and chronic glomerulonephritis. Among the glomerulonephritides, IgA nephropathy occupies an important position in the differential diagnosis of glomerular hematuria because it often presents with hematuria characterized with episodic gross hematuria and because it is perhaps the most common glomerulonephritis in certain countries, including Japan.

Since its original description by Berger and Hinglais in 1968 (1), IgA nephropathy has been recognized as a distinct and the most common form of primary glomerular disease in the world. The term *IgA nephropathy* is synonymous with *isolated glomerulonephritis with mesangial IgA deposits, idiopathic IgA mesangial nephropathy,* IgA glomerulonephritis, and *Berger's disease.* The characteristic histologic feature of IgA nephrophthy is diffuse mesangial deposition of immunoglobulins, especially IgA as a predominent species, with less intense deposition of IgG and of a complement component C_3. Other glomerulonephritides with the mesangial IgA deposition, such as Henoch-Schoenlein purpura syndrome, systemic lupus erythematosus, and alcoholic liver cirrhosis, should be differentiated by the absence of associated signs and symptoms of systemic diseases. The prognosis of this disease was thought to be good in initial short-term studies, but subsequent reports based on long-term observations showed a variable outcome, including a relatively high incidence (10–20%) of progression to end-stage renal failure.

EPIDEMIOLOGY

IgA nephropathy is perhaps the most common glomerular disease in Australia, Southern Europe (France, Italy, and Spain), and Asia (Japan Singapore). The incidence of IgA nephropathy in all biopsied patients with primary glomerulonephritis ranges from 20% to 25% in Southern Europe and Australia, and 30–40% in Asia. It seems to be uncommon in USA, Britain, and the Netherlands. Whether the observed geographic variation in the incidence of this disease reflects the influence of genetic or environmental factors in its pathogenesis is unclear. It should be pointed out, however, that the high incidence in Japan and Singapore may be related to performing routine renal biopsy in otherwise asymptomatic patients picked up by periodic urinalysis done in some school children and in the healthy population.

IgA nephropathy is most commonly found in the second and third decades and affects males two to four times more often than females. Familial IgA nephropathy has been reported but is quite rare.

CLINICAL FEATURES

In 20–30% of patients, the clinical onset is characterized by the sudden appearance of gross hematuria. In the rest of the cases, the clinical onset is more insidious, with mild-to-moderate proteinuria and/or microscopic hematuria being detected on routine urinalysis. Recurrent bouts of macroscopic hematuria may be seen in about 30% of the cases. These episodes are often preceded by nonspecific upper respiratory infections, with a latent period of usually less than 2–3 days. This *synpharyngitic* hematuria may be accompanied by fever, malaise, fatigue, generalized muscle aches, and loin pain. Other signs of *acute nephritic syndrome* are absent, thus there is usually no associated elevation of BUN, hypertension, edema, or massive proteinuria. Between these attacks of synpharyngitic hematuria, which occur at variable intervals, the majority of patients have intermittent persistent microscopic hematuria.

Mild-to-moderate proteinuria, both persistent and intermittent, is found in the majority of patients, the amount of proteinuria usually being < 1.0 m/24 hr. Nephrotic range proteinuria may be seen in 4–6% of the patients. It should be emphasized that many patients with recurrent macroscopic hematuria undergo unnecessary urological investigation before the recognition of granular and red-cell casts in the urinary sediment, indicating the glomerular origin of hematuria and proteinuria. There is no family history of renal disease, nor signs or symptoms of systemic disease. Renal function and blood pressure are usually normal at the onset. A small number of patients may present with rapidly progressive glomerulonephritis, or acute renal failure complicating local or systemic infections.

LABORATORY FINDINGS

There are no characteristic serologic, biochemical, or hematologic abnormalities in IgA nephropathy. In spite of the remarkable mesangial deposition of C_3 in most cases, the serum complement profile reveals normal levels of Cl_q, C_4, C_3, properdin, and C_3 proactivator. Serum IgA concentration may be increased and exceeds the upper normal limit in 50% of cases. Serum IgG and IgM levels are within normal limits.

At the time of synpharygnitic hematuria, a variety of specific bacterial or viral antigens may be isolated, but no common infective antigens could be identified by microbiological investigations (2). Laboratory tests for collagen vascular diseases are consistently negative. The circulating immune complexes (ICs) could be detected by solid-phase Cl_q, Raji cell radioimmunoassays (3) and by other more specific methods (4, 5). The presence of ICs may be correlated with clinical evidence of disease activity but not with the high concentration of serum IgA. Thus, the immunogenetics of this disease have not been confirmed. An increased frequency of HLA BW35 and DR4 antigens has been reported by some investigators (6, 7).

PATHOLOGY

The glomerular lesions by light microscopy are variable. The glomeruli may be normal, may contain a focal-segmental proliferation of mesangial cells and matrix, or may demonstrate a mild-to-moderate generalized to diffuse mesangial hypercellularity. Diffuse and/or segmental glomerulosclerosis, partial capsular adhesions, and focal epithelial crescents may be present. Tubulointerstitial lesions tend to parellel the degree of glomerular changes, and focal tubular atrophy, interstitial fibrosis, and chronic interstitial inflammatory changes may be found with a relatively high frequency. Arteriolar hyalinosis is also common (8).

The glomerular immunofluorescence pattern is essentially identical in most cases, in spite of the variation seen in light microscopy. The glomeruli contain a generalized to diffuse granular mesangial deposition of IgA, forming the characteristic pattern of this disease. Intense mesangial deposits of IgA are usually accompanied by C_3 and properdin, and less frequently IgG and IgM. IgD, IgE, C_4, and Cl_q have not been identified in the mesangial deposits. The presence of properdin in a distribution similar to that with IgA and C_3 may imply activation of the complement system by the alternative pathway (9).

Finely granular electron-dense mesangial deposits are typically situated between the mesangial cells and the basement membrane in electron microscopic examinations. In younger patients, these mesangial deposits are typically large and globular, and may be recognized by light microscopy as hyaline nodules. Subendothelial, intramembranous, and subepithelial deposits may occur but are less frequent (10).

DIFFERENTIAL DIAGNOSIS

Since the morphologic changes identified by light and electron microscopy are relatively nonspecific, the immunofluorescent identification of mesangial IgA deposits is essential for the diagnosis. In addition to IgA nephropathy, mesangial IgA deposition can also be found in the nephritides associated with systemic lupus erythematosus, Henoch–Schoenlein purpura, alcoholic liver cirrhosis, and other specific conditions. These diseases must be excluded by appropriate clinical and laboratory examinations.

The increased serum IgA level and the synpharygnitic macroscopic hematuria are strong but not conclusive evidence for the diagnosis.

PATHOGENESIS

IgA nephropathy is presumed to be mediated by an immunologic mechanism. This is supported by the presence of granular deposits of IgA and C_3 in glomeruli by immunofluorescence microscopy and of mesangial electron-dense deposits by electron microscopy. Increased levels of IgA-containing circulating ICs (4), the recurrence of the disease in the transplanted kidney from a healthy donor to a recipient with end-stage renal failure due to IgA nephropathy (11), and the production of experimental IgA nephropathy by injection of polymeric IgA-containing ICs (12) all strongly support an immunologic mechanism of this disease.

The persistent presence of IgA-containing ICs in the blood is an important prerequisite for their subsequent mesangial deposition. It has been suggested that a defect in the regulation of IgA production and its clearance may underlie the elevated circulating IgA levels. Indeed, available data show increased numbers of circulating IgA-bearing lymphocytes, both in patients and in members of their families (13, 14) and an increase in the ratio of circulating helper/suppressor T cells (OKT4/OKT8) due to a decrease in suppressor T lymphocytes and an increase in helper T lymphocytes (15). A defective generation of IgA-specific suppressor cells and increased production of IgA-specific helper Tα cells have also been reported (16). An impairment of the immune clearance of polymeric IgA has been described in this disease. Thus, a defective reticulophagocytic function (17), a defective Fc-receptor function of the mononuclear phagocytic system (18), and depressed phagocytic activity of polymorphonuclear leucocytes (19) have been reported.

IgA is the principal immunoglobulin defense system directed against viral and bacterial antigens in exocrine secretions. Episodes of synpharyngitic hematuria and other signs of acute exacerbation of IgA nephropathy are usually associated with mucosal infections. Therefore, it is probable that this disease may be triggered by an infection of respiratory or gastrointestinal mucosa. Whether the ICs deposited in the mesangium are derived from mucosal IgA with corresponding viral or bacterial antigens has not been proved, but it has been suspected that idiopathic IgA nephropathy is a glomerulonephritis due to deposition of IgA ICs, probably originating in the migratory lymphocytes from the secretory tissues in response to stimulation by many common exogenous bacterial or viral antigens.

PROGNOSIS

About 70% of patients with IgA nephropathy have normal renal function with mild urinary abnormalities and mild histologic changes in the glomeruli. These patients have a good prognosis and show no deterioration of renal function during their lives. For this group of patients, therefore, no treatment is necessary. The remainder of the patients may progress to renal failure, most of them following a long insidious course of many years, from one to three decades. Few patients show a very rapid decline of renal function with a clinical picture of rapidly progressive glomerulonephritis. Considering that the true onset of the disease can considerably antedate the apparent clinical onset, it is presumed that the renal survival is higher than the actuarial estimation of approximately 50% in 20 years (20).

Although it is difficult to predict the prognosis of individual patients, certain clues indicate the likelihood of a progressive course. These include the following findings at the onset: old age, moderate-to-massive proteinuria, hypertension, decreased glomerular filtration rate, and the presence of crescents and/or segmental sclerosis in renal biopsy.

TREATMENTS

Because of its rather good prognosis, aggressive therapeutic approaches may not be necessary in the majority of patients with IgA nephropathy. In order to eradicate the possible offending mechanism of the disease, i.e., upper respiratory infection, some investigators performed tonsillectomies in patients with IgA nephropathy and reported an increased rate of clinical remission (21). Whether this aggressive surgical intervention is warranted awaits further studies.

Use of steroids and immunosuppressive drugs has been advocated for two subgroups of patients: one with a rapidly progressive course terminating in renal failure (8) and another with an overlapping syndrome of IgA nephropathy and lipoid nephrosis, a very rare combination (22). In the former a combination of intensive steroid therapy, including IV pulse-dose and cyclophosphamide administration, is often effective, and in the latter steroids may be effective, as might be expected.

A prospective study in patients with IgA nephropathy with moderate proteinuria treated with long-term steroids showed the therapy may be effective in reducing proteinuria and in maintaining renal function (23). Patients with persistent moderate proteinuria of between 1.0 and 2.0 g/day, a level generally considered to be one of the most reliable prognostic indices for the early stage of the progressive course, were selected. In one group of patients, prednisolone was given at an initial dose of 40 mg per day for 4 weeks, and the dose of prednisolone was gradually tapered, usually by 5 mg each 3–6 months. Most of the patients received the steroid for 1–3 years. After the course of steroids, all patients received nonsteroidal antiinflammatory and/or antiplatelet drugs until completion of the study. Results of the treatment were compared with the control group of patients who received a nonsteroidal antiinflammatory drug (indomethacin, 75 mg/day) and/or and antiplatelet drug (dipyridamole, 300 mg/day) only. At the start of the study, the mean creatinine clearance and 24-hour urinary protein excretion were similar in both groups. At the end of the study, creatinine clearance in the control group deteriorated and proteinuria remained unchanged, whereas in the steroid group creatinine clearance remained at the initial level and proteinuria improved markedly. These results suggest that treatment with steroids may be beneficial in IgA nephropathy, especially in those with a moderate degree of proteinuria and preserved renal function. Accordingly, these investigators suggest an indication for treatment with steroids in IgA nephropathy includes creatinine clearance values of 70 ml/min or higher, moderate proteinuria between 1.0 and 2.0 g/day, and histologic alterations showing a trend toward progressive glomerular and tubulointerstitial sclerotic changes.

Another controlled study of mesangial proliferative glomerulonephritis including IgA nephropathy treated with a combined therapy of cyclophosphamide, dipyridamole, and warfarin was reported recently (24). The treatment group was given a combination of cyclophosphamide (1.5 mg/kg body weight/day) for 6 months, dipyridamole (300 mg/day) for 36 months, and warfarin (doses to maintain thrombotests between 30% and 50% of normal) for 36 months; additional medications for hypertension, as well as diuretics for edema, were included as needed. Patients in the control group were given only antihypertensives and/or diuretics as indicated. There was no significant difference in the distribution between the treatment and control group of patients showing segmental sclerosis and global sclerosis by initial biopsies. The results showed that the patients in the treatment group have significantly less proteinuria and more stable renal function, whereas those in the contol group had a significant deterioration of renal function with no decrease in proteinuria. In addition, the regimen of dipyridamole and low-dose warfarin without cyclophosphamide seems effective in the preservation of renal function.

Danazol®, an anabolic steroid, which may increase circulating complement and thus may solubilize immune deposits, has been used with some clinical benefits (25).

Trials with phenytoin based upon its alleged effects on lowering serum IgA concentrations have been conducted in Spain and Australia (26, 27). Although the serum levels of IgA were reduced, no significant effects on any other clinical, morphologic, or immunopathologic features of the disease were demonstrated. It may be that the drug was not effective in reducing the concentration of circulating IgA-containing ICs.

As described already, some defects in the regulation of IgA production caused by an abnormally activated mucosal immune system might be responsible for the accumulation of IgA-containing circulating ICs, with their subsequent deposition in the glomerular mesangium. Blocking and elimination of the accumulating ICs in the circulation are thought to be important. Future developments, thus, may include a selective pharmacologic blockade of the effects of T cells or of activation of IgA-producing B cells by specific immunosuppressive agents or monoclonal antibodies and removal of IgA-circulating ICs through periodic selective plasma exchanges with immunoadsorbents.

For the treatment of end-stage renal disease caused by IgA nephropathy, chronic hemodialysis and renal transplantation are indicated, as for other end-stage renal diseases. However, the recurrence of mesangial IgA deposits in the transplanted kidney is common.

ACKNOWLEDGMENTS

I would like to thank Dr. Kiyoshi Kurokawa for critical reading and editing of the manuscript.

REFERENCES

1. Berger J, Hinglais N: Les dépôts intercapillaires d'IgA-IgG. J Urol Néphrol 74:694–695, 1968.
2. Woodroffe AJ, Gormly AA, McKenzie PE, Wootton AM, Thompson AJ, Seymour AE, Clarkson AR: Immunologic studies in IgA nephropathy. Kidney Int 18:366–374, 1980.
3. Tung KSK, Woodroffe AJ, Ahlin TD, Williams RC, Wilson CB: Applications of the solid phase C1q and Raji cell radioimmunoassays for the detection of circulating immune complexes in glomerulonephritis. J Clin Invest 62:61–72, 1978.
4. Hall RP, Stachura I, Cason J, Whiteside TL, Lawley TJ: IgA-containing circulating immune complexes in patients with IgA nephropathy. Am J Med 74:56–63, 1983.
5. Valentijn RM, Kauffman RH, Dela Reveliere GB, Daha MR, Van Es LA: Presence of circulating macromolecular IgA in patients with hematuria due to primary IgA nephropathy. Am J Med 74:375–381, 1983.
6. Berthoux FC, Gagne A, Sabatier JC, Ducret F, Le Petit JC, Marcelin M, Mercier B, Bizard CP: HLA-BW35 and mesangial IgA glomerulonephritis. N Engl J Med 298:1034–1035, 1978.
7. Nomoto Y, Endoh M, Miura M, Suga T, Tomino Y, Sakai H, Nose Y, Tsuji K: IgA nephropathy associated with HLA-DR4 antigen. Am J Nephrol 4:184–187, 1984.
8. D'Amico G, Imbasciati E, Barbiano di Belgioioso G, Bertoli S, Fogazzi G, Ferrario F, Fellin G, Ragni A, Colasanti G, Minetti L, Ponticelli C: Idiopathic IgA mesangial nephropathy. Clinical and histological study of 374 patients. Medicine 64:49–60, 1985.
9. Götze O, Müller-Eberhard HJ: The C3 activator system: An alternate pathway of complement activation. J Exp Med 134:905–1085, 1971.
10. Clarkson AR, Seymour AE, Thompson AJ, Haynes WDG, Chan YL, Jackson B: IgA nephropathy: A syndrome of uniform morphology, diverse clinical features and uncertain prognosis. Clin Nephrol 8:459–471, 1977.
11. Berger J, Yaneva H, Nabarra B, Barbanel C: Recurrence of mesangial deposition of IgA after renal transplantation. Kidney Int 7:232–241, 1975.
12. Rifai A, Small PA, Teague PO, Ayoub EM: Experimental IgA nephropathy. J Exp Med 150:1161–1173, 1979.
13. Nomoto Y, Sakai H, Arimori S: Increase of IgA-bearing lymphocytes in peripheral blood from patients with IgA nephropathy. Am J Clin Path 71:158–161, 1979.
14. Sakai H Nomoto Y, Arimori S, Komori K, Inouye H, Tsuji K: Increase of IgA bearing peripheral blood lymphocytes in families of patients with IgA nephrophthy. Am J Clin Path 72:452–456, 1979.
15. Egido J, Blasco R, Sancho J, Illescas M, Hernando L: Abnormalities of immune regulation in patients with IgA mesangial glomerulonephritis. Proc Eur Dial Transpl Assoc 19:642–647, 1983.
16. Sakai H, Endon M, Tomino Y, Nomoto Y: Increase of IgA specific helper Tα cells in patients with IgA nephropathy. Clin Exp Immunol 50:77–82, 1982.
17. Lawrence S, Pussell BA, Charlesworth JA: Mesangial IgA nephropathy: Detection of defective reticulophagocytic function in vivo. Clin Nephrol 19:280–283, 1983.
18. Roccatello D, Coppo R, Piccoli G: Monocyte-macrophage system function in primary IgA nephropathy. Contr Nephrol 40:130–136, 1984.
19. Sato M, Kinugasa E, Ideura T, Koshikawa S: Phagocytic activity of polymorphonuclear leukocytes in patients with IgA nephropathy. Clin Nephrol 19:166–171, 1983.
20. Droz D, Noël LH: Ré-evaluation du prognostic des glomérulonephrites á dépôts intracapilaires d'IgA. Semin Nephrol Pédiat 1983:26–31, 1983.
21. Lagrue G, Sandreux T, Laurent J, Hirbec G: Is there a treatment of mesangial IgA glomerulonephritis? Clin Nephrol 16:161, 1981.
22. Mustonen J, Pasternack A, Rantala I: The nephrotic syndrome in IgA glomerulonephritis: Response to corticosteriod therapy. Clin Nephrol 20:172–176, 1983.
23. Kobayaski Y, Fujii K, Hiki Y, Tateno S: Steroid therapy in IgA nephropathy: A prospective pilot study in moderate

proteinuric cases. *Q J Med New Series* 61, 234:935–943, 1986.
24. Woo KT, Edmondson RPS, Yap HK, Wu AYT, Chiang GSC, Lee EJC, Pwee HS, Lim CH: Effects of triple therapy on the progression of mesangial proliferative glomerulonephritis. *Clin Nephrol* 27:56–64, 1987.
25. Tomino Y, Sakai H, Miura, Suga T, Endoh M, Nomoto T: Effect of danazol on solubilization of immune deposits in patients with IgA Nephropathy. *Am J Kidney Dis* 14:135–140, 1984.
26. Egido J, Rivera F, Sancho J, Barat Am, Hernando L: Phenytoin in IgA nephropathy: A long-term controlled trial. *Nephron* 38:30–39, 1984.
27. Clarkson AR, Seymour AE, Woodroffe AJ, McKenzie PE, Chan L, Wootton AM: Controlled trial of phenytoin therapy in IgA nephropathy. *Clin Nephrol* 13:215–218, 1980.

CHAPTER 23

Urinary Tract Infections

MARVIN FORLAND

INTRODUCTION

The management of infections of the urinary tract provides a continuing challenge to the physician for a variety of reasons. They are common — an estimated 10–20% of women will experience one. They may be painfully symptomatic or entirely silent. They tend to recur, in some with near-incapacitating frequency. Approaches to therapy have been shifting, with emphasis on shorter duration of treatment on one end of the spectrum and longer on the other. Finally, perspective on their long-term risks is being clarified, with reassurance for most, but with definition of the populations in whom their consequences may be critical.

PATHOPHYSIOLOGY

Except for the presence of small numbers of organisms in the anterior urethra, the urinary tract is normally sterile. The detection of organisms elsewhere in the urinary tract indicates the presence of infection. Cystitis-urethritis denotes restriction of infection to the lower tract. Pyelonephritis implies spread to the upper collecting system and renal parenchyma. Acute pyelonephritis usually presents clinically with fever and costovertebral angle tenderness, often accompanied by irritative lower tract symptoms of dysuria, urgency, and frequency. Chronic pyelonephritis is a form of tubulointerstitial nephritis that is the consequence of bacterial proliferation and must be separated from other predominantly interstitial diseases of diverse etiology. Prostatitis indicates infection of the prostate gland and may be acute and symptomatic or chronic and covert. Asymptomatic infection is common and a variety of localizing techniques suggest as many as half such patients have upper tract involvement. Clinical signs and symptoms, except for fever, are usually poorly reliable indicators of localization because of the frequent relative silence of upper tract involvement (1). Hence, there is great interest in immunologic (2) or enzymatic markers (3) that can provide noninvasive evidence of localization.

The prevalence of asymptomatic bacteriuria in women increases from slightly more than 1% in schoolgirls, to 6–7% during pregnancy, and 10–12% among elderly women. Except in the newborn period, urinary infections are considerably less common in males; however, the prevalence rises markedly after age 40, usually as a consequence of prostatic obstruction or renal calculi.

The initial step in the development of infection in the kidney generally is believed to be the establishment of lower tract infection. Renal involvement, pyelonephritis, is a consequence of the ascendancy of bacteria to the kidney through the collecting system. A miliary-type infection as a result of bacteremia may occur, most characteristically with staphylococcal and *Candida* sepsis. Lymphatic transmission of organisms to the kidney is of doubtful pathogenic significance.

The organisms most frequently responsible for urinary tract infection are the Enterobacteriaceae with *E. coli* comprising the single most significant pathogen. These organisms are usually serologically identical to *E. coli* isolated from the patient's stool (4). *Chlamydia trachomatis*, an obligate, intracellular, gram-negative bacteria, also has been recognized as a cause of dysuria and frequency, associated with pyuria and sterile routine bacterial cultures (5). With recurrent infection, more resistant strains of gram-negative organisms appear, including *Klebsiella, Enterobacter, Pseudomonas*, and *Proteus*. Gram-positive microorganisms account for 5–10% of urinary tract infections, commonly *Streptococcus fecalis* (enterococci) and *Staphylococcus aureus*. Coagulase-negative, novobiocin-resistant *Staphylococcus saprophyticus* has been identified recently as a frequent cause of urinary tract infection, particularly in young women (6).

Establishment of infection reflects the net balance between organism virulence factors and the patient's defensive capacity. Characteristics of microorganisms that may play roles in their pathogenicity include cell-wall antigenicity (7), ability to adhere to cell membranes (8), urease production (9), and capacity to persist as cell-free protoplasts (10).

An initial step in the infective sequence postulated by some (11) but not all investigators (12) is the introital carriage of Enterobacteriaceae. Such colonization has been found by some to occur with greater frequency in women with recurrent urinary tract infections and to precede their episodes of symptomatic or asymptomatic bacteriuria. Factors implicated in promoting such colonization include high pH (> 4.4) of vaginal secretions (13) and greater adherence of organisms to vaginal epithelial cells (14). The report of decreased production of specific cervicovaginal antibody (15) has been contested (16). Mild uretheral trauma is a means of promoting ascendancy of organisms (17); sexual intercourse has been demonstrated to result in an increase in urinary colony counts of more than one log in 30% of coital episodes in approximately half of the women studied (18). An increased risk of urinary tract infection has been reported in women using diaphragms, possibly related to increased vaginal colonization (19). The bladder provides protection against such spread through its vigorous emptying mechanism, as well as an intrinsic antibacterial factor not present in voided urine. It has recently been described as a pH-dependent acid glycosaminoglycan lining the normal bladder wall and capable of acting as a nonspecific antiadherence factor (20). Impaired emptying or ureterovesical reflux resulting in residual urine may be sufficient to overwhelm intrinsic defenses and to lead to infection. The ability of bacteria to ascend the ureters independent of ureterovesical reflux has been demonstrated in experimental animals (21). The medullary area of the kidney appears to be the initial site of bacterial proliferation in ascending infection. The unique physiologic milieu of the region compromises a number of usual defense mechanisms; its relatively low blood flow, oxygen content, and pH may impair the delivery and activity of phagocytes. Its hypertonicity may impair phagocytic ability, inhibit complement activity, and promote protoplast formation (22). Finally, ammonia may inactivate the fourth component of complement and locally impair immunologically mediated defense mechanisms (23). In addition to the protective effect of the longer male urethra, a prostatic factor with bactericidal activity has been described that appears to be a zinc-containing compound (24).

DIAGNOSIS

Urine culture

Confirmation of the presence of a urinary tract infection is dependent upon growth of a significant number of bacteria from a properly collected urine specimen. Contamination of voided specimens by organisms from the anterior urethra, or vulvovaginal area in women, is the major source of diagnostic confusion. The introduction of quantitative microbiology to urine culture assessment in the mid-1950s was a major contribution toward resolving the problem of contamination versus infection (25, 26). Employing voided, clean-catch, midstream urine specimens, Kass and associates found more than 95% of patients with clinical acute pyelonephritis had urinary bacterial counts of 100,000 colonies/ml or greater. In survey studies, urine specimens with counts below 100,000/ml usually contained saprophytic organisms and were from subjects without histories of urinary tract symptoms. A second culture rarely grew the same organism. In contrast, when bacterial counts reached or exceeded 100,000 colonies/ml, the organisms were usually pathogens, the majority of patients had a history of urinary symptoms, and results were reproducible on repeated culture.

The reproducibility of results of a clean-catch midstream specimen is approximately 85%. Identification of the same organism on two consecutive specimens yields approximately 95% reproducibility on subsequent collection. Consequently, the clean-catch midstream specimen has gained wide acceptance as a collection method of choice, avoiding the potential risks of introducing organisms by bladder catheterization. It is critical to appreciate that many of these studies defining the significance of colony counts were performed on asymptomatic subjects utilizing clean-catch collections. Recent studies of symptomatic women indicated the criterion of 10^5 bacteria/ml urine would exclude approximately half of those women whose urine contains organisms on a suprapubic aspiration or bladder catheterization. In symptomatic women the predictive criterion of 10^2/ml of coliform organism was high (0.88) and was considered to be of optimal sensitivity and specificity for clinical decision making (27). These findings are highly relevant to our understanding of the urethral syndrome, as often this may represent instances of low colony-count cystitis-urethritis (vide infra). In the symptomatic patient significant growth from a single specimen provides adequate diagnostic confirmation. In the asymptomatic patient, a second, confirmatory specimen should be obtained before considering treatment or evaluation. The collected urine must be cultured immediately or refrigerated until processed by the laboratory to prevent bacterial proliferation and misleadingly high colony counts. The properly processed negative culture is a definitive finding. With borderline results in the asymptomatic patient (> 10,000– < 100,000 colonies/ml) or when questions remain concerning the reliability of the collection, a catheter-obtained or suprapubic aspiration specimen may resolve the problem.

Growth of 100 or more colonies/ml of pathogenic organisms from a catheter-obtained specimen or suprapubic aspirate is also evidence of infection. The necessity of obtaining urine cultures in women presenting with acute dysuria and pyuria in the absence of known risk factors for pyelonephritis has been questioned (28). The appreciation of the significance of low colony-count bacteriuria and the minimal benefit of antibacterial sensitivity testing in this group, which is usually promptly responsive to treatment, supports this position in settings where followup for both patient and physician is readily available.

Other laboratory findings

Urinalysis findings may strongly suggest the presence of urinary tract infection. Pyuria, > 5 WBCs/hpf, is an indication of urinary tract inflammation, and consequently a nonspecific finding. Pyuria may be absent on routine sediment examination in up to half of patients with documented bacteriuria. Quantitation of urinary white cells with a counting chamber has been reported as a more reproducible technique than simple slide microscopy of the centrifuged specimen. Ten leukocytes/mm^3 or more, in uncentrifuged urine, correlates well with significant bacteriuria in symptomatic men and women (29). Dipsticks detecting leukocyte esterase activity are also available as a semiquantitative means of detecting pyuria. When asymptomatic pyuria persists in the absence of positive routine bacterial cultures or evidence of glomerulonephritis, urine cultures for *Mycobacterium tuberculosis* are mandatory (30). Recent studies indicate dysuria and pyuria with negative routine cultures are frequently a result of *Chlamydia trachomatis* infection. White cell casts in the presence of infection suggest parenchymal involvement, as do the recently described bacteria casts (31).

The presence of bacteria on oil-immersion microscopic examination of an unspun, clean-catch specimen using carefully cleansed glassware correlated well with culture growth of > 100,000 colonies/ml and is useful initial screening procedure (32). Gram staining facilitates observation of the organisms and their identification.

A variety of chemical tests based on bacterial metabolic activity are available commercially to facilitate the office diagnosis of urinary tract infection. None are ideal and our preference remains with microscopic examination and culture techniques. A number of simplified culture methods, commercially produced, make adequate bacterial quantitation available conveniently and at a reasonable cost. Dip-slide techniques, using a glass slide coated with agar medium (33), and the filter paper method (34) are readily performed with the availability of a small incubator and are easily interpreted.

COMPONENTS OF THE DISORDER REQUIRING MANAGEMENT

Infection

Antibiotic therapy is the mainstay in the treatment of active infection, and the basic principles of selection are similar to those for other sites of infection. Usually the narrowest spectrum of antibacterial activity is sought, combined with the least potential toxicity. The urinary concentration achieved by the antibacterial agent appears to be a critical determinant for therapeutic efficacy, but blood levels are also important, particularly with complicating bacteremia or relapse of infection, that is, prompt recurrence post-therapy with the same organism. Because of the broad range of presentations of urinary tract infections, the determination of the antibiotic agent of choice and the route of administration are also governed initially by the patient's clinical condition, as will be reviewed subsequently (see *Clinical Patterns of Genitourinary Infection*). Sensitivity studies provide useful guidelines when treatment can be deferred, as with asymptomatic bacteriuria or when the response to treatment is not prompt. The physician must be cognizant of local variations in bacterial antibiotic sensitivities, particularly within hospital settings. In addition, patterns of organism sensitivity may change in response to local preferences for specific antibiotics. Table 1 is a summary of characteristic patterns of antibiotic sensitivities based on both personal experience and published studies.

The importance of the renal excretory route is of particular consequence in selecting antibiotic agents in the patient with a urinary tract infection and renal insufficiency. Attention must be directed toward selecting an agent that achieves effective renal and urinary concentrations while avoiding potentially serious side effects due to impaired renal excretory function. Selection of antibiotic agents and modification of their dosage with renal insufficiency has been summarized recently by Bennett et al. (35)

Pain

Irritative lower urinary tract symptoms are frequently the presenting complaint in patients with either upper or lower tract infection. A diagnostically useful distinction has been suggested between *internal dysuria* perceived by the patient as inside the body and characteristic of urethritis, and *external dysuria*, pain induced by the stream of urine irritating the inflamed vaginal labia and experienced with vaginitis (28). Phenazopyridine hydrochloride is a useful oral urinary analgesic for symptomatic relief of internal dysuria. Often it is prescribed in a subeffective dosage: the recommended dose is 200 mg three times daily. It should be continued only while the patient is symptomatic, rarely more than 3–4 days. It colors the urine a vivid red-orange and staining of clothing is difficult to remove. Headache

Table 1. Characteristic antimicrobial sensitivities of common pathogens

Organisms	Sulfonamide	Nitrofurantoin	Ampicillin	Cephalexin, cefactor	Cefamandole	Moxalactam	Tetracycline	Gentamicin	Tobramycin	Amikacin	Carbenicillin	Sulfa-trimethaprim	Norfloxacin
E. coli	+	+	±	+	+	+	+	+	+	+	+	+	+
Klebsiella	±	−	−	+	+	+	+	+	+	+	−	+	+
Enterobacter	+	−	−	−	+	+	+	+	+	+	+	+	+
Proteus mirabilis	+	−	+	+	+	+	−	+	+	+	+	+	+
Proteus (indole positive)	−	−	−	−	±	+	−	+	+	+	+	+	+
Pseudomonas	−	−	−	−	−	−	−	+	+	+	±	−	+
Enterococcus	−	±	+	−	−	−	−	+	−	−	±	−	+

+ = >75% of isolates sensitive.
± = 60–75% sensitive.
− = <60% sensitive.

and gastrointestinal upset are the most frequent adverse reactions. Its use is contraindicated in patients with renal or hepatic failure.

Occasionally marked costovertebral angle pain and tenderness with acute pyelonephritis may necessitate administration of codeine or meperidine. Pain is particularly prominent when infection complicates obstruction due to renal calculus passage or papillary necrosis and may be an important diagnostic clue to their presence.

Volume depletion

High fever, anorexia, nausea and vomiting, and a transient urinary concentration impairment, individually or in combination, may produce significant extracellular volume depletion in the patient with acute pyelonephritis. Assessment of the state of hydration through the usual physical examination findings, including measurement of postural blood pressure variation, are necessary. Serum electrolytes and BUN or serum creatinine are additional useful guides toward evaluating the possible necessity for intravenous fluids and the quantitation of water and sodium replacement.

Fluid intake

The clinical efficacy of water diuresis in the management of urinary tract infections has yet to be demonstrated. Experimental models show wide host species and pathogen variations, with outcomes ranging from prevention of infection (36) to increased susceptibility and accelerated progression (37). Conceptually, a water diuresis with more frequent voidings should minimize bladder dwelltime, lower bacterial concentrations, and facilitate intrinsic bladder defenses. Decreasing renal medullary tonicity should assist leukocytic migration and phagocytosis, and possibly promote complement activity. However, possible deleterious consequences can be postulated as readily; these include dilution of both administered antimicrobial drugs and normally present antibacterial substances, decreased urinary acidification, and possibly promotion of ureterovesical reflux from the more frequently distended bladder.

Alterations in renal function

Impairment in the maximal renal concentrating ability is a frequent finding in patients with an upper tract infection (38). The rapidity of its restoration following effective antibiotic therapy has raised the possibility that it may be a functional defect related to the presence of the bacteria and their products (39). Its clinical consequences are usually minimal. Persistent impairment in the maximal urinary concentrating ability is an early finding in chronic tubulointerstitial nephritis, including chronic pyelonephritis, and may be a significant contributor toward volume depletion.

Elevation in BUN or creatinine reflecting a fall in the glomerular filtration rate (GFR) suggests upper tract infection, unless the cystitis-urethritis is superimposed on an underlying renal parenchymal disease. With acute pyelonephritis mild elevations may reflect the previously described effects of volume depletion. Consideration must be given to such impairment indicating an underlying renal anatomic abnormality associated with transient obstruction and/or chronic parenchymal damage.

With chronic pyelonephritis, alterations in tubular function that usually precede a clinically significant decline in GFR include impairment in urinary acidification. This characteristically results in a hyperchloremic acidosis, often associated with the early development of hyperkalemia (40). A similar laboratory picture may be seen in patients with long-standing diabetes mellitus, independent of their previous history or findings of urinary infection (41). This decrease in reserve may lead to presentation with a more serious acidosis with a superimposed acute pyelonephritis. Careful monitoring of serum potassium levels and consideration of administration of sodium bicarbonate, as well as volume replacement, are necessary.

Further evaluation of the urinary tract to rule out an underlying predisposing anatomic abnormality or to assess the presence of scarring or functional impairment of an individual kidney generally is considered indicated in women with recurrent infections or acute pyelonephritis and in males with an initial episode that is not clearly prostatic in origin. Several clinical series recently have questioned this practice in women because of a quite low yield of positive finding (42, 43). Clearly the request for intravenous pyelography and invasive procedures such as voiding cystography or cytoscopy must be justifiable to both the physician and the patient, and might best be reserved for women with risk factors associated with parenchymal abnormalities, including elevated serum creatinine, fever, and a history of renal calculi.

There are a number of clinical settings or courses related to urinary tract infection in which prompt radiologic or urologic assessment is warranted. The development of oliguria in the absence of severe volume depletion or other prerenal factors suggests bilateral obstruction with a prompt need for ultrasound studies and/or cystoscopy and retrograde pyelography. Pain in the urinary tract suggesting obstruction or frank colic, possibly related to stone or papilla passage, indicates a need for intravenous pyelography if overall renal function is maintained. Failure to respond to appropriate antibiotic therapy with continued pain, and particularly fever for greater than 48–72 hours, suggests the possibilities of obstruction or a perirenal abscess (44). Ultrasonography or computerized tomography are sensitive means for detecting acute focal bacterial nephritis, frank abscess formation, or extension or rupture of the infection into the perinephric space (45). Massive or persistent gross hematuria warrants cystoscopy, intravenous pyelography, and possibly angiography as a subsequent step.

Of less immediate urgency is the need for thorough evaluation of urinary infection in infancy or early childhood. Long-term studies indicate renal scarring usually is established before age 5, with ureterovesical reflux playing an important etiologic role (46). Hence intravenous pyelography and voiding cystourethrography are needed to demonstrate ureteral abnormalities and possible intrarenal reflux as soon as possible (see Vesicoureteral Reflux (VUR)).

Alteration of urinary pH

Lowering of urinary pH maximizes the intrinsic antibacterial activity of normal urine. This is most readily accomplished by the maintenance of higher concentrations of normally excreted organic acids, such as hippuric and β-hydroxybutyric acid, in undissociated form. This permits nonionic diffusion across the bacterial wall. The time-honored therapeutic effect of cranberry juice is achieved by increasing hippuric acid excretion.

Alteration of urinary pH also can promote the local effectiveness of some antimicrobial agent. Acidification is necessary for the effectiveness of methenamine salts, which act through release of formaldehyde into urine at low pH. Administered mandelic and hippuric acid also are most inhibitory of bacterial growth in acid urine. The effectiveness of tetracycline and nitrofurantoin are increased by urinary acidification. Ascorbic acid, 500 mg four times a day, or methionine in divided dosage of 2–12 g daily, are both effective and usually well-tolerated acidifying agents. Individual dosage should be established by the patient with the use of pH-indicator paper.

The effectiveness of the aminoglycoside antibiotics — streptomycin, gentamicin, tobramycin, and amikacin — are promoted by urinary alkalinization. The antibacterial spectrum of erythromycin can be broadened to include most of the enteric bacteria causing urinary infection by maintaining an alkaline urine (47). Sodium bicarbonate in divided dosage of 4–12 g daily can achieve this. Urinary pH manipulation clearly is not necessary in all patients, but may be useful in a refractory therapeutic situation. A 20% increase in therapeutic success has been reported through more careful management of urinary pH (48).

CLINICAL PATTERNS OF GENITOURINARY INFECTION

Acute, uncomplicated infections

In a patient presenting with an initial episode of lower urinary tract symptoms — frequency, dysuria, and hesitancy without fever or flank pain — *E. coli* is usually the responsible organism if the culture is positive. If the organism was not acquired in the hospital or was not introduced by instrumentation, it generally will respond promptly to treatment with a sulfonamide. As considered earlier (see Diagnosis), the necessity for urine culture in such patients who also demonstrate pyuria has been questioned. However culture confirmation is of importance when an underlying "subclinical" pyelonephritis is a consideration. This includes patients with risk factors such as preexisting renal disease, diabetes mellitus, symptoms for greater than 5 days, and past history of acute pyelonephritis (28). With a symptomatic patient, treatment should be initiated promptly and before the return of the culture report. Sulfonamide therapy, such as sulfisoxazole, has the advantages of broad efficacy with both minimal cost and risk of side effects.

A careful pelvic examination is an important part of the evaluation of a woman with urinary tract symptoms. Common conditions that may mimic or help initiate urinary tract infection include trichomonal, monilial or *Gardnerella vaginalis* vaginitis, Bartholin and Skene gland infection, urethral carbuncle, meatal stenosis, or postmenopausal atrophic vaginitis (49).

Followup cultures may be useful in ensuring the adequacy of therapy. Urine cultures should be sterile within 48–72 hours after initiation of therapy and thus can provide a useful form of in-vivo sensitivity testing if resolution is not prompt. The cost effectiveness of routine post-treatment cultures at 2-week, 6-week, and 6-month intervals in patients with acute lower tract infections has been challenged, as the majority of recurrences are reinfections and are evident by the symptoms (50).

A series of recent studies have demonstrated the efficacy of single-dose antibiotic treatment in acute, uncomplicated cystitis. Agents employed in a single dose have included amoxicillin (3 g) (51), trimethaprim-sulfamethoxazole (1–2 g) (52), and kanamycin (500 mg IM) (53). Advantages of this approach include decreased cost, diminished exposure to drug sensitization, and minimal dependency on patient compliance. Patient selection in several studies has been based on the presence or absence of antibody coating of urinary bacteria. However, relapse has been so prompt in those with upper tract localization, that relapse after therapeutic trial with a single dose has been suggested as a means of selecting patients for conventional therapy. At the present time, single-dose therapy should be restricted to those patients whose site of infection is localized by conventional techniques or, in their absence, afebrile, otherwise healthy younger women with lower tract symptoms of brief duration who can be reliably followed (54).

Acute pyelonephritis

The patient presenting with acute pyelonephritis usually complains of fever, frequently chills, and often flank pain or tenderness, all of which may or may not be associated with lower urinary tract symptoms. Treatment with a bacterial agent that achieves significant renal and urinary concentrations is necessary. Oral ampicillin or amoxicillin are effective against most of the common gram-negative pathogens and are reasonable initial choices for a patient with an apparently uncomplicated infection. However, if the patient develops acute pyelonephritis while in the hospital or has underlying structural or functional urinary tract abnormalities, or evidence of possible gram-negative shock, extremely high fever, unstable blood pressure, or decreasing renal function, parenteral medication is necessary. In the hospitalized patient, blood cultures should always be obtained prior to the initiation of treatment to facilitate bacterial identification.

Gentamicin intramuscularly is the drug of choice in the latter situation because of its broad bactericidal spectrum against gram-negative organisms, including *Pseudomonas*, and its lesser, though by no means negligible degree of ototoxicity and nephrotoxicity as compared to kanamycin. Ampicillin is a useful second drug to ensure coverage against enterococci. If the clinical response is prompt and cultures indicate that the organism is sensitive to ampicillin, this agent may be continued for the 10- to 14-day course and gentamicin may be discontinued. Gentamicin-resistant strains of *Pseudomonas aeruginosa* are becoming progressively more common, and tobramycin is the most effective agent in their management. Other gram-negative rods that are gentamicin resistant are often also tobramycin resistant, but are susceptible to amikacin. Parenteral trimethaprim-sulfamethoxazole and second- or third-generation cephalosporins are among the other alternatives for the hospitalized patient with acute pyelonephritis. Vancomycin provides broad coverage for the less frequent gram-positive coccal infections.

Recurrent infection

Recurrences of urinary tract infections following treatment are often classified as either relapses or recurrences (55). Relapses are prompt recurrences within days or weeks, with the same species and serotype organism. Reinfections are the result of different organisms, and the recurrence develops at a variable, often lengthy, time interval. Relapses have been considered to represent manifestation of an incompletely eradicated upper tract focus and reinfection to indicate limitation to the lower tract. These concepts have been undergoing reevaluation. Some localization studies have not supported a major association of relapse with upper tract infection (56), and reinfection appears to be the predominant recurrence pattern, independent of the initial or previous site of infection (57). Relapses may be related to the persistence post-treatment of the same predominant fecal and hence perineal organism.

The importance of organism identification and sensitivity testing is increased with recurrent infection, since the more resistant gram-negative organisms emerge as the principal pathogens and are more refractory to treatment. Frequent recurrences of infections accompanied by irritative lower tract symptoms may occur, although evaluation may fail to demonstrate anatomic or functional lesions or association with sexual activity. Cultures are usually positive, with varying serotypes of *E. coli* or species of gram-negative organisms. The value of sustained full-dosage therapy beyond 2 weeks has not been established in this setting (58, 59). Patient-initiated, single-dose trimethaprim-sulfamethoxazole has been used in selected women with frequently recurring infections who can reliably recognize early symptoms (60). While the nature of the altered local resistance to infection is still undergoing elucidation, prophylactic therapy and regular perineal cleansing with antibacterial-treated swabs may be useful.

Prophylactic therapy, as first employed, consisted of the long-term use of methenamine mandelate or hippurate along with a acidifying agent such a methionine (26). The dosage was adjusted to maintain urinary pH at 5.5 or lower. This regimen has the advantages of not promoting the development of resistant organisms or altering fecal flora, but it is a cumbersome program for the patient. Considerable success has been achieved with the use of nitrofurantoin (50–100 mg) or trimethoprim-sulfamethoxazole (40–80/200–400 mg) as a single bedtime dose (61–63). This approach is easily followed and may be continued for 6–12 months in a patient with very frequent uncomfortable recurrences.

When a direct relationship between sexual activity and frequent episodes of cystitis appears to be present, a number of relatively simple measures may be effective. Postcoital voiding following rinsing the urethral area with soap solution may be helpful in eliminating potentially ascending organisms. If this does not reduce recurrences, it can be combined with the use of a single oral dose of sulfonamide, ampicillin, or nitrofurantoin following intercourse (64).

A number of nonsecific measures have been suggested but lack the support of controlled studies. These include the avoidance of possibly irritating bubble-bath preparations, substitution of showering for tub bathing, and the use of vaginal tampons rather than sanitary napkins.

Urethral syndrome

The terms *urethral syndrome* or *frequency and dysuria syndrome* have been used to characterize the approximately 50% of women seen with these complaints who fail to grow 100,000 colonies/ml of bacteria on repeated urine cultures (65). This is clearly a heterogeneous group defined in a varying manner by individual clinical investigators (66). With the appreciation of the frequency and significance of low colony-count bacteriuria in an acute symptomatic lower tract infection (see Diagnosis), it is evident that in most women this does not represent a distinct clinical condition and should be diagnosed and managed as a lower urinary tract bacterial infection.

A small group remains defined by repeated sterile urine cultures and no evidence of inflammation. Frequency is often more severe than dysuria, and evidence for impedance to flow should be evaluated urologically. Diazepam (Valium®) has been suggested as an effective agent in the group with frequency and normal voiding dynamics, acting perhaps through a bladder-relaxing mechanism rather than its better-described psychopharmacologic activity (67). Dysuria with pyuria must alert the physician to the possibility of genitourinary tuberculosis (30). Reports of a high yield of *Chlamydia trachomatis* isolates from such patients using cell culture techniques for isolation of the organisms would support the use of tetracycline as an empiric agent of choice (5).

A summary of differential diagnostic considerations in dysuria is included in Table 2.

Prostatitis

Presentation with urinary tract symptoms in the male raises the additional diagnostic consideration of prostatitis (68). Acute bacterial prostatitis is usually characterized by fever, lower tract symptoms, and frequently low back pain with or without a perineal component. Rectal examination reveals a very tender, enlarged, indurated, and irregular gland. Massage for culture is contraindicated to avoid the risk of bacterial dissemination. Cystitis is almost invariably present, and urine culture will yield the infecting, usually gram-negative organism. The response is generally prompt to treatment with agents efficacious in the therapy of acute pyelonephritis, related perhaps to the increased permeability to antibiotics of the acutely inflamed gland.

Chronic bacterial prostatitis may be asymptomatic until complicated by development of a secondary cystitis. Segmented urine collections with quantitative cultures indicate prostatic origin when expressed prostatic fluid (EPS) and post-massage urine collections (voided bladder 3) (VB_3) grow greater numbers of pathogens than the initial urethral (VB_1) and bladder (VB_2) samples (69). Achievement of effective concentration of antimicrobial agents in prostatic fluid in the absence of acute inflammation is impaired, because most drugs normally employed in the treatment of gram-negative infection are acid salts. Consequently, they are largely dissociated at plasma pH, making them lipid insoluble and poorly penetrable across epithelial membranes. Others, such as nalidixic acid, are largely protein bound. Trimethoprim is a lipid-soluble base with a pKa of 7.31; therefore, it traverses readily across epithelial cells by non-ionic diffusion (70). Prostatic fluid concentrations exceed plasma concentrations because of trapping of the ionic form of trimethoprim formed due to the relative acidity of prostatic fluid (pH 6.4). Trimethoprim has been most extensively used in combination with sulfamethoxazole and a series of studies indicate fewer recurrences when treatment is continued for 6–12 weeks (71, 72). In these studies, segmented cultures were used as an indicator of prostatic invasion or antibody-coated bacteria as a marker of invasion of uroeptihelium. Table 3 provides a summary of antimicrobial agents used in treating genitourinary infections.

Chronic bacteriuria

In most clinical practices, a group of patients can be identified who fail to respond to conventional courses of treatment, develop resistant organisms during prophylactic therapy, or promptly recur following discontinuation of long-term treatment. Such characteristics usually indicate discrete anatomic or functional abnormalities of the urinary tract — cystocele in the elderly woman, calculus disease, chronic prostatic obstruction, or the protracted use of an indwelling catheter. If definitive treatment cannot resolve the underlying abnormality, it is usually best to consider the patient to have chronic bacteriuria. Potent and possibly toxic antibiotics should be reserved for symptomatic episodes with the potential for development of life-threatening sepsis.

Table 2. The differential diagnosis of dysuria

I. Urinary tract infection

    Enterobacteriaceae and other gram-negative organisms
    Gram-positive organisms
    Chlamydia trachomatis
    Mycobacterium tuberculosis
    Adenovirus II
    Cytomegalovirus
    Schistosoma hematobium

II. Vaginitis

  A. Bacteria
    Chlamydia trachomatis
    Gardnerella vaginalis
    Neisseria gonorrhoeae
    Treponema pallidum (endourethral chancre)

  B. Fungi
    Candida albicans

  C. Protozoa
    Trichomonas vaginalis

III. Genital infection

    Herpes simplex (genitalis)
    Condyloma accuminata
    Parurethral glands

IV. Estrogen deficiency

V. Interstitial cystitis (Hunner's ulcer)

VI. Bladder tumor

VII. Chemical irritants

    Douches
    Deodorant aerosols
    Contraceptive jellies
    Bubble bath
    Medications: cyclophosphamide

VIII. Impedance to flow

    Chronic fibrosis after trauma
    Impaired synergy — bladder contraction and sphincter relaxation
    Meatal stenosis or stricture
    Transient urethral edema
    Urethral carbuncle or diverticuli

IX. Regional disease

    Crohn's disease
    Diverticulitis
    Radium implant of cervix
    Behcet's syndrome
    Reiter's syndrome

Table 3. Antimicrobial agents used in the treatment of genitourinary infections

Agent	Adult dosage	Comment
Sulfonamide (sulfisoxazole)	1 g qid	Single-dose therapy: 1–2 g PO
Nitrofurantoin	100 mg qid	Contraindicated with renal insufficiency
Trimethoprim	100 mg bid	Single-dose therapy: 400 mg PO
Trimethoprim/sulfamethoxazole	160 mg/800 mg bid	Single-dose therapy: 160/800 mg or 320/1600 mg PO; efficacious in low dosage for recurrence prophylaxis; an agent of choice for prostatitis
Norfloxacin	400 mg bid	A fluoroquinolone with a broad spectrum of activity against gram-positive and gram-negative aerobic bacteria
Methenamine mandelate	1 g qid	Limited to prophylaxis following definitive therapy; use with acidifying agents such as ascorbic acid or methionine
Ampicillin	250–500 mg qid	Single-dose therapy: 3.5 g PO; can be given orally, IV or IM
Amoxicillin	250–500 mg tid	Superior absorption after oral administration with less frequent diarrhea; single-dose therapy: 3.0 g PO
Cephalexin	250–500 mg qid	First-generation cephalosporin; serum levels relatively low for treatment of systemic infection
Cefamandole	1–2 g IV or IM, q 4–6 h	Second-generation cephalosporin; expanded coverage for gram-negative bacilli
Moxalactam	1–2 g IV, q 6–8 h	Third-generation cephalosporin; enhanced effectiveness against gram-negative bacilli, less against gram-positive
Tetracycline	250–500 mg qid	Effective against *Chlamydia trachomatis*; late fetal or early childhood dental staining
Gentamicin	3–5 mg/kg/day IM or IV q 8 h	Shares potential renal and ototoxicity of the aminoglycosides
Tobramycin	3–5 mg/kg/day IV q6–8 h; IM q 8 h	Useful for gentamicin-resistant strains of *Pseudomonas*
Amikacin	15 mg/kg/day IM or IV q 8–12 h	Often effective against non-*Pseudomonas*, gentamicin-resistant gram-negative organisms
Carbenicillin indanyl	2 tablets qid (764 mg)	Parenteral carbenicillin preparation available

PREVENTION OF URINARY TRACT INFECTION

A number of clinical circumstances have been identified in which the risks of urinary tract infection or symptomatic exacerbation appear to be significantly increased. Awareness of these circumstances and appropriate management should decrease the risk of development of symptomatic infection and its potential for serious complications.

Indwelling catheters

An estimated 40% of hospital-acquired infections originate in the urinary tract, in large part due to the use of indwelling urethral catheters. Preventive systemic antibiotic therapy only encourages the emergence of resistant organisms and is not recommended for use in the patient with an indwelling catheter. Antibiotics should be reserved for the development of urinary symptoms or other evidence of sepsis arising from the genitourinary tract.

The usual hospital use of an indwelling catheter is a week or less, and its septic risks can be minimized by several simple measures (73). Sterile, closed drainage systems have been demonstrated to help minimize the problem of infection for the bedridden patient. The collection bag should always be positioned below the level of the bladder, and the portal for external drainage should be located at the bottom of the bag to minimize the possibility of backflow and postemptying residua. The use of daily meatal care regimens utilizing povidone-iodine solution and ointment, or green soap, has been questioned (74). Evidence of higher rates of bacteriuria with such treatment has been reported, possibly related to the adverse effect of urethral manipulation. Urine specimens for cultures and other studies should be obtained by aspiration of freshly flowing urine from the distal end of the catheter with a number 21 needle after thorough cleansing of the catheter segment with an antibacterial solution.

Intermittent irrigation with saline or antibiotic solutions is of little value in the prevention or treatment of bacterial urinary infections. Continuous bladder irrigation with a three-way catheter system using neomycin-polymixin solutions has been proposed as an effective supplement to a closed drainage system (75). A controlled study of this system showed a mean daily increment in infection of 5% in both the treatment and control groups (76). The suppressive role of the irrigation solution appeared to be counteracted by the increased rate of disconnections due to the extra junction used for irrigation; the latter also led to more resistant strains.

Vesicoureteral reflux (VUR)

Vesicoureteral reflux is the retrograde flow of urine from bladder to ureter. It has been characterized as both the cause and consequence of urinary tract infection. VUR is not normally found in infancy and its congenital presence appears related to trigonal muscular weakness or intrinsic defects of the submucosal ureter. It often accompanies such underlying ureteral abnormalities as complete ureteral duplication, ectopic ureteral orifice, or a ureterocoele. The presence of cystitis may compromise a previously "border-line" vesticoureteral valve due to the development of local edema, with prompt resolution following clearing of the infection (77)

VUR promotes renal infection through a number of pathophysiologic mechanisms. These include the presence of residual urine, a more available ascending pathway to the kidney, and a possible damaging mechanical effect ("water hammer") upon renal tissue that is independent of infection. Intrarenal reflux, the appearance of contrast material in the renal parenchyma during voiding cystourethrography, has been demonstrated in the multipapillary kidney of miniature pigs in which partial urethral obstruction has been created to produce elevated voiding pressures (78). Renal scars resembling chronic pyelonephritis then develop in areas of intrarenal reflux, independent of infection. However, the significance of reflux alone in the absence of infection in the development of human scarring that is characteristic of chronic pyelonephritis and progressive renal disease (reflux nephropathy) remains a topic of controversy (79).

VUR has been found to be present on radiographic evaluation in 35–50% of children with urinary tract infection and has been correlated with younger age of diagnosis and more critical clinical illness (80). Reports of its occurrence in adults have ranged widely from 8% in a bacteriuric population to as high as 50% in patients with recurrent infection. Approximately one third of children and adults with VUR have evidence of renal scarring, and when parenchymal scarring is observed in childhood VUR is almost invariably present. The de-novo development of scarring is rarely observed in adults, and the Cardiff–Oxford studies indicate that such scarring is usually initiated before age five (46).

Ureteral dilatation appears to be a critical determinant of prognosis, and VUR will usually remit in its absence in the majority of children if infection can be prevented. The capacity for the submucosal ureteral segment to lengthen with age and for its muscle cells to proliferate and mature permits the development of valvular competency. Conservative management of VUR consists of maintaining the urinary tract free of infection with long-term, low-dosage prophylactic antimicrobial agents and the institution of a triple-voiding program at 2-minute intervals to minimize residual urine. Approximately 90% of children maintained with this regimen will achieve normal renal growth without scarring (81). Surgery appears indicated with diagnosis within the first 3 years of life, particularly in males, with the presence of marked ureteral dilatation, development of scarring in association with marked reflux, infection refractory to medical management, and evidence of a periureteral diverticulum. Surgery usually achieves its immediate goal of correction of reflux in 90% of patients, and less than 5% develop postoperative obstruction, which may necessitate reoperation. Postsurgical reinfection rates of 10–15% have been described but are usually benign following restoration of valvular competency.

Asymptomatic bacteriuria

The reproducible finding of significant bacterial growth on urine cultures obtained in the evaluation of patients with nonrenal complaints or on screening studies ranges in prevalence from 1.2% among schoolgirls to as high as 10–12% of women over age 60. The occurrence is higher among women than men and is frequently associated with gynecologic abnormalities in older women and prostatic hypertrophy in men. A careful history often reveals minimal symptoms and the term *covert bacteriuria* has been preferred by some to asymptomatic bacteriuria.

The clinician's major concerns with the finding of asymptomatic bacteriuria are the potential for development of symptomatic infection and the possibility of underlying anatomical abnormalities, which may result in progressive renal impairment. In Kunin's study of bacteriuric schoolgirls, 22% had VUR on cystourethrograms (82). Recurrence of infection followed the initial course of conventional therapy in 80%, but approximately 20% went into long-term remission after each successive course of therapy (83). Careful followup and repeated treatment achieved what Kunin has termed successful *fractional extraction* of a segment of patients with each subsequent course of treatment. While the Cardiff–Oxford studies have demonstrated the dangers of scarring are mainly in the age group below 5 years (46), Kunin has pointed out the bacteriuric schoolgirls are at greater risk for recurrence following marriage and careful followup appears indicated (83).

Evidence to suggest renal parenchymal involvement in a significant segment of patients with asymptomatic bacteriuria has included an increased prevalence of IVP abnormalities (84), impairment in urinary concentrating ability (85), elevation in serum antibodies to bacterial components (86), and the still disputed findings of higher mean arterial blood pressure and an increased incidence of hypertension (87, 88). In a number of studies, particularly in the elderly, bacteriuria has been associated with an unexplained increased mortality rate (89).

In the absence of contraindications, it has been our policy to treat patients with asymptomatic bacteriuria with a 10- to 14-day course of an antibacterial agent selected by sensitivity testing. We recommend diagnostic evaluation in a manner similar to the patient with recurrent urinary tract infection. Although authorities disagree on the necessity for treatment of all patients with asymptomatic bacteriuria, three subsets necessitate careful consideration. These include infection in young males and in the presence of pregnancy or diabetes mellitus (see the next two sections on pregnancy and diabetes mellitus).

Pregnancy

The incidence of asymptomatic bacteriuria in pregnancy is approximately 6–7% (90). Bacteriuria will usually be

include diabetes mellitus or renal calculi but may also include all the other conditions predisposing to recurrent urinary tract infections (44). Presentation is most often with unilateral flank pain and fever, which may or may not have been preceded by symptomatic genitourinary infection. A flank or abdominal mass will be found in approximately half the patients. Laboratory findings are characteristic of urinary tract infection, and blood cultures have been reported as positive in 20–40%. An important clinical clue to the presence of a perinephric abscess is the tendency to a longer duration of signs and symptoms as compared to uncomplicated acute pyelonephritis. Symptoms are usually present in excess of 5 days, and fever tends to continue for 5 days or longer after the initiation of antibiotic therapy, in contrast to the rapid resolution with uncomplicated pyelonephritis.

Radiologic studies usually are critical to the diagnosis. Abnormalities of the chest x-ray on the side of the abscess occur in approximately 20%, and plain film of the abdomen reveals changes in about 50%. Retrograde pyelography or IVP will demonstrate abnormalities in 65–85% of patients. Ultrasonography and computerized tomography have both facilitated and made safer the detection of intrarenal and perinephric abscesses. Both are sensitive means of demonstrating a characteristic perirenal fluid or gas collection (45).

Evidence of renal localization may be minimal clinically, and the diagnosis has been made postmortem in as high as 30% of reported series. Successful management depends on the rapidity of diagnosis and effective establishment of surgical drainage. Mortality in reported series ranges 45–59% (44).

Papillary necrosis

Renal papillary necrosis is the partial or total loss of papillae and their adjacent medullary region. Renal infection appears to play a secondary precipitating role following the establishment of localized areas of ischemia due to preexisting renal disease. Urinary obstruction and diabetes mellitus are the most frequent coexisting processes, but analgesic abuse nephropathy with papillary necrosis and interstitial nephritis is being recognized with increasing frequency (100–101). About one third of these latter patients will have secondary infections. Other associations include fulminant acute pyelonephritis, sickle-cell anemia, alcoholism, and Balkan nephropathy. The process is found in 1–1.5% of autopsies and increases in frequency with advancing age.

The highly variable clinical manifestations of papillary necrosis may be grouped into three patterns. It may present as an acute febrile illness with chills, renal colic, progressive azotemia, and ultimately oliguria with renal failure if the process is bilateral. Obstruction, diabetes mellitus, or severe acute pyelonephritis are the usual settings for this course. Papillary necrosis may be seen as a chronic recurrent renal disease with infection, gross hematuria, intermittent colic, and ureteric obstruction due to papillary sequestration. Finally, the insidious progression of chronic renal insufficiency with anemia may occur with analgesic abuse in the absence of symptomatic secondary infection or urinary passage of papillae.

Diagnosis is readily confirmed by the passage of tissue, however, in approximately one third of patients, the tissue passage may not be recognized. Intravenous or retrograde pyelography may reveal characteristic filling defects or the "ring sign" of a sequestered papilla (102).

Treatment is similar to acute pyelonephritis, with emphasis on excluding or remedying an obstruction. Ureteric impaction with a sloughed papilla may often be effectively relieved with endoscopic surgery utilizing a Dormia ureteric stone basket.

Calculi

Renal calculi may lead to or result from a urinary tract infection. Areas of localized intrarenal obstruction resulting from calculus formation appear to decrease resistance to bacterial proliferation. Thus, renal calculus disease independent of etiology is often complicated by acute episodes of symptomatic urinary tract infection as well as chronic pyelonephritis.

Calculus formation may result from urinary infection when the responsible organism has the capability to split urea and to create a persistently alkaline urine. The precipitation of magnesium-ammonium-phosphate (struvite) is promoted by the alkaline urine and a high ammonium concentration, and may result in stone formation. Such infection stones are usually associated with *Proteus mirabilis* infection, but may also be caused by *Klebsiella* and certain *E. coli* with the capacity for urea splitting. Bacteria may persist in the interstices of removed stones, and their lack of accessibility to antimicrobial agents is probably responsible for the frequent recurrence of infection following therapy. The use of long-term prophylactic antibacterial therapy has been shown to maintain sterile urine, to prevent symptoms and to stabilize or improve renal function in some patients with idiopathic stone formation, however, stone growth may continue and infection recurs during or shortly after discontinuation of prophylaxis in most patients (103). Surgical intervention is frequently necessary to control recurrent infection by removing these struvite calculi (104). An oral regimen of acetohydroxamic acid, a urease inhibitor, has been reported to inhibit the growth of struvite stones in patients with chronic infections with urea-splitting organisms (105). The frequency of adverse reactions is high, and its use is recommended primarily in patients in whom surgery is contraindicated or in the immediate postoperative period to aid in the dissolution of small stone particles.

CHRONIC PYELONEPHRITIS

Clinical investigations through the last two decades have clarified the role of bacterial infection in the pathogenesis of progressive renal insufficiency (106–109). Chronic pyelonephritis is recognized as only one form of chronic tubulointerstitial nephritis; it is the variant related to chronic bacterial infection. A similar clinical and histologic picture may result from a wide diversity of metabolic, immune-mediated, or toxic etiologies (101). In addition, chronic pyelonephritis is now appreciated to evolve as a consequence of associated anatomic and/or metabolic abnormalities that compromise the intrinsic ability of the genitourinary tract to effectively clear infection. A number of the particular management problems seen with chronic pyelonephritis, such as a renal-concentrating defect and hyperchloremic acidosis, have been considered (see Alterations in Renal Function). Progressive renal insufficiency and renal hypertension are reviewed elsewhere in this book.

The relative benignity of uncomplicated urinary tract infection in relationship to progressive renal damage provides reassurance for most patients with this problem. Nonetheless, sepsis and stone formation remain potential consequences of an initially uncomplicated urinary tract infection. These hazards and the major incapacitation often associated with recurrent infections justify a carefully considered approach to both the treatment and prevention of nonobstructive infection.

REFERENCES

1. Fairley KF: The routine determination of the site of infection in the investigation of patients with urinary tract infection. In: P Kincaid-Smith, KF Fairley, eds, *Renal Infection and Renal Scarring*. Mercedes, Melbourne, pp 107–116, 1970.
2. Thomas VL, Forland M: The significance of antibody-coated bacteria in urinary tract infections. *Kidney Int* 21:1–7, 1982.
3. Applemelk BJ, MacLaren DM: Localization of urinary-tract infection with urinary lactic dehydrogenase isoenzymes. *Lancet* 1:1417–1418, 1981.
4. Schwartz H, Schirmer HKA, Post B, et al.: Correlation of *Escherichia coli* occurring simultaneously in the urine and stool of patients with clinically significant bacteriuria: Serotyping with group-specific O antisera. *J Urol* 101:379–382, 1969.
5. Stamm WE, Wagner KF, Ansel R, et al.: Causes of the acute urethral syndrome in women. *N Engl J Med* 303:409–415, 1980.
6. Horvelius B, Mardh P-A: *Staphylococcus saprophyticus* as a common cause of urinary tract infections. *Rev Infect Dis* 6:328–337, 1984.
7. Glynn AA, Brumfitt W, Howard CJ: K antigens of *Escherichia coli* and renal involvement in urinary tract infections. *Lancet* 1:514–516, 1971.
8. Jacobson SH, Lins LE, Svenson SB: P-fimbriated *Escherichia coli* in adults with acute pyelonephritis. *J Infect Dis* 152:426–427, 1985.
9. Musher DM, Griffith DP, Yawn D, et al.: Role of urease in pyelonephritis resulting from urinary tract infection with *Proteus. J Infect Dis* 131:177–181, 1975.
10. Guze LB, Kalmanson GM: Persistence of bacteria in 'protoplast' form after apparent cure of pyelonephritis in rats. *Science* 143:1340–1341, 1964.
11. Stamey TA, Sexton CC: The role of vaginal colonization with enterobacteriaceae in recurrent urinary infections. *J Urol* 113:214–217, 1975.
12. Cattell WR, McSherry MA, Northeast A, et al.: Periurethral enterobacterial carriage in pathogenesis of recurrent urinary infection. *Br Med J* 4:136–139, 1974.
13. Stamey TA, Timothy MM: Studies of introital colonization in women with recurrent urinary tract infections. I. Role of vaginal pH. *J Urol* 114:261–263, 1975.
14. Schaeffer AF, Jones JM, Dunn JK: Association of in vitro *Escherichia coli* adherence to vaginal and buccal epithelial cells with susceptibility of women to recurrent urinary-tract infections. *N Engl J Med* 304:1062–1066, 1981.
15. Stamey TA, Wehner N, Mihara G, et al.: The immunologic basis of recurrent bacteriuria: Role of cervicovaginal antibody in enterobacterial colonization of the introital mucosa. *Medicine* 57:47–56, 1978.
16. Kurdydyk LM, Kelly K, Harding GKM, et al.: Role of cervicovaginal antibody in the pathogenesis of recurrent urinary tract infection in women. *Infect Immunol* 29:76–82, 1980.
17. Bran JL, Levison ME, Kaye D: Entrance of bacteria into the female urinary bladder. *N Engl J Med* 286:626–629, 1972.
18. Buckley RM Jr, McGuckin M, MacGregor RR: Urine bacterial counts after sexual intercourse. *N Engl J Med* 298:321–324, 1978.
19. Fihn SD, Latham RH, Roberts P, et al.: Association between diaphragm use and urinary tract infection. *JAMA* 254:240–245, 1985.
20. Parsons CL: Bladder surface glycosaminoglycan: Efficient mechanism of environmental adaptation: *Urology (Supplement)* 27:9–14, 1986.
21. Vivaldi E, Cotran R, Zangwill DP, et al.: Ascending infection as a mechanism in pathogenesis of experimental nonobstructive pyelonephritis. *Proc Soc Exp Biol Med* 102:242–244, 1959.
22. Chernew I, Braude AI: Depression of phagocytosis by solutes in concentrations found in the kidney and urine. *J Clin Invest* 41:1945–1953, 1962.
23. Beeson PB, Rowley D: The anti-complementary effect of kidney tissue. *J Exp Med* 110:685–697, 1959.
24. Fair WR, Wehner N: The prostatic antibacterial factor: Identity and significance. In: H Marberger, H Haschek, HKA Schirmer, et al., eds *Prostatic Disease*. Alan R Liss, New York, pp 383–403, 1976.
25. Kass EH: Asymptomatic infections of the urinary tract. *Trans Assoc Am Phys* 69:56–63, 1956.
26. Kass EH: Bacteriuria and the diagnosis of infections of the urinary tract; with observations on the use of methionine as a urinary antiseptic. Arch Intern Med 100:709–714, 1957.
27. Stamm WE, Counts GW, Running KR, et al.: Diagnosis of coliform infection in acutely dysuric women. *N Engl J Med* 307:463–468, 1982.
28. Komaroff AL: Urinalysis and urine culture in women with dysuria. *Ann Intern Med* 104:212–216, 1986.
29. Stamm WE: Measurement of pyuria and its relation to bacteriuria. *Am J Med* 75(1B):53–58, 1983.
30. Simon HB, Weinstein AJ, Pasternak MS, et al.: Genitourinary tuberculosis: Clinical features in a general hospital population. *Am J Med* 63:410–420, 1977.
31. Lindner LE, Jones RN, Haber MH: A specific urinary cast in acute pyelonephritis. *Am J Clin Pathol* 73:809–811, 1980.
32. Kunin CM: The quantitative significance of bacteria visualized in the unstained urinary sediment. *N Engl J Med* 265:589, 1961.

33. Cohen S, Kass EH: A simple method for quantitative urine culture. *N Engl J Med* 277:176–180, 1967.
34. Dodge WF, West EF, Fras PA, et al.: Detection of bacteriuria in children. *J Pediatr* 74:107–110, 1969.
35. Bennett WM, Aronoff GR, Morrison G, et al.: Drug prescribing in renal failure: Dosing guidelines for adults. *Am J Kidney Dis* 3:155–193, 1983.
36. Levison SP, Kaye D: Response of enterococcal pyelonephritis to furosemide-induced diuresis alone and in combination with ampicillin. *J Infect Dis* 127:626–631, 1973.
37. Freedman LR: Experimental pyelonephritis. XIII. On the ability of water diuresis to induce susceptibility to *E. coli* bacteriuria in the normal rat. *Yale J Biol Med* 39:255–266, 1967.
38. Ronald AR, Cutler RE, Turck M: Effect of bacteriuria on renal concentrating mechanisms. *Ann Intern Med* 70:723–733, 1969.
39. Clark H, Ronald AR, Cutler RE, et al.: The correlation between the site of infection and maximal concentrating ability in bacteriuria. *J Infect Dis* 120:47–53, 1969.
40. Lathem W: Hyperchloremic acidosis in chronic pyelonephritis. *N Engl J Med* 258:1031–1036, 1958.
41. Schambelan M, Sebastian A, Hulter HN: Mineralocorticoid excess and deficiency syndromes. *Contemp Issues Nephrol* 2:232–268, 1978.
42. Fowler JE Jr, Pulaski ET: Excretory urography, cystography, and cystoscopy in the evaluation of women with urinary-tract infection: A prospective study. *N Engl J Med* 304:462–465, 1981.
43. Fairchild TN, Shuman W, Berger RE: Radiographic studies for women with recurrent urinary tract infections. *J Urol* 128:344–345, 1982.
44. Morgan WR, Nyberg LM: Perinephric and intrarenal abscesses. *Urol* 26:529–536, 1985.
45. June CH, Browning MD, Smith LP, et al.: Ultrasonography and computed tomography in severe urinary tract infection. *Arch Intern Med* 145:841–845, 1985.
46. Cardiff–Oxford Bacteriuria Study Group: The sequelae of covert bacteriuria in schoolgirls. *Lancet* 1:889–893, 1978.
47. Sabath LD, Gerstein DA, Loder PB, et al.: Excretion of erythromycin and its enhanced activity in urine against gram-negative bacilli with alkalinization. *J Lab Clin Med* 72:916–923, 1968.
48. Brumfitt W, Percival A: Adjustment of urine pH in the chemotherapy of urinary tract infection. *Lancet* 1:186–190, 1962.
49. Schultz HJ, McCaffrey LA, Keys TF, et al.: Acute cystitis: A prospective study of laboratory tests and duration of therapy. *Mayo Clin Proc* 59:391–397, 1984.
50. Komaroff AL, Pass TM, McCue JD, et al.: Management strategies for urinary and vaginal infections. *Arch Intern Med* 138:1069–1073, 1978.
51. Rubin RH, Fang LST, Jones SR, et al.: Single dose amoxicillin therapy for urinary tract infection: Multicenter trial using antibody-coated bacteria localization technique. *JAMA* 244:561–564, 1980.
52. Ludwig P, Buckwold F, Harding G, et al.: Single-dose therapy of acute cystitis in adult females: Prospective randomized comparison of four regimens. In: JD Neison, C Grassi, eds, *Current Chemotherapy and Infectious Disease.* Proceedings of the 11th International Congress on Chemotherapy, 19th Interscience Conference on Antimicrobial Agents and Chemotherapy, American Society of Microbiology, Washington DC, pp 1297–1298, 1980.
53. Ronald AR, Boutros P, Mourtada H: Bacteriuria localization and response to single-dose therapy in women. *JAMA* 235:1854–1856, 1976.
54. Stamm WE: Single-dose treatment of cystitis. *JAMA* 244:591–592, 1980.
55. Turck M, Ronald AR, Petersdorf RG: Relapse and reinfection in chronic bacteriuria. II. The correlation between site of infection and pattern of recurrence in chronic bacteriuria. *N Engl J Med* 278:422–427, 1968.
56. Cattell WR, Charlton CAC, McSherry A, et al.: The localization of urinary tract infection and its relationship to relapse, reinfection and treatment. In: W Brumfitt, AW Asscher, eds, *Urinary Tract Infection.* Oxford University Press, London, pp 206–214, 1973.
57. McGeachie J: Recurrent infection of the urinary tract: Reinfection or recrudescence? *Br Med J* 1:952–954, 1966.
58. Kincaid–Smith P, Fairley KF: Controlled trial comparing effect of two and six weeks' treatment in recurrent urinary tract infection. *Br Med J* 2:145–146, 1969.
59. Forland M, Thomas VL: The treatment of urinary tract infections in women with diabetes mellitus. *Diabetes Care* 8:499–506, 1985.
60. Wong ES, McKevitt M, Running K, et al.: Management of recurrent urinary tract infections with patient-administered single-dose therapy. *Ann Intern Med* 102:302–307, 1985.
61. Harding GKM, Ronald AR: A controlled study of antimicrobial prophylaxis of recurrent urinary infection in women. *N Eng J Med* 291:597–601, 1974.
62. Stamey TA, Condy M, Mihara G: Prophylactic efficacy of nitrofurantoin macrocrystals and trimethoprim-sulfamethoxazole in urinary infection. *N Engl J Med* 296:780–783, 1977.
63. Harding GKM, Buckwold FJ, Marrie TJ, et al.: Prophylaxis of recurrent urinary tract infection in female patients: Efficacy of low-dose thrice-weekly therapy with trimethoprim-sulfamethoxazole. *JAMA* 242:1975–1977, 1979.
64. Vosti KL: Recurrent urinary tract infections: Prevention by prophylactic antibiotics after sexual intercourse. *JAMA* 231:934–940, 1975.
65. Brooks D, Maudar A: Pathogenesis of the urethral syndrome in women and its diagnosis in general practice. *Lancet* 2:893–898, 1972.
66. Charlton CAC, Cattell WR, Canti G, et al.: The nonurethral syndrome. In: W Brumfitt, AW Asscher, eds, *Urinary Tract Infection.* Oxford University Press, London, pp 173–177, 1973.
67. Cattell WR, Brooks HL, McSherry MA, et al.: Approach to the frequency and dysuria syndrome. *Kidney Int* 8:S138–S143, 1975.
68. Meares EM Jr: Prostatitis. *Ann Rev Med* 30:279–288, 1979.
69. Meares EM Jr, Stamey TA: Bacteriologic localization patterns in bacterial prostatitis and urethritis. *Invest Urol* 5:492–518, 1968.
70. Stamey TA, Bushby SRM, Bragonje J: The concentration of trimethoprim in prostatic fluid: Non-ionic diffusion or active transport? *J Infect Dis* 128:S686–S690, 1973.
71. Smith JW, Jones SR, Reed WP, et al.: Recurrent urinary tract infections in men: Characteristics and response to therapy. *Ann Intern Med* 91:544–548, 1979.
72. Gleckman R, Crowley M, Natsios GA: Therapy of recurrent invasive urinary-tract infections of men. *N Engl J Med* 301:878–880, 1979.
73. Stamm WE: Guidelines for prevention of catheter-associated urinary tract infections. *Ann Intern Med* 82:386–390, 1975.
74. Burke JP, Garibaldi RA, Britt MR, et al.: Prevention of

74. catheter-associated urinary tract infections: Efficacy of daily meatal care regimens. *Am J Med* 70:655–658, 1981.
75. Martin, CM, Bookrajian EN: Bacteriuria prevention after indwelling urinary catheterization: A controlled study. *Arch Intern Med* 110:703–711, 1962.
76. Warren JW, Platt R, Thomas RJ, et al.: Antibiotic irrigation and catheter-associated urinary-tract infection. *N Engl J Med* 299:570–573, 1978.
77. Kunin CM: Tendency of vesico-ureteric reflux to disappear coincident with specific antimicrobial therapy. In: P Kincaid-Smith, KF Fairley, eds, *Renal Infection and Renal Scarring*. Mercedes, Melbourne, pp 287–292, 1970.
78. Hodson CJ, Maling TMJ, McManamon PJ, et al.: The pathogenesis of reflux nephropathy (chronic atrophic pyelonephritis). *Br J Radiol* 13(Suppl):1–26, 1975.
79. Torres VE, Velosa JA, Holley KE, et al.: The progression of vesicoureteral reflux nephropathy. *Ann Intern Med* 92:776–784, 1980.
80. Smellie JM, Normand ICS: Bacteriuria, reflux and renal scarring. *Arch Dis Child* 50:581–585, 1975.
81. Normand C, Smellie J: Vesicoureteric reflux: The case for conservative management. In: J Hodson, P Kincaid-Smith, eds, *Reflux Nephropathy*. Masson Publishing, New York, pp 281–286, 1979.
82. Kunin CM: A ten year study of bacteriuria in schoolgirls: Final report of bacteriologic, urologic and epidemiologic findings. *J Infect Dis* 122:382–393, 1970.
83. Kunin CM: The natural history of recurrent bacteriuria in schoolgirls. *N Engl J Med* 282:1443–1448, 1970.
84. Manners BTB, Grob PR, Dulake C, et al.: The interrelationships of asymptomatic bacteriuria, acute bacterial pyelonephritis and bacterial cystitis in women. In: W Brumfitt, AW Asscher, eds, *Urinary Tract Infection*. Oxford University Press, London, pp 186–194, 1973.
85. Kaitz AL: Urinary concentrating ability in pregnant women with asymptomatic bacteriuria. *J Clin Invest* 40:1331–1338, 1961.
86. Percival A, Brumfitt W, DeLouvois J: Serum-antibody levels as an indication of clinically inapparent pyelonephritis. *Lancet* 2:1027–1033, 1964.
87. Miall WE, Kass EH, Ling J: Factors influencing arterial pressure in the general population in Jamaica. *Br Med J* 2:497–506, 1962.
88. Kass EH: Horatio at the orifice: The significance of bacteriuria. *J Infect Dis* 138:546–557, 1978.
89. Kass EH: Bacteriuria and excess mortality: What should the next steps be? *Rev Infect Dis* 7:762S–766S, 1985.
90. Ampel WM, Zinner SH: Bacterial urinary tract infection in pregnancy. In: B Francois, P Perrin, eds, *Urinary Infection. Insights and Prospects*. Butterworth, London, pp 141–160, 1983.
91. Condi AP, Brumfitt W, Reeves DS, et al.: The effects of bacteriuria in pregnancy on fetal health. In: W Brumfitt, AW Asscher, eds, *Urinary Tract Infection*. Oxford University Press, London, pp 108–116, 1973.
92. Williams JD, Reeves DS, Brumfitt W, et al.: The effects of bacteriuria in pregnancy on maternal health. In: W Brumfitt, AW Asscher, eds, *Urinary Tract Infection*. Oxford University Press, London, pp 103–107, 1973.
93. Harris R, Thomas V, Shelokov A: Asymptomatic bacteriuria in pregnancy: Antibody-coated bacteria, renal function, and intrauterine growth retardation. *Am J Obstet Gynecol* 126:20–25, 1976.
94. Forland M, Thomas V, Shelokov A: Urinary tract infections in patients with diabetes mellitus: Studies on antibody-coating of bacteria. *JAMA* 238:1924–1926, 1977.
95. McCabe WR: Gram-negative bacteremia. *Adv Intern Med* 19:135–158, 1974.
96. Wolff S: Biological effects of bacterial endotoxins in man. *J Infect Dis* 128:S259–S264, 1973.
97. Winslow EJ, Loeb HS, Rahimtoola SH, et al.: Hemodynamic studies and results of therapy in 50 patients with bacteremic shock. *Am J Med* 54:421–432, 1973.
98. Sprung CL, Caralis PV, Marcial EH, et al.: The effects of high-dose corticosteroids in patients with septic shock. A prospective controlled study. *N Engl J Med* 311:1137–1143, 1984.
99. Kass EH: High-dose corticosteroids for septic shock. *N Engl J Med* 311:1178–1179, 1984.
100. Gloor FJ: Changing concepts in pathogenesis and morphology of analgesic nephropathy as seen in Europe. *Kidney Int* 13:27–33, 1978.
101. Murray T, Goldbery M: Chronic interstitial nephritis etiologic factors. *Ann Intern Med* 82:453–459, 1975.
102. Lindvall N: Radiological changes of renal papillary necrosis. *Kidney Int* 13:93–106, 1978.
103. Chinn RH, Maskell R, Mead JA, et al.: Renal stones and urinary infection: A study of antibiotic treatment. *Br Med J* 2:1411–1413, 1976.
104. Silverman DE, Stamey TA: Management of infection stones: The Stanford experience. *Medicine* 62:44–51, 1983.
105. Williams J, Rodman J, Peterson C: A randomized double-blind study of acetohydroxamic acid in struvite nephrolithiasis. *N Engl J Med* 311:760–764, 1984.
106. Kleeman SET, Freedman LR: The finding of chronic pyelonephritis in males and females at autopsy. *N Engl J Med* 263:988–992, 1960.
107. Kimmelstiel P, Kim OJ, Beres JA, et al.: Chronic pyelonephritis. *Am J Med* 30:589–607, 1961.
108. Freedman LR: Chronic pyelonephritis at autopsy. *Ann Intern Med* 66:697–710, 1967.
109. Huland H, Busch R: Chronic pyelonephritis as a cause of end stage renal disease. *J Urol* 127:642–643, 1982.

CHAPTER 24

Vesicoureteral Reflux and Reflux Nephropathy

PRISCILLA KINCAID-SMITH

INTRODUCTION

For many years the treatment of vesicoureteral reflux has been regarded as an area that concerned the urologist and not the nephrologist. It has been assumed that treatment of this condition, if indicated, was surgical. However, the place of surgery in the treatment of vesicoureteral reflux remains controversial. The importance of medical management in the control of infection and of other complications has gained considerable support over recent years.

The link between a form of renal scarring called *chronic atrophic pyelonephritis* and the presence of vesicoureteral reflux in childhood was established largely through the studies of Hodson. Hodson drew attention to the association of these two conditions and subsequently demonstrated how intrarenal reflux determined the site of segmental scar formation (1-3). Subsequent studies in children confirmed the importance of intrarenal reflux in determining the site of scar formation(4).

There is now abundant evidence that focal scars (Figure 1) develop largely during early childhood. The more diffuse parenchymal loss occasionally seen in severe reflux may resemble obstructive atrophy (Figures 2 and 3), but it occurs in the absence of obstruction and could have a congenital component (5). Intrarenal reflux, which determines the site of scarring, was only found in 16 patients from a large series of 386 children examined in Christchurch, and it was not observed in any child over the age of four (4). Documentation of fresh scar formation in children over the age of five or in adults is sparse. The term *reflux nephropathy* is used to cover all the forms of renal parenchymal damage seen in association with vesicoureteral reflux. The gross morphologic change illustrated in Figure 1 is well accepted as reflux-related scarring. The mechanism of scar formation and the relative roles of reflux and infection in producing scars has still not been fully elucidated.

Recently, it has become apparent that an adult with unilateral parenchymal scarring may develop progressive impairment of renal function and progressive loss of parenchyma in the contralateral "spared" kidney (6-12). When end-stage renal disease develops in adolescents or adults with reflux nephropathy, progression to renal fai-

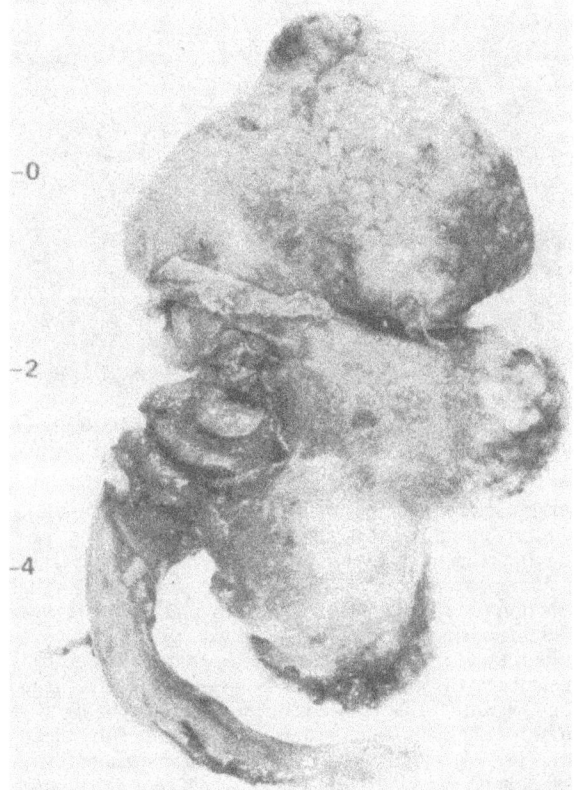

Figure 1. Coarse irregular parenchymal scarring in a 6-cm kidney removed from a 25-year-old man shortly after he commenced hemodialysis. The irregular pattern of scarring and the dilated and hypertrophied ureter are both characteristic of chronic atrophic pyelonephritis, the lesion associated with vesicoureteral reflux.

lure is almost invariably related to a progressive glomerular lesion (6-12). In a few cases, uncontrolled hypertension or overwhelming bacterial infection may contribute to

364 Therapy of Renal Diseases and Related Disorders

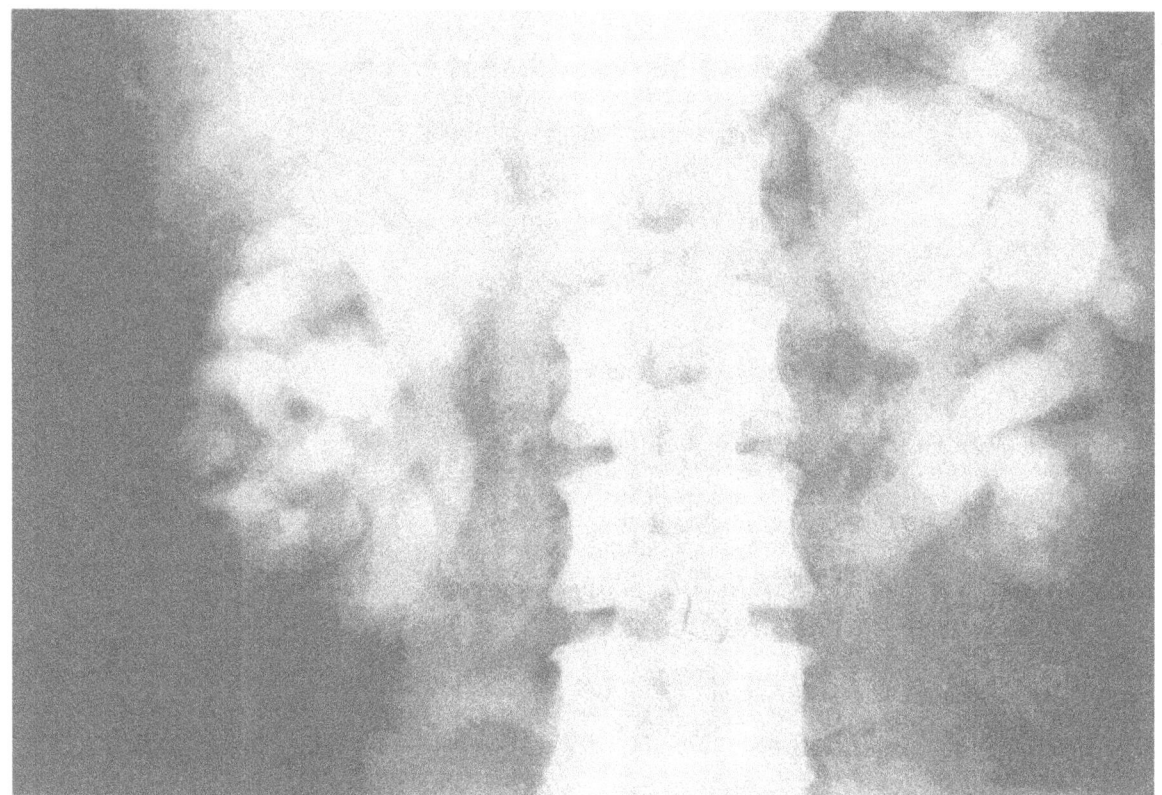

Figure 2. Diffuse parenchymal loss and dilatation of the collecting system in an asymptomatic 27-year-old woman who presented with proteinuria. No obstruction was present. The micturating cystourethrogram of this patient is shown in Figure 3.

progression. Generally, the long-term prognosis in adults with unilateral reflux nephropathy is good (12), but proteinuria marks the onset of a glomerular lesion and heralds a poor prognosis and progressive deterioration of renal function (6–12). Serial studies in individual patients show that increasing microscopic hematuria accompanies proteinuria and the urine deposit shows glomerular red cells resembling those seen in other forms of glomerular bleeding (Figure 4), in contradistinction to morphologically uniform red cells, which are seen in nonglomerular bleeding (13, 14). The parenchymal lesions associated with reflux have many different facets, which require separate consideration in the context of therapy.

COMPONENTS OF THE DISORDERS THAT MAY REQUIRE MANAGEMENT

Infection

There is no doubt that urinary tract infection plays a central role in the development of focal parenchymal scars in reflux nephropathy. Documentation of the development of this type of scar has almost invariably been associated with proven infection (5, 15, 16). The details in two children who developed progressive scars over a period when no infection was documented were reported by Rolleston and colleagues (4). It is noteworthy that only two and four urine tests, respectively, were available over 3 and 5 year follow-up periods in these two children. Furthermore, no account was taken of possible occult infection with organisms such as anaerobes or ureaplasmas. Bacteriuria may disappear spontaneously in young girls (17). As many as 38% of untreated children were free of bacteriuria at follow-up in one study (18). Hence, the two children quoted by Rolleston and colleagues (4) in whom scars developed in the absence of infection may well have had asymptomatic infection, which could have resolved spontaneously during the long periods in which no urine examinations were done.

There is thus slender evidence that focal-scar formation occurs in children in the absence of infection. Infants who present in the first few months of life with a thin rim of parenchyma and extreme calceal dilatation may show radiologic and functional deterioration in the absence of infection (5, 15).

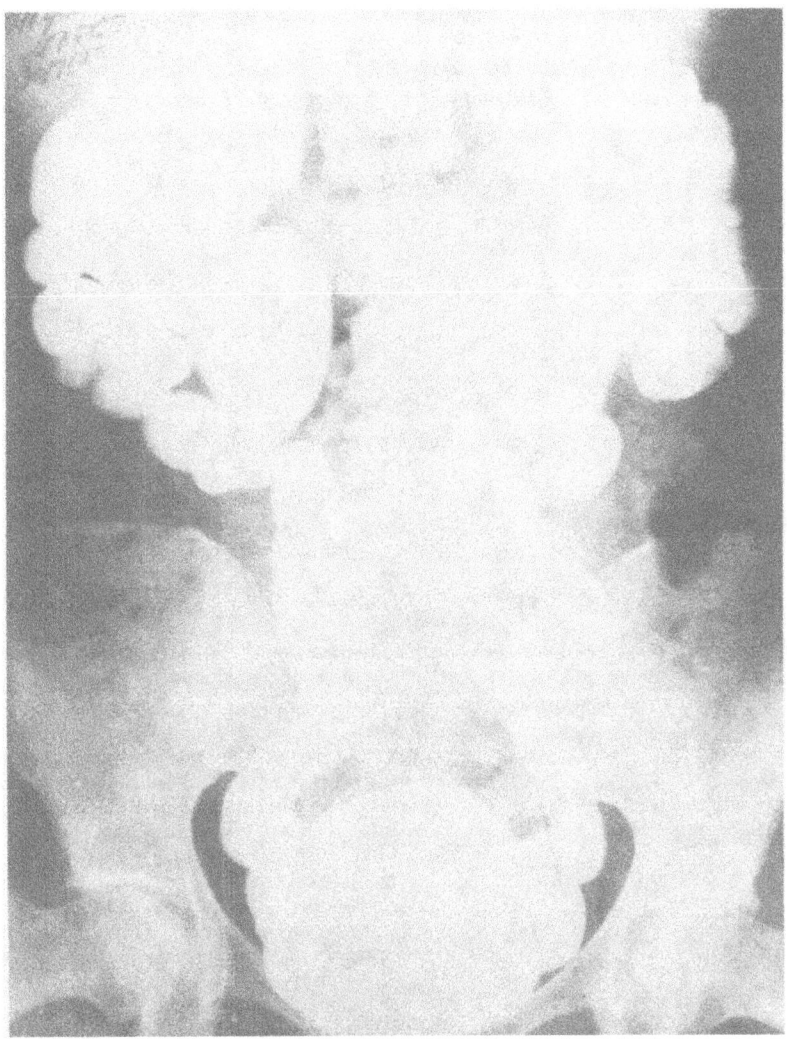

Figure 3. Micturating cystourethrogram showing extreme dilatation of the pelvicalyceal system during micturition in the 21-year-old patient whose intravenous pyelogram is shown in Figure 11.

Vesicoureteral reflux is equally distributed between male and female infants (19). At the time of the first detection of reflux in infancy, 20% of kidneys already show associated focal parenchymal scars. These are more numerous in children with gross reflux (19). Two factors thus appear to influence segmental scar formation in vesicoureteral reflux — the grade of reflux and the presence of infection. The site of a scar and the very typical pattern of sharply defined irregular parenchymal scars (see Figure 1) is determined by the site of intrarenal reflux (3). A single episode of intrarenal reflux with infected urine may lead to rapid scarring in the affected area of parenchyma (3).

The role of infection in the more diffuse "back pressure atrophy" type of parenchymal scarring (see Figures 2 and 3) is less well defined in humans, particularly where this lesion is demonstrated during early infancy (15). Episodes of infection in such patients can, however, be shown to be associated with a loss of renal function, and with each episode there may be an irreversible further deterioration in renal function (Figure 5).

Infection with atypical microorganisms such as anaerobes and mycoplasmas could be involved in progressive deterioration of renal function in patients with reflux nephropathy. Sterile urine cultures using conventional

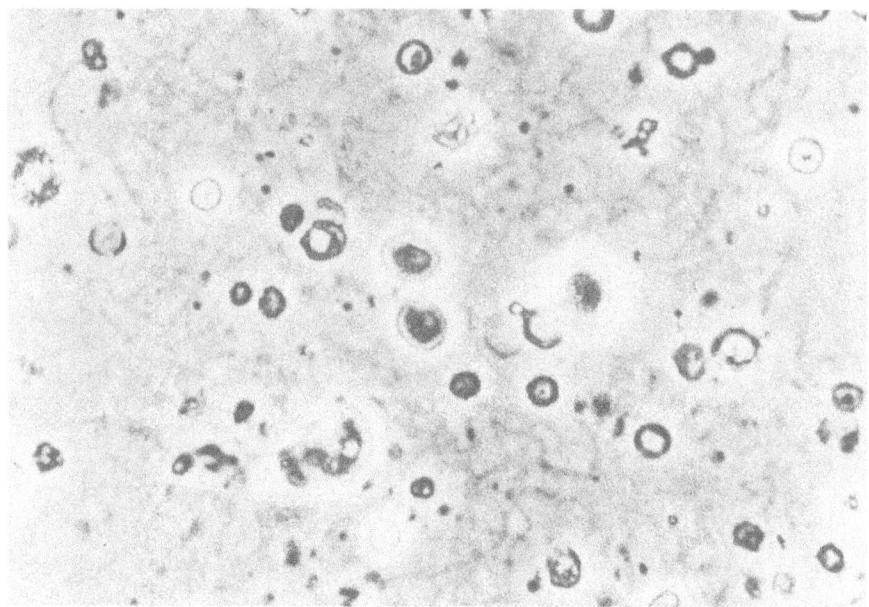

Figure 4. Dysmorphic red cells characteristic of those seen in glomerular disease (13, 14). The appearance of such cells in the urine deposit in a patient with reflux nephropathy indicates the development of glomerular lesions.

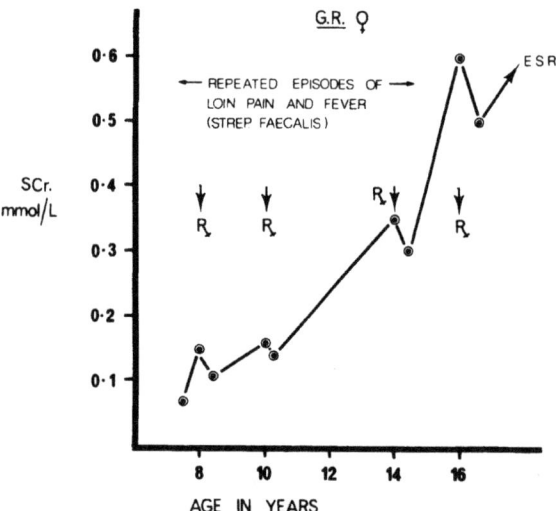

Figure 5. Course in a young girl who deteriorated from normal renal function to end-stage renal failure over a period in which repeated renal infections occurred. The occasional attendances were due to patient (parental) non compliance. The patient had bilateral reflux with a thin rim of renal parenchyma, but repeated infections and lack of continuing treatment were the likely major cause for deterioration in function: SCr = serum creatinine; Rx = course of treatment for documented infection; Strep = *Streptococcus*; ESRF = end-stage renal failure.

techniques led to a search for atypical and fastidious microorganisms. The presence of pyuria accompanying deterioration in some patients strongly suggested that infection may be present (20). Urine aspirated from the bladder in patients with reflux nephropathy will yield a positive culture in a high percentage of cases, even when a midstream urine has shown no evidence of conventional urinary tract pathogens. The organisms found will depend upon the microbiologic techniques used.

A variety of different organisms have been cultured in these studies (20–22), and they may play a part in causing progression. Recent interest has focused on mycoplasma organisms. Ureaplasmas are detected in the bladder aspirates in 37% of patients with reflux nephropathy, compared with 3% of controls. They are also more commonly present in patients with impaired renal function due to reflux nephropathy (21). The role of unusual organisms in producing progressive infection has not yet been established, but their isolation from kidneys and bladder urine in patients with progressive impairment of function certainly warrants further study.

Overall, therefore, infection plays a very important part in the progression of reflux-related scarring during childhood, and this is very well documented in the common form of focal scarring that is illustrated in Figures 1 and 6. Of all the factors that influence progressvie deterioration in reflux nephropathy, infection is the one that can be most easily treated, and it should be prevented by continuous antibacterial agents in children with vesicoureteric reflux.

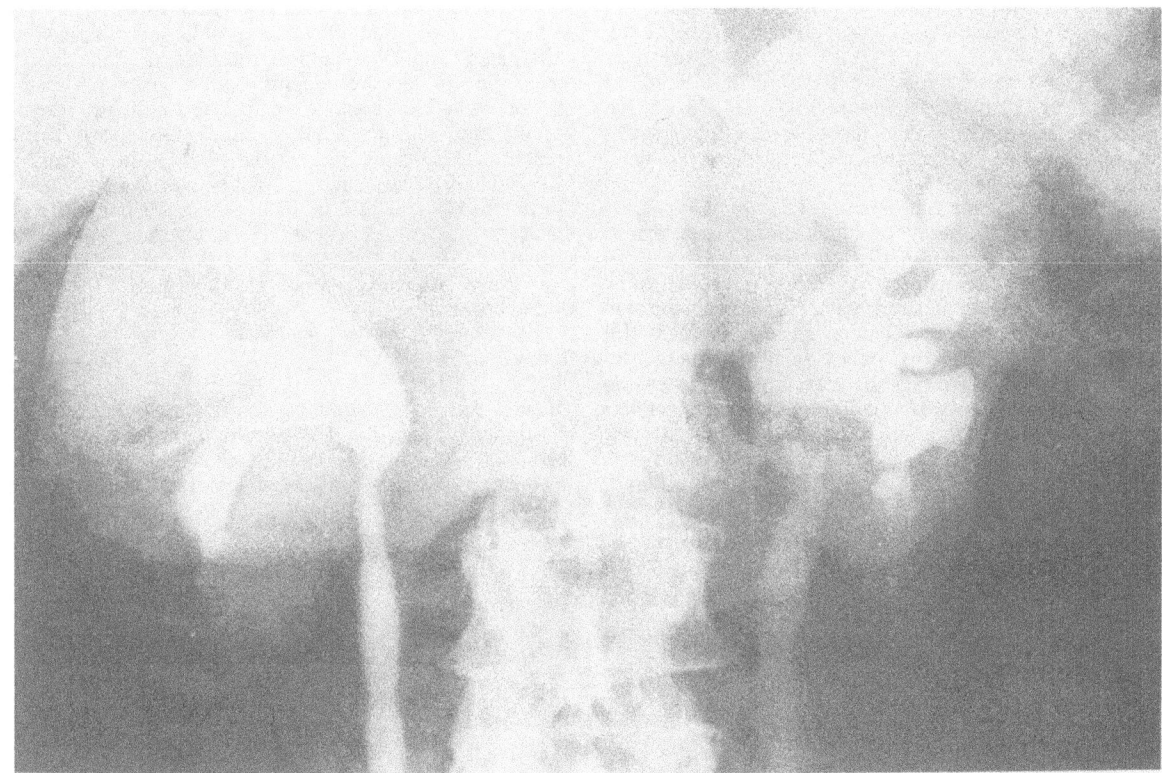

Figure 6. Coarse irregular scarring of the renal parenchyma of the left kidney together with clubbing of calyces in relation to areas of parenchymal loss — typical features of reflux-related scarring.

Hypertension

Hypertension commonly accompanies reflux nephropathy or chronic atrophic pyelonephritis. Autopsy studies show a prevalence of hypertension ranging from 65% to 75% (Table 1) (23–27). Hypertension is often severe; among patients dying of malignant hypertension, the classical scarring of chronic atrophic pyelonephritis is found in 15–27% of cases (Table 2) (24, 28–30). Children with renal scarring of the reflux type have a definite risk of developing hypertension and may develop severe hypertension (31–33). Reflux nephropathy is the underlying cause of hypertension in 60% of children with severe hypertension (34). There is some evidence that the mechanism involved in hypertension in childhood may be related to a high plasma renin activity (32, 35). Poutasse (36) and Dillon and Smellie (37) have reported cures of hypertension by removal of segmental areas in the kidney from which renal-vein samples showed high renin levels. Children who have reflux-related parenchymal scarring but no hypertension may also have raised plasma renin

Table 1. Hypertension in chronic pyelonephritis

	Ref no.	Percent
Longcope	23	66.0
Weiss & Parker	24	75.0
Kincaid-Smith	25	66.0
Brod	26	66.0
Bengtsson	27	65.0

Table 2. Chronic pyelonephritis in patients dying of malignant hypertension

	Ref no.	Percent
Weiss & Parker	24	18.20
Heptinstall	28	16.0
Kincaid-Smith	29	27.0
Kimmelstiel	30	15.0

368 Therapy of Renal Diseases and Related Disorders

levels (35). Hypertension is often refractory to treatment, and children with hypertension have a high risk of developing renal failure (31, 33). Among adults with reflux nephropathy, 40% have a diastolic blood pressure over 90 mmHg, and severe hypertension with a diastolic blood pressure over 120 mmHg is present in 10% (11, 38). These figures are much lower than those from autopsy series shown in Table 1, but, as they are derived from clinical studies, this is to be expected.

The possible angiotensin-dependent nature of hypertension in reflux nephropathy has implications in relation to treatment. The suggestion that the vascular lesions in chronic pyelonephritis caused hypertension through causing ischemia of the renal parenchyma (25) has gained some support from more recent animal studies. In pigs with chronic reflux nephropathy, only a small percentage develop hypertension. All pigs that developed hypertension showed well-marked vascular lesions in the kidney, similar to those associated with areas of ischemic tubular atrophy and hypertension in humans (25). These scars in pigs with sterile reflux have recently been studied in more detail.

Perivascular fibrosis consisting of dense collagen is proposed as a cause of ischemia (39). These studies, together with those that show elevated plasma renin activity in children (31, 35, 36), support the view that the hypertension in chronic pyelonephritis or reflux nephropathy may be related to excessive renin secretion by the scarred parenchyma, but no definitive study has clearly documented this as a causal relationship. Bailey and colleagues (40) found a renal-vein renin ratio over 1.5 in 3 of 17 normotensives and in 2 of 12 hypertensive patients with unilateral reflux nephropathy. This would appear to support the concept that the scarred renal parenchyma may secrete excessive amounts of renin, but they concluded otherwise.

Reflux of urine

There seems no real doubt that intrarenal reflux is one factor predisposing to the development of the coarse segmental scars in the renal parenchyma that are illustrated in Figure 1 and are shown radiographically in

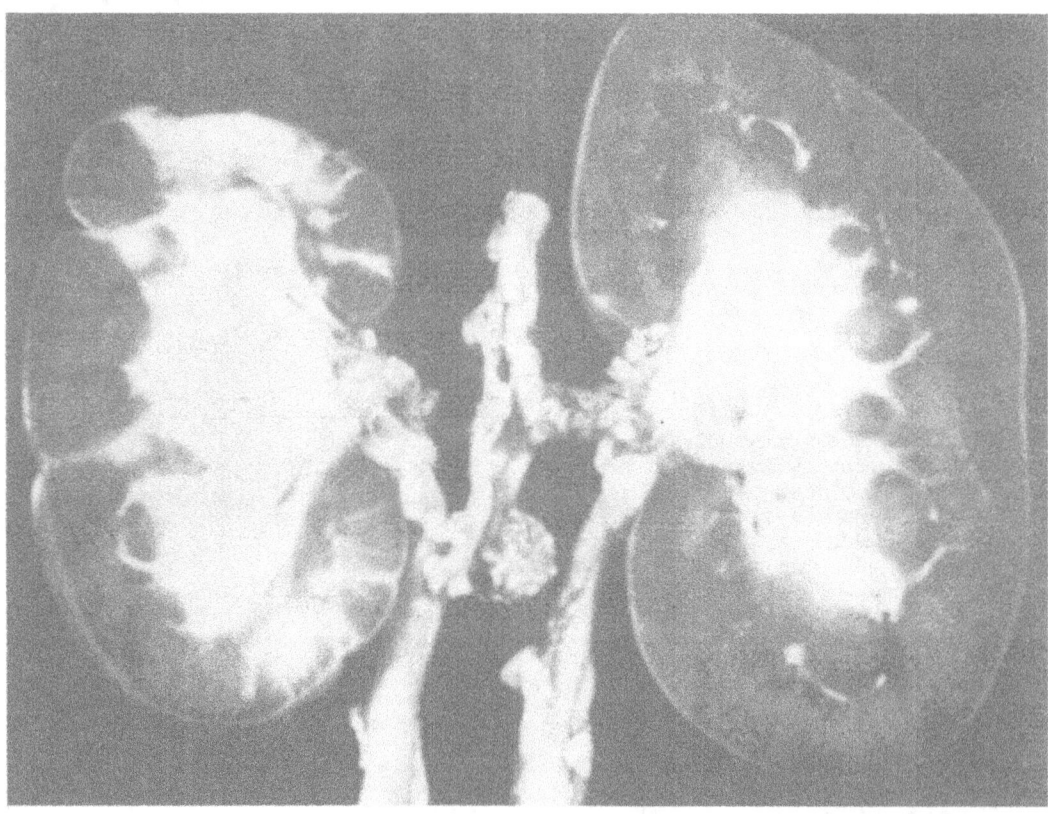

Figure 7. Renal scarring on the right side resulting from sterile vesicoureteral reflux. The kidney shows scars at upper and lower poles in areas that previously showed intrarenal reflux. "Slit scars" are also seen on the lateral surface that are rather similar to the "slit scar" on the lateral surface in Figure 1. From Hodson (3) with permission.

Figure 6. The role of infection in the development of such scars is discussed above (see Infection). A simple approach to the problem of reflux nephropathy might be that surgical correction of the reflux could prevent scar formation. There are, however, many reasons why we cannot adopt this simple view of reflux, and these are discussed in the section, Surgical management — the controversy.

When vesicoureteral reflux of urine is associated with high bladder voiding pressure, and hence a high pressure is transmitted to the pelvis of the kidney, the reflux itself may well play a part in causing parenchymal loss. Hodson (3) developed a model of reflux nephropathy in the pig with an associated high bladder pressure achieved by placing a clip on the urethra in young pigs. The pressure generated in the bladder in this model were often above 35 mmHg, which Hodson regarded as the critical pressure for scar formation. Hodson has demonstrated unequivocally that coarse focal scars that are virtually identical with those seen in humans, developed in localized areas in pigs in which the urine was constantly sterile (Figure 7) (3). Recent studies have confirmed and extended this work (39, 41), and Ransley, who originally disputed the development of scars in association with sterile vesicoureteral reflux, has recently confirmed Hodson's findings, using a high bladder-pressure model in the pig (42).

The fact that scar formation occurs with sterile reflux in the pig kidney has been widely quoted as demonstrating that sterile reflux itself can cause reflux nephropathy in humans, but the importance of the urethral obstruction and high voiding pressures in these pigs is often overlooked. In the models that Hodson and Ransley have used, there seems little doubt that a high bladder pressure is an essential factor in the production of reflux-related scars when the urine is sterile. The significance of these studies in relation to vesicoureteral reflux in the child remains uncertain. Far more needs to be known about the pressure generated in the bladder and transmitted to the pelvis before it can be assumed that sterile reflux is able to cause parenchymal scarring in humans. When there is an obstructive lesion in the urethra associated with reflux, it is likely that pressures approaching those achieved in the pig reflux studies can be transmitted from the bladder to the renal pelvis and that parenchymal scarring may occur in the absence of infection. There has been little clinical documentation of such cases, but the voiding disorders discussed below provide some examples of the association of high bladder pressure and reflux.

The concept of intrarenal reflux as an explanation for the sharply demarcated scars of reflux nephropathy was first introduced by Hodson (2). It is now well accepted that segmental parenchymal scars form in areas of intrarenal reflux. This has been best documented in pigs (3) and confirmed in humans (4). Using contrast medium, it can be shown that the urine enters through the papilla and refluxes back to the outer cortex. The route that the urine takes has still not been clearly elucidated. It undoubtedly enters via the ducts of Bellini, and some remains within tubules and may be found refluxing back as far as the glomerulus (3). When labeled with barium, it can be shown that refluxing urine finds its way into the interstitium and hence to local lymph nodes (3). Lymphatic channels in the cortex are prominent in refluxing kidneys (43).

The factors that govern the entry of urine into the papilla have been clearly described by Ransley and colleagues (44). Compound papillae, which are most frequently found at the upper pole of the kidney, are particularly liable to show intrarenal reflux. The origins in the duct of Bellini are slit-like on a normal, single papilla and gape, particularly in the middle ducts in a compound papilla. It is these gaping ducts that most readily permit reflux of urine into the renal parenchyma (44). With progressive scarring, and particularly with high pressures, normal papillae may become deformed and ducts of Bellini that were previously resistant to intrarenal reflux may gape open and permit the reflux of urine. The role of the urine or its constituents, such as Tamm Horsfall protein, in the interstitium in causing parenchymal scars has not been clearly defined. There is, however, much current interest in this question (41, 45–49). A compelling case has been made for the participation of Tamm Horsfall protein in the pathogenesis of the lesions seen in sterile scars in the pig (39). When intrarenal reflux occurs in the presence of an infected urine, acute pyelonephritis is restricted to the affected segment. Hodson has coined the term *acute lobar nephronia* to describe this. Rapid scarring may follow such an event, even if it results from a single episode of intrarenal reflux with infected urine (3).

Voiding disorders

Voiding studies in the 1950s and 1960s revealed a high incidence of vesicoureteral reflux in children with urinary tract infection, and many assumed that obstruction at the bladder neck may be the cause. An early study by Stephens and Lenaghan (50) presented compelling evidence against the view that bladder neck obstruction may be responsible for reflux. They found no radiographic evidence to suggest bladder neck or urethral obstruction. They measured pressures during filling and voiding in three groups of children – normals, those with proven urethral obstruction (mainly prostatic valves), and those with idiopathic vesicoureteral reflux. There was no difference in voiding pressure between the normal group and those with idiopathic vesicoureteral reflux. The group with obstructive lesions showed high voiding pressures. In the latter group, there was no correlation between the height of the pressure and the presence of reflux. Only a third showed reflux. In adult men with bladder neck obstruction, only 13% show reflux (51). In a further study at Stanford, Zatz (52) measured voiding and intraabdominal pressures in 30 girls with infection. There was no difference between the 15 who showed reflux and the 15 who did not. Puppies normally reflux between 1 and 6 months of age, and this reflux ceases spontaneously. Imposing severe urethral obstruction on refluxing young puppies did not prevent the spontaneous cessation of reflux in any case

(53). All these studies argue against the role of bladder neck obstruction in vesicoureteral reflux.

Recent studies have again focused attention on the possible causal relationships between dysfunctional voiding patterns in the bladder and vesicoureteral reflux and renal scarring. Koff and colleagues (54) investigated 53 children with recurrent urinary tract infection. Over 50% of ureters in this group showed reflux. The children were aged 2.5–17 years and 42% had had febrile pyelonephritic episodes; 68% had had urinary incontinence with frequency, urgency, and precipitate micturition. All children underwent combined cystometry and periurethral muscle sphincter electromyography, and all showed uninhibited detrusor contractions. Under light nitrous oxide anesthesia, these detrusor contractions were associated with sphincter relaxation and micturition. When awake, the same children experienced a sense of urgency with the onset of an uninhibited detrusor contraction; however, they did not usually void urine. Instead, an intense abrupt rise in periurethral muscle sphincter activity occurred with a coincidental sharp rise in intravesical pressure (54).

Allen (55) reported similar studies on a group of children with functional voiding disorders characterized mainly by poor coordination between detrusor activity and external urethral sphincter activity. Fifty percent showed vesicoureteral reflux at the time of the study and several developed reflux during follow-up.

Van Gool (56) also found a high incidence of detrusor sphincter dyssynergia associated with high bladder pressure when the urge to void was resisted. He found that urinary tract infection itself could induce a range of disorders associated with detrusor sphincter hyperactivity associated with high bladder pressures, urgency, and frequency. These studies emphasize the need for more careful studies of bladder pressures and sphincter contractions in children with urinary tract infections. The potential influence of high bladder pressures on the renal parenchyma is clearly apparent from the data quoted above in pigs. Studies in adult women with voiding disorders have also revealed a detrusor hyperreflexia in 43% of patients (57). It is worth emphasizing that the hyperactivity of the sphincter is a functional, not a structural, abnormality and that the old concept of vesical neck obstruction has been clearly and definitively laid to rest (58, 59). Van Gool has

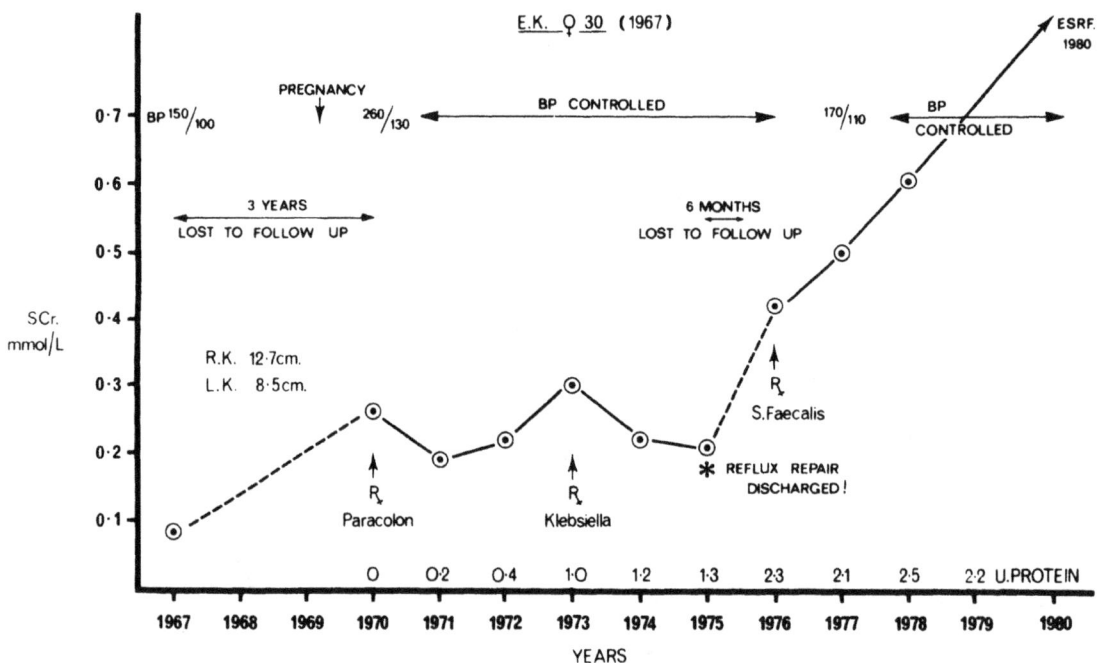

Figure 8. Course in a woman who presented in 1967 at age 30 and developed end-stage renal failure in 1980. This patient had unilateral scarring of the coarse reflux-related type that was complicated by severe hypertension following pregnancy and by intermittent infection. Urinary infection was associated with a temporary impairment of renal function in 1970 and 1973, but renal function improved following treatment on each occasion. Over a period of 6 months following discharge by the surgeon after the repair of left-sided vesicoureteral reflux, renal function deteriorated abruptly. On this occasion, there was no improvement following the treatment of infection and deterioration has continued. Hyalinosis/sclerosis glomerular lesions were first demonstrated in 1971 and proteinuria gradually increased thereafter: ESRF = end-stage renal failure; SCr = serum creatinine; BP = blood pressure; RK = right kidney; LK = left kidney; Rx Paracolon = treatment for paracolon infection; Rx Klebsiella = treatment for *Klebsiella* infection; Rx S. faecalis = treatment for *S. faecalis* infection.

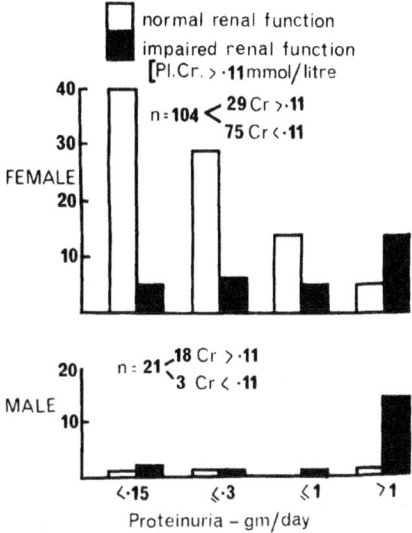

Figure 9. The relationship between proteinuria and impaired renal function in 145 adults with reflux nephropathy. Pl. Cr. = plasma creatinine; Cr = creatinine.

recently extended and expanded his observations on bladder sphincter dysfunction in children with and without vesicoureteric reflux and reports good results from cognitive bladder training (60).

Proteinuria and the nephrotic syndrome

Although factors such as uncontrolled hypertension, recurrent infection, and pregnancy can cause deterioration in renal function in reflux nephropathy, there is now overwhelming evidence that the usual mechanism involved in progression in adults is a secondary glomerular lesion (6–12, 61–65). We first described a progressive glomerular lesion in biopsies from the contralateral kidney in what appeared radiologically to be unilateral reflux nephropathy in 1972 (6, 7). The course in one of the early patients with unilateral disease is recorded in Figure 8. We subsequently documented a glomerular lesion in a large series of patients with reflux nephropathy and proposed that this lesion was the cause of progression (8–11).

Clinically glomerular microscopic hematuria (13, 14) may be present in the urine, but frequently the glomerular erythrocyte count is only just outside the normal range, although the count of urinary casts is elevated. The appearance of the glomerular lesion in reflux nephropathy

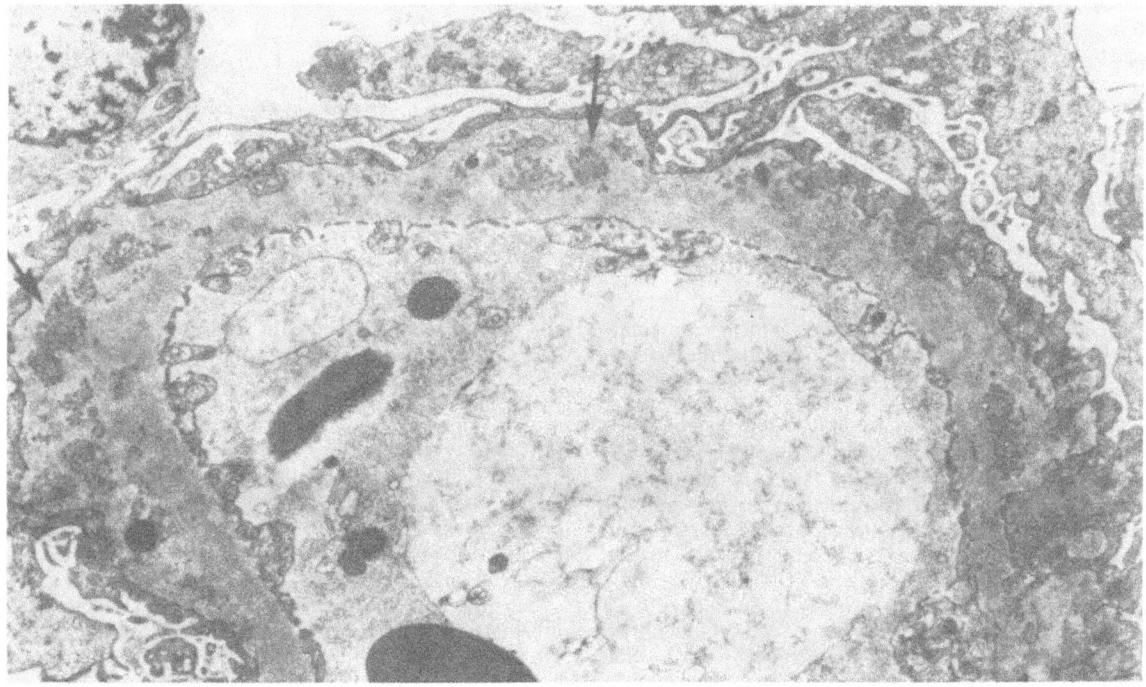

Figure 10. Electron micrograph from a patient with reflux nephropathy, and the light and fluorescent microscopy pattern of membranous glomerulonephritis. On electron microscopy the deposits within the basement membrane consist of collections of small spherical particles (arrows). While these are seen in other biopsies, they have been a particular feature in reflux-associated glomerular lesions (22) (× 8000).

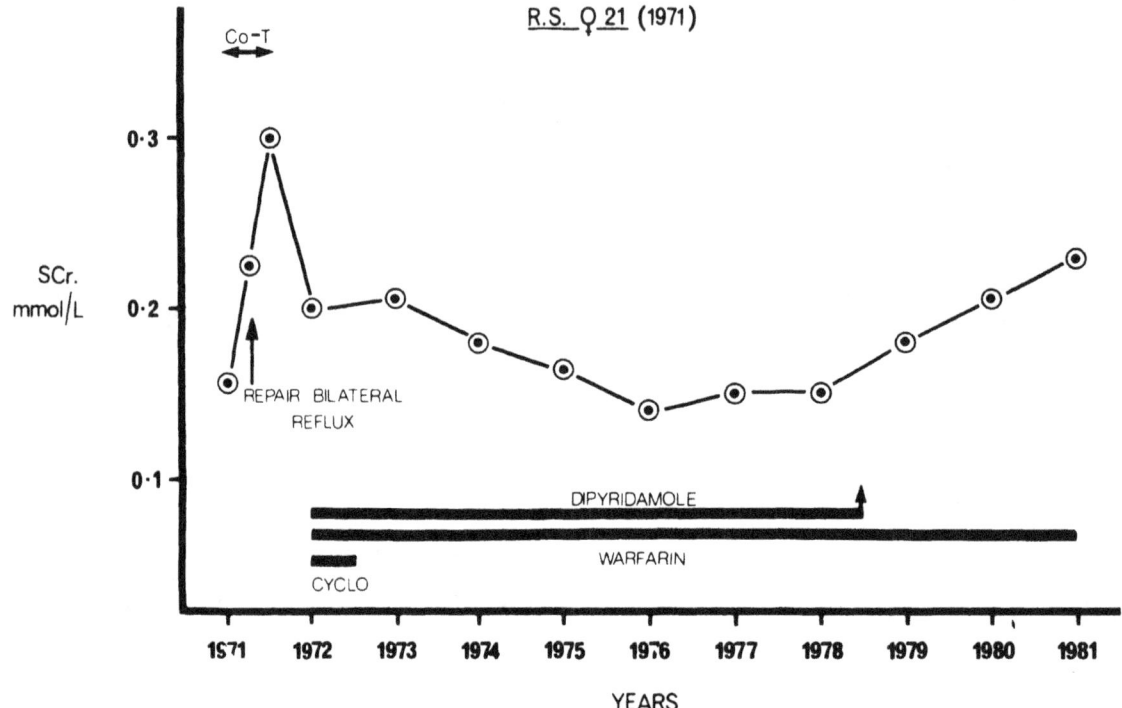

Figure 11. Course in a 21-year-old women who presented in 1971 with rapidly deteriorating renal function that reached a level of 0.3 mm/l over a period of 4 months. Treatment with co-trimoxazole (Co-t) was thought to be a contributing factor. Rapid improvement in renal function followed the withdrawal of co-trimoxazole. Bilateral vesicoureteral reflux repair in 1971 did not halt the functional deterioration. A biopsy at that time showed diffuse membranous glomerulonephritis, and this was treated by a 6-month course of cyclophosphamide, 100 mg/day, and more prolonged treatment with warfarin and dipyridamole. The membranous lesion had disappeared in a biopsy in 1974. Renal function has improved and stabilized over 6 years, but has shown some recent deterioration following withdrawal of dipyridamole. This is a benign course that would usually be expected in a patient with impaired renal function and proteinuria and reflux nephropathy. SCr = serum creatinine; Co-T = co-trimoxazole; CYCLO = cyclophosphamide.

is associated with the development of significant proteinuria (> 0.15 g in 24 hours). Figure 9 shows that the amount of protein in the urine correlates with the degree of impairment in renal function.

Glomerular lesions are not invariably of the focal and segmental hyalinosis and sclerosis morphologic variety. A small percentage of biopsies show other forms of glomerulonephritis. Our own series has included a small number with mesangial IgA glomerulonephritis and membranous glomerulonephritis (10), which could be due to the coexistence of two different lesions.

In some series, however, as many as 10% have been recorded as showing membranous glomerulonephritis (RSNanra, personal communication). This suggests that there may be an underlying immunologic mechanism causing glomerular lesions. The course may be more benign in patients with a membranous glomerular lesion.

Figure 10 shows the electron microscopy in one such patient, and Figure 11 illustrates the benign course in a patient with reflux nephropathy and underlying membranous glomerulonephritis that responded to treatment.

The most logical explanation of the common glomerular lesion, namely, focal and segmental hyalinosis and sclerosis, in reflux nephropathy is that it corresponds to the so-called 5/6 nephrectomy or renal ablation experimental model (66). The major weakness in attributing this lesion to a loss of renal mass (65) is that it occurs in patients with normal-sized (Figure 8) or even hypertrophied contralateral kidneys who have unilateral radiologic scarring (Figure 12 and 13).

Since the first edition of this book it has become apparent that diffuse interstitial parenchymal lesions are present in the areas of preserved or hypertrophied nephrons in reflux nephropathy (67, 68). Needle biopsies from patients with known reflux nephropathy can be distiguished on blind histologic analysis from biopsies of other forms of renal disease on the basis of interstitial abnormalities, such as interstitial scarring around glomeruli ($p < 0.002$), perig-

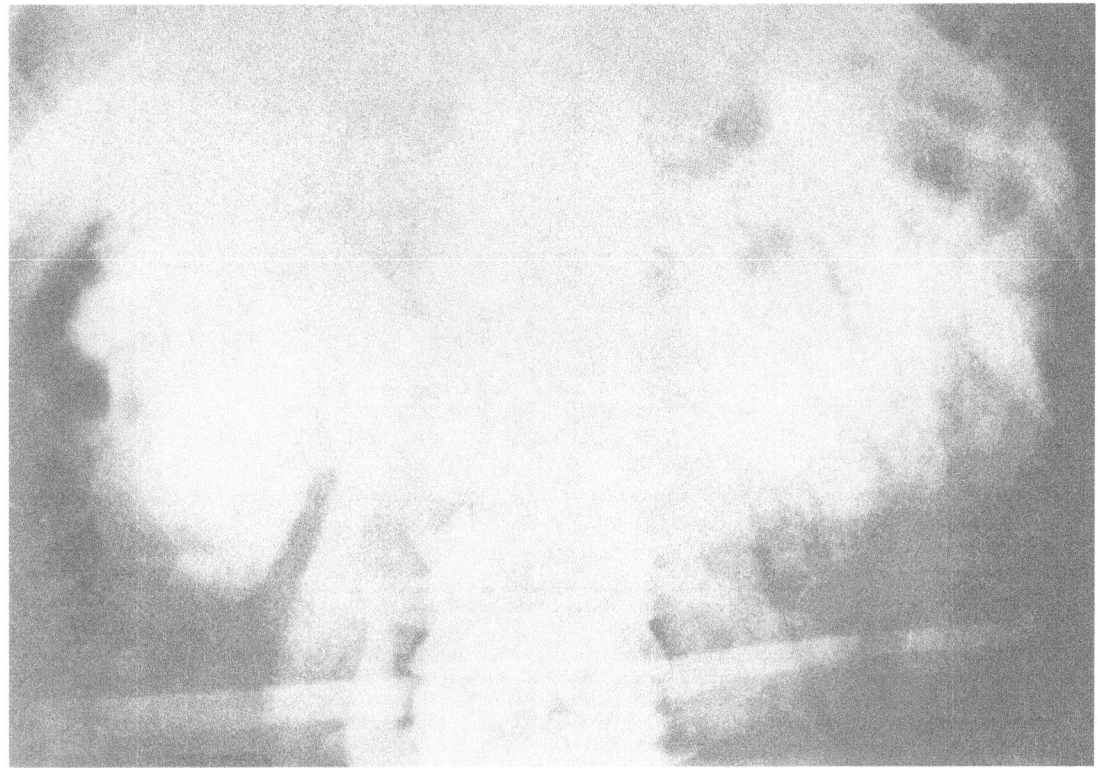

Figure 12. Large (16-cm) right kidney and small scarred left kidney in a woman aged 27 whose course is illustrated in Figure 13.

lomerular fibrosis (p < 0.0001), streaky areas of cortical fibrosis (p < 0.02), dense collagen scars (p < 0.005), and interstitial inflammatory cell infiltration (p < 0.001) (68).

Because these were needle biopsies and hence not selected from scarred areas, these data suggest that diffuse interstitial changes of the type indicated above are diffusely distributed in the cortex in reflux nephropathy.

Because these lesions are detected in adults with no evidence of radiologic parenchymal scarring in the kidney that was biopsied (6–10), and because they are also found in kidneys that show vesicoureteric reflux but no radiologic scars in either kidney (67), these observations suggest that the number of nephrons lost in this diffuse scarring process, together with obvious radiologic scarring, account for significantly more than the apparent 50% renal parenchymal loss.

Focal and segmental glomerulosclerosis and proteinuria have been described in patients with unilateral agenesis (69) and in solitary functioning kidneys (70), hence it is not necessary to seek evidence of loss of more than 50% of the renal parenchyma to explain glomerular lesions, nonetheless in reflux nephropathy it appears that the parenchymal loss is more diffuse and more extensive than is suggested by the presence of radiologic scarring.

Glomeruli are markedly hypertrophied in biopsies from patients with reflux nephropathy, and the glomerular size correlates with the creatinine clearance (Figure 14). Glomerular size also correlates with renal size, and hence with the degree of parenchymal loss detected by radiologic studies (Figure 15).

The greater the degree of glomerular hypertrophy, the greater the impact of hemodynamic factors such as hyperfiltration and hyperperfusion, which are proposed by Hostetter et al. (71) to cause progressive glomerulosclerosis following the reduction of renal mass.

Renal insufficiency

There are some special features about renal insufficiency that are seen in association with reflux nephropathy. A salt-losing tendency may be present, and this is one of the renal conditions that may occasionally mimic Addison's disease.

If the patient is first seen when uremic, the invariable presence of proteinuria, glomerular red cells (see Figure 4), and casts in the urine suggests glomerular disease, and only careful imaging studies will reveal the characteristic pattern of parenchymal scarring. Such patients are often

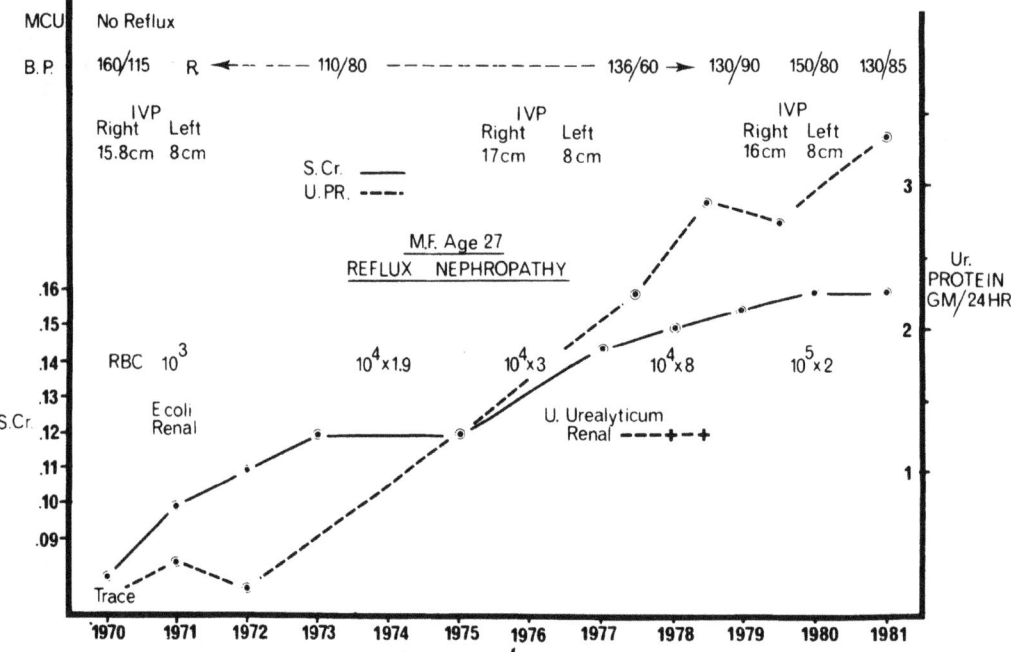

Figure 13. Course over 11 years in a patient with a small scarred left kidney and hypertrophied right kidney whose recent intravenous pyelogram is shown in Figure 12. Urine protein, urinary red cells, and serum creatinine all climbed steadily. In 1981, typical hyalinosis/sclerosis glomerular lesions were detected in an open biopsy from the 16-cm kidney. R. = treatment; B.P. = blood pressure; S.Cr. = serum creatinine; U.PR. = urine protein; RBC = red blood cells/ml of urine; MCU = micturating cystourethrogram; IVP = intravenous pyelogram; E coli renal = *E. coli* renal infection; U. Urealyticum Renal = series of positive cultures for *Ureaplasma urealyticum* renal in localization.

diagnosed as having glomerulonephritis because of reluctance to carry out radiographic studies in patients with advanced renal failure. Arteriography may be helpful in revealing a typical pattern of coarse parenchymal scarring, a picture quite different from the smooth, contracted kidneys of chronic glomerulonephritis. Advances in imaging techniques will facilitate the documentation of renal parenchyma in the future.

Patients with reflux nephropathy present with renal failure at an earlier age than other patients (72). Two thirds of the patients developing end-stage renal failure due to reflux nephropathy in our unit are under the age of 35 years, whereas the mean age of all patients who developed end-stage renal failure in this unit over the same period of time was 42 years (72). Reflux nephropathy accounted for 18% of end-stage renal failure cases in this unit over the period when bilateral nephrectomies were being carried out in all patients. This permitted a specific morphologic diagnosis in each patient (7). The proportion of males developing end-stage renal failure due to reflux nephropathy is greater than would be expected from the far greater preponderance of females in all clinical series. In an earlier study of 68 adults attending this unit, 83% were women and only 17% were men. Impaired renal

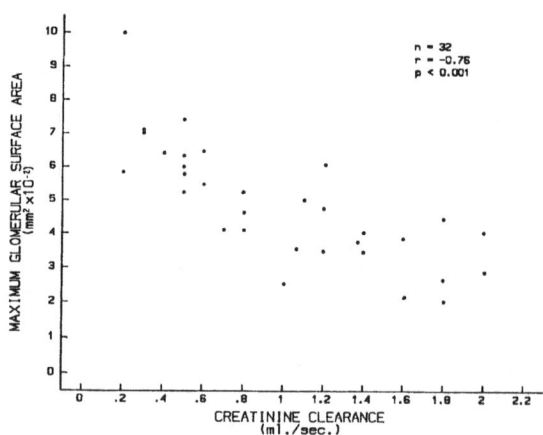

Figure 14. Relationship between maximum glomerular size and creatinine clearance in a series of biopsies in patients with reflux nephropathy.

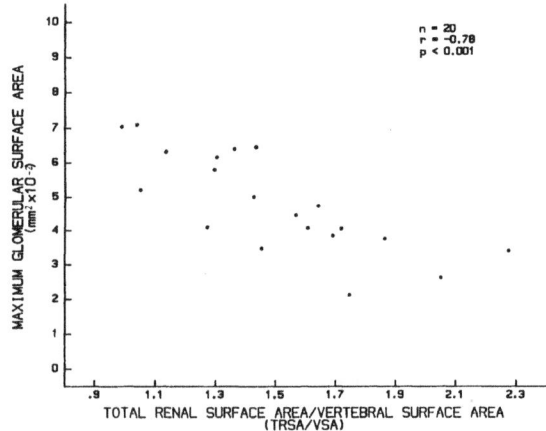

Figure 15. Relationship between maximum glomerular size and renal size, as expressed by the total renal surface area divided by the area of the first three lumbar vertebrae in intravenous pyelograms (glomerular size was measured on renal biopsy).

function was, however, far more frequent in males, and 6 of 7 males had a serum creatinine above 0.15 mm/1 on presentation (12). Figure 9 illustrates that in a much larger series of patients impaired renal function was far more often present in males. In the same hospital, 32% of patients developing end-stage renal failure due to reflux nephropathy were men and 68% females. In some studies, vesicoureteral reflux has been equally distributed between the sexes in patients with end-stage renal failure (73). In a recent 15–30 year follow-up of children who presented with reflux nephropathy, the diffuse form of reflux nephropathy associated with a narrow rim of surviving parenchyma was an important prognostic factor in males. Twenty-eight of 30 males were available for follow-up: eight had developed renal failure, six of these showing the diffuse type of parenchymal lesion with a thin rim of parenchyma (unpublished observations).

PREVENTION OF REFLUX NEPHROPATHY

It is likely that the type of reflux nephropathy that mimics obstruction in which there is a very dilated system with a thin rim of parenchyma cannot usually be prevented, because it is commonly present in the first studies done in infants and is regarded by some as a congenital lesion (5). Van Gool (60), however, showed some convincing tracings of intravenous pyelograms showing increasing dilation of the pelvis and calices, and diffuse parenchymal loss developing in children with meningomyelocoele. Generalized calieactasis developed in association with high-pressure vesicoureteric reflux and infection, and Van Gool implied that it can be prevented in the context of abnormalities associated with spina bifida. Hodson's recent studies (74) on experimental reflux nephropathy in the pig also clearly demonstrated that gross generalized damage with dilatation of calices and considerable parenchymal thinning can occur as a result of sterile high-pressure reflux in the pig. It is important to distinguish this lesion clearly from obstructive atrophy, which is quite different and is much milder than high-pressure reflux nephropathy (75). These experimental results suggest that diffuse scarring associated with high-pressure reflux in children may be preventable in some circumstances.

The coarsely scarred kidney (see Figure 1) is, however, an acquired lesion, and it should be possible to prevent this form of scarring. The small scarred kidney illustrated in Figure 1 results from two processes, one of which is failure to grow and the other is the development of coarse scars.

Infection plays a major role, not only in coarse scar formation, as discussed above, but also in retarding normal growth. Neonatal pyelonephritis will retard renal growth irrespective of the presence or absence of vesicouretric reflux (76). The renal growth pattern in these children remained abnormal for up to 4 years after a single episode of infection. Table 3 shows the results of another large study (77) in which renal growth was normal in almost all children in whom no infection occurred, but slow in a high percentage of cases where infection was documented. Asscher and Chick (78) found that the reflux of heat-killed *E. coli* caused a focal scar in the kidney and retarded growth of the kidney, and suggested that the effect on growth may be mediated by endotoxin.

Almost all coarse scars develop before the age of 7, and all of those documented in a recent large collaborative study were associated with an episode of infection (79). Theoretically, therefore, it should be possible to prevent both coarse scar formation and retarded growth by preventing infection in children with vesicoureteric reflux. In practice, however, 22% of infants already have renal parenchymal scars at first presentation (80). A high prop-

Table 3. Renal growth in relation to urinary tract infection episodes (256 periods of observation)

Renal growth	Urinary tract infection	No urinary tract infection
Slow	31	9
Normal	68	148
Total	99	157

$p < 0.001$.
From Normand & Smellie (77) with permission.

Table 4. Renal growth in relation to previous scarring

Renal growth	Scarred kidney	Nonscarred kidney
Slow	5	3
Normal	14	91
Total	19	94

$p < 0.01$.
From Edwards et al. (85) with permission.

Table 5. Radiologic renal parenchymal loss during follow-up

Management	No. of kidneys		Follow-up	Progressive radiologic parenchymal loss
Edwards et al. (85)				
Continuous prophylaxis	Unscarred	(94)	7–15 years	1 (1.06%)
	Scarred	(19)		1 (5.2%)
Lenaghan et al. (84)				
Multiple micturition	Unscarred	(76)	5–18 years	16 (21%)
Intermittent medication	Scarred	(44)		29 (66%)
Friedland (86)				
Intermittent medication	Treated medically (40)		Mean = 3.8 years	17 (42.5%)
	Treated surgically (37)		3.3 years postsurgery	16 (43.2%)

ortion develop further scars and have impaired renal growth (80).

The presence of scars in the kidney has been shown by several groups to be associated with slow renal growth (Table 4). To prevent both scar formation and to avoid the retardation of renal growth (which occurs with both scars and with episodes of pyelonephritis), it is necessary to prevent renal infection. The great contrast in the percentage of cases that demonstrate progressive evidence of scarring radiologically observed by different groups is likely to relate to the care with which infection is treated.

Three studies are contrasted in Table 5. Smellie's group (77, 81), using long-term continuous chemoprophylaxis with the trimethoprin sulphamethoxazole combination, documented very little progressive scarring. Two studies in which intermittent medication was given only for symptomatic infection showed a much higher percentage of scar formation (83, 84).

The Birmingham prospective trial of treatment of vesicoureteric reflux provides important new information on scar formation (82). To prevent scar formation in reflux nephropathy, it would be necessary to screen for the presence of vesicoureteric reflux by some simple noninvasive technique and to treat those with reflux using long-term chemoprophylaxis to prevent urinary tract infection and hence scar formation. The Birmingham prospective study results (82) offer some hope that scars do not develop in children on continuous chemoprohylaxis.

SPECIFIC THERAPEUTIC APPROACHES

Control of infection

OVERT INFECTION WITH CONVENTIONAL URINARY TRACT PATHOGENS

Continuous antibacterial treatment to prevent recurrent infection and to render the urine sterile must undoubtedly be regarded as the single most important aspect of therapy at the present time. Using this method, Smellie and colleagues (16, 77, 81, 83) have achieved excellent results in

Table 6. Birmingham reflux study group: Progressive scars

	Operative 49 children	Nonoperative 47 children
0–2 years	25%	33%
0–5 years	2.5%	7.5%

terms of a low incidence of new scars and normal renal growth.

The striking differences between Smellie's results using continuous antibacterial medication as a prophylactic measure and two other series of cases where intermittent medication was administered for episodes of infection (Table 5) suggests that the aim should be to maintain a sterile urine in these children and to not use intermittent treatment when episodes of symptomatic infection occur.

Friedland (86) and the previous publication from the same group, as well as Filly and colleagues (83), published a key paper in which a group of medically treated and surgically treated patients were compared. As shown in Table 5, the degree of scarring was the same in both groups. Both were managed with intermittent medication and followed for 3.3 years and 3.8 years, respectively.

The best data comes from the prospective trial in Birmingham. Unpublished data from this trial provided by Professor R.H.R. White show no difference in the rate of scarring in the operative or nonoperative groups either between 0 and 2 years or between 2 and 5 years (Table 6). Both groups were on chemoprophylaxis and no new scars developed in either group beyond 2 years.

There are two aspects of the control of urinary tract infection in these patients. The first is eradication of the infection, and the second is maintaining the urine in a sterile condition. For eradication of infection, any of the conventional antibacterial agents to which the infecting organism is sensitive may be used. There is no evidence that prolonging the course of treatment beyond 1 week is advantageous in eradicating infection (87, 88). With 1 week or 6 weeks of treatment, infection is eradicated in almost all cases. Single-dose treatment, valuable in uncomplicated urinary tract infection, is probably not desirable in patients with vesicoureteral reflux. There is some evidence that a single dose of an antibacterial agent is less likely to eradicate infection when radiologic abnormalities such as pyelonephritic scars are present (89). Eradication of infection should therefore be carried out with a conventional dosage of an appropriate antibacterial agent for 5–7 days. To prevent a recurrence of the infection and to maintain sterile urine after the infection has been eradicated, a drug that is not likely to render fecal enterobacteria resistant should be used. The drug combination that eradicates virtually all common urinary tract pathogens from the fecal flora is the combination of trimethoprim and sulphonamides (90, 91). It was demonstrated many years ago that the use of sulphonamides alone produces resistant strains in the bowel flora and does not prevent recurrences that are caused by organisms resistant to sulphonamides (92). Trimethoprim alone may well be as effective as the combination of trimethoprim with sulphonamide. It is likely that some of the more serious side effects of this medication, such as Stephens Johnson's syndrome and acute renal failure, are due to the sulphonamide component of the combination (93, 94), and there is good justification for careful trials of trimethoprim alone as a long-term prophylactic agent, particularly in children with vesicoureteral reflux who remain on treatment for years. A small dose (one quarter of the regular daily dose) taken at night is usually recommended. If the drug is taken on alternate nights, it still offers protection (95).

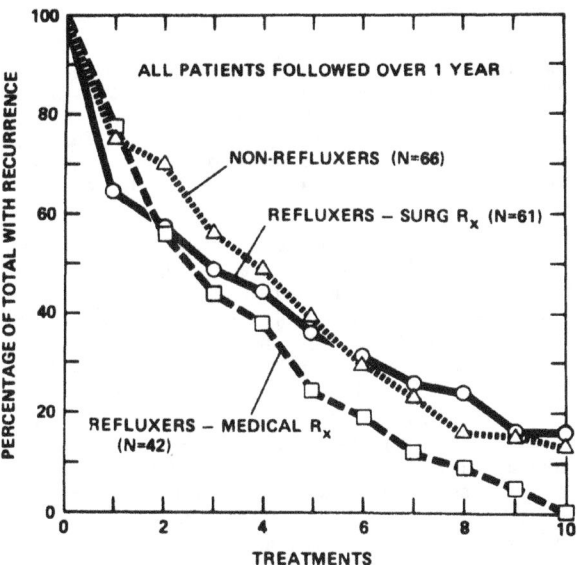

Figure 16. Urinary tract infection in girls. Extraction percentage following each infection. Results of short-term antibacterial therapy in three groups of children with recurrent bacteriuria: 66 without ureteral reflux, 42 with ureteral reflux treated with medical therapy alone, and 61 with reflux corrected surgically. Results as plotted indicate a similar cure rate in each of three groups after each treatment of an infection. Reproduced with permission from Stamey (91).

Table 7. Surgical correction of vesicoureteric reflux: Birmingham study group 1982

Break-through infection in patients	
Operative	Nonoperative
12/49	11/47

Nitrofurantoin is now usually used in the macrocrystalline form, Macrodantin®, because of the lower incidence of gastrointestinal side effects using the latter form (96). This is another drug that does not cause the emergence of resistant strains in the fecal flora and hence is an effective long-term prophylactic agent. Cephalexin is the third antibacterial agent and the only antibiotic that is not associated with the development of resistant strains, presumably because of its absorption high up in the bowel, so that it does not persist in high concentrations in the colon (TA Stamey, personal communication).

Smellie's group advocate continuation of prophylactic antibacterial treatment through childhood in children with reflux nephropathy. It is the need for this long-term supervision to prevent infection that has led many to believe that surgical repair of vesicoureteral reflux is preferable to medical management. It is important to stress that surgical correction does not, however, reduce the rate of subsequent episodes of infection (Figure 16) and does not prevent subsequent scarring (83, 86), which was identical in medically treated children and in those managed by reimplantation of the ureter. The prospective Birmingham study has confirmed that the rate of break-through infections is the same in the operative and nonoperative groups (Table 7).

There is clear evidence that both scar formation and impaired growth are related to infection and much less convincing evidence that they are influenced by persisting vesicoureteral reflux in the absence of infection. Because successful repair of vesicoureteral reflux has not been shown to diminish the risks of subsequent scar formation, it is stressed that careful long-term supervision aimed at the prevention of recurrent urinary tract infection is important in both the medically and surgically treated groups. Surgical reimplantation of the ureter does not exonerate the physician from careful long-term supervision to ensure that urinary infection does not recur.

CONTROL OF OCCULT INFECTION WITH ANAEROBES AND UNUSUAL ORGANISMS

As indicated above, urine aspirated from the bladder may yield a growth of anaerobic organisms and other atypical bacteria (22). Mycoplasmas have been cultured from bladder urine in 37% of patients with reflux nephropathy (21). *Ureaplasma urealyticum*, the organism most frequently cultured, may be difficult to eradicate. It may be sensitive to erythromycin, tetracycline, and to the new drug, rosearmycin (DF Birch, personal communication). In individual patients, an unexpectedly good course may be seen when drugs such as the tetracyclines are used for the long-term

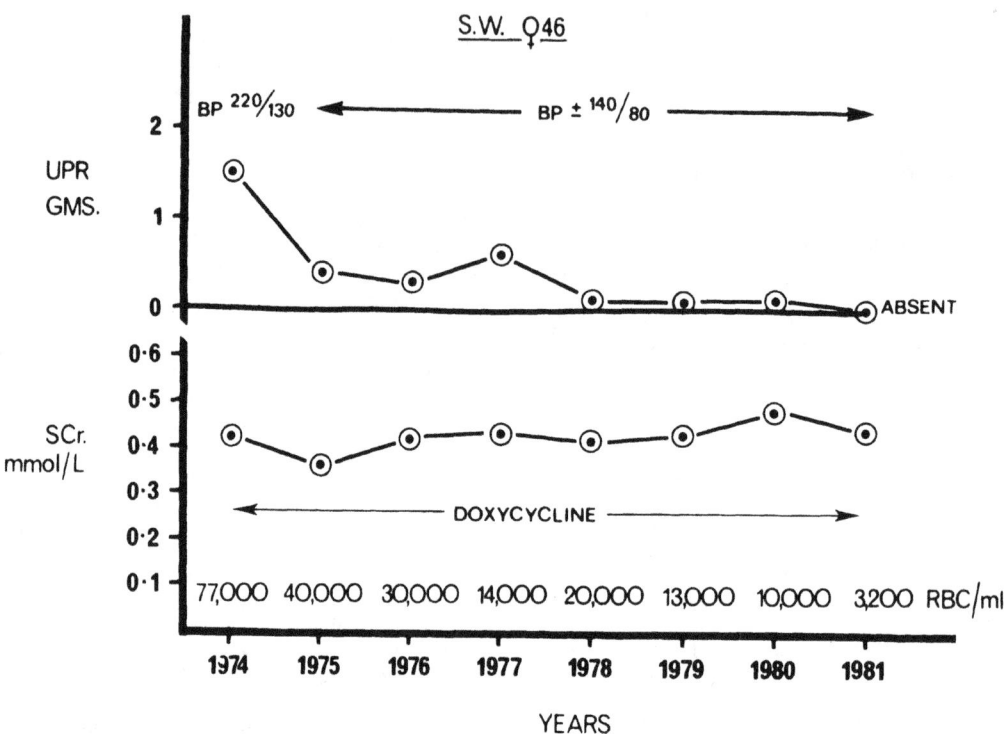

Figure 17. Course in a 46-year-old woman referred in 1974 with severe hypertension and impaired renal function. Although her renal function was severely compromised at the outset, it has remained relatively stable over 7 years. Urine protein has fallen and the reduction in the number of erythrocytes in the urine over the same period suggest that the glomerular lesion has become less active. This course is unusual in advanced reflux-associated nephropathy, but the lesions were clearly those of bilateral chronic atrophic pyelonephritis and were not associated with analgesia. Management included carefull blood pressure control and continuous doxycycline. This was first given for an occult anaerobic streptococcal infection and subsequently continued to prevent recurrences. UPR = urine protein, g/l; SCr. = serum creatinine; RBC/ml = erythrocytes/ml.

control of atypical bacteria (Figure 17). It may be relevant that the patient whose course is illustrated in Figure 17 was treated with tetracycline, which could have been effective against ureaplasma infection as well as the anaerobic *Streptococcus*, which was cultured in 1974. Disappearance of proteinuria and erythrocytes from the urine as well as stable renal function over 7 years after the serum creatinine has reached 0.4 mm/l is very unusual in reflux nephropathy.

Hypertension

THE PLACE OF NEPHRECTOMY FOR CONTROL OF HYPERTENSION IN THE CASE OF A UNILATERAL SCARRED PYELONEPHRITIC KIDNEY

Enthusiasm for surgical removal of kidneys in patients with unilateral reflux nephropathy has waned considerably since the introduction of effective drugs for the control of the blood pressure. In childhood, severe resistant hypertension may still prove a problem and warrant nephrectomy.

Renal vein renin estimations from main and segmental renal veins have been advocated as a guide to the likely outcome of surgery in such patients (36). Recent careful documentation of the levels of renal-vein renin and the outcome of surgery has been carried out at the Hospital for Sick Children in London. Hypertension was cured in 66% of 22 children subjected to surgery on the basis of high renin levels in the main renal veins or in segmental branches. The remaining patients all had significant improvement in blood pressure levels (37). These excellent results warrant consideration of surgical removal of scarred areas of parenchyma in patients, particularly children, in whom the control of hypertension is difficult.

DRUG TREATMENT FOR HYPERTENSION

The renal parenchyma may be very considerably reduced in an adult with bilateral reflux nephropathy. Hypertrophy of the remaining areas of normal glomeruli and tubules may be extreme, and is one of the factors responsible for the irregular surface of a pyelonephritic kidney (see Figure 1). Particular attention should be given to maintaining the blood pressure at normal levels in patients with greatly reduced renal parenchyma. Escape from control for quite a short period can lead to the development of malignant hypertension and end-stage renal failure, presumably because of the very considerable reduction in the renal reserve. Treatment with oral contraceptive agents or pregnancy, may lead to fulminating malignant hypertension in this group of patients (97, 98).

Drugs used in the control of hypertension in patients with reflux nephropathy do not differ overall from those used in essential hypertension, except in the context of severe resistant hypertension, which is particularly likely to develop in childhood or in the post-partum period in patients with reflux nephropathy.

If the blood pressure is resistant to control with conventional agents, the powerful vasodilators, oral diazoxide and minoxidil, will usually quickly bring the blood pressure under control (99–101). The majority of adults can be controlled using a combination of a thiazide with a beta-adrenergic blocking agent and a peripheral vasodilator such as prazosin. Some patients with severe hypertension in whom renal function is deteriorating in the presence of uncontrolled hypertension may remain stable for long periods when the blood pressure is adequately controlled (Figure 17).

Selective beta-adrenergic blocking agents produce less reduction in glomerular filtration rate than nonselective agents, and nadolol may increase the renal blood flow (102). A combination of drugs such as thiazide, prazosin, and methyl dopa will achieve adequate control in most patients, and these drug combinations do not cause reduction in renal blood flow or in the glomerular filtration rate.

There is no doubt that the new converting-enzyme inhibitors are the drugs of choice in the treatment of hypertension in reflux nephropathy. This group of drugs produces a modest increase in the glomerular filtration rate (103), but the most compelling reason for using them relates to the effect on the progression of the glomerular lesion discussed below.

In a few patients with reflux nephropathy, a rapid deterioration in renal function may occur when a converting-enzyme inhibitor is given (Figure 18) (106). This sudden rise in serum creatinine is quickly reversed when the converting-enzyme inhibitor is stopped. This suggests an underlying hemodynamic mechanism, such as has been described in bilateral renal artery stenosis (64, 105). The diffuse narrowing of peripheral vessels in the kidney in patients with hypertenison due to reflux nephropathy (25) and the similarity between the course of the patient illustrated in Figure 18 and the course in a patient with renal artery stenosis suggests that the same mechanism is involved. It is proposed that glomerular filtration pressure is maintained by angiotensin-dependent narrowing in efferent arterioles, and when this is blocked by converting-enzyme inhibition the glomerular filtration rate falls. This hemodynamic change is quickly reversed by cessation of the drug.

Proteinuria and the nephrotic syndrome

Although treatment of a specific glomerular lesion has been associated with apparent improvement, in a few patients (see Figure 11) there is a good correlation between the impairment of renal function and proteinuria (see Figure 9), and the appearance of proteinuria is usually followed by progression to renal failure over 10–15 years.

The recognition that the typical glomerular lesion of focal and segmental hyalinosis and sclerosis in reflux nephropathy almost certainly reflects a reduction in renal mass has opened up a number of therapeutic possibilities that may stabilize the course in patients with reflux nephropathy or slow the rate of progression.

The different types of intervention that have been shown to influence progression in the renal ablation model in animals are

1. Low protein diet (107)
2. Reduction of intraglomerular pressure by converting-enzyme inhibitors (108)
3. Anticoagulant and antiplatelet agents — heparin, warfarin, dipyridamole, and aspirin (109–111)
4. Thromboxane synthetase inhibition (111)

1. *Low-protein diet.* This method, which has been shown to prevent or slow the progression of the glomerular lesion in the renal ablation model in animals, may well have a wide application in renal disease in humans. Preliminary studies have demonstrated the benefit of protein restriction in progressive deterioration in renal function in humans (112, 113)

2. *Reduction of intraglomerular pressure using converting-enzyme inhibitors.* Brenner's group has demonstrated that converting-enzyme inhibitors prevent the development of glomerular capillary hypertension and limit glomerular injury in the renal ablation model in rats (108). Although there are many current studies in progress, this benefit has not yet been conclusively demonstrated in humans, but reflux nephropathy is

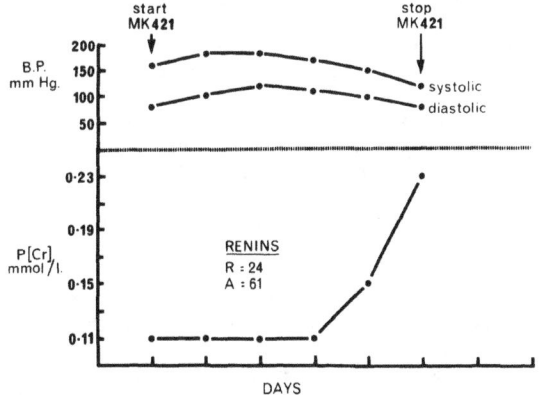

Figure 18. Course in a 38-year-old woman with reflux nephropathy and no renal artery stenosis. P[Cr] = plasma creatinine; B. P. = blood pressure; MK421 = enalapril.

clearly an area in which there is great potential for the study of the effects of converting-enzyme inhibitors on progressive glomerular damage. Reflux nephropathy is the best example in humans of a common disease in which a glomerular lesion develops as a consequence of a reduction of the renal mass.

3. *Anticoagulant and antiplatelet agents.* Benefit in the renal ablation model has been demonstrated with heparin, warfarin, and dipyridamole and aspirin. This suggests that platelets and coagulation may be involved in the progression of the glomerular lesion. Appropriate trials of these drugs have not been carried out in humans.

4. *Thromboxane synthetase inhibitors.* This group of drugs, like antiplatelet drugs, have been shown to have a beneficial effect in animals with a progressive glomerular lesion due to renal ablation. This suggests that platelets may be involved in the pathogenesis of the glomerular lesion. No studies have been done in humans.

Surgical management — the controversy

The demonstration by Stephens, many years ago (114), that vesicoureteral reflux usually disappears spontaneously during childhood caused him to advocate conservative management for vesicoureteral reflux. His early observations have been adequately substantiated by others. Normand and Smellie (77) have recently reported that vesicoureteral reflux disappears during childhood from 79% of refluxing ureters. They further demonstrated that even gross reflux associated with ureteric dilatation disappears in as many as 41% of cases (85). Because of this, the justification for surgical correction of vesicoureteral reflux must be very carefully considered.

It should be stressed again that surgical correction of reflux does not absolve the attending physician from responsibility of arranging careful long-term follow-up after the operation to control infection. A quote from Stamey's recent monograph, "Pathogenesis and Treatment of Urinary Tract Infections" (115), serves to emphasize this: "The more severe the reflux and the worse the renal scarring, the more closely the child must be followed bacteriologically whether reimplanted or not." This view of a well-respected urologist emphasizes the need for careful control of infection in these children, irrespective of prevailing attitudes about whether surgical intervention should or should not be undertaken.

POTENTIAL BENEFITS OF SURGERY FOR VESICOURETERAL REFLUX

Can surgery prevent infection?

If surgery could be shown to prevent infection and could avoid the need for long-term control of infection in childhood, then an operation could be justified on this indication alone. It has been clearly established that reimplantation of the ureters does not reduce the rate of recurrent episodes of infection (see Figure 16). The recent controlled trial of surgical treatment in reflux nephropathy has given a clear answer to this question. Both operative and nonoperative groups were placed on continuous chemoprophylaxis with trimethoprim sulphonamide tablets. Break-through infections occurred with equal frequency in the two groups (see Table 7).

Can surgery prevent segmental scar formation?

Coarse segmental scar formation is rare after the age of five, hence, if surgery has a place in the prevention of scar formation, repair of reflux would need to be carried out in infancy, as advocated by McRae and colleagues (116). Scars form as a result of infection and there is little if any evidence in humans that scars form in the absence of infection (see Infection). Continuous control of infection has been shown to be associated with a very low incidence of new scar formation (see Table 5) (16, 79, 85). It has been demonstrated that the risk of developing a scar is the same in a surgically treated group as it is in groups treated with intermittent antibacterial treatment (83, 86), and both of these are substantially higher than the rate of new scar formation observed by Smellie's group using continuous antibacterial agents (see Table 5) (16, 79, 85). This suggests that the benefit of surgery in preventing subsequent scar formation is small. The best data on this again comes from the Birmingham controlled trial of surgery in reflux nephropathy. There was no significant difference in the occurrence of scars in the operative and nonoperative groups at either 2 or 5 years (see Table 6). No new scars developed in either group after 2 years, demonstrating again in this prospective study the efficacy of chemoprophylaxis in preventing new scar formation.

Surgical treatment of vesicoureteral reflux — the current status.

When reimplantation of ureters has been undertaken, it has usually been done in the hope of preventing further infection and further scar formation (117, 118). Controversy has arisen because reflux disappears from 79% of refluxing ureters during childhood and because scar formation is very rare with careful conservative management (16, 79, 85). The further evidence that the same degree of scarring occurs after surgical correction as occurs in patients managed conservatively (83, 86) makes it difficult to defend reimplantation of refluxing ureters at the present time.

McRae and colleagues (116) advocate surgery in infants with gross reflux in whom they claimed restoration of a normal growth. Because infection alone can have a profound impact on renal growth in infants (76), this question can really only be answered by a controlled study. The question of prevention of scar formation by surgical correction is also the subject of controlled studies. Three controlled trials are currently being carried out: one at the Hospital for Sick Children in London, one in Birmingham, and an international study being conducted in the United States and Germany. The preliminary results of the Birmingham study have been published (82). These show no significant differences in renal function, renal growth, or scar formation up to 5 years after entry.

The prospective controlled trial of surgical correction of reflux at the Hospital for Sick Children in London is now in its eighth year. This study comparing two groups of infants with severe reflux — one treated by surgical repair of vesicoureteral reflux and the other managed conservatively — has not yet shown any difference between the two groups. In both groups, urinary tract infection is under constant supervision and control (42). The results of the international study are not yet available.

Management during pregnancy

Vesicoureteral reflux or reflux nephropathy is often first diagnosed during pregnancy. Complications of pregnancy are frequent and may be serious (84, 119). Twenty-seven percent of adult women in our study developed their first symptoms during pregnancy. Urinary tract infection and hypertension were the most frequent complications of pregnancy (12).

Scarring of the type seen with vesicoureteral reflux was the most frequent lesion found in association with asymptomatic bacteriuria detected by screening pregnant women for infection. This type of scarring accounted for over half the radiologic abnormalities detected in this study (120). Nineteen percent of women with pregnancy bacteriuria had undoubted reflux-type parenchymal scars, and a further 20% had probable reflux nephropathy. Over 50% of all intravenous pyelograms in women with pregnancy bacteriuria were abnormal. Calculating on the basis of the number of classical parenchymal scars detected in the screened population of 4000 normal pregnant women, this suggests that vesicoureteral reflux is not a rare disease and may be present in a little under 1% of women.

Investigation of women who develop symptomatic urinary tract infection during pregnancy will reveal a high percentage of patients with radiologic evidence of coarse parenchymal scars. Because we now know that reflux nephropathy may progress in adults, the investigation of women who develop symptomatic or asymptomatic infection during pregnancy is desirable as a means of identifying this group of "at-risk" patients.

Women with bilateral small scarred kidneys due to reflux nephropathy and impaired renal function have a significant risk of developing malignant hypertension and renal failure during pregnancy (97, 119). A marked rise in serum urea and creatinine may occur during pregnancy, and resistant malignant hypertension is a common mode of rapid progression to end-stage renal failure in the postpartum period.

It is likely that this progression after pregnancy is due to similar occlusive vessel changes to those seen in postpartum thrombotic microangiopathy (119). Because thrombosis is the mechanism underlying such vessel lesions, we have used treatment with heparin and by plasma exchange in an attempt to prevent these vessel lesions (121).

JUDGING THE EFFICIENCY OF MANAGEMENT

Reflux nephropathy has a different impact in the child and the adult. In the child, benefits of therapy can be assessed largely by the prevention of scar formation and the preservation of normal renal growth rates. Very careful measurements of the renal parenchyma and comparison with normal expected growth curves must be carried out in assessing the damage (122).

Careful assessment of renal function of the two kidneys has been used by some groups (123). In adults, renal function tests provide a more accurate assessment of the efficiency of management than repeated radiographic studies, because scar formation is rare and progression is due to diffuse parenchymal disease. Accurate assessment of urine protein provides the most accurate guide to prognosis, and once it appears a deteriorating course is likely. Only an occasional patient will show a gradual decline in the amount of protein in the urine, and in such patients renal function may stabilize even when severely impaired (see Figure 17).

PROGNOSTIC FACTORS

In infancy, the severity of the reflux is an important prognostic factor. The more severe the reflux, the greater the degree of initial scarring and subsequent scarring (80, 85). The degree of parenchymal scarring is important in both children and adults. Children with parenchymal scars are likely to develop more scars in the same kidney (see Table 5). Patients with advanced bilateral scarring may develop end-stage renal failure during childhood. They may also develop severe hypertension during childhood.

In adults, in addition to the extent of parenchymal scarring, the major prognostic factor is the presence of proteinuria, which indicates that a secondary glomerular lesion has developed. This is the usual mode of progression to renal failure in adults. Some patients with considerably reduced renal parenchyma bilaterally may remain stable, whereas others with a normal kidney on one side may progress to end-stage renal failure.

Severe hypertension is an important prognostic factor in both children and adults. Modern antihypertensive medication has improved the outlook in such patients.

REFERENCES

1. Hodson CJ, Edwards D: Chronic pyelonephritis and vesicoureteric reflux. *Clin Radiol* 11:219–231, 1960.
2. Hodson CJ: The mechanism of scar formation in chronic pyelonephritis. In: Kincaid-Smith P, Fairley KF (eds) Renal Infection and Renal Scarring. Mercedes, Melbourne, 1971, p 327.
3. Hodson CJ, Maling TM, McManamon PJ, Lewis MG: The pathogenesis of reflux nephropathy (chronic atrophic pyelonephritis). *Br J Radiol* (Suppl 13): 1–26, 1975.
4. Rolleston GL, Maling TM, Hodson CJ: Intrarenal reflux and the scarred kidney. *Arch Dis Child* 49: 531–539, 1974.
5. Heale WF: Age of presentation and pathogenesis of reflux

nephropathy. In: CJ Hodson, P Kincaid-Smith, eds, *Reflux Nephropathy*. Masson Publishing, New York, p 140, 1979.
6. Kincaid-Smith P: Discussion: Classification of glomerulonephritis. In: P Kincaid-Smith, TH Mathew, EL Becker, eds, *Glomerulonephritis: Morphology, Natural History and Treatment*. John Wiley & Sons, New York, p 155, 1973.
7. Kincaid-Smith P: The prevention of renal failure. In: *Proceedings of the 6th International Congress of Nephrology, Vol 3*. Mexico, 1972. Karger, Basel, pp 100–118, 1974.
8. Kincaid-Smith P: Glomerular lesions in atrophic pyelonephritis and reflux nephropathy. *Kidney Int 8* (Suppl 4): 81–83, 1975.
9. Kincaid-Smith P: *The Kidney: a Clinicopathological Study*. Blackwell Scientific Publications, London, p 354, 1975.
10. Kincaid-Smith P: Glomerular and vascular lesions in chronic atrophic pyelonephritis and reflux nephropathy. In: J Hamburger, J Crosnier, MH Maxwell, eds, *Advances in Nephrology*. Year Book Medical, Chicago, pp 3–17, 1975.
11. Kincaid-Smith P, Becker GJ: Reflux nephropathy in the adult. In: CJ Hodson, P Kincaid-Smith, eds, *Reflux Nephropathy*. Masson Publishing, New York, pp 21–28, 1979.
12. Kincaid-Smith P, Becker GJ: Reflux nephropathy and chronic atrophic pyelonephritis: A review. *J Infect Dis* 138:774–780, 1978.
13. Fairley KF, Birch DF: Haematuria: Glomerular or nonglomerular. *Lancet* 2:845, 1979.
14. Fairley KF, Birch DF: Haematuria: A simple method for identifying glomerular bleeding. *Kidney Int* 21:105-108, 1981.
15. Heale WF, Ferguson RS: The pathogenesis of renal scarring in children. In: EH Kass, W Brumfitt, eds, *Infections of the University of Chicago Press, Chicagoo*, p 201, 1978.
16. Smellie J, Edwards D, Hunter N, Normond ICS, Prescod N: Vesicoureteric reflux and reflux scarring. *Kidney Int* 8 (Suppl 4):65–72, 1975.
17. Kunin CM: Emergence of bacteriuria, proteinuria and symptomatic urinary tract infections among a population of school girls followed for 7 years. *Paediatrics* 41:968, 1968.
18. Cardiff-Oxford Bacteriuria Study Group: Sequelae of covert bateriuria in schoolgirls. A four year follow-up study. *Lancet* 1:889-893, 1978.
19. Rolleston GL: The significance and management of vesicoureteric reflux in infancy. Part 2. Radiological aspects. In: P Kincaid-Smith, KF Fairley, eds, *Renal Infection and Renal Scarring*. Mercedes, Melbourne, p 246, 1971.
20. Fairley KF, Butler HM: Sterile pyuria as a manifestation of occult bacterial pyelonephritis with special reference to intermittent bacteriuria. In: P Kincaid-Smith, KF Fairley, eds, *Renal Infection and Renal Scarring*. Mercedes, Melbourne, p 51, 1971.
21. Birch DF, Fairley KF, Pavillard RE: Unconventional bacteria in urinary tract disease: *Ureaplasma urealyticum*. *Kindney Int* 19:58–64, 1981.
22. Fairley KF, Becker GJ, Butler HM, McDowall DRM, Leslie DW: Diagnosis in the difficult case. *Kidney Int* 8:S12-S19, 1975.
23. Longcope WT: Chronic bilateral pyelonephritis: Its origin and its association with hypertension. *Ann Intern Med* 11:149, 1937.
24. Weiss S, Parker F Jr: Pyelonephritis: Its relation to vascular lesions and to arterial hypertension. *Medicine* 18:221, 1939.
25. Kincaid-Smith P: Vascular obstruction in chronic pyelonephritic kidneys and its relation to hypertension. *Lancet* 2:1263–1269, 1955.
26. Brod J: Chronic pyelonephritis. *Lancet* 1:1973, 1956.
27. Bengtsson U, Hogdahi A-M, Hood B: Chronic non-obstructive pyelonephritis and hypertension: A long-term study. *J Med* 37:361, 1968.
28. Heptinstall RH: Malignant hypertension: A study of 51 cases. *J Pathol Bacteriol* 65:423, 1953.
29. Kincaid-Smith P, McMichael J, Murphy EA: The clinical course and pathology of hypertension with papilloedema (malignant hypertension). *J Med (New Series 27)*: 117–153, 1958.
30. Kimmelstiel P, Kim OJ, Beres JA, Wellmann K: Chronic pyelonephritis. *Am J Med* 30:589, 1961.
31. Holland HN, Kotchen T, Bhathena D: Hypertension in children with chronic pyelonephritis. *Kidney Int 8* (Suppl 5):243–251, 1975.
32. Holland NH: Reflux nephropathy and hypertension. In: W Hodson, P Kincaid-Smith, eds, *Reflux Nephropathy*. Masson publishing, New York, p 257, 1979.
33. Andersen HJ, Jacobsson B, Larsson H, Winberg J: Hypertension, asymmetric renal parenchymal defect, sterile urine and high E. coli antibody titre. *Br Med J* 3:14–18, 1973.
34. Still JL, Cottom D: Severe hypertension in childhood. *Arch Dis Child* 42:34–39, 1967.
35. Savage JM, Dillon MJ, Shah V, Barratt TM, Williams D: Renin and blood pressure in children with renal scarring and vesicoureteric reflux. *Lancet* 2:441–444, 1978.
36. Poutasse F, Stecker J Jr, Ladage LE, Sperber E: Malignant hypertension in children secondary to chronic pyelonephritis: Laboratory and radiological indications for partial or total nephrectomy. *J Urol* 119:264–267, 1978.
37. Dillon MJ, Smellie JM: Peripheral plasma renin activity, hypertension and renal scarring in children. In: CJ Hodson, RH Heptinstall, J Winberg, eds, *Reflux Nephropathy Update 1983*. Karger, Basel. *Contr Nephrol* 39:68–80, 1984.
38. Kincaid-Smith P: Clinical implications of reflux in the adult. In: W Zurukzoglu, M Papadimitriou, M Pyrpasopoulos, M Sion, C Zamboulis, eds, *Proceedings of the 8th International Congress of Nephrology*, Athens, 1981. Karger, Basel, pp 359–362, 1981.
39. Heptinstall RH, Hodson CJ: Pathology of sterile reflux in the pig. In: CJ Hodson, RH Heptinstall, J Winberg, eds, *Reflux Nephropathy Update 1983*. Karger, Basel. Contr Nephrol 39:344–357, 1984.
40. Bailey RR, McRae CU, Maling TM, Tisch G, Little PJ: Renal vein renin concentration in the hypertension of unilateral reflux nephropathy. *J Urol* 120:21–23, 1978.
41. Hodson CJ: Sterile reflux. In: W Zurukzoglu, M Papadimitriou, M Pyrpasopoulos, M Sion, C Zamboulis, eds, *Proceedings of the 8th International Congress of Nephrology*, Athens, 1981. Karger, Basel, pp 368–373, 1981.
42. Ransley PG: The renal papilla, intrarenal reflux and chronic pyelonephritis. In: W Zurukzoglu, M Papadimitriou, M Pyrpasopoulos, M Sion, C Zamboulis, eds, *Proceedings of the 8th International Congress of Nephrology*, Athens, 1981. Darger, Basel, pp 363–367, 1981.
43. Kincaid–Smith P, Hodson CJ: Lesions in the pig kidney with chronic reflux nephropathy. In: CJ Hodson, P Kincaid-Smith, eds, *Reflux Nephropathy*. Masson Publishing, New York, pp 197–212, 1979.
44. Ransley AG, Risdon RA: Reflux and renal scarring. *Br J Radiol* (Suppl 14):1978.
45. Cotran RS, Hodson CJ: Extratubular localization of Tamm-Horsfall protein in experimental reflux nephropathy in the pig. In: Hodson CJ, Kincaid-Smith P (eds) *Reflux Nephropathy*. Masson Publishing, New York, p 213, 1979.
46. Hoyer JR: Tubulointerstitial immune complex nephritis in

rats immunized with Tamm-Horsfall protein. *Kidney Int* 17:284–292, 1980.
47. Fasth A, Hanson LA, Fodal U, Peterson H: Antibodies to Tamm-Horsfall protein associated with urinary tract infections in girls. *J Pediatr* 95:54–60, 1979.
48. Hoyer JR, Ishidate T: Pathophysiology of Tamm-Horsfall protein in tubulointerstitial nephritis. In: W Zurukzoglu, M Papdimitriou, M Pyrpasopoulos, M Sion, C Zamboulis, eds, *Proceedings of the 8th International Congress of Nephrology*, Athens, 1981. Karger, Basel, pp 783–789, 1981.
49. Fasth A, Jodal U: Autoantibodies against Tamm-Horsfall Protein: Their usefulness as indicators of presence of renal damage and reflux. In: W Zurukzoglu, M Papadimitriou, M Pyrpasopoulos, M Sion, C Zamboulis, eds, *Proceedings of the 8th International Congress of Nephrology*, Athens, 1981. Karger, Basel, pp 790–796, 1981.
50. Stephens FD, Lenaghan D: The anatomical basis and dynamics of vesicoureteral reflux. *J Urol* 87:669, 1962.
51. Morillo MM, Orandi A, Fernandes M, Draper JW: Vesicoureteral reflux in male adults with bladder neck obstruction. *J Urol* 89:389, 1963.
52. Zatz LM: Combined physiologic and radiologic studies of bladder function in female children with recurrent urinary tract infection. *Invest Urol* 3:278, 1965.
53. Lenaghan D, Cussen LJ: Vesicoureteral reflux in pups. *Invest Urol* 5:449, 1968.
54. Koff SA, Lapides J, Piazza DH: The uninhibited bladder in children: A cause for urinary obstruction, infection and reflux. In: CJ Hodson, P Kincaid-Smith, eds, *Reflux Nephropathy*. Masson Publishing, New York, pp 161–170, 1979.
55. Allen TD: Vesicoureteral reflux as a manifestation of dysfunctional voiding. In: CJ Hodson, P Kincaid-Smith, eds, *Reflux Nephropathy*. Masson Publishing, New York, p 171, 1979.
56. Van Gool JD: Bladder infection and pressure. In: CJ Hodson, P Kincaid-Smith, eds, *Reflux Nephropathy*. Masson Publishing, New York, p 181, 1979.
57. Godec CJ, Eshq J, Cass AS: Correlation among cystometry, urethral pressure profilometry and pelvic floor electromyograpjy in the evaluation of female patients with voiding dysfunction symptoms. *J Urol* 124:678–682, 1980.
58. Shopfner CE: Roentgenological evaluation of bladder neck obstruction. *Am J Roentegenol* 100:162–176, 1967.
59. Stamey TA: Urinary infections in infancy and childhood. In: *Pathogenesis and Treatment of Urinary Tract Infections*. Williams & Wikins, Baltimore, p 310, 1980.
60. Van Gool JD, Kuitjen RH, Donckerwolcke RA, Messer AP, Vijverberg M: Bladder-sphincter dysfunction, urinary infection and vesico-ureteral reflux with special reference to cognitive bladder training. In: CJ Hodson, RH Heptinstall, J Winberg, eds, *Reflux Nephropathy Update 1983*. Karger, Basel. Contr Nephrol 39:190–210, 1984.
61. Aladjem M, Schoeneman MJ, Bennett B, Levitt S, Spitzer A, Greifer T: Focal segmental glomerulosclerosis with proteinuria and chronic interstitial nephritis. *N Y State J Med*:579, 1978.
62. Bhatena DB, Weiss JH, Holland NH, McMorrow RG, Curtis JJ, Lucas Ba, Luke EG: Focal and segmental glomerular sclerosis in reflux nephropathy (chronic pyelonephritis). *Am J Med* 68:886–892, 1980.
63. Senekjian HO, Stinebaugh BJ, Mattioli CA, Suki WN: Irreversible renal failure following vesicoureteral reflux. *JAMA* 241:169, 1979.
64. Torres VE, Velosa JA, Holley KE, Kelalis PP, Stickler GB, Kurtz SB: The progression of vesicoureteral reflux nephropathy. *Ann Intern Med* 92:776, 1980.
65. Cotran RS: Pathogenetic mechanisms in the progression of reflux nephropathy: The roles of glomerulosclerosis and extravasation of Tamm-Horsfall protein. In: W Zurukzoglu, M Papadimitriou, M Pyrpasopoulos, M Sion, C Zamboulis, eds, *Proceedings of the 8th International Congress of Nephrology*, Athens, 1981. Karger, Basel, pp 374–381, 1981.
66. Shimamura T, Morrison AB: A progressive glomerulosclerosis occurring in partial five-sixth nephrectomized rats. *Am J Pathol* 79:95–106, 1975.
67. Kincaid–Smith P: Glomerular lesions in atrophic pyelonephritis (RN). In: P Kincaid-Smith, J Hodson, eds, *Reflux Nephropathy*. Masson Publishing, New York, pp 268–272, 1979.
68. Kincaid-Smith P: Diffuse parenchymal lesions in reflux nephropathy and the possibility of making a renal biopsy diagnosis in reflux nephropathy. In: GM Berlyne, S Giovanetti, eds, *Contributions to Nephrology*. Karger, Basel, 1984, 39:111–115.
69. Kiprov DD, Colvin RB, McCluskey RT: Focal and segmental glomerulosclerosis and proteinuria associated with unilateral renal agenesis. *Lab Invest* 46:275–281, 1982.
70. Bhatena DB, Julian BA, McMorrow RG, Baehler RW: Focal sclerosis of hypertrophied glomeruli in solitary functining kidneys of humans. *Am J Kid Dis* 5:226–232, 1985.
71. Hostetter TH, Olson JL, Rennke HG, Venkatachatan MA, Brenner BM: Hyperfiltration in remnant nephrons: A potentially adverse response to renal ablation. *Am J Physiol* 241:585–592, 1981.
72. Kincaid-Smith P: Pyelonephritis, chronic interstitial nephritis and obstructive uropathy. In: J Hamburger, ed, *Nephrology*. John Wiley & Son, New York, pp 553–582, 1979.
73. Bakshardeh K, Charles L, Carrion H: Vesicoureteral reflux and end stage renal disease. *J Urol* 116:557–558, 1976.
74. Hodson CJ, Twohaill SA: The time factor in the development of sterile renal scarring following high-pressure vesicoureteral reflux. In: CJ Hodson, RH Heptinstall, J Winberg, eds, *Reflux Nephropathy Update 1983*. Karger, Basel. Contr Nephrol 39:358–369, 1984.
75. Hodson CJ, Craven JD: Experimental obstructive nephropathy in the pig. *Br J Urol* 14 (Suppl 6):3-57, 1969.
76. Winberg J, Claesson I, Jacobsson B, Jodal U, Petersen H: Renal growth after acute pyelonephritis in childhood: An epidemiological approach. In: CJ Hodson, P Kincaid-Smith, eds, *Reflux Nephropathy*. Masson Publishing, New York, p 309, 1979.
77. Normand C, Smellie J: Vesicoureteric reflux: The case for conservative management. In: CJ Hodson, P Kincaid-Smith, eds, *Reflux Nephropathy*. Masson Publishing, New York, p 281, 1979.
78. Asscher AW, Chick S: Increased susceptibility of the kidney to ascending *Escherichia coli* infection following unilateral nephrectomy. *Br J Urol* 44:202, 1972.
79. Smellie JM, Ransley PG, Normand ICS, Prescod N, Edwards D: Development of new renal scars: A collaborative study. *Br Med J* 290:1957–1960, 1985.
80. Rolleston GL, Shannon FT, Utley WLF: Relationship of infantile vesicoureteric reflux to renal damage. *Br Med J* 1:460, 1970.
81. Smellie JM, Gruneberg RN, Leakey EN, Atkin W: Long-term low dose co-trimoxazole in prophylaxis of childhood urinary tract infection — clinical aspects. *Br Med J* 2:203–206, 1976.

82. Birmingham Reflux Study Group: Prospective trial of operative versus non-operative treatment of severe vesicoureteric reflux: Two years' observation in 96 children. *Br Med J* 287:171–174, 1983.
83. Filly RA, Friedland GW, Goven DE, Fair WR: Development and progression of clubbing and scarring in children with recurrent urinary tract infections. *Radiology* 113:145–153, 1974.
84. Lenaghan D, Whitaker JG, Jensen F, Stephens FD: The natural history of reflux and long-term effects of reflux on the kidney. *J Urol* 115:728–730, 1976.
85. Edwards D, Normand ICS, Prescod N, Smellie JM: Disappearance of vesicoureteric reflux during long-term prophylaxis of urinary tract infection in children. *Br Med J* 2:285–288, 1977.
86. Friedland GW: Post-reimplantation renal scarring. In: CJ Hodson, P Kincaid-Smith, eds, *Reflux Nephropathy*. Masson Publishing, New York, p 323, 1979.
87. Kincaid-Smith P, Friedman A, Nanra RS: Controlled trials of treatment in urinary tract infection. In: P Kincaid-Smith, KF Fairley, eds, *Renal Infection and Renal Scarring*. Mercedes Publishing Services, Melbourne, pp 165–174, 1971.
88. Kincaid-Smith P, Fairely KF: Controlled trial comparing effect of two and six weeks treatment in recurrent urinary tract infection. *Br Med J* 2:145–146, 1969.
89. Fairley KF, Whitworth JA, Kincaid-Smith P, Durman O: Single dose therapy in the management of urinary tract infection. *Med J Aust* 2:75–76, 1978.
90. Stamey TA: General and specific principles of therapy. In: *Pathogenisis and Treatment of Urinary Tract Infections*. Williams & Wilkins, Baltimore, p 569, 1980.
91. Stamey TA: Urinary tract infections in women. In: *Pathogenesis and Treatment of Urinary Tract Infections*. Williams & Wilkins, Baltimore, p 143, 1980.
92. Lincoln K, Lidin-Janson G, Winberg J: Treatment trials in urinary tract infection with special reference to the effect of antibodies on the faecal flora. In: P Kincaid-Smith, KF Fairley, eds, *Renal Infection and Renal Scarring*. Mercedes, Melbourne, p 151, 1971.
93. Richmond JM, Whitworth JA, Fairley KF, Kincaid-Smith P: Co-trimoxazole nephrotoxicity. *Lancet* 1:493, 1979.
94. Kalowski S, Nanra RS, Mathew TH, Kincaid-Smith P: Deterioration in renal function in association with Co-trimoxazole therapy. *Lancet* 1:394–397, 1973.
95. Harding GKM, Buckwald FJ, Marrie TJ, Thompson L, Light RB, Ronald AR: Prophylaxis of recurrent urinary tract infection in female patients. *JAMA* 242 (18):1975–1977, 1979.
96. Kalowski S, Radford N, Kincaid-Smith P: Crystalline and macrocrystalline nitrofurantoin in the treatment of urinary tract infection. *N Engl J Med* 290:385–387, 1974.
97. Fairley KF: Hypertension and renal disease in pregnancy. In: W Zurukzoglu, M Papadimitriou, M Pyrpasopoulos, M Sion, C Zamboulis, eds, *Proceedings of the 8th International Congress of Nephrology*, Athens, 1981. Karger, Basel, pp 440–444, 1981.
98. Fairley KF: Hypertension associated with oral contraceptive agents and hypertension in pregnancy. In: P Kincaid-Smith, JA Whitworth, eds, *Hypertension: Mechanisms and Management*. ADIS Science Press, Sydney, pp 112–116, 1982.
99. Fang P, MacDonald IM, Laver M, Hua A, Kincaid-Smith P: Oral diazoxide in uncontrolled malignant hypertension. *Med J Aust* 2:621–624, 1974.8
100. Kincaid-Smith P, Fang P, Laver MC: A new look at the treatment of severe hypertension. *Clin Sci Mol Med* 45:75S–87S, 1973.
101. Kincaid-Smith P: The treatment of resistant hypertension. *Drugs 11* (Suppl 1):78–86, 1976.
102. Hollenbers NK, Douglass FA, McKinstry DW, Williams GH, Borucki LJ, Sulivan JM: Beta-adrenoreceptor blocking agents and the kidney: Effect of nadolol and proparanolol on the renal circulation. *Br J Clin Pharmacol* 7 (Suppl 2):219S–225S, 1979.
103. Hollenberg NK, Swartz SL, Dian R, Passan BS, Williams GH: Increased glomerular filtration rate after converting enzyme inhibition in essential hypertension. *N Engl J Med* 301:9–12, 1979.
104. Hricick DE, Brownong PJ, Kopelman R, Goorno WE, Madias NE, Dzau VJ: Captopril-induced functional renal insufficiency in patients with bilateral renal-artery stenoses or renal-artery stenosis in a solitary kidney. *N Engl J Med* 308:373–376, 1983.
105. Curtis JJ, Luke RG, Whelchel JD, Diethelm AG, Jones P, Dustan HP: Inhibition of angiotensin-converting enzyme in renal transplant recipients with hypertension. *N Engl J Med* 308:377–381, 1983.
106. Kincaid-Smith P: Role of ACE inhibitors in treatment of hypertension — experience with renovascular hypertension. In: Doyle AE, Bearn AG (eds) *Hypertension and the Angiotensin System: Therapeutic Approaches*. Raven Press, New York, pp 233–240, 1984.
107. Meyer TW, Hostetter TH, Rennke HG, Noddin JL, Brenner BM: Preservation of fenal structure and function by long term protein restriction in rats (abstract). *Kidney Int* 23:218, 1983.
108. Meyer TW, Anderson S, Rennke HG, Brenner BM: Control of glomerular hypertension retards progression of established glomerular injury in rats with renal ablation (abstract). *Kidney Int* 27:247, 1985.
109. Purkeson ML, Hoffsten PE, Klahr S: Pathogenesis of the glomerulopathy associated with renal infarction in rats. *Kidney Int* 9:407–417, 1976.
110. Purkeson ML, Joist JH, Greenberg JM, Kay D, Hoffsten PE, Klahr S: Inhibition by anticoagulant drugs of the progressive hypertension and uremia associated with renal infarction in rats. *Thromb Res* 26:227–240, 1982.
111. Purkeson ML, Joist JH, Yates J, Klahr S: Role of hypertension and coagulation in the glomerulopathy of rats with subtotal renal ablation. In: *Abstracts IX International Congress on Nephrology*, Los Angeles, p 359A, 1984.
112. Gretz N, Korb E, Strauch M: Low-protein diet supplemented by keto acids in chronic renal failure: A prospective controlled study. *Kidney Int* 24 (Suppl.26):S263–S267, 1983.
113. Rosman JB, Ter Wee PM, Meijer S, Piers-Becht TPM, Slutter WJ, Donker AJM: Prospective randomised trial of early dietary protein restriction in chronic renal failure. *Lancet* 2:1291–1296, 1984.
114. Stephens FD, Lenaghan D: The anatomical basis and dynamics of vesicoureteral reflux. In: R Webster, ed, *Congenital Malformations of the Rectum, Anus and Genito-Urinary Tracts*. E & S Livingstone, London, p 147, 1963.
115. Stamey TA: Urinary infections in infancy and childhood. In: *Pathogenesis and Treatment of Urinary Tract Infections*. Williams & Wilkins, Baltimore, p 335, 1980.
116. McRae CU, Shannon FT, Utley WLF: Effect on renal growth of reimplantation of refluxing ureters. *Lancet* 1:1310, 1974.
117. Bauer SB, Willischer MK, Zammuto PJ, Retik AB: Long-term results of anti-reflux surgery in children. In: CJ Hod-

son, P Kincaid-Smith, eds, *Reflux Nephropathy*. Masson Publishing, New York, p 287, 1979.
118. Hendren WH: A ten year experience with ureteral reimplantation in children. In: P Kincaid-Smith, KF Fairley, eds, *Renal Infection and Renal Scarring*. Mercedes, Melbourne, p 269, 1971.
119. Kincaid-Smith P, Fairley KF: The changing spectrum of acute renal failure in pregnancy and the post-partum period. In: GM Berlyne, ed, *Contributions to Nephrology*, Vol 25. Karger, Basel, p 159–165, 1981.
120. Kincaid-Smith P, Bullen M: Bacteriuria in pregnancy. *Lancet* 1:395–399, 1965.
121. d'Apice AJF, Reti LL, Pepperell RJ, Fairley KF, Kincaid-Smith P: Treatment of severe pre-eclampsia by plasma exchange. *Aust NZ J Obstet Gynaecol* 20:231–235, 1980.
122. Hodson CJ: Reflux nephropathy: Scoring the damage. In: CJ Hodson, P Kincaid-Smith, eds, *Reflux Nephropathy*. Masson Publishing, New York, pp 29–27, 1979.
123. Aperia A, Broberger O, Ekengren K, Wikstad I: The relationship between renal area and renal function in well defined childhood nephropathies. *Acta Radiol Diagn* 19:186–196, 1977.

CHAPTER 25

Genitourinary Tuberculosis

JAMES E. GOW

INTRODUCTION

Tuberculosis is a disease that has been known for many thousands of years, because the remains of ancient skeletons have shown the characteristic changes of tuberculosis. It is a disease that used to carry a high mortality, indeed, very little progress was made until the discovery of the antituberculous drugs, particularly streptomycin in 1943, isoniazid in 1952, and rifampicin in 1966.

The term *genitourinary tuberculosis* was first suggested by Wildbolz in 1937, when he demonstrated that renal tuberculosis and tuberculous epididymitis were not isolated diseases, but different manifestations of the same blood-borne infection, which could attack any organ in the body.

INVESTIGATIONS

When genitourinary tuberculosis is suspected, a careful series of investigations should be carried out. The diagnosis is confirmed by the isolation of *Mycobacterium tuberculosis* from the urine. This test is performed by inoculating the deposit of at least three, but preferably five, consecutive early morning specimens of urine onto a series of artificial culture media, three with and three without pyruvate, the latter to exclude the rare cases of bovine tuberculosis that still do occur, especially in Third World countries. It is important that each specimen of urine is inoculated daily, and that they are not all pooled together and are left until the third or fifth day, otherwise the results will be certain, because of the effect certain that biochemical substances in the urine exert on the *Mycobacterium tuberculosis* if they remain in contact for any length of time. A direct smear is never accepted, because such nonpathogenic organisms as *Bacillus smegma* are acid-and-alkaline-fast and can give a false-positive result. Guinea-pig inoculation tests are now not necessary, except on the very rare occasions when the disease is clinically suspected, yet the urine culture remains consistently negative, as artificial culture methods normally give equally good results. If the urine is positive, standard drug sensitivity tests are performed.

A full blood count is carried out, and the erythrocyte sedimentation rate, and urea and electrolyte values are estimated. Furthermore, if calcification is present on direct abdominal x-ray, a full biochemical profile of calcium metabolism is essential.

Radiography

A straight x-ray of the whole urinary tract is important, as it may show calcification in the renal areas, ureter, seminal vesicles, or even in the prostate. A plain x-ray of the chest is also necessary to exclude evidence of old or active disease.

Intravenous urogram

The introduction of the high-dose intravenous urogram has transformed the investigation of renal tract pathology and has made retrograde pyelography in genitourinary tuberculosis usually unnecessary. Tomography may be combined if more precise information of a renal lesion is needed. The extent of the disease in the kidney, either early or severe, is readily disclosed, and is an important factor in the planning of treatment.

Furthermore, an image intensifier will permit a dynamic study of any diseased ureter, particularly in the area of the pelviureteric junction. It can also give an indication of the amount of fibrosis that is present by the absence or presence of ureteric peristalsis.

Retrograde pyelography

Retrograde pyelography is only indicated when there is a stricture of the lower end of the ureter. A bulb catheter is used and the injection of the dye is monitored by an image intensifier. This will identify the length of the stricture and the condition of the ureter proximal to the obstruction. If no dye passes up the ureter and ultrasound shows a hydronephrotic kidney, a percutaneous nephrostomy is necessary to establish the extent of the disease.

Arteriography

Arteriography and radioisotope investigations are rarely required and should only be performed if there is a definitive indication, the main one for arteriography being the suspected coincidental presence of a renal tumor, that for radioisotope investigations being the necessity to know, when bilateral disease is present, how much each kidney is contributing to the total renal function.

Endoscopy

Endoscopy is of little importance in making the diagnosis of genitourinary tuberculosis, but does, however, help in assessing the extent of the bladder disease and its response to treatment. It must always be carried out under general anesthesia with a muscle relaxant, otherwise hemorrhage may be severe and may obscure any detailed view of the bladder.

A bladder biopsy should never be carried out, because of the danger of disseminating the disease, causing a miliary spread. Granulations surrounding the ureteric orifice may be resected by diathermy if it is necessary to have a clear view of the orifice for the purpose of catheterization.

MANAGEMENT

In the developed countries, there is evidence that the incidence of tuberculosis has been falling since the turn of the century and is diminishing at the rate of 5% per annum (1). This means that, under the present conditions of human resistance and environment, the disease will eventually be eradicated, although it will take many years. If, however, modern chemotherpy is added to the natural falling incidence, it is estimated that the decrease in the incidence will be about a further 8%. The addition of these two percentages will mean that in the Western world the disease will be completely eradicated by the end of the century.

In the developing countries, however, the situation is different, as there is very little natural immunity and therefore no downward trend over the last 10 years. In fact, there will be a slight increase in the number of infected cases as case finding improves. It is therefore of vital importance that in the developing countries chemotherapy is applied efficiently, continuously, and for the appropriate length of time. Compliance is the major factor in successful treatment, and if patients cannot be guaranteed to take the drugs, then in these areas either it should be administered daily, under supervision, or the patients should be admitted to hospital to ensure that all the drugs are taken in the correct amount at the right time.

In the Western world it is no longer necessary to treat patients in hospital, except for socioeconomic conditions in which it is impossible to look after the patient at home or the symptoms are excessively severe.

Patients are seen weekly as outpatients. Liver function tests are carried out to detect early liver toxicity, and the urine is inspected to ensure that rifampicin is being taken regularly, because if not, the urine will be the normal yellow color instead of orange/brown.

If surgery is planned, it should be carried out within the first 8 weeks of intensive chemotherapy, the optimum time being 6 weeks after the drug regime has started.

CHEMOTHERAPY

Antituberculous drugs are divided into two groups, primary and secondary agents. (Table 1). The primary agents are rifampicin, isoniazid, pyrazinamide, and streptomycin, all of which are bacteriocidal. The secondary agents are ethambutol, ethionamide, and cycloserine.

Rifampicin

Rifampicin is highly active against *Mycobacterium tuberculosis*, having an MIC of $0.02 \mu g/ml$. It is lipid soluble and is excreted in the urine, giving a lethal concentration for more than 36 hours after a single oral dose of 600 mg.

Isoniazid

Isoniazid is active against *M. tuberculosis* in concentrations of $0.05-0.2 \mu g/ml$. It is metabolized in the liver, but over 70% is excreted by the kidneys. There is no cross-resistance with rifampicin.

Pyrazinamide

Pyrazinamide has an activity of $20 \mu g/ml$ against *M. tuberculosis*, which is increased considerably in an acid medium. It is metabolized by the liver, but some is excreted by the kidney, so that after a single oral dose of 1 g there is a lethal concentration in the urine for more than 36 hours.

Streptomycin

Streptomycin has an MIC against *M. tuberculosis* of $8 \mu g/ml$. It rapidly diffuses into body tissues and is excreted in the urine. A concentraton of $200-400 \mu g/ml$ is obtained in the urine for more than 24 hours after a single 1-g instramuscular injection.

Ethambutol

Ethambutol is active against *M. tuberculosis* and has an MIC of $2 \mu g/ml$. It is also active against strains resistant to

Table 1. Classification of antituberculous drugs

Classification	Agent	Activity
Primary agents	Streptomycin Isoniazid Pyrazinamide Rifampicin	Bacteriocidal
Secondary agents	Ethambutol Cycloserine	Bacteriostatic

isoniazid. Approximately 80% is excreted in the urine and lethal concentrations remain for 24 hours after a single oral dose of 1 g.

Up to the early 1970s the standard method of treatment had been streptomycin, isoniazid, and PAS in various combinations for periods up to 2 years, the philosophy being to prevent the emergence of resistant strains of organisms and to reduce the relapse rate. Now, however, the approach has changed and physicians are seeking to sterilize lesions by the use of the modern, powerful antituberculous drugs. Since rifampicin was discovered in 1966 and was found to be as effective as isoniazid, research into short-course treatment has been intensified, as it was realized that if the courses could be shortened then there would be an immense saving in time and resources, both for the patient and the medical staff.

To understand the reason for using short-course treatment it is mandatory to appreciate the mechanisms of the drugs, actions. The understanding of short-course chemotherapy was based initially on experimental work at the Pasteur Institute, carried out by Professor Grosset (2). Grosset summarized the experiments as follows:
1. Pyrazinamide and rifampicin are potent sterilizing drugs.
2. The most vital sterilizing combinations are isoniazid and pyrazinamide and isonizid plus rifampicin.
3. Adding streptomycin and ethambutol has very little additional to offer to the sterilizing capacity of the two previous combinations.

Mitchison (3) pointed out that there were four bacterial populations. (Figure 1). The first is a population of *Mycobacterium tuberculosis* that divided rapidly. These are killed by all the bacteriocidal drugs. The second are those that metabolize intermittently and that probably metabolize for periods of less than a few hours. These are only killed by rifampicin, because this drug has a rapid action, so that its bacteriocidal activities start within a period of 3 hours, whereas with isoniazid there is a period of up to 24 hours before the maximum effect is exerted.

The third group are those that exist in the acid environment of the macrophages. These are destroyed by pyrazinamide, because its activity is greatly increased in an acid medium and because it readily enters into macrophages.

The fourth group are the dormant organisms, which are not affected by any antibiotics or are very unlikely to cause any disease.

As a result of this experimental work, various drug combinations have been clinically studied in the treatment of pulmonary tuberculosis. The British Thoracic Association (4) showed that treatment regimes that did not contain pyrazinamide were definitely inferior to those that did. There are now many effective 6 month regimes, all of which have in common the initial use of rifampicin, isoniazid, and pyrazinamide in various combinations. In patients in which the organism is sensitive to these three agents, it is likely that no further drugs are required; but if there is bacterial resistance to any of them, either streptomycin or ethambutol can be added. The result of these trials showed a relapse rate of between 1% and 4%.

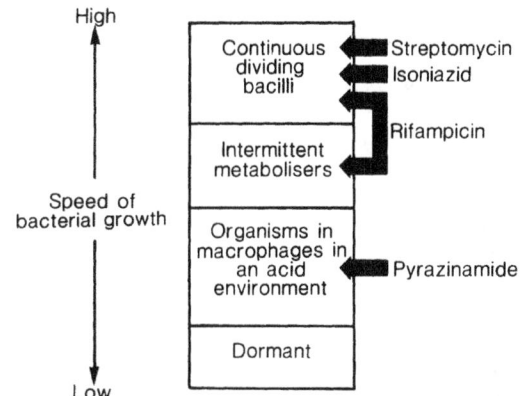

Figure 1. Different bacterial populations within lesions in humans. [Modified from Mitchison (3)] with permission.

All these investigations were carried out in cases with pulmonary tuberculosis, because there were far greater numbers of these patients in whom the various drug regimes could be tried. They all showed that, for the pulmonary disease, 6 months was the minimum time for chemotherapy.

How do these results affect the genito-urinary disease? There are certain aspects of genito-urinary tuberculosis that make it likely to respond better to short-course chemotherapy than the pulmonary infection. Indeed, courses shorter than the 6 month have now become a standard practice. The reasons why the genito-urinary disease will respond better are
1. There are far fewer organisms, sometimes one 100-fold less in renal than in pulmonary disease, and the organisms from the kidney are invariably excreted intermittently.
2. There are high concentrations of pyrazinamide, isoniazid, and rifampicin in the urine.
3. Isoniazid and rifampicin pass easily into renal cavities, in concentrations high enough to kill any *M. tuberculosis*.
4. All the suggested drugs penetrate the kidneys, ureters, bladder, and prostate in concentrations that are lethal to the *M. tuberculosis*.

Various regimes of treatment have been tried, all based on pulmonary tuberculosis trials, but for shorter periods of time. The two recommended regimes for this disease, which have given excellent results, are shown in Table 2. There is now accumulating evidence that isoniazid, rifampicin, and pyrazinamide are as effective three times a week as when they are taken daily. Nevertheless, it is suggested that, until this evidence has been further confirmed, the drug regime of pyrazinamide, isoniazid, and rifampicin daily for 2 months, followed by isoniazid and rifampicin three times a week for a further 2 months, should be adopted. However, in Third World countries, especially if there is satisfactory compliance, the three-times-a-week

Table 2. Alternative regimes

1. *Pyrazinamide*
   25 mg/kg body wt/day
   Maximum dose 2 g daily
   Isoniazid
   300 mg daily   600 mg 3 times a week
   Followed by
   Rifampicin
   450 mg daily   900 mg 3 times a week
   2 months   2 months
2. *Streptomycin*
   1 g daily
   Isoniazid
   300 mg daily   600 mg 3 times a week
   Followed by
   Rifampicin
   450 mg daily   900 mg 3 times a week
   Pyrazinamide
   25 mg/kg body wt/day
   Maximum dose 2 g daily
   2 months   2 months
3. *Pyrazinamide*
   25 mg/kg body wt/day
   Maximum dose 2 g daily
   Isoniazid   600 mg
   Rifampicin   450 mg
   3 times a week for 4 months

treatment can be used, as there is a considerable savings in cost.

Streptomycin can be added in the initial 2 months of intensive therapy if there is any suggestion of resistance to any of the other three drugs or if there are intense symptoms relating to the bladder. Occasionally, patients with extensive disease come with an infected bladder of small capacity. They have frequency, nocturia, hematuria, and occasionally intense pain. The addition of streptomycin may help these patients over the initial severe phase. In the author's series, all the urines of the last 150 patients have been sterilized at the end of 2 months. There has only been one relapse, which responded to a further 3 months of treatment, as the organism was sensitive to all three drugs. This patient admitted that she had not been taking the drugs regularly (7).

USE OF STEROIDS

In a further attempt to reduce the length of time of chemotherapy, it has been suggested that steroids should be added to the primary treatment. However, after extensive trials, there was no evidence after 6 weeks of the combination of prednisolone and chemotherapy that the sterilizing capacity of the regimes was improved. It is, however, justified to add steroids in the case of very extensive genitourinary disease, especially when the bladder is severely affected, as this may help to alleviate the severe symptoms. High doses of prednisolone are required, 20 mg three times a day, as McAllister (5) showed that when prednisolone was added to regimes, including rifampicin, the amount of available active drug was reduced by 66%.

TOXICITY

All the antituberculous drugs may produce toxic phenomena, but these are rarely serious and occur in only about 3% of cases. The two main types of toxicity are a hypersensitivity reaction and jaundice.

HYPERSENSITIVITY

All the antituberculous drugs can produce hypersensitive reactions. Streptomycin and rifampicin cause the main problems and are the only two that are of any real significance. The clinical appearances are an irritable macro rash, which may or may not be accompanied by fever. More serious reactions can occur: Conjunctivitis, generalized lymphadenopathy, gastrointestinal disturbance, generalized aching of limbs, and rarely, Stephen Johnson syndrome.

Management

The minor reactions can be treated by antihistamines, and do not usually cause the treatment to be stopped. If, however, the reaction becomes severe, then all the treatment should be suspended until the symptoms have subsided. Once the patient is back to normal, the management should comprise the identification of the drug and the resumption of the satisfactory chemotherapy as soon as possible.

To identify the drug likely to be the cause, each drug is challenged in turn so that the one responsible can be identified and, if appropriate, the dose reduced. Challenging doses are outlined in Table 3.

Hepatotoxicity

It is important to understand that a transient increase in liver enzymes occurs almost invariably during the treatment of tuberculosis with any chemotherapeutic drugs.

Table 3. Challenge doses for detecting hypersensitivity to antituberculous drugs

	Challenge dose	
Drug	Day 1	Day 2
Isoniazid	50 mg	300 mg
Rifampicin	75 mg	300 mg
Pyrazinamide	250 mg	1000 mg
Streptomycin	125 mg	500 mg
Ethambutol	100 mg	500 mg
Cycloserine	125 mg	250 mg

Adapted from Girling DJ: Drugs 23:56, 1982, with permission.

Once the drugs are stopped, the concentrations rapidly return to normal. It should also be appreciated that the three most important drugs — pyrazinamide, rifampicin, and isoniazid — are all metabolized in the liver, and therefore it is likely that there will be some cases in which damage occurs that is sufficient to produce jaundice.

MANAGEMENT

When jaundice appears, all the drugs should be stopped. If the jaundice is due to the drugs, recovery is rapid, and once the serum bilirubin has returned to normal the drugs are recommenced, but it is usually advisable to reinstate the course with the drugs taken three times a week rather than daily. In these cases the weekly estimation of the liver function tests is especially important.

Other rare reactions

Izoniazid can cause neurologic disturbances, which are readily controlled by pyridoxine, 25 mg daily. There is also diminished absorption if the patient is taking antacids, in which case a higher dose must be given. Rifampicin can give rise to purpura and rarely to acute renal failure. It also decreases the effect of oral coagulants, corticosteroids, and digoxin. Pyrazinamide can cause nausea, anorexia, and painful joints. Streptomycin is ototoxic. This is dose related and is reversible if the reaction is discovered in time and the drug withdrawn. Ethambutol can cause retrobulbar neuritis, and should be stopped if eye symptoms are noticed. These changes are also dose related, so the drug must be carefully regulated at all times and, if necessary, stopped completely. As this drug is being used less and less, the importance of this serious complication is diminishing.

Rifampicin and the contraceptive pill

Rifampicin may cause failure of oral contraceptive steroid therapy if it is not appreciated that when estrogens are taken with rifampicin, there is a rapid breakdown of the estrogen, so that the levels fall below those required for adequate contraception. If the contraceptive pill is being taken during treatment with rifampicin, then the dose of the estrogen should be considerably increased. It is, however, better to advise the patient to adopt some other method of contraception. The metabolism of estrogen returns to normal within 4 weeks after the cessation of treatment.

Antituberculous drugs and renal failure

Streptomycin and ethambutol are excreted almost unchanged in the urine, whereas rifampicin, pyrazinamide, and isoniazid are all metabolized in the liver, so that dose reduction with these latter three drugs does not have to be as drastic as with streptomycin and ethambutol. Table 4 shows the recommended doses in the presence of various degrees of renal insufficiency, based on the creatinine clearance, which is the most accurate and reliable method to work out the best dose regime.

SURGERY

Surgery has still an important part to play in the management of genitourinary tuberculosis; especially since with short-course regimes, it is essential to remove the diseased tissue, as it is not only sound surgical practice, but also allows the drugs to act on the remaining existing small foci of infection, an infection that can almost certainly be sterilized. Surgery is divided into two groups: removal of diseased tissue and reconstructive surgery.

Removal of diseased tissue

NEPHRECTOMY

The indications for nephrectomy are a nonfunctioning kidney with or without calcification, extensive disease, together with hypertension and coincidental renal carcinoma. There is strong evidence (6), that, despite sterilizing regimes, and even when the urine is sterile, 50% of the kidneys that were removed showed active tuberculosis on histologic examination. This surgery should be carried out within the first 6 weeks of the intensive course of treatment.

NEPHROURETERECTOMY

Nephroureterectomy is rarely indicated. As much of the ureter as possible is removed through the nephrectomy

Table 4. Recommended doses in the presence of various degrees of renal insufficiency

Drug	Dose	Frequency of administration Creatinine clearance (ml/min)		
		> 100 ml/min	50–10 ml/min	< 10 ml/min
Isoniazid	300 mg	1 × 24 hr	1 × 36–48 hr	1 × 60–72 hr
Rifampicin	450 mg	1 × 24 hr	1 × 24 hr	1 × 48 hr
Pyrazinamide	25 mg/kg body wt	1 × 24 hr	1 × 24 hr	1 × 48 hr
Streptomycin	1 g	1 × 24 hr	1 × 72 hr	1 × 96 hr
Ethambutol	25 mg/kg body wt	1 × 24 hr	1 × 48 hr	1 × 72 hr

incision. This is all that is required, because it is very rare for the residual stump of the ureter to cause any complications, as it becomes completely fibrosed.

PARTIAL NEPHRECTOMY

The indications for this operation are becoming less and less. It is now very rarely carried out and is performed only when there is extensive calcification located in one pole. The operation again should be carried out during the first 6 weeks of intensive treatment.

EPIDIDYMECTOMY

The need for this procedure is now rare, but it is required when there is a caseating abscess with a discharging sinus that is not responding to chemotherapy. Another indication is a firm swelling of the epididymis that is not improved with chemotherapy, because there is the possible risk of coincidental carcinoma. The author has seen two such cases. Involvement of the testis is exceptional and only 5% of the cases require orchidectomy.

CAVERNOTOMY

This procedure has no place in the modern management of genitourinary tuberculosis, because with modern x-ray techniques, on the rare occasions that an abscess forms, it can be aspirated under the control of an image intensifer.

RECONSTRUCTIVE SURGERY

Stricture of the ureter

Stricture of the ureter occurs most commonly at the ureterovesical junction. The second most common place is the pelviureteric junction, and lastly, at the midureter. Very rarely are all areas involved, but in these cases the kidney is usually grossly diseased. Pelviureteric strictures should be repaired as soon as possible, under a screen of chemotherapy. The kidney should always be drained, preferably by a small pyelostomy tube, so that the pelvis can be irrigated with a mixture of 5% rifampicin and 1% isoniazid.

A double-J stent is a considerable asset to the surgical technique and can be left in situ for 4 weeks or longer before being removed endoscopically. The pyelostomy drain is removed in 2–3 weeks, depending on the extent of the renal disease.

Stricture of the lower end of the ureter

These occur in approximately 9% of patients. Most strictures are narrow and short, rarely more than 2 in. in length. The initial management should always be chemotherapy, especially if at cystoscopy there is edema around the ureteric orifice, as edema alone can produce quite a severe ureteric obstruction. The management should be to start the normal course of chemotherapy and to take a 25-minute full-size intravenous urogram film weekly. This will show the whole of the renal tract and will allow the lesion to be assessed. If there is no improvement after the third week of chemotherapy, steroids should be added, such as prednisolone, 20 mg tds. The weekly full-length 25-minute film should continue to be taken, so that progress can be monitored.

If there is no improvement after 6 weeks, reimplantation of the ureter is necessary. The reimplantation should always be reflux preventing, either directly into the bladder or, if the stricture is too long, then by either a Boari flap or psoas hitch.

Strictures of the middle third of the ureter

These are very rare, but if found can be satisfactorily treated by means of either the Davies intubation technique or the double-J stent, which is left in situ for 6 or 8 weeks.

Augmentation cystoplasty

This is required when there is an acutely inflamed bladder of small capacity, which gives the patient intolerable frequency, pain, urgency, and hematuria. Such a bladder is never likely to recover with chemotherapy, as once it reaches this stage there is invariably intramural fibrosis. Either the ileum, cecum, or colon can be used. the author prefers the cecum, because it has given satisfactory results over a number of years and has the advantage that if reimplantation of the ureters is required, either for stenosis or for reflux, this can be carried out into the termial ileum, again using a reflux-preventing technique.

Urinary diversion

Urinary diversion is now very rarely necessary and is only indicated when there is a history of psychiatric disturbance, enuresis, or incontinence. Once incontinence is present, the chances of successful treatment by augmentation cystoplasty are extremely unlikely, indeed, in the author's experience it is a contraindication to this procedure.

Follow-up

All patients should be followed up for a period of 1 year. Intravenous urogram and three or five early morning specimens of urine should be taken at 6 months and a year. Provided that these are satisfactory, the patient is discharged and told to report back to his or her general practitioner if any symptoms related to the renal tract recur.

If calcification is present, however, especially calcification in the kidney, the patient should be followed in the same way as any other patient with a calculus. Our policy is to see patients for at least 10 years on an annual basis after the first year. On each visit a straight x-ray of the whole renal tract is taken, to exclude any deterioration in

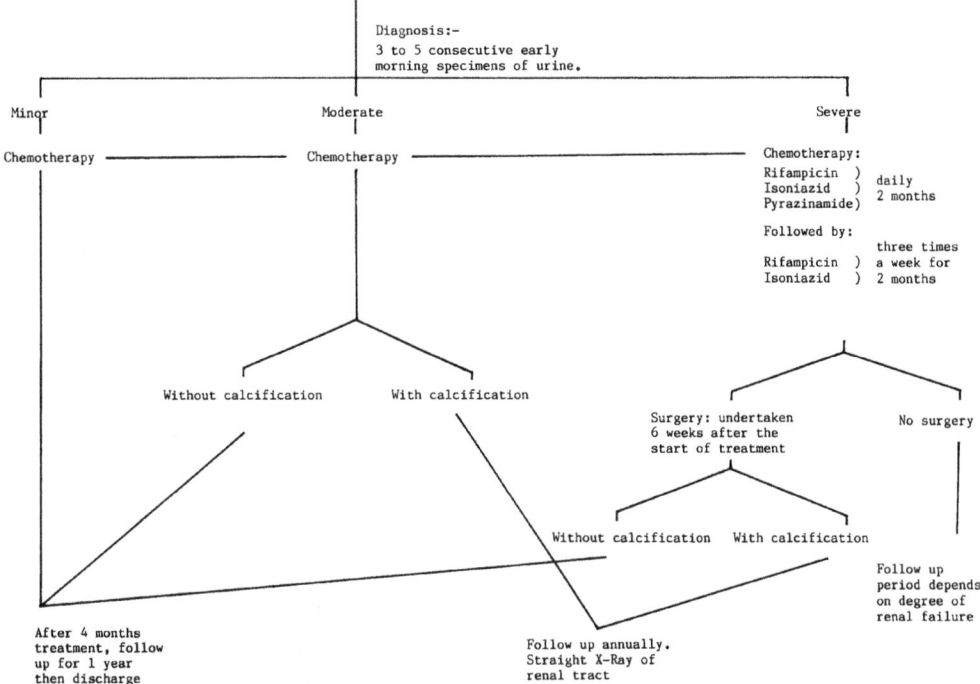

Figure 2. Algorithm for genitourinary tuberculosis.

the condition of the kidney. If there is an obvious increase in the calcification, an intravenous urogram is carried out.

Surgical treatment will depend on the nature of the calcification, its extent, progression, and effect on the kidney. An algorithm outlines the modern management of genitourinary tuberculosis (Figure 2).

REFERENCES

1. Sutherland I: Recent studies in the epidemiology of tuberculosis based on the risk of being infected by the tubercle bacillus. *Adv Tuberc Res* 19:1, 1976.
2. Grosset J: The sterilising value of rifampicin and pyrazinamide in experimental short course chemotherapy. *Tubercle* 59:287, 1978.
3. Mitchison DA: Treatment of tuberculosis. *JR Coll Physic* (London) 14:91, 1980.
4. British Thoracic Association: Short course therapy in pulmonary tuberculosis. *Lancet* 1:1182, 1980.
5. McAllister WAC, Thompson PJ, Al-Habet SM, Rogers HJ: Rifampicin reduces effectiveness and bio-availability of prednisolone. *Br Med J* 286:923, 1983.
6. Osterhage HR, Fischer U, Barbensak K: Positive histological tuberculous findings despite stable sterility of the urine on culture. *Eur Urol* 6(2):116, 1980.
7. Gow JG, Barbosa S: Genito-urinary tuberculosis — a study of 1117 cases over a period of 34 years. *Br J Urol* 56:449, 1984.

CHAPTER 26

Systemic Lupus Erythematosus

SUSAN L. ANDREW & DAVID P. HUSTON

INTRODUCTION

Systemic lupus erythematosis (SLE) is an autoimmune disease of unknown etiology (1–3). Clinical features of SLE include fatigue, fever, dermatitis, photosensitivity, alopecia, arthritis, serositis, hematologic abnormalities, mucosal ulcerations, Raynaud's phenomenon, neurologic disease, and glomerulonephritis. Serologic features include false-positive VDRL; antibodies to nuclear constituents, leukocytes, and erythrocytes; circulating immune complexes; and depressed complement levels. The diagnosis of SLE should be made if a patient fulfills four or more of the criteria proposed by the American Rheumatism Association (4). Although genetic (5), hormonal (6), and environmental (7) factors have been implicated in the etiology and modification of disease activity, immunologic abnormalities are postulated as essential in the pathogenesis of disease (8, 9). A number of effector and regulatory T-cell defects (10–14), as well as monocyte defects (15, 16), have been described. Cytokine abnormalities have also been found; for example, lymphocytes from some patients with SLE are unable to produce or respond to interleukin-2 normally (17, 18). However, the hallmark of SLE is polyclonal B-cell hyperactivity with hypergammaglobulinemia, the presence of large amounts of autoantibodies, and the resultant formation of immune complexes (19–22). Many of the clinical manifestations of SLE appear to be secondary to inflammatory reponses initiated by these immune complexes (23–25), of which the DNA-anti-DNA complexes are of particular importance (26–35). The immune complexes may be formed in situ in the involved tissues as well as deposited by entrapment of complexes preformed in the general circulation (25, 28, 30–33). For example, some antibodies that bind DNA also crossreact with antigens expressed by glomerular basement membrane (34, 35). Whether the hyeractive B-cell state that leads to production of these autoantibodies is due to an endogenous B-cell defect versus a T-cell regulatory abnormality remains controversial (9–14, 17, 18, 21, 22, 29).

Many features of SLE are ameliorated with the administration of anti-inflammatory agents. Although nonsteroidal antiinflammatory drugs or the 4-aminoquinoline (antimalarial) drugs occasionally modify some of the manifestations of SLE, many patients require corticosteroid therapy (36, 37). Prior to the availability of corticosteroids in the early 1950s, patients with SLE frequently died within the first 2 years of their disease (38–40). Since then, corticosteroids have provided an effective therapy for the acute fulminating form of the disease (41, 42), with recent survival figures approaching 90% at 5 years (37, 41, 43–47) and 55–75% at 15 years (42, 48). Antibiotics, antihypertensive drugs, and intensive care units have also probably prolonged survival. However, despite these improved survival patterns, renal involvement remains an ominous finding in SLE (49–51).

NEPHRITIS-RELATED COMPLICATIONS

Renal insufficiency

The incidence of lupus nephritis varies from 40% to 70% of SLE cases, based on clinical criteria (52–58). Such criteria include proteinuria; hematuria; active urine sediments with red cells, white cells, and casts; and a decline of renal function. There is a significant amount of silent lupus nephritis in that renal histology assessments have demonstrated close to 90% incidence of nephritis with SLE (54, 59–61). Recent reviews on survival patterns of SLE patients report approximately a 12% 5-year mortality; those with clinical evidence of nephritis have demonstrated a 20–40% 5-year mortality (48–51). Claims that assessment of glomerular histopathology helps to prognosticate the eventual outcome of renal disease have increasingly led to the inclusion of a renal biopsy in the evaluation of the SLE patient with clinical nephritis (49, 62–66).

A wide spectrum of histologic changes have been observed in the renal biopsies of SLE patients. Attempts to devise a clinically useful histologic classification have been numerous. The World Health Organization Committee on Morphological Classification and Nomenclature of Renal Diseases and the International Committee for Nomenclature and Nosology of Renal Disease has classified lupus nephritis, based on light microscopy, as a) mesangial, b) focal proliferative, c) diffuse proliferative, d) membrano-proliferative, or e) membranous glomerulonephritis (67). Descriptions of where immune deposits are located help to distinguish between the light microscopic categories. The pathogenesis of renal disease in lupus nephritis is felt to be related to these deposits (31, 59, 63). Immune complex deposition may occur by precipitation from the circulation or actual in-situ formation (31–35). Deposition of circulating immune complexes is enhanced by inadequate extrarenal clearance of the complexes (32, 68–71). Defective mononuclear phagocytosis has been described in patients with SLE (15, 16) and could decrease clearance of antigen-antibody complexes, thereby leading to mesangial deposition. Qualitative differences in immune complexes themselves, such as size and charge, also affect deposition (27–32, 70, 72). Large latticed and cationic complexes tend to deposit more readily. Deposits that are formed by precipitation are thought to locate initially in the mesangial or subendothelial regions (31, 32). Subepithelial deposits may represent immune complexes formed in situ by antibodies that recognize glomerular antigens (31–35). Regardless of the mechanism behind immune complex deposition, damage is the consequence of complement activation by these deposits (31, 32). Determination of the location and pattern of immunoglobulin and complement deposition is facilitated by immuofluorescent microscopy (60). The precise ultrastructural localization of the sites of immune-complex deposition are further characterized by electron microscopy (73). Several studies (59–63, 67, 74) have correlated the immunofluroescent and electron microscopy findings with the five light microscopy categories of lupus nephritis and renal function (Table 1).

Proliferation of mesangial cells and an increased mesangial matrix with electron-dense deposits and immunofluorescence staining only in the mesangium are characteristics of mesangial glomerulonephritis (61, 63. 75). This lesion is found in approximately 20% of lupus patients and usually correlates with clinically mild or no renal dysfunction. The extramesangial lupus glomerulonephritides include focal proliferative, diffuse proliferative, membranoproliferative, and membranous glomerulonephritis (67, 76). Focal is distinguish from diffuse proliferative disease under light microscopy by less than 50% of the glomeruli having endothelial cell proliferation, irregular thickening of capillary loops, and active inflammation. If the capillary loops are uniformly thickened with evidence of endothelial proliferation and inflammation, and extension of the mesangial cells toward the capillary loops with splitting of the basement membrane, the lesion is called *membranoproliferative*. Five to 22% of lupus nephritis patients have local proliferative, 25–65% have diffuse proliferative, and 7–35% have membranoproliferative glomerulonephritis (54, 66, 74, 76). Transition from one to another of these lesions has been well documented (50, 77–80). In general, patients with diffuse proliferative or membranoprolifera-

Table 1. Histologic assessment of lupus nephritis

WHO classification of lupus glomerulonephritis	Light microscopy	Electron microscopy	Immunofluorescent microscopy
Mesangial	Mesangial matrix enlarged	No or few mesangial deposits	Mesangial staining only
Focal proliferative	Mesangial matrix enlarged + < 50% of glomeruli have segmental endothelial cell proliferation, segmental thickening of capillary loops, and occasional area of necrosis	Mesangial deposits + subendothelial, intramembranous, and/or subepithelial cell deposits + segmental thickening of the basement membrane	Staining of mesangium + segmental peripheral staining
Diffuse proliferative	Mesangial matrix enlarged + > 50% of glomeruli have endothelial cell proliferation, usually with a diffuse glomerular distribution and segmental thickening of capillary loops and areas of necrosis	Mesangial deposits + subendothelial, intramembranous, and/or subepithelial cell deposits + segmental thickening of the basement membrane	Staining of mesangium + diffuse granular peripheral staining, usually with focal areas of intense staining
Membranoproliferative	Mesangial matrix enlarged + diffuse endothelial cell proliferation with uniform thickening of capillary loops and segmental necrosis	Mesangial deposits + subendothelial, intramembranous, and/or subepithelial cell deposits + interposition of mesangial cells in the thickened basement membrane	Staining of mesangium + diffuse granular peripheral staining, usually with focal areas of intense staining
Membranous	Minimal mesangial matrix enlargement or endothelial cell proliferation + uniformly thickened capillary loops	Few mesangial or subendothelial cell deposits; predominantly intramembranous and/or subepithelial cell deposits	Variable, usually not intense, staining of mesangium or capillary loops

tive glomerulonephritis have the most severe clinical evidence of renal disease and the worst prognosis. In the past approximately 50% progress to renal failure within 5 years (49, 76). Most patients with this prognosis have the nephrotic syndrome at the time of diagnosis of nephritis (49, 81). However, not all patients with the nephrotic syndrome have clinical or histologic progression of nephritis (49), and more recent studies suggest a more favorable prognosis with cytotoxic drug therapy (66). Histologically, the presence of subendothelial electron-dense deposits represents active disease with the potential for deterioration of renal function. Subepithelial and/or intramembranous electron-dense deposits, without subendothelial deposits, may represent a more indolent state with a lower likelihood of clinical or histologic progression (61, 75, 78, 82). Membranous glomerulonephritis accounts for less than 8% of lupus nephritis (76). Characteristically it is associated with the nephrotic syndrome, subepithelial and intramembranous electron-dense deposits, and slow clinical and/or histologic progression (54, 73, 74).

There is a significant incidence of intrarenal vasculopathy in lupus nephritis patients. Associated with vasculitis is a deterioration of renal function as well as accelerated hypertension. The presence of intrarenal vasculitis may therefore imply a worse prognosis (83).

Interstitial changes are often observed in patients with any of the five light microscopic categories of lupus nephritis (50, 73, 74, 76). Only recently has inclusion of these changes in the assessment of lupus nephritis been suggested (76, 83–85). The inclusion of interstitial changes in the overall assessment of lupus nephritis may result in more reliable scoring systems for therapeutic prognostication (83, 84). The prognosis for the occasional lupus patient with only interstitial disease is unknown.

The Nephrology Service at the NIH has supported the use of a semiquantitative scoring system, originally described by Pirani et al. (86) in 1964, as a sensitive measure of activity for lupus nephritis. This scoring system (0–3⁺ for each variable) establishes an activity index and a chronicity index (83, 84). Those histologic abnormalities that are potentially reversible contribute to the activity index and include a) proliferative changes, b) necrosis/ karyorrhexis, c) cellular crescents, d) leukocyte infiltration, e) hyaline thrombi, and f) interstitial inflammation. Any histologic abnormalities that are irreversible make up the chronicity index, which is the sum of scores for a) sclerotic glomeruli, b) fibrous crescents, and c) tubular atrophy and interstitial fibrosis. Evidence supports using this scoring mechanism as an adjunct to the WHO classification of lupus nephritis in order to better describe, prognosticate, and direct therapy at certain types of renal pathoglogy (64, 65).

Proteinuria

While a primary emphasis of concern with lupus nephritis is progression to renal failure, other renal-related manifestations often dominate the clinical pattern. Proteinuria, a poor prognostic sign with regard to renal failure

Table 2. Prognostic implications of proteinuria*

Developed clinical nephritis	Developed nephrotic syndrome	% survival after diagnosis of SLE		
		5 year	10 year	15 year
No	—	94	88	84
Yes	—	80	64	58
—	No	81	68	58
—	Yes	79	64	57
Yes	Early onset	74	48	44
Yes	Late onset	88	75	73

* Abstracted from Wallace et al. (49).

(Table 2), often leads to peripheral edema, pleural effusions, and/or bowel edema. Frequently, peripheral edema is the patient's presenting and major renal-related chronic complaint. Proteinuria suggests a membranous component to the lupus nephritis. Massive proteinuria without an active urine sediment is characteristic of the membranous class of lupus glomerulonephritides, and such patients also may be at an increased risk for developing thromboembolic events (51, 87–90). However, proteinuria in the absence of an active urine sediment can also be seen with any histologic category of glomerular lesion. Amyloidosis, which very rarely occurs in SLE patients, secondary to amyloid A protein deposition, may also be manifest as proteinuria (91–94).

Hypertension and atherosclerosis

Hypertension is often present in SLE patients with clinically active glomerulonephritis (48, 95). The histologic presence of glomerulosclerosis, in addition to glomerulonephritis, in many such patients suggests that hypertension also contributes to renal compromise. The presence of hypertension and nephritis has been associated with a poor prognosis (48, 51, 55).

Accelerated atherosclerosis-related complications have also become evident in lupus nephritis patients (51, 96, 97). Associated with the atherosclerosis are deaths due to cardiovascular and cerebrovascular disease (Table 3). In one study, vascular-related complications accounted for almost 60% of the nonrenal mortality in treated lupus nephritis patients surviving for more than 2 years (51). The exact cause for the accelerated atherosclerosis and increased incidence of thrombotic events in lupus nephritis patients is unknown, but may be related to endothelial damage by immune-complex-activated mediators of inflammation, the effects of therapeutic doses of corticosteroids on carbohydrate metabolism, the unexplained presence of elevated serum cholesterol levels (51, 55, 97–100), and/or the presence of lupus anticoagulant (101, 102).

Infection and immunization

The most frequent nonrenal cause of death in lupus patients within the first 2 years after diagnosis of nephritis is

Table 3. Nonrenal deaths in patients with lupus nephritis*

Nonrenal causes of death	% of nonrenal causes of death (years after diagnosis of nephritis)	
	< 2 years	> 2 years
Vascular related	21	59
Infection	42	14
Extrarenal SLE	32	9
Other	5	18

* Abstracted from Karsh et al. (51).

infection (51, 76). Approximately 40% of such patients die from infection (Table 3). However, survival for at least 2 years decreases the risk of infectious death to less than 15%. The temporally related mortality secondary to infection probably correlates best with the extent of immuosuppression. The responsible organisms are diverse and include routinely pathogenic bacteria, fungi, and protozoa, plus the rarely pathogenic organisms that are observed in immunocompromised hosts. Although a plethora of immunologic defects are found in SLE patients on no medications, these infections are considered primarily a complication of pharmacologic immunosuppression.

Attempts to protectively immunize SLE patients with nonliving vaccines such as Pneumovax® (pneumococcal vaccine polyvalent, MSD) have demonstrated near-normal antibody responses (103). However, the protective effect of these vaccines in SLE patients, and especially those on immunosuppressive drugs, is unknown. Regarding live vaccines, most physicians will withhold their use in SLE patients receiving immunosuppressive therapy.

Fetal and maternal morbidity and mortality

In contrast to earlier reports indicating poor maternal and fetal outcomes with pregnancy in SLE patients (104, 105), recent analyses portray a more favorable prognosis if the lupus is clinically quiescent for at least 6 months prior to conception (106–109). Intrapartum or postpartum flares occur in approximately one half of the women who exhibit clinically active disease within 6 months of conception. Up to 15% of these mothers who flare may die, and less than two thirds of the fetuses survive. In women with clinically inactive SLE during the 6 months preconception, maternal flares occur less than one third of the time, with death a rarity, and live births approximating 90%. Conversely, if SLE is first manifest intrapartum or postpartum, the maternal and fetal prognoses are similar to those for women with active disease preconception. The major determinant of maternal/fetal prognosis is the severity of clinical disease activity.

Independent of clinical disease activity, azotemia and the nephrotic syndrome have been implicated as significant risk factors in pregnant SLE mothers (108). In separate studies, fetal loss approached 50% in SLE patients when the serum creatinine was greater than 1.5 mg/dl and/or the serum albumin was less than 3.0 gm/dl. Lately much has been said concerning pregnancy, fetal outcome, and the presence of lupus anticoagulant, which is an antiphospholipid antibody associated with thrombotic events (101, 102, 110–111). Of importance pathogenically is the interaction of this antibody in vitro with platelet factor 3 and the subsequent inhibition of prothrombin activator complex formation (102). More recently, the presence of this antibody has been associated with fetal distress, preeclampsia, and spontaneous abortion in pregnant lupus patients (102, 110). In addition, paitents with a high incidence of spontaneous abortion, and who do not necessarily have SLE, have been found to have antiphospholipid antibodies (111). It remains unclear whether the presence of these antiphospholipid antibodies is of predictive or pathogenic importance in pregnant lupus patients. The only significant developmental abnormality in full-term infants of SLE mothers has been an increased incidence of congenital heart block (112, 113); its relationship to intrapartum maternal disease activity is unknown.

THERAPY

Experience in murine models

Therapeutic approaches to SLE can emphasize either prophylaxsis or treatment. Spontaneous murine models of autoimmunity have been helpful in evaluating potential therapeutic modalities (Table 4). (NZBxNZW)F_1 mice have been particularly useful since they develop lupus

Table 4. Therapy of murine lupus nephritis[1]

Treatment	Effects on survival of (NZBxNZW)F_1 mice		
	Before nephritis	Early nephritis	Established nephritis
Ribavirin	+[2]	+	ND[3]
Androgens	+	+	0[4]
ConA-induced factors	+	+	−[5]
Prostaglandins	+	+	ND
Diet (eicosapentaenoic acid)	+	+	+
Antithymocyte globulin	+	+	0
Tolerance of nucleic acids	+	0	0
Corticosteroids	+	+	0
Cytotoxic drugs	+	+	0
Selective lymphoid irradiation	ND	+	+
Monoclonal antibodies	+	+	+
Cyclosporine	+	+	+

[1] Abstracted from references 117, 119, 121–125, 127–157.
[2] Prolonged survival.
[3] Not done.
[4] No effect.
[5] Shortened survival.

nephritis (114–117). Murine models of SLE have suggested that autoimmunity can be genetically modified (118–120). However, the outbred nature of humans and the limited understanding of human immunogenetics do not yet allow us either to predict who will develop SLE or to genetically modulate the disease. Thus, genetic studies are currently directed more toward an understanding of pathogenesis than treatment.

The implication of a viral etiology has led to therapeutic trials with the antiviral agent ribavirin in (NZBxNZW)F_1 mice (121). Ribavirin-treated mice had less proteinuria, decreased titers of anti-DNA antibodies, and lived longer; however, the beneficial effects may have been due to the immunosuppressive properties of the drug.

The exacerbations of SLE during pregnancy and the increased incidence of SLE in females have implicated a role for sex hormones in the modulation of disease activity (56). Similarly, female (NZBxNZW)F_1 mice develop renal disease earlier in life than the male mice (115, 119). Castration and reconstitution experiments in (NZBxNZW)F_1 mice have helped delineate the effects of androgens and estrogens on autoimmune renal disease (122–124). While treatment with the antiestrogen, Nafoxidine, had some beneficial effects on autoimmunity in (NZBxNZW)F_1 mice (123), androgens significantly retarded the development of glomerulonephritis (122, 124). This beneficial effect was observed in both castrated or sham-operated females and in castrated males that were treated with testosterone by subcutaneous capsule implantation. Castrated or sham-operated females not given testosterone did equally poorly; castrated males not given testosterone had a 50% increased mortality. The exact mechanism by which testosterone affects antoimmunity is unknown. Sex hormones may act either directly as physiologic adjuvants and suppressors, or indirectly in a complex immune-endocrine network (124). Dehydroisoandrosterone, which has itself no known intrinsic androgenic effect, prevents formation of autoantibodies and prolongs survival when fed to (NZBxNZW)F_1 mice (125). This "adrenal androgen" may exert its effect through active metabolites. A recent study found that female patients with active SLE had low levels of plasma androgens (126). Regardless of the mechanism, these results suggest that sex hormones may become an important therapeutic regimen for the modulation of autoimmunity. Routine clinical application must await the completion of controlled human trials with attenuated androgens. Such trials are particularly important due to a reported exacerbation of SLE in a patient treated with danazol for C1 esterase inhibitor deficiency (127).

A number of studies have suggested that treatment of (NZBxNZW)F_1 mice with exogenous suppressor factors (128, 129) or prostaglandins (130, 131) may prolong survival. Likewise, antithymocyte globulin (132, 133), selective lymphoid irradiation (134), and induction of tolerance to nucleic acids (135, 136) have retarded the development of glomerulonephritis in these mice. Of these various modalities the most clinically applicable is selective irradiation to the major lymph nodes, spleen, and thymus. This approach is similar to that used for Hodgkin's disease, and the short- and long-term complications should also be similar. Clinical trials of selective lymphoid irradiation are underway in SLE. Long-term followup will be necessary to determine whether or not beneficial effects in autoimmune disease are longlasting or transient.

More recently, attempts to modulate murine lupus nephritis have employed dietary manipulations. A diet either deficient in essential fatty acids (137) or enriched in eicosapentaenoic acid (138, 139) administered to autoimmune mice with renal disease has resulted in less severe glomerulonephritis and prolonged survival. In addition, there appears to be reversal of kidney pathology in affected mice given eicosapentaenoic acid (139). Eicosapentaenoic acid is metabolized by the same enzymes that metabolize arachidonic acid. Eicosapentaenoic acid is metabolized to trienoic prostanoids in contrast to the dienoic prostanoids, which are produced when arachidonic acid is the precursor substrate. The dienoic prostanoids have different effects than the trienoic prostanoids and may be what ultimately leads to the therapeutic efficacy of eicosapentaenoic administration (140). Alteration of dietary fatty acid intake may prove to be a relatively benign therapeutic approach to lupus nephritis.

The most extensive therapeutic studies in (NZBxNZW)F_1 mice have employed corticosteroids and/or cytotoxic drugs. The effectiveness of treatment was affected by the extent of disease at the initiation of therapy. Comparisons of mice a) prior to the onset of nephritis, b) during the active stages of nephritis, and c) with advanced nephritis have demonstrated the difficulty in interpreting results. Prior to the onset of nephritis, high-dose corticosteroids, low-dose corticosteroids plus azathioprine, or bolus cyclophosphamide had minimal but favorable effects (141–148); neither low-dose corticosteroids nor azathioprine singly had a demonstrable effect (142, 143). During the active stages of early and moderately severe nephrities, high-dose corticosteroids, azathioprine, and/or cyclophosphamide with or without low-dose corticosteroids, or especially bolus cyclophosphamide, had dramatic beneficial effects on renal histology and survival (144–148); low-dose corticosteroids alone had no effect. Only minimal benefit was observed with any regimen started in mice with advanced nephritis (142–144). In summary, these studies suggested that murine lupus nephritis was most effectively treated during its early stages with either a) a combination of daily prednisone, azathioprine, and cyclophosphamide or b) bolus cyclophosphamide. Bolus cyclophosphamide was most effective.

Modulation of immune responses with monoclonal antibodies has also become a popular therapeutic concept in clinical immunology. The delayed onset of nephritis in (NZBxNZW)F_1 mice given anti-DNA monoclonal antibodies was reported (149–152). Such monoclonal antibodies may alter the properties of pathogenic immune complexes and/or induce antiidiotypic antibodies for downregulation of anti-DNA antibody production. Monoclonal antibodies directed at T cells were used in the treatment of three strains of autoimmune mice (153). One strain of mouse (MLR/lpr) responded well to monoclonal antibody therapy with retardation of renal disease and prolongation of life. Another mouse strain (NZBxNZW)F_1 was unaffected by therapy, and the third mouse strain (BXSB) developed fatal anaphylaxis when monoclonal antibody therapy was administered. These results were interesting in that different mouse models of lupus nephritis responded differently to therapy, implying that there are differences in the pathogenicity of disease between these mouse strains. Selective depletion of T-cell subsets in (NZBxNZW)F_1 mice, the mouse strain unaffected by total T-cell depletion, was recently studied for therapeutic efficacy (145). Anti-L3T4 is a monoclonal antibody that recognizes the murine homologue of the human CD4 molecule. Anti-L3T4 binds to and impairs the function of T cells with class II major histocompatibility complex-restricted cellular interactions, and thereby can inhibit helper/inducer T-cell function. Anti-L3T4 was injected weekly into (NZBxNZW)F_1 mice and resulted in depletion of 90% of the circulating L3T4$^+$ lymphocytes. Therapeutically, this resulted in reduction of antibodies to double-stranded DNA, improvement in renal function, and prolongation of life in these mice. Thus, monoclonal antibodies directed against T-cell subsets in mice have been shown to both prevent and reverse nephritis (153, 154). Perhaps a similar mechanism (elimination of T-cell help) accounts for the favorable results with cyclosporine therapy for nephritis of autoimmune mice (155–157). The effects of either antibody or cyclosporine therapy on humans with lupus are under investigation.

Therapy of lupus glomerulonephritis

Considering the current concepts on the pathogenesis of lupus nephritis (9–24), supression of the immune system seems a logical approach. While considerable attention has been paid to the use of corticosteroids, with or without cytotoxic drugs, conclusive evidence for therapeutic efficacy is lacking. The difficulties in interpreting and comparing therapeutic studies include a) a lack of control groups, b) severity and duration of disease at study entry, c) previous therapy, d) inadequately defined histologic classifications of nephritis, e) variable followup, and f) variability of the disease. The poorly understood multifactorial pathogenesis of SLE further confuses attempts to construct adequate therapeutic trials. Therefore, assessment of therapeutic studies on lupus nephritis must be done cautiously.

CORTICOSTEROIDS

No controlled trials with corticosteroids in SLE have ever been performed. However, the beneficial effects of corticosteroids on many extrarenal manifestations of SLE have been well recognized for a long time (38, 40). It therefore seems unlikely that a trial of corticosteroids versus no corticosteroids will ever occur. Given this constraint, virtually all therapeutic studies of lupus nephritis have compared their results to percorticosteroid historic controls and/or low-dose corticosteroid-treated controls. In a retrospective statistical analysis of the effects of corticosteroid treatment on the survival of SLE patients, as reported in 52 papers from 1936 to 1966, efficacy in promoting survival was only observed among very ill patients (158). A specific benefit to patients with nephritis was also only observed when their overall clinical condition placed them in the seriously ill category.

Perhaps the most widely accepted control group today is patients treated with high-dose daily oral corticosteroids, as popularized by Pollack et al. (159) and Baldwin et al. (81). Doses usually vary from 60 to 100 mg prednisone equivalent per day until remission, or for up to 6 months. Chronic doses greater than 1 mg prednisone equivalent/kg/day are associated with increased steroid-related morbidity without documented greater efficacy. Based on favorable experience with the management of renal transplant rejection (160, 161), high-dose intravenous pulse methylprednisolone has also been advocated for the treatment of lupus nephritis (162–165). There have been no major controlled trials of pulse steroids in the management of SLE. Uncontrolled trials generally show rapid improvement in renal function in those patients who respond to therapy (162–167). The responding patients tend to have had a recent antecedent deterioration in their clinical course. Unfortunately, the response rate to pulse steroid therapy has generally been incomplete, and the majority of patients have relapses despite being on maintenance low-dose steroids (164–167). One group treated relapses with addditional pulses of steroids and showed that this was effective in most instances (164). While efficacy for high-dose intravenous pulse corticosteroids in the treatment of lupus nephritis is not yet proven, it may prove to be a useful adjunct to other forms of therapy.

CYTOTOXIC DRUGS

Cytotoxic drugs are usually reserved for the lupus patient a) who cannot tolerate corticosteroids or who suffers from intolerable steroid side effects, b) whose extrarenal disease is not controlled with corticosteroids, or c) whose renal function is deteriorating and/or whose renal histology reveals diffuse proliferative or membranoproliferative glomerulonephritis. The patients with an intermediate chronicity index in particular should receive cytotoxic therapy (168). Of the available cytotoxic drugs, the greatest experience has been with alkylating agents (nitrogen mustard, cyclophosphamide and chlorambucil) and purine analogues (6-mercaptopurine and azathioprine). There have been numerous reviews of "controlled" and uncontrolled experiences with these agents. However, every study, regardless of efforts to be carried out in a "controlled" manner, suffers from the heterogeneity of lupus itself. Different approaches have been used for assessment of these conflicting reports: a) comparison of short-term and long-term effects of various drug regimens and b) comparison of renal survival patterns over 5 years or longer.

Table 5 contrasts therapeutic outcomes observed from studies done from 1971 to 1986 (76, 168–175), comparing

Table 5. Prednisone alone versus prednisone with oral cytotoxic agents

Study (ref #)	Year	Months studied	Prednisone alone		Prednisone and azathioprine		Prednisone and cyclophosphamide	
			Total[1]	Failure[2]	Total[1]	Failure[2]	Total[1]	Failure[2]
Sztejnbok (169)	1971	12–48	14	6 (43)	12	0 (0)	—	—
Donadio (165)	1972	6	11	2 (18)	7	0 (0)	—	—
Cade (171)	1973	1–72	15	9 (60)	13	6 (46)	—	—
Donadio (172)	1974	36	9	0 (0)	7	0 (0)	—	—
Hahn (173)	1975	18–24	13	3 (23)	11	2 (18)	—	—
Donadio (174)	1977	6–70	26	7 (27)	—	—	24	7 (29)
NIH (76)	1979	58–43	23	7 (30)	19	6 (32)	15	4 (26)
NIH (168)	1983	85	15	7 (47)	20	5 (25)	18	4 (22)
NIH (175)	1986	85	28	10 (36)	19	6 (32)	18	4 (22)

[1] Total number of patients in each treatment group.
[2] Number (percent of total) of patients who progressed to renal failure or died.

corticosteroids with or without the immunosuppressive drugs azathioprine (1–4 mg/kg/day) or cyclophosphamide (1–4 mg/kg/day). Statistical analysis of the various regimens gives mixed results. Only Sztejnbok et al. (169) and Cade et al. (171) concluded that corticosteroids plus azathioprine was better than corticosteroids alone for the treatment of lupus nephritis. The remaining studies observed no significant differences between these regimens. Likewise, analysis by Wallace et al. (55), in a retrospective 15-year review of nonrandomized therapies for lupus nephritis, yielded no significant differences in survival between patients treated with corticosteroids alone and those treated with corticosteroids plus azathioprine. Most studies examining the use of low-dose oral cyclophosphamide plus low-dose prednisone versus prednisone only also showed no significant differences between treatment groups. However, because of the small numbers of patients in these groups, statistical significance could not truly be ascertained. Data from studies such as in Table 5 were pooled and analyzed by Felson et al. to try to improve the power of the statistical findings (176). Their analysis showed that patients on immunosuppressive drugs did better with less renal deterioration, less end-stage renal disease, and less mortality stemming from renal disease than did patients on corticosteroids alone.

Table 6 shows the therapeutic outcomes of an NIH study at 42 and 85 months of followup. The study compares low-dose oral corticosteroids alone to a) combination low-dose oral corticosteroids plus low-dose oral cyclophosphamide (1 mg/kg/day) and low-dose azathioprine (1 mg/kg/day) versus b) intravenous cyclophosphamide (500–1000 mg/m^2 every 3 months) (175, 177). This study revealed statistically significant improvement in outcome for patients treated with intravenous cyclophosphamide and corticosteroids as compared to those patients treated with corticosteroids alone. The combination regimen of oral cyclophosphamide, azathioprine, and corticosteroid showed a trend of improved outcome over corticosteroid use alone, but the results were not found to be statistically significant. In a double-blind crossover study, 14 lupus patients with diffuse proliferative glomerulonephritis were treated for 1 year with a) prednisone plus azathioprine or b) prednisone, azathioprine, and cyclophosphamide (178). Triple-drug use showed no significant advantage over the prednisone and azathioprine regimen. In summary, there now exists statistically significant evidence for the efficacy of intravenous cyclophosphamide in the management of SLE. The efficacy of other regimens using immunosuppressive agents is not as clear-cut, and the morbidity from these agents, as outlined in Table 7, is not insignifiant

Table 6. Comparison of oral and intravenous immunosuppressive therapy

Study (ref #)	Year	Prednisone		Triple oral[1]		Intravenous cyclophosphamide	
		Total[2]	Failure[3]	Total[2]	Failure[3]	Total[2]	Failure[3]
NIH (177)	1982[4]	13	1 (8)	16	1 (6)	12	2 (17)
NIH (175)	1986[5]	28	10 (36)	22	2 (9)	20	1 (5)

[1] Triple oral regimen consisted of prednisone, azathioprine, and cyclophosphamide.
[2] Total number of patients in treatment group.
[3] Number (percent of total) of patients who progressed to renal failure or died.
[4] Mean length of followup was 42 months.
[5] Mean length of followup was 85 months.

Table 7. Morbidity associated with cytotoxic drugs commonly used to treat lupus nephritis

Morbid effect	Purine analogues (azathioprine)	Alkylating agents (cyclophosphamide)
Bone marrow suppression	++	+++
Risk of infection	+	+
Hepatitis	+	Rare
Pancreatitis	+	0
Pulmonary fibrosis	0	Rare
Hemoorrhagic cystitis	0	++ (rarely, bladder cancer)
Alopecia	0	++
Inappropriate antidiuretic hormone secretion	0	Rare
Gonadal dysfunction	0	++
Lymphoreticular malignancies	+	+

(179–183). Hence, the decision to use these agents must be weighed against the overall clinical picture of each patient.

TOTAL LYMPHOID IRRADIATION

In an uncontrolled study, total lymphoid irradiation was administered to ten patients with lupus nephritis who were refractory to prednisone used with or without azathioprine therapy (184). By 6 weeks after therapy, overall renal function and various immunological parameters had improved in all patients. After 1 year, there continued to be renal improvement in eight patients. The side effects were significant in all patients, and complications included neutropenia, viral and bacterial infections, and thrombocytopenia. Another study, using total lymphoid irradiation on just two patients, was considered a failure both because of persistent disease activity and unacceptable side effects, which included septicenia, bronchopneumonia, and death in one patient (185). Although these reports are preliminary, taken together they suggest that the morbidity of total lymphoid irradiation outweighs the actual benefits and that cytotoxic drugs as immunosuppressive agents are more beneficial in lupus therapy.

CYCLOSPORINE

The use of cyclosporine in preventing transplant rejection has become widespread (186, 187). The immunosuppression mediated by cyclosporine is felt to arise from its ability to inhibit T-cell helper function by suppressing the synthesis and release of IL-2 (188). Cyclosporine has been used in limited clinical trials for treatment of systemic lupus erythematosus. Isenberg et al. gave cyclosporine (10 mg/kg/day) to five patients with active SLE, none of whom could tolerate the drug for more than 7 weeks due to side effects, which included nephrotoxicity (189). In this short period only two of the patients had improvement in any aspect of their lupus. In a larger uncontrolled trial (190), cyclosporine (5 mg/kg/day) was given along with corticosteroids to 20 patients who were followed for up to 28 months, with a mean of 9 months. Seventeen of the patients had a favorable therapeutic result. This study has since been expanded to included 41 cases of severe SLE. Five patients on the cyclosporine/steroid regimen either showed no clinical improvement or had intolerable side effects, and so discontinued the cyclosporine; the remaining 36 patients have been followed for a mean of 14 months (191). Another study (192) treated seven lupus patients with a combination of plasmapheresis as well as cyclosporine (2.5 mg/kg/day). Five of these patients needed several courses of plasmapheresis. This small study yielded no conclusions about the use of cyclosporine in the treatment of lupus. In summary, larger, long-term double-blind trials with cyclosporine therapy need to be performed prior to making any decisions regarding the efficacy of cyclosporine as a therapeutic agent in SLE.

PLASMAPHERESIS

Plasmapheresis was first reported as a treatment of SLE in 1976 (193). Since then, numerous uncontrolled trials of plasmapheresis in SLE have been reported (192, 194–217) with variable success. The major difficulties in interpreting the reported results, in addition to the lack of controls, have been a) the spontaneous waxing and waning nature of SLE, b) changes in medications and their doses, c) the use of different plasma replacement solutions, d) different amounts of plasma removed, e) erratic plasmapheresis schedules, and f) a lack of strict criteria for study entry. While some patients with mild extrarenal manifestations of SLE reportedly improved with plasmapheresis in conjunction with noncytotoxic drug therapy, most patients had also been receiving cytotoxic drugs. The reported benefits from plasmapheresis have been postulated to be due to a reduction of autoantibodies and circulating immune complexes that are inadequately cleared by a saturated reticuloendothelial system (194, 200, 208, 209, 211, 213, 218, 219). However, improvement has been noted in some patients without detectable reduction of autoantibodies or circulating immune complexes for more than 1 or 2 weeks postplasmapheresis (207, 208). An additional benefit attributed to plasmapheresis, in conjunction with cytotoxic drug therapy, has been the reestablishment of normal immunoregulatory mechanisms (210).

A review of the reports on plasmapheresis therapy of lupus nephritis reveals that all patients who substantially improved were also receiving cytotoxic agents (197, 198, 200, 213, 217). It therefore becomes difficult to discriminate between the effects of cytotoxic drugs and those of plasmapheresis. Clark et al. did a pilot study on the effects of monthly plasmapheresis on the renal function of lupus patients with nephritis (218). In addition to taking azathioprine and/or corticosteroids, 12 patients with diffuse proliferative glomerulonephritis were randomized to receive, or not receive, a 4-l plasma exchange every month, for up to 2 years. While the authors were cautious in their interpretation of the data, the patients receiving plasmapheresis did have better preservation of renal function, reduced disease activity, fewer hospital admissions, and less need for corticosteroids and/or azathioporine; accompanying the clinical improvement was a reduction in serologic abnormalities. A multicenter, randomized controlled study on plasmapheresis of lupus nephritis patients over a 3-year period was subsequently undertaken (219). Twenty patients received 4-l plasmaphereses every 3–4 weeks, and 19 others were not treated with plasmapheresis. The patients receiving plasmapheresis had an overall improvement in renal function as compared to the other treatent regimens. In a unique report, one patient with SLE and diffuse proliferative glomerulonephritis was treated with daily corticosteroids and cyclophosphamide, and a course of affinity apheresis. The patient's plasma was passed over sequential columns, the first containing immobilized DNAase and the second containing immobilized DNA. This treatment resulted in an abrupt decline of detectable circulating immune complexes and anti-DNA antibodies. There was a rapid improvement in renal function, with a substantial reduction in subendothelial deposits in a post-treatment renal biopsy, as compared to the pretreatment biopsy (220). Unfortunately, this patient died several months later from an infection, so no further followup is available. In another report (217), two patients with active systemic lupus and glomerulonephritis, despite corticosteroid therapy, were plasmaphered approximately 3-l daily for 3 days, then given three daily infusions of 12 mg cyclophosphamide/kg. Thereafter they were maintained on 2 mg cyclophosphadmide/kg orally plus low-dose oral corticosteroids. Both patients had clinical remission and preservation of renal function at 14 months followup.

Despite the many reports attributing a therapeutic effect to plasmapheresis in the management of SLE, only recently have there been double-blind assessments of plasmapheresis. A study done at the NIH was designed to evaluate the efficacy of plasmapheresis for extrarenal SLE (221). A total of 20 patients were randomized and studied. Only SLE patients with extrarenal manifestations of disease that were unresponsive to nonsteroidal antiinflammatory and/or corticosteroids drugs were studied.

None of the patients were on cytotoxic drugs, and none of the patients had a renal biopsy. Analysis of the data revealed that plasmpheresis resulted in significant transient improvement of immunochemical parameters of the disease (222). Several cellular functions were abnormal in these patients, but they remained unaffected by plasmapheresis (223). Consistent with only a transient immunochemical effect, no significant differences in clinical disease activity were observed between the two groups.

If plasmapheresis has a therapeutic role in SLE, then, as suggested by uncontrolled studies, it may best serve as an adjunct to cytotoxic drug therapy. We have been comparing the potential efficacy of monthly intravenous cyclophosphamide ($750\,\text{mg/m}^2$) with or without intense plasmapheresis in patients taking less than 0.5 mg prednisone/kg/day. These patients all have deteriorating renal function and diffuse proliferative glomerulonephritis. Our regimen represents a more aggressive use of bolus cyclophosphamide therapy than that reported by the NIH (175, 177). Bolus cyclophosphamide is given for a total of 6–12 months, then discontinued (224). Patients randomized to also receive plasmapheresis undergo five daily 3-l plasmaphereses starting 48 hours after each of the first three monthly boluses of cyclophosphamide. Our results (Table 8), after studying 20 patients, suggest that plasmapheresis may be a useful adjunct to cytotoxic drug therapy for severe lupus nephritis. The addition of 1 g boluses of methylprednisolone daily for 3 days after cyclophosphamide infusion has not improved therapeutic responses. More patients and longer follow up will be necessary before bolus cyclophamide and plasmpheresis therapy can be recommended as efficacious. A cooperative 5-year study assessing the effects of plasmapheresis and oral cyclophosphamide on the survival of patients with lupus nephritis is also currently in progress.

CURRENT RECOMMENDATIONS FOR THERAPY OF LUPUS NEPHRITIS

Two fundamental questions remain unresolved: a) which patients with lupus nephritis should be treated with immunosuppressive drugs, and b) what is the appropriate therapy? The first question has been argued extensively,

Table 8. Assessment of plasmapheresis as an adjunct to monthly bolus cyclosphosphamide therapy of patients with diffuse proliferative glomerulonephritis[1]

Treatment[2]	Serum creatinine (mg/dl)			Creatinine clearance (ml/min)			Proteinuria (g/24 hr)		
	Entry	3 mos	%Δ	Entry	3 mos	%Δ	Entry	3 mos	%Δ
Intravenous cyclophosphamide ($750\,\text{mg/m}^2\text{/mo}$)	2.0	3.0	+50	44	39	−12	6.6	6.0	−10
Intravenous cyclophosphamide & plasmapheresis	2.3	1.2	−48	39	75	+92	9.3	5.7	−39

[1] Data are expressed as the mean for all patients in each treatment group.
[2] The intravenous cyclophosphamide group without plasmapheresis consisted of eight patients, and the group also receiving plasmapheresis consisted of 12 patients. All patients were taking approximately 20 mg prednisone/day.

with some basing their decision on renal histology and others on clinical findings. Eiser et al. (225) have demonstrated that some lupus patients without any clinical evidence of nephritis have diffuse proliferative glomerulonephritis on biopsy, but the risk for rapid progression to renal failure in silent nephritis appears small. Conversely, progressive renal compromise over the short term is usually associated with a) diffuse proliferative glomerulonephritis, b) nephrotic syndrome, and c) an active urine sediment. Renal deterioration is less well correlated with serologic titers of autoantibodies, immune complexes, and complement (49, 69, 76, 78, 226). Lacking definitive criteria of whom to treat, educated decisions must be made by the physician in charge. This deicision must take into account both the risks of not treating and the drug-related morbidity. If the renal histology will alter the choice of drugs, then a biopsy should be obtained. A conservative approach (Table 9) that is widely used (85, 175, 224) employs only low or moderate doses of corticosteroids (<0.5 mg/kg/day) for stable patients with longstanding lupus nephritis and normal creatinine clearance. High-dose corticosteroids (1 mg prednisone/kg/day) plus or minus several daily intravenous boluses of methylprednisolone (1 g/day) are employed if the patient demonstrates the nephrotic syndrome and/or progressive renal compromise despite several weeks to months of high-dose corticosteroids. The NIH experience shows that intravenous cyclophosphamide (500–1000 mg/m^2) every 3 months, indefinitely, is efficacious for lupus nephritis (175). Plasmapheresis should currently be restricted to research protocols or for progressive disease despite cytotoxic drug therapy (217, 227).

OTHER CONSIDERATIONS

Hypertension is associated with the more severe cases of lupus nephritis (83, 95). However, only scant information suggests that hypertension forebodes a poorer renal prognosis (33, 36, 40, 51, 55, 83). Nevertheless, aggressive control of blood pressure may represent a major factor in improved survival curves.

Some drugs, such as hydralazine and procainamide, can induce a lupuslike syndrome (228). Drug-induced lupus usually resolves after withdrawal of the offending agent and is not associated with nephritis. Interestingly, these drugs are not contraindicated in patients with preexisting lupus. For example, hydralazine may be used to treat hypertension in a lupus patient without increased risk of exacerbating the spontaneous autoimmune disease.

Ultraviolet light is an exacerbating factor in some lupus patients, and flaring of renal disease has been reported following prolonged sun exposure (2). This may reflect accelerated turnover of DNA in ultraviolet-light-damaged skin. Therefore, lupus patients should be instructed to avoid prolonged ultraviolet light exposure (sun, sun lamps, etc.) and encouraged to use sun-blocking agents.

Nonsteroidal antiinflammatory drugs (NSAIDs) are frequently used for fever, arthritis, and other manifestations of lupus. NSAID use may obviate the need for steroids. Therefore, the effect of NSAIDs on renal function determinations is an important consideration in the evaluation of patients with lupus nephritis (229–231). A decline in glomerular filtration soon after initiation of NSAID therapy may reflect a pharmacologic effect on intrarenal arachidonic acid metabolism, and thereby prostaglandin synthesis, resulting in altered cortical renal blood flow. Discontinuation of the NSAIDs for 1 week should result in an improved glomerular filtration if the decline was due to NSAIDs.

One of the most difficult therapeutic dilemmas arises in patients who are pregnant or considering pregnancy. Despite retrospective analyses, there is no foolproof way to prognosticate the effects of pregnancy on a given patient. However, based on the Yale review (109), most physicians will strongly advise against pregnancy if there has been evidence of active disease in the preceding 6 months. Otherwise, counseling as to the unknown potential for the development of a life-threatening exacerbation of lupus is indicated. The patient and family can then weigh the potential risks against their desire for the patient to become pregnant. Should a lupus patient become pregnant and her lupus exacerbate, corticosteroids may be used in an attempt to control disease activity. Although cytotoxic drugs have teratogenic potential and may cause fetal loss, Tozman et al. (107) and Zulman et al. (108) have con-

Table 9. Current recommendations for therapy of lupus nephritis*

Clinical status	Drug	Dose
Longstanding nephritis and stable renal function	Prednisone	≤ 0.5 mg/kg/day to control extrarenal disease activity
Recent-onset nephritis or deteriorating renal function	Prednisone $\pm$ Methylprednisone	1 mg/kg/day $\times$ 1 month 1 g IV bolus/day $\times$ 3 days
Progressive deterioration of renal function despite several weeks of high-dose prednisone	Prednisone + Cytotoxic therapy	≤ 0.5 mg/kg/day to control extrarenal disease activity Oral azathioprine 1 mg/kg/day + cyclophosphamide 1 mg/kg/day or Intravenous cyclophosphamide 750–1000 mg/m^2 monthly $\times$ 6 months versus every 3 months chronically
	$\pm$ Plasmapheresis	3-l exchanges as an adjunct to initiation of cytotoxic therapy

* Abstracted from Coggins (85), Austin et al. (175) and Tsokos et al. (223).

curred that fetal anomalies have not been associated with cytotoxic drug therapy. Nevertheless, cytotoxic drugs should be discontinued for at least 6 months prior to conception, and pregnancy in the context of cytotoxic drug therapy requires counseling of the patient regarding teratogenic drug potential. The potential for sex-hormone modulation of SLE and the exacerbations of disease observed with pregnancy argues against the use of birth control pills in lupus patients (232). Birth control measures other than birth control pills should be used. Before treating male lupus patients with alkylating cytotoxic drugs, storage of sperm in a sperm bank should be considered, and similar consideration for storage of ova from women may be a viable option in the near future.

MONITORING THERAPEUTIC EFFECT

Attempts to identify parameters that accurately reflect lupus nephritis activity have been, for the most part, unrewarding. Likewise, the clinical variability of lupus nephritis and the lack of a proven efficacious treatment make it difficult to monitor the effects of any treatment regimen. Despite statistically significant correlation with clinical or histologic evidence of nephritis, no serologic or immunologic test has been widely accepted as a reliable index for lupus nephritis. Lacking a reliable extrarenal parameter to monitor, most physicians rely on renal parameters. Unfortunately, none of the conventional markers for nephritis are optimal for monitoring disease activity. An active urine sediment may be seen with masangial nephritis (76), diffuse proliferative glomerulonephritis may exist with an inactive urine sediment (225), and transition between the conventional histologic categories of lupus nephritis is well documented (63, 80, 224, 233). Proteinuria, although a poor prognostic sign (49, 226), does not necessarily correlate with the severity of the renal lesion on biopsy (76).

The glomerular filtration rate represents the sum of renal damage plus compensatory reserve renal function (84). Lacking a marker for renal reserve, improvements in glomerular filtration may not necessarily represent preservation of inflamed renal parenchyma. Even renal biopsies, when evaluated within conventional frameworks of classification, have been unreliable predictors of the eventual renal outcome, although adding the Pirani scoring system has helped somewhat. Attempts to establish correlates with simpler, more benign serologic or immunologic tests will be needed. However, until definitive evidence in support of specific parameters is established to assess the effects of therapy, the monitoring physician should, as a minimum, follow the glomerular filtration rate. Adjusting therapy to preserve renal function is the obvious primary goal.

SUMMARY

The management of lupus nephritis is extremely controversial. This stems from unsatisfactory prognostic measures and inaccurate parameters for following disease activity. Despite the amelioration of many signs and symptoms of SLE and lupus nephritis by corticosteroids, improved survival curves have not been correlated with steroids. Intravenous cyclophosphamide therapy has improved survival curves, but the morbidity and mortality associated with immunosuppressive therapy is substantial. Therefore, in one's efforts to manage the patient with lupus nephritis, attention should be paid to the unproven benefits versus the known risks of therapy. While plasmapheresis, cyclosporine, diet, or monoclonal antibodies may hold promise, careful scrutiny of controlled therapeutic trials will be essential to determine their efficacy.

ACKNOWLEDGMENTS

This research was supported in part by NIH grants #RO1-AI24644, #PO1-AI21289, and #RR-00350. The expert secretarial assistance of Mrs. Sarah Petrash in the preparation of this manuscript is greatly appreciated.

REFERENCES

1. Osler W: On the visceral manifestations of the erythema group of skin disease. *Am J Med Sci* 127:1, 1904.
2. Dubois EL (ed): *Lupus Erythematosus: A Review of the Current Status of Discoid and Systemic Lupus Erythematosus and their Variants*, 2nd revised ed. University of Southern California Press, Los Angeles, 1976.
3. Fries JF: The clinical aspects of systemic lupus erythematosus. *Med Clin North Am* 61:229, 1977.
4. Tan EM, Cohen AS, Fries JF, et al.: Special article: The 1982 revised criteria for the classification of systemic lupus erythematosus. *Arthritis Rheum* 25:1271, 1982.
5. Winchester RJ, Nunez-Roldan A: Some genetic aspects of systemic lupus erythematosus. *Arthritis Rheum* 25:833, 1982.
6. Lahita RG, Bradlow L, Fishman J, et al.: Estrogen metabolism in systemic lupus erythematosus: Patients and family members. *Arthritis Rheum* 25:843, 1982.
7. Pincus T: Studies regarding a possible function for viruses in the pathogenesis of systemic lupus erythematosus. *Arthritis Rheum* 25:847, 1982.
8. Messner RP. Lindstrom FD, Williams RC Jr: Peripheral blood lymphocyte cell surface markers during the course of systemic lupus erythematosus. *J Clin Invest* 52:3046, 1973.
9. Fauci, AS, Steinberg AD, Haynes BF, et al.: Immunoregulatory abberrations in systemic lupus erythematosus. *J Immunol* 121:1473, 1978.
10. Paty JG Jr, Sienknecht CW, Townes AS, et al.: Impaired cell-mediated immunity in systemic lupus erythematosus (SLE): A controlled study of 23 untreated patients. *Am J Med* 59:769, 1975.
11. Abdou NI, Sagawa A, Pascual E, et al.: Suppressor T cell abnormality in idiopathic systemic lupus erythematosus. *Clin Immunol Immunopathol* 6:192, 1976.
12. Smolen JS, Chused TM, Leiserson WM, et al.: Heterogeneity of immunoregulatory T cell subsets in systemic lupus erythematosus: Correlation with clinical features. *Am J Med* 72:783, 1982.
13. Winfield JB, Shaw M, Yamada A, et al.: Subset specificity

of antilymphocyte antibodies in systemic lupus erythematosus. II. Preferential reactivity with T4$^+$ cells is associated with relative depletion of autologous T4$^+$ cells. *Arthritis Rheum* 30:162, 1987.
14. Morimoto C, Steinberg AD, Letvin N, et al.: A defect of immunoregulatory T cell subsets in systemic lupus erythematosus patients demonstrated with anti-2H4 antibody. *J Clin Invest* 79:762, 1987.
15. Philips R, Lomnitzer R, Wadee AA, et al.: Defective monocyte function in patients with systemic lupus erythematosus. *Clin Immunol Immunopathol* 34:69, 1985.
16. Shirakawa F, Yamashita U, Suzulci H: Decrease in HLA-DR positive monocytes in patients with systemic lupus erythematosus (SLE). *J Immunol* 134:3560, 1985.
17. Murakawa Y, Takada S, Ueda T, et al.: Characterization of T lymphocute subpopulations responsible for deficient Interleukin-2 activity in patients with systemic lupus erythematosus. *J Immunol* 134:187, 1985.
18. Linder–Israeli M, Bakke A, Quismorio FP, et al.: Correction of interleukin-2 production in patients with systemic lupus erythematosus by removal of spontaneously activated suppressor cells *J Clin Invest* 75:762, 1985.
19. Koffler D, Carr RI, Angello V, et al.: Antibodies to polynucleotides in human sera, antigenic specificity and relation to disease. *J Exp Med* 134:294, 1971.
20. Notman DD, Kurata N, Tan EM: Profiles of antinuclear antibodies in systemic rheumatic diseases. *Ann Intern Med* 83:464, 1975.
21. Blease M, Grayson J, Steinberg AD: Increasaed immunoglobulin-secreting cells in the blood of patients with active systemic lupus erythematosus. *Am J Med* 69:345, 1980.
22. Zubler RH, Huang Y, Miescher PA: Mcchanisms of physiologic B cell responses and B cell hyperactivity in systemic lupus erythematosus. *Springer Semin Immunopathol* 9:195, 1986.
23. Koffler D, Agnello V, Thoburn R, et al.: Systemic lupus erythematosus: Prototype of immune complex nephritis in man. *J Exp Med* 134 (Suppl):169, 1971.
24. Bretjens J, ossi E, Albini B, et al.: Disseminated immune deposits in lupus erythematosus. *Arthritis Rheum* 20:962, 1977.
25. Suzuki Y, Oite T, Shimizu F, et al.: Solubilization of immune complex deposits by native 7S IgG molecules in lupus glomerulonephritis — a possible antigen excess effect on rheumatoid factor-IgG complexes. *Clin Exp Immunol* 58:663, 1984.
26. Harbeck RJ, Bardana EJ, Kohler PF, et al.: DNA:anti-DNA complexes: Their detection in systemic lupus erythematosus sera. *J Clin Invest* 52:789, 1973.
27. Sano H, Morimoto C: Isolation of DNA from DNA/anti-DNA immune complexes in systemic lupus erythematosus. *J Immunol* 126:538, 1981.
28. Morimoto C, Sano H, Abe T, et al.: Correlation between clinical activity of systemic lupus erythematosus and the amounts of DNA in DNA/anti-DNA antibody immune complexes. *J Immunol* 139:1960, 1982.
29. Datta SK, Patel H, Berry D: Induction of a cationic shift in IgG anti-DNA autoantibodies, role of T helper cells with the classical and novel phenotypes in three murine models of lupus nephritis. *J Exp Med* 165:1252, 1987.
30. Chetrit EB, Dunsky EH, Wollner S, et al.: In vivo clearance and tissue uptake of an anti-DNA monoclonal antibody and its complexes with DNA. *Clin Exp Immunol* 60:159, 1985.
31. Couser WG: Mechanisms of glomerular injury in immune-complex disease. *Kidney Int* 28:569, 1985.
32. Wener MH, Mannik M: Mechanisms of immune deposit formation in renal glomeruli. *Springer Semin Immunolpathol* 9:219, 1986.
33. Gay S, Losman MJ, Koopman WJ, et al.: Interaction of DNA with connective tissue matrix proteins reveals preferential binding to type V collagen. *J Immunol* 135:1097, 1985.
34. Isenberg DA, Collins C: Detection of cross-reactive anti-DNA antibody idiotypes on renal tissue-bound immunoglobulins from lupus patients. *J Clin Invest* 76:287, 1985.
35. Madaio MP, Carlson J, Cataldo J. et al.: Murine monoclonal anti-DNA antibodies bind directly to glmerular antigens and form immune deposits. *J Immunol* 138:2883, 1987.
36. Rudnicki RD, Gresham GE, Rothfield NF: The efficacy of antimalarials in systemic lupus erythematosus. *J Rheumatol* 2:323, 1975.
37. Urman JD, Rothfield NF: Corticosteroid treatment of sytemic lupus erythematosus. *JAMA* 238:2272, 1977.
38. Carey RA, Harvey AM, Howard JE: The effect of adrenocroticotropic hormone (ACTH) and cortisone on the course of disseminated lupus erythematosus and periarteritis nodosa. *Bull Johns Hopkins Hosp* 87:425, 1950.
39. Klemperer P, Pollack AD, Baehr G: Pathology of disseminated lupus erythematosus. *Arch Pathol* 32:569, 1941.
40. Pickering G, Bywaters EGL, Danielli JF, et al.: Treatment of systemic lupus erythematosus with steroids. Report to the medical research council by the collagen diseases and hypersenitivity panel. *Br Med J* 2:915, 1961.
41. Feinglass EJ, Arnett FC, Dorsch CA, et al.: Neuropsychiatric manifestations of systemic lupus erythematosus: Diagnosis, clinical spectrum, and relationship to other features of the disease. *Medicine* 55:323, 1976.
42. Kaplan S: Treatment of systemic lupus erythematosus. *Arthritis Rheum* 20 (Suppl):175, 1977.
43. Merrell M, Shulman LE: Determination of prognosis in chronic disease, illustrated by sytemic lupus erythematosus. *J Chron Dis* 1:12, 1955.
44. Kellum RE, Haserick JR: Systemic lupus erythematosus: A statistical evaluation of mortality based on a consecutive series of 299 patients. *Arch Intern Med* 113:200, 1964.
45. Dubois EL, Wierzchowiecki MD, Cox MB, et al.: Duration and death in system lupus erythematosus: An analysis of 249 cases. *JAMA* 227:1399, 1974.
46. Leonhardt T: Long-term prognosis of systemic lupus erythematosus. *Acta Med Scand* 445:440, 1966.
47. Estes D, Christain CL: The natural history of systemic lupus erythematosus by prospective analysis. *Medicine* 50:85, 1971.
48. Cameron JS, Turner DR, Ogg CS, et al.: Systemic lupus with nephritis: A long-term study. *Q J Med* 48:1, 1979.
49. Wallace DJ, Podell T, Weiner J, et al.: Systemic lupus erythematosus — survival patterns: Experiences with 609 patients. *JAMA* 245:934, 1981.
50. Pollak V, Pirani CL, Schwartz F: Thc natural history of renal manifestations of systemic lupus erythematosus. *J Lab Clin Med* 53:493, 1964.
51. Karsh J, Klippel JH, Balow JE, et al.: Mortality in lupus nephritis. *Arthritis Rheum* 22:764, 1979.
52. Cohen AS, Reynolds WE, Franklin EC, et al.: Preliminary criteria for the classification of systemic lupus erythematosus. *Bull Rheum Dis* 21:643, 1971.
53. David P, Atkins BC, Josse RG, et al.: Criteria for classification of SLE. *Br Med J* 3:88, 1973.
54. Sinniah R, Feng PH: Lupus nephritis: Correlation between light, electron microscopic and immunofluorescent findings

and renal function. *Clin Nephrol* 6:340, 1976.
55. Wallace DJ, Podell TE, Weiner JM: Lupus nephritis: Experience with 230 patients in a private practice from 1950 to 1980. *Am J Med* 72:209, 1982.
56. Dubis EL, Tuffanelli DL: Clinical manifestations of systemic lupus erythematosus: Complete analysis of 520 cases. *JAMA* 190:104, 1964.
57. Rothfield NF, McClusky RT, Baldwin DS: Renal disease in systemic lupus erythematosus. *N Engl J Med* 269:537, 1963.
58. Meislin AG, Rothfield N: Systemic lupus erythematosus in childhood. *Pediatrics* 42:37, 1968.
59. Dillard MG, Tillman RL, Sampson CC: Lupus nephritis: Correlation between the clinical course and presence of electron-dense deposits. *Lab Invest* 32:261, 1975.
60. Koffler D, Agnello V, Carr I, et al.: Variable patterns of immunoglobulin and complement deposition in the kidneys of patients with systemic lupus erythematosus. *Am J Pathol* 56:305, 1969.
61. Dujovne I, Pollak VE, Pirani CL, et al.: The distribution and character of glomerular deposits in systemic lupus erythematosus. *Kidney Int* 2:33, 1972.
62. Pollak VE,, Pirani CL: Pathology of the kidney in systemic lupus erythematosus: Serial renal biopsy studies and the effects of therapy on kidney lesions. In; Dubois EL, ed, *Lupus Erythematosus*, 2nd ed. Univ. of Southern California Press, Los Angeles, 1974.
63. Baldwin, DS, Gluck, MC, Lowenstein J, et al.: Lupus nephritis: Clinical course as related to morphologic forms and their transitions. *Am J Med* 62:12, 1977.
64. Austin HA, Muenz LR, Joyce KM, et al.: Diffuse proliferative lupus nephritis: Identification of specific pathologic features affecting renal outcome. *Kidney Int* 25:689, 1984.
65. Austin HA, Muenz LR, Joyce KM, et al.: Prognostic factors in lupus nephritis contribution of renal histologic data. *Am J Med* 75:382, 1983.
66. Stamenkovic T, Farre H, Donath A, et al.: Renal biopsy in SLE irrespective of clinical finding: Long term follow-up. *Clin Nephrol* 26:109, 1986.
67. Siegel NJ, Hayslett JP: Renal involvement in systemic lupus erythematosus. In: WN Suki, G Eknoyan, eds. *The Kidney in Systemic Diseases*, 2nd ed. John Wiley, New York, 1981.
68. Haakenstad AO, Mannik M: Saturation of the reticuloendothelial system with soluble immune complexes. *J Immunol* 112:1939, 1974.
69. Gershwin ME, Steinberg AD: Qualitative characteristics of anti-DNA antibodies in lupus nephritis. *Arthritis Rheum* 17:947, 1974.
70. Southemier RD, Gilliam JN: DNA antibody class, subclass, and complement fixation in systemic lupus erythematosus with and without nephritis. *Clin Immunol Immunopathol* 10:459, 1978.
71. Winfield JB, Faiferman I, Koffler D: Avidity of anti-DNA antibodies in serum and IgG glomerular eluates from patients with systemic lupus erythematosu. *J Clin Invest* 59:90, 1977.
72. Sano H, Morimoto C: DNA isolated from DNA/anti-DNA antibody immune complexes in systemic lupus erythematosus is rich in guanine-cytosine content. *J Immunol* 128:1341, 1982.
73. Pirani CL, Olesnicky L: Role of electronmicroscopy in the classification of lupus nephritis. *Am J Kidney Dis* 2 (Suppl 1): 150, 1982.
74. Comerford FR, Cohen AS: The nephropathy of systemic lupus erythematosus. An assessment of clinical, light, and electron microscopic criteria. *Medicine* 46:425, 1967.
75. Grishman E, Porush JG, Lee SL, et al.: Renal biopsies in lupus nephritis. *Nephron* 10:25, 1973.
76. Decker JL, Steinberg Ad, Reinertsen JL, et al.: Systemic lupus erythematosus: Evolving concepts. *Ann Intern Med* 91:587, 1979.
77. Zimmerman SW, Jenkins PG, Shelp WP, et al.: Progression from mineral or focal to diffuse proliferative lupus nephritis. *Lab Invest* 32:665, 1975.
78. Baldwin DG, Gallo GR, Lupus nephritis. *Clin Rhem Dis* 1:639, 1975.
79. Mery JP, Morel–Maroger L, Boelaert J, et al.: Evolution anatomoclinique des glomerulites diffuses et focales au course du lupus erythemateux dissemine. *J Urol Nephrol* 4–5:321, 1973.
80. Ginzler EM, Nicastri AD, Chun–Kuo C, et al.: Progression of mesangial and focal to diffuse lupus nephritis. *N Engl J Med* 291:693, 1974.
81. Baldwin DS, Lowenstein J, Rothfield NF, et al.: The clinical course of proliferative and membranous forms of lupus nephritis. *Ann Intern Med* 73:929, 1970.
82. Farquhar MG, Palade GE: Functional evidence for the existence of a third cell type in the renal glomerulus. *J Cell Biol* 13:55, 1962.
83. Tsumagari T, Fukumoto S, Kinjo M, et al.: Incidence and significance of intrarenal vasculopathies in patients with systemic lupus erythematosus. *Human Path* 16:43, 1985.
84. Balow JE: Therapeutic trials in lupus nephritis — problems related to renal histology, monitoring of therapy, and measures of outcome. *Nephron* 27:171, 1981.
85. Coggins CH: Overview of treatment of lupus nephropathy. *Am J Kidney Dis* 2:197, 1982.
86. Pirani CL, Pollak VE, Schwartz FD: The reproducibility of semiquantitative analysis of renal histology. *Nephron* 1:230, 1964.
87. Symchych PS, Perrin EV: Thrombosis of main pulmonary artery in nephrosis. Thromboembolism as a complication of nephrosis. *Am J Dis Child* 110:636, 1965.
88. Appel GB, Williams GS, Meltzer JI, et al.: Renal vein thrombosis, nephrotic syndrome, and systemic lupus erythematosus. *Ann Intern Med* 85:310, 1976.
89. Cade R, Spooner G, Juncos L, et al.: Chronic renal vein thrombosis. *Am J Med* 63:387, 1977.
90. Kant KS, Pollak VE, Weiss MA, et al.: Glomerular thrombosis in systemic lupus erythematosus: Prevalence and significance. *Medicine* 60:71, 1981.
91. Schleissner LA, Sheehan WW, Orselli RC: Lupus erythematosus in a patient with amyloidosis, adrenal insufficiency, and subsequent immunoblastic sarcoma. *Arthritis Rheum* 19:249, 1976.
92. King RW, Falls WF: Renal amyloidosis development in a case of systemic lupus erythematosus. *Clin Nephrol* 6:467, 1976.
93. Webb S, Segura F, Cervantes F, et al.: Systemic lupus erythematosus and amyloidosis. *Arthritis Rheum* 22:554, 1979.
94. Huston DP, McAdam PWJ, Balow JE: Amyloidosis in systemic lupus erythematosus. *Am J Med* 70:320, 1981.
95. Budman DR, Steinberg AD: Hypertension and renal disease in systemic lupus erythematosus. *Arch Intern Med* 136:1003, 1976.
96. Urowitz MB, Bookman AM, Koehler BE, et al.: The bimodal mortality pattern of systemic lupus erythematosus. *Am J Med* 60:221, 1976.
97. Bulkley BH, Roberts WC: The heart in systemic lupus erythematosus and the changes induced in it by cortico-

steroid therapy. *Am J Med* 58:243, 1975.
98. El-Shaboury AH, Hayes TM: Hyperlipidemia in asthmatic patients receiving long-term steroid therapy. *Br Med J* 2:85, 1973.
99. Hardin NJ, Minick R, Murphy GE: Experimental induction of atherosclerosis by the synergy of allergic injury to arteries and lipid rich diet. *Am J Pathol* 73:301, 1973.
100. Minick CR, Stemerman MB, Insull W: Role of endothelium and hypercholesterolemia in intimal thickening and lipid accumulation. *Am J Pathol* 95:131, 1979.
101. Glueck HI, Kant KS, Weiss MA, et al.: Thrombosis in systemic lupus erythematosus: Relation to the presence of circulating anticoagulants. *Arch Intern Med* 145:1389,1985.
102. Petri M, Rheinschmidt M, Whiting–O'Keefe Q, et al.: The frequency of lupus anticoagulant in systemic lupus erythematosus. *Ann Intern Med* 106:524, 1987.
103. Klippel JH, Karsh J, Stahl NI, et al.: A controlled study of pneumococcal polysaccharide vaccine in systemic lupus erythematosus. *Arthritis Rheum* 22:1321, 1979.
104. Friedman EA, Rutherford JW: Pregnancy and lupus erythematosus. *Obstet Gynecol* 8:601, 1956.
105. Garsenstein M, Pollak VE, Karl RM: Systemic lupus erythematosus and pregnancy. *N Engl J Med* 267:165, 1962.
106. Houser MT, Fish AJ, Tagatz GE, et al.: Pregnancy and systemic lupus erythematosus. *Am J Obstet Gynecol* 138:409, 1980.
107. Tozman ECS, Urowitz MB, Gladman DD: Systemic lupus erythematosus and pregnancy. *J Rheumatol* 7:624, 1980.
108. Zulman JI, Talal N, Hoffman GS, Epstein WV: Problems associated with the management of pregnancies in patients with systemic lupus erythematosus. *J Rheumatol* 7:37, 1980.
109. Hayslett JP, Lynn RI: Effect of pregnancy in patients with lupus nephropathy. *Kidney Int* 18:207, 1980.
110. Lockshin MD, Druzin ML, Goli S, et al.: Antibody to cardiolipin as a predictor of fetal distress or death in pregnant patients with systemic lupus erythematosus. *N Engl J Med* 313:152, 1985.
111. Branch DW, Scott JR, Kochenous NK, et al.: Obstetric complications associated with the lupus anticoagulant. *N Engl J Med* 313:1322, 1985.
112. Chameides L, Truex RC, Vetter V, Rashkind WJ, et al.: Association of maternal systemic lupus erythematosus with congenital complete heart block. *N Engl J Med* 294:687, 1977.
113. McCue CM, Mantakas ME, Tingelstad JB, Rubby S: Cogenital heart block in newborns of mothers with connective tissue disease. *Circulation* 56:82, 1977.
114. Helyer BJ, Howie JB: Renal disease associated with positive lupus erythematosus tests in cross-bred strains of mice. *Nature* 197:197, 1963.
115. Burnet FM, Holmes MC: The natural history of the NZB/NZW F_1 hybrid mouse; a laboratory model of systemic lupus. *Aust Ann Med* 14:185, 1965.
116. Lambert PH, Dixon FJ: Pathogenesis of the glomerulonephritis of NZB/W mice. *J Exp Med* 127:507, 1968.
117. Huston DP, Steinberg AD: Animal models of human systemic lupus erythematosus. *Yale J Biol Med* 52:289, 1979.
118. Raveche ES, Novotony EA, Hansen, CT, et al.: Genetic studies in NZB mice: V. Recombinant inbred lines demonstrate that separate genes control autoimmune phenotype. *J Exp Med* 153:1187, 1981.
119. Steinberg AD, Raveche ES, Laskin CA, et al.: Systemic lupus erythematosus: Insights from animal models. *Ann Intern Med* 100:714, 1984.
120. Kotzin BL, Palmer E: The contribution of NZW genes to lupus-like disease in (NZBxNZW)F_1 mice. *J Exp Med* 165:1237, 1987.
121. Klassen LW, Budman DR, Williams GW, et al.: Ribarvin: Efficacy in the treatment of murine autoimmune disease. *Science* 195:787, 1977.
122. Roubinian JR, Papoian R, Talal N: Androgenic hormones modulate autoantibody responses and improve survival in murine lupus. *J Clin Inves* 59:1066, 1977.
123. Duvic M, Steinberg AD, Klassen LW: Effect of antiestrogen, Nafoxidine, on NZB/W autoimmune disease. *Arthritis Rheum* 21:414, 1978.
124. Melez KA, Reeves JP, Steinberg AD: Regulation of the expression of autoimmunity in NZBxNZW F_1 mice by sex hormones. *J Immunopharm* 1:27, 1978.
125. Lucas JA, Ahmed SA, Casey ML, et al.: Prevention of autoantibody formation and prolonged survival in New Zealand Black/New Zealand White F_1 mice fed dehydroisoandrosterone. *J Clin Invest* 75:2091, 1985.
126. Lahita RG, Bradlow HL, Ginzler E, et al.: Low plasma androgens in women with systemic lupus erythematosus. *Arthritis Rheum* 30:241, 1987.
127. Fretwell MD, Altman LC: Exacerbation of a lupus erythematosus-like syndrome during treatment of non-C1-esterase-inhibitor-dependent angioedema with danazol. *J Allergy Clin Immunol* 69:306, 1982.
128. Krakauer RS, Strober W, Rippeon DL, et al.: Prevention of autoimmune disease in experimental systemic lupus erythematosus by the administration of soluble immune response suppressor. *Science* 196:56, 1977.
129. Reinertsen JL, Steinberg AD: *In vivo* immune response suppression by the supernatant from concanavalin A-activated spleen cells. *J Immunol* 19:217, 1977.
130. Zurier RB, Sayadoff DM, Torrey SB, et al.: Prostaglandin E_1 treatment of NZB/W mice. II. Prevention of glomerulonephritis. *Arthritis Rheum* 20:1449, 1977.
131. Zurier RB: Prostaglandins, immune responses, and murine lupus. *Arthritis Rheum* 25:804, 1982.
132. Denman, AM, Denman EJ, Holborow EJ: Effects of antilymphocyte globulin on kidney disease in (NZBxNZW)F_1 mice. *Lancet* 2:841, 1966.
133. Denman AM, Russell AS, Loewi G, et al.: 6 Immunopathology of New Zealand Black mice treated with antilymphocyte globulin. *Immunology* 20:973, 1971.
134. Kotzin BL, Strober S: Reversal of NZB/NZW disease with total lymphoid irradiation. *J Exp Med* 150:371, 1979.
135. Steinberg AD, Talal N: Suppression of antibodies to nucleic acids with polyinosinic polycytidylic acid and cyclophosphamide in murine lupus. *Clin Exp Immunol* 7:687, 1971.
136. Borel H, Bastian D, Cooper B, et al.: A possible new therapy of systemic lupus erythematosus (SLE). *Ann NY Acad Sci* 475:296, 1986.
137. Hurd ER, Johnston JM, Okita JR, et al.: Prevention of glomerulonephritis and prolonged survival in New Zealand Black/New Zealand White F_1 hybrid mice fed an essential fatty acid deficient diet. *J Clin Invest* 67:476, 1981.
138. Prickett JD, Robinson DR, Steinberg AD: Dietary enrichment with the polyunsaturated fatty acid eicosapentaenoic acid prevents proteinuria and prolongs survival in NZB/NZW F_1 mice. *J Clin Invest* 68:556, 1981.
139. Robinson DR, Prickett JF, Makoul GT, et al.: Dietary fish oil reduces progresion of established renal disease in (NZBxNZW)F_1 mice and delays renal disease in BXSB and MRL/l strains. *Arthritis Rheum* 29:539, 1986.
140. Fischer, S. Weber PC: Prostaglandin I_3 is formed *in vivo* in man after dietary eicosapentaenoic acid. *Nature* 307:165, 1984.
141. Casey TP: Systemic lupus erythematosus in NZBxNZW

hybrid mice treated with the corticosteroid drug betamethasone. *J Lab Clin Med* 71:390, 1968.
142. Gelfand MC, Steinberg AD: Therapeutic studies in NZB/W mice. II. Relative efficacy of azathioprine, cyclophosphamide, and methylprednisone. *Arthritis Rheum* 15:247, 1972.
143. Hahn BH, Bagby MK, Hamilton TR, et al.: Comparison of therapeutic and immunosuppressive effects of azathioprine, prednisolone and combined therapy in NZB/NZW mice. *Arthritis Rheum* 16:163, 1973.
144. Steinberg AD, Gelfand MC, Hardin JA, et al.: Therapeutic studies in NZB/W mice. II. Relationship between renal status and efficacy of immunosuppressive drug therapy. *Arthritis Rheum* 18:9, 1975.
145. Casey, TP: Immunosuppression by cyclophosphamide in NZBxNZW mice with lupus nephritis. *Blood* 32:436, 1968.
146. Horowitz RE, Dubois EL, Weiner J, et al.: Cyclophosphamide treatment of mouse systemic lupus erythematosus. *Lab Invest* 21:199, 1969.
147. Russell PJ, Hicks JD, Burnet FM: Cyclophosphamide treatment of kidney disease in (NZBxNZW)F_1 mice. *Lancet* 1:1279, 1966.
148. Russell PJ, Hicks JD: Cyclophosphamide treatment of renal disease in (NZBxNZW)F_1 hybrid mice. *Lancet* 1:440, 1968.
149. Andrzejenski C Jr, Stollar BD, Lalor TM, et al.: Hybridoma autoantibodies to DNA. *J Immunol* 124:1499, 1980.
150. Hahn BH, Ebling F, Freeman S, et al.: Production of monoclonal murine antibodies to DNA by somatic cell hybrids. *Arthritis Rheum* 23:942, 1980.
151. Rauch J, Lafer E, Andrzejewski C, et al.: Monoclonal lupus autoantibodies. *Arthritis Rheum* 25:744, 1982.
152. Hahn B: Characteristics of pathogenic subpopulations of antibodies to DNA. *Arthritis Rheum* 25:747, 1982.
153. Wofsy D, Ledbetter JA, Hendler PL, et al.: Treatment of murine lupus with monoclonal anti-T cell antibody. *J Immunol* 134:852, 1985.
154. Wofsy D, Seaman WE: Reversal of advanced murine lupus in NZB/NZW F_1 mice by treatment with monoclonal antibody to L3T4. *J Immunol* 138:3247, 1987.
155. Gunn HC: Successful treatment of autoimmunity in (NZBxNZW)F_1 mice with cyclosporin and (Nva^2)-cyclosporine: I. Reduction of autoantibodies. *Clin Exp Immunol* 64:226, 1986.
156. Gunn HC, Ryffel B: Successful treatment of autoimmunity in (NZBxNZW)F_1 mice with cyclosporine and (Nva^2)-cyclosporine: II. Reduction of glomerulonephritis. *Clin Exp Immunol* 64:234, 1986.
157. Balow JE, Austin HA, Tsokos GC, et al.: Lupus nephritis. *Ann Intern Med* 106:79, 1987.
158. Albert DA, Hadler NM, Ropes MW: Does corticosteroid therapy effect the survival of patients with systemic lupus erythematosus? *Arthritis Rheum* 22:945, 1979.
159. Pollack VE, Pirani CL, Kark RM: Effect of large doses of prednisone on the renal lesions and life span of patients with lupus glomerulonephritis. *J Lab Clin Med* 57:495, 1961.
160. Bell PRF, Calman KC, Wood RFM et al.: Reversal of acute clinical and experimental organ rejection using doses of intravenous methylprednisolone, *Lancet* 1:876, 1971.
161. Mussche MM, Ringoir SMG, Lameire NN: High intravenous doses of methylprednisolone for acute cadaveric renal allograft rejection. *Nephron* 16:287, 1976.
162. Cathcart ES, Scheinberg MA, Idelson BA, et al: Beneficial effects of methylprednisolone "pulse" therapy in diffuse proliferative lupus nephritis. *Lancet* 1:163, 1976.
163. Nebout T, Sobel A, Lagrue G: Intravenous methylprednisolone pulses in diffuse proliferative lupus nephritis (letter). *Lancet* 1:909, 1977.
164. Ponticelli C, Zucchelli P, Banfi G, et al.: Treatment of diffuse proliferative lupus nephritis by intravenous high-dose methylprednisolone. *Q J Med* 201:16, 1982.
165. Dosa S, Mallick NP, Lawler W, et al.: The treatment of lupus nephritis by methylprednisolone pulse therapy. *Postgrad Med J* 54:628, 1978.
166. Kimberly RP, Lockshin MD, Sherman RL, et al.: High-dose intravenous methylprednisolone pulse therapy in system lupus erythematosus. *Am J Med* 70:817, 1981.
167. Ballou SP, Khan MA, Kushner I: Intravenous pulse methylprednisolone followed by alternate day corticosteroids therapy in lupus erythematosus: A prospective evaluation. *J Rheumatol* 12:944, 1985.
168. Carette S, Klippel JH, Decker JL, et al.: Controlled studies of oral immunosuppressive drugs in lupus nephritis. A long-term followup. *Ann Intern Med* 99:1, 1983.
169. Sztejnbok M, Stewart A, Diamond H, et al.: Azathioprine in the treatment of systemic lupus erythematosus: A controlled study. *Arthritis Rheum* 14:639, 1971.
170. Donadio JV Jr, Holley KE, Wagoner RD, et al.: Treatment of lupus nephritis with prednisone and combined prednisone and azathioprine. *Ann Intern Med* 77:829, 1972.
171. Cade R, Spooner G, Schlein E, et al.: Comparison of azathioprine, prednisone, and heparin alone or combined in treating lupus nephritis. *Nephron* 10:37, 1973.
172. Donadio JV Jr. Holley KE, Wagoner RD, et al.: Further observations on the treatment of lupus nephritis with prednisone and combined prednisone and azathioprine. *Arthritis Rheum* 17:573, 1974.
173. Hahn BH, Kantor OS, Osterland CK: Azathioprine plus prednisone compared with prednisone alone in the treatment of systemic lupus erythematosus: Report of a prospective controlled trial in 24 patients. *Ann Intern Med* 83:597, 1975.
174. Donadio JV Jr, Holley KE, Ferguson RH, et al.: Treatment of diffuse proliferative lupus nephritis with prednisone and combined prednisone and cyclophosphamide. *N Engl J Med* 299:1151, 1978.
175. Austin HA, Klippel JH, Balow JE, et al.: Therapy of lupus nephritis. Controlled trial of prednisone and cytotoxic drugs. *N Engl J Med* 314:614, 1986.
176. Felson DT, Anderson J: Evidence for the superiority of immunosuppressive drugs and prednisone over prednisone alone in lupous nephritis. *N Engl J Med* 311:1528, 1984.
177. Dinant HJ, Decker JL, Klippel JH, et al.: Alternative modes of cyclophosphamide and azathioprine therapy in lupus nephritis. *Ann Intern Med* 96:728, 1982.
178. Ginzler E, Diamond H, Guttadauria M, et al.: Prednisone and azathioprine compared to prednisone plus low-dose azathioprine and cyclophosphamide in the treatment of diffuse lupus nephritis. *Arthritis Rheum* 19:693, 1976.
179. Schein PS, Winokur SH: Immunosuppressive and cytotoxic chemotherapy: long-term complications. *Ann Intern Med* 82:84, 1975.
180. Gerber NL, Steinberg AD: Clinical use of immunosuppressive drugs: Parts 1 and 2. *Drugs* 11:14, 1976.
181. Plotz PH, Klippel JH, Decker JL, et al.: Bladder complications in patients receiving cyclophosphamide for systemic lupus erythematosus or rheumatoid arthritis. *Ann Intern Med* 91:221, 1979.
182. Bacon AM, Rosenberg SA: Cyclophosphamide hepatotoxicity in a patient with systemic lupus erythematosus. *Ann Intern Med* 97:62, 1982.
183. Decker JL: Cytotoxic drug benefit/risk ratio: Often too close to encourage use. *Workshops in Rheumatology* 3(8):1, 1982.
184. Strober, S, Field E, Hoppe RT, et al.: Treatment of intract-

able lupus nephritis with total lymphoid irradiation. *Ann Intern Med* 102:450, 1985.
185. Ben-Chetrit E, Gross DJ, Braverman A, et al.: Total lymphoid irradiation in refractory systemic lupus erythematosus. *Ann Intern Med* 105:58, 1986.
186. The Canadian Multicentre Transplant Study Group: A randomized clinical trial of cyclosporine in cadaveric renal transplantation. *J Engl J Med* 309:809, 1983.
187. Merion RM, David MD, White DJ, et al.: Cyclosporine: Five years experience in cadaveric renal transplantation. *N Engl J Med* 310:148, 1984.
188. Borel JF, Ryffel B: Mechanism of action of ciclosporin: A continuing puzzle. In: R Schindler, ed, *Cyclosporin in Autoimmune Diseases*. First International Symposium. Springer-Verlag, Basel, p 24, 1985.
189. Isenberg DA, Snaith ML, Morrow WJ, et al.: Cyclosporin A for the treatment of systemic lupus erythematosus. *Int J Immunopharmacol* 3:63, 1981.
190. Miescher PA, Miescher A: Combined ciclosporin-steroid treatment of systemic lupus erythematosus. In: R Schindler, ed, *Cyclosporin in Autoimmune Diseases*. First International Symposium. Springer-Verlag, Basel, p 337, 1985.
191. Miescher PA: Treatment of systemic lupus erythematosus. *Springer Semin Immunopathol* 9:271, 1986.
192. Bambauer R, Jutzler GA, Pees H, et al.: Cyclosporine (CyA) and therapeutic plasma exchange in steroid-resistant SLE. In: R, Schindler, ed, *Cyclosporine in Autoimmune Diseases*. First International Symposium. Springer-Verlag, Basel, p 346, 1985.
193. Jones JV, Cumming RH, Bucknall RC, Asplin CM: Plasmapheresis in the management of acute systemic lupus erythematosus? *Lancet* 1:709, 1976.
194. Jones JV, Cumming RH, Bacon PA, et al.: Evidence for a therapeutic effects of plasmapheresis in patients with systemic lupus erythematosus. *Q J Med* 48:555, 1979.
195. Moran CJ, Parry HF: Plasmapheresis in systemic lupus erythematosus. *Br Med J* 1:1573, 1977.
196. Schlansky R, DeHoratius RJ, Pincus T, Tung KSK: Plasmapheresis in systemic lupus erythematosus. *Arthritis Rheum* 24:49, 1981.
197. Lockwood CM, Pussell B, Wilson CB, Peters DK: Plasma exchange in nephritis. *Adv Nephrol* 8:383, 1979.
198. Lockwood CM, Peter DK: Plasma exchange in glomerulonephritis and related vasculitides. *Ann Rev Med* 31:687, 1979.
199. Schildermans F, Dequeker J, DePutte IV: Plasmapheresis combined with corticosteroids and cyclophosphamide in uncontrolled active systemic lupus erythematosus. *J Rheumatol* 6:687, 1979.
200. Lockwood CM, Rees AJ, Pussell B, et al.: Experience of the use of plasma exchange in the management of potentially fulminating glomerulonephritis and SLE. *Exp Hematol* 5:117s, 1977.
201. Hubbard HC, Portnoy B: Systemic lupus erythematosus in pregnancy treated with plasmapheresis. *Br J Dermatol* 101:87, 1979.
202. Isbister JP, Ralston M, Wright: Fulminant lupus pneumonitis with acute renal failure and RBC aplasia. *Arch Intern Med* 141:1081, 1981.
203. Fitchen JJ, Cline MJ, Saxon A, et al.: Serum inhibitors of hemopoiesis in a patient with aplastic anemia and systemic lupus erythematosus: Recovery after plasma exchange. *Am J Med* 66:537, 1979.
204. McKenzie PE, Taylor AE, Woodroffe AJ, et al.: Plasmapheresis in glomerulonephritis. *Clin Nephrol* 12:97, 1979.
205. Rossen RD, Hersh EM, Sharp JT, et al.: Effect of plasma exchange on circulating immune complexes and antibody formation in patients with cyclophosphamide and prednisone. *Am J Med* 63:647, 1977.
206. Young DW, Thompson RA, McKenzie PH: Plasmapheresis in hereditary angioneurotic edema and systemic lupus erythematosus. *Arch Intern Med* 140:127, 1980.
207. Blacklock HA, Hill RS, Bridle M, et al.: Therapeutic plasmapheresis by continuous flow centrifugation. *N Z Med J* 92:145, 1980.
208. Parry HF, Moran CJ, Smith ML, et al.: Plasma exchange in systemic lupus erythematosus. *Ann Rehum Dis* 40:224, 1981.
209. Jones JV, Robinson MF, Parciany RK, et al.: Therapeutic plasmapheresis in systemic lupus erythematosus: Effect on immune complexes and antibodies to DNA. *Arthritis Rehum* 24:1113, 1981.
210. Abdou NI, Lindsley HB, Pollock A, et al.: Plasmapheresis in active SLE: Effects on clinical serum, and cellular abnormalities. Case report. *Clin Immunol and Immunopathol* 19:44, 1981.
211. Lockwood CM, Worlledge S, Nichols A, et al.: Reversal of impaired splenic function in patients with nephritis or vasculitis (or both) by plasma exchange. *N Engl J Med* 300:524, 1979.
212. Habersetzer R, Samtleben W, Blumenstein M, et al.: Plasma exchange in systemic lupus erythematosus. *Int J Artific Organs* 6:39, 1983.
213. Vangelista A, Frasca H, Orsi C, et al.: Short-term plasmapheresis in acute lupus nephritis. *Int J Artific Organs* 6:43, 1983.
214. Hamblin, TJ, Smith DS: Long-term exchange (a feasible treatment in systemic lupus erythematosus and other diseases). *La Ricerca Clin Lab* 13:95, 1983.
215. Moriconi L, Ferri C, Fanara G, et al.: Plasma exchange in the treatment of lupus nephritis. *Int J Artific Organs* 6:35, 1983.
216. Schena FP, Manno C, Carabellese S, et al.: Plasma exchange in systemic lupus erythematosus. *Int J Artific Organs* 6:29, 1983.
217. Schroeder JO, Haus HE, Loffler H: Synchronization of plasmapheresis and pulse cyclophosphamide in severe systemic lupus erythematosus. *Ann Intern Med* 107:334, 1987.
218. Clark WF, Lindsay RM, Cattran DC, et al.: Monthly plasmapheresis for systemic lupus erythematosus with diffuse proliferative glomerulonephritis. A pilot study. *Can Med Assoc J* 125:171, 1981.
219. Clark WF, Cattran DC, Balfe JW, et al.: Chronic plasma exchange in systemic lupus erythematosus nephritis. *Proc Eur Dial Transplant Assoc* 20:629, 1983.
220. Terman DS, Buffaloe G, Mattioli C, et al.: Extracorporal immunoadsorption: Initial experience in human systemic lupus erythematosus. *Lancet* 2:824, 1979.
221. Wei N, Klippel JH, Huston DP, et al.: Randomized trial of plasma exchange in mild systemic lupus erythematosus. *Lancet* 1:17, 1983.
222. Huston DP, Wei N, Klima E, Hall RP, et al.: Immunochemical effects of plasmapheresis in systemic lupus erythematosus (SLE). *Arthritis Rheum* 24 (Suppl): 92, 1981.
223. Tsokos GC, Balow JE, Huston DP, et al.: Effect of plasmapheresis on T and B lymphocyte functions in patients with systemic lupus erythematosus: A double blind study. *Clin Exp Immunol* 48:449, 1982.
224. Huston, DP, White MJ, Mattioli C, et al.: A controlled trial of plasmapheresis and cyclophosphamide therapy of lupus

nephritis. *Arthritis Rheum* 26 (Suppl): 33, 1983.
225. Eiser AR, Katz SM, Swartz C: Clinically occult diffuse proliferative lupus nephritis. *Arch Intern Med* 139:1022, 1979.
226. Ginzler EM, Diamond HS, Weiner M, et al.: A multicenter study of outcome in systemic lupus erythematosus. I. Entry variable as predictors of prognosis. *Arthritis Rheum* 25:601, 1982.
227. Health Technology Assessment Reports: Apheresis in the treatment of systemic lupus erythematosus (SLE) Vol 17, 1985.
228. Reidenberg MM: The chemical induction of systemic lupus erythematosus and lupus-like illnesses. *Arthritis Rheum* 24:1004, 1981.
229. Simon LS, Mills JA: Nonsteroidal anti-inflammatory drugs. *N Engl J Med* 302:1179, 1980.
230. Zipser RD, Henrich WL: Implications of nonsteroidal anti-inflammatory drug therapy. *Am J Med* 80 (SIA):78, 1986.
231. Karsh J, Kimberly RP, Stahl NI, et al.: Comparative effects of aspirin and ibuprofen in the management of systemic lupus erythematosus. *Arthritis Rheum* 23:1401, 1980.
232. Jungers P, Dougados M, Pellissier C, et al.: Influence of oral cotraceptive therapy on the activity of systemic lupus erythematosus. *Arthritis Rheum* 25:618, 1982.
233. Mahajan SK, Ordoney NG, Spargo BH, et al.: Changing histopathology patterns in lupus nephropathy. *Clin Nephrol* 10:1, 1978.

CHAPTER 27

Vasculitic Diseases of the Kidney

JAMES E. BALOW & HOWARD A. AUSTIN III

POLYARTERITIS

Introduction

Polyarteritis is characterized by inflammatory, necrotizing, and thrombotic lesions of blood vessels that result in ischemia of affected tissues. The clinical manifestations of polyarteritis are extremely heterogenous and include a variable mix of nonspecific constitutional features and focal deficits according to the severity and distribution of the involved vasculature (1–7). It is unknown whether the diversity of clinical and pathologic manifestations relates to a multiplicity of etiologies for the polyarteritis syndrome or to differences in individual host responses to common stimuli.

There are few clues to the etiology or pathogenesis of polyarteritis (8, 9). Rarely, hypersensitivity reactions to drugs, vaccines, or other exogenous agents may cause polyarteritis; empiric elimination of potentially inciting agents should be advised whenever possible. Most cases of polyarteritis are idiopathic and immunologic mechanisms can only be inferred. Studies of pathogenesis are also hampered by the paucity of relevant experimental models. Although immune complexes have been postulated to cause vasculitic lesions, their role is controversial (10); circulating immune complexes have been found in patients with active polyarteritis, but the evidence is not compelling that they are pathogenic, since affected sites, including glomeruli, rarely show significant immune deposits (11, 12). The presence of hepatitis B surface antigen (HBsAg) in 10–40% of patients is provocative. However, its presence is predictive of neither the clinical manifestations nor the course of the disease, and HBsAg often persists after remission of polyarteritis. Recently, an autoantibody to cytoplasmic antigens of neutrophilic leukocytes has been described in patients with active Wegener's granulomatosis and polyarteritis (13–16). It is not known whether these autoantibodies are involved in the pathogenesis of the vasculitic lesions, but measurement of titers appears to be helpful in assessment of disease activity and management.

Classification

Polyarteritis is usually divided into two categories according to the predominant size of vessel involvement (17). Classic polyarteritis (or polyarteritis nodosa) mainly affects medium-sized arteries and may result in nodular aneurysms whose presence may facilitate the diagnosis by arteriography (18). Microscopic polyarteritis affects predominantly glomerular capillaries and is commonly associated with necrotizing and crescentic glomerulonephritis on renal biopsy. The designation of these two categories should be viewed as a practical clinical approach that is useful to describe the predominant renal manifestations of polyarteritis; this classification scheme does not imply a difference in pathogenesis, and overlapping of these categories is relatively common.

Several vasculitic diseases involving the kidney are separated from polyarteritis on the basis of clinical and/or pathologic differences (1, 19). These include Wegener's granulomatosis, allergic angiitis and granulomatosis (Churg–Strauss disease), and Takayasu's arteritis. Overlap syndromes with features of more than one of these conditions and/or cutaneous vasculitis are relatively common (20, 21). The interrelationships among these vasculitic diseases remain unclear.

Medical specialties vary in their preferences for the lumping and splitting of vasculitic diseases. In nephrology and nephropathology, there is a growing tendency to report together patients with microscopic polyarteritis, Wegener's granulomatosis, and a no-immune-deposit form of necrotizing and crescentic glomerulonephritis (22–26). It is important to be cognizant of differences in patient populations in the various reports appearing in the literature.

Diagnostic considerations

Polyarteritis is typically manifested clinically by fever, malaise, weight loss, arthralgias, and vague myalgias. The presence of focal vasculitic skin lesions, mononeuritis multiplex, fluctuating gastrointestinal signs, and/or renal disease hasten the diagnosis. Diagnostic efforts should be focused on involved organs, utilizing radiologic and histologic studies of vascular pathology. Blind biopsies of clinically unaffected tissues are generally unrewarding. Arteriography can be particularly helpful in diagnosis, even in the absence of visceral dysfunction. Renal, hepatic, and mesenteric arteriography may show aneurysms, vessel tapering, or beading; there is a somewhat higher yield of abnormalities of the renal vasculature in hypertensive than in normotensive individuals with polyarteritis.

Renal manifestations

At least two thirds of patients with polyarteritis have renal involvement, although kidney disease is rarely a presenting manifestion, even in microscopic polyarteritis (22). In classic polyarteritis, renal cortical ischemia, thrombosis, and/or infarcts may occur. Severe renin-mediated hypertension is seen during either the active acute stage or the healing chronic phase of polyarteritis (27, 28). Spontaneous rupture of visceral aneurysms can present life-threatening complications. This should underscore the need to vigorously control hypertension in patients with polyarteritis, especially those with documented aneurysms. Mild proteinuria may be present without the usual signs of active glomerulonephritis. Insidious renal insufficiency may progress due to chronic ischemia and hypertension.

Typical renal pathologic changes of microscopic polyarteritis include focal, segmental proliferative, and necrotizing glomerulonephritis. In severe cases, crescent formation may be prominent and may lead to rapidly progressive renal failure. The proportion of glomeruli affected by crescents has a graded effect on the prognosis (22, 23). Extraglomerular vasculitis is commonly found at autopsy, but may elusive in ordinary needle biopsies and rarely produces diagnostic arteriographic changes in patients with the predominantly microscopic form of polyarteritis (22, 23).

Clinical course

The patient with polyarteritis may present with an insidious chronic illness with few or subtle clinical signs of major organ system dysfunction, a situation often contributing to late diagnosis. On the other hand, about one half of patients have an initially aggressive and progressive disease with a risk of serious morbidity and mortality due to vital organ system involvement. The majority of deaths from polyarteritis occur within the first few months and tend to be due to complications of active extrarenal vasculitis (22, 23, 29–31).

If the patient survives the early phase of disease, the subsequent course in a few may proceed to total remission, but the majority develop chronic or relapsing disease, requiring long-term immunosuppressive drug therapy. Morbidity and mortality in late phases are often due to complications of prolonged corticosteroid treatment and to vascular compromise resulting from hypertension and the sclerosis of healed vasculitic lesions. The overall expected survival rate at 5 years is approximately 60% for patients with either classic or microscopic polyateritis (22–24, 29–32). Those patients with smoldering disease have a substantially worse prognosis than those who remit with effective therapy (22).

Therapeutic intervention

Polyarteritis is considered to be mediated by immunologic factors and hence regimens of immunosuppressive and antiinflammatory drugs form the basis of primary therapy. However, diverse medical and surgical complications of multisystem involvement often require the use of entire therapeutic armamentarium available in clinical medicine. A discussion of the treatment of complications of vascular insults to specific viscera is beyond the scope of this presentation.

A composite of cumulative survival data extracted from several published series on patients with predominantly classic polyarteritis is shown in Figure 1. The effects of the major forms of immunosuppressive drug therapies are compared to the natural history of untreated polyarteritis. The shaded areas represent the range of outcomes indicated in the combined series. Aspects of the individual series will be considered in subsequent discussions of the different forms of therapy of polyarteritis.

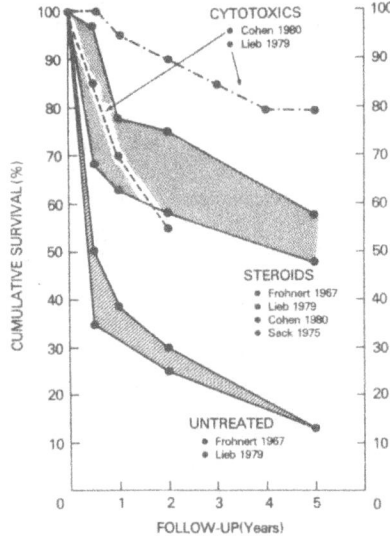

Figure 1. Prognosis related to treatment of polyarteritis. Composite curves have been constructed from several reported series as indicated. Shaded areas represent the extremes of survival in patients who were untreated or in those receiving corticosteroid therapy. Separate survival curves for two series reporting the effects of cytotoxic drugs are shown: The results of Cohen et al. (31) indicated no advantage of cytotoxic drug treatment over corticosteroids, while the series by Lieb et al. (30) indicates a favorable effect of cytotoxic drug therapy (see text).

CORTICOSTEROID THERAPY

The strongest support for the use of high-dose corticosteroids comes from the report by Frohnert and Sheps (32). In an analysis of 130 patients with polyarteritis evaluated at the Mayo Clinic between 1946 and 1962, these authors noted that the group of patients receiving corticosteroids had a survival of 48%, while the untreated group had a meager 13% survival after 5 years of followup. It should be emphasized that this was not a prospective or randomized therapeutic study, and consequently the 20 untreated patients may not have been comparable to the corticosteroid-treated group. Many of the untreated patients had not been treated because they were atypical and eluded early diagnosis (9 of 20 had been diagnosed only after coming to autopsy). In spite of the limitations of this retrospective analysis, corticosteroid therapy appeared to improve survival when compared to the untreated patients at the same institution, as well as to other historical controls. This study has remained as one of the strongest supports for the standard use of early high-dose corticosteroids in polyarteritis.

In a similar retrospective study reported in 1979, Leib and associates noted than patients treated with corticosteroids had a 58% 2-year survival, compared to a 25% survival in a small group of untreated patients at the same center (30). Indeed, estimates of the 2-year survival of corticosteroid-treated patients from several uncontrolled series (29–32) range between 57% and 75%, as shown in Figure 1.

The historic suggestion that corticosteroids may have a deleterious effect on vasculitic lesions, or may even actually produce a vasculopathy indistinguishable from systemic necrotizing vasculitis itself, is no longer seriously considered. On the other hand, recurrent or prolonged use of corticosteroids regularly and predictably induces a myriad of side effects, some of which may be indistinguishable from the underlying vasculitic disease.

CYTOTOXIC DRUG THERAPY

Although there is little debate that corticosteroids add substantively to the management and longevity of patients with polyarteritis, several investigators have turned to other immunosuppressive agents to improve therapeutic results and particularly to reduce the complications of long-term corticosteroid therapy. Favorable reports have appeared that indicate an improvement in 2-year survival to 80–90% in patients treated with azathioprine (30) or cyclophosphamide (30, 33). In a study from the National Institutes of Health, 17 patients with systemic vasculitis who were unresponsive to or were having complications from previous corticosteroid therapy were treated with oral cyclophosphamide (33). Sustained remissions were achieved in 14 of the 17 patients, including regression of vascular aneurysms in certain cases (34). It is important to recognize, however, that this study does not directly address the therapy of early or acute polyarteritis, and does not specifically emphasize the effect of cytotoxic therapy on survivorship. The patients had predominantly chronic disease, having been on corticosteroids for a mean duration of 22 months. Nonetheless, the evidence of improved rates and quality of remissions and the reduction of corticosteroid toxicity are important points to be taken from this study.

Echoing the claim for a favorable effect of cytotoxic agents is the report of Lieb and colleagues (30). They treated 22 patients with polyarteritis with a variety of cytotoxic drugs (mainly azathioprine) and noted a 95% 2-year survival rate, compated to 65% in patients treated with corticosteroids and to 25% in untreated patients (Figure 1). It must be emphasized that this was not a prospective study, and it did not address the treatment of early acute polyarteritis; patients ultimately treated with cytotoxic drugs had received corticosteroids for a mean period of 7 months. The authors were not able to determine which of the cytotoxic drugs used was the most efficacious.

Opposing views of the benefits of cytotoxic drugs have been presented. In a report by Cohen and colleagues of 53 patients with polyarteritis studied at the Mayo Clinic (31), survival was not improved when azathioprine or cyclophosphamide were instituted (Figure 1). However, these drugs were usually started after patients had exhibited poor responses to standard corticosteroid therapy.

Unfortunately, both of these reports represent uncontrolled studies, and one must strongly suspect that unrecognized selection biases could have led the authors to opposing views of the role of cytotoxic drugs on survivorship.

The efficacy of cytotoxic drugs in the early treatment of polyarteritis has not been well studied. Preliminary evidence by Lockshin et al. suggests that cyclophosphamide has not improved the high early mortality of polyarteritis treated with corticosteroids alone (35). Again, it is not clear whether the selection of disproportionately ill patients for cyclophosphamide treatment may have contributed to the unfavorable results. Only a prospective trial will ascertain whether the early addition of cytotoxic drugs to standard corticosteroid therapy is capable of reducing the morbidity of acute polyarteritis.

PLASMA EXCHANGE THERAPY

A proper perspective on the role of plasma exchange in polyarteritis cannot be formulated from available data. Plasma exchange may offer the greatest potential in early aggressive vasculitis, but its expense and its contribution to an infection diathesis in patients already at high risk of infection from corticosteroids and from visceral complications of active vasculitis should caution against its routine use. Plasma exchange is mostly used as an adjunctive therapy in patients with severe polyarteritis that is inadequately controlled with standard immunosuppressive drug therapy alone.

A recent controlled study of the effects of plasma exchange in a group of patients with microscopic polyarteritis, Wegener's granulomatosis, and idiopathic crescentic glomerulonephritis showed no benefit of the addition of plasma exchange to standard immunosuppressive therapy, except in patients who presented with advanced renal insufficiency (36). Plasma exchange seems to be an effective therapeutic adjunct to standard immunosuppressive drug therapy in patients with fulminant glomerulonephritis due to polyarteritis.

PRACTICAL THERAPEUTIC GUIDELINES

In the absence of compelling evidence from prospective therapeutic trials, what is a reasonable approach to the treatment of polyarteritis? Corticosteroids certainly must be considered the mainstay of early therapy in the patient with predominantly rheumatic components of polyarteritis. Conventional doses of prednisone, e.g., 1.0 mg/kg/day, should be promptly initiated in the face of active systemic diseases. The response of the constitutional manifestations of polyarteritis is usually dramatic. Tapering to alternate-day prednisone therapy within approximately 8 weeks is a laudable goal. The duration and dose of maintenance corticosteroids should be as short and as low as possible to control disease activity and to minimize the long-term side effects. Too frequently, clinicians are reluctant to begin tapering corticosteroids when the desired clinical remission has been achieved, for fear of relapse. Our position is that it is no more acceptable to allow passively the emergence of insidious corticosteroid complications than to risk a flare of disease by repeatedly testing for the lowest dose of corticosteroid effective for disease control. Patients with chronic relapsing or smoldering polyarteritis may be particularly well suited for cytotoxic drug treatment, as the risks thereof are often less than those of repeated an/or prolonged corticosteroid therapy.

Patients with potentially catastrophic visceral involvement from polyarteritis, particularly nervous system, cardiac, gastrointestinal, and/or renal disease, are usually treated early with prednisone and adjunctive immunosuppressive therapy. The latter may include pulse methylprednisolone (22, 37, 38), cytotoxic drugs, and/or plasma exchange. At present there is no evidence that megadose corticosteroid pulses, e.g., methylprednisolone $1.0 g/m^2$, hold any advantage over conventional doses of corticosteroids. However, methylprednisolone pulse therapy has emerged as the preferred initial therapy in patients with rapidly progressive glomerulonephritis due to microscopic polyarteritis. These patients are usually given maintenance therapy, which includes conventional high (but tapering) doses of prednisone, as well as daily oral cyclophosphamide.

The cytotoxic drug of choice for certain patients with polyarteritis cannot be rigidly defended. Cyclophosphamide is the most widely used drug because of the evidence that it is more potent than azathioprine in suppressing experimentally induced immune responses and in achieving clinical remission of a variety of immunologically mediated diseases. Azathioprine is most often used as substitution therapy in those patients unable to tolerate cyclophosphamide or for long-term maintenance therapy in those who have responded to cyclophosphamide but wish to minimize exposure to this drug.

Cyclophosphamide therapy is routinely initiated at a dose of 2.0 mg/kg/day (the use of intermittent pulse doses of intravenous cyclophosphamide has not been established for the treatment of polyarteritis). Patients must be willing and able to comply with the compulsive monitoring of white blood counts necessary for the safe administration of cytotoxic drug therapy. The doses of cyclophosphamide should be adjusted to maintain the leukocyte count above $4000/mm^3$. Dose reduction should be instituted as soon as downward trends in white blood cell counts are identified, since leukopenia may progress for a week or more after a reduction in the cyclophosphamide dose. Proper management of leukocyte counts minimizes the risk of infection (except for *Herpes zoster*, which virtually never disseminates).

The risk of hemorrhagic cystitis should be minimized by instructing the patient to ingest cyclophosphamide as a single morning dose and to force fluids to approximately 3 l per day, along with frequent voiding.

In the absence of drug intolerance, it is our practice to wait until a complete remission of polyarteritis has been sustained for approximately 12 months before cyclophosphamide is discontinued.

Renal failure outcomes

A portion of patients with either classic or microscopic polyarteritis progresses to end-stage renal failure. Severe hypertension due to chronic vascular insufficiency of the kidneys is regularly seen in azotemic patients and often requires very aggressive antihypertensive therapy. Bilateral nephrectomy should rarely be considered with currently available antihypertensive drugs. Renal replacement therapy by chronic dialysis and/or transplantation presents no particular problems in patients with end-stage renal failure secondary to polyarteritis, except for their possibly having an increased risk of vascular access complications. The potential for the recurrence of polyarteritis in a renal graft appears to be small (39).

WEGENER'S GRANULOMATOSIS

Introduction

Wegener's granulomatosis is a form of systemic vasculitis with specific clinical and pathologic features. The clinical syndrome includes chronic inflammatory disease with vasculitis and granulomas of the upper and lower respiratory tract plus necrotizing glomerulonephritis (40–43). The etiology and pathogenesis of Wegener's granulomatosis are unknown, but the recent detection of autoantibodies to cytoplasmic antigens of neutrophilic leukocytes is a provocative observation (13–16). These antibodies are of unknown significance in the pathogenesis of Wegener's granulomatosis, but their titers appear to correlate with disease activity.

Prognostic features

As with most systemic diseases, extrarenal symptoms and signs tend to dominate the clinical manifestations. It is imperative that all patients with suspected Wegener's granulomatosis be carefully monitored for evidence of early renal disease, which untreated often explosively progresses to serve necrotizing and crescentic glomerulonephritis with renal failure. Occasionally, glomerulonephritis may be the presenting feature of Wegener's granulomatosis (44).

The risk of progression to end-stage renal disease in a cohort of patients with Wegener's granulomatosis treated at the National Institutes of Health is shown in Figure 2. In the total group of 44 patients with renal involvement early in the course of Wegener's granulomatosis, the probability of developing end-stage renal failure was 17% at 5 years and 33% at 10 years. Patients presenting early in their course with proteinuria ≥ 2.5 g/day or rapidly progressive glomerulonephritis had a significantly worst prognosis.

Therapeutic considerations

Historically, patients with Wegener's granulomatosis and renal involvement have had a mean survival at 1 year of 20% in untreated patients (45) and 34% in patients receiving corticosteroid therapy (46). Since the institution of cytotoxic drugs, patient survival has improved to 86% at 1 year and 68% at 5 years in experience gained at several institutions (40–48).

CYTOTOXIC DRUG THERAPY

Cyclophosphamide is the most widely used cytotoxic drug for Wegener's granulomatosis. Patients with mild to moderately active Wegener's granulomatosis may be started on conventional schedules of oral cyclophosphamide at 2.0 mg/kg/day and tapered appropriately to keep blood leukocytes above 4000/mm^3. Patients with unusually aggressive disease (particularly, severe crescentic glomerulonephritis) are initially given intravenous cyclophosophamide in doses of 4–5 mg/kg/day for 3 days followed by oral maintenance doses of approximately 2.0 mg/kg/day. After induction of remission, azathioprine is sometimes used as a substitute drug for maintenance in patients unable or unwilling to continue cyclophosphamide therapy.

CORTICOSTEROID THERAPY

Conventional high-dose prednisone (1.0 mg/kg/day) is usually initiated in the early phases of Wegener's granulomatosis. This is particularly important in patients with severe inflammation and/or extensive granulomas (e.g., orbital, central nervous system, coronary, serosal), in those with necrotizing and/or crescentic glomerulonephritis, and in those with debilitating constitutional symptoms. However, corticosteroids rarely should be used a sole therapy unless the diagnosis is in doubt. It is our practice to begin tapering to alternate-day prednisone after 4–6 weeks, by which time cyclophosphamide can be expected to have its full immunosuppressive effect. From this point forward, alternate-day prednisone can be tapered to cessation in those patients acheiving complete remission, or varying doses of alternate-day prednisone may be continued for treatment of residual constitutional symptoms. In certain patients with persistently active disease who tolerate only 50 mg/day or less of cyclophosphamide because of neutropenia, alternate-day prednisone can be reinstituted. This generally improves peripheral leukocyte counts via a salutary effect of prednisone on bone marrow granulopoiesis (41) and allows a larger therapeutic dose of cyclophosphamide to be administered. Parenthetically, care should always be taken that leukocyte counts are not obtained within the first 8 hours after a dose of prednisone, as there may be a misleading and transient leukocytosis in this period, apparently due to the effect of corticosteroids on leukocyte margination.

Undesirable side effects from immunosuppression with cyclophosphamide certainly occur. Some are predictable, such as suppression of gonadal function and bone marrow reserve; some can be minimized, such as cystitis, by scrupulous attention to a high fluid intake plus frequent bladder emptying. Chronic cyclophosphamide administration imposes a small but significant diathesis for malignancy (49), which should be explained to the patient before starting therapy. *Herpes zoster* is a potential problem in patients on cyclophosphamide, but dissemination is extremely rare.

Although these issues of cytotoxic drug side effects must be seriously considered, they must be balanced against the potentially devastating relapses of Wegener's granulomatosis in patients inadequately treated to sustained remission. Definition of the adequate duration of remission is difficult, but we have had some patients develop fulminant

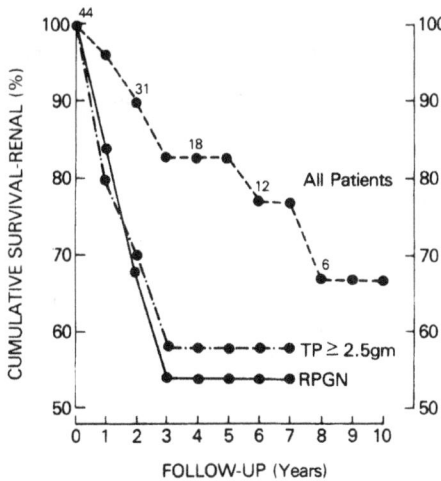

Figure 2. Cumulative renal survival in patients with Wegener's granulomatosis. The curves represent the probability of escaping end-stage renal failure at various intervals of follow up after diagnosis. Also shown are the changes in renal prognosis in patients with urinary total protein (TP) excretion ≥ 2.5 g/day or rapidly progressive glomerulonephritis (doubling or more of serum creatinine monthly) early in the course of Wegener's granulomatosis, before cytotoxic drug therapy was initiated.

renal failure when cyclophosphamide was discontinued prematurely. Consequently, our current practice is to continue cyclophosphamide (usually without concomitant corticosteroids) for a minimum of 1 year of sustained remission of Wegener's granulomatosis (41).

Implicit in these considerations is the difficulty of defining active disease in Wegener's granulomatosis. A major problem is encountered in distinguishing active vasculitic disease from recurrent infections (usually *Staphylococcus aureus*) of the sinuses and nasopharynx due to the loss of normal mucosal defenses. Repeated courses of antistaphylococcal antibiotics and surgical drainage procedures are required in some patients with these problems. There have been provocative suggestions that infectious complications may actually stimulate vasculitic disease activity (50) and that antibiotic therapy may induce a remission of Wegener's granulomatosis (51). The latter contention has not been verified.

OTHER THERAPIES

Antimetabolite drugs, such as 6-mercaptopurine and methotrexate, and other alkylating drugs, such as nitrogen mustard and chlorambucil, have been used in Wegener's granulomatosis (reviewed in 1,40). No direct comparisons of the efficacy of any of these drugs to cyclophosphamide have been made.

Recently, plasma exchange therapy has been used in active Wegener's granulomatosis, mainly as a rapid stopgap measure until cytotoxic drugs could become effective (42). It is unknown whether plasma exchange therapy adds to the effects of drug therapy in Wegener's glomerulonephritis, but it is often used in patients with fulminant glomerulonephritis and in those with suboptimal responses to prednisone and cyclophosphamide.

Cyclosporin A is being tested under investigational protocols for use in the management of refractory cases of Wegener's granulomatosis.

Renal failure

Temporary dialysis support may be needed in certain patients with fulminant glomerulonephritis (52, 53). Reversal of acute renal failure depends on the degree of glomerular crescent formation, the extent of glomerular architectural disruption due to necrosis, and the extent of underlying chronic glomerular and tubulointerstitial disease. Although our experience indicates that the majority of patients with the first episode of rapidly progressive glomerulonephritis usually recovers adequate renal function, relapses of glomerulonephritis are associated with a high risk of persistent renal failure.

No specific manifestation of Wegener's granulomatosis appears to present a unique problem in patients requiring renal replacement therapy. Patients who have had a chronic or relapsing course may continue to have symptoms of Wegener's granulomatosis during maintenance dialysis. Cyclophosphamide therapy may be required during chronic dialysis in some patients to control extrarenal disease.

Kidney transplantation should certainly be considered for renal replacement therapy in Wegener's granulomatosis (54, 55). Generally, it is advisable to maintain patients on chronic dialysis until their disease is in complete remission (preferably off drug therapy) and any residual complications of pulmonary disease (e.g., tracheal stenosis, lung cavities) have resolved. Experience to date indicates that the results of transplantation in Wegener's granulomatosis are comparable to those of patients with primary nephropathies. Treatment with azathioprine and corticosteroids for normal transplant management is usually effective to prevent the recurrence of Wegener's granulomatosis. The recurrence of glomerulonephritis apparently due to Wegener's granulomatosis has been documented (55–57), but is apparently rare; azathioprine may be replaced by cyclophosphamide in patients with reactivation of Wegener's granulomatosis.

HENOCH–SCHÖNLEIN NEPHRITIS

Introduction

Henoch–Schönlein syndrome is a form of systemic necrotizing vasculitis associated with IgA-containing circulating immune complexes and manifestations of skin, joint, renal, and gastrointestinal involvement that may occur in any combination and in any order (7, 58–61). Pediatric patients are chiefly affected; other forms of systemic necrotizing vasculitis are more common in the adult age group (1). The expected outcome of Henoch–Schönlein syndrome is favorable, including patients with nephritis. Even in selected series from referral centers, the majority of patients with Henoch–Schönlein nephritis follow a relatively benign course, often without specific therapy (58, 62). The actuarial survival of 135 patients with Henoch–Schönlein nephritis seen at Guy's Hospital was approximately 90% at 10 years (63).

Renal involvement

In series of patients with Henoch–Schönlein syndrome reported from referral centers, the incidence and severity of the renal disease are highly variable. Adults may have a higher prevalence of glomerulonephritis (approximately 50%) than do children (approximately 30%) with this syndrome (64). Moreover, in some but not all studies, adults appear to have a higher rate (13–14%) of progression to end-stage renal failure than do children (5%) with Henoch–Schönlein nephritis (58, 64, 65). The risk of renal failure may be lower in unselected pediatric patient populations (66).

Henoch–Schönlein nephritis, when present, usually appears within 3 months after the initial skin and/or visceral manifestations; rarely, the nephritis may precede the extrarenal components and may occasionally dominate the clinical presentation (58, 61, 67). In general, there is no consistent relationship between the severity of nephritis and the severity of the extrarenal manifestations of the Henoch–Schönlein syndrome (58, 62, 67). Henoch–Schönlein nephritis is manifested by microscopic hematuria and proteinuria in essentially all patients. The prevalence of the acute nephritic syndrome and/or the nephrotic syndrome in the total population of patients with Henoch–Schönlein nephritis is unclear, but approachs 40% of patients in referral centers (58, 62, 68).

The pathologic manifestations of Henoch–Schönlein nephritis vary from mild mesangial proliferation to diffuse proliferative and crescentic glomerulonephritis. The pattern of immune complex deposition assessed by immunofluorescence and electron microscopy bears great similarity to that of systemic lupus erythematosus, with deposits predominantly in the mesangium and variably in subendothelial and subepithelial locations in complicated cases (69). Complexes containing IgA have been demonstrated in the circulation, skin, and glomeruli, and are suspected to have a pathogenetic role in this form of vasculitis (59, 63, 70–74).

Prognostic considerations

The typical patient with Henoch–Schönlein syndrome has a self-limiting illness with complete recovery within 3–6 weeks. Severe gastrointestinal bleeding, bowel infarction, and/or intussusception can occasionally present serious complications of acute disease. Glomerular disease is the major determinant of long-term prognosis. Renal involvement per se is not an adverse prognostic sign in most cases of Henoch–Schönlein syndrome. However, clinically and pathologically defined subsets of patients have been shown to be at increaed risk of developing end-stage renal failure in many but not all studies of Henoch–Schönlein nephritis (68, 75).

Using composite data from several published series (58, 62, 66, 68, 76), the status of patients at the latest followup has been assessed in relationship to their presenting clinical features of renal disease (Figure 3). As noted, greater than 75% of all patients presenting with microscopic hematuria, proteinuria, or even uncomplicated nephrotic syndrome completely remitted or had minimal abnormality after several years of followup. On the other hand, of 55 patients presenting with the nephrotic syndrome complicated by various combinations of hypertension, azotemia, oliguria, and/or hypoproteinemia, greater than 40% were azotemia at the last followup; 30% of patients had reached end-stage renal disease, usually within 3 years of the onset of Henoch–Schönlein nephritis. Persistence of the nephrotic (or nephritic-nephrotic) syndrome for approximately 1 year or more after presentation has been associated with an increased risk of chronic renal insufficiency (77).

A composite series of patients (58, 62, 66, 68) was also used to analyze the prognostic value of early renal histology. All patients with minor glomerular lesions on light microscopy had complete remission or minimal urinary abnormalities at the latest followup. Features associated with a less favorable prognosis include: diffuse endocapil-

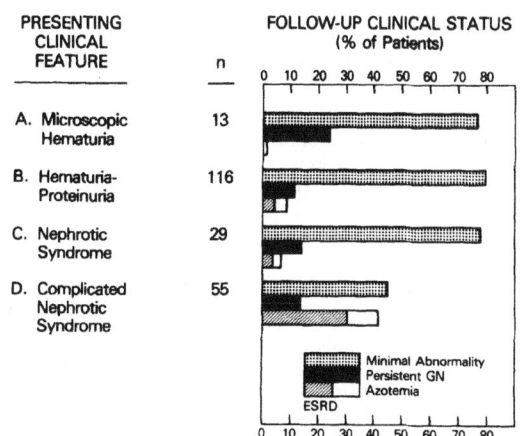

Figure 3. Prognosis of Henoch–Schönlein nephritis according to clinical features. Results are based on composite data on 213 patients collected from four separate published reports (58, 62, 66, 76). The definition of complicated nephrotic syndrome varied somewhat among these reports, but mostly indicated the presence of renal functional impairment.

lary proliferation, widespread segmental necrosis and/or sclerosis, extensive crescent formation, as well as subendothelial and subepithelial electron-dense deposits (58, 74, 78–80). The level of circulating immune complexes containing IgA has been correlated with the extent of crescent formation (81). In several studies, the percentage of glomeruli affected by crescents emerged as a powerful prognostic feature (Figure 4). Patients whose initial nephritis was complicated by increasing cellular crescents had a progressively higher risk of developing persistent azotemia. Indeed, two thirds of patients with greater than 75% cellular crescents progressed to end-stage renal disease. Finally, no patient with proliferative glomerulonephritis and 100% cellular crescents escaped renal fai-

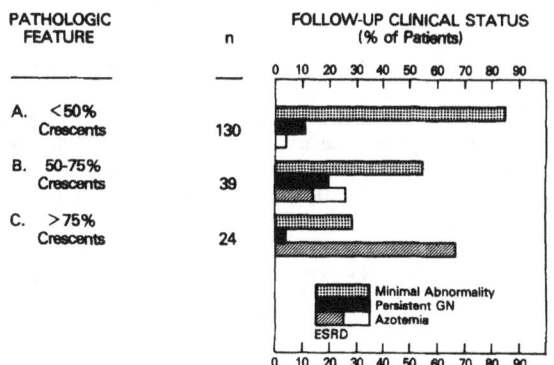

Figure 4. Prognosis of Henoch–Schönlein nephritis according to the severity of renal pathology. The results are based on composite data from 193 patients collected from three separate reports (58, 62, 66).

lure, regardless of the type of therapeutic intervention (58). This survey underscores the potential prognostic value of histologic features of renal biopsy in Henoch–Schönlein nephritis. Unfortunately, because of the retrospective nature of this analysis, neither the indications for, nor the effect of, immunosuppressive therapy on any particular type of renal manifestation of Henoch–Schönlein nephritis was identified.

Therapeutic approaches

The majority of patients with Henoch–Schönlein syndrome do not require specific therapy because of the probability of spontaneous remission. Concern for an etiologic role of drug hypersensitivity should prompt the withdrawal of any drugs that are not absolutely required for underlying medical problems. Dietary manipulation is rarely indicated, as food allergy has not been documented to be responsible for the Henoch–Schönlein syndrome. Prophylactic antibiotics are not indicated in patients with frequent relapses, as there is no convincing evidence that streptococcal infections are related to recurrences of Henoch–Schönlein syndrome.

Antiinflammatory drugs, including aspirin, are used for the treatment of the arthritis component of the Henoch–Schönlein syndrome, which may last several months. Corticosteroids are recommended in severe cases of joint and gastrointestinal involvement. Dramatic improvement of abdominal colic and gastrointestinal hemorrhage can occur, and corticosteroids may decrease the risk of intussusception. As there is little evidence that corticosteroids alter the duration of illness or the relapse rate, high-dose prednisone should be rapidly tapered to alternate-day therapy and discontinued as soon as the patient's wellbeing can be maintained by less toxic forms of antiinflammatory drug therapy. Fortunately, the episodic and/or self-limited nature of Henoch–Schönlein syndrome reduces the need for chronic corticosteroids and/or cytotoxic drugs and, therefore, makes their long-term toxicity a comparatively unusual problem.

The approach to therapy of Henoch–Schönlein nephritis is complicated by certain considerations that cannot be easily integrated. On one hand, it is recognized that many patients are likely to have a spontaneous remission of their nephritis. On the other hand, certain clinical and pathologic features of Henoch–Schönlein nephritis (described above) appear to indicate an adverse prognosis in spite of intense therapeutic intervention. The challenge to the clinician is to identify patients whose prognosis is intrinsically neither too benign nor too malignant in order that drug therapy could reasonably be expected to influence the course of the nephritis. Thus, reserving immunosuppressive therapy for patients with 100% glomerular crescents and progressive renal failure is unlikely to be productive in Henoch–Schönlein nephritis. At the same time, the benefit of treatment of early Henoch–Schönlein nephritis may be quite obscure if prevention of renal failure is used as the measure of therapeutic efficacy. Intermediate measures of outcome (e.g., changes in renal histology) have not been adequately applied to the therapy of Henoch–Schönlein nephritis, but may offer an attractive alternative in a condition where progression to renal failure is an infrequent event.

Published results of the therapy of Henoch–Schönlein nephritis must be carefully interpreted in light of the issues raised above. In a large series from Hopital Necker in Paris, Levy and colleagues suggested that immunosuppressive treatment of patients with greater than 50% of glomeruli affected by crescents may be beneficial, although the relative advantage in preventing renal failure was not statistically significant (58). Other uncontrolled studies of immunosuppressive therapy have also been favorable in achieving renal functional and pathologic improvement in some cases (67, 82, 83). However, certain reports have conveyed skepticism about the role of immunosuppression in Henoch–Schönlein nephritis (84, 85). In a series of reports from Guy's Hospital in London, experience with multiple-drug regimens, including corticosteroids, cytotoxic agents, anticoagulants, and antiplatelet drugs, failed to convince the authors of a favorable effect of any particular treatment of Henoch–Schönlein nephritis (62, 63, 86, 87). It seems possible that the group receiving cytotoxic drug therapy may have been unfavorably weighted with a disproportionate number of patients with advanced renal histologic changes (62).

Observations from an uncontrolled experience suggest that high-dose intravenous pulse methylprednisolone may be beneficial for patients with severe Henoch–Schönlein nephritis (88). Furthermore, we have begun to test an alternative approach of giving cyclophosphamide as single monthly intravenous infusion $(0.5-1.0 \, g/m^2)$ for seven doses followed by every 3 monthly infusions, comparable to an approach under investigation for severe lupus nephritis.

Anecdotal reports have indicated that plasma exchange may be useful in the treatment of Henoch–Schönlein nephritis (89, 90). However, the lack of controls and the use of adjunctive therapies make interpretation of these results difficult. Randomized collaborative trials are needed to determine the value of these therapeutic interventions.

When patients with severe Henoch–Schönlein nephritis are encountered, therapy with prednisone and cyclophosphamide is usually initiated. Intravenous pulse methylprednisolone and/or plasma exchange also warrant consideration as adjunctive therapy. Although no definitive list of indications can be constructed, such therapy would be reasonable for patients with greater than 50% cellular crescents and for those with the nephrotic syndrome complicated by hypertension, azotemia, oliguria, and/or hypoproteinemia in an attempt to decrease the risk of progressive renal failure (Figures 3 and 4). Whether there is benefit in attempting to treat less severely active glomerular lesions with comparable immunosuppressive therapy cannot be ascertained at the present time. Prospective studies with patient stratification into clinically and/or pathologically defined subsets are necessary to resolve these questions.

End-stage renal failure

No unusual management problems are anticipated in those patients progressing to renal failure. There are no published data to indicate whether the risk of recurrent Henoch–Schönlein syndrome is affected by uremia. Kidney transplantation is certainly an acceptable alternative to chronic dialysis. There is some risk of recurrent Henoch–Schönlein nephritis in the graft, particularly in patients having a rapidly progressive course of renal disease. It seems prudent, therefore, to delay renal transplantation until the patient has had remission of the Henoch–Schönlein syndrome for several months (91). Hopefully, refinement of tests for specific circulating immune complexes (59) and/or cell-mediated immunologic disturbances will provide clearer identification of the pathogenesis and measures of disease activity in Henoch–Schönlein nephritis, including risk factors for recurrence in the engrafted kidney.

REFERENCES

1. Cupps TR, Fauci AS: *The Vasculitides*. WB Saunders, Philadelphia, 1981.
2. Fan PT, Davis JA, Somer T, Kaplan L, Bluestone R: A clinical approach to systemic vasculitis. *Semin Arthritis Rheum* 9:248–304, 1980.
3. Fauci AS, Haynes BF, Katz P: The spectrum of vasculitis. Clinical, pathologic, immunologic and therapeutic considerations. *Ann Intern Med* 89:660–676, 1978.
4. Scott DG, Bacon PA, Elliott PJ, Tribe CR, Wallington TB: Systemic vasculitis in a district general hospital 1972–1980: Clinical and laboratory features, classification and prognosis of 80 cases. *Q J Med* 51:292–311, 1982.
5. Conn DL, Hunder GG: Necrotizing vasculitis. In: WD Kelly, ed, *Textbook of Rheumatology*, 2nd ed. WB Saunders, Philadelphia, pp 1137–1166, 1984.
6. Serra A, Cameron JS: Clinical and pathologic aspects of renal vasculitis. *Semin Nephrol* 5:15–33, 1985.
7. Balow JE: Renal vasculitis. *Kidney Int* 27:954–964, 1985.
8. Soter NA, Austen KF: Pathogenetic mechanisms in the necrotizing vasculitides. *Clin Rheum Dis* 6:233–253, 1980.
9. Brentjens JR, Andres G: Immunopathogenesis of renal vasculitis. *Semin Nephrol* 5:3–14, 1985.
10. Leib ES, Hibrawi H, Chia D, Blaker RG, Barnett EV: Correlation of disease activity in systemic necrotizing vasculitis with immune complexes. *J Rheumatol* 8:258–265, 1981.
11. Spargo BH, Seymour AE, Ordenez NG: Vasculitis. In: *Renal Biopsy Pathology with Diagnostic and Therapeutic Implications*. John Wiley and Sons, New York, pp 205–218, 1980.
12. Ronco P, Verroust P, Mignon F, Kourilsky O, Vanhille P, Meyrier A, Mery JP, Morel–Maroger L: Immunopathological studies of polyarteritis nodosa and Wegener's granulomatosis: A report of 43 patients with 51 renal biopsies. *Q J Med* 52:212–223, 1983.
13. Davies DJ, Moran JE, Niall JF, Ryan GB: Segmental necrotizing glomerulonephritis with antineutrophil antibody: Possible arbovirus aetiology? *Br Med J* 285:606, 1982.
14. van der Woude FJ, Rasmussen N, Lobatto S, Wiik A, Permin H, van Es LA, van der Giessen M, van der Hem GK, The TH: Autoantibodies against neutrophils and monocytes: Tool for diagnosis and marker of disease activity in Wegener's granulomatosis. *Lancet* 1:425–429, 1985.
15. Lockwood CM, Bakes D, Jones S, Whitaker KB, Moss DW, Savage CO: Association of alkaline phosphatase with autoantigen recognised by circulating anti-neutrophil antibodies in systemic vasculitis. *Lancet* 1:176–720, 1987.
16. Savage C, Winearls CG, Jones S, Marshall PD, Lockwood CM: Prospective study of radioimmunoassay for antibodies against neutrophil cytoplasm in diagnosis of systemic vasculitis. *Lancet* 1:1389–1393, 1987.
17. Davson J, Ball J, Platt R: The kidney in periarteritis nodosa. *Q J Med* 17:175–202, 1948.
18. Travers RL, Allison DJ, Brettle RP, Hughes GRV: Polyarteritis nodosa: A clinical and angiographic analysis of 17 cases. *Semin Arthritis Rheum* 8:184–199, 1979.
19. McCluskey RT, Fienberg R: Vasculitis in primary vasculitides, granulomatoses, and connective tissue disease. *Hum Pathol* 14:305–315, 1983.
20. Leavitt RY, Fauci AS: Polyangiitis overlap syndrome. Classification and prospective clinical experience. *Am J Med* 81:79–85, 1986.
21. Pischel KD, Zvaifler NJ: Simultaneous occurrence of polyarteritis nodosa and leukocytoclastic vasculitis. *J Rheumatol* 11:542–544, 1984.
22. Serra A, Camerson JS, Turner DR, Hartley B, Ogg CS, Neild GH, Williams DG, Taube D, Brown CB, Hicks JA: Vasculitis affecting the kidney: Presentation, histopathology and long-term outcome. *Q J Med* 53:181–207, 1984.
23. Savage CA, Winearls CG, Evans DJ, Rees AJ, Lockwood CM: Microscopic polyarteritis: Presentation, pathology and prognosis. *Q J Med* 56:467–483, 1985.
24. Heilman RL, Offord LP, Holley KE, Velosa JA: Analysis of risk factors for patient and renal survival in crescentic glomerulonephritis. *Am J Kidney Dis* 9:98–107, 1987.
25. Croker BP, Lee T, Gunnells JC: Clinical and pathologic features of polyarteritis nodosa and its renal-limited variant: Primary crescentic and necrotizing glomerulonephritis. *Hum Pathol* 18:38–44, 1987.
26. Velosa JA: Idiopathic crescentic glomerulonephritis or systemic vasculitis. *Mayo Clin Proc* 62;145–147, 1987.
27. Pickering TG, Lockshin MD, Eisenmenger WJ: Renin-dependent hypertension in polyarteritis nodosa. *Br Med J* 282:1758–1981.
28. O'Connell MT, Kubrusly DB, Fournier AM: Systemic necrotizing vasculitis seen initially as hypertensive crisis. *Arch Intern Med* 145:265–267, 1985.
29. Sack M Cassidy JT, Bole GG: Prognostic factors in polyarteritis. *J Rheumatol* 2:411–420, 1975.
30. Leib ES, Restivo C, Paulus HE: Immunosuppressive and corticosteroid therapy of polyarteritis nodosa. *Am J Med* 67:941–947, 1979.
31. Cohen RD, Conn DL, Ilstrup DM: Clinical features, prognosis and response to treatment in polyarteritis. *Mayo Clin Proc* 55:146–155, 1980.
32. Frohnert PP, Sheps SG: Long-term follow-up study of periarteritis nodosa. *Am J Med* 43:8–14, 1967.
33. Fauci AS, Katz P, Haynes BF, Wolff SM: Cyclophosphamide therapy of severe systemic necrotizing vasculitis. *N Engl J Med* 301:235–238, 1979.
34. Fauci AS, Doppman JL, Wolff SM: Cyclophosphamide-induced remissions in advanced polyarteritis nodosa. *Am J Med* 64:890–894, 1978.
35. Lockshin MD: Treatment of vasculitis with cyclophosphamide (letter). *N Engl J Med* 301:1123, 1979.
36. Pusey CD, Lockwood CM: Plasma exchange for glomerular disease. In: RR Robinson, ed, *Nephrology*, Vol II. Springer-Verlag, New York, pp 1474–1485, 1984.

37. Neild GH, Lee HA: Methylprednisolone pulse therapy in the treatment of polyarteritis nodosa. *Postgrad Med J* 53:382–387, 1977.
38. Bolton WK: Use of pulse methylprednisolone in primary and multisystem diseases. In: RR Robinson, ed, *Nephrology*, Vol. II. Springer–Verlag, New York, pp 1464–1473, 1984.
39. Montalbert C, Carvallo A, Broumand B, Noble D, Anstine LA, Currier CB: Successful renal transplantation in polyarteritis nodosa. *Clin Nephrol* 14:206–209, 1980.
40. Appel GB, Gee G, Kashgarian M, Hayslett JP: Wegener's granulomatosis: Clinical-pathological correlations and long-term course. *Am J Kidney Dis* 1:27–37, 1981.
41. Fauci AS, Haynes BF, Katz P, Wolff SM: Wegener's granulomatosis: Prospective clinical and therapeutic experience with 85 patients for 21 years. *Ann Intern Med* 98:76–85, 1983.
42. Pinching AJ, Lockwood CM, Pussell BA, Rees AJ, Sweny P, Evans DJ, Bowley N, Peters DK: Wegener's granulomatosis: Observations on 18 patients with severe renal diseases. *Q J Med* 52:435–460, 1983.
43. Weiss MA, Crissman JD: Renal biopsy findings in Wegener's granulomatosis: Segmental necrotizing glomerulonephritis with glomerular thrombosis. *Hum Pathol* 15:943–956, 1984.
44. Woodworth TG, Abuelo JG, Austin HA III, Esparaza A: Severe glomerulonephritis with late emergence of classic Wegener's granulomatosis. Report of 4 cases and review of the literature. *Medicine* 66:181–191, 1987.
45. Walton EW: Giant cell granuloma of the respiratory tract (Wegener's granulomatosis). *Br J Med* 2:260–270, 1968.
46. Hollander D, Manning RT: The use of alkylating agents in the treatment of Wegener's granulomatosis. *Ann Intern Med* 67:393–398, 1967.
47. Reza MJ, Dornfield L, Goldberg LS, Bluestone P, Pearson CM: Wegener's granulomatosis. Long-term follow-up of patients treated with cyclophosphamide. *Arthritis Rheum* 18:501–506, 1975.
48. van der Woude FJ, Hoorntje SJ, Weening JJ, van Overbeek JJ, van der Hem GK: Renal involvement in Wegener's granulomatosis. Report of three unusual cases. *Nephron* 32:185–187, 1982.
49. Ambrus JL, Fauci AS: Diffuse histiocytic lymphoma in a patient treated with cyclophosphamide for Wegener's granulomatosis. *Am J Med* 76:745–747, 1984.
50. Pinching AJ, Rees AJ, Pussell BA, Lockwood CM, Mitchison RS, Peters DK: Relapses in Wegener's granulomatosis: The role of infection. *Br Med J* 281:836–838, 1980.
51. DeRemee RA, McDonald TJ, Weiland LH: Wegener's granulomatosis: Observations on treatment with antimicrobial agents. *Mayo Clin Proc* 60:27–32, 1985.
52. Dahlberg PJ, Newcomer KL, Yutuc WR, Kalfayan B: Renal failure in Wegener's granulomatosis: Recovering following dialysis and cyclophosphamide-prednisone therapy. *Am J Med Sci* 287:47–50, 1984.
53. ten Berge IJ, Wilmink JM, Meyer CJ, Surachno J, ten Veen KH, Balk TG, Schellekens PT: Clinical and immunological follow-up of patients with severe renal disease in Wegener's granulomatosis. *Am J Nephrol* 5:21–29, 1985.
54. Fauci AS, Balow JE, Brown R, Chazan J, Steinman T, Sahyoun AI, Monaco AP, Wolff SM: Successful renal transplantation in Wegener's granulomatosis. *Am J Med* 60:437–440, 1976.
55. Kuross S, Davin T, Kjellstrand CM: Wegener's granulomatosis with severe renal failure: Clinical course and results of dialysis and transplantation. *Clin Nephrol* 16:172–180, 1981.
56. Steinman TI, Jaffe BF, Monaco AP, Wolff SM, Fauci AS: Recurrence of Wegener's granulomatosis after kidney transplantation. Successful reinduction of remission with cyclophosphamide. *Am J Med* 68:458–460, 1980.
57. Curtis JJ, Diethelm AG, Herrera GA, Crowell WT, Whelchel JD: Recurrence of Wegener's granulomatosis in a cadaver renal allograft. *Transplantation* 36:452–454, 1983.
58. Levy M, Broyer M, Arsan A, Levy-Benoilila D, Habib R: Anaphylactoid purpura nephritis in childhood: Natural history and immunopathology. *Adv Nephrol* 6:183–228, 1976.
59. Kauffmann RH, Herrmann WA, Meyer CJ, Daha MR, van Es LA: Circulating IgA-immune complexes in Henoch–Schonlein purpura. A longitudinal study of their relationship to disease activity and vascular deposition of IgA. *Am J Med* 69:859–866, 1980.
60. Meadow SR: The prognosis of Henoch–Schoenlein nephritis. *Clin Nephrol* 9:87–90, 1978.
61. Cybulsky AV, Jothy S, Seely JF: Late development of purpura in a patient with glomerulonephritis. *Can Med Assoc J* 130:149–152, 1984.
62. Counahan R, Winterborn MH, White RH, Heaton JM, Meadow SR, Bluett NH, Swetschin H, Cameron JS, Chantler C: Prognosis of Henoch-Schonlein nephritis in children. *Br Med J* 2:11–14, 1977.
63. Cameron JS: The nephritis of Schonlein–Henoch purpura: Current problems. In: P Kincaid–Smith, AJF d'Apice, RC Atkins, ed, *Progress in Glomerulonephritis*. John Wiley and Sons, New York, p 283, 1979.
64. Crumb CK: Renal involvment in Schonlein–Henoch syndrome. In: WN Suki, ed, *The Kidney in Systemic Disease*. John Wiley and Sons, New York, pp 43–55, 1976.
65. Kalowski S, Kincaid–Smith P: Glomerulonephritis in Henoch–Schonlein syndrome. In: P Kincaid–Smith, TH Mathew, EL Becker, ed, John Wiley and Sons, New York, pp 1123–1137, 1973.
66. Koskimies O, Mir S, Rapola J, Vilska J: Henoch–Schonlein nephritis: Long-term prognosis of unselected patients. *Arch Dis Child* 56:482–484, 1981.
67. Hurley RM, Drummond KN: Anaphylactoid purpura nephritis: Clinicopathological correlations. *J Pediatr* 81:904–911, 1972.
68. Austin HA III, Balow JE: Henoch–Schonlein nephritis: Prognostic features and the challenge of therapy. *Am J Kidney Dis* 2:512–520, 1983.
69. Antonovych TT, Mostofi FH: *Atlas of Kidney Biopsies*. Armed Forces Institute of Pathology, Washington DC, pp 201–235, 1980.
70. Levy M, Broyer M, Habib R: Pathology and immunopathology of Schonlein–Henoch glomerulonephritis. In: P Kincaid-Smith, AJF d'Apice, RC Atkins, eds, *Progress in Glomerulonephritis*. John Wiley and Sons, New York, p 261, 1979.
71. Levinsky RJ, Barratt TM: IgA immune complexes in Henoch–Schonlein purpura. *Lancet* 2:1100–1103, 1979.
72. Hall RP, Lawley TJ, Heck JA, Katz SI: IgA-containing circulating immune complexes in dermatitis herpetiformis, Henoch–Schonlein purpura, systemic lupus erythematosus and other diseases. *Clin Exp Immunol* 40:431–437, 1980.
73. Baart de la Faille-Kuyper EH, Kater L, Kuijten RH, Kooiker CJ, Wagennar SS, Van der Zouwen P, Mees EJ: Occurrence of vascular IgA deposits in clinically normal skin of patients with renal disease. *Kidney Int* 9:424–429, 1976.
74. Heaton JM, Turner DR, Cameron JS: Localization of glomerular "deposits" in Henoch–Schnolein nephritis. *Histopathology* 1:93–104, 1977.
75. Lee HS, Koh HI, Kim MJ, Rha HY: Henoch–Schonlein nephritis in adults: A clinical and morphological study. *Clin Nephrol* 26:125–130, 1986.

76. Bar-on J, Rosenmann E: Schonlein–Henoch syndrome in adults: A clinical and histological study of renal involvement. *Israel J Med Sci* 8:1702–1715, 1972.
77. Farine M, Poucell S, Geary DL, Baumal R: Prognostic significance of urinary findings and renal biopsies in children with Henoch–Schonlein nephritis. *Clin Pediatr* 25:257–259, 1986.
78. Sinniah R, Feng PH, Chen BT: Henoch–Schonlein syndrome: A clinical and morphological study of renal biopsies. *Clin Nephrol* 9:219–228, 1978.
79. Roth DA, Wilz DR, Thiel GB: Schonlein–Henoch syndrome in adults. *Q J Med* 55:145–152, 1985.
80. Yoshikawa N, White RH, Cameron AG: Prognostic significance of the glomerular changes in Henoch–Schonlein nephritis. *Clin Nephrol* 16:223–229, 1981.
81. Coppo R, Basolo B, Martina G, Rollino C, De Marchi M, Giacchino F, Mazzucco G, Messina M, Piccoli G: Circulating immune complexes containing IgA, IgG and IgM in patients with primary IgA nephropathy and with Henoch–Schonlein nephritis. Correlation with clinical and histologic signs of activity. *Clin Nephrol* 18:230–239, 1982.
82. White RH, Cameron JS, Trounce JR: Immunosuppressive therapy in steroid-resistant proliferative glomerulonephritis accompanied by the nephrotic syndrome. *Br Med J* 2:853–860, 1966.
83. Michael AF, Vernier RL, Drummond KN, Levitt JI, Herdman RC, Fish AJ, Good RA: Immunosuppressive therapy of chronic renal disease. *N Engl J Med* 276:817–828, 1967.
84. Medical Research Council Working Party: Controlled trial of azathioprine and prednisone in chronic renal disease. *Br Med J* 2:239–241, 1971.
85. Fillastre JP, Morel-Maroger L, Richet G: Schonlein–Henoch purpura in adults. *Lancet* 1:1243–1244, 1971.
86. Brown CB, Wilson D, Turner D, Cameron JS, Ogg CS, Chantler C, Gill D: Combined immunosuppressive and anticoagulation in rapidly progressive glomerulonephritis. *Lancet* 2:1166–1172, 1974.
87. Cameron JS, Gill D, Turner DR, Chantler C, Ogg CS, Vosnides G, Williams DG: Combined immunosuppression and anti-coagulation in rapidly progressive glomerulonephritis. *Lancet* 2:923–925, 1975.
88. Rose GM, Cole BR, Robson AM: The treatment of severe glomerulopathies in children using dose intravenous methylprednisolone pulses. *Am J Kidney Dis* 1:148–156, 1981.
89. McKenzie PE, Taylor AE, Woodroffe AJ, Seymour AE, Chan YL, Clarkson AR: Plasmapheresis in glomerulonephritis. *Clin Nephrol* 12:97–108, 1979.
90. Kauffmann RH, Houwert DA: Plasmapheresis in rapidly progressive Henoch–Schoenlein glomerulonephritis and the effect on ciruclating IgA immune complexes. *Clin Nephrol* 16:155–160, 1981.
91. Cameron JS: Glomerulonephritis in renal transplants. *Transplantation* 34:237–245, 1982.

CHAPTER 28

Noninflammatory Vascular Diseases of the Kidney

GARABED EKNOYAN

INTRODUCTION

The kidneys are highly vascularized organs that normally receive 20–25% of the cardiac output. The arterial network of the kidney is highly specialized and is adapted to the regulatory functions of this organ. It is not unusual, therefore, to encounter functional and structural changes in the kidneys in diseases of the vasculature of any etiology. The compromise in renal function that ensues, in turn, adversely affects the course of the primary vascular disease. Conversely, the successful therapy of either the underlying vascular disease or the consequent deterioration of renal function will favorably alter the course of the other. This chapter deals only with the noninflammatory vascular diseases that compromise renal blood flow and alter renal function. The specific entities to be covered are: essential hypertension, malignant hypertension, renovascular hypertension, scleroderma, embolic diseases, and renal vein thrombosis.

ESSENTIAL HYPERTENSION

That hyperentsion produces vascular damage that can be arrested by appropriate antihypertensive therapy has been confirmed by several carefully controlled studies (1–3). The end organs most frequently damaged by hypertensive vascular disease are the brain, heart, and kidneys. The development of renal dysfunction in essential hypertension and the overall relationship between the kidney and hypertension has been the focus of extensive study that has established a pivotal role of the kidney in all forms of elevated blood pressure (4–6). The three principal mechanisms by which the kidney influences arterial blood pressure are: a) release of renin and activation of the renin-angiotensin system, b) maintenance of sodium balance and extracellular fluid volume, and c) the release of vasodilator substances (Figure 1). In fact, renal parenchymal or vascular disease are the most common causes of secondary hypertension, each accounting for about 4–5% of patients with hypertension, the bulk of whom, over 90%, will have essential hypertension (7). The elevated blood pressure of this latter group, over time, will result in sclerotic changes of the renal vascular so that many patients with essential hypertension will develop renal insufficiency. The incidence and degree of renal involvement in patients with essential hypertension varies, with higher incidence and more severe involvement in those with higher levels of blood pressure (8) and in blacks (9). As renal damage and hypertension progress, it will become difficult to determine which one of them was the initiating event, particularly in the absence of a reliable past history and previous laboratory data.

In patients with renal parenchymal disease, some degree of elevated arterial pressure is present in about three fourths of the cases and may well be the presenting find in some (10). Hence, a careful urinalysis is important and the physician should look for renal parenchymal disease in all patients who present with hypertension. Determination of the underlying renal lesion is important, both to decide whether specific therapy of the kidney disease is indicated and to help clarify the pathogenesis and, therefore, the appropriate treatment of the elevated arterial pressure. Diseases that affect the vasculature, whether involving the major vessels (renovascular disease) or the smaller vessels (polyarteritis, scleroderma), usually raise arterial pressure by a disproportionate rise in the renin-angiotensin system. In these, the rise in blood pressure occurs earlier in the course of the disease, is more severe in degree, and pursues a more fulminant course. Diseases that affect the microvasculature of the glomeruli usually elevate the arterial pressure by an inappropriate retention of sodium. Thus, the expanded extracellular volume becomes the major cause of hypertension, although some degree of increased pressor activity also contributes to the hypertension. Diseases that affect the tubules and interstitium develop hypertension late in the course of parenchymal disease, when renal failure is advanced and a tendency for sodium retention develops. In any case, the principal etiology of hypertension in parenchymal renal diseases, be they primarily glomerular or tubulointerstitial, is extracellular fluid volume expansion, and the hypertension in most such cases is largely volume dependent (4–6, 10–12).

Whereas the severity of hypertension varies considerably during the course of diseases of the kidney, as a rule

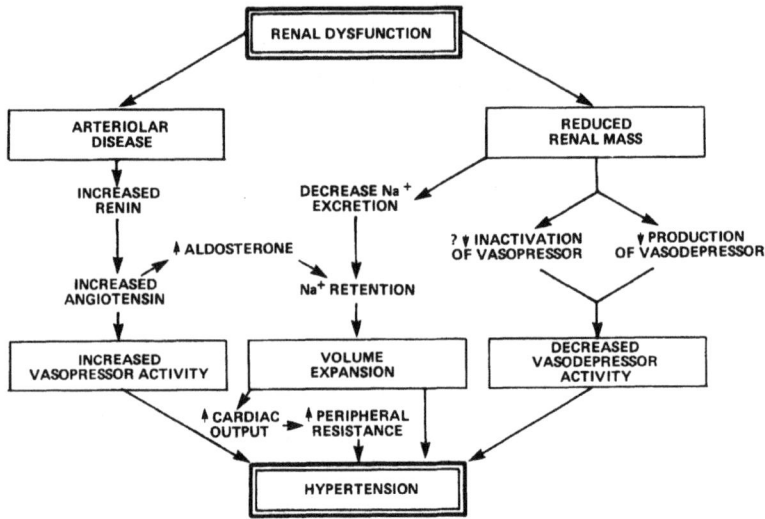

Figure 1. Role of the kidney in the pathogenesis of hypertension.

it tends to increase with progression of the renal insufficiency. Additionally, whatever the initiating mechanism of hypertension may have been in the first place, as renal function deteriorates and the ability to maintain salt and water homeostasis becomes compromised, the elevated blood pressure becomes more and more dependent upon the expanded intravascular volume. This will be the case in 80–85% of patients as renal function deteriorates. This constitutes the group of patients whose hypertension is salt sensitive, in the majority of whom the hypertension will respond to diuretics or the attainment of dry weight on dialysis. In the remainder, intrarenal ischemia and consequent stimulation of the renin-angiotensin mechanism is the major course of hypertension. It is in this latter group of patients that hypertension persists in spite of dry weight attained by dialysis or loop diuretics (13–14), but shows a dramatic response to inhibition of the angiotensin-converting enzyme (15). It must be noted, however, that an abnormal relationship between sodium and the renin–angiotensin system has been demonstrated in hypertensive individuals with renal parenchymal disease, and that even in those patients with volume-dependent hypertension, renin levels remain inappropriately elevated (16, 17). Thus, in most patients with chronic renal failure, the elevated blood pressure is due to both volume overload and renin excess, although the contribution of each will vary from one patient to the other (18). Consequently, the separation of hypertension into volume- or renin-dependent forms in an individual patient represents an oversimplification, and to overemphasize the treatment of one extreme or the other will be to the detriment of the patient. In arriving at a therapeutic regimen, both volume control and inhibition of the renin-angiotensin system must be taken into consideration. In this regard, it must be kept in mind that increased sympathetic nerve activity may also contribute to the pathogenesis of hypertension in patients with renal failure. Blood levels of norepinephrine are increased in renal failure independent of the presence or absence of hypertension, and are normalized following the initiation of maintenance dialysis, again independent of the presence or absence of hypertension (19). Inhibition of the sympathetic nervous system effectively lowers the blood pressure along with that of the plasma norepinephrine level of patients with renal failure.

Hypertensives, with or without underlying renal disease, are at greater risk of developing coronary heart disease, congestive heart failure, or cerebrovascular disease. The reduction in these cardiovascular morbid events, as well as in the renal parenchymal damage due to hypertension, by adequate control of blood pressure of these individuals is now well established (1–3, 8). In addition, the presence of hypertension exerts a detrimental effect on the course of parenchymal renal disease (5, 6, 20), and the control of the blood pressure exerts a salutary influence on the rate of decline in renal function in hypertensives with renal parenchymal disease (5, 6, 20–22). Experimental evidence for this clinical observation has been advanced (23), and the hemodynamically mediated alterations in the microvasculature of the kidney as a cause of the progressive sclerosis and functional deterioration of the kidney has been demonstrated (24).

Assessment of renal function is important in planning the therapy of hypertensives. As functional mass diminishes, the effectiveness of some agents (thiazides) diminishes, while the pharmacokinetics of those dependent upon renal clearance is altered (Table 1), and the use of others (spironolactone, triamterene, amiloride) becomes contraindicated.

Restriction of the dietary intake of salt must be an integral component of the management of all hypertensives,

Table 1. Pharmacokinetics of drugs used in the treatment of hypertension

	Usual daily dosage				Half-life hours		
	mg	Frequency	Route of excretion*	Protein binding	Normal	Renal failure	Dosage modification in renal failure
1 DIURETICS							
1.1 *Thiazide group* (195, 196)							
Hydrochlorothiazide	25–100	1–2	R	60–75	1–2	4–6	Ineffective at GFR < 30
Trichlomethiazide	2–4	1–2	R	60–75	1–2	4–6	Ineffective at GFR < 30
Metolazone (197, 198)	2.5–10	1	R	70–80	8	?	No dosage modification
Chlorthalidone	25–50	1	R		40–65	Prolonged	Ineffective at GFR < 30
1.2 *Loop diuretics*							
Furosemide (199, 200)	20–120	2–4	R	95	5–2	2–4	Larger doses necessary
Ethacrynic acid (201)	50–200	2–4	R	90	2–4	2–4	Larger doses necessary
Bumetanide (202, 203)	0.5–4	2–4	R	95	1–2	2–3	Larger doses necessary
1.3 *Potassium saving*							
Spironolactone (204)	25–400	3–4	H	98	10–35	10–35	Avoid at GFR < 30
Triamterene (205)	100–200	2	R < 10, H	50	2	10	Avoid at GFR < 30
Amiloride (206)	5–20	1–2	R	Low	6–9	Prolonged	Avoid at GFR < 30
2 ADRENERGIC INHIBITORS							
2.1 Methyldopa (208, 209)	250–3000	1–3	R 60, H	< 20	2–4	4	HD, PD, metabolites accumulate; reduce to 50% for GFR < 20
2.2 Clonidine (210, 211)	0.1–2.4	1–2	R 40–50	20–40	7–16	4	Reduce to 50% for GFR < 50; to 30% for GFR < 20
2.3 Reserpine (212, 213)	0.1–0.5	1	H	40	50–100	Prolonged	No dosage modification
2.4 Guanabenz (214)	4–32	2	R 70–80	90	6	Prolonged	No dosage modification
2.5 Guanfacine (215)	1	1	R 40	70	10–20	20–30	Reduce to 50% for GFR < 20
3 BETA BLOCKERS (216, 217)							
3.1 Atenolol	50–100	1	R 85	< 5	6–9	40–120	HD, replace 50% dose. Reduce to 50 with GFR < 50; to 25–50% with GFR < 20
3.2 Metoprolol	50–400	2–3	R 5–10	10	2–4	2–4	HD, reduce to 75% with GFR < 20
3.3 Pindolol	10–60	2–3	R 35	60	3–4	3–4	Increased sensitivity; reduce dosage to 50–75%
3.4 Propranolol	40–480	2–3	H	60–90	3–6	3–6	Active metabolites accumulate, reduce dose
3.5 Timolol	10–20	1–2	R 20, H	10	4–6	4–6	No dose modification
3.6 Nadolol	40–640	1	R 60, H	25–30	16–24	25–45	HD, replace 50% dose; reduce dose to 50–75% with GFR < 50; to 25–50% for GFR < 20
4 ALPHA BLOCKERS							
4.1 Prazosin (41)	1–20	1–2	R < 20, H	97	2–3	?	No dose modification
5 VASODILATORS							
5.1 Hydralazine (40, 218, 219)	50–300	2–3	H	90	3	16	No dose modification
5.2 Minoxidil (220, 221)	5–100	1–2	H	0	4	4	HD, PD; replace after dialysis. No dose modification
6 CONVERTING-ENZYME INHIBITORS							
6.1 Captopril (222)	50–450	2–3	R 40–50	30	2–3	20–30	HD, PD, metabolites accumulate; reduce to 20–30% with GFR < 50; 10–20% with GFR < 20
6.2 Enalapril (223)	5–20	1–2	R 60	50–60	11–14	Prolonged	HD, PD, reduce to 30% for GFR < 50; to 15% for GFR < 20

Table 1. (Cont.).

	Usual daily dosage		Route of excretion*	Protein binding	Half-life hours		Dosage modification in renal failure
	mg	Frequency			Normal	Renal failure	
7 CALCIUM-CHANNEL BLOCKERS (55)							
7.1 Nifedipine	10	3	H	92–80	4–5	5–7	No dose modifcation, metabolites accumulate
7.2 Verapramil	80–120	2–3	H	90	3–7	2–4	Reduce to 50–75% with GFR < 10%, metabolites accumulate
7.3 Diltiazem	30	3–4	H	70–80	2–8	2–4	No dose modification

* R = renal excretion; H = hepatic elimination. The number after these letters refer to the percent of total dose excreted by that route.
+ GFR = glomerular filtration rate; HD = removal of drug by hemodialysis; PD = removal of drug by peritoneal dialysis. The numbers refer to the percent of the normal dose that is recommended at each level of renal dysfunction.

particulary in those with renal insufficiency or evidence of salt-sensitive hypertension. The threshold concentration to obtain a definite effect has been set at 35 mEq/day. Increasing the intake to 50 mEq/day results in weight gain and an increment in the blood pressure (25). Restriction of sodium intake to 75 mEq/day generally allows for a palatable diet that is effective in lowering the blood pressure in some (26). The addition of a thiazide diuretic is a common next step in those that fail to respond to such modest salt restriction alone. As renal insufficiency progresses and the serum creatinine levels attain 2–3 mg/dl, a more rigid sodium restriction regimen (50–75 mEq/day) becomes necessary. In addition, at these levels of renal function, thiazides — except for metolazone — become ineffective and the use of more potent loop diuretics will be necessary: furosemide (40 mg), bumetanide (1 mg) given twice or thrice daily, or metolazone 2.5–5 mg given once daily (10, 11, 27). Metolazone, although a thiazide diuretic, remains effective at glomerular filtration rates of < 30 ml/min because of its proximal tubular effect (28). The effective dosage of loop diuretics generaly correlates inversely with the levels of renal function, and the dosage will have to be increased as renal failure progresses. In patients who become refractory to large doses of loop diuretics, the addition of metolazone will prove effective because of the proximal effect of metolazone. This must be done carefully and under close supervision to avoid severe volume depletion. As kidney function deteriorates to end-stage renal failure, diuretics will no longer suffice to control volume-dependent hypertension, but the maintenance dialysis instituted for the renal failure will be adequate to handle volume overload.

Beta-adrenergic receptor blockers may be effective in patients with renin-dependent hypertension. Their blood-pressure lowering effect is due to: a) β_1 receptor blockade of the heart with consequent reduction of cardiac output and rate; b) suppression of renal renin release and, therefore, the reduction of the pressor effect of angiotensin; and c) inhibition of the central vasomotor center (29). The multiple effects of these agents in lowering blood pressure, as well as the salutary effect they exert on post-myocardial infarction patients (30, 31), has resulted in the emergence of these agents as first-line drugs in the management of hypertension. However, caution must be exerted in their use in patients with borderline renal function, peripheral vascular disease, insulin-dependent diabetes mellitus, and elevated serum potassium levels (hyporeninemic hypoaldosteronism) (29, 32). A decrease in cardiac output is a common effect of all beta blockers, but a reduction in the glomerular filtration rate and renal perfusion has been demonstrated with propranolol but not with other beta blockers (11, 32–34). Beta-adrenergic blocking agents, particularly those that are nonselective, inhibit muscle gluconeogenesis and can predispose to hypoglycemia in insulin-dependent diabetics and malnourished uremics (33). Their ability to interfere with the adrenergic-mediated intracellular transport of potassium results in hyperkalemia, especially in the presence of hyporeninemic hypoaldosteronism or exogenous potassium administration (29, 35). The excretion of these agents varies (Table 1); of note is that of nadolol, which is excreted largely unchanged by the kidney and will require dosage adjustment in renal failure.

The centrally acting antihypertensive agents — methyldopa, clonidine, guanabenz, and guanfacine — exert their effect through stimulation of the central alpha$_2$ receptors, thus reducing sympathetic outflow from the central vasomotor center (36–38). The first three in this group of antihypertensive agents are effective in lowering the blood pressure over a wide dose-response curve. Guanfacine has a fixed response at a dosage of 1 mg/day, which appears to be equal to that of the half-maximal effect of the others (38).

Because vasodilators trigger compensatory mechanisms, increased heart rate, salt retention, and elevated plasma renin, they are not effective in the control of hypertension when used alone. On the other hand, the addition of a vasodilator to hypertensives whose volume-dependent component and renin-angiotensin vasoconstriction has been controlled by other agents can be most effective (34). These agents should be added to the regimen of all those with uncontrolled hypertension. Over the years, hydralazine, in doses of 200–400 mg/day, has been most successful in this regard (40). The introduction of prazosin, an alpha-adrenergic blocking agent, has added a new dimension to vasodilator therapy because of its reported lower sympathetic stimulatory effect and, therefore, fewer side effects (41), although this was unsubstantiated in a randomized double-blind clinical trial comparing prazosin to hydralazine (42). The vasodilator that has had the greatest impact in the management of severe refractory hypertension is minoxidil (43, 44). It is the most potent oral vasodilator currently available. As with other vasodilators, it is associated with sodium retention and reflex tachycardia and must be used in conjunction with a potent diuretic and a centrally acting antihypertensive or a beta blocker.

The availability of orally effective angiotensin-converting enzyme inhibitors has added a new dimension to the therapy of hypertension. Although inhibition of angiotensin II formation appears to be the major mechanism of action of these agents, inhibition of bradykinin breakdown or stimulation of vasodepressors may also play a role (11, 45–47). An especially attractive feature of these agents has been the experimental demonstration of their ability to favorably alter intraglomerular capillary hemodynamics and thereby provide protection from progressive renal injury (24, 48, 49). Preliminary studies indicate that this protective effect may also be observed in hypertensive patients with reduced renal function (48). Such a protective effect has also been adduced from the reduction of the proteinuria noted in diabetic patients with diabetic nephropathy (50, 51). The potential of these agents in retarding the progression of renal disease is currently the subject of intense scrutiny. An acute progressive deterioration of renal function has been noted to occur with these agents in patients with bilateral renal artery stenosis, renal artery stenosis in a solitary kidney and in the presence of severe sclerosis in the intrarenal vasculature (52, 53). A similar effect may occur when these agents are administered in conjunction with potent diuretics. Another serious side effect is the development of hyperkalemia in patients with hyporeninemic hypoaldosteronism and in those with exogenous potassium supplementation (54). Hence, it is important to monitor renal function and serum potassium levels shortly after the institution of therapy with converting-enzyme inhibitors.

Table 2. Cardinal features of hypertensive crisis

1. Elevated blood pressure, usually > 190/130 mmHg
2. Hypertensive encephalopathy
   Headaches, restlessness, irritability, stupor, convulsions, coma, nystagmus, focal seizures
3. Retinopathy
   Hemorrhages, exudates, papilledema
4. Rapidly progressive renal failure
   Proteinuria, hematuria, RBC casts
5. Cardiomyopathy
   LVH, CHF, pulmonary edema, MI, arrhythmias
6. Endocrinopathy
   Increased renin, aldosterone

Renal excretion is the major clearance route of these agents, and the appropriate reduction of their dosage is essential in the presence of reduced renal function.

The calcium-channel antagonists, first introduced for their antianginal and antiarrhythmic properties, have now established themselves as a new group of antihypertensive agents. They are particulary effective in salt-sensitive hypertension, do not seem to cause the salt retention noted with other direct vasodilators, and increase renal blood flow (55, 56). A salutary effect of these agents on the progressive nature of renal disease has been demonstrated in experimental animals and in humans (56).

ACCELERATED AND MALIGNANT HYPERTENSION

Severe elevations of blood pressure (diastolic > 130 mmHg) will cause generalized vascular damage, which accounts for the systemic manifestations (Table 2) and rapid deterioration of these patients. Of these, the development of hypertensive crisis is the most dramatic and the one that demands immediate therapy (57–60). The drugs most useful to reduce arterial pressure in hypertensive emergencies are summarized in Table 3. The choice among these drugs must be determined by the suitability of their hemodynamic effect to the existing clinical situation (57–61). Nitroprusside is the most potent and predictable agent where immediate reduction of the blood pressure is necessary (57, 62). Diazoxide, used in a rapidly injected bolus dose of 100 mg every 30 minutes or infused at 15 mg/min over 20–30 minutes, can also be used effectively to achieve individual titration (27, 63). Oral clonidine, at an initial dose of 0.2 mg, followed by 0.1 mg hourly doses for up to 6 hours or until the desired blood pressure has been attained, may be sufficient in the control of severe hypertension without the necessity of resorting to intravenous therapy (64). Oral and sublingual nifedipine is another effective approach that circumvents intravenous therapy (65). With a peak effect attained at 30 minutes, it is quite easy to determine rapidly whether increased dosing or additional therapy is necessary. As a direct vasodilator, however, nifedipine dilates cerebral blood vessels and may cause an increased intracranial pressure, which could be detrimental in patients with hypertensive encephalopathy. Labetolol, a combined alpha-and beta-adrenergic blocking agent, is also effective orally, although its intravenous administration is the generally used route in the management of severe hypertension (66). Angiotensin-converting enzyme inhibitors have been effectively used in hypertensive emergencies (67). The availability of enalaprilat in the intravenous formulation permits its use in patients unable to take medication orally (68).

The essential structural lesions of severe hypertension are endothelial swelling and the sudden appearance of minute disruptions in the intima of the terminal arterioles, which ultimately result in patchy disruption and necrosis of the medial muscle fibers. The inflammatory reaction designed to repair the initial disruptions forms the character-

Table 3. Drug treatment of hypertensive emergencies

Drug	Mode of action	Onset	Peak	Duration	Dosage
Diazoxide (Hyperstat)	Direct arteriolar vasodilation	1–2 min	3–5 min	4–24 hr	IV bolus of 50–150 mg every 5 min or infusion at 7.5–30 mg/min
Sodium nitroprusside (Nipride)	Direct arteriolar vasodilation	0.5–1 min	1–2 min	3–5 min	IV drip (0.1 g/l) at 0.03–0.5 µg/min or 0.5–8 µg/kg/min
Hydralazine (Apresoline)	Direct arteriolar vasodilation	10–20 min	20–40 min	3–8 hr	10–50 mg IM or IV every 3–6 hr
Methyldopa (Aldomet)	Decreased sympathetic activity	1 hr	2 hr	4–8 hr	500 mg IV every 2 hr for 4 doses
Reserpine	Catecholamine depletion at adrenergic nerve endings	2–3 hr	3–4 hr	6–24 hr	0.25–8 mg IM every 4–12 hr
Trimethaphan camsylate (Arfonad)	Ganglionic blockade	1–2 min	2–5 min	10 min	IV drip at 0.5–5 mg/min
Labetolol (Trandate, Normodyne)	α- and β-adrenergic blockade	2–5 min	5 min	3–6 hrs	2–8 mg/min or 20–80 mg/10 min IV up to maximum of 300 mg
Propranolol (Inderal)	β-adrenergic blockade	2–10 min	30 min	2–12 hr	1–10 mg IV load, 3 mg/hr maintenance
Nifedipine (Procardia)	Calcium-channel blockade	5–15 min	30 min	3–6 hr	10–20 mg chewed, sublingual or swallowed
Clonidine (Catapres)	Sympatholytic	30–60 min	2 hr	6–8 hr	0.2 mg then 0.1 mg/hr orally, up to 0.8 mg total
Captopril (Capoten)	Angiotensin-converting enzyme inhibition	15–30 min	30 min	4–6 hr	6.25–50 mg PO

istic early *fibrinoid necrosis* that later progresses to the proliferative cellular intimal thickening, narrowed lumen, fragmented elastica, and scarred media and adventitia of *endarteritis fibrosa* (69–71). The rapid control of blood pressure in the early phases of development of the vascular lesions will prevent and usually reverse the progressive irreversible end-organ damage that might otherwise ensue (21, 22, 72–74). The early and rapid reduction in blood pressure necessary to circumvent this eventuality will be associated with an initial reduction in renal perfusion pressure and, therefore, of the glomerular filtration rate (73). In cases where uremia develops, dialysis may have to be instituted while the blood pressure is maintained under control. With chronic therapy, the initial deterioration in renal blood flow and the glomerular filtration rate, brought about by the acute reduction of perfusion pressure, will subside even after prolonged uremia (75, 76), except in those where the lesion has progressed to irreversible vascular damage with renal arteriolar scarring and obstructive lesions (21, 22). Failure to adequately control the blood pressure, under the erroneous notion of maintaining adequate perfusion pressure, will result in the invariable progression of the vascular lesion to its irreversible progressive stage in all.

If parenteral therapy has been instituted because of the presence of hypertensive encephalopathy (Tables 2 and 3), therapy with oral agents must be initiated as soon as possible (Table 1). A variety of oral regimens have been effectively used in the initial treatment of severe hypertension, including clonidine, methyldopa, labetolol, nifedipine, angiotensin-converting enzyme inhibitors, prazosin, hydralazine, and minoxidil (27, 77). In all instances these must be administered frequently and in increasing doses until the pressure is well under control. Whether oral or parenteral therapy is instituted, the use of a loop diuretic will almost always become necessary. Combination therapy with either converting-enzyme inhibition, beta-adrenergic blockade, adrenergic-suppressing drugs, or vasodilators together with loop diuretics and dialysis, when necessary, will ultimately improve renal function or at least arrest its progressive deterioration (72–76). The need for bilateral nephrectomy or nonsurgical renal artery embolization, while effective in the treatment of these cases (13, 78, 79), has been obviated by the availability of the potent vasodilator minoxidil (43, 44, 80). Exacerbation of angina pectoris and pericardial effusion has been observed in about 3% of patients treated with minoxidil, with pericardial tamponade developing in some. These serious side effects notwithstanding, the potential disadvantages of nephrectomy so far as depriving the body of any residual excretory (urine output) and endocrine (erythropoietin, vitamin D hydroxylation) function of the diseased kidney far outweigh its effectiveness, now that satisfactory reduction of blood pressure can be achieved (75, 76, 81).

RENOVASCULAR HYPERTENSION

Strictly defined, renovascular hypertension is elevation of arterial pressure due to obstruction or narrowing of a renal artery, with the implication that correction of the vascular lesion or removal of the ischemic kidney will result in the restoration of blood pressure to normal levels. Whereas such a restrictive definition renders the diagnosis of true renovascular hypertension one that can be made only in retrospect, it does help to emphasize two important points. The first is that renal artery stenosis may be present in the absence of hypertension. The second is that the presence of renal artery stenosis is not always the cause of elevated blood pressure. The available data would suggest that renal artery stenosis is present in over 10% of the hypertensive population, only one third of whom have renovascular hypertension. Stated otherwise, renovascular hypertension accounts for about 3–4% of the cases of hypertension (82–86). Its importance arises not from its prevalence but from its potential for total cure and the preservation of renal function if it is diagnosed and treated early (85).

The principal causes of stenosis of the main renal arteries are fibromuscular dysplasia and atherosclerosis. The former accounts for two thirds of the cases of renovascular hypertension; is a lesion of older age, usually over 50 years; and is commonly present in those with systemic evidence of generalized atherosclerosis with end-organ involvement, being more common in those with an associated history of smoking. Both forms are more common among whites than blacks (82–87).

The history, physical findings, and laboratory results can be extremely useful in suggesting renovascular hypertension. As a rule the following are suggestive of renovascular hypertension: the hypertension is of shorter duration, the family history is negative for hypertension, the retinal findings are more prominent, the level of blood pressure is higher and accelerated or malignant hypertension are common, the blood urea nitrogen is elevated, the urinary sediment is abnormal (proteinuria, hematuria, casts), and the serum potassium is low. The presence of an epigastric or a flank blowing bruit, particularly when both a systolic and diastolic component are present, and especially in a young individual, is an invaluable clue, although its absence does not rule out renovascular lesions (83–88).

Rapid sequence intravenous pyelography and radioisotope renography have both been used as screening tests for renovascular hypertension (84, 85, 89). The advantage of both procedures is their relative simplicity. Their major disadvantage is the 15–20% of false-positive and negative results and, more importantly, their failure to establish whatever lesion is detected as the cause of the elevated blood pressure (85, 86, 90, 91). The measurement of a random plasma renin is of more limited use, as it will be elevated in only half of those with renovascular hypertension, whereas it is increased in about 10–20% of those with essential hypertension (85–87, 90).

The conclusive diagnosis of renovascular hypertension depends on the radiographic demonstration of the vascular lesions, and the assessment of its functional significance in producing renin-angiotensin assessed from the depressor response to angiotensin blockers. The infusion of graded doses of the angiotensin II blocker, saralasin, or the oral administration of the converting-enzyme inhibitor, captopril, while frequent blood measurements are made, has been successfully used by some (85, 86, 92). The theoretical attractiveness of this procedure notwithstanding, its sensitivity and specificity do not appear to be superior to that of rapid sequence pyelography, as it is truly positive in only 85% of cases and is falsely positive in 8.5% (86, 88). Others have advocated the response to chronic administration of an oral angiotensin-converting enzyme inhibitor alone for a period of 2–4 weeks (93, 94). Given the multiple effects of these agents in lowering blood pressure (enhancement of kinins and increased prostaglandin), the limitations of this approach are evident. A further limitation of such an approach is the state of sodium balance of the patient at the time of testing. Neither enalapril nor captopril dramatically lower the blood pressure in salt-loaded subjects, whereas both are effective when the extracellular volume is depleted (87, 88, 95).

In the final analysis, the cause and effect relationship between an anatomic lesion and hypertension is dependent upon the demonstration of an anatomic lesion by arteriography and the functional significance of the lesion by the hypersecretion of renin from the affected kidney. As a rule, an increase of renin of 1.5 times or more on the affected side is highly suggestive of a significant lesion (96). The usefulness of this test, however, is limited by a fairly high-negative rate of about 50% (86, 97). The value of renal vein renin can be enhanced by sampling from the vena cava and taking this value as equal to the level of arterial renin, since renin is cleared primarily by the liver. When this is done, the V-A renin should approach zero on the affected side, where V is the renal vein and A the arterial renin activity. The sensitivity and specificity can be further improved by the calculation of the increment of renin contributed by each kidney from the formula: (V-A)/A. An increment of at lease 50% on one side indicates hypersecretion, while an increment of less than 25% on the other side infers contralateral suppression (98). The measurement of plasma renin activity after angiotensin-converting enzyme inhibition with oral captopril has been reported to add to the discriminatory value of renal vein and peripheral renin evaluation (94, 99, 100).

Digital subtraction angiography has added a new dimension to the diagnosis of renovascular hypertension and can be performed in conjunction with renal-vein renin determinations (85–88). Essentially after renal vein samples are obtained, the cathether is left in the vena cava and dye is injected for imaging. Whether this can ultimately replace renal arteriography remains to be seen.

The traditional therapy of renovascular hypertension has been surgical repair or nephrectomy. The recent introduction of percutaneous transluminal renal angioplasty has provided an alternative effective means of treating renal artery stenosis due to fibromuscular dysplasia or unilateral nonostial atheroma, which avoids the risks and limits the cost of the surgical procedure (99). Given the equivocal results of most tests on renovascular hypertension, in patients with strong evidence of renovascular hypertension (based on history, physical examination, and routine laboratory data), a direct approach with renal arteriography coupled with renal angioplasty, if a lesion is present, provides the most direct and efficient approach (100). As a rule the best results of angioplasty are obtained with fibromuscular dysplasia affecting a short segment of the main renal artery. Renal angioplasty is not without risk. Reported complications include renal embolization, arterial rupture, thrombosis or aneurysm, restenosis of the dilated vessel, and contrast-dye-induced renal failure (101, 102). With proper patient selection, the results of both procedures, with regard to cure rates, are similar (100–103). About 50–65% are cured, 10–15% improve, and 10–15% fail to respond (85–88). The success rate with either procedure is diminished in the presence of a small atrophic kidney (< 9 cm), parenchymal renal disease, and intrarenal vascular lesions.

Not all patients with renovascular hypertension respond to angioplasty or are suitable candidates for surgery. Factors favoring medical treatment are listed in Table 4. Beta-receptor blockade has been effective in lowering blood pressure in patients with elevated plasma renin activity (104). The availability of converting-enzyme inhibitors, with their more specific action on the renin-angiotensin system, has added a new and more effective agent to the medical management of these patients (85, 86, 105). Elevation of the serum creatinine level (106) and cases of acute renal failure (107) have been reported after converting-enzyme inhibition therapy. Patients at particular risk are those with volume depletion, bilateral renal artery stenosis, stenosis of a solitary kidney, or unilateral stenosis with contralateral severe nephrosclerosis. Therapy with converting-enzyme inhibitors should be instituted under careful observation and at the lowest dose necessary to control blood pressure. Inordinate and precipitious deterioration of renal function following institution of converting-enzyme inhibition therapy should always lead to the suspicion of, and the quest for, the presence of renovascular hypertension. Since volume depletion induces reactive rises in renin and augments the azotemia that might be caused by these agents, concomitant diuretic therapy is best avoided and, if necessary, is used with caution and at the lowest doses possible to control edema or hypertension.

Table 4. Factors favoring the medical therapy of renovascular hypertension

---

1. Patient
   Age > 50 years
   Coexisting diseases that increase operative risk (COPD, ASHD)
   Personality conducive to cooperation and compliance
2. Vascular lesion
   Atherosclerosis, generalized and severe
   Extensive enough that nephrectomy could be the only surgical procedure
   Bilateral except if stenosis is severe enough to cause loss of renal function
3. Clinical findings
   Doubtful functional significance of lesion, i.e., equivocal renal vein renin activity
   Long duration of hypertension with left ventricular hypertrophy and coronary artery disease
   Good response to drug therapy

SCLERODERMA — PROGRESSIVE SYSTEMIC SCLEROSIS

Scleroderma or progressive systemic sclerosis (PSS) is a chronic disease of unknown etiology characterized by excessive collagen deposition and vascular changes in different organ systems (108–110). Its most common and classical clinical manifestations are the cutaneous changes that begin as edema, thickening, tightness, erythema, and altered pigmentation, followed by a sclerotic stage in which the skin becomes smooth, waxy, and shiny; ultimately trophic changes with thinning of the epidermis and ulcers of the digits develop. The striking morphologic feature of the involved organs is noted in the vascular changes, consisting of extensive intimal proliferation and fibrosis, which results in luminal narrowing, medial thinning and adventitial collagen deposition in the arteries, and ultimately the fibrinoid necrosis of the small arteries and arterioles (108–111). A distinction between scleroderma, a disorder affecting the skin alone, and systemic sclerosis, a generalized disease with some skin manifestations, has been made by some, but these terms are used synonymously by most. Over two thirds of the cases occur among whites, usually affecting adults in their third to fifth decade, and the disease is three to four times as common in women as in men (112).

Vascular involvement manifests itself as Raynaud's phenomenon, which may precede the skin lesions and the diagnosis of scleroderma by several years. The most frequently involved organs are the gastrointestinal tract, lungs, heart, and kidneys. Disturbances in esophageal motility and small bowel motility with consequent dysphagia and malabsorption are present in the majority of patients, and, together with the skin changes, are the characteristic presenting features that lead to the diagnosis of scleroderma (108–112). Renal involvement, while rarely present at the onset of the disease, usually occurs within 3 years of the development of the other classic signs and symptoms (108–113). The renal lesions consist of cortical wedge-shaped microinfarcts due to the characteristic vascular lesion of scleroderma that affects the interlobular arteries and the afferent and efferent arterioles (110, 111). Glomerular involvement is focal, affecting anywhere from 3% to 60% of the glomeruli, and consists of localized areas of basement membrane thickening. Morphologic evidence of renal involvement is present in 85% of all cases of progressive systemic sclerosis. Clinical evidence of renal involvement, however, will be evident in only half of these, and the lesions will be found at autopsy in the other half with no overt clinical renal disease. Renal involvement manifests itself in one of two forms. About half of those whose kidneys are affected, or 14–20% of patients with PSS, will develop a rapidly progressive oliguric renal failure eventuating in uremia, which has been termed *scleroderma renal crisis*. This is usually accompanied by severe hypertension, which dominates the clinical manifestations and presents a picture classical of a malignant hypertensive crisis (Table 2). In others, clinically evident renal disease is manifestated by proteinuria, which is rarely in the nephrotic range, a measurable reduction in the glomerular filtration rate, modest azotemia, and occasionally mild-to-moderate hypertension (110, 113–116).

Until about a decade ago, the syndrome of severe uncontrolled hypertension and rapidly progressive renal failure, termed *scleroderma renal crisis*, had been considered uniformly fatal, accounting for half of the overall death rate in scleroderma (112, 113, 117). Reports of survival after nephrectomy and dialysis provided a new hope in the early 1970s (118–120). Because of reports of vascular-access problems and decreased peritoneal clearances (118–121), transplantation after bilateral nephrectomy has been proposed as a better alternative in the management of patients with scleroderma renal crisis (122–124). The availability of new antihypertensive agents has favorably altered this otherwise dismal outcome.

The malignant hypertension that develops in PSS is pressor in origin and is renin-angiotensin dependent. In all cases with scleroderma renal crisis, the plasma renin activity is elevated, the renal blood flow is reduced, and renal arteriograms reveal cortical ischemia and vasospasm (113, 120, 125, 126). The hyperreninemia is consequent to the reduced renal blood flow caused by the obstructive lesion of scleroderma affecting the renal vasculature. The rationale for nephrectomy, to relieve the malignant hypertension, consists then of the high plasma renin activity found during the renal scleroderma crisis (125, 126) and the suggestive evidence that the high renin-angiotensin activity may accelerate not only the hypertension and renal failure, but also other systemic manifestations of PSS (125–127).

In fact, the clinical manifestations and course of patients with scleroderma renal crisis is quite similar to that of patients with hypertension of any etiology. Its response to antihypertensive therapy is no different from that of malignant hypertension, and evidence that control of hypertension results in reversal of renal failure in PSS has been advanced (128–131). The initial group of patients were treated with diazoxide, hydralazine, and propranolol (128–130). The availability of the converting-enzyme inhibitors has added a new and more specific approach to treatment that appears to be particularly effective (131–132). Because of the high renin state characteristic of the disease, it is important to initiate converting-enzyme inhibitors at low doses and titrated gradually to attain the desired blood pressure. Minoxidil, another orally effective potent vasodilator, is also a valuable addition to the management of these individuals, as well as for malignant hypertension (43, 129). Favorable results have also been reported with prazosin and calcium-channel blockers (130). As with malignant hypertension, the initial reduction of blood pressure may result in the further deterioration of the glomerular filtration rate, and despite good pressure control the renal failure may be progressive (132). In such instances, the patients should be maintained on dialysis, as recovery of some degree of renal function may ultimately occur after several months of treatment (120). For the same reasons detailed under Malignant Hypertension, nephrectomy should be avoided in PSS. Those who fail to respond to control of hypertension and dialysis can be transplanted (123, 124). There is, however, evidence of recurrence of the lesion in transplanted kidneys (120). Particularly rewarding are reports that survival from scleroderma renal crisis appears to be accompanied by improvement of the cutaneous mainfestitations and regression of Raynaud's phenomenon (110, 130). While the reasons for these are not readily evident, a detrimental effect of the hyperreninemic state, which accompanies scleroderma renal crisis, on the systemic manifestations of scleroderma has been implicated (127, 130).

While evidence in plasma renin activation precedes the development of scleroderma renal crisis, and the characteristic changes of fibrinoid necrosis of the capillary loops and intimal hyperplasia of the interlobular arteries are indistinguishable from those encountered in malignant hypertension, it is important to note that scleroderma renal crisis is a different disease and cannot be dismissed as just another form of malignant hypertension. In the first place, malignant hypertension and scleroderma renal crisis occur in only 15% of cases, whereas renal involvement is much more common, being clinically evident in 40% and present at autopsy in 75–80% of cases of PSS (110, 114–117). Secondly, progressive renal failure can occur in scleroderma without the development of hypertension (110, 114–117, 120, 130). Thirdly, some of those who develop renal failure with normal plasma renin activity and blood pressure may have accompanying evidence of microangiopathic hemolyic anemia, indicative of vascular narrowing (108, 110, 114–117, 120, 130). Fourthly, whereas the vascular lesions of malignant hypertension are primarily limited to the afferent arterioles, the lesions of scleroderma are present in both the afferent and efferent arterioles (110, 120). Thus, the rewarding experience with control of the blood pressure on the course of the scleroderma crisis notwithstanding, the disease remains one of undetermined etiology, with only a limited number of cases developing severe renal involvement. Whether the use of angiotensin-converting enzyme blockade can be beneficial in those without renal failure remains to be seen. In all cases, supportive therapy for the care of the skin lesions, physical medicine, and appropriate nutritional support must be an integral part of the management. (134).

On the basis of rather tenuous evidence, and autoimmune etiology of PSS has been suggested (135). The use of plasmapheresis in conjunction with low-dose steroid has been shown to be effective in the control of some of the manifestations of scleroderma (136). Whether this form of therapy can be useful for the renal failure patients without hypertension remains to be seen.

RENAL EMBOLIZATION/EMBOLIC DISEASE OF THE KIDNEY

The renal arteries and its branches are end arteries and the occlusion of any of them will result in renal infarction. The symptoms and signs that develop, and the degree of renal function loss that ensues, will depend on the size and extent of vascular obstruction. Emboli may originate from cardiovascular thrombi, endocardial vegetations, tumors, fat, or atheromatous plaques (137, 138). They may be large enough to obstruct the main renal arteries, but more frequently are small in size and obstruct the peripheral small vessels. In over two thirds of the cases of renal artery embolization, there will be coexistent evidence of embolization to extrarenal organs, predominantly to the spleen, the lung, and the brain (137).

Large-vessel embolization

As a rule, larger emboli originate from the heart. The source are mural thrombi in the left ventricle following myocardial infarction; left atrial thrombi in rheumatic heart disease with mitral stenosis, particularly if associated with atrial fibrillation; bacterial or marantic vegetations of the endocardium; and clots formed on prosthetic heart valves (139–141). The characteristic clinical finding in a patient with an embolus to the main renal artery or a major branch is the sudden onset of pain on the afflicted side, followed shortly thereafter by the development of tenderness in the kidney area. Flank pain may be severe but usually is mild or absent (142, 143). Hypertension, which may be transient or persistent, will develop in some. The incidence of hypertension in renal embolic disease is uncertain, but its presence can be construed as evidence of some blood flow, since the hypertension of renal infarction is hyperreninemic in origin and requires that there be some renal blood flow (142–145). Fever and leukocytosis occur within 48 hours, but are present in only half the cases. The urinalysis is negative or noncontributory in most, with microhematuria and mild proteinuria present in a third of the cases (142, 143). Strikingly elevated LDH levels, in association with only a small or no increase in alkaline phosphatase or liver anzymes, are said to be strongly suggestive of renal infarcts, particularly if LDH is also elevated in the urine (144, 145). LDH peaks at 2–4 days after infarction, begins to decline after the fourth day, but remains elevated in half the cases (142), although if emboli are bilateral or occur in an individual with one kidney, severe renal failure and anuria will occur (147, 148). On the other hand, segmental infarction of the kidney may result in little reduction in renal function and may not be clinically detectable.

Prompt diagnosis and surgical repair is important in symptomatic cases, as the prognosis for the return of renal function in cases of total occlusion is poor unless the flow is reestablished promptly. Normothermic human renal tissue has been reported to lose viability after 2 hours of arterial occlusion (149). Renal function has been restored following surgical intervention as long as 2–7 days after the insult (138, 143, 151). Collateral circulation develops very rapidly after occlusion and in slow or partial occlusion will maintain viability of the organ. Even with sudden occlusion, the subcortical area and medullary rim may remain viable due to blood supply from the capsular, ureteral, and pelvic vessels.

While renal scintigram and flow studies may be suggestive of the diagnosis, renal arteriography is the most important radiographic study to perform, as it both confirms the diagonsis and accurately locates the embolus (139, 143). It is, therefore, expedient to proceed to aortography and selective renal angiography. In addition to confirming the diagnosis, such an approach provides the means of transcatheter embolectomy (152) and of local fibrinolytic therapy (153). Roentgenographic features that suggest that revascularization is likely to restore function are normal-sized kidneys, a faint nephrogram effect, visualization of renal veins on delayed films, and evidence of collateral circulation. Back-bleeding from the kidney when the renal artery is surgically opened is also a favorable prognostic indicator. Discoloration of the kidney at the time of surgery should not be accepted as unequivocal evidence for nephrectomy. Viability is best judged by the appearance and consistency of the kidney after arterial flow has been restored. Every effort should be made to preserve the kidney.

In patients who are poor surgical candidates, recovery of renal function has been reported with anticoagulation (154, 155). In fact, in one study of patients with unilateral embolization where surgical treatment was compared to anticoagulation and supportive measures, mortality rates were greater in the surgically treated group (156).

Small-vessel embolization

Small emboli lodging in terminal vessels that are 150–300 µm in diameter may be bacterial, fat, or atheromatous in origin (138). The development of renal findings in patients with endocarditis or fracture of a long bone will usually suggest the diagnosis of the former two. It is patients will atheroembolic emboli who may present with puzzling findings.

Atheroembolic emboli may be large and manifest as specific organ involvement, or they may be small or manifest as multiple-system involvement. The latter is the more common form, occurring predominantly in the elderly, with evidence of extensive atherosclerotic disease, and is predominantly a disease of men (157, 158). The organ most commonly involved is the kidney (159, 160). The initial lesion is that of endothelial injury, followed by histiocytic or giant cell reaction, endothelial proliferation and intimal fibrosis, often complicated by thrombosis (159–161). The consequent ischemic infarcts that result account for the clinical evidence of renal involvement that develops. If involvement is spotty, few clinical manifestations develop and the lesions will go unrecognized, as evidenced by the much higher incidence of atheromatous emboli at autospy than are suspected clinically (157–160). On the other hand, if sufficient parenchymal damage occurs, renal function will deteriorate, presenting as acute renal failure or slowly progressive renal failure over several months (159, 160). Atheromatous emboli occur spontaneously, or after aortic surgery and angiography. Most patients with postoperative atheroembolic kidney disease will develop acute renal failure and will require dialysis (159, 160, 162). On the other hand, in those that develop embolization after angiography, the course of renal of failure is more insidious, but nevertheless is progressive to end-stage renal failure within a few months at most (159, 160, 163). Atheroembolic disease has also been reported as a rare complication of warfarin therapy (164). Although the mechanism by which warfarin induces atheroemboli is unknown, it has been attributed to its interference with the healing of ulcerated atherosclerotic plaques. It does appear to worsen atheroembolic disease and should be avoided or discontinued once a diagnosis is established (165).

The diagnosis should be suspected whenever sudden or otherwise unexplained renal failure and hypertension develops in older patients (159, 160). The hypertension is hyperreninemic in origin (166). The multiple organ involvement by atheroemboli should suggest the multisystemic nature of the disease (157, 158, 167). The finding of recurrent refractile crystals in the retinal vessels can help establish the diagnosis. Typically, these lodge at vascular bifurcations and frequently can be dislodged by tapping or pushing on the eye (167, 168). The skin may also be involved, with plaquelike reddened lesions that are elevated and tender, very reminiscent of periarteritis nodosa (158, 167). Actually, periarteritis nodosa or a vasculitis are the most confusing entities in the differential diagnosis of atheroembolic disease, particularly since eosinophilia and an elevated sedimentation rare are common in atheroembolic disease (169). The eosinophilia is transient, lasting only a few days, and of variable degree, ranging from 6% to 18% of the total leukocyte count (170). Hypocomplementemia is another useful diagnostic clue of atheroembolic disease (171). A biopsy of the skin or muscle, however, will quickly establish the diagnosis by the demonstration of the vascular cholesterol clefts (172). Atheromatous embolization cannot be proven by arteriography but may be demonstrated in renal biopsy specimens (159, 160). While the value of renal biopsy has been questioned by some, when the disease is symptomatic there is likely to be sufficient emboli to the kidney present to be appreciated in a random biopsy (161). Still, a sampling error exists, and the diagnosis cannot be excluded, even if the biopsy is negative.

The prognosis for recovery of renal function is poor, and often dialysis is the only alternative available to these patients. Elevated blood pressure, if present, is hyperreninemic in origin and should be treated accordingly. Steroids, low molecular weight dextran, intraarterial vasodilators, and anticoagulants have been tried without any beneficial effect (159, 163, 169). Actually, the implication has been made that anticoagulation should not be used since it inhibits thrombus deposition on the ulcerated atheromatous plaques, thereby favoring the release of further cholesterol emboli (168). Avoiding dislodgement of atheromatous material by proper clamping at surgery and minimal manipulation of the catheter during aortography remain the preventive measures of choice in all candidates at risk of atheroembolic disease.

RENAL VEIN THROMBOSIS

Thrombosis of the renal veins develops in a variety of clinical conditions such as an extension of vena caval thrombosis, an invasion of renal veins by tumor cells in abdominal carcinomatosis, a result of surgical or blunt trauma, and a complication of renal disease (173, 174). In the latter category, there is a well-documented association between renal vein thrombosis (RVT) and the nephrotic syndrome. The earlier notion that RVT precedes the nephrotic syndrome (174–176), and hence serves as the initiating event, has been refuted. The overwhelming evidence now available indicates that RVT develops as a complication of preexisting renal diseases associated with the nephrotic syndorme. and a hypercoagulable state (177–180).

In adults, membranous nephropathy is the renal lesion most commonly associated with RVT and the nephrotic syndrome (177–181). In a prospective study of 33 patients with the nephrotic syndrome and renal vein thrombosis, the etiology of the nephrotic syndrome was membranous nephropathy in 60% of the cases, membranoproliferative glomerulonephritis in 18% of the cases, lipoid nephrosis in 3% of the cases, and systemic diseases with renal involvement in 13% of the cases (178). The systemic diseases commonly associated with RVT are systemic lupus erythematosus, sarcoidosis, amyloidosis, periarteritis nodosa, sickle cell anemia, and diabetes mellitus (179–182). In children, and more specifically in neonates, RVT differs from that encountered in adults in that it is rarely accompanied by the nephrotic syndrome and is often related clinically to dehydration or to an intercurrent illness (183, 184).

The clinical presentations of RVT are varied and depend upon the rapidity of the venous thrombosis and upon the extent of the occlusion (78, 185). Sudden or rapid thrombosis of the renal vein may result in severe noncolicky lumbar pain, usually characterized as a dull fullness, enlargement of the kidneys, varying degrees of transient hematuria, deterioration of renal function, and worsening of the preexisting proteinuria (178, 181, 185). None of these features are consistent, nor is hypertension a prominent feature of RVT, and when present it may be related to the underlying renal disease. Survival of the kidney depends upon the development of venous collaterals before the thrombotic occlusion is complete. Rapid deterioration of renal function may occur if bilateral occlusion persists without reestablishment of venous drainage by collaterals. In cases of gradual or partial RVT, any functional derangement may be transitory, producing nonspecific clinically undetected findings (178–181, 185). Although a slow, mild progressive deterioration of renal function has been attributed to chronic RVT (178), there is no good evidence that this may be different from that due to the natural course of the underlying renal disease. Thus, the initial symptomatology and prognosis of patients who develop RVT depends on the adequacy and the possibility of reestablishing venous drainage. The subsequent prognosis is related to the occurrence of pulmonary emboli and the course of the underlying disease (171–182). Pulmonary emboli account for the major morbidity and mortality of patients with RVT (171–182). Actually, thromboembolic phenomena occur in patients with the nephrotic syndrome, particularly in those due to membranous nephropathy, just as frequently as in the absence of RVT (173, 181, 186) because of the hypercoaguable state that characterizes the nephrotic state (187–189). In fact, it is this hypercoagulable state that has been implicated as the cause of RVT (177–181).

The radiographic criteria on the basis of which the diagnosis of RVT can be suspected are enlargement or nonvisualization of the kidney, notching of the ureter, and pelvocalyceal distortion or stretching (185, 190). None of these, however, are specific (191). Inferior venocavagraphy and selective renal vein phlebography are more useful and, if positive, will establish the diagnosis (190). It is important to note that a negative venogram does not exclude the diagnosis and the procedure is not without risk. In fact, the manipulation of the catheter and forceful injection of contrast material into the veins has been implicated as a cause for embolization due to the dislodgement of thrombi (180, 181). Angiography is an accurate and useful procedure because of the different phases of renal circulation that can be demonstrated (190). Ultrasonography and computer-enhanced subtraction angiography may prove to be potentially useful procedures (192, 193).

Once the diagnosis is confirmed, a decision must be made to treat with anticoagulants. Convincing evidence has been presented that treatment with anticoagulants reduces the incidence of new embolic episodes and often reverses the deterioration of renal function that might have occurred with an acute RVT (177, 178, 181, 182). Treatment should begin with heparin, in an amount that is sufficient enough to maintain a clotting time of 2–2.5 times greater than normal, for a period of 1–2 weeks; followed by several months of oral anticoagulant therapy. The preferred duration of oral anticoagulant therapy varies from 2 to 6 months, depending to a great extent on patient compliance and the bleeding complications encountered. For patients with recurrent embolic phenomenon or RVT, longer periods of oral anticoagulant therapy are necessary. Throughout the period of anticoagulation, patients should be carefully monitored for evidence of bleeding, initially from the site of the venography procedure and subsequently from the gastrointestinal tract. In the occasional oliguric patient, supportive dialytic therapy may be necessary during the acute phase of the disease. Appropriate treatment of the underlying renal disease, depending on the biopsy findings, should accompany treatment of the thromboembolic problems.

Surgical thrombectomy may be useful in patients with acute bilateral thrombosis who are not otherwise expected to survive the acute episode or when pulmonary emboli recur despite adequate anticoagulation (184). Fibrinolytic agents are useful in the treatment of RVT but are not without danger (194).

REFERENCES

1. Veterans Administration Cooperative Study on Antihypertensive Agents. Effects of treatment on morbidity in hypertension. I. Results in patients with diastolic blood pressure averaging 115 through 129 mmHg. *J A M A* 202:1028–1034, 1967.
2. Veterans Administration Cooperative Study on Antihypertensive Agents. Effects of treatment on morbidity in hypertension. II. Results in patients with diastolic blood pressure averaging 90–114 mmHg. *J A M A* 213:1143–1152, 1970.
3. Hypertension Detection and Follow-Up Cooperative Group. Five-year findings of the hypertension detection and follow-up program. I. Reduction in mortality of persons with high blood pressure, including mild hypertension. *J A M A* 242:2652–2671, 1979.
4. Kaplan NM: The role of the kidney in hypertension. *Hypertension* 1: 456–461, 1979.
5. Ferris TF: The kidney and hypertension. *Arch Intern Med* 142:1889–1895, 1982.
6. Suki WN: The kidney in hypertension. *Contr Nephrol* 7:290–308, 1977.
7. Berglund G, Andersson O, Wilhelmsen L: Prevalence of primary and secondary hypertension: Studies in a random population sample. *Br Med J* 2:554–558, 1976.
8. Moyer JH, Heider C, Pevey K, Ford RV: The vascular status of a heterogeneous group of patients with hypertension, with particular emphasis on renal function. *Am J Med* 24:164–176, 1958.
9. Rostand, SG, Kirk KA, Rutsky EA, Pate BA: Racial differences in the indicence of treatment for end-stage renal disease. *N Engl J Med* 306:1276–1279, 1982.
10. Russell RP, Whelton PK: Hypertension in chronic renal failure. Clinical presentation, prognosis, pathophysiology and treatment. *Am J Nephrol* 3:185–192, 1983.
11. Sullivan JM, Johnson JG: The management of hypertension in patients with renal insufficiency. *Sem Nephrol* 3:40–51, 1983.
12. Lifschitz MD: Hypertension in chronic renal failure. *Contemp Issues Nephrol* 4:222–246, 1981.
13. Vertes V, Cangano JL, Berman LB, Gould A: Hypertension in end-stage renal disease. *N Engl J Med* 280:978–980, 1969.
14. Weidmann P, Maxwell MH, Lupu AN, Lewin AJ, Massry SG: Plasma renin activity and blood pressure in terminal renal failure. *N Engl J Med* 285:757–762, 1971.
15. Zuccheli P, Santoro A, Zuccala A: Genesis and control of hypertension in hemodialysis patients. *Semin Nephrol* 8:163–168, 1988.
16. Davies DL, Schalekampp MA, Beevers DG, Brown JJ, Briggs JD, Lever AF, Medina AM, Morton JJ, Robertson JIS, Tree M: Abnormal relation between exchangeable sodium and the renin-angiotensin system in malignant hypertension and in hypertension with chronic renal failure. *Lancet* 1:683–687, 1973.
17. Warren DJ, Ferris TF: Renin secretion in renal hypertension. *Lancet* 1:149–163, 1970.

18. Weidmann P, Beretta-Piccoli C, Steffen F, Blumberg A, Reubi F: Hypertension in terminal renal failure. *Kidney Int* 9:294-301, 1976.
19. Campese VM, Romoff MS, Levitan D: Autonomic nervous system dysfunction in uremia. *Kidney Int* 19:246-253, 1981.
20. Morgenson CE: Progression of nephropathy in long-term diabetes with proteinuria and effect of initial antihypertension treatment. *Scand J Clin Lab* 36:384-388, 1976.
21. Woods JW, Blythe WB: Management of malignant hypertension complicated by renal insufficiency. *N Engl J Med* 277:57-61, 1967.
22. Woods JW, Blythe WB, Huffines WD: Management of malignant hypertension complicated by renal insufficiency. *N Engl J Med* 291:10-14, 1974.
23. Okuda S, Onoyama K, Fujimi S, Oh Y, Nomoto K, Omae T: Influence of hypertension on the progression of experimental autologous immune complex nephritis. *J Lab Clin Med* 101:461-470, 1983.
24. Brenner BM: Hemodynamically mediated glomerular injury and the progressive nature of kidney disease. *Kidney Int* 23:647-655, 1983.
25. Freis ED: Does moderate sodium restriction lower blood pressure? *Hypertension* 8:265-266, 1986.
26. Ram CVS, Garrett BN, Kaplan NM: Moderate restriction and various diuretics in the treatment of hypertension. Effects on potassium wastage and blood pressure control. *Arch Intern Med* 141:1015-1919, 1981.
27. Kaplan NM: Management strategies in hypertension. *Contemp Issues Nephrol* 4:339-366, 1981.
28. Suki WN, Dawoud F, Eknoyan G, Martinez MM: Effects of metolazone on renal function in normal man. *J Pharm Exp Ther* 180:6-12, 1972.
29. Frishman WH: β-adrenoreceptor antagonists: New drus and new indications. *N Engl J Med* 305:500-506, 1981.
30. The Norwegian Multi-Center Study Group. Timolol-induced reduction in morality and reinfarction in patients surviving acute myocardial infarction. *N Engl J Med* 304:801-807, 1981.
31. Braunwald E, Muller JE, Kloner RA, Maroko PR: Role of beta-adrenergic blockade in the therapy of patients with myocardial infarction. *Am J Med* 74:113-123, 1983.
32. Weber MA, Drayer JIM: Renal effects of beta-adrenoreceptor-blockade. *Kidney Int* 18:686-699, 1980.
33. Wright AD, Barber SG, Kendall MJ: Beta-adrenoreceptor blocking drugs and blood sugar control in diabetes mellitus. *Br Med J* 1:159-161, 1979.
34. Greenblatt DJ, Koch-Wesser J: Adverse reactions to propranolol in hospitalized patients. A report from the Boston Collaborative Drug Surveillance Program. *Am Heart J* 86:478-485, 1973.
35. Rosa RM, Silva P, Young JB, Brown RS, Rowe JW, Epstein FH: Adrenergic modulation of extrarenal potassium disposal. *N Engl J Med* 302:431-434, 1980.
36. Frohlich ED: Methyldopa. Mechanism and treatment 25 years later. *Arch Intern Med* 140:954-959, 1981.
37. Pettinger WA: Clonidine, a new antihypertensive drug. *N Engl J Med* 293:1179-1180, 1975.
38. Saameli K, Jerie P, Scholtysik G: Guanfacine and other centrally acting drugs in antihypertensive therapy: Pharmacological and clinical aspects. *Clin Exp Hypertension* 4:209-219, 1982.
39. Chidsey CA, Gottlieb TB: The pharmacological basis of antihypertensive therapy: The role of vasodilator drugs. *Prog Cardiovasc Dis* 17:99-113, 1974.
40. Koch-Wesser J: Hydralazine. *N Engl J Med* 295:61-65, 1981.
41. Graham RM, Pettinger WA: Prazosin. *N Engl J Med* 300:232-236, 1979.
42. Veterans Administration Cooperative Study Group on Antihypertensive Agents. Comparison of prazosin with hydralazine in patients receiving hydrochlorothiazide. A randomized, double-blind clinical trial. *Circulation* 64:772-779, 1981.
43. Keusch GW, Weidmann P, Campese V, Lee DBN, Upham AT, Massry SG: Minoxidil therapy in refractory hypertension. Analysis of 155 patients. *Nephron* 21:1-15, 1979.
44. Mitchell JC, Graham RM, Pettinger WA: Renal function during long-term treatment of hypertension with minoxidil. Comparison of benign and malignant hypertension. *Ann Intern Med* 93:676-681, 1980.
45. Ram CVS: Clinical application of therapeutic advances. Captopril. *Arch Intern Med* 142:914-916, 1982.
46. Rubin B, Antonaccio MJ, Horowitz ZP: Captopril: A new orally active inhibitor of angiotensin-converting enzyme and antihypertensive agent. *Prog Cardiovasc Dis* 21:183-187, 1978.
47. Vidt DG, Bravo EL, Fouad FM: Captopril. *N Engl J Med* 306:214-219, 1982.
48. Bauer JH, Reams GP, Lal SM: Renal protective effect of strict blood pressure control with enalapril therapy. *Arch Intern Med* 147:1397-1400, 1987.
49. Zatz R, Anderson S, Meyer TW, Dunn BR, Rennke HG, Brenner BM: Lowering arterial blood pressure limits glomerular sclerosis in rats with renal ablation and in experimental diabetes. *Kidney Int* 31 (Suppl 20):S123-S129, 1987.
50. Hostetter TH, Rennke HG, Brenner BM: The case for intrarenal hypertension in the initiation and progression of diabetic and other glomerulopathies. *Am J Med* 73:375-380, 1982.
51. Bjorck S, Nyberg G, Mulec H, Granerus G, Herlitz H, Aurell M: Beneficial effects of angiotensin converting-enzyme inhibition on renal function in patients with diabetic nephropathy. *Br Med J* 293:471-474, 1986.
52. Levenson DJ, Dzau VJ: Effects of angiotensin-converting enzyme inhibition on renal hemodynamics in renal artery stenosis. *Kidney Int* 31 (Suppl 20):S173-S179, 1987.
53. Mujais SK, Fouad FM, Textor SC, Tarazi RC, Bravo EL, Hart N, Gifford RW: Transient renal dysfunction during initial inhibition of converting enzyme in congestive heart failure. *Br Heart J* 52:63-71, 1984.
54. Textor SC, Bravo E, Fouad FM: Hyperkalemia in azotemic patients during angiotensin-converting enzyme inhibition and aldosterone reduction with captopril. *Am J Med* 73:719-725, 1982.
55. Ram CVS: Calcium antagonists in the treatment of hypertension. *Am J Med Sci* 290:118-133, 1985.
56. Loutzenhiser R, Epstein M: Effects of calcium antagonists on renal hemodynamics. An editorial review. *Am J Physiol* 249:F616-F621, 1985.
57. Koch-Wesser J: Hypertensive emergencies. *N Engl J Med* 290:211-214, 1974.
58. Keith TA: Hypertension crisis. Recognition and management. *J A M A* 237:1570-1577, 1977.
59. Carry CL: Current treatment of malignant hypertension. *J A M A* 232:1367-1369, 1975.
60. Ram CVS: Hypertensive encephalopathy — recognition and management. *Arch Intern Med* 138:1851-1853, 1978.
61. Bhatia SK, Frohlich ED: Hemodynamic comparison of agents useful in hypertensive emergencies. *Am Heart J*

85:367–373, 1973.
62. Cohn JH, Burke LP: Nitroprusside. *Ann Intern Med* 91:752–757, 1979.
63. Ram CVS, Kaplan NM: Individual titration of diazoxide dosage in the treatment of severe hypertension. *Am J Cardiol* 43:627–630, 1979.
64. Houston MC: Treatment of hypertensive emergencies and urgencies with oral clonidine loading and titration. A review. *Arch Intern Med* 146:586–589, 1986.
65. Haft JI, Litterer WE: Chewing nifedipine to rapidly treat hypertension. *Arch Intern Med* 144:2357–2359, 1984.
66. Wilson DJ, Wallin JD, Vlachakis ND, Freis ED, Vidt DG, Michelson EL, Langford HG, Flamenbaum W, Poland MP: Intravenous labetalol in the treatment of severe hypertension and hypertensive emergencies. *Am J Med* 74:95–102, 1983.
67. Brollaz J, Waeber B, Brunner HR: Hypertensive crisis treated with orally administered captopril. *Eur J Clin Pharmacol* 25:145–149, 1983.
68. Reams GP, Lal SM, Whalen JJ, Bauer JH: Enalaprilat — an intravenous substitute for oral enalapril therapy. *J Clin Hypertension* 3:245–253, 1986.
69. Byrom FB: The evolution of acute hypertensive arterial disease. *Prog Cardiovasc Dis* 17:31–37, 1974.
70. MacMahon HE: Malignant nephrosclerosis — A reappraisal. *Pathol Ann* 3:297–334, 1968.
71. Allison PR, Bleeham N, Brown W, Pickering GW, Robb-Smith AHT, Russell RP: The production and resolution of hypertensive vascular lesions in the rabbit. *Clin Sci* 33:39–51, 1967.
72. Pickering G: Reversibility of malignant hypertension. Follow-up of three cases. *Lancet* 1:413–418, 1971.
73. Mroczek WJ, Davidov M, Gavrilovich L, Finnerty F: The value of aggressive therapy in the hypertensive patient with azotemia. *Circulation* 40:893–904, 1969.
74. Friedlander MM, Rubinger D, Popovtzer MM: Improved renal function in patients with primary renal disease after control of severe hypertension. *Am J Nephrol* 2:12–14, 1982.
75. Eknoyan G, Siegel MB: Survival from anuria due to malignant hypertension. *JAMA* 215:1122–1125, 1971.
76. Dichoso CC, Minuth ANW, Eknoyan G: Malignant hypertension: Recovery of kidney function after renal allograft failure. *Arch Intern Med* 135:300–303, 1975.
77. Ram CVS, Hyman D: Hypertensive crisis. *J Intensive Care Med* 2:151–162, 1987.
78. Mahoney JF, Gibson GR, Shiel AGR, Storey BG, Stokes GS, Stewart JH: Bilateral nephrectomy for malignant hypertension. *Lancet* 1:1036–1038, 1972.
79. McCarron DA, Rubin RJ, Varnes BA, Harrington JT, Nillan EG: Therapeutic bilateral renal infarction in end-stage renal disease. *N Engl J Med* 294:652, 1976.
80. Pettinger WA, Mitchell JC: Minoxidil. An alternative to nephrectomy for refractory hypertension. *N Engl J Med* 289:167–171, 1973.
81. Mroczek WJ: Malignant hypertension: Kidneys too good to be extirpated. *Ann Intern Med* 80:754–757, 1974.
82. Maxwell MH, Bleifer KH, Franklin SJ, Varady PO: Demographic analysis of the study. *JAMA* 220:1195–1204, 1972.
83. Simon N, Franklin SS, Bleifer KH, Maxwell MH: Characteristics of renovascular hypertension. *JAMA* 220:1209–1218, 1972.
84. Hunt JC, Sheps SG, Harrison EG, Strong CG, Bernatz PE: Renal and renovascular hypertension. A reasoned approach to diagnosis and management. *Arch Intern Med* 133:988–999, 1974.
85. Working Group on Renovascular Hypertension: Detection, evaluation, and treatment of renovascular hypertension. Final report. *Arch Intern Med* 147:820–829, 1987.
86. Jacobson HR: Ischemic renal disease: An overlooked clinical entity? *Kidney Int* 34:729–743, 1988.
87. Grim CE, Weinberger MH: Renal artery stenosis and hypertension. *Semin Nephrol* 3:52–64, 1983.
88. Dzau VJ, Gibbons GH, Levin DC: Renovascular hypertension: An update on pathophysiology, diagnosis and treatment. *Am J Nephrol* 3:172–184, 1983.
89. Brookstein JJ, Abrams HL, Buenger RE, Lecky J, Franklin SS, Reis MD, Bleifer KH, Klatte EC, Varady PD, Maxwell MH: Urography in unilateral renovascular disease. *JAMA* 220:1225–1230, 1972.
90. Grim CE, Luft FC, Weinberger MH, Grim CM: Sensitivity and specificity of screening tests for renal vascular hypertension. *Ann Intern Med* 91:617–622, 1979.
91. McNeil BJ, Varady PD, Burrows BA, Adelstein SJ: Measures of clinical efficacy: Cost effectiveness calculation in the diagnosis and treatment of hypertensive renovascular disease. *N Engl J Med* 293:216–221, 1975.
92. Hollenberg NK, Williams GH, Adams DF, Moore T, Brown C, Boruki LJ, Leung F, Bavli S, Solomon HS, Passan D, Dluhy R: Response to saralasin and angiotensin role in essential and renal hypertension. *Medicine* 58:115–127, 1979.
93. Case DB, Atlas SA, Laragh JH, Sealey JE, Sullivan PA, McKinstry DN: Clinical experience with blockade of the renin-angiotensin aldosterone system by an oral converting enzyme inhibitor (SQ14225, captopril) in hypertensive patients. *Prog Cardiovasc Dis* 21:195–206, 1978.
94. Staessen J, Wilms G, Baert A, Fagard R, Lynen P, Suy R, Amery A: Blood pressure during long-term converting-enzyme inhibition predicts the curability of renovascular hypertension by angioplasty. *Am J Hypertension* 1:208–214, 1988.
95. Navis G, de Jong PE, Donker AJM, van der Hem GK, de Zeeuw D: Moderate sodium restriction in hypertensive subjects: Renal effects of ACE-inhibition. *Kidney Int* 31:815–819, 1987.
96. Sealey JE, Buhler FR, Laragh JH, Vaughan D: The physiology of renin secretion in essential hypertension: Estimation of renin secretion rate and renal plasma flow from peripheral and renal vein renin levels. *Am J Med* 55:391–401, 1973.
97. Marks LS, Maxwell MH: Renal vein renin. Value and limitations in the prediction of operative results. *Urol Clin North Am* 2:311–325, 1975.
98. Vaughan ED, Buehler FR, Laragh JH, Sealey JE, Baer L, Bard RH: Renovascular hypertension: Renin measurements to indicate hypersecretion and contralateral suppression, estimate renal blood flow, and score for surgical curability. *Am J Med* 65:402–414, 1973.
99. Sos TA, Pickering TG, Sniderman K, Saddekin S, Case DB, Silane MF, Vaughan ED, Laragh JH: Percutaneous transluminal renal angioplasty in renovascular hypertension due to atheroma or fibromuscular dysplasia. *N Engl J Med* 309:274–279, 1983.
100. Madias NE: Renovascular hypertension. *Nephrology Lett* 3:27–42, 1986.
101. Martin LG, Price RB, Casarekka WJ, Stones PJ, Wells SO, Zellmer RA, Chuang VP, Silbiger ML, Berkman WA: Percutaneous angioplasty in clinical management of renovascular hypertension: Initial and long-term results. *Radiology* 155:629–633, 1985.

102. Krener HTK, de Jong PE, de Zeeuw D, Donker AJM, Schuur KH, van der Hem GK: Restenosis prevalence and long-term effects on renal function after percutaneous transluminal renal angioplasty. *Nephron* 44 (Suppl 1):64–67, 1986.
103. Geyskes GG: Treatment of renovascular hypertension with percutaneous transluminal renal angioplasty. *Am J Kid Dis* 12:253–265, 1988.
104. Buhler FR, Laragh JH, Vaughan ED, Brunner HR, Gavras H, Baer L: The antihypertensive action of propranolol. Specific anti-renin responses in high and normal renin forms of essential, renal, renovascular and malignant hypertension. *Am J Cardiol* 32:511–522, 1973.
105. Case DB, Atlas SA, Marion RM, Laragh JH: Long-term efficacy of captopril in renovascular and essential hypertension. *Am J Cardiol* 49:1440–1446, 1982.
106. Aldigier JC, Ploum P, Guyene TT, Thibonnier M, Carval P, Menard J: Comparison of the hormonal and renal effects of captopril in severe essential and renovascular hypertension. *Am J Cardiol* 49:1447–1452, 1982.
107. Hricik DE, Browning PJ, Kopelman R, Goorno WE, Madias NE, Dzau VJ: Captopril-induced functional renal insufficiency in patients with bilateral renal-artery stenosis or renal artery stenosis in a solitary kidney. *N Engl J Med* 308:373–376, 1983.
108. Orabona ML, Albano O: Systemic progressive sclerosis. *Acta Med Scandinav* 333 (Suppl):1–170, 1958.
109. Winkelmann RK: Classification and pathogenesis of scleroderma. *Mayo Clin Proc* 46:83–91, 1971.
110. Eknoyan G, Suki WN: Renal vascular phenomena in systemic sclerosis. *Semin Nephrol* 5:34–45, 1985.
111. Norton WL, Nardo JM: Vascular disease in progressive systemic sclerosis (scleroderma). *Ann Intern Med* 73:317–324, 1970.
112. Medsger TA, Masi AT, Rodnan GP, Benedek TG, Robinson H: Survival with systemic sclerosis (scleroderma): A life-table analysis of demographic and clinical factors in 309 patients. *Ann Intern Med* 75:369–376, 1971.
113. Cannon PJ, Hassar M, Case DB, Casarella WJ, Sommers SC, LeRoy C: The relationship of hypertension and renal failure in scleroderma (progressive systemic sclerosis) to structural and functional abnormalities of the renal cortical circulation. *Medicine* 53:1–46, 1974.
114. Hannigan CA, Hannigan MH, Scoh EL: Scleroderma of the kidneys. *Am J Med* 20:793–797, 1956.
115. Rodnan GP, Schreiner GE, Black RL: Renal involvement in progressive systemic sclerosis (generalized scleroderma). *Am J Med* 23:445–462, 1957.
116. Fisher ER, Rodnan GP: Pathologic observations concerning the kidney in progressive systemic sclerosis. *Arch Pathol* 65:29–39, 1958.
117. Medsger TA, Masi AT: Survival with scleroderma-II: A life-table analysis of clinical and demographic factors in 358 male U.S. veteran patients. *J Chron Dis* 26:647–660, 1973.
118. Richardson JA: Hemodialysis and kidney transplantation for renal failure from scleroderma. *Arthritis Rheum* 16:265–271, 1973.
119. Shapiro CB, Lerner NE, Achad AS, Abramson R, Stein RM: Malignant hypertension and uremia in scleroderma: Efficacy of nephrectomy and hemodialysis. *Clin Nephrol* 8:321–323, 1977.
120. Dichoso CC: The kidney in progressive systemic sclerosis (scleroderma). In: WN Suki, G Eknoyan, eds, *The Kidney in Systemic Disease*, 2nd ed. John Wiley & Sons, New York, pp 109–128, 1981.
121. Brown ST, Ahearn DJ, Nolph KD: Reduced peritoneal clearance in scleroderma increased by intraperitoneal isoproterenol. *Ann Intern Med* 78:891–894, 1973.
122. Oliver JA, Cannon PJ: The kidney is scleroderma. *Nephron* 18:141–150, 1977.
123. LeRoy EC, Fleischmann RM: The management of renal scleroderma: Experience with dialysis, nephrectomy and transplantation. *Am J Med* 64:974–978, 1978.
124. Keane WF, Danielson B, Raij L: Successful renal transplantation in progressive systemic sclerosis. *Ann Intern Med* 85:199–202, 1976.
125. Stone RA, Tisher CC, Hawkins HK, Robinson RR: Juxtaglomerular hyperplasia and hyperreninemia in progressive systemic sclerosis complicated by acute renal failure. *Am J Med* 56:119–123, 1974.
126. Kovalchik MT, Guggenheim SJ, Silverman MH, Robertson JS, Steigerwald JC: The kidney in porgressive systemic sclerosis: A prospective study. *Ann Intern Med* 89:881–887, 1978.
127. Gavras H, Gavras I, Cannon PH, Brunner HR, Laragh JH: Is elevated plasma renin activity of prognostic importance in progressive systemic sclerosis? *Arch Intern Med* 137:1554–1558, 1977.
128. Moorthy AV, Wu MJ, Bierne GJ, Sundstrom WS: Control of hypertension and acute renal failure in scleroderma without nephrectomy. *Lancet* 1:563–564, 1978.
129. Mitnich PD, Fieg PU: Control of hypertension and reversal renal failure in scleroderma. *N Engl J Med* 299:871–872, 1978.
130. Wasner C, Cooke CR, Fries JF: Successful medical treatment of scleroderma renal crisis. *N Engl J Med* 299:873–875, 1978.
131. Lopez–Overjero JA, Saal SD, D'Angelo WA, Cheigh JS, Stenzel KH, Laragh JH: Reversal of vascular and renal crisis of scleroderma by oral angiotensin-converting enzyme blockade. *N Engl J Med* 300:1417–1419, 1979.
132. Whitman HH, Case DB, Laragh JH, Christian CL, Botstein G, Maricq H, LeRoy EC: Variable response to oral angiotensin-converting-enzyme blockade in hypertensive scleroderma patients. *Arthritis Rheum* 25:241–248, 1982.
133. Waldo R: Prazosin relieves Raynaud's vasospasm. *J A M A* 241:1037, 1979.
134. Winkelmann RK, Kierland RR, Perry HO, Muller SA, Sams WM: Management of scleroderma. *Mayo Clin Proc* 46:128–134, 1971.
135. Rodnan GP: Progressive systemic sclerosis (scleroderma). In: Samler, ed, *Immunological Diseases*, Vol. II. Little, Brown, Boston, pp 1109–1141, 1978.
136. Dau PC, Kahleh MB, Sagebiel RW: Plasmapheresis and immunosuppressive drug therapy in scleroderma. *Arthritis Rheum* 24:1128–1136, 1981.
137. Hoxie HJ, Coggin CB: Renal infarction: Statistical study of 205 cases and detailed report of an unusual case. *Arch Intern Med* 65:587–594, 1940.
138. Peterson NE, McDonald DF: Renal embolization. *J Urol* 100:140–145, 1968.
139. Foley WJ, Kraft RO: Renal artery embolectomy. *Arch Surg* 103:748–751, 1971.
140. Gill TJ, Dammin GJ: Paradoxical embolism with renal failure casued by occlusion of the renal arteries. *Am J Med* 25:780–787, 1958.
141. Case Record of the Massachusetts General Hospital (Case 32-1962). *N Engl J Med* 266:1054–1062, 1962.
142. Shabanah FH, Conolly JE, Martin DC: Acute renal artery occulusion. *Surg Gyn Obst* 131:489–494, 1970.

143. Besarab A, Brown RS, Rubin NT, Salzman E, Wirthlin L, Steinman T, Atlia RR, Skillman JJ: Reversible renal failure following bilateral renal artery occlusive disease. Clinical features, pathology, and the role of surgical revascularization. *J A M A* 235:2838–2841, 1976.
144. Arakawa K, Torii S, Kibuchi Y, Nakamura M: Delayed renin release in renal infarction. *Arch Intern Med* 129:958–962, 1972.
145. Arakawa K, Torri S, Naito S, Minohara A, Vemura N, Nakamura M: Plasma renin activity as a more specific diagnostic aid for renal infarction. *Arch Intern Med* 125:830–834, 1970.
146. London IL, Hoffsten P, Perkoff GT, Pennington TG: Renal infarction. Elevation of serum and urinary lactic dehydrogenase (LDH). *Arch Intern Med* 121:87–90, 1968.
147. Duncan DA, Dexter RN: Anuria secondary to bilateral renal-artery embolism. *N Engl J Med* 266:971–973, 1962.
148. Smith SP, Hamburger RJ, Donohue JP, Grim CE: Occlusion of the artery to a solitary kidney. Restoration of renal function after prolonged anuria. *J A M A* 230:1306–1307, 1974.
149. Kerr WK, Kyle VN, Kerestici AG, Smythe CA: Renal hypothermia. *J Urol* 84:236–242, 1960.
150. Brest AN, Bower R, Heider C: Renal functional recovery following anuria secondary to renal artery embolism. *J A M A* 187:540–542, 1964.
151. Perkins RP, Jacobsen DS, Feder FP, Lipchik EO, Fine PH: Return of renal function after late embolectomy. *N Engl J Med* 276:1194–1195, 1967.
152. Millan VG, Sher MH, Deterling RA, Packard A, Morton JR, Harrington JT: Transcatheter thromboembolectomy of acute renal artery occlusion. *Arch Surg* 113:1086–1092, 1978.
153. Fischer CP, Konnach JW, Cho KJ, Eckhauser FE, Stanley JC: Renal artery embolism: Therapy with intra-arterial streptokinase infusion. *J Urol* 125:402–404, 1981.
154. Lessman RK, Johnson SF, Coburn JW, Kaufman JJ: Renal artery embolism. Clinical features and long-term follow-up of 17 cases. *Ann Intern Med* 89:477–482, 1978.
155. Parker JM, Lord JO: Renal artery embolism. A case report with return of complete function of the involved kidney following anticoagulant therapy. *J Urol* 106: 339–341, 1971.
156. Moyer JD, Rao CN, Widrich WC, Olsson CA: Conservative management of renal artery embolus. *J Urol* 109:138–143, 1973.
157. Flory CM: Arterial occlusions produced by emboli from eroded aortic atheromatous plaques. *Am J Path* 21:549–565, 1945.
158. Retan JW, Miller RE: Microembolic complications of atherosclerosis. Literature review and report of a patient. *Arch Intern Med* 118:534–545, 1966.
159. Kassirer JP: Atheroembolic renal disease. *N Engl J Med* 280:812–818, 1969.
160. Smith MC, Ghose M, Henry AR: Clinical spectrum of renal cholesterol embolization. *Am J Med* 71:174–180, 1981.
161. Jones DB, Iannaccone PM: Atheromatous emboli in renal biopsies. An ultrastructural study. *Am J Path* 78:261–270, 1975.
162. Thurbleck WM, Castleman B: Atheromatous emboli to the kidneys after aortic surgery. *N Engl J Med* 257:442–477, 1957.
163. Harrington JT, Sommers SC, Kassirer JP: Atheromatous emboli with progressive renal failure. Renal arteriography as the probably inciting factor. *Ann Intern Med* 68:152–160, 1968.
164. Hyman BT, Landas SK, Ashman RF, Schleper RL, Robinson RA: Warfarin-related purple toes syndrome and cholesterol microembolization. *Am J Med* 82:1233–1237, 1987.
165. Bruns FJ, Segel DP, Adler S: Control of cholesterol embolization by discontinuation of anticoagulant therapy. *Am J Med Sci* 275:105–108, 1978.
166. Handler FP: Clinical and pathologic significance of atheromatous embolization with episodes on the etiology of renal hypertension. *Am J Med* 20:366–373, 1956.
167. Richardson JH, Alderfer HH, Reid JD: Response of eye and brain to microemboli. *Ann Intern Med* 57:1013–1017, 1962.
168. Case Records of Massachusetts General Hospital (Case 25–1967). *N Engl J Med* 276:1368–1377, 1967.
169. Richards AM, Eliot RS, Kanjub VI, Bloemendaal RD, Edwards JE: Cholesterol embolism. A multisystem disease masquerading as polyarteritis nodosa. *Am J Cardiol* 15: 696–707, 1965.
170. Kasinath BS: Eosinophilia as a clue to the diagnosis to the diagnosis of atheroemboli renal disease. *Arch Intern Med* 147:1384–1385, 1987.
171. Cosio F, Zager R, Sharma H: Atheroembolic renal disease causes hypocomplementemia. *Lancet* 2:118–121, 1985.
172. Anderson WR, Richards AM, Evaluation of lower extremity muscle biopsies in the diagnosis of atheroembolism. *Arch Path* 86:535–541, 1968.
173. Baum NH, Moriel E, Carlton CE: Renal vein thrombosis. *J Urol* 119:443–448, 1978.
174. Harrison CV, Milne MD, Steiner RE: Clinical aspects of renal vein thrombosis. *Q J Med* 25:285–298, 1956.
175. McCarthy LJ, Titus JL, Daugherty GW: Bilateral renal vein thrombosis and the nephrotic syndrome in adults. *Ann Intern Med* 58:837–857, 1963.
176. Baird WL, Buchanan DP: The nephrotic syndrome following thrombosis of the inferior vena cava. *Am J Med* 32:128–130, 1962.
177. Llach F, Arieff AI, Massry SG: Renal vein thrombosis and nephrotic syndrome. A prospective study of 36 adult patients. *Ann Intern Med* 83:8–14, 1975.
178. Llach F, Papper S, Massry S: The clinical spectrum of renal vein thrombosis: Acute and chronic. *Am J Med* 69:819–827, 1980.
179. Harrington JT, Kassirer JP: Renal vein thrombosis. *Ann Rev Med* 33:255–262, 1982.
180. Llach F: Hypercoagulability, renal vein thrombosis, and other thrombotic complications of nephrotic syndrome. *Kidney Int* 28:429–439, 1985.
181. Trew PA, Biava CG, Jacobs RP, Hopper J: Renal vein thrombosis in membranous glomerulonephropathy. Incidence and association. *Medicine* 57:69–82, 1978.
182. Rosenmann E, Pollak VE, Pirani CL: Renal vein thrombosis in the adult — a clinical and pathologic study based on renal biopsies. *Medicine* 47:269–335, 1968.
183. McFarland JB: Renal venous thrombosis in children. *Q J Med* 34:269–290, 1965.
184. Arneil GC, MacDonald AM, Murphy AV, Sweet EM: Renal venous thrombosis. *Clin Nephrol* 1:119–131, 1973.
185. Wegner GP, Crummy AB, Flaherty TT, Hipona FA: Renal vein thrombosis. A roentgenographic diagnosis. *J A M A* 209:1661–1667, 1969.
186. Kirulata HG, Bruce AW, Jarzylo SV, Morrin PAF: The protean manifestations of renal vein thrombosis in the adult. *J Urol* 115:634–638, 1976.
187. Kanfer A, Kleinknecht D, Broyer M, Josso F: Coagulation

studies in 45 cases of nephrotic syndrome without uremia. *Thromb Diath Haemorrh* 24:562–571, 1970.
188. Kendall AG, Lohmann RC, Dossetor JB: Nephrotic syndrome: A hypercoagulable state. *Arch Intern Med* 127:1021–1027, 1971.
189. Thomson C, Forbes CD, Prentice CRM, Kennedy AC: Changes in blood coagulation and fibrinolysis in the nephrotic syndrome. *Q J Med* 43:399–407, 1974.
190. Hipona FA, Crummy AB: The roentgen diagnosis of renal vein thrombosis; clinical aspects. *Am J Roentgen Rad Ther Nucl Med* 93:122–131, 1966.
191. Mulhern CB, Arger PH, Miller WT, Chait A: The specificity of renal vein thrombosis. *Am J Roentgen Rad Ther Nucl Med* 125:291–299, 1975.
192. Rosenfield AT, Zeman RK, Cronan JJ, Taylor KJW: Ultrasound in experimental and clinical renal vein thrombosis. *Radiology* 137:735–741, 1980.
193. Zerhouni EA, Barth KH, Ziegelman SS: Demonstration of venous thrombosis by computer tomography. *Am J Roentgen Rad Ther Nucl Med* 134:753–758, 1980.
194. Frantantoni JD, Ness P, Simon TL: Thrombolytic therapy. Current status. *N Engl J Med* 293:1073–1076, 1975.
195. Hobbs DC, Twomey TM: Kinetics of polythiazide. *Clin Pharmacol Ther* 23:241–246, 1978.
196. Beerman B, Groschinsky-Grind M: Pharmacokinetics of hydrochlorothiazide in man. *Eur J Clin Pharmacol* 12:297–303, 1977.
197. Dargie HJ, Allison ME, Kennedy AC, Gray AJ: High dose metolazone in chronic renal failure. *Br Med J* 1:196–198, 1972.
198. Tilsone WJ, Dargie JH, Dargie EN, Morgan HG, Kennedy AC: Pharmacokinetics of metolazone in normal subjects and in patients with cardiac or renal failure. *Clin Pharmacol Ther* 16:322–329, 1974.
199. Beerman B, Dalen E, Lindstron B: Elimination of furosemide in healthy subjects and in those with renal failure. *Clin Pharmacol Ther* 22:70–78, 1977.
200. Rane A, Villeneuve JP, Stone WJ, Wilkenson JR, Branch RA: Plasma binding and disposition of furosemide in the nephrotic syndrome and in uremia. *Clin Pharmacol Ther* 24:199–207, 1978.
201. Schwartz FD, Pillay V, Kark RM: Ethacrynic acid: Its usefulness and untoward effects. *Am Heart J* 79:427–428, 1970.
202. Davies DL, Lant AF, Millard NR, Smith AJ, Ward JW, Wilson GM: Renal action, therapeutic use and pharmacokinetics of the diuretic bumetanide. *Clin Pharmacol Ther* 15:141–155, 1974.
203. Barclay JE, Lea HA: Clinical and pharmacokinetic studies of bumetanide in chronic renal failure. *Postgrad Med J* 51 (Suppl):3–46, 1975.
204. Karin A: Spironolactone: Disposition, metabolism, pharmacodynamics and bioavailability. *Drug Metab Rev* 8:151–188, 1978.
205. Knaut H, Schnippenkotter I, Wais U, Geissler H, Grebian B, Mutschler E: Diuretic activity and renal elimination of triamterene and metabolites in renal insufficiency. *Kidney Int* 13:528–529, 1978.
206. Schwartz A, Seller R, Onesti G, Kim, Swartz C, Brest AN: Pharmacodynamic effects of a new potassium-sparing diuretic, amiloride. *J Clin Pharmacol* 9:217–223, 1969.
207. Stenbock O, Myhre E, Rugstad HE, Arnold E, Hanson T: Pharmacokinetics of methyldopa in healthy man. *Eur J Clin Pharmacol* 12:117–123, 1977.
208. Myhre E, Brodwall EK, Stenbock O, Hanson T: Plasma turnover of methyldopa in advanced renal failure. *Acta Med Scand* 191:343–347, 1972.
209. Yeh BK, Dayton PG, Waters WC: Removal of alpha methyldopa (Aldomet) in man by dialysis. *Proc Soc Exp Biol Med* 135:840–843, 1970.
210. Dollery CT, David DS, Draffon GH, Dargie JH, Dean CR, Reid JL, Clare RA, Murray S: Clinical pharmacology and pharmacokinetics of clonidine. *Clin Pharmacol Ther* 19:11–17, 1976.
211. Hulter HN, Licht JH, Ienicki LP, Singh S: Clinical efficacy and pharmacokinetics of clonidine in hemodialysis and renal insufficiency. *J Lab Clin Med* 93:223–231, 1979.
212. Stitzel RE: The biological fate of reserpine. *Pharmacol Rev* 28:179–208, 1976.
213. Zoster TT, Johnson GE, DeVeber GA, Paul H: Excretion and metabolism of reserpine in renal failure. *Clin Pharmacol Ther* 14:325–330, 1973.
214. Baure JH: Effects of guanabenz therapy on renal function and body fluid composition. *Arch Intern Med* 143:1163–1167, 1983.
215. Carchman SH, Crowe JT: Steady-state plasma levels and pharmacokinetics of guanfacine in hypertensive patients with normal renal function. *Clin Pharmacol Ther* 37:186–192, 1985.
216. Wilkinson R: B-blockers and renal function. *Drugs* 23:195–206, 1982.
217. Johnsson G, Regardh CG: Clinical pharmacokinetics of B-adrenoreceptor blocking drugs. *Clin Pharmacokinet* 1:233–263, 1976.
218. Reidenberg MM, Drayer D, De Marco AL, Bello CT, Hydralazine elimination in man. *Clin Pharmacol Ther* 14:970–977, 1973.
219. Talseth T: Studies on hydralazine: Elimination and steady-state concentration in patients with impaired renal function. *Eur J Clin Pharmacol* 10:311–317, 1976.
220. Gottlieb TB, Thomas RC, Chedsey CA: Pharmacokinetic studies of minoxidil. *Clin Pharmacol Ther* 13:436–441, 1972.
221. Lowenthal DT, Mutterperl RE, Zinns G: Bioavailability, pharmacokinetics and pharmacodynamics of minoxidil in chronic renal failure (abstract). *Clin Pharmacol Ther* 21:109, 1977.
222. Rommel AJ, Pieridew AM, Heald A: Captopril elimination in chronic renal failure. *Clin Pharmacol Ther* 27:282, 1980.
223. Todd PA, Heel RC: Enalapril. A review of its pharmacodynamic and pharmacokinetic properties, and therapeutic use in hypertension and congestive heart failure. *Drugs* 31:198–248, 1986.

CHAPTER 29

Thrombotic Microangiopathy

ELLIN LIEBERMAN

BACKGROUND

The hemolytic uremic syndrome (HUS) and thrombotic thrombocytopenic purpura (TTP) are examples of thrombotic microangiopathy (1–4) characterized by endothelial damage of small- to medium-sized arteries with localization of fibrin deposits (5). In HUS, the focus of organ damage is the kidney (5–7), whereas in TTP the major sites of organ involvement are the brain, heart, spleen, pancreas, and, to a lesser extent, the kidney (7–9). However, overlap of clinical and morphologic features of HUS and TTP has created problems in distinguishing these two vasculopathies (1, 6, 7, 9–11). Accordingly, the view has emerged that HUS and TTP basically reflect a microangiopathic process and are considered by some under the combined term *HUS/TTP* (10).

Classic and prototypic descriptions of HUS and TTP provide different clinical profiles for these disorders, depending on the severity and spectrum of target organ damage, but they share many clinical, laboratory, and morphologic features (1, 5–11). Recognition of the similarities and differences between HUS and TTP is essential so that phenomena that influence management and outcome can be considered (1, 5, 9, 10, 12–16).

HEMOLYTIC UREMIC SYNDROME

Epidemiology

HUS has been recognized since Gasser's description in 1955 (1); it has been described throughout the world and is endemic in temperate zones (6, 17–19). HUS occurs both in sporadic (20) and epidemic forms (21); sporadic or atypical cases tend to have an unfavorable prognosis (22).

HUS has occurred after exposure to a wide variety of viruses (24, 25), a rickettsia-like organism (25), and bacteria (21, 26–28). Recent reports have emphasized the significance of *Eschericha coli* organisms that produce vero-cell cytotoxin (verotoxin) and are known as VTEC (verotoxin-producing *E. coli*) (27, 28). Impressive evidence has accumulated that worldwide epidemics of HUS have been associated with 0157:H7 VTEC (28) and toxin-producing shigella (26, 28), which have direct cytotoxic effects on endothelial cells (28). Other bacteria associated with HUS are neuraminidase-producing organisms (29). However, one outbreak in Canada failed to identify any infectious agent or exogenous toxin (30). Several instances of compromised hosts developing HUS have also been recorded (31). It thus appears that many agents may trigger HUS in the epidemic form; it remains unclear what initiates the syndrome in individuals without antecedent infections and in those with familial forms of the disease.

Pathogenesis

The endothelium has emerged as the target organ that plays an essential role in the pathogenesis of HUS. Prototypical HUS is a disorder in a susceptible host triggered by an infection and mediated by altered endothelial-platelet-plasma interactions. Classic or epidemic forms of HUS are initiated by infections, most often enteric pathogens that produce endotoxins that are directly injurious to the gastrointestinal tract (32) and also to the renal vasculature (32), thus providing a focus for platelet adhesion, release of platelet alpha and dense granule contents (33, 34), aggregation (35), and the generation of thromboxane A_2 from platelets (36). Markers for endothelial damage include high molecular weight von Willebrand (vWF) multimers and altered prostacyclin (PGI_2) production. The roles of vWF multimers and diminished PGI_2 are either controversial or unsubstantiated (10, 12). A perpetuating cycle with further adhesion, clumping, and secretion of platelet contents ensues until platelet exhaustion occurs (37).

Concurrently, as a consequence of platelet activation, the hemostatic protein cascade also becomes activated, ultimately leading to local fibrin deposition. Fibrin deposition obstructs arterial lumina and when red cells traverse obstructing fibrin bands, microangiopathic hemolytic anemia (MAHA) occurs (38, 39). Defective fibrinolysis has also been implicated because the kidney ordinarily can lyse fibrin clots; however, in HUS renal biopsy specimens characteristically reveal widespread fibrin deposition (10). Bergstein et al. (40) studied normal renal tissue exposed to normal sera and to sera from HUS patients; they found that fibrinolysis was inhibited by HUS sera.

Support for the view that HUS may either directly or indirectly result from an immunologic insult is drawn from disparate lines of evidence. Some patients with TTP have an IgG antibody that binds to endothelium and induces platelet aggregation (41, 42). Similar studies are not available from children with prototypical HUS. Furuse et al. (43) reported high concentrations of circulating immune complexes early in the course of HUS. Kaplan et al. (44) reported reduced IgG and increased IgM and IgA. Studies of the complement system have revealed that early components of the classic pathway are reduced in some patients with epidemic HUS (45) and in some families with autosomal recessive HUS (46). The C5-C9 membrane attack complex remains intact. In addition, alternative complement pathway activation has been proposed because of the presence of C3Nef (47), and of the presence of factor B or its breakdown products (48). Some renal biopsy specimens have also revealed the deposition of IgM and C3 in glomeruli (5, 49) and of C3 and IgM in renal arteries (10). The final and perhaps the most persuasive evidence that HUS results from immunologic mechanisms is the similarity between its pathology and that of renal allografts that have undergone hyperacute rejection (10, 50).

Pathology

The original description of renal findings found at autopsy was by Gasser (1), who reported renal cortical necrosis. Subsequently the histologic findings have been detailed; Habib (5) has defined the classic lesion as thrombotic microangiopathy. Three patterns have emerged: cortical necrosis, thrombotic microangiopathy with primarily glomerular involvement, and thrombotic microangiopathy with primarily arterial involvement (10). Patients with predominantly arterial lesions tend to have atypical HUS, are older, and have a less favorable outcome (10, 22). Affected arterioles and arteries demonstrate intimal edema, intimal proliferation, thrombosis, and necrosis. Immunofluorescent microscopy demonstrates fibrinogen along capillary walls and in vessel lumina. Occasionally granular deposits of C3 and IgM are found long the walls of glomerular capillaries (5) or in arterial walls (49).

Clinical features of hemolytic uremic syndrome

HUS has been described in all age groups (5, 10, 15), with a preponderance in the young (5, 28, 31), although a high fatality rate in the eldest and most frail have recently been described (51). HUS is endemic in many parts of the world (5, 19, 31, 52), with epidemics occurring worldwide (28); other forms of HUS include sporadic or atypical cases (20), recurrent cases (10, 53-55), and familial cases (46, 56).

Familial occurrence of HUS was highlighted by Kaplan et al. in 1975 (56); family members who became ill at less than 20 days after the index case (group I) had a good prognosis (i.e., 10 of 53 died); those who became ill after 1 year or longer had a less favorable outcome (i.e., 19 of 28 died). Most likely the former group represents familial spread of the disease, whereas the latter had inherited forms of HUS. Subsequently, patients with HUS and with TTP were described in families, consistent with an autosomal recessive pattern of inheritance (57-59). Finally, descriptions consistent with an HUS autosomal dominant pattern of inheritance have been published (60). No marker for either the autosomal recessive or autosomal dominant form of these disorders has as yet been identified (10, 28), and both forms have a poor prognosis, regardless of treatment.

The classical epidemic form of HUS affects young children and is well described (5, 20, 31, 44). The severity of symptoms and signs reflects the extent of the renal microvascular process. The renal and hematologic manifestations result from the severity of the endothelial injury. There may be variable involvement of other organ systems, such as the gastrointestinal tract, the liver, the pancreas, the central nervous system, and the heart (10, 11, 31, 61).

Laboratory studies

HEMATOLOGIC

The essential laboratory finding is the demonstration of microangiopathic hemolytic anemia (MAHA). Other routine hematologic abnormalities include thrombocytopenia in about 75% of cases, leukocytosis with a left shift, and reticulocytosis of 2% to 25%. Walters et al. (62) emphasized that classic HUS is more often associated with an elevated white cell count in contrast to normal or low white counts in those with atypical (sporadic) forms of HUS. In patients who are urinating, hematuria and mild proteinuria are common. In a minority with rapid and severe hemolysis, hemoglobinuria may be detected. The combination of MAHA and acute renal failure developing in a child with prodromal gastroenteritis (in the majority) or with an upper respiratory infection (in the minority) suggests the likelihood of HUS.

Additional hematologic findings include: an increase in platelet size, shortened platelet half-life, and, depending on the status of intravascular coagulation, either normal, increased, or decreased levels of fibrinogen, factor V, and factor VIII (63-65). Fibrin degradation products (FDP) are often increased and the protamine paracoagulation test (ppp) for circulating fibrin monomers may be positive.

The unfavorable prognostic factors listed in Table 1 are summarized from worldwide literature. Because the severity of HUS differs throughout the world and tends to be mildest in temperate zones, these factors must be interpreted in the context of epidemiologic variations attributable to geography. At Childrens Hospital of Los Angeles (CHLA), the major factors related to prognosis are anuria of 72 hours or longer, hypertension at the time of presentation, and familial or recurrent disease. These findings have been associated with residual renal impairment regardless of age, delay in determining diagnosis, or initiation of treatment. Children older than 2

Table 1. Hemolytic uremic syndrome: Unfavorable prognostic factors

Age
Older children, adults, pregnancy-related, elderly

History
Upper respiratory infection; no antecedent infection
Familial involvement (1 year or more apart)
Recurrent with acute renal failure
Greater than 72 hours of anuria at presentation

Physical findings and course
Hypertension
Severe CNS changes
Need for 5 or more blood transfusions
Prolonged anuria

Table 2. Hemolytic uremic syndrome: (Hospital for Sick Children, London, 1980–85[a]): Comparison of epidemic and sporadic cases (n = 69)

Characteristic	Epidemic (typical)	Sporadic (atypical)
Number	60 (87%)	9 (13%)
Age-mean (range) yr.	2.5 (0.4–13.7)	6.0 (0.1–13.5)
Summer presentation	47 (78%)	1 (11%)
Prodrome	Diarrhea	Respiratory/nil
Acute dialysis	51 (85%)	7 (78%)
Death	2 (3%)	2 (22%)
Renal sequelae	5 (9%)	5 (71%)[b]
Relapse	0	7 (78%)
Pathology	Glomerular	Arteriolar

[a] Modified from Barratt et al., 1987.
[b] Percent of survivors.

years of age tended to be sicker. Poor prognosis has been associated at other centers with major central nervous system findings, especially seizures (28). Features comparing typical with atypical HUS are presented in Table 2 to emphasize the poor prognostic features associated with the latter.

Treatment of hemolytic uremic syndrome

Sophistication in the management of fluid and electrolyte abnormalities coupled with dialysis has accounted for the marked improvement in the mortality rates in children. Since the initial report of Gasser (1), acute mortality in pediatric centers has been recorded as low as 4.5% (44). At CHLA in more than 100 patients since 1972 (66), two children died during the acute phase: one was a child with multiple anomalies for whom the family wished supportive therapy discontinued, and the second was a child who had not received heparin nor antiplatelet agents and died with an intracranial bleed. An additional two children who had required chronic dialysis have died: the first as a result of uncontrolled hypertension and the second from a failed renal allograft. The second patient was the offspring of a mother who had died following HUS several years earlier.

Data concerning the outcome in children were reviewed from 1964 through 1980 by Gomperts and Lieberman (68) and by Miller (62) to determine whether or not specific forms of therapy might further lower acute morbidity and mortality, or alter the incidence of residual renal disease. Prior to 1965 acute mortality was as high as 50%, whereas it was reduced to as low as 5% in some areas of the world between 1964 and 1980. Therapeutic strategies that have been employed without significant short or long-term benefits in children include corticosteroids (61), heparin (68), streptokinase (69), antiplatelet agents (70, 71), and prostacyclin (10, 72).

Since 1980 plasma infusion or plasma exchange (PE) with fresh-frozen plasma as substitution has been advocated as helpful in the treatment of children and adults with HUS. The lines of evidence supporting the use of PE include: removal of toxins, removal of antigen and/or antibody directly injurious to vascular endothelium, removal of injured red blood cells, removal of inhibitors of PGI_2 production or of fibrinolysis, and finally removal of factor(s) that might enhance abnormal platelet aggregation. Coupling PE with plasma infusion (PI) might be advantageous by providing missing factors to support PGI_2 production, by providing missing PGI_2, by providing factor(s) needed for fibrinolysis, or by providing factors to enhance platelet aggregation.

Published literature concerning PE and PI in pediatrics is sparse. Of 17 children with a single episode of HUS, PI alone was used in 10; PE, PI and antiplatelet therapy in 5, PE in 1, and PE and PI in 1 (73–78). Of these 17, 13 survived without apparent residua, 4 with residua, and none died. The follow-up was less than 2 years; whether or not chronic renal failure or end-stage renal disease will be prevented remains unclear.

Rizzoni and colleagues (79) conducted a controlled trial of plasma infusion in 32 anuric children with HUS. All 32 were observed within 8 days of illness, required dialysis, had not been previously transfused in excess of 25 ml/kg, and had not received anticoagulants nor antiplatelet therapy. The study group initially received plasma (30 ml/kg) and then 10 ml/kg until the platelet count exceeded 150,000. The average number of infusion days was 9.7. The control group received supportive therapy and packed red blood cells. When possible a surgical renal biopsy was obtained within 35 days of illness. Of the 17 study patients, 11 were less than 3 years old and 6 were older. No significant differences between the two groups were found after 24 months of follow-up. Renal biopsies were comparable in the two groups, except that none of the study group had evidence of vascular injury. In contrast, a French study of 79 children with HUS suggested that 39 treated with PI fared better than the controls (80). The results in the acute phase were comparable. Subsequently, the plasma creatinine was slightly higher in the untreated group at 6 months. Of 54 kidney biopsies (27 from each group), none of the treated group had renal cortical necrosis, whereas 7 of the control group did. The explanation for the differences between the Italian study (80) and the French study (81) is not clear.

Treatment of *recurrent* HUS in children by PE, PI, with or without antiplatelet agents has been described in very few children (53–56) and adults (81). Clearly individuals of all ages with recurrent HUS undergo a different course than those with single episodes. Their prognosis is unfavorable. Women who develop recurrent HUS in association with pregnancy are at even higher risk (15). More information concerning the mechanisms involved in recurrent HUS is needed before recommendations regarding plasma exchange and plasma infusion can be based on scientific criteria. Meanwhile, empirically, because this form of HUS has such a poor prognosis, PE and PI are being performed as a life-saving maneuver.

Weiner (15) reviewed the salient features of HUS and TTP during and after pregnancy. Treatment of both syndromes yielded dismal results until the introduction of plasma therapy, i.e., plasma infusion with or without plasmapheresis. However, the favorable impact of such intervention was much more impressive for TTP than post partum HUS (PHUS). His review of 40 publications with PHUS included 62 cases, of whom 58 were diagnosed post partum. The overall maternal mortality rate was 55%. Treatment with plasma therapy benefitted three survivors, as compared with 34 of 59 who died without plasma. Weiner recommends plasma therapy and dialysis for pregnant patients with TTP or HUS. Moreover, his additional recommendations include glucocorticoids, antiplatelet agents, and splenectomy for both conditions. These additional approaches may be appropriate for critically ill patients with TTP who have not responded to plasma exchange and infusion, but they have not benefitted children nor adults with HUS.

Sheth and colleagues (82) presented data on three children with HUS who received high-dose immunoglobulin (400 mg/kg/day infused over 6 hours × 5 days). Following infusion, platelet agglutinating factor (PAF) disappeared. Platelet counts rose consistently to normal levels with infusion and all three children achieved normal renal function within 1 to 4 weeks. Because HUS in children often resolves without intervention, these data are difficult to interpret. A controlled trial incorporating sufficient numbers of patients and observations is needed before determining the value of high-dose intravenous gamma globulin therapy for HUS.

Transplantation

The issue of renal transplantation and HUS is complicated by several factors. Acute transplant rejection may be accompanied by microangiopathic hemolytic anemia (MAHA), renal dysfunction, and renal biopsy changes that are indistinguishable from those found in patients with HUS (83). Folman et al. (84) summarized the reports of nine adult transplant recipients whose primary diagnosis was not HUS, who had not received cyclosporine (CsA), and who developed clinical features of HUS. MAHA developed in 8 of 9 between 7 days and 20 months; one was septic and died with septic shock. The remainder had histologic evidence of vascular rejection.

Van Buren et al. (85) in 1985 described de novo HUS in three adults who received CsA for immunosuppression. One of three grafts was lost to chronic rejection and 1 of 3 patients received intravenous CsA and had high CsA blood levels. The renal tissue from all three showed vascular glomerulopathy consistent with a microangiopathic process.

Schlanger et al. (86) described 100 patients with graft dysfunction among 200 graft recipients; 9 of the 100 with graft dysfunction developed HUS while receiving CsA. Among the nine, six lost their grafts and three retained their grafts with resolution of HUS after withdrawal of CsA. None had evidence of rejection on renal biopsy.

A survey of the literature (5, 10, 85, 87–92) concerning HUS and transplantation is presented in Table 3. Of 26 patients, 40 grafts were performed; 22 were LRD, 13 were cadaveric grafts, and details of 5 from Habib (5) were not available. In the report of Hebert et al. (92), patients no. 5 and no. 9 had recurrent HUS prior to transplantation. Of the 26 patients, azathioprine (Aza) was used for immunosuppression for 32 grafts, CsA for 3 grafts, and details were not included for 5 (5), although CsA was not in wide use for pediatrics in 1982. Of the total group of 26, using both clinical and morphologic criteria. HUS recurred in 16 grafts among 11 patients. In the Minnesota series (92), patient no. 5 with recurrent HUS had nonrecurrence with Aza and recurrence with CsA, whereas patient no. 9 had no recurrence with Aza immunosuppression.

The vasculotoxic effects of cyclosporine have led to the caveat that CsA should not be used in patients with HUS. The possibility that familial and recurrent forms of HUS represent a high risk for posttransplant recurrence has not been emphasized. Unpublished data from Gianantonio (28) and Lieberman (93) have indicated that CsA may be used in epidemic HUS without exacerbating underlying HUS. In summary, regardless of which immunosuppressive regimen is used, HUS patients, especially those with recurrent or familial forms, are at high risk for recurrence, and all strategies that improve graft outcome should be employed.

THROMBOTIC THROMBOCYTOPENIC PURPURA

Thrombotic thrombocytopenic purpura (TTP) is a syndrome characterized by microangiopathic hemolytic anemia (MAHA), thrombocytopenia, fluctuating neurologic abnormalities, fever, and renal dysfunction, which varies from mild to severe (9). Amorosi and Ultmann's review documented the high mortality associated with TTP (8); since then remarkable progress in treatment has resulted in a dramatic reduction in mortality (14). Recent reviews (10, 14) have focused on the overlapping features of HUS and TTP, on new developments related to pathogenesis (94), and on the results of treatment (14).

Unlike primary or classic HUS, patients with TTP may present without an antecedent infection, although preceding infections have been implicated. Kwaan (95) summarized the secondary causes of TTP: pregnancy and puerperium, cancer, tissue transplantation, connective tissue disorders, immune complex disease, drugs, and

Table 3. HUS and renal transplantation

Author year (Ref.)	Pt. no.	Age (yr)	Sex	Graft no.	LRD/CAD	Imm. Rx	HUS appear. (clinical)	Biopsy proven	Course	Outcome
Gerilli 1972	1	5/12	F	1	CAD	Aza, ALG	0	None	No recurrence	Good function
(88)	2	8	F	1	LRD	Aza, ALG	0	None	No recurrence	Graft lost
				2	LRD	Aza, ALG	12 hrs	None	HUS resolved	Good function
Folman	1	2	M	1	CAD	Aza	0	0	No recurrence	Graft lost
1977 (84)				2	CAD	Aza	$4\frac{1}{2}$ mos	+	Recurrence	Graft lost
				3*	CAD	Aza	10 wks	+	Recurrence	Graft lost
				4*	CAD	Aza	2–3 wks	+	Recurrence	Patient died
Leithner	1	32	M	1	CAD	Aza	0	0	No recurrence	Graft lost
1982 (87)				2	CAD	CsA	14–21 days	+	Recurrence	Graft lost
Hamilton 1982 (89)	1	12	F	1	CAD	CsA	0	0	No recurrence	Graft dysfunction
Habib 1982	1			1			0	0	No recurrence	Graft dysfunction
(5)	2			1			0	0	No recurrence	Graft lost
	3			1			0	+	No recurrence	Graft lost
	4			1			0	+	No recurrence	Graft lost
				2			0	0	No recurrence	Good function
Stevenson 1982 (90)	1	22	M	1	CAD	Aza	12 days	+	Recurrence	Good function
CPC N Eng J Med Strom 1986 (91)	1	$8\frac{1}{2}$	F	1	LRD	Aza	13 mos.	+	Recurrence	Graft lost
		GROUP I								
Hebert 1986 (92)	1	2 7/12	F	1	LRD	Aza, ALG	13 mos.	+	Recurrence	Graft lost
		3 3/12		2	CAD	Aza, ALG	2 mos.		Recurrence	Graft lost
	2	52	M	1	LRD	Aza, ALG	4 days	+	Recurrence	Stable function
	3	1 11/12	F	1	LRD	Aza, ALG	None		No recurrence	Graft lost
		3 7/12		2	LRD	Aza, ALG	8 days	+	Recurrence	Cr. 1.1
	4	18 2/12	F	1	LRD	Aza, ALG	2 mos.	+	Recurrence	Graft lost
		18 8/12		2	LRD	Aza, ALG	None	None	No recurrence	Graft lost
	5	4 8/12	F	1	CAD	Aza, ALG	None	None	No recurrence	Graft lost
		5 2/12		2	CAD	Aza, ALG	None	None	No recurrence	Graft lost
		6 1/12		3	LRD	CsA	1 day	+	Recurrence	Died
	*	(12	M	1	LRD	Aza, ALG	8 days		Recurrence	Graft lost)
	*	(38	F	1	LRD	Aza, ALG	2 days		Recurrence	Graft lost)
		GROUP II								
	6	1 9/12	M	1	LRD	Aza, ALG	0	0	No recurrence	Graft lost
		2 10/12		2	LRD	Aza, ALG	0	None	No recurrence	Graft lost
		4		3	LRD	Aza, ALG	0	None	No recurrence	BP, Cr 2.0
	7	7 3/12	F	1	LRD	Aza, ALG	0	+	No recurrence	Graft lost
		8 7/12		2	LRD	Aza, ALG	0	0	No recurrence	BP, Cr. 2.3
	8	1 10/12	M	1	LRD	Aza, ALG	0	0	No recurrence	Cr 1.0
		GROUP III								
	9	3 9/12	F	1	LRD	Aza, ALG	0	0	No recurrence	Cr. 0.5
	10	5 8/12	F	1	LRD	Aza, ALG	0	0	No recurrence	Cr. 1.0
	11	31	M	1	LRD	Aza, ALG	0	0	No recurrence	Cr. 1.4
	*	(1 5/12	M	1	LRD	Aza, ALG	0		No recurrence	Good function)
Remuzzi 1987 (10)	1	41	M	1	CAD	Aza	7 wks	+	Recurrence	Cr. 8.

* Information from addendums in Folman's and Hebert's articles has been included.

toxins. The distinction of TTP from HUS often appears arbitrary because of their overlapping clinical and laboratory features. On the other hand, the management of TTP or TTP-like syndromes is significantly different from that of most cases of HUS, such that an attempt will be made in this section to provide a rationale for the therapy of TTP.

Clinical features of thrombotic thrombocytopenic purpura

Excellent reviews with accumulated case studies are recommended for further information (10, 12, 14, 15, 97). Although Moschcowitz (98) is credited with describing the disorder now kown as TTP, several years elapsed before the major clinical features were identified and the name *thrombotic thrombocytopenic purpura* was applied by Singer and his group (99), who described the triad of thrombocytopenia, hemolysis, and neurologic manifestations. Subsequently, fever and renal involvement were also recognized as features, so that the triad became a pentad (99). Ridolfi and Bell (13) noted that the triad was present in 74% and the pentad in 40% of 258 patients. Kwaan's (96) recent review summarized presenting findings from four series. The frequency of neurologic symptoms varied from 52% to 92%; of hemorrhage (especially petechiae) from 38% to 74%; fever from 14% to 87%, and of pallor from 6% to 17%. Nonspecific constitutional symptoms occur in 15% or less. Occasionally the major presenting feature is abdominal pain caused by pancreatitis (96). The duration of symptoms prior to presentation is characteristically days. Renal invovement as reflected by proteinuria and hematuria is common (100), although a recent report emphasizes that severe renal involvement may be present (9).

Typical laboratory studies reveal Coombs negative microangiopathic hemolytic anemia (MAHA), thrombocytopenia, reticulocytosis, increased blood levels of unconjugated bilirubin, increased levels of lactic dehydrogenase (LDH), hemoglobinemia, and decreased plasma haptoglobin. Thrombocytopenia is characteristically severe, although mild to moderate depression may occur at presentation with increasing thrombocytopenia developing with progression of disease. LDH is currently used in conjunction with hemoglobin levels and reticulocyte counts as clinical indicators of the severity of hemolysis (97). hemostatic studies reveal normal prothrombin time, normal partial thromboplastin time, and occasionally elevated fibrin degradation products (FDP). The protamine monosulfate test for fibrin monomers may be positive.

Pathology and pathogenesis

TTP is characterized by widespread small-vessel thromboocclusive lesions as the key pathologic abnormality. Widespread thrombi occluding capillaries and arterioles (not veins) have been found in all organs including heart, pancreas, adrenal, kidney, brain, pituitary gland, liver, and spleen (102). Histologic analysis of thrombotic vascular lesions demonstrates that the characteristic vascular lesion is a hyaline thrombus composed of fibrin and platelets (96). Immunofluorescent studies have shown that the lesions have positive reactions for fibrin, platelet antigen, and von Willebrand factor (vWF) (102).

Analysis of the pathologic lesions does not shed light on the sequence of events leading to widespread thrombus formation. The most plausible explanation, with many parallels to current thinking concerning HUS, is that there is a primary endothelial injury leading to thrombus formation in the microvasculature, followed by secondary platelet adhesion and aggregation or disseminated intravascular aggregation/agglutination as a primary event, resulting in endothelial damage (96). Table 4 summarizes the mechanisms thought to have a role in the development of TTP.

Table 4. Pathogenetic mechanisms of TTP

Vasculopathy	
Localized absence of fibrinolytic activity	Localized defect shown; decreased levels of plasminogen activator; not 1° event because fibrin formation is 2° to vessel damage
Antiendothelial antibodies	Conflicting data exist; complement activation does not occur in TTP; endothelial cell surface proteins may be defective
Vessel wall prostaglandin (PGI_2) deficiency	Conflicting data; may be epiphenomenon
Disseminated intravascular platelet aggregation	
Platelet-associated immunoglobulin	IgG or antibodies to IgG may inhibit platelet clumping
Circulating immune complexes	Role of immune complexes not defined. Complexes found in nonimmune thrombocytopenias as well.
Platelet aggregating factor	Factor, yet to be delineated, may lead to agglutination in TTP; factor could be derived from immune-mediated reaction. Results are inconsistent.
Plasma prostaglandin deficiency	PGI_2 metabolite levels variable; could be problem in decreased synthesis or increased destruction; abnormalities found in other disorders. Data inconclusive.
Large von Villebrand multimers	Role of large vWF multimers controversial
PAF-inhibitor abnormality	Possible that inhibitors of PAF activity exist in plasma; more study required.

Modified from Shepherd & Bukowski (14).

Therapeutic approach to thrombotic thrombocytopenic purpura

During the past decade, the management of TTP has resulted in a profound improvement in morbidity and mortality for the majority of patients (14). In contrast to the dismal outlook before 1960 when TTP was almost always fatal (8), the overall survival rate is currently approximately 80% (14) for those patients who are not post partum (15) nor suffering from a malignancy (103). Changes in morbidity and mortality are attributed to intervention with plasma infusion (14) and/or plasma exchange using fresh-frozen plasma (but not albumin-containing solutions as replacement) and support with dialysis if volume overload develops or if renal function deteriorates. The regimen that is most widely recommended is outlined in Figure 1. The overall improvement in clinical outcomes is not disputed; controversy exists as to why either plasma infusion or plasma exchange confers clinical benefits. The review by Shepard and Bukowski (14) examines therapy in

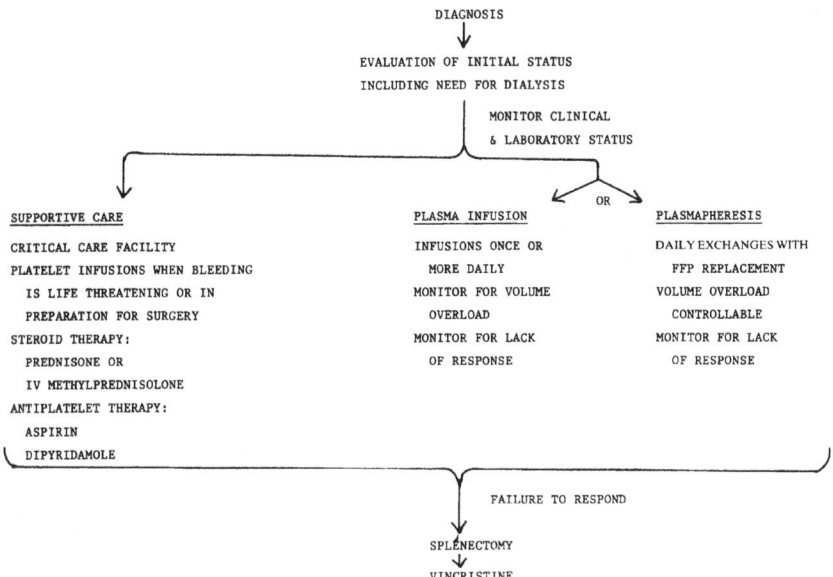

Figure 1. Integrated flow diagram for the clinical management of acute TTP.

the light of theories of pathophysiology of TTP and implications for treatment.

Prior to the widespread use of plasma therapy, whole-blood exchange transfusions were advocated. Shepard and Bukowski included 17 patients from the Cleveland Clinic Foundation along with 16 additional published cases (14). These data indicate that approximtely 50% achieved a good clinical response; however, those who failed such therapy within 48 hours required plasma infusion or exchange. No persuasive evidence exists that whole-blood exchange transfusions should be the first modality applied to patients with TTP.

The value of plasma infusions for therapy of acute TTP was highlighted in 1977 by Bukowski and colleagues (104) and Byrnes and Khurana (105). Subsequent reports corroborated the initial studies and indicated that between 60% and 70% of affected patients responded favorably (106–108). Why plasma infusion is beneficial remains moot. Aster (109) suggested that TTP may represent a heterogeneous disorder such that more than one mechanism may be causally related (109). The results of plasma infusion in 24 patients were also included in the Shepard and Bukowski review (14). In addition to their study, there are many publications describing experience with plasma infusion in adults with TTP (10). The literature is flawed, however, by the lack of controlled trials (10), by descriptions of cases or series that are not comparable, and by inclusion of multiple therapeutic interventions. Currently a Canadian collaborative trial designed to compare plasmapheresis with plasma infusion alone is underway (110).

Plasma exchange or plasmapheresis using fresh-frozen plasma (FFP) as replacement therapy has been advocated as a two-tiered approach. Removal of unknown agents plus plasma volume reduction by replacement of less than 100% of removed plasma with FFP might offer the ideal regimen.

From 1980 through 1986, plasmapheresis has been advocated as the treatment of choice; remissions have reached 70% (111). Nonetheless some patients fail to respond and in these desperately ill cases splenectomy (111) and vincristine (111) with or without antiplatelet therapy has been advocated. The potential for fatal bleeding and sepsis are well recognized; nevertheless, the use of these interventions in experienced hands may result in superior survival and remission rates.

ACKNOWLEGEMENT

We are indebted to Cari Adams for her excellent secretarial assistance.

REFERENCES

1. Gasser C, Gautier E, Steck A, Siebenmann RE, Oechslin R. Hamolytisch-Uramische Syndromes: bilaterale Nierenrindennekrosen bei akuten erworbenchenschr hamolytischen Anamien. *Schweiz Med Wochnschr* 85:905–909, 1955.
2. Symmers W. Thrombotic microangiopathic haemolytic anaemia. *Br Med J* 2:897–903, 1952.
3. Rossi EC, Carone FA, Del Greco F. Hemolytic-uremic syndrome and platelet-endothelial interactions. In: Remuzzi

G, Mecca G, De Gaetano G, eds. *Hemostasis, Prostaglandins and Renal Disease.* Raven, New York, 1980, pp 1–329.
4. Gianantonio C, Vitacco M, Mendilaharzu F, Rutty A, Mendilaharzu J. The hemolytic-uremic syndrome. *J Pediatr* 64: 478–491, 1964.
5. Habib R, Levy M, Gagnadoux M-F, Broyer M. Prognosis of the hemolytic uremic syndrome in children. *Adv Nephrol* 11:99–128, 1982.
6. Lieberman E, Heuser E, Donnell GN, Landing BH, Hammond GD. Hemolytic-uremic syndrome. Clinical and pathological considerations. *N Engl J Med* 275:227–236, 1966.
7. Brain MC, Neame PB. Thrombotic thrombocytopenic purpura and the hemolytic uremic syndrome. *Semin Thromb Hemostas* 8:186–197, 1982.
8. Amorosi EL, Ultmann JE. Thrombotic thrombocytopenic purpura: Report of 16 cases and review of the literature. *Medicine* 45:139–159, 1966.
9. Eknoyan G, Riggs SA. Renal involvement in patients with thrombotic thrombocytopenic purpura. *Am J Nephrol* 6: 117–131, 1986.
10. Remuzzi G. HUS and TTP: Variable expression of a single entity. *Kidney Int* 32:292–308, 1987.
11. Upadhyaya K, Barwick K, Fishaut M, Kashgarian M, Siegel NJ. The importance of nonrenal involvement in hemolytic-uremic syndrome. *Pediatrics* 65:115–120, 1980.
12. Remuzzi G. Thrombotic thrombocytopenic purpura and allied disorders. In: Verstraete M, Vermylen J, Lijnen HR, Arnout J, eds, *Thrombosis and Haemostasis 1987.* International Society on Thrombosis and Haemostasis, Leuven University Press, Leuven, 1987, pp 673–708.
13. Ridolfi RL, Bell WR. Thrombotic thrombocytopenic purpura. Report of 25 cases and review of the literature. *Medicine* 60:413–428, 1981.
14. Shepard KV, Bukowski RM: The treatment of thrombotic thrombocytopenic purpura with exchange transfusions, plasma infusions and plasma exchange. *Semin Hematol* 24: 178–193, 1987.
15. Weiner CP. Thrombotic microangiopathy in pregnancy and the post partum period. *Semin Hematol* 24:119–129, 1987.
16. Kaplan BS, Proesmans W. The hemolytic uremic syndrome of childhood and its variants. *Semin Hematol* 24:148–160, 1987.
17. Kaplan BS, Katz J, Krawitz S, Lurie A. An analysis of the results of therapy in 67 cases of the hemolytic-uremic syndrome. *J Pediatr* 78:420–425, 1971.
18. Tune BM, Leavitt TJ, Gribble TJ. The hemolytic-uremic syndrome in California: A review of 28 nonheparinized cases with long-term follow-up. *J Pediatr* 82:304–310, 1973.
19. Kibel M, Barnard PJ. The hemolytic-uremic syndrome. A survey in South Africa. *S Afr Med J* 42:692–698, 1966.
20. Levin M, Elkon KB, Nokes TJC, Buckle AM, Dillon MJ, Hardisty RM, Barratt TM. Inhibitor of prostacyclin production in sporadic haemolytic uraemic syndrome. *Arch Dis Childh* 58:703–708, 1983.
21. Spika JS, Parsons JE, Nordenberg D, Wells JG, Gunn RA, Blake PA: Hemolytic uremic syndrome and diarrhea associated with *Escherichia coli* 0157:H7 in a day care center. *J Pediatr* 109:287–291, 1986.
22. Barratt TM, Dillon MJ, Hardisty RM, Levin M, Nokes TJC, Smith C, Stroobant P, Walters MDS. The role of platelets and platelet-derived growth factors in the pathogenesis of haemolytic-uraemic syndrome. In: Murakami K, Kitagawa T, Yabuta K, Sakai T, eds. *Recent Advances in Pediatric Nephrology.* Excerpta Medica, Amsterdam, 1987, pp 577–580.
23. Glasgow LA, Balduzzi P. Isolation of coxsackie virus group A, type 4, from a patient with hemolytic-uremic syndrome. *N Engl J Med* 273:754–756, 1965.
24. Ray CG, Tucker VL, Harris DJ, Cuppage FE, Chin TDY. Enteroviruses associated with hemolytic-uremic syndrome. *Pediatrics* 46:378–388, 1970.
25. Mettler NE. Isolation of a microtatobiote from patients with hemolytic-uremic syndrome and thrombotic thrombocytopenic purpura and from mites in the United States. *N Engl J Med* 281:1023–1027, 1969.
26. Koster F, Levin J, Walker, Tung KSK, Gilman RH, Rahaman MM, Majid MA, Islam S, Williams RC Jr. Hemolytic-uremic syndrome after shigellosis. *N Engl J Med* 298:927–933, 1978.
27. Karmali MA, Steele BT, Petric M, Lim C. Sporadic cases of haemolytic-uraemic syndrome associated with faecal cytotoxin and cytotoxin-producing *Escherichia coli* in stools. *Lancet* 1:619–620, 1983.
28. An International Symposium and Workshop on Verocytotoxin-Producing Infections. July 12–15, 1987, Toronto, Canada.
29. Hamilton DV, Black AJ, Darnborough J, Bird GWG. Haemolytic-uraemic syndrome and T-activation of red blood cells. *Clin Lab Haematol* 5:109–112, 1983.
30. Steele BT, Arbus GS, Rance CP. An outbreak of hemolytic uremic syndrome associated with ingestion of fresh apple juice. *J Pediatr* 101:963, 1982.
31. Lieberman E. Hemolytic-uremic syndrome. *J Pediatr* 80: 1–6, 1972.
32. Bolande RP, Kaplan BS. Experimental studies on the hemolytic-uremic syndrome. *Nephron* 39:228–236, 1985.
33. Niewiarowski S, Varma KG. Biochemistry and physiology of secreted platelet proteins. In: Colman RW, Hirsch J, Marden VJ, Salzman EW, eds. *Hemostasis and Thrombosis: Basic Principles and Clinical Practice.* JB Lippincott, Philadelphia, 1982, pp 421–430.
34. George JN, Nurden AT, Phillips DR. Molecular defects in interactions of platelets with the vessel wall. *N Engl J Med* 311:1084–1098, 1984.
35. Jorgensen KA. Platelets and renal disease. *Danish Med Bull* 28:116–122, 1981.
36. Moncada S, Vane JR. Arachidonic acid metabolites and the interactions between platelets and blood-vessel walls. *N Engl J Med* 300:1142–1147, 1979.
37. Fong JSC, Kaplan BS. Impairment of platelet aggregation in hemolytic uremic syndrome: Evidence for platelet "exhaustion". *Blood* 60:564–570, 1982.
38. Brain MC, Dacie JV, Hourihane OB. Microangiopathic hemolytic anemia: The possible role of vascular lesions in pathogenesis. *Br J Haematol* 8:358–374, 1962.
39. Heptinstall RH. Hemolytic uremic syndrome, thrombotic thrombocytopenic purpura, and systemic scleroderma (progressive systemic sclerosis). In: Heptinstall RH, ed. *Pathology of the Kidney*, Little, Brown, Boston, 1983, pp 907–961.
40. Bergstein JM, Kuederli U, Bang NU. Plasma inhibitor of glomerular fibrinolysis in the hemolytic-uremic syndrome. *Am J Med* 73:322–327, 1982.
41. Burns ER, Zucker-Franklin D. Pathologic effects of plasma from patients with thrombotic thrombocytopenic purpura on platelets and cultured vascular endothelial cells. *Blood* 4:1030–1037, 1983.
42. Wall RT, Harker LA. The endothelium and thrombosis. *Ann Rev Med* 31:361–371, 1980.
43. Furuse A, Hattori S, Matsuda I. A case of hemolytic uremic syndrome with high concentration of circulating immune

complex in the initial stage. *Int J Pediatr Nephrol* 4:123–126, 1983.
44. Kaplan BS, Thomson PD, deChadarevian J-P. The hemolytic uremic syndrome. *Pediatr Clin North Am* 23:761–777, 1976.
45. Kaplan BS, Thomson PD, MacNab GM. Serum complement levels in the haemolytic uraemic syndrome. *Lancet* 2:1505–1506, 1973.
46. Carreras L, Romero R, Requescens C, Oliver AJ, Carrera M, Clavo M, Alsina J. Familial hypocomplementemic hemolytic-uremic syndrome with HLA-A3, B7 haplotype. *JAMA* 245:602–604, 1981.
47. Barre P, Kaplan BS, deChadarevian J-P, Drummond KN. Hemolytic uremic syndrome with hypocomplementemia, serum C3NeF, and glomerular deposits of C3. *Arch Pathol Lab Med* 101:357–361, 1977.
48. Kim Y, Miller K, Michael AF. Breakdown of C3 and factor B in hemolytic-uremic syndrome. *J Lab Clin Med* 89:845–850, 1977.
49. Gonzalo A, Mampaso F, Gallego N, Bellas C, Sequi J, Ortuno J. Hemolytic-uremic syndrome with hypocomplementemia and deposits of IgM and C3 in the involved renal tissue. *Clin Nephrol* 16:193–199, 1981.
50. Myburgh JA, Cohen I, Gecelter L, Meyers AM, Abrahams C, Furman KI, Goldberg B, van Blerk PJP. Hyperacute rejection in human-kidney allografts — Shwartzman or Arthus reaction? *N Engl J Med* 281:131–135, 1969.
51. Carter AO, Borczyk AA, Carlson JAK, Hockin JC, Krishnan C, Korn DA. An outbreak of *Escherichia coli* 0157:H7 associated hemorrhagic colitis in a nursing home. Presented at an International Symposium and Workshop on Verocytotoxin-Producing Infections, July 12–15, 1987, Toronto, Canada.
52. Van Wieringen PMV, Monnens LAH, Schretlen EDAM. Haemolytic-uraemic syndrome. Epidemiological and clinical study. Arch Dis Childh 49:432–437, 1974.
53. Sweny P, Winning A, Gross MLP, Moorhead JF. Plasmapheresis in the haemolytic-uraemic syndrome in children. *Br Med J* 282:2137, 1981.
54. Bergada E, Torras A, Puig L, Arrizabalaga P, Revet L. Plasmapheresis-dependent recovery from recurrent hemolytic-uremic syndrome. *Int J Artif Org* 6:79–80, 1983.
55. Feldhoff CM, Luboldt W, Bussmann K, Schror K. Plasma exchanges in frequently recurrent hemolytic-uremic syndrome in a child. *Int J Pedatr Nephrol* 4:239–242, 1983.
56. Kaplan BS, Chesney RW, Drummond KN. Hemolytic uremic syndrome in families. *N Engl J Med* 292:1090–1093, 1975.
57. Qazi GH, Schutta EJ. Haemolytic uraemic syndrome in sibs. *Arch Dis Childh* 52:337–338, 1977.
58. Edelsten AD, Tuck S. Familial haemolytic uraemic syndrome. *Arch Dis Childh* 53:255–256, 1978.
59. Kirchner KA, Smith RM, Gockerman JP, Luke RG. Hereditary thrombotic thrombocytopenic purpura: Microangiopathic hemolytic anemia, thrombocytopenia, and renal insufficiency occurring in consecutive generations. *Nephron* 30:28–30, 1982.
60. Hogewind BL, de la Riviere GB, Van Es LA, Veltkamp JJ. Familial occurrence of the haemolytic uraemic syndrome. *Acta Med Scand* 207:73–77, 1980.
61. Miller K, Kim Y. Hemolytic uremic syndrome. In: Holliday MA, Barratt TM, Vernier RL, eds. *Pediatric Nephrology*, 2nd ed. Williams & Wilkins, Baltimore, 1987, pp 482–491.
62. Walters MDS, Matthei IU, Smith C, Levin M, Dillon MJ, Barratt TM. Laboratory evidence of heterogeneity of haemolytic uraemic syndrome (abstract). Presented at an International Symposium and Workshop on Verocytotoxin-Producing Infections, July 12–15, 1987, Toronto, Canada.
63. Katz J, Lurie A, Kaplan BS, Krawitz S, Metz J. Coagulation findings in the hemolytic-uremic syndrome of infancy: Similarity to hyperacute renal allograft rejection. *J Pediatr* 78:426–434, 1971.
64. Kisker CR, Rush RA. Absence of intravascular coagulation in the hemolytic-uremic syndrome. *Am J Dis Child* 129:223–226, 1975.
65. Monnens L, Kleynen F, van Munster P, Schretlen E, Bonnerman A. Coagulation studies and streptokinase therapy in the haemolytic-uraemic syndrome. *Helv Paediatr Acta* 27:45–54, 1972.
66. Lieberman E, unpublished.
67. Gomperts Ed, Lieberman E. Hemolytic uremic syndrome and thrombotic thrombocytopenic purpura. In: Suki WN, Massry SG, eds. *Therapy of Renal Diseases and Related Disorders*. Martinus Nijhoff, Boston, 1984, pp 297–313.
68. Monnens L, van Collenburg J, de Jong M, Zoethout H, van Wieringen P. Treatment of the hemolytic-uremic syndrome. Comparison of the results of heparin treatment with the results of streptokinase treatment. *Helv Paediatr Acta* 33:321–328, 1978.
69. Bergstein JM, Edson JR, Michael AF Jr. Fibrinolytic treatment of the haemolytic-uraemic syndrome. *Lancet* 1:448–449, 1972.
70. Arenson EB Jr, August CS. Preliminary report: Treatment of the hemolytic-uremic syndrome with aspirin and dipyridamole. *J Pediatr* 86:957–961, 1975.
71. O'Regan S, Chesney RW, Mongeau J-G, Robitaille P. Aspirin and dipyridamole therapy in the hemolytic-uremic syndrome. *J Pediatr* 97:473–476, 1980.
72. Webster J, Rees AJ, Lewis PJ, Hensby CN. Prostacyclin deficiency in haemolytic-uraemic syndrome. *Br Med J* 281:271, 1980.
73. Beattie TJ, Murphy AV, Willoughby MLN. Plasmapheresis in the haemolytic-uraemic syndrome in children. *Br J Med* 282:1667–1668, 1981.
74. Denneberg T, Friedberg M, Holmberg L, Mathiasen C, Nilsson KO, Takolander R, Walder M. Combined plasmapheresis and hemodialysis treatment of severe hemolytic-uremic syndrome following campylobacter colitis. *Acta Paediatr Scand* 71:243–245, 1982.
75. Kalmin ND, Himot ED. Plasmapheresis in a child with the hemolytic-uremic syndrome. *Transfusion* 23:139–142, 1983.
76. Misiani R, Appiani AC, Edefonti A, Gotti E, Bettinelli A, Giani M, Rossi E, Remuzzi G, Mecca G. Haemolytic uraemic syndrome: Therapeutic effect of plasma infusion. *Br Med J* 285:1304–1306, 1982.
77. Thysell H, Oxelius V-A, Norlin M. Successful treatment of hemolytic uremic syndrome and thrombotic thrombocytopenic purpura with fresh frozen plasma and plasma exchange. *Acta Med Scand* 212:285–288, 1982.
78. Weyl M, Rivard GE, O'Regan S, Robitaille P. Hemolytic uremic syndrome; treatment with plasma, vitamin E and cod liver oil. *Int J Pediatr Nephrol* 4:243–245, 1983.
79. Rizzoni G, Pavanello L, Claris-Appiani A, Edefonti A, Facchin P, Franchini F, Gusmano R, Imbasciati E, Perfumo F, Remuzzi G. Treatment of children with hemolytic uraemic syndrome (HUS) with plasma: A multicenter controlled trial. *Pediatr Nephrol* 1:C14, 1987.
80. Loirat C, Sonsino E, Hinglais N, Landais P, Jais JP, Fermanian J. Treatment of hemolytic uremic syndrome (HUS) with fresh frozen plasma (FFP) — A prospective trial from the French Society of Pediatric Nephrology. *Pediatr Nephrol* 1:C52, 1987.

81. Hauglustaine D, Van Damme B, Vanrenterghem Y, Michielsen P. Recurrent hemolytic uremic syndrome during oral contraception. *Clin Nephrol* 15:148–153, 1981.
82. Sheth KJ, Gill JC, Leichter H. High dose immunoglobulin (IG) infusions in hemolytic uremic syndrome (HUS) (abstract). American Society Nephrology, December 1986, Washington D.C.
83. Hutton MM, Prentice CRM, Allison MEM, Duguid WP, Kennedy AC, Struthers NW, McNicol GP. Renal homotransplant rejection associated with microangiopathic haemolytic anaemia. *Br Med J* 3:87–88, 1970.
84. Folman R, Arbus GS, Churchill B, Gaum L, Huber J. Recurrence of the hemolytic uremic syndrome in a 3½ year-old child, 4 months after second renal transplantation. *Clin Nephrol* 10:121–127, 1978.
85. Van Buren D, Van Buren CT, Flechner SM, Maddox AM, Verani R, Kahan BD. De novo hemolytic uremic syndrome in renal transplant recipients immunosuppressed with cyclosporine. *Surgery* 98:54–62, 1985.
86. Schlanger RE, Henry ML, Sommer BG, Ferguson RM. Identification and treatment of cyclosporine-associated allograft thrombosis. *Surgery* 100:329–333, 1986.
87. Leithner C, Sinzinger H, Pohanka E, Schwartz M, Kretschmer G, Syre G. Recurrence of haemolytic uraemic syndrome triggered by cyclosporin A after renal transplantation. *Lancet* 1:1470, 1982.
88. Cerilli GJ, Nelsen C, Dorfmann L. Renal homotransplantation in infants and children with the hemolytic-uremic syndrome. *Surgery* 71:66–71, 1972.
89. Hamilton DV, Calne RY, Evans DB. Haemolytic-uraemic syndrome and cyclosporin A. *Lancet* 2:151–152, 1982.
90. Stevenson JA, Dumke A, Glassock RJ, Rajfer J, Cohen AH. Thrombotic microangiopathy: Recurrence following renal transplant and response to plasma infusion. *Am J Nephrol* 2:227–231, 1982.
91. Case 15–1986, Case Records of the Massachusetts General Hospital. *N Eng J Med* 314:1032–1040, 1986.
92. Hebert D, Sibley RK, Mauer SM. Recurrence of hemolytic uremic syndrome in renal transplant recipients. *Kidney Int* 30:S51–S58, 1986.
93. Lieberman E, personal communication.
94. Kwaan HC. Pathogenesis of thrombotic thrombocytopenic purpura. *Semin Thrombos Hemostas* 5:184–198, 1975.
95. Kwaan HC. Miscellaneous secondary thrombotic microangiopathy. *Semin Hematol* 24:141–147, 1987.
96. Kwaan HC. Role of fibrinolysis in thrombotic thrombocytopenic purpura. *Semin Hematol* 24:101–109, 1987.
97. Kwaan HC. Clinicopathologic features of thrombotic thrombocytopenic purpura. *Semin Hematol* 24:71–81, 1987.
98. Moschcowitz E. Hyaline thrombosis of the terminal arterioles and capillaries: A hitherto undescribed disease. *Proc NY Pathol Soc* 24:21–24, 1924.
99. Singer K. Thrombotic thrombocytopenic purpura. *Adv Intern Med* 6:195–234, 1954.
100. Lukes RJ, Rath CE, Steussy CN, Mailliard J. Thrombotic thrombocytopenic purpura — Clinical and pathological findings in 49 cases (abstract). *Blood* 17:366, 1961.
101. Kennedy SS, Zacharski LR, Beck JR. Thrombotic thrombocytopenic purpura: Analysis of 48 unselected cases. *Semin Thrombos Hemostas* 6:341–349, 1980.
102. Lian E C-Y. Pathogenesis of thrombotic thrombocytopenic purpura. *Semin Hematol* 24:82–100, 1987.
103. Murgo AJ. Thrombotic microangiopathy in the cancer patient including those induced by chemotherapeutic agents. *Semin hematol* 24:161–177, 1987.
104. Bukowski RM, King JW, Hewlett JS. Plasmapheresis in the treatment of thrombotic thrombocytopenic purpura. *Blood* 50:413–417, 1977.
105. Byrnes JJ, Khurana M. Treatment of thrombotic thrombocytopenic purpura with plasma. *N Engl J Med* 297:1386–1389, 1977.
106. Bryness JJ. Plasma infusion in the treatment of thrombotic thrombocytopenic purpura. *Semin Thromb Hemost* 7:9–14, 1981.
107. Bukowski RM. Thrombotic thrombocytopenic purpura: A review. *Prog Hemost Thromb* 6:287–337, 1982.
108. Machin SJ. Clinical annotation: Thrombotic thrombocytopenic purpura. *Br J Haematol* 56:191–197, 1984.
109. Aster RH. Plasma therapy for thrombotic thrombocytopenic purpura: Sometimes it works, but why? *N Engl J Med* 312:985–987, 1985.
110. Rock GA, Members of Canadian Plasma Exchange Study Group. A clinical research project to study plasma exchange and plasma infusion in treatment of thrombotic thrombocytopenic purpura. In: Tindall: Progress in Clinical and Biological Research: *Therapeutic Apheresis and Plasma Perfusion.* Alan R Liss, New York, 1982, pp 307–315.
111. Liu ET, Linker CA, Shuman MA. Management of treatment failures in thrombotic thrombocytopenic purpura. *Am J Hematol* 23:347–361, 1986.

CHAPTER 30

Renal Involvement in Dysproteinemias

DOMINIQUE GANEVAL & JEAN-PIERRE GRÜNFELD

INTRODUCTION

Within the term *dysproteinemia* are included a number of diseases characterized by B-cell proliferation with cell secretion of immunoglobulins (Ig) detected in the serum and/or urine. The two main diseases in this group are multiple myeloma and Waldenström's disease. In AL amyloidosis, the amyloid substance is derived from Ig light chains. Frequently monoclonal Ig component or light chains (also called Bence Jones proteins, BJP) are found in the serum or urine. Other chemical types of amyloid substances have been identified and have been shown to derive from (or be associated with) serum components [serum A amyloid (SAA), protein, prealbumin or $beta_2$ microglobulin; see below]. Some considerations on the management of amyloidosis have therefore been included in this chapter.

The clinical manifestations of dysproteinemias are related to three mechanisms: a) proliferation of lymphoplasmacytic cells (infiltrating kidneys and contributing to renal failure in very rare cases); b) B-cell production of mediators, such as the osteoclast activating factor (OAF), causing bone destruction and hypercalcemia, or factors inhibiting polyclonal Ig synthesis; and c) production by lymphoplasmacytic cells of Ig or light chains (LCs) with peculiar physicochemical properties. Renal involvement is mainly related to the latter mechanism, and renal toxicity of free LC has been well demonstrated. Light chains that are of low molecular weight (22,000 daltons as monomers to 44,000 as dimers) filter through glomerular capillaries and are almost totally reabsorbed and catabolized by tubular epithelial cells. Some LCs produced in excessive amounts exert direct tubular toxicity and/or precipitate into the tubular lumens, leading to Bence Jones (BJ) cast nephropathy (myeloma kidney). In AL amyloidosis, the LCs secreted are processed by macrophages, acquire a beta-pleated sheet configuration and form amyloid fibrils that deposit in many tissues, including the kidneys. In light chain deposit disease (LCDD), unstable LCs deposit in the form of a granular nonamyloid material. The type of deposition probably depends on the specific physicochemical properties of the LCs produced, but the mechanisms involved are still poorly known. In rare cases, the Ig itself contributes to renal toxicity, such as in mixed essential cryoglobulinemia or in the hyperviscosity syndrome induced by high serum levels of IgM in Waldenström's disease.

MULTIPLE MYELOMA

Renal involvement is frequent in multiple myeloma. In the largest series, comprising 869 patients, proteinuria was found in 88% of patients (half of them having Bence Jones proteinuria) and renal insufficiency was an initial finding in 55% of cases (1). In other series the initial incidence of renal failure is lower, approximately 20% (2, 3). However, renal insufficiency will develop in 30–50% of myeloma patients (4, 5). The development of renal failure is considered a poor prognosis factor. Mean survival is shorter in myeloma patients with renal failure than in those without renal failure (2).

Symptomatic measures

HYPERCALCEMIA

Hypercalcemia is found in 20–30% of patients with myeloma (2, 3, 5). It is a direct consequence of increased bone resorption due to OAF production by myeloma cells. However, the absolute level of serum calcium is also influenced by other factors, such as renal function. The development of severe hypercalcemia is facilitated by preexistent renal failure. Hypercalcemia also leads to renal loss of salt and water, and thus to prerenal azotemia.

Correction of hypercalcemia includes first rehydration by intravenous saline infusion. High-dose furosemide, combined with water and electrolyte compensation, is often recommended in the treatment of hypercalcemia when normal plasma volume has been restored. This measure is less effective when GFR is decreased, since the filtered load of calcium is reduced. In case of end-stage renal failure, hemodialysis can lower the serum calcium level, but its effect is of short duration. Two drugs, prednisone and mithramycin, can be used, even when renal function is impaired. Prednisone at high doses (approximately 1 mg/kg/day) is usually sufficient to correct or strongly reduce hypercalcemia. If prednisone is ineffective or insufficient, IV mithramycin may be indicated (20 µg/kg in 500 ml 5% dextrose, with a 25% decrease of the dose when GFR is below 20 ml/min). It acts within 24–48 hours, with an effect that usually lasts for several days. In some cases, a second injection of mithramycin may be necessary. Inorganic phosphate, which may be helpful in patients with normal renal function, must not be given when renal insufficiency is present. Bisphosphonates, which inhibit bone resorption by osteoclasts (6, 7), have been used with success in tumor-induced hypercalcemia and in a few cases of hypercalcemia occurring in myeloma. Aminohydroxypropylidene diphosphonate (or ADP) is administered IV at a dose of 15 mg per day, dissolved in 250–500 ml isotonic saline solution, over 2 hours; the infusions are repeated daily until normalization of the serum calcium concentration is achieved, but not for more than 10 days (7). Salmon calcitonin (400 IU subcutaneously, every 8 hours) may also be effective.

HYPERURICEMIA

Hyperuricemia can develop, although rarely, after chemotherapy or spontaneously. When the serum uric acid level is very high (> 650µM/l or 10 mg/dl), IV urate-oxydase (1000 U per day or every 12 hours) is rapidly effective through its uricolytic effect. However, hyperuricemia should be prevented by administration of allopurinol, if necessary, and its consequences should be suppressed by adequate hydration and alkalinization.

Chemotherapy

Cytotoxic agents associated with prednisone, or more complex chemotherapy in patients with a high tumor mass (8; Table 1) or resistant to conventional treatment (Table 2), have been shown to be effective and to increase the median survival to approximately 2–4 years. Examples of chemotherapy are indicated in Table 2. The list is not exhaustive. Other protocols are available. Prophylactic antacid treatment and antibiotics may be associated. Leukocyte and platelet counts should be determined at midcourse and just before each course. The response to chemotherapy is evaluated after three courses. It is defined as a 50% decrease in the serum M component or in the BJ proteinuria in BJ myelomas.

The duration of chemotherapy is still controversial. In responders, chemotherapy is prolonged over at least 24 months. No definite information is available in myeloma patients with renal failure. In these patients, we usually do not interrupt chemotherapy if tolerance is satisfactory.

The favorable effect of chemotherapy on myeloma nephropathy has not been adequately emphasized. In our experience, 85% of the patients presenting with renal failure that persisted after symptomatic management had improved or stabilized renal function during the first month after chemotherapy, and the beneficial effect on renal function was maintained in almost all patients as long as the response to chemotherapy persisted.

Chemotherapy protocols are rather similar in renal patients and in myeloma patients without renal involvement. However, the degree of renal failure should be taken into acount in the use of some drugs (Table 3).

The alkylating agent most used when there is renal failure is cyclophosphamide. In the patient with normal renal function, cyclophosphamide exerts little nephrotoxicity. Hemorrhagic cystitis is rare; it occurs only with doses above 50 mg/kg, is more frequent with ifosfamide, and is linked to a metabolite, acroleine. Hyperhydration avoids accumulation of acroleine in the bladder and the risk of hemorrhagic cystitis. Concomitant use of 2-mercaptoethane-sodium sulfonate (mesna), which binds to acroleine, also decreases this risk. Although there is a certain degree of retention of active metabolites of cyclophosphamide in renal failure patients (9), this drug can be used in these patients without decreasing the dose.

Melphalan is the most widely used drug for treating myeloma without renal involvement. Melphalan is not nephrotoxic (10). Its use in renal failure patients was limited for a long time, however, because myelotoxicity appeared to be increased in these patients (11), although the body distribution and renal excretion of melphalan in patients with renal failure had never been well studied. Recently kinetic studies of melphalan in the renal failure patient confirmed earlier observations, showing a progressive increase in the half-life of the drug that parallels the decrease in creatinine clearance (G. Fredj, unpublished results). This should suggest a progressive decrease of the dose of melphalan as renal failure increases, for example, by 25% when GFR is < 60 ml/min and by 50% when it is < 20 ml/min. If severe leukopenia or thrombopenia are not observed after the initial dose, subsequent doses can be increased progressively. Since absorption of melphalan varies from patients to patient, determination of the serum melphalan concentration should be of value in individual patients.

Table 1. Staging system for multiple myeloma patients

Criteria \ Stage	I Pts with all of the following	II	III Pts with one or more of the following
Hemoglobin	> 10 g/100 ml		< 8.5 g/100 ml
Serum calcium	Normal	Neither I	> 3 mM/l
X-ray	Normal	nor III	Advanced lytic bone lesions
M component			
IgG	< 50 g/l		> 70 g/l
IgA	< 30 g/l		> 50 g/l
BJ proteinuria	< 4 g/day		> 12 g/day
Subclassification	A: serum creatinine value < 177 µM/l B: serum creatinine value ≥ 177 µM/l		

From Durie and Salmon (8).

Table 2. Examples of chemotherapy protocols for multiple myeloma[1]

Drugs	Dose (per day)	Route of administration	Duration (in days)	Interval between courses (in weeks)
First-line chemotherapy				
Melphalan	8 mg/m^2	PO	1–4	4
or cyclophosphamide	800 mg/m^{2}[2]	IV	1	
	or			3 or 4
	200 mg/m^2	PO	1–4	
+ prednisone	40 mg/m^2	PO	1–4	3 or 4
Combinations of chemotherapy[3]				
VMCP				
Vincristine	1 mg/m^2	IV	1	
Melphalan	5–6 mg/m^2	PO	1–4	4
Cyclophosphamide	100–125 mg/m^2	PO	1–4	
Prednisone	40 mg/m^2	PO	1–4	
VMBCP				
Vincristine	1 mg	IV	1	
BCNU	20 mg/m^2	IV	1	
Melphalan	6 mg/m^2	PO	2–6	5
Cyclophosphamide	400 mg/m^2	IV	1	
Prednisone	40 mg/m^2	PO	1–6	
Therapy for resistant disease				
VBAP				
Vincristine	2 mg	IV	1	
BCNU	30 mg/m^2	IV	1	3 or 4
Adriamycin	30 mg/m^2	IV	1–4	
Prednisone	40 mg/m^2	PO	1–4	
VAD[4]				
Vincristine	0.4 mg	Continuous IV infusion	1–4	
Adriamycin	9 mg/m^2	Continuous IV infusion	1–4	4
Dexamethasone	40 mg	IV or PO	1–4 9–12 17–20	

[1] The doses are indicated for patients with normal GFR. When GFR is reduced, the doses of some drugs should be decreased (see Table 3).
[2] In case of gastric intolerance, IV infusion of cyclophosphamide may be administered in two half-doses on day 1 and day 2.
[3] Combination chemotherapy is usually indicated for patients with a high tumor mass and for patients with no initial response to alkylating agents.
[4] Dosage for VAD protocol must be reduced by 50% for the first course in patients who already received other chemotherapy and then increased, if possible, for the next course.

Prednisone doses should not be modified in the case of renal failure. Attention should be focused on prevention and follow-up of infectious complications because of the decreased immunologic defenses due both to renal failure and to chemotherapy.

Many other cytotoxic drugs can be used in treatment of myeloma. Among the most frequently used are adriamycin® (doxorubicin) and BCNU® (carmustine). Adriamycin is nephrotoxic in some animals, provoking the nephrotic syndrome with minimal glomerular changes after a single injection, but nephrotoxicity in humans appears to be infrequent, and it is not known whether it is dose dependent, as is myocardial toxicity. Because of its cardiotoxicity, it is recommended not to exceed a cumulative dose of 500 mg/m^2. In renal failure patients, the dose of Adriamycin is not reduced, except in the case of a severe decrease in glomerular filtration (creatinine clearance < 10 ml/min), in which administering 75% of the normal dose has been recommended (12). The dosage should also be decreased in patients with associated liver dysfunction. BCNU is the most often used nitrosourea agent in myeloma and is usually given in combination with another drug. Active metabolites of BCNU are largely but not exclusively eliminated by the renal route, and the doses of this drug need not be decreased in renal failure patients.

Chemotherapy does not induce a cure of myeloma, and most patients ultimately die of their disease or of a complication. Progress remains to be made for the in-vitro prediction of drug sensitivity. New therapeutic protocols must be tested, such as recombinant alpha interferon,

Table 3. Drugs currently used for treatment of myeloma patients and adjustments for renal failure

Drug	Major excretion route	Adjustement for renal failure % of theoretical dose			Remarks
		Glomerular filtration rate (ml/min)			
		>60	20–60	<20	
Cyclophosphamide (C)	Hepatic (renal: 5–20% unchanged, major route for metabolites)	Unchanged	Unchanged	Unchanged or 75%	IV C often better tolerated than oral C by pts with renal failure; removed by hemodialysis
Melphalan	Nonrenal and renal $T_{\frac{1}{2}}\uparrow$ in renal failure	Unchanged	75%	50%	Interpatient variable absorption; hypersensitivity reactions reported after IV administration; myelotoxicity enhanced in renal failure
Vincristine	Biliary (renal <12%)	Unchanged	Unchanged	Unchanged	
Doxorubicin (Adriamycin)	Hepatic (renal <15%)	Unchanged	Unchanged	Unchanged or 75%	Dosage should be decreased in patients with associated liver dysfunction. Dose-related cardiotoxicity. Dose-related nephrotoxicity?
BCNU (carmustine)	Renal (metabolites) (hepatic)	Unchanged	Unchanged	Avoid?	
Prednisone		Unchanged	Unchanged	Unchanged	

Antineoplastic drugs, and especially combination of drugs, should be carefully monitored in patients with renal failure. It may be beneficial to lower the first dosage and then increase it, if possible, for the next course. Dehydration (i.e., by vomiting) must be avoided during therapy.

monoclonal antibodies, systemic irradiation, or high-dose melphalan combined with bone marrow transplantation (5).

Renal failure

Renal failure in myeloma is essentially due to both reabsorption of excessive amounts of LCs, resulting in a toxic effect on tubular epithelial cells, and precipitation of LCs in the tubular lumens with Tamm–Horsfall protein (THP) and subsequent formation of tubular casts. The finding of THP in the glomeruli of some patients may be ascribed to tubular obstruction by casts and to reflux of tubular fluid to the glomerulus (13, 14). The resulting tubular atrophy and interstitial fibrosis cause chronic renal damage. Other mechanisms, such as amyloidosis or LCDD, are rarely involved in the pathogenesis of chronic renal failure.

Tubular casts may develop slowly and lead to progressive renal failure. On the other hand, if certain circumstances favor intratubular precipitation of LCs, cast formation is abrupt, and massive and acute renal failure (ARF) ensues. Thus there is no fundamental difference between chronic and acute renal failure in myeloma. It is more clinically relevant to distinguish reversible and irreversible renal failure.

The key role played by LCs in inducing renal failure explains why more than 50% of myeloma patients with renal failure have LC myeloma and an even higher percentage have Bence Jones proteinuria (15, 16). Unknown physicochemical properties account for renal toxicity of some LCs. It had been postulated that LCs with an isoelectric point (pI) greater than 5.6 could be more nephrotoxic, but further studies showed that the pI of LCs per se does not play a crucial role in the formation of casts (17).

The aim in treating renal insufficiency is triple: a) to stop or decrease the production of Ig and LC by plasma cells. This is the role of chemotherapy (see above); b) to avoid or decrease the renal excretion of LCs as long as they are produced by plasma cells. Removal of LCs has been attempted by peritoneal dialysis or hemodialysis using highly permeable membranes, and especially by plasma exchange; and c) to avoid intratubular precipitation of LCs.

ACUTE RENAL FAILURE (ARF)

In the presence of urinary excretion of LCs, any factor capable of provoking a decrease in the tubular fluid flow rate or pH is also capable of triggering ARF. The most frequent circumstances that may induce ARF are hypercalcemia, all other causes of dehydration, infection, and the use of potentially nephrotoxic drugs, such as nonsteroidal antiinflammatory drugs and aminoglycosides (14, 18–20). The use of radiologic contrast media is responsible for ARF, either directly or indirectly by interacting with the THP, when such substances are used without precaution in patients with unknown myeloma.

The prognosis of ARF in myeloma has long been considered as very poor (1–3) but considerable progress has

Table 4. Outcome of myeloma patients with acute deterioration of renal function (recent series)

Reference	Number of patients	Triggering factors						HD PD	PE	Reversible renal failure	
		Drugs	Sepsis*	D	HCA	Contrast media	Other			n	(%)
18	10	2	5	6			2	3		6	(60%)
23	13	3	6	4	4	1	2	4		4	(30%)
24	19				2			19	10	10	(53%)
14	34	9	5	22	13	3		15	15	16	(47%)
Necker series	31	3	5	8	7	3	4	10	9	17	(54%)

* Urinary tract infection excluded.
D = dehydration; HCA = hypercalcemia; HD = hemodialysis; PD = peritoneal dialysis; PE = plasma exchange.

been made in recent years, with a resulting increase in the percentage of partial or complete recoveries of renal function and a decrease in the percentage of deaths (15, 18, 21–25; Table 4). In our series and in the study by Rota et al., the deterioration of renal function was totally or partially reversible in about half of the patients with severe renal failure occurring in the course of myeloma.

Symptomatic measures

In addition to the treatment of hypercalcemia, hyperuricemia, and/or sepsis, the extracellular fluid volume should be rapidly restored, if necessary. Then abundant and alkaline diuresis should be induced. In nonoliguric patients, abundant fluid intake (> 2–3 l per day) is easily achieved by the oral or intravenous route. Four to 8 g of sodium bicarbonate per day are necessary to maintain the urinary pH > 7. The amounts of sodium and water should be reduced in patients with heart failure or persistent oliguria.

Removal of circulating LCs

Chemotherapy, when effective, reduces the plasma cell clone and then the secretion products. It should be started as soon as the diagnosis of myeloma is established. However, an immediate effect cannot be expected. It has therefore been attempted to decrease the pool of circulating monoclonal proteins more rapidly. Plasma exchange, also used for treatment of hyperviscosity, has been effective in removing high quantities of LCs (21, 26). Recently, in a randomized study on 19 myeloma patients with acute or rapidly progressive renal failure, the improvement in renal function and survival was better in the group treated by plasmapheresis and hemodialysis than in the group treated by peritoneal dialysis without plasma exchange (24).

Dialysis

Hemodialysis is currently recommended. Peritoneal dialysis does not appear to have a clear advantage over hemodialysis, and its infectious risk is higher. Dialysis should be pursued as long and as frequently as necessary. The recovery time may be very long, as shown in the study by Rota et al. (14), ranging from 9 to 210 days (mean, 77) in patients with completely reversible renal failure, and from 28 days to 11 months in those with partially reversible renal failure. The patients with complete recovery subsequently had a survival time (23.4 months) near that reported for myeloma patients with a similar tumor mass but without renal failure (14). In a recent Italian cooperative study, survival at 1 year was higher in the patients who regained renal function than in those in whom renal function did not improve (25).

These results indicate that rapid and active treatment of renal failure is essential when acute deterioration is suspected.

CHRONIC RENAL FAILURE

In nonterminal renal failure, the therapy includes sustained alkaline diuresis and chemotherapy. Some authors have stated that in this condition high diuresis is more important than urine alkalinization (16). Symptomatic management alone, before the beneficial effect of chemotherapy may be obtained, improves or stabilizes renal function in most cases (15, 16). The possible effect of plasma exchange in early or slowly progressive renal failure has not yet been tested.

Therapy has distinctly improved the prognosis of myeloma with chronic renal failure. In older series, the mean survival time ranged from 2 to 12 months. Our own results are illustrated in Figure 1. The median survival rate for all patients is 23 months. Two main prognostic factors emerge: the level of serum creatinine (SCr) at presentation and the response to chemotherapy. In the patients with SCr < 600 µM/l, the median survival is 37 months, whereas it is only 13 months in those with SCr ≥ 600/µM/l. The median surival is 38 months in responders versus 19 months in nonresponders, and this is independent of the SCr at presentation (Figure 1).

Renal replacement therapy has obviously played an important role in improvement of the prognosis in patients with acute deterioration of renal function (see above) and in those with end-stage renal failure (ESRF) (27, 28). Dialysis is indicated: a) when renal failure is discovered at the same time as myeloma, in order to provide the time interval required for a response to chemotherapy; b) in all cases where the response to chemotherapy is obtained and the extrarenal involvement is not too severe and

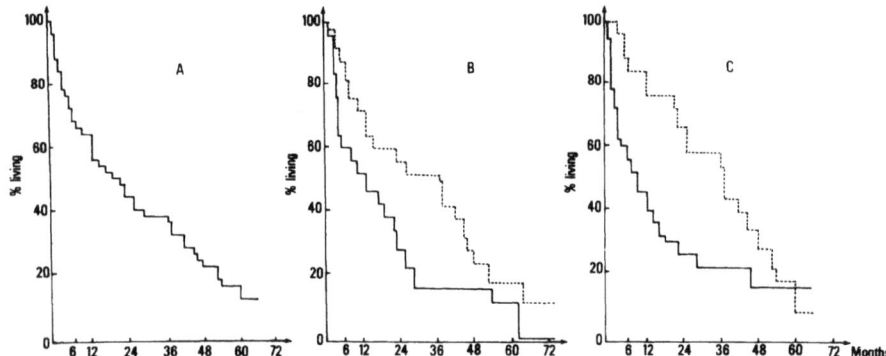

Figure 1. Prognosis in 57 patients with multiple myeloma and renal failure. On the left panel (A), survival curve for all patients; median = 23 months. On the intermediate panel (B), survival according to serum creatinine level (S_{Cr}) at presentation. .... S_{Cr} < 600 µM/l (n = 32), median = 37 months; — $S_{Cr} \geq$ 600 µM/l (n = 25), median = 13 months. On the right panel (C), influence of response to chemotherapy on survival. .... responders (n = 24, mean S_{Cr} at presentation = 707 µM/l), median = 38 months. — nonresponders (n = 31, mean S_{Cr} at presentation = 751 µM/l), median = 19 months. Response is defined as a 50% decrease in serum M component or in daily BJ proteinuria (BJ myeloma).

extensive. It should be kept in mind that renal involvement does not parallel the extent and severity of bone marrow and skeletal involvement.

In 1979, the EDTA registry recorded 143 myeloma patients treated by regular dialysis (29). Hemodialysis is the most commonly used method. It may be difficult in severely thrombopenic patients. Although survival of myeloma patients treated by regular hemodialysis improved in recent years (27, 28), it is obviously much shorter than that of the whole dialysis population, or even of those at risk, such as diabetics and elderly patients (28). The 1-year survival rate is, however, 53%, compared to 66% for patients with myeloma who do not have renal failure (28). In two reported cases, hemodialysis could be discontinued after 13 and 16 months respectively, because of amelioration of renal function (30, 31).

Kidney transplantation has been performed in myeloma patients in remission (32–35) but these cases are rare. Only three living transplant patients were included in the EDTA registry in 1979 (29).

PREVENTION OF RENAL FAILURE

Sustained alkaline diuresis should be recommended in myeloma patients. They should also be aware of potentially nephrotoxic factors, such as dehydration, sepsis, or drugs (radiologic contrast media, antibiotics, and nonsteroidal antiinflammatory drugs). A possible beneficial effect of pneumococcal vaccination has been suggested (36). Hypercalcemia or coincidental acute tubular necrosis should be promptly recognized and treated in order to avoid massive Bence Jones cast formation and passage from reversible to irreversible renal failure.

WALDENSTRÖM'S MACROGLOBULINEMIA

Waldenström's macroglobulinemia is defined as a lymphoplasma cell proliferative disorder with secretion by the malignant cells of a monoclonal IgM protein. The IgM molecule has a cryoprecipitating character in 10–20% of cases.

Extrarenal clinical manifestations included asthenia, weight loss, infections, neurologic symptoms, or symptoms linked to the lymphoid cell proliferation, i.e, hepatomegaly, splenomegaly, and lymphadenopathy. The hyperviscosity syndrome is frequent and may be responsible for bleeding, blurred vision, headache, somnolence, and coma.

In contrast to that in multiple myeloma, significant renal involvement is rare in Waldenström's macroglobulinemia (37). Proteinuria, usually moderate, is found in about 30% of patients. In some patients it is heavy with the nephrotic syndrome. Bence Jones proteinuria is found in up to 60% of cases (38), most often in small amounts. Renal insufficiency may occur, but evolution to ESRF is uncommon. In some patients dehydration may be responsible for oliguric acute episodes.

Renal involvement is characterized by glomerular subendothelial deposits or "thrombi," without cellular proliferation (39–41). The deposits contain the IgM monoclonal protein without other immunoglobulins (39) or IgM associated with other immunoglobulins and C3 (42, 43). Although Bence Jones proteinuria is frequent, BJ casts are very uncommon and when present no macrophagic cellular reaction is found (39). Other lesions observed in macroglobulinemia include amyloidosis (AL type) and light chain deposition disease (see below).

The treatment of macroglobulinemia differs little in patients with or without renal involvement. Chlorambucil, 6–8 mg, or cyclophosphamide, 100–150 mg, are given daily by the oral route. More than two thirds of patients respond to this treatment. In others a combination of several cytotoxic agents plus prednisone may be effective. Acute leukemia has developed in some treated patients, and chemotherapy is usually discontinued after 2 or 3 years if a positive response has occurred (44). The mean survival of patients with macroglobulinemia is about 6 years.

Acute oliguric episodes must be treated by rehydration if necessary and are usually reversible. The hyperviscosity syndrome necessitates urgent treatment with plasma exchanges, which may rapidly reverse the symptoms.

LIGHT CHAIN NEPHROPATHIES

M-component consisting of intact Ig or of BJ proteinuria without apparent cause (i.e., in the absence of myeloma, Waldenström's macroglobulinemia, and AL amyloidosis) has long been referred to as "benign" monoclonal gammopathy. In recent years, it has been shown that malignancy (e.g., overt myeloma) or amyloidosis can appear in these patients, sometimes after 10–20 years of followup. Thus, it was proposed to use the term *monoclonal gammopathy of undertermined significance* (MGUS) to designate such apparently isolated "idiopathic" or "benign" gammopathies (45). Some of these cases are associated with renal manifestations.

Tubular dysfunction

Acquired Fanconi syndrome (a proximal tubular disorder characterized by glycosuria, hyperaminoaciduria, increased phosphate clerance, and tubular acidosis) has been observed in patients with BJ proteinuria, mainly of the kappa type. In many of these patients, myeloma occurs later, usually after a long period of followup (up to 15 years). The Fanconi syndrome requires symptomatic management, including administration of bicarbonate or citrate to correct acidosis, and of vitamin D to prevent osteomalacia.

Distal tubular acidosis has also been observed, alone or associated with the Fanconi syndrome. Nephrogenic diabetes insipidus can be present in rare patients with either isolated BJ proteinuria or myeloma (46). Tubular dysfunction is ascribed to tubular toxicity of LCs, as has been shown in vitro (47).

Light chain deposition disease (LCDD)

LCDD has been recently identified. About 100 patients with LCDD have so far been reported, but the exact frequency of the disease is possibly underestimated. The disease is characterized by the deposition of an amorphous, nonamyloid substance in organs (48, 49). In the kidney the deposition takes place along the tubular basement membranes and in glomeruli. The diagnosis is based on the immunofluorescent demonstration of monoclonal LC (mostly kappa) tissular deposits (40, 50, 51). The precise mechanism of LC deposition is not known, but structural and chemical abnormalities of LCs (abnormal length, polymeric, and highly glycosylated), which have been demonstrated in some patients (40, 51, 52), could play a role in the pathogenesis.

Renal involvement is a constant feature of LCDD. It is the presenting symptom and the major manifestation in most if not in all patients (48, 51, 53, 54). Renal manifestations are proteinuria, either mild or heavy with the nephrotic syndrome, and renal failure, which is frequent, early, and usually rapidly progressive to ESRD (48–50, 52, 53).

Extrarenal involvement in LCDD was demonstrated by Randall et al. in 1976 (50). From the data reported in the literature and from our own experience, deposition of LCs in various organs is extremely frequent. However, deposits can be scarce or present only in the vessel walls, with no or few clinical symptoms. In contrast, in some patients the deposits are diffuse and massive, leading to severe clinical consequences. Among organs, the liver (55) and heart are the most frequently involved.

In about 80% of cases, LCDD occurs in patients with overt myeloma, occult myeloma presenting with renal disease, or rarely another lymphoproliferative disease. However in 20% of cases, no malignancy can be detected at presentation. These patients may or may not have small amounts of BJ proteinuria. In the latter cases, with no detectable malignant disease, the course is variable. In some patients, myeloma develops after a short interval. However, many remain free of malignancy for a long period of time, up to 10 years for one patient in our series with the longest followup who never received chemotherapy.

Since the disease is linked to the production of LCs by one plasma cell clone, the logical treatment of LCDD is chemotherapy, whether myeloma is present or not. Available data (48, 56, 57) show that chemotherapy (i.e., melphalan or cyclophosphamide associated with prednisone, as in myeloma), associated with symptomatic measures, has a favorable stabilizing effect on the course of renal insufficiency. In the absence of, or in delayed, chemotherapy most patients progress rapidly to ESRD. The effect of chemotherapy on extrarenal deposition of LCs is more difficult to assess given the uncertainties with regard to its natural history.

In patients with LCDD and myeloma, chemotherapy is indicated, as in classic myeloma. In contrast, in patients with LCDD but without detectable myeloma, therapy should be discussed. When renal failure is moderate, we usually recommend chemotherapy, with the hope of preventing or delaying the progression of renal involvement. In patients with ESRD, we initiate chemotherapy only when there is evidence of extrarenal manifestations, likely due to LC deposition. Since overt myeloma may appear after a long time interval, patients with LCDD should be carefully followed up.

Kidney transplantation has been performed in a few patients with LCDD. Recurrence of the disease was reported in two patients (57, 58).

RENAL INVOLVEMENT IN AMYLOIDOSIS

Chemical and clinical classification

Chemical analysis of amyloid fibrils has led to a new classification of amyloidosis, (59) as shown in Table 5. The incidence of renal involvement differs in AA and AL amyloidosis. Renal involvement is found in almost all cases of AA amyloidosis. In contrast, a renal localization

Table 5. Chemical classification of amyloid fibril proteins and their association with the various clinical types of amyloidosis

Clinical type	Chemical type	Amyloid protein
Primary (idiopathic) amyloidosis, systemic or localized	AL	Aκ, Aλ
Amyloidosis associated with myeloma	AL	Aκ, Aλ
Secondary (reactive) amyloidosis	AA	AA
Heredofamilial amyloidosis		
Autosomal recessive		
FMF	AA	AA
Autosomal dominant		
Familial amyloid polyneuropathy	AF_p	Prealbumin variant
Familial amyloid cardiomyopathy	AF_c	Prealbumin-like
Hereditary cerebral hemorrhage with amyloidosis	AF_b	γ-trace-like
Muckle–Wells syndrome	AA	AA
Senile cardiac amyloidosis	AS_c	Prealbumin-like
Alzheimer's disease		β-protein
Down syndrome (trisomy 21)		β-protein
Endocrine amyloidosis		
Medullary thyroid carcinoma	AE_t	(Pro-?)calcitonin
Dialysis-associated amyloidosis	AH	$β_2$-microglobulin-like

Adapted from Husby and Sletten (59).
p = peripheral nerves (polyneuropathy); c = cardiac; b = brain; t = thyroid.

is observed in only approximatively 30% of the cases of primary AL amyloidosis. AL amyloidosis complicates 5–15% of the cases of myeloma and its incidence is higher in BJ myeloma. Amyloidosis is demonstrated in < 5% of myelomas with renal involvement (51).

Clinical presentation and diagnosis

Renal amyloid deposition may be asymptomatic. This latent phase may last months or years. This has been documented in some patients with familial Mediterranean fever (FMF) or in autopsy specimens in Type I familial amyloid polyneuropathy. Subsequently, renal involvement results in proteinuria, the nephrotic syndrome, and renal failure, leading to ESRD. Tubular defects are rarely prominent. The blood pressure remains normal or low in most cases, but some patients become hypertensive when renal failure develops. The rate of renal progression depends on the type of amyloidosis. In primary AL amyloidosis, patient survival is short, about 1 to 2 years, or even less in patients with congestive heart failure due to amyloidosis (44), and in these patients renal involvement is not a prominent prognostic factor (44). In AA amyloidosis complicating FMF, ESRD is reached after a mean time interval of 7 years, but the rate of progression differs from one subject to another. The renal prognosis is difficult to make. Spontaneous remission of the nephrotic syndrome (60, 61) after surgery for cancer (62) or after treatment of an infectious disease leading to secondary amyloidosis (63, 64) has been reported. The presence or absence of the nephrotic syndrome is not correlated with the amount of amyloid deposition in glomeruli. Similarly the rate of progression to renal failure is not correlated with glomerular deposition and is more closely dependent on the extent of tubular atrophy and interstitial fibrosis (65–69).

The diagnosis of amyloidosis is based on the demonstration of the amyloid substance in a tissue specimen. Renal biopsy provides definite diagnosis and information on the severity of the renal changes. However, since amyloidosis is a systemic disease, biopsies of other organs may be valuable. Rectal biopsy gives positive results in 80–90% of the cases of amyloidosis with renal involvement, provided that the biopsy sample contains arterioles in the submucosal layer. Liver biopsy entails a significant risk of bleeding. It has been shown recently that aspiration and examination of subcutaneous abdominal fat could provide a simple and highly informative means of diagnosis (70, 71).

Typing of the amyloid substance necessitates chemical analysis. However, simple methods have been devised and provide useful information. The Wright technique differentiates AA amyloid (sensitive to potassium permanganate, i.e., Congo-red staining disappears after pretreatment with $KMnO_4$) and and AL amyloid (Congo-red stainng resistant to $KMnO_4$). Immunofluorescence study with anti-AA and anti-LC antibodies is also valuable. When concordant results are found with $KMnO_4$ and IF techniques, the amyloid substance can be reliably classified (72), and this may be helpful for further investigations, prognosis, and treatment.

Treatment

To evaluate the effects of therapy, it should be kept in mind that renal amyloidosis is more "resistant" than other localizations (such as liver or splenic amyloidosis); the nephrotic syndrome may undergo remission, whereas kidney amyloid deposits persist, and thus repeat biopsy is necessary to ascertain the benefit of treatment. To our knowledge, complete disappearanc of renal amyloid deposits has never been reported.

ERADICATION OF THE CAUSE IN SECONDARY AMYLOIDOSIS

Eradication of suppuration or removal of kidney carcinoma have been followed in some patients by remission of clinical manifestations and, more rarely, by the decrease of kidney deposits (74–76). In two patients, partial resolution of amyloid was accompanied by alterations of the persisting deposits and of the membranes of the glomerular capillaries (73, 74). In contrast, rapid deterioration of renal function has been reported in other patients after surgical eradication of the causative suppuration (77). The postoperative period should be carefully supervised, most particularly to prevent the development of renal vein thrombosis (see below).

Treatment of the underlying inflammatory process can halt or reverse the progression of amyloidosis. Secondary amyloidosis is a rare complication in psoriasis. A favorable response to treatment with etretinate and ultraviolet light A was recently reported in a single patient. The nephrotic syndrome disappeared, the xylose absorption test normalized, and arthritis became inactive. The authors state that "amyloid deposits were no longer detectable," but kidney biopsy was not performed (78).

Prevention of secondary amyloidosis should be attempted in high-risk patients, such as paraplegics or children with cystic fibrosis, by adequate control of recurrent infection.

COLCHICINE

Colchicine administration (1–2 mg per day) has been shown to be highly effective in reducing or suppressing attacks of FMF. Complete remission is achieved in about 75% of the patients. Children usually require the full adult colchicine dosage (61). Colchicine can be administered in pregnant patients. Pras et al. recommend amniocentesis and advise therapeutic abortion when fetal abnormality is revealed. In most cases, pregnancy results in the delivery of normal live infants (61). It has been subsequently demonstrated that colchicine therapy has a preventive effect on amyloidosis in FMF patients and that it may decrease renal amyloid deposits in such patients with renal amyloidosis (Figure 2). In contrast, colchicine does not affect the renal course when the renal function is already altered (79).

The mechanism of action of colchicine is not yet elucidated (80–82). Suppressor T-cell activity and chemotaxis are decreased in FMF patients, and these abnormalities are reversed by colchicine therapy. Colchicine has been reported to inhibit casein-induced amyloidosis in mice (experimental amyloidosis is always of the AA type) and to block the synthesis and secretion of SAA protein from hepatocytes of mice (81). By interfering with microtubule cell function, it may also alter the processing of amyloid precursors by macrophages. Because of a possible role of macrophages in the pathogenesis of AA amyloidosis and of the presumed processing of immunoglobulins by macrophages prior to tissue deposition in AL amyloidosis, it has been suggested that colchicine may also inhibit amyloid formation in AL amyloidosis (82).

From these clinical and experimental data, colchicine therapy has been attempted in types of amyloidoses other than FMF-associated amyloidosis. Based on comparison with historic control subjects, colchicine has been said to be valuable in improving the survival of patients with primary (AL) amyloidosis (82). A trial comparing melphalan-prednisone (M-P) versus colchicine has been performed in patients with primary systemic amyloidosis (see below). Surprisingly, no clinical trial is available in AA amyloidosis other than FMF-associated amyloidosis.

IMMUNOSUPRESSIVE THERAPY

Since AL amyloid substance is derived from LC fragments and AL amyloidosis is often associated with M-component or BJ proteinuria, it was logical to direct therapy against the plasma cell clone that produces LCs, although in primary amyloidosis the plasma cell clone has a lower rate of proliferation than in myeloma.

Immunosuppressive regimens have included M-P and, in some cases, D-penicillamine. Clinical remission has been observed in a few isolated cases (83–85), but complete regression of liver amyloidosis has been documented in only one patient (86). The results of two prospective randomized trials are available. In 1978, Kyle and Greipp compared M-P to placebo in 55 patients with primary amyloidosis. The survival rate did not differ significantly between the two groups. In two patients receiving Me-Pr, the nephrotic syndrome disappeared. The progression to renal failure was similar in both groups. The presence of congestive heart failure heralded a very poor prognosis (87). In 1985, Kyle et al. compared M-P (initial doses, melphalan, 0.15 mg/kg; prednisone, 0.8 mg/kg per day × 7 days, every 6 weeks) versus colchicine (0.6 mg twice a day, increased by 0.6 mg daily each week until abdominal cramp or diarrhea developed). Since this was a crossover trial, interpretation of the results is difficult. No difference in survival was found. However, additional analysis suggested that M-P was potentially superior to colchicine. On the other hand, the survival was better in patients with amyloid congestive heart failure who received M-P. Of note, serum M protein decreased or disappeared in almost one third of the patients treated with M-P. Urinary protein excretion decreased in 21 of the 39 patients with the nephrotic syndrome, and the serum creatinine level remained stable in approximately 50% of them. Finally, four patients receiving M-P developed acute nonlymphocytic leukemia, probably from the alkylating agent (88).

Satisfactory treatment for primary amyloidosis does not exist. The trials by Kyle and coworkers do not show a strong beneficial effect of M-P on renal amyloidosis. In some cases, the nephrotic syndrome may disappear or be attenuated, but the progression to renal failure does not seem to be favorably influenced. The risk/benefit ratio should be carefully weighed.

DIMETHYLSULFOXIDE (DMSO)

It has been shown that DMSO can break amyloid fibrils in vitro and in animals (89–90). In humans an amyloid-like fibrillar substance has been observed in the urine of patients with amyloid nephropathy after a single injection of DMSO (91). Because of these data, treatment with DMSO was tried in few amyloid patients, but no clear benefit of this treatment has emerged. Improvement of renal function observed in a few patients could be due to an indirect phenomenon rather than an effect on amyloid itself (92). Moreover, treatment was poorly accepted

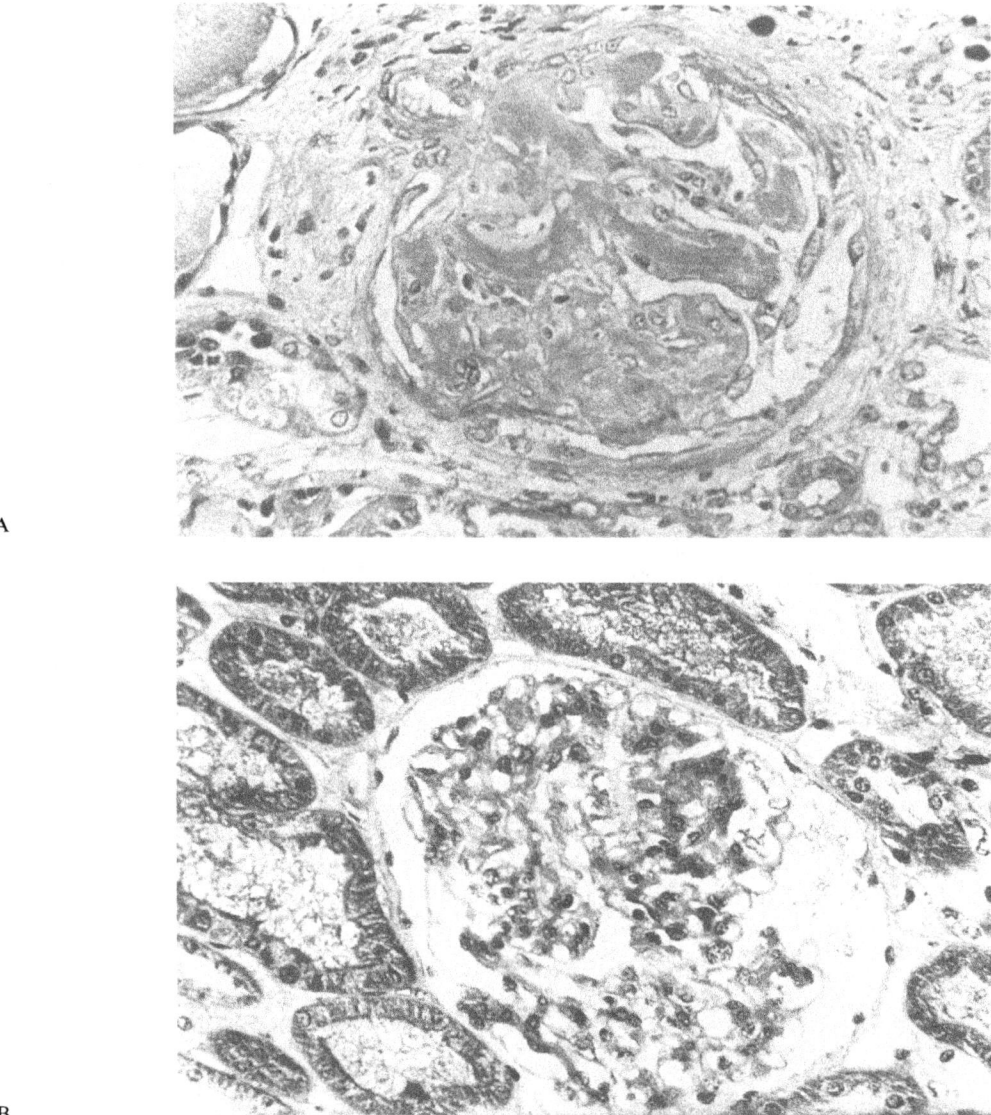

Figure 2. Repeated biopsies in a 24-year-old female with familial Mediterranean fever and renal amyloidosis. At the time of diagnosis, proteinuria was 6 g/day with the nephrotic syndrome, and renal function was normal. A percutaneous renal biopsy showed amyloid deposits in all glomeruli and in vessel walls (A). Colchicine was then given at a continuing daily oral dose of 1 mg. Proteinuria progressively decreased and totally disappeared after 4 years. A second renal biopsy, 5 years after starting colchicine (B) showed nearly normal glomeruli with only very small, hardly discernable amyloid deposits. Light microscopy, ×400. (Kindly provided by Dr. L.H. Noël.)

by patients and their families because of the unpleasant breath odor typical of DMSO ingestion (92).

SYMPTOMATIC MANAGEMENT

The nephrotic syndrome may be severe, with a marked decrease in the serum albumin concentration, hypovolemia, and extensive edema. Rapid volume depletion by potent diuretics should be avoided, especially in elderly patients. Albumin infusion should be associated with progressive administration of diuretics in these patients. In contrast with most cases of primary glomerulonephritis, severe nephrotic syndrome with nutritional consequences and the risk of thromboembolic complications may persist in patients with amyloidosis and renal failure, even in ESRD. "Medical bilateral nephrectomy" has been proposed in some of these patients by embolization of both renal arteries.

There are conflicting data on the incidence of renal vein thronbosis in amyloidosis with the nephrotic syndrome. It ranges from 2% to 51% (93). The risk of vein thrombosis (both renal and extrarenal) is inversely correlated with the level of serum albumin. In patients with severe hypoalbuminemia (< 1.8–2.0 g/dl), diuretics should be used with caution to avoid rapid plasma volume concentration, and continuous treatment by anticoagulants or antiplatelet drugs is recommended by some authors (93).

Acute renal failure has been reported in some patients with stable or slowly progressive amyloid disease, with or without preexistent renal failure, after general anesthesia and surgery (77). Reversal is rare and is usually partial.

Treatment of end-stage renal failure necessitates regular dialysis and/or kidney transplantation. In patients with heart involvement and congestive heart failure, peritoneal dialysis may be indicated. In many others, regular hemodialysis has been used. The 1979 EDTA registry records 550 patients with amyloidosis receiving replacement therapy. No information is available on the respective numbers of AA and AL amyloidosis, but the latter group was probably much smaller (29). Survival of patients with amyloidosis — except for a few series (94) — is shorter than that of the entire dialysis population (95–97). The first results of kidney transplantation in amyloidosis have been disappointing, mainly because of the high incidence of infectious complications (98–100). The most recent series provide a more optimistic view (101, 102). Severe infection can be avoided, and the incidence of rejection is surprisingly low. The recurrence of amyloidosis in the transplanted kidney has been reported in 16 cases, but without a rapid alteration of renal function (102). Prevention of recurrence in FMF patients may be provided by colchicine administration (101, 102). However, there is no evidence that colchicine prevents extension of extrarenal amyloid deposits, that are present before transplantation. Survival over 10 years may be expected in transplanted patients with AA amyloidosis (102).

Identification of cardiac amyloid involvement is of great importance. Cardiac complications (cardiac rhythm disorders and congestive heart failure) are the main causes of death in dialysis and transplanted patients with amyloidosis (102, 103). AL amyloidosis with heart involvement has a very poor prognosis. The two-dimensional echocardiogram provides the most valuable information: A combination of increased myocardial echogenicity and increased atrial thickness is highly suggestive of amyloidosis (104). Patients with cardiac involvement often have extreme sensitivity to digoxin, which has been ascribed to increased binding to amyloid fibrils (105). A similar mechanism may explain the aggravation of congestive heart failure by calcium-channel blocking agents in patients with cardiac amyloidosis (105).

Acquired factor X deficiency has been reported in amyloidosis. This disorder may lead to life-threatening bleeding. Improvement has been observed after splenectomy and, more recently, after daily administration of prednisone and intermittent administration of melphalan (106).

No information is so far available concerning the therapy of amyloidosis derived from beta$_2$-microglobulin in dialysis patients. The carpal tunnel syndrome requires surgical treatment. It has been suggested that dialysis with highly permeable and biocompatible membranes might prevent (or delay) amyloid formation (107). This hypothesis needs to be tested in prospective studies.

CRYOGLOBULINEMIAS

Classification and clinical characteristics of cryoglobulinemias (or cryoimmunoglobulinemias) are indicated in Table 6. We will focus on mixed Type II and Type III cryoglobulinemias, and most particularly on mixed IgM-IgG essential cryoglobulinemia. The latter group represents approximately 30% of mixed cryoglobulinemias (108).

Extrarenal manifestations comprise purpura, Raynaud's phenomenon, urticaria, arthralgia, fever, neuritis, and hepatosplenomegaly. Renal involvement, found in 10–60% of cases, is characterized by glomerular changes:

Table 6. Cryoglobulinemias: Classification and clinical correlations

Type	Main characteristics	Associated diseases
I. Monoclonal cryoglobulin	IgM, IgG, IgA, Bence Jones protein; no antibody activity > 500 mg/dl in most cases	Multiple myeloma, Waldenström's macroglobulinemia
II. Mixed cryoglobulin with a monoclonal component	IgM–IgG mainly (rarely IgA–IgG); monoclonal IgM has anti-IgG activity and usually rheumatoid factor activity > 500 mg/dl in 40%	Sjögren's syndrome, Waldenström's macroglobulinemia, Lymphoma *essential*
III. Mixed polyclonal cryoglobulin	IgM–IgG mainly; anti-IgG activity < 100 mg/dl in 80%	Chronic infections (Hepatitis B virus, Epstein–Barr virus), SLE–systemic vasculitis; Neoplasia *essential*

From Brouet et al. (108).

diffuse endocapillary proliferation, double-contour appearance, intraluminal "thrombi" and subendothelial deposits (both containing IgM and IgG), monocyte infiltration, and, more rarely, segmental and focal crescents, and arteriolar fibrinoid necrosis (109–110).

Renal manifestations usually consist of proteinuria and hematuria, with mild renal failure and hypertension. The acute nephritic syndrome, simulating acute glomerulonephritis, is found in approximately 25% of cases, the nephrotic syndrome in 20%, and ARF in less than 5% (110). Serum $C1_q$, C4, and CH50 levels are depressed, whatever the activity of the disease. The high incidene of HB infection has been stressed in some series; in others, EBV infection has been frequently found (110).

The renal course is less severe than was initially thought. Remissions occur in one third of patients. In another third, urinary abnormalities persist and do not progress to renal failure. Recurrent exacerbations develop in 20% of cases. Chronic renal failure is found in 10% of patients and only 3% progress to ESRD. The main causes of extrarenal death are infection, liver failure, and cardiovascular accidents (110). In a large series collected in Italy, the probability of patient survival at 10 years was 70% (111). Poor prognosis was correlated with the following features: severity and diffusion of the extrarenal manifestations, hypertension, acute exacerbations of the renal disease, nephrotic acute nephritic syndrome, and the severity of interstitial fibrosis, tubular atrophy, and exudative glomerular changes.

No prospective randomized therapeutical trial is available in mixed essential cryoglobulinemia. Aggressive therapy is indicated to control severe renal exacerbations, most particularly when extrarenal manifestations of angiitis are associated. In these cases, the treatment usually includes IV pulse methylprednisolone and plasma exchanges combined with prednisone and cyclophosphamide (at the usually recommended dosages; see 112, 113). There is no evidence that such a treatment is needed in patients with milder symptoms and in the more chronic forms. The risks of aggressive therapy should be balanced with the estimated benefits. Overzealous therapy of mild forms should be avoided.

REFERENCES

1. Kyle RA: Multiple myeloma. Review of 869 cases. *Mayo Clin Proc* 50:29–40, 1975.
2. Galton DAG, Peto R: Report on the first myelomatosis trial. Part I. Analysis of presenting features of prognostic importance. *Br J Haematol* 24:123–139, 1973.
3. Alexanian R, Balcerzak S, Bonnet JD, Gehan EA, Haut A, Hewlett JS, Monto RW: Prognostic factors in multiple myeloma. *Cancer* 36:1192–1201, 1975.
4. Fang LST: Light-chain nephropathy. *Kidney Int* 27:582–592, 1985.
5. Kyle RA: Multiple myeloma: Current therapy and a glimpse of the future. *Scand J Haematol* 35:38–47, 1985.
6. Van Breukelen FJM, Bijvoet OLM, Van Oosterom AT: Inhibition of osteolytic bone lesions by (3-amino-l-hydroxypropylidene)1, 1-bisphosphonate (APD). *Lancet* 1:803–805, 1979.
7. Harinck HIJ, Bijvoet OLM, Plantingh AST, Body JJ, Elte JWF, Sleeboom HP, Wildiers J, Neijt JP: Role of bone and kidney in tumor-induced hypercalcemia and its treatment with bisphosphonate and sodium chloride. *Am J Med* 82:1133–1142, 1987.
8. Durie BGM, Salmon SE: A clinical staging system for multiple myeloma. Correlation of measured myeloma cell mass with presenting clinical features, response to treatment, and survival, *Cancer* 36:842–854, 1975.
9. Powis G: Effect of human renal and hepatic disease on the pharmacokinetics of anticancer drugs. *Cancer Treat Rev* 9:85–124, 1982.
10. Weiss RB, Poster DS: The renal toxicity of cancer. Chemotherapeutic agents. *Cancer Treat Rev* 9:37–52, 1982.
11. Cornwell GG III, Pajak TF, McIntyre OR, Kochwa S, Dosik H: Influence of renal failure on myelosuppressive effects of melphalan: Cancer and leukemia group B experience. *Cancer Treat Rep* 66:475–481, 1982.
12. Reich SD: Clinical correlations of adriamycin pharmacology. *Pharmacol Ther Part C* 2:239–249, 1978.
13. Cohen AH, Border WA: Myeloma kidney. An immunomorphogenetic study of renal biopsies. *Lab Invest* 42:248–256, 1980.
14. Rota S, Mougenot B, Baudoin B, De Meyer-Brassur M, Lemaitre V, Michel C, Mignon F, Rondeau E, Vanhille P, Verroust P, Ronco P: Multiple myeloma and severe renal failure: A clinicopathologic study of outcome and prognosis in 34 patients. *Medicine* 66:126–137, 1987.
15. Ganeval D, Cathomen M, Noel LH, Grunfeld JP: Kidney involvement in multiple myeloma and related disorders. *Contr Nephrol* 33:210–222, 1982.
16. MRC Working Party on Leukaemia in Adults: Analysis and management of renal failure in fourth MRC myelomatosis trial. *Br Med J* 288:1411–1416, 1984.
17. Melcion C, Mougenot B, Baudouin B, Ronco P, Moulonguet–Doleris L, Vanhille Ph, Beaufils M, Morel-Maroger L, Verroust P, Richet G: Renal failure in myeloma: Relationship with isoelectric point of immunoglobulin light chains. *Clin Nephrol* 22:138–143, 1984.
18. Cohen DJ, Sherman WH, Osserman EF, Appel GB: Acute renal failure in patients with multiple myeloma. *Am J Med* 76:247–256, 1984.
19. Craig JB, Powell BL: Multiple myeloma. *Arch Intern Med* 144:863–864, 1984.
20. Wu MJ, Kumar KS, Kulkarni G, Kaiser H: Multiple myeloma in naproxen-induced acute renal failure. *N Engl J Med* 317:170–171, 1987.
21. Misiani R, Remuzzi G, Bertani T, Licini R, Levoni P, Crippa A, Mecca G: Plasmapharesis in the treatment of acute renal failure in multiple myeloma. *Am J Med* 66:684–688, 1979.
22. Coward RA, Mallick NP, Delamore IW: Should patients with renal failure associated with myeloma be dialysed? *Br Med J* 287:1575–1578, 1983.
23. Diaz MA, Feliu J, Garcia Alegria J, Medrano J, Picazo ML, Barbado FJ, Ordonez A, Gil A, Vasques JJ: Fracaso renal agudo y mieloma mùltiple: Anàlisis de trece casos. *Med Clin (Barc)* 85:650–652, 1985.
24. Pasquali S, Cagnoli L, Rovinetti C, Rigotti A, Zucchelli P: Plasma exchange therapy in rapidly progressive renal failure due to multiple myeloma. *Int J Artif Organs* 8:27–30, 1985.
25. Pozzi C, Pasquali S, Donini U, Casanova S, Banfi G, Tiraboschi G, Furci L, Porri MT, Ravelli M, Lupo A,

Schena FP, Brunati C, Imbasciati E, Locatelli F: Prognostic factors and effectiveness of treatment in acute renal failure due to multiple myeloma: A review of 50 cases. *Clin Nephrol* 28:1–9, 1987.
26. Feest TG, Burge PS, Cohen SL: Successful treatment of myeloma kidney by diuresis and plasmapheresis. *Br Med J* 1:503–504, 1976.
27. Johnson WJ, Kyle RA, Dahlberg PJ: Dialysis in the treatment of multiple myeloma. *Mayo Clin Proc* 55:65–72, 1980.
28. Cosio FG, Pence TV, Shapiro FL, Kjellstrand CM: Severe renal failure in multiple myeloma. *Clin Nephrol* 15:206–210, 1981.
29. Brunner FP, Brynger H, Chantler C, Donckerwolcke RA, Hathway RA, Jacobs C, Selwood NH, Wing AJ: Combined report on regular dialysis and transplantation in Europe, IX. In: *Proc Eur Dial Trans Assoc* 16:2–73, 1978.
30. Brown WW, Hebert LA, Piering WF, Pisciotta AV, Leman J Jr, Garancis JC: Reversal of chronic end-stage renal failure due to myeloma kidney. *Ann Intern Med* 90:793–794, 1979.
31. Dahlberg PJ, Newcomer KL, Yutuc WR, Smith MJ: Myeloma Kidney: Improved renal function following long-term chemotherapy and hemodialysis. *Am J Nephrol* 3:242–243, 1983.
32. Humphrey RL, Wright JR, Zachary JB, Sterioff S, De Fronzo RA: Renal transplantation in multiple myeloma. *Ann Intern Med* 83:651–653, 1975.
33. De Lima JJG, Kourilsky O, Meyrier A, Morel-Maroger L, Sraer JD: Kidney transplant in multiple myeloma. Early recurrence in the graft with sustained normal renal function. *Transplantation* 31:223–224, 1981.
34. Briefel GR, Spees EK, Humphrey RL, Hill GS, Saral R, Zachary JB: Renal transplantation in a patient with multiple myeloma and light chain nephropathy. *Surgery* 93:579–584, 1983.
35. Walker F, Bear RA: Renal transplantation in light-chain multiple myeloma. *Am J Nephrol* 3:34–37, 1983.
36. Lazarus HM, Lederman M, Lubin A, Herzig RG, Schiffman G, Jones P, Wine A, Rodman HM: Pneumococcal vaccination: The response of patients with multiple myeloma.
37. Morel-Maroger L, Beaufils M, Richet G: The kidney in dysproteinemias. In: J Hamburger J, Crosnier J, JP Grunfeld, ed, *Nephrology*. John Wiley and Sons, New York, pp 711–726, 1979.
38. Morel-Maroger L, Basch A, Danon F, Verroust P, Richet G: Pathology of the kidney in Waldenström's macroglobulinemia. *N Engl J Med* 283:123–129, 1970.
39. Morel-Maroger L, Verroust P: Glomerular lesions in dysproteinemias. *Kidney Int* 5:249–252, 1974.
40. Gallo GR, Feiner HD, Buxbaum JN: The kidney in lymphoplasmacytic disorders. In: SC Sommers, PP Rosen eds, *Pathology Annual* Appleton-Century-Crofts, Norwalk, CT, Part 1, Vol 17, pp 291–317, 1982.
41. Hill GS: Multiple myeloma, amyloidosis, Waldenström's macroglobulinemia, cryoglobulinemias, and benign monoclonal gammopathies. In: RH Heptinstall, ed, *Pathology of the Kidney*, Little, Brown, Boston pp 993–1067, 1983.
42. Martelo OJ, Shultz DR, Pardo V, Perez-Stable E: Immunologically-mediated renal disease in Waldenström's macroglobulinemia. *Am J Med* 58:567–575, 1975.
43. Faraggiana T, Parolini C, Previato G, Lupo A: Light and electron microscopic findings in five cases of cryoglobulinemic glomerulonephritis. Virchows Arch A [Path Anat Histol] 384:29–44, 1979.
44. Kyle RA: Diagnosis and management of multiple myeloma and related disorders. *Prog Hematol* 14:257–282, 1986.
45. Kyle RA: Monoclonal gammopathy of undetermined significance: Natural history in 241 cases. *Am J Med* 64:814–826, 1978.
46. Smithline N, Kassirer JP, Cohen JJ: Light-chain nephropathy renal tubular dysfunction associated with light-chain proteinuria. *N Engl J Med* 294:71–74, 1976.
47. Preuss HG, Hammack WJ, Murdaugh HV: The effect of Bence Jones protein on the in vitro function of rabbit renal cortex. *Nephron* 5:210–216, 1967.
48. Ganeval D, Noel LH, Preud'Homme JL, Droz D, Grunfeld JP: Light-chain deposition disease: Its relation with Al-type amyloidosis. *Kidney Int* 26:1–9, 1984.
49. Noel LH, Droz D, Ganeval D, Grunfeld JP: Renal granular monoclonal light chain deposits: Morphological aspects in 11 cases. *Clin Nephrol* 21:2163–2169, 1984.
50. Randall RE, Williamson WC, Mullinax F, Tung MY, Still WJS: Manifestations of systemic light chain deposition. *Am J Med* 60:293–299, 1976.
51. Ganeval D, Mignon F, Preud'Homme JL, Noel LH, Morel-Maroger L, Droz D, Brouet JC, Mery J Ph, Grunfeld JP: Visceral deposition of monoclonal light chains and immunoglobulins: A study of renal and immunopathologic abnormalities. In: J Hamburger J, Crosnier J, JP Grunfeld, MH Maxwell, eds, *Advances in Nephrology*, Vol 11, Year Book Medical Publishers, Chicago pp 25–63, 1982.
52. Preud'Homme JL, Morel-Maroger L, Brouet JC, Cerf M, Mignon F, Guglielmi P, Seligmann M: Synthesis of abnormal immunoglobulins in lymphoplasmacytic disorders with visceral light chain deposition. *Am J Med* 69:703–710, 1980.
53. Seymour AE, Thompson AJ, Smith PS, Woodroffe AJ, Clarkson AR: Kappa light chain glomerulosclerosis in multiple myeloma. *Am J Pathol* 101:557–580, 1980.
54. Tubbs RR, Gephardt GN, McMahon JT, Hall PF, Valenzuela R, Vidt DG: Light chain nephropahty. *Am J Med* 71:263–269, 1981.
55. Droz D, Noel LH, Carnot F, Degos F, Ganeval D, Grunfeld JP: Liver involvement in nonamyloid light chain deposits disease. *Lab Invest* 50:683–689, 1984.
56. Gipstein RM, Cohen AH, Adams DA, Adams T, Grabie MT: Kappa light chain nephropathy without evidence of myeloma cells. Response to chemotherapy with cessation of maintenance hemodialysis. *Am J Nephrol* 2:276–281, 1982.
57. Gerlag PGG, Koene RAP, Berden JHM: Renal transplantation in light chain nephropathy: Case report and review of the literature. *Clin Nephrol* 25:101–104, 1986.
58. Case Records of the Massachusetts General Hospital (Case 1-1981): *N Engl J Med* 304:33–43, 1981.
59. Husby G, Sletten K: Chemical and clinical classification of amyloidosis 1985. *Scand J Immunol* 23:253–265, 1986.
60. Mery J Ph, Mostefa S: Remission in renal amyloidosis. *Ann Intern Med* 83:581, 1975.
61. Pras M, Gafni J, Jacob ET, Cabili S, Zemer D, Sohar E: Recent advances in Familial Mediterranean Fever. In: JP Grunfeld, MH Maxwell, eds, *Advances in Nephrology*, Vol 13, Year Book Medical Publishers, Chicago, pp 261–270, 1984.
62. Karsenty G, Ulmann A, Droz D, Carnot F, Grunfeld JP: Clinical and histological resolution of systemic amyloidosis after renal cell carcinoma removal. *Nephron* 40:232–234, 1985.
63. Lowenstein J, Gallo G: Remission of the nephrotic syndrome in renal amyloidosis. *N Engl J Med* 282:128–132, 1970.
64. Michael J, Jones NF: Spontaneous remissions of nephrotic

syndrome in renal amyloidosis. *Br Med J* 1:1592–1593, 1978.
65. Thoenes W, Schneider HM: Human glomerular amyloidosis with special regard to proteinuria and amyloidogenesis. *Klin Wochenschr* 58:667–680, 1980.
66. Dikman SH, Churg J, Kahn T: Morphologic and clinical correlates in renal amyloidosis. *Hum Pathol* 12:160–169, 1981.
67. Janssen S, Van Rijswijk MH, Meijer S, Ruinen L, Van Der Hem GK: Clinical evaluation of AA and AL amyloid disease. In: J Marrink, MH Van Rijswijk, eds, *Amyloidosis*. Martinus Nijhoff, Boston, pp 61–72, 1986.
68. Fain O, Ganeval D, Roija L, Kreis H, Noel LH, Barbanel C, Vantelon J, Hannedouche T: Prognostic factors in 63 patients with amyloidosis and renal involvement (abstract). XXIVth Congr Europ Dial Transpl Assoc Europ Renal Assoc Berlin (West), in press, 1987.
69. Pasqualis, Zucchelli P, Cagnoli L, Confalonieri R, Pozzi C, Banfi G, Lupo A, Bertani T: Renal histological lesions and clinical syndromes in multiple myeloma. *Clin Nephrol* 27:222–228, 1987.
70. Libbey CA, Skinner M, Cohen AS: Use of abdominal fat tissue aspirate in the diagnosis of systemic amyloidosis. *Arch Intern Med* 143:1549–1552, 1983.
71. Duston MA, Skinner M, Shirahama T, Cohen AS: Diagnosis of amyloidosis by abdominal fat aspiration. Analysis of four years' experience. *Am J Clin Pathol* 87:756–761, 1987.
72. Noel LH, Droz D, Ganeval D: Immunohistochemical characterization of renal amyloidosis. *Am J Clin Pathol* 87:756–761, 1987.
73. Gise HV, Helmchen U, Mikeler E, Bruning L, Walther CH, Christ H, Mackensen S, Bohle A: Correlations between the morphological and clinical findings in a patient recovering from secondary generalised amyloidosis with renal involvement. *Virchows Arch A* [Path Anat Histol] 379:119–129, 1978.
74. Falck HM, Tornroth T, Skifvars B, Wecelius O: Resolution of renal amyloidosis secondary to rheumatoid arthritis. *Acta Med Scand* 205:651–656, 1979.
75. Triger DR, Joekes AM: Renal amyloidosis. A fourteen year follow-up. *Q J Med* 42:15–40, 1973.
76. Dikman SH, Kahn T, Gribetz D, Churg J: Resolution of renal amyloidosis. *Am J Med* 63:430–433, 1977.
77. Jacquot Ch, D'Auzac Ch, Loirat Ph, Bariety J: Aggravation foudroyante d'amylose rénale après chirurgie. Trois observations. *Nouv Press Med* 10:3389–3395, 1981.
78. Ekenstam E, Michaelsson G, Hallgren R: Response of secondary amyloidosis in psoriasis to treatment with etretinate and ultraviolet light. *Br Med J* 293:733–734, 1986.
79. Zemer D, Pras M, Sohar E, Modan M, Cabili S, Gafni J: Colchicine in the prevention and treatment of the amyloidosis of Familial Mediterranean Fever. *N Engl J Med* 314:1001–1005, 1986.
80. Cohen AS, Shirahama T, Sipe JD, Skinner M: Amyloid proteins, precursors, mediator, and enhancer. *Lab Invest* 48:1–4, 1983.
81. Shirahama T, Cohen AS: Blockage of amyloid induction by colchicine in an animal model. *J Exp Med* 140:1102–1107, 1974.
82. Cohen AS, Rubinow A, Anderson JJ, Skinner M, Mason JH, Libbey C, Kayne H: Survival of patients with primary (AL) amyloidosis. Colchicine-treated cases from 1976 to 1983 compared with cases seen in previous years (1961 to 1973). *Am J Med* 82:1182–1190, 1987.
83. Cohen HJ, Lessin LS, Hallal J, Burkholder P: Resolution of primary amyloidosis during chemotherapy. Studies in a patient with nephrotic syndrome. *Ann Intern Med* 82:466–473, 1975.
84. Buxbaum JN, Hurley ME, Chuba J, Spiro T: Amyloidosis of the AL type. Clinical, morphologic and biochemical aspects of the response to therapy with alkylating agents and prednisone. *Am J Med* 67:867–878, 1979.
85. Kyle RA, Wagoner RD, Holley KE: Primary systemic amyloidosis. Resolution of the nephrotic syndrome with melphalan and prednisone. *Arch Intern Med* 142:1445–1447, 1982.
86. Gertz MA, Kyle RA: Response of primary hepatic amyloidosis to melphalan and prednisone: A case report and review of the literature. *Mayo Clin Proc* 61:218–223, 1986.
87. Kyle RA, Greipp PR: Primary systemic amyloidosis: Comparison of melphalan and prednisone versus placebo. *Blood* 52:818–827, 1978.
88. Kyle RA, Greipp PR, Garton JP, Gertz MA: Primary systemic amyloidosis. Comparison of melphalan/prednisone vs. colchicine. *Am J Med* 79:708–716, 1985.
89. Kedar (Keizman) I, Greenwald M, Ravid M: Treatment of experimental murine amyloidosis with dimethylsulphoxide. *Eur J Clin Invest* 7:149–150, 1977.
90. Kisilevsky R, Boudreau L, Foster D: Kinetics of amyloid deposition. II. The effects of dimethylsulfoxide and colchicine therapy. *Lab Invest* 48:60–67, 1983.
91. Ravid M, Kedar (Keizman) I, Sohar E: Effect of a single dose of dimethylsulphoxide on renal amyloidosis. *Lancet* 2:730–731, 1977.
92. Ravid M, Shapira J, Lang R, Kedar I: Prolonged dimethylsulphoxide treatment in 13 patients with systemic amyloidosis. *Ann Rheum Dis* 41:587–592, 1982.
93. Cameron JS: Coagulation and thromboembolic complications in the nephrotic syndrome. In: JP Grunfeld, MH Maxwell, eds, *Advances in Nephrology*, Vol 13, Year Book Medical Publishers, Chicago, pp 75–114, 1984.
94. Ben Ari J, Zlotnik M, Oren A, Berlyne GM Dialysis in renal failure caused by amyloidosis of Familial Mediterranean Fever. A report to ten cases. *Arch Intern Med* 136:449–451, 1976.
95. Jones NF Renal amyloidosis: Pathogenesis and therapy. *Clin nephrol* 6:459–464, 1976.
96. Hamblin TG: the kidney in myeloma. *Br J Med* 292:2–3, 1976.
97. Wheeler DC, Feehally J, Burton P, Walls J: The kidney in myeloma. *Br Med J* 292:339, 1986.
98. Cohen AS, Bricetti AB, Harringto JT, Mannick: Renal transplantation in two cases of amyloidosis. *Lancet* 2:513–516, 1971.
99. Jacob ET, Bar-Nathan N, Shapira Z Renal transplantation in the amyloidosis of Familial Mediterranean Fever. *Arch Intern Med* 139:1135–1138, 1979.
100. Kuhlback B, Falck H, Tornroth T, Wallenius M, Lindstrom BL, Pasternack A: Renal transplantation in amyloidosis. *Acta Med Scand* 205:169–172, 1979.
101. Jacob ET, Siegal B, Bar-Nathan N, Gafni J: Improving outlook for renal transplantation in amyloid nephropathy. *Transpl Proc* 14:41–45, 1982.
102. Cuvelier R, Pirson Y, Cosyns JP, Squifflet JP, Alexandre GPJ, Van Ypersele De Strihou C: Transplantation rénale en cas d'amylose. *Néphrologie* 7:63–66, 1986.
103. Kyle RA, Greipp PR: Amyloidosis (AL). Clinical and laboratory features in 229 cases. *Mayo Clin Proc* 58:665–683, 1983.
104. Falk RH, Plehn JF, Deering T, Shick EC Jr, Boinay P,

Rubinow A, Skinner M, Cohen AS: Sensitivity and specificity of the echocardiographic features of cardiac amyloidosis. *Am J Cardiol* 59:418–422, 1987.
105. Gertz MA, Skinner M, Connors LH, Falk RH, Cohen AS, Kyle RA: Selective binding of nifedipine to amyloid fibrils. *Am J Cardiol* 55:1646, 1985.
106. Camoriano JK, Greipp PR, Bayer GK, Bowie EJW: Resolution of acquired factor X deficiency and amyloidosis with melphalan and prednisone therapy. *N Engl J Med* 316:1133–1135, 1987.
107. Van Ypersele De Strihou C, Honhon B, Vandenbroucke JM, Huaux JP, Noel H, Maldague B: Dialysis amyloidosis. In: JP Grunfeld, MH Maxwell, eds, *Advances in Nephrology*, Vol 17. Year Medical Book Publishers, Chicago, pp 401–421, 1988.
108. Brouet JC, Clauvel, JP, Danon F, Klein M, Seligmann M: Biological and clinical significance of cryoglobulins. A report of 86 cases. *Am J Med* 57:775–788, 1974.
109. Cordonnier D, Vialtel P, Renversez J CH, Chenais F, Favre M, Tournoud A, Barioz C, Bayle F, Dechelette E, Denis Mc, Couderc P: Renal disease in 18 patients with mixed type II IgM-IgG cryoglobulinemia: Monoclonal lymphoid infiltration (2 cases) and membranoproliferative glomerulonephritis (14 cases). In: J Hamburger, J Crosnier, JP Grunfeld, MH Maxwell, eds, *Advances in Nephrology*, Vol 12, Year Book Medical Publishers, Chicago, pp 177–204, 1983.
110. D'Amico G, Colasanti G, Ferrario F, Sinico AR, Bucci A, Fornasier A: Renal involvement in essential mixed crylgolbulinemia: A peculiar type of immune-mediated renal disease. In: JP Grunfeld, MH Maxwell, eds, *Advances in Nephrology*, Vol 17. Year Book Medical Publishers, Chicago, pp 219–239, 1988.
111. Tarantino A, Montagnino G, Baldassari A, Barbiano DI Belgio–Joso G, Colasanti G, Montoli A, Bucci A, Ponticelli C: Prognostic factors in essential mixed cryoglobulinemia nephropathy. In: *Antiglobulins, Cryoglobulins and Glomerulonephritis*. C Ponticelli, L Minetti, G D'Amico, eds, Martinus Nijhoff, Boston pp 219–225, 1986.
112. Pusey CK, Schifferli JA, Lockwood CM: Use of plasma exchange in the management of mixed essential cryoglobulinemia. *Artif Organs* 5:183–187, 1981.
113. De Vecchi A, Montagnino G, Pozzi G, Tarantino A, Locatelli F, Ponticelli C: Intravenous methylprednisolone pulse therapy in essential mixed cryoglobulinemia nephropathy. *Clin Nephrol* 19:221–22, 1983.

CHAPTER 31

Hyperuricemic Nephropathy

EDWARD R. AHRENS & THOMAS H. STEELE

INTRODUCTION

Clinical relationships between uric acid and the human kidney have long been a topic of perennial interest (1). In this chapter we shall review the different types of renal involvement caused by uric acid or urate, and summarize the available treatment modalities.

ACUTE URIC ACID NEPHROPATHY

Pathogenesis

The term *uric acid nephropathy* refers to a syndrome of acute renal failure developing as a consequence of florid hyperuricemia (2, 3). Severe hyperuricemia results in increased concentrations of uric acid and urate within the renal tubules. During progressive acidification along the nephron, tubule fluid pH may decrease to values that are less than the first pK_a of uric acid. The latter, in the range of 5.4–5.5 (4, 5), is well within the range of urinary pH changes, indicating that substantial urinary uric acid can be nonionized. Nonionized uric acid is sparingly soluble in acid solutions (4, 6), and supersaturation of the urine with respect to uric acid can easily occur. This predisposes to uric acid precipitation and can lead to the obstruction of terminal nephron segments by crystals. Consequently, an *intrarenal hydronephrosis* caused by crystal deposition is the most likely pathogenetic factor underlying acute uric acid nephropathy (2).

Intramedullary deposition of uric acid and monosodium urate has been induced experimentally in the rat by Conger et al. (7). Decreased whole kidney and superficial nephron glomerular filtration rates, as well as increased proximal and distal tubule hydraulic pressures, resulted. Hydraulic pressures in the efferent arterioles and peritubular capillaries were increased, as was the renal vascular resistance. Those change in vascular resistance could have reflected the deposition of sodium urate crystals within the renal vasculature. More likely, they may have been caused by extravascular compression secondary to increased renal tissue pressure, a common finding during urinary tract outflow obstruction.

In order to produce acute renal failure, high concentrations of uric acid must be present within the renal tubules. Emmerson and Row, studying a patient with hyperuricemia and renal failure secondary to uric acid overproduction, correlated the degree of renal failure with the filtered load of urate (8). Jenkins and Rieselbach demonstrated that normal persons can tolerate substantial hyperuricemia without detrimental effects on renal function (9). They increased the serum urate by increasing uric acid production secondary to RNA ingestion and simultaneously inhibiting the tubular secretion of urate with pyrazinamide. In that setting, the urinary uric acid excretion did not increase despite hyperuricemia, and renal function remained unaffected. Consequently, hyperuricemia per se is probably insufficient to cause actue renal failure by itself. Coexisting hyperuricosuria is also required.

Clinical setting and diagnosis

Uric acid nephropathy frequently occurs in association with hematologic malignancies, especially acute leukemias and non-Hodgkin's lymphomas. Although it may occur spontaneously in settings of rapid cell turnover (10, 11), the syndrome usually appears following the initiation of either radiotherapy (12) or chemotherapy (2). Rapid cell destruction and nucleic acid degradation into uric acid form the basis for the pathogenesis. A good example is Burkitt's lymphoma, in which chemotherapeutic destruction of large amounts of tumor occurs rapidly (13, 14). More rarely, uric acid nephropathy has been described as a complication of other neoplasms such as anaplastic carcinoma (15) and invasive breast carcinoma (16).

Uric acid nephropathy has been implicated in the acute renal failure occurring in patients with hypoxanthine-guanine phosphoribosyl transferase (HGPRT) deficiency (17), and occasionally after beginning the use of uricosuric agents or the uricosuric diuretic, ticrynafen (18). During the lowering of the serum urate by any of these agents, the urinary uric acid increases rapidly. A similar mechanism is thought to underlie the renal insufficiency and flank pain associated with the use of suprofen, a recently released and withdrawn nonsteroidal antiinflammatory agent (19, 20). Uric acid nephropathy also has been implicated in the pathogenesis of a type of oliguric renal failure in newborns secondary to excretion of large amounts of uric acid (21). Finally, uric acid nephropathy may contribute to acute renal failure after major motor seizures (22), although rhabdomyolysis also contributes to renal failure in that setting.

The symptoms are nonspecific and may reflect uremia, electrolyte imbalance, or dehydration. Patients usually are oliguric, but may be completely anuric if uric acid crystals or calculi completely obstruct urine outflow (23–25). The renal failure of acute uric acid nephropathy is often reversible (26). Serum urate values may range from 10 to 87 mg/dl (0.6–5.2 mM/l) (27, 28), often exceeding 20 mg/dl (1.2 mM/l). In a number of reports, the serum urate has been measured by nonspecific colorimetric techniques and may have been overestimated because of interfering subtances retained in uremia (29, 30).

Although finding uric acid crystals in the urine can be helpful diagnostically, the presence of crystals is a variable finding. Crystalluria also may be absent in the acute renal failure occasionally associated with the initial administration of uricosuric agents. In addition to uric acid, monosodium urate and ammonium urate have been identified in renal calculi and may possibly function as potentially pathogenic crystals in acute renal failure (31).

The question frequently arises as to whether hyperuricemia is the cause or result of renal failure. Kelton et al. examined urinary uric acid/creatinine concentration ratios in patients with acute renal failure due to various etiologies (32). The patients who were thought to have acute uric acid nephropathy had ratios greater than unity, presumably reflecting increased urate production. Recently it has been reported that high urinary uric acid/creatinine ratios may occur in catabolic patients with acute renal failure associated with infectious diseases causing fever and in other patients with jaundice (33). This test therefore appears to be less specific than was originally thought.

The pathogenesis underlying acute renal failure often is likely to be multifactorial, and the relative contribution made by uric acid often is unclear. For example, in the *tumor lysis syndrome*, the cell death of large tumors may result in extreme hyperphosphatemia as well as hyperuricemia (13, 14). Hyperphosphatemia could contribute independently to the pathogenesis of acute renal failure by promoting the intrarenal precipitation of calcium phosphate (34).

Treatment of acute uric acid nephropathy

URINARY ALKALINIZATION

The deposition of uric acid crystals within terminal nephron segments appears to result from a diminished pH and an increased uric acid concentration in tubule fluid. Because the relative concentration of nonionized uric acid decreases and its solubility increases in alkaline solutions, urinary alkalinization traditionally has been utilized in acute uric acid nephropathy. Nonetheless, the utility of urine alkalinization has been questioned recently. Conger and Falk were unable to demonstrate a beneficial effect of alkalinization per se in experimental uric acid nephropathy in the rat (35). In addition, the solubility of monosodium urate decreases progressively as the pH increases (4). Although sodium urate crystals are seen only infrequently in urine, intrarenal monosodium urate precipitation presumably would likely affect renal function adversely.

Urinary alkalinization to the pH range of 6.5–7.0 can be accomplished by administration of the carbonic anhydrase inhibitor acetazolamide, 250–500 mg every 4–6 hours, together with sodium bicarbonate or a citrate-containing solution such as Shohl's solution, which is metabolized to bicarbonate. The amount of base required is likely to be at least 50 mmol per 24 hours and may be much more. Acetazolamide and bicarbonate can be administered intravenously if needed. This combination of carbonic anhydrase inhibition with supplemental alkali can be quite useful. Acetazolamide promotes the urinary excretion of sodium (as sodium bicarbonate) and is useful in those patients predisposed to develop circulatory overload and pulmonary congestion.

Acetazolamide alone can produce a mild metabolic acidosis, but it usually will not further exacerbate an existing metabolic acidosis. It is ineffective at eliciting bicarbonaturia in advanced renal failure. In patients with hypocalcemia, rapid intravenous administration of alkali may result in increased neuromuscular irritability and tetany. Also, the intratubular precipitation of calcium phosphate could be promoted by a high urine pH. Finally, acetazolamide, a sulfonamide derivative, may itself cause acute renal failure through a hypersensitivity mechanism (36).

SOLUTE AND WATER DIURESIS

Promotion of diuresis and increased solute excretion have been utilized ever since early attempts at treatment of uric acid nephropathy (37). Indeed, it is difficult to alkalinize the urine rapidly without eliciting concomitant increases in urine flow and solute excretion. In their rat model of experimental hyperuricemic nephropathy, Conger and Falk selectively varied tubule fluid flow rates, utilizing either solute or water diuresis, and independently induced urine alkalinization (35). High tubule flow and solute excretion rates were protective of the glomerular filtraton rate and prevented much of the intrarenal urate deposition. Urinary alkalinization alone did not protect renal function and did not prevent intrarenal uric acid and urate crystal deposition.

Urine flow and solute excretion may be increased utilizing mannitol or a loop diuretic such as furosemide or bumetanide (38). In contrast to mannitol, loop diuretics have the advantage of not expanding the extracellular fluid volume, a property that can be helpful in avoiding circulatory overload and pulmonary congestion. The use of furosemide, together with the replacement of urinary solute and water losses, may transform oliguric real failure to nonoliguric renal failure and accord an improved prognosis (39, 40). In severely oliguric patients, however, all attempts at eliciting diuresis may be ineffective. Because the consequences of therapeutic maneuvers are not predictable at the time of their initiation, it is best to avoid volume expansion with mannitol until it is clear that a diuresis can be evoked.

If mannitol is utilized, an initial dosage of 25-50 g intravenously can be followed by a constant infusion at a dosage of approximately 100-150 g per 24 hours. Furosemide, 40-200 mg, or bumetanide, 1-5 mg, can be given intravenously every 4-6 hours. If urinary fluid and electrolyte losses are not replaced and extracellular volume depletion occurs, the diuresis evoked by these loop agents usually will terminate within a few hours.

INHIBITION OF URIC ACID SYNTHESIS

Allopurinol is utilized in order to decrease the body urate pool and to secondarily reduce the amounts of urate filtered and secreted by the kidneys. allopurinol has become the standard therapy for *preventing* acute uric acid nephropathy (41). This drug inhibits the enzyme xanthine oxidase, which catalyzes two oxidations (of hypoxanthine and xanthine) immediately prior to the formation of uric acid. Although xanthine is sparingly soluble, there have been only a few instances of xanthine precipitation and calculus formation during allopurinol therapy (42, 43). This probably reflects the fact that the combined molar amounts of xanthine and hypoxanthine excreted during allopurinol therapy normally are less than the preceding amount of urinary uric acid (44). Through feedback inhibition, increased hypoxanthine levels depress the rate of de-novo purine biosynthesis and secondarily the rate of uric acid formation. Allopurinol also acts to promote purine salvage (45). The increased xanthine levels produced by allopurinol may lead to falsely low estimates of the serum urate concentration (46).

Allopurinol usually is given at a daily dose of 300 mg or less. Commonly it is initiated 1-3 days prior to chemotherapy for hematologic malignancies or other conditions in which bulk tumor necrosis may be anticipated. Once uric acid nephropathy is established, allopurinol is considerably less effective than if it has been used as a preventive measure. Intravenous allopurinol apparently has little advantage over the oral preparation (47).

Allopurinol usually is well tolerated in patients with normal renal function. However, serious toxicity can occur in patients with renal failure (48). Both allopurinol and its pharmacologically active metabolite, oxipurinol, are retained in renal failure (49). Elevated serum levels of oxipurinol, the renally excreted major metabolite of allopurinol, correlate well with the development of toxic side effects (50, 51). In the extreme, these may include a diffuse erythematous desquamative skin rash (toxic epidermal necrolysis), fever, hepatic dysfunction, eosinophilia, and declining kidney function. An allergic hepatitis has been described as a separate entity (52). The clinical syndrome and the results of skin an renal biopsies have suggested the presence of vasculitis (53). Although a number of deaths have occurred, most patients have recovered following early withdrawal of the drug. Dosage suggestions for patients with compromised renal function, based upon studies of the renal clearnace of oxipurinol, have been published (48). Pharmacokinetic data for allopurinol are available (54-56). Although the manufacturer recommends a dosage reduction when the creatinine clearance falls to 20 ml/min, it may be prudent to reduce the dosage of allopurinol in patients with less severe disease.

Allopurinol should also be used with great care in patients receiving azathioprine (Imuran®) (57). The dose of azathioprine should be reduced by about two thirds because of an allopurinol-mediated reduction in the metabolism of this immunosuppressive agent.

HEMODIALYSIS

This treatment modality can be utilized effectively to accelerate the removal of uric acid from the body (58). With a large dialyzer, the uric acid clearance can range from 70 to 145 ml/min and can result in decreasing the serum urate concentration by 50% during a 6-hour dialysis (58, 59). Kjellstrand et al. demonstrated somewhat greater uric acid clearances with large parallel-plate dialyzers compared to hollow-fiber and coil units (58). In contrast to hemodialysis, peritoneal dialysis is only marginally effective at accelerating urate removal. Peritoneal urate clearances have been reported to range from only 7 to 15 ml/min (60, 61).

URICOLYTIC THERAPY

Allantoin, the end product of purine catabolism in mammals other than humans and the great ape, is far more soluble than is uric acid, and its renal clearance is equal to the glomerular filtration rate (62). It is the oxidation product of urate and is produced by the action of the enzyme uricase (urate oxidase). In human trials conducted in France, parenteral uricase derived from fungi rapidly decreased the serum urate and urinary uric acid, concomitantly increasing the serum and urine concentrations of allantoin (63-65). Uricase has been utilized in preexisting renal failure secondary to uric acid nephropathy, and also has seemed beneficial in preventing uric acid precipitation in patients with malignancies undergoing chemotherapy. However, repeated injection of the enzyme can lead to allergic manifestations, including anaphylaxis (63). Because there is a delay in the onset of action of allopurinol, uricolytic therapy may prove advantageous in early uric acid nephropathy if newer enzyme preparations with fewer side effects prove to be safe (66, 67).

OTHER ASPECTS OF URIC ACID NEPHROPATHY

In patients becoming rapidly oliguric or anuric during the development of acute uric acid nephropathy (68, 69), retrograde pyelography has occasionally revealed bilateral obstruction of the ureters with uric acid crystals or calculi (25, 70). Ureteric catheterization and irrigation with alkaline solutions have been utilized to dissolve these precipitates (71). Other causes of oliguria or anuria can include leukemic or lymphomatous infiltration of the kidneys, hypercalcemic nephropathy, and renal outflow obstruction secondary to blood clots. Finally, nephrotoxic antibiotics, sepsis, and hypotension with ischemia can contribute to renal failure. Patients with uric acid nephropathy require the same type of intensive medical and nutritional support as do patients with other types of acute renal failure.

CHRONIC HYPERURICEMIC NEPHROPATHY

Uric acid and the kidney in gout

Acute or rapidly progressing renal failure is an infrequent complication in patients with gout. Occasionally, however, gouty patients with marked uric acid overproduction and high-grade hyperuricemia develop acute renal failure (8). Accelerated renal failure also has been reported in familial gout. This type of renal involvement probably occurs secondary to renal monosodium urate deposition and has occurred with unusual frequency in young females (72).

In gout accompanied by either the overproduction of uric acid or complicated by progressive renal failure, reducing the rate of uric acid formation is the most rational form of therapy. In normal adults consuming an average diet and with a normal glomerular filtration rate, the 24-hour urinary uric acid excretion can be utilized as an estimate of urate production. This parameter usually is 800 mg (4.9 mM) per 24 hours or less (73). Measuring the urinary uric acid/creatinine concentration ratio in untimed urine specimens has been proposed as a substitute for inconvenient 24-hour collections (74). However spot urine testing apparently does not correlate well with the 24-hour urinary uric acid excretion in individual patients, thereby limiting its usefulness (75).

In gouty patients with urate overproduction and normal renal function, allopurinol can be administered as a single daily dose of 300 mg, although a higher dosage is sometimes needed. In the presence of renal disease, the dosage of allopurinol should be reduced, as already discussed. However, in the majority of patients with gout, the 24-hour urinary uric acid excretion lies within normal limits. In such uric acid "normoproducers," the data suggest that the renal tubular secretion of urate is sluggish (76). However, the rate of reabsorption of secreted urate also could be abnormally high in these patients (77).

Although individuals with gout appear to have a special predilection to develop hypertension and arteriosclerotic vascular complications (78, 79), renal insufficiency is not particularly common. The older rheumatologic literature, prior to the longstanding availability of hypouricemic agents, contains descriptions of patients developing chronic renal insufficiency and often dying with massive intrarenal tophaceous deposits (80). A number of reports described slowly progressive renal failure associated with the presence of interstitial fibrous, nephrosclerosis, and medullary deposits of urate crystals (81, 82). Those findings led to the notion that gouty nephropathy, characterized by the renal interstitial precipitation of urate and secondary stimulation of fibrosis, is a relatively common cause of chronic renal failure.

However, very little correlation appears to exist between the presence of medullary urate deposits and a history of gout. Linnane et al. found renal urate deposits in 8.4% of 1733 autopsies performed in Brisbane, Australia over a 12-month period (83). Although a history of gout was present in a higher percentage of patients with renal urate deposition, nearly 90% of patients with urate deposits had no history of gout. Gout also may occur as a complication of established chronic renal impairment, especially adult polycystic kidney disease (84) and medullary cystic disease (85). Whether gout and renal urate deposition influence the rate of deterioration of renal function in those situations is uncertain.

Longitudinal studies involving large numbers of gouty patients have revealed that renal insufficiency in uncommon (86, 87). When renal failure is observed, hypertension and atherosclerotic disease are common coexistent factors that have an increased prevalence in gouty patients. Epidemiologic studies suggest that while hypertension, atherosclerosis, and diabetes mellitus are found commonly in gouty subjects, there appears to be no causative rolve of gout or hyperuricemia (88, 89). Families have been described who present with both severe gout and associated progressive renal insufficiency at an early age (72, 85, 90). Usually an autosomal dominant form of inheritance is suggested. It presently is thought that, in at least some cases, the primary inherited disorder may be the occurrence of interstitial nephritis. Hyperuricemia and gout could then develop as a consequence of renal disease (91). Chronic lead intoxication has been implicated in the pathogenesis of chronic renal failure associated with gout, although the role of lead in that setting in controversial (92).

The foremost rationale for reducing the serum urate in gout lies in preventing or decreasing the frequency of attacks of acute gouty arthritis (93). Traditionally, uricosuric agents have been used widely for this purpose. They decrease the serum urate by inhibiting the renal tubular reabsorption of urate (94). Early in the course of treatment, the urinary uric acid excretion increases, but subsequently falls toward the pretreatment level as the serum urate is reduced (95). Although there is little substantive evidence to suggest that traditional uricosuric drugs can cause acute uric acid nephropathy, the older literature contains references to renal colic occurring soon after the onset of drug administration (94). Accordingly, uricosuric agents should be prescribed at initial dosages of 25–50% of the usual maintenance dose and increased until the desired reduction of serum urate occurs. Typical daily maintenance dosages are 1–2 g of probenecid or 200–800 mg of sulfinpyrazone, given in divided doses. In patients with significant renal disease or others in whom uricosuric agents are ineffective, allopurinol can be utilized, employing the guidelines discussed above.

The initiation of treatment with uricosuric agents or allopurinol increases the risk of acute gouty arthritis (93). Therefore, one may stabilize the gouty patient with anti-inflammatory agents prior to prescribing agents that lower the serum urate (96). Colchicine, 0.5–0.6 mg once or twice daily, usually is effective at preventing attacks of gouty arthritis during the early weeks of allopurinol or uricosuric therapy. In order to do this, colchicine should be started several days prior to beginning the latter types of agents and should be continued for about 6 weeks. At a low dosage, colchicine does not cause gastrointestinal or other side effects in normal persons. However, even low maintenance doses of this drug can cause a disabling neuromyopathy in patients with renal failure and should be used with caution in that setting (97).

Asymptomatic hyperuricemia

What is to be done with hyperuricemic individuals who do not have gout? Patients with diuretic-treated hypertension constitute the largest single group of hyperuricemic persons, and it appears that fewer than 10% are destined to develop gouty arthritis (98). Most diuretics used for treating hypertension can cause hyperuricemia by reducing the renal urate clearance, probably by facilitating tubular urate reabsorption secondary to diuretic-induced volume depletion (99).

Older data from the Framingham Study have suggested that persons with a serum urate greater than 9 mg/dl (0.54 mM/l) are at a substantially increased risk of developing acute gouty arthritis (100). However, those studies suffered from the lack of a prospective design and from only small numbers of patients. More recently, Fessel and colleagues have followed asymptomatic hyperuricemic individuals prospectively (101). They observed that individuals with a serum urate greater than 9 mg/dl (0.54 mM/l) were not at significantly great risk of gouty attacks or renal calculi than were hyperuricemic patients with lower serum urate concentrations. Those results were recently confirmed by Campion et al. (87). An association did exist between hyperuricemia and the development of modest increases in the plasma glucose and blood pressure (101). Body weights correlated strongly with the latter, suggesting that hyperuricemia per se probably was not an independent risk factor. However, another report from the same group suggested that hyperuricemia is predictive of future cardiovascular disease, independently of the body weight (102).

Urate precipitation can occur selectively in the renal medullas of otherwise normal persons (103) and also in the kidneys of nongouty patients with advanced renal failure (104, 105). Fessel has reported a very low risk of developing renal function abnormalities in persons with hyperuricemia unless the serum urate was greatly elevated (106). Those observations agree with other data indicating that deterioration in renal function of patients with untreated gout is likely to be very modest (107, 108).

The routine patient with asymptomatic low-grade hyperuricemia probably should not be treated for that abnormality (109). In general, current recommendations are to withhold treatment until the occurrence of gouty arthritis or uric acid nephrolithiasis (110). At urate concentrations near the upper limit of normal (7 mg/dl; 0.42 mM/l), the serum becomes saturated with respect to monosodium urate (111). At higher serum urate levels, monosodium urate is "metastable" in the sense that it can precipitate from supersaturated serum if a suitable nucleating site is available. With further hyperuricemia, spontaneous precipitation of monosodium urate could at least theoretically take place. The urate level at which spontaneous urate precipitation might commence is not known, but a value of about twice the upper limit of normal seems a reasonable estimate. Accordingly, there may be some utility in lowering the serum urate in asymptomatic individuals with *extreme* hyperuricemia, perhaps when the serum urate values exceed 12 mg dl (0.7 mM/l).

In patients with hyperuricemia secondary to diuretics, the serum urate can be reduced by uricosuric agents without impairing the antihypertensive efficacy of the diuretic (112). Several years ago, there was considerable interest and preliminary activity related to the development of pharmaceutical agents possessing a combination of diuretic and uricosuric activities in order to permit the treatment of hypertension by diuretics without the putative risks of hyperuricemia. Those agents were discussed in the first edition of this book (113). Since that time, there has been very little further development of such drugs, and it seems unlikely that any will become widely available in the near future.

REFERENCES

1. Steele TH: Urate excretion in man, normal and gouty. In: WN Kelley, IM Weiner, eds, *Uric Acid. Handbook of Experimental Pharmacology*, Vol 51. Springer-Verlag, Berlin, pp 257–286, 1978.
2. Rieselbach RE, Bentzel CJ, Cotlove E, Frei E III, Freireich J: Uric acid excretion and renal function in the acute hyperuricemic of leukemia. *Am J Med* 37:876–884, 1964.
3. Conger JD: Acute uric acid nephropathy. *Semin Nephrol* 1:69–74, 1981.
4. Wilcox WR, Khalaf A, Weinberger A, Kippen I, Klinenberg JR: Solubility of uric acid and monosodium urate. *Med Biol Eng Comput* 10:522–531, 1972.
5. Finlayson B, Smith A: Stability of the first dissociable proton of uric acid. *J Chem Eng Data* 19:94–97, 1974.
6. Yü T-F, Gutman A: Uric acid nephrolithiasis in gout: Predisposing factors. *Ann Intern Med* 67:1133–1148, 1967.
7. Conger JD, Falk SA, Guggenheim SJ, Burke TJ: A micropuncture study of the early phase of acute urate nephropathy. *J Clin Invest* 58:681–689, 1976.
8. Emmerson BT, Row PG: An evaluation of the pathogenesis of the gouty kidney. *Kidney Int* 8:65–71, 1975.
9. Jenkins P, Rieselbach RE: Unique characteristics of the mechanism for reabsorption of filtered versus secreted urate (abstract). *Proc Am Soc Clin Invest* 36A, 1974.
10. Passwell J, Boichis H, Cohen BE: Hyperuricemic nephro-

pathy. *Am J Dis Child* 120:154–156, 1970.
11. Kanwar F, Maraligod J: Leukemic urate nephropathy. *Arch Pathol* 99:467–472, 1975.
12. Merrill D, Jackson H: The renal complications of leukemia. *N Engl J Med* 228:271–276, 1943.
13. Cohen LF, Balow JE, Magrath IT, Poplack DG, Ziegler JL: Acute tumor lysis syndrome. *Am J Med* 68:486–491, 1980.
14. Tsokos GC, Balow JE, Spiegel RJ, Magrath, IT: Renal and metabolic complications of undifferentiated and lymphoblastic lymphomas. *Medicine* 60:218–229, 1981.
15. Crittenden DR, Ackerman GL: Hyperuricemic acute renal failure in disseminated carcinoma. *Arch Intern Med* 137:97–99, 1977.
16. Ultmann JE: Hyperuricemia in disseminated neoplastic disease other than lymphomas and leukemias. *Cancer* 15:122–129, 1962.
17. Emmerson BT, Thompson L: The spectrum of hypoxanthineguanine phosphoribosyl transferase deficiency. *Q J Med* 42:423–440, 1973.
18. Bennett WM, Van Zee BE, Hutchings R, Cohen LH, Norby LH, Champion C, Spargo B, Selby T: Acute renal failure from ticrynafen. *N Engl J Med* 301:1179–1181, 1979.
19. Wolfe SM: Suprofen-induced transient flank pain and renal failure. *Engl J Med* 316:1025, 1987.
20. Suprofen labelling revised. *FDA Drug Bulletin* 16;15–16, 1986.
21. Ahmadian Y, Lewy P: Possible urate nephropathy of the newborn infant as a cause of transient renal insufficiency. *J Pediatr* 91:96–100, 1977.
22. Warren DJ, Leitch AG, Leggett RJE: Hyperuricemic acute renal failure after epileptic seizures. *Lancet* 2:385–387, 1975.
23. Holland P, Holland N: Prevention and management of acute hyperuricemia in childhood leukemia. *J Pediatr* 72:358–366, 1972.
24. Yolken RH, Miller DR: Hyperuricemia and renal failure — presenting manifestations of occult hematologic malignancies. *J Pediatr* 89:775–777, 1976.
25. Lear H, Oppenheimer GD: Anuria following radiation therapy in leukemia. *JAMA* 143:806–807, 1950.
26. Watts RWE, Watkins PJ, Mathias JQ: Allopurinol and acute uric acid nephropathy. *B Med J* 1:205–208, 1966.
27. Kritzler RA: Anuria complicating the treatment of leukemia. *Am J Med* 25:532–538, 1958.
28. Alsarraf D, Reese L: Management of acute renal failure due to marked hyperuricemia. *Can Med Assoc J* 106:352–354, 1972.
29. Howorth PJN, Zilva JF: Determination of uric acid levels in uraemia by enzymatic and colorimetric techniques. *J Clin Pathol* 21:192–195, 1968.
30. Caraway WT: Non-urate chromogens in body fluids. *Clin Chem* 15:720–726, 1969.
31. Prien EL, Prien EL Jr: Composition and structure of urinary stone. *Am J Med* 45:654–672, 1968.
32. Kelton J, Kelley WN, Holmes EW: A rapid method for the diagnosis of acute uric acid nephropathy. *Arch Intern Med* 138:612–615, 1978.
33. Tangsanga K, Boonwichit D, Lekhakula A, Sitprija V: Urine uric acid and urine creatinine ratio in acute renal failure. *Arch Intern Med* 144;934–937, 1984.
34. Kanfer A, Richet G, Roland J, Chatelet F: Extreme hyperphosphatemia causing acute anuric nephrocalcinosis in lymphosarcoma. *B Med J* 1:1320, 1979.
35. Conger JD, Falk SA: Intrarenal dynamics in the pathogenesis and prevention of acute urate nephropathy. *J Clin Invest* 59:127–128, 1978.
36. Higenbottam T, Ogg CS, Saxton HM: Acute renal failure from the use of acetazolamide (Diamox). *Postgrad Med J* 54:127–128, 1978.
37. Barry KG, Hunter RH, Davis TE, Crosby WA: Acute uric acid nephropathy. *Arch Intern Med* 111:452–459, 1963.
38. Handa SP: Acute renal failure in association with hyperuricemia. *South Med J* 64:676–678, 1971.
39. Anderson RJ, Linas SL, Berns As, Henrich WL, Miller TR, Gabow PA, Schrier RW: Non-oliguric acute renal failure. *N Engl J Med* 296:1134–1138, 1977.
40. Schrier RW: Acute renal failure. *Kidney Int* 15:205–216, 1979.
41. DeConti RC, Calabresi P: Use of Allopurinol for prevention and control of hyperuricemia in patients with neoplastic disease. *N Engl J Med* 274:481–486, 1966.
42. Bard PR, Silverberg DS, Henderson JF, Ulan RA, Wensel RH, Banerjee TK, Little AS: Xanthine nephropathy in a patient with lymphosarcoma treated with allopurinol. *N Engl J Med* 283:354–357, 1970.
43. Albin A, Stephens BG, Hirata T, Wilson K, Williams HE: Nephropathy, xanthinuria, and orotic aciduria complicating Burkitt's lymphoma treated with chemotherapy and allopurinol. *Metabolism* 21:771–778, 1972.
44. Elion GB: Allopurinol and other inhibitors of urate synthesis. In: WN Kelley, IM Weiner, eds, *Uric Acid. Handbook of Experimental Pharmacology*, Vol 51. Springer-Verlag, Berlin, pp 485–514, 1978.
45. Edwards NL, Recker D, Airozo D, Fox IH: Enhanced purine salvage during allopurinol therapy: An important pharmacologic property in humans. *J Lab Clin Med* 98:673–682, 1981.
46. Hande KR, Perini F, Putterman G, Elin R: Hyperxanthinemia intefers with serum uric acid determinations by the uricase method. *Clin Chem* 25:1492–1494, 1979.
47. Kann HE Jr, Wells JH, Gallelli JF, Schein PS, Cooney DA, Smith ER, Seegmiller JE, Carbone PP: The development and use of an intravenous preparation of allopurinol. *Am J Med Sci* 256:53–63, 1968.
48. Hande K, Noone R, Stone W: Severe allopurinol toxicity description and guildines for prevention in patients with renal insufficiency. *Am J Med* 76:47–56, 1984.
49. Elion GB, Yü T-F, Gutman AB, Hitchings GH: Renal clearance of oxipurinol, the chief metabolite of allopurinol. *Am J Med* 45:69–77, 1968.
50. Kantor G: Toxic epidermal necrolysis, azotemia, and death after allopurinol therapy. *JAMA* 212:478–479, 1970.
51. Simmonds HA, Cameron JS, Morris GS, Davies PM: Allopurinol in renal failure and the tumour lysis syndrome. *Clin Chim Acta* 160:189–195, 1986.
52. Al-Kawas FH, Seeff LB, Berendson RA, Zimmerman HJ, Ishak KG: *Ann Intern Med* 95:588–590, 1981.
53. Utsinger P: Allopurinol hypersensitivity: Granular deposition of IgM at the dermal-epidermal junction. *Am J Med* 61:287–294, 1976.
54. Hande K, Reed E, Chabner B: Allopurinol kinetics. *Clin Pharm Ther* 23:598–605, 1978.
55. Applebaum SJ, Mayersohn M, Dorr RT, Perrier D: Allopurinol kinetics and bioavailability. *Cancer Chemother Pharmacol* 8:93–98, 1982.
56. Berlinger WG, Park GD, Spector R: The effect of dietary protein on the clearance of allopurinol and oxypurinol. *N Engl J Med* 313:771–776, 1985.
57. Friedman H, Grasela T: Adenine arabinoside and allopurinol: Possible adverse drug interaction. *N Engl J Med*

304:423, 1981.
58. Kjellstrand CM, Campbell DC, von Haritzsch B, Buselmeier TJ: Hyperuricemic acute renal failure. *Arch Intern Med* 133;349–359, 1974.
59. Steinberg SM, Galen MM, Lazarus JM, Lowrie EG, Hampers CL, Jaffe N: Hemodialysis for acute anuric uric acid nephropathy. *Am J Dis Child* 130:956–958, 1975.
60. Maher JF, Ruth CE, Schreiner GE: Hyperuricemia complicating leukemia. *Arch Intern Med* 123:198–200, 1969.
61. Deger G. Waggoner R: Peritoneal dialysis in acute uric acid nephropathy. *Mayo Clin Proc* 47:189–192, 1972.
62. Greger R, Lang F, Deetjen P: Handling of allantoin by the rat kidney. clearance and micropuncture data. *Pflügers Arch* 357:201–207, 1975.
63. Zittoon R, Dauchy F, Teillaud C, Barthelemy M, Bouchard P: Le traitment des hyperuricémies en hématologie par l'unst-oxydase et l'allopurinol. *Ann Med Interne* 127:479–482, 1976.
64. Feuillu A, Herve JP, Pogamp PL, Garre M, Chevet D: Traitement de l'hyperuricémie secondaire de l'insuffisance rénale chronique per uricolyse enzymatique. *Thérapie* 35: 734–749, 1980.
65. Brogard JM, Stahl A, Stahl J: Enzymatic uricolysis and its use in therapy. In: WN Kelly, IM Weiner, eds, *Uric Acid, Handbook of Experimental Pharmacology*, Vol 51. Springer-Verlag, Berlin, pp 515–524, 1978.
66. Abuchowski A, Karp D, Davis FF: Reduction of plasma urate levels in the cokerel with polyethylene glycol-uricase. *J Pharmacol Exp Ther* 219:352–354, 1981.
67. Davis S, Park YK: Hypouricaemic effect of polyethylene glycol modified urate oxidase. *Lancet* 2:281–283, 1981.
68. Fitzgerlad RH, Wallace KM, Baker A: Acute obstructive uric acid nephropathy after treatment of neoplastic adenopathy. *South Med J* 74:424–426, 1981.
69. Bedrna J, Polcak J: Alcuter harnleiter verschluss nach bestrahlung chronischer leukämien mit röntgenstrahlen. *Med Klin* 25:1700–1701, 1929.
70. Kravitz SC, Diamond HD, Craver LF: Uremia complicating leukemia chemotherapy. *JAMA* 146:1595–1597, 1951.
71. Eason AA, Sharlip ID, Spaulding JT: Dissolution of bilateral uric acid calculi causing anuria. *JAMA* 240:670–671, 1978.
72. Simmonds HA, Warren DJ, Cameron JS, Potter CF, Farebrother DA: Familial gout and renal failure in young women. *Clin Nephrol* 14;176–182, 1980.
73. Coe FL: *Nephrolithiasis Pathogenesis and Treatment*. Yearbook Medical Publishers, Chicago, pp 95–115, 1978.
74. Simkin PA, Hoover PL, Paxson CS, Wilson WF: Uric acid excretion: Quantitative assessment from spot, midmorning serum and urine samples. *Ann Intern Med* 91:44–47, 1979.
75. Wortmann RL, Fox IH: Limited value of uric acid to creatinine ratios in estimating acid excretion. *Ann Intern Med* 93:822–825, 1980.
76. Rieselbach RE, Sorensen LB, Shelp WD, Steele TH: Diminished renal urate secretion per nephron as a basis for primary gout. *Ann Intern Med* 73:359–366, 1970.
77. Steele TH, Boner G: Origins of the uricosuric response. *J Clin Invest* 51:1368–1375, 1973.
78. Jacobs DR: The coronary drug project research group: Serum uric acid: Its association with other risk factors and with mortality in coronary heart disease. *J Chron Dis* 29: 557–569, 1976.
79. Viozzi FJ, Bluhm GB, Riddle JM: Gout and arterial thrombosis. *Henry Ford Med J* 20:119–214, 1972.
80. Talbott JH, Terplan KL: The kidney in gout. *Medicine* 38:405–462, 1960.
81. Barlow K, Beilin L: Renal disease in primary gout. *J Med* 37:79–98, 1968.
82. Modern F, Meister L: The kidney of gout, a clinical entity. *Med Clin North Am* 36:941–952, 1952.
83. Linnane J, Barry A, Emmerson B: Urate deposits in the renal medulla. *Nephron* 29:216–222, 1981.
84. Yü T-F: Cystic diseases of the kidney and gout. *Arch Intern Med* 138:1609, 1978.
85. Thompson GR, Weiss JJ, Goldman RT, Rigg GA: Familial occurrence of hyperuricemia, gout and medullary cystic disease. *Arch Intern Med* 138:1614–1617, 1978.
86. Yü T-F, Berger L. Impaired renal function in gout, its association with hypertensive vascular disease and intrinsic renal disease. *Am J Med* 72:95–100, 1982.
87. Campion E, Glynn R, Delabry M. Asymptomatic hyperuricemia. Risks and consequences in the normative aging study. *Am J Med* 82:421–426, 1987.
88. Brand F, McGee D, Kannel W, Stokes J, Castell W. Hyperuricemia as a risk factor of coronary heart disease: The Framingham Study. *Am J Epid* 121:11–18, 1985.
89. Reunanen A, Takkunen H, Knekt P, Aromaa A. Hyperuricemia as a risk factor for cardiovascular mortality. *Acta Med Scand* 668(Suppl):49–59, 1982.
90. Massari P, Usa C, Barnes R, Poxigikas P, Weller J. Familial hyperuricemia and renal disease. *Arch Intern Med* 140: 680–684, 1980.
91. Richmond J, Kincaid-Smith P, Whitworth J, Becker G. Familial gout and renal failure. *Arch Dis Child* 56:699–704, 1981.
92. Foley RJ, Weinman EJ: Review: Urate nephropathy. *Am J Med Sci* 288:208–211, 1984.
93. Kelley WN: Pharmacologic approach to the maintenance of urate homeostasis. *Nephron* 14:99–115, 1975.
94. Gutman AB: Uricosuric drugs, with special reference to probenecid and sulfinpyrazone. *Adv Pharmacol Chemother* 4:91–142, 1966.
95. Reese OG Jr, Steele TH: Renal transport of urate during diuretic-induced hypouricemia. *Am J Med* 60:973–979, 1976.
96. Wallace SL, Ertel NH: Pharmacology of drugs used in treatment of acute gout. In: WN Kelley, IM Weiner, eds, *Uric Acid, Handbook of Experimental Pharmacology*, Vol 51. Springer-Verlag, Berlin, pp 525–556, 1978.
97. Kuncl RW, Duncan G, Watson D, Alderson K, Rogawski MA, Peper M: Colchicine myopathy and neuropathy. *N Engl J Med* 316:1562–1568, 1987.
98. Steele TH: Diuretic-induced-induced hyperuricemia. In: WN Kelley, ed, *Crystal-Induced Arthropathies*. Clinics in Rheumatic Diseases. Saunders, London, pp 37–50, 1977.
99. Manuel MA, Steele TH: Changes in renal urate handling after prolonged thiazide treatment. *Am J Med* 57:741–746, 1974.
100. Hall AP, Barry PE, Dawber TR, McNamara PM: Epidemiology of gout and hyperuricemia: A long-term population study. *Am J Med* 42:27–37, 1967.
101. Fessel WJ, Siegelaub AB, Johnson ES: Correlates and consequences of asymptomatic hyperuricemia. *Arch Intern Med* 132:44–54, 1973.
102. Fessel WJ: High uric acid as an indicator of cardiovascular disease. Independence from obesity. *Am J Med* 68:401–404, 1980.
103. Cannon PJ, Symchych PS, DeMartini FE: The distribution of urate in human and primate kidney. *Proc Soc Exp Biol Med* 129:278–285, 1968.

104. Verger D, Leroux-Robert C, Ganter P, Richet G: Les tophus goutteux de la medullaire rénale des urémiques chroniques. *Nephron* 4:356-370, 1967.
105. Östberg Y: Renal urate deposits in chronic renal insufficiency. *Acta Med Scand* 183:197-201, 1968.
106. Fessel WJ: Renal outcomes of gout and hyperuricemia. *Am J Med* 67:74-82, 1979.
107. Yü T-F, Berger L: Renal disease in primary gout: A study of 253 gout patients with proteinuria. *Semin Arthritis Rheum* 4:293-305, 1975.
108. Berger L, Yü T-F: Renal function in gout: IV. An analysis of 525 gouty subjects including long-term follow-up studies. *Am J Med* 59:605-613, 1975.
109. Liang MH, Fries JF: Asymptomatic hyperuricemia: The case for conservative management. *Ann Intern Med* 88:666-670, 1978.
110. Kelley W, Fox I. Gout and related disorders of purine metabolism. In: W Kelley, E Harris, S Ruddy, C Sledge, ed, *Textbook of Rheumatology*, 2nd. WB Saunders, Philadelphia pp 1359-1358, 1985.
111. Loeb JN: The influence of temperature on the solubility of monosodium urate. *Arthritis Rheum* 15:189-192, 1972.
112. Smilo RP, Beisel WR, Forsham PH: Reversal of thiazide-induced transient hyperuricemia by uricosuric agents. *N Engl J Med* 267:1225-1227, 1962.
113. Smith WE, Steele TH: The hyperuricemic nephropathies. In: WN Suki, SG Massry, eds, *Therapy of Renal Diseases and Related Disorders*, 1st ed. Martinus Nijhoff, Boston, pp 327-333, 1984.

CHAPTER 32

Renal Disorders in Liver Disease

MURRAY EPSTEIN

INTRODUCTION

Cirrhosis of the liver is a common clinical condition that afflicts a major portion of the population of the United States. The importance of this disease is underscored by reports indicating that the age-adjusted death rate (14.8 deaths/100,000 population) for cirrhosis has increased by 67% between 1950 and 1969, ranking it as the tenth leading cause of death in the United States (1). At least 600,000 Americans (3.6 of every 1000 adults in the U.S. population) are estimated to have cirrhosis, but many think this figure greatly underestimates the prevalence of this disorder. Since most patients with cirrhosis have ascites and edema during the course of the disease, the impact of ascites on health care is enormous. Included among the numerous complications that affect the course of cirrhosis are derangements of renal function. Since several studies have indicated that renal failure occurs in 50–75% of patients dying of cirrhosis (2, 3), extrapolation of these data underscore the clinical importance of this complication.

The interrelationship of liver disease and simultaneous kidney disease has been recognized for hundreds of years (4). Unfortunately, liver-kidney interrelationships are exceedingly complex and at times not fully appreciated. Providing an overview of such a large and complex subject has made it necessary to select the information presented and to establish rather arbitrary priorities concerning which areas receive more detailed discussion. In the present review, emphasis will be placed on abnormalities of renal sodium and water handling, the acute azotemic syndromes, hemodialysis-associated hepatitis, and the glomerulonephritides of liver disease.

Renal sodium handling

CLINICAL FEATURES

It is well appreciated that patients with Laennec's cirrhosis manifest a remarkable capacity for sodium retention; indeed, such patients frequently excrete urine that is virtually free of sodium (5–8). Extracellular fluid accumulates excessively and eventually becomes evident as clinically detectable ascites and edema. It should be emphasized that such fluid retention is primarily a function of the acquisition of sodium; cirrhotic patients who are unable to excrete sodium will continue to gain weight and to accumulate ascites and edema as long as the dietary sodium content exceeds the maximal urinary sodium excretion. If access to sodium is not curtailed, the relentless retention of sodium may lead to the accumulation of vast amounts of ascites (on occasion up to 20 l). Weight gain and ascites formation promptly cease, however, when the sodium intake is limited.

The abnormality of renal sodium handling in cirrhosis should not be regarded as a static and unalterable condition. Rather, cirrhotic patients may undergo a spontaneous diuresis followed by a return to avid salt retention (5, 8). While a significant number of patients who are maintained on a sodium-restricted dietary program may demonstrate a spontaneous diuresis, there is inadequate information about the incidence with which this occurs. Sometimes spontaneous diuresis occurs within a few days, but more often within 1 or 2 weeks after hospital admission. There is no reliable way of predicting which patients will demonstrate it and which will not.

While many clinicians have tended to view ascites as an indicator of deterioration of the underlying hepatic disease, it should be recognized that this caveat does not always hold true. Sometimes the onset of ascites can be related directly to an increased dietary sodium intake and is more a reflection of salt loading than of progressive alterations in hepatic function. Occasionally a history of increased intake of salt loading than of salted foods in the period prior to entry to the hospital can be elicited, while other patients resort to the use of sodium-containing remedies such as antacids. Even when such precipitating events are ruled out, it is evident that there is a poor relationship between abnormalities in renal sodium handling and the presence or absence of "compensation." As discussed elsewhere (6), it is not possible to predict the presence or magnitude of the impairment of renal sodium handling in the cirrhotic patient merely on the basis of the absence of ascites and/or edema.

Portions of this chapter are adapted with permission from Epstein M: Renal sodium handling in liver disease. In: *The Kidney in Liver Disease*, 3rd ed. Williams & Wilkins, Baltimore, pp 3–30, 1988.

Finally, it should be emphasized that the primary renal excretory abnormality causing fluid retention is a disturbance of sodium, rather than water excretion. Some sodium-retaining patients with ascites and edema are capable of excreting large volumes of dilute urine in response to the administration of large amounts of water without sodium. However, when sodium is administered, it is not excreted.

PATHOGENESIS

The pathogenetic events leading to the deranged sodium homeostasis of cirrhosis are exceedingly complex and remain the subject of continuing controversy. The present chapter is not intended to comprise an exhaustive review of the diverse alterations in liver structure and function, and the perturbations in circulatory homeostasis that may contribute to the renal sodium retention of liver disease. Rather, the discussion will consider the role of a diminished "effective" blood volume and the effectors that respond to these hemodynamic alterations, eventuating in renal sodium retention. It is hoped that this discussion will constitute a suitable framework for considering the therapy of ascites and edema in liver disease.

Role of diminished "effective" volume

Traditionally, it has been proposed that ascites formation in cirrhotic patients begins when a critical imbalance of Starling forces in the hepatic sinusoids and splanchnic capillaries causes an excessive amount of lymph formation, exceeding the capacity of the thoracic duct to return this lymph to the general circulation. Consequently, excess lymph accumulates in the peritoneal space as ascites, with a subsequent contraction of the circulating plasma volume. Thus, as ascites develops, there is a progressive redistribution of plasma volume. While total plasma volume may be increased in this setting, the physiologic circumstance may mimic a reduction in plasma volume (a reduced "effective" plasma volume). The diminished "effective" volume is thought to constitute an afferent signal to the renal tubule to augment salt and water reabsorption. Thus, the traditional formulation suggests that the renal retention of sodium was a secondary rather than a primary event.

In this context, it is important to underscore that the term *effective plasma volume* refers to that part of the total circulating volume that is effective in stimulating volume receptors. The concept is somewhat elusive, since the actual volume receptors remain incompletely defined. A diminished "effective" volume may reflect subtle alterations in systemic hemodynamic factors, such as decreased filling of the arterial tree, a diminished central blood volume, or both. Since the stimulus is unknown and the afferent receptors are incompletely elucidated, alterations in the "effective" volume must be defined in a functional manner, such as the kinetic response to volume manipulation. In an earlier editorial, evidence has been marshalled by utilizing the clinical investigative model of head-out water immersion in support of this concept (9, 10).

Over the past two decades, an alternative hypothesis has been proposed. Lieberman and Reynolds and their associates (11, 12) proposed the overflow theory for ascites formation. In contrast to the traditional formulation, the overflow theory suggests that the primary event is the inappropriate retention of excessive sodium by the kidneys, with a resultant expansion of plasma volume. In the setting of abnormal Starling forces (both portal venous hypertension and a reduction in plasma colloid osmotic pressure) in the portal venous bed and hepatic sinusoids, the expanded plasma volume is sequestered preferentially in the peritoneal space with ascites formation. According to this formulation, therefore, renal sodium retention and plasma volume expansion precede rather than follow the formation of ascites.

Since the promulgation of the overflow theory of ascites formation, controversy has centered on which of the two hypotheses is correct (10, 13). Although I believe that the presently available evidence favors a prominent role for a diminished effective volume in mediating the avid sodium retention of many cirrhotic patients, it is important to underscore that these two formulations (i.e., diminished effective volume and overflow theory) may not be mutually exclusive. It is worth remembering that virtually all the available clinical studies of deranged sodium homeostasis were carried out at a time when decompensation was well established, with little information available during the incipient stage of sodium retention. Thus, it is possible to reconcile these two ostensibly differing formulations by viewing the pathogenesis of abnormal sodium retention in cirrhosis as a complex clinical constellation in which differing forces participate in varying degrees as the derangement in sodium homeostasis evolves. It is conceivable that a primary defect in renal sodium handling may assume a more prominent role in the early stages of cirrhosis, and a more diminished effective volume may constitute the major determinant of sodium retention in many patients, once the derangement is established.

The effectors of renal sodium retention

The initial attempts to explain the abnormalities of renal sodium handling focused on the decrement in the glomerular filtration rate (GFR) that occurs frequently in patients with advanced liver disease (5). A number of observations indicate, however, that a decrease in GFR cannot constitute the major determinant of the abnormalities in renal sodium handling. Many observers have reported that derangements in renal sodium reabsorption have been observed even in the face of supranormal GFR (7, 14). The weight of evidence demonstrates that the renal sodium retention accompanying cirrhosis is attributable primarily to enhanced tubular reabsorption rather than to alterations in the filtered load of sodium.

The mediators of the enhanced tubular reabsorption of sodium in cirrhosis and their relative participation in the avid sodium retention have not been elucidated completely. Several hormonal, neural and hemodynamic mechanism(s) have been suggested. Those mechanism(s) for which there is some evidence, and their interrelationships, are summarized schematically in Figure 1.

The demonstration that cirrhotic patients manifest in-

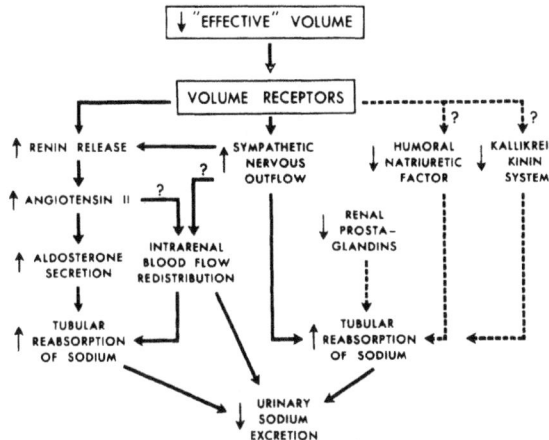

Figure 1. Schematic drawing of possible mechanisms whereby a diminished "effective" volume results in sodium retention. The heavy arrows indicate pathways for which evidence is available, the dashed lines represent proposed pathways, the existence of which remains to be established. Modified with permission from Epstein M. Renal sodium handling in liver disease. In: *The Kidney in Liver Disease*, 3rd ed. Williams & Wilkins, Baltimore, pp 3–30, 1988.

creased levels of aldosterone in the urine and plasma prompted many observers to propose that aldosterone is a major determinant of sodium retention. A number of recent studies have questioned the validity of such a formulation, suggesting that the elevated plasma aldosterone (PA) levels and the sodium retention of cirrhosis are *pari passu* events and are not necessarily etiologically related. As discussed in a recent review (6), dissociations between sodium excretion and PA have been demonstrated repeatedly in cirrhotic patients. Taken together, the evidence presently available, therefore, favors the postulate that the hyperaldosteronism of cirrhosis is a permissive factor only and that the predominant component of the abnormal renal sodium handling is a diminished distal delivery of filtrate. Only when distal filtrate delivery is enhanced by an experimental or pharmacologic maneuver does aldosterone exert a major role in renal sodium handling in cirrhosis.

The demonstration that hyperaldosteronism cannot account completely for sodium retention in cirrhosis has prompted a search for other hormonal mediators that participate in this derangement. Within the past several years, increasing evidence has accumulated suggesting that renal prostaglandins constitute important contenders in this regard. The administration of inhibitors of prostaglandin synthetase (both indomethacin and ibuprofen) has been reported to induce significant decrements in GFR and renal plasma flow (ERPF) in patients with alcoholic liver disease (15, 16). Of interest, the decrement in renal hemodynamics varied directly with the degree of sodium retention, i.e., the patients with the most avid sodium retention manifested the largest decrements in GFR (16). Taken together, these observations suggest that renal prostaglandins constitute critical modulators of renal function during conditions or disease states involving volume contraction, including cirrhosis. According to this formulation, any impairment of renal prostaglandin synthesis, such as the administration of prostaglandin synthetase inhibitors, would potentiate renal sodium retention.

THE MANAGEMENT OF ASCITES AND EDEMA IN LIVER DISEASE

The role of diuretics

As a consequence of the events enumerated above, the renal retention of sodium eventuates as clinically manifest ascites and edema. Ascites is associated with many unwanted side effects in patients with liver disease (18). Conn has proposed a causal relationship between ascites and both high portal pressure and gastroesophageal reflux (18). According to this fomulation, ascites enhances the possibility of variceal bleeding by favoring both rupture of varices and reflux, with a resultant erosion of the varices. While such a relationship had not been clearly established, such formulations underscore the general clinical notion that ascites per se is detrimental and requires relief. Furthermore, it has been suggested that ascites is the *sine qua non* of spontaneous bacterial peritonitis (19). Finally, the frequent association of ascites with the development of the hepatorenal syndrome raises the possibility that ascites may play an important role in its pathogenesis.

While ascites is indeed the "...root of much evil" (18), the decision to relieve ascites with diuretic agents should not be automatic. On the other hand, several studies suggest that diuretic therapy in the cirrhotic patient may be associated with a substantial risk of adverse effects. Sherlock surveyed diuretic-related complications occurring in a group of cirrhotic patients treated from 1962 to 1965 and reported an incidence of encephalopathy varying from 22% to 26% (depending on the diuretic used), hyponatremia varying from 40% to 49%, and azotemia (BUN > 40 mg/100 ml) ranging from 20% to 40% (20). The incidence of hypokalemia was marked (as high as 64%), and this complication persisted, albeit at a much lessened frequency, in spite of concomitant administration of potassium-sparing diuretics such as spironolactone and amiloride. While it may be argued that this 16-year-old survey may be unrepresentative and that this study was uncontrollable in nature, recent prospective reports from drug surveillance programs suggest that diuretic-induced complications still constitute formidable problems even today (21, 22). Such reports commend our consideration of nondiuretic approaches to the management of ascites.

A rational approach to management

The initial goal of any treatment program should be an attempt to obtain weight loss resulting from a spontaneous diuresis in association with consistent and scrupulous adherence to a well-balanced diet with rigid dietary sodium restriction (250 mg/day). It should be emphasized that the sodium intake prescribed for cardiac patients (1200–1500 mg daily) is not sufficiently restrictive for the cirrhotic patient who continues to gain weight on such a regimen. Since cirrhotic patients often excrete as little as 5–10 mEq of sodium per day, it is evident that a 1500 mg sodium diet (i.e., 65 mEq sodium) will result in a net positive sodium balance of 420 mEq/week, with an attendant weight gain of 3 kg.

While the frequency with which such dietary management successfully relieves ascites is unsettled, such a diet should be prescribed to all hospitalized patients, since it is impossible to predict which patients will respond favorably. When the response to dietary management is inadequate, or when the imposition of rigid dietary sodium restriction is not feasible due to cost or unpalatability of the diet, the use of diuretic agents may be considered.

The rational basis of diuretic therapy lies in an understanding of the mechanism(s) and sites of action of the diuretic agent, coupled with an understanding of the pathophysiology of sodium retention in cirrhosis. Since the attributes and efficacy of the varying diuretic agents have been reviewed in detail elsewhere (23, 24), this chapter will focus solely on therapeutic considerations that are unique to the cirrhotic patient. When diuretics are used, the therapeutic aim is a slow and gradual diuresis that does not exceed the capacity for mobilization of ascitic fluid. Shear et al. (26) have demonstrated that ascites absorption averages about 300–500 ml/day during spontaneous diuresis and has as its upper limits 700–900 ml/day. Thus, any diuresis that exceeds 900 ml/day (in the ascitic patient without edema) must perforce be mobilized at the expense of the plasma compartment, with resultant volume contraction.

Finally, the dangers of diuretic-associated hypokalemia should be emphasized. Since total body potassium depletion is often associated with cirrhosis (27), the use of any diuretic that acts proximally to the distal potassium-secretory site may result in profound hypokalemia. Because of the frequently observed temporal relationship between diuretic therapy and the induction of hepatic encephalopathy, and the probability that the enhanced renal ammonia production of hypokalemia may be related to the encephalopathy (27), great care should be exercised in monitoring potassium derangements in the cirrhotic patient receiving diuretics. The overriding consideration, however, in diuretic therapy is that its use for the sole indication of cosmetic improvement is clearly contraindicated.

PARACENTESIS

The role of paracentesis in the treatment of ascites, with or without simultaneous plasma volume expansion, remains controversial. The potential renal benefit of a reduction of ascitic fluid volume includes diminished intraabdominal pressure with possible relief of inferior vena cava obstruction and augmentation of cardiac output. The improvement in renal function, when it occurs, is transient, and because the abnormal hydraulic pressures that sustain ascites formation are not altered by paracentesis, continued fluid removal is necessary and may result in progressive depletion of intravascular volume with subsequent deterioration in cardiac function and renal perfusion. Nevertheless, recent reports indicate that paracentesis may induce a more favorable response than previously thought (28–30).

TREATMENT WITH EXTRACORPOREAL DEVICES

Ascites reinfusion

Because sodium retention in cirrhosis is linked to increased renal tubular sodium reabsorption in response to a contracted "effective" plasma volume, a physiologic approach to its correction has been to expand plasma volume (5). A profound diuresis often follows infusions of colloid solutions, such as albumin or plasma, to patients with severe ascites. An inexpensive alternative method of expanding plasma volume is to withdraw ascitic fluid with a peritoneal catheter and reinfuse it into the systemic circulation. An effective diuresis is often obtained, especially when ascites reinfusion is used concomitant with diuresis (33). This approach, however, is time consuming, awkward, and is occasionally associated with fever, coagulopathy, and bacteremia.

In 1971, the Rhodiascit machine was introduced to facilitate ascites reinfusion in patients with severe ascites. This device consists of sterile disposable I.V. tubing, a pump, and a membrane that concentrates the ascitic fluid two- to fourfold prior to its reinfusion to a peripheral vein. Experience with this procedure has been extensive in Europe, but it has not achieved widespread use in the United States (34). Complications include fever, sepsis, congestive heart failure, coagulopathy, and gastrointestinal bleeding. No controlled trials have compared the Rhodiascit technique with conventional diuretic management in terms of morbidity, mortality, and cost.

Several practical considerations preclude use of the Rhodiascit machine in all massively ascitic patients. Although this procedure is capable of rendering patients nearly ascites free and can be repeated at monthly intervals, its use may be attended by the aforementioned complications. The presence of severe heart disease may result in a worsening of congestive failure due to the large (200–400 ml/hr) volumes reinfused. Thus, the presence of severe renal failure, which might limit a protective increase in urine flow rate, is a relative contraindication. Severe hepatic decompensation with prolongation by greater than 3–5 seconds of the prothrombin time (PT) or the presence of encephalopathy renders the prognosis poor. The ascites problem must then be put in perspective with the other aspects of the patient's liver failure. A careful review of the coagulation status, including PT, activated partial thromboplastin time, fibrinogen, thrombin time, platelet count bleeding time, and euglobulin lysis time, should be performed in conjunction with a diagnostic paracentesis in the 24–48 hours prior to infusion.

Procedure. On the morning of the procedure, using local anesthesia, an intraabdominal pediatric dialysis catheter is placed. The machine is primed with normal saline, the pump started, and finally the postmembrane concentrate (when the initial saline has drained through the tubing system) is reinfused via a peripheral intravenous line. By means of pressure and resistance adjustments, a hydrostatic head of pressure is maintained in the membrane chamber to effect concentration of the ascitic fluid. Since the pore size permits passage only of molecules with a molecular weight less than 45,000, the dialysate is a clear fluid with a protein concentration of less than 5 mg/dl. The concentrations of sodium, chloride, and potassium are similar to those of the patient's plasma. The infusion is continued from 4 to 15 hours, depending on patient need and tolerance of the infusion.

As an example of the efficacy of this procedure, Inoue et al. (35) reported their experience in the treatment of intractable ascites by continuous reinfusion of sterile, cell-free, concentrated ascites. Their apparatus consisted of a cellulose acetate hollow-fiber filter and a polyacrylonitrile hollow-fiber ultrafilter with their respective pumps.

Role of LeVeen shunt

One of the recent advances in the management of the patient with ascites and edema formation is the availability of the LeVeen peritoneovenous (P-V) shunt (36–38). Since the underlying abnormality in patients with ascites and sodium retention is not solely an excess of fluid, but rather a maldistribution of ECF, much attention has focused on developing procedures that might redistribute body fluid between compartments, so that the central compartment is replenished at a time when ascites is decreasing. Earlier attempts at autogenous reinfusion of ascites have proven too cumbersome a technique to constitute a useful form of therapy. In 1974, LeVeen and associates resolved many of the technical problems associated with maintaining shunt patency by developing a one-way valve activated by a pressure gradient (36). The success of the new valve in facilitating continuous P-V shunting of ascitic fluid and the technical simplicity of its insertion has resulted in its widespread acceptance. Recently, an additional ascites valve based on a modification of the hydrocephalus valve has been introduced, i.e., the Denver shunt (37).

There is no question that peritoneovenous shunting has been demonstrated to constitute a highly efficacious means to relieve massive ascites rapidly. Nevertheless, the role of the peritoneovenous shunt in altering the natural history of refractory ascites is unclear. Despite its widespread usage, little specific data are currently available concerning either the efficacy of the peritoneovenous shunt or its appropriate use in the treatment of ascites. Furthermore, there is increasing awareness that the widespread utilization of the P-V shunt has been attended by a wide array of complications (37–43). As noted in an earlier editorial (38), once again we seem to have erred. We are quick enough to develop and apply new techniques, but not in any hurry to evaluate them rigorously.

Another factor that should be weighed in any decision on the suitability of shunting is the question of patient compliance. It should be emphasized that the patient's cooperation and compliance is a requisite ingredient in the successful application of the peritoneovenous shunt. If a patient has intractable ascites on the basis of noncompliance, it is unlikely that he or she will be benefited by a peritoneovenous shunt; rather, the patient is very likely to have recurrent "intractable" ascites, which is aggravated by the superimposed complication of an intraperitoneal and intravenous foreign body. Furthermore, it should be remembered that a functioning peritoneovenous shunt is not a panacea. In most patients, diuretics and dietary sodium restriction continue to constitute a requisite part of the therapeutic regimen (37). Respiratory exercises initiated in the postoperative period may have to be continued for an indefinite period of time, even after the patient's abdominal muscles regain their tone. An abdominal binder may be necessary for a prolonged period of time. Failure to comply with any of these facets of the regimen may completely obviate the benefits of peritoneovenous shunting with a recurrence of ascites.

In this author's opinion, given the constraints mentioned above, the P-V shunt should be used less frequently and with greater forethought than is the case today. The shunt should be reserved for ascitic patients whose conditions are truly refractory to a regimen of moderate doses of diuretic, with concomitant dietary sodium restriction following an adequate trial. Such patients with intractable ascites may be less common than we have been led to believe. Greenlee et al. (39) reported on their extensive experience on the management of ascites over a 40-month period and observed that only 4.5% of cirrhotic patients with ascites failed to respond to intensive medical therapy (diuretics together with dietary sodium restriction) with a decrease in ascites. Furthermore, cognizance of the numerous ancillary requirements for successful functioning of the shunt, including continuing diuretics and dietary sodium restriction, respiratory exercises, and an abdominal binder, mandates that the procedure be reserved for compliant patients.

Dialytic ultrafiltration of ascites

An alternative approach to the patient with refractory ascites has been ultrafiltration of ascitic fluid with reinfusion of the concentrate into the peritoneal cavity (44, 45). This procedure, like that using the Rhodiascit machine, removes salt and water from ascitic fluid without loss of protein. In contrast, volume overload does not occur because the ascitic fluid is not reinfused into the vascular compartment. Two catheters (or one double-lumen catheter) are inserted into the peritoneal cavity. Ascitic fluid is removed through one of the catheters by means of a roller pump and circulated through the ultrafilter. The concentrated, protein-rich, ascitic fluid is then returned to the abdominal cavity.

Ultrafiltration of ascites is associated with small but significant increases in cardiac output and stroke volume. In addition, the patient's responsiveness to diuretics may improve dialytic ultrafiltration of ascites.

Dialysis and hemofiltration

Intermittent forms of therapy have been the classical means of support in renal failure: isolated ultrafiltration for fluid management and intermittent hemodialysis for electrolyte, acid/base, and azotemic control. More recently, variations of these basic procedures have led to combinations of therapy that enhance patient stability and allow for greater control of biochemical and volume variables.

Currently, continuous extracorporeal therapeutic modalities have been applied to various selected patients (46, 47). These methods permit an enhanced level of fluid and solute removal in association with hemodynamic stability, and have been applied to the sicker, unstable patient with multiorgan failure. In addition, fluid balance is improved, permitting a higher intake to be achieved with much less risk of fluid overload. Increased experience with these therapies, as well as greater awareness of their capabilities, have prompted several groups to apply them to the treatment of the renal complications of liver disease.

Intermittent hemodialysis has been used for the treatment of ascites. This procedure, however, may be attended by hemodynamic instability and bleeding, and fluid removal is difficult. Recently, slow continuous ultrafiltration (SCUF), continuous arteriovenous hemofiltration (CAVH), and continuous arteriovenous hemodialysis (CAVHD) have been introduced for the removal of fluids and solutes in critically ill patients with hemodynamic instability. These procedures utilize small filters with a membrane that is highly permeable to water and low molecular weight solutes. With SCUF and CAVH, the patient's own blood pressure is usually sufficient to maintain filtration, and a high rate of fluid removal (0.4–12 l/hr) can be achieved. We recently (48) utilized CAVU for the treatment of refractory ascites in a patient with advanced liver cirrhosis. The procedure safely induced a negative fluid balance of 4 l and restored the sensitivity to diuretics without causing hypotension, bleeding, or decreases in renal function.

This author believes that SCUF or CAVH may prove to have a valuable role in the management of some patients with massive ascites. Since information concerning these emerging modalities is not yet readily available to clinicians, a brief overview of these techniques follows.

CAVH requires the use of either temporary access to the circulation (via femoral catheters) or a semipermanent Scribner shunt. Blood propelled by the patient's own arterial pressure flows through a low-resistance hemofilter and returns to the patient through the venous limb.

Heparinization of the device is necessary to prevent clotting.

The ultrafiltrate formed is collected into a plastic bag. According to the need for fluid removal, part of the ultrafiltrate is replaced by intravenous administration of a solution such as isotonic NaCl or Ringer's lactate. Replacement fluid can be infused together with heparin through a port that is either proximal to the hemofilter (predilution) or distal to the venous limb (postdilution).

Treatment continues around the clock until ultrafiltration is no longer needed. It is not unusual for a patient to be treated for several days. For example, using the postdilution technique with CAVH, urea clearance approximates the amount of filtrate that is replaced. Thus, clearance would be about 12 l/day.

In conclusion, the optimal treatment of truly intractable ascites has not been established. The dialytic techiques discussed above are easier to institute and may occasionally result in a return of responsiveness to diuretics. On the other hand, the peritoneal-venous shunt (PVS) provides a more permanent solution but entails more risk and expense. Additional controlled studies will be necessary in order to establish the optimal therapeutic modality in these patients.

The choice of dialytic technique in the management of

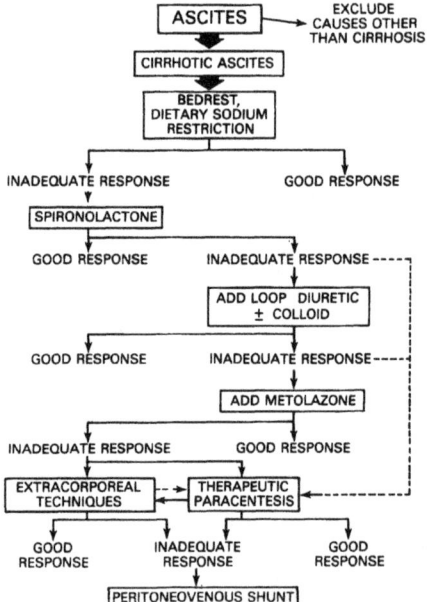

Figure 2. Algorithm for the comprehensive management of cirrhotic ascites. The solid lines represent therapeutic options and sequences that are believed to be well established. The interrupted lines indicate uncertainty regarding the appropriate positioning of therapeutic paracentesis in the therapeutic sequence. Reproduced with permission from M. Epstein (ed): *The Kidney in Liver Disease*, 3rd ed. Williams & Wilkins, Baltimore p 549, 1988.

intractable ascites also remains undefined. Each of them has specific advantages and limitations. As mentioned, ascites infusion with the Rhodiascit machine (or similar devices), although effective in ascites removal, may be complicated by sepsis, coagulopathy, and fluid overload. Dialytic ultrafiltration of ascites avoids infusion of fluid into the vascular compartment and may be ineffective in the long term. Finally, CAVH avoids the insertion of a peritoneal catheter and intravascular infusion of ascites, but requires temporary vascular access, careful monitoring, and certainly requires further experience.

In summary, the algorithm presented in Figure 2 is suggested for the management of cirrhotic ascites. Approximately 10% of cirrhotic patients with ascites can be managed with bedrest and sodium restriction. The importance of good nutrition and abstaining from alcohol should be emphasized. The next step is the use of spironolactone in doses up to 400–600 mg/day. Combined diuretic therapy (spironolactone plus loop diuretics with or without the addition of metolazone) may induce a response in some patients but risks substantial complications. Simultaneous administration of colloid may help reduce the chance of hyponatremia and volume contraction. In some patients, especially those with peripheral edema, therapeutic paracentesis may be a reasonable alternative. For the patient who is truly refractory to the above maneuvers, the therapeutic choices include extracorporeal techniques and the peritoneovenous shunt. The former include ascites reinfusion, dialytic ultrafiltration of ascites, or continuous arteriovenous hemofiltration.

SYNDROMES OF ACUTE AZOTEMIA

Introduction

Acute renal failure occurs with increased frequency in patients with hepatic and biliary disease. While acute azotemia may often represent classic acute renal failure, cirrhotic patients may also develop a unique form of renal failure for which a specific cause cannot be elucidated — the *hepatorenal syndrome* (HRS). The following section will review the spectrum of acute azotemic syndromes, initially discussing the hepatorenal syndrome, and subsequently acute intrinsic renal failure (ATN) in the setting of hepatic and biliary disease.

THE HEPATORENAL SYNDROME

Progressive oliguric renal failure commonly complicates the course of patients with advanced hepatic disease (47, 48). While this condition has been designated by many names, including *functional renal failure* and the *renal failure of cirrhosis*, the more appealing albeit less specific term, *hepatorenal syndrome* (HRS) has been utilized commonly to describe this syndrome. For the purposes of this discussion, the hepatorenal syndrome may be defined as unexplained renal failure occurring in patients with liver disease in the absence of clinical, laboratory, or anatomic evidence of other known causes of renal failure.

Clinical features

The essential features of the HRS were first described by Austin Flint in a surprisingly up-to-date report published over a century ago (51). A review of the clinical features of HRS reveals marked variability regarding both the clinical presentation and the clinical course (49, 52). The HRS occurs usually in cirrhotic patients who are alcoholic, although cirrhosis is not a *sine qua non* for the development of HRS. HRS may complicate other liver diseases, including acute hepatitis (53) and hepatic malignancy (54). Numerous reports have emphasized the development of renal failure following events that reduce the effective blood volume, including abdominal paracentesis, vigorous diuretic therapy, and gastrointestinal bleeding, although it can occur in the absence of an apparent precipitating event. In this context, several careful observers have recently noted that HRS patients seldom arrive in the hospital with preexisting azotemia (49). Rather, HRS seems to develop in the hospital, raising questions as to whether events in the hospital might precipitate this syndrome. Virtually all HRS patients have ascites, which is often tense, and clinical stigmata of portal hypertension are usually present. The degree of jaundice is extremely variable, and it is noteworthy that occasionally renal failure may develop at a time when the serum bilirubin concentration is decreasing. Although the majority of reports suggest that the HRS occurs in patients who manifest evidence of severe hepatocellular disease, it is quite apparent that the HRS can occur with minimal jaundice and with little evidence of severe hepatic dysfunciton (55). The majority of patients have a modest decrease in systemic blood pressure, but profound hypotension occurs usually as a terminal event.

The overwhelming majority of patients with HRS die, and recoveries are sufficiently rare to be considered worthy of reporting (56). It should be noted, however, that the mortality of this syndrome may be exaggerated by the very concept, which holds that if the patient survives the episode of acute azotemia, this per se constitutes evidence that such patients did not have the hepatorenal syndrome.

HRS patients manifest a rather characteristic urine excretory pattern, voiding urine that is practically sodium free and retaining the capacity to concentrate urine to a modest degree. As seen in Table 1, the biochemical characteristics of the urine in such patients is indistinguishable from that seen in the setting of hypovolemia. Such observations underscore the importance of considering hypovolemia in any diagnostic evaluation of azotemia in the setting of liver disease.

Pathogenesis

There is compelling support for the concept that the renal failure of HRS is functional in nature. Despite the severe derangement of renal function, pathologic abnormalities

Table 1. Differential diagnosis of acute azotemia in the patient with liver disease: Important differential urinary findings

	Prerenal azotemia	Hepatorenal syndrome	Acute renal failure
Urine sodium concentration (mEq/l)	< 10	< 10	< 30
Urine/plasma creatinine	> 30 : 1	> 30 : 1	< 20 : 1
Urine osmolality	At least 100 mOsm > plasma	At least 100 mOsm > plasma	Equal to plasma osmolality
Urine sediment	Normal	Unremarkable	Cellular debris

are minimal and inconsistent. Furthermore, tubular functional integrity is maintained during the renal failure, as manifested by avid sodium reabsorption and relatively unimpaired concentrating ability. Finally, more direct evidence is derived from the demonstration that kidneys transplanted from patients with HRS are capable of resuming normal function in the recipient (57).

Despite extensive study, the precise pathogenesis of the HRS remains obscure. Our laboratory has applied the ^{133}Xe washout technique and selective renal arteriography to the study of the HRS and demonstrated a significant reduction in the calculated mean blood flow and a preferential reduction in cortical perfusion (58). In addition, cirrhotic patients manifested marked vasomotor instability, which was characterized not only by a variability between serial xenon washout studies, but also by instability within a single curve (58). This phenomenon has not been encountered in renal failure of other etiologies. In addition, Epstein and coworkers carried out simultaneous renal arteriography to delineate further the nature of hemodynamic abnormalities. Selective renal arteriograms disclosed marked beading and tortuosity of the interlobar and proximal arcuate arteries, and an absence of both distinct cortical nephrograms and of vascular filling of the cortical vessels (58). Postmortem angiography carried out on the kidneys of five patients studied previously during life disclosed a striking normalization of the vascular abnormalities with reversal of all vascular abnormalities in the kidneys (58). The peripheral vasculature filled completely, and the previously irregular vessels became smooth and regular (58). These findings provide additional strong evidence for the functional basis of the renal failure, operating through active renal vasoconstriction.

Although renal hypoperfusion with preferential renal cortical ischemia has been shown to underlie the renal failure of HRS, the factors responsible for sustaining the reduction in cortical perfusion and the suppression of filtration in HRS have not been elucidated. Several major hypotheses have been proposed that implicate or suggest a number of mediators, including: a) activation of the renin-angiotensin system, b) an increase in sympathetic nervous system activity, c) alterations in the endogenous release of prostaglandins, d) changes in the kallikrein-kinin system,

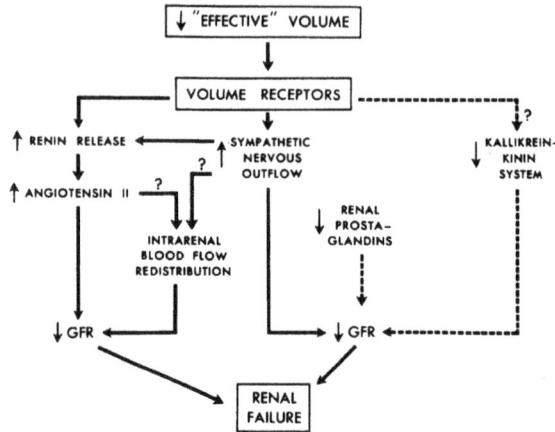

Figure 3. Schematic representation of possible mechanism whereby a diminished "effective" volume in the patient with liver disease might modulate a number of hormonal and neural effectors, eventuating in renal failure. The solid arrows indicate pathways for which evidence is available. The dashed lines represent proposed pathways, the existence of which remains to be established.

and e) endotoxemia. These proposed mechanisms and their possible interrelationships are summarized schematically in Figure 3.

ACUTE INTRINSIC RENAL FAILURE

Although much attention has been directed to the HRS, it should be borne in mind that cirrhotic patients are not less vulnerable than noncirrhotic patients to the development of acute intrinsic renal failure (ATN). Indeed, a review of several published series disclosed that among liver disease patients who developed renal failure, the etiology of the renal failure was more commonly ATN than the HRS (59). The increased frequency of ATN may relate to the hypotension, bleeding dyscrasias, infection, and multiple metabolic disorders that complicate the course of these patients. Finally, the association between obstructive jaundice and ATN merits comment. Dawson noted that of patients undergoing operation for the relief of obstructive jaundice, the incidence of acute renal failure was many times greater than that encountered in a comparable group of non-jaundiced patients (60). It was further noted that the greater the degree of jaundice, the greater the risk of ATN. It should be noted, however, that there is a lack of unanimity of opinion regarding the uniqueness of the association of biliary tract disease and ATN (61).

Differential diagnosis

The abrupt onset of oliguria in a cirrhotic patient does not necessarily imply the presence of HRS. Prerenal causes are important to differentiate, particularly since they constitute reversible conditions if recognized and treated in the incipient phase. Volume contraction or cardiac pump failure may present as a "pseudohepatorenal" syndrome. Furthermore, as already mentioned, it is not uncommon for patients with alcoholic cirrhosis to develop classic ATN. In many instances the differentiation from HRS can be made readily by recognition of the precipitating event and by characteristic laboratory findings. Table 1 lists laboratory features helpful in differentiating the three principal causes of acute azotemia in the patient with liver disease. The most uniform finding in the urine of HRS patients is a strikingly low sodium concentration, usually less than 10 mEq/l, and occasionally as low as 2–5 mEq/l. Similarly, prerenal azotemia is associated with low urinary sodium concentrations. In contrast, patients with oliguric ATN frequently have urinary sodium concentrations exceeding 30 mEq/l, and usually even higher. Both HRS and prerenal azotemia exhibit a well-maintained urinary concentrating ability, characterized by a urine to plasma osmolality ratio (U/Posm) > 1.0, whereas ATN patients excrete an isoosmotic urine. The urine to plasma creatinine ratio (U/P creatinine) is > 30 in both prerenal failure and HRS, whereas U/P creatinine is < 20:1 in ATN. Proteinuria is absent or minimal in HRS.

In summary, the finding of a low urinary sodium concentration in the presence of oliguric acute renal failure precludes the diagnosis of ATN. Only when prerenal failure and ATN are excluded, can one establish the diagnosis of HRS.

Treatment

The management of the HRS has been discouraging in view of the absence of any effective treatment modality until now. Since knowledge about the pathogenesis of HRS is inferential and incomplete, therapy to the present time has been supportive. Accumulating evidence, however, has pointed to a very significant iatrogenic component in the pathogenesis of this syndrome.

The initial step in management (Table 2) is not to equate decreased renal function with HRS, but rather to search diligently for and to treat correctable causes of azotemia such as volume contraction, cardiac decompensation, and urinary tract obstruction. The diagnosis of

Table 2. Principles of management of the patient with hepatorenal syndrome

I. General measures
   1. Try not to make the diagnosis
   2. *Primum non nocere*
II. Specific therapeutic measures
   1. Ascites reinfusion
   2. Infusion of vasodilators
      a. Prostaglandins A_1 and E
      b. Dopamine
   3. Portacaval shunting
   4. Dialysis
   5. Hepatic transplantation
   6. Le Veen (peritoneovenous) shunt

Table 3. Drugs that may adversely affect renal function in the patient with liver disease

1. Nonsteroidal antiinflammatory drugs
2. Diuretics
3. Demeclocycline
4. Lactulose

ATN (vasomotor nephropathy) should be considered, since cirrhotic patients with ATN may recover if supported with dialytic therapy (49).

While we commonly invoke the caveat of *primum non nocere*, it takes on greater meaning than it had in earlier times. Our increasing knowledge of the effects of numerous drugs in the setting of liver disease has now amplified the myriad ways whereby such agents may actually induce acute renal failure in the cirrhotic patient (Table 3). Thus, it is well established that nonsteroidal antiinflammatory drugs, which inhibit prostaglandin synthetase activity, are all capable of inducing detrimental effects on renal function in the patient with liver disease and ascites (15, 16). Similarly, the broad-spectrum antibiotic, demeclocycline, has been shown to be capable of inducing acute azotemia in the patient with cirrhosis and ascites (62–64). Finally, we should be cognizant of the fact that drugs that may be indicated for the management of complications of liver disease (i.e., lactulose for the treatment of hepatic encephalopathy) are capable of inducing profound hypovolemia with resultant azotemia. Clearly, we are encountering ever-increasing "diseases of medical progress" in the management of the patient with advanced liver disease.

Once the correctable causes of renal functional impairment are excluded, the mainstay of therapy is careful restriction of sodium and fluid intake. While a number of specific therapeutic measures have been attempted, none have proved to be of practical value (see Table 2). Attempts at volume expansion with different exogenous expanders have resulted in only transient improvement in renal hemodynamics and function without significant improvement in the outcome. Similarly, attempts at reinfusion of ascites utilizing peritoneal fluid that has been concentrated have not provided any lasting improvement.

In view of the prominent role assigned to renal cortical ischemia in the pathogenesis of HRS, it is not altogether surprising that there have been numerous attempts to treat HRS with vasodilators. The widest experience has been with the infusion of prostaglandins A and E (64, 65) and dopamine (66). While such therapeutic manipulations have occasionally resulted in salutary effects on renal function, the benefits have not been sustained.

TREATMENT OF HRS WITH INVASIVE PROCEDURES

Dialytic techniques

Although dialysis has been reported to be ineffective in the management of HRS (67), it may be helpful and is warranted in certain patients (*vide infra*).

Peritoneal dialysis

There are few published data concerning the treatment of HRS with peritoneal dialysis (68–70). Of a total of 47 patients with fulminant hepatic failure and HRS treated with peritoneal dialysis, there were only four survivors. In patients with cirrhosis, only 1 of 35 patients survived. Ring-Larsen et al. (68) reported 12 patients with cirrhosis and five with acute hepatic insufficiency and HRS who were treated with peritoneal dialysis in order to correct hyponatremia. Several patients had hepatic encephalopathy. Despite correction of the electrolyte abnormalities, all of the patients died within a few days.

Included among the difficulties in instituting peritoneal dialysis in the HRS are a) coagulopathy requiring surgical rather than percutaneous placement of the catheter; b) ascites, making the exchanges more inefficient and augmenting protein losses; and c) insufficient rates of solute clearance.

Hemodialysis and ultrafiltration

Several investigators have reported that hemodialysis is ineffective in the management of HRS (67, 71–73). Our own recent experience, however, suggests that such a condemnation should be qualified (74). Although most of the published literature indeed suggests a dismal prognosis for patients with chronic end-stage liver disease, our experience and that of others (70) suggests that in carefully selected patients, i.e., patients with acute hepatic dysfunction, in whom there is reason to believe that the underlying liver disease may reverse (making long-term survival and even spontaneous recovery of renal function possible), dialytic therapy is indicated.

Potential advantages and disadvantages of dialysis in patients with decompensated liver disease (Table 4). The possible beneficial effects of dialysis in the setting of the hepatorenal syndrome include correction of fluid, electrolyte, and acid-base abnormalities; correction of the platelet defect of uremia; and removal of toxic metabolites that may contribute to hepatic (such as ammonia, mercaptans, amino acids, and octopamine) and/or uremic encephalopathy. Potential disadvantages include dialysis-induced hypotension, increased risk of infection, worsening of coagulopathy, and changes in drug-protein binding.

Dialysis may correct pulmonary edema in patients requiring fluids for the treatment of shock or coagulopathy. In addition, the removal of excess fluid may permit the daily administration of adequate amounts of parenteral nutrition.

Portacaval shunt

In 1970, Schroeder et al. (75) reported the recovery of a 42-year-old woman with HRS following side-to-side portacaval anastomosis. This group has subsequently performed a portacaval shunt in an additional four patients with HRS with a reversal of the azotemia in 3 of the 4 patients (Schroeder et al., personal communication). A similar reversal of HRS has been reported by Ariyan et al. (76) in an elderly patient with cirrhosis of unknown etiology following side-to-side portacaval anastomosis. Although these beneficial effects have been attributed to a hemodynamic redistribution with the "normalization" of a diminished "effective" blood volume, such a hypothesis remains to be validated. In summary, while preliminary results are encouraging, careful consideration will be required to establish criteria and indications for future therapeutic attempts at treating HRS with "decompression," and consideration should be given to a controlled prospective study for delineating the role of this therapeutic modality in the treatment of HRS.

Peritoneovenous shunts. In 1974, Leveen and associates introduced peritoneovenous shunts (PVS) for the treatment of refractory ascites (36). Recently, there has been a flurry of enthusiasm for the use of the peritoneovenous shunt (LeVeen shunt) in the management of HRS (37, 77). Since the underlying abnormality is thought to be a maldistribution of ECF with a resultant diminished "effective" blood volume (30), attention had focused on developing procedures that might redistribute body fluids between compartments, so that the central compartment is replenished at a time when ascites is decreasing. Earlier attempts at autogenous reinfusion of ascites have proven to be too cumbersome to constitute a useful form of therapy. With the development of a one-way valve activated by a pressure gradient that facilitates continuous shunting of ascitic fluid (28), this valve has been utilized in patients with HRS. Recently, there have been a number of reports suggesting a reversal of the HRS following P-V shunting (37, 77). Subsequently, these authors reported five long-term survivals in nine patients with HRS treated with the PVS (77). Other reports that followed (78–81) claimed long-term survival rates approaching 40%. Nevertheless, careful scrutiny of the reported cases reveals that diagnosis of HRS was frequently inadequately documented and that many of the original cases were included in subsequent series (38). The only clear-cut beneficial results in patients with carefully established HRS were those of Schroeder et al. (78). Four of their five cases

Table 4. Theoretical advantages and disadvantages of dialysis in combined renal and hepatic failure

Advantage	Disadvantage
Correction of fluid and electrolyte disturbances	Dialysis-induced hypotension
Improvement in platelet function	Increased risk of infection
Improvement in hepatic coma	Worsening of coagulopathy
Normalization of plasma amino acid levels	Lack of correction of ascites
Facilitated administration of nutritional supplements	
Removal of endotoxin fragments	Changes in drug-protein binding

treated in this manner experienced long-term survival; nevertheless, all of their patients exhibited creatinine clearances greater than 50 ml/min prior to shunting, suggesting that they were treated at a very early stage of the HRS.

Only two prospective randomized studies of the role of PVS in the treatment of HRS have been performed (81, 82). Linas et al. (81) prospectively compared the effects of the PVS (n = 10) or medical therapy (n = 10) on renal function and mortality in 20 patients with HRS associated with alcoholic liver disease. After 48–72 hours, body weight and serum creatinine were increased with medical therapy and decreased (from 3.6 ± 0.4 to 3.0 ± 0.5; $p < 0.05$) in patients with the shunt. Despite improvement of renal function, only one patient with the PVS had a prolonged survival (210 days). In the remainder, survival was 13.0 ± 2.2 days, compared with 4.0 ± 0.6 days with medical therapy.

The preliminary results of the VA Cooperative Study are also available (82). Although there were seven long-term survivals in a group of 14 patients treated with PVS, the results were not statistically significant when compared with the results of a group of 19 patients undergoing medical therapy. The mean half-life of patients treated with the shunt did not differ significantly from that of controls. Of note, the group of patients with the HRS was carefully selected, and patients with severe complications of chronic liver disease were excluded. From the above information, it can be concluded that the role of the PVS in the treatment of HRS has not been established. Although some patients exhibit an improvement in renal function, further controlled studies with larger numbers of patients are necessary to access the effect of the PVS on long-term survival, quality of life, and the incidence of complications.

Hepatic transplantation

This is the ultimate modality of therapy that results in correction not only of the HRS (83), but also of many of the metabolic complications of advanced liver disease. Obviously the procedure is complicated, expensive, and performed in only a few centers around the world.

Alcoholic cirrhosis is the most common form of cirrhosis in North America and many parts of Western Europe, and is the leading cause of hepatic mortality and morbidity. Despite the magnitude of the problem, alcoholics have made up only a tiny percentage of patients who have undergone liver transplantation. The major deterrent has been concern that alcoholics would not be abstinent post-transplantation and would not maintain the disciplined life style and aftercare necessary for successful management.

A recent report by Starzl et al. (84) has placed this question in a new light. The latter investigators reported that of 41 alcoholic cirrhotics treated in the cyclosporine (CsA) era, 73% were alive at 1 year and 68% at between 1 to 3 years. These results are no different from those obtained in 625 adult patients who received liver transplants for other reasons. These newer considerations suggest that we may wish to reassess the role of hepatic transplantation in the management of selected patients with the hepatorenal syndrome.

Water immersion

We are often asked in consultation if water immersion might be tried as a therapeutic maneuver for a patient who has been diagnosed as having the HRS. There has been an increasing awareness that the underlying abnormality in patients with decompensated cirrhosis is not solely an excess of total body fluid, but to a greater extent a maldistribution of extracellular fluid. Consequently, much attention has been focused on developing procedures to redistribute body fluids, not only between compartments, as with the PVS, but also within the vascular compartment.

Studies from our laboratory have provided substantial evidence that head-out water immersion markedly augments central blood volume (85, 86). To the extent that diminished effective blood volume constitutes a major determinant of renal sodium retention in established liver disease, one might justifiably speculate on the use of water immersion as a means of replenishing the contracted effective volume. Although at first glance such a proposal appears attractive, repeated use of water immersion would be a time-consuming and costly procedure, requiring the continuous attendance of paramedical personnel. These clinically fragile patients, when exposed to the marked hemodynamic alterations that attend immersion, require close medical monitoring. Finally, a patient could only reasonably be immersed for a small percentage of the day, and it is unknown if this confers a lasting beneficial effect.

The "chronic" effect of water immersion on central blood volume is unknown. Certainly, water immersion constitutes a powerful and highly productive means of investigating deranged volume homeostasis in many edematous disorders, including cirrhosis. We believe, however, that at the present time, pending carefully controlled investigative studies, its application as therapy in managing patients with decompensated cirrhosis is inappropriate.

In summary, the following schema is recommended for the evaluation and management of acute renal failure in cirrhosis (Figure 4). The three important diagnostic considerations are prerenal azotemia, acute tubular necrosis, and the hepatorenal syndrome. The fractional excretion of sodium (FE_{NA}) or the urinary sodium concentration in a spot urine, and the pulmonary capillary wedge pressure (PCWP) or the central venous pressure (CVP) may help to distinguish among these diagnostic possibilities. There is, however, considerable overlap between the three categories, and often patients present with more than one diagnosis. For example, patients with HRS often exhibit acute tubular necrosis, and HRS and prerenal failure often coexist. In fact, the response to colloid infusion is the only feature that helps to differentiate the latter two conditions. Of note, because of the low peripheral resistance associated with cirrhosis, volume expansion frequently does not result in a marked increase in CVP or PCWP. Intensive hemodialysis and/or hemoperfusion is indicated for the

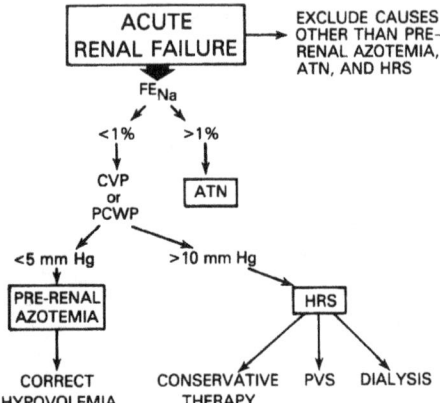

Figure 4. Algorithm for the evaluation and management of a cirrhotic patient with acute renal failure. Reproduced with permission from M. Epstein (ed): *The Kidney in Liver Disease*, 3rd ed. Williams & Wilkins, Baltimore p 113, 1988.

management of HRS complicating acute (reversible) liver injury. In patients with chronic cirrhosis, dialysis may maintain the patient until a suitable liver donor is found. Otherwise, good risk patients may be treated by the peritoneovenous shunt.

HEMODIALYSIS-ASSOCIATED HEPATITIS

With the advent of long-term dialysis as the standard treatment for end-stage renal disease, hepatitis became a seemingly inevitable accompaniment of this therapeutic approach. The magnitude of the problem can be gauged by briefly considering the following data.

In 1971 hepatitis B virus infection was endemic in 43% of the 367 dialysis centers of 24 European countries; the hepatitis B virus carrier rate at these centers was between 20% and 40%, and the infection rate among staff members was close to 30% (87, 88). The situation was even worse in the United States, where a survey of 65 dialysis centers by the National Center for Disease Control (CDC) disclosed that 82% had cases of hepatitis during 1966–1970 (89). A 1972 serologic survey of the cumulative prevalence of hepatitis B surface antigen (HBsAg) and antibody (HBsAb) in 15 U.S. centers indicated an infection rate of 55.2% among patients and 33.9% among staff (90).

Although a variety of measures have been undertaken to reduce the incidence of hepatitis B infection, one of the most promising approaches centers on the physical isolation of HBsAg-positive carriers. Thus, in 1974, a report from England noted a profound reduction in hepatitis in response to such isolation techniques (91). In 1979 there were only four cases of hepatitis from Great Britain reported to the Registry of the European Dialysis and Transplant Association of 1144 patients treated in hospitals. In contrast there were 586 cases reported of the 6624 patients treated in France, where geographic isolation was not routine (92). More recently, Najem et al. (93) reported on the experience of five hemodialysis centers in New Jersey with regard to the use of an isolation hemodialysis center. They demonstrated a marked decrease in the incidence of hepatitis B infection by isolation of antigen-positive patients. In the latter study, isolation was achieved by the use of a geographically separate isolation unit. An alternative isolation approach would be the isolation to a specifically restricted part of the dialysis unit with separate staff and equipment.

The situation is complicated by the increasing frequency of hepatitis due to the non-A, non-B viruses, for which effective testing procedures were not yet available. Should there be a second isolation unit for these patients? In the absence of test for antibody, it would be difficult to staff such units.

Although the vaccine for hepatitis B infection may solve the problem for patients infected with this virus. While extensive testing with such a vaccine has already been completed among healthy adults (94), the question of whether the findings observed in healthy subjects are applicable to other groups with an increased risk of acquiring HBV infection remains to be determined. The answer will depend in great part upon their anti-HBs response after vaccination. In light of a decreased immune response in many uremic patients, the results could not be predicted. In a recent report, however, preliminary data have become available. Stevens et al. (95), assessed the antibody responses to hepatitis B vaccine in a large group of hemodialysis patients. Although the female hemodialysis patients seemed to behave as well as healthy adults, the male patients had a much lower antibody response rate and lower titres. Thus, by extrapolation from the results of a trial in homosexual men, up to 26% of the male dialysis patients may remain unprotected, even after the full vaccine course. What actually happens will be revealed by the efficacy trial now in progress.

In the meantime, what steps toward control should be undertaken? In a recent editorial, Dean and Chalmers proposed that no new dialysis units should be allowed to be open in well-populated regions unless a separate and adequately sized unit for HBAg-positive patients is available (96). They concluded that there is no longer any excuse for continuing to treat such patients in proximity to uninfected staff and patients.

While this might constitute an ideal approach, fiscal and administrative constraints may preclude the feasibility of such an approach in most areas. An alternative approach that we have adopted with success in our own unit is offered for consideration (Table 5). In essence, we have demonstrated that rigid surveillance measures and dialysis of HBsAg-positive patients in an isolation room has been successful in minimizing dialysis-associated hepatitis in our unit. The specific measures of our program (as proposed by Dr. E. Schiff) are detailed in Table 5 for the reader's consideration.

Table 5. Infection control for viral hepatitis in a dialysis unit

Surveillance

1. Candidates for dialysis and potential employees should be screened for HBsAg, anti-HBc, anti-HBs, SGOT, and SGPT.
2. The status of HBsAg and SGOT should be known on visiting and home patients. A call to the visiting patient's unit may be necessary.
3. Patients who are negative for HBsAg, anti-HBc, and anti-HBs should be tested monthly for HBsAg, anti-HBc, SGOT, and SGPT; and every 3 months for anti-HBs.
4. Staff members who are HBsAg, anti-HBc, and anti-HBs negative should be tested every 3 months.
5. Patients and staff members confirmed on two consecutive tests as being anti-HBs positive and HBsAg negative should be tested for anti-HBs yearly.
6. Patients and staff members confirmed on two consecutive tests as being HBsAg positive should be tested every 3 months or more frequently if clinically indicated.
7. Patients and staff members who develop anti-HBc only should be tested monthly until anti-HBs develops or for 6 months in the case of staff.
8. New employees who are HBsAg positive should be reassigned to other units in the hospital.

Record keeping

1. The patient dialysis record should have
   a. Lot number of blood transfusion.
   b. Statement about blood leak, blood spills, and replacement of malfunctioning machine.
   c. The number and location of machine used for antigen treatment.
   d. The name of staff member connecting and disconnecting the patient.

Education

1. Continuing education program should be planned each year.

Control and prevention

1. HBsAg-positive patients should be isolated and dialyzed on machine reserved for HBsAg-positive patients.
2. After starting dialysis on a patient in an isolation room, staff should care only for those patients and may also care for anti-HBs-positive patients. Only in an emergency should they care for patients who have no serologic evidence of viral B infection (negative anti-HBs, anti-HBc, HBsAg).
3. Patients should be assigned to a bed number.
4. Patients should be assigned a supply tray.
5. Clamps should be disinfected for 20 minutes in cidex after all patient treatments.
6. Disposable gloves should be worn by staff when handling the patient, dialysis equipment, and accessories for their own protection. This should include taking blood pressure, administering N/S, or touching machine knobs. All of this is done for staff protection. For patient protection, the gloves should be changed between patients to prevent cross-contamination. Gloves should be worn when handling blood specimens and testing hematocrit.
7. It is good practice to wear protective glasses if splattering of blood is possible, for example, when dismantling artificial kidney from machine and to mask for possible blood aerosol.
8. Protective clothing should be worn in the unit.
9. Hepatitis precautions should be practiced in isolation room.
10. Nondisposable equipment and supplies should be sterilized after all patient treatments. Control knobs on the machine, all surface areas, and equipment should be cleaned after all patient treatments.
11. In single-path delivery system, the machine should be sterilized for 20 minutes between treatments. For recirculating single path, the machine should be cleaned between treatment according to procedure.
12. Linens should be used and changed between each treatment on beds and chairs.
13. Filters should be used and changed between treatments.
14. The staff lounge should be used for eating, drinking, and smoking.
15. Patients should not share food or ashtrays.
16. After a blood spill, the staff should immediately clean the area with one-stroke disinfectant. Blood should not be left on the floor, walls, equipment, or other surfaces. During cleaning, gloves should be worn.
17. Specimens for HBsAg-positive patients should be labeled and charts labeled.
18. Outpatients should have a selection of one meal on the unit. Inpatients should have an early breakfast and lunch on unit.
19. All new patients and visitors should have treatment on machines labeled for acute treatment until HBsAg and SGPT reports are received.
20. Any patient with SGPT or SGOT elevations should receive treatment on machine labeled for acute treatment and repeat test. If test remains elevated, patient will be placed in isolation and dialyzed on a machine reserved for non-B hepatitis.
21. Any patient with new HBsAg-positive report should be placed on acute treatment machine and should repeat the test. If test is positive for two consecutive times, the patient should be placed in isolation and dialyzed on a machine reserved for HBsAg-positive patients.
22. Patient with repeatedly HBsAg-positive reports should remain in an isolation room. Patient converting to negative HBsAg should have developed anti-HBs before being removed from isolation.
23. Patient with negative HBsAg and increased enzymes should remain in isolation until three consecutive SGPT reports within normal limits are received.
24. Patient who has received blood transfusions should have SGPT drawn every 2 weeks for 6 months.
25. Beds, chairs, stands, blood pumps, overbed tables, and heparin pumps should be cleaned between patient treatments.
26. Floors should be mopped after each shift.

GLOMERULAR CHANGES IN LIVER DISEASE

Glomerular changes occur primarily in patients with cirrhosis and acute hepatitis B virus infection.

Cirrhosis

Over 30 years ago, the first report of glomerular changes in patients with cirrhosis of the liver appeared. Subsequent studies have demonstrated that glomerular changes are quite common in patients with cirrhosis of the liver. Eknoyan has surveyed the available literature and noted that glomerular abnormalities were present in over 95% of the 116 biopsy studies reported in the literature (97). He suggested that the higher incidence of changes observed in biopsy specimens as compared with autopsy series may be a reflection of the better preservation of the tissue specimens and the higher resolution provided by electron microscopy, as the changes seen may be minor and go undetected when viewed by light microscopy alone. On a histopathologic basis, it is possible to distinguish two types of glomerular abnormalities: a) forms without proliferation and b) forms with proliferation.

The changes without proliferation are characterized by sclerosis and an increase in the mesangial matrix. Electron microscopy reveals electron-dense deposits that are mainly mesangial, but frequently extend into the subendothelial stage. It has been suggested that IgA constitutes the main immunoglobulin in the deposits, often accompanied by IgG and/or IgM. These glomerular changes are usually not associated with urinary abnormalities. However, some of these patients present with proteinuria, microscopic hematuria, or both.

GLOMERULAR CHANGES WITH PROLIFERATION

These changes are characterized by slight mesangial hypercellularity, endocapillary and extracapillary proliferation, and mesangial interposition, giving a pattern similar to that of membranoproliferative glomerulonephritis. IgA is again the major immunoglobulin, but the deposits are endomembranous. The cases with endocapillary proliferation present with a clinical picture similar to that of acute glomerulonephritis. Patients with membranoproliferative glomerulonephritis may have no urinary abnormalities or present with proteinuria and microscopic hematuria.

The pathogenesis of these glomerular changes and the relationship to the underlying hepatic disease is unsettled. While it is, of course, possible for a patient with cirrhosis to develop glomerulonephritis unrelated to his or her hepatic disease, the available evidence suggests that the glomerular changes are related to the liver disease per se. Since the major immunoglobulin in the glomerular deposits in cirrhotic patients is IgA, and since this immunoglobulin is quite uncommon in acute glomerulonephritis, it seems likely that the majority of cases of proliferative glomerulonephritis encountered in cirrhotic patients are related to the presence of hepatic disease. It has been proposed that the immunoglobulin deposits in the kidneys of these patients are the result of precipitation in the glomeruli of either aggregated immunoglobulins or circulating complexes.

Viral hepatitis

Renal morphologic and functional alterations have been reported in patients with acute and chronic viral hepatitis. In the majority of patients with acute viral hepatitis, renal function is only mildly impaired. The most common findings include a modest degree of proteinuria, hematuria, and a mild reduction in GFR. While a reduction in the renal concentrating ability has been suggested, more recent studies point to unimpaired renal concentrating ability in these patients.

Renal biopsies in patients with acute viral hepatitis reveal mild proliferative glomerulonephritis. Immunofluorescence discloses the presence of IgG, IgM, IgA, and complement as discrete nodular deposits with electron-dense deposits, primarily near the mesangial areas on electron microscopy. Although follow-up information in most of these patients is relatively limited, preliminary indications suggest that most patients with acute viral hepatitis manifest a return to normal renal function as far as GFR and proteinuria are concerned.

Hepatitis B virus infection

In contrast to acute viral hepatitis, more severe impairment of renal function has been reported in patients with persistent HB_sAg antigenemia associated with chronic active hepatitis.

Over the past decade, convincing evidence has been marshalled that infection with hepatitis B virus (HBV) may initiate an immunologic process responsible for the development of glomerular changes and chronic renal disease. Infection with the HBV nearly always produces immune reactions. Antibodies may be formed to any of the antigenic particles listed and have been termed *anti-HB_c*, *anti-HB_s*, and *anti-HB_e*. Using different methods of detection, circulating immune complexes have been demonstrated in the acute and chronic forms of infection with the virus, with HB_sAg being the more commonly identified inciting agent (98). This immune complex phenomena has been incriminated as the causative mechanism of the extrahepatic manifestations of viral hepatitis in the skin, joints, small arteries and arterioles, and renal glomeruli (99).

Since the first report of the association between HBV and membranous nephropathy in 1971 (100), there have been additional cases reported in the literature, strongly suggesting that HBV, through the immune response elicited by one of its antigens, is causally related to the development of glomerular changes in humans. Recently, Eknoyan has critically examined the clinical and laboratory data from 54 of the cases reported in sufficient detail to permit extraction of this information (97).

The characteristic glomerular lesion in such cases with

progressive deterioration of renal function has been a membranoproliferative or epimembranous glomerulonephritis. Clinically, these patients present with proteinuria, nephrotic syndrome, or renal failure. It appears, therefore, that the glomerulonephritides associated with HB_sAg hepatitis are due to an immune-complex mediated glomerulonephritis. This glomerulonephritis could be initiated either by the deposition of the HB_sAg itself in the glomerular basement membrane, or alternatively and more likely, by the circulating immune complexes formed by the binding of HB_sAg to specific antibodies in the serum and their subsequent deposition in the glomerular basement membrane. It appears that the severity of the renal lesion and its accompanying clinical disease may depend on the duration of HB_sAg-antigenemia. The prognosis of the glomerulonephritis in patients with persistent HB_sAg remains to be delineated.

The treatment of HBV-associated glomerulonephritis is unsatisfactory. In the handful of cases in which treatment with steroids or immunosuppressive drugs were attempted, therapy does not seem to have been effective. There is currently no evidence that would favor the institution of steroids or immunosuppressive agents for treatment of the renal lesions, other than what might be necessitated to treat the chronic active hepatitis that might be present in some patients.

SUMMARY

In summary, it is apparent that the renal functional abnormalities in patients with advanced liver disease constitute complex pathophysiologic constellations with numerous and diverse causes. In this chapter, the pathophysiology of several of these renal functional abnormalities has been reviewed, including deranged renal sodium and water handling, the acute azotemic syndromes, and hemodialysis-associated hepatitis. Based on these pathophysiologic considerations, an approach to the therapy of these diverse renal disorders has been proposed.

REFERENCES

1. Mortality Trends for Leading Causes of Death, United States — 1950–1969. Vital and Health Statistics, Ser. 20:26, p 4. *DHEW publication (HRA)* 74–1853.
2. Clermont RJ, Vlahcevic ZR, Chalmers TC, Adham NF, Curtis GW, Morrison RS: Intravenous therapy of massive ascites in patients with cirrhosis II. Long-term effects on survival and frequency of renal failure. *Gastroenterology* 53:220–228, 1967.
3. Epstein M: Treatment of refractory ascites. *N Engl J Med* 321:1675–1677, 1989.
4. Brown J: The philosophical transaction of the Royal Society, Vol. III. 1685, p 248.
5. Epstein M: Renal sodium handling cirrhosis. In: M Epstein, ed, *The Kidney in Liver Disease*, 3rd ed. Williams and Wilkins, Baltimore, pp 3–30, 1988.
6. Epstein M: The sodium retention of cirrhosis: A reappraisal. *Hepatology* 6:312–315, 1986.
7. Klinger EL Jr, Vaamonde CA, Vaamonde LS, Lancestremere RG, Morosi HJ, Frisch E, Papper S: Renal function changes in cirrhosis of the liver. *Arch Intern Med* 126:1010–1015, 1970.
8. Gabuzda GJ: Cirrhosis, ascites, and edema. Clinical course related to management. *Gastroenterology* 58:546–553, 1970.
9. Epstein M: Renal effects of head-out water immersion in man: Implications for an understanding of volume homeostasis. *Physiol Rev* 58:529–581, 1978.
10. Epstein M: Renal sodium handling in cirrhosis: A reappraisal. *Nephron* 23:211–217, 1979.
11. Lieberman FL, Denison EK, Reynolds TB: The relationship of plasma volume, portal hypertension, ascites and renal sodium retention in cirrhosis: The overflow theory of ascites formation. *Ann NY Acad Sci* 170:202–212, 1970.
12. Lieberman FL, Ito S, Reynolds TB: Effective plasma volume in cirrhosis with ascites. Evidence that a decreased value does not account for renal sodium retention, a spontaneous reduction in glomerular filtration rate (GFR) and a fall in GFR during drug-induced diuresis. *J Clin Invest* 48:975–981, 1969.
13. Levy M, Wexler MJ, McCaffrey C: Sodium retention in dogs with experimental cirrhosis following removal of ascites by continuous peritoneovenous shunting. *J Lab Clin Med* 94:933–946, 1979.
14. Chaimovitz C, Szylman P, Alroy G, Better OS: Mechanism of increased renal tubular sodium reabsorption in cirrhosis. *Am J Med* 52:198–202, 1972.
15. Boyer TD, Zia P, Reynolds TB: Effect of indomethacin and prostaglandin A_1 on renal function and plasma renin activity in alcoholic liver disease. *Gastroenterology* 77:215–222, 1979.
16. Zipser RD, Hoefs JC, Speckart PF, Zia PK, Horton R: Prostaglandins: Modulators of renal function and pressor resistance in chronic liver disease. *J Clin Endocrinol and Metab* 48:895–900, 1979.
17. Epstein M, Lifschitz M: Renal eicosanoids as determinants of renal function in liver disease. *Hepatology* 7:1359–1367, 1987.
18. Conn HO: Diuresis of ascites: Fraught with or free from hazard. *Gastroenterology* 73:619–621, 1977.
19. Conn HO, Fessel JM: Spontaneous bacterial peritonitis in cirrhosis. Variations on a theme. *Medicine* 50: 161–197, 1971.
20. Sherlock S: Ascites formation in cirrhosis and its management. *Scand J Gastroenterol* 7 (Suppl):9–15, 1970.
21. Naranjo CA, Pontigo E, Valdenegro C, Gonzalez G, Ruiz J, Busio V: Furosemide-induced adverse reactions in cirrhosis of the liver. *Clin Pharm Therap* 25:154–160, 1979.
22. Spino M, Sellers EM, Kaplan HL, Stapleton C, MacLeod SM: Adverse biochemical and clinical consequences of furosemide administration. *Can Med Assoc J* 118:1513–1518, 1978.
23. Brater DC: Pharmacokinetics and pharmacodynamics in cirrhosis. In: M Epstein, ed, *The Kidney in Liver Disease*, 3rd ed. Williams & Wilkins, Baltimore, pp 551–571, 1988.
24. Berger BE, Warnock DG: Clinical uses and mechanisms of action of diuretic agents. In: BM Brenner, FC Rector, eds, *The Kidney*. WB Saunders, Philadelphia, pp 433–455, 1986.
25. Epstein M: Diuretic therapy in liver disease. In: M Epstein, ed, *The Kidney in Liver Disease*, 3rd ed. Williams & Wilkins, Baltimore, pp 537–550, 1988.
26. Shear L, Ching S, Gabuzda GJ: Compartmentalization of ascites and edema in patients with hepatic cirrhosis. *N Engl J*

Med 282:1391–1396, 1970.
27. Gabuzda GJ, Hall PW III: Relation of potassium depletion to renal ammonium metabolism and hepatic coma. *Medicine* 45:481–490, 1966.
28. Arroyo V, Gines P, Planas R, Panes J, Rodes J: Paracentesis in the management of cirrhotics with ascites. In: M Epstein, ed, *The Kidney in Liver Disease*, 3rd ed. Williams & Wilkins, Baltimore, pp 578–592, 1988.
29. Kao HW, Rakov NE, Savage E, Reynolds TB: The effect of large volume paracentesis on plasma volume — A cause of hypovolemia? *Hepatology* 5:403–407, 1985.
30. Pockros PJ, Reynolds TB. Rapid diuresis in patients with ascites from chronic liver disease: The importance of peripheral edema. *Gastroenterology* 90:1827–1833, 1986.
31. Simon DM, McCain JR, Bonkovsky HL, Wells JO, Hartle DK, Galambos JT: Effects of therapeutic paracentesis on systemic and hepatic hemodynamics, and on renal and hormonal function. *Hepatology* 7:423–429, 1987.
32. Flint A: A clinical report of hydro-peritoneum, based on an analysis of forty-six cases. *Am J Med Sci* 45:306–339, 1863.
33. Eknoyan G, Martinez-Maldonado M, Yuim JJ, Suki WN: Combined ascitic fluid infusion and furosemide in the management of ascites. *N Engl J Med* 282:713–717, 1970.
34. Wilkinson SP, Davidson AR, Henderson J, Williams R: Ascites reinfusion using the Rhodiascit apparatus: Clinical experience and coagulation abnormalities. *Postgrad Med* 51:585–587, 1975.
35. Inoue N, Yamazaki Z, Oda T, Sugiura M, Wada T: Treatment of intractable ascites by continuous reinfusion of the sterilized, cell-free and concentrated ascitic fluid. *Trans Am Soc Artif Intern Organs* 23:699–702, 1977.
36. LeVeen HH, Christoudias G, Ip M, Luft R, Falk G, Grosberg S: Peritoneo-venous shunting for ascites. *Ann Surg* 180:580–590, 1974.
37. Epstein M: Role of the peritoneovenous shunt in the management of ascites and the hepatorenal syndrome. In: M Epstein, ed, *The Kidney in Liver Disease*, 3rd ed. Baltimore, Williams & Wilkins, pp 593–612, 1988.
38. Epstein M: The LeVeen shunt for ascites and hepatorenal syndrome. *N Engl J Med* 302:628–630, 1980.
39. Greenlee HB, Stanley MM, Reinhardt GF: Long term results in 52 alcoholic cirrhotics with intractable ascites treated with peritoneovenous shunts (LeVeen): 24–64 months follow-up. *Arch Surg* 116:518–526, 1981.
40. Smadja C, Franco D: The LeVeen shunt in the elective treatment of intractable ascites in cirrhosis. A prospective study on 140 patients. *Ann Surg* 201:488–493, 1985.
41. Kostroff KM, Ross DW, Davis JM: Peritoneo-venous shunting for cirrhotic versus malignant ascites. *Surg Gynecol Obstet* 161:204–208, 1985.
42. Rubenstein D, McInnes I, Dudley FJ: Morbidity and mortality after peritoneo-venous shunt surgery for refractory ascites. *Gut* 26:1070–1073, 1983.
43. Greig PD, Langer BD, Blendis LM: Complications after peritoneovenous shunting for ascites. *Am J Surg* 139:125–131, 1980.
44. Adler AJ, Feldman J, Friedman EA, Berlyne GM: Use of extracorporeal ascites dialysis in combined hepatic and renal failure. *Nephron* 30:31–35, 1982.
45. Raju SF, Achord JL: The effects of dialytic ultrafiltration and peritoneal reinfusion in the management of diuretic resistant ascites. *Am J Gastroenterol* 79:308–312, 1984.
46. Lauer A, Saccaggi A, Ronco C, Belledonne M, Glabman S, Bosch JP: Continuous arteriovenous — hemofiltration in the critically ill patient: Clinical use and operational characteristics. *Ann Intern Med* 99:455–460, 1983.
47. Paganini E: Continuous replacement modalities in acute renal dysfunction. In: M Paganini, ed, *Acute Continuous Renal Replacement Therapy*. Martinus Nijhoff, Boston, 1986.
48. Epstein M, Perez GO, Bedoya LA, Molina R: Continuous arteriovenous ultrafiltration in cirrhotic patients with ascites or renal failure. *Int J Artif Organs*, 9:253–256, 1986.
49. Epstein M: Hepatorenal syndrome. In: M Epstein, ed, *The Kidney in Liver Disease*, 3rd ed. Williams & Wilkins, Baltimore, pp 89–118, 1988.
50. Epstein M: Hepatorenal syndrome. In: JE Berk, ed, *Gastroenterology*, 4th ed. WB Saunders, Philadelphia, pp 3138–3149, 1985.
51. Flint A: A clinical report on hydro-peritoneum, based on an analysis of forty-six cases. *Am J Med Sci* 45:306–339, 1863.
52. Epstein M: The Kidney in Liver Disease. In: SG, Massry, RB Glassock, eds, *Textbook of Nephrology*. Williams & Wilkins, Baltimore, pp 966–977, 1989.
53. Ritt DJ, Whelan G, Werner DJ, Eigenbrodt EH, Schenker S, Combes B: Acute hepatic necrosis with stupor or coma. *Medicine* 48:151–172, 1969
54. Vesin P, Roberti A, Viguie RR: Defaillance renale fonctionnelle terminale chez des malades atteints de cancer du foie, primitif ou secondaire, Semin Hop Paris 26:1216–1220, 1965.
55. Epstein M, Oster JR, De Velasco RE: Hepatorenal syndrome following hemihepatectomy. *Clin Nephrol* 5:128–133, 1976.
56. Goldstein H, Boyle JD: Spontaneous recovery from the hepatorenal syndrome. Report of four cases. *N Engl J Med* 272:895–898, 1965.
57. Koppel MH, Coburn JW, Mims MM, Goldstein H, Boyle JD, Rubini ME: Transplantation of cadaveric kidneys from patients with hepatorenal syndrome. Evidence for the functional nature of renal failure in advanced liver disease. *N Engl J Med* 280:1367–1371, 1969.
58. Epstein M, Berk DP, Hollenberg NK, Chalmers TC, Abrams HL, Merrill JP: Renal failure in the patient with cirrhosis. The role of active vasoconstriction. *Am J Med* 49:175–185, 1970.
59. Shear L, Kleinerman J, Gabuzda GJ: Renal failure in patients with cirrhosis of the liver. I. Clinical and pathologic characteristics. *Am J Med* 39:184–198, 1965.
60. Dawson JL: The incidence of postoperative renal failure in obstructive jaundice. *Br J Surg* 52:663–665, 1965.
61. Bismuth H, Kuntziger H, Corlette MB: Cholangitis with acute renal failure. *Ann Surg* 181:881–887, 1975.
62. Oster JR, Epstein M, Ulano HB: Deterioration of renal function with demeclocycline administration. *Curr Ther Res* 20:794–801, 1976.
63. Carrilho F, Bosch J, Arroyo V, Mas A, Viver J, Rodes J: Renal failure associated with demeclocycline in cirrhosis. *Ann Intern Med* 87:195–197, 1977.
64. Arieff AI, Chidsey CA: Renal function in cirrhosis and the effects of prostaglandin A_1. *Am J Med* 56:695–703, 1974.
65. Zusman RM, Axelrod L, Tolkioff-Rubin N: The treatment of the hepatorenal syndrome with intrarenal administration of prostaglandin E_1. *Prostaglandins* 13:819–830, 1977.
66. Bennett WM, Keffe E, Melnyk C, Mahler D, Rosch J, Porter GA: Response to dopamine hydrochloride in the hepatorenal syndrome. *Arch Intern Med* 135:964–971, 1975.
67. Perez GO, Epstein M, Oster JR: Role of dialysis and ultrafiltration in the treatment of the renal complications of liver disease. In: M Epstein, ed, *The Kidney in Liver Dis-*

ease, 3rd ed. Williams & Wilkins, Baltimore, pp 613–624, 1988.
68. Ring-Larsen H, Clausen E, Ranek L: Peritoneal dialysis in hyponatremia due to liver failure. *Scand J Gastroenterol* 8:33–40, 1973.
69. Jacobson S, Bell B: Recognition and management of acute and chronic hepatic encephalopathy. *Med Clin North Am* 57:1569–1577, 1973.
70. Wilkinson SP, Weston MJ, Parsons V, Williams R: Dialysis in the treatment of renal failure in patients with liver disease. *Clin Nephrol* 8:287–292, 1977.
71. Klinger EL Jr, Cronin RJ: Renal failure in cirrhosis of the liver; Observations during intermittent hemodialysis. Abstracts *Am Soc Artif Intern Organs* :26, 1972.
72. Coratelli P, Passavanti G, Munno I, Fumarola D, Amerio A: New trends in hepatorenal syndrome. *Kidney Int* 17:S143–S147, 1985.
73. Ellis D, Avner ED: Renal failure and dialysis therapy in children with hepatic failure in the perioperative period of orthotopic liver transplantation. *Clin Nephrol* 25:295–303, 1986.
74. Perez GO, Oster JR, Epstein M: Role of dialysis and ultrafiltration in the treatment of renal complications of liver disease. In: M Epstein, ed, *The Kidney in Liver Disease*, 3rd ed. Williams & Wilkins, Baltimore, 1988.
75. Schroeder ET, Numann PJ, Chamberlain BE: Functional renal failure in cirrhosis. Recovery after portacaval shunt. *Ann Intern Med* 72:923–928, 1970.
76. Ariyan S, Sweeney T, Kerstein MD: The hepatorenal syndrome. Recovery after portacaval shunt. *Ann Surg* 181: 847–849, 1975.
77. Kinney MJ, Schneider A, Wapnick S, Grosberg S, LeVeen HH: The 'hepatorenal' syndrome and refractory ascites: Successful therapy with the LeVeen-type peritoneal-venous shunt and valve. *Nephron* 23:228–232, 1979.
78. Schroeder ET, Anderson GH, Smulyan H: Effect of a portacaval or peritoneovenous shunt on renin in the hepatorenal syndrome. *Kidney Int* 15:54–61, 1979.
79. Fullen WD: Hepatorenal syndrome: Reversal by peritoneovenous shunt. *Surgery* 82:337–341, 1977.
80. Schwartz ML, Vogel SB: Treatment of hepatorenal syndrome. *Am J Surg* 139:370–373, 1980.
81. Linas SL, Schaefer JW, Moore EE, Good JT Jr, Giansiracusa R: Peritoneovenous shunt in the management of the hepatorenal syndrome. *Kidney Int* 30:736–740, 1986.
82. Stanley MM, Ochi S, Lee KK, Nemchausky BA, Greenlee HB, Allen JI, Allen MJ, et al.: Peritoneovenous shunting as compared with medical treatment in patients with alcoholic cirrhosis and massive ascites. *N Engl Med* 321:1632–1638, 1989.
83. Iwatsuki S, Popovtzer MM, Corman JL, Ishikawa M, Putnam CW, Katz FH, Starzl TE: Recovery from "hepatorenal syndrome" after orthotopic liver transplantation. *N Engl J Med* 289:1155–1159, 1973.
84. Starzl TE, VanThiel D, Tzakis AG, Iwatsuki S, Todo S, Marsh JW, Koneru B, et al.: Orthotopic liver transplantation for alcoholic cirrhosis. *JAMA* 260:2542–2544, 1988.
85. Epstein M. Renal effects of head-out water immersion in man: Implications for an understanding of volume homeostasis. *Physiol Rev* 58:529–581, 1978.
86. Levinson R, Epstein M, Sackner MA, Begin R: Comparisons of the effects of water immersion and saline infusion on central hemodynamics in man. *Clin Sci Mol Med* 52:343–350, 1977.
87. Soulier JP, Jungers P, Zingraff J: Virus B hepatitis in hemodialysis centers. *Adv Nephrol* 6:383–405, 1976.
88. Kleinknecht D, Courouce AM, Delons S, et al.: Prevention of hepatitis B in hemodialysis patients using hepatitis B immunoglobulin: A controlled study. *Clin Nephrol* 8:373–376, 1977.
89. Marmion BP, Tonkin RW: Control of hepatitis in dialysis units. *Br Med Bull* 38:169–179, 1972.
90. Szmuness W, Prince AM, Grady GF, et al.: Hepatitis B infection: A point-prevalence study in 15 U.S. hemodialysis centers, *JAMA* 227:901–906, 1974.
91. Decrease in the incidence of hepatitis in the dialysis units associated with prevention programmes. Public Health Laboratory Service Survey. *Br Med J* 4:751–754, 1974.
92. Kramer P, Brunner FP, Brynger H: Combined report on regular dialysis and transplantation in Europe, X, 1979. Read before the Proceedings of the European Dialysis and Transplant Association, Prague, June 11, 1980.
93. Najem GR, Louria DB, Thind IS, Lavenhar MA, Cocke DJ, Baskin SE, Miller AM, Frankel HJ, Notkin J, Jacobs MG, Weiner B: Control of hepatitis B infection: The role of surveillance and an isolation hemodialysis center. *JAMA* 245:153–157, 1981.
94. Editorial. Hepatitis B vaccine. *Lancet* 2:1229–1230, 1980.
95. Stevens CE, Szmuness W, Goodman AI, Weseley SA, Fotino M: Hepatitis B vaccine. Immune responses in haemodialysis patients. *Lancet* 2:1211–1213, 1980.
96. Deane N, Chalmers TC: Hepatitis and hemodialysis revisited. *JAMA*: 245:171–172, 1981.
97. Eknoyan GA: Glomerular abnormalities in liver disease. In: M Epstein, ed, *The Kidney in Liver Disease*, 3rd ed. Williams & Wilkins, Baltimore, pp 154–181, 1988.
98. Takekoshi Y, Tanaka M, Miyakawa Y, Yoshizawa, Takahashi K, Mayumi M: Free "small" and IgG-associated "large" hepatitis B_e antigen in the serum and glomerular capillary walls of two patients with membranous glomerulonephritis. *N Engl J Med* 300:814–819, 1979.
99. Gocke DJ: Extrahepatic manifestations of viral hepatitis. *Am J Med Sci* 270:49–52, 1975.
100. Combes B, Stastny P, Shorey J, Eigenbrodt EH, Barrera A, Hull AR, Carter NW: Glomerulonephritis with deposition of Australia antigen-antibody complexes in glomerular basement membrane. *Lancet* 2:234–237, 1971.

CHAPTER 33

Renal Complications of Pregnancy

JOHN M. DAVISON, ADRIAN I. KATZ & MARSHALL D. LINDHEIMER

INTRODUCTION

Clinicians may be consulted on the advisability of conception or continuing a pregnancy in women with renal problems, and advice is too often based on anecdotal clinical experience. To give sound advice, the clinician must appreciate that a pregnant woman is physiologically different from a nonpregnant individual, and that during pregnancy there are progressive changes in the renal system that must be understood if we are to detect, diagnose, and manage disease.

THE KIDNEY IN NORMAL PREGNANCY

Anatomic changes

Kidney length increases approximately 1 cm during normal pregnancy. More striking, however, are the anatomic changes in the calyces, renal pelvis, and ureter, which dilate markedly, often giving the erroneous impression of obstructive uropathy (1, 2).

These anatomic changes have important clinical implications:
1. Dilatation of the urinary tract may lead to collection errors in tests based on timed urine volume (e.g., 24-hour creatinine or protein excretion).
2. Urinary stasis within the ureters may contribute to the propensity of pregnant women with asymptomatic bacteriuria to develop frank pyelonephritis.
3. Acceptable norms of kidney size should be increased by 1 cm if estimated during pregnancy or immediately after delivery, and since dilatation of the ureters persists into the puerperium, elective radiologic examination of the urinary tract should be deferred until about 12 weeks after delivery.

Functional changes

RENAL HEMODYNAMICS

The glomerular filtration rate (GFR) and effective renal plasma flow (ERPF) increase to levels about 50–60% above nonpregnant values. These increases occur shortly after conception (3), and all increments are maximal in the second trimester (4, 5). There is often a reduction in GFR of 15% during the final month of the third trimester (measured as 24-hour creatinine clearance), and this must be taken into account, especially when assessing the course of pregnancy in a women with known renal disease (6) (Figure 1).

Since GFR increases without substantial alterations in the production of creatinine and urea, plasma levels of these solutes decrease. Creatinine levels fall from a nonpregnant level of 73 to 65 µM/l in the first trimester, to 51 M/l in the second trimester, and to 47 M/l in the third trimester (7). Some of the fall in plasma urea may be due to reduced protein degradation (increased anabolism) as well as increased clearance of this solute.

Average plasma urea levels of 3.5, 3.3, and 3.1 mM/l in successive trimesters, rising to 4.3 mM/l 6 weeks postpartum, have been described (8).

Awareness of these physiologic changes is important, since values considered normal in nonpregnant women may reflect decreased renal function during pregnancy. Plasma levels of creatinine and urea exceeding 75 M/l and 4.5 mM/l, respectively, should alert the clinician to investigate renal function further.

A number of other changes in normal pregnancy may be due to augmented renal hemodynamics, including increased excretion of nutrients and protein (9). With regard to nutrient excretion, particularly glucose, there is evidence that tubular reabsorption is also less efficient (10). Increased protein excretion may be due to increased glomerular plasma flow. Proteinuria should not be considered abnormal until it exceeds twice the upper limits of normal (usually 150–250 mg/24 hr in nonpregnant individuals). Increasing proteinuria in women with known chronic renal disease does not necessarily signify deterioration.

VOLUME HOMEOSTASIS

Most healthy women gain approximately 12.5 kg during the first pregnancy and 1 kg less during subsequent pregnancies. This increment in weight consists largely of fluid, as total body water increases 6–8 l, 4–6 l, of which are

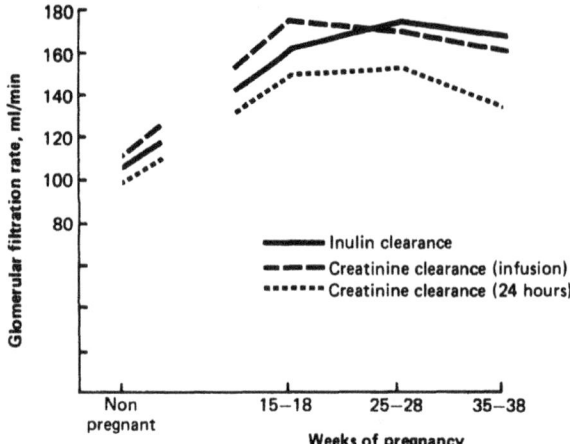

Figure 1. Mean GFR (by three methods) in ten healthy women during pregnancy and 8–12 weeks after delivery. [Modified from Davison and Hytter (4) with permission].

extracellular. There are also increases in plasma volume (which is greatest during the second trimester when increments approach 50%) and in fluid within fetal and maternal interstital spaces, which are greatest in late pregnancy. During most normal pregnancies, there is also a gradual cumulative retention of about 900 mM of sodium, distributed between the products of conception and the maternal extracellular space (11–13).

The alterations in maternal intravascular and interstitial spaces produce a "physiologic hypervolemia." Nevertheless, the mother's volume receptors sense these changes as normal, and when salt restriction or diuretic therapy limits this physiologic expansion, the maternal response resembles that of salt-depleted nonpregnant subjects (11, 13). The meaning or importance of these changes is unknown: It has been reported that multigravidas considered "poor reproducers" have smaller imcrements in both plasma volume and GFR when compared with multigravidas who have delivered normal-sized babies (14) and in pregnancies of women who subsequently aborted (3).

BLOOD PRESSURE REGULATION

Mean blood pressure decreases early in pregnancy, and by the second trimester diastolic levels are about 10 mmHg lower than before the patient became pregnant (11, 12). Blood pressure then increases slowly, approaching prepregnancy values shortly before delivery. Since cardiac output rises quickly in the first trimester (reaching values that are 30–40% greater than those before pregnancy) and remains relatively constant thereafter, the fall in blood pressure at this time must be due to marked decrease in peripheral vascular resistance. This is greatest in the uterine vasculature, which eventually develops into a large, low-resistance shunt. However, other organ systems, especially the kidneys and skin, participate in the generalized vasodilation that is characteristic of normal pregnancy. The rise of blood pressure toward nonpregnant levels during the third trimester suggests that increasing vasoconstrictor tone is a feature of late normal pregnancy, and if the clinician is not aware of this pattern of change diagnostic errors may ensue.

ASYMPTOMATIC BACTERIURIA

In this condition there is an absence of symptoms of acute urinary tract infection at a time when true bacteriuria exists.

Diagnostic pitfalls

URINE COLLECTION AND EXAMINATION

Pregnant women often complain of or will admit to symptoms of urgency, frequency, dysuria, and nocturia occurring singly or in combination. These symptoms are not in themselves diagnostic of urinary tract infection and can be elicited from women with sterile urine (15, 16).

The growth of bacteria on qualitative culture of the urine may represent either true bacteriuria (the multiplication of bacteria within the urinary tract) or contamination of the urine with urethral or perineal organisms at the time of collection. True bacteriuria can be separated from contamination on the basis of colony counts from a freshly obtained midstream urine specimen (MSU), with 10^5 colonies/ml of urine as the divided line (17). Two consecutive clean-voided specimens containing the same organism in numbers greater than 100,000 colonies/ml of urine represents true bacteriuria, as does a single suprapubic aspiration with any bacterial growth (11, 16, 17).

The use of the clean-catch technique is satisfactory, provided that each clinic determines the number of cultures needed to achieve a reasonable level of confidence (95 or greater) that bacteriuria exists. The use of antiseptic solutions for vulvar cleansing should be avoided, as contamination of the urine may result in a false-negative culture. A plain soap solution or distilled water is satisfactory. It is important to advise the patient that at least three wipes of the vulva are necessary before voiding.

A number of presumptive tests based on changes of chemical indicators are available, but the dependability of these varies greatly.

Site of infection

Investigators have utilized a multitude of tests, including ureteral catheterization, bladder washout technique renal biopsy, urine concentration tests, determination serum antibody titres, and, more recently, identification antibody-coated bacteria in the urine, as a means of differentiating between upper and lower tract infection (reviewed in 11, 16, 17, 18). This differentiation is of importance, as upper tract infection is more likely to recur and may require more intense therapy and surveillance. In practice, however, no single test is sufficiently precise to give complete confidence in localizing infection, but concentration tests are easy to perform in an outpatient setting, and more precision can be obtained if the clinical laboratory also attempts to analyze urine for the presence of antibody-coated bacteria.

Clinical implications

INCIDENCE

The reservoir of young women with asymptomatic bacteriuria acquired during childhood has been estimated at 5%, but only 1.2% are infected at any one time (19, 20). The incidence rises after puberty and varies from 2% to 10%, depending on the technique employed for testing and the socioeconomic status of the patients.

In pregnancy, significant asymptomatic bacteriuria will usually be found at the first antenatal visit. Less than 1.5% of women with originally sterile urine will acquire bacteriuria later in pregnancy (17).

IMPORTANCE OF DIAGNOSIS

Up to 40% of the infected group will develop an acute symptomatic urinary tract infection (15–18, 20), and treatment will prevent approximately 50–70% of all cases of acute urinary tract infection. However, about 2% of those with negative cultures will develop acute infections. Thus of the 90–98% that have no evidence of asymptomatic bacteriuria at the booking visit (and therefore are not treated), the number who are actually at risk of developing acute urinary tract infection is quite significant and accounts for about 30–50% of all acute urinary tract infection in pregnancy. (Figure 2).

Any other postulated benefits of eradication of asymptomatic bacteriuria are unsubstantiated, and the avavilable data suggest that the association with increases in fetal loss, prematurity, preeclampsia, or anemia is unproven (11, 12, 20–24). It is likely that up to 30–40% of pregnant women with asymptomatic bacteriuria have upper urinary tract infection, and these women may be a special population at greatest risk of pregnancy problems and acute urinary infection. Indeed, underlying chronic pyelonephritis may be present in some cases and may be responsible for the reported increased incidence of prematurity, fetal loss, and preeclampsia.

Lastly, there is a view that screening for asymptomatic bacteriuria is not justified, because only a small proportion of bacteriuric patients develop urinary infections, and most patients with infections do not have bacteriuria on routine screening (25). Furthermore, it has been shown that a positive history of previous urinary tract infection is almost as effective in predicting urinary infection in pregnancy (26). Accordingly, it is argued that combining the finding of bacteriuria with a history of urinary infection signifies the greatest risk of infection in pregnancy, with such women being ten times more likely than those with neither feature of developing a clinical infection and four times more likely than those with asymptomatic bacteriuria alone (26, 27).

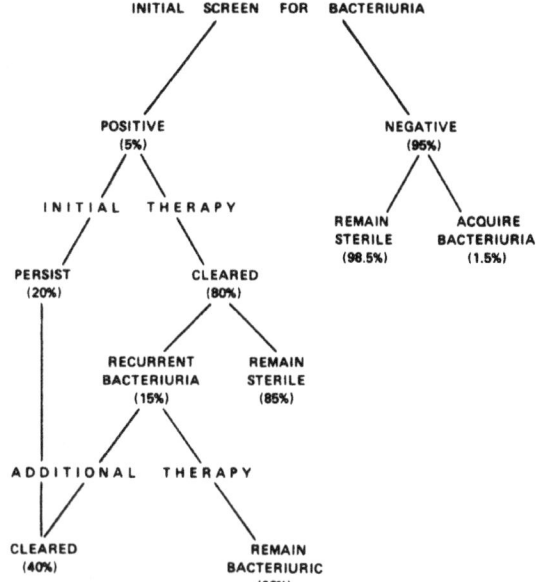

Figure 2. Natural history of asymptomatic bacteriuria and the effects of treatment during pregnancy. Approximate percentages given in brackets.

Management

CHOICE OF DRUG

The choice of drug should be based on the sensitivity of the isolated organisms. Short-acting sulphonamides or nitrofurantoin derivatives are usually the initial therapy (16–18). Other antibiotics are reserved for the treatment of failures and for symptomatic infection. Ampicillin and the cephalosporins produce few known adverse reactions in the fetus and can safely be used throughout pregnancy. Tetracyclines are contraindicated because of staining of the teeth of infants by binding with orthophosphates, as well as the rare maternal complication of acute fatty liver of pregnancy. (See Acute fatty liver of pregnancy). If sulphonamides are still being prescribed in late pregnancy, they should be withheld during the last 2–3 weeks, since they compete with bilirubin for albumin binding sites, increasing the risk of fetal hyperbilirubinemia and kernicterus. Nitrofurantoin used during the last few weeks may precipitate hemodialysis due to erythrocyte phosphate dehydrogenase deficiency in the newborn.

DURATION OF THERAPY

Opinions differ on the optimal duration of therapy in patients with asymptomatic bacteriuria (11). Continuous antibiotic therapy was once recommened from the time of diagnosis until after delivery, based on the belief that the relapse rate can be high because of problems of renal parenchymal involvement. However, as at least 60% of patients have bladder involvement alone, administration of short-term therapy (2 weeks) is satisfactory. Furthermore, if patient follow-up is meticulous, there appears to be no advantage in using continuous long-term administration of antibiotics, and the possible hazards of such therapy to the fetus are avoided (16). With the explosion of new antibiotics that have been introduced during this decade, many have been administered to pregnant women. The clinician should limit antibiotic use to those with a proven record during pregnancy. (Categories have been established for all drugs and are listed yearly in *Physicians Desk Reference*, Medical Economics.)

Follow-up urine cultures should be obtained 1 week after therapy is discontinued and then at regular intervals throughout the pregnancy (suggest every 4 weeks).

RELAPSES AND REINFECTION

Relapse is the recurrence of bacteriuria caused by the same organism, usually within 6 weeks of the initial infection. Reinfection is the recurrence of bacteriuria involving a different strain of bacteriuria, after successful eradication of the initial infection. Most patients with a reinfection pattern have infections limited to the bladder, usually occurring at least 6 weeks after therapy.

Approximately 25% of patients will have a recurrence during pregnancy, and a second course of treatment should be given, based on a repeat culture with sensitivity testing (see Figure 2). Since *E. coli* causes the majority of initial infections as well as recurrences, it is sometimes desirable to employ an *E. coli* serotyping system to precisely distinguish different strains. In the group of patients who relapse or who are resistant to the first course of therapy, only about 40% will have the asymptomatic bacteriuria cleared with subsequent therapy.

Long-term management

NEED FOR FOLLOW-UP

As the interval between treatment of bacteriuria in pregnancy and postpartum follow-up becomes longer, the influence of the bacteriuria becomes less noticeable. Ten or more years after an initial episode of bacteriuria of pregnancy, the prevalance of bacteriuria (25%) in women not treated during pregnancy is virtually the same as in those women who were treated (29%). Women who never had bacteriuria during pregnancy have rates of bacteriuria of around 5%. Thus a single course of treatment during the index pregnancy does not appear to protect against persistent or recurrent bacteriuria years later.

There are few prospective studies available, but there is no evidence that persistent asymptomatic bacteriuria in women with normal urinary tracts causes long-term renal damage or that treatment reduces the incidence of chronic renal disease (15–17).

POSTPARTUM EVALUATION

There is no consensus of opinion regarding the need for a postpartum evaluation, including intravenous urography. It is known that 20% of all patients with asymptomatic bacteriuria have radiologic abnormalities, and the percentage is increased among patients with acute infections and/or infections difficult to eradicate during pregnancy (28).

The significance of this is not so certain (29). It may indicate a predisposition to infection, it may result from infection, or it may be unrelated to infection. Most abnormalities are minor and neither resulted from nor caused the renal infection (28).

An intravenous urogram should be performed on one occasion to document a nonobstructed urinary tract in women who have had asymptomatic bacteriuria during pregnancy and who fulfill the addition following criteria:
1. Difficulty in eradicating the bacteriuria
2. Episode(s) of acute symptomatic urinary tract infection
3. History of acute symptomatic urinary tract infections prior to pregnancy
4. Persistence/recurrence of asymptomatic bacteriuria or acute infection postpartum.

In this way about 90% of women with major urinary tract abnormalities will be detected (29).

ACUTE SYMPTOMATIC URINARY TRACT INFECTION

Perspective

Where there is symptomatic urinary tract infection (UTI), two clinical syndromes are recognized: lower UTI or cystitis and upper UTI or acute pyelonephritis (15). The latter is the most common renal complication of pregnancy, occurring in 1–2% of all pregnancies. It has been blamed as a cause of intrauterine growth retardation, congenital abnormalities, and fetal death, and can certainly cause premature labor (16, 21, 22).

Acute cystitis

This occurs in about 1% of pregnant women, 60% of whom have a negative initial screening. The symptoms are often difficult to distinguish from those due to pregnancy itself. Features indication a true infection include hematuria, dysuria, and suprapubic discomfort, as well as a positive urine culture. The bacteriology is the same as in women with asymptomatic bacteriuria. Similar treatment is recommended, with the aims of abolishing symtoms and preventing the occurrence of acute pyelonephritis. Finally, it is too early to gauge that sccess of single-dose therapy for gravidas with cystitis, and we continue to recommend a standard couse of treatment.

Acute pyelonephritis

The differential diagnosis includes other urinary tract pathology: other causes of pyrexia, such as respiratory tract infection, viremia, or toxoplasmosis (appropriate serologic screening should be performed); and other causes of acute abdominal pain, such as acute appendicitis, biliary colic, gastroenteritis, uterine fibroid degeneration, or abruptio placentae.

Acute appendicitis can be a difficult diagnosis to make, especially in the third trimester. Usually at the onset of the appendicitis the pain is referred to the center of the abdomen, vomiting is not a marked feature, the pyrexia is not as high, as in acute pyelonephritis, and rigors rarely occur.

Pneumonia on the affected side should present no difficulties if attention is paid to the type of respiration, the respiratory rate, and the physical signs in the chest. It should be noted, however, that the so-called adult respiratory distress syndrome (ARDS), with accompanying liver and hematopoietic dysfunction, can be a significant complication of pyelonephritis (16, 30) (Table 1).

Management

A midstream urine should be sent for culture and sensitivities immediately. Treatment should be aggressive and should be undertaken in a hospital setting, and good nursing case is mandatory.

Table 1. Comparison of clinical factors with acute pyelonephritis in pregnancy with and without respiratory distress

	With respiratory distress (n = 15)	Without respiratory distress (n = 30)
Duration of symptoms[a]	2.6 days	2.5 days
Duration of pyrexia[a]	3.2 days	1.9 days
Maximum temperature	39.7°	39.1°
Tachypnea (>28/min)	100%	16%
Blood creatinine >90 µM/l	57%	20%
Hematocrit (%)[a]		
Initial	30.1	32.3
Decrement	4.9	4.7
Platelets ($\times 10^9$/l)[a]		
Initial	215,000	277,000
Lowest	153,000	242,000
<100,000	40%	0
Highest leukocytes ($\times 10^9$/l)[a]	18,100	14,000
Positive blood culture	43%	22%
Preterm labor	21%	4%

[a] Mean values.
Modified from Cunningham et al. (16) with permission.

FLUID BALANCE

The patient may be dehydrated due to vomiting and sweating, and may require intravenous fluid therapy. Regulation assessment of renal function and plasma urea and electrolytes should be undertaken. Although the infection attack is said to have little effect on renal hemodynamics in nonpregnant patients, such attacks during pregnancy have been observed to cause transient but marked decrements in creatinine clearance (31).

CHOICE AND DURATION OF THERAPY

Dogmatic statements cannot be made regarding the type of antimicrobial therapy for acute urinary tract infection, and the appropriate duration of regimens is also debatable (15). Treatment should aim at administering the most effective drug to eradicate a particular infection without exposing the fetus to an unnecessarily harmful agent.

Antibiotics producing high blood levels and resulting in high renal parenchymal concentrations are favored. Two antibiotics that give appropriate blood levels are ampicillin and cephalosporins. *E. coli*, the most common organism isolated in urinary infections, is usually sensitive to these antibiotics. Until the patient is afebrile, it is preferable to give intravenous antibiotics, and then to adminster them orally thereafter.

The duration of treatment should be 2 weeks for low-tract symptomatic infection and a minimum of 1 month for acute pyelonephritis. Antibiotic sensitivity should be reviewed within 48 hours. In patients showing clinical deterioration or whose urine cultures reveal bacteria resistance to the selected antibiotic, a repeat urine culture is necessary and alternative antibotic therapy should be considered. In severely ill patients, blood specimens should be taken for culture.

After the completion of treatment, urine for culture should be taken at every antenated visit for the rest of the pregnancy. Since upper tract infections tend to recur, and given the seriousness of such disease in pregnant women (11), mandelamine may be given as "suppressive therapy" until term.

GRAM-NEGATIVE SEPSIS

This can occur in severely ill patients with acute pyelonephritis, but the situation is commonly associated with instrumentation of an infected urinary tract. An aminoglycoside antibiotic is best, because it is effective against nearly all of the gram-negative urinary bacteria.

Enterococci less commonly cause bacteriemia but, because of the resistance of aminoglycosides, ampicillin can be used combined with an aminoglycoside until culture results are available.

ACUTE RENAL AND PYELONEPHRITIS

This is discussed elsewhere (see Acute renal failure and pyelonephritis in this chapter).

Table 2. Clinical entities associated with pregnancy-induced urinary tract dilatation

Clinical entity	Clinical features
Overdistension syndrome	Flank pain, renal colic
Pyelonephritis	Flank pain, fever, bacteriuria
Urinary tract rupture	
Retroperitoneal	
Parenchymal	Flank pain
	Mass: abscess, hematoma
	Anemia/hypotension due to blood loss Hematuria
Collecting system	Flank pain
	Mass: perinephric or subcapsular urinoma
	Hematuria (microscopic)
Intraperitoneal	Peritonitis
Parenchymal	Flank pain
Collecting system	Anemia/hypotension due to blood loss Hematuria

Table 3. Rupture of the urinary tract

Traumatic	
Nontraumatic	
Parenchymal	Tumor, especially hamartoma
	Abscess
	Vasculities: polyarteritis nodosa
	Cystic disease
	Congenital: tuberous sclerosis
Nonparenchymal	Obstruction due to urolithiasis,
Pregnancy related	infection, reflux, or stricture

NONTRAUMATIC RUPTURE OF THE URINARY TRACT

There is a broad spectrum of the so-called overdistension syndrome (32). Obstruction may occur at varying levels at or above the pelvic brim (Table 2). The intrusion or unremitting pain and hematuria upon the course of the "overdistension syndrome" or peylonephritis suggest rupture of the urinary trace (Table 3). Furthermore, urinary tract rupture can masquerade as other obstetric and surgical abdominal catastrophes, including appendicitis, pelvic abscess, cholecystitis, urolithiasis, or abruptio placentae. Prompt recognition may prevent a small tear and urine leak, treatable by postural or tube drainage, from extending and/or expanding. Rupture of the renal parenchyma, with hemorrhagic shock, formation of a flank mass, or distension of urinary tract contents intraperitoneally compels prompt surgical intervention, usually with nephrectomy.

ACUTE RENAL FAILURE

Acute renal failure is a clinical syndrome characterized by a sudden and marked decrease in glomerular filtration, rising plasma urea and creatinine levels, and usually by a decrease in urine output to below 400 ml in 24 hours. As a clinical diagnosis, the term only describes the functional state of the kidneys, without distinguishing between the different forms of underlying pathology (33–35). For the most part, acute renal failure occurs in persons with previously healthy kidneys, but it may also complicate the course of patients with preexisting renal disease.

Before anuria or oliguria are ascribed to acute renal failure, obstruction of the renal outflow must be excluded, usually by infusion urography if investigation is needed. This is particularly pertinent in an obstetric practice, since it is all too easy to unwittingly damage the urinary tract when performing emergency surgery for obstetric disasters, such as postpartum hemorrhage, which are themselves causes of acute renal failure.

Perspective

Recently there has been a marked decline in the number cases of acute renal failure related to obstetrics, and the current incidence is probably less than 0.01% (33, 34). These decreases have been attributed chiefly to declines in the number of septic abortions, and improvements in perinatal care, with clinicians ready to intervene quickly and aggressively in situations that could potentially lead to renal failure. Such situations include placental abruption, acute pyelonephritis, preeclampsia, postpartum hemorrhage, and any disease that may lead to systemic infection, dehydration, and/or hypotension (33–36).

Pregnant women are more prone than nonpregnant women to develop cortical necrosis, especially the incomplete ("patchy") variety (33, 34). The reasons for this disposition remain unknown. Two entities associated with pregnancy and idiopathic postpartum renal failure (hemolytic uremic sydrome) are fortunately rare.

Diagnosis and investigation

A carefully taken history and physical examination may reveal a background of abortion, severe hyperemesis, gravidarum, hemorrhage, sensitization to drugs, incompatible blood transfusion, or preeclampsia. Once the diagnosis of acute renal failure has been considered to be a possibility then exploration of the multiple causes must be pursued. A full initial assessment is essential (described in detail elsewhere in this book), remembering that postpartum a decision will be received regarding the timing and route of delivery.

Diagnostic pitfalls

It is difficult and often impossible to decide on the etiology of the acute renal failure. Total anuria or altering periods of anuria and polyuria strongly suggest obstruction, but normal urine volumes do not exclude obstruction. Complete anuria and/or evidence of disseminated intravascular coagulation are suggestive of acute cortical necrosis, but this diagnosis can only be firmly established by renal biopsy.

The differential diagnosis between functional renal insufficiency caused by dehydration or hypotension (prerenal failure) and acute tubular or cortical necrosis is of practical importance, as their therapies are diametrically different.

Management

The management of acute renal failure is detailed elsewhere in this book, and while the principles behind the therapies are similar in gravid and nonpregnant women, certain precautions warrant emphasis.

INSENSIBLE FLUID LOSSES

Insensible loss may be increased in pregnancy, but there are few data on this. It is not known whether or not the catabolic effects of acute renal failure are similar in pregnant and nonpregannt women. Thus the tendency to aim for daily weight losses of 0.3–0.5% kg may be excessive in gravidas, especially in the final trimester, where fetal weight gain may be 0.3 kg per week. Given those uncertainties, frequent careful clinical assessment may be the only source of signs suggesting dehydration or volume overload.

PREGNANCY-SPECIFIC LABORATORY VALUES

Abnormal laboratory values should be interpreted in terms of "pregnancy norms." For example, normal values for arterial pH, sodium, and bicarbonate are 7.44, 135 mM/l, and 20 mM/l, respectively, where pCO_2 is only 28–30 torr.

Dialysis

Both peritoneal dialysis and hemodialysis have been used in patients with obstetric renal failure. Some authors (37) prefer the peritoneal route and comment that ". . . neither pelvic peritonitis nor an enlarged uterus is a contraindication to the method." We agree and consider the procedure safe if the catheter is inserted high in the abdomen under direct vision through a small incision. Since both routes are safe, the choice should be determined by the underlying clinical condition (i.e., peritoneal dialysis is certainly preferable in the patient with septic shock or any other hypotensive complications) and by the facilities available in a given unit. If protracted dialysis is projected in a woman with an immature fetus (i.e., at 24 weeks of gestation), chronic ambulatory peritoneal dialysis should be considered, as it keeps rapid fluid and metabolic perturbations to a minimum when compared with other modes of therapy (38).

Since urea, creatinine, and many other metabolites that accumulate in uremia cross the placenta, dialysis should be undertaken early in gravidas, with the aim of maintaining urea around 10 mM/l (serum urea nitrogen at 30 mg%). Thus the advantage of each dialysis proposed for nonpregnant patients becomes even more germane for gravidas and makes the argument for "prophylactic" dialysis more compelling. During dialysis itself, the fluid balance must be closely monitored, being careful to avoid excessive shifts in the fluid compartments that could compromise uteroplacental perfusion. If the pregnancy is near maturity, delivery should be effected as soon as the mother's condition has been stabilized.

FORMS OF ACUTE RENAL FAILURE FOUND IN PREGNANCY

Renal failure in septic abortion or septic shock

PERSPECTIVE

Until recently a common source of septicemia associated with pregnancy was septic abortion with pyelonephritis, chorioamnionitis, and puerperal sepsis, occurring less frequently (36). Only occasionally was the abortion spontaneous, although detailed questioning may be required to elicit evidence that abortifacients have been used. The advent of liberal abortion laws and progress in antibiotic therapy have led to marked declines, and even an apparent disappearance, of this life-threatening syndrome. However, the clinician should not be lulled into a false sense of security given the ever-present potential of antibiotic-resistant bacterial stains and the movements in some countries towards repealing therapeutic abortion policies.

PATHOLOGY

There are many reasons why acute renal failure should be associated with septic abortion. The patient is both dehydrated and hypotensive, a combination that leads to considerable renal ischemia. Hemoglobinuria (due to hemolysis) and disseminated intravascular coagulation are often present, and soap and lysol, common abortifacients, have specific nephrotoxic effects (34). The severity of renal dysfunction associated with clostridial infections suggests to some that clostridia produces a specific nephrotoxin (39). The marked hemolysis caused by bacteria and chemical abortifacients is, however, sufficient to provoke the renal shutdown. Most pregnancy sepsis is due to gram-negative bacteria, and clostridia is responsible for only 0.5% of patients developing shock.

DIAGNOSIS AND INVESTIGATION

The presentation can be quite dramatic, especially in cases of clostridia and *E. coli* infections. There can be an abrupt rise in temperature (to 40°C), often associated with myalgias, vomiting, and diarrhea, the latter occasionally being bloody.

Once symptoms commence, hypotension, tachypnea, and progression to frank shock occur rapidly. The patients are usually jaundiced, with a particular bronzelike color ascribed to the association of jaundic, with cutaneous vasodilation, cyanosis, and pallor. Despite the presence of fever, the extremities are often cold and display purplish areas, which may be precursors of small patches of necrosis on the toes, fingers, or nose.

There is laboratory evidence of severe anemia due to hemolysis and hyperbilirubinemia of the indirect type. There are also alterations in clotting factors, which suggest disseminated intravascular coagulation (DIC). Leukocytosis ($25.000/mm^3$) with marked shifts to the left is the rule, and platelets are often difficult to detect on a blood smear. Thrombocytopenia of less than $50,000/mm^3$ is often observed. Hypocalcemia that is severe enough to provoke tetany can occur (40).

An abdominal x-ray may demonstrate air in the uterus or abdomen, the result of gas-forming organisms and/or perforation of the uterus. Despite an obvious toxic and septicemic picture, bacterial identification may be difficult. The situation can be further confused because clostridia are normally present in the female genital tract.

Full initial assessment should be conducted as discussed for acute renal failure, with the following addition points being important:

1. *Blood sugar*. Diabetes must be excluded. Blood from a finger prick should not be used if there is poor skin perfusion.
2. *Acid-base status*. The patient may be hypotoxic, through ventilation-perfusion inequality. The carbon dioxide level is usually low in order to compensate for the increasing metabolic acidosis. An elevated carbon dioxide level is unusual, but may simply imply deterioration in the level of consciousness with loss of respiratory drive or, in a few cases, preceding respiratory failure or depression due to drugs. A metabolic acidosis is generally related to inadequate oxygenation peripherally, anaerobic metabolism, and the onset of lactic acid adidosis. An increasing and irreversible metabolic acidosis following initial resuscitation is a bad prognostic sign.
3. *Coagulation indices*. Hypercoagulability may be seen early and can alternate with hypocoagulability. Hematologic evidence of disseminated intravascular coagulation (DIC) correlates with the severity of the shock and poor peripheral oxygenation. The potential for blood loss in septic abortion increases the susceptibility to DIC.

It is important that DIC not be mistaken for coagulation problems that follow massive transfusion. The usual evidence of DIC is oozing from venepuncture sites and skin hemorrhages. Thrombocytopenia alone is common in sepsis.

4. *Sophisticated investigations*. Occasionally baseline assessment is insufficient for hemodynamic evaluation. More elaborate investigations may be needed, such as wedge pressure (PCWP), etc., and this requires skilled personnel as well as specialized equipment (see Assessment of fluid balance). Therefore, should a patient fail to respond to volume replacement or be severely shocked, metabolic correction and antibiotic treatment must be conducted in an intensive therapy unit.

DIAGNOSTIC PITFALLS

The clinician may be misled by an asymptomatic patient admitted with an incomplete abortion who rapidly develops shock and prostration within hours. Generalized muscular pains, often most intense in the thorax and abdomen, may lead to confusion with intraabdominal inflammatory processes; this is especially true when a history of provoked abortion is denied or not sought for, since heavy vaginal bleeding is often not a prominent feature. Knowledge of recent treatment with antibiotics or other drugs is important if one is to diagnose bacterial resistance, suppressed infection, and drug-modified physiology.

MANAGEMENT

Severely ill patients are best managed in an intensive care unit. The initial steps include vigorous supportive therapy and the use of antibiotics in high doses. The use of clostridia antitoxin, the role of steroids, and the place of surgical intervention are controversial. Some favor the radical surgical approach, performing an abdominal hysterectomy where a patient is responding poorly to fluid (41). There is the view, however, that modern antibiotic therapy is usually capable of localizing the infection in the pelvis and eventually eradicates it from the uterus (40), bearing in mind that many young women with a septic abortion may want a pregnancy in the future.

Volume and metabolic control

It is essential to restore an adequate circulating volume as soon as possible, and the volume infused must be regulated according to central venous pressure (CVP) or right atrial pressure readings. An increase in urine output above 40 ml/hr is an excellent prognostic sign.

The fluid selected for volume replacement will depend upon whether there is an obvious electrolyte deficit, possible albumin depletion, or if fluid is merely required to increase the circulating volume. Colloid is the solution of choice for volume replacement. Should the urine output improve, potassium supplementation may be necessary.

It is of interest that in an appreciable number of these cases anuria may persist for up to 3 or more weeks (42). Often it is just when the patient is thought to have cortical rather than tubular necrosis that the polyuria phase commences. Some women with septic abortion do develop cortical necrosis, perhaps due to the severity of the ischemic insult or to massive DIC.

Bacteriologic control

Appropriate antibiotic therapy is essential, but in the shocked patient it is of secondary value to the restoration of adequate organ perfusion. Before antibiotics are given, the appropriate specimens for aerobic and anaerobic cultures must be taken. A bactericidal antibiotic may produce temporary clinical deterioration, because of breakdown of bacteria and endotoxin release. This is an additional reason for performing basic resuscitation procedures before starting antibiotic therapy.

The antibiotic should be as specific as possible: A narrow-spectrum antibiotic is preferable in patients in whom the source of infection can be isolated and microscopy is diagnostic. There is still controversy about the best drug combination in patients suffering from suspected gram-negative sepsis. In patients without antibiotic therapy, it is reasonable to commence with a combination of a cephalosporin and metronidazole. Should the shock be severe and a resistant *Klebsiella* or coliform be suspected, or a *Pseudomonas* or *Proteus* infection, gentamicin should be included, Once the sensitivities are available, the antibiotic therapy may be modified. The dosage of gentamicin must be regulated according to daily peak and trough levels. Antibiotics should be given intravenously in the first instance, changing, once the shock phase is over, to intramuscular administration, if considered preferable.

Hemotologic control

It is important to observe the clotting indices sequentially. A steady deterioration may be seen with the diagnosis of DIC, and this is commonly associated with overall clinical deterioration. Active treatment is not required where there are minor changes in the coagulation indices and there is no clinical evidence of bleeding, and where shock is rapidly corrected.

Should the clotting factors continue to deteriorate in spite of the preceding resuscitative measures, fresh-frozen plasma should be given. Heparin should be considered if there is a further fall in the fibrinogen titre, especially where the source of sepsis is not readily treatable.

A persistent thrombocytopenia (platelet count of less than 40,000/mm^3) and capillary oozing in spite of replacement of clotting factors is an indication for an infusion of platelets or platelet-enriched plasma.

Other measures

Hyperbaric oxygen and exchange transfusion have both been used to treat clostridial sepsis, but the results are too fragmentary to recommend specific protocols.

Digotoxin should be used (provided the plasma potassium is normal) when there is evidence of myocardial failure or the patient develops atrial flutter or fibrillation. Other drugs that may affect the hemodynamic state include dopamine hydrochloride, isoprenaline, and phentolamine mesylate, and their use must be based on changes found when monitoring the hemodynamic situation generally (42).

Acute renal failure and preeclampsia/eclampsia

PERSPECTIVE

Preeclampsia, characterized by hypertension, proteinuria, and edema, and at times coagulation abnormalities, affects 5–10% of all pregnancies (11); it usually occurs in nulliparas, invariably after the 20th gestational week. There is no doubt that some cases labeled as preeclampsia progressing to renal failure have been incompletely or improperly classified. This is because when considering hypertension it is difficult to distinguish clinically between the different etiologic categories — preeclampsia, hypertension secondary to renal disease, essential hypertension, and combinations of these separate pathologic states (43, 44). In multiparous patients the diagnosis of pure preeclampsia should be suspect (43, 44).

PATHOLOGY AND ITS RELATIONSHIP TO MANAGEMENT

Preeclampsia is accompanied by a characteristic renal lesion in which the glomeruli enlarge and become ischemic due to swelling of the intracapillary cells — glomerular endothelioses and mesangiosis (11, 43, 44). Most preeclamptics experience moderate decreases in GFR, but occasionally this decrease is accompanied by acute renal failure.

The kidney failure is usually due to acute tubular necrosis, but acute cortical necrosis may also occur (33–36). It is possible that acute tubular necrosis is the obligatory outcome of glomerular cell swelling, which can lead to complete abliteration of the capillary lumen. This appears unlikely, as the extent of the morphologic lesion correlates poorly with eclampsis and is exquisitely sensitive to the vasoactive influence of angiotensin II and catecholamines; these vasoconstrictors may play a role in the genesis of the acute renal failure.

The preeclampsia patient has vasoconstriction and hemoconcentration, and has a reduced intravascular volume (11, 12). The decrement usually precedes the development of the hypertension, and the susceptibility of hypertensive pregnant women to develop prerenal azotemia when salt restricted and/or prescribed diuretics is well known. It is therefore possible that these patients (who also have an increased incidence of placental abruption) may be more susceptible than healthy women to the adverse renal effects of antepartum and intrapartum hemorrhage.

MANAGEMENT

When antepartum preeclampsia is accompanied by severe renal dysfunction, the therapy of choice is termination of the pregnancy.

Acute renal failure and pyelonephritis

As noted previously (see Acute symptomatic urinary tract infection in this chapter), acute pyelonephritis is the most common renal complication during pregnancy. In the absence of complicating features, such as obstruction, calculi, papillary necrosis, and analgesic nephropathy, acute pyelonephritis is an extremely rare cause of acute renal failure in nonpregnant subjects, but this association appears to be more frequent in pregnant women (33–35).

The reason is obscure. It is known that in pregnant women acute pyelonephritis is accompanied by marked decrements in GFR, as well as significant increments in plasma creatinine levels (31), and this is in contrast to the situation in nonpregnant patients. It has been suggested that the vasculature in pregnancy may be more sensitive to the vasoactive effect of bacterial endotoxins (33, 35).

Acute fatty liver of pregnancy

PERSPECTIVE

Acute fatty liver of pregnancy (also called obstetric pseudo acute yellow atrophy) is a rare complication of pregnancy and is characterized by jaundice and severe hepatic dysfunction in late pregnancy or the early postpartum period (45).

PATHOLOGY

The renal failure appears to be due to hemodynamic factors, as in the "hepatorenal syndrome," but some cases have been associated with intravascular coagulation (33–36). Some believe that tetracyclines may precipitate this condition, but this antibiotic is no longer used in obstetric practice. In addition, reversible urea-cycle enzyme deficiencies (orthinine transcarbamylase and carbamyl phosphate synthetase) resembling those seen in Reye's syndrome have been described (34–46, 47). It has been suggested that this condition may be an adult form of Reye's syndrome that is provoked by the metabolic stress of pregnancy (47).

DIAGNOSIS AND INVESTIGATION

A typical patient presents with fever, abdominal pain, nausea, and vomiting, then rapidly develops severe jaundice and hepatic encephalopathy (34–48). Common misdiagnoses are septicemia or preecamplasia with liver involvement (49, 50). It has been suggested hat acute fatty liver and preeclampsia coexist approximately 20% of the time, and even higher incidence have been proposed (34, 51).

Serum transaminases are only minimally increased (if at all) in a patient with marked hyperbilirubinaemia and severe hepatic failure. Alkaline phosphatase and amylase levels are occasionally elevated, and hyperammonemia has been recorded (34, 35). A substantial number of patients manifest laboratory evidence of disseminated intravascular coagulation. Serum urate levels may be elevated out of proportion to the degree of renal dysfunction: In fact, hyperuricemia may precede the clinical presentation (52).

MANAGEMENT

Treatment consists of termination of the pregnancy and supportive therapy for hepatic and renal failure. The efficacy of termination, however, has not been proven.

The mortality rate is high, with death resulting primarily from hepatic rather than renal failure. The more recent literature, however, suggests that the prognosis for this condition has improved and more survivors are being recorded (34).

Idiopathic postpartum renal failure or hemolytic uraenine syndrome

PERSPECTIVE AND PATHOLOGY

Idiopathic postpartum renal failure or hemolytic uraenine syndrome (HUS) is a rare and frequently fatal syndrome that is characterized by the onset of renal failure in the puerperium. It has been given a variety of names, including postpartum malignant sclerosis and irreversible postpartum renal failure (34, 35).

It is characterized by the onset of renal failure 3–10 weeks into the puerperium (34, 35, 53, 54) after the patient has had an uneventful pregnancy and delivery. She then develops marked axotemia and severe hypertension, frequently associated with microangiopathic hemolytic anemia and platelet aggregation, with formation of the microthrombi in the terminal portions of the renal vasculature. It should be remembered that renal failure, microangiopathic hemolytic anemia, and thrombocytopenia may be associated in pregnant women with various entities such as severe preeclampsia, the so-called HELLP syndrome (Hemolysis, Elevated Liver enzymes, Low Platelets), acute fatty liver of pregnancy (AFLP), and thrombotic thrombocytopenic purpura. Distinction between HUS and some of these antenatal disorders may be difficult, since they may overlap into the postpartum period. Although there is a wide clinical spectrum, correct identification is necessary, since specific investigations and/or therapy are needed in some.

The pathophysiology is unknown and the controversies about management reflect this uncertainly (55–57). It has a poor prognosis: A review of 49 patients with HUS revealed that death occurred in 61%, complete recovery of renal function in 9.5%, and 12% had terminal renal failure requiring maintenance dialysis (56).

It has been suggested that enothelial damage is the key lesion in HUS. This may involve the Sanarelli-Schwartman reaction (58), the action of an *E. coli*-produced Vero-cell toxin (Verotoxin) (59), and/or platelet aggregation and deposition. Genetic and environmental factors have been implicated as in post-pill HUS, idiopathic HUS, and thrombocytopenic purpura. Of interest is a report of two HLA-identical sisters, one of whom developed postpartum HUS and the other post-pill HUS (60). A pathogenic role for immunologic factors has been proposed as transient hypocomplementemia can occur.

MANAGEMENT

There is uncertainly concerning the management of this condition (33–36, 56), as many patients succumb despite treatment with dialysis; immunosuppression; and heparin, streptokinase, dipyridamole, acetylsalicylic acid, or corticosteroids, alone or combined.

Other forms of management have evolved in recent years and have been used with some success (reviewed in 33–35). A supposed lack of prostacyclin (PGI_2), a powerful vasodilator and potent endogenous inhibitor of platelet aggregation, can be counteracted by exchange transfusion or even plasma infusion alone. Prolonged PGI_2 infusions have been tried with the aim of restoring the deficiency, thus controlling the hypertension and reversing the platelet consumption.

It has been argued that DIC is of pathogenic significance, with placental thromboplastin being released during labor. The extension of this argument is that antithrombin III (AT-III) may have a protective effect and can be given as a concentrate to correct the low plasma AT-III concentrations sometimes found at the onset of the syndrome. This approach needs further evaluation. Lastly, renal transplantation may be successful, but there is a chance of recurrence of the HUS lesion in the allograft.

Cortical necrosis in pregnancy

PERSPECTIVE AND PATHOLOGY

Renal cortical necrosis, a pathologic entity characterized by tissue death throughout the cortex with sparing of the medullary portions, occurs more readily in gravidas than in nonpregnant individuals. (34). Acute cortical necrosis may develop in patients with intravascular coagulation, which sometimes complicates septic abortion, with overwhelming septicemia; but it is actually more common in the third trimester or the puerperium, when septic complications occur less often. Multigravidas beyond the age of 30 are more likely to develop cortical necrosis, which tends to be associated with specific obstetric complications, mainly placental abruption, less commonly unrecognized longstanding intrauterine death, and on occasion, preeclampasia (35). It has been considered the clinical counterpart of the experimental Sanarelli–Schwartman reaction (58).

While cortical necrosis may involve the entire renal cortex, resulting in irreversible renal failure, it is the "patchy" variety that occurs more often in pregnancy (33–35). This is characterized by an initial episode of severe oliguria, which lasts much longer than in uncomplicated acute tubular necrosis, followed by a variable return of function and a stable period of moderate renal insufficiency. Years later, for reasons still obscure, renal function decreases again in some of these patients, often leading to end-stage renal failure.

DIAGNOSIS

The differential diagnosis between acute tubular and cortical necrosis may be difficult, since severe oliguria and/or anuria may be present in both. More accurate diagnosis is based on renal biopsy and possibly selective arteriography (33–35). With arteriography a cortical nephrogram is absent in complete necrosis and a striated or heterogeneous appearance is evident in the "patchy" variety. Obviously, renal biopsy may miss the lesion in women with "patchy" cortical necrosis, and the diagnosis should always be entertained in women with incomplete functional recovery.

MANAGEMENT

Management of cortical necrosis is similar to that outlined for acute renal failure in general. Severe hypertension may occur in these cases and should be treated as described elsewhere in this book.

Obstructive uropathy

Obstruction of the ureters by the enlarged pelvic organs is extremely uncommon but does not occur, especially in gravidas, with a solitary kidney and in those with polyhydramnios (34, 61). The effects of dehydramnios are very occasionally added by a fetal abdominal mass (62). If postural maneuvers fail to relieve the obstruction, then surgical intervention may be required (63).

IMPORTANT CONSIDERATIONS IN MANAGEMENT OF RENAL DISEASE IN PREGNANCY

Obstetric renal failure: Some conclusions

1. Acute renal failure can occur during pregnancy in a variety of situations that are similar to those causing sudden renal dysfunction in nonpregnant patients. Pathology peculiar to pregnancy, however, must always be considered. Acute fatty liver (AFLP) can be complicated by renal failure, and its early recognition with prompt treatment could reduce the fetal and maternal mortality rate. HUS is also associated with a high morbidity and mortality.
2. The need to get on and treat acute renal failure is important, but the need to reach and have an early (histologic) diagnosis of its cause must not be forgotten (64).
3. Treatment of sudden renal failure resembles that in nonpregnant populations and aims at retarding the appearance of uremic symptomatology, acid-base and electrolyte disturbances, and volume problems (i.e., overhydration when the patient has oliguria and dehydration during the polyuria phase).
4. There must be constant awareness of the propensity of patients with acute renal failure to become infected, a complication that can be quite serious in pregnant women.
5. Some of the problems can be dealt with by judicious conservative management, but if such an approach is unsuccessful, dialysis must be promptly used.
6. Dialysis in patients with acute renal failure can be prescribed "prophylactically," that is, prior to the appearance of electrolyte and/or proton imbalance, or uremic symptoms. Furthermore, as urea, creatinine,

and (presumably) a variety of metabolic wate products cross the placenta, "prophylactic" dialysis could be more compelling in pregnant women with immature fetuses and in whom temporaziation is desired. A policy of "buying time" without modifying the underlying pathology should be continually reviewed.

7. The method of dialysis (peritoneal or hemodialysis) should be dictated by the facilities available and by clinical circumstances. Peritoneal dialysis is effective and safe, as long as the catheter is inserted high in the abdomen under direct vision through a small incision. It probably minimizes rapid metabolic pertubations.
8. Controlled anticoagulation during hemodialysis should be similar with heparin to that used in nongravid patients (i.e., maintainence of between 150 and 180 seconds). Volume shifts during hemodialysis must be minimized to avoid impairment of uteroplacental blood flow.
9. In addition to dialysis, potent antihypertensive therapy, and blood transfusion (if necessary), other specific approaches, such as plasm infusion, plasma exchange, and antiplatelet drugs, may be of value.
10. Increments in uterine activity or the onset of labor can occur during or immediately after dialysis. Therefore, when possible, early delivery (as dictated by fetal maturity) should be undertaken.
11. At or after delivery, blood losses should be replaced quickly to the point of slight overtransfusion, because any hemorrhage may be underestimated.
12. The neonate can be subject to rapid dehydration because increased levels of urea and other solutes within the fetal circulation precipate an osmotic diuresis in the neonate shortly after birth.

RENAL FUNCTION AND THE IMPACT OF PREGNANCY

There are different obstetric and remote prognoses in women with different degrees of renal insufficiency, and therefore the impact of pregnancy should be considered by categories of functional renal status prior to conception (Tables 4 and 5).

Preserved/mildly impaired renal function

Women with chronic renal disease, but normal or only mildly decreased prepregnancy renal function (plasma creatinine < 125 μM/l), usually have a successful obstetric

Table 4. Categories of pregnancy functional renal status

Category	Plasma creatinine (μM/l)
Preserved/mildly impaired renal function	<125
Moderate renal insufficiency	125–250
Severe renal insufficiency	>250

Table 5. Pregnancy prospects for women with chronic renal disease

Renal status	Problems in pregnancy	Successful obstetric outcome	Problems in long term
Mild	22%	95% (82%)	<5% (8%)
Moderate	41%	90% (56%)	25% (77%)
Severe	84%	48% (8%)	53% (92%)

Estimates based on 911 women/1284 pregnancies (1973–1987) that attained at least 28 weeks gestation. Figures in parentheses refer to prospects when complications developed prior to 28 weeks gestation.

outcome, and pregnancy does not adversely affect the course of their disease (65–77). Although true for most patients, some authors suggest that this statement be tempered somewhat in lupus nephropathy, membranoproliferative glomerulonephritis, focal glomerular sclerosis, and perhaps IgA and reflux nephropathies, which appear more sensitive to intercurrent pregnancy (78).

Most show increments in GFR, but less than those of normal pregnant women (Figure 3). Increased proteinuria is common, occurring in 50% of pregnancies (although rarely in women with chronic pyelonephritis), and it can be massive (often exceeding 3 g in 24 hours), with nephrotic edema. The prevalence of hypertension, renal function abnormalities, and proteinuria, as well as their severity, are considerably lower between pregnancies and during

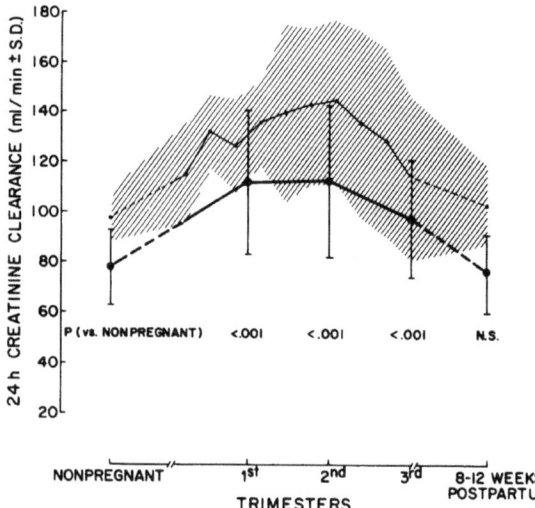

Figure 3. Serial 24 hr creatinine clearance (mean ± 1 SD) during 33 pregnancies (26 women) complicated by chronic renal disease (solid line). Measurements from ten healthy women (mean ± 1 SD) shown by hatched area. [From Katz et al. (72) with permission].

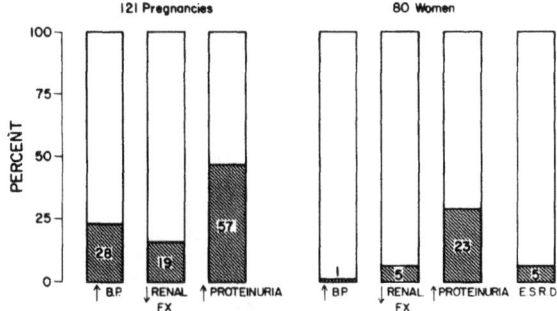

Figure 4. Course of renal disease in 89 women during pregnancy and the puerperium (three columns on left) and in 80 women under review after pregnancy (four columns on right). Numbers within columns are individual pregnancies (on left) and individual women (on right). Fx = function. ESRD = end-stage renal disease.

long-term follow-up (Figure 4). When renal failure does supervene, it usually reflects in inexorable course of a particular renal disease.

Another study of the influence of pregnancy (69) revealed an immediate loss of renal function in 29 patients whose creatinine levels were less than 135 μM/l. In contrast, 4 of 8 patients with initial creatinine levels above 145 μM/l experienced further significant increases during pregnancy, which were complicated in most cases. Four patients in this group progressed to end-stage renal failure within 18 months of delivery.

The customary recommendation has been that pregnancy is best avoided in women who have lost 50% of their kidney function. Recent studies, however, have reopened the question. Hou and her colleagues (80) recorded a successful obstetrical outcome in 92% of the pregnancies in 22 women with creatinine levels of 150–240 μM/l whose pregnancies were allowed to go beyond the second trimester. Many of these patients had escalating hypertension, and in 25% there was an accelerated decline in renal function. It is now recognized that uncontrolled hypertension is a very important factor in the overall deterioration (76, 80–85).

Severe renal insufficiency

Most women in this category (plasma creatinine > 250 μM/l) are amenorrheic and/or anovulatory (86). The likelihood of conception, let alone having a normal pregnancy and delivery, is low but not, as some have been misled to believe, impossible. The risk of severe maternal complications is greater than the probability of a successful obstetric outcome (82) (Table 5).

Realistically, these patients should not take additional health risks. The aim should be to preserve what little renal function remains and/or to achieve renal rehabilitation via a dialysis and transplant program, after which the question of pregnancy can be considered, if appropriate.

GENERAL MANAGEMENT PLAN FOR RENAL DISEASE IN PREGNANCY

Antenatal care

There is good evidence that one of the main factors in reducing maternal and perinatal morbidity and mortality is good antenatal care. The value of such care is greatly enhanced the earlier in the pregnancy it is commenced, with repetition at regular intervals, so that trends may be detected and the significance of an abnormal observation. Where patients have renal disease, the following aims are important:
1. Assessment of the size and development of fetus and placental function
2. Assessment of maternal renal function and also nutritional status in heavily proteinuric patients
3. Detection of hypertension and assessment of its severity
4. Detection of superimposed preeclampsia

With an uncomplicated antenatal course, the patient can be seen at 2-weekly intervals until about 32 weeks, and weekly thereafter. Hospital admission is recommended in the following circumstances:
1. Signs of intrauterine growth retardation and/or deterioration of placental function
2. Deterioration of renal function, as evidenced by decrements in creatinine clearance or increasing plasma creatinine levels
3. An onset of, or marked increase in, proteinuria that persists
4. Development of diastolic blood pressure levels at or above 95 mmHg in the second, or 100 mmHg in the third, trimester. Readings should be taken on two or more occasions separated by an interval of at least 6 hours
5. Suspicion of preeclampsia

Evaluation during pregnancy: Question of continuing a pregnancy

When the question of renal disease is raised for the first time during a pregnancy, it is essential to try to establish a diagnosis and a course of management that will be helpful to both the mother and fetus. When a patient presents with hypertension, proteinuria, and decreased renal function, parenchymal renal disease is difficult to distinguish from preeclampsia. Obviously a previous history of renal disorders, abnormal urine analysis, a family history of renal disease, or a history of a systemic illness known to involve the kidneys is helpful, but in the last analysis parenchymal renal disease and preeclampsia may coexist.

The evaluation of the patient and subsequent blood and urine testing are similar to those of nonpregnant women with an unknown renal disorder, but the exact diagnosis usually has to wait for further postpartum assessment. Such patients should be hospitalized and their pregnancies allowed to continue if renal function is serious in preeclampsia, however, the pregnancy should be terminated if further deterioration occurs. Interim hemodialysis has been used to "temporarize" (87, 88), but we believe such a course is too risky for the mother's well-being.

The role of renal biopsy in antenatal management

In pregnancy, the experience with renal biopsy is sparse, mainly because clinical circumstances rarely justify the minimal risks of biopsy at this time, and the procedure is usually deferred to the postpartum period (18). Clinical anecdotes, as well as specific reports of excessive bleeding and other complications in pregnant women, have led some to consider pregnancy a relative contraindication to renal biopsy (89), although others have not observed any increased morbidity (90). When the biopsy is performed in the immediate puerperium in subjects with well-controlled blood pressure and normal coagulation indices, the morbidity is certainly similar to that reported in nonpregnant patients (91).

A recent report by Packham and Fairley (92) on 111 biopsies in pregnant women, all preterm, confirmed and extended the impression that the risks of the procedure resemble those in the nonpregnant population. In fact, their incidence of transient gross hematuria, 0.9% (all patients undergoing biopsy have microscopic hematuria unless the kidney has been missed), was considerably lower than in nonpregnant patients, where it is 3–5%. Such excellent statistics no doubt reflect the experience and technical skills of the unit. Statistics have also been improved by refinement of the prebiopsy evaluation, which includes verifying that the patient is not significantly hypertensive and has not ingested drugs that interfere with clotting (i.e., aspirin) for at least 7–10 days prior to the procedure, as well as the usual tests to exclude bleeding diatheses.

Given this recent information, it is in order to restate that pregnancy adds little or no risk to the procedure. However, because complications do occur, it is still important to have specific indications for renal biopsy in pregnancy. Packham and Fairley (92) suggest that closed (percutaneous) needle biopsy should be undertaken quite often, because they believe that certain glomerular disorders are adversely influenced by pregnancy, and that this effect might be blunted by specific therapy, such as anti-platelet agents. The consensus goes against such broad indications and reiterates that renal biopsy should be performed infrequently during pregnancy (91). Even in nonpregnant populations, the reasons for renal biopsy are not clearly defined, and experts categorize indications as "most useful," "possible useful," and of "little or no use" (93).

There are, however, a few widely agreed specific indications for renal biopsy during pregnancy:
1. When there is a sudden deterioration of renal function prior to 32 weeks gestation without obvious cause. This is because certain forms of rapidly progressive glomerulonephritis may respond to aggressive treatment with steroid "pulses," chemotherapy, and/or perhaps plasma exchange, when diagnosed early.
2. When there is symptomatic nephrotic syndrome occurring prior to 32 weeks gestation. While some might consider a therapeutic trial of steroids in such cases, it is best to determine beforehand whether the lesion is likely to respond to steroids, because pregnancy is itself a hypercoagulable state prior to worsening by such treatment. On the other hand, proteinuria alone in a normotensive woman with well-preserved renal function, and who has neither marked hypoalbuminemia nor intolerable edema, would mean that the patient should be examined at more frequent intervals and biopsy should be deferred to the postpartum period. This is because the consensus among most investigators (72–78) is that the prognosis is determined primarily by the level of renal function and the presence or absence of hypertension. A similar approach applies to the management of pregnancies with asymptomatic microscopic hematuria of pregnancies with asymptomatic microscopic hematuria alone when neither stone nor tumor is suggested by ultrasonography.
3. When the presentation is characterized by "active urinary sediment" (red and white blood cells and casts), proteinuria, and "borderline" renal function in a patient who had not been evaluated in the past, this is a controversial area, it could be argued that diagnosis of a collagen disorder, such as scleroderma or periarteritis, would be grounds for termination of the pregnancy, or that classification of the type of lesion in a woman with SLE would determine the type and intensity of therapy. The first two diseases are only infrequently diagnosed by renal biopsy, and a normotensive woman with stable renal function and neither systemic involvement nor laboratory evidence of these collagen disorders should be watched closely without intervening. Biopsy may be indicated, however, in the latter condition, i.e., in selected patients with SLE and lupus nephropathy of uncertain histopathology.

Serial assessment of fetal well-being is essential, because renal disease can be associated with intrauterine growth retardation and, when complications do arise, the judicious moment for intervention is influenced by fetal status (94, 95). Current technology should minimize intrauterine fetal death as well as neonatal morbidity and mortality. Regardless of gestational age, most babies weighing 1500 g or more survive better in a special care nursery than in a hostile intrauterine environment. More and more, there is reliance on deliberate preterm delivery if there are signs of impending intrauterine fetal death, if renal function deteriorates substantially, if uncontrollable hypertension supervenes, or if eclampsia occurs. It must be realized, however, that "buying time" for the immature fetus, for example, by attempting to control escalating hypertension, is really only controlling a sign without really modifying the underlying disorder.

Assessment of renal function during pregnancy

Serial data on renal function are needed to supplement routine antenatal observations. Specialized tests involving infusion procedures are usually not available, and their use is primarily for clinical research. Tests that are available for use in routine clinical practical include the estimation and determination of creatinine, electroytes, and urate, and the determination of creatinine clearance. The test does not measure absolute GFR as creatinine secreted by the renal tubules, but it is a reliable index, and in the last analysis the assessment of renal function requires serial surveillance of creatinine clearance (see Figures 1 and 3). Urate levels and rnal reabsorption urate are significantly higher in pregnancies complicated by preeclampsia or intrauterine growth retardation (96, 97). Above a critical level of 350 µM/l, there is significant perinatal mortality in hypertensive patients (98). However, physiologic variability is such that for serum concentrations, a single random measurement is of no value (99, 100), but serial measurements may be useful in monitoring the progress in preeclampsia (101).

When reporting renal function values, it must be remembered that correcting data to a standard body surface of $1.73\,m^2$ (and thus, by implication, to a standard kidney size) is not applicable in pregnancy (18). In order to investigate any individual's renal function, serial tests should be performed, and where possible, compared with her nonpregnant values.

If renal function deteriorates during any stage of pregnancy, reversible causes should be sought, such as urinary tract infection or obstruction, subtle dehydration, or electrolyte imbalance, perhaps secondary to inadvertant diuretic therapy. Failure to detect a reversible cause for the decrease is grounds for recommending ending the pregnancy by elective delivery.

Near term, a 15% decrement in function (which affects plasma creatinine minimally) is permissible (6). If hypertension accompanies any observed decrease in renal function, the outlook is usually more serious; immediate decisions may be required regarding elective delivery. Where renal function deteriorates markedly but hypertension is absent the role of hemodialysis is controversial (11, 87, 88, 102). We prefer to terminate such pregnancies regardless of the stage of gestation.

Decision regarding delivery

Preterm delivery (less than 37 completed weeks of pregnancy) adds to the hazards of intrauterine growth retardation, so pregnancy should be prolonged to this stage. If pregnancy procedes satisfactorily, it is probably advisable to induce labor at 38 weeks, because prolonging the pregnancy beyond this time can be associated with a greater risk of placental failure and intrauterine death. Moreover, the fetus should be relatively free of risks if the expected date of delivery is correct.

Delivery before 38 weeks may be necessary if renal function deteriorates markedly, if there are signs of impending intrauterine death, if uncontrollable hypertension supervenes, of if severe preeclampsia occurs.

Patients should be delivered where full facilities and personnel are available for fetal monitoring, operative delivery, and neonatal resuscitation.

Decisions regarding treatment of hypertension

In deciding what, if any, treatment is appropriate for hypertension, several factors should be taken into consideration (103, 104).

LEVEL OF HYPERTENSION UNDER CONSIDERATION

There is no widespread agreement concerning classification. From the clinical point of view, it is a question of establishing a dividing line that is useful from the point of view of management. Some authorities do not treat women in the third trimester until diastolic levels surpass 110 mmHg, while we would consider treating such women when levels exceed 100 mmHg (103–107). All cases must be assessed individually; a teenage gravida whose first trimester recordings were in the vicinity of 90–110/50–60 mmHg may require treatment of diastolic blood pressures above 90 mmHg (107).

Patients with labile blood pressures should not be ignored, as they often appear with severe and sustained hypertension in late pregnancy (108, 109).

UNDERLYING CAUSE OF THE HYPERTENSION

When considering hypertension, it is difficult to distinguish clinically between the different etiologic categories — preeclampsia, hypertension, secondary to the chronic renal disease, essential hypertension, and combinations of these separate pathologic states (11, 43). Except for the occasional availability of biopsy, reliance is placed on clinical assessment. The most common cause of marked hypertension in pregnancy is severe preeclampsia, which may of course by superimposed on the chronic renal disease. Preeclampsia (more common in primigravidae) is characterized by hypertension, proteinuria, edema, and, at times, coagulation abnormalities and is the most serious of the hypertensive complications of pregnancy. If it is neglected it may rapidly progress to a life-threatening convulsive phase, eclampsia.

An unusual but important feature of very severe preeclampsia is the appearance of nocturnal hypertension (110, 111). This reserves the usual diurnal-nocturnal changes seen in both pregnant and nonpregnant individuals in whom the lowest blood pressures are seen during sleep. Any regime of hypotension management may need to anticipate nocturnal hypertension by a variable schedule, with the lowest doses given at night.

EFFECT OF HYPERTENSION ON MATERNAL COMPLICATION RATE

In long-term studies, a reduction of arterial blood pressure by antihypertensive agents has proved to be of benefit in nonpregnant patients with chronic hypertension. It is not relevant, however, to make a comparison with mild hypertension in pregnancy, because pregnant women are young, the exacerbating stimulus is finite, and the complications to be avoided are rare at these blood pressure levels. The risks of hypertension in pregnancy are closely related to the fundamental question of its relation to preeclampsia. Diastolic levels of 105 mmHg or higher must always be treated, since gravidas with such pressures have been known to develop cerebral hemorrhage, cardiac failure, and occasionally renal failure.

EFFECT ON PERINATAL MORBIDITY AND MORTALITY

Most the specific risks of moderate hypertension appear to be mediated through superimposed preeclampsia. Without this complication, pregnant women with mean arterial pressures as high as 105 mmHg have a perinatal outcome that is similar to gravidas who remain normotensive.

DETRIMENTAL EFFECTS OF TREATMENT

It has been argued that hypertension is compensatory and is necessary for an adequate blood flow to vital organs. Hypertension largely depends on arteriolar constriction, and if that is reduced specifically, then the resistance to flow decreases and perfusion is maintained at lower pressures. The effect on the uteroplacental circulation is an important consideration when deciding whether or not to reduce the blood pressure of a pregnant woman with hypertension (107).

There is little evidence with which to rationalize with certainty the use of antihypertensive agents on the basis of improvement of the lifeline to the fetus, and there are two approaches. Some believe that the uterine artery behaves like a rigid conduit or is in a maximally dilated state, that reductions in maternal blood pressure concomitantly decrease uteroplacental perfusion, and that large reductions in maternal blood pressure should be guarded against, especially near term (112). Others believe that uteroplacental blood flow autoregulates rapidly and therefore recommend aggressive lowering of blood pressure (113, 114). Obviously, the best approach to treatment will not be known until there is resolution of this controversy. Assuming that this autoregulation does occur in humans, it might be asked how quickly it takes place, since the fetus may be compromised by trivially brief periods of ischemia.

EFFECT ON LONG-TERM MATERNAL PROGNOSIS

In the absence of chronic pathology, the ultimate prevalence of hypertension among primigravidae who develop severe preeclampsia is not greater than that in unselected women matched for age and rate (12, 115), In multiparous women who have severe preeclampsia, it is the antecedent hypertension that has predisposed them to it, rather than the preeclampsia that led to chronic hypertension. Recurrent hypertension in pregnancy is indicative of a high risk of later chronic hypertension. Women who remain normotensive throughout successive pregnancies are at very low risk of developing chronic hypertension (43).

Role of antihypertensive therapy

Treatment of hypertension is not considered until diastolic levels are 95 mmHg or greater in the second, and 100 mmHg or above in the third, trimester. Antihypertensive agents can be useful (Table 6) in the following situations (103).

CONTROL OF BLOOD PRESSURE IN CHRONIC HYPERTENSION

If is patient is stabilized effectively with drugs that are not specifically contraindicated in pregnancy, these medications should be continued during pregnancy. Some, including our group, will discontinue diuretics.

TEMPORIZATION IN A CASE OF PREECLAMPSIA

In an attempt to temporize, where hospitalization alone has had no effect in a case of preeclampsia and 1 or 2 weeks will enhance the chances of neonatal survival, it is justified to prescribe antihypertensive agents. Despite lowering the blood pressure, the other changes of preeclampsia will progress, as the treatment merely suppresses one manifestation of the disorder. More often than not the blood pressure is refractory to treatment "escapes," and the pregnancy must be interrupted for both maternal and fetal reasons (11, 12, 103).

MANAGEMENT REGIMES FOR HYPERTENSION IN PREGNANCY

Role of bedrest

It is difficult to enfore strict bedrest but, compared with activities at home, women in hospital are more sedentary. Furthermore, the elegant studies at Dallas, where hypertensive nulliparas are housed in a minimum care environment, amply demonstrate that this type of care alone dramatically reduces blood pressure (107, 116). Time represents amelioration of the vasospasm, rather than the cure of the disease. Even if there is not much reduction in the symptoms of severe preeclampsia, and with evidence of favorable fetal growth, pregnancy should be allowed to continue.

Role of sedation

Nonspecific sedation does not control blood pressure, and it is useless to resort to this approach. Phenothiazines may provoke convulsions and diazepam (Valium® has adverse effects in the neonatal period (see Use of epidural anaesthesia in labor).

Methyldopa (Aldomet®)

This is one of the first drugs used in a controlled setting to treat gestational hypertension (104, 117, 118). Methyldopa acts centrally, and an adequate therapeutic response

Table 6. Antihypertensive drugs in pregnancy

Drug	Use
Alpha-receptor agonists	Methyldopa (0.5–3 g/day) is most extensively used in the U.S.; safety and efficacy supported in randomized trials. Neonatal tremors have been reported; other side effects as in nongravid population. Trials with clonidine in progress embryopathy has been described in animals, and this drug is not currently recommended.
Beta-receptor antagonists	These agents, currently undergoing extensive testing, appear safe and efficacious. Atenolol (50–100 mg/day), metoprolol (50–225 mg/day), and propranolol (40–240 mg/day) used more frequently to date. Fetal and neonatal bradycardia and hypoglycemia reported, and animal data suggest the possibility of a decreased ability of the fetus to tolerate hypoxic stress.
Alpha- and beta-receptor angagonists	Labetalol, currently undergoing extensive testing, appears as effective as methyldopa. Possible association with premature separation of placenta under investigation.
Arteriola vasodilators	Hydralazine (50–200 mg/day) used frequently as adjunct therapy with methyldopa and beta-receptor antagonists. Fragmentary experience with minoxidil, thus not recommended at present.
Converting-enzyme inhibitors	Captopril associated with fetal death in several animal species. Should not be used in pregnancy.
Diuretics	Most authorities discourage their use, though some continue these medications if prescribed prior to gestation. We would prescribe diuretics when blood pressure control remains poor despite other agents, fetus is immature, and pregnancy termination is the only alternative.
Miscellaneous	Calcium-channel blockers (nifedipine) and serotonin antagonists (ketanserin) are currently under investigation. Use of ganglion-blocking agents (cause meconium ileus) and nitroprusside (see text) are not recommended.

From Lindheimer, Katz (111) with permission.

can be achieved by oral adminstration within 6–12 hours, provided a large initial loading dose of 750–1000 mg is used. Given the lability of the blood pressure of some gravidas, we utilize lower doses initially. Most increase dosage to a maximum of 2 g/day, but Redman and associates at Oxford (104) have successfully treated pregnant women with doses up to 3–4 g/day.

Sedation is almost the rule in the first 48 hours of the regime. As the blood pressure falls, a transient episode of oliguria is common. This can cause anxiety about further renal deterioration, a complication easily discounted by determining creatinine clearance.

SIDE EFFECTS

If patients are confined to bed, the common initial problems of dizziness and lethargy are not encountered. Depression, nightmares, salt and water retention, cholestatic jaundice, rashes, and blood dyscrasia have all been reported as rare problems.

The most significant "allergic" reaction is the indication of a positive Coomb's test, usually after 6 months or more of treatment, and thus it is not usually a problem in pregnancy. There is also the rare appearance of hemolytic anemia, from which deaths have been reported.

PRECAUTIONS

The safety of methyl dopa in pregnancy has been established by controlled and uncontrolled observations (117–120). It crosses the placenta, but no serious adverse fetal effect has yet been documented, although treatment should not be started, if possible, between 16 and 20 weeks gestation to avoid possible effects on fetal head growth (121, 122).

Patients with renal impairment may accumulate methyl dopa, and hypotension may therefore be a problem. It should not be given to women with a history of depression.

Hydralazine

Hydralazine acts by directly relaxing vascular smooth muscle, affecting arterioles more than veins. Systolic and diastolic blood pressures are decreased, as well as causing reflex tachycardia and increased stroke volume and cardiac output. Hydralazine can be given orally, 25–75 mg 6-hourly.

Toxic effects are common and include symptoms that mimic impending eclampsia, such as headaches, tremors, nausea, and vomiting; these may complicate decisions about management. Vasodilatation may produce a hot, flushed skin and nasal congestion. More rarely urticaria, paresthesia, and drug fever have been reported.

Long-term administration can cause a syndrome resembling systemic lupus erythematosus, including the development of antinuclear antibodies. Again, this is not a problem in pregnancy, and this complication is rare if total daily dosage does not exclude 300 mg. Some individuals may be unusually sensitive to hydralazine because of a genetically reduced capacity to metabolize the drug by acetylation — "slow acetylators." Finally, neonatal thrombocytopenia has been noted in the neonate, albeit rarely.

Whether it is related to the drug or the preeclampsia per se remains to be delineated (123).

Methyldopa with hydralazine

Oral hydralazine on its own is a weak antihypertensive drug, but its action is potentiated by that of methyldopa, which abolishes the very unpleasant reflex tachycardia induced by hydralazine. If blood pressure control is not satisfactory on maximum methyldopa therapy, then 25–75 mg oral hydralazine can be also given 6-hourly.

Beta-adrenoceptor blocking agents

The use of beta-adrenoceptor blocking agents (beta blockers) in pregnancy is controversial, although they are widely used for the management of hypertension in nonpregnant patients.

The first effect of their use is often a reduction in cardiac output and not a lowering of blood pressure. This would imply that there is an increase in peripheral resistance, and only after more prolonged adminstration does this return to normal. Blood pressure then falls because cardiac output remains depressed. However, beta blockers also inhibit renin secretion, and since levels of this enzyme are increased in both normal and hypertensive pregnant women (compared with nonpregnant subjects), beta blockers might be more effective in pregnancy.

Many different agents are available, and they have been used in pregnancy for the treatment of conditions other than hypertension, i.e., cardiac arrhythmias (124), hyperthyroidism (125), and hypertrophic obstructive cardiomyopathy (126). There are several controlled studies (127, 128), and in one, in particular (128), it has been claimed that beta blockade not only controls maternal hypertension, but also prompts plasma volume expansion, causing the apparently better fetal growth in the beta blocker-treated group.

Beta blockers cross the placenta with a speed that is dependent on lipid solubility. However, despite trials, little is known about the effects of beta blockade on the fetus. Congenital abnormalities have not been reported, but intrauterine growth retardation and fetal bradycardias, as well as neonatal hypoglycemia, bradycardia, respiratory depression, and meconium ileus, have been reported (129–133). Nevertheless, trials published to date find no statistical effects on the newborn (106, 107). Because of some $beta_2$ blockade of uterine muscle, premature or precipitated labor might be expected to be a complication of treatment, but the larger series are reassuring on the point.

Combined alpha-and beta-adrenoceptor blocking agents

Peripheral resistance is decreased by alpha-adrenoceptor blockage, and the reflex sympathetic drive, normally induced by peripheral vasodilation, is prevented by the cardiac beta-blocking effect.

In the United Kingdom labetalol (Trandate®) is a popular drug for the treatment of nonpregnant hypertension of the moderate and severe variety. It has been claimed that use of labetalol in pregnancy achieves a more satisfactory control of blood pressure, with no adverse side effects (134). The usual initial dose is 400 mg orally per day, which can be doubted after 3 days if satisfactory blood pressue control has been occurred. It can be increased to a total of 1200 mg daily. Side effects are unually minor and include headache and tremulousness. One disturbing feature is the observation of an increase in retroplacental dots, noted in the ongoing study at Oxford (135).

Role of diuretics

Diuretics have been prescribed during pregnancy to prevent treat preeclampsia, to alleviate excessive gain, or asymptomatic edema, and to treat symptomatic heart disease (136). Several detailed reviews on the use and abuse of diuretics in pregnancy with emphasis on the thiazides, have been published (11, 12, 107), and we agree that saliuretic therapy does more harm than good during gestation. Nevertheless, several investigators still claim that diuretic therapy is important in the management of hypertensive disorders in pregnancy and that "loop diuretics" (such as frusemide) are important in treating severe hypertension late in gestation, especially in acute emergencies (11, 111, 137).

Prophylactic thiazide therapy has been reported to reduce the incidence of preeclampsia in certain susceptible populations, but these claims could not be confirmed (11, 12, 107). In fact, more recent information derived from a large epidemiologic survey suggests that diuretics given to pregnant patients who have neither hypertension nor renal disease (presumably women with gestational edema or "abnormal" weight gain) may increase perinatal mortality (138).

Saliuretic drugs are successful in mobilizing edema fluid, but it is unclear whether such therapy will favorably influence the course of preeclampsia. In fact, there is anectodal evidence that some of the more fulminant instances of this syndrome occur in "dry" preeclampsia (11, 106, 107). Furthermore, diuretics are not without risk. Maternal complications due to saliuretic therapy have included pancreatitis, volume contraction, alkalosis, decreased carbohydrate intolerance, severe hypokalemia, and death. Arrhythmias, bleeding diathesis, hyponatremia, and perhaps intrauterine growth retardation have occurred in the neonate.

Thiazides decrease the abnormal vascular reactivity to angiotensin II that is characteristic of preeclampsia. However, these drugs also reduce the metabolic and placental clearances of dehydroepiandrosterone sulphate, which is considered by some to reflect a decrease in the fetoplacental circulation (of function) (139).

It remains to be established whether the normal increment in maternal extracellular volume is required for optimal uteroplacental perfusion. In one report, the authors demonstrated that diuretics limited the "physiologic hypervolemia" in normotensive women who subsequently delivered infants of lower weight than those in the control group. It should also be noted that in preeclampsia, where intravascular volume is already decreased, the administration of diuretics has been accompanied by signs of serious fluid and electrolyte depletion in prepartum women, as well as hypotension and shock after delivery.

Cardiac output has alternatively been described as decreased, unchanged, and increased in preeclampsia. since plasma volume and placental perfusion are already decreased, unchanged, and increased in preeclampsia. The most convincing studies in our opinion are those of Groenendisk et al, (reviewed in 140), which demonstrated both decreased cardiac output and low pulmonary capillary wedge pressures in preeclamptics. Since plasma volume and placental perfusion are already decreased in these women, and cardiac "compensation" is already maximal, further volume depletion could conceivably lead to decreases in cardiac output and placental perfusion.

Because diuretic agents have yet to be proved beneficial and the risks associated with their use are substantial, there are few unequivocal indications for diuretic therapy during gestation. The only patients for whom we prescribe saliuretics unhesitatingly are pregnant women, and possibly for the treatment of the rare complication of preeclampsia, pharyngolaryngeal edema (141).

Role of anticoagulant therapy

There have been isolated and conflicting reports on the use of heparin in the management of preeclampsia (142). The risk of anticoagulants in patients whose hypertensive disease may be associated with cerebral bleeding, and subscapular hematoma of the liver is too great to allow controlled studies. However, those who believe that most the pathologic manifestations of preeclampsia are attributable to disseminated intravascular coagulation have suggested such trials.

Role of volume expansion therapy

PERSPECTIVE

This has been suggested as a form of treatment where preeclampsia supervenes. The decrease in plasma volume, the occasional low central venous pressure, and the possibility that vasoconstriction may be due to overcompensation of the sympathetic or other pressor systems to intravascular volume depletion all provide the basis for a controversy. One view is that decreasing intravascular volume is the primary event that may be responsible for the rise in blood pressure. Another view, that of the traditional hypertension experts, is that decrements in volume are secondary to vasoconstriction, and they warn that treatment with volume expanders is dangerous.

PRESENT SITUATION

On reviewing the literature, the findings are equivocal and unconvincing. The ongoing experience of Gallery and associates (143) is an exception. These authors have carefully studied hospitalized hypertensive pregnant women whose blood pressure remained elevated despite 48 hours of bedrest. Plasma volume and extracellular spaces were measured with Evans blue dye and mannitol, respectively, and the patients were infused 500 ml of commercial stable-protein substitute over 15–20 mg. Rapid decreases in both systolic and diastolic pressures of intravascular and extracellular compartments demonstrated that the decrement in pressure was accompanied by restoration of an initially low plasma volume to values normal for pregnancy, the increment in intravascular volume being due to mobilization of fluid from the interstitial space. The authors acknowledge the possibility that the decrement in pressure may be due to contamination of the plasma protein infusate with vasodilatory peptides (i.e., bradykinin) but believe that if such were the case the decrease in blood pressure should be transient, while that observed by them persisted for 48 hours.

For the moment, there should be caution against plasma expansion therapy for several reasons. Myocardial performance may be compromised in severe preeclampsia. Volume expansion, especially with saline, may enhance vascular reactivity. Furthermore, infusion of crystalloids alone decreases the oncotic pressure, which is already quite low in most preeclamptics. Since central volumes and pressures tend to rise postpartum, the liberal use of saline may result in decrements in oncotic levels to a point where pulmonary and/or cerebral edema could ensure (144, 145). It is of interest that many of the complications occur during the first postpartum day when oncotic pressure is reaching its nadir and pulmonary capillary wedge pressure, initially low in preeclampsia, is rising. Therefore crystalloid therapy during labor should be kept to below 75 ml/hr (146).

Role of prostaglandin therapy

There is a suggestion that preeclampsia is a state of generalized prostaglondin (PGI) deficiency and increased thromboxane A_2 (TXA_2) production (107). Dietary supplementation with essential fatty acid precursors has been reported not to decrease the incidence of preeclampsia, but large studies are needed. Similarly, the results of direct infusion of PGI in women with severe preeclampsia have not been encouraging. The short plasma half-life of PGI necessitates continuous infusion and, although PGI_2 infusions are effective in lowering blood pressure, there are side effects, including weakness, nausea, headache, hypotension, and bradycardia. Fetal demise may occur, perhaps as a result of reduced uteroplacental perfusion secondary to maternal peripheral vasodilation.

It would seem that the incidence of preeclampsia is lower in women who take any aspirin in pregnancy compared with those who do not (147). It has been suggested that low-dose aspirin (< 100 mg/day), which inhibits the cyclooxygenase enzyme of TXA_2-generating platelets more effectively than the cyclooxygenase of PGI_2-generating endothelial cells, may therefore be beneficial in preeclampsia, but there has not been general agreement on the dose of aspirin needed.

A role for prophylactic treatment has been suggested for pregnant women who might develop preeclampsia, bearing in mind that the disease process itself starts early in pregnancy, well in advance of hypertension (148). Aspirin with or without a variety of antithrombotic drugs has been used (dipyramidole, dazoxiben) in women with histories of recurrent fetal loss and hypertension, with successful obstetric outcome (149–151).

Control of severe hypertension

The objectives of successful management of severe preeclampsia are to prevent convulsions, to lower blood pressure to a level that is not imminently dangerous, to maintain maternal well-being and to deliver an undamaged surviving infant.

The treatment of acute severe hypertension and the treatment of actual of impending eclamptic fits should be considered as two parallel but separate medical problems (11, 12, 106, 107) (Table 7).

The aim of therapy is to lower diastolic blood pressure to levels of about 100 mmHg, based on an unproved assumption that more drastic reductions jeopardize fetal survival in some individuals (i.e., teenagers) with very low first-trimester blood pressure levels. The diastolic pressure may be decreased 10–15 mmHg more. The use of a single medication is preferable, because both its efficacy and its toxicity are easily identified, so that sudden decrements of pressure to levels that are dangerous to fetal survival are avoided; also the ideal medication is one in which the decrement in pressure can be controlled and percipitious decrements can be avoided.

USE OF HYDRALAZINE

A loading dose of 5–10 mg can be given intravenously. Thereafter, 40–60 mg dissolved in a liter of dextrose can be infused at a rate that keeps the diastolic blood pressure around 100 mmHg, or 10 mg doses can be repeated at 20 minute intervals. The onset of action of action of hydralazine takes 20 minutes and its effect lasts 2–3 hours. Since peak action, however, is at 45 minutes, vigilance to avoid an "overshoot" is required.

Some individuals are unduly sensitive to the drug, so if there is time, a test dose of 5 mg can be given to prevent marked hypotension. The clinician must be aware that one of the side effects of hydralazine is severe headache, mimicking fulminating preeclampsia.

USE OF DIAZOXIDE

This is a potent agent that rapidly decreases blood pressure in hypertensive gravidas (152). The recommended mode of administration is intravenous injection of 300 mg. This large dose, however, is rarely necessary and may cause dangerous hypotension (153) (Figure 5). Instead it is adequate to give a titrated dose, and therefore the patient should have an indwelling intravenous catheter through which 30 mg boluses of diazoxide can be injected periodically. Blood pressure can be measured every 2 minutes in the other arm and diazoxide discontinued when the desired blood pressure is attained (154).

A reflex tachycardia accompanies the induced fall of blood pressure, but this can be prevented by sympathetic blocking agents, thereby enchancing the effect of diazoxide. If the patient is already on methyldopa, she will need less diazoxide, and this is an advantage in preventing diazoxide side effects.

It has been argued that the hypotensive action of diazoxide is too drastic and that sometimes blood pressure will be reduced to shock levels. There is also the risk of uterine atony, with arrest of labor and reduction of uterine blood flow. After repeated administration of diazoxide, it is essential to check for hyperglycemia in both the mother and neonate.

USE OF NIFEDIPINE

This calcium-channel blocker inhibits the slow-channel influx of calcium ions in vascular 5-month muscle. Walters and Redman (155) have shown that after a single oral dose of 5–10 mg, a significant reduction in mean systolic and diastolic pressures ensued within 30 minutes and persisted for 4–8 hours. There were no serious side effects or sequelae, but the authors concluded that further studies were needed on this category of drug (particularly its use concurrently with other drugs) before firm recommendations could be made. There are currently several studies

Table 7. Guidelines for treating severe hypertension near term or during labor

I	Degree to which blood pressure should be decreased is disputed. Levels between 90 and 105 mmHg are recommended (see text). In the final analysis, maternal well-being and the individual clinician's experience will dictate choice of therapy.
II	a. Parenteral hydralazine is the drug of choice. Use low doses (start with 5 mg, then 5–10 mg q 20–30 minutes) in order to avoid precipitous decreases. Side effects include tachycardia and headache. Neonatal thrombocytopenia reported. b. Diazoxide recommended for the occasional patient refratory to hydralazine. Use 30-mg miniboluses, as material nvascular collapse and death have been associated with the customary 300-mg dose. Side effects include arrest of labor and neonatal hyperglycemia. c. Do not use nitroprusside (fetal cyanide poisoning reported), ganglion-blocking agents (meconium ileus), or loop diuretics (e.g., furosemide) (see text).
III	Parenteral MgSO$_4$ is drug of choice in the United States for preventing impending eclamptic convulsions. Therapy should continue 12 (and sometimes 24) hours into the puerpeium, as one third of preeclamptics convulse postpartum.

Modified from Lindheimer and Katz (111) with permission.

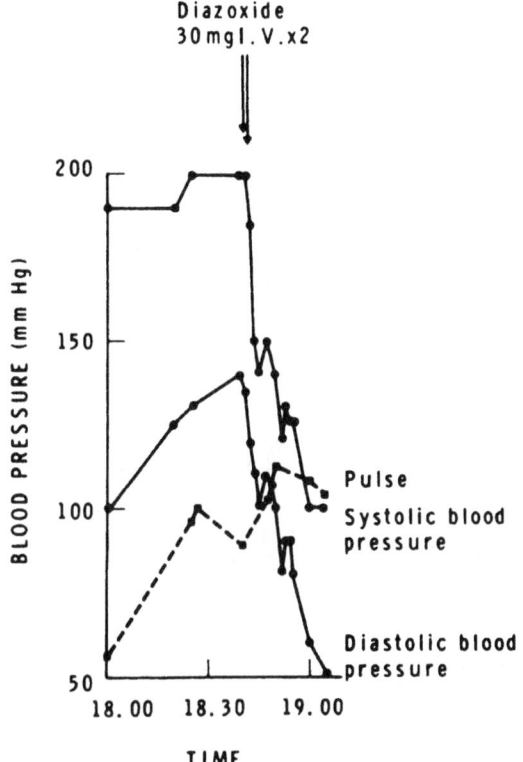

Figure 5. Patients already taking methyldopa had a placental abruption at 18.00 hours with immediate intrauterine death. Rapid reduction of blood pressure achieved by two 3 mg I.V. boluses of diazoxide. [From Redman (111) with permission].

in progress comparing the use of nifedipine and other calcium-channel blocking agents in situation where parenteral hydralazine is utilized.

USE OF OTHER ANTIHYPERTENSIVE AGENTS

Sodium nitroprusside is a very potent vasodilator. There are, however, great risks of excessive hypotension, reduced uteroplacental blood flow, and cyanide toxicity (in both the mother and fetus). Opinions vary as to its usefulness and safety (156). We do not recommend its use. Serotonin (type II) receptor blockers (e.g., ketanserin) have been used with variable success (157). Experimental studies have been revealed that intravenous serotonin that is less than that released from platelets can cause hypertension, dema, and antidiuresis.

Use of magnesium sulphate to prevent eclampsia

The use of this regime has been popularized by Pritchard (116), who admits that his approach is empirical, but its remarkable success justifies its clinical application. Magnesium sulphate is not given for its antihypertensive effects, which are minimal, but to prevent the convulsive phase of preeclampsia-eclampsia.

Many of the actions of magnesium sulphate have been attributed to effects on the central nervous system, as well as skeletal muscle paralysis. There are arguments as to whether or not it simply peripherally blocks the motor response to cortical dysfunction, which, in the abscence of such a peripheral block, would be evidenced as a fit. There are some data to suggest that magnesium sulphate induces central suppression of neuronal burst firing (159). A recent theory is that magnesium may enhance placental prostacyclin production (160).

The regime used by Pritchared (116) is as follows:
1. Initially 20 ml 20% magnesium sulphate ($MGSO_4$) (4 g) is intravenously given at 1 g/min along with two 10 ml 50% $MgSO_4$ (5 g) doses given deep into each buttock.
2. Thereafter 10 ml 50% $MgSO_4$ (5 g) is given deep intramuscularly every 4 hours into alternate buttocks.
3. It is important to check that the patellar reflex is still present, that urine flow exceeds 100 ml per 4 hours, and that respiration is not depressed.
4. With this regime, the initial plasma magnesium levels are 7–9 mM/l, subsiding to 4–5 mM/l and stabilizing. Signs of impending toxicity include the loss of respiratory movements with signs of hypoxia. The effective antidote is 10 ml 10% calcium gluconate (1 g).

Use of sedation to prevent eclampsia

Impending eclampsia or eclampsia demands the administration of an agent known to increase the cerebral seizure threshold. It is extremely dangerous to resort to nonspecific sedation. Phenothiazines may provoke convulsions, whilst opiates, by inducing vomiting or depressing respiration, can only dangerously exacerbate the patient's problems.

Chlormethiazole (Heminevrin®) is frequently used in the United Kingdom and is usually administered intravenously as an 0.8% solution at approximately 50 drops/min initially, taking care to ensure that the patient is always rousable. Thereafter the infusion rate can be reduced to 10–15 drops/min.

Diazepam (Valium®) is sometimes used, intramuscularly and intravenously (bolus injection and infusion), despite evidence of adverse side effects in the neonatal period (161). As Valium is only slowly metabolized by the newborn, significant circulating levels persist for up to 8 days after delivery.

A dose of 20–30 mg or more administered before or during labor can delay breathing at birth and produce shallow and inadequate respirations thereafter. In addition, floppiness, impaired thermogensis, and poor sucking ability are well-documented side effects, and symptoms due to withdrawal of Valium have been described. Another anticonvulsant that is used is epanutin. Magnesium sulphate alone is used routinely in the United States.

Use of epidural anesthesia in labor

The role of epidural anesthesia in the acutely hypertensive patient prior to delivery is controversial (106, 116, 162, 163). These patients are vasoconstricted and hypovolemic and, although autonomic nervous sytem blockage may reverse the hypertension, a severe degree of hypotension may ensue because of the hypovolemia. Avoidance or alleviation of this hypotension by intravenous fluid loading may help, but the consequences throughout an already grossly altered cardiovascular system, and particularly the perfusion of the uteroplacental circulation, are not known. There is no doubt, however, that epidural anesthesia is an effective method of pain relief without significant transfer of central nervous system depressants to the fetus.

Blood transfusion policy in hypertensive emergencies

A woman with a shrunken intravascular compartment is less tolerant of blood loss than is the normal pregnant woman (164). Blood replacement must therefore be initiated sooner, and at the same time very carefully, to guard against the dangers of underfilling and overfilling. Close monitoring of the central venous pressure (CVP) is helpful, especially where there is oliguria.

SPECIFIC PROBLEMS IN RELATION TO CERTAIN TYPES OF RENAL DISEASE

Table 8 summarizes the course of pregnancy in a number of types of renal disease.

Acute glomerulonephritis

Acute post-streptococcal glomerulonephritis complicating pregnancy is very rare, but does occur (165) and can be misdiagnosed as preeclampsia.

Chronic glomerulonephritis

It is difficult to evaluate the prognosis of chronic glomerulonephritis during pregnancy, primarily because most reports are poorly documented, often failing to list the degree of functional impairment, the blood pressure prior to conception, and the histology of the so-called glomerulonephritis.

Investigators in Australia (79, 166–168) have stated that pregnancy tends to aggravate most glomerular diseases because of the hypercoaguable state that accompanies pregnancy; in particular, they claim that crescentric glomerular lesions occur more readily. Their experience is that such patients are more prone to superimposed preeclampsia or hypertensive crises early in pregnancy. Another view is that kidney function decreases most often in patients in whom hypertension is severe; nonetheless, most pregnancies are successful (11, 72, 73, 78).

Table 8. Pregnancy and specific renal diseases

Renal disease	Effects
Chronic glomerulonephritis	Usually no adverse effect in the absence of hypertension. One view is that glomerulonephritis is adversely affected by the coagulation changes of pregnancy.
Systemic lupus erythematosus (SLE)	Controversial; prognosis most favorable is disease in remission prior to conception. Steroids should be increased postpartum.
Scleroderma	If onset during pregnancy, then can be rapid overall deterioration. Reactivation of quiescent scleroderma may occur post-partum.
Periarteritis nodosa	Fetal prognosis is dismal and maternal death often occurs.
Diabetic nephropathy	No adverse effect on the renal lesion, but there is increased frequency of infection, edema, and/or preeclampsia.
Pyelonephritis	Bacteriuria in pregnancy can lead to exacerbation.
Reflux nephropathy	Risks of sudden escalating hypertension and worsening of renal function.
Urolithiasis	Infections can be more frequent, but ureteral dilatation and stasis do not seem to affect natural history.
Polycystic disease	Renal impairment and hypertension usually minimal in childbearing years.
Permanent urinary diversion	Often associated with other malformations of the urogenital tract. Urinary tract infection common during pregnancy. Renal function may undergo reversible decrease. No significant obstructive problem, but caesarean section could be needed for abnormal presentation.
After nephrectomy, solitary and pelvic well tolerated	Might be associated with other malformations of urogenital tract. Pregnancy dystocia rarely occurs with pelvic kidney.

FOCAL GLOMERULOSCLEROSIS

Increased proteinuria and hypertension during pregnancy are frequent but are usually reversible. The renal lesion may be accelerated by pregnancy, but this is rare if the prepregnancy renal function is normal (84, 78). Overall fetal loss rates are about 25%.

MEMBRANOUS NEPHROPATHY

If renal function is satisfactory and stable, and hypertension is absent or under control, then the outlook is good. Pregnancy does not further aggravate the renal lesion.

DIFFUSE PROLIFERATIVE GLOMERULONEPHRITIS

This label covers a heterogeneous group of patients with prolonged proteinuria. Hypertension proteinuria invariably worsen during pregnancy, but the rate of subsequent progression into renal failure is not hastened. Fetal loss rates average 15%.

MEMBRANOPROLIFERATIVE GLOMERULONEPHRITIS

It is difficult to assess whether the course of membranoproliferative glomerulonephritis (MPGN), which is usually not good, is worsened by pregnancy. Certainly hypertension arising in pregnancy invariably persists afterwards, and even when the prepregnancy status is "mild" (plasma creatinine $< 125 \mu M/l$), pregnancy can have an overall deleterious effect. Fetal loss rates may be as high as 50% Some women with persistent hypocomplementemia have a circulating antibody "C3 nephritis factor" and placental transmission, and transient neonatal hypocomplementemia (without long-term sequelae) have been described (170).

MESANGIAL IgA NEPHROPATHY (IgA-CN)

The risk of hypertension during pregnancy is probably higher than for other subtypes, and its persistence after delivery can be problematic. If prepregnancy status is "moderate" (plasma creatinine $125-250 \mu M/l$), then progressive renal failure after delivery is highly likely, but there is no way of knowing whether this may have happened anyway. Fetal loss rates are around 15%, except in the Melbourne series (168). IgA-GN is associated with HLA-Bw35, and in some cases it may be an inheritable disease, but as yet the genetic counseling implications are unclear.

MINIMAL CHANGES GLOMERULONEPHRITIS

This is also called *minimal-changed nephrotic syndrome*. Most women of childbearing age are in stable remission with "mild" status, and pregnancy is well tolerated without risk of relapse. For women who are "frequent relapsers," prednisone can be continued throughout pregnancy, but some decide to stop therapy and to take a calculated risk of further relapse during pregnancy.

Hereditary nephritis

Pregnancy in these women is usually successful from a renal viewpoint but can be complicated by bleeding problems, usually due to disordered platelet morphology and function (171). This heterogenous group, sometimes called *familiar GN*, raises the question of renal disease transmission to the next generation, a problem not seen with any of the primary GNs, except possibly IgA-GN. The inheritance of Alport's syndrome (familial GN with deafness) is usually through less-affected females and typically has greater expression in males. Benign familial hematuria syndrome is inheritable sometimes as an autosomal dominant disease (172).

Systemic lupus erythematosis

This relatively common disease has a predilection to the childbearing age group, and coincidence with pregnancy poses complex clinical problems due to the profound disturbance of the immunologic system, multiple organ involvement in systemic lupus erythematosis (SLE), and the complicated immunology of pregnancy itself (173). Transient improvements, no change, and a tendency to relapse have all been reported.

Any decisions regarding the status of the disease and the importance to the patient and her partner of having a baby should be made on an individual basis. The majority of pregnancies succeed, especially when the maternal disease to conception, even if there were severe pathologic changes in the original renal biopsy and heavy proteinuria in the early stages of the disease (174, 175). Continued signs or disease activity or increasing renal dysfunction certainly increase the likelihood or a complicated pregnancy. SLE nephropathy may sometimes become manifest during pregnancy, and when accompanied by hypertension and renal dysfunction it may be mistaken for preeclampsia.

Some patients have a definite tendency to relapse, occasionally severely in the puerperium, and therefore some think it prudent to prescribe or increase steroids at this time (18, 176). Rarely a particularly severe postpartum syndrome may develop, consisting of pleural effusion, pulmonary infiltration, fever, ECG abnormalities, and even cardiomyopathy, with extensive IgG, IgM, Ig, and C3 deposition in the myocardium (177). Others, including some using case control data (178), do not believe in the "stormy puerperium" and do not automatically increase steroid therapy after delivery (174, 178, 179).

There can be placental transmission of lupus serum factors (perhaps the so-called LE-anticoagulant) (180). The LE-anticoagulant was first described in a patient with SLE, but it has since been observed in other conditions and even without any identifiable disorder (181). Intrauterine death is common in women with circulating LE-anticoagulant, and the placentae in such cases show extensive thrombotic and arteriosclerotic changes. Because treatment with steroids and aspirin can lead to successful pregnancies, it is important to screen for LE-anticoagulant in all women with SLE, and perhaps also in those with a history of recurrent intrauterine death or thrombotic episodes, in order to identify this particular cohort.

An increased incidence of congenital cardiac anomalies occurs in the offspring of women with SLE and other maternal connective-tissue disease, even when maternal pathology appears quiescent (182). This association appears to be related to the transplacental passage of maternal antibody (anti-Ro) (SS-A) to soluble tissue ribonucleoprotein, which is detectable in almost all cases of isolated congenital complete heart block (183). Antibody deposition may initiate an immune inflammatory response and autopsies on neonates who die of congenital heart block in SLE mothers reveal fibrosis and calcification of the antiventricular node and bundle of HIS, endocardial fibroelastosis, cardiomyopathy, and occasionally multiple structural cardiac abnormalities (184). The critical damage presumably occurs during organogenesis of the heart at 6 weeks gestation, and paradoxically, the mother's heart is usually unaffected. The fetal heart may therefore be more vulnerable to antibody-mediated damage than the mature heart, it may possess phase-specific antigens or it may lack blocking maternal antibodies (IgA or IgM not transferred to the fetus), which could stop an IgA antibody from causing maternal damage. Maternal lupus may become apparent, clinically and serologically, many years after the birth of a baby with heart block (185).

Prospective attempts to reduce the effects of the anti-Ro antibody in the fetus (and possibly the mother) have involved high-dose steroid regimens (prednisone, 1 mg/kg/day) supplemented with plasmaphoresis (186) and antiplatelets, as well as thromboxane-suppressing drugs. Success is very rare, however, and when achieved it is interesting that the anti-Ro antibody was never absent from the maternal serum and was also detected in cord blood.

Systemic sclerosis

Scleroderma is a term that includes a heterogeneous group of limited and systemic conditions causing hardening of the skin. Systemic sclerosis (SS) implies involvement of both the skin and other sites, particularly certain internal organs. Renal involvement is thought to occur in about 60% of patients with SS, usually within 3–4 years of diagnosis.

The combination of SS and pregnancy is unusual, because it occurs most often in the fourth and fifth decades, and patients with SS are usually infertile. The presentation may be the sudden onset of malignant hypertension, rapidly progressive renal failure, or slowly worsening proteinuria and/or azotemia. Where SS has its onset in pregnancy, there is a much greater tendency for deterioration.

The extent of systemic involvement is probably more important than the duration of the disease, and limited mild disease carries a better prognosis. Patients with scleroderma and no evidence of renal involvement prior to conception can develop severe kidney disease in pregnancy. There are also instances when pregnancy has been uneventful and successful, but marked reactivation occurred unexpectedly in the puerperium (187). Most maternal deaths involve rapidly progressive scleroderma with severe pulmonary complications, multiple infections, hypertension, and/or renal failure.

Sclerosis usually spares the abdominal wall skin, but there is one report of hydronephrosis, presumed to be secondary to thickened skin and decreased abdominal wall compliance, in a twin pregnancy complicated by polyhydramnios (188).

Periarteritis nodosa

The outcome of pregnancy in women with renal involvement due to periarteritis nodosa is very poor, largely because of the associated hypertension, frequently of a malignant nature (11). Although a few successful pregnancies have been reported, in most cases the fetal prognosis is dismal, and many have ended with maternal death. This may merely reflect the nature of the disease itself, but it is important when making decisions about pregnancy. Early therapeutic termination has less maternal risk (189).

Diabetic nephropathy

Because many patients have been diabetic since childhood, they probably already have microscopic changes in their kidneys (190, 191). Maternal hazards and perinatal loss are twice as common in diabetics with clinically overt renal disease as in those without.

During pregnancy, diabetic women have an increased prevalence of covert bacteriuria (and may be more susceptible to urinary tract infection), preeclampsia, peripheral edema, and occasionally severe, but transient, nephrotic syndrome (192). Most women with transient, nephrotic syndrome (192). Most women with diabetic nephropathy demonstrate the normal GFR increments and pregnancy does not accelerate renal deterioration (191, 193).

Whether or not hypertension should be treated more aggressively, especially preconception, is open to question (194). Diabetes already causes glomerular hyperfiltration, which theoretically may be further exacerbated by pregnancy if renal autoregulation fails to prevent excessive transmission of arterial pressure to the glomerular capillaries. Normalizing pressures may help to prevent (further) glomerular damage. The use of microalbuminuria as a predictor of diabetic nephropathy is controversial.

Pyelonephrotis (tubulointerstitial disease)

Acute pyelonephritis is dealt with separately in this. With chronic pyelonephritis (tubulointerstitial disease), the prognosis in pregnancy is similar to that for patients with glomerular disease, in that outcome is best in patients with adequate renal fucntion and normal blood pressure. Compared with the nonpregnant state, there is an increased frequency of symptomatic infections in pregnant women, but overall they have a more benign antenatal course than do women with glomerular disease (78).

Reflux nephropathy

This term is used to describe renal morphologic and functional changes that are the urodynamic consequence of vesicoureteric and intrarenal reflux, often complicated by recurrent infection. There are glomerular lesion (focal and segmental hyalinosis and sclerosis) as well as parenchymal atrophy and scarring. It is one of the most frequent renal diseases in women of childbearing age, a third of case are clinically unmasked by pregnancy, and up to 30% of women developing end-stage renal failure have reflux nephropathy and are usually less than 40 years.

It is frequently associated with hypertension and moderate to severe renal dysfunction features, which can adversely affect the pregnancy outcome (84, 85, 196). Specific obstetric worries in these patients include severe fetal untrauterine growth retardation and the risk of sudden, rapid worsening of hypertension and renal function with accelerated progression to renal failure.

Urolithiasis

The prevalence of urolithiasis in pregnancy is 0.03–0.35% (196, 197). Renal and ureteric calculi are one of the most common causes of nonuterine abdominal pain that is severe enough to necessitate hospital admission during pregnancy (198, 199).

Management should be conservative initially, with adequate hydration, appropriate antibiotic therapy, and pain relief with systemic analgesics (200). The use of continuous segmental (T11-L2) epidural block has been advocated, as in nonpregnant patients with ureteric colic, and may even favorably influence the spontaneous passage of stone(s) (201). With good pain relief, the patient micturates without difficulty, moves without assistance, and is less at risk from thromboembolic problems than if drowsy, nauseated, and bedridden with pain.

When there are complications that might need surgical intervention, then pregnancy should not be a detrminant to intravenous urography (IVU), even though there is a valid reluctance on the part of the clinician to consider radiologic investigation. The specific criteria that should be sought before undertaking an IVU are a) microscopic haematuria, b) recurrent urinary tract symptoms, and c) sterile urine culture when pyelonephritis is suspected, the presence of any two of which indicates a diagnosis of calculi in 60% of women (202).

Alternative management, avoiding x-rays during pregnancy, has recently been proposed, which involves the cystoscopic placement of an internal ureteral tube or stent, between the bladder and kidney under local anesthesia (203). The stent retains its positions because it has a pigtail of J-like curve at each end, and to prevent encrustation it can be changed every 8 weeks. Early empirical use for presumed stone obstruction in pregnant women with flank pain could be helpful, especially when hydration, analgesia, and antibiotics do not resolve pain and/or fever. When the pregnancy is over, the usual x-ray films should be obtained and standard management resumed.

In patients with cystinuria, assiduous maintainence of high fluid intake is the mainstay of management. Athough D-penicillamine appears relatively safe, it should only be used for severe causes, where urinary cystine excretion is known to be very high (204).

Polycystic kidney disease

This entity is the commonest single-gene genetic disease of humans, with an incidence of perhaps about 1 in 1000. Most cases do not have clinical manifestations until the fourth the fifth decade of life — only 17% are diagnosed by the age of 25 (205). It may therefore remain undetected during pregnancy, but careful questioning for a history of familial problems and the use of ultrasonography may lead to earlier detection.

Patients do well when functional impairment is minimal and hypertension is absent, as is often the case in the childbearing years. Compared to the pregnancies of sisters unaffected by this autosomal-dominant disease, they do have an increased incidence of hypertension late in pregnancy (20% vs. 2%) and a slightly higher perinatal mortality (206).

If one or the other parent has polycystic renal disease, they may seek genetic counseling. There will be 50% chance pf transmitting the disease to their offspring. DNA probe techniques are now being developed so that antenatal diagnosis may be possible by chronic villus sampling, allowing women to undergo selective termination of pregnancy (207).

Permanent urinary diversion

The surgical approach is still used in the management of patients with congenital lower urinary tract defects, but its place in the treatment of neurogenic bladders has declined since the introduction of self-catheterization. With an ileal conduit, elevation and compression by the expanding uterus can cause outflow obstruction, whereas with a uterosigmoid anastomosis, actual ureteral obstruction may occur (208). The changes usually reverse after delivery.

The most common complication of pregnancy is urinary infection. Premature labor occurs in 20%, and the use of prophylactic antibiotics throughout pregnancy may reduce its incidence. A decline in renal function may occur, invariably related to infection and/or intermittent obstruction.

The mode of delivery is dictated by obstetric factors. Abnormal presentation accounts for a caesarian section rate of 25%, related no doubt to minor genital tract abnormalities. Vaginal delivery is safe, but as the continence of a urethrosigmoid anastomosis depends on an intact anal sphincter, this must be protected with a mediolateral episiotomy.

The solitary kidney

Some patients have either a congenital absence of one kidney or marked unilateral hypoplasia. Most, however, have had a previous nephrectomy because of pyelonephritis (with abscess or hydronephrosis), unilateral tuberculosis, congenital abnormalities, or a tumor. Occasionally the woman may have been a living-related kidney donor (209). It is important to know the indication for and the time since the nephrectomy (199). There is no difference whether the right or left kidney remains, as long as it is located in the normal anatomic position.

In patients with an infectious and/or structural renal problem, sequential prepregnancy assessment should be undertaken to detect persistent infection. If the function is normal and stable, most women seem to tolerate pregnancy well, despite the superimposition of GFR increments on already hyperfiltering nephrons.

Ectopic kidneys (usually pelvic) are more vulnerable to infection and are associated with decreased fetal salvage, probably of associated malformations of genital tract (199). If infection occurs in a solitary kidney during pregnancy and does not quickly respond to antibiotics, then termination may have to be considered for the preservation of renal function. Pregnancy in women who have survived childhood treatment for a nephroblastoma (Wilm's tumor) has a 30% perinatal loss, perhaps because of the late effects of radiotherapy on the uterus (210).

Nephrotic syndrome and pregnancy

The most common cause of the nephrotic syndrome in late pregnancy is preeclampsia (43, 211). This form has a poorer fetal prognosis than pregnancy-induced hypertension, with less heavy proteinuria, but maternal prognosis is similar.

Other causes of the nephrotic syndrome in pregnancy include membranous nephropathy, proliferative or membranoproliferative glomerulonephritis, lipid nephrosis, lupus nephropathy, hereditary nephritis, diabetic nephropathy, renal vein thrombosis, amyloidosis, and secondary syphilis. Some of these conditions do not respond to, and may even be aggravated by, corticosteroids, which underscores the importance of establishing a tissue diagnosis before initiating therapy (Table 9).

If renal function is adequate and hypertension is absent, there should be few complications during pregpregnancy; however, several of the "physiologic changes" occurring during gestation may simulate aggravation or exacerbation of the disease. For example, increments in renal hemodynamics, as well as an increase in renal vein pressure, may enhance protein excretion. The levels of serum albumin usually decrease by 5–10 g/l in normal pregnancy, and the further decreases that can occur in the nephrotic syndrome may enhance the tendency toward fluid retention. Despite edema, diuretics should not be given, as these patients have a decreased intravascular volume and this therapy could further compromise uteroplacental perfusion or aggravate the increased tendency to thrombotic episodes. (see Table 9).

While the majority of these pregnancies succeed and are maintained to term, there is a report that infants of normotensive mothers who had heavy proteinuria during pregnancy manifest impaired neurologic and mental development (212).

Renal disease and pregnancy: Some conclusions

1. A balance must be struck between the anticipated pregnancy outcome and the impact pregnancy might have on the remote prognosis (75). Crucial determinants are prepregnancy renal functional status, the absence or presence of hypertension (and its management), and the renal lesion itself. Better fetal surveillance, more timely delivery, and improvements in neonatal care have also contributed to better perinatal outcome.
2. The absence of severe hypertension/renal insufficiency before pregnancy is favorable. If dysfunction is moderate, there is still a fair chance that pregnancy will succeed, but the risks are much greater. If a woman with chronic renal disease wishes to have children, the sooner she sets about it the better, because renal function with in any case diminish with age.
3. The pregnancy outcome in the presence of focal glomerular sclerosis, membranoproliferative glomerulonephritis, the collagen disorders, and IgA and reflux nephropathies is controversial.
4. Proteinuria is common during pregnancy (many over 3 g/24 hrs) (72).
5. Severe hypertension is a much greater adverse feature

Table 9. Manifestations and management of nephrotic syndrome in pregnancy

Manifestation	Effect of pregnancy	Management
Proteinuria	Increments in renal hemodynamics as well as increases in renal-vein pressure may enhance protein excretion and simulate aggravation of disease.	High protein diet (3 g/kg body weight). Infusion of salt-poor albumin may be beneficial for patient with decreasing renal function secondary for marked oligemia, and for those with postural hypotension.
Hypoalbuminemia	Serum albumin levels usually decrease by 5–10 g/l in normal pregnancy. Further decreases in nephrotic patients may enhance tendency towards fluid retention.	
Edema	Usually increases during pregnancy.	Avoid diuretics, which may increase the hypovolemia and compromise uteroplacental perfusion.
Infectious complications	May be a high incidence of infectious complications in nephrotic pregnant women.	Screen frequently for asymptomatic bacteriuria. Treat any infection vigorously.
Thrombotic episodes	Pregnancy is a hypocoagulable state. Some claim that there are more frequent thrombotic episodes in pregnant patients with nephrotic syndrome.	Not usually anticoagulated prophylactically. If anticoagulation is required, heparin, which does not cross the placenta, is preferred.
Hyperlipidemia	Cholesterol and free fatty acids usually increase during pregnancy.	Treatment rarely required in pregnancy. Most lipid-lowering agents not tested in this situation.

than low but stable renal function. Beware of controlling a sign without modifying the basic disorder.
6. Deteriorating renal function, even without hypertension, is a cause for concern.
7. Pregnancy does not appear to cause any detioration or to otherwise affect the rate of progression of the disease beyond what might be expected in the nonpregnant state, provided kidney dysfunction was minimal and hypertension is absent prepregnancy. An important factor in the prognosis of nonpregnant patients may be the sclerotic effects that hyperfiltration and increased glomerular pressure have on the residual (intact) glomeruli of kidneys of these women). The situation may be more precocious in the presence of a single diseased kidney, where presumably hyperfiltration and glomerular pressure are greater. Theoretically progressive loss of renal function can ensue in pregnancy, as many women with underlying disease still increase their GFR. Thus it is encouraging that data from animal models suggest that this is not the case in pregnancy (213, 214). Nevertheless, in some women with renal disease there can be an unpredicted, accelerated, and irreversible renal decline in pregnancy or immediately afterwards. The mechanisms are unknown and more human and animal research in needed (78, 214, 215).

MANAGEMENT OF PREGNANCY IN PATIENTS UNDERGOING CHRONIC HEMODIALYSIS

It is over 20 years since the first description of conception and successful delivery in a patient on chronic hemodialysis (216), and since then further case reports and registry data have been published (11, 38, 217).

Any optimism must be tempered by remembering that clinicians are reluctant to publish their failures, and consequently the true incidence of unsuccessful pregnancies in women on hemodialysis cannot be determined. There is no doubt that the high surgical abortion rate of these patients indicates that those who became pregnant do so accidentally, probably because they are unaware that pregnancy is a possibility (38).

Pregnancy counseling

In spite of their irregular or absent menstruation and impaired fertility, women on hemodialysis should use birth control if they wish to avoid pregnancy (38, 86). There are substantial arguments against pregnancy and these should be pointed out, not the least of which are the risks to the patient and the greatly reduced likelihood of a successful outcome.

Early pregnancy assessment

An early diagnosis of pregnancy is difficult. Irregular menstruation is common and a missed period will usually be ignored (86). The main mistake the clinician will make is not even to consider the possibility of pregnancy. As urine pregnancy tests are unreliable (218), even if there is any urine available, then early diagnosis and the estimation of gestational age is best accomplished by ultrasound.

Pregnancy management

For a successful outcome, scrupulous attention must be paid to blood pressure control, fluid balance, increased dialysis , and provision of good nutrition. This will place many demands on the hospital team, as well as the patient's family, and might even be considered to be a misuse of scarce resources and manpower.

DIALYSIS STRATEGY DURING PREGNANCY

Some patients show increments in GFR, despite the fact that the level of renal function is too poor to sustain life without hemodialysis (216). Women with residual renal function and satisfactory daily urine volumes in whom biochemical control is easier are more likely to become pregnant.

From our limited experience, the planning of dialysis strategy should have the following aims:
1. Maintain plasma urea at less than 20 mM/1; some would argue around 10 mM/l. It has been suggested that intrauterine death is likely if levels are much in excess of 20 mM/1 (219), but in one case report success was achieved despite levels of 25 mM/l for many weeks.
2. Avoid hypertension during dialysis. In late pregnancy the gravid uterus and the supine posture may aggravate this by decreasing venous return.
3. Ensure rigid control of blood pressure.
4. Ensure minimal fluctuations in fluid balance and limit volume changes. Dialysis and uterine contractions are associated (220).
5. Limit interdialysis weight gain to about 1 kg until late pregnancy.

Inevitably this means increased hours and frequency of dialysis, in some instances requiring an increase in time spent of as much as 50%. There is no doubt that frequent dialysis renders dietary management and control of weight gain much easier, but the logistical problems caused might need to be solved by a combination of home and hospital dialysis.

ANEMIA

Increasing anemia can cause concern for maternal and fetal welfare. Patients are usually anemic and blood transfusion may be needed (221). Anemia is greatest in anephric patients (38). Caution is needed because transfusion may exacerbate hypertension and might also impair the ability to control circulatory overload, even with extra dialysis. Fluctuations in blood volume can be minimized, however, if packed red cells are transfused during dialysis.

Unnecessary blood sampling should be guarded against in the face of anemia, and in any case, lack of venepuncture sites can be a problem. The protocol for various tests usually performed in a particular unit should be followed, removing no more blood per venepuncture than is absolutely necessary. Screening for Australia antigen is mandatory.

HYPERTENSION

Blood pressure tends to be labile, and because these patients have such abnormal lipid profiles and possibly accelerated atherogenesis, it is difficult to predict the cardiovascular capacity to tolerate pregnancy. Normal blood pressure, however, is reassuring. Unfortunately hypertension is a common problem, though it may be possible to control this by ultrafiltration. Any other measures must be carefully assessed in the light of possible side effects.

ATTENTION TO NUTRITION

Despite more frequent dialysis, relatively free dietary intake should be discouraged. An oral intake of at least 70 g protein, 1500 mg calcium, 50 mMl potassium, and 80 mMl sodium per day is advised, and oral supplements of dialyzable vitamins should be given. Vitamin D supplements can be difficult to judge in patients who have had parathyroidectomy. All this poses logical risks for fetal nutrition, in addition to the fact that the exact impact of the uremic environment is difficult to assess.

FETAL SURVEILLANCE AND DELIVERY

What has been said about fetal surveillance in relation to chronic renal disease in pregnancy applies here. Cesarean section should only be necessary for purely obstetric reasons, although it could be argued that an elective caesarean section in all cases would minimize potential problems during labor. In fact, preterm labor is generally the rule, and the role of caesarean section in this situation needs to be carefully considered.

MANAGEMENT OF PREGNANCY IN PATIENTS UNDERGOING CHRONIC AMBULATORY PERITONEAL DIALYSIS

Experience with gestation in women undergoing chronic ambulatory peritoneal dialysis (CAPD) is just beginning. Psychosocial problems are common and can influence libido and potency (222). Nevertheless, young women have been managed with this approach, and a few successful pregnancies have been reported (223). Although anticoagulation and some of the fluid balance and volume complications of hemodialysis are avoided in these women, they nevertheless face the same obstetric problems — abruptio placentae, hypertension, premature labor, and sudden intrauterine death. Furthermore, it should be remembered that peritonitis can be a severe complication of CAPD and accounts for the majority of therapy failures (224, 225). If peritonitis was to occur during pregnancy, there would not only be a confusing diagnostic picture, but a whole series of subsequent treatment problems (226).

There are reports of gynecologic sequelae in these patients. Reflux of menstrual blood can occur through the intraperitoneal catheter under normal circumstances, as well as due to endometriosis (227).

MANAGEMENT OF PREGNANCY IN RENAL TRANSPLANT PATIENTS

Perspective

Renal transplantation usually reverses the abnormal reproductive function of hemodialyzed women. The resumption of regulation menstruation and ovulation correlates closely with the level of function achieved by the graft (228). With the increase in the number of transplanted women of childbearing age, clinicians are now more likely to be faced with the risk of counseling such patients as to whether or not they should conceive, as well as managing the pregnancies of those who are already pregnant. Indeed, it has been estimated that 1 of every 50 women of childbearing age having a functional renal transplant become pregnant (229).

A recent review (230) that brought together the experience of such pregnancies emphasized that it is difficult to assess the exact incidence of the various management problems because some of the data in the literature are imcomplete and many more pregnancies than those reported have occurred (231-236). Excluding the large Denver series (231), where 75% of patients had received kidneys from living donors, only 20% of births occurred in recipients of living-donor grafts. Despite the publication of numerous case reports, several series, and registry data from North America and Europe, little has been done to establish guidelines on the managment of the transplant recipient who conceives. In some instances pregnancy is not diagnosed until the second, or even the third, trimester, and many patients are under the impression that they could not conceive. Medical concern seems to center on the management of the pregnancy, rather than the advisability of the initial conception.

Pregnancy counseling

Management starts by counseling all couples who want a child, discussing the implications of pregnancy, as well as long-term prospects (Table 10).

PREPREGNANCY ASSESSMENT

Patients should be assessed on the basis of the following general guidelines (230):
1. Good general health for 2 years after transplantation
2. Stature compatible with good obstetric outcome
3. No proteinuria
4. No significant hypertension
5. No evidence of graft rejection

Table 10. Pregnancy prospects for renal allograft recipients

Problems in pregnancy	Successful obstetric outcome	Problems in long term
46%	92% (73%)	11% (24%)

Estimates based on 849 women in 1141 pregnancies who attained at least 28 weeks gestation (1961–1987). Figures in parentheses refer to prospects when complications developed prior to 28 weeks gestation.

6. No evidence of pelvicalyceal distention on a recent excretory urogram
7. Plasma creatinine of 180 M/l or less (preferably less than 124 M/l)
8. Drug therapy: prenidsone, 15 mg/day or less and azathioprine 2 mg/kg/day or less (criteria for cyclosporin A remains to be determined but are quoted anecdotally at 10 mg/kg/day or less, or even a change from cyclosporine-A to azathioprine before or in early pregnancy).

After full prepregnancy assessment, advice can then be given, but it can only be advice. since patients must ultimately decide for themselves what degree of risk is acceptable. If the situation is tackled prospectively, the final decision is in the nature of an agreement rather than a judgement.

LONG-TERM PROSPECTS

Major concern is that the mother may not survive or remain well enough to raise the child she bears. Average survival figures of large numbers of patients from all over the world (230, 237, 238) indicate that between 60% and 80% of recipients of kidneys from living donors are alive 5 years after transplantation, and with cadaveric kidneys the figure is 40–50%. Functional survival of the allograft at 5 years is 45–65% in recipients of living-donor kidneys and 30–35% in recipients of cadaveric organs. Despite these statistics, many patients will choose parenthood in an effort to renew a normal life and possibly in defiance of the sometimes negative attitudes of the medical establishment. Furthermore, new advances in immunosuppression might possibly improve statistics in the future.

Pregnancy management

Patients must be monitored as high-risk cases. Management requires attention to serial assessment of renal function, diagnosis and treatment of rejection, biologic pressure control, early diagnosis or prevention of anemia, and treatment of any infection, as well as meticulous assessment of fetal well-being.

Antenatal visits should be 2-weekly up to 32 weeks and weekly thereafter. Monthly are following tests should be undertaken:
1. Full blood count, including platelets
2. Plasma, creatinine, electrolytes, and urate levels
3. 24-hour creatinine clearance and protein excretion
4. Midstream urine specimen for microscopy and culture test.

Liver function tests, plasma protein, calcium and phosphate levels, and cytomegalovirus (CMV) and titres should be checked at 6-weekly intervals. Immunosuppressive therapy is usually maintained at prepregnancy levels, but adjustment will be needed if there are decreases in the maternal white cell and platelet counts. Hematinics should be prescribed if the various hemotological indices indicate deficiency.

EARLY PREGNANCY PROBLEMS

Ectopic pregnancy has been reported and it would seem that it occurs in at least 0.5% of all conceptions (240). The diagnosis can be difficult in these patients, because irregular bleeding and amenorrhea may accompany deteriorating renal function or even intrauterine pregnancy. Transplant patients might be at slightly a high risk of ectopic pregnancy because of pelvic adhesive due to previous urologic surgery, peritoneal dialysis, or intrauterine contraceptive devices. The main clinical problem is that symptoms secondary to genuine pelvic pathology are erroneously attributed to the transplantation because of its location near the pelvis (239).

ALLOGRAFT FUNCTION

Serial data on renal function are needed to supplement routine antenatal observations. Specialized tests, invariably infusion procedures, are usually impractical, but serial surveillance of creatinine clearance is essential. The following points are important:
1. The increase in GFR, characteristic of early pregnancy and maintained thereafter, is evident in transplant recipients, even though the allograft is ectopic, denervated, potentially damaged by previous ischemia, and immunologically different from both the recipient and her fetus (240) (Figure 6).
2. The better the renal function before pregnancy, the greater is the increment in GFR during pregnancy.
3. There can be a transient reduction in GFR during the late third trimester (228–230), and such a change does not usually represent a deteriorating situation with permanent impairment.
4. In 15% of patients, significant renal function impairment develops during pregnancy and may persist following delivery (228, 230). However, as a gradual decline in allograft function is a common occurrence in nonpregnant patients, it is difficult to delineate the specific role of pregnancy. Subclinical chronic rejection, with a decline in renal function, may occur as a late result of tissue damage after acute rejection or when immunosuppression has not been adequate.
5. Proteinuria occurs near term in about 40% of patients, but disappears postpartum and, in the absence of hypertension, is not significant (240).

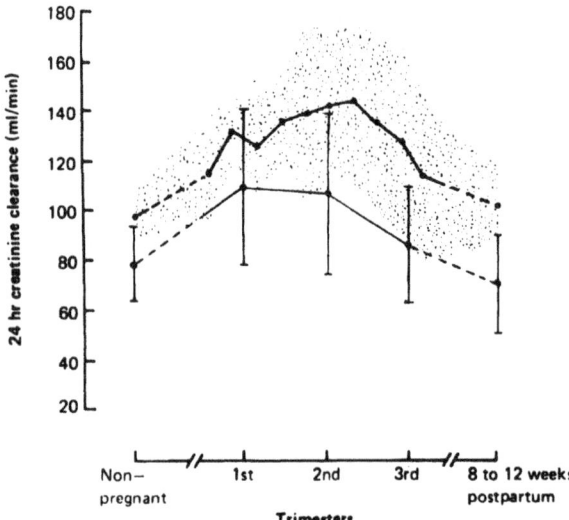

Figure 6. Weekly 2 hr creatinine clearances (GFR) over conception and in pregnancy in five women with renal transplants. The upper solid line represents the mean and stippled area the range for eight healthy women over the same period of time.

ALLOGRAFT REJECTION

It has been reported that serious rejection episodes occur in 9% of women with pregnancies lasting into the third trimester (reviewed in 230). While this incidence of rejection is no greater than expected for nonpregnant transplant patients, it must be considered unusual, because it has always been assumed that the privileged immunologic state of pregnancy would benefit the transplant. Furthermore, there are reports of the reduction or cessation of immunosuppressive therapy during pregnancy without rejection spisodes (241, 242).

Chronic rejection may be a problem in all recipients, having a progressive subclinical course. If this is somehow influenced by pregnancy, there does not appear to be any consistent factor(s) serving to predict which patients will develop rejection episodes, as they are unrelated to prior episodes, the transplant-pregnancy time interval, and problems in previous pregnancies or HLA types.

Rejection occasionally occurs in the puerperium, and this may be the result of the return to a normal immune state (despite immunosuppression) or possibly a rebound effect from the altered immunoresponsiveness associated with pregnancy.

The following points are important:
1. Rejection at any time is difficult to diagnose.
2. If any of the clinical hallmarks are present — fever, oliguria, or deteriorating renal function, often associated with renal enlargement and tenderness — then the diagnosis should be considered.
3. Without renal biopsy rejection cannot be distinguished from acute pyelonephritis, recurrent glomerulopathy, and possibly severe preeclampsia. Renal biopsy is therefore indicated before embarking upon antirejection therapy.

HYPERTENSION AND PREECLAMPSIA

The appearance of hypertension in the third trimester and its relationship to deteriorating renal function, and the possibility of chronic underlying pathology and preeclampsia, is a diagnostic problem. Preeclampsia is diagnosed clinically in about 30% of pregnancies. In at least one instance where eclampsia supervened, its development was rapid (243).

FETAL WELL-BEING

These patients need meticulous monitoring of fetal growth, best performed by ultrasound measurements. Where there is evidence of intrauterine growth retardation, the possibility of congenital CMV infection should be considered (244).

IMMUNOSUPPRESSIVE THERAPY DURING PREGNANCY

On surveying the literature, there appear to be no predominant or frequent developmental abnormalities. Azathioprine is teratogenic in animals, but only in large doses, so that the risks of modest doses (150 mg per day or less) taken by patients with stable renal function may not be excessive (245). Similarly, congenital abnormalities result from very large doses of steroids in experimental animals, but the consensus is that the risk to the fetus from the doses used after transplantation is small.

Changes in therapy must not jeopardize overall suppression, and there are some reports of therapy being reduced or stopped during pregnancy without invoking rejection (241, 242). At no point after transplantation, however, is it prudent to stop all immunosuppressive therapy, barring serious drug toxicity. Gravidas may become more sensitive to the hepatotoxic effects of azathioprine, and liver function tests should be monitored during pregnancy (230). With the advent of cyclosporin-A, new assessments are needed. Preliminary evidence suggests that it may be more effective than conventional drugs (246), but experience in pregnancy is sparse (230, 247–249). Many of the side effects of this agent may, potentially vary in human pregnancy (230).

Delivery

Preterm delivery is common (45–60%) because of intervention for obstetric reasons, and the common occurrence of premature rupture of membranes or premature labor. Premature labor is commonly associated with poor renal function, and this may be a contributory factor in transplant patients (67). In some, however, there is no obvious explanation, and it has been postulated that long-term steroid therapy may weaken connective tissues and contribute to the increased incidence of premature rupture of membranes (230).

Augmentation of steroids is necessary to cover the stress of delivery. Vaginal delivery should be the aim, and there is no evidence that there is mechanical injury to the transplanted kidney. Unless there are specific obstetrical problems (250), then spontaneous onset of labor is to be encouraged. Indications should be undertaken if there are specific indications.

MANAGEMENT DURING LABOR

Careful monitoring of maternal fluid balance, cardiovascular status, and temperature is essential, and aseptic technique is mandatory for every procedure. Prophylactic antibiotics must be given before any surgical procedure, however trivial. Surgical induction of labor by amniotomy and episiotomy warrants antibiotic cover (251).

Pain relief is conducted as for healthy women. If there are problems with acute hypertension, then management should be as previously outlined (see Treatment of severe preeclampsia).

ROLE OF CESAREAN SECTION

Although obstructed labor due to the position of the graft has been reported (252), the kidney does not usually obstruct the birth canal (see Figure 7). Cesarean section is only necessary for purely obstetrical reasons, although from the literature it appears that more sections than might be expected have been performed, presumably reflecting fear of the unknown, rather than certainty that vaginal delivery would be hazardous for mother and/or child.

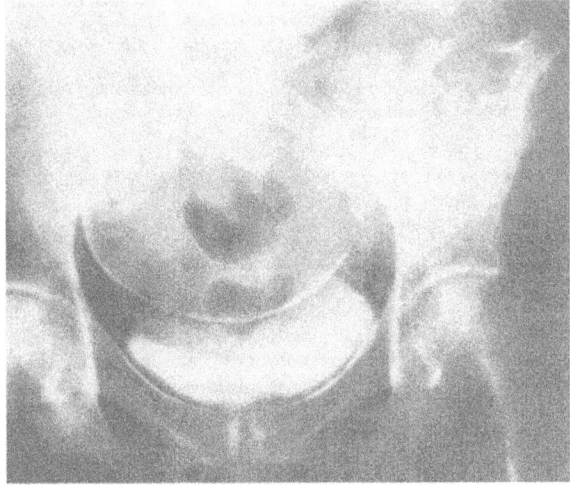

Figure 7. Single shot intravenous urogram performed at 36 weeks gestation in a pregnant patient with a renal transplant patient in the left iliac fossa.

The following are important when making a final decision on the route of delivery:
1. Transplant patients may have pelvic osteodystrophy related to their previous renal failure (and dialysis) or prolonged steroid therapy, particularly before puberty (253). For instance, avascular necrosis, particularly of the femoral head, is a common problem, occurring in 20% of all transplant patients. Patients with pelvic problems should be recognized antenatally and delivered by caesarean section if there is cephalopelvic disproportion.
2. Some authors have recommended that if there is any question of disproportion or kidney compression on simultaneous intravenous urogram and x-ray, pelvimetry should be performed at 36 weeks gestation (Figure 7) (242).
3. When a cesarean section is performed a lower surgical approach is usually feasible, but previous urologic surgery may make this difficult (254, 255).

Pediatric management

IMMEDIATE PROBLEMS

Over 50% of liveborns have no neonatal problems. Preterm delivery is common (45–60%), small-for-dates infants are delivered in about 15% of cases, and occasionally the two problems occur together. Their management is the same as in neonates of nontransplant mothers, but there are some problems peculiar to the offspring of the group of patients. (Table 11). Thymic atropy, transient leukopenia bone marrow hypoplasia, reduced blood levels of IgA and IgM, septicemia, hypoglycemia, and hypocalcemia have all been reported (179, 180, 191, 193, 199, 203, 204). Cord-blood samples taken at delivery should all be aimed at excluding any serious problems.

Adrenocortical insufficiency due to the maternal steroid therapy increases the risk of overwhelming neonatal infection. Occasionally the neonate collapses, showing overwhelming infection, after delivery, and adrenocortical insufficiency should be suspected (231). Once the diagnosis

Table 11. Factors causing neonatal problems in offspring of renal allograft patients

---
Preterm delivery/small for gestational age
Respiratory distress syndrome
Depressed hematopoiesis
Lymphoid/thymic hypoplasia
Adrenocortical insufficiency
Septicemia
CMV infection
Hepatitis-B surface antigen carrier state
Congenital abnormalities
Immunologic problems
   Reduced lymphocyte PHA reactivity
   Reduced T lymphocytes
   Reduced immunoglobulin levels
Chromosome aberrations in leukocytes
---

is entertained, the proper therapy consists of steroids, antibiotics, gamma globulin, and appropriate electrolyte solutions.

LONG-TERM PROBLEMS

If azathioprine causes chromosome aberrations in fetal lymphocytes (257), however transient, the fear is that these anomalies may not be temporary in other tissues not studied. The sequelae could be the future development of malignancies and/or fertility problems in the offspring (258). It is imperative that any child exposed to immunosuppressive therapy have a careful evaluation of the immune system and a long-term follow-up (207, 208, 259, 260).

Postnatal assessment

These patients have the same problems that affect healthy women. In addition, because they are receiving immunosuppressive therapy, they have a risk of developing de-novo malignancy that is 35 times higher than normal (230, 261), and the female genital tract is no exception. There are reports of cervical changes ranging from cellular atypia through carcinoma in situ to invasive squamous cell carcinoma (262). Consequently, a cervical smear is mandatory as the postnatal review, and regular gynecological assessment should be organized if it was not already underway prepregnancy.

Renal transplants and pregnancy: Some conclusions

1. The reproductive endocrinology of uremia is complex and has been reviewed elsewhere (86). Suffice it to say that renal transplantation is usually quickly followed by improvements in reproductive function.
2. The possibility of conception in women of childbearing age emphasizes the need for compassionate and comprehensive counseling. Couples who want a child should be encouraged to discuss all the implications, including long-term maternal survival prospects.
3. Therapeutic abortion is an option taken by 1 in every 5 women.
4. The spontaneous abortion rate is about 16%, the same as for the normal population. Of the conceptions that go beyond the first trimester, over 90% end successfully.
5. In most women, renal function is augmented during pregnancy, but permanent impairment occurs in 15% of pregnancies. In others there may be a transient deterioration in late pregnancy (with or without proteinuria).
6. There is a 30% chance of developing hypertension, preeclampsia, or both.
7. Preterm delivery occurs in 45–60%, and intrauterine growth retardation occurs in at least 20% of pregnancies.
8. Despite its pelvic location, the transplanted kidney very rarely produces dystocia and is not injured during vaginal delivery. A cesarean section should be reserved for obstetric reasons only.
9. Neonatal complications include respiratory distress syndrome, leucopenia, thrombocytopenia, adrenocortical insufficiency, and infection. No predominant or frequent developmental abnormalities have been described, and the data on progress in infancy and childbearing are encouraging.
10. Further data are needed to improve the understanding and management in the following areas: prepregnancy assessment criteria, the mechanisms of gestational renal dysfunction and proteinuria, the side effects and implications of immunosuppression in pregnancy, and the remote effects of pregnancy on both maternal renal prognosis and the offspring.

REFERENCES

1. Bailey RR, Rolleston GL: Kidney length and ureteric dilatation in the puerperium. *J Obstet Gynaecol Br Commonw* 78:55–61, 1971.
2. Rasmussen PE, Nielsen FR: Hydronephrosis during pregnancy: A literature review. *Eur J Obstet Gynecol* 27:249–259, 1988.
3. Davison JM, Noble MCB: Serial changes in 24-hour creatinine clearance during normal menstrual cycles and the first trimester of pregnancy. *Br J Obstet Gynaec* 88:10–17, 1981.
4. Davison JM, Hytter FF: Glomerular filtration during and after pregnancy. *J Obstet Gynaec Br* 81: 588–589, 1974.
5. Dunlop W: Serial changes in renal haemodynamics during normal human pregnancy. *Br J Obstet Gynaec* 88:1–9, 1981.
6. Davison JM, Dunlop W, Ezimokhai M: Twenty-four hour creatinine clearance during the third trimester of normal pregnancy. *Br J Obstet Gynaec* 87:106–109, 1980.
7. Kuhlback B, Widelm O: Plasma creatinine in normal pregnancy. *Scand J Clin Lab Invest* 18:654–658, 1966.
8. Robertson EG, Cheyne GA: A plasma biochemistry in relation to oedema of pregnancy. *J Obstet Gynaec Br Commonw* 79:769–776, 1972.
9. Davison JM: Renal nutrient excretion. *Clin in Obstet Gynaecol* 2:365–380, 1975.
10. Dunlop W, Davison JM: Renal haemodynamics and tubular function in human pregnancy. *Clin Obstet Gynecol (Bailliere)* 1:769–786, 1987.
11. Lindheimer MD, Katz AI: The kidney in pregnancy. In: BM Brenner, FC Rector JR, eds, *The Kidney* WB Saunders, Philadelphia, pp 1253–1295, 1986.
12. Chesley LC: In: *Hypertensive disorders in Pregnancy*. Appleton-Century-Crofts, New York, 1978.
13. Boron M. Sodium and plasma volume regulation in normal and hypertensive pregnancy: A review of physiology and clinical implication. *Clin Exp.*
14. Gibson HM: Plasma volume and glomerular filtration rate in pregnancy and their relationship to fetal growth. *J Obstet Gynaec Br Commonw* 80:1067–1074, 1973.
15. Cunningham FG: Urinary tract infections complicating pregnancy. *Clin Obst Gyaec (Balliere)* 1:891–908, 1987.
16. Cunningham FG, Lucas MJ, Hankins GDV: Pulmonary injury complicating antepartum pyelonephritis. *Am J Obstet Gynec* 156:797–807, 1985.
17. McFadyen IR, Eykyn SJ, Gardner NHN, Vanier TM, Bennett AE, Mayo ME, Lloyd-Daview RW: Bacteriuria of

pregnancy. *J Obstet Gynaec Br* 80:385–405, 1973.
18. Lindheimer MD, Katz AI: Kidney function and disease in pregnancy. *Lea and Febiger, Phieadelphia* 1977, Chapter 4.
19. Kunin CM: The natural history of recurrent bacteriuria in schoolgirls. *N Engl J Med* 282:1443–1448, 1970.
20. Whalley PJ: Bacteriuria of pregnancy. *Am J Obstet Gynecol* 97:723–738, 1967.
21. Roark ML: Renal infection and pregnancy outcome. *Am J Obstet Gynec* 141:709–716, 1981.
22. Condie AP, Brumfitt W, Reeves DS, Williams JD: The effects of bacteriuria in pregnancy on fetal health. In: W Brumfitt, AW Asscher, eds, *Urinary Tract Infection*. Oxford University Press, London, pp 108–116, 1973.
23. Davison JM, Sprott MS, Selkon JB: The effect of covert bacteriuria in schoolgirls on renal function at 18 years and during pregnancy. *Lancet* 2:652–655, 1984.
24. Sacks SH, Verrier Jones K, Roberts R, Asscher AW, Ledingham JGG: Effect of symptomless bacteriuria in childhood on subsequent pregnancy. *Lancet* 2:991–994, 1987.
25. Lawson DH, Miller AWF: Screening for bacteriuria in pregnancy: A critical reappraisal. *Arch Intern Med* 132:925–928, 1973.
26. Chng PK, Hall MH: Antenatal pradication of urinary tract infection in pregnancy. *Br J Obstet Gynaecol* 89:8–11, 1982.
27. Campbell-Brown M, McFadyen IR, Seal DV, Stephenson ML: Is screening for bacteriuria in pregnancy worthwhile? *Br Med J* 294:1579–1582, 1987.
28. Gower PE, Haswell B, Sidaway ME, de Wardener HE: Follow-up of 164 patients with bacteriuria of pregnancy. *Lancet* 1:990–994, 1968.
29. Briedahl P, Hurst PE, Martin JD, Vivian AB: The postpartum investigation of pregnancy bacteriuria. *Med J Aust* 2:1174–1177, 1972.
30. Pruett K, Faro S: Pyelonephritis associated with respiratory distress. *Obstet Gynecol* 69:444–446, 1987.
31. Whalley PJ, Cunningham FG, Martin FG: Transient renal dysfunction associated with acute pyelonephritis of pregnancy. *Obstet Gynecol* 46:174–179, 1975.
32. Meyers SJ, Lee RV, Munchauer RW: Dilatation and non-traumatic rupture of the urinary tract during pregnancy: A review. *Obstet Gynecol* 66:809–815, 1983.
33. Grunfeld JP, Pertuiset N: Acute renal failure in pregnancies. *Am J Kid Dis* 9:359–362, 1987.
34. Lindheimer MD, Katz AI, Ganeval D, Grunfeld JP: Renal failure in pregnancy. In: BM Brenner, JH Lazarus, eds, 2nd ed, Churchill-Livingstone, New York, 19 .
35. Pertuiset N, Grunfeld J-P: Acute renal failure in pregnancy. *Clin Obstet Gynaecol* (Ballière) 1:873–890, 1987.
36. Chugh KS, Singhal PC, Sharma BK, Pal Y, Mathew MT, Dhall K, Data BN: Acute renal failure of obstetrics origin. *Obstet Gynecol* 48:642–646, 1976.
37. Miller RB, Tassitro CR: Peritoneal dialysis. *N Eng J Med* 281:945–947, 1969.
38. Hou S: Peritoneal and hemodialysis in pregnancy. *Clin Obstet Gynaecol* (Baillière) 1:1009–1025, 1987.
39. Richet G, Alagille D: La proteolyse precoce au course anuries hemolytiques du postabortum. *Rev Fran Clin Biol* 2:475–479, 1975.
40. Hawkins OF, Sevitt LH, Fairbrother PF, Tothil AU: Management of chemical septic abortion with renal failure, use of conservative regimen. *N Engl J Med* 292:722–725, 1975.
41. Bartlett RH, Yahia C: Management of septic ab. with renal failure: Report of five consecutive cases in five survivors. *N Engl J Med* 281:747–750, 1969.
42. Hanson GC: Shock and infection. In: Hanson GC (eds) The Medical Management of the Critically Academic Press, London, 1978, pp 367–373.
43. Fisher K, Luger A, Spargo BH, Lindheimer MD: Hypertension in pregnancy: Clinical-pathological correlation and remote prognosis. *Medicine* 60:267–274, 1981.
44. Gaber LW, Spargo BH, Lindheimer MD: Renal Pathology in preeclampsia. *Clin Obstet Gynaecol* (Balliere) 1:971–995, 1987.
45. Sheehan H: The pathology of acute yellow atrophy delayed chloroform poisoning. *J Obstet Gynaecol Br:* 47–56, 1940.
46. Weber FL, Snodgrass PJ, Powell DE, Rao P, Hoffman Brady RG: Abnormalities of hepatic mitochrondrial of cycle enzyme activities and hepatic ultrastructure in a fatty liver of pregnancy. *J Lab Clin Med* 94:27, 1979.
47. Reye RDK, Morgan G, Banal J: Encephalopathy and degeneration of the viscera. A disease entity in children. *Lancet* 2:749–752, 1963.
48. Long RG, Scheur PJ, Sherlock S: Pre-eclampsia presenting with deep jaundice. *J Clin Pathol* 30:212–216, 1979.
49. Aarnoudse JG, Houthoff HJ, Weits J, Vellenga E, Huisjes HJ: A syndrome of liver damage and intravascular coagulation in the last trimester of normotensive pregnancy. A clinical and histopathological study. *Br J Obst Gynaecol* 94:145–155, 1986.
50. Hague WM, de Swiet M: A syndrome of liver damage and intravascular coagulation in the late trimester of normotensive pregnancy. A clinical and histopathological study. *Br J Obstet Gynaecol* 93:1113–1114, 1986.
51. Riely CA, Latham PS, Romero R, Duffy TP. Acute fatty liver of pregnancy: A reassessment based on observations in nine patients. *Ann Intern Med* 106:703–706, 1987.
52. Quigley MM: Acute obstetric yellow atrophy presenting as idiopathic hyperuricaemia. *Southern Med J* 67:142–146, 1974.
53. Editorial: Haemolytic uraemic syndrome. *Lancet* 2:1078–1079, 1984.
54. Hayslett JP: Postpartum renal failure: *N Engl J Med* 312:1556–1559, 1985.
55. Sun NCJ, Johnson SJ, Sung DTW, Woods JE: Idiopathic postpartum renal failure: Review and case report of a successful renal transplantation. *Mayo Clin Proc* 50:395–401, 1975.
56. Segonds A. Louradour N, Suc JM, Orfila C: Postpartum hemolytic uremic syndrome: A study of three cases and review of the literature. *Clin Nephrol* 12:229–242, 1979.
57. Drummond KN: Hemolytic uremic syndrome — then and now. *N Engl J Med* 312: 116–118, 19 .
58. Conger JD, Falk SA, Gugengenheim SJ: Glomerular dynamics and morphologic changes in the generalised Schwartzman reaction in postpartum rats. *J Clin Invest* 67:1334–1346, 1981.
59. Karmali MA, Petric M, Steele BT, Lim C: Sporadic cases of haemolytic-uraemic syndrome associated with faecal cytotoxin and cytotoxin-producing *Escherichia coli* in stools. *Lancet* 1:619–629, 1983.
60. Kaplan AL, Smith JP, Tillman AJB: Healed acute and chronic nephritis in pregnancy. *Am J Obstet Gynecol* 83:1519–1525, 1962.
61. Vintzileos AM, Turner GW, Campbell WA, Weinbaum PJ, Ward SM, Nochimson DJ: Polyhydramnios and obstructive renal failure: A case report and review of the literature. *Am J Obstet Gynecol* 152:883–885, 1985.
62. Seeds JW, Cefalo RC, Herbert WNP, Bowes WA: Hydramnios and maternal renal failure: Relief with fetal therapy. *Obstet Gynecol* 64:268–295, 1984.

63. Meares EM: Clinical implications of ureteral reflux in pregnancy. *Clin Obstet Gynecol* 21:863–873, 1978.
64. Warren DJ: Acute renal failure: Diagnosis of cause within hours. *Br Med J* 294:1569, 1987.
65. Werko L, Bucht H: Glomerular filtration rate and renal blood flow in patients with chronic diffuse glomerulonephritis during pregnancy. *Acta Med Scand* 153:177–186, 1956.
66. Kaplan AL, Smith JP, Tillman AJB: Healed acute and chronic nephritis in pregnancy. *Am J Obstet Gynecol* 83:1519–1525, 1962.
67. Felding CF: Obstetric aspects in women with histories of renal disease. *Acta Obstet Gynecol Scand* 48:2–43, 1969.
68. Strauch BS, Hyslet JP: Kidney disease and pregnancy. *Br Med J* 4:578–582, 1974.
69. Bear RA: Pregnancy in patients with renal disease: A study of 44 cases. *Obstet Gynecol* 48:13–18, 1976.
70. Leppert P, Tisher CC, Shu-Chung SC, Harlan WR: Antecedent renal disease and the outcome of pregnancy, *Ann Int Med* 90:747–751, 1979.
71. Klockars M, Saarikes S, Ilonen E, Kuhlback BC: Pregnancy in patients with renal disease. *Acta Med Scand* 207:207–214, 1980.
72. Katz AI, Davison JM, Hayslett JP, Singson E, Lindheimer MD: Pregnancy in women with kidney disease. *Kidney Int* 18:192–206, 1980.
73. Surian M, Imbasciati E, Cosci P, Banfi G, Barbiano Di Belgiojoso G, Brancaccio D, Minetti L, Ponticelli C: Glomerular disease and pregnancy: A study of 123 pregnancies in patients with primary and secondary glomerular disease. *Nephrology* 36:101–195, 1984.
74. Abe S, Amagasaki Y, Konishi K, Kato E, Sakaguchi H, Iyorie S: The influence of antecedent renal disease on pregnancy. *Am J Obstet Gynecol* 94:145–155, 1985.
75. Katz AI, Lindheimer MD: Does pregnancy aggravate primary glomerular disease? *Am J Kidney Dis* 6:261–265, 1985.
76. Jungers P, Forget D, Henry-Amar M, Albonzo G, Fournier P, Vischer V, Diaz D, Noel LH, Grunfeld J-P: Chronic kidney disease and pregnancy. *Adv Nephrol* 15:103–141, 1986.
77. Barcelo P, Lopez-Lillo J, Caberto L, Del Rio G: Successful pregnancy in primary glomerular disease. *Kidney Int* 30:914–919, 1986.
78. Lindheimer MD, Katz AI: Gestation in women with kidney disease: prognosis and management. *Clin Obstet Gynecol* (Baillière) 1:921–937, 1987.
79. Kincaid-Smith, PS, Whitworth JA, Fairley KF: Mesangial IgA nephropathy in pregnancy. *Clin Exp Hypertens* 2:821–838, 1980.
80. Hou SH, Grossman SD, Madias NE: Pregnancy in women with renal disease and moderate renal insufficiency. *Am J Med* 78:185–194, 1985.
81. Imbasciati E, Pardi G, Bozetti P, Massa E, Capetta P, Airoldi ML, Pagliari B, Ambroso GC: Pregnancy in women with chronic renal failure. In: *Proc. IVth World Congr. Int. Soc. Study of Hypertension in Pregnancy* 1984, R78A.
82. Imbasciati E, Pardi G, Capetta P, Albroso G, Bozzetti P, Pagliari B, Ponticelli C: Pregnancy in women with chronic renal failure. *Am J Nephrol* 6:193–198, 1986.
83. Hou S: Pregnancy in women with chronic renal disease. *N Engl J Med* 312:836–839, 1985.
84. Jungers P, Forget D, Houillier P, Henry-Amar M, Grunfeld J-P: Pregnancy in IgA nephropathy, reflux nephropathy and focal glomerular schlerosis. *Am J Kidney Dis* 9:334–338, 1987.
85. Jungers P, Joillier P, Forget D: Reflux nephropathy and pregnancy. *Clin Obstet Gynaecol* (Baillière) 1987.
86. Lim VS: Reproductive endocrinology in uremia. *Clin Obstet Gynaecol* (Baillière) 1:997–1008, 1987.
87. Mitra S, Vertes V, Roza O, Berman LB: Periodic hemodialysis in pregnancy. *Am J Med Sci* 259:333–339, 1970.
88. Goldsmith JH, Menzies DN, De Boer CH, Caplan W: Delivery of healthy infants after five week's dialysis treatment for fulminating toxaemia of pregnancy. *Lancet* 2:738–740, 1971.
89. Schecoitz LJ, Friedman EA, Pollak VE: Bleeding after renal biopsy in pregnancy. *Obstet Gynecol* 26:295–304, 1965.
90. Lindheimer MD, Spargo BH, Katz AI: Renal biopsy in pregnancy-induced hypertension. *J Reprod Med* 15:189–194, 1975.
91. Lindheimer MD, Davison JM: Renal biopsy during pregnancy: "To b . . . or not to b . . . ?" *Br J Obstet Gynaecol* 94:932–934, 1987.
92. Packham D, Fairley KF: Renal biopsy: Indications and complications in pregnancy. *Br J Obstet Gynaecol* 94:935–939, 1987.
93. Cutler RD, Striker GE: Renal biopsy. In: *Textbook of Nephrology*. Massry SG, Glassock RJ, eds, Williams & Wilkins, Baltimore 10:14–19
94. Thacker SB, Berkelman R: Assessing the diagnostic accuracy and efficacy of selected antepartum fetal surveillance techniques. *Obstet Gynecol Survey* 41:121–141, 1986.
95. Vintzileos AM, Campbell WA, Nochimson DJ, Weinbaum PJ: The use and misuse of the biophysical profile. *Am J Obstet Gynecol* 156:527–533, 1987.
96. Dunlop W, Furness C, Hill LM: Maternal haemoglobin concentration, haematocrit and renal handling of urate in pregnancies ending in the births of small-for-dates infants. *Br J Obstet Gynaecol* 85:838–940, 1978.
97. Dunlop W, Hill LM, landon MJ, Oxley A, Jones P: Clinical relevance of coagulation and renal changes in preeclampsia. *Lancet* 2:346–349, 1978.
98. Redman CWG, Beilin LJ, Bonnar J, Wilkinson RH: Plasma urate measurements in precid. fetal death in hypertensive pregnancy. *Lancet* 1:1370–1375, 1976.
99. Chesley LC, Valenti C: The evalation of tests to differentiate pre-eclampsia from hypertensive disease. *Am J Obstet Gynecol* 75:1165–1173, 1958.
100. Hill LM, Furness C, Dunlop W: Diurnal variation of serum urate in pregnancy. *Br Med J* 2:1250, 1977.
101. Beilin LJ, Redman CWG, Bonnar J: Hypertension in pregnancy. In: JGG Ledingham, ed, *Advanced Medicine*, Vol 10. Pitman Medical, Landon, p 3–20.
102. Naik RB, Clark AD, Warren DJ: Acute proliferative glomerulonephritis with crescents and renal failure in pregnancy successfully managed by intermittent haemodialysis. *Br J Obset Gynaecol* 86:819–822, 1979.
104. Redman CWG: Therapy of non-preeclampsic hypertension in pregnancy. *Am J Kidney Dis* 9:324–327, 1987.
105. Lindheimer MD, Katz AI: Hypertension and pregnancy. In: J Genest, O Kuchel, D Hamlet, M Cantin, eds, *Hypertension. Pathophysiology and Treatment*. McGraw Hill, New York, 19 , pp 889–913.
106. Lindheimer MD, Katz AI: Hypertension and pregnancy. *N Eng J Med* 313:675–80, 1985.
107. Davison JM, Lindheimer MD: Hypertension and pregnancy In: *Diseases of the Kidney*. RW Schrier, CW Gottschalk, eds, Little, Brown, Boston, pp 1653–1686, 1987.
108. Tillman AJB: The effect of normal and toxemic pregnancy on blood pressure. *Am J Obstet Gynecol* 70:589–603, 1955.

109. Page EW, Christianson R: The impact of mean arterial pressure in the middle trimester upon the outcome of pregnancy. *Am J Obstet Gynecol* 125:740–746, 1976.
110. Seligman SA: Diurnal blood-pressure variation in pregnancy. *J Obstet Gynaecol Br Commonw* 78:417–422, 1971.
111. Redman CWG: The use of antihypertensive drugs in hypertension in pregnancy. *Clin Obstet Gynaecol* 4:685–699, 1977.
112. Woods JR Jr, Brinkman CR III: The treatment of gestational hypertension. *J Reprod Med* 15:195–200, 1975.
113. Ferris TF: Toxemia of pregnancy: A model of human hypertension. *Cardiovas Med* 2:887–886, 1977.
114. Slavin MJ: Renal function and hypertension associated with pregnancy. *J Am Obstet Assoc* 80:258–263, 1980.
115. Chesley LC: Hypertension in pregnancy: Definitions, familial factor and remote prognosis. *Kidney Int* 18:234–240, 1980.
116. Pritchard JA: Management of pre-eclampsia and eclampsia. *Kidney Int* 18:259–266, 1980.
117. Redman CWG, Beilin LJ, Bonnar J, Ounsted MK: Fetal outcome in trial of antihypertensive treatment in pregnancy *Lancet* 2:753–756, 1976.
118. Redman CWG, Beilin LJ, Bonnar J: Treatment of hypertension in pregnancy with methyl dopa: Blood pressure control side effects. *Br J Obstet Gynaecol* 84:419–426, 1977.
119. Kincaid-Smith P, Bullen M, Mills J: Prolonged use of methyl dopa in severe hypertension in pregnancy. *Br Med J* 1:174–276, 1966.
120. Leather HM, Humphreys DM, Baker P, Chadd MA: A controlled trial of hypotensive agents in hypertension in pregnancy. *Lancet* 2:488–490, 1968.
121. Moar VA, Jeffries MA, Mutch LMM, Ounsted MK, Redman CWG: Neonatal head circumference and the treatment of maternal hypertension. *Br J Obstet Gynaecol* 85:933–937, 1978.
122. Ounsted MK, Moar VA, Good PJ, Redman CWG: Hypertension during pregnancy with and without specific treatment: the children at the age of 4 years. *Br J Obstet Gynaecol* 87:19–24, 1980.
123. Widerlov E, Karlman I, Starsater J. Hydralazine-induced neonatal thrombocytopenia. *N Engl J Med* 303:1235, 1980.
124. Schroeder JS, Harrison DC: Repeated cardioversion during pregnancy: Treatment of refractory paroxysmal atrial tachycardia during three successive pregnancies. *Am J Cardio* 27:445–445, 1971.
125. Burrow GN: Hyperthyroidism during pregnancy. *N Engl J Med* 298:150–153, 1978.
126. Turner GM, Oakley CM, Dixon HG: Management of pregnancy complicated by hypertrophic obstructive cardiomyopathy. *Br Med J* 4:281–284, 1968.
127. Tunstall ME: The effect of propanolol on the onset of breathing at birth. *Br J Anaesth* 41:792–794, 1969.
128. Gallery EDM, Saunders DM, Hymyor SM, Gyory AZ: Randomized comparison of methyl dopa and oxprenolol for treatment of hypertension in pregnancy. *Br Med J* 1:1591–1594, 1979.
129. Gladstone GR, Gersony WM: Propanolol administration during pregnancy: Effects on the fetus. *J Paediat* 86:962–946, 1975.
130. Cottril CM, McAllister RG, Bettes L, Noonan JA: Propanolol administration during pregnancy, labour and delivery: Evidence for transplacental drug transfer and impaired neonatal drug disposition. *J Paediat* 91:812–814, 1977.
131. Habib A, McCarthy JS: Effects on the neonate of propanolol administered during pregnancy. *J Paediat* 91:808–811, 1977.
132. Lieberman BA, Stittat GM, Cohen SL, Beard RW, Picker GD, Belsey E: The possible adverse effect of propanolol on the fetus in pregnancies complicated by sever hypertension. *Br J Obstet Gynaecol* 85:678–683, 1978.
133. Dumez Y, Tchobroutsky C, Hornych H, Amiel-Tison C: Neonatal effects of maternal administration of acebutolol. *Br Med J* 2:1077–1079, 1981.
134. Lamming GD, Broughton Pipkin F, Symonds ED: Comparison of the alpha and beta blocking drug. Labetolol and methyldopa in the treatment of moderate and severe pregnancy-induced hypertension. *Clin Exp Hyper* 2:865–895, 1980.
135. Redman CWG: A controlled trial of the treatment of hypertension in pregnancy: Labetalol compared with Methyldopa. In: A Riley, EM Symonds, eds, *The Investigation of Labetalol in the management of Hypertension in Pregnancy*. Excerpta Medica, Amsterdam pp 101–110, 1982.
136. Collins R, Yusuf S, Peto R: Overview of randomized trials of diuretics in pregnancy. *Br Med J* 290:17–23, 1985.
137. Finnerty JA: Hypertension and pregnancy. In: J Genest, E Koiw, O Kuchel, eds, *Hypertension*. McGraw Hill, New York, pp 866–873, 1977.
138. Christianson R, Page EW. Diuretic drug and pregnancy. *Obstet Gynecol* 48:647–52, 1976.
139. Gant NF, Worley RJ: *Hypertension in Pregnancy: Concepts and Management*. Appleton-Century-Crofts, New York, 1980
140. Wallenbery HCS. Haemodynamics in hypertensive pregnancy. In: *Handbook of Hypertension, Vol 10, Hypertension in Pregnancy* SC Rubin, ed, Elsevier, Amsterdam, pp 66–101, 1988.
141. Heller PJ, Schneider EP, Marx GF: Pharyngolaryngeal edema as a presenting symptom in pre-eclampsia. *Obstet Gynecol* 62:523–524, 1985.
142. Howie PW, Prentice CRM, Forbes CD: Failure of heparin therapy to affect the clinical course of severe pre-eclampsia. *Br J Obstet Gynaecol* 82:711–717, 1975.
143. Gallery EDM, Delprada W, Gyory AZ: Antihypertensive effect of plasma volume expansion in pregnancy-associated hypertension. *Aust NZ J Med* 2:20–24, 1981.
144. Cotton DB, Gonik B, Spillman T: Intrapartum to postpartum changes in colloid osmotic pressure. *Am J Obstet Gynecol* 149:174–178, 1984.
145. Zinaman M, Rubin J, Lindheimer MD: Serial plasma oncotic pressure levels and echoencephalography during and after delivery in severe pre-eclampsia. *Lancet* 1:1245–1257, 1985.
146. Hankins GP, Wendel GD, Cunningham FG, Leveno KG: Longitudinal evaluation of hemodynamic changes in eclampsia. *Am J Obstet Gynecol* 150:506–509, 1984.
147. Crandon AJ, Isherwood DM: Effect of aspirin on incidence of pre-eclampsia. *Lancet* 1:356–358, 1979.
148. Lindheimer MD, Katz AI: Pre-eclampsia: Pathophysiology, diagnosis and management. *Ann Rev Med* 40:233–250, 1989.
149. Beaufils M, Uzan S, Donsimoni R, Colan JC: Prevention of pre-eclampsia by early antiplatelet therapy. *Lancet* 1:840–842, 1985.
150. Van Asche FA, Spitz B, Vermylen J, Deckmijn H: Preliminary observations on treatment of pregnancy-induced hypertension with a thromboxane synthesase inhibitor. *Am J Obstet Gynecol* 148:216–218, 1984.
151. Wallenburg HCS, Dekker GA, Makovitz JW, Rotmans P: Low-dose aspirin prevents pregnancy-induced hypertension

and pre-eclampsia in angiotensin-sensitive primigravidae. *Lancet* 1:1–4, 1986.
152. Morris JA, Arce JJ, Hamilton CJ, Davidson EC, Maidman JE, Clark JH, Bloom RS: The management of severe pre-eclampsia and eclampsia with intravenous diazoxide. *Obstet Gynecol* 49:675–680, 1977.
153. Newman J, Weiss B, Rabello Y, Calbel L, Freeman RK: Diazoxide for the acute control of severe hypertension complicating pregnancy: A pilot study. *Obstet Gynecol* (Suppl): 50S–55S, 1979.
154. Dudley DKL. Minibolus diazotide in the management of severe hypertension in pregnancy. *Am J obstet Gynecol* 151:196–200, 1985.
155. Walters BNJ, Redman CWG: Treatment of severe pregnancy associated hypertension with the calcium antagonist nifedipine. *Br J Obstet Gynaecol* 91:330–332, 1984.
156. Shoemaker CT, Meyers M: Sodium introprusside for control of severe hypertensive disease of pregnancy: A case report and discussion of potential toxicity. *Am J Obstet Gynecol* 149:171–174, 19 .
157. Montenegro R, Knuppel RA, Shah D: The effect of serotonergic blockade in postpartum pre-eclampsia patients. *Am J Obstet Gynecol* 153:130–134, 1985.
158. Donaldson JO: *Neurology in Pregnancy*. WB Saunders and Company. Philadelphia, 1978.
159. Borgers LF, Gucer G. Effect of magnesium on edi foci. *Epilepsis* 29:81–91, 1978.
160. Watson KV, Moldow CF, Ogburn PL, Jacob JH. Magnesium sulfate: Rationale for its use in pre-eclampsia. *Proc Natl Acad Sci* USA 83:1075–1078, 1985.
161. Cree JE, Meyer J, Hailey DM: Diazepam in laborat. Metabolism and effect on the clinical condition and mogenesis of the newborn. *Br Med J* 4:251–254, 1978.
162. Crawford JS: Epidural analgesia in pregnancy hypertension. *Clin Obstet Gynecol* 4:735–749, 1977.
163. Joyce TH III, Debnath KS, Baker EA: Pre-eclampsia relationship of CVP and epidural analgesia. *Anesthesiology* 51:S297, 1979.
164. Tatum HJ, Mule JG: Puerperal vasomotor coll. patients with toxemia of pregnancy: A new concept etiology and a rational plan of treatment. *Am J Gynecol* 71:492–498, 1956.
165. Nadler N, Salinas-Madrigal L, Charles AG, Pollak VE: Acute glomerulonephritis during late pregnancy. *Obstet Gynecol* 34:277–283, 1969.
166. Kincaid-Smith P, Fairley KF, Bullen M: Kidney disease and pregnancy. *Med J Aust* 2:1155–1159, 1967.
167. Kincaid-Smith P, Whitwort JA, Fairley KF: Mes. IgA nephropathy in pregnancy. *Clin Exp Hyper* B2:821–838, 1980.
168. Fairley KF, Whittworth JA, Kincaid-Smith P: Glomerulonephritis and pregnancy. In: P Kincaid-Smith, TH Mathew, EL Becker, eds, *Glomerulonephritis* (Part II), 1973, pp 997–1011.
169. Kincaid-Smith P, Fairley KF: Renal disease in pregnancy. Three controversial areas: Mesangial IgA nephropathy, focal glomerular sclerosis (focal and segmental hyalinosis and sclerosis) and reflux nephropathy. *Am J Kidney Dis* 9:328–333, 1987.
170. Cameron JS, Hicks J: Pregnancy in patients with pre-existing glomerular disease. *Contr Nephrol* 37:1459–155, 1984.
171. Grunfeld J-P, Noel LH, Hafez S, Droz D: Renal prognosis in women with hereditary nephritis. *Clin Nephrol* 23:267–270, 1985.
172. Rogers PW, Kurtzman NA, Bunn SM: Familial benign essential hematuria. *Arch Int Med* 131:257–259, 1973.
173. Mor-Josef S, Navot D, Rabinowitz R, Sehenker JG: Collagen disease in pregnancy. *Obstet Gynecol Surv* 39:67–83, 1984.
174. Editorial: Effect of transplantation on non-renal effects of renal failure. *Br Med J* 284:221–222, 1982.
175. Jungers P, Dougados M, Pellissies C: Lupus nephropathy and pregnancy. *Arch Intern Med* 142:771, 1982.
176. Leikin JB, Arof HM, Pearlman LM: Acute lupus pneumonitis in the postpartum period. A case history and review of the literature. *Obstet Gynecol* 68:293–315, 1986.
177. Kochenour NK, Branch WD, Rote NS, Scott JR: A new postpartum syndrome associated with antilipid antibodies. *Obstet Gynecol* 69:460–468, 1987.
178. Lockshin MD, Reinitz E, Druzin ML, Murrman M, Estes D. Lupus pregnancy: Case control prospective study demonstrating absence of lupus exacerbation during or after pregnancies. *Am J Med* 72:893–89, 1984.
179. Hayslett JP, Reece EA: Systemic lupus erythematosus in pregnancy. *Clin Perinatal* 12:539–50, 1985.
180. Editorial: Lupus anticoagulant. *Lancet* 1:1157–1158, 1984.
181. Lubbe WF, Butler WS, Palmer SJ, Liggins GC: Lupus anticoagulant in pregnancy. *Br J Obstet Gynaecol* :357–363, 1984.
182. Singsen BH, Akhter JE, Weinstein MM, Sharp GC: Congenital complete heart block and SSA antibodies *Am J Obstet Gynecol* 152:655–659, 1985.
183. Scott JS, Maddison PJ, Taylor PV, Esscher E, Sotto O, Skinner RP: Connective-tissue disease, antibodies to ribonucleoprotein and congenital heart block. *N Engl J Med* 309:209–212, 1983.
184. Taylor PV, Scott JS, Gerlis LM, Esscher E, Scott O: Maternal antibodies against fetal cardiac antigens in congenital complete heart block. *N Engl J Med* 315:667–672, 1986.
185. Kasinath BS, Katz AI: Delayed maternal lupus after delivery of offspring with congenital heart block. *Arch Int Med* 142:1217–1298, 1983.
186. Barclay CS, French MAH, Ross LD, Sokol RJ: Successful pregnancy following steroid therapy and plasma exchange in a woman with anti-Ro (SS-A) antibodies. Case report. *Br J Obstet Gynaecol* 94:369–371, 1987.
187. Smith CA: Progressive systemic sclerosis and post-partum renal failure complicated by peripheral gangrene. *J Rheum* 9:455–460, 1982.
188. Moore M, Saffon JE, Barof HSB: Systemic sclerosis and pregnancy complicated by obstructive uropathy. *Am J Obstet Gynecol* 153:893–895, 1985.
189. Nagey DA, Fortier KJ, Linden J: Pregnancy complicated by periarteritis nodosa: Induced abortion as an alternative. *Am J Obstet Gynecol* 147:103–195, 1983.
190. Cousins L: Pregnancy complications among diabetic women: Review 1965–1985. *Obstet Gynec Surv* 42:140–149, 1987.
191. Hayslett JP, Reece EA: Managing diabetic patients with nephropathy and other vascular complications. *Clin Obstet Gynaecol* (Baillière) 1S:939–954, 1987.
192. Patterson KR, Lunan CB, MacCuish AC: Severe transient nephrotic syndrome in diabetic pregnancy. *Br Med J* 291:1612, 1985.
193. Reece EA, Coustan DR, Hayslelt JP: Diasctic nephropathy. Pregnancy performance and fetomaterual outcome. *Am J Obstet Gynecol* 159:56–66, 1988.
194. Parving H-H, Andersen AR, Smidt UM, Hommonel E, Mathiesen ER, Svendsen PA: Effect of antihypertensive treatment on kidney function in diabetic nephropathy. *Br*

Med J 294:1443-1447, 1987.
195. Becker GJ, Ihle BO, Fairley KF, Bastos M, Kincaid-Smith: Effect of pregnancy on moderate renal failure in reflux nephropathy. *Br Med J* 294:796, 1986.
196. Kincaid-Smith P, Fairley KF: Renal disease in pregnancy: Three controversial areas: mesangial IgA nephropathy, focal glomerular scherosis (Focal and sequental hyalinosis and sclerosis) and reflux nephropathy. *Am J Kid Dis* 9:328-333, 1987.
197. Maikranz P, Coe FL, Parks J, Lindheimer MD: Nephrolithiasis and gestation. *Clin Obstet Gynaecol* 1987.
198. Scott JR, Cruikshank DP, Kochenour NK, Pitkin RM, Warenski JC: Fetal platelet counts in the obstetric management of immunologic thrombocytopenic purpura. *Am J Obstet Gynecol* 136:495-499, 1980.
199. Klein EA: Urologic problems of pregnancy. *Obstet Gynecol Surv* 39:605-615, 1983.
200. Strong DW, Murcheson RJ, Lynch DF. The management of renal calculi during pregnancy. *Surg Gynecol Obstet* 146:604-608, 1978.
201. Ready BL, Johnson ES: Epidural block for treatment of renal colic during pregnancy. *Can Anaes Soc J* 28:77-79, 1981.
202. Miller DR, Kakkis J: Prognosis, management and outcome of obstructive renal disease in pregnancy. *J Reprod Med* 27:199-201, 1982.
203. Loughlin KR, Bailey RB: Internal ureteral stents for conservative management of ureteral calculi during pregnancy. *N Engl J Med* 315:1647-1649, 1986.
204. Gregory MC, Mansell MA: Pregnancy and cystinuria. *Lancet* 2:1158-1160, 1983.
205. Bear JC, McManamon P, Morgan P: Age at clinical onset and at ultrasongraphic detection of adult polycystic kidney disease: Data for genetic counseling. *Am J Med Genetics* 18:45-59, 1984.
206. Milutinoivic J, Fialkow PJ, Agodoa LY: Fertility and pregnancy complications in women with autosomal dominant polycystic kidney disease. *Obstet Gynecol* 61:566-570, 1983.
207. Reeders ST, Zerres K, Gal A, Hogenkamp T, Propping P, Schmidt WM, Waldherr R, Dolata MM, Davies KE, Weatherall DJ: Prenatal diagnosis of autosomal dominant polycystic kidney disease with a DNA probe. *Lancet* 2:6-7, 1986.
208. Barrett RJ, Peters WA: Pregnancy following urinary diversion. *Obstet Gynecol* 62:582-56, 1983.
209. Buszta C, Steinmuller DR, Nogick AC, Schreiber MJ, Cunningham R, Popowniak KL, Streem SB, Steinhilber D, Brun WE: Pregnancy after donor nephrectomy. *Transplantation* 40:651-655, 1985.
210. Li FP, Gimbrere K, Gelber RD: Outcome of pregnancy in survivors of Wilm's tumor. *J Am Med Assoc* 257:216-219, 1987.
211. First MR, Ooi BS, Wellington J, Pollak VE: Pre-eclampsia with the nephrotic syndrome. *Kidney Int* 13:16a, 1978.
212. Rosenbaum AI, Churchill JA, Shakhasashiri ZA: Neuropsychologic outcome of children whose mothers had proteinuria during pregnancy. *Obstet Gynecol* 33:118-123, 1969.
213. Baylis C: The determination of renal hemodynamics in pregnancy. *Am J Kidney Dis* 9:260-264, 1987.
214. Baylis C: Renal disease in gravid animal models. *Am J Kidney Dis* 9:350-353, 1987.
215. Baylis C: Glomerular filtration and volume regulation in gravid animal models. *Clin Obstet Gynaecol* (Baillière) 1:789-813, 1987.
216. Confortini P, Galanti G, Ancona G, Giongo A, Lorenzini E: Full term pregnancy and successful delivery in a patient on chronic haemodialysis. In: JS Cameron, ed, *Proceedings of the European Dialysis and Transplant Association*. Pitman Medical, London, pp 74-78, 1971.
217. Registration Committee of the European Dialysis and Transplant Association: Successful pregnancies in women treated by dialysis and kidney transplantation. *Br J Obstet Gynaecol* 87:839-845, 1980.
218. Hogan WJ, Price JW: Proteinuria as a cause of false positive results in pregnancy tests. *Obstet Gynecol* 29:585-589, 1967.
219. Tenney B, Dandrow RV: Clinical Study of hypertension disease in pregnancy *Am J Obstet Gynecol* 81:8-15, 1961.
220. Ackrill P, Goodwin FJ, March FP, Stratton D, Wagman H: Successful pregnancy in patient on regular dialysis. *Br Med J* 2:172-174, 1975.
221. Rigenbach M, Renger B, Beavais P, Imbs FJ, Eschbach J, Frey G: Grossesse er accouchment d'un enfant vivant diez une patiente traitte par haemodialyse iterative. *J Urol Nephrol* (Paris) 84:360-366, 1979.
222. Borgeson BD: Continous ambulatory dialysis (CAPD): Some psychosocial observations. *Dialysis Transpl* 11:54-56, 1982.
223. Kioko EM, Shaw KM, Clark AD, Warren DJ: Successful pregnancy in a diabetic patient treated with continuous ambulatory peritoneal dialysis. *Diabetes Care* 6:298-300, 1983.
224. Goodship THJ, Heaton A, Rodger SC, Ward MK, Wilkinson R, Kerr DNS: Factors affecting development of peritonitis in continuous ambulatory peritoneal dialysis. *Br Med J* 298:1485-1486, 1984.
225. Gotloib L, Shustak A, Varka I, Haas R, Mines M, Weiss Z: What is the acute incidence of peritonitis in maintenance peritoneal dialysis? A prospective study. *Artif Organs* 9:160-163, 1985.
226. Rubin J, Rogers WA, Taylor HM, Everett ED, Prowant BF, Fruto LV, Nolph KD: Peritonitis during continuous ambulatory peritoneal dialysis. *Ann Intern Med* 92:7-13, 1980.
227. Blumenkrantz MJ, Gallagher N, Bashore RA, Tenckhoff MD: Retrograde menstruation in women undergoing chronic peritonel dialysis. *Obstet Gynecol* 57:667-670, 1981.
228. Merkatz IR, Schwartz GH, David DS, Stenzel KH, Riggio RR, Whitsell JC: Resumption of female reproductive function following renal transplantation. *JAMA* 216:1749-1754, 1971.
229. Editorial: Pregnancy after renal transplantation. *Br Med* 1:733-734, 1976.
230. Davison JM: Pregnancy in renal allograft recipients: prognosis and management. *Clin Obstet Gynaecol* (Baillière) 1:1027-1045, 1987.
231. Penn I, Makowski EL, Harris PL: Parenthood following renal transplantation. *Kidney Int* 187:221-233, 1980.
232. Meier PR, Makowski EL: Pregnancy in the patient with a renal transplant. *Clin Obstet Gynecol* 27:902-913, 1984.
233. Lau RJ, Scott JR: Pregnancy following renal transplantation. *Clin Obstet Gynecol* 27:902-913, 1984.
234. O'Donnell D, Sevitz H, Seggie JL, Meyers AM, Botha JR, Myburgh JA: Pregnancy after renal transplantation. Australia *NZ J Med* 15:320-332, 1985.
235. Hadi HA: Pregnancy in renal transplant recipients: A review. *Obstet Gynecol Surv* 41:264-271.
236. Penn I: Pregnancy following renal transplantation. In: VE Andreucci, ed, *The Kidney in Pregnancy* Martinus Nijhoff, Boston, pp 195-204, 1985.
transplantation followed by successful pregnancies. *Obstet*

Gynecol 43:732–737, 1974.
253. Ibels LS, Alfrey AC, Huffer WE: Aseptic necrosis of bone
237. The 13th report of the human renal transplant registry. *Transpl Proc* 9:9–26, 1977.
238. *U.K. Transplant Service Annual Report*, 1981, pp 26–36.
239. Scott JR, Cruikshank D, Corry RJ: Ectopic pregnancy in kidney transplant patients. *Obstet Gynecol* 51:565–585, 1978.
240. Davison JM: The effect of pregnancy on kidney function in renal allograft recipients. *Kidney Int* 27:74–79, 1985.
241. Kaufmann JJ, Dignam W, Goodwin WE, Martin DC, Goldman R, Maxwell MH: Successful normal childbirth after kidney homotransplantation. *J Am Med Assoc* 200:162–165, 1967.
242. Rifle G, Traeger J: Pregnancy after renal transplantation: an international review. *Transpl Proc* (Suppl 1) 723–728, 1975.
243. Williams PF, Jelen J: Eclampsia in a patient who had had a renal transplant. *Br Med J* 2:972, 1979.
244. Evans TJ, McCollum JPK, Valdimasson H: Congenital cytomegalovirus infection after maternal renal transplantation. *Lancet* 1:1359–1360, 1975.
245. Gross A, Fein A, Serr DM, Nebel L: The effect of imuran on implantation and early embryonic development in rats. *Obstet Gynecol* 50:713–718, 1976.
246. Calne RY: Cyclosporin in cadaveric renal transplantation: 5 year follow-up of a multicentre trial. *Lancet* 2:506–507, 1987.
247. Blumenkrantz MJ, Gallagher N, Bashore RA, Tenckhoff MD: Retrograde menstruation in women undergoing chronic peritoneal dialysis. *Obstet Gynecol* 57:667–670, 1981.
248. Flechner SM, Katz AR, Rogers AJ, van Buren C, Kahan BD: The presence of cyclosporine in body tissues and fluids during pregnancy. *Am J Kidney Dis* 5:6–63, 1985.
249. Davison JM: Renal transplantation and pregnancy. *Am J Kidney Dis* 9:374–380, 1987.
250. Maclean AB, Sharp F, Briggs JD, MacPherson SG: Successful triplet pregnancy following renal transplantation. *Scottish Med J* 25:320–322, 1980.
251. Myerowitz RL, Medeiros AA, O'Brien TF: Bacterial infection in renal homotransplant recipients: A study of fifity-three bacteremic episodes. *Am J Med* 53:308–314, 1972.
252. Nolan GH, Sweet RL, Laros RK, Roure CA: Renal cadaver following renal transplantation: Experience in 194 transplant recipients and review of the literature. *Medicine* (Baltimore) 57:25–45, 1978.
254. Faber M, Kennison RD, Jackson HT, Sbarra AJ, Widnere JB: Successful pregnancy after renal transplantation. *Obstet Gynecol* 48:2–4, 1976.
255. Coyne SS, Walsh JW, Tisnado J, Brewer WH, Sharpe AR, Amendola MA, Mendez-Picon G, Lee HM: Surgically correctable renal transplant complications: An integrated clincial and radiologic approach. *Am J Radiol* 136:1113–1119, 1981.
256. Davison JM, Lindheimer MD: Pregnancy and renal transplantation: Look before you leap. *Int J Artif Organs* 12:144–146, 1989.
257. Price HV, Salaman JR, Laurence KM, Langmaid H: Immunosuppressive drugs and the fetus. *Transplantation* 21:294–298, 1976.
258. Reimers TJ, Sluss PM: 6-mercaptopurine treatment of pregnant mice: Effects on second and third generations. *Science* 201:65–67, 1978.
259. Korsch BM, Klein JD, Negrete VF, Henderson DJ, Fine RN: Physical and psychological follow-up on offspring of renal allograft recipents. *Pediatrics* 65:275–283, 1980.
260. Rasmussen P, Fasth A, Ahlmen J, Brynger H, Iwarson S, Kjellmer I: Children of female renal transplant recipients. *Acta Paediat Scand* 70:869–875, 1981.
261. Hoover R, Fraumeni JR: Risk of cancer in renal transplant recipients. *Lancet* 2:55–57, 1973.
262. Poreco R, Penn I, Droegemneller W, Greer B, Makowski EL: Gynecologic malignancies in immunosuppressed organ homograft recipients. *Obstet Gynecol* 45:359–364, 1975.
263. Keller AJ, Irvine WJ, Jordan JJ, London NB: Phytohemagglutin in induced lymphocyte transformation in oral contraceptive users. *Obstet Gynecol* 49:83–91, 1976.
264. Taylor ES: Editorial comments. *Obstet Gynecol Surv* 30:739, 1975.
265. Rao VK, Smith EJ, Alexander JW: Thromboembolic disease in renal allograft recipients. *Arch Surg* 111:1090–1092, 1976.
266. Tatum HJ: Clinical aspects of intrauterine contraceptive circumspection. *Fetil and Stenl* 28:3–27, 1976.
267. Thompson HE: The intrauterine device and tuboovar. abscess. *Am J Obstet Gynecol* 123:338–348, 1975.

CHAPTER 34

Diabetic Nephropathy

ELI A. FRIEDMAN

INTRODUCTION

Diabetes mellitus may be complicated by diverse renal disorders (Table 1) ranging from an increased susceptibility to serious intrarenal infections such as renal carbuncle, to progressive microvasculopathy and macrovasculopathy of renal arteries, culminating in renal insufficiency. Throughout the industrialized world, the glomerulopathy termed *diabetic nephropathy* is the third most common cause of treatment for end-stage renal disease (ESRD). Uremia associated with diabetes in the United States accounts for the largest defined subset of federally supported patients with ESRD; 12.2% of Medicare-funded uremic patients who are currently treated by maintenance hemodialysis or renal transplantation are diabetic. While "glomerulonephritis" (28.4%) and "hypertension" (17.4%) are reported more frequently in the American registry (1), these diagnoses are usually employed as synonyms for unexplained kidney failure associated with small kidneys in the majority of patients so labeled.

The actual number of Americans afflicted with diabetes has been esimated to range between 4% and 9% depending on the age, sex, and race of the population studied. According to the 1976–1980 National Health and Nutrition Examination Survey (NINHS), the prevalence of diabetes in adults aged 20–74 is 6.6%, meaning that more than 8 million Americans are diabetic (2). There is a rising prevalence of diabetes with aging, to the extent that in the NINHS report, 17.7% of those aged 65–74 are diabetic. Although a number of disorders that induce hyperglycemia and glycosuria are categorized as diabetes mellitus, two main varieties of diabetes encompass nearly all patients seen in practice.

The most prevalent form of diabetes — accounting for 80–90% of all patients labeled as diabetic — is non-insulin-dependent diabetes mellitus (NIDDM or Type II). NIDDM characteristically occurs in older adults (also termed *maturity onset diabetes*), who are overweight at the onset of hyperglycemia and have normal or elevated plasma insulin levels. Approximately 10–20% of American diabetics have insulin-dependent diabetes mellitus (IDDM or Type I). IDDM is believed to be the consequence of immune destruction of the beta cells of the islets of Langerhans, causing insulinopenia. Usually occurring in children and young adults, individuals with IDDM (also termed *juvenile diabetes*) are ketosis prone and are of normal weight at onset. Whether a result of reclassification of patients who previously would have been counted as dying from a myocardial infarction of stroke, or reflective of a true increase, the reported incidence of renal failure attributed to diabetic nephropathy is increasing in the United States (3). The proportion of new diabetics begun on ESRD therapy has increased most among black Americans. Throughout the United States and Canada, in 1988, diabetic nephropathy is the diagnosis applied to a minimum of 20%, and as many as 45%, of new dialysis patients, depending on the state or province. In hemodialysis facilities serving some native western American Indian tribes, more than 90% of patients carry the diagnosis of diabetic nephropathy.

NATURAL HISTORY OF NEPHROPATHY: CAN DIABETES BE PREVENTED OR CURED?

Najarian and coworkers' demonstration that rehabilitation follows renal transplantation in appropriately selected patients with diabetic nephropathy stimulated intensive inquiries into the pathogenesis of diabetic microvasculopathy (4). Both IDDM and NIDDM are genetically predetermined, although the relative importance of inheritance in each type is incompletely understood (5). Detection of anti-islet and anti-insulin antibodies in IDDM prior to expression of hyperglycemia supports the thesis that in susceptible individuals (especially HLA type DR3 and DR4) an immune iletitis destroys insulin synthesis, leading to insulinopenia, the principal defect necessitating insulin therapy. Among 566 siblings of patients with IDDM followed for up to 10 years, IDDM developed at an overall prevalance of 11% for second cases in families — the triad of HLA identity, iselt-cell-antibody positivity, and impaired insulin secretion identified children at high risk of IDDM (6). Immunomodulation, currently consisting of administration of immunosuppessive drugs (cyclosporine, antithymocyte globulin) has restored sufficient endogenous insulin production to maintain euglycemia for

Table 1. Renal disorders associated with diabetes

Infectious
  Bacteriuria
  Pyelonephritis
  Renal carbuncle
Toxic
  Contrast-media-induced nephropathy
Neurogenic
  Cystopathy (hydronephrosis)
Vascular
  Nephrosclerosis
  Atheromatous embolic disease
  Renal artery stenosis
Microvasculopathic
  Diffuse intercapillary glomerulosclerosis
  Nodular intercapillary glomerulosclerosis

months to as long as 1 year (7). Still clearly investigational, immunotherapy for IDDM, if administered while islet injury is reversible (within weeks of the onset of hyperglycemia), holds the promise of "curing" some patients. A high incidence of nephrotoxicity observed in patients with uveitis or heart transplants immunosuppressed with cyclosporine (8, 9) tempers enthusiasm for long-term cyclosporine treatment in IDDM, as well as for immunosuppressive trials in noninsulinopenic individuals judged at risk of IDDM on the basis of anti-islet antibodies.

Although anti-islet antibodies have been detected in a minority ($< 5\%$) of NIDDM patients (10), the case for an immune pathogenesis in this type of diabetes is unproven. Prevention (delay) of the precipitation of overt diabetes (hyperglycemia-glycosuria) in those with a strong family history of NIDDM may be effected by maintaining a normal or subnormal weight, although there is little data to sustain this conjecture.

RENAL FUNCTIONAL PERTURBATIONS

In most patients, years of abnormal renal function precede the onset of proteinuria or azotemia, the first clinical signs of diabetic nephropathy. Typically, functional (clinically silent) changes occur in both the eye and kidney during the first years of IDDM. Leakage from retinal capillaries and microalbuminuria (vide infra) herald the respective onset of retinopathy and glomerulopathy. Extensive histopathologic evidence of microvasculopathy may be discovered in kidney biopsies from adolescent IDDM patients who have a consistently normal blood urea nitrogen (BUN) and creatinine levels associated with a normal to supernormal glomerular filtration rate (GFR).

MICROALBUMINURIA

Albumin excretion in healthy individuals varies between 2.5 and 26 mg/24 hr, with a geometric mean of about 9.5 mg/24 hr; almost all values (92%) fall below 18 mg/24 hr. Diabetics with Albustix® positive tests for protein excrete > 250 mg/24 hr, of which about 50% is albumin, i.e., the lower limit of *macroalbuminuria*, since albumin excretion rates between 26 and 250 mg/24 hr have been termed *microalbuminuria* by various investigators. Microalbuminuria is defined as a daily albumin excretion of 100–250 mg.

The importance of detecting small amounts of proteinuria in diabetics lies in the demonstration that microalbuminuria in either IDDM or NIDDM identifies a subset of diabetics likely to progress to clinical nephropathy. Elevated urinary albumin excretion at any time in the course of diabetes mellitus, without clinical proteinuria (albumin excretion > 1 g/24 hr), signals a likely progression of renal disease; the risk of developing renal insufficiency is approximately 20 times greater in diabetics with even small amounts of urinary albumin excretion than in those free of this finding. There appears to be a gradual but continuous increase in albumin excretion during the years between the onset of microalbuminuria and the development of a typical nephrotic syndrome (> 3.5 g/24 hr). Diabetics remaining Albustix negative for proteinuria after 30 years appear to be spared the subsequent risk of nephropathy. Detection of small amounts of albumin in an otherwise "well" diabetic is viewed by Viberti et al. as "a powerful indicator of late renal disease that is amenable to correction by improved degrees of glycemic control and possibly by careful maintenance of 'normal' BP levels (11)." There is no uniform thinking on whether screening for microalbuminuria has advanced from an investigational tool to a standard of practice. Once microalbuminuria is detected, however, diabetatologists agree that careful regulation of the blood glucose level and normalization of hypertensive blood pressures are appropriate. Because these two components of care are applicable to all diabetics in every stage of their disease, any special importance of microalbuminuria as a guide to therapy requires further validation.

PROTEINURIA

Whether or not preceded by microalbuminuria, proteinuria (greater than microalbuminuria) discovered by dipstick, heat, and acetic acid, or by sulfosalicylic acid testing, is first noted in routine urine samples after 10–15 years of IDDM, and at any time after the onset in NIDDM. Constant or "fixed" proteinuria occurs in about one half of diabetics by the 20th year of insulin treatment. Fixed proteinuria in IDDM is an ominous sign, harbinging impending azotemia, usually within 1–5 years. The meaning of *fixed proteinuria* in NIDDM is less clear. Older patients may have nephrosclerosis, which causes proteinuria on its own, in addition to diabetic nephropathy.

Albuminuria in excess of 500 mg daily is a constant correlate of advanced glomerulosclerosis, the end point of renal damage in diabetes (vide infra). Technical differences in protein measurement probably account for the varying proportion of diabetics found to be proteinuric.

Proteinuria has been reported to vary in all diabetics after 6 months to 39 years, or only after 10 or more years of insulin dependence. So-called "fixed" proteinuria may be neither constant nor irreversible. Illustrating this point is the observation by Jerums et al., who followed six IDDM patients, aged 31–59 years, whose duration of diabetes ranged from 0 to 33 years, that "remission and progression of proteinuria may occur frequently in the same individual... (12)" Consistent with this view is the sharp decline in proteinuria that follows treatment with captopril (13) or administration of insulin via a permanent intraperitoneal device (14). Other urinary proteins have been measured in diabetes. Urinary beta$_2$-microglobulin, for example, has been used to approximate GFR in IDDM. There is no established specific treatment for proteinuria per se in diabetes.

NEPHROTIC SYNDROME

Clinical presentation of diabetic nephropathy typically relates to fluid accumulation in a nephrotic syndrome. Urinary protein excretion in excess of 3.5 g/day in association with hypoalbuminuria defines a nephrotic syndrome in IDDM and NIDDM. Insidious weight gain of 10–20 kg over weeks to months, due to retention of salt and water, may expand intravascular volume, simulating intrinsic heart disease. Coincident diabetic retinopathy frequently becomes symptomatic in a nephrotic diabetic, inducing changes in visual acuity or obscured sight due to vitreous hemorrhage at the time that edema fluid accumulates. Although diabetics develop other causes of glomerulopathy as frequently as nondiabetics, it is reasonable to presume that massive (> 3.5 g/day) proteinuria in a diabetic of 10 or more years duration is caused by diabetic nephropathy, especially when retinopathy is extensive (proliferative retinopathy, vitreous hemorrhages). There is seldom a need for a percutaneous renal biopsy to confirm the presumed diagnosis in a nephrotic diabetic. In cases when the fundi are normal, or the findings on microscopic urinalysis are unusual (red cell casts, for example), a renal histologic diagnosis is helpful.

Within months to several years after the onset of nephrosis, the diabetic typically experiences a ceaseless decline in renal reserve, manifesting the signs of progressive renal insufficiency, including anemia, cold intolerance, nausea, and a reduced capacity for mentation. The interval between the start of nephrosis and lapses into renal insufficiency in untreated diabetics rarely exceeds 4 years. During this penultimate phase in the natural history of nephropathy, the nephrotic diabetic is sicker than a nondiabetic with an equivalent degree of edema and hypoalbuminemia. Sampietro et al. recently demonstrated that glycosylated albumin more readily permeated the microcirculation of the hamster cheek pouch than did normal albumin, a phenomenon that, if true in the human, would explain why the nephrotic diabetic is more liable to symptomatic volume overload than other diabetics with equivalent hypoalbuminemia (15). Muscle weakness, peripheral motor neuropathy, cardiomyopathy, and/or coronary artery disease inducing heart failure magnify the diabetic's stress in coping with multiple organ failure. Profound depression is provoked at this stage by a seemingly unending series of enervating diabetic complications, typically including vitreous hemorrhages, nocturnal diarrhea, gastroparesis, and foot ulceration and infection.

Treatment options of proven value that are applicable to the nephrotic diabetic are limited. Although there is debate over the value of "strict" glucose regulation once clinical manifestations of vasculopathy are evident, most diabetologists concur in the wisdom of reducing hypertensive blood pressures to normal. There may be a special advantage to the use of converting-enzyme inhibitors (captopril and enalapril in the United States), which, in preliminary studies, have been shown to reduce proteinuria while preserving GFR (16). Restricting dietary protein is advocated as a means of lowering a supranormal GFR, which, in animal models of diabetes, has been linked to glomerular sclerosis. Cohen et al. found that a protein restricted diet [median 47 (38–57) g/day] fed to eight normotensive IDDM patients, reduced median overnight albumin excretion from 23.0 to 15.4 µg/min (17). A 12-month trial of a 40-g high-biologic-value protein diet was administered by Evanoff et al. to eight Type I diabetics who manifested both a decrease in mean urinary protein excretion and a slowed rate of renal functional decline (7 of 8 patients) (18). Appreciating the lack of a controlled prospective trial of a restricted protein diet in diabetic nephropathy, the author nevertheless prescribes a 40-g protein diet for proteinuric patients with either IDDM or NIDDM.

No currently available therapeutic regimen uniformly halts the progression of diabetic nephropathy. Totally compliant diabetics adherent to a low-protein diet while maximizing blood glucose and blood pressure regulation still evince diminishing GFR with time — uremia is the inescapable end point of nephropathy.

Lacking identification of a single, pathogenetic mechanism to explain the initiation and/or progression of microvasculopathy in diabetes, clinicians are presently evaluating a number of *partial* or *incomplete* therapeutic regimens. Pharmacologic interventive measures under investigation include: a) reduced production of polyols (sorbitol) by inhibiting aldose reductase with sorbinil (19), b) blockade of prostaglandin synthesis with indomethacin (20), c) restoration of erythrocyte flexibility with pentoxifylline (21), d) impeding platelet activation with a combination of aspirin and dipyridamole (22). It should be kept in mind that a clinical trial of (a) through (d) above has been reported in only small groups of patients, precluding any generalization as to their merit.

COURSE OF NEPHROPATHY

Many IDDM patients with nephropathy follow a well-described sequence of renal abnormalities: a) initial glomerular hyperfiltration; b) reversible proteinuria (with or without microalbuminuria); c) fixed "massive" proteinuria; d) renal failure (23). Recently reported preliminary studies in NIDDM suggest that a similarly ordered sequence occurs in those individuals who develop renal insufficiency. Complicating the interpretation of studies of renal function in NIDDM of recent onset is the fact that, when compared with IDDM, the typical patient with NIDDM is older, has systemic atherosclerosis, and may have suffered strokes and heart attacks, each variable in itself a cause of kidney damage. Renal evaluation in NIDDM, to a greater extent than in IDDM, thus requires recognition of diabetic and nondiabetic components of renal injury.

DISTINGUISHING DIABETIC FROM NONDIABETIC NEPHROPATHY

There is usually litle diagnostic challenge posed by the evaluation of a nephrotic and/or azotemic diabetic. Typically, diabetics progressing toward uremia manifest sequential microalbuminuria, proteinuria, nephrotic range proteinuria, azotemia, and, finally, renal insufficiency. The probability that intercapillary glomerulosclerosis is the main morphologic glomerular abnormality is very great when the anticipated serial course has ben followed; a renal biopsy is not indicated. On the other hand, should signs atypical for diabetic glomerulopathy be noted, such as gross hematuria, azotemia in the absence of proteinuria, and nephrotic-range (> 3 g per 24 hr) proteinuria in a relatively new (< 5-year duration) diabetic, further renal investigation — including percutaneous renal biopsy — is appropriate.

GLOMERULAR PATHOLOGY IN DIABETES

Kimmelsteil and Wilson first described nodular intercapillary glomerulosclerosis in kidneys from NIDDM patients studied at autopsy (24), a lesion that remains specific for diabetics and is present in about half of diabetic kidneys examined at autopsy. KW nodules are noted in both IDDM and NIDDM, and first appear as an increase in the glomerular mesangial matrix that grows into single or multiple spherical lesions encroaching on patent capillary loops. The more prevalent glomerular abnormality in IDDM and NIDDM, diffuse intercapillary glomerulosclerosis, begins as a thickened glomerular basement membrane, associated with an enlarging mesangium filled with amorphous material that stains with periodic acid-Schiff (PAS). Nodular intercapillary glomerulosclerosis, although a specific finding a diabetic nephropathy, can be mimicked by membranoproliferative (lobular) glomerulonephritis, myeloma kidney, or idiopathic membranous glomerulonephritis. Complete study of the renal biopsy specimen, including fluorescence and electron microscopy, should clarify the distinction between diabetes and other glomerular disorders,

Light and ultrastructural investigations of the diabetic kidney have focused on alterations in the mesangium, glomerular basement membrane (GBM), and small blood vessels. Biopsies obtained from azotemic diabetics consistently show mesangial expansion, GBM thickening, and afferent and efferent glomerular arteriolonephrosclerosis. As the duration of diabetes lengthens, glomeruli become obliterated by a mixture of diffuse and nodular intercapillary glomerulosclerosis.

Mauer et al. applied semiquantitative light microscopy and quantitative electron microscopic stereologic morphometry to the analysis of renal biopsies obtained from 45 IDDM patients, noting a "weak relationship" between mesangial expansion and GBM thickness. It was not possible for Mauer et al. to define a close correlation between GBM thickening and decreased GFR, the amount of albuminuria, or the level of hypertension. Mesangial expansion, by contrast, did correlate with the severity of clinical diabetic nephropathy. Based on these relationships, Mauer et al. theorize that mesangial expansion could promote glomerular functional deterioration by restricting glomerular capillary vasculature and its filtering surface (25).

DURATION AND NEPHROPATHY

Renal failure develops in a shorter time in older onset NIDDM patients than in childhood-onset IDDM. Based on a retrospective computation of the interval between the onset of diabetes and the first hemodialysis in diabetics in Brooklyn, Lowder et al. found that IDDM patients with a mean age of 32.2 years were diabetic for a mean of 20.5 years before requiring hemodialysis, while NIDDM patients with a mean age of 63.1 years started hemodialysis in a mean of 13.3 years after developing diabetes (26). Although investigators may disagree on the extent to which the duration determines the severity of glomerulopathy, there is concurrence in the view that Albustix-positive proteinuria, hypertension, and declining glomerular filtration rate are signs of far-advanced renal lesions. Proteinuria and azotemia signify extensive glomerular destruction.

HYPERFILTRATION

Glomeruli in diabetics are injured by a least two different mechanisms, protein denaturation by high ambient glucose levels, and the adverse effect of intraglomerular hypertension (discussed below). The earliest effect of hyperglycemia in IDDM is induction of a "supernormal" GFR, a phenomenon termed *hyperfiltration*. Normalization of a greater than normal GFR by continuous infusion of insulin by a wearable pump will reduce the GFR to normal. Kidney size, glomerular diameter, tubular size, and glomerular capillary filtration surface area are all increased by about one third in IDDM. A multicenter trial is in progress in the United States to determine whether strict glucose control will retard the development of diabetic vasculopathy, including retinopathy and glomerulopathy (27).

Evidence accumulated in rat models of human diabetes suggests that euglycemia will indeed prove salutory to the diabetic. Control of hyperglycemia in streptozotocin-induced diabetic rats by insulin treatment, or iselt of Langerhans transplants, interdicts subsequent glomerulopathy (28). Rats made hyperglycemic by streptozotocin also develop renal and glomerular hypertrophy. In the induced-diabetic rat, correction of hyperglycemia by insulin treatment or islet of Langerhans transplantation prevents renal and glomerular enlargement. Extrapolation from rat to human, however, may be misleading. Glomerular lesions of mesangial expansion, GBM thickening, and segmental sclerosis in streptozotocin-induced diabetic rats do not progress to the nodular and diffuse intercapillary glomerulosclerosis that are typical of human diabetic nephropathy. Furthermore, rats made diabetic with streptozotocin do not become uremic.

Hyperfiltration and associated intrarenal hypertension may, as promulgated by Brenner's group, be responsible for continuing glomerular pathologic injury in diabetes (and other chronic kidney disorders) (29). Supporting this view are experiments in which normal rats, after an 80% nephrectomy, evince compensatory changes in remaining nephrons that are similar to those observed in rats with streptozotocin-induced diabetes. Increased single-nephron glomerular flow and pressure have been measured in rats with a reduced nephron mass (30). It is argued that these increases in pressure and flow alter glomerular permselectivity (solute-handling properties), initially causing proteinuria and later causing morphologic changes. Kidneys in streptozotocin-induced diabetic rats have an expanded mesangium and a thickened GBM. GBM thickening and a reduced filtration surface area are followed by development of focal and segmental glomerular sclerosis, a lesion found in induced diabetes in the rat that is not typical of human glomerulosclerosis. Even if hyperfiltration is shown to be uniformly present in the early years of human diabetes, hyperglycemia may still be indicated as the main factor responsible for glomerular injury. According to the syllogism that hyperglycemia causes hyperfiltration, which, in turn, induces glomerulopathy, hyperglycemia causes glomerulopathy, it follows that establishment of euglycemia should preempt the development of glomerulopathy in new-onset IDDM. Furthermore, experiments in rodents that support the hyperfiltration hypothesis of glomerulosclerosis may not be translatable to the glomerulopathy of human diabetes. Reducing the nephron mass in dogs, for example, does not lead to progressive renal insufficiency, whether a high- or low-protein diet is fed (31).

DIETARY PROTEIN

Protein feeding acutely increases renal function as a prelude to digesion. GFR in normal subjects rises $2\frac{1}{2}$ hours after a large protein meal by a maximum of about 40%. Subtracting baseline GFR from the maximal GFR after protein load yields what has been termed the *renal reserve* (32). Renal reserve amounts to about 34 ml/min in normal subjects and is progressively lost in patients with nephropathy. It has been reasoned that since an elevated GFR, whether produced by hyperglycemia or protein feeding, is injurious to the glomerular integrity, limitation of dietary protein might be a wise precaution in diabetes and other disorders in which renal functional decline may be predestined. Restriction of dietary protein slows the rate of progression of glomerulosclerosis in the streptozotocin-induced diabetic rat. Induced-diabetic rats fed a 50% protein diet develop elevated glomerular filtration and ultrafiltration pressures. Zatz et al. found that proteinuria was present at 6 months and glomerulosclerosis by 12 months in rats made diabetic. Treatment with enalapril, an angiotensin-converting enzyme inhibitor, reduced mean arterial pressure in rats from 115 to 98 mmHg, and, like protein restriction, prevented increases in ultrafiltration and GFR while maintaining normal glomerular histology (33). Several trials, only one of which was prospective and controlled, of restrictive protein feeding in patients with varying kidney diseases suggest that the rate of loss of GFR can be slowed, and uremia can be delayed for months to years (34). Caution in acceptance of the limited trials of protein-restricted diets has been advocated, as have guidelines for future experimentation to determine the place, if any, for protein restricted (0.6 g/kg protein intake) diets.

Transfiguration of rat and human studies of the effect of ingested protein on the progression of renal insufficiency into a dietary prescription for nephrotic and non-nephrotic diabetics is difficult. In one study, serum albumin levels actually rose in six nephrotic patients (including one diabetic) fed a protein-restricted diet (35). Until pertinent clinical trials are completed, it seems wise to limit the protein prescription to 40–60 g/day for nonazotemic proteinuric diabetics. Once creatinine clearance falls below 40 ml/min, a further reduction to about 40 g/day, or to the extent tolerated, seems rational, although admittedly it is a recommendation unsubstantiated by data.

RENAL FAILURE

Severe glomerular damage may be present in diabetes without an overt sign of renal malfunction. Renal biopsies in asymptomatic adolescents with IDDM have shown advanced intercapillary glomerulosclerosis while the GFR was normal (or supernormal). Appreciating that years of unchecked hypertension and hyperglycemia are common to many diabetics, the onset of fixed proteinuria should not be viewed as the start of diabetic nephropathy but, rather, its first clinical sign. The retention of nephrotic edema fluid in diabetics is evident at higher serum albumin levels (3.0–3.4 g/dl) than in nondiabetics, due to a "leaky capillary syndrome," which may be the consequence of transcapillary migration of glycosylated albumin (14). Nephrotic diabetics typically excrete 4–8 g of protein daily, but daily urinary protein losses may rise to as much as 20–30 g. Fluid retention in the nephrotic diabetic is often massive; weight loss postdiuresis reveals unappreciated fluid accumulations of 10–30 kg in leg edema, ascites, and pleural effusions. Because of this fluid burden, severe hypertension, fatigue, and breathlessness force the patient into an existence as an invalid.

Intensive diuresis during the nephrotic stage of diabetic nephropathy contracts intravascular volume, sometimes resulting in prerenal azotemia. Prerenal azotemia is distinguishable from renal azotemia by the disproportionate elevation in plasma urea level (with a normal or minimally elevated plasma creatinine concentration) in the former condition. Insidiously, as residual renal function deteriorates, azotemia ensues. Diabetics are sicker at every level of renal insufficiency than are nondiabetics with equivalent renal malfuction. Concurrent diabetic macrovasculopathy expressed as coronary artery disease, cerebrovascular disease, or peripheral vascular disease may divert attention from worsening symptomatic renal insufficiency. Diabetics whose GFR has fallen below 20 ml/min become catabolic, depressed, and are subject to multiple intercurrent illnesses. The diabetic with a creatinine clearance of 15 ml/min is confined to bed by a minor respiratory illness that is easily tolerated by a nondiabetic with equivalent renal function. It follows that dialytic therapy is usually required at a higher level of residual renal function in a diabetic than in a nondiabetic. Maintenance hemodialysis, for instance, is rarely initiated in a nondiabetic while the creatinine clearance remains above about 5 ml/min (approximately equivalent to a serum creatinine of 10–15 mg/dl). Nephropathic diabetics, by contrast, whose creatinine clearance falls to about 10 ml/min (serum creatinine concentration of approximately 5 mg/dl) are usually too sick to attempt work, home, or school responsibilities without dialytic support. In both IDDM and NIDDM, diminished renal catabolism of insulin (and other small peptide hormones) may cause episodic profound hypoglycemia following the injection of formerly safely tolerated doses of insulin.

TREATMENT STRATEGY

Any hope for the efficacy of protocols designed to retard or prevent glomerular injury in diabetes requires their introduction during those *silent* years of hyperglycemia that are associated with few signs and symptoms. Aggressive regulation of blood glucose and blood pressure initiated after extensive glomerular destruction has occurred has little likelihood of restoring normal renal function. Sclerotic glomeruli do not regenerate.

Management of hypertension

In rat models of induced diabetes, intrarenal hypertension appears to be at least as important as hyperglycemia in the pathogenesis of glomerulosclerosis. Reduction of blood pressure in the hypertensive streptozotocin-induced diabetic rat protects against glomerular sclerosis and proteinuria, even though hyperglycemia is untreated. Hypertension jeopardizes the integrity of the kidney, heart, and eye at every stage of diabetes. Several studies in IDDM have shown that normalization of hypertensive blood pressures unquestionably slows the rate of decline of creatinine clearance by about 5 ml/min per year (36). Normalization of hypertensive blood pressure is the cornerstone of preuremic management of diabetic nephropathy. Potent antihypertensive drugs are available to permit effective treatment of all nephropathic diabetics. Selection of the specific combination of diuretics, vasodilators, calcium channel blockers, and renin antagonists for an individual patient is a pragmatic exercise that may take months to complete. Recent evidence derived from the streptozotocin-induced diabetic rat and patients with IDDM indicates that the angiotensin converting enzyme (ACE) inhibitors may have special application in the management of hypertensive diabetes (37). By reducing intrarenal hypertension, consequent to relaxation of efferent glomerular arterioles, ACE inhibitors such as enalapril and captopril may blunt a key pathogenetic mechanism responsible for glomerular damage.

Intravascular volume expansion contributes to hypertension in hypoproteinemic diabetics. Accordingly, diuretics are an essential component of the hypertensive regimen. As in the nondiabetic, a thiazide diuretic is appropriate so long as the residual GFR exceeds 50 ml/min. When GFR declines below about 25% of normal, thiazide diuretics become inefficacious and must be replaced by a loop diuretic such as furosemide. Doses of furosemide as high as 480 mg daily may be required when the creatinine clearance is less than 20 ml/min in order to maintain a nephrotic diabetic free of edema. Metolazone, a long-acting thiazide, in daily doses of 5–20 mg, often affects diuresis when administered with furosemide in hypoalbuminemic nephrotic azotemic diabetics unresponsive to furosemide alone.

LIMIT OF CONSERVATIVE THERAPY

It is usually possible in diabetic nephropathy to project the need for dialysis or a kidney transplant a year or longer in advance. The course of renal functional decline may be charted as the reciprocal of serum creatinine against time (38). As a generalization, uremia therapy should be initiated when the creatinine clearance falls to 5–10 ml/min; a creatinine clearance of < 5 ml/min is an absolute indication for ending conservative treatment. Periodic discussions between the azotemic diabetic and his nephrologist to review the rate of renal deterioration will avoid surprise and panic when the moment for uremia therapy has to be faced.

Conservative therapy may be terminated abruptly by a medical catastrophe such as a myocardial infarction, stroke, or sepsis. Typically, however, dialysis is mandated by more gradual deterioration, manifested as weight loss, worsening hypertension, and inability to perform work or home responsibilities. It is rational to end conservative management when further deterioration, especially of visual acuity and the cardiovascular system, appears inevitable.

LONG-TERM PLANNING

Our experience indicates that few diabetics when first seen for nephrosis or azotemia have an understanding of the present or probable future course of their kidney disease. The patient, when first advised of the gravity of his or her condition by the nephrologist may react with disbelief, anger, confusion, hostility, and/or a desire to flee to seek a less threatening opinion. Acceptance of the knowledge that renal failure is likely in months to years frequently results in a transient (sometimes permanent) reactive depression that taxes the patient's social support system. While selecting uremia therapy — peritoneal or hemodialysis, or renal transplantation — (Table 2) attention must be devoted to the presence of depression as well as consideration of the patient's family, social, and economic circumstances. Despite its advantages, for example, home hemodialysis is not applicable to a blind diabetic who lives alone. CAPD, however, has been successfully performed by blind diabetics (39). Similarly, the desire for an intrafamilial kidney transplant must be based on the availability of healthy and willing family donors. Construction of a "life plan" for treatment of uremia in a diabetic requires careful blending of the patient's wishes and his or her real life circumstances. For some diabetics, especially after a stroke or other major macrovascular complication, election of a "no-treatment" option (meaning near-term death in uremia) may appear a rational choice. A blind, legless diabetic suffering multiple daily episodes of angina and explosive nocturnal diarrhea may view the *gift* of a transplant as proffering minimal benefit. Depressed diabetics who manifest the "giving-up-given-up" syndrome (40) sometimes respond favorably to visits by rehabilitated dialysis patients or transplant recipients by reversing their decision to die. Providing that a thorough attempt has been made to inform the patient of the probable outcome, it is unwise to coerce a diabetic to accept dialysis or kidney transplantation when life is preceived as having minimal or negative value. Noncompliance to dietary and drug regimens by a reluctant patient is tantamount to passive suicide.

KIDNEY TRANSPLANTATION

In Brooklyn, of 232 diabetics undergoing maintenance hemodialysis in 14 facilities in 1986, only 27% were able to perform any activity beyond self-care (26), Poor rehabilitation was also noted in a national survey of CAPD patients in 1987 (41). The reasons for suboptimal rehabilitation of diabetics treated by dialysis are not clearly defined, though continuing vascular complications — especially in the eye and heart — and a generalized *failure to thrive* afflict most individuals so treated. By contrast, approximately half of diabetic recipients of a renal transplant are able to return to home, school, or occupational responsibilities for at least 3 years. Of all currently employed treatments for the uremic diabetic, living related donor kidney transplantation provides the highest probability of return to the preuremia lifestyle. Selected IDDM patients in individual transplant center reports have achieved better than 90% survival 5 years after a related donor transplant (42). Substantial improvement has also affected the outcome of cadaver donor kidney transplants following replacement of azathioprine by cyclosporin for immunosuppression (43). Patient and renal graft survival in diabetic recipients of cadaver transplants at the University of Minnesota are equal to results in nondiabetic patients (44).

Patient and renal graft 1-year survival in uremic patients with IDDM can be as high as 92% and 85%, respectively. In Norway, Iowa, Wisconsin, and Minnesota, coincident cadaveric renal and pancreas transplants are now the treatment of choice for the patient with IDDM in renal failure (45). Perusal of the International Pancreas Transplant Registry indicates that 1-year pancreas allograft survival exceeds 60% and that no additional burden to patient or renal graft survival is imposed by a simultaneous pancreas transplant (46). Immunosuppressive regimens for pancreas and kidney transplants are now based on so-called triple therapy, meaning a combination of prednisone, azathioprine, and cyclosporin (47). Rejection episodes are treated with either monoclonal antibody directed against thymic derived t lymphocytes or increased doses of corticosteroids administered as intravenous boluses.

Kidneys obtained from nondiabetics when transplanted into diabetics risk injury due to: a) allograft rejection, b) immunosuppressive drug-induced nephrotoxicity, and c) recurrent diabetic glomerulopathy. Distinguishing the singular effect of recurrent diabetes from other causes of renal damage has been difficult and confusing. Mauer and his associates have shown that both streptozotocin-induced diabetic rats and human diabetic transplant recipients manifest glomerular mesangial proliferation and basement membrane thickening in allografts within months to years post-transplantation (48). Whether proteinuria — the cardinal sign of diabetic glomerulopathy in native kidneys — is a marker for recurrent diabetic

Table 2. Options in therapy for the uremic diabetic

Hemodialysis
   Home hemodialysis
   Facility hemodialysis
Peritoneal dialysis
   Intermittent (IPD)
   Continuous ambulatory (CAPD)
   Continuous cyclic (machine) (CCPD)
Kidney transplantation
   Living donor kidney
   Cadaver donor kidney
Hemofiltration (Europe)

glomerulopathy in renal allografts is unknown. Proteinuria in the immediate post-transplant period may occur transiently during acute rejection episodes in diabetic and nondiabetic recipients. Persistent proteinuria > 3.0 g/day is present in about 10% of nondiabetic renal allograft recipients and has been related to recurrent glomerulonephritis, chronic rejection, or drug toxicity (cyclosporine nephrotoxicity is not associated with proteinuria). Proteinuria in kidney graft recipients is a serious finding, as most patients with significant proteinuria lose their kidneys within 5 years.

Recurrent diabetic glomerulopathy in transplants progresses at a variable rate, in an undetermined proportion of patients, to a second episode of end-stage renal failure attributed to typical nodular and diffuse intercapillary glomerulosclerosis (49).

COMPREHENSIVE CARE

Guidance in the selection of treatment for the diabetic with renal insufficiency must perforce be drawn from uncontrolled studies of small numbers of patients. There are no reports of prospective controlled trials in which the relative merits of dialysis (hemodialysis or CAPD) versus kidney transplantation have been assessed. While extrapolations employing the Cox Proportional Hazard statistical technique have been drawn to compare kidney transplantation with maintenance hemodialysis and CAPD, the statistical technique is artificial and cannot overcome the inherent bias of a younger (by a mean of 10–20 years) transplant group being compared with older dialysis patients. That such analyses find renal transplantation superior to either hemodialysis or CAPD in sustaining life and promoting rehabilitation may or may not be a valid inference that requires a controlled study to confirm.

No uniform criteria for scoring rehabilitation in ERSD patients have been accepted. Life quality can be rated in four major categories of variables: sociodemographic variables, medical variables, objective indicators of the quality of life, and subjective indicators of the quality of life. For purposes of comparative study, differences between patients in the severity of concurrent illnesses can be scored in a "comorbity index" (Table 3). A score of 0 to 3 according to severity (0 = absent, 1 = of minor import, 2 = moderate, 3= severe) can be assigned to each of the listed comorbid disorders. The sum of all fractional scores then comprises the comorbidity index at the time of rating.

Our observation of diabetics treated by dialysis and renal transplantation has fostered the belief that a transplant is preferable because of markedly enhanced rehabilitation. We advise that uremic diabetics under the age of 50 years be offered a kidney transplant as *first-choice therapy* unless a contraindication to surgery or immunosuppression is present. Tests and evaluating procedures that are helpful in quantifying the extent of systemic illness in a diabetic under consideration for a kidney transplant are listed in Table 4. To avoid post-transplant frustration and disappointment, the patient should be given a realistic

Table 3. Co-morbid factors Affecting outcome of uremia therapy in diabetics

1. Angina or myocardia infarction
2. Other cardiovascular problems, hypertension, congestive heart failure, cardiomyopathy
3. Respiratory disease
4. Gastrointestinal problems, gastroparesis, obstipation, nocturnal diarrhea
5. Neurologic problems, cerebrovascular accident, or stroke residual
6. Musculoskeletal disorders, including renal bone disease
7. Infections excluding vascular access-site or peritonitis
8. Hepatitis, hepatic insufficiency
9. Hematologic problems other than anemia
10. Spinal abnormalities, lower back problems, or arthritis
11. Vision loss
12. Limb amputation
13. Mental or emotional illness (psychosis, neurosis, depression)

Each factor can be scored from 0 to 3 (0 = absent, 1 = mild — of minor import to patient's life, 2 = moderate, 3 = severe). By proportional hazard analysis, the relative significance of each variable can be isolated from the other 12.

Table 4. Pretransplant evaluation of co-morbid risk factors

1. Cystometrogram, urine culture, residual volume
2. Electrocardiogram, exercise stress test
3. Coronary angiography
4. Vital capacity
5. Visual acuity, fluorescein angiography
6. Metabolic radiographic bone survey
7. Podiatric assessment
8. Dental assessment
9. Social worker and nurse educator's assessment of potential for self-care

appraisal of the degree to which independent living may be possible should be transplant succeed. Coronary artery disease, gastroparesis, neuropathy, and the need for antihypertensive drugs will persist. Even a perfect kidney transplant cannot restore function to blinded eyes or amputated legs.

Diabetes in its late, complicated stages is a difficult and enervating disorder. The patient and physician locked in a struggle against an inexorable disease learn that at every phase of treatment for renal insufficiency, the fragility of the diabetic must be kept in mind. Minor stresses tolerated by nondiabetic uremic patients may, in a diabetic, precipitate a metabolic or septic crisis. Planning for minor surgery, radioactive scans, and post-transplant hemodialyses must take into account the necessity for synchronizing insulin injections with meals, a practical consideration that is often ignored in the scheduling of radiographic and other studies *that separate a diabetic given insulin in the morning from the food that will prevent hypoglycemia.* Emotional crises in the patient and family are to be anticipated when a childhood diabetic prepares to start dialysis. Intrafamilial conflicts, parent-child guilt interrelationships, and frustration over the failure to stem a downward course all culminate in the nephrologist's office. By the time that uremia suprevenes, the usual diabetic has met and left a number of practitioners and has been scolded repeatedly for noncompliance with an incomprehensible regimen only dimly understood by the health care team. Over the past 5 years, for example, the diabetic diet has been modified from a high- to low-protein diet and its lipid content has been sharply altered. Availability, patience, and a willingness to listen to the diabetic's fears over an uncertain future usually suffices to weather the rough seas encountered during uremia therapy. Faced with relating to and understanding his or her cardiologist, opthalmologist, endocrinologist, vascular surgeon, radiologist, podiatrist, and transplant surgeon, the uremic diabetic needs an advocate and friend, a role suited to the empathetic nephrologist.

In the 1980s, renal failure in diabetes has responded to treatment in the majority of cases for at least several years. Interest in insulin replacement by islets or pancreas grafts, the pathogenesis of microvasculopathy, and simplification of drug therapy for hypertension, should improve diabetes therapy within the next decade. Immunosuppressive regimens based on cyclosporin derivatives and monoclonal antibodies that avoid corticosteroids should permit reduced morbidity post kidney transplant. Perhaps most intriguing of the initiatives directed towards the therapy of diabetes is the attempt to halt and/or reverse insulinopenia in IDDM shortly after the onset of hyperglycemia by immunomodulation. Clarification of the underlying genetics and precipitating stresses responsible for clinical IDDM and NIDDM are objectives attainable before this century closes. Their pursuit adds excitement to the care of a ubiquitous disease that was previously regarded as hopeless in its later stages.

REFERENCES

1. Sugimoto T, Rosansky SJ: The incidence of treated end stage renal disease in the Eastern United States: 1973–1979. *Am J Public Health* 74:14–16, 1984.
2. Harris MI, Hadden WC, Knowler WC, Bennett PH: Prevalence of diabetes and impaired glucose tolerance and plasma glucosel levels in U.S. population aged 20–74 yr. *Diabetes* 36:523–534, 1987.
3. Sievers ML, Fisher JR: *Diabetes in America*. National Diabetes Data Group, National Institutes of Health, Washington DC, 1985.
4. Sutherland DER, Fryd DS, Simmons RL, Kjellstrand CM, Ramsay RC, Goetz FC, Mauer SM, Najarian JS: Long-term diabetic renal transplants. In: EA Friedman, L'Esperance, eds, Diabetic Renal Retinal Syndrome. Grune & Stratton, New York, pp 353–371, 1980.
5. Selden RF, Skoskiewicz MJ, Russel PS, Goodman HM: Regulation of insulin-gene expression. Implications for gene therapy. *N Engl J Med* 317:1067–1076, 1987.
6. Ginsberg-Fellner F, Rubinstein P, Notkins AL: Ten-year longitudinal study of children at high risk of insulin dependent diabetes (letter). *N Engl J Med* 317:1352–1353, 1987.
7. Colman PG, Eisenbarth GS: Immunotherapy in type I diabetes. Approaches to prevention and treatment. *Postgrad Med* 81:146–155, 1987.
8. Palestine AG, Austin HA, Balow JE, Antonovych TT, Sabnis SG, Preuss HG, Nussenblatt RB: Renal histopathologic alterations in patients treated with cyclosporine for uveitis. *N Engl J Med* 314:1293–1298, 1986.
9. Chomette G, Auriol M, Beaufils H, Rottemberg J, Cabrol C: Morphology of cyclosporine nephrotoxicity in human heart transplant recipients. *J Heart Transplant* 5:273–278, 1986.
10. Kobayashi T, Sugimoto T, Itoh T, Kosaha K, Tanaka T, Suwa S, Sato K, Tsuji K: The prevalence of islet cell antibodies in Japanese insulin-dependent and non-insulin-dependent diabetic patients studied by indirect immunofluorescence and by a new method. *Diabetes* 35:335–340, 1986.
11. Viberti GC, Macintosh D, Bilous RW, Pickup JC, Keen H: Proteinuria in diabetes mellitus: Role of spontaneous and experimental variation of glycemia. *Kidney Int* 21:714–720, 1982.
12. Jerums G, Cooper ME, Seeman E, Murray RML, McNeil JJ: Spectrum of proteinuria in Type I and Type II diabetes. *Diabetes Care* 10:419–427, 1987.
13. Taguma U, Kimamoto U, Futaki G, Hitoshi U, Hiromichi M, Makoto I, Hisashi T, Hiroshi S, Yasuhiko S: Effect of captopril on heavy proteinuria in azotemic diabetics. *N Engl J Med* 313:1617–20, 1985.
14. Stephen RL, Maxwell JG, Kablitz C, Jacobson SC, Hanover B, Tyler F: *Proc Eur Dial Transpl Assoc* 20:692–699, 1983.
15. Sampietro T, Bertuglia S, Colantuoni A, Bionda A, Lenzi S, Donato: Increased permeability of hamster microcirculation to glycosylated albumin. *Lancet* 2:994–996, 1987.
16. Marre M, Leblanc H, Leobardo S, Thanh-Tam G, Menard J, Passa P: Converting enzyme inhibition and kidney function in normotensive diabetic patients with persistent microalbuminuria. *Br Med J* 294:1448–1452, 1987.
17. Cohen D, Dodds R, Viberti G: Effect of protein restriction in insulin dependent diabetes at risk of nephropathy. *Br Med J* [Clin Res] 294:795–798, 1987.
18. Evanoff GV, Thompson CS, Brown J, Weinman EJ: The effect of dietary protein restriction on the progression of diabetic nephropathy. A 12-month follow-up. *Arch Int Med* 147:492–495, 1987.
19. Raskin P, Rosenstock J: Aldose reductase inhibitors and diabetic complications. *Am J Med* 83:298–306, 1987.
20. Hommel E, Mathiesen E, Arnold-Larsen S, Edsberg B, Olsen UB, Parving HH: Effects of indomethacin on kidney function in type 1 (insulin-dependent) diabetic patients with nephropathy. *Diabetologia* 30:78–81, 1987.
21. Ferrari E, Fioravanti M, Patti AL, Viola C, Solerte SB: Effects of long-term treatment (4 years) with pentoxifylline on haemorheological changes and vascular complications in diabetic patients. *Pharmatherapeutica* 5:26–39, 1987.
22. Nath KA. Platelet participation in renal diseases. The Kidney (Published by National Kidney Foundation) 20:1–6, 1987.
23. Friedman EA, Peterson CM (eds): *Diabetic Nephropathy*. Martinus Nijhoff, Boston, 1986.
24. Kimmelstiel P, Wilson C: Intercapillary lesions in the

glomeruli of the kidney. *Am J Pathol* 12:83–98, 1936.
25. Mauer SM, Chavers BM: A comparsion of kidney disease in type I and type II diabetes. *Adv Exp Med Biol* 189:299–303, 1985.
26. Lowder GM, Perri NA, Friedman EA: Demographics, diabetes type, and degree of rehabilitation in diabetic patients on maintenance hemodialysis in Brooklyn. *J Diabetic Complications*, in press, 1988.
27. The DCCT Research Group: The diabetes control and complications trial (DCCT). Design and methodologic considerations for the feasibility phase. *Diabetes* 35:530–45, 1986.
28. Mauer SM, Brown DM, Steffes MW: Studies on the reversibility of kidney changes in experimental diabetes in the rat. *Acta Endocrinol* (Suppl) 242:29–30, 1981.
29. Zatz R, Brenner BM: Pathogenesis of diabetic microangiopathy. The hemodynamic view. *Am J Med* 80:443–453, 1986.
30. Anderson S, Meyer TW, Rennke HG, Brenner BM: Control of glomerular hypertension limits glomerular injury in rats with reduced renal mass. *J Clin Invest* 76:612–619, 1985.
31. Finco DR, Crowell WA, Barsanti JA: Effects of three diets on dogs with induced chronic renal failure. *Am J Vet Res* 46:646–653, 1985.
32. Bosch JP, Lauer A, Glabman S: Short-term protein loading in assessment of patients with renal disease. *Am J Med* 77:873–879, 1984.
33. Zatz R, Dunn BR, Meyer TW, Anderson S, Rennke HG, Brenner BM: Prevention of diabetic glomerulopathy by pharmacological amelioration of glomerular capillary hypertension. *J Clin Invest* 77:1925–1930, 1986.
34. Ciavarella A, DiMizio G, Stefoni S, Borgnino LC, Vannini P: Reduced albuminuria after dietary protein restriction in insulin-dependent diabetic patients with clinical nephropathy. *Diabetes Care* 10:407–413, 1987.
35. Kaysen GA, Gambertoglio J, Jimenez I, Jones H, Hutchison FN: Effect of dietary protein intake on albumin homeostasis in nephrotic patients. *Kidney Int* 29:572–577, 1986.
36. Mogensen CE: Progression of nephropathy in long-term diabetics with proteinuria and effect of initial antihypertensive treatment. *Scand J Clin Lab Invest* 36:383–388, 1976.
37. Passa P, LeBlanc H, Marre M: Effects of enalapril in insulin-dependent diabetic subjects with mild to moderate uncomplicated hypertension. *Diabetes Care* 10:200–204, 1987.
38. Rutherford WE, Blondin J, Miller JP, Greenwalt AS, Vavra JD, Chronic progressive renal disease: Rate of change of serum creatinine concentration. *Kidney Int* 11:62–70, 1977.
39. Flynn CT, Shadur CA: A comparsion of continuous ambulatory peritoneal dialysis in diabetic and nondiabetic patients. *Am J Kidney Dis* 1:15–23, 1981.
40. Engle GL: A life setting conducive to illness. The giving-up–given-up complex. *Bull Menninger Clin* 32:355–365, 1968.
41. Lindblad AS, Nolph KD, Novak JW, Friedman EA: A survey of the NIH CAPD registry population with end-stage renal disease attributed to diabetic nephropathy. *J Diabetic Complications*, in press, 1988.
42. Burlingham WJ, Grailer A, Sparks–Mackety EM, Sondel PM, Sollinger HW: Improved renal alograft survival following donor-specific transfusions. II. In vitro correlates of early (DST-type) rejection episodes. *Transplantation* 43:41–44, 1987.
43. Terasaki PI, Himaya NS, Cecka M, Cicciarelli J, Cook DJ, Ito T, Iwaki Y, Mickey MR, Takiff H, Tiwari JL, Toyotome A. Overview. In: Terasaki PI, ed, *Clinical Transplants 1986*. UCLA Tissue Typing Laboratory, Los Angeles, pp 367–398, 1986.
44. Sutherland DER, Morrow CE, Fryd DS, Ferguson R, Simmons RL, Najarian JS: Improved patient and primary renal allograft survival in uremic diabetic recipients. *Transplantation* 34:319–325, 1982.
45. Sollinger HW, Stratta RJ, Kalayoglu M, Belzer FO: The University of Wisconsin experience in pancreas transplantation. *Transplant Proceed* 19 (Suppl 4):48–54, 1987.
46. Sutherland DE, Moudry KC: Pancreas Transplant Registry: History and analysis of cases 1966 to October 1986. *Pancreas* 2:473–488, 1987.
47. Slapak M: Triple and quadruple immunosuppressive therapy in organ transplantation. *Lancet* 2:958–960, 1987.
48. Mauer SM, Steffes MW, Connett J, Najarian JS, Sutherland DE, Barbosa J: The development of lesions in the glomerular basement membrane and mesangium after transplantation of normal kidneys to diabetic patients. *Diabetes* 32:948–52, 1983.
49. Maryniak RK, Mendoza N, Clyne D, Balakrishnan K, Weiss MA: Recurrence of diabetic nodular glomerulosclerosis in a renal transplant. *Transplantation* 39:35–38, 1985.

CHAPTER 35

Renal Cystic Disorders

JARED J. GRANTHAM, JOANN B. RECKLING & SHARON L. SLUSHER

INTRODUCTION

Renal cystic disorders encompass a relatively large group of diseases typified by the formation of one or more fluid-filled cavities within the kidneys. Cysts can arise in all parts of the kidney. Renal cysts may develop in utero or they may be acquired after birth. They may be congenital or hereditary. Cysts may be slightly larger than a single nephron structure (i.e., a few microns in diameter) in their formative stage, or they may be so large as to compress the abdominal viscera. Renal cysts may be innocent occupants or they may compromise function, causing severe renal failure. Cysts may be the primary renal disorder or they may appear in association with nonrenal disorders.

In this chapter we discuss the management of various renal cystic disorders, including adult and infantile polycystic kidney disease, medullary cystic disease and nephronophthisis, medullary sponge kidney, multicystic kidney, acquired cysts, and simple cysts. The management of cystic disorders largely involves recognizing the specific lesions, alleviating symptoms, recognizing their genetic propensity and the potential for other system problems such as cerebral aneurysm, diverticulitis, hepatic cysts, slowing the onset of renal function changes, maintaining vigilance for malignant changes, utilizing appropriate counseling strategies, and understanding the prognosis. We have reviewed selected references from the literature and surveyed 29 dialysis and transplant centers, to which we add our personal experiences and those of our colleagues who care for patients with cystic disorders. Several reviews have been published that the reader may wish to consult for discussions of the pathology and pathogenesis of these fascinating disorders (1–5).

POLYCYSTIC KIDNEY DISEASE IN THE ADULT

Introduction and background

The adult form of polycystic kidney disease may be recognized in utero, shortly after birth, or after several decades of "normal" life. Consequently, designation of this disorder as an "adult" type of polycystic disease is not strictly correct. Since this cystic disorder has been recognized to have a strong hereditary transmission by an autosomal dominant mechanism (6), we will refer to it as *autosomal dominant polycystic kidney disease* (ADPKD).

ADPKD occurs in virtually all cultures on all the continents throughout the world. Although variably expressed, the gene for this disorder has a high degree of penetrance. It has been estimated by Dalgaard (6) that all individuals possessing the gene will demonstrate clinical evidence of the process by 80 years of age. In the United States it has been estimated that between 1 in 500 and 1 in 1000 persons have ADPKD, i.e., about 500,000 citizens. In 1981 we surveyed 24 dialysis and transplant centers in this country involving 2083 ESRD patients (Table 1). These patients appeared to be distributed evenly throughout the United States. This survey is congruent with more extensive data from national and international registries from 1980 to 1984 (7), which report that 5.9–12% of dialysis patients have polycystic kidney disease. It is easy to figure that the annual expenditure for the dialysis treatment of ADPKD may exceed $200,000,000.

Table 2 lists some of the clinical features of ADPKD. This disorder is held to be bilateral with rare exceptions (8–14). Some physicians claim that ADPKD may arise as a spontaneous mutation, but this has never been rigorously documented. In ADPKD the cysts are diffusely scattered through the renal parenchyma with islands of normal tissue between the cysts in early cases (Figure 1), and the cysts arise from all segments of the nephron and collecting system, as established by microdissection and ultrastructure studies (37–40). The cysts appear to function in several ways, like the nephrons from which they are derived (41, 42). There may be abnormalities in other organs. Liver cysts have been reported in approximately 20–75% of patients (6, 43–46). Pancreatic cysts have been detected in a few instances. Hiatal and inguinal hernias may have an increased incidence in ADPKD patients, and an increased incidence of diverticular disease has been observed in one series of dialyzed ADPKD patients (47–49). Cerebral artery aneurysms are found in approximately 10–20% of patients (6, 43). A variety of other cardiovascular abnormalities, including abdominal aortic aneurysms (50, 51) and cardiac valvular abnormalities (45, 52), have been

Table 1. Incidence of ADPKD in United States dialysis units. Response from 24 centers grouped geographically according to time zones.

Time zone	Number of centers surveyed	Total patients surveyed	Patients with ADPKD	% of dialyzed patients
Eastern	5	407	18	4.4%
Central	14	1400	112	8.0%
Mountain	2	85	6	7.1%
Pacific	3	146	13	8.9%
Totals	24	2038	149	7.3%

Table 2. Characteristics of ADPKD

1. Cystic disease recognized prenatally, at birth or at any age (15–36)
2. Autosomal dominant pattern of inheritance (6)
3. Bilateral involvement of the kidneys with rare exceptions (8–14)
4. Diffuse involvement of the kidneys with cysts.
5. Cysts arise from all segments of the nephron and collecting system (37–40)
6. Involvement of other organs:
    a. Liver cysts in 20–75% (6, 43–46)
    b. Pancreatic cysts
    c. Hiatal and inguinal hernias
    d. Diverticular disease (47–49)
    e. Cerebral artery aneurysms (6, 43)
    f. Aneurysms of abdominal aorta (50, 51)
    g. Cardiac valvular abnormalities (45, 52)
    h. Arachnoid cysts (53)
7. Progression to end-stage renal failure in one half of cases (54, 55)

reported, but the significance of these is unclear. Arachnoid cysts have been reported (53). One of the most devastating features is the fact that ADPKD undergoes a relentless progression to end-stage renal failure in a high percentage of patients.

Components of ADPKD that require management

BASIC FLUID AND ELECTROLYTE MANAGEMENT

Patients with early forms of ADPKD may have a diminished ability to maximally concentrate the urine (56–58). Nocturia may be the only symptom caused by this defect. No specific therapy is indicated. Patients with normal creatinine clearances can conserve sodium normally (59). A tendency to "waste" sodium is usually not seen until a significant decrease in creatinine clearance has occurred (59). Prior to the development of end-stage renal failure, most patients with ADPKD can be managed rather simply with respect to salt and water intake. The patients should be advised to drink a reasonable amount of water (1–2 l/day). Only if the patients have renal calculi or infection are higher volume intakes indicated. In a few patients with arterial hypertension, sodium restriction may be necessary. Physicians should be prescribe low-salt diets for all ADPKD patients with hypertension and/or renal insufficiency, however. Azotemic ADPKD patients may be unable to adapt their renal excretion to a strenuously restricted sodium intake. These patients may develop severe volume contraction and worsening of their renal insufficiency. Probably the best way to manage these patients is to determine the amount of salt in the diet during one or two regular office visits. If the patients have no hypertension, congestive heart failure, or edema, no modification of sodium intake is necessary. On the other hand, if the patients tend to retain sodium and water, the intake of sodium should probably be cut back to approximately 1 mEq/kg body weight (BW). This modest limitation of sodium intake will usually give a suitable baseline from which the physician can judge the need for further sodium restriction or addition of diuretic substances. All patients should be cautioned that should they have intestinal flu or other ailments that cause the loss of body fluids through the intestinal tract or the skin, they have an increased risk of aggravating their underlying renal condition. These patients should be advised to see their physicians when they have intercurrent illnesses that might predispose them to severe salt and water depletion.

Patients who are approaching the end stage of their disease may have hyperchloremic metabolic acidosis. The mechanism of this form of acidosis is not clearly understood. It can be ameliorated to some extent by reducing the acid ash content of the diet and by supplementing the diet with sodium bicarbonate. Patients with ADPKD and moderate renal insufficiency occasionally have difficulty in eliminating potassium. Whether this is due to a renal defect or reflects failure of the colonic mechanism to adaptively increase potassium excretion is not known. This problem may require some decrease in the potassium intake or, alternatively, the addition of a small amount of polystyrene sulfonate resin to the diet. Maintaining soft and regular bowel movements is another important way of assisting the patient in maintaining a reasonable potassium balance.

DIETARY MANAGEMENT

In patients with relatively normal renal function, modification of the diet to decrease protein and phosphate intake may be helpful in slowing the progression of renal failure (60), but controlled prospective studies need to be done to demonstrate the actual effectiveness of this treatment in ADPKD patients. When ADPKD patients approach the end stage of their disease, they require diets similar to any patient with renal insufficiency. These patients often have hiatal hernia and should be instructed to eat frequent, small amounts of food, to elevate the head of their bed, and to avoid eating immediately prior to retiring. Constipation is also a nagging problem for some patients and can usually be combated by eating a diet with increased fiber content and using stool softeners or mineral oil.

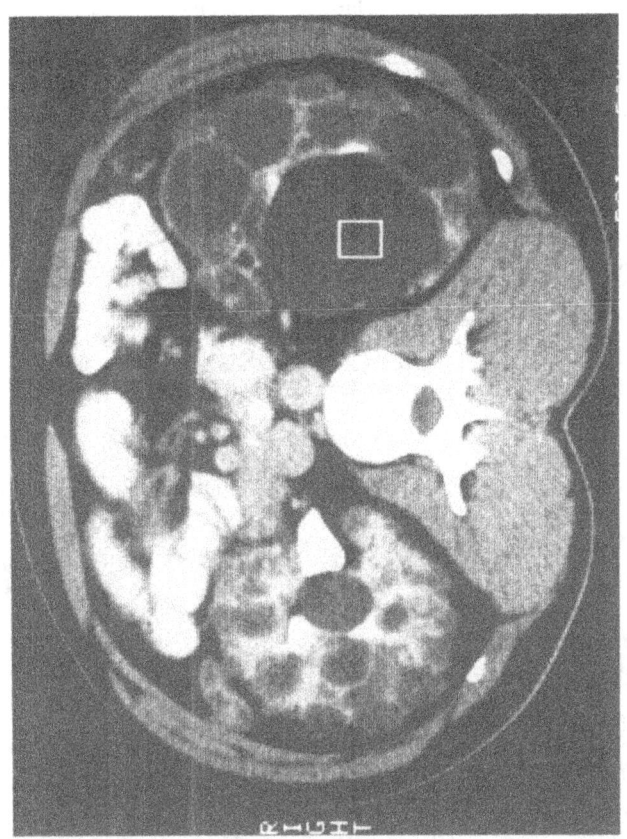
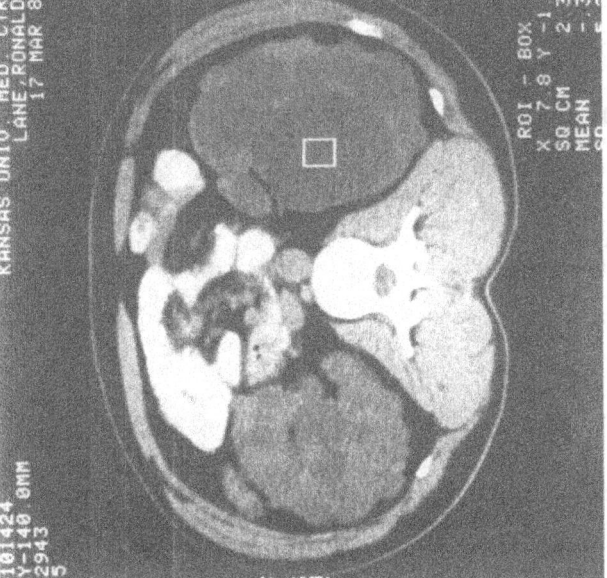

Figure 1. Computer assisted tomography appearance of ADPKD. View is from the patient's feet. *Left:* Without intravenous contrast enhancement (gut contains gastrografin contrast material). *Right:* Appearance after intravenous infusion of urographic contrast material. The left kidney contains several large cysts with scant areas of functional parenchyma between the cysts. The cysts in the right kidney are smaller than in the left. The right contains more functional parenchyma than the left.

PHYSICAL ACTIVITY AND LIFESTYLE

Most patients with ADPKD require no modification in physical activity or lifestyle until they approach the end stage of their illness. In some instances, however, patients will be unusually susceptible to physical trauma to the abdomen. Cyst rupture has been caused by seat belt constraints in automobiles and airplanes (61, 62). In male patients with massive kidneys, we recommend the use of suspenders rather than constrictive belts. Patients with ADPKD probably should not participate in strenuous athletic events such as wrestling, boxing, football, and horseback riding. Although there is no evidence to suggest that recurrent cyst rupture will adversely affect renal function, the constant bouts of pain secondary to cyst rupture can probably be avoided by tailoring the physical activity of these patients.

PAIN

Pain in one or both kidneys is the most common initial complaint in patients with ADPKD (6) and recurs frequently during the course of the disease (45). The pain may be of a dull aching quality, a vague sense of heaviness, or knifelike and stabbing. The pain may be disabling when chronic, often leading to analgesic abuse and dependence on narcotics. The exact etiology of renal pain in ADPKD has not been established but is thought to arise from stretching of the renal capsule, excessive weight causing traction on the pedicle, or compression of adjacent organs.

In addition to being an important symptom of ADPKD, thought to be caused by enlarging cysts, pain can signal the presence of other concurrent renal or nonrenal disease processes. Renal pain may result from intrarenal or perinephric hemorrhage, obstruction, infection, or neoplasms. Pain similar to ADPKD pain may be produced by diverticulitis, liver cysts, or an enlarging abdominal aneurysm (63).

In addition to patient history, physical examination, and urine and blood studies, radiologic studies including sonography, abdominal computer-assisted tomography (CT), and occasionally magnetic resonance imaging (MRI) are useful techniques for evaluating pain in patients with ADPKD (64–66).

When concurrent renal or nonrenal disease is ruled out by appropriate measures, pain from polycystic kidneys should be treated conservatively. Management strategies for pain control range from mild analgesics on a temporary basis to helping patients cope with long-term chronic pain, using available resources such as a pain clinic. Caution must be used when prescribing narcotics or nephrotoxic analgesics, as well as drugs that alter platelet function (63).

Occasionally pain may be associated with the massive enlargement of one or more cysts in the kidney. Pain of polycystic kidney disease can be relieved by percutaneous aspiration of the fluid from massively enlarged cysts. Alternatively, chronic pain attributed to cyst enlargement has been relieved by open surgical aspiration and internal drainage of the cysts. The Rovsing procedure, which was largely abandoned for the treatment of polycystic kidney disease (67–70) was reintroduced in China as a means of controlling the progression of hypertension and for the relief of pain related to the massive enlargement of cystic kidneys (71). Bennett et al (72) have recently reported reducing the size of individual cysts by percutaneous cyst aspiration or by surgical reduction. The results of these studies are impressive and suggest that the Rovsing procedure, carefully performed, should be evaluated again in a few controlled trials. It would seem, therefore, that patients who experience chronic persistent pain and who have no explanation other than the fact that certain cysts in the kidneys have enlarged to a massive extent, might benefit from percutaneous or direct intraabdominal aspiration of fluid from the cysts or surgical amputation of cyst domes.

HEMATURIA AND HEMORRHAGE

Hematuria is a common objective sign in patients with ADPKD (6, 45, 73–76). The patient usually experiences the sudden appearance of blood in the urine, which may persist as macroscopic or microscopic hematuria for several days. Hemorrhage with accompanying pain can occur when medium-size blood vessels rupture and cause extravasation of blood either into cysts or, rarely, into perinephric tissue. Cyst rupture into the pelvis of the kidney results in hematuria.

The excretion of blood in the urinary tract has been associated with the development of clots in the renal pelvis and ureters, obstructing urine flow. If the obstruction is not relieved spontaneously, or by forced diuresis, it may be necessary to insert a retrograde catheter to move the clot along. Alternatively, a surgical approach, removing clots and the domes of the cysts, may be indicated if the obstruction cannot be relieved by less invasive maneuvers (77, 78). We found no reports to indicate that lytic enzymes had ever been infused into the urinary tract, either retrograde or antegrade, in an attempt to dissolve established clots in the urinary tract.

Occasionally protracted and massive bleeding persists. In patients who have reasonably normal renal function, every effort should be made to preserve kidney function. If a bleeding vessel can be identified, renal artery embolization may be considered before open surgical intervention. Percutaneous transcatheter arterial infarction with a variety of materials (autologous clot, gelatin sponges, Gianturco coils, detachable balloons, and polyvinyl alcohol) may be considered (63, 79). Material selection depends upon the degree of permanence and the degree of embolic selectivity desired, and use of superselective embolization allows cessation of hemorrhage from a segmental renal artery while sparing other viable areas of parenchyma. Most patients will experience a postinfarction syndrome of pain, fever, and nausea that usually lasts 12–96 hours and is treated medically. Transcatheter infarction should probably not be used in patients who have established infection within polycystic kidneys. One instance of apparent successful control of bleeding in an

ADPKD patient by the oral administration of epsilon aminocaproic acid has been reported (80), but its use for the control of hemorrhage from ADPKD is questionable because of its known thrombotic complications (63).

Arteriovenous fistula has been found in at least one polycystic kidney and has resulted in hematuria and acute renal failure (81). The fistula was closed by a surgical procedure and the clinical symptoms abated.

All hematuria from polycystic kidneys should not be considered a *direct* consequence of the cystic lesions. For example, a patient with ADPKD developed hematuria and a precipitous decrease in renal function secondary to the superimposition of acute glomerulonephritis (82). The nephrotic syndrome has also been reported in patients with ADPKD, and though it may not have a direct pathogenetic relation to cystic disease, the nephrotic syndrome may occur from time to time purely on a chance basis. This means, of course, that in patients with ADPKD who experience hematuria for the first time, or if recurrent hematuria persists at some point for an unusually long time, the urine sediment should be examined carefully. Further in this regard, oval fat bodies in the urine do not necessarily mean that the patient has a glomerular disorder. We aspirated fluid from several so-called hemorrhagic cysts in a patient with polycystic kidney disease. Examination of the cyst sediment revealed a large number of oval fat bodies (doubly refractile bodies on polarizing microscopy). We believe this finding indicates that blood within cysts may lead to the formation of oval fat bodies by the viable tubule cells lining the cyst wall, much in the same manner that renal tubular epithelial cells form oval fat bodies in the nephrotic syndrome. We have found oval fat bodies in the voided urine of a large fraction of patients with ADPKD (83).

Perinephric hemorrhage is a rare complication of ADPKD (65). It may be associated with intense discomfort and obvious changes in the configuration of the abdomen upon direct physical examination, as well as clinical evidence of blood loss (66). Computed tomography is the optimal method for evaluation of perinephric hemorrhage, but occasionally MRI may be helpful to supplement CT findings and to differentiate hemorrhagic cysts from carcinomas. Spontaneous or traumatic hemorrhage in or about cystic kidneys can usually be treated by simple bed rest and analgesics, although persistent or recurrent hematuria can result in anemia and can require more aggressive measures. Most patients recognize this problem as a transient disorder once they have been carefully counseled by a physician. Correction of underlying coagulopathies and blood replacement may be necessary, and patients undergoing hemodialysis may require modification of the anticoagulant regimen during bleeding episodes (66). Only when bleeding and hypotension persist despite fluid and blood replacement is intervention required. Transcatheter renal arterial embolization or nephrectomy may then be necessary. In patients in whom persistent pain and bleeding occurs, one must consider renal infection, stones, or malignant tumors. Thus renal pain that changes in character and that lasts more than a few days, especially associated with prolonged hematuria, should be evaluated by a physician.

INFECTION

Experimental animals with renal cysts are especially susceptible to the development of pyelonephritis (84). Humans appear to be highly susceptible as well, and renal infection is common in patients with ADPKD, affecting up to 75% of the patients (85).

Upper urinary tract infections, involving renal parenchyma and cysts, produce pain and localized tenderness (86). Although urinary tract infection can develop as a consequence of hematogenous dissemination of microorganisms, patients with polycystic kidney disease usually acquire upper urinary tract infections by an ascending mechanism. Female patients appear to be especially susceptible to upper tract infections, probably reflecting the fact that females in the general population are more likely than males to develop urinary tract infections secondary to colonization of the lower urinary tract. Permanent upper tract infection in men can often be traced to an invasive procedure such as urinary catheterization, cystoscopic examination, or a retrograde urological procedure. In our experience polycystic kidneys are commonly infected unilaterally, although bilateral parenchymal infection occurs occasionally.

Parenchymal and cyst infections are devastating complications, and early differential diagnosis is difficult but important. A recent study by Schwab (86) revealed a distinction between cyst and renal parenchymal infections in their response to therapy. Cyst infections frequently do not respond to aminoglycosides and penicillins despite favorable sensitivities, but require treatment with lipid-soluble antibiotics, whereas parenchymal infections respond to initial antibiotic therapy within 5 days.

When a suspected infection is accompanied by renal pain, fever, leukocytosis, pyuria, and positive blood or urine cultures, diagnosis of an upper urinary tract infection is virtually assured. But when a single cyst is infected, bacteriuria may be undetectable because the contribution of bacteria from one infected cyst to the overall urine is minuscule. Patients with diffuse parenchymal disease may shed sufficient organisms into the urine to significantly elevate the colony count. Schwab et al. (86, 87) report that cyst infections had a higher percentage of positive blood cultures, while parenchymal infections showed more WBC casts and positive urine cultures.

Renal ultrasound is of no value in the detection of infection (87). CT scan cannot differentiate between hemorrhagic or infected cysts nor define parenchymal infection, but infected cysts may be recognized from increased thickness of the wall on CT scan (88). Gallium scans are helpful when positive, but have a high false-negative rate (87). Case reports indicate indium-111 leukocyte scans may be useful (89, 90), but a systematic study needs to be done. Thus, a clear constellation of symptoms and signs to differentiate parenchymal from cyst infection is found infrequently, and one must begin treatment based upon empirical judgments, changing therapy based on the patient response. Schwab et al. (87) conclude that failure to respond to standard antibiotic therapy, despite favorable sensitivities, may be the most useful criterion for the diagnosis of cyst infection.

Very little has been known about the organisms responsible for infections in polycystic kidneys, but the recent study by Schwab (86) revealed that gram-negative enterics were the causative organisms in 92% of the cyst and 100% of the parenchymal infections. The usual antibiotic treatment combination of ampicillin and an aminoglycoside was effective in this series in all the parenchymal infections but in only one of the cyst infections, even though sensitivities were favorable. Use of lipid-soluble antibiotics eradicated 83% of the cyst infections. This response is believed to be due to the high membrane penetrability of the drugs.

We have observed low oxygen tension ($pO_2 < 40$ mmHg) in several cysts from a polycystic kidney. This raises the possibility that anaerobic organisms might grow in such an environment.

Several investigators (91–98) have evaluated the penetration of antibiotics into proximal and distal cysts of patients with ADPKD (Table 3). Cysts have been grouped into gradient and non-gradient varieties depending on the sodium concentration of the fluid (40, 41). Nongradient cysts are characterized by loose or leaky cellular junctions, similar to normal proximal tubular cells. Gradient cysts are characterized by tight cellular junctions typical of distal tubular epithelia. Most antibiotics appear to enter nongradient cysts to some extent, with levels approaching those in the plasma detected occasionally, whereas in gradient cysts antibiotic levels are frequently low. Since it is believed that antibiotics pass through the wall of cysts rather than entering the cavity by glomerular filtration, it is hypothesized that only lipid-soluble antibiotics can enter distal cysts in sufficient concentrations to eradicate infecting organisms.

This poses a therapeutic problem because many antibiotics that are effective against gram-negative aerobes are lipid insoluble and polar. Antibiotics that have been shown to enter cyst fluid are, in general, ineffective against the most likely pathogens. Thus it is suggested that one may begin antibiotic therapy with ampicillin or a cephalosporin and an aminoglycoside. If no response occurs after 5 days, convert to a lipid-soluble agent such as chloramphenicol, ciprofloxacin, clindamycin, trimethoprim, or metronidazole if in-vitro sensitivities are favorable. Drawbacks to using lipid-soluble antibiotics as initial therapy are the limited number of available antibiotics and the possibility of selecting resistant organisms. Most clinicians choose the parenteral as opposed to the oral route for giving the antibiotics.

Occasionally the infection may be so serious and intractable that nephrectomy is necessary. This drastic step should be used as a last resort, and only after the patient has received parenteral antibiotics for relatively long periods of time and the possibility of urinary tract obstruction has been excluded. When intrapelvic urinary stones exist, infection is difficult or impossible to eradicate until the stones are removed. In patients who experience a decrease in signs and symptoms, some physicians would continue oral antibiotics for an indefinite period of time. We are aware of two patients with recurrent Klebsiella infections who required continuous suppressive antibiotics for 2 years to maintain an asymptomatic state.

We advise all of our patients about routine hygiene measures. For women we recommend showers rather than tub baths, frequent voiding, good perineal hygiene, and voiding immediately after intercourse. We make a special point to advise all patients with ADPKD to refuse urinary tract instrumentation procedures unless absolutely necessary (99).

NEOPLASTIC CHANGES

The frequency and malignant potential of renal neoplasms in ADPKD is currently being studied (100). Case reports (101–106) of renal cell carcinoma occurring in patients with ADPKD exist, but it is unclear whether this is a chance or true association. In seven patients, bilateral renal malignancies were found (107). Evidence of an increased incidence of malignant changes in acquired cystic disease in long-term dialysis patients is being reported. Thus neoplastic changes in cysts must be given consideration in differential diagnosis when new symptoms arise in ADPKD.

Pain may be the first sign of malignancy within the kidney. Pain in association with fever, weight loss, anemia, and a striking change in the configuration of the kidney must raise the suspicion of renal malignancy. The most reliable diagnostic signs of malignancy include speckled calcifications within the parenchyma of the kidney (108), the appearance of a solid mass structure by sonography (109), the appearance of tissue with a high computed tomography (CT) number (88, 110), and a typical arteriogram appearance upon infusion of urographic contrast material into the renal artery (106, 111–113). MRI is

Table 3. Penetration of antibiotics into cysts of patients with ADPKD

Type of antibiotic	Degree of accumulation in cysts	
	Nongradient*	Gradient*
Aminoglycoside (91, 93, 97)		
Gentamicin	+	0
Tobramycin	0	0
Cephapirin (91)	+	+
Ticarcillin (91)	+	0
Clindamycin (93)	+	+++
Trimethoprim (96)	+	+++
Sulfamethoxazole (96)	+	0
Ciprofloxacin (98)	+	+++
Chloramphenicol (94)	?	?
Metronidazole (97)	+	+

* Nongradient cysts have sodium levels near those of plasma; gradient cysts have lower sodium levels (< 40 mEq/l) (40, 41).

useful in differentiating between hemorrhagic and neoplastic masses when CT and sonography are indeterminate (65). We suggest that if a unilateral carcinoma is detected in a patient with ADPKD, removal of both kidneys may be warranted.

HYPERTENSION

Arterial hypertension of a mild-to-moderate degree develops in approximately one half of patients with ADPKD at some time in the course of the disease (6, 73–76, 114, 115), although malignant hypertension is exceptional. Hypertension often antedates measurable functional renal impairment by several years (116, 117), with one study (45) noting a frequency of 62% in nonazotemic persons with polycystic kidney disease. Hypertension is thought to accelerate renal destruction in some patients (61).

The pathogenesis of hypertension in ADPKD is still poorly understood. Renal artery stenosis has been observed in two patients with ADPKD (118, 119). The hypertension was improved in one of them after correcting the stenotic lesion. Most often, however, a proximate cause for the hypertension cannot be found. Since solitary renal cysts may cause hypertension by compressing renal vasculature, thus producing increased amounts of renin, angiotensin, and aldosterone (vide infra), physicians have looked carefully at the role of these hormones in the hypertension of ADPKD. Several studies indicated that the renin-angiotension-aldosterone axis is intact in patients with ADPKD (120, 121). While in one study (122) saralasin, an inhibitor of angiotension II, had no effect on the blood pressure of ADPKD patients, making it seem unlikely that renin release mediates the hypertension in these patients, another (123) contradicts this finding. Studies indicate that hypertension may be mediated by ECF volume (124, 125), but the evidence for this is not certain. Thus more work is needed to resolve these problems.

Most hypertensive ADPKD patients respond to conventional therapy, the backbone of which is a reduction in the sodium intake. Modest reduction to 50–75 mM of NaCl per day can be tolerated by most patients. If salt restriction alone fails, one may add a peripheral sympatholytic agent (labetalol, prazosin, propranolol, metoprolol), a central sympatholytic agent (clonidine, methyldopa), or an arteriolar dilator (hydralazine, minoxidil, nifedipine, verapamil). For those patients who cannot adhere to a reduced salt intake, diuretics (metolazone, chlorthalidone, hydrochlorothiazide) may be needed to enhance the effectiveness of the other agents. Although there is no proof, we are concerned that diuretics used for long periods may reduce the removal of salt and water from cysts, causing them to enlarge at a rate faster than usual. Thus, we prefer to withhold diuretics if at all possible.

ANEURYSM OF CEREBRAL AND ABDOMINAL VESSELS

In ADPKD, intracranial aneurysms are thought to be secondary to a developmental defect in the arterial wall. Death from spontaneous rupture of a cerebral aneurysm occurs in patients with ADPKD. Little is known about the natural history of cerebral aneurysms. They may rupture in relatively young patients with ADPKD, but most are discovered over the age of 30.

The aneurysms are occasionally found, before they rupture, during evaluations for headache or cranial nerve paralysis. Wiebers et al. (126) studied the natural history of unruptured intracranial saccular aneurysms in the general population. The size of the aneurysm was the best indicator of future rupture. None of the aneurysms smaller than 1 cm in diameter ruptured, whereas 27% of aneurysms over 1 cm in diameter ruptured. This study indicates that in ADPKD asymptomatic aneurysms smaller than 1 cm in diameter are less threatening than larger lesions.

De la Monte et al. (127) studied risk factors for the development and rupture of intracranial berry aneurysms in the general population and noted that, in addition to size, rupture of berry aneurysm was positively correlated with long-term analgesic use, especially aspirin, excessive ethanol consumption, fatty changes in the liver, and the presence of multiple aneurysms. Aneurysm rupture was negatively correlated with treatment with insulin to control diabetes mellitus, leanness, chronic pancreatitis, malignant tumors, and moderate or severe coronary or renal atherosclerosis.

Whether all patients with ADPKD should be evaluated at some time for cerebral aneurysm remains controversial (128–130), but most specialists agree that routine screening in asymptomatic patients *without* a family history of intracranial aneurysm is not recommended. Family clustering of intracranial aneurysms may exist (131, 132), raising the possibility of a greater risk for some patients. In patients in whom CT examination of the abdomen (with contrast) is planned, it is reasonable to include a view of the head at the same time. Lesions larger than 1 cm in diameter may be detected this way, but MRI is superior to CT for aneurysm screening in patients with a strong family history of strokes.

Aneurysm of the abdominal aorta has been reported in four patients with ADPKD (50, 51), and we have observed this complication in one case. Other cardiovascular abnormalities, including systolic murmurs in nonhypertensive patients (45), cardiac valvular abnormalities, annuloaortic ectasia (133), and ruptured chordae tendinae, have also been noted (52, 134). These findings, together with the cranial lesions, suggest that a generalized connective tissue defect in several structures (arteries, renal rubules, bile ducts, pancreatic ducts, colon, cardiac valves) may be a common denominator of ADPKD.

NEPHROLITHIASIS

The fact that patients with ADPKD develop stones within the parenchyma and collecting system has been known since the classic studies of Dalgaard (6). Radioopaque urinary stones can usually be demonstrated by simple abdominal radiographic procedures. Radiolucent stones (uric acid) can be revealed only by contrast studies or by computed tomography. The localization of stones to the

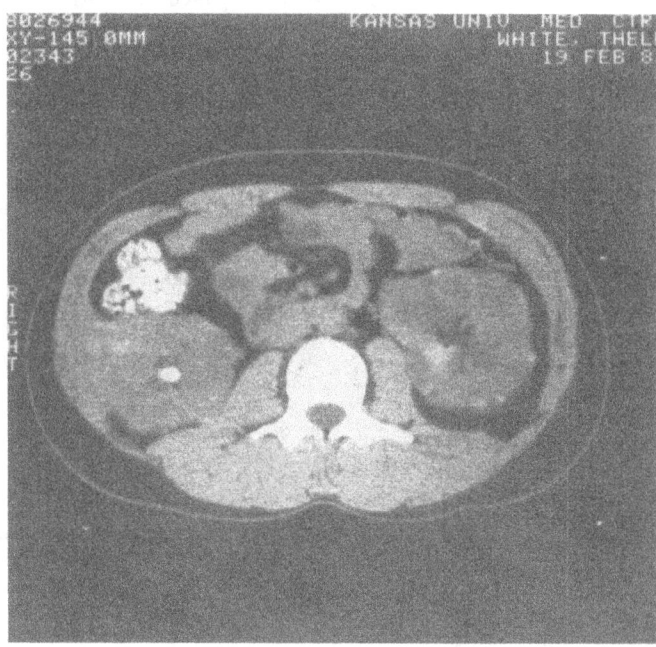

Figure 2. CT scan of abdomen. Calculus is evident in pelvis of right kidney. Calcifications of renal parenchyma scattered throughout both kidneys.

collecting portion of the kidney is feasible when CT scans are done with contrast enhancement (Figure 2). A systematic analysis of the nature of urinary stones has recently been made in 30 patients with ADPKD (135) and it revealed that the stones consisted of uric acid (56.6%), calcium oxalate (46.6%), calcium phosphate (20%), and struvite (10%). The most common metabolic abnormality in these patients was hypocitric aciduria, with the urine pH in first-voided morning specimens significantly lower than that of a control population. Based on the composition of the stones, the frequency of hypocitric aciduria, and the low urine pH, possibly related to the defect in excretion of ammonia described in ADPKD, the investigators suggest that metabolic, along with mechanical, factors are responsible for the frequent occurrence of nephrolithiasis in this disease.

Patients with ADPKD and renal lithiasis deserve the same metabolic work-up as any patient. An evaluation for hypercalciuria and hyperuricosuria is a reasonable way to start. For patients with stones, a high fluid intake is recommended (> 2 l/day).

Stones may lodge in various portions of the collecting system and cause obstruction. In the pelvis and ureter, they can usually be removed surgically if they do not pass spontaneously. Stones in the calyces are more difficult to remove surgically. The authors are aware of one anecdotal report of a stone treated successfully with lithotripsy in a patient with ADPKD, but further investigation needs to be done in this area. Stones and urinary tract infection are a devastating combination. If the stone cannot be removed, pain and inflammation can be controlled in some patients by using antibiotics continuously. Resistant organisms generally appear in such cases. Occasionally the urine bacteria colony count can be reduced by drugs such as mandelamine and furadantin, even when the organisms appear to be moderately resistant by in-vitro tests.

GASTROINTESTINAL PROBLEMS

Patients with far advanced kidney cystic disease often have severe abdominal discomfort not originating in the kidneys (136). Liver cysts appear in approximately 20–75% of the patients and occasionally the liver can be massively enlarged, especially in females. A CT scan of a cystic liver is shown in Figure 3. Liver cysts may undergo hemorrhagic distension and cause acute discomfort. They may become infected. Liver cysts may cause obstruction of the major bile ducts and jaundice (137, 138). In the adult form of polycystic kidney disease, liver cysts may become so numerous that they cause portal hypertension, esophageal varices, and severe hemorrhoids (139–142). Gastrointestinal hemorrhage may arise from these venous sources. Instances of hepatocellular insufficiency in patients with ADPKD are few, as the synthetic functions appear to be maintained for a long period of time, but as patients live longer on dialysis, the possibility of liver complications is

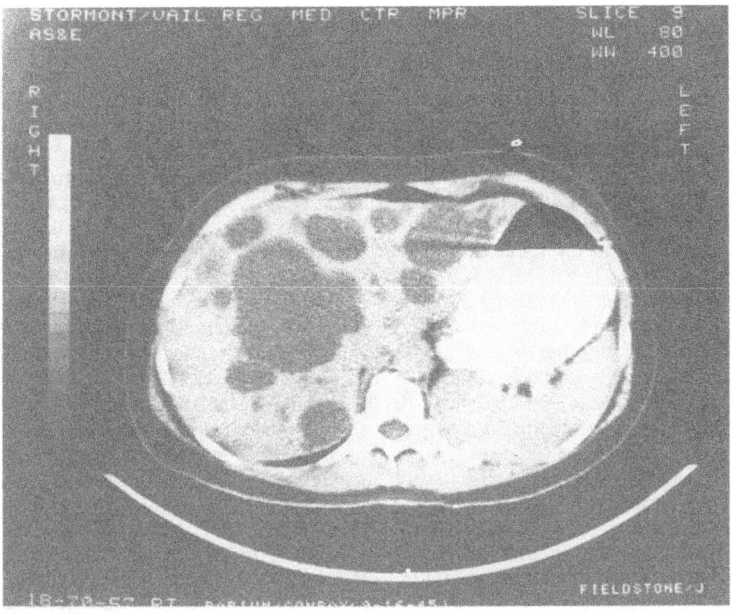

Figure 3. CT appearance of polycystic liver in a patient with ADPKD. Cysts are scattered throughout the liver. The spleen is not cystic.

increasing (46). Cholangiocellular carcinoma has been reported in two uremic patients with polycystic kidney and liver disease (143), and primary hepatocellular carcinoma has been reported in one renal transplant recipient (144).

Constipation, presumably with increased intraluminal bowel pressure, is a significant problem in patients with adult polycystic disease. In those with massively enlarged kidneys and livers, there is very little room left in the abdominal cavity for the intestinal tract. Female patients may feel as though they are chronically pregnant. Patients who have developed renal failure have further contributing factors toward constipation: restricted fluid intake, required phosphate binders, and possibly autonomic nervous system dysfunction. The possible increased incidence of diverticulosis in this population is an added risk factor for intestinal perforation, and signs and symptoms of this life-threatening complication may be masked. Striking in one series (48) was the timing and severity of presentation of intestinal perforation in renal failure patients as compared to the general population. Over one half had free perforation of diverticula into the peritoneal cavity, with minimal surrounding inflammation. Therefore it is suggested that constipation be avoided if possible to attempt to decrease diverticular disease. One group of investigators noted that hepatic cysts and symptomatic cerebral aneurysms were more common in ADPKD patients with diverticulosis (48), but this needs confirmation. There appears to be a high incidence of hiatus hernia in ADPKD patients.

PREGNANCY

ADPKD does not appear to have any adverse effect on the ability of female patients to become pregnant (145). Affected males also appear capable of fathering offspring in a normal fashion. Patients with no symptomatic or objective findings of polycystic kidney disease at the time that they become pregnant usually have reasonably normal pregnancies, although they appear to be at increased risk for developing hypertension (145, 146). Urinary tract infections do not occur more frequently in patients with polycystic kidney disease than in other pregnant women, but if a given patient has urinary tract infections in one pregnancy, she will probably have recurrent urinary tract infections in subsequent pregnancies (145). Patients who have significant hypertension, proteinuria, or renal insufficiency at the time that they become pregnant have an increased number of complications during pregnancy (147). Pregnancy appears to have no deleterious effect on the course of ADPKD, and the number of pregnancies does not affect the rate of progression toward renal failure (145, 146, 148).

PROGNOSIS

At the present time there is no accurate way to judge the prognosis in those patients who have no significant degree of renal impairment at the time they are evaluated. Dalgaard (6) suggested that patients within a family developed renal failure at about the same age. Many exceptions to this "rule" have been found, so that family history is not always helpful. Once patients have begun to show a significant decrease in creatinine clearance, the prognosis for the progression of the disease can be judged relatively accurately from the relationship between the reciprocal of plasma creatinine concentration ($1/p_{cr}$) and time (149). Barring intercurrent infections, ureteral obstruction, or other abnormalities, the patients generally experience a chronic persistent loss of a fixed amount of creatinine clearance each year. This is reflected by a linear decline in $1/p_{cr}$ versus time (54, 150).

It is important to note that the $1/p_{cr}$ versus time relationship is probably valid only when the serum creatinine level begins to rise appreciably. In other words, some patients may experience perfectly normal glomerular filtration rates and plasma creatinine levels for up to 40 years (55). However, when the creatinine clearance begins to fall and the serum creatinine rises, it appears that in uncomplicated cases there is a persistent loss of a relatively fixed amount of creatinine clearance per unit of time.

There are no therapies directed specifically at the polycystic disease process that are generally held to be of benefit. Reducing the protein content of the diet may slow progression slightly (61). Surgical aspiration of surface cysts on the kidney (Rovsing's procedure) has been reported to increase rather than decrease the progression to renal insufficiency. However, recent reports (71, 72) suggest that ultrasound-guided percutaneous aspiration of cyst fluid, or careful surgical "cyst decapitation" relieves pain and hypertension, and may also retard the progression to end-stage renal disease. This therapeutic approach should be studied in greater detail.

DIALYSIS AND TRANSPLANTATION

Hemodialysis has been used to treat patients with end-stage polycystic kidney disease for nearly three decades. Reports from dialysis and transplant registries in Europe, Canada, and the United States indicate that from 5.9–12% of the patients have ADPKD (7).

Patients with adult polycystic kidney disease appear to do better in hemodialysis programs than do patients with other renal disease (151, 152). This is probably due in large measure to the fact that these patients have rather high hematocrit values. Also their urinary volumes may be higher than those in patients with other renal diseases, thus minimizing fluid overload problems (107).

Polycystic kidneys may atrophy during long duration of treatment by hemodialysis (153, 154), but reports of an increase in size do exist (155). Patients in hemodialysis programs do not appear to develop nonrenal infections, hemorrhage, or other routine complications any more commonly than nonazotemic patients. It should be noted that hypertension shortly after initiating the dialysis procedure has been reported in two patients to be secondary to compression of the inferior vena cava by massively enlarged kidneys (156). This problem was averted by removing the kidneys.

One of the special problems of ADPKD patients in the hemodialysis programs is repeated fistula closure secondary to thrombosis, probably due to the relatively high hematocrit and the viscosity values of their blood. Some ADPKD patients have persistent hypotension in interdialytic and intradialytic periods, but this may not be a unique trait. The mechanism of the hypotension is unknown and the therapy is empiric. The patients will occasionally respond to the liberalization of salt intake, mineralocorticoid supplementation, and the liberal use of albumin during the dialysis procedure. Urinary tract bleeding secondary to cyst rupture may occasionally be intensified by the use of heprain. in these instances, regional heparinization, the use of a low-dose regimen, or, more recently, the use of heparin-free citrate regional anticoagulation (157) is often helpful.

Peritoneal dialysis, either intermittent peritoneal dialysis or chronic ambulatory peritoneal dialysis, has been used to treat patients with ADPKD. The role of these treatments in patients with polycystic kidney disease remains uncertain. Although many ADPKD patients have large kidneys and livers, and additional fluid in the peritoneal cavity may be very uncomfortable, it is being used successfully in some centers. Others report a high incidence of spontaneous intestinal perforation (158) and discourage its use. Because of the large volume of the kidneys, inadvertant puncture of the bowel and of blood vessels during catheter insertion may be a problem. This complication can be avoided if a direct surgical approach is used rather than the trocar method of introducing the peritoneal catheter.

Renal transplantation is now used routinely to treat patients with end-stage renal disease with ADPKD (159–167). Related living donors have been used at several transplantation centers. The possibility of siblings with identical HLA specificities also possessing the ADPKD gene has been addressed. Although specific histocompatability testing data have not been reported in living, related transplantation groups, in a few instances "A" match kidneys were transplanted. This suggests that siblings with identical HLA specificities do not necessarily possess the ADPKD gene. In a study of 2548 cadaveric renal transplant recipients of whom 108 had ADPKD (168), gene frequency analysis revealed no HLA-A or -B antigen linkage with polycystic disease. One series (166) involving 22 patients showed an increased frequency of HLA-A3 (54%) and HLA-B7 (45%). Each of these tissue-typing specificities would be expected to appear in 26% of the normal population. Despite this latter observation, it seems unlikely that the ADPKD gene and the HLA gene share the same chromosome, since linkage analysis has localized the mutant gene on chromosome 16 (169).

Use of donor-specific blood transfusions from living, related donors and deliberate preliminary blood transfusions in cadaver transplant candidates appears to increase graft survival and is being used regularly in some centers.

Some clinicians have advocated the use of hemodialysis as the primary, if not the sole, means of taking care of patients with end-stage ADPKD (151). This opinion is based on the observation that the hemodialysis survival rate for patients with ADPKD is extremely good. On the other hand, renal transplantation has been used effectively in patients with ADPKD. Post-transplant survival rates in such patients appear to be equal to those in patients with other renal disorders requiring renal transplantation. Deaths have been reported in the immediate post-transplant period and later on in patients with ADPKD. The most common cause of death in this group of patients is sepsis, as in other patients. Unusual causes of death include cerebral vascular accident secondary to a ruptured aneurysm and peritonitis secondary to ruptured colonic diverticula. Infection of hepatic cysts has been reported post-transplantation (170). Splenomegaly has been observed in approximately 12% of patients with polycystic kidney disease who come to transplantation. This is usually due to portal hypertension and hypersplenism. This important problem must be found before the transplant is done, since hypersplenism intensifies the response to immunosuppressive therapy.

The original cystic kidneys have been observed to shrink in size after successful renal transplantation (171). Whether or not the original polycystic kidneys should be removed is one of the major problems confronting transplant surgeons. In a 1981 survey of 29 dialysis and transplant centers in the United States, a variety of opinions regarding this question were expressed (Table 4). Five programs required that all ADPKD patients be nephrectomized. Twenty-two centers nephrectomized only those patients with symptomatic problems such as pain, infection, hemorrhage, positive urine culture, or a recent history of pyelonephritis. Two centers avoided nephrectomy if at all possible. It is clear from this survey that there are no hard or fast rules with respect to the criteria for ADPKD-recipient nephrectomy.

Table 5 summarizes some of the guides that may be used to determine the need for pretransplant nephrectomy.
1. Recurrent infection manifested by pyuria, flank pain, leukocytosis, or sepsis seems a clear indication for pretransplant nephrectomy. If the infectious process has been dormant for a number of years, then one might choose to leave the kidneys in place.

Table 4. Preferences of 29 dialysis-transplant centers in the U.S. regarding pretransplant nephrectomy of polycystic kidneys

	Number of centers
1. All patients with ADPKD nephrectomized before renal transplantation	5
2. Only patients with symptomatic problems related to polycystic kidneys nephrectomized before renal transplantation (renal pain, renal infection, renal hemorrhage, postive urine culture, recent history of pyelonephritis)	22
3. Other (do not nephrectomize)	2

Table 5. Indications for pretransplant nephrectomy in ADPKD

1. Recurrent urinary tract infection
2. Intractable pain
3. Renal neoplasm
4. Persistent gross hematuria
5. Nephrolithiasis
6. Pyuria
7. Positive gallium scan
8. Compression of inferior vena cava

2. Intractable abdominal pain may be a relative indication for pretransplant nephrectomy. In some centers Rovsing's operation has been performed prior to transplantatio to alleviate pain. This operation does not appear to add any complications to the subsequent transplant procedure and gives the patient the benefit of a high hematocrit and other favorable features of residual renal function should the allograft fail.
3. The appearance of a tumor in a kidney is certainly an indication for pretransplant nephrectomy (101–104). Since tumors in polycystic kidneys do not uncommonly appear in both kidneys, bilateral nephrectomy is indicated if a tumor is found in one kidney (105–106). While the risk of malignancy might be viewed as reason to remove all cystic kidneys before transplantation, the incidence of this complication is relatively low. Careful CT, sonographic, and arteriographic evaluation of the cystic kidneys in asymptomatic patients before transplantation should reveal most occult neoplasms.
4. Gross hematuria that persists during the dialysis routine is an indication for pretransplant nephrectomy.
5. Nephrolithiasis with demonstrated calculi in the renal collecting system is an indication for pretransplant nephrectomy.
6. Persistent pyuria in the absence of culturable organisms is a relative indication for pretransplantation nephrectomy.
7. A positive gallium scan suggests active parenchymal infection, necessitating nephrectomy if transplantation is planned in the near future.
8. Compression of the vena cava by large kidneys is an indication for pretransplant nephrectomy.

Prevention and counseling

Prevention is one way to decrease the incidence of ADPKD, but it can be realized only by prospectively identifying those with the disorder before they bear children. Recent advancements in presymptomatic diagnostic techniques have made such identification possible for young adults, and the discovery of the genetic locus for ADPKD (169, 172, 173) may eventually provide reliable prenatal diagnosis. However, before presymptomatic screening is undertaken, geneticists caution that important socioeconomic, psychological, and ethical implications of test results must be considered (174).

The family history is a crucial part of the counseling

process. In the authors' experience, many family members are unwilling to reveal the fact that they or other members in their family have had this particular disease, and in those families with known disease not all are willing to be tested. Guilt and denial are prominent coping patterns in families of patients with ADPKD (175). Often patients do not learn that they have the ADPKD gene until they have passed into or beyond their child-bearing period (176). A study of Sahney et al. (177) showed that only 23% of patients with ESRD secondary to ADPKD knew their disorder was hereditary at the time of diagnosis, and in only 18% was genetic counseling suggested. Studies of attitudes toward prenatal or presymptomatic testing in this disease and in Huntington's disease (176, 178) confirm that even when early diagnosis is possible, not everyone wishes to have such information.

If a patient or family does decide to proceed with screening, they must be aware that problems can result from either a positive or a negative diagnostic result. For the patient who is not found to have the renal disease, the future is clear — there is virtually no chance the disease will be passed on. Yet even this information can have an intense impact on unaffected members of a family, a situation described by psychologists as "survivor guilt" (174, 179).

For the young patient discovered to have early ADPKD, several psychological and socioeconomic problems have been recognized. Perhaps the most difficult problem is the fact that nothing can be done to prevent the progression of the disease at this time. Certainly, the patient can be made aware of some of the complications that are important in patients with polycystic kidney disease, including infection, hypertension, aneurysm, and stone formation. But taking measures to minimize risk factors for these complications is a small comfort to a patient who is told early in life that renal dialysis or transplantation may be needed within the next 20 or 30 years. Adverse effects such as personal feelings of depression or unworthiness, or, alternatively, an inappropriately casual attitude may occur, possibly resulting in disruption of the family, divorce, or marital stress. Especially in younger persons, stigmatization in attracting a mate may occur, and the issue of disclosure arises (179, 180). Furthermore, the early discovery in the young person of a potentially disabling or life-threatening disease may affect future employability and insurability. These factors must be carefully discussed with the patients prior to the time that they are screened for polycystic kidney disease, as well as during the course of the disease, as the perception of risks may change with time (177, 180).

If patients are able to make a decision, i.e., they have the rights of majority in the state in which they are being counseled and decide they want to undergo diagnostic studies to determine if they have ADPKD, then it is reasonable to proceed with physical examination, sonography and possibly CT scanning, urinalysis, and measurements of plasma creatinine and urea. If sonography is unequivocally positive, there is no need to do additional studies, especially with a family history of ADPKD. On the other hand, if sonography is negative or equivocal, we recommend computer-assisted tomography with and without contrast enhancement. With the newer CT instruments it is possible to identify cysts smaller than 0.5 cm in diameter within the kidneys. Recent studies using combined sonography and CT scanning indicate that the presence of the disease in young persons can probably be established with a high degree of certainty (45, 88, 181–187). If sonography and CT scanning do not reveal diffuse cystic involvement of both kidneys and the liver is normal, then patients may be advised with reasonable certainty that they do not have the disorder.

Although significant advances have occurred in genetic testing, the 3'HVR marker currently available has an error rate of approximately 5%, and in our view it will not lead to certain diagnosis in adults with an accuracy greater than CT scanning. As markers closer to the mutant gene are identified, patients and their family members can be diagnosed with greater certainty.

For adults with a positive diagnosis of early ADPKD, it becomes a personal decision as to whether or not to have their own biologic children or to find other means for having a family. Since ADPKD is an autosomal disorder, patients with the gene may expect that each child will have a 50/50 chance of having or not having the gene. Although the possibility of sonographic or genetic prenatal diagnosis is increasing, it is not yet reliable. Newer sonographic techniques reveal cysts in fetal kidneys, in some cases as early as the second trimester, but definitive diagnosis may remain uncertain (36, 188–191). Thus, the multifaceted aspects of diagnosis, prevention, and treatment of ADPKD demand effective education and counseling for individuals both prior to and at the time of diagnosis, as well as during the course of the disease.

POLYCYSTIC DISEASE, INFANTILE

Introduction and background

Infantile polycystic kidney disease is a rare disorder occurring once in every 16,000 live births. The disorder is transmitted as an autosomal recessive trait, thus it is almost never recognized in either parent. We prefer the abbreviation ARPKD to signify infantile *autosomal recessive polycystic kidney disease* in contrast to ADPKD. Since both asymptomatic parents must have the recessive gene, each offspring of the carrier parents has a 1 in 4 chance of having the full-blown disease. Blyth and Ockenden (192) suggested that ARPKD may appear in four distinctive clinical forms, although subsequent investigators (193, 194) have suggested that the disease actually represents a continuum of renal and hepatic disease. According to the widely used Blyth and Ockenden classification, based on the degree of histologic change in the kidneys and liver, in the *perinatal* form the infants are born with large palpable polycystic kidneys and seldom survive for more than a few days. The liver shows minimal periportal fibrosis. In the *neonatal* form the kidneys are enlarged at birth with dilatation of approximately 90% of the renal tubules. There is mild fibrosis of the liver in this form. These patients usually die within a few months after birth. In the *infantile* form fewer numbers of nephrons appear to be cystic than in more aggressive perinatal and neonatal forms, and the fibrosis in the liver appears to be somewhat greater. These patients may live to be several years of age. In the *juvenile* form only about 10% of the tubules appear to be cystic, but there is very severe fibrosis of the liver that is frequently associated with portal hypertension and hypersplenism. Patients with the juvenile form of polycystic ARPKD may live into the second and third decade.

In the perinatal and neonatal forms the pathologic changes in the kidneys are distinctive and are usually not confused with other cystic disorders. The kidneys are bilaterally enlarged and maintain their reniform appearance. The kidneys have a sponge quality owing to the linear distention of the nephrons causing a radial pattern of cyst formation. There is no normal parenchyma in these cystic kidneys. In older patients with ARPKD the pathologic changes may be difficult to differentiate from ADPKD. In the older patients macrocysts form throughout the kidney, causing calyceal distortion and an irregular bumpy appearance to the surface of the kidney (192, 195). The livers of the patients often show initial periportal fibrosis and occasional cysts in the liver and kidneys (196–199). Severe portal hypertension with esophageal varices, and massively enlarged spleens with hypersplenism, are encountered frequently. Liver biopsy showing periportal fibrosis is perhaps the best way to distinguish ARPKD from ADPKD in young adults.

Those investiagtors preferring to discuss ARPKD in terms of a continuum of renal and hepatic disease note that it varies in the severity and consequences of renal and liver involvement, and demonstrates a spectrum of radiologic and pathologic change. Infants with severe disease present with respiratory distress, congestive heart failure, or hypertension (194), and seldom survive for more than a few days. The liver shows typical platelike hamartomatous bile duct proliferation associated with a mild increase in portal connective tissue involving all portal areas (194). In less severely affected patients the renal involvement is less, but the liver involvement demonstrates the same bile duct proliferation with more prominent portal fibrosis. Early tissue diagnosis, including both renal and liver biopsies, is useful in separating patients with ARPKD from many other inherited and sporadic malformation syndromes.

Newer radiographic techniques provide valuable diagnostic data in infants and young children, as well as antenatally. Intravenous nephrotomography may be of some value, but sonography appears to be a more important diagnostic tool presently available for initial screening purposes (189–191, 195, 198, 200). Sonography is noninvasive and uses no ionizing radiation. Typical sonograms show enlarged kidneys with increased echogenicity in the cortex and medulla. The sonograms also show poor definition of the collecting system and rather fuzzy delineation of the kidneys from surrounding tissues. Antenatal sonographic findings of ARPKD appear at an extremely variable gestational age, from 18 to 30 weeks (189, 190). They include the presence of oligohydramnios, absent urinary bladder, bilateral renal enlargement as measured by the kidney circumference/abdominal circumference ratio, and the typical hyperechogenic appearance of the kidneys (189). Caution must be used in using this data for therapeutic decisions, however, as both false-positives and false-negatives have been reported (190). In juvenile patients macrocystic changes can be observed. Computer-assisted tomography has also been used in patients with ARPKD for diagnostic purposes (201). This procedure is limited to those patients who are able to cooperate during the performance of the test, which eliminates most children under the age of 3 years. Computer-assisted tomography carries a significant radiation hazard in patients at this age of development. Nonetheless, this diagnostic technique can be used, especially with contrast enhancement, to delineate the fine details of the renal architecture in patients with a doubtful diagnosis.

Glomerular cystic disease

Glomerular cystic disease is a rare disorder that presents a diagnostic dilemma. It characteristically has been described as a cystic disorder with dilatation of Bowman's space, the glomerular cysts containing abortive or primitive-appearing glomeruli, and with little or no tubular involvement (202, 203). At one time believed virtually indistinguishable clinically from ARPKD (204, 205), recently cases of GCD with an autosomal dominant inheritance pattern have been reported (203, 206), as well as cases in adults (203, 207, 208). Furthermore, improved fetal ultrasonographic technology has increased early detection of renal cystic diseases, and because glomerular cysts occur in several disease processes and infant malformation syndromes (202), controversy exists regarding the existence of a separate glomerulocystic disease category. Are the glomerular cysts simply variant manifestations of other diseases, or are they an entity unto themselves? If GCD is a separate entity, the rarity of clinical recognition at this time deprives us of knowledge of its natural history. Therefore more research must be done before prevention and counseling strategies can be recommended. What has been reported is summarized as follows: Ultrasonographic features of GCD can be confused with ARPKD, although the cysts in ARPKD are limited to the distal nephron. Ultrasound is **not** diagnostic, but requires histologic confirmation when clinical examination and family screening fail to reveal the diagnosis. Renal macrocysts and hepatic cysts may be found in GCD as well as ARPKD. Renal size in GCD may diminish as the child grows.

Components of the disease that require management

HYPERTENSION

Arterial hypertension has been observed in many patients with ARPKD. Although the proximate cause of hypertension is not known, most patients respond favorably to salt restriction and the usual antihypertensive drugs (diuretics, vasodilators). Aggressive control of hypertension is thought to be essential in preventing or delaying the deterioration of renal function (194).

EDEMA

Patients with ARPKD frequently have edema and impaired renal and/or hepatic function. The edema may be treated by a combination of salt restriction and diuretic substances, usually requiring the potent loop diuretics such as furosemide, bumetanide, or ethacrynic acid.

HEPATIC INSUFFICIENCY

Patients with ARPKD usually develop signs of portal hypertension and hepatic insufficiency between the ages of 5 and 10 years. Consequently, ARPKD patients should undergo relatively frequent assessments for hepatic dysfunction and portal hypertension. Esophageal and gastric varices, and hypersplenism, have been observed routinely in patients with this disorder. Gastrointestinal hemorrhage may be life threatening. Patients with large spleens secondary to portal hypertension may have hypersplenism with leukopenia, thrombocytopenia, and anemia. Portacaval and splenorenal shunts have been successful in such children, although there is a high incidence of surgical morbidity in patients undergoing the shunting procedures. Consequently, hemodialysis facilities must be available in case there is worsening of the renal failure caused by the surgical procedure. Removal of the spleen may be necessary to assist with the management of immunosuppressive therapy.

URINARY TRACT INFECTION

Patients with ARPKD are unusually susceptible to urinary tract infection, as are other patients with renal cystic disorders. With this in mind, clinicians should be extremely careful about instrumenting the urinary tract in patients known to have ARPKD. With the advent of the newer noninvasive techniques, retrograde ureteral catheterization and bladder catheterization can probably be avoided. Suprapubic bladder aspiration, rather than urethral catheterization, is the preferred method for culturing the urine. There have been no large series or even anecdotal clinical reports regarding the specific treatment of urinary tract infection in patients with ARPKD. An approach to therapy similar to that discussed in respect to ADPKD seems reasonable.

RENAL INSUFFICIENCY

Patients with ARPKD develop renal insufficiency at variable times during the course of the disease. A significant proportion of patients with ARPKD live to be young adults. In those patients who live beyond the perinatal and neonatal periods, renal insufficiency may develop insidiously. It should be noted that after the first year of life the physical findings in ARPKD are less specific than during the first year. The enlarged kidneys appear to decrease in relative size, and this process appears to be associated with the slowly progressive renal insufficiency, anemia, renal osteodystrophy, and hypertension. These patients experience growth retardation, as do most patients in the pediatric age group who have progressive renal insufficiency. Improvement in growth appears to be directly related to improvement in renal function. Although no specific growth-promoting measures are known, increasing the caloric intake of children in chronic hemodialysis programs has resulted in linear growth rates that are more nearly normal (194, 209). In patients who are not candidates for chronic hemodialysis, nausea and vomiting and dietary restrictions are important causes of growth failure.

The management of chronic renal failure in children with ARPKD follows the same general guidelines for any patient with established chronic renal insufficiency. Complications such as hyperkalemia, hypertension, and infection must be treated promptly. Hyperkalemia can be treated by reducing the potassium content of the diet, by using oral resins that bind potassium in the intestine, and in acute emergencies by infusing glucose, insulin, and bicarbonate intravenously. Infections are treated by first identifying the organism and then choosing bactericidal antibiotics. Blood pressure is controlled by sodium restriction and vasodilator drugs.

Renal osteodystrophy can be ameliorated by reducing intestinal phosphate absorption with oral aluminium hydroxide gel, increasing oral calcium intake, in combination with derivatives of vitamin D (1,25 hydroxy cholecalciferol). The serum calcium and phosphate levels should be monitored at regular intervals.

Children with ARPKD should probably be accepted for dialysis and transplantation on the same terms as other children with chronic renal insufficiency. ARPKD patients, however, must be classified as high-risk candidates for hemodialysis, peritoneal dialysis, and renal transplantation in view of the fact that the fibrotic liver disorder is progressive and there is no known substitution therapy available except liver transplantation. These patients also appear to have some increased susceptibility to infection and to show rather poor wound healing, possibly as a consequence of their longstanding disease. Older patients with ARPKD may be suitable candidates for dialysis and transplantation, provided there are no other associated disorders that might compromise their care.

The Ehlers–Danlos syndrome has been reported in patients with ARPKD and is associated with berry aneurysms in the cerebral vasculature and dissecting aneurysms in the thoracic and abdominal aorta (210). There does not appear to be an increased incidence of renal tumors in patients with ARPKD, in contrast to ADPKD. Wilms tumor has been reported in one instance in association with ARPKD (211). Pneumothorax and pneumomediastinum are relatively frequent problems encountered in neonatal patients with ARPKD, but there is no evidence that these pulmonary complications occur in older patients.

Prevention and counseling

Parents who give birth to a child with ARPKD may want to know the risk of the disease in future offspring. On a statistical basis, each child has a 1 in 4 chance of having the disease and a 1 in 2 chance of being a "carrier". Persons with the disease who live long enough to become parents face a low risk of having children with the disease, provided their mates are not immediate or distant relatives.

In families with more than one affected sibling, the clinical course and pathologic expression of renal disease may be dissimilar. Even twins have demonstrated very different courses (194). Therefore it appears that therapeutic decisions antenatally, as well as with infants, must be made with care. In some situations the diagnosis of a severe form of the disease can be made before 24 weeks of pregnancy, when the option of elective termination of pregnancy is available. Diagnostic criteria include the association of a positive family history, bilaterally enlarged kidneys, oligohydramnios, absence of a urinary bladder, and the typical kidney texture (189). Serial sonographic examinations are recommended after an original negative scan, as the disease may manifest itself later in the pregnancy. In infants, some authors think that therapeutic decisions should be based on tissue diagnosis, rather than on an earlier sibling's course (194).

CYSTIC DISEASE OF THE RENAL MEDULLA

There appear to be at least three distinct diseases in humans that primarily involve the tubular structures in the renal medulla. The diseases are associated with variable enlargement of the distal tubules and collecting ducts (212, 213), and are associated with interstitial fibrosis and inflammation of a variable extent. *Medullary cystic disease* and *juvenile nephronopthisis* are familial disorders that, in the view of several authors, are separable and distinct disease entities. Both of these conditions progress to end-stage renal failure. By contrast, *medullary sponge kidney* is a relatively benign condition and occurs only occasionally in members of the same family. To facilitate discussion of the management of these disorders, we include medullary cystic disease and juvenile nephronophthisis together. Medullary sponge kidney is discussed separately.

Juvenile nephronopthisis-medullary cystic disease

INTRODUCTION AND BACKGROUND

The relationship between juvenile nephronophthisis and medullary cystic disease is not clearly defined (214–223). Some authors emphasize their identity and others stress their differences. There may very well be two genetic disorders, autosomal recessive juvenile nephronopthisis and autosomal dominant medullary cystic disease, which are distinguishable by their familial patterns of inheritance and by the age of onset of symptomatology and renal dysfunction. Some authors suggest these diseases are analogous to polycystic disease; namely, the *childhood* type (juvenile nephronopthisis is an autosomal recessive disorder) and the *adult* type (medullary cystic disease) is an autosomal dominant process. Because we, too, are unable to distinguish between the two processes in this discussion, we will use the compromise appellation, medullary cystic disease-nephronophthisis complex (JN-MCD), as suggested by Gardner (224).

The medullary process is characterized by multiple small cysts in the outer medulla of the kidney and less frequently in the cortex. The cysts arise from collecting ducts (212, 225). This disorder has been associated with hyperplasia of the juxtaglomerular apparatus (220), Fanconi syndrome (226), hepatic fibrosis (222, 223), a predilection for patients with red and blond hair (227, 228), in association with various retinal abnormalities (222, 224), central nervous system abnormalities (221, 222), hyperuricemia and gout (223, 229), salt depletion, anemia, hypertension, and azotemia. The diagnosis of the JN-MCD complex should be suspected in patients who have end-stage renal disease in childhood or in azotemic adults with a familial history of renal disease. The diagnosis can be verified in several ways. Excretory urography has been used effectively (230, 231). The defect is usually seen as an inhomogeneous streaky nephrogram confined to the medulla due to accumulation of contrast material in the collecting ducts. Renal arteriography was advocated as a conclusive diagnostic approach in the older literature. Recently, however, sonography and computer-assisted tomography have been added to the diagnostic armamentarium, especially for those patients with relatively small medullary cysts that cannot be diagnosed unequivocally by the usual urographic procedures. Needle biopsy is not recommended for diagnosis (217, 220).

Within a family structure the disease appears to be inherited in a relatively uniform way. For example, patients who acquire the late manifestations of renal insufficiency in childhood usually have a form of the disease that is transmitted as an autosomal recessive trait. The typical clinical representation for the juvenile form is that of a child who is usually age 4–10 years with a history of polydipsia, polyuria, pallor, lethargy, and growth retardation. These patients not uncommonly reach the end stage of the disease process before the age of 20 years. In the adult form the clinical presentation is not unlike that in the juvenile patients, with the exception that growth retardation and a long history of anemia and other manifestations of end-stage renal disease are usually not found. Medullary cystic disease has been discovered in adults in their sixth and seventh decade (217, 231). These patients may pass through a period in which they have urinary concentrating defects sufficient to cause serious sodium wastage, hyponatremia, and extracellular fluid volume contraction. The authors remember one of these patients well for the fact that he ate approximately 20 g of rock salt and drank 5–6 l of fluid each day to maintain blood pressure in an acceptable range. Fractional excretion of sodium in the urine, estimated by C_{Na}/C_{inulin}, was approximately 50% in this patient.

It is unusual for patients with the JN-MCD complex to have flank pain, hypertension, hematuria, or renal calculi. This is in contrast to patients with polycystic kidney disease and medullary sponge kidney.

COMPONENTS THAT REQUIRE MANAGEMENT

Sodium wasting

It has been suggested that salt wasting is a cardinal sign of the JN-MCD complex. This may be true during certain periods of a patient's life, but it is usually a transient condition just preceding the development of end-stage renal disease. Presumably the renal salt-wasting is secondary to anatomic abnormalities in the distal collecting ducts and other nephron structures in the medulla, although the cysts themselves may not be directly responsible. The salt wasting is occasionally associated with hyperreninemia and juxtaglomerular celll hyperplasia (219, 226). More than likely the JG hyperplasia is secondary to the salt depletion.

Salt wasting is managed by determining the amount of sodium replacement needed to maintain a conscious upright posture and blood pressure. Some patients require vast quantities of sodium chloride and water to maintain sodium balance. Should oral intake be interrupted for some reason, intravenous salt and water replacement is mandatory. As the disease progresses to end stage, it is not uncommon for patients to retain sodium and become hypertensive as residual functioning nephrons decrease. At this point, the sodium and water intake must be reduced to prevent ECF volume expansion. When acidosis occurs, the diet should be altered to reduce acid residues, and oral sodium bicarbonate should be given in addition to NaCl. The acidosis and hyperkalemia encountered in this disorder are probably due to a significant defect in the distal tubule handling of sodium, potassium, and hydrogen ions. These disorders are corrected by altering the dietary intake of potassium and hydrogen ion, and by using ion exchange resins that bind potassium.

Anemia

The anemia may be profound and may appear earlier than is usual for other diseases leading to renal insufficiency. No specific therapy for the anemia of JN-MCD complex is known. Erythrocytosis has been described in one patient with medullary cystic disease (226).

Renal insufficiency

The onset of renal insufficiency in this disorder is usually insidious and is not unique, except for the occasional patient with salt wasting. Two patients with medullary cystic disease were followed up to 100 months using the $1/P_{cr}$ relationship as an indication of prognosis (149). The relationship was linear in these two patients, indicating that a constant amount of creatinine clearance was lost per unit time.

Clinical infection of the kidney appears to be relatively uncommon in the JN-MCD complex, and it does not appear to be a major factor in the development of chronic renal failure. Secondary hyperparathyroidism, renal osteodystrophy, and neuropathy may be observed. At the end stage, renal insufficiency can be managed by dialysis and/or renal transplantation. No recurrence of the disease in transplanted kidneys has been reported (221, 222).

Prevention and counseling

The uncertain genetic transmission of the JN-MCD complex is a severe ignorance that is especially felt when advising family members of the propensity for genetic transmission and in the selection of donors for renal transplantation. Avasthi et al. (219) suggest that if the transplant recipient's renal morphology suggests chronic interstitial nephritis and a live, related transplant is considered, an extensive search should be made to detect renal disease within the family.

Medullary sponge kidney

INTRODUCTION AND BACKGROUND

Medullary sponge kidney (tubular ectasia) is found in approximately 1 of every 200 citizens in this country. The disease is characterized by dilatations of the papillary collecting ducts in one or more papillae of the kidneys. The disease is usually bilateral, but it may occur in a single kidney and may involve one or more papillae within a kidney. The disease is associated with hematuria, gross and microscopic, which may be recurrent. Infections of the urinary tract often are the first signs of an underlying abnormality. Nephrolithiasis with renal colic, loin pain, and excretion of small stones is one of the more prominent features of medullary sponge kidney. The stones form in the ectatic portions of the collecting ducts. They may consist of calcium oxalate, calcium phosphate, and other types of calcium salts.

Renal function has been examined in a number of patients with medullary sponge kidney (233–238). The disease seldom progresses to end-stage renal failure, although reduced glomerular filtration rates have been observed. The most commonly recognized functional abnormalities include defective urinary solute concentrating ability, inability to reduce the urinary pH to a minimum value of 5.5, and systemic acidosis secondary to renal tubular acidosis (239–241).

COMPONENTS THAT REQUIRE MANAGEMENT

Renal tubular acidosis

Type I renal tubular acidosis has been described in several patients with medullary sponge kidney (234–236, 239–

241). In these cases the medullary sponge kidney is usually associated with urolithiasis. The renal tubular acidosis has not been characterized beyond recognition that it is of the classic "distal" type. Alkali therapy is usually sufficient to correct the systemic acidosis. Patients with incomplete renal tubular acidosis, i.e., those who have a defect in urinary acidification but who have normal plasma bicarbonate levels and pH, probably do not require bicarbonate therapy. The impact of bicarbonate therapy in patients with complete and incomplete renal tubular acidosis of the distal type on the pathogenesis of nephrolithiasis has not been examined critically. Since oral alkali will increase rather than decrease the urinary pH, there might be some risk of promoting calculus formation in patients who have calcium phosphate stones in the ectatic tubules.

Nephrolithiasis

Nephrolithiasis is a common clinical problem for patients with medullary sponge kidney. In 612 recurrent stone formers, Backman et al. (242) diagnosed medullary sponge kidney from typical findings on pyelography in 3.6% of the patients. Yendt and colleagues (243) investigated 1035 patients with calcium urolithiasis. They used strict criteria for the performance of intravenous urograms and did not accept poor-quality radiographs in their evaluations. By this rigorous process they claim that 13% of renal stone formers have medullary sponge kidney. In normal patients the incidence of tubular ectasia was only 2% using the same rigorous diagnostic techniques. O'Neill, Breslau, and Pak (244) reported a 3.6% incidence of medullary sponge kidney in their group of stone formers. Although the incidence appears to vary among different groups of stone formers, it is clear that medullary sponge kidney is frequently associated with renal lithiasis. The possible relationship between hyperparathyroidism and medullary sponge kidney has been emphasized in numerous publications (245–250). It is postulated that renal calcium loss causes a reduction in plasma ionized calcium concentration, which in turn stimulates the secretion of parathyroid hormone. It is thought that this process may ultimately cause the formation of parathyroid adenomas.

O'Neill et al. (224) have critically examined the excretion of calcium in patients with medullary sponge kidney and other stone-forming disorders. Absorptive hypercalciuria was the most common abnormality in patients with medullary sponge kidney, occurring in 59%. Only three patients (18%) had hypercalciuria due to renal calcium "leak." None of the other patients had primary hyperparathyroidism. In the opinion of O'Neill et al. (244), patients with medullary sponge kidneys and renal stones have the same spectrum of metabolic abnormalities as the overall population of stone formers, and it is their belief that these patients should be so evaluated and treated.

Yendt et al. (243) interpreted their results somewhat differently and suggested that calcium and phosphorus metabolism is different in patients with tubular ectasia than in those without ectasia, and further speculated that the pathogenesis of both the hypercalciuria and the stone formation may be different in these two groups of patients (i.e., medullary sponge kidney patients vs. regular stone formers). Moreover, they showed that the plasma calcium levels were significantly increased after prolonged treatment with thiazide diuretics in patients with medullary sponge kidney. Backman et al. (242) agree with O'Neill et al. (244) that patients with medullary sponge kidneys have defective tubular function no more often than other recurrent stone formers. Thus, it seems reasonable to suggest that patients with medullary sponge kidneys and nephrolithiasis should be evaluated in the same manner as other stone-forming patients who do not have this disorder.

Asymtomatic patients incidentally found to have medullary sponge kidney require no specific therapy and should visit a family physician yearly for routine urinalysis. As a general rule, patients with nephrolithiasis should excrete about 2 l of urine each day. This maneuver reduces the propensity for calcium salts to precipitate in the distal portions of the collecting ducts and pelvis of the kidney. Patients with hypercalciuria may benefit from long-term therapy with thiazide diuretics. For patients with calcium urolithiasis and normal urinary calcium excretion, oral phosphate therapy may be useful. There are no reports of an increased incidence of hyperuricosuria in patients with medullary sponge kidney, but of course this possibility should be looked for in the routine evaluation of such a patient. If hyperuricosuria is observed a trial of allopurinol may slow the formation of urinary stones.

In some instances the persistence of renal stone formation in kidneys with medullary sponge disease has been associated with significant morbidity from the pain of urolithiasis and urinary tract infection with persistent bacteriuria (251–253). In some of these cases, especially those in which the tubular ectasia is unilateral or segmental, a unilateral or partial nephrectomy has been used to treat the disorder (254, 255). Partial nephrectomy has been associated with the cure and sustained freedom from nephrolithiasis, urolithiasis, and urosepsis. Since medullary sponge kidney is usually a bilateral disorder, partial or complete nephrectomy should be undertaken cautiously and only after careful evaluation of renal function in the remaining kidney indicates sufficient function to maintain life.

Patients with medullary sponge kidney appear to be more susceptible to urinary tract infections (253, 256). Consequently, routine preventive measures seem to be warranted, especially in female patients.

PROGNOSIS AND COUNSELING

Most patients discovered incidentally to have medullary sponge kidney can be advised that the disorder is benign and that they can anticipate no serious morbidity or mortality from the disorder. Nephrolithiasis can be a difficult problem in symptomatic patients (257).

A clear familial transmission of this disease has not been established. However, if there is a history of medullary sponge disease in the family, detailed investigation is advisable to determine a potential genetic pattern of transmission (258).

MULTICYSTIC KIDNEY

Introduction and background

Congenital multicystic kidneys are dysplastic structures with disturbed differentiation in which the renal parenchyma is replaced by cysts of various sizes. The typical kidney is characterized by many cysts varying in size and held together by loose connective tissue. The renal calyces, the renal pelvis, and the proximal portion of the ureter are usually atretic, or even absent. The disease is usually unilateral but on occasion it can involve both kidneys. Although bilateral multicystic kidneys usually cause death shortly after birth, the bilateral disorder is seen rarely in adults (259).

The disease is usually discovered in childhood when an infant or child is found to have a unilateral flank mass. Less commonly it is found incidentally during adult life when radiographs of the abdomen are taken for other purposes. The cysts may calcify, a typical appearance being a rimlike deposit of calcium. The radiologic triad (260) for the diagnosis of multicystic kidney disease includes: a) unilateral nonfunctioning kidney associated with a flank mass or shell-like calcification on the plain film; b) absent or atretic proximal ureter on the retrograde pyelogram; and c) absent or hypoplastic renal artery, no collateral arterial supply, and no nephrogram on the abdominal aortogram.

Multicystic kidney can be identified in patients by sonography (261) and computer-assisted tomography (262). Multicystic kidney has been identified in the fetus in utero by ultrasonography (263–265) and can be distinguished from hydronephrosis by the following criteria (265). In multicystic dysplasia, the reniform contour of the kidney is lost, the parenchyma is replaced by multiple, randomly positioned cysts of various sizes, visible tissue is distributed in small islands between the cysts, and no communication between the cysts is detectable. In hydronephrosis, the reniform contour remains, and fluid-filled spaces are anatomically arranged and communicate with each other. Interestingly, the multicystic kidney may change appearance in utero, growing larger and then smaller. The change in size is hypothesized to correlate with the kidney's ability to filter plasma, growing larger while filtration function occurs, and then diminishing in size as function decreases (265).

Components that require management

Pain in the region of the mass is the most frequent presenting complaint in adults (266). Urinary tract infection, hematuria, and hypertension are infrequent presenting signs. Renal abnormalities in the contralateral kidney may be found, these being ureteropelvic obstruction and hydronephrosis most commonly. Malignant tumors have been found in several dysplastic kidneys (267–270). The finding of these tumors has precipitated a management debate regarding removal of the nonsymptomatic tumors in the neonate.

Historically, most multicystic kidneys have been discovered by surgical exploration and were removed at discovery, often in infancy. With the advent of improved sonographic techniques, surgical exploration has decreased, thus requiring a decision regarding an elective surgical procedure for removal of the multicystic kidney. Furthermore, because so many of these kidneys have been removed historically, there is incomplete data regarding development of complications from their presence. Thus there is active debate as to whether or not surgical intervention is always necessary. If the patient has no pain, no infection, and no hypertension or other problems potentially related to the multicystic kidney, it seems reasonable to leave the kidney in place. On the other hand, if there is pain, hypertension, or other abnormalities such as hematuria or pyuria to suggest secondary involvement of the kidney, it probably should be removed. Since malignant degeneration apparently occurs only rarely in multicystic kidneys, one cannot use this as a compelling reason for removing all multicystic kidneys.

ACQUIRED CYSTIC DISEASE

Introduction and background

Dunnill, Millard, and Oliver (271) reported in 1977 that patients maintained on hemodialysis for relatively long periods of time may develop multiple cysts in their remnant kidneys. Despite initial skepticism about this report, the observation has been confirmed repeatedly throughout the world (272). Study (273–276) of clinical characteristics and diagnostic methods has revealed that this acquired cystic disease occurs in patients undergoing peritoneal dialysis as well as hemodialysis, increases markedly in incidence in patients dialyzed for more than 3 years (over 50% in some series), and occurs more frequently in males. It often decreases after renal transplantation and does not occur in a functioning transplanted kidney (277–279). The cause of the cysts is unknown, although it is hypothesized that since hemodialysis and peritoneal dialysis are relatively imperfect substitutes for normally functioning kidneys, certain insufficiently eliminated substances accumulate and promote the production of renotropic factors, which in turn stimulate cyst formation and, on occasion, renal tumors. Complications of acquired cystic disease include life-threatening spontaneous retroperitoneal hemorrhage, microscopic hematuria, matrix stone formation, and development of malignant disease in the renal parenchyma (275, 280–284). Cysts do not develop in other organs.

The cysts may vary from less than 0.5 cm to over 3 cm in diameter and may contain clear fluid or hemorrhagic material (272). They may be detected by computed tomography or sonography (272, 274, 279, 285, 286), although one group of investigators (274) has reported a low level of diagnostic accuracy for both CT and ultrasound in the detection of renal cysts. We prefer CT because, frequently, shrunken end-stage kidneys are difficult to visualize sonographically and CT is more sensitive than sonography in detecting small renal tumors. Selective renal arteriography may be helpful in further evaluation of renal tumors detected by CT or sonography, but the accuracy of this technique has not been established firmly. Such cysts have also been demonstrated at autopsy (275, 287).

Ishikawa et al. (285) used computer-assisted tomography to study the fate of the remnant end-stage kidney in 96 chronically hemodialyzed patients. Kidney volume decreased progressively for up to 3 years after the start of dialysis. However, after about 4 years of dialysis, there was a striking increase in the average volume of the remnant kidneys. Multiple cysts were found in 43.5% of patients on dialysis for less than 3 years and in 79.3% of patients dialyzed more than 3 years. There was a striking epithelial hyperplasia within the cysts and in some frank adenocarcinoma was found. The results have been repeatedly confirmed (272, 279, 286–292).

Components that require management

The striking incidence of cyst development in patients undergoing chronic maintenance hemodialysis or peritoneal dialysis is a rather disturbing development, especially since the pathogenesis of the cyst formation appears to involve hyperplasia of the tubular epithelium in the remnant kidneys. Reports of the incidence of renal adenocarcinoma in acquired cystic disease vary (272, 275, 279–285, 289, 291–294), precipitating a quandry regarding routine screening in dialysis patients. If these kidneys are prone to develop malignant changes, it is curious that a higher incidence of adenocarcinoma has not been reported in remnant kidneys by more dialysis and transplant centers. Although a few highly aggressive metastatic tumors have occurred, the majority of neoplasms have been found at autopsy or upon examination of surgically removed kidneys (275). Furthermore, while one might suppose that immunosuppressed patients would have a greater risk for developing malignancy, we are aware of only a few anecdotal reports in transplant programs. In a recent systematic study of the relationship between renal cystic disease and renal neoplasia, Ishikawa (295) reported an incidence of renal adenocarcinoma significantly greater than would be expected in the average Japanese citizen.

In view of current limited economic resources, some authors (275) question the efficacy of periodic screening by CT, yet more data needs to be collected regarding the risk of clinically significant renal cancer. In the absence of compelling data we suggest that it is prudent to routinely screen by sonography patients dialyzed for longer than 3 years. If the sonogram reveals cystic disease, a CT scan with contrast enhancement is indicated. Suspicious masses can be further evaluated by MRI. Because renal cell carcinomas grow slowly in most cases and their metastatic potential is impossible to predict, difficult management decisions are precipitated by the discovery of a small tumor.

All would agree that symptomatic renal tumors more than 3.0 cm should be resected. Bilateral nephrectomy would seem advisable in prospective renal transplant recipients with renal tumors, regardless of their size. Tumors smaller than 3 cm in diameter have been observed to metastasize, so removal of such a mass requires careful evaluation and sound clinical judgment.

Since the loss of renal mass associated with bilateral nephrectomy may increase the transfusion requirements and thereby jeopardize comfort and lifestyle, removal of cystic kidneys containing no tumor masses should probably be reserved for those patients who are candidates for renal transplantation or those who develop significant clinical signs and symptoms of acquired cystic disease. These include bilateral or unilateral flank pain, gross or microscopic hematuria, urinary tract infection, ureteral colic due to clots obstructing one or more ureters, and a palpable abdominal mass. Surgical excision is the preferred therapy, although renal infarction by intraarterial installation of coagulant material may be worthwhile for high-risk surgical candidates. When a few rather large renal cysts are associated primarily with flank pain, percutaneous aspiration of the fluid and cytologic examination might be a reasonable temporizing measure.

SIMPLE CYSTS

Introduction and background

So-called simple cysts are the most common cystic abnormality encountered in human kidneys. They may be solitary or multiple. The wall is lined by a single layer of flat epithelium. The fluid is chemically similar to an ultrafiltrate of plasma (296–298). In one study employing computed tomography of the upper abdomen in which the kidneys were not the primary organ of interest, at least one renal cyst was identified in 64 out of 670 patients (299, 300). Autopsy studies indicate that as many as one or more cysts may be present in nearly one-half of those persons 50 years of age or older (301). Simple cysts do not appear to be associated with any decrease in renal function (302).

Early work in this century suggested that simple cysts may develop in the parenchyma of the kidney as a consequence of ischemia (303). More recent information indicates that, as with other cystic structures in the cortex and medulla, the so-called simple cysts probably develop from tubular epithelium (304–306). Electrolyte gradients typical of proximal and distal cysts have not been found, in contrast to ADPKD (41). Simple cysts appear to be relatively impermeable to small molecular weight solutes injected into the blood of patients (296, 298). The hydrostatic pressure is approximately 22 cm H_2O (307). The few ultrastructural studies of the epithelium from simple cysts indicate that they are lined by simple cuboidal epithelium that has no distinctive features. Some cysts have grown to enormous size and have contained several liters of fluid.

Most cysts are found on routine urographic examination. With increased use of abdominal sonography and CT scanning, more and more simple cysts are being recognized in children as well as in adults. The most common problem encountered in the evaluation of the simple cysts is the differentiation from a malignant mass. With a lesion that is seen so commonly, especially in adult patients, one can appreciate the enormous economic impact that might be felt if all simple cysts were evaluated as potential malignancies. Steg (308, 309) reviewed 1342 cases of renal cyst in adult and found 13 cancers. Interestingly, only four tumors were in contact with the cyst itself, the others being spacially removed from the cyst. Five tumors were in the opposite kidney! Steg emphasizes that the risk of failure to recognize cancer associated with a cyst is very small. McClennan et al. (310) have suggested a reasonable scheme for the evaluation of patients with a renal mass discovered by urography, a protocol that is in general agreement with the strategy proposed by Sagel et al. (311) involving the use of CT scanning in the evaluation of renal mass lesions (Figure 4). Most radiologists agree that ultrasonic examination is the first logical step following the identification of an indeterminate mass on urography. Whereas some radiologists suggested just a few years ago that the next step might be to perform cyst puncture to confirm a benign etiology, McClellan et al. (310) argue that cyst puncture may not be necessary in view of the high probability that CT scanning will reveal the correct diagnosis. The criteria for the CT diagnosis of benign cysts are (310, 311): a) homogeneous attenuation value near water density, b) no enhancement with intravenous contrast material, c) no measurable thickness of the cyst wall, and d) a smooth interface with renal parenchyma. If the mass does not meet the CT criteria for a benign cyst, i.e., the cyst falls into an indeterminant or solid category, surgical exploration is recommended.

When cyst puncture is performed the character of the fluid aspirated from the cyst is especially important. Simple cyst fluid is usually straw colored and clear, and is free of erythrocytes, leukocytes, and atypical cells. By contrast, fluid aspirated from cystic malignant tumors is usually bloody or dark coloured, has a high lipid content (cholesterol and total lipids), and contains malignant cells on cytologic examination.

At the present time it does not appear that rigid criteria have been adapted for the use of CT scanning, sonography, arteriography, and cyst puncture in the work-up of patients with renal mass lesions. Clearly, all of these techniques have some value in their own right in selected cases. Moreover, the quality of the equipment and the expertise of the radiologist also figure prominently in the approach to the renal mass in individual institutions. There is insufficient information determined prospectively to decide whether or not CT scanning can *completely* supplant ultrasound and angiographic evaluation of renal mass lesions. Until such studies are done it seems reasonable to use arteriography, ultrasound, and CT scanning together in the evaluation of questionable cystic lesions of the kidney.

Components that require management

INCIDENTAL UROGRAPHIC DISCOVERY

As noted above, benign simple cysts will be found with increased frequency as diagnostic methods improve for defining the structure of the kidneys by screening techniques. In asymptomatic patients with a few small cysts in the kidney discovered by urography or CT scanning, further evaluation is probably not indicated if there is no fever, leukocytosis, hematuria, or renal discomfort. Followup examinations at periodic intervals by sonography may be worthwhile in determining the natural history of this disease, as well as noting significant changes in the cysts or development of solid lesions. A recent study (312) using serial sonographic examination of simple renal cysts indicates that the tendency of simple renal cysts is to progress in number rather than in size. Renal masses may be found to contain calcium that is visible by radiologic studies. 1–2% of simple cysts, and perhaps 10% of renal cell carcinomas, contain calcium (108). Calcium located within the body of the mass is a strong indicator of malignancy, whereas in simple cysts the calcium appears to be on the periphery of the mass lesion. The important "rule" deriving from the Mayo Clinic study is that calcification within a renal mass lesion should be considered to reflect malignancy until proven otherwise.

Steg (309) has pointed out the great diversity in the therapeutic approach. In this study of 1342 cases, 1 patient out of 2 was operated on, and 1 out of 6 operations was a nephrectomy. The mortality rate was 1.2% and complications occurred in 10% of the patients. Steg suggests that too many cysts are treated surgically considering the small chance of finding cancer and the relatively high morbidity and mortality rates.

SIMPLE CYSTS IN CHILDREN

Although not nearly as common as in adults, children have been found to have simple renal cysts (313–318). In the newborn this may be associated with posterior urethral valves (319, 320). Proteinuria has been associated with renal cysts in children (321). In the infant or younger child the most common presenting feature of simple cysts is a palpable abdominal mass. Hematuria has been described in children with simple cysts in the kidney, especially following trauma to the abdomen.

HYPERTENSION

Solitary intrarenal cysts have been found to cause hypertension in a few patients (318, 322–328). The plasma renin activity is usually increased in these patients, and following successful aspiration of the fluid or operative removal of the cyst the hypertension may disappear. These solitary renal cysts are thought to produce hypertension by compressing adjacent vessels in the kidney, causing selective ischemia and increased renin production.

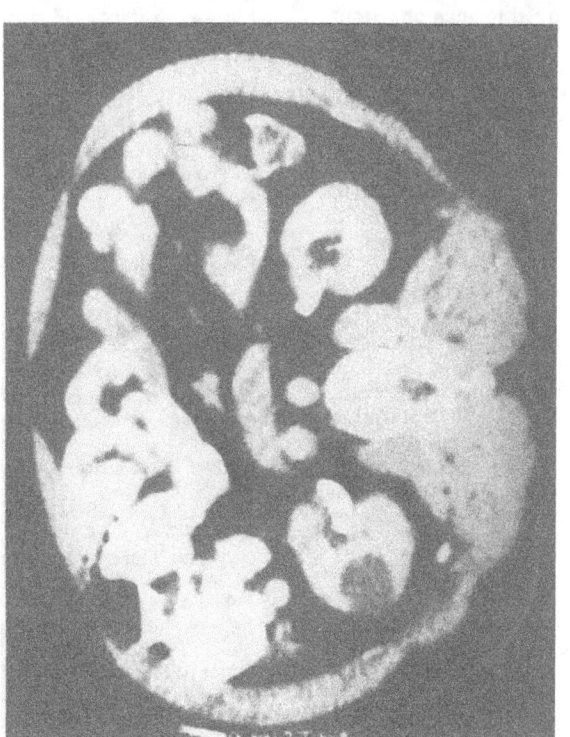

Figure 4. Left: CT appearance of a solitary simple renal cyst in the right kidney. Contrast enhancement was used. *Right*: Appearance of the cyst by conventional intravenous urography.

INFECTED SIMPLE CYSTS

Several examples of infected simple renal cysts have been reported (329–333). These lesions are usually associated with flank pain, pyuria, fever, and leukocytosis. The differentiation of an infected renal cyst from an abscess of the kidney may be difficult. Some clinicians have suggested that the clinical triad of acute pyelonephritis and a vascular mass lesion in the kidney with ipsilateral pleural effusion is characteristic of this condition. The most common organisms encountered are *E. coli*, staphylococcus, and *Proteus* species. Tuberculosis was cultured from a cyst in one patient (334). An operative approach is usually taken to treat the infected cysts, although the fluid can be drained by percutaneous aspiration (335, 336). Conservative treatment has not been specifically evaluated in the therapy of infected simple cysts.

ADDITIONAL PROBLEMS CAUSED BY RENAL CYSTS

Simple renal cysts may cause calyceal obstruction (337–341). When this is encountered it is suggested that the cyst be drained or enucleated to relieve the obstruction and the potential for urinary tract infection. Hematuria and massive pyelovenous reflux has been observed secondary to a benign renal cyst (340). Such a lesion may be difficult to differentiate from renal malignancy.

In one instance a renal cyst enlarged to such an extent that it caused afferent loop obstruction and acute pancreatitis (342). The obstruction was successfully relieved by resecting the portion of the cyst wall extrinsic to the kidney and by mobilizing the duodenal loop into its normal location.

Benign renal cysts have been associated with erythrocytosis, and in a few instances increased amounts of erythropoietin have been isolated from the cyst fluid (343–345). In one patient the erythrocytosis remitted after decompression of the cysts (346).

The management of simple renal cysts can take several forms. Most intermediate-sized cysts may be aspirated percutaneously (347–349). In some instances sclerosing agents or, alternatively, radiocontrast material has been instilled into the cyst cavity in an attempt to prevent recurrence (350–352). Large cysts (greater than 500 ml in volume) are usually drained surgically.

In at least one center, a stiff-walled needlescope is inserted into the cavity of cysts percutaneously in order to examine the walls for the presence or absence of tumor masses (353).

ACKNOWLEDGMENT

The authors wish to thank the PKR Foundation for support.

REFERENCES

1. Gardner KD: *Cystic Diseases of the Kidney*. John Wiley and Sons, New York, 1976.
2. Grantham JJ: Polycystic renal disease. In: LE Earley, CW Gottschalk, eds, *Strauss and Welt's Diseases of the Kidney*, 3rd ed. Little, Brown, Boston, pp 1123–1146, 1979.
3. Gardner KD Jr: Medullary cystic diseases: The nephronophthisis-cystic renal medulla complex and medullary sponge kidney. In: LE Earley, CW Gottschalk, eds, *Strauss and Welt's Diseases of the Kidney*, 3rd ed. Little, Brown, Boston, pp 1147–1166, 1979.
4. Welling LW, Grantham JJ: Cystic and developmental diseases of the kidney. In: BM Brenner, FC Rector, eds, *The Kidney*, 3rd ed. WB Saunders, Philadelphia, pp 1341–1376, 1986.
5. Grantham JJ, Gardner KD (eds): *Problems in Diagnosis and Management of Polycystic Kidney Disease*. PKR Foundation, Kansas City, MO, 1985.
6. Dalgaard OZ: Bilateral polycystic disease of the kidneys. A followup of two hundred and eighty four patients and their families *Acta Med Scandinav* 158–328 (Suppl): 1–255, 1957.
7. Ito Y, Singh S, Pollack VE: Efficacy of dialysis treatment. In: Grantham JJ, Gardner KD, eds, *Problems in Diagnosis and Management of Polycystic Kidney Disease*. PKR Foundation, Kansas City, MO, pp 160–168, 1985.
8. Sellers AL, Winfield A, Rosen V: Unilateral polycystic kidney disease. *J Urol* 107:527–529, 1972.
9. Cole AT, Gill WB: Dual renal cell carcinomas in a unilateral polycystic kidney. *J Urol* 109:182–185, 1973.
10. Bear RA: Solitary kidney affected with polycystic disease: A report of 2 cases. *J Urol* 111:566–567, 1974.
11. Lee JKT, McClennan BL, Kissane JM: Unilateral polycystic kidney disease. *Am J Roent* 130:1165–1167, 1978.
12. Kossow AS, Meek JM: Unilateral adult polycystic kidney disease. *J Urol* 127:297–300, 1982.
13. Porch P, Noe HN, Stapleton FB: Unilateral presentation of adult-type polycystic kidney disease in children. *J Urol* 135:744–746, 1986.
14. Gutnik LM, Coury A, Raszkowski R: A patient with known unilateral renal cysts who developed epigastric pain, nausea and vomiting. *S Dak J Med* 39:31–32, 1986.
15. Hoeffel JC, Jacottin G, Bourgeois JM: Renal cysts in childhood: A descriptive classification with clinical notes. *Clin Pediatr* 10:701–705, 1971.
16. Kaye C, Lewy PR: Congenital appearance of adult-type (autosomal dominant) polycystic kidney disease. *J Pediatr* 85:807–810, 1974.
17. Petereit MF: Adult renal polycystic disease in the juvenile patient demonstrated by nephrotomography. *S Dakota J Med* 27:25–56, 1974.
18. Bengtsson U, Hedman L, Svalander C: Adult type of polycystic kidney disease in a new-born child. *Acta Med Scand* 197:447–450, 1975.
19. Stickler GB, Kelalis PP: Polycystic kidney disease. Recognition of the "adult form" (autosomal dominant) in infancy. *Mayo Clin Proc* 50:547–548, 1975.
20. Ross DG, Travers H: Infantile presentation of adult-type polycystic kidney disease in a large kindred. *J Pediatrics* 87:760–763, 1975.
21. Fellows RA, Leonidas JC, Beatty EC Jr: Radiologic features of "adult type" polycystic kidney disease in the neonate. *Pediat Radiol* 4:87–92, 1976.
22. Ritter R, Siafarikas K: Hemihypertrophy in a boy with renal polycystic disease: Varied patterns of presentation of renal polycystic disease in his family. *Pediatric Radiol* 5:98–102, 1976.
23. Kaplan BS, Rabin I, Nogrady MB, Drummond KN: Autosomal dominant polycystic renal disease in children. *J Pediatr* 90:782–783, 1977.

24. Loh JP, Haller JO, Kassner EG, Aloni A, Glassberg K: Dominantly-inherited polycystic kidneys in infants: Association with hypertrophic pyloric stenosis. *Pediat Radiol* 6:27–31, 1977.
25. Shokeir MHK: Expression of "adult" polycystic renal disease in the fetus and newborn. *Clinical Genetics* 14:61–72, 1978.
26. Eulderink F, Hogewind BL: Renal cysts in premature children. Occurrence in a family with polycystic kidney disease. *Arch Pathol Lab Med* 102:592–594, 1978.
27. Fryns JP, Van Den Berghe H: "Adult" form of polycystic kidney disease in neonates. *Clinical Genetics* 15:205–206, 1979.
28. Chevalier RL, Garland TA, Buschi AJ: The neonate with adult-type autosomal dominant polyscytic kidney disease. *Int J Ped Nephrol* 2:73–77, 1981.
29. Zerres K, Weiss H, Bulla M, Roth B: Prenatal diagnosis of an early manifestation of autosomal dominant adult-type polycystic kidney disease. *Lancet* 30:988, 1982.
30. Anton PA, Abramowsky CR: Adult polycystic renal disease presenting in infancy: A report emphasizing the bilateral involvement. *J Urology* 128:1290–1291, 1982.
31. Hayden CK Jr, Swischuk LE, Davis M, Brouhard BH: Puddling: A distinguishing feature of adult polycystic kidney disease in the neonate. *Am J Roentg* 142:811–812, 1984.
32. Zerres K, Hansmann M, Knopfle G, Stephan M: Prenatal diagnosis of genetically determined early manifestation of autosomal dominant polycystic kidney disease?: *Hum Genet* 71:368–369, 1985.
33. Valdes-Dapena M, Huff DS, Arey JB: Adult polycystic renal disease in a young child. *Pediatr Path* 4:151–155, 1985.
34. Fryns JP, Vandenberghe K, Moerman F: Mid-trimester ultrasonographic diagnosis of early manifesting "adult" form of polycystic kidney disease: *Hum Genet* 74:461, 1986.
35. Taitz LS, Brown CB, Blank CE, Steiner GM: Screening for polycystic kidney disease: Importance of clinical presentation in the newborn. *Arch Dis Childhood* 62:45–59, 1987.
36. Sedman A, Bell P, Manco-Johnson M, Schrier R, Warady BA, Heard EO, Butler-Simon N, Gabow P: Autosomal dominant polycystic kidney disease in childhood: A longitudinal study: *Kidney Int* 31:1000–1005, 1987.
37. Lambert PP: Polycystic disease of the kidney: A review. *Arch path* 44:34–58, 1947.
38. Potter EL: *Normal and Abnormal Development of the Kidney.* Year Book Medical Publishers, Chicago, 1972.
39. Baert L: Hereditary polycystic kidney disease (adult form): A microdissection study of two cases at an early stage of the disease. *Kidney Int* 13:519–525, 1978.
40. Cuppage FE, Huseman RA, Chapman A, Grantham JJ: Ultrastructure and function of cysts from human adult polycystic kidneys. *Kidney Int* 17:372–381, 1980.
41. Huseman R, Grady A, Welling D, Grantham JJ: Macropuncture study of polycystic disease in adult human kidneys: *Kidney Int* 18:375–385, 1980.
42. Martinez-Maldonado M: Functional aspects: Electrolyte and uric acid excretion with a comment on stone formation. In: JJ Grantham, KD Gardner, eds, *Problems in Diagnosis and Management of Polycystic Kidney Disease.* PKR Foundation, Kansas City, MO, pp 70–80, 1985.
43. Hartnett J, Bennett W: Extrarenal manifestations of cystic renal disease. In: KD Gardner, eds, *Cystic Diseases of the Kidney.* John Wiley and Sons, New York, pp 201–219, 1976.
44. Milutinovic J, Fialkow PJ, Rudd TG, Agodoa LY, Phillips LA, Bryant JI: Liver cysts in patients with autosomal dominant polycystic kidney disease. *Am J Med* 68:741–743, 1980.
45. Gabow PA, Ikle DW, Holmes JH: Polycystic kidney disease: Prospective analysis of nonazotemic patients and family members. *Ann Int Med* 101:238–247, 1984.
46. Grunfeld J-P, Albouze G, Jungers P, Landais P, Dana A, Droz D, Moynot A, Lafforgue B, Boursztyn E, Franco D: Liver changes and complications in adult polycystic kidney disease. *Adv Nephrology* 14:1–20, 1985.
47. Scheff RT, Zuckerman G, Harter H, Delmez J, Koehler R: Diverticular disease in patients with chronic renal failure due to polycystic kidney disease. *Ann Intern Med* 92:202–204, 1980.
48. Starnes HF Jr, Lazarus JM, Vineyard G: Surgery for diverticulitis in renal failure. *Dis Colon Rectum* 28:827–831, 1985.
49. Kupin W, Norris C, Levin NW, Johnson C, Joseph C: Incidence of diverticular disease in patients with polycystic kidney disease (PCKD). *ICN Abstracts* 10:43, 1987.
50. Chapman JR, Hilson AJW: Polycystic kidneys and abdominal aortic aneurysms. *Lancet* 1:646–647, 1980.
51. Montoliu J, Torras A, Revert L: Polycystic kidneys and abdominal aortic aneurysms. *Lancet* 1:1133–1134, 1980.
52. Hossack KF, Leddy CL, Schrier RW, Gabow PA: Incidence of cardiac abnormalities associated with autosomal dominant polycystic kidney disease (ADPKD). *ASN Abstracts* 46A, 1986.
53. Allen A, Wiegmann TB, MacDougall ML: Arachnoid cyst in a patient with autosomal-dominant polycystic kidney disease. *Am J Kid Dis* 8:128–130, 1986.
54. Franz KA, Reubi FC: Rate of functional deterioration in polycystic kidney disease. *Kidney Int* 23:526–529, 1983.
55. Churchill DN, Bear JC, Morgan J, Payne RH, McManamon PJ, Gault MH: Prognosis of adult onset polycystic kidney disease re-evaluated. *Kidney Int* 26:190–193, 1984.
56. Martinez-Maldonado M, Yium JJ, Eknoyan G, Suki WN: Adult polycystic kidney disease: Studies of the defect in urine concentration. *Kidney Int* 2:107–113, 1972.
57. D'Angelo A, Mioni G, Ossi E, Lupo A, Valvo E, Maschio G: Alterations in renal tubular sodium and water transport in polycystic kidney disease. *Clin Neph* 3:99–105, 1975.
58. Preuss H, Geoly K, Johnson M, Chester A, Kliger A, Schreiner G: Tubular function in adult polycystic kidney disease. *Nephron* 24:198–204, 1979.
59. Martinez-Maldonado M, Yium JJ, Suki WN, Eknoyan G: Electrolyte excretion in polycystic kidney disease: Interrelationship between sodium, calcium, magnesium, and phosphate. *J Lab & Clin Med* 90:1066–1075, 1977.
60. Maschio G, Oldrizzi L, Rugiu C, Valvo E, Lupo A, Tessitore N, Loschiavo C, Fabris A, Gammaro L, Panzetta GO: Dietary management. In: JJ Grantham, KD Gardner, eds, *Problems in Diagnosis and Management of Polycystic Kidney Disease.* PKR Foundation, Kansas City, MO, pp 87–92, 1985.
61. Amend WJ, Galen M: Polycystic kidney disease and seatbelts (letter). *Annals Int Med* 79:287, 1973.
62. Whelton A: Seat belts and polycystic kidneys (letter). *Lancet* 2:273–274, 1978.
63. Sholder A, Grayhack JT: Management of pain and hemorrhage. In: JJ Grantham, KD Gardner, eds, *Problems in Diagnosis and Management of Polycystic Kidney Disease.* PKD Foundation, Kansas City, MO, pp 111–120, 1985.
64. Hilpert PL, Friedman AC, Radecki PD, Caroline DF, Fishman EK, Meziane MA, Mitchell DG, Kressel HY: MRI of hemorrhagic renal cysts in polycystic kidney disease. *Am J Radiol* 146:1167–1172, 1986.
65. Levine E, Grantham JJ: Perinephric hemorrhage in autosomal dominant polycystic kidney disease: CT and MR findings. *J Comp Assist Tomog* 11:108–111, 1987.

66. Levine E, Grantham JJ, MacDougall ML: Spontaneous subcapsular and perinephric hemorrhage in end-stage kidney disease: Clinical and CT findings. *Am J Roentg* 148:755–758, 1987.
67. Walters W, Brassach WF: Surgical aspects of polycystic kidney: Report of 85 surgical cases: *Surg Gyn Obst* 58:647–650, 1934.
68. Bricker NS, Patton JF: Renal-function studies in polycystic disease of the kidneys: With observations on the effects of surgical decompression. *N Eng J Med* 256:212–214, 1957.
69. Milam JH, Magee JH, Bunts RC: Evaluation of surgical decompression of polycystic kidneys by differential renal clearances. *J Urol* 90:144–149, 1963.
70. Brassach WF: Clinical data of polycystic kidney. *Surg Gyn Obst* 23:697–702, 1916.
71. Shangzhi H, Shiyuan A, Heming J, Rong Y, Yufeng C: Cyst decapitating decompression operation in polycystic kidney. *Chinese Med J* 93:773–778, 1980.
72. Bennett WM, Elzinga L, Golper TA, Barry JM: Reduction of cyst volume for symptomatic management of autosomal dominant polycystic kidney disease. *J Urol* 137:620–622, 1987.
73. Brassach WF, Schacht FW: Pathological and clinical data concerning polycystic kidney. *Surg Gyn Obst* 57:467–475, 1933.
74. Higgins CC: Bilateral polycystic kidney disease: Review of ninety-four cases. *Arch Surg* 65:318–329, 1952.
75. Simon HB, Thompson GJ: Congenital renal polycystic disease: A clinical and therapeutic study of three hundred sixty-six cases: *JAMA* 159:657–662, 1955.
76. Mitcheson HD, Williams G, Castro JE: Clinical aspects of polycystic disease of the kidneys. *Br Med J* 1:1196–1199, 1977.
77. Lue Y-B, Anderson EE, Hartwell H: The surgical management of polycystic renal disease. *Surg Gyn Obstet* 122:45–49, 1966.
78. Barbaric ZL, Spataro RF, Segal AJ: Urinary tract obstruction in polycystic renal disease. *Radiology* 125:627–629, 1977.
79. Harley JD, Shen FH, Carter SJ: Transcatheter infarction of a polycystic kidney for control of recurrent hemorrhage. *Am J Roentgenol* 134:818–820, 1980.
80. Rao KV: Use of epsilon aminocaproic acid in protracted bleeding from polycystic kidneys: A case report. *J Urol* 136:887–888, 1986.
81. Chisholm GD: An arteriovenous fistula in a polycystic kidney: A cause of acute renal failure and hematuria. *J Urol* 96:854–857, 1966.
82. Licina MG, Adler S, Bruns FJ: Acute renal failure in a patient with polycystic kidney disease. *JAMA* 245:1664–1665, 1981.
83. Duncan KA, Cuppage FE, Grantham JJ: Urinary lipid bodies in polycystic kidney disease. *Am J Kid Dis* 5:49–53, 1985.
84. Bricker NS: Experimental polycystic disease and susceptibility to pyelonephritis. 14th Annual Conference on the kidney. Little, Brown, Boston, 1963.
85. Bennett WM: Evaluation and management of renal infection. In: JJ Grantham, KD Gardner, eds, *Problems in Diagnosis and Management of Polycystic Kidney Disease*. PKR Foundation, Kansas City, MO, pp 98–105, 1985.
86. Schwab SJ, Bander SJ, Klahr S: Renal infection in autosomal dominant polycystic kidney disease. *Am J Med* 82:714–718, 1987.
87. Schwab SJ, Bander S: Diagnosis of cyst infection in polycystic kidney disease (PKD). *ASN Abstracts* 59A, 1986.
88. Levine E, Grantham JJ: The role of computed tomography in the evaluation of adult polycystic kidney disease. *Am J Kidney Dis* 1:99–105, 1981.
89. Fortner A, Taylor A Jr, Alazraki N, Datz FL: Advantage of Indium-111 leukocytes over ultrasound in imaging an infected renal cyst. *J Nucl Med* 27;1147–1149, 1986.
90. Tsang V, Hilson A, Sweny P: Indium-111 white blood cell scan for infectious complications of polycystic renal disease (letter). *J Nucl Med* 27:1376, 1986.
91. Muther RS, Bennett WM: Cyst fluid antibiotic concentrations in polycystic kidney disease: Differences between proximal and distal cysts. *Kidney Int* 20:519–522, 1981.
92. Waters WB, Hershman H, Klein LA: Management of infected polycystic kidneys. *J Urol* 122:383–385, 1979.
93. Schwab SJ, Hinthorn D, Diederich D, Cuppage F, Grantham JJ: pH-dependent accumulation of clindamycin in a polycystic kidney. *Am J Kidney Dis* 3:63–66, 1983.
94. Schwab SJ: Efficacy of chloramphenicol in refractory cyst infections in autosomal dominant polycystic kidney disease: *Am J Kidney Dis* 5:258–261, 1985.
95. Schwab S: Experience with chloramphenicol in refractory renal infection. In: JJ Grantham, KD Gardner, eds, *Problems in Diagnosis and Management of Polycystic Kidney Disease*. PKR Foundation, Kansas City, MO, pp 106–110, 1985.
96. Schwab SJ, Weaver ME: Penetration of trimethoprim and sulfamethoxazole into cysts in a patient with autosomal-dominant polycystic kidney disease: *Am J Kidney Dis* 7:434–438, 1986.
97. Bennett WM, Elzinga L, Pulliam JP, Rashad AL, Barry JM: Cyst fluid antibiotic concentrations in autosomal-dominant polycystic kidney disease: *Am J Kidney Dis* 6:400–404, 1985.
98. Elzinga L, Rashad A, Golper TA, Bennett WM: Antibiotic activity in cyst fluid of patients with cystic kidney disease (CKD). *ICN Abstracts* 41, 1987.
99. Rothermel FJ, Miller FJ Jr, Sanford E, Drago J, Rohner TJ: Clinical and radiographic findings of focally infected polycystic kidneys. *Urol* 9:580–585, 1977.
100. Gregoire JR, Torres VE, Holley KE, Farrow GM: Renal epithelial hyperplastic and neoplastic proliferation in autosomal dominant polycystic kidney disease. *Am J Kidney Dis* 9:27–38, 1987.
101. Tan KH, Donner R, Oe PL: Renal carcinoma associated with polycystic kidneys: Occurrence after chronic hematuria and hypertension. *J Urol* 118:322, 1977.
102. Ng RCK, Suki WN: Renal cell carcinoma occurring in a polycystic kidney of a transplant recipient. *J Urol* 124:710–712, 1980.
103. Kumar S, Cederbaum AI, Pletka PG: Renal cell carcinoma in polycystic kidneys: Case report and review of literature. *J Urol* 124:708–709, 1980.
104. Regan RJ, Abercrombie GF, Lee HA: Polycystic renal disease: Occurrence of malignant change and role of nephrectomy in potential transplant recipients. *Br J Urol* 49:85–91, 1977.
105. Roberts PF: Bilateral renal carcinoma associated with polycystic kidneys. *Br Med J* 3:273–274, 1973.
106. Sogbein SK, Moors DE, Jindal SL: A case of bilateral renal cell carcinoma in polycystic kidneys. *Can J Surg* 24:193–194, 1981.
107. Novick AC, Ho-Hsieh H: Renal transplantation. In: JJ Grantham, KD Gardner, eds, *Problems in Diagnosis and Management of Polycystic Kidney Disease*. PKR Founda-

tion, Kansas City, MO, pp 172–179, 1985.
108. Daniel WW, Hartman GW, Witten DM, et al.: Calcified renal masses. *Radiol* 103:503–508, 1972.
109. Rosenfield AT, Lipson MH, Wolf B, Taylor KJW, Rosenfield NS, Hendler E: Ultrasonography and nephrotomography in the presymptomatic diagnosis of dominantly inherited (adult-onset) polycystic kidney disease. *Radiol* 135:423–427, 1980.
110. Goulandris N, Stringaris C, Xatzilias P, Petsinis C, Giannopoulos A, Triantaphyllou D, Dimopoulos C: Computed tomography in the diagnosis of renal cystic disease. *J Neph, Urol Andrology* 1:65–67, 1980.
111. Howard RM, Young JD Jr: Two malignant tumors in a polycystic kidney. *J Urol* 102:162–164, 1969.
112. McFarland WL, Wallace S, Johnson DE: Renal carcinoma and polycystic disease. *J Urol* 107:530–532, 1972.
113. Tegtmeyer CJ, Cail W, Wyker AW Jr, Gillenwater JY: Angiographic diagnosis of renal tumors associated with polycystic disease. *Radiology* 126:105–109, 1978.
114. Schacht FW: Hypertension in cases of congenital polycystic kidney. *Arch Intern Med* 47:500–509.
115. Reubi F: Hypertension. In: JJ Grantham, KD Gardner, eds, *Problems in Diagnosis and Management of Polycystic Kidney Disease*. PKR Foundation, Kansas City, MO, pp 121–128, 1985.
116. Hansson L, Karlander LK, Lundgren W, Peterson LK: Hypertension in polycystic kidney disease. *Scand J Urol Nephrol* 8:203–205, 1974.
117. Nash DA: Hypertension in polycystic kidney disease without renal failure. *Arch Int Med* 137:1571–1575, 1977.
118. Messerli FH, DeCarvalho GR, Mills NL, Frohlich ED: Renal artery stenosis and polycystic kidney diseases. *Intern Med* 138:1282–1283, 1978.
119. Traub YM, Rosenfeld JB: Renal artery occlusion and malignant hypertension in polycystic kidney disease. *J Urol* 124:279–280, 1980.
120. Shapiro AP, Leenan FHH, Galla SJ, Redmond DP, Vagnucci AH, McDonald RH Jr. Blood pressure regulation during chronic renal failure due to polycystic renal disease. *Acta Physiol Latinoam* 24:432–435, 1974.
121. Leenen FH, Galla SJ, Redmond DP, Vagnucci AH, McDonald RH, Shapiro AP: Relationships of the renin-angiotensin-aldosterone system and sodium balance to blood pressure regulation in chronic renal failure of polycystic kidney disease. *Metabolism* 24:589–603, 1975.
122. Anderson RJ, Miller PD, Linas SL, Katz FH, Holmes JH: Role of the renin-angiotensin system in hypertension of polycystic kidney disease. *Min Elect Metab* 2:137–141, 1979.
123. Danielsen H, Pedersen EB, Nielsen AH, Herlevsen P, Kornerup HJ, Posborg V: Expansion of extracellular volume in early polycystic kidney disease. *Acta Med Scand* 219:399–405, 1986.
124. Calabrese G, Vegalli G, Cristofano C, Barsotti G: Behaviour of arterial pressure in different stages of polycystic kidney disease. *Nephron* 32:207–208, 1982.
125. Valvo E, Gammaro L, Tessitore N, Panzetta G, Lupo A, Loschiavo C, Oldrizzi L, Fabris A, Rugiu C, Ortalda V, Maschio G: Hypertension of polycystic kidney disease: Mechanisms and hemodynamic alterations. *Am J Nephrol* 5:176–181, 1985.
126. Wiebers DO, Whisnant JP, O'Fallon WM: The natural history of unruptured intracranial aneurysms: *N Engl J Med* 304:696–726, 1981.
127. de la Monte SM, Moore GW, Monk MA, Hutchins GM: Risk factors for the development and rupture of intracranial berry aneurysms. *Am J Med* 78:957–964, 1985.
128. Levey AS, Pauker SG, Kassirer JP: Occult intracranial aneurysms in polycystic kidney disease: When is cerebral arteriography indicated? *N Engl J Med* 308(17):986–993, 1983.
129. Levey AS: Cerebral aneurysms. In: JJ Grantham, KD Gardner, eds, *Problems in Diagnosis and Management of Polycystic Kidney Disease*. PKR Foundation, Kansas City, MO, pp 135–144, 1985.
130. Wiebers DO: Management of unruptured intracranial aneurysms. In: JJ Grantham, KD Gardner, eds, *Problems in Diagnosis and Management of Polycystic Kidney Disease*. PKR Foundation, Kansas City, MO, pp 145–153, 1985.
131. Torres VE, Forbes GS, Wiebers DO, Erickson SB, Smith LH: Value of routine screening for intracranial aneurysms (ICA) in autosomal dominant polycystic kidney disease (ADPKD). *ICN Abstracts* 10:45, 1987.
132. Kaehny W, Bell P, Earnest M, Stears J, Gabow P: Family clustering of intracranial aneurysms (ICA) in autosomal dominant polycystic kidney diseases (ADPKD). *ASN Abstracts* 47A, 1986.
133. Nunez L, O'Connor LF, Pinto AG, Gil–Aguado M, Gutierrez M: Annuloaortic ectasia and adult polycystic kidney: A frequent association. *Chest* 90:299–300, 1986.
134. Leier CV, Baker PB, Kilman JW, Wooley CF: Cardiovascular abnormalities associated with adult polycystic kidney disease. *Ann Intern Med* 100:683–688, 1984.
135. Torres VE, Erickson SB, Smith LH, Wilson DM, Hattery RR: The association of nephrolithiasis and autosomal dominant polycystic kidney disease: *ICN Abstracts* 10:44, 1987.
136. Ulreich S, Burrell MI, Lowman RM: Radiology of the gastrointestinal abnormalities seen in patients with adult hepatorenal polycystic disease. *Clin Radiol* 29:547–552, 1978.
137. Wittig JH, Burns R, Longmire WP: Jaundice associated with polycystic liver disease: *Am J Surg* 136:383–386, 1978.
138. Ergun H, Wolf BH, Hissong SL: Obstructive jaundice caused by polycystic liver disease. *Radiology* 136:435–436, 1980.
139. Katzen NG: Fatal hepatic polycystic disease. *Br Med J* 1:839–840, 1964.
140. DelGuercio E, Greco J, Kim KE, Chinitz J, Swartz C: Esophageal varices in adult patients with polycystic kidney and liver disease. *N Engl J Med* 289:678–679, 1973.
141. Ratcliffe PJ, Reeders S, Theaker JM: Bleeding oesophageal varices and hepatic dysfunction in adult polycystic kidney disease. *Br Med J* 288:1330–1331, 1984.
142. McGarrity TJ, Koch KL, Rasbach DA: Refractory ascites associated with polycystic liver disease. *Dig Dis Sci* 31:217–220, 1986.
143. Landais P, Grunfeld J-P, Droz D, Drueke T, Albouze G, Gogusev J, Chaveau D, Moynot A: Cholangiocellular carcinoma in polycystic kidney and liver disease. *Arch Intern Med* 144:2274–2276, 1984.
144. Gardner BP, Evans DB: Primary hepatocellular carcinoma arising in a renal transplant recipient with polycystic disease. *Postgraduate Med J* 59:120–121, 1983.
145. Milutinovic J, Fialkow PJ, Agodoa Ly, Philips LA, Bryant JI: Fertility and pregnancy complications in women with autosomal dominant polycystic kidney disease. *Obstet Gynecol* 61:566–570, 1983.
146. Jungers P, Forget D, Henry–Amar M, Albouze G, Fournier P, Vischer U, Droz D, Noel LH, Grundfeld JP: Chronic kidney disease and pregnancy. *Adv Nephrol* 15:103–141, 1986.

147. Oken DE: Chronic renal diseases and pregnancy: A review. *Am J Obstet Gynecol* 94:1023–1043, 1966.
148. Ambroso GC, Como G, Imbasciati E: Pregnancy in patients by polycystic kidney. A retrospective study in 56 women. *ICN Abstract* 10:40, 1987.
149. Mitch WE, Walser M, Buffington GA, Lemann J: A simple method of estimating progression of chronic renal failure. *Lancet* 2:1326–1327, 1976.
150. Rutherford WE, Blondin J, Miller JP, et al.: Chronic progressive renal disease: Rate of change of serum creatinine concentration. *Kidney Int* 11:62–70, 1977.
151. Chester AC, Argy WP Jr, Rakowski TA, Schreiner GE: Polycystic kidney disease and chronic hemodialysis. *Clin Nephrol* 10:129–133, 1978.
152. Neff MS, Eiser AR, Slifkin RF, Baum M, Baez A, Gupta S, Amarga E: Patients surviving 10 years of hemodialysis. *Am J Med* 74:996–1004, 1983.
153. Thaysen JH, Christensen E, Alarcon–Zurita A, Movild B: Involution of polycystic kidneys during active treatment of terminal uremia. *Acta Med Scand* 197:257–60, 1975.
154. Thaysen JH, Thomsen HS: Involution of polycystic kidneys during replacement therapy of terminal renal failure. *Acta Med Scand* 212:389–394, 1982.
155. Ishikawa I, Tateishi K, Kitada H, Shinoda A: Regression of adult type polycystic kidneys during chronic intermittent hemodialysis. Is it a universal phenomenon? *Nephron* 36:147, 1984.
156. Raulerson JD, Juncos LI, Fuller TJ, Cade R: Obstruction of the inferior vena cava complicating hemodialysis in polycystic kidney disease. *South Med J* 72:1389–1392, 1979.
157. Pinnick RV, Wiegman TB, Diederich DA: Regional citrate anticoagulation for hemodialysis in the patient at high risk for bleeding. *N Engl J Med* 308:258–261, 1983.
158. Graham AN, Neale TJ, Hatfield PJ, Morrison RBI, Meech PR, Jacobson A, Faircloth C: Endstage renal failure due to polycystic kidney disease managed by continuous ambulatory peritoneal dialysis. *NZ Med J* 99:491–493, 1986.
159. Lazarus JM, Bailey GL, Hampers CL, Merrill JP: Hemodialysis and transplantation in adults with polycystic renal disease. *JAMA* 217:1821–24, 1971.
160. Amamoo DG, Woods JE, Anderson CF: Renal transplantation in end stage polycystic renal disease. *J Urol* 112:443–44, 1974.
161. Mendez R, Mendez RG, Payne JE, Berne TV: Renal transplantation: In adult patients with the end stage polycystic kidney disease. *Urology* 5:26–28, 1975.
162. Salvatierra O Jr, Wolfson M, Cochrum K, Amend W, Belzer FO: End stage polycystic kidney disease: Management by renal transplantation and selective use of preliminary nephrectomy. *J Urology* 115:5–7, 1976.
163. Wolfson M, Amend WJC, Cochrum KC, Belzer FO, Salvatierra O Jr: Transplantation in end-stage polycystic kidney disease. *Dialysis Transplan* 5:66–102, 1976.
164. DeBono DP, Evans DB: The management of polycystic kidney disease with special reference to dialysis and transplantation. *Q J Med* 46:353–363, 1977.
165. Wallenius M, Kuhlback B, Brotherus JW: Renal transplantation in polycystic kidney disease. *Scand J Urol Nephrol* 12:75–77, 1978.
166. Williams G, Mitcheson HD, Castro JE: Transplantation for polycystic kidney disease. *Urology* 12:628–630, 1978.
167. Pechan W, Novick AC, Braun WE, Nakamoto S, Popowniak K, Steinmuller D: Management of end stage polycystic kidney disease with renal transplantation. *J Urology* 125:622–624, 1981.
168. Sanfilippo FP, Vaughn WK, Peters TG, Bollinger RR, Spees EK: Transplantation for polycystic kidney disease. *Transplantation* 36:54–59, 1983.
169. Reeders ST, Breuning MH, Davies KE, Nicholls RD, Jarman AP, Higgs DR, Pearson PL, Weatherall DJ: A highly polymorphic DNA marker linked to adult polycystic kidney disease on chromosome 16. *Nature* 317(10):542–544, 1985.
170. Bourgeois N, Kinnaert P, Vereerstraeten P, Schoutens A, Toussaint C: Infection of hepatic cysts following kidney transplantation in polycystic disease. *World J Surg* 7:629–631, 1983.
171. Martin DC, Goodwin WE: Renal transplantation in polycystic renal disease. *JAMA* 202:654–657, 1967.
172. Zerres K, Volpel MC, Weib B: Cystic kidneys: Genetics, pathologic anatomy, clinical picture, and prenatal diagnosis. *Hum Genet* 68:104–135, 1984.
173. Reeders ST, Zerres K, Gal A, Hogenkamp T, Propping P, Schmidt W, Waldherr R, Dolata MM, Davies KE, Weatherall DJ: Prenatal diagnosis of autosomal dominant polycystic kidney disease with a DNA probe. *Lancet* 2:6–8, 1986.
174. Rowley PT: Implications of the new genetics: Diagnostic dilemmas: Symposium summary. *Am J Hum Genet* 38:784–787, 1986.
175. Manjoney DM, McKegney FP: Individual and family coping with polycystic kidney disease: The harvest of denial. *Int J Psychiatry* 9:19–31, 1978.
176. Zerres K,, Stephan M: Attitudes to early diagnosis of polycystic kidney disease. *Lancet* 2:1395, 1986.
177. Sahney S, Weiss L, Levin N: Genetic counseling in adult polycystic kidney disease. *Am J Med Genetics* 11:461–468, 1982.
178. Evers-Kiebooms G, Cassiman JJ, Van den Berghe H: Attitudes toward predictive testing in Huntington's disease: A recent survey in Belgium. *J Med Genet* 24:275–279, 1987.
179. Schimke RN: Huntington's disease: Medical problem and ethical dilemma. *Midwest Medical Ethics Newsletter* 3:1, 6, 1986.
180. Schimke RN: A genetic approach. In: JJ Grantham, KD Gardner, eds, Problems in Diagnosis and Management of Polycystic Kidney Disease. PKR Foundation, Kansas City, MO, pp 187–193, 1985.
181. Pickens RL: Early diagnosis of polycystic kidney disease. *Urology* 2:188–190, 1973.
182. Lufkin EG, Alfrey AC, Trucksess ME, Holmes JH: Polycystic kidney disease — earlier diagnosis using ultrasound. *Urology* 4:5–12, 1974.
183. Begleiter ML, Smith TH, Harris DJ: Ultrasound for genetic counselling in polycystic kidney disease. *Lancet* 2:1073–1074, 1977.
184. Milutinovic J, Fialkow PJ, Phillips LA, Agodoa LY, Bryant JI, Denney JD, Rudd TG: Autosomal dominant polycystic kidney disease: Early diagnosis and data for genetic counseling. *Lancet* 1:1203–1205, 1980.
185. Milutinovic J, Agodoa LCY, Culter RE, Striker GE: Autosomal dominant polycystic kidney disease. Early diagnosis and consideration of pathogenesis. *Am J Clin Pathol* 73:740–747, 1980.
186. Chester AC, Geoly K, Schreiner GE, Preuss HG: Early diagnosis of polycystic kidney disease. *Am Fam Physician* 23:175–181, 1981.
187. Bear JC, McManamon P, Morgan J, Payne RH, Lewis H, Gault MH, Churchill DN: Age at clinical onset and at ultrasonographic detection of adult polycystic kidney disease: Data for genetic counselling. *Am J Med Genet* 18:45–

53, 1984.
188. Fryns JP, Vandenberghe K, Moerman F: Mid-trimester ultrasonographic diagnosis of early manifesting "adult" form of polycystic kidney disease. *Hum Genet* 74:461, 1986.
189. Romero R, Cullen M, Jeanty P, Grannum P, Reece EA, Venus I, Hobbins JC: The diagnosis of congenital renal anomalies with ultrasound II. Infantile polycystic kidney disease. *Am J Obstet Gynecol* 150:259–262, 1984.
190. Luthy DA, Hirsch JH: Infantile polycystic kidney disease: Observations from attempts at prenatal diagnosis. *Am J Med Genetics* 20:505–517, 1985.
191. Fong KW, Rahmani MR, Rose TH, Skidmore MB, Connor TP: Fetal renal cystic disease: Sonographic-pathologic correlation. *Am J Radiol* 146:767–773, 1986.
192. Blyth H, Ockenden BG: Polycystic disease of kidneys and liver presenting in childhood. *J Med Genetics* 8:257–284, 1971.
193. Mauseth R, Lieberman E, Heuser ET: Infantile polycystic disease of the kidneys and Ehlers–Danlos syndrome in an 11-year-old patient. *J Pediatr* 90:81–83, 1977.
194. Gang DL, Herrin HT: Infantile polycystic disease of the liver and kidneys. *Clin Nephrol* 25:28–36, 1986.
195. Boal DK, Teele RL: Sonography of infantile polycystic kidney disease. *Am J Roentgenol* 135:575–580, 1980.
196. Landing BH, Wells HT: Anatomy of the hepatic lesion of infantile polycystic disease. *Pediatr Univ Tokyo* 18:112–119, 1970.
197. Bradford WD, Bradford JW, Porter FS, Sidbury JB Jr: Cystic disease of liver and kidney with portal hypertension. A cause of sudden unexpected hematemesis. *Clin Pediatrics* 7:299–306, 1968.
198. Broussin JAB, Cadier L, Diard F: Aspects echographiques des polykystoses hepato-renales recessives chez l'enfant. *J Radiol* 61:243–249, 1980.
199. Thaler MM, Ogata ES, Goodman JR, Piel CF, Korobkin MT: Congenital fibrosis and polycystic disease of liver and kidneys. *Am J Dis Child* 126:374–380, 1973.
200. Metreweli C, Garel L: The echographic diagnosis of infantile renal polycystic disease. *Eur Soc Pediatr Radiol* 23:103–107, 1982.
201. Howie JL, Nicholson RL: Ct evaluation of infantile polycytic disease. *J Can Assoc Radiol* 31:202–203, 1980.
202. Fitch SJ, Stapleton FB: Ultrasonographic features of glomerulocystic disease in infancy: Similarity to infantile polycystic kidney disease. *Pediatr Radiol* 16:400–402, 1986.
203. Carson RW, Bedi D, Cavallo T, DuBose TD Jr: Familial adult glomerulocystic kidney disease. *Am J Kidney Dis* 9:154–165, 1987.
204. Vlachos J, Tsakraklidis V: Glomerular cysts: An unusual variety of "polycystic kidneys" Report of two cases. *Am J Dis Child* 114:379–384, 1967.
205. Krous HF, Richie JP, Sellers B: Glomerulocystic kidney: A hypothesis of origin and pathogenesis. *Arch Pathol Lab Med* 101:462–463, 1977.
206. Melnick SC, Brewer DB, Oldham JS: Cortical microcystic disease of the kidney with dominant inheritance: A previously undescribed syndrome. *J Clin Pathol* 37:494–499, 1984.
207. Oh Y, Onoyama K, Kobayashi K, Nanishi F, Mitsuoka W, Ohchi N, Tsuruda H, Fujishima M: Glomerulocystic kidneys: Report of an adult case. *Nephron* 43:299–302, 1986.
208. Reznik VM, Griswold WT, Mendoza SA: Glomerulocystic disease — a case report with 10 year follow-up. *Int J Ped Neph* 3:321–323, 1982.
209. Landing BH, Gwinn JL, Lieberman E: Cystic diseases of the kidney in children. In: KD Gardner, eds, *Cystic Diseases of the Kidney*. John Wiley and Sons, New York, pp 187–200, 1976.
210. Mauseth R, Lieberman E, Heuser ET: Infantile polycystic disease of the kidneys and Ehlers–Danlos syndrome in an 11-year-old patient. *J Pediatr* 90:81–83, 1977.
211. Lahiri B, Lahiri VL, Agrawal BM: Wilms' tumour with polycystic kidney. *Br J Urol* 51:411, 1979.
212. Sherman FE, Studnicki FM, Fetterman GH: Renal lesions of familial juvenile nephronophthisis examined by microdissection. *Am J Clin Path* 55:391–400, 1971.
213. Baert L: Microdissection findings of medullary sponge kidney. *Urology* 11:637–640, 1978.
214. Mangos JA, Opitz JM, Lobeck CC, Cookson DU: Familial juvenile nephronophthisis: An unrecognized renal disease in the United States. *Pediatrics* 34:337–345, 1964.
215. Goldman SH, Walker SR, Merigan TC Jr, Gardner KD Jr, Bull JMC: Hereditary occurrence of cystic disease of the renal medulla. *N Engl J Med* 274:984–992, 1966.
216. Strauss MB, Sommers SC: Medullary cystic disease and familial juvenile nephronophthisis: Clinical and pathological identity. *N Engl J Med* 277:863–864, 1967.
217. Gardner KD Jr: Evolution of clinical signs in adult-onset cystic disease of the renal medulla. *Ann Int Med* 74:47–54, 1971.
218. Giangiacomo J, Monteleone PL, Witzleben CL: Medullary cystic disease vs. nephronophthisis. A valid distinction? *JAMA* 232:629–631, 1975.
219. Avasthi PS, Erickson DG, Gardner KD Jr: Hereditary renal-retinal dysplasia and the medullary cystic disease-nephronophthisis complex. *Ann Intern Med* 84:157–161, 1976.
220. van Collenburg JJM, Thompson MW, Huber J: Clinical, pathological and genetic aspects of a form of cystic disease of the renal medulla: Familial juvenile nephronophthisis (FJN). *Clin Nephrol* 9:55–62, 1978.
221. Steele BT, Lirenman DS, Beattie CW: Nephronophthisis. *Am J Med* 68:531–538, 1980.
222. Cantani A, Bamonte G, Ceccoli D, Biribicchi G, Farinella F: Familial juvenile nephronophthisis; a review and differential diagnosis. *Clin Pediatr* 25:90–95, 1986.
223. Burke JR, Inglis JA, Craswell PW, Mitchell KR, Emmerson BT: Juvenile nephronophthisis and medullary cystic disease — the same disease (report of a large family with medullary cystic disease associated with gout and epilepsy). *Clin Nephrol* 18:1–8, 1982.
224. Gardner KD Jr: Nephronophthisis and renal medullary cystic disease. In: KD Gardner Jr, eds, *Cystic Diseases of the Kidney*. John Wiley and Sons, New York, pp 173–185, 1976.
225. Pascal RP: Medullary cystic disease of the kidney: Study of a case with scanning and transmission electron microscopy and light microscopy. *Am J Clin Path* 59:659–665, 1973.
226. Fyhrquist FY, Klockars M, Gordin A, Tornroth T, Kock B: Hyperreninemia, lysozymuria, and erythrocytosis in Fanconi syndrome with medullary cystic kidney. *Acta Med Scand* 207:359–365, 1980.
227. Rayfield EJ, McDonald FD: Red and blonde hair in renal medullary cystic disease. *Arch Intern Med* 130:72–75, 1972.
228. Editorial: Renal cysts and red hair. *Br Med J*: 631–632, 1973.
229. Thompson GR, Weiss JJ, Goldman RT, Rigg GA: Familial occurrence of hyperuricemia, gout, and medullary cystic disease. *Arch Intern Med* 138:1614–1617, 1978.
230. Burgener FA, Spataro RF: Early medullary cystic disease:

A urographic diagnosis? *Radiology* 130:321–322, 1979.
231. Link DP, Hansen S, Palmer J: High dose excretory urography and medullary cystic disease of the kidney. *Am J Roentgenology* 133:303–305, 1979.
232. Swenson RS, Kempson RL, Friedland GW: Cystic disease of the renal medulla in the elderly. *JAMA* 228:1401–1404, 1974.
233. Morris RC, Yamauchi H, Palubinskas AJ, Howenstine J: Medullary sponge kidney. *Am J Med* 38:883–891, 1965.
234. Granberg PO, Lagergren C, Theve NO: Renal function studies in medullary sponge kidney. *Scand J Urol Nephrol* 5:177–180, 1971.
235. Feest TG: Medullary sponge kidney: Abnormalities of renal tubular and glomerular function, and their relationship to clinical features. In: GHB Robinson, eds, *Dialysis, Transplants, & Nephrology. Proceeding of the European Dial & Transplant Association*. Pittman Medical, London, pp 511–517, 1978.
236. Higashihara E, Nutahara K, Tago K, Ueno A, Niijima T: Medullary sponge kidney and renal acidification defect. *Kidney Int* 25:453–459, 1984.
237. Higashihara E, Nutahara K, Tago K, Ueno A, Niijima T: Unilateral and segmental medullary sponge kidney: Renal function and calcium excretion. *J Urol* 132:743–745, 1984.
238. Green J, Szylman P, Sznajder II, Winaver J, Better OS: Renal tubular handling of potassium in patients with medullary sponge kidney: A model of renal papillectomy in humans. *Arch Intern Med* 144:2201–2204, 1984.
239. Deck MDF: Medullary sponge kidney with renal tubular acidosis: A report of 3 cases. *J Urol* 94:330–35, 1965.
240. Popa M, Stanescu V: Renal tubular acidosis and hypergammaglobulinaemic purpura in a 10 year old girl with roentgenographic signs suggesting medullary sponge kidney. *Acta Paediatr Scand* 58:290–294, 1969.
241. Kumagai I, Matsuo S, Kato T: A case of incomplete renal tubular acidosis (type I) associated with medullary sponge kidney followed by nephrocalcinosis. *J Urol* 123:250–252, 1980.
242. Backman U, Danielson BG, Fellstrom B, Johansson G, Ljunghall S, Wikstrom B: Clinical and laboratory findings in patients with medullary sponge kidney. In: *International Meeting on Urolithiasis, 1980*. Plenum, New York, 1980.
243. Yendt ER, Jarzylo S, Finnis WA, Cohanim M: Medullary sponge kidney (tubular ectasia) in calcium urolithiasis. In: *International Meeting on Urolithiasis, 1980*. Plenum, New York, 1980.
244. O'Neill M, Breslau NA, Pak CY: Metabolic evaluation of nephrolithiasis in patients with medullary sponge kidney. *JAMA* 245:1233–1236, 1981.
245. Stella FJ, Massry SG, Kleeman CR: Medullary sponge kidney associated with parathyroid adenoma: A report of two cases. *Nephron* 10:332–336, 1973.
246. Gremillion DH, Kee JW, McIntosh DA: Hyperparathyroidism and medullary sponge kidney — a chance relationship? *JAMA* 237:799–780, 1977.
247. Rao DS, Frame B, Block MA, Parfitt AM: Primary hyperparathyroidism: A cause of hypercalciuria and renal stones in patients with medullary sponge kidney. *JAMA* 237:1353–1355, 1977.
248. Rao DS, Frame B, Block MA, Parfitt AM: Hyperparathyroidism and medullary sponge kidney (letter). *JAMA* 238:1912–1913, 1977.
249. Diabal PW, Jordan RM, Dorfman SG: Medullary sponge kidney and renal-leak hypercalciuria: A link to the development of parathyroid adenoma? *JAMA* 241:1490–1491, 1979.
250. Hellman DE, Kartchner M, Komar N, Mayes D, Pitt M: Hyperaldosteronism, hyperparathyroidism, medullary sponge kidneys, and hypertension. *JAMA* 244:1351–1353, 1980.
251. Macdougall JA, Prout WG: Medullary sponge kidney — clinical appraisal and report of twelve cases. *Br J Surg* 55:130–133, 1968.
252. Huland H, Lewin K, Stamey TA: Unilateral medullary sponge kidney — cause of persistent bacteriuria. *Urology* 8:373–377, 1976.
253. Parks JH, Coe FL, Strauss AL: Calcium nephrolithiasis and medullary sponge kidney in women. *N Engl J Med* 306:1088–1107, 1982.
254. Beck AD: Medullary sponge kidney: Report of a case showing progressive enlargement of renal calculi. *Aust Radiol* 14:298–301, 1970
255. Modarelli RO, Wettlaufer JN: Surgically documented segmental medullary sponge kidney: Case report. *J Urol* 117:244–245, 1977.
256. Harrison AR, Rose GA: Medullary sponge kidney. *Urolog Res* 7:197–207, 1979.
257. Butler MR, O'Flynn JD, Devine HF: Medullary sponge kidney: Review of the literature and presentation of 33 cases. *J Irish Med Assoc* 66:5–13, 1973.
258. Kuiper JJ: Medullary sponge kidney in three generations: *NY State J Med* 71:2665–2669, 1971.
259. Flower CDR, Kitchener PG: Multicystic kidney — an example of bilateral involvement in an adult. *Br J Radiol* 51:543–545, 1978.
260. Kyaw MM: The radiological diagnosis of congenital multicystic kidney: Radiological triad. *Clin Radiol* 25:45–62, 1974.
261. Sumner TS, Thomas J, Friedland GW, Crowe J, Parker B, Resnick M: Preoperative diagnosis of unilateral multicystic kidney with hydropelvis. *Urology* 11:519–522, 1978.
262. Takao R, Amamoto Y, Matsunaga N, Tasaki T, Kakimoto S, Ito M, Fujii H, Futagawa S, Sekine I: Computed tomography of multicystic kidney: Case report. *J Comput Assist Tomog* 4:548–549, 1980.
263. Older RA, Hinman CG, Crane LM, Cleeve DM, Morgan CL: In utero diagnosis of multicystic kidney by gray scale ultrasonography. *Am J Roentgenol* 133:130–131, 1979.
264. Friedberg JE, Mitnick JS, Davis DA: Antepartum ultrasonic detection of multicystic kidney. *Radiology* 131:198, 1979.
265. Hashimoto BE, Filly RA, Callen PW: Multicystic dysplastic kidney in utero: Changing appearance in US. *Radiology* 159:107–109, 1986.
266. Ambrose SS: Unilateral multicystic renal disease in adults: Birth Defects. *Orig Art Ser* 13:349–353, 1977.
267. Barrett DM, Wineland RE: Renal cell carcinoma in multicystic dysplastic kidney. *Urology* 15:152–154, 1980.
268. Birken G, King D, Vane D, Lloyd T: Renal cell carcinoma arising in a multicystic dysplastic kidney. *J Ped Surg* 20:619–621, 1985.
269. Hartman GE, Smolik LM, Shochat SJ: The dilemma of the multicystic dysplastic kidney. *Am J Dis Child* 140:925–928, 1986.
270. Stanisic TH: Review of 'The dilemma of the multicystic dysplastic kidney' (editorial). *Am J Dis Child* 140:865, 1986.
271. Dunnill MS, Millard PR, Oliver D: Acquired cystic disease of the kidneys: A hazard of long-term intermittent maintenance haemodialysis. *J Clin Path* 30:868–877, 1977.

272. Grantham JJ, Levine E: Acquired cystic disease: Replacing one kidney disease with another. *Kidney Int* 28:99–105, 1985.
273. Ishikawa I, Onouchi Z, Saito Y, Tateishi K, Shinoda A, Suzuki S, Kitada H, Sugishita N, Fukuda Y: Sex differences in acquired cystic disease of the kidney on long-term dialysis. *Nephron* 39:336–340, 1985.
274. Narasimhan N, Golper TA, Wolfson M, Rahatzad M, Bennett WM: Clinical characteristics and diagnostic considerations in acquired renal cystic disease. *Kidney Int* 30:748–752, 1986.
275. Hughson MD, Buchwald D, Fox M: Renal neoplasia and acquired cystic kidney disease in patients receiving long-term dialysis. *Arch Pathol Lab Med* 110:592–601, 1986.
276. Thomson BJ, Allan PL, Winney RJ: Acquired cystic disease of kidney: Metastatic renal adenocarcinoma and hypercalcaemia. *Lancet* 2:502–503, 1985.
277. Thompson BJ, Jenkins DAS, Allan PL, Winney RJ: Acquired cystic disease of the kidney: An indication for renal transplantation? *Br Med J* 293:1209–1210, 1986.
278. Ishikawa I, Yuri T, Kitada H, Shinoda A: Regression of acquired cystic disease of the kidney after successful renal tranplantation. *Am J Nephrol* 3:310–314, 1983.
279. Levine E, Grantham JJ, Slusher SL, Greathouse JL, Krohn BP: CT of acquired cystic kidney disease and renal tumors in long-term dialysis patients. *Am J Roentgenol* 142:125–131, 1984.
280. Hughson MD, Hennigar GR, McManus JFA: Atypical cysts, acquired renal cystic disease, and renal cell tumors in end stage dialysis kidneys. *Lab Invest* 42:475–480, 1980.
281. Rudge CJ: Acquired cystic disease of the kidney: Serious or irrelevant? *Br Med J* 293:1186–1187, 1986.
282. MacDougall ML, Welling LW, Wiegmann TB: Renal adenocarcinoma and acquired cystic disease in chronic hemodialysis patients. *Am J Kidney Dis* 9:166–171, 1987.
283. Ruggenenti P: Acquired renal cystic disease and renal adenocarcinoma in long-term dialysis patients. *Int J Artif Org* 8:303–306, 1985.
284. Gardner KD: Acquired renal cystic disease and renal adenocarcinoma in patients on long-term hemodialysis. *N Engl J Med* 310:390, 1984.
285. Ishikawa I, Saito Y, Onouchi A, Kitada H, Suzuki S, Kurihara S, Yuri T, Shinoda A: Development of acquired cystic disease and adenocarcinoma of the kidney in glomerulonephritic chronic hemodialysis patients. *Clin Nephrol* 14:1–6, 1980.
286. Bommer J, Waldherr R, van Kaick G, Strauss L, Ritz E: Acquired renal cysts in uremic patients — in vivo demonstration by computed tomography. *Clin Nephrol* 14:299–303, 1980.
287. Elliott HL, MacDougall AI, Buchanan WM: Acquired cystic disease of kidney. *Lancet* 2:1359, 1977.
288. Scanlon MH, Karasick SR: Acquired renal cystic disease and neoplasia: Complications of chronic hemodialysis. *Radiology* 147:837–838, 1983.
289. Turani H, Levi J, Zevin D, Kessler E: Acquired cystic disease and tumors in kidneys of hemodialysis patients. *Israel J Med Sci* 19:614–618, 1983.
290. Ratcliffe PJ, Dunnill MS, Oliver DO: Clinical importance of acquired cystic disease of the kidney in patients undergoing dialysis. *Br Med J* 287: 1855–1858, 1983.
291. Brendler CB, Albertsen PC, Goldman SM, Hill GS, Lowe FC, Millan JC: Acquired renal cystic disease in the end stage kidney: Urological implications. *J Urol* 132:548–552, 1984.
292. Gehrig JJ Jr, Gotteiner TI, Swenson RS: Acquired cystic disease of the end-stage kidney. *Am J Med* 79:609–620, 1985.
293. Pateras VR: Malignancy in chronic dialysis patients. *Int J Artif Org* 8:301–302, 1985.
294. Gardner KD Jr, Evan AP: Cystic kidneys: An enigma evolves. *Am J Kidney Dis* 3:403–413, 1984.
295. Ishikawa I: Malignant potential of renal cell carcinoma in chronic hemodialysis patients. *ICN Abstract* 10:146, 1987.
296. Bricker NS, Patton JF: Cystic disease of the kidneys — A study of dynamics and chemical composition of cyst fluid. *Am J Med* 18:207–219, 1955.
297. Clarke BG, Hurwitz IS, Dubinsky E: Solitary serous cysts of the kidney: Biochemical, cytologic and histologic studies. *J Urol* 75:772–775, 1956.
298. Steg A: Renal cysts. II. Chemical and dynamic study of cystic fluid. *Eur Urol* 2:164–167, 1976.
299. Williamson B Jr, Hattery RR, Stephens DH, Sheedy PF II: Computed tomography of the kidneys: *Semin Roentgenol* 13:249–255, 1978.
300. Love L, Reynes CJ, Churchill R, Moncada R: Third generation CT scanning in renal disease. *Radiol Clin North Am* 17:77–90, 1979.
301. Ackerman LV, Rosai J: *Surgical Pathology.* CV Mosby, St. Louis, MO, p 639, 1974.
302. Roth JK Jr, Roberts JA: Benign renal cysts and renal function. *J Urol* 123:625–628, 1980.
303. Hepler AB: Solitary cysts of the kidney: A report of seven cases and observations on the pathogenesis of these cysts. *Surg Gynecol Obstet* 50:668–687, 1930.
304. Baert L, Steg A: On the pathogenesis of simple renal cysts in the adult. A microdissection study. *Urol Res* 5:103–108, 1977.
305. Baert L, Steg A: Is the diverticulum of the distal and collecting tubules a preliminary stage of the simple cyst in the adult? *J Urology* 118:707–710, 1977.
306. Baert L, Steg A: Diverticula on distal tubule, simple renal cysts, and ureteral obstruction. Causal relationship. *Urology* 11:221–224, 1978.
307. Derezic D, Cecuk L: Possible role for enzyme inhibition in controlling kidney cysts. *Lancet* 1:217, 1978.
308. Steg A: Renal cysts in adults. III. Clinical aspect and diagnostical approach, based on the analysis of 1342 cases. *Eur Urol* 2:209–212, 1976.
309. Steg A: Renal cysts in adults. IV. Therapeutic problems. *Eur Urol* 2:213–215, 1976.
310. McClennan BL, Stanley RJ, Melson GL, Levitt RG, Sagel SS: CT of the renal cyst: Is cyst aspiration necessary? *Am J Roent* 133:671–675, 1979.
311. Sagel SS, Stanley RJ, Levitt RG, Geisse G: Computed tomography of the kidney. *Radiology* 124:359–370, 1977.
312. Dalton D, Neiman H, Grayhack JT: The natural history of simple renal cysts: A preliminary study. *J Urol* 135:905–908, 1986.
313. Ahmed S: Simple renal cysts in childhood. *Br J Urol* 44:71–75, 1972.
314. Firstater M, Farkas A: Simple renal cyst in a newborn. *Br J Urol* 45:366–369, 1973.
315. Redman JF, Scriber LJ, Bissada NK: Simple renal cyst in a child. *J Ped Surg* 11:117–119, 1976.
316. Gordon RL, Pollack HM, Popky GL, Duckett JW Jr: Simple serous cysts of the kidney in children. *Ped Radiol* 131:357–361, 1979.
317. Siegel MJ, Mcalister WH: Simple cysts of the kidney in children. *J Urol* 123:75–78, 1980.
318. Pearl M, Klein S: Simple renal cyst and hypertension.

Annales de Radiologie 29:421–423. 1986.
319. Baert L: Cystic kidneys, renal dysplasia and microdissection data in 5 children with congenital valvular urethral obstruction. *Eur Urol* 4:382–387, 1978.
320. Farkas A, Firstater M, Johnston JH: Neonatal solitary renal cysts associated with posterior urethral valves. *J Pediatr Surg* 14:132–137, 1979.
321. Noe HN, Larimer PJ: Simple renal cyst manifest by proteinuria in children. *J Urol* 118:854–855, 1977.
322. Rockson SG, Stone RA, Gunnells JC Jr: Solitary renal cyst with segmental ischemia and hypertension. *J Urol* 112:550–552, 1974.
323. Churchill D, Kimoff R, Pinsky M, Gault MH: Solitary intrarenal cyst: Correctable cause of hypertension. *Urology* 6:485–488, 1978.
324. Kala R, Fyhrquist F, Halttunen P, Rauste J: Solitary renal cyst, hypertension and renin. *J Urol* 116:710–711, 1976.
325. Rose HJ, Pruitt AW: Hypertension, hyperreninemia and a solitary renal cyst in an adolescent. *Am J Med* 61:579–582, 1976.
326. Mang HYL, Markovic PR, Chow S, Maruyama A: Solitary intrarenal cyst causing hypertension: With plasma renin activity study before and after cyst aspiration. *NY State J Med* 78:654–656, 1978.
327. Renders GAM, Moonen WA, DeBruyne FMJ: Resolution of hypertension after percutaneous puncture of a solitary renal cyst. *Acta Urol Belg* 47:555–559, 1979.
328. Luscher TF, Wanner C, Siegenthaler W, Vetter W: Simple renal cyst and hypertension: Cause or coincidence? *Clin Nephrol* 26:91–95, 1986.
329. Limjoco UR, Strauch AE: Infected solitary cyst of the kidney: Report of a case and review of the literature. *J Urol* 96:625–630, 1966.
330. Deliveliotis A, Zorzos S, Varkarakis M: Suppuration of solitary cyst of the kidney. *Br J Urol* 39:472–478, 1967.
331. Altemus R, Salazar H, Rotheram EB Jr: Infected solitary cyst of the kidney: A case report with selective renal angiography. *Vasc Dis* 5:125–129, 1968.
332. Stables DP, Jackson RS: Management of an infected simple renal cyst by percutaneous aspiration. *Br J Radiol* 47:290–292, 1974.
333. Patel NP, Pitts WR Jr, Ward JN: Solitary infected renal cyst: Report of 2 cases and review of the literature. *Urology* 11:164–167, 1978.
334. Livingstone B: Tuberculous infection of a serous cyst of the kidney: Short case report. *Br J Urol* 45:702, 1973.
335. Mindell HJ: Percutaneous renal cyst puncture: Unusual results in 2 cases. *J Urol* 114:332–336, 1975.
336. Sagalowsky A, Solotkin D: Infected renal mass successfully treated by ultrasound-guided needle aspiration. *Southern Med J* 73:957, 1980.
337. Reid RE: Pyelocalyceal obstruction due to a renal cyst. *J Natl Med Assoc* 58:342–344, 1966.
338. Evans AT, Coughlin JP: Urinary obstruction due to renal cysts. *J Urol* 103:277–280, 1970.
339. Notley RG: Calyceal obstruction due to parapelvic cyst (abridged). *Proc R Soc Med* 64:66, 1971.
340. Smith DC, Rich DH, Barnes RW: Hematuria and massive calycovenous reflux secondary to benign renal cyst. *Urology* 9:698–700, 1977.
341. Hinman F Jr: Obstructive renal cysts. *J Urol* 119:681–683, 1978.
342. Bubrick MP, Hitchcock CR: Renal cyst causing afferent loop obstruction and acute pancreatitis. *Am Surgeon* 41:440–443, 1975.
343. Gernert JE, Stein J, Bischoff AJ: Solitary renal cysts: Experience with 100 cases. *J Urol* 100:251–253, 1968.
344. Weiner MA: Renal mass associated with polycythemia. *JAMA* 207:1339–1341, 1969.
345. Koplan JP, Sprayregan S, Ossias AL, Zanjani ED: Erythropoietin-producing renal cyst and polycythemia vera: Clarification of their relationship. *Am J Med* 54:819–824, 1973.
346. Vertel RM, Morse BS, Prince JE: Remission of erythrocytosis after drainage of a solitary renal cyst. *Arch Intern Med* 120:54–58, 1967.
347. Wahlqvist L, Grumstedt B: Therapeutic effect of percutaneous puncture of simple renal cyst; follow-up investigation of 50 patients. *Acta Chir Scand* 132:340–347, 1966.
348. Kyaw MM, Newman H: Percutaneous puncture of renal cysts for diagnosis and treatment. *J Can Assoc Radiol* 24:150–156, 1973.
349. Thompson IM Jr, Kovac A, Geshner J: Ultrasound followup of renal cyst puncture. *J Urol* 124:175–178, 1980.
350. Raskin MM, Roen SA, Viamonte M Jr: Effect of intracystic pantopaque on renal cysts. *J Urol* 114:678–679, 1975.
351. Raskin MM, Poole DO, Roen SA, Viamonte M Jr: Percutaneous management of renal cysts: Results of a four-year study. *Radiology* 115:551–553, 1975.
352. Mindell HJ: On the use of pantopaque in renal cysts. *Radiology* 119:747–748, 1976.
353. Pollack HM, Goldberg BB: Percutaneous needle endoscopy of renal cysts. *Radiology* 118:723–724, 1976.

CHAPTER 36

Renal Disorders in Sickle Hemoglobinemia

STEPHANIE LEAR & ROBERT M. ROSA

INTRODUCTION

Sickle hemoglobinemia, a term that refers to the presence of sickle hemoglobin (Hb-S) in either the heterozygous or homozygous form, has been associated with numerous and widely varying forms of disordered renal function, the majority of which are ultimately a consequence of the sickling process. In the presence of hypoxia, acidosis, or hyperosmolality (which causes red cells to shrink, thereby increasing the intracellular hemoglobin concentration), the rate of gelation and tactoid formation increases and red cells become sickled (1–5). When this morphologic change occurs in the capillary bed there is an increase in blood viscosity. Resistance to blood flow is thereby increased, passage of red cells through capillaries is further delayed, and more deoxygenation and sickling ensue. This process, which has been described as "a vicious cycle of erythrostasis" (6), can eventually lead to ischemia and infarction of tissue. In the relatively hypoxic, acidic, and hyperosmolar environment of the renal medulla, such a process will eventually produce obliteration of the vasa recta, focal scarring, medullary interstitial fibrosis, papillary necrosis, and tubular atrophy, which are the pathologic hallmarks of sickle-cell nephropathy (7–11). It is this widespread pathologic disruption of renal medullary anatomic integrity that accounts for most of the renal disorders that afflict patients with sickle hemoglobinemia.

DISORDERS OF RENAL FUNCTION

Hyposthenuria

The most prevalent abnormality of sickle-cell nephropathy is the inability of the kidney to excrete a concentrated urine. This observation was initially made by Herrick in the very first case of sickle-cell anemia reported: "the urine was amber in color, specific gravity 1.010 to 1.014, slightly increased in amount — 2000 c.c." (12). This defect in urinary concentrating ability is more severe in the homozygous than the heterozygous state, but in both it worsens with age (13–15). The maximal urinary concentration of Hb-SS patients older than 10 years of age is in the range of 400–450 mOsm/kg H_2O and does not decline further with age, whereas the maximal urinary concentration of Hb-AS patients is closer to normal in early childhood and declines progressively with age until by the fifth decade it approaches a similar range.

The hyposthenuria of sickle-cell nephropathy is not caused by either an impaired release of antidiuretic hormone or an impaired renal response to antidiuretic hormone, since Hb-SS patients have a normal capacity to reabsorb free water ($T^c_{H_2O}$) under conditions of solute loading (16, 17). Tubular transport of sodium is also not different from that of normal subjects under conditions of sodium loading or when the tubular sodium load is low (water diuresis) (18). The normal capacity to reabsorb free water strongly suggests that the impaired ability to concentrate urine maximally is a consequence of damage to the medulla and papillae in sickle-cell nephropathy. Papillectomy in rats, which selectively removes nephrons originating in the juxtamedullary cortex, produce a similar dissociation in water metabolism (19). The best interpretation of this observation is that the cortical nephrons with short loops of Henle are primarily responsible for $T^c_{H_2O}$ during solute loading, while the juxtamedullary nephrons with long loops of Henle that enter the papillae are required for achieving maximal urinary osmolality.

The ability to restore normal renal concentrating ability in young children with sickle-cell anemia by multiple transfusions of normal red blood cells (13, 20) would suggest that the hyposthenuria may have both a functional and a histopathologic component. Early in life, sickling within the vasa recta of the hyperosmotic medulla and papillae, with its attendant increase in blood viscosity, may impair oxygen and substrate delivery to renal tubular cells and limit the reabsorption of chloride and sodium necessary to trap solute and produce a maximally concentrated urine (5). With advancing age, repetitive episodes of sickling and energy deprivation would produce the irreversible medullary interstitial and papillary infarction and fibrosis characteristically observed. Finally, the ability to dilute urine normally in sickle-cell nephropathy (13, 14, 18) is not surprising, since this is predominantly a function of the cortical diluting segment of the cortical nephrons.

Hematuria

Hematuria in patients with sickle hemoglobinemia is a common and occasionally dramatic event. It is usually painless and may occur after heavy exertion or flank trauma, and may persist for weeks to months, producing life-threatening anemia (9, 21, 22). Although the incidence of hematuria in patients with sickle hemoglobinemia is unknown, hematuria has been reported to occur much more commonly in patients with Hb-AS than in those with Hb-SS, Hb-SC, or sickle-thalassemia (23, 24). This apparent increased incidence in patients with Hb-AS is probably a result of the much greater prevalence of Hb-AS in the population. The often-stated predilection for males over females may represent sampling bias.

Hematuria complicating sickle-cell nephropathy occurs at any age and is almost always unilateral, the left kidney being the source four times more frequently than the right (23), an observation that remains without adequate explanation. The etiology of the hematuria is undoubtedly related to the environment of the renal medulla, which fosters the sickling process. Studies of kidneys removed because of unilateral hematuria have demonstrated congestion and hemorrhage in the renal pelvis and severe stasis in the peritubular capillaries of the medulla, with peritubular hemorrhage and extravasation of blood into the tubules (9). Microradioangiographic studies have also demonstrated almost a complete absence of vasa recta in patients with sickle-cell anemia and a partial loss of vasa recta in patients with Hb-AS (7). If the juxtamedullary microvascular pattern of humans is similar to that of the dog and the rat, in which the efferent vessels divide to form the vasa recta and the peritubular capillaries of the juxtamedullary nephrons as well as nutrient vessels for the renal pelvic mucosa (25, 26), then an explanation for the hematuria is apparent. Progressive obliteration of vasa recta from infarction due to sickling might increase the flow and congestion in the peritubular and pelvic branches, leading to the hemorrhagic pattern observed. Such a mechanism might also account for the marked enlargement and engorgement of juxtamedullary glomeruli that is characteristic (8, 11, 27, 28).

Patients with sickle-cell nephropathy and hematuria have almost a 50% likelihood of rebleeding at some future time (23). Since filling defects in the renal pelvis and calyces caused by clotted blood are one of the most common radiographic findings in this setting, many patients underwent nephrectomies unnecessarily before the association between sickle hemoglobin and hematuria was appreciated because of concern that the filling defects represented neoplasms. Unexplained hematuria in a black patient is, therefore, a mandate to test for the presence of sickle hemoglobin.

Papillary necrosis and renal infarction

Thrombosis of the medullary vasculature from sickling very commonly produces papillary necrosis, which is usually asymptomatic and is discovered by intravenous pyelography. In some cases the incidence of radiographically diagnosed papillary necrosis approximates 50%, even in patients with no urologic symptoms (29–31). Various patterns of urographic papillary abnormalities have been described that are felt to be consistent with papillary necrosis. These abnormalities include linear streaks of contrast material extending laterally from the forniceal angle, cavities in the forniceal angle, total obliteration of the forniceal angle with papillary effacement, and central cavities in the papillae (30). Other abnormalities commonly observed by radiographic studies of patients with sickle hemoglobin are poor visualization of the collecting system, blunting of the calyces, parenchymal scarring, and arterial pruning (32–34). In addition to papillary necrosis, sickling may produce renal cortical infarcts and, rarely, large perinephric hematomas (35–38).

Vasodilatory prostaglandins are ordinarily produced in abundance in the renal medulla. Ischemic damage to the inner medulla as a result of sickling might be expected to impair the synthesis of vasodilator prostaglandins. Although urinary PGE_2 excretion was found to be normal during conditions of diuresis and antidiuresis in patients with sickle-cell anemia, urinary $PGF_{2\text{-alpha}}$ levels were significantly decreased (39). In addition, a normal vasopressin-prostaglandin relationship has been demonstrated in sickle-cell anemia (40).

There is also evidence to suggest that stimulation or synthesis of erythropoietin is submaximal in sickle cell patients, even without overt renal insufficiency (41). This observation is consistent with the theory that the site of erythropoietin production is the renal medulla.

Urinary tract infections

The incidence of asymptomatic bacteriuria during pregnancy and the puerperium is much greater in women with sickle-cell trait or sickle-cell anemia than in women without sickle-cell hemoglobin (42, 43). Further, those pregnant women with sickle hemoglobin and asymptomatic bacteriuria are more likely to develop an overt urinary tract infection during pregnancy. While it is contended that this may correlate with the increased incidence at autopsy of "pyelonephritis" in patients with Hb-AS (44), the pathologic changes seen in sickle-cell nephropathy could easily be misinterpreted as pyelonephritis. At present, it is uncertain whether this population with urinary tract infection is at increased risk for spontaneous abortion, premature delivery, or perinatal death (43, 45).

Defect in acidification and potassium excretion

A mild, incomplete form of distal renal tubular acidosis occurs in patients with Hb-SS and Hb-SC disease, though not in patients with Hb-AS and normal glomerular filtration rates (46–50). When challenged with a standard ammonium chloride load, these patients cannot maximally acidify their urine, and titratable acid and total hydrogen excretion are lower than in normal controls. Ammonia excretion appears to be appropriate for the urine pH in most reported studies. Oral administration of phosphate does not correct the defect, although titratable acid and hydrogen secretion increase when phosphate is given with the ammonium chloride load. Urine can be maximally acidified, however, with infusion of sodium sulfate (47). There is no definite evidence that bicarbonate reabsorption is abnormal (47).

While patients with sickle-cell anemia and normal glomerular filtration rates are not normally acidotic (51), hyperchloremic metabolic acidosis with hyperkalemia has been described in patients with Hb-SS, Hb-AS, and Hb-SC, usually in the setting of impaired glomerular filtration (52, 53). While some of these patients have hypoaldosteronism with or without hyporeninism to account for the acidosis and hyperkalemia in conjunction with decreased filtration, impaired renal excretion of an acute potassium load has also been described in sicklemic patients with normal glomerular filtration rates and normal renins and aldosterones (50). Given the importance of the contribution of the distal tubule and the collecting duct in acid and potassium excretion (56), the state of functional papillectomy in these patients is undoubtedly responsible for these defects.

Renal metabolism of uric acid, phosphate, and magnesium

Although uric acid overproduction is common in patients with sickle-cell anemia, gout is not (57–59). Despite overproduction, young adults with sickle-cell anemia are usually normouricemic because renal urate clearance is enhanced. The enhanced urate clearance may be related to the increased effective renal plasma flow (C_{PAH}) observed early in the course of sickle-cell nephropathy (15, 59, 60) and to improved tubular secretion of uric acid. Diminished resorption of secreted urate might also account for the increased urate clearance. With increasing age, urate clearance declines, as does renal function and the incidence of hyperuricemia increases (61).

Some patients with sickle-cell anemia have elevated serum phosphorus and magnesium levels with a normal serum calcium and normal glomerular filtration rate. In such patients, the maximal tubular reabsorption of phosphate per deciliter of glomerular filtrate (T_mP/GFR) is increased while urinary calcium is decreased. An interesting explanation for this curious collection of electrolyte abnormalities is that such patients may be mildly volume contracted from their hyposthenuria. Volume depletion would tend to enhance proximal tubular resorption of sodium, calcium, and magnesium. Increased renal calcium resorption would tend to suppress parathyroid hormone release, there by increasing T_mP/GFR (62). Another indicator of enhanced proximal tubular reabsorptive activity has been noted in sickle-cell anemia; there is increased uptake of beta$_2$-microglobulin, which correlates with phosphate reabsorption (40).

Of interest, an increased frequency of painful crises has been noted in sickle-cell patients with hyperphosphatemia as compared to those with normal serum phosphate levels. Although the reason for this observation is not clear, the mechanism may involve the effect of serum phosphate on erythrocyte 2,3-DPG metabolism and the hemoglobin-oxygen dissociation curve (63).

Glomerular disease

While increased values of GFR and effective renal plasma flow have been observed in infants with Hb-SS (15, 60), these values are generally normal in young adults (13–15, 64) and may be decreased in some older patients (65, 66). The etiology of the supranormal filtration rate and renal plasma flow is not understood, but a course of transfusion either to correct the anemia or to achieve almost complete replacement of Hb-S by Hb-A does not reduce these values (20).

Proteinuria is a common finding in sickle-cell anemia. The actual prevalence may be as high as 30% although the amount is usually not greater than 500 mg/l (67). Protein excretion in the nephrotic range, though uncommon, occurs more frequently than can be ascribed to chance alone (68–76). The clinical course of the nephrotic syndrome seen in patients with sickle-cell anemia is variable. Proteinuria varies from moderate to severe, glomerular filtration rate may be normal or markedly decreased, and occasionally end-stage chronic renal failure may occur in less than 1 year (68, 70). Hypertension may also accompany the nephrotic syndrome (68, 75), and one case of renal vein thrombosis has been documented (76). Three patients with sickle-cell trait who developed chronic renal failure, which in two instances was preceded by nephrotic-range proteinuria, have also been described (77).

The most consistent finding on light microscopy in patients with nephrotic syndrome and sickle-cell anemia is a membranoproliferative glomerulonephritis with reduplication of the glomerular basement membrane and mesangial proliferation (73, 75). Other findings include segmental or diffuse sclerosis of the glomeruli, interstitial fibrosis, tubular atrophy and dilatation, and intimal thickening and hyalinization of the vasculature. Serum complement levels, however, are characteristically normal.

Electron microscopy reveals mesangial cytoplasmic processes sandwiched in between the lamina densa of the glomerular basement membrane and the endothelium. The finding of electron-dense deposits in the glomeruli or mesangium has been variable (70, 73, 75).

Immunofluorescent studies have also yielded varying results. While studies of some patients reveal no significant staining on immunofluorescence (65), others demonstrate immunoglobulin and complement components distributed in a granular pattern along the glomerular basement membrane in all of the patients studied (75), suggesting immune-complex glomerular disease. The nature of a possible immune-complex glomerulonephritis has been somewhat clarified by the discovery of a cold-insoluble complex of renal tubular antigen and antibody in the blood of a patient with immune-complex membranoproliferative glomerulonpehritis and sickle-cell anemia (78). The cryoprotein contained IgG, IgM, and renal tubular epithelial antigen. Subsequently, a patient with sickle-cell anemia and membranoproliferative glomerulonephritis was found to have renal tubular epithelial antigen in association with IgG, IgM, Cl_q, and C_3 in a granular pattern along the glomerular basement membrane (79). Most recently, a patient with Hb-AS and significant, but not nephrotic-range, proteinuria had cryoprecipitable complexes of renal tubular epithelial antigen and antibody in the serum and deposits of renal tubular epithelial antigen, immunoglobulins, and complement localized in the glomerular basement membrane. Immunoglobulin, complement, and renal tubular epithelial antigen were also present in the proximal tubules (80).

Despite the morphologic and immunologic data acquired, the pathogenesis of proteinuria in patients with sickle-cell nephropathy has not been well established. The presence of electron-dense particles, thought to represent complexes of iron and protein, in glomerular cells (predominantly in the mesangium) led to speculation that iron released during hemolysis of sickled cells might be responsible for the proteinuria (70). This hypothesis is based on the observation that saccharated iron-oxide injections produce proteinuria in rabbits (86, 87). An alternate explanation might be that ischemia in the renal microcirculation from sickling could lead to the release of renal tubular epithelial antigens producing circulating antigen-antibody immune complexes with ultimate glomerular complex deposition and nephritis (78–80).

The development of renal failure, often associated with the nephrotic syndrome after an early phase of hyperfiltration, is also consistent with the hypothesis of glomerular hyperfiltration described in the remnant kidney model (28). Progressive ischemia and infarction caused by sickling in the medullary microvasculature is probably the proximate cause of loss of functioning renal tissue, resulting in compensatory hyperfiltration in the remaining nephrons. This hypothesis is supported by histologic studies in children with sickle-cell disease that demonstrate glomerular enlargement (10, 81, 82) and by a recent study of children with sickle-cell disease who underwent renal biopsy because of persistent proteinuria or the nephrotic syndrome (83). Renal biopsy in 8 of 13 children demonstrated glomerulosclerosis, and the remaining five showed mesangial proliferation. In addition, there are case reports of the nephrotic syndrome in sickle-cell anemia due to focal glomerulosclerosis (81, 83–85). In light of the increased glomerular surface area and hyperfiltration found in young patients with sickle-cell anemia, it is reasonable to postulate that, like the experimental models of subtotal renal ablation, hyperfiltration per se may result in glomerulosclerosis and renal insufficiency.

Whatever the mechanism, end-stage renal failure, often preceded by the nephrotic syndrome, is a well-known complication of sickle-cell anemia (68, 70, 74, 88). Indeed, the number of patients with sickle-cell anemia who develop chronic renal failure and uremia may be increasing in this country, since it is likely that the treatment of infection, the most common cause of death during the first decade of life (89), is improving. This contention is supported by a recent study that found that renal failure was the second most common cause of death in 52 patients with sickle-cell anemia and was more common in adults than in children (90).

Other disorders

Acute renal failure associated with rhabdomyolysis and disseminated intravascular coagulation has been reported in military recruits with the sickle-cell trait following vigorous exercise (91, 92). It is speculated that patients with Hb-AS may be more at risk for this complication than those with Hb-SS, since the former can achieve more vigorous degrees of exercise than the latter. Such exercise, if associated with sufficient degrees of dehydration, hypotension, and increased blood viscosity, might accelerate the rate of sickling with subsequent muscle infarction, leading to acute renal failure. Finally, a patient with sickle-cell disease has been described who suffered extensive marrow infarction with peripheral fat embolization to the brain, lungs, and kidneys. Uremia developed and death ensued. Postmortem analysis revealed fat globules in the glomerular capillaries and in some of the capillaries of the renal tubules (93).

PREVENTION

The inheritance of Hb-S follows classic Mendelian genetics. It is estimated that approximately 8% of all black Americans have sickle-cell trait. While the incidence of sickle-cell anemia can be estimated to be approximately 1 in 625, it is difficult to predict the actual prevalence of sickle-cell anemia in the entire black population since the lifespan of these patients is not known (94). At the present time, prevention of inheritance of Hb-S rests entirely upon broad screening programs and subsequent genetic counseling of those harboring the gene.

THERAPY

General considerations

While there are numerous interesting and diverse disorders of renal function in sickle-cell nephropathy, some have no or minimal clinical consequence and, therefore, require no treatment. Hyposthenuria, for example, will not lead to dehydration if there is free access to water unless there are excessive fluid losses, vomiting, or diarrhea. The average solute load of 600–800 mOsm per day can readily be excreted in a urine volume of about 2 l per day. Should nonrenal fluid loss be excessive because of concurrent illness or a hot climate, fluid intake should be increased to more than 2 l/day.

The mild impairment in urinary acidification and in potassium excretion were discovered under conditions of acid or potassium loading (46–48, 50). Spontaneous hyperchloremic metabolic acidosis and hyperkalemia have been documented, although usually in the setting of a decreased glomerular filtration rate, stress, or a painful crisis (52, 53). Treatment consists of volume expansion, sodium polystyrene sulfonate administration when indicated, and appropriate tests to exclude aldosterone deficiency. The abnormalities in the renal metabolism of uric acid, phosphate, calcium, and magnesium in patients with sickle-cell nephropathy described above have no known clinical significance. The incidence of urolithiasis is not increased in this population.

Hematuria

Hematuria in patients with sickle-cell nephropathy can be a dramatic and, occasionally, life-threatening event. Initial treatment should be directed toward lowering the osmolality of the renal medulla, since modest decrements in osmolarity, by expanding red cell size, will lower the intracellular concentration of Hb-S and decrease the tendency of cells to sickle (2–4, 95). This goal may be best achieved by the administration of water by mouth or hypotonic solutions intravenously (e.g., 5% dextrose) in conjunction with either loop diuretics or mannitol to achieve a high rate of urine flow. Sodium bicarbonate may also be useful by increasing the medullary pH and, possibly, by helping to lower the medullary osmolarity (96). Conventional therapy for protracted renal bleeding is exchange transfusion, a modality that should be reserved for the most serious cases because of the growing concern over transmission of hepatitis and human immunodeficiency viruses. While administration of epsilon-aminocaproic acid has been advocated by some (97, 98), its potential hazards warrant its use only should the aforementioned therapies fail. Nephrectomy should be considered only as a last resort in patients with life-threatening bleeding refractory to all other therapy.

Finally, it should be stated that patients with Hb-S and protracted, severe hematuria should be investigated, as should other patients with abnormal bleeding, for the presence of a coagulation disorder. To date, five patients with sickle-cell trait and hematuria have been found to have coexisting von Willebrand's disease. In this situation, cryoprecipitate should be administered to stop bleeding (99, 100).

Papillary necrosis and urinary tract infection

While papillary necrosis is an extremely common radiographic finding in patients with sickle-cell disease, it is asymptomatic in the majority of instances (29–31). The recognition of papillary necrosis becomes important, however, in the setting of a septic patient with pyelonephritis who fails to respond to appropriate antibiotic therapy. Ultrasound examination of the kidneys is then mandatory to look for obstruction that may require surgical intervention. If the ultrasound examination is nondiagnostic, intravenous pyelography should be done to look for obstruction.

Although the incidence of asymptomatic bacteriuria during pregnancy and puerperium is much greater in women with sickle-cell trait or sickle-cell anemia, and such people are more likely to develop and overt urinary tract infection, it is less certain that the incidence of "pyelonephritis" is greater in this population (42–45). Sickle-cell nephropathy alone may produce both radiologic and pathologic evidence that is indistinguishable from pyelonephritis caused by bacterial invasion of the kidney. Despite this caveat and the uncertainty about whether this population is at increased risk for fetal morbidity or mortality (42, 43, 45), it seems reasonable to recommend very close surveillance for evidence of urinary infection in this population.

In theory, papillary necrosis and scarring might be prevented or minimized if the interstitial milieu of the renal papilla was rendered isotonic rather than hypertonic over long periods of time through sustained water diuresis, thus reducing the tendency to sickling of red blood cells in the vasa recta. Such prolonged forcing of fluids is difficult to achieve in practice, and there are no prospective data bearing on its efficacy in the prevention of renal complications. The propensity of erythrocytes with SS hemoglobin to sickle in a hypertonic, anoxic environment should, however, serve as a rationale to avoid dehydration whenever possible in children with sickle-cell disease, since this may predispose to sickling and consequent erythrostasis in a hypertonic renal medulla. Nonsteroidal antiinflammatory agents that inhibit prostaglandin synthesis should likewise be avoided, since they may further reduce blood flow to the papilla and exacerbate ischemic damage.

Recently, two experimental and theoretically appealing approaches to decrease red cell sickling by expanding red cell volume have been reported. The first involves the production of sustained dilutional hyponatremia, achieved by the administration of DDAVP, increased fluid intake, and sodium restriction (95). A second experimental strategy involves the use of cardiac glycosides to inhibit Na-K-ATPase, thereby promoting an increase in intracellular cation and water content, with concomitant increases in red cell volume (103). Further in vitro studies and clinical trials are warranted.

Glomerular disease

End-stage chronic renal failure, often preceded by the nephrotic syndrome, is being described with increasing frequency in patients with Hb-S, particularly in those who are homozygous (68, 70, 74, 77, 88). As suggested, this phenomenon may be a consequence of a prolonged life span as the result of more effective treatment of infection, the leading cause of death in the first decade of life in this population (89, 90).

Although steroids, ACTH, and cyclophosphamide have all been administered in an attempt to ameliorate the proteinuria or to retard the deterioration of renal function in these patients, there is no convincing evidence of the benefit of such therapies (69, 70, 72, 75). Therapy for ESRD in patients with sickle-cell anemia involves all conventional modalities of renal replacement, including hemodialysis, peritoneal dialysis, and transplantation. Initial concerns about increased clotting of the dialysis membrane precipitated by sickling have not been substantiated, though thrombosis of the vascular access may be a recurrent problem (75, 88, 101). Successful transplantation of both cadaveric and living, related-donor renal allografts in sickle-cell patients has been reported in a growing number of centers. However, the reemergence of numerous severe painful crises after transplantation was reported, and these were best explained by the simultaneous rise in hematocrit (101). In spite of good renal function after transplantation, a defect in urinary concentration has been noted (102).

ACKNOWLEDGMENT

Supported in part by a grant from the General Clinical Research Centers Branch of the Division of Research Resources of the National Institutes of Health, Grant MO1 RR 01032.

REFERENCES

1. Murayama M: Molecular mechanism of red cell "sickling." *Science* 153:145–149, 1966.
2. Greenberg MS, Kass EH, Castle WB: Studies on the destruction of red blood cells. XII. Factors influencing the role of S hemoglobin in the pathologic physiology of sickle cell anemia and related disorders. *J Clin Invest* 36:833–843, 1957.
3. May A, Huehns ER: The concentration dependence of the oxygen affinity of haemoglobin S. *Br J Haematol* 30:317–335, 1975.
4. Bookchin RM, Balazs T, Landau LC: Determinants of red cell sickling: Effects of varying pH and of increasing intracellular hemoglobin concentrations by osmotic shrinkage. *J Lab Clin Med* 87:597–616, 1976.
5. Perillie PE, Epstein FH: Sickling phenomenon produced by hypertonic solutions: A possible explanation for the hyposthenuria of sicklemia. *J Clin Invest* 42:570–580, 1963.
6. Ham TH, Castle WB: Relation of increased hypotonic fragility and of erythrostasis to the mechanism of hemolysis in certain anemias. *Trans Assoc Am Physicians* 55:127–132, 1940.
7. Statius van Eps LW, Pinedo-Veels C, de Vries GH, de Koning J: Nature of concentrating defect in sickle-cell nephropathy: Microradioangiographic studies. *Lancet* 1:450–452, 1970.
8. Sydenstricked VP, Mulherin WA, Houseal RW: Sickle cell anemia. Report of two cases in children, with necropsy in one case. *Am J Dis Child* 26:132–154, 1923.
9. Mostofi FK, Vorder Bruegge CF, Diggs LW: Lesions in kidneys removed for unilateral hematuria in sickle-cell disease. *Arch Pathol* 63:336–351, 1957.
10. Pitcock JA, Muirhead EE, Hatch FE, Johnson JG, Kelly BJ: Early renal changes in sickle cell anemia. *Arch Pathol* 90:403–410, 1970.
11. Buckalew VM Jr, Someren A: Renal manifestations of sickle cell disease. *Arch Intern Med* 133:660–669, 1974.
12. Herrick JB: Peculiar elongated and sickle-shaped red blood corpuscles in a case of severe anemia. *Arch Intern Med* 6:517–521, 1910.
13. Keitel HG, Thompson D, Itano HA: Hyposthenuria in sickle cell anemia: A reversible renal defect. *J Clin Invest* 35:998–1007, 1956.
14. Schlitt L, Keitel HG: Pathogenesis of hyposthenuria in persons with sickle cell anemia or the sickle cell trait. *Pediatrics* 26:249–254, 1960.
15. Statius van Eps LW, Schouten H, ter Haar Romeny-Wachter CC, la Porte-Wijsman LW: The relation between age and renal concentrating capacity in sickle cell disease and hemoglobin C disease. *Clin Chem Acta* 27:501–511, 1970.
16. Levitt MF, Hauser AD, Levy MS, Polimeros D: The renal concentrating defect in sickle cell disease. *Am J Med* 29:611–622, 1960.
17. Whitten CF, Younes AA: A comparative study of renal concentrating ability in children with sickle cell anemia and in normal children. *J Lab Clin Med* 55:400–415, 1960.
18. Hatch FE, Culbertson JW, Diggs LW: Nature of the renal concentrating defect in sickle cell disease. *J Clin Invest* 46:336–345, 1967.
19. Lief PD, Sullivan A, Goldberg M: Physiological contributions of thin and thick loops of Henle to the renal concentrating mechanism. *J Clin Invest* 48:52a, 1969.
20. Statius van Eps LW, Schouten H, la Porte-Wijsman LW, Struyker Boudier AM: The influence of red blood cell transfusions on the hyposthenuria and renal hemodynamics of sickle cell anemia. *Clin Chim Acta* 17:449–461, 1967.
21. Abel MS, Brown CR: Sickle cell disease with severe hematuria simulating renal neoplasm. *JAMA* 136:624–625, 1948.
22. Goodwin WE, Alston EF, Semans JH: Hematuria and sickle cell disease: Unexplained, gross unilateral, renal hematuria in negroes, coincident with the blood sickling trait. *J Urol* 63:79–96, 1950.
23. Lucas WM, Bullock WH: Hematuria in sickle cell disease. *J Urol* 83:733–741, 1960.
24. Sharpe AR Jr, Fox PG Jr, Dodson AI Sr: Unilateral renal hematuria associated with sickle cell C disease and sickle cell trait: Study of five patients and review of literature. *J Urol* 81:780–783, 1959.
25. Moffat DB, Fourman J: The vascular pattern of the rat kidney. *J Anat* 97:543–553, 1963.
26. Thorburn GD, Kopald HH, Herd JA, Hollenberg M, O'Morchoe CCC, Barger AC: Intrarenal distribution of nutrient blood flow determined with Krypton^{85} in the unanesthetized dog. *Circ Res* 13:290–307, 1963.
27. Bernstein J, Whitten CF: A histological appraisal of the kidney in sickle cell anemia. *Arch Pathol* 70:407–418, 1960.
28. Hostetter TH, Olson JL, Rennke HG, Venkatachalam MA, Brenner BM: Hyperfiltration in remnant nephron: A potentially adverse response to renal ablation. *Am J Physiol* 241:F85–F93, 1981.
29. Harrow BR, Sloane JA, Liebman NC: Roentgenologic demonstration of renal papillary necrosis in sickle-cell trait. *N Engl J Med* 268:969–976, 1963.
30. Eckert DE, Jonutis AJ, Davidson AJ: The incidence and manifestations of urographic papillary abnormalities in patients with S hemoglobinopathies. *Radiology* 113:59–63, 1974.
31. Pandya KK, Koshy M, Brown N, Presman D: Renal papillary necrosis in sickle cell hemoglobinopathies. *J Urol* 115:497–501, 1976.
32. Margulies SI, Minkin SD: Sickle cell disease. The roentgenologic manifestations of urinary tract abnormalities in adults. *Am J Roentgen Rad Ther and Nucl Med* 107:702–710, 1969.
33. Khademi M, Marquis JR: Renal angiography in sickle-cell

disease. A preliminary report correlating the angiographic and urographic changes in sickle-cell nephropathy. *Radiology* 107:41–46, 1973.
34. Karayalcin G, Dorfman J, Rosner F, Aballi AJ: Radiological changes in 127 patients with sickle cell anemia. *Am J Med Sci* 271:132–144, 1976.
35. Kimmelstiel P: Vascular occlusion and ischemic infarction in sickle cell disease. *Am J Med Sci* 216:11–19, 1948.
36. Femi–Pearse D, Odunjo EO: Renal cortical infarcts in sickle-cell trait. *Br Med J* 3:34, 1968.
37. Miller WA, Peck D, Lowman RM: Perirenal hematoma in association with renal infarction in sickle cell trait. *Radiology* 92:351–352, 1969.
38. Sickles EA, Korobkin M: Perirenal hematoma as a complication of renal infarction in sickle-cell trait. *Am J Roentgenol* 122:800–803, 1974.
39. De Jong PE, Saleh AW, DeZeeuw D, Donker AJM, van Der Hem GK, Pratt JJ, Sewrahsingh GS, Statius van Eps LW: Urinary prostaglandins in sickle cell nephropathy: A defect in 9-ketoreductase activity? *Clin Nephrol* 22:212–213, 1984.
40. De Jong PE, Saleh AW, DeZeeuw D, Donker AJM, van Der Hem GK, Statius van Eps LW: Prostaglandin-vasopressin interaction in sickle cell nephropathy (abstract). *Kidney Int* 23:277, 1983.
41. Sherwood JB, Goldwasser E, Chilcote R, Carmichael LD, Nagel RL: Sickle cell anemia patients have low erythropoietin levels for their degree of anemia. *Blood* 67:46–49, 1986.
42. Whalley PJ, Martin FG, Pritchard JA: Sickle cell trait and urinary tract infection during pregnancy. *JAMA* 189:903–906, 1964.
43. Pathak UN, Tang K, Williams LL, Stuart KL: Bacteriuria of pregnancy: Results of treatment. *J Inf Dis* 120:91–95, 1969.
44. Amin UF, Ragbeer MS: The prevalence of pyelonephritis among sicklers and nonsicklers in an autopsy population. *West Ind Med J* 21:166, 1972.
45. Whalley PJ, Pritchard JA, Richards JR Jr: Sickle cell trait and pregnancy. *JAMA* 186:1132–1135, 1963.
46. Ho Ping Kong H, Alleyne GAO: Defect in urinary acidification in adults with sickle-cell anemia. *Lancet* 2:954–955, 1968.
47. Ho Ping Kong H, Alleyne GAO: Studies on acid excretion in adults with sickle-cell anemia. *Clin Sci* 41:505–518, 1971.
48. Goossens JP, Statius van Eps LW, Schouten H, Giterson AL: Incomplete renal tubular acidosis in sickle cell disease. *Clin Chim Acta* 41:149–156, 1972.
49. Oster JR, Lee SM, Lespier LE, Pellegrini EL, Vaamonde CA: Renal acidification in sickle cell trait. *Arch Intern Med* 136:30–35, 1976.
50. DeFronzo RA, Taufield PA, Black H, McPhedran P, Cooke CR: Impaired renal tubular potassium secretion in sickle disease. *Ann Intern Med* 90:310–316, 1979.
51. Ho Ping Kong H, Alleyne GAO: Acid-base status of adults with sickle-cell anemia. *Br Med J* 3:271–273, 1969.
52. Battle D, Itsarayoungyven K, Arruda JAL, Kurtzman NA: Hyperkalemic hyperchloremic metabolic acidosis in sickle cell hemoglobinopathies *Am J Med* 72:188–192, 1982.
53. DeFronzo RA. Hyperkalemia and hyporeninemic hypoaldosteronism. *Kidney Int* 17:118–134, 1980.
54. Yoshino M, American R, Brautbar N: Hyporeninemic hypoaldosteronism in sickle cell disease. *Nephron* 31:242–244, 1982.
55. Rosansky SJ, Kennedy M: Sickle cell trait with episodic acute renal failure and Type IV renal tubular acidosis (letter). *Ann Intern Med* 93:643, 1980.
56. Finkelstein FO, Hayslett JP: Role of medullary structures in the functional adaptation of renal insufficiency. *Kidney Int* 6:419–425, 1974.
57. Gold MS, Williams JC, Spivack M, Grann V: Sickle cell anemia and hyperuricemia. *JAMA* 206:1572–1573, 1968.
58. Diamond H: Renal handling of uric acid in sickle cell anemia. *Adv Exp Med Biol* 41B:759–762, 1973.
59. Diamond HS, Meisel A, Sharon E, Holden D, Cacatian A: Hyperuricosuria and increased tubular secretion of urate in sickle cell anemia. *Am J Med* 59:796–802, 1975.
60. Etteldorf JN, Tuttle AH, Clayton GW: Renal function studies in pediatrics. I, Renal hemodynamics in children with sickle cell anemia. *Am J Dis Child* 83:185–191, 1952.
61. Diamond H, Meisel A, Holden D, Sharon E, Cacatian A, Virdi R: Hypcruricemia in Sickle Cell Anemia. In: JI Hercules, AN Schecter, WA Eaton, RE Jackson, eds, *Proceedings, First National Symposium on Sickle Cell Anemia*, Department of Health, Education, and Welfare, Bethesda, MD, Publication No. 75–723, p 371, 1974.
62. de Jong PE, de Jong–van den Berg LTW, Statius van Eps LW: The tubular reabsorption of phosphate in sickle-cell nephropathy. *Clin Sci Mol Med* 55:429–434, 1978.
63. Smith EC, Valike KS, Woo JE, O'Donnell JG, Gordon DL, Westerman MP: Serum phosphate abnormalities in sickle cell anemia. *Proc Soc Exp Biol Med* 168:254–258, 1981.
64. Hatch FE Jr, Azar SH, Ainsworth TE, Nardo JM, Culbertson JW: Renal circulatory studies in young adults with sickle cell anemia. *J Lab Clin Med* 76:632–640, 1970.
65. Etteldorf JN, Smith JD, Tuttle AH, Diggs LW: Renal hemodynamic studies in adults with sickle cell anemia. *Am J Med* 18:243–248, 1955.
66. Morgan AG, Serjeant GR: Renal function in patients over 40 with homozygous sickle cell disease. *Br Med J* 282:1181–1183, 1982.
67. Henderson AB: Sickle cell anemia. Clinical study of fifty-four cases. *Am J Med* 9:757–765, 1950.
68. Berman LB, Schreiner GE: Clinical and histologic spectrum of the nephrotic syndrome. *Am J Med* 24:249–267, 1958.
69. Berman LB, Tublin I: The nephropathies of sickle-cell disease. *Arch Intern Med* 103:602–606, 1959.
70. McCoy RC: Ultrastructural alterations in the kidney of patients with sickle cell disease and the nephrotic syndrome. *Lab Invest* 21:85–95, 1969.
71. Miller RE, Hartley MW, Clark EC, Lupton CH Jr: Sickle cell nephropathy. *Ala J Med Sci* 1:233–238, 1964.
72. Sweeney MJ, Dobbins WT, Etteldorf JN: Renal disease with elements of the nephrotic syndrome associated with sickle cell anemia. A report of 2 cases. *J Pediatr* 60:42–51, 1962.
73. Elfenbein IB, Patchefsky A, Schwartz W, Weinstein AG: Pathology of the glomerulus in sickle cell anemia with and without nephrotic syndrome. *Am J Pathol* 77:357–376, 1974.
74. Walker BR, Alexander F, Birdsall TR, Warren RL: Glomerular lesions in sickle cell nephropathy, *JAMA* 215:437–440, 1971.
75. Pardo V, Strauss J, Kramer H, Ozawa T, McIntosh RM: Nephropathy associated with sickle cell anemia: An autologous immune complex nephritis. II. Clinicopathologic study of seven patients. *Am J Med* 59:650–659, 1975.
76. Strom T, Muehrcke RC, Smith RD: Sickle cell anemia with the nephrotic syndrome and renal vein obstruction. *Arch Intern Med* 129:104–108, 1972.
77. Nicholson GD, Amin UF, Brooks SEH, Alleyne GAO: End-stage renal failure in sickle cell trait. *West Ind Med J*

28:235–239, 1979.
78. Strauss J, Koss M, Griswold W, Chernack W, Pardo V, McIntosh RM: Cryoprecipitable immune complexes, nephropathy, and sickle-cell disease (letter). *Ann Intern Med* 81:114–115, 1974.
79. Strauss J, Pardo V, Koss MN, Griswold W, McIntosh RM: Nephropathy associated with sickle cell anemia: An autologous immune complex nephritis. I. Studies on nature of glomerular-bound antibody and antigen indentification in a patient with sickle cell disease and immune deposit glomerulonephritis. *Am J Med* 58:382–387, 1975.
80. Ozawa T, Mass MF, Guggenheim S, Strauss J, McIntosh RM: Autologous immune complex nephritis associated with sickle cell trait: Diagnosis of the haemoglobinopathy after renal structural and immunological studies. *Br Med J* 1:369–371, 1976.
81. Buckalew VM, Someren A: Renal manifestations of sickle cell disease. *Arch Intern Med* 133:660–669, 1974.
82. Bernstein J, Whitten CF: A histological appraisal of the kidney in sickle cell anemia. *Arch Pathol* 70:407–418, 1970.
83. Tejani A, Nicastri A, Chen CK, Sen D, Phadke K, Adamson O: Renal lesions in sickle cell nephropathy in children. *Nephron* 39:352–356, 1985.
84. McCoy RC: Ultrastructural alterations in the kidney with sickle cell disease and the nephrotic syndrome. *Lab Invest* 21:85–95, 1969.
85. Lippner-Markenson AJ, Chandra M, Lewy JE, Miller DR: Sickle Cell anemia, the nephrotic syndrome and hypoplastic crisis in a sibship. *Am J Med* 64:719–723, 1978.
86. Ellis JT: Glomerular lesions and the nephrotic syndrome in rabbits given saccharated iron oxide intravenously. *J Exp Med* 103:127–144, 1956.
87. Ellis JT: Glomerular lesions in rabbits with experimentally induced proteinuria as disclosed by electron microscopy. *Am J Pathol* 34:559–560, 1958.
88. Friedman EA, Sreepada Rao TK, Sprung CL, Smith A, Manis T, Bellevus R, Butt KMH, Levere RD, Holden DM: Uremia in sickle-cell anemia treated by maintenance hemodialysis. *N Engl J Med* 291:431–435, 1974.
89. Powers DR: Natural history of sickle cell disease — the first ten years. *Semin Hemat* 12:267–285, 1975.
90. Gerry JL Jr, Bulkley BH, Hutchins GM: Clinicopathologic analysis of cardiac dysfunction in 52 patients with sickle cell anemia. *Am J Cardiol* 42:211–216, 1978.
91. Koppes GM, Daly JJ, Coltman CA Jr, Butkus DE: Exertion-induced rhabdomyolysis with acute renal failure and disseminated intravascular coagulation in sickle cell trait. *Am J Med* 63:313–317, 1977.
92. Kark JA, Posey DM, Schumacher HR, Ruehle CJ: Sickle cell trait as a risk factor for sudden death in physical training. *N Engl J Med* 317:781–787, 1987.
93. Evans PV, Symmes AT: Bone marrow infarction with fat embolism and nephrosis in sickle cell disease. *J Indiana Med Assoc* 50:1101–1105, 1957.
94. Motulsky AG: Frequency of sickling disorders in U.S. blacks. *N Engl J Med* 288:31–33, 1973.
95. Rosa RM, Bierer BE, Thomas R, Stoff JS, Kruskall M, Robinson S, Bunn HF, Epstein FH: A study of induced hyponatremia in the prevention and treatment of sickle-cell crisis. *N Engl J Med* 303:1138–1143, 1980.
96. Knochel JP: Hematuria in sickle cell trait: The effect of intravenous administration of distilled water, urinary alkalinization, and diuresis. *Arch Intern Med* 123:160–165, 1969.
97. Immergut MA, Stevenson T: The use of epsilon amino caproic acid in the control of hematuria associated with hemoglobinopathies. *J Urol* 93:110–111, 1965.
98. Sweeney WM: Aminocaproic acid, inhibitor of fibrinolysis. *Am J Med Sci* 249:576–589, 1965.
99. Brody JI, Levison SP, Jung CJ: Sickle cell trait and hematuria associated with von Willebrand syndromes. *Ann Intern Med* 86:529–533, 1977.
100. Weinger RS, Benson GS, Villarreal S: Gross hematuria associated with sickle call trait and von Willebrand's disease. *J Urol* 122:136–137, 1979.
101. Chatterjee SN, National study on natural history of renal allografts in sickle cell disease or trait. *Nephron* 25:199–201, 1980.
102. Spector D, Zachary JB, Sterioff S, Millan J: Painful crises following renal transplantation in sickle cell anemia. *Am J Med* 64:835–839, 1978.
103. Izumo H, Lear S, Williams M, Rosa R, Epstein FH: Sodium-potassium pump, ion fluxes, and cellular dehydration in sickle cell anemia. *J Clin Invest* 79:1621–1628, 1987.

CHAPTER 37

Inherited Renal Tubular Disorders

RUSSELL W. CHESNEY

INTRODUCTION

A number of clinical syndromes have been described that have as their basic foundation a defect in some transport function of the renal tubule (Table 1). Using this paradigm, one can define conditions in which single or multiple substances are lost, in which ions or organic solutes are lost, and in which the whole body pools of these substances are altered because of excessive urinary excretion. The basic pathophysiologic mechanisms underlying these transport disorders are described elsewhere (1–4). The purpose of this chapter is to describe the current form of therapy in these conditions.

AMINOACIDURIAS

Several of the aminoacidurias including *iminoglycinuria*, in which excessive amounts of L-proline, hydroxy-L-proline, and glycine are found in the urine, are benign traits and require no therapy (5). In *dicarboxylic aminoaciduria*, no specific clinical features are apparent and thus no therapy is recommended (6).

Hartnup disease is a condition with massive aminoaciduria of the neutral monomamino-monocarboxylic amino acids, as well as intestinal malabsorption of the same compounds. Because of tryptophan malabsorption, affected patients develop the features of pellagra (7) since they cannot produce adequate nicotinamide. The appreciable clinical features in this disorder can be alleviated by nicotinamide (40–150 mg daily) or an American diet containing green leafy vegetables. Provision of nicotinamide heals the red scaly rash and improves the neurologic problems (7).

Renal and urinary tract stores develop in *cystinuria*, an autosomal recessive disorder in which the poorly soluble disulfide amino acid is excreted into the urine in increased amounts (7). This heterogeneous condition is found in 1 in 12,000 persons worldwide and thus is a moderately frequent cause of nephrolithiasis. The treatment of *cystinuria* has been modified by several recent advances. As always, the initial goal is to lower the urinary concentration of cystine below its solubility limit (8). A high fluid intake will generally accomplish this task, since it dilutes urinary cystine. However, this form of therapy requires strict compliance and ingestion of liquids around the clock, with nocturnal rising to empty the bladder and imbibition of additional fluid. In general, patients are also recommended to take oral alkali, such as $NaHCO_3$ 650 mg q 6–8 hr, since cystine solubility is also pH dependent. The urinary solubility of cystine rises steeply at a pH higher than 7.5 (9).

If these measures fail, the next line of therapy is oral D-penicillamine. D-penicillamine (dimethylcystine) is a mercapton that undergoes an in-vivo disulfide exchange reaction with cystine, thereby causing the urinary excretion of a more soluble penicillamine-cystine mixed disulfide. In parallel, the concentration of cystine in the urine of a cystinuric subject actually falls (8). Although treatment with oral D-penicillamine at 1–2 g/day in the adult and 30 mg/kg in the child is highly effective in reducing urinary cystine excretion below 200–300 mg/24 hr, patient tolerance is poor and side effects are disturbingly frequent (10). Serious side effects requiring abandonment of the use of this agent occur in 30–50% of patients. The major side effects are skin rash, membranous or linear IgG anti-GBM antibody-induced nephropathy, nausea, emesis, impairment or loss of smell or taste, and pemphigus (8, 10).

Because of these serious side-effects, several additional sulfhydryl compounds that could potentially lower urinary cystine content by mixed disulfide formation have been considered. The greatest experience has been gained in the use of 2-mercapto-propionylglycine (α-MPG). α-MPG leads to mixed disulfide formation and is 1½ times as effective as D-penicillamine in reducing free cystine and in increasing the quantity of mixed disulfide appearing in the urine (11). α-MPG also results in considerable side effects, including nausea, emesis, and rash, but at a significantly lower rate than with D-penicillamine use. Further, development of the nephrotic syndrome is rare (10). The final dose of α-MPG needed to reduce urinary cystine varies from 100 to 2000 mg daily but is usually lower than the dose of D-penicillamine. Although many patients experience side effects, it is seldom necessary to discontinue therapy and only 6% of patients who are receiving α-MPG

Table 1. Therapy of renal tubular disorders

1. Introduction
2. Aminoacidurias
    Hartnup's disease
    Cystinuria
3. Glucosurias
4. Renal tubular acidosis
    Type I
    Type II
    Type IV
    Pseudohypoaldosteronism
5. Phosphaturias
    X-linked hypophosphatemic rickets
    Hypophosphatemic bone disease
    Hypophosphatemia with hypercalciuria
    Oncogenous or tumoral rickets
    Adult sporadic hypophosphatemic rickets
6. Magnesurias
7. Fanconi syndrome
8. Bartter syndrome

because of D-penicillamine toxicity are forced to stop α-MPG (10). It is anticipated that α-MPG will soon receive FDA approval and will undoubtedly add importantly to the therapy of cystinuria and to the prevention of stone formation.

The report that glutamine can induce a marked reduction in urinary cystine excretion has been difficult to confirm (13). Reinvestigation of the anticystinuric influence of glutamine in cystinuric patients demonstrates that glutamine will reduce urinary cystine excretions only in association with a high dietary sodium intake (14). When dietary sodium intake is restricted to 150 mM daily, no anticystinuric effect of glutamine is noted. However, the low sodium diet itself reduced the urinary excretion of both lysine and cystine. This study suggests that L-glutamine therapy would not likely be of benefit in patients on a normal diet. It also indicates that sodium restriction may lower urinary cystine excretion.

Surgery for large staghorn calculi or obstructing stones can be potentially avoided by the use of percutaneous ultrasonic lithotripsy (15) or by extracorporeal shock-wave lithotripsy (16). The former technique uses an ultrasonic probe passed up the ureter during a cystoscopic examination and is 97% effective in removing the obstructing calculus. Extracorporeal shock-wave lithotripsy employs a totally external technique, with patients placed in a special bath, anesthetized, and then undergoing thousands of precisely directed shock waves. The main shortcomings are hematuria, failure of stone passage, and mild-to-moderate obstruction, but nearly all patients pass the stone fragments with mild colic. Shock-wave lithotripsy is an outpatient procedure, but requires an expensive device and considerable space for the waterbath setup. However, this technique will undoubtedly change the pattern of therapy for cystinuric patients with staghorn calculi (17).

The condition *hypercystinuria* probably requires no therapy, since patients do not excrete as much cystine as patients with classical cystinuria (7). Other conditions such as *histidnuria*, *Oasthouse syndrome* (urinary and intestinal methionine malabsorption), *glycinuria*, and *dicarboxylic aminoaciduria* do not require therapy.

GLYCOSURIAS

The *renal glycosurias* are a group of conditions where excessive urinary excretion of glucose occurs in the absence of hyperglycemia. The glycosurias occur because of abnormal renal tubular reabsorption of glucose (18). The clinical course of the primary renal glycosurias is benign, since this disorder does not result in progressive renal disease nor in any serious metabolic consequences. Thus, no form of therapy is indicated. However, it is important to distinguish the primary renal glycosurias from diabetes mellitus, since patients with the glycosurias do not require insulin therapy.

RENAL TUBULAR ACIDOSIS

The renal tubular acidoses are a group of disorders in which a systemic hyperchloremic metabolic acidosis arises because the excretion of hydrogen ions into the urine and the reabsorption of bicarbonate by different nephron sites is impaired. Currently, three major forms of renal tubular acidosis (RTA) are recognized (19): distal or Type I RTA, isolated proximal or Type II RTA, and hyperkalemic or Type IV RTA. Those renal tubular acidoses associated with other tubulopathic conditions, such as the Fanconi syndrome, will be discussed elsewhere (Table 2).

Type I or distal RTA

Type I RTA can arise from at least six pathophysiologic events: an isolated secretory defect for H^+, acid backleak, a voltage-dependent defect in distal Na^+ transport, a rate-dependent defect in H^+ secretion, selective aldosterone deficiency, and aldosterone resistance (20). The treatment of Type I RTA should be aimed at correction of systemic metabolic acidosis, which is best accomplished by the administration of oral sodium bicarbonate. The therapy of distal RTA in children is difficult since their bicarbonate needs may vary between 1 and 3 mg/kg/24 hr (21). Some young children may require higher doses of bicarbonate; thus it is convenient to provide the medication in a solution containing 1.0 mEq/ml of solution (4). If the sodium bicarbonate cause bloating, sodium citrate may be more palatable. If children experience profound hypokalemia, a mixture of sodium and potassium citrate may be advisable. In adults and older children, sodium bicarbonate at a dose of 1 mEq/kg/24 hr will suffice. Sodium bicarbonate should be provided in four to five divided doses since urinary bicarbonate losses occur around the clock. Complete correction of the hyperchloremic metabolic acidosis wil correct growth retardation in children (22),

Table 2. Features and therapy of renal tubular acidosis

	Distal	Proximal	Hyperkalemic
Form	Type I	Type II	Type IV
Sex Predominance	Female	Male	Equal
Serum potassium concentration	Reduced	Normal	Increased
Urine pH	> 6.2	< 6.2 if acidotic	< 6.2 if acidotic
Hypercalciuria	Yes	No	No
Osteomalacia	Yes	No	Not usual
NaHCO$_3$ mEq/kg/24 hr			
Child	2–3+	10–15	
Adult	1.0	—	
Vitamin D	Yes	No	No
Prognosis	Lifelong	Transient	May resolve if obstructive type No resolution if due to hyporeninemia

and since hypercalciuria ceases, osteomalacia will also be corrected (23). Since osteomalacia/rickets may only heal slowly using oral alkali alone, some authorities recommend the use of vitamin D, such as dihydrotachysterol at 0.2–0.6 mg/daily (20). In patients with nephrolithiasis and hypercalciuria, hypocitraturia is invariable (24). In most cases, correction of metabolic acidosis with oral bicarbonate therapy will reverse hypercalciuria (20). Some patients with hypercalciuria and hypocitraturia will require larger doses of bicarbonate to correct these defects.

Type II or proximal RTA

Type II RTA is a rare condition in which 15% or more of filtered bicarbonate of the serum bicarbonate level is normalized. This can represent a load of 10–15 mEq/kg/24 hr (25). Because of this huge dose requirement, Edelmann (25) suggests that sodium bicarbonate alone be used. One measuring tablespoonful of baking soda contains 44 mEq NaHCO$_3$ hr, thus, this will be the daily requirement for a child of 3–4 kg. Since patients with Type II RTA do not have hypokalemia or hypercalciuria, there is no need to provide additional potassium or citrate (25). Again, another feature of isolated Type II RTA is the absence of osteomalacia, thus, no vitamin-D therapy is required. A failure of high-dose sodium bicarbonate therapy to ameliorate metabolic acidosis has been noted in some patients with Type II RTA, presumably due to the creation of state of volume expansion (26, 27). The infusion of high-dose sodium bicarbonate has resulted in a reduction in the bicarbonate threshhold (27). In these patients the concomitant administration of a thiazide diuretic, such as hydrochlorthiazide at 2.0 mg/kg/24 hr, will lead to mild extracellar volume contraction and improved renal tubular reabsorption of bicarbonate (25, 26).

Hyperkalemic renal tubular acidosis or Type IV RTA

Type IV RTA is a complex disorder of numerous etiologies including isolated aldosterone deficiency, glucocorticoid and mineralocorticoid deficiency, pseudohypoaldosteronism, urinary tract obstruction, renal transplant, systemic lupus erythematosus, and chronic interstitial nephritis (28). Other conditions such as obstructive uropathy and diabetes mellitus can result in severe hyperkalemia with renal tubular acidosis (29). Many of these disorders have in common a state of chronic renal insufficiency and either aldosterone deficiency or hyporesponsiveness, and a serum potassium concentration of > 5.5 mEq/l is the rule.

Classical pseudohypoaldosteronism

Classical pseudohypoaldosteronism is a condition described 30 years ago in which there exist renal tubular NaCl wasting, hyperkalemia, and normal renal and adrenal function (30). The salt wasting will not respond to exogenous mineralocorticoids unless excess NaCl is provided in the diet. This hyperkalemic state occurs in infancy and NaCl losses of 10–15 mEq/kg/24 hr, despite hypovolemia and hyponatremia, are common (31). The administration of glucocorticoids, DOCA, or fluorinated glucocorticoids (which have extensive mineralocorticoid activity), even in large doses, do little to reverse hyponatremia and hyperkalemia (32). The most effective therapy is supplementary sodium chloride in the diet based on the magnitude of urinary losses (mEq/kg/day) (32, 33). Salt supplements normalize growth and correct serum sodium and chloride concentrations, despite the finding of persistently elevated renin and aldosterone concentrations. Patients can usually have their salt supplements discontinued after infancy without effects and patients continue to grow at a normal rate (31).

Hyporeninemic hypoaldosteronism

Hyporeninemic hypoaldosteronism is a common condition in adults with chronic renal insufficiency and tubulointerstitial nephropathy, particularly in relation to diabetes mellitus or systemic lupus erythematosus (34). Hyperkalemia and hyperchloremic metabolic acidosis are due to isolated aldosterone deficiency caused by hyporeninism. The treatment of this condition consists of a low potassium diet and high levels of fluorinated steroids (34). This use of high doses of fluorinated glucocorticoids can both correct the hyperkalemia and enhance proton secretion (35). In a variety of hyperkalemic forms of distal renal tubular acidosis, increasing distal nephron sodium delivery, thus increasing transepithelial voltage potential, can enhance both potassium and/or proton into the tubular lumen (4). This can sometimes be accomplished by increased sodium intake or by the use of diuretics, particularly loop diuretics, depending on the clinical status of the patient. Finally, these patients should generally limit their intake of potassium-rich foods and avoid potassium-sparing diuretics such as triamterene, amiloride, and aldactone.

PHOSPHATURIAS

Phosphorus is the predominant mineral anion that is found in bone (75-85% of total body phosphate) and is also essential for nearly all life processes such as DNA metabolism, energy storage (ATP, GTP, etc.), maintenance of cell membrane stability, second messenger activity (cAMP, inositol phosphates), and cellular intermediary metabolites (glycolysis, gluconeogenesis). Since phosphate is a key anion for these biologic systems, physiologic processes designed to maintain phosphate homeostasis are important. The renal proximal tubule is the major nephron site that regulates phosphate homeostasis (36). A number of clinically distinguishable phosphaturic syndromes have been defined (37), all of which result in hypophosphatemic osteomalacia. If these conditions present during childhood, the result is undermineralization of the growth plate, bone structural weakness, widened metaphyses, and the radiologic appearance of rickets.

Since the pathogenesis of the major phosphaturic syndromes differ, their treatment is also quite different (Tables 3 and 4).

Primary hypophosphatemic rickets on X-linked hypophosphatemic rickets

This X-linked dominant disorder is the most common of the phosphateric syndromes and involves a dual renal tubular disorder — a defect in Na^+-PO_4^- contransport across the brush border surface of the proximal tubule and a reduction in the conversion of 25-(OH)D to 1,25-$(OH)_2D$ by the proximal tubule cell mitochondria (38, 39). Current information suggests that the best form of treatment is a combination of oral phosphate supplements alone with twice daily oral 1,25-$(OH)_2D_3$ at a dose of 65 ng/kg/24 hr (40, 41). This therapy has been shown to improve Ca and PO_4 retention, but phosphate doses must be given every 4-5 hours since the renal phosphate leak persists. Therapy is needed for the life of the patient. Not only is the rachitic growth-plate lesion improved, but endosteal bone trabecular lesions improve, a change not apparent when using vitamin D_2 (42). Oral phosphate can be administered as Joulie's solution (43) or as neutral

Table 3. Types of primary hypophosphatemic rickets

Condition	Inheritance pattern	Associated finding	Salient clinical features	Age detected	Therapy
1. X-linked hypophosphatemic rickets; also called vitamin D-dependent rickets or familial hypophosphatemic rickets	X-linked dominant, rarely autosomal dominant or autosomal recessive	Occasional patient with parathyroid adenomas or hyperplasia	Bowing of lower segment, short stature, no myopathy; usually affects males more severely	9-13 months	Oral phosphate, 1-4 g/24 hr given 4-5 times each day; 1,25-$(OH)_2D$ at 65-75 ng/kg/24 hr
2. Hypophosphatemic nonrachitic bone disease	Autosomal dominant or sporadic		No radiologic evidence of rickets; disease is milder & short stature may appear in late adolescence	3 years to adult	Oral phosphate and vitamin D; may be healed by 1,25-$(OH)_2D$
3. Hereditary hypophosphatemic rickets with hypercalciuria	Autosomal recessive; consanguinity	High calcitriol level; increased intestinal Ca absorption; hypercalciuria, low urinary cAMP	Rickets, short stature, osteomalacia, sexes equally affected	Early childhood	Oral phosphate reverses biochemical features
4. Oncogenous rickets with phosphaturia	Sporadic or autosomoal dominant, autosomal recessive	Sometimes neurofibromatosis, polyostotic fibrous dysplasia, epidermal nevus syndrome	Rickets is healed by removal of tumor where measured serum 1,25-$(OH)_2D$ values are low	Birth onwards	Oral phosphate and 1,25-$(OH)_2D$ will reverse hypophosphatemia; surgery may be curative if tumor is totally removed
5. Adult sporadic hypophosphatemic osteomalacia	Sporadic	Glycinuria	Severe bone pain, vertebral flattening, Looser zones, severe myopathy & weakness	Adult	Oral phosphate plus vitamin D in any form

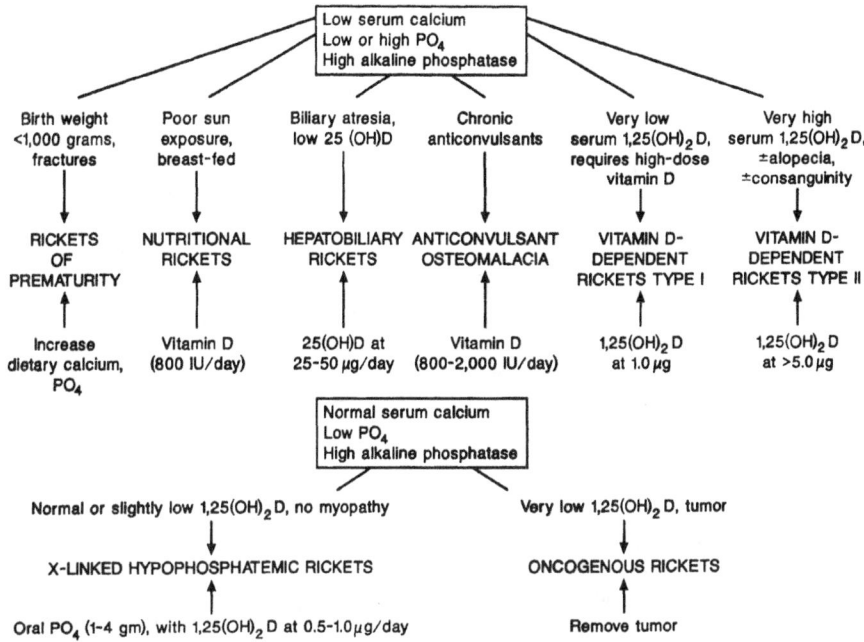

Figure 1. Primary hypophosphatemic rickets on X-linked hypophosphatemic rickets.

phosphate. This form of therapy should be given during childhood. No long-term studies in adults have indicated its role in adult victims of this disorder; however, some studies indicate that calcification of ligaments and joints can occur in untreated adult patients (44), suggesting the possible need for therapy in adult life. Four additional primary phosphaturic conditions have been distinguished that are chemically different (Table 3, Figure 1).

Hypophosphatemic

Hypophosphatemic nonrachitic bone disease is an autosomal dominant or possibly sporadic disorder in which hypophosphatemia is milder than in X-linked hypophosphatemia and rickets are absent (45). The T_mPO_4/GFR is normal in hypophosphatemic patients and serum 1,25-$(OH)_2D_3$ is normal. Therapy with vitamin D_2 and oral phosphate salts appear to mineralize bone. Oral 1,25-$(OH)_2D_3$ can be used instead of vitamin D_2 or D_3 (45).

Hereditary hypophosphatemic rickets with hypercalcemia

This is a familial disorder with rickets, short stature, phosphaturia, hypercalciuria (8 mg/kg/24 hr of calcium), and augmented intestinal calcium and phosphate absorption (46). As distinct from X-linked hypophosphatemic rickets, where serum 1,25-$(OH)_2D$ values are reduced, and from hypophosphatemic bone disease, where values are normal, the circulating values are two to five times normal. It has been speculated that this disorder represents a renal phosphate leak that results in hypophosphatemia that is sufficient to increase 1,25-$(OH)_2D_3$ synthesis. These higher vitamin-D metabolite concentrations result in increased intestinal calcium absorption, suppression of PTH secretion, and hypercalciuria. Since 1,25-$(OH)_2D_3$ concentrations in plasma are elevated, vitamin-D therapy is not indicated and long-term oral phosphate will reverse the biochemical features of this rare disorder.

Oncogenous rickets with phosphaturia

This ia a sporadic disorder in which tumors of mesenchymal origin appear to elaborate a substance that promotes phosphaturia and hypophosphatemic osteomalacia (47). These mesenchymal tumors may be found in soft tissue or in bone. The levels of 1,25-$(OH)_2D_3$ in plasma are extremely low and rise to normal values within a few hours of removal of the tumor (48). Therapy with 1,25-$(OH)_2D$ at 2.5–3.0 µg daily and oral phosphate at 1–4 g daily will improve calcium and phosphate balance and will sometimes result in bone healing. This therapy should be used in cases where the tumor is inoperable or where surgery must be postponed. Clearly, however, the best form of therapy is removal of the tumor.

Adult sporadic osteomalacia

Hypophosphaturic osteomalacia arising de novo in adults is termed *adult sporadic osteomalacia* (49). The diagnosis is made by history of muscle bone and joint pains or "the princess-on-the-pea syndrome," and its common signs are a myopathy, Looser–Milkman zones, and collapsed "codfish" vertebrae (50). Pathogenesis is uncertain but does not involve hyperparathyroidism or hypercalcitoninemia, nor changes in vitamin-D metabolism (37). Although 1,25-$(OH)_2$D therapy will improve intestinal calcium absorption, this therapy alone will not heal osteomalacia and completely reverse hypophosphatemia. Treatment with vitamin D and oral phosphate supplements will improve all signs and symptoms. The doses of vitamin D provided are 1–2 mg/day for 1,25-$(OH)_2$D, 50–100 mg/day for 25(OH)D, and 100,000–300,000 U IV/day of vitamin D_2, in addition to several grams of oral phosphate. With rare exceptions (51), phosphate and vitamin D must be given for life. Due to the overlap in findings in this syndrome and in those with oncogenic rickets, a thorough search for a tumor is needed.

MAGNESURIAS

Magnesium depletion is an uncommon mineral disorder that is frequently overlooked because of the complex clinical setting and the associated clinical setting with which it arises. Renal magnesium wasting can be a primary inherited disorder (52, 53) or may be associated with several clinical disorders (54). Renal magnesium wasting can be associated with diabetic ketoacidosis, hyperaldosteronism, hypercalciuria (and the use of loop diuretics), Bartter syndrome, and the therapeutic use of cisplatin and aminoglycoside antibiotics (54).

A typical feature of magnesium deficiency is hypocalcemia related to impaired function of the parathyroid gland. Hypomagnesemia also contributes to the development of hypocalcemia by altering end-organ responsiveness to parathyroid hormone (55). Further intravenous magnesium supplements to magnesium-deficient, hypocalcemic patients has been shown to augment the serum values for PTH (56). Magnesium may also be an important factor in the action and/or metabolism of vitamin D in that some hypomagnesemic patients may respond to 1α-vitamin D metabolites only after corrections of serum magnesium values (57). Finally, serum concentrations of 1,25-$(OH)_2$D are reduced in magnesium-depleted patients (57, 58). Thus, the mineral abnormalities can include reduced serum magnesium, calcium, 1,25-$(OH)_2D_3$, and PTH concentrations, all of which may be restored by infusion of or oral ingestion of magnesium. Therapy with magnesium oxide at 1–5 g (50–250 mEq) daily will cause the following changes: increased serum and urine magnesium and calcium, reduced phosphate in serum and increased in urine, and increased serum 1,25-$(OH)_2D_3$ and PTH (59). Although the doses of oral magnesium needed to correct magnesium-deficiency vary from patient to patient, and depending on the underlying cause of renal magnesium wasting (60), improved magnesium homeostasis can usually be achieved. As with the renal phosphaturia syndromes, magnesium should be taken several times a day since urinary magnesium hyperexcretion is occurring continuously and since in renal magnesium wasting patients will continue to excrete large quantities of magnesium until they are magnesium depleted. Finally, renal magnesium wasting can occur in conjunction with varying degrees of renal insufficiency (59), and those patients may also require oral vitamin D analogs and calcium salts. A dose of 0.25–1.0 µg of 1,25-$(OH)_2$D may be required as well as calcium lactate or carbonate (59).

FANCONI SYNDROME

The Fanconi syndrome is a generalized proximal tubulopathy affecting a varying number of proximal tubule transport systems that occurs in conjunction with a number of hereditary or acquired conditions (61) (Table 4). Patients always show hyperexcretion of substances that are reabsorbed and diminished excretion of substances that are secreted (1–4). Depending on the underlying disorder leading to tubular disease, the manifestations of the Fanconi syndrome may differ. Typically, tubular dysfunction involves glucosuria, phosphaturia, generalized aminoaciduria, proteinuria, polyuria, and Type II renal tubular acidosis. Other substances that are frequently excreted in increased quantities are uric acid, sodium, potassium, magnesium, citrate, and low molecular weight proteins of under 45,000 daltons. Because of phosphaturia, hypophosphatemia, and renal insufficiency, a variety of bone disorders, including rickets, osteomalacia, osteoporosis, and osteitis fibrosa, may be found (62). Because of the severity of osteomalacia in adult patients with the Fanconi syndrome, intense bone pain and muscle weakness are common presenting features (63). Hypokalemic symptoms, including muscle weakness, growth failure, dehydration, unexplained fevers due to volume depletion, and profound metabolic acidosis, are other clinical features (61, 62).

The therapy of the Fanconi syndrome is either generalized or specific depending on the etiology. Symptomatic therapy includes the provision of large doses of alkali (often as high as 10–15$_m$Eq $NaHCO_3$/kg/24 hr), phosphate supplements given four to five times daily, a vitamin D analog, adequate water, and adequate sodium and potassium replacement to correct volume depletion and signs of hypokalemia.

Patients with cystinosis have several additional specific needs. Cystine deposition within the cornea leads to photophobia, which may be improved with dark glasses, wetting solutions, and the possibility of cysteamine eye drops, which can dissolve cystine deposits (64). Since the defect in this disorder involves reduction in the rate of efflux of cystine, but not cysteine, from within a lysosomal compartment (64), the oxidized (S-S) form of this sulfur amino acid remains trapped and intralysomal crystals form. At least two cystine-depleting agents, cysteamine and pantothine (its precursor), can be used to deplete lysosomes, since they form mixed disulfides with cystine, which are freely permeable across the lysosomal membrane. The reduced form (-SH) is thereby free to exit the lysosome as well and intracellular cystine values fall (65).

Table 4. Familial and hereditary disorders associated with the Fanconi syndrome

Primary or idiopathic (no identifiable associated disorder)
1. Familial
2. Sporadic

Hereditary
1. Cystinosis (Lignac–Fanconi disease)
2. Lowe syndrome
3. Hereditary fructose intolerance
4. Tyrosinemia, Type 1 (tyrosinosis)
5. Galactosemia
6. Glycogen storage disease
7. Wilson disease
8. Others
   hereditary mitochondrial myopathy with lactic acidemia
   metachromatic leukodystrophy
   subacute necrotizing encephalomyelopathy (Leigh syndrome)
   hereditary nephritis (Alport syndrome)
   medullary cystic disease

Adapted from Brewer (61).

The results of the National Collaborative Cysteamine Study indicate that 98 patients receiving cysteamine show a real slowing of their progression toward renal failure and an improved linear growth pattern as compared to more than 100 historic control cystinotic subjects (66). A recent analysis of 88 patients followed for more than 10 years identified not only uremia, but also hepatomegaly, splenomegaly, neurologic disease, progressive ocular disease, and continuing poor growth patterns despite a functioning renal allograft (67). These results suggest the need for continuing cysteamine therapy, but this point has not been shown by controlled trials.

Due to cystine crystals, hypothyroidism is common in cystinosis and thus low-dose thyroxine is needed to prevent the features of this endocrinopathy (61). The dose of L-thyroxine should be sufficient to suppress TSH values into the normal range. Cystinotic patients have also been shown to be carnitine deficient, since they lose massive amounts of this acyl-transporting substance (68) and oral therapy may reverse muscle carnitine depletion and histologic features of this deficiency.

The final caveat in treating cystinotic subjects is that it represents a lifelong disorder with continuing cystine deposition. The long-term involvement of organs other than the kidney are only now being appreciated since long-term survivors of a renal tranplantation are available for study (66, 67).

In *Lowe's syndrome* — an X-linked disorder involving cataracts, glaucoma, growth impairment, hypotonia, mental retardation, and features of the Fanconi syndrome (69) — treatment is largely directed at correcting features of the Fanconi syndrome. Renal dysfunction begins with tubular dysfunction but can progress to chronic renal failure. Tubular dysfunction actually diminishes because of the decline in the glomerular filtration rate. Patients with this syndrome usually die of renal insufficiency or infection but have a lifelong need for opthalmologic evaluations.

In patients with *galactosemia* caused by autosomal recessive, inherited galactose-1-phosphate uridyl transferase deficiency, the Fanconi syndrome develops but is reversible when patients are placed on a galactose- and lactose-free diet (70). Maintenance of a lifelong galactose-free diet is required.

Tyrosinosis leads to hepatomegaly, cirrhosis, and the Fanconi syndrome, due presumably to an autosomal recessive defect in fumarylacetoacetate fumaryl hydrolase with the accumulation of succinylacetone and succinylacetoacetate (71). This disorder usually results in death in children due to cirrhosis and/or hepatoblastomas; a low-tyrosine, low-phenylalanine diet can treat the Fanconi syndrome and prevent rickets, but it does not prevent cirrhosis from developing. Thus, the definitive form of therapy is a liver transplant (72).

Hereditary fructose intolerance is the autosomal recessive disorder caused by a deficiency of aldolase B activity in the liver renal cortex and small intestine, resulting in the accumulation of fructose-1-phosphate (73). Diagnosis is by the aversion to sweets, the lack of caries, and the hepatomegaly in these patients (61). The development of the Fanconi syndrome is temporally related to exposure to fructose. Thus, treatment is to avoid ingestion of this sugar. As in galactosemia, the development of the Fanconi syndrome may take only a few hours and patients become profoundly ill. Patients quickly recognize the advantage of avoiding these sugars.

The Fanconi syndrome can be seen in certain children with an as yet *untyped glycogen storage disease*. These patients present with hepatomegaly, massive glycosuria, and, as in idiopathic Fanconi syndrome, patients have glucose and galactose intolerance (74, 75). These patients are profoundly growth retarded, and their treatment consists of controlling the symptoms of the Fanconi syndrome. These patients improve with age.

Wilson's disease represents the hepatocellular disorder that presents with hepatomegaly and the Fanconi syndrome. It is an autosomal recessive disorder of copper metabolism that results in abnormally elevated copper deposits in the brain, liver, and kidney (76). Patients with Wilson's disease also have, in addition to their proximal RTA, findings that can only be explained as distal RTA; urinary calculi are common (77). Hypoparathyroidism has also been described in a single patient with Wilson's disease, possibly related to copper deposits within the parathyroid gland (78). The therapy of Wilson's disease consists of D-penicillamine at doses commonly used in cystinuria (79). The side effects of D-penicillamine are troublesome and are well described in the section on cystinuria. Whenever D-penicillamine cannot be used, triethylene tetramine dihydrochloride can be used without fear of the same allergic manifestations (79).

A variety of acquired conditions result in the Fanconi syndrome (Table 5). Most prominent among these are the syndromes associated with multiple myeloma and other dysproteinemias. The current dogma states that proximal

Table 5. Acquired disorders associated with the Fanconi syndrome

1. Disorder of protein metabolism/excretion
   Multiple myeloma
   Benign monoclonal gammopathy
   Light chain nephropathy
   Amyloidosis
   Sjogren syndrome
   Nephrotic syndrome
2. Immunologic disorders
   Interstitial nephritis with anti-TBM antibody
   Renal transplantation
   Malignancy
3. Drug related
   Outdated, degraded tetracycline
   Methyl-3-chromone
   6-mercaptopurine
   Gentamicin and aminoglycoside antibiotics
   Valproic acid
   Streptozotocin
   Isophrthalanilide
4. Heavy metal exposure
   Cadmium
   Lead
   Mercury
   Uranium
   Cisplatinum
5. Other toxin exposure
   Paraquat poisoning
   Lysol burn
   Toluene inhalation (glue sniffing)
6. Other renal disorder
   Balkan nephropathy
   Paroxysmal nocturnal hemoglobinuria
   Renal vein thrombosis hemoglobinuria
7. Vitamin-D disorders with secondary hyperparathyroidism
   Vitamin-D deficiency
   Vitamin-D-dependent rickets

Adapted from Brewer (61).

tubular damage is related to the massive filtration and reabsorption of kappa light chains (80). The Fanconi syndrome may develop insidiously over years in patients who ultimately develop the complete features of multiple myeloma. Therapy of the underlying dysproteinemia will generally cause disappearance of tubular dysfunction.

When the Fanconi syndrome appears in conjunction with the nephrotic syndrome, it usually is found in association with focal sclerosing glomerulonephropathy; however, tubular atrophy and interstitial fibrosis are prominent (81). The treatment of this form of the nephrotic syndrome is unsatisfactory, and thus the features of the Fanconi syndrome continue until renal failure ensues. The Fanconi syndrome can occur in conjunction with tubulointerstitial nephritis, which may sometimes be on an allergic basis (82). Removal of the offending allergin, if identified, can reverse features of the syndrome (61). Unfortunately, however, many patients with tubulointerstitial nephritis and circulating antitubular basement membrane antibodies develop progessive renal failure (61).

The Fanconi syndrome that occurs after a renal allograft is usually indicative of an acute rejection episode and resolves following antirejection therapy (83).

A variety of drugs and heavy metals can be associated with the nephrotic syndrome, which is reversible upon removal of exposure to the offending toxin. Perhaps the most famous of these is the syndrome in association with anhydro-4-epitetracycline, a degradation product of tetracycline exposed to air, heat, dampness, and retention of drug beyond the expiration date (84). Exposure to methyl-3-dicromone, a compound chemically similar to tetracycline, can cause the syndrome (85). A variety of heavy metals, including platinum, uranium, mercury, lead, and cadmium, may lead to the syndrome, and in the case of lead and cadmium, chelation therapy with calcium-EDTA or BAL are indicated (86, 87).

Finally, the Fanconi syndrome has been described secondary to vitamin D deficiency. In some cases, therapy with vitamin D will reverse secondary hyperparathyroidism, phosphaturia, aminociduria, and proximal RTA (88). If this syndrome occurs with vitamin D-dependency rickets Types I or II, $1,25-(OH)_2D$ therapy may reverse the proximal tubulopathy (37).

BARTTER SYNDROME

Bartter syndrome is defined by hyperplasma of the juxtaglomerular appartus, increased circulating angiotensin II concentrations, normal blood pressure with diminished pressor response to infused angiotensin II, hyperaldosteronism, hypokalemic alkalosis, and vasopressin-resistant polyuria (89). It is apparent that this condition is a very heterogenous disorder in that most patients present in childhood or adolescence, but a presentation over the age of 40 has occurred (90). The inheritance pattern is sporadic or autosomal recessive (91). Children may also present with growth failure as well as the weakness, muscle cramps, polyuria, abdominal pain, and delayed or slowed mentation seen in all Bartter syndrome patients (89). The laboratory features are also heterogeneous in that patients show variable degrees of excessive urinary losses of potassium, sodium, chloride, magnesium, calcium, and kallikrein, and increased production and excretion of prostaglandin E_2 (89, 92). With the finding of abnormalities in the concentration of prostaglandins in plasma and urine, it became the vogue to consider that a defect in prostaglandins was the primary defect (93). Elevated prostaglandin values could explain vasodilation, a lack of responsiveness to pressors, the inhibition of chloride transport in the loop of Henle, and potassium hyperexcretion and metabolic alkalosis.

However, prostaglandin inhibition does not always correct the defect in patients with Bartter syndrome, and continued use of prostaglandin inhibitors may not result in continuing therapeutic benefit (94). Moreover, in disorders that mimic familial Bartter syndrome, such as bulimia, chronic diuretic abuse, and chloride-deficient formula-induced disease, the same plasma and urine profile is evident (95). Recent studies suggest at least five pathogenic sequences to produce Bartter syndrome (53, 96, 97). First, patients may have isolated potassium transport defects with normal sodium and chloride reabsorption. Second, chloride and sodium transport defects may occur at multiple sites along the nephron. Potassium loss would be the result of enhanced sodium-potassium exchange in the distal tubule and increased urine flow within the tubule lumen. Third, and perhaps the most common, is a defect in chloride and thus in sodium transport by the thick ascending limb of the loop of Henle. Potassium wasting would occur by the same mechanism as in the second pathogenic sequence. Fourth, magnesium- wasting syndromes can lead to virtually all the features of Bartter syndrome, with prominent renal potassium wasting (53, 59). Fifth, patients with increased production of prostaglandins E_2 and $F_{2\alpha}$ can have abnormalities of chloride reabsorption and hypokalemia as a result of renal hyperprostaglandinism (97, 98). These patients do not have juxtaglomerular hyperplasia, but show hypertrophy of prostaglandin-producing cells (97) or dense cytoplasm, compact mitochondria, pyknotic nuclei, and hypertrophy of the basement membrane (99). This latter group of patients do not have abnormal chloride reabsorption.

The therapy of Bartter syndrome can be very difficult. Potassium supplementation is needed and large quantities of oral KCl may be required. Prostaglandin inhibitors, of which indomethacin has been the most often used, have short-lived effects when used alone, unless the patients have one of the renal hyperprostaglandinuric syndromes (97–99). These prostaglandin inhibitors appear to work best in most patients if they are considered as an adjunct therapy that limits the need for KCl supplements (100). If magnesium wasting is present, then clearly magnesium supplementation is also indicated.

In some patients, the use of supplemental KCl and treatment with a prostaglandin synthease inhibitor may not fully correct hypokalemia, which is the first aim of therapy. A potassium-sparing diuretic such as triameterene or amiloride in the usual doses can then be added (101).

These therapeutic approaches, if constantly applied, can usually result in improved growth and development in children and can usually improve the life of adult patients with Bartter syndrome.

ACKNOWLEDGMENTS

This work was supported in part by NIH grant #DK37223-04 and by a grant from Miles Laboratories.

REFERENCES

1. Scriver CR, Chesney RW, McInnes RR: Genetic aspects of renal tubular transport. Diversity and topology of carriers. *Kidney Int* 9:149–171, 1976.
2. Schneider JA: Hereditary disorders of tubular function. In: BM Tune, SA Mendoza, eds, *Pediatric Nephrology. Contemporary Issues in Nephrology*, 12th issue, Churchill-Livingston, New York, pp 85–109, 1984.
3. Chesney RW: Defects of renal tubular transport. In: SG Massry, R Glassock, eds, *Textbook of Nephrology*. Elsevier, North Holland, pp 3.178–3.190, 1983.
4. Chesney RW, Friedman AL: Isolated renal tubular disorders. In: RW Schrier, CW Gottschalk, eds, *Diseases of the Kidney*, 4th ed., pp 663–688, 1988.
5. Scriver CR: Familial iminoglycinuria. In: JB Stanbury, JB Wyngaarden, DS Frederickson, JL Goldstein, MS Brown, eds, *The Metabolic Basis of Inherited Disease*, 5th ed. McGraw-Hill, New York, pp 1792–1803, 1983.
6. Melanan SB, Dallaire L, Lemieux B, Robitaille P, Portier M: Dicarboxylic aminoaciduria: An inborn error of amino acid conservation. *J Pediatr* 94:422–427, 1977.
7. Foreman JW, Segal S: Aminoacidurias. In: HC Gorick, VM Buckalew Jr, eds, *Renal Tubular Disorders. Pathophysiology, Diagnosis and Management*. Marcel Dekker, New York, pp 131–157, 1985.
8. Segal S, Thier SO: Cystinuria. In: JB Stanbury, JB Wyngaarden, DS Frederickson, JL Goldstein, MS Brown, eds, *The Metabolic Basis of Inherited Disease*, 5th ed. McGraw-Hill, New York, pp 1174–1791, 1983.
9. Pak CYC, Fuller CJ: Assessment of cystine solubility in urine and of heterogeneous nucleation. *J Urol* 129:1066–1074, 1983.
10. Pak CYC, Fuller C, Sakhaee K, Zerwekh JE, Adams BV: Management of cystine nephrolithiasis with alpha-mercaptopropinyl-glycine. *J Urol* 136:1003–1008, 1986.
11. Harbar JA, Cusworth DC, Lawes LC, Wrong OM: Comparison of 2-mercaptopropronyl-glycine and D-penicillamine in the treatment of cystinuria. *J Urol* 136:146–149, 1986.
12. Rodman JS, Blackburn P, Williams JJ, Brown A, Poapiaxhil MA, Peterson CM: The effect of dietary protein on cystine excretion in patients with cystinuria. *Clin Nephrol* 22:273–278, 1984.
13. Skovby F, Rosenberg LE, Thiers SO: No effect of L-glutamine on cystinuria. *N Engl J Med* 302:236–237, 1980.
14. Jaeger P, Portmann L, Saunders A, Rosenberg LE, Thier SO: Anticystinuric effects of glutamine and of dietary sodium restriction. *N Engl J Med* 315:1120–1123, 1986.
15. Bass RB, Beard JH, Cooner WH, Mosley BR, Pond HS, Rutherford CL, Jr: Percutaneous ultrasonic lithotrypsy in the community hospital. *J Urol* 133:1586–1587, 1985.
16. Brannen GE, Bush WH: Percutaneous ultrasonic versus surgical removal of kidney stones. *Surg Gynecol Obstet* 161:473–478, 1985.
17. Grantham JR, Millner MR, Kande JV, Findlayson B, Hunter PT, Newman RC: Renal stone disease treated with extracorporeal shock wave lithotrypsy: Short term observations in 100 patients. *Radiology* 158:203–206, 1986.
18. Wen SF: Glycosurias In:HC Gonick, VM Buckalew Jr, eds, *Renal Tubular Disorders, Pathophysiology, Diagnosis and Management*. Marcel Dekker, New York, pp 131–157, 1985.
19. McSherry E: Renal tubular acidosis in childhood. *Kidney Int* 20:799–809, 1981.
20. Batlle DC, Kurtzman NA: The defect in distal (Type I) renal tubular acidosis. In: HC Gonick, VM Buckalew Jr, eds, *Renal Tubular Disorders, Pathophysiology, Diagnosis and Management*. Marcel Dekker, New York, pp 281–305, 1985.
21. Buckalew VM Jr, Carvana RJ: The pathophysiology of distal (Type I) renal tubular acidosis. In: HC Gonick, VM

Buckalew Jr, eds, *Renal Tubular Disorders, Pathology Diagnosis and Management*. Marcel Dekker, New York, pp 357–386, 1985.
22. McSherry E: Acidosis and growth in nonuremic renal disease. *Kidney Int* 14:349–354, 1978.
23. Brenner RJ, Spring DB, Sebastian A, McSherry EM, Genant HK, Palubinskas AJ, Morris RC Jr: Incidence of radiographically evident bone disease, nephrocalcinosis and nephrolithiasis in various types of renal tubular acidosis. *N Engl J Med* 307:217–222, 1982.
24. Buckalew VM Jr, Purvis ML, Shulman MG, Herndon CN, Rudman D: Hereditary renal tubular acidosis. Report of 64 member kindred with variable clinical expression including idiopathic hypercalciuria. *Medicine* 53:229–254, 1954.
25. Edelmann CM Jr: Isolated proximal (Type II) renal tubular acidosis. In: HC Gonick, VM Buckalew Jr, eds, *Renal Tubular Disorders. Pathophysiology, Diagnosis and Management*. Marcel Dekker, New York, pp 261–280, 1985.
26. Donckerwolcke RA, Van Stekelenburg GJ, Tiddens HA: Therapy of bicarbonate-losing renal tubular acidosis. *Arch Dis Child* 45:774–779, 1970.
27. Boyer M, Proesmans W, Royer P: La titration des bicarbonates chez l'enfant normal et au cours de diverses nephropathies. *Rev Ethudes Clin Biol* 14:556–568, 1969.
28. Sebastian A, Schambelan M, Hulter HN, Maher T, Kurtz I, Biglieri EG, Rector FC Jr, Morris RC Jr: Hyperkalemic renal tubular acidosis. In: HC Gonick, VM Buckalew Jr, eds, *Renal Tubular Disorders, Pathophysiology, Diagnosis and Management*. Marcel Dekker, New York, pp 307–356, 1985.
29. Batlle DC, Arruda JAL, Kurtzman NA: Hyperkalemic distal renal tubular acidosis associated with obstructive uropathy. *N Engl J Med* 304:373–380, 1981.
30. Cheek DB, Perry JW: A salt wasting syndrome in infancy. *Arch Dis Child* 33:252–256, 1958.
31. Chesney RW: Renal tubular disorders. In: HC Gonick, ed, *Contemporary Nephrology*. Yearbook Medical Publishers, Chicago, 11:107–138, 1988.
32. Armanini D, Kuhnle U, Strasser T, Dorr H, Butenandt T, Weber PC, Stockigt JR, Pearce P, Funder JW: Aldosterone-receptor deficiency in pseudohypoaldosteronison. *N Engl J Med* 313:1178–1181, 1985.
33. Oberfield SE, Levine LS, Carey RM, Bejark B, New MI: Pseudohypoaldosteronism: Multiple target organ unresponsiveness to mineralocorticoid hormones. *J Clin Endocrinol Metab* 48:228–234, 1979.
34. De Fronzo RA: Hyperkalemia and hyporenienemic hypoaldosteronism. *Kidney Int* 29:186–202, 1980.
35. Schambelain M, Sebastian A, Biglieri EG: Prevalence, pathogenesis and functional significance of aldosterone deficiency in hyperkalemic patients with chronic renal insufficiency. *Kidney Int* 17:89–94, 1980.
36. Massry SG, Fredley RM, Coburn JW: Excretion of phosphate and calcium: Physiology of their renal handling and relation to clinical medicine. *Arch Intern Med* 131:828–859, 1973.
37. Chesney RW: Phosphaturic syndromes. In: H Gonick, VM Buckalow Jr, eds, *Renal Tubular Disorders*. Marcel Dekker, New York, pp 201–238, 1985.
38. Tenenhouse HS: Effect of age and the X-linked *hyp/y* mutation on renal adaptation to vitamin D and calcium deficiency. *Can Biochem Physiol* 81A:367–371, 1985.
39. Tenenhouse HS: Abnormal renal mitochondrial 25-hydroxyvitamin D-1α-hydroxylase activity in the vitamin D and calcium deficient X-linked *hyp/y* mouse. *Endocrinology* 113:816–818, 1983.
40. Drezner MK, Lyles KW, Haussler MR, Harrelson JM: Evaluation of a role for 1,25-dihydroxyvitamin D_3 in the pathogenesis and treatment of X-linked hypophosphatemic rickets and osteomalacia. *J Clin Invest* 66:1020–1032, 1980.
41. Chesney RW, Mazess RB, Rose P, Hamstra AJ, DeLuca HF, Breed AL: Long-term influence of calcitrol (1,25-dihydroxyvitamin D) and supplemental phosphate in X-linked hypophosphatemic rickets. *Pediatrics* 71:559–567, 1983.
42. Marie PJ, Glorieux FM: Histromorphometric study of bone remodeling in hypophosphatemic vitamin D-resistant rickets. *Metab Bone Dis Rel Res* 3:31–39, 1981.
43. Glorieux FH, Scriver CR, Reade TM, Goldman H, Roseborough A: Use of phosphate and vitamin D to prevent dwarfism and rickets in X-linked hypophosphatemic rickets. *N Engl J Med* 287:481–485, 1972.
44. Polisson RB, Martinez SJ, Khoury M, Harrell RM, Lyles KW, Friedman N, Harrelson JM, Reisner E, Drezner MK: Calcification of entheses associated with X-linked hypophosphatemic osteomalacia. *N Engl J Med* 313:1–6, 1985.
45. Scriver CR: On phosphate transport and genetic screening, "understanding backward-living forward" in human genetics: William Allen Memorial Award Address. *Am J Hum Genet* 31:243–248, 1979.
46. Terder M, Modai D, Samuel R, Arie R, Malabe A, Bab I, Gabizon D, Lieberman VA: Hereditary hypophosphatemic rickets with hypercalciuria. *N Engl J Med* 312:611–616, 1985.
47. Harrison HE, Harrison HC: Rickets and osteomalacia. In: *Major Problems in Clinical Pediatrics: Disorders of Calcium and Phosphate Metabolism in Childhood and Adolescence*. WB Saunders, Philadelphia, vol. xx, pp 141–256, 1979.
48. Drezner MK, Feinglos MN: Ostemalacia due to 1,25-dihydroxycholecalciferol deficiency. *J Clin Invest* 60:1046–1053, 1977.
49. Dent CE, Stamp TCB: Hypophosphatemic osteomalcia presenting in adults. *Q J Med* 40:303–329, 1971.
50. Lundberg E, Bergengren H, Lundquist B: Mild phosphate diabetes in adults. *Acta Med Scand* 204:93–96, 1978.
51. Dent CE, Friedman M: Hypophosphatemic osteomalacia with complete recovery. *Br Med J* 1:1676–1679, 1964.
52. Booth BE, Johanson A: Hypomagnesiemia due to renal tubular defect in reabsorption of magnesium. *J Pediatr* 84:350–354, 1974.
53. Evans RA, Carter JN, George CRP, et al.: The congenital magnesium losing kidney. *Q J Med* 197:39–52, 1981.
54. Agus ZS, Wasserstein A, Goldfarb S: Disorders of calcium and magnesium homeostasis. *Am J Med* 72:473–488, 1982.
55. Rude RK, Oldham SB, Singer FR: Functional hypoparathyroidism and parathyroid hormone end-organ resistance in human magnesium deficiency. *Clin Endocrinol* 5:209–214, 1976.
56. Duran MJ Borst GC, Osburne RC, Eil C: Concurrent renal hypomagnesemia and hypoparathyroidism with normal parathormone responsiveness. *Am J Med* 76:151–154, 1984.
57. Ralston S, Boyle IT, Cowan RA, Creau GP, Jenkins A, Thomson WS: PTH and vitamin D responses during treatment of hypomagnesiemia hypoparathyroidism. *Acta Endocrinol* 103:535–538, 1983.
58. Rude RK, Adams JS, Ryzen E, Endres DB, Niimi H, Horst RL, Haddad JG, Singer FR: Low serum concentrations of 1,25 dehydroxyvitamin D in human magnesium deficiency. *J Clin Endocrinol Metab* 61:933–940, 1985.
59. Zelikovic I, Dabbagh S, Friedman AL, Goelzer ML, Chesney RW: Severe renal osteodystrophy without elevated serum immunorective parathyroid hormone concentrations in hypomagnesiemia due to renal magnesium wasting.

Pediatrics 79:403–409, 1987.
60. Allen DB, Friedman AL, Greer FR, Chesney RW: Hypomagnesemia masking the appearance of elevated parathyroid hormone concentrations in familial pseudohypoparathyroidism. Am J Med Genet 31:153–158, 1988.
61. Brewer ED: The Fanconi syndrome: Clinical disorders. In: HC Gonick, VM Buckalew Jr, eds, Renal Tubular Disorders. Marcel Dekker, New York, pp 475–544, 1985.
62. Chesney RW: Etiology and pathogenesis of the Fanconi syndrome. Miner Electrolyte Metab 4:303–316, 1980.
63. Wallis LA, Engle RL: The adult Fanconi syndrome II: Review of eighteen cases. Ann J Med 22:13–23, 1957.
64. Gahl WA: Cystinosis coming of age. Adv Pediatr 33:95–126, 1986.
65. Schneider JA: Therapy of cystinosis. N Engl J Med 313:1473–1474, 1985.
66. Gahl WA, Thoene JG, Schneider JA, Mendoza SA, Schulman JG: Results of the national collaborative cystamine study: Improvement in linear growth and slowed progression of renal failure. N Engl J Med 366:971–977, 1987.
67. Gahl WA, Schneider JA, Thoene JG, Chesney RW: Course of nephropathic cystinosis after 10 years of age. J Pediatr 109:605–608, 1986.
68. Bennardini I, Rizzo WB, Dalakas M, Berner J, Gahl WA: Plasma and muscle free carnitine deficiency due to renal Fanconi syndrome. J Clin Invest 75:1124–1130, 1985.
69. Abassi V, Lowe CU, Calcagno PL: Oculo-cerebro-renal syndrome. A review. Am J Dis Child 115:145–168, 1968.
70. Segal S: Disorders of galactose metabolism. In: JB Stanbury, JB Wyngaarden, DS Frederickson, JL Goldstein, MS Brown, eds, The Metabolic Basis of Inherited Disease, 5th ed. McGraw-Hill, New York, pp 166–191, 1983.
71. Lindblad B, Lindstedt S, Steen G: On the enzymic defects in hereditary tyrosinemua. Proc Natl Acad Sci USA 74:4641–4645, 1977.
72. Scriver CR, Silverberg M, Clow CL: Hereditary tyrosinemia and tyrosyluria: Clinical report of four patients. Can Med Assoc J 97:1047–1050, 1967.
73. Steinmann B, Gitzelmann R: The dignosis of hereditary fructose intolerance. Helv Pediatr Acta 36:297–316, 1981.
74. Chesney RW, Kaplan BS, Teitel D, Colle E, McInnes RR, Goldman M, Scriver CR: Metabolic abnormalities in the idiopathic Fanconi syndrome: Studies of carbohydrate metabolism in two patients. Pediatrics 67:113–118, 1981.
75. Brodehl J, Gelessen K, Hagge W: The Fanconi syndrome in hepatorenal glycogen storage disease in progress. In: G Peiters, Roch–Rainel F, eds, Nephrology. Springer-Verlag, New York, pp 241–243, 1969.
76. Strickland GT, Lew ML: Wilson's disease, clinical and laboratory manifestations in 40 patients. Medicine 54:113–137, 1975.
77. Bearn AG, Yu TF, Gutman AB: Renal function in Wilson's disease. J Clin Invest 36:1107–1114, 1957.
78. Walshe JM: Effect of penicillamine on failure of renal acidification in Wilson's disease. Lancet 1:775–779, 1985.
79. Walshe JM: Treatment of Wilson's disease with trientine (trithlene tetramine) dihydrochloride. Lancet 1:643–647, 1982.
80. Maldonado JE, Velosa JA, Kyle RA, Wagoner RD, Molley KE, Salassa RM: Fanconi syndrome in adults. A manifestation of a latent form of myeloma. Am J Med 58:354–364, 1975.
81. Burke EC, Holley KE, Stickler GB: Familial nephrotic syndrome with nephrocalcinosis and tubular dysfunction. J Pediatr 82:202–206, 1973.
82. Bergstein JM, Litman N: Interstitial nephritis with anti-tubular-basement-membrane antibody. N Engl J Med 292:875–878, 1975.
83. Friedman AL, Chesney RW: Fanconi's syndrome in renal transplantation. Am J Nephrol 1:45–47, 1981.
84. Mavromatis F: Tetracyline nephropathy. JAMA 193:10: 191–194, 1965.
85. Otter J, Vis HL: Acute reversible renal tubular dysfunction following intoxication with methyl-3-chromone. J Pediatr 73:422–425, 1968.
86. Chrisolm JJ: Increased lead absorption and lead poisoning. In: RE Behrman, Vaughn VC, eds, Nelson Textbook of Pediatrics, 11th ed. WB Saunders, Philadelphia, pp 1801–1804, 1983.
87. Hoakawa Y, Abe J, Tamaka S: Bone changes in experimental chronic cadmium poisoning. Arch Environ Health 26:241–244, 1973.
88. Chesney RW, Harrison HE: Fanconi syndrome following bowel surgery and hepatitis reversed by 25-hydroxycholecalciferol. J Pediatr 86:857–861, 1975.
89. Gill JR Jr: Bartter's syndrome. In: HC Gonick, Buckalew VM Jr, eds, Renal Tubular Disorders. Marcel Dekker, New York, pp 457–473, 1985.
90. Tomko DJ, Yeh BPY, Falls WF Jr: Bartter's syndrome. Study of a 52 year old man with evidence for a defect in proximal tubular sodium reabsorption and comments on therapy. Am J Med 61:111–117, 1976.
91. Pererra RR, Von Wersch J: Inheritance of Bartter syndrome. Am J Med Genet 15:79–84, 1983.
92. White MG: Bartter's syndrome. A manifestation of renal tubular defects. Arch Intern Med 129:41–47, 1972.
93. Gill JR, Frohlich JC, Bowden RE, Taylor AA, Keiser HR, Seyberth HV, Oates JA, Bartter FC: Bartter's syndrome: A disorder characterized by high urinary prostaglandins and dependence of hyperreninemia on prostaglandin synthesis. Am J Med 61:43–51, 1976.
94. Halushka PV, Wohltmann H, Privitera PJ, Hurwitz G, Margolius HS: Bartter's syndrome: Urinary prostaglandin E-like material and kallikrein; indomethacin effects. Ann Intern Med 87:281–286, 1977.
95. Veldhius JD, Bardin CW, Demers LM: Metabolic mimcry of Bartter's syndrome to covert vomiting. Am J Med 66:361–363, 1979.
96. Stein JH: The pathogenic spectrum of Bartter's syndrome. Kidney Int 28:85–93, 1985.
97. Seyberth HW, Rascher W, Schweer H, Kuhl PG, Mehls O, Scharer K: Congenital hypokalemia with hypercalcemia in preterm infants. A hyperprostaglandinuric tubular syndrome different from Bartter syndrome. J Pediatr 107:694–698, 1985.
98. Hornuch I, Huet de Barochez Y, Bariety J, Branca GF, Vigeral P, Girard JF, Kazatchkine M, DeGennes JL, Truffert J, Bocquet L, Paris M: Bartter's syndrome with normal sodium chloride reabsorption during indomethacin treatment. Nephron 46:137–143, 1987.
99. Gullner HC, Bartter FC, Gill JR Jr, Bickman PS, Wilson CB, Tiwari JL: A subship with hypokalemic alkalosis and renal proximal tubulopathy. Arch Intern Med 143:1534–1537, 1983.
100. Fishman MP, Telfer N, Zia P, Speckart P, Golub M, Rude R: Role of prostaglandins in the pathogenesis of Bartter's syndrome. Am J Med 60:785–797, 1976.
101. Griffing GT, Melby JC: The therapeutic use of a new potassium-sparing diuretic, amiloride and converting enzyme inhibitor, MK421, in preventing hypokalemia associated with primary and secondary hyperaldosteronism. Clin Exper Hypertens A5:779–801, 1983.

CHAPTER 38

Cancers of the Kidney and Urinary Tract

PETER T. SCARDINO & MADELINE CANTINI

INTRODUCTION

Over the past two decades we have witnessed a remarkable change in the management of cancer. While the results of treatment with each modality—surgery, radiotherapy, chemotherapy, and immunotherapy—have improved, the most dramatic successes have resulted from combining two or more of these approaches. Integrated, multimodal therapy can now offer substantial control of testicular cancers, lymphomas, Wilms' tumors, and others, and has yielded dramatic improvements for osteogenic and soft-tissue sarcomas and for breast, ovarian, and head and neck cancers (1). Improved management of malignant tumors of the urinary tract has also contributed to these advances. Combinations of surgery and chemotherapy are commonly used now for transitional cell carcinomas of the renal pelvis, ureter, and bladder. Topical applications of chemotherapy, combined with surgical resection, have become highly effective in controlling superficial bladder tumors. Surgery, radiotherapy, and endocrine therapy are effective for some prostate cancers, but combinations of these modalities now appear to offer even more successful control. Innovative efforts are underway to develop combinations of chemotherapy, surgery, radiotherapy, and endocrine therapy to treat advanced bladder and prostatic cancers.

In addition, our understanding of the natural history of these malignancies has steadily improved, so that therapy can more appropriately be geared to the threat of the tumor. Diagnostic tests, such as computed tomography scanning, magnetic resonance imaging, ultrasonography, flow cytometry and image analysis, and biochemical tumor markers, have improved our ability to detect, stage, and monitor these tumors. Innovative surgical techniques now offer the patient with bladder and prostate cancer an opportunity for an improved quality of life by preserving normal sexual and urinary function.

In this chapter, we will review the therapy of the major malignant tumors of the urinary tract in light of these recent changes and outline their current management. Much has been accomplished, but further improvements in our ability to prevent and to cure these lethal tumors will require a deep commitment to continuing research into their causes and treatment.

MALIGNANT TUMORS OF THE KIDNEY

The most common malignant tumor of the kidney is renal cell carcinoma, often inappropriately referred to as "hypernephroma." It arises from proximal tubular cells (2). The etiology of renal cell carcinoma is unknown, although it is most common among tobacco users (3, 4). Because similar tumors have been induced in laboratory animals given estrogens, an endocrinologic etiology has been presumed, but remains unsubstantiated in humans (4). A chromosomal basis for this tumor has been postulated based on a familial renal cell carcinoma with a chromosomal translocation. Patients with von Hippel-Landau syndrome are at high risk for multiple renal cell carcinomas (5–7).

The peak incidence of renal cell carcinoma occurs in patients between the ages of 50 and 60, but these tumors can be found in any age group, even infants and children. The incidence in males is 2.7 times greater than in females. In 1990 over 19,000 new cases will be diagnosed and 8000 people will die from renal cell carcinoma in the United States (8). There is less geographic or racial variation for renal cell carcinoma than for the other urinary tract tumors (4, 5).

These tumors are bilateral in only 2% of cases. Histologically, they can be subclassified by cell type as either clear cell, granular cell, or sarcomatoid, each associated with a progressively poorer prognosis (7, 9). The grade or degree of anaplasia also affects the prognosis (9). Renal cell carcinoma tends to be highly vascular, an important feature in diagnosis, although 10–25% are hypovascular, and 5–6% are avascular on angiography. Invasion of vessels is quite common, with extension into the main renal vein in 34% and the vena cava in 10% (10). Interestingly, extension of a tumor thrombus into large veins is the rule rather than actual invasion of the wall of the vein. Massive extension of tumor thrombus into the supradiaphragmatic vena cava and the right atrium can occur (Figure 1).

594 *Therapy of Renal Diseases and Related Disorders*

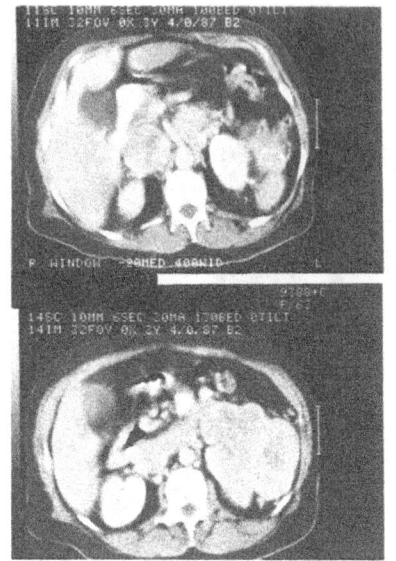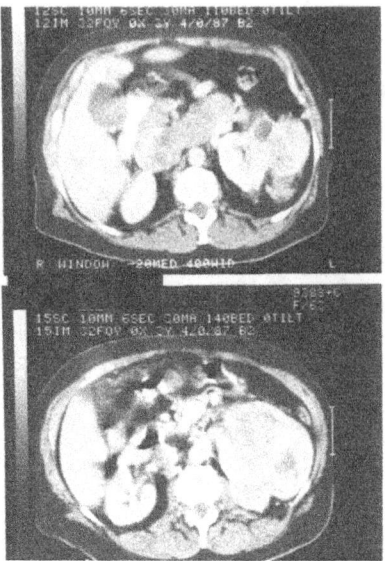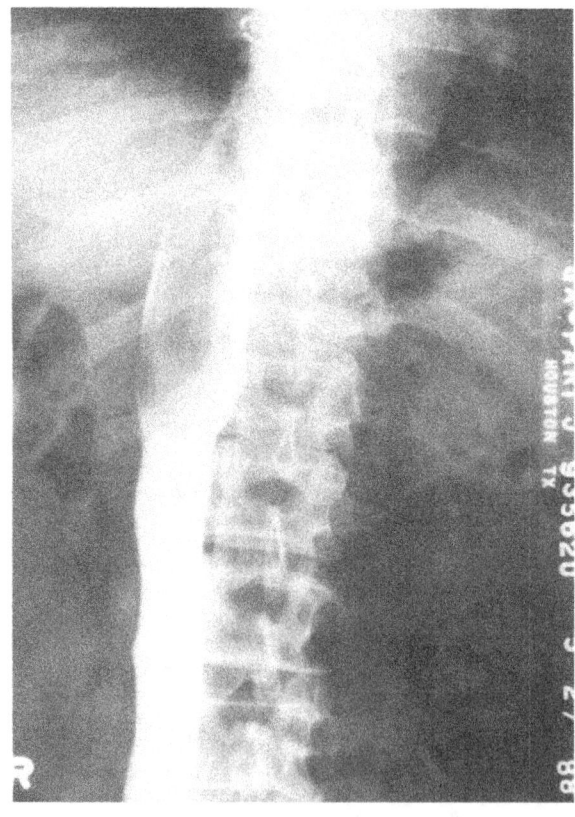

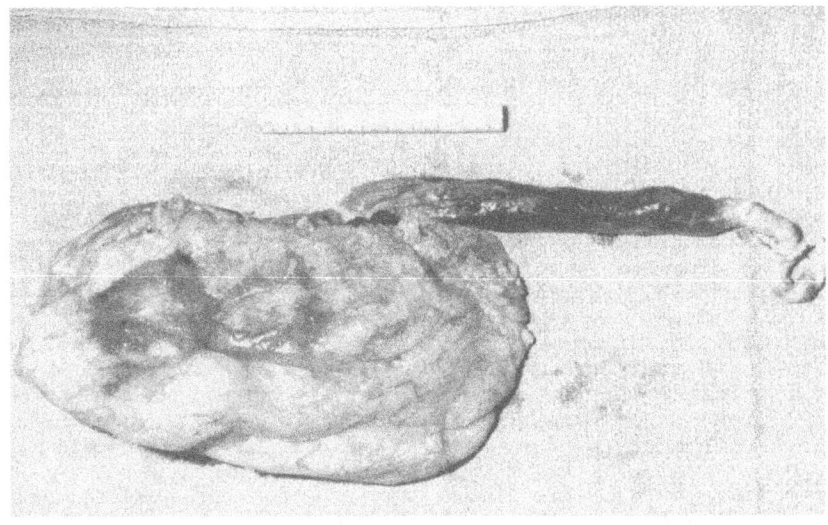

Figure 1. Renal cell carcinoma. A: Computed tomography scan (CT) shows a large left renal mass with extension of tumor thrombus into the inferior vena cava. B: Venocavogram shows a large tumor thrombus in the inferior vena cava extending above the diaphragm into the right atrium. C: The surgical specimen with the tumor thrombus attached to the left kidney.

Because of the protected position of the kidney high in the retroperitoneum, renal tumors often grow silently to a large size, averaging 7 cm. They tend to expand locally, compressing the surrounding normal parenchyma into a "pseudocapsule," penetrating the true renal capsule or renal hilum to invade the perinephric fat in half the cases. Lymphatic dissemination is common, with regional nodes involved in 25% of operable cases. Distant metastases are found in 30% of patients at first presentation and will eventually occur in 60–70% of remaining patients. The most common cause of death from these tumors is not local growth but widespread metastases. Metastases occur to the lungs (55%), lymph nodes (38%), liver (35%), bone (33%), adrenal (19%), contralateral kidney (8%), and brain (7%) (5–7, 9).

The natural history of renal cell carcinoma is unpredictable. Similar to breast cancer, the disease may evolve very slowly; a patient has been reported whose first evidence of metastases was 31 years after nephrectomy (11)! Yet the overall 5-year survival rate is only 40% for patients with operable tumors and 3% for those with metastases at diagnosis. Spontaneous remissions, although well documented, are extremely rare, with only 5 in over 1340 well-studied cases (6).

Benign renal adenomas have been a source of controversy, but most authorities now agree that the size of the tumor alone (i.e., < 2.5 cm) is not a reliable reason for excluding malignancy, and standard histologic and clinical criteria should be used to differentiate an adenoma from a carcinoma (5, 7). The special case of renal oncocytoma, a well-differentiated solid tumor consisting entirely of unique "oncocytes," appears to behave as a benign tumor (12).

Diagnosis and staging

Renal-cell carcinoma may present with a wide spectrum of signs and symptoms, and is often thought of as the "great mimic" (Table 1). The local mass is most often associated with hematuria (59%), flank pain (41%), and a palpable abdominal mass (45%), although this classic triad occurs in only 9% (8). Systemic symptoms may be related to metastases or to the frequent paraneoplastic syndromes associated with this tumor (13), including fever, weight

Table 1. Initial signs and symptoms of renal cell carcinoma

Sign or symptom	Frequency
Hematuria	59%
Flank pain	41%
Palpable mass	45%
All three (hematuria, pain, mass)	9%
Weight loss	28%
Anemia	21%
Symptoms of metastases	10%
Fever	7%
Erythrocytosis	3%
Hypercalcemia	3%
Varicocele	2%
Incidental radiographic finding	7%

After Skinner et al. (9) with permission.

loss, anemia, erythrocytosis, hypercalcemia, hepatopathy, hypertension, as well as a variety of symptoms directly related to metastases. In over a third of patients, the tumor is discovered incidentally during a radiologic investigation for other causes. For such patients, the prognosis is significantly better (14).

The essential diagnostic test is the excretory urogram (intravenous pyelogram or IVP) preferably with nephrotomograms, which should be routinely performed in any patient who has hematuria and who is more than 40 years old. If a renal mass appears cystic, renal ultrasonography can confirm the diagnosis. Fine-needle aspiration with cystography and cytology, although extremely accurate, is no longer used routinely because of the small risk of needle tract seeding and the high accuracy of computed tomography (CT) scanning. If a renal mass is calcified, solid, or equivocal, CT scanning is performed. Magnetic resonance imaging (MRI) offers little advantage over CT scanning. Aortography, with selective renal angiography, previously routine, is now reserved for patients in whom either the diagnosis or the extent of the tumor remains equivocal, preoperative assessment of the arterial distribution is desired for partial nephrectomy, or for the rare patient who is to undergo angiographic infarction. The renal vein should be visualized to rule out venous extension preoperatively in all patients with large tumors and in most with right-sided tumors, because of the short right renal vein. In some patients, perhaps 3%, radiologic studies will not yield a diagnosis, and surgical exploration is essential.

The staging system most widely used for renal cell carcinoma is based on the surgical findings and the pathologic extent of the tumor (Table 2). However, a major flaw in the system comes from the classification within stage III when the renal vein is involved. Skinner and others have shown that renal-vein involvement per se does not substantially worsen the prognosis (15); hence stage III should be reserved for those with nodal metastases.

Therapy

The only proven effective therapy for renal cell carcinoma is radical surgical excision. The fundamental principles of cancer surgery apply. Since radiographic diagnosis is reliable, diagnostic biopsy is rarely necessary and is usually contraindicated because of possible tumor spillage and local recurrence. Adequate exposure of the origin of the renal artery and vein requires a generous incision, which can be midline or transverse upper abdominal or thoracoabdominal (Figure 2). We prefer the extended subcostal incision or thoracoabdominal in most cases. Standard flank incisions are inappropriate for radical nephrectomy, since the kidney must be excessively handled before the vessels are ligated. For lower pole tumors or those of limited size, an incision above the eleventh rib, remaining extrapleural and extraperitoneal, is also satisfactory.

Partial nephrectomy or "enucleation" of tumors has recently been advocated. Although long-term results in patients with a solitary kidney appear to be comparable

Table 2. Staging system and approximate 5-year survival for renal cell carcinoma

Stage	Definition	Survival at 5 years
I	Confined to the kidney	65%
II	Invasion into perinephric fat	47%
III	Extension into renal vein, inferior vena cava, or metastases to regional lymph nodes	51%
IV	Distant metastases	8%

After Skinner et al. (9) with permission.

with those for radical nephrectomy, stage for stage, this limited operation is more morbid than total nephrectomy, risks local recurrence, and should be reserved for patients with impaired renal function or a solitary kidney.

Radical nephrectomy implies removal *en bloc* of the kidney, the surrounding fat both within and around Gerota's fascia, the adrenal gland, and the hilar lymph nodes. Regional lymph node dissection should be considered as well, removing all node-bearing tissue surrounding the great vessels from the diaphragm and superior mesenteric artery superiorly to the bifurcation of the great vessels inferiorly. Since lymph nodes are involved in 25% of operable tumors and this procedure can be done with little additional morbidity, and the 5- and 10-year survival rates range as high as 51% and 17%, respectively, for patients with positive nodes, we generally perform regional lymphadenectomy (8, 14) except in patients with substantial aortic atherosclerosis. Extension of tumor into the vena cava does not preclude successful resection. Even direct extension to the right atrium can be removed *en bloc* by utilizing a technique of total body hypothermia and circulatory arrest with temporary exsanguination in conjunction with cardiopulmonary bypass, which permits surgery to proceed in a bloodless field (15, 16).

Overall survival after radical nephrectomy is 57% at 5 years and 44% at 10 years. Survival is directly related to the stage and grade. Five and 10-year survival rates have been reported as high as 70% and 55%, respectively, for stage I, 64% and 30% for stage II, and 51% and 17% for stage III.

Radiotherapy, either alone or combined with nephrectomy, has been marginally active and is no longer used.

Although formerly nephrectomy was considered essential, even in patients with metastases, abundant data now attest the fruitlessness of this approach. Except for symptomatic palliation (pain, bleeding), nephrectomy alone improves neither the survival nor the quality of life for these patients (6, 7). An exception may be the occasional patient with a solitary treatable metastasis in whom aggressive therapy of both the primary tumor and metastasis may be justified.

There is no consistently effective therapy for metastases nor adjuvant therapy for patients who are at high risk for recurrence after nephrectomy (7). Fewer than 10% of patients will respond to chemotherapy. In-vitro chemo-

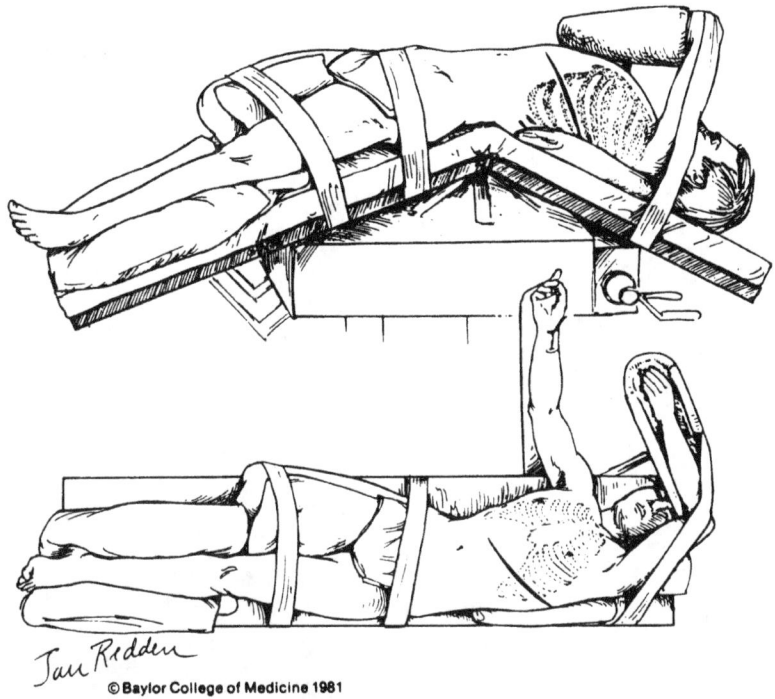

Figure 2. The left torque-flank position is ideal for left radical nephrectomy with retroperitoneal lymphadenectomy. Wide exposure is available. An intraperitoneal and extraperitoneal dissection is possible through this incision.

sensitivity testing has not improved these results. Hormonal therapy is often used, but objective responses are rare and subjective responses are short lived. Immunotherapy has been widely used in this disease, with interferon the most commonly used agent. Response rates vary from 10% to 40%, but no increase in survival has been documented (17). A novel approach has been the use of immunotherapy with interleukin-2, often used in combination with lymphokine-activated killer (LAK) cells (adoptive immunotherapy), which provides objective and sometimes durable responses in nearly 50% of patients (18).

NEOPLASMS OF THE RENAL PELVIS AND URETER

Malignant tumors of the renal pelvis and ureter arise predominantly from the transitional epithelial cells lining these urinary conduits. They are rare, accounting for less than 1% of all genitourinary tumors. The most common tumor of these structures is transitional cell carcinoma (95%), similar histologically though worse prognostically than bladder cancer (19–23). The peak age of incidence of transitional cell carcinoma is 50–70. In children, these epithelial tumors are invariably polypoid and benign (20). In adults, renal pelvic and ureteral tumors occur with equal frequency, although ureteral tumors per se have a strong predilection for the lower one third of the ureter.

Multiplicity of tumors, both in time and in location (polychronotropy), is a hallmark of transitional cell carcinoma. The large epithelial surface of the bladder is also lined with transitional cells, and there is a strong association of upper-tract tumors with bladder cancer. Half of all patients with a transitional cell carcinoma of the renal pelvis or ureter will have a similar tumor in the urinary bladder. The bladder tumors may occur before, during, or after the diagnosis of the primary upper tract tumor. Fortunately, bilateral upper tract tumors are far less common, occurring in only 2% of cases, and are often low grade and amenable to local resection (19–22).

Transitional cell carcinomas occur with increased frequency in chronic phenacetin users (24) and in patients with Balkan nephropathy (25). Squamous cell carcinoma is associated with chronic inflammation and irritation of the urinary tract epithelium from calculi or other agents. The etiology is otherwise not known, although the patterns of occurrence are similar to that for bladder cancer.

Diagnosis and staging

Hematuria, either gross or microscopic, is seen in 80–100% of patients with upper-tract tumors. Nearly half will present with pain, colicky or constant. Occasionally a mass

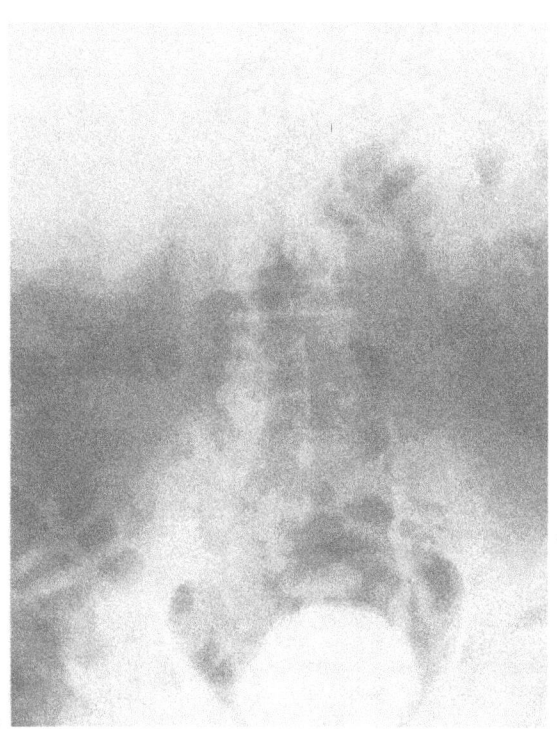 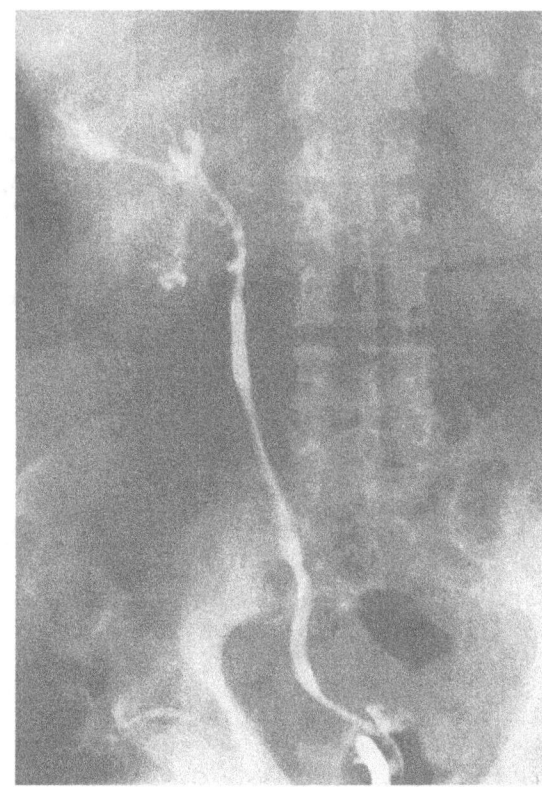

Figure 3. A: IVP in an elderly woman with gross hematuria. The right kidney is not visualized. B: Retrograde pyelogram demonstrates an obstructing ureteral transitional cell carcinoma.

is palpable, but this is usually due to an obstructed hydronephrotic kidney. When ureteral tumors are discovered on IVP during routine follow-up of a patient with bladder cancer, half of the patients are asymptomatic at the time (19–22).

In a patient with hematuria, excretory urography must be performed in such a way as to demonstrate the collecting system in its entirety. The most common finding is a filling defect in the renal pelvis, demonstrated in 50–70% of the pyelograms. Nearly 25% of patients with documented ureteral or renal pelvic tumors have an IVP misinterpreted as "normal" initially, because an area that did not fill out was ascribed to peristalsis. In a third of cases, the involved kidney will not excrete contrast media adequate for visualization (Figure 3).

Cystoscopy is essential in these patients to rule out a bladder cancer, to localize the site of bleeding if gross hematuria is present, and to allow retrograde ureteropyelograms to visualize fully the upper collecting systems. A radiolucent filling defect suggests a tumor, although the differential diagnosis includes blood clot, radiolucent calculus, ectopic or sloughed papilla, vascular impressions, extrinsic compression due to a renal parenchymal tumor, fungus ball, benign stricture, air bubble, pyelitis or ureteritis cystica, venous varicosities or tortuous arterial collaterals, granulomatous lesion, benign tumor, or metastases from other malignancies (19–22).

Urinary cytology is helpful if positive, but false-negative rates range from 22% to 67%. Accuracy is increased by retrograde catheterization and lavage with saline, but even with high-grade (III or IV) lesions 10% will still have negative or equivocal cytologic findings. Brush biopsy of the lesion is often possible with modern, steerable catheters, and it adds considerably to diagnostic accuracy. The recent development of both rigid and flexible ureteroscopes allows direct retrograde visualization of the ureter, making possible tissue diagnosis and improved preoperative staging and grading (Figure 4). Ureteroscopy should only be considered in selected cases, since the procedure carries the risks of perforation, with the possibility of intraperitoneal or retroperitoneal seeding. To rule out a renal pelvic tumor, particularly in a patient with a solitary kidney or renal insufficiency in whom a nephro-ureterectomy would carry extreme morbidity, or when the index of suspicion is low but a tumor cannot otherwise be ruled out, percutaneous antegrade nephroscopy with biopsy,

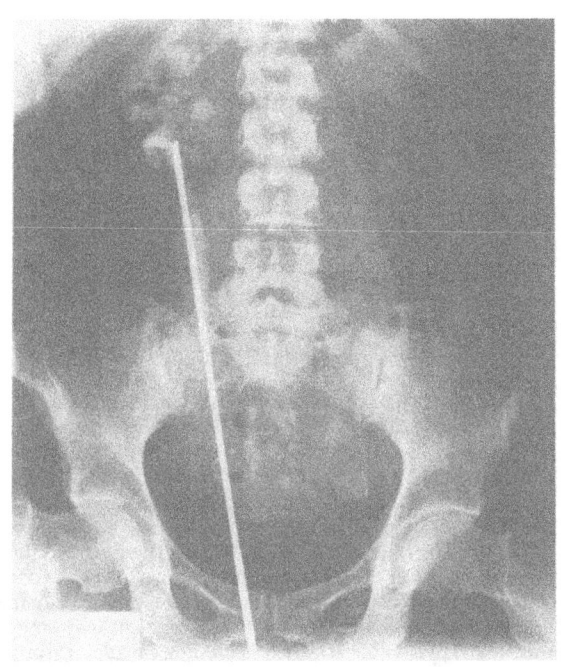
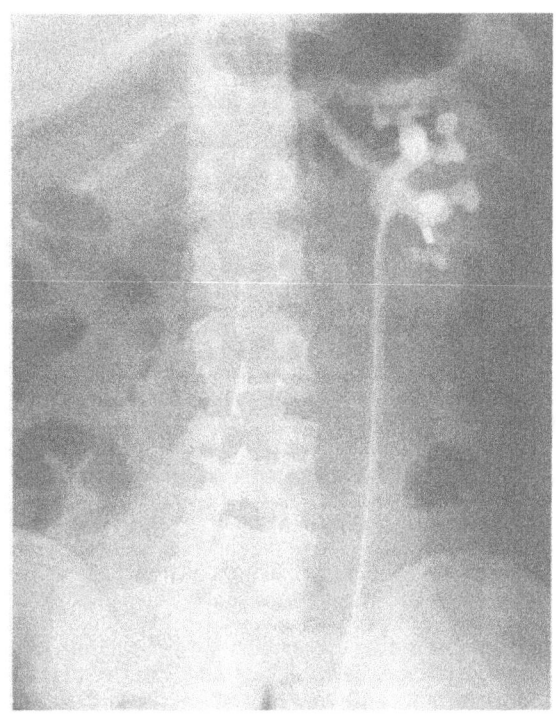

Figure 4. A: The rigid ureteroscope has been passed from the bladder to the right renal pelvis (outlined by contrast media) to view a right upper ureteral filling defect. B: The flexible ureteroscope is particularly useful for viewing all of the calyces. + Courtesy of Dr. Donald P. Griffith.

and even electrofulguration of a renal pelvic tumor, can be performed (19, 22).

Prognosis for renal pelvic and ureteral tumors depends on the grade and stage of the lesion (19–22, 26). The staging system most widely used is identical to that for bladder cancer (Table 3) and is based on the depth of invasion. Approximately 50% of tumors are invasive into muscle or beyond. Carcinoma in situ (intraepithelial neoplasia) occurs in the upper urinary tract as well as the bladder, frequently in association with overt tumors, but also as an isolated lesion. The widespread distribution of intraepithelial neoplastic changes, evident only on histologic examination, may be responsible for the frequent recurrence seen after conservative resection of renal pelvic and ureteral tumors (27).

Therapy

The standard therapy for a documented renal pelvic or ureteral carcinoma is radical nephrectomy (as for renal cell carcinoma) along with total ureterectomy. The ureter should be excised widely, with as much periureteral tissue as possible, down to the urinary bladder. The bladder should be opened and a wide cuff (1–2 cm in radius) around the ureteral orifice excised. The rationale for this approach is the improved survival reported, the high recurrence rate if a ureteral stump is left after nephrectomy, and the difficulty in detecting recurrence in such a blind stump (19–23, 28, 29). The mortality from such an operation, even in the elderly patients who develop these tumors, has been very low in the past 15 years (1%).

Regional lymphadenectomy, when the patient's condition permits, is prudent for the reasons indicated above (see Therapy for renal cell carcinoma) (23). The exception to radical nephroureterectomy is the patient with a low-grade, low-stage, papillary transitional cell carcinoma of the distal ureter. If the proximal collecting system can be adequately demonstrated to be feee of tumor, then distal ureterectomy with ureteroneocystostomy gives excellent long-term results (19, 21). Conservative resection of higher ureteral and renal pelvic tumors may be appropriate in selected cases when a focal, low-grade, low-stage tumor is documented preoperatively (19), especially in patients with compromised renal function. The peculiar reasoning that limited resection of high-grade, high-stage tumors is all that is necessary, since these tumors are rarely curable anyway, represents unfounded nihilism and is not supported by published statistics. (20–23, 26, 28, 29).

With optimal surgical therapy, 5-year survival is 70–100% for noninvasive (stage O and A) tumors, 30–50%

Table 3. Staging systems and approximate 5-year survival for transitional cell carcinoma of the bladder, renal pelvis, and ureter

Stage			Survival at 5 years	
North American	TNM	Definition	Bladder	Pelvis/ureter
CIS	TIS	Carcinoma in situ	—	—
O	T_1	Papillary tumor not invading through basement membrane	95%	95%
A	T_1	Invasion into lamina propria	80%	80%
B	T_2, T_{3a}	Invasion into muscle	40%	40%
C	T_{3b}	Invasion into fat	20%	25%
D_1	N_{1-3}	Regional nodal metastases	15%	—
D_2	M_1	Distant metastases	5%	0%

for stage B (invasion into muscularis), 20–30% for stage C (into surrounding fat or renal parenchyma), and 0% for stage D (metastases). Transitional cell carcinoma is radiosensitive, but in bladder cancer there is good evidence that radiotherapy alone is an inferior therapeutic approach. Radiotherapy has not been used as a primary curative modality for these tumors. Combining radical surgery with postoperative radiotherapy in high-risk patients may decrease the risk of local recurrence in ureteral carcinoma (21), but has been largely supplanted by adjuvant chemotherapy. Transitional cell carcinomas are somewhat sensitive to chemotherapy, with cisplatin the most widely used agent, either alone or in combination (21). Immunotherapy has received few therapeutic trials.

CARCINOMA OF THE BLADDER

Carcinoma of the bladder is one of the more common tumors of the urinary tract. In 1990, it will affect 49,000 people in the United States and will account for approximately 9,700 deaths (8). There is a constant age-related increase in the incidence of carcinoma of the bladder, and interestingly there is a significantly increased incidence of carcinoma of the bladder in women born after 1920, suggesting that cigarette smoking is an etiologic factor. This same rise in incidence is noted in carcinoma of the lung in women. The male/female ratio in the United States is 2.7:1 (30).

Carcinoma of the bladder provides us with one of the better examples of the effect of environmental carcinogens. It is well documented that exposure to aniline dyes is associated with a significant increase in the incidence of bladder cancer, and an excess of cases have occurred among people employed as rubber workers, textile weavers, dye workers, hairdressers, petroleum workers, etc. Prior pelvic irradiation and analgesic abuse predispose to bladder cancer. There is a higher incidence of and mortality from bladder cancer among cigarette smokers, but cigar and pipe smoking have not been associated with an increased risk. It is estimated that 48% of bladder cancer cases result from cigarette smoking (31). Tryptophan metabolites and artificial sweeteners have been implicated in the causation of carcinoma of the bladder, but at this point the data have not conclusively implicated these compounds. The long latency time between the onset of use of a carcinogen and the development of bladder cancer will not resolve this issue in the near future.

Ninety percent of bladder tumors are transitional cell carcinomas, usually papillary and often multicentric. Six to eight percent are squamous cell carcinomas, and only approximately 2% are adenocarcinomas. Benign bladder tumors are extremely rare.

The prognosis for bladder cancer correlates most closely with the stage and grade of the lesion. Stage depends solely upon the depth of invasion of the tumor into the bladder wall and is the best guide to prognosis and appropriate therapy (Table 3). As the tumor invades through the basement membrane into the lamina propria, the muscularis, and the perivesical fat, the incidence of lymph nodal and distant metastases increases and the prognosis worsens (32). In general, the prognosis is worse for sessile as opposed to papillary tumors, and for lymphatic and/or vascular invasion. The tumors are graded by the degree of cellular atypia and nuclear abnormalities. A modification of Broder's classification stratifies tumors into three grades — well, moderate, and poorly differentiated. Although the grade correlates with stage, in a proportion of patients these two prognostic features are discordant (33–35).

A confusing manifestation of bladder cancer has been carcinoma in situ, perhaps best termed *intraepithelial neoplasia*, analogous to the similar, well-characterized lesion in the uterine cervix. Traditionally, carcinoma in situ refers to a high-grade, flat, intraepithelial transitional cell carcinoma that has not invaded the basement membrane. It has a tendency to be diffuse or multifocal, to produce irritative voiding symptoms, and to be particularly aggressive. Some 50% of patients with carcinoma in situ will develop an invasive, potentially lethal bladder tumor within 5 years (36). If carcinoma in situ is found in the bladder along with a superficial noninvasive papillary tumor, 86% of patients will develop an invasive bladder tumor within 5 years (37).

Since the prognosis and the therapy of bladder cancer depend on an accurate assessment of the natural history and lethal potential of the tumor, efforts have been made to further characterize these tumors. The presence or absence of cell-surface blood group antigens on noninvasive papillary transitional-cell carcinomas appears to correlate strongly with the subsequent behavior of the tumor (38).

Bladder cancer has a marked tendency toward multicentricity and recurrence (polychronotropy). Since the entire urinary tract is lined by transitional epithelium, the patient with a bladder cancer is at higher risk for a similar renal pelvic, ureteral, or urethral tumor (33–35).

Diagnosis and staging

The cardinal presenting event in carcinoma of the bladder is hematuria, gross or microscopic, which is seen in more than 70% of patients. Painless hematuria occurring throughout the urinary stream is the most common presenting sign or symptom, but urinary frequency, urgency, dysuria, and pelvic pain also occur. A third of patients will have an associated urinary tract infection, and this symptom complex is all too often dismissed as "hemorrhagic cystitis." Approximately 30% of patients will have irritative voiding symptoms as the only presenting complaint. This frequently signifies muscle invasion, but it may also suggest the presence of carcinoma is situ (33).

The essential diagnostic tests are the excretory urogram (IVP), cystoscopy, and bimanual examination under anesthesia. Any suspicious or apparent lesion within the bladder should be biopsied. A patient who presents with unexplained vesical irritative symptoms or unexplained hematuria should have bladder lavage with saline for cytology and biopsies of even normal-appearing bladder to rule out the presence of carcinoma in situ. Exfoliative cytology is becoming more accurate and is in more widespread use as a screening procedure. Whereas a positive cystology must be pursued aggressively, the study is not yet of sufficient accuracy to be used to exclude the presence of carcinoma without cystoscopic examination and biopsy.

Flow cytometry has become another potentially useful technique in the diagnosis and follow-up of patients with urothelial malignancies. Limiting factors in the use of this technique include the cost of the equipment, the requirement for highly trained personnel, and technical problems ranging from specimen collection and cell fixation to cellular contaminants to the difficulty of distinguishing DNA from RNA. Several recent studies have investigated the overall accuracy of flow cytometry of voided urine or bladder lavage specimens compared with conventional cytology. Flow cytometry and urine cytology were found to be of comparable accuracy in predicting the presence of tumor (83% vs. 78%). When flow cytometry and urine cytology were combined, the diagnostic yield increased to 95%. The false-positive rate in patients with no evidence of disease was reported to be as high as 38%. Although flow cytometry may be comparable to urine cytology, its specificity using current criteria for aneuploidy remains questionable. (39, 40).

The IVP is important to rule out upper-tract tumors and to identify obstruction. Ureteral obstruction suggests either a ureteral tumor or invasion of a bladder tumor into the muscularis. If a tumor is identified cystoscopically, careful bimanual examination of the bladder in a well-anesthetized patient, both before and after the tumor is resected, can help to determine whether the tumor invades muscle, and if so, whether it is fixed to the pelvic sidewall or is mobile.

These initial studies enable the clinician to classify a bladder tumor into one or two groups: either superficial, requiring conservative therapy, or invasive, requiring aggressive therapy. If a tumor appears papillary and superficial and no mass is palpable, it should be resected transurethrally in its entirety and biopsies should be obtained from other areas of the bladder. However, if a tumor appears sessile, deeply invasive, and a mass is palpable, then a deep biopsy should be performed, along with biopsies of the remaining bladder epithelium. Further management will depend on the stage and grade of the primary tumor, the presence of other epithelial abnormalities, such as carcinoma in situ, and the particular circumstances of the individual patient (age, general health, prior history of bladder cancer) (41).

A patient with a low-grade, low-stage superficial tumor needs no other staging studies before therapy can proceed. An extensive "metastatic work-up" is invariably fruitless and unnecessarily expensive. Patients with high-grade or high-stage tumors should undergo further studies to document the extent of the tumor. Other than a complete history, physical examination, chest film, blood counts, and renal and liver function tests, there is no universal agreement on which studies are either necessary or appropriate. Bladder cancer tends to metastasize to the regional lymph nodes (obturator, hypogastric, external iliac, common iliac), liver, lungs, and bones most frequently. Bone scans are used by some, but the yield is low unless the patient has bone pain or an elevated alkaline phosphatase. Liver scans have not been helpful when used routinely. Bipedal lymphography has not been routine but can be used, along with computed tomography scanning, to assess pelvic lymph nodes in the very high risk patient. Suspicious nodes can be biopsied with a thin needle to confirm metastases, thereby avoiding an exploratory operation. Perhaps the most inefficient and inaccurate staging study has been the computed tomography scan to assess the local extent of the tumor. Several studies have now shown that the CT scan cannot accurately differentiate superficial from muscle-invasive tumors, nor can it accurately distinguish "fixed" inoperable cancers from other extensive but operable tumors. Hence, the image obtained is curiously interesting but of little practical consequence to the patient and should not be routinely performed.

Therapy

Treatment is based primarily on the stage of the tumor, with histologic grade playing a role in borderline cases, i.e., a superficial tumor might be treated with more radical therapy if it is poorly differentiated (41).

Fortunately, most bladder tumors, approximately 70%, are superficial low-grade papillary lesions, which can be easily and effectively treated with transurethral resection and fulguration of the base of the tumor. The patient is then followed with periodic cystoscopic examinations to rule out recurrent tumors. A typical follow-up schedule would call for repeat cystoscopy every 3 months for three consecutive negative exams, then every 6 months for two negative exams, then annually for life. With the improvement of flexible endoscopes, flexible cystocopy is a useful technique for office monitoring of this patient population, eliminating the need for anesthesia. Laser therapy has also been used in the treatment of small superficial bladder tumors, but the disadvantage is that the tumor tissue is destroyed, which does not allow for histologic information.

In patients who demonstrate a proclivity to recurrence of superficial tumors, topical chemotherapy or immunotherapy has been effective in diminishing or preventing these recurrences. Thiotepa, adriamycin, mitomycin-C, and BCG are among the most effective agents, and are usually instilled intravesically weekly for 6 weeks, then monthly for 6 months, although treatment schedules vary with each agent (42). Some large tumors cannot be completely resected, and these same intravesical agents can be used therapeutically to destroy or reduce the residual superficial tumor. One can expect complete disappearance of tumor in one third of patients, a substantial reduction (partial response) in one third, and no response in the remaining one third. The drugs can be used sequentially (42).

Carcinoma in situ is by definition a superficial (i.e., noninvasive) bladder cancer, but its diffuse and occult nature makes transurethral resection or fulguration difficult. Topical instillation of chemotherapeutic or immunotherapeutic (BCG) agents has been reported effective in eradicating these lesions, particularly when the disease is more focal and the symptoms minimal. Recent studies with intravesical interferon show an overall complete response rate of 44% with negligible toxicity. Further studies are being conducted comparing intravesical interferon with other treatments. At present, it appears that intravesical BCG is more effective than chemotherapeutic agents. The more aggressive nature of this tumor, especially if the lesion is diffuse or the patient severely symptomatic, or if it is found associated with overt papillary superficial tumors, mandates close follow-up and repeated cytology and bladder biopsies (36, 42, 43).

More aggressive therapy, i.e., total cystectomy, may be necessary for superficial bladder cancer or carcinoma in situ if optimal conservative therapy fails to control the lesion. Some authorities advocate early agressive therapy for diffuse symptomatic carcinoma in situ or for papillar tumor associated with carcinoma in situ. If the epithelial lining of the deep prostatic ducts become malignant, conservative therapy will not be effective and total cystoprostatectomy will be required (36).

When a tumor begins to invade the muscular wall of the bladder, a major surgical procedure must be carried out if the patient is to be offered the best hope of long-term survival. Partial cystectomy is an attractive alternative to total cystectomy. However, because of the multicentric nature of bladder cancer and its tendency to occur near the bladder neck and ureteral orifices, partial cystectomy can be performed as a curative procedure in only approximately 5% of patients with invasive lesions. To be suitable, a patient must have a solitary initial lesion on the dome or posterior wall of the bladder, with negative biopsies throughout the remaining bladder wall. Partial cystectomy is then performed only if the lesion invades the muscularis or is inaccessible to transurethral resection, is high grade, or is in a diverticulum (44).

Most bladder tumors that cannot be managed conservatively require total cystectomy (45). The operation involves removal of the urinary bladder and distal ureters, and in the male, the prostate and seminal vesicles as well. Total urethrectomy is performed if the tumor extends into the urethra or the prostate, or if there is diffuse carcinoma in situ. Careful dissection to preserve the pelvic nerves, which innervate the corpora cavernosa and are responsible for penile erections, mean that cystoprostatectomy (without urethrectomy) can be performed with preservation of erectile potency in selected patients, whereas before men were uniformly impotent after this procedure. However, wide dissection around the bladder, with removal of all perivesical fat and with early ligation of the lateral and posterior vascular pedicles, remain essential hallmarks of a safe, adequate cancer operation. Formerly this operation carried a 10–15% mortality rate, but in the past decade this has been reduced to 1–2% (46).

Since bladder cancer frequently metastasizes to the pelvic lymph nodes, a pelvic lymph node dissection has become the standard initial phase of the operation. Even in the presence of positive nodes, a cystectomy offers palliation to many patients and cure for some (46).

The value of radiotherapy in bladder cancer remains controversial. Interstitial implantation of radium has been used in European centers for localized tumors with excellent results (47). External beam radiotherapy alone for invasive tumors has been compared to preoperative radiotherapy plus cystectomy by Miller and Johnson in a randomized controlled clinical trial. The 5-year survival rate was 16% for radiotherapy alone and 46% for the combined therapy (48). Whitmore (49) and Johnson (34) have particularly championed the combined approach, which is now the subject of two national cooperative clinical trials comparing the combination to surgery alone. However, the only completed randomized study comparing these two regimens showed no significant difference (50, 51). Recent reports of series using cystectomy plus pelvic lymph node dissection show results equal to those of combined therapy (52). Currently, with either approach, one can expect 5-year survival rates after cystectomy of approximately 50% for patients with negative nodes. Most patients who relapse after therapy do so with distant metastases, so that future improvement in survival rates will require more effective systemic adjuvant therapy.

Transitional cell carcinoma has been shown to be responsive to chemotherapy, with cisplatin the most active and widely used drug. Methotrexate has also shown activity, as have combinations of cisplatin, cytoxan, adriamycin (CISCA) and cisplatin plus methotrexate (53). The M-VAC (methotrexate, vinblastine, adriamycin, and cisplatin) regimen was developed by Yagoda and associates, who have reported overall response rates of 71% and complete responses in 50% of patients (54). With response rates in the range of 40%, these drugs may prove useful as neoadjuvant therapy prior to definitive regional surgery or radiation therapy, or as adjuvant therapy after cystectomy for high-risk patients.

An exciting avenue of investigation involves the combined use of regional intra-arterial chemotherapy combined with radiotherapy, either for patients with inoperable local tumors or as an alternative to cystectomy. Preliminary results indicate that some local tumors can be eradicated with this combination.

When the bladder is removed for cancer, urinary diversion is necessary. The most widely used technique has been ureteroileal cutaneous diversion, which can also be performed using the Kock continent pouch technique (55). Direct ureterocutaneous anastomosis is ill advised, except for short-term diversion of the inoperable patient, because of the high incidence of stenosis and obstruction. Ureterosigmoidostomy avoids a cutaneous stoma, but requires frequent voiding per rectum day and night, and is associated with a somewhat higher incidence of postoperative complications, such as obstruction and pyelonephritis. Modern stomal appliances and peristomal care have reduced the morbidity of the cutaneous stoma but have caused distressing alterations of body image (56). There recently has been an explosion of interest in techniques for urinary tract reconstruction that obviate the need for an external urinary appliance and completely restore the continuity of the urinary tract to allow voiding per urethra while maintaining continence. An increased understanding of intestinal physiology has led the way for new techniques of replacing the bladder with bowel segments in order to ensure a low-pressure system within the reservoir until the maximum capacity is reached (Figure 5). The indication for this procedure should be limited to selected patients with little chance of extension to the urethra.

PROSTATIC CANCER

The prostate has become the leading site of cancer and prostatic cancer the second leading cause of cancer deaths in men, making it a major public health problem in Western countries. In 1990, 106,000 new cases will be diagnosed in the United States and 30,000 men will die of the disease (8). The lifetime risk of developing prostatic cancer for a 50-year-old man in 1985 was estimated at 9.5% and the risk of dying from the disease 2.9% (57). Histologic evidence of prostatic cancer can be found in over 30% of men over 50 years old who die of unrelated causes, making it the most common malignancy in human beings (58, 59).

Although prostatic cancer is considered a disease of "old age," it can be found in 29% of men age 50–59 who die of urelated causes (58). Another common misconception is that prostatic cancer is "curable" with a simple endocrine manipulation. A fourth of the patients with this

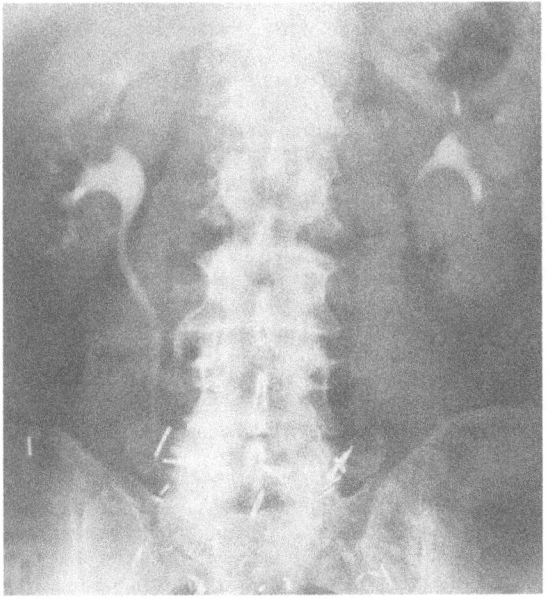
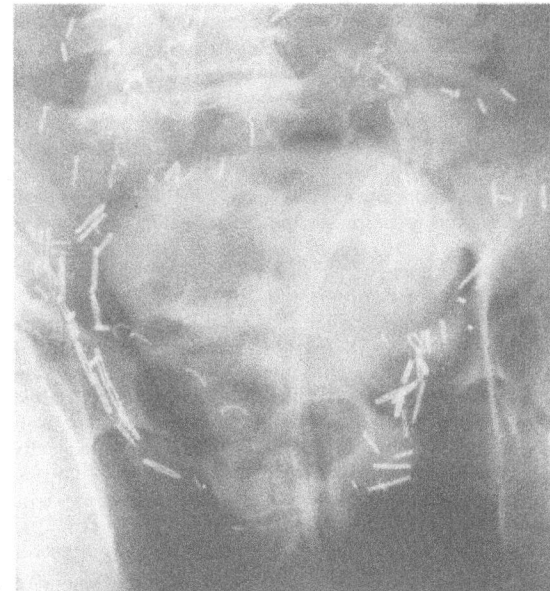

A B

Figure 5. Excretory urogram (A) and cystogram (B) taken 6 months after replacement of the urinary bladder with a "neobladder" constructed from detubularized ileum. The capacity is 500 cc and the patient is continent.

tumor have metastases at the time of diagnosis, and the median survival with endocine therapy (androgen deprivation) is less than 3 years. This brief review will outline our current understanding of the natural history, diagnosis, staging, and therapy of prostatic cancer and point to new avenues that promise better treatment for these patients in the future. More complete reviews have recently been published (60).

Natural history

The etiology of prostatic cancer remains uncertain. Recent evidence implicates cadmium exposure of workers in the battery manufacturing industry, but only a small number of cases can be attributed to this cause. The hormonal milieu is important, since men castrated at an early age seem not to develop prostatic cancer. The marked discepancy in incidence among countries (i.e., low in the Orient, high in Europe and North America) suggests both a genetic (racial) predisposition and an environmental cause. The incidence increases in Japanese immigrants to the United States and is higher still in second-generation immigrants. Dietary factors, such as animal fats, have been postulated as etiologic agents (31).

More than 95% of prostatic malignancies are adenocarcinomas, arising from the prostatic acini. These tumors may assume a variety of histologic patterns, ranging from well-differentiated glands that are difficult to distinguish from the normal prostate to solid or cribiform patterns with almost no recognizable glands. The prognosis correlates strongly with the grade, or degrees of differentiation, of the tumor (61).

The pattern of growth of prostatic cancer is quite diverse (62). Most tumors arise in the periphery of the gland, spread diffusely throughout the prostate, extend locally through the prostatic capsule into the periprostatic tissue, and infiltrate around or into the seminal vesicles. Locally advanced tumors may invade the bladder neck and trigone, causing bladder outlet obstruction or ureteral obstruction with hydronephrosis. At any point in its local growth, a tumor may metastasize via the lymphatics to the pelvic lymph nodes or via the bloodstream to the bones, lungs, liver, or other soft-tissue sites. There is a general correlation between the size of the primary tumor, its grade, and the risk of metastases (63).

Since these adenocarcinomas arise from prostatic acini, it is not surprising that they produce and secrete proteins found in the normal epithelial cells, including prostatic acid phosphatase (PAP) and prostate-specific antigen (PSA). Acid phosphatase was the first clinically useful biochemical tumor marker and served as an objective indicator of response to orchiectomy in Nobel laureate Charles Huggins' discovery that this malignant tumor would respond to androgen deprivation (64). Total acid phosphatase measurements are imprecise. Most current laboratories assay the prostatic fraction only, referred to as PAP (prostatic acid phosphatase), by either an enzymatic or a radioimmunoassay technique. PAP and PSA can be localized within tissue sections with an immunoperoxidase stain utilizing specific antisera. Also, since other tumors have rarely been associated with PAP or PSA production, identification of either of these markers within tumor tissue strongly suggests that the tumor is prostatic in origin (65).

Diagnosis and staging

The classic test for detecting prostatic cancer is the digital rectal examination (66). Most palpable tumors arise in the posterior periphery of the gland, adjacent to the anterior rectal wall, causing nodular "rock hard" induration, irregularity of the gland, or obliteration of the median or lateral sulci. Though never proven by controlled trials, early detection of prostatic cancer through routine digitial rectal examination of males over 40 is believed to be the most important method to achieve a substantial reduction in the death rate from prostatic cancer. It behooves all physicians to insist that such patients undergo annual rectal examination with careful palpation of the prostate. Prostatic cancer tends to remain clinically silent for a long period, and it is this asymptomatic group of patients in whom the tumor is usually confined to the prostate and therefore potentially curable (67).

Symptoms suggesive of prostatic cancer include a recent change in voiding habits, gross or microscopic hematuria, perineal or rectal pain, lower extremity lymphedema from lymphatic metastases, bony pain within the axial skeleton, and constitutional symptoms of anorexia, weight loss, and fatigue.

Transrectal prostatic ultrasongraphy offers a new imaging modality to aid in the diagnosis of prostatic malignancies. Many prostatic tumors are less echogenic than the normal peripheral zone of the prostate (Figure 6) (68, 69). Limited studies comparing transrectal ultrasonography (TRUS) to digital rectal examinations (DRE) in screening patients for prostate cancer have suggested that ultrasonography is more sensitive in identifying early disease. TRUS has been shown to detect prostate cancer in approximately 3% of men over the age of 60% compared with approximately 1% detected with DRE (70, 71). Further clinical investigations of TRUS are being conducted to establish the overall sensitivity and specificity rates, and thus to determine whether this imaging technique is warranted in screening large groups of patients.

Although biochemical markers such as PAP have been touted as potential screening tests for prostatic cancer, the radioimmunossay for prostatic acid phosphatase, the so-called male PAP test, recommended by commercial vendors for routine screening has proved disappointing because of a high false-positive rate (72–74). Among patients admitted for transurethral resection of benign prostatic hypertrophy, about 10% have an elevated PAP by the radioimmunoassay (75), and patients in acute urinary retention have a 25% incidence of positive PAP (74).

More recently, prostate-specific antigen has been investigated as a method of screening or early detection. Described by Wang and associates in 1979 as an antigen associated only with prostatic tissue, PSA was subsequent-

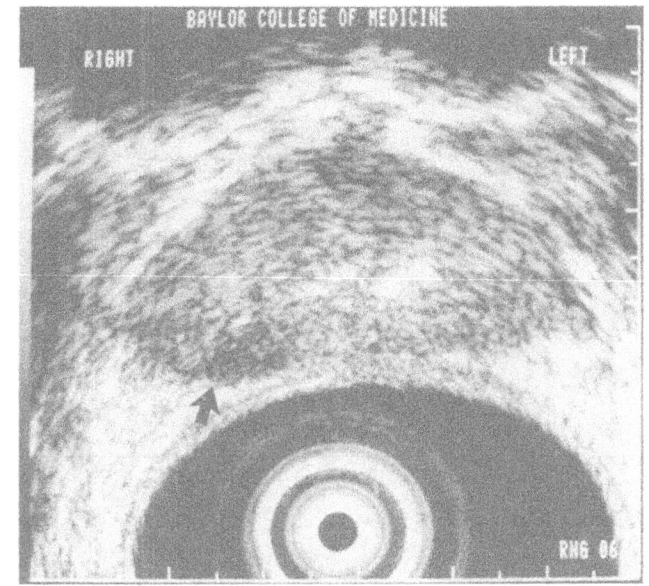

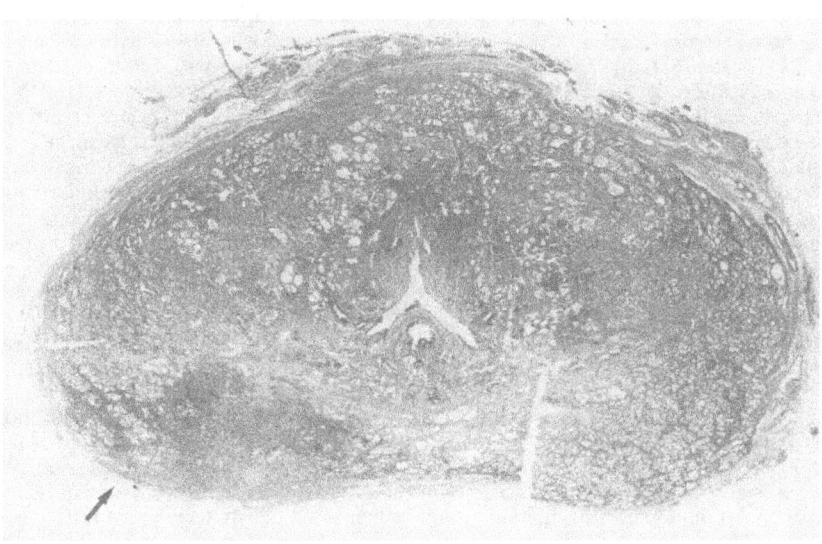

Figure 6. Transrectal ultrasound of the prostate. Transverse image (A) shows a dark (hypoechoic) area in the right peripheral zone (arrow) representing the cancer as seen in the whole-mount histologic section (B). (H + E, reduced from 3.5x). Reproduced with permission from Shinohara K et al. (69).

ly detected in prostate cancer, benign prostatic hyperplasia (BPH), and seminal fluid (76, 77). Studies comparing the levels of elevated PSA in patients with BPH, which is much more prevalent than prostate cancer, and various stages of prostate cancer demonstrate a lack of specificity of PSA and a lack of sensitivity for early stage disease, which make the use of PSA as a "stand-alone" screening test problematic (75, 78–88). Despite these problems, PSA levels are useful in an early detection program when combined with digital rectal examination and transrectal ultrasonography (71, 89). Patients who have a suspicious digital rectal examination or transrectal ultrasonography

Table 4. Staging systems and approximate 10-year survival rate for prostatic cancer

Stage		Definition	Survival at 10 years
North American[89]	TNM[92]		
A	T_A	Incidental pathologic finding after surgery for prostatic obstruction	70%
A_1	T_{A1}	Focal, ≤ three low-power fields, well differentiated	80%
A_2	T_{A2}	Diffuse or less well differentiated	55%
B	T_B	Palpable tumor confined to the prostate	60%
B_{1N}	T_{B1}	≤ 1.5 cm nodule surrounded by normal prostate on three sides, one lobe	75%
B_1	T_{B2}	> 1.5 cm, one lobe	60%
B_2	T_{B3}	Both lobes	40%
C	T_C	Extension beyond prostate (indicates B stage also)	30%
C_1		Invasion into seminal vesicle, ≤ 6 cm (or ≤ 70 g)	40%
C_2		> 6 cm (or > 70 g)	15%
D	N_{1-3}, M_1	Metastases	15%
D_1	N_{1-3}	Regional nodal metastases	20%
D_2	M_1	Distant metastases	10%

are much more likely to have cancer if their PSA level is elevated (89, 90).

Staging of prostatic cancer in the United States has usually been by the American urological system proposed by Whitmore (Table 4) (91). However, the TNM classification proposed by the International Union Against Cancer (UIAC) is now recommended by the American Joint Committee for Cancer Staging and End Results Reporting, and a modification of the TNM system has been accepted by a committee of the Organ System Program of the National Cancer Institute as the official staging system to be adopted in the United States (92).

The classification of nonpalpable tumors found incidentally at the time of transurethral prostatectomy (TURP) for apparent benign prostatic hypertrophy (BPH) as "stage A" (or T_A) has been a source of some confusion and controversy (93). Nearly 1 in 4 patients is classified as stage A at diagnosis (94). Some 10–14% of patients with no palpable evidence of prostatic cancer on rectal examination are found incidentally to have adenocarcinoma in the prostatic tissue removed for the relief of bladder outlet obstruction (95). We know that autopsy studies of men over age 50 who have no clinical evidence of prostatic cancer reveal that 30% (increasing with age) have adenocarcinoma in the prostate (60). How then are we to interpret the biologic potential of such incidentally found tumors? Several recently published series support the concept that when the tumor is well differentiated and occupies no more than three microscopic high-power fields (93), or 5% of the tissue removed (96) the risk of progression is low. Such tumors have been termed A_1 (T_{A1}), and metastases are almost never found in the pelvic lymph nodes (97). For such patients, the risk of local growth or distant dissemination is low during the first 5–10 years, but with time the risk increases, so that young men (less than 60 years old) may best be served by immediate treatment rather than observation (98).

More diffuse or less well-differentiated tumors (stage T_{A2}) have a less favorable prognosis. In our experience at Baylor with 98 such patients, 27% had metastases to the pelvic lymph nodes, as determined by node dissection, and 43% developed progressive disease by 5 years, despite treatment with definitive radiotherapy (99). Hence, nonpalpable prostatic cancer may assume a pattern of insignificant growth with little risk to the host or one of insidious, rapid progression with life-threatening potential. Exactly how to determine the potential of a given tumor is an important question for future investigation (93).

The diagnosis of prostatic cancer is established by biopsy. A transrectal or transperineal large-core (14-gauge) needle biopsy has been the standard approach, but can be quite uncomfortable and often requires anesthesia. Fine-needle aspiration biopsy, as advocated by the Scandinavians who have performed thousands of aspirates, is considered a safe and comfortable procedure, which can be performed as an office procedure in a nonanesthetized patient, but accurate diagnosis is dependent on a trained cytopathologist (100). Recently a spring-loaded biopsy "gun" combined with a small 18-gauge needle has proved highly successful for obtaining multiple biopsies of the prostate under ultrasound or direct finger guidance (68, 101). The procedure can be performed in the office without the use of anesthesia and provides greater accuracy than blind biopsy techniques (102).

Once the diagnosis is established, staging studies include serum acid phosphatase, prostate specific antigen, creatinine and urea nitrogen, and hemoglobin levels. Transrectal ultrasonography of the prostate and the new magnetic resonance imaging with an endorectal coil have proved particularly valuable for documenting the local extent of the tumor (103). A chest film, excretory urogram, or other imaging study of the upper urinary tracts, and a radioisotopic bone scan should also be obtained. Focal radiographs or tomograms of abnormalities detected on bone scan will help to eliminate benign lesions, but the hallmark of bony metastases is increased uptake within the axial skeleton on

Table 5. Frequency of elevated serum levels of acid phosphatase (PAP) and prostate-specific antigen (PSA) in patients with prostatic cancer

Clinical stage	Marker elevation (%)	
	PAP	PSA
T_A	5	50
T_B	20	65
T_C	35	85
N^+, M^+	80	98

Table 6. Incidence of pelvic lymph nodal metastases in each clinical stage of prostatic cancer

Stage		Percent with nodal metastases
A		15
	A_1	0
	A_2	27
B		25
	B_{1N}	14
	B_1	19
	B_2	30
C		50
	C_1	44
	C_2	80

bone scan in an area that appears radiographically normal. Acid phosphatase is a useful staging and prognostic marker. Persistent elevation almost invariably means occult metastases, but a fourth of patients with bony metastases will have a normal acid phosphatase level (Table 5). PSA levels are elevated in most patients with prostatic cancer, and the frequency of elevated levels increases with increasing stage (Table 5) (81, 83, 88).

Metastases to the pelvic lymph nodes are common in all stages of prostatic cancer except A_1 (Table 6) (97). Accurate radiographic techniques for identifying pelvic nodal metastases are not available. Both CT scanning and lymphography have a high incidence of false-positive, false-negative, and equivocal results compared with pelvic lymph-node dissection. Staging pelvic-node dissection is a simple procedure, with a low incidence of morbidity and mortality (99). It has become widely used in patients who are otherwise candidates for definitive therapy with total prostatectomy, radioactive gold, or iodine implantation, but is not generally recommended before external beam radiotherapy because of the increased morbidity associated with the combination of pelvic-node dissection and full pelvic irradiation.

Therapy

The treatment of prostatic cancer depends primarily on the stage of the tumor. Tumors confined to the prostate and immediate periprostatic tissue (TA and TB) can be treated successfully by radical prostatectomy (67). Radical surgery is effective only if the tumor is completely removed with the specimen. Many investigators have begun to use prostate sonography for staging prostatic cancer. In a series of 100 patients with localized prostatic cancer, we compared the stage based on transrectal ultrasonography with the stage on digital rectal exam and judged the accuracy of each staging technique with reference to the surgical or pathologic stage of the tumor. Ultrasonography added useful information and proved to be more reliable than DRE in determining whether a tumor was confined to the prostate or extended outside of the prostate (not confined). Staging pelvic lymph-node dissection most accurately detects nodal metastases and therefore should be done before radical prostatectomy. Historically, the morbidity of radical prostatectomy had been high, with a 15% risk of incontinence and almost invariable erectile impotence. Recent developments enable experienced surgeons to perform the operation with a small (2%) risk of severe incontinence and a high probability of the preservation of potency (104). The decrease in morbidity of the procedure, combined with an increased accuracy of staging, has reawakened interest in surgical excision of the prostate whenever it appears that the tumor can be completely removed (67). PSA levels should become undetectable in patients following radical prostatectomy; otherwise residual or recurrent disease should be suspected (88, 90).

In the majority of patients, however, the tumor has extended beyond the prostatic capsule and irradiation therapy may be more suitable. Radiotherapy can be delivered by external beam alone, ^{125}I implantation, or a combination of radioactive gold (^{198}Au) implantation and external beam irradiation. More experience is available with external beam therapy, which Bagshaw pioneered in the 1950s, than with the implant techniques (105). With external beam irradiation, no operative procedure is necessary and wide fields can be employed. A dosage of at least 6500–7000 rad is necessary to control stage B and C tumors, respectively. At these dosages, complications such as radiation cystitis and proctitis do occur. In an effort to deliver a curative dose of irradiation with fewer complications, several investigators have turned to the implantation of radioactive isotopes. Carlton et al. have successfully employed implantation with ^{198}Au seeds followed by limited external beam therapy for a total dose of 8000–8900 rad (99). Whitmore and Hilaris have used radioactive ^{125}I seeds (106). There are no controlled trials to document the relative merits of these techniques. Our own data indicate an 80% 5-year and a 57% 10-year actuarial disease-free survival rate for patients with localized carcinoma of the prostate and negative pelvic lymph nodes when treated with ^{198}Au implantation plus external beam irradiation (99).

The modern era of systemic treatment of cancer was born in 1940 with the pioneering work of Huggins, who demonstrated that prostatic cancer responds to hormonal manipulation. An effective manipulation requires androgen deprivation, either through bilateral orchiectomy or the administration of agents that will effectively block androgen production by the testes. Estrogens are usually administered in the form of diethylstilbestrol, 1 mg three times a day. Several controlled trials have shown that orchiectomy and estrogen therapy are equally effective. Despite obvious psychologic concerns, orchiectomy seems preferable to estrogen therapy because of the decreased morbidity. Estrogens cause gynecomastia, fluid retention, and a 9% risk of serious thromboembolic complications during the first year. A variety of new agents have become available, and of these the LHRH analogues have been the focus of extensive clinical testing. In clinical trials there was no difference in time to progression between patients treated with DES (3 mg/day orally) and leuprolide (1 mg/day subcutaneously) (107). Some have raised concern about the role of adrenal androgens in patients who have been selectively deprived of testicular androgens alone. The concept of complete androgen blockade led to a large randomized prospective study conducted by the National Cancer Institute comparing leuprolide plus placebo versus leuprolide plus the antiandrogen flutamide. The combination did result in a statistically significant increase in the time to progression and in the survival time, although the quantitative differences were small (less than 3 months and less than 6 months, respectively) (108). Other forms of endocrine therapy are being explored, but hormonal therapy is palliative—most patients will eventually die of their disease—and it is best reserved for patients with otherwise incurable prostate cancer. The median survival with any hormonal manipulation is less than 3 years (109).

Clinical trials of the National Prostatic Cancer Project have studied numerous chemotherapeutic agents alone and in combination, and, as yet, none of these drugs have shown a reproducible level of objective response. Combinations of hormonal and chemotherapy are under investigation but so far have proved of no value when compared with endocrine therapy alone (110).

SUMMARY

The management of neoplasms of the urinary tract has changed substantially in the past decade. A wealth of data regarding the natural history, diagnosis, staging, and treatment of these tumors has emerged, justifying the publication of three texts devoted solely to genitourinary cancer, and a generation of subspecialists has emerged in the medical centers who are thoroughly trained in urologic oncology. Even more rapid change can be expected in the next decade, so that optimum care of patients with these potentially lethal tumors will increasingly depend upon their referral to a central facility that is staffed and equipped to provide the multimodal therapy required.

REFERENCES

1. DeVita VT Jr, Hellman S, Rosenberg SA (eds): *Cancer: Principles and Practice of Oncology*, 2nd ed. JB Lippincott, Philadelphia, 1982.
2. Wallace AC, Nairn RC: Renal tubular antigens in kidney tumors. *Cancer* 29:977–981, 1972.
3. Bennington JL, Laubsch FA: Epidemiologic studies on carcinoma of the kidney: Association of renal adenocarcinoma with smoking. *Cancer* 21:1069, 1986.
4. Morrison AS, Cole P: Epidemiology of urologic cancers. In: N Javadpour, ed, *Principles and Management of Urologic Cancer*. Williams and Wilkins, Baltimore, pp 1–27, 1979.
5. Bennington JL, Beckwith JB: Tumors of the kidney, renal pelvis and ureter. In: *Atlas of Tumor Pathology, Fascide 12*, Washington, DC, Armed Forced Institute of Pathology, 1975.
6. DeKernion JB, Berry D: The diagnosis and treatment of renal cell carcinoma. *Cancer* 45:1947–1956, 1980.
7. Paulson DF, Perez CA, Anderson T: Cancer of the kidney and ureter. In:VT DeVita Jr, S Hellman, SA Rosenberg, eds, *Cancer: Principles and Practice of Oncology*, 2nd ed, JB Lippincott, Philadelphia, pp 895–915, 1985.
8. Silverberg E, Boring CC, Squires TS: Cancer statistics, 1990. *CA* 40:9–26, 1990.
9. Skinner DG, Colvin RB, Vermillion CD, Pfister RC, Leadbetter WF: Diagnosis and management of renal cell carcinoma. A clinical and pathological study of 309 cases. *Cancer* 28:1165–1177, 1971.
10. Goncharenko V, Gerlock AJ Jr, Kadir S, Turner B: Incidence and distribution of venous extension in 70 hypernephromas. *Am J Radiol* 133:263–265, 1979.
11. Kradjian RM, Bennington JL: Renal carcinoma: Recurrent 31 years after nephrectomy. *Arch Surg* 90:192–195, 1965.
12. Lieber MM, Tomera KM, Farrow GM: Renal oncocytoma. *J Urol* 125:418–485, 1982.
13. Marshall FF, Walsh, PC: Extrarenal manifestations of renal cell carcinoma. *J Urol* 117:439–440, 1977.
14. Nishijima Y, Noguchi R, Ishikawa S, Nemoto R, Kanoh N, Koiso K: Renal cell carcinoma as an incidental finding by ultrasonography and computed tomography (abstract). *J Urol* 139:423A, 1988.
15. Skinner D, Lieskovsky G, Pritchett T: In: D Skinner, G Lieskovsky, eds, *Diagnosis and Management of Genitourinary Cancer*. WB Saunders, Philadelphia, 1988.
16. Marshall FF, Reitz BA, Diamon DA: A new technique for management of renal cell carcinoma involving the right atrium: Hypothermia and cardiac arrest. *J Urol* 131:103–107, 1984.
17. Quesada JR, Swanson DA, Trindade A, Gutterman JV: Renal cell carcinoma: Antitumor effects of leukocyte interferon. *Cancer Res* 43:940–947, 1983.
18. Rosenberg SA, et al.: Observations on the systemic administration of autologous lymphokine activated killer cells and recombinant interleukin-2 to patients with metastatic cancer. *N Engl J Med* 313:1485, 1985.
19. Gittes, RF: Tumors of the ureter and renal pelvis. In: JH Harrison, RF Gittes, AD Perlmutter, T Stamey, PC Walsh, eds, *Campbell's Urology*, 4th ed. WB Saunders, Philadelphia, pp 1010–1032, 1979.
20. Bergman H, Hotchkiss RS: Ureteral tumors. In: H Bergman, ed, *The Ureter*, 2nd ed. Springer-Verlag, New York, pp 271–300 1981.
21. Johnson, DE: Renal pelvic and ureteral tumors: In: DE Johnson, MA Boileau, eds, *Genitourinary Tumors: Fundamental Principles and Surgical Techniques*. Grune and Stratton, New York, pp 353–370, 1982.
22. Clayman RV, Lange PH, Fraley, EE: Cancer of the upper urinary tract. In: N Javadpour, ed, *Principles and Management of Urologic Cancer*, 2nd ed. Williams and Wilkins,

Baltimore, pp 544–559, 1983.
23. Richie JP: Management of ureteral tumors. In: DG Skinner, JB deKernion, eds, *Genitourinary Cancer*. WB Saunders, Philadelphia, pp 150–165, 1978.
24. Lomax-Smith JD, Seymour AE: Neoplasia in analgesic nephropathy. A urothelial field change. *Am J Surg Pathol* 4:565–572, 1980.
25. Petkovic SD: Treatment of bilateral renal pelvis and ureteral tumors. *Eur Urol* 4:391–400, 1979.
26. Cummings KB, Correa RJ, Gibbons RP: Renal pelvic tumors. *J Urol* 113:158–162, 1977.
27. Mahadevia PS, Karwa GL, Koss LG: Mapping of urothelium in carcinomas of the renal pelvis and ureter. *Cancer* 51:890–897, 1983.
28. Cummings KB: Nephroureterectomy: Rationale in the management of transitional cell carcinoma of the upper urinary tract. *Urol Clin North Am* 7:569–578, 1980.
29. Johansson S, Wahlqvist L: A prognostic study of urothelial renal pelvic tumors. *Cancer* 43:2525–2531, 1979.
30. Cancer Statistics, 1983. *Cancer* 33:9–25, 1983.
31. Morrison AS, Cole P, Maclure KM: Epidemiology of urologic cancers. In: N Javadpour, ed, *Principles and Management of Urologic Cancer*. Williams and Wilkins, Baltimore, pp 12–31, 1983.
32. Skinner DG: Current state of classification and staging of bladder cancer. *Cancer Res* 37:2838–2842, 1977.
33. DeKernion JB, Skinner DG: Epidemiology, diagnosis and staging of bladder cancer. In: DG skinner, JB DeKernion, eds, *Genitourinary Cancer*. WB Saunders, Philadelphia, pp 213–231, 1978.
34. Johnson DE, Boileau MA: Bladder Cancer: Overview. In: DE Johnson, MA Boileau, eds, *Genitourinary Tumors: Fundamental Principles and Surgical Techniques*. Grune and Stratton, New York, pp 399–447, 1982.
35. Gittes, RF: Tumors of the bladder. In: JH Harrison, RF Gittes, AD Perlmutter, T Stamey, PC Walsh, eds, *Campbell's Urology*, 4th ed. WB Saunders, Philadelphia, pp 1033–1070, 1979.
36. Utz, DC, DeWeerd JH: The management of low-grade low-stage carcinoma of the bladder. In: DG Skinner, JB DeKernion, eds, *Genitourinary Cancer*. WB Saunders, Philadelphia, pp 256–268, 1978.
37. Heney NM, Daly J, Prout GR et al.: Biopsy of apparently normal urothelium in patients with bladder cancer. *J Urol* 120:559, 1978.
38. Newman AJ Jr, Carlton CE Jr, Johnson S: Cell surface A, B, or O(H) blood group antigens as an indication of malignant potential in stage A bladder carcinoma. *J Urol* 124:27–29, 1980.
39. Murphy WM, Emerson LD, Chandler RW et al.: Flow cytometry versus urinary cytology in the evaluation of patients with bladder cancer. *J Urol* 136:815–819, 1986.
40. deVere White RW, Olson CR, Dietrich AD: Flow cytometry: Role in monitoring transitional cell carcinoma of the bladder. *Urology* 28:15–20, 1986.
41. Skinner DG: Current perspectives in the management of high-grade invasion of invasive bladder cancer. *Cancer* 45:1866–1874, 1980.
42. Soloway MS: The management of superficial bladder cancer. *Cancer* 45:1856–1865, 1980.
43. Utz DC, Farrow CM, Rife CC, Segura JW, Zincke H: Carcinoma in situ of the bladder. *Cancer* 45:1842–1848, 1980.
44. Utz DC, Schmitz SE, Fugelo PD, Farrow GM: A clinicopathologic evaluation of partial cystectomy for carcinoma of the urinary bladder. *Cancer* 32:1075, 1973.
45. Skinner, DG, Kauffman JJ: The management of invasive and high grade bladder cancer. In: DG Skinner, JB DeKernion, eds, *Genitourinary Cancer*. WB Saunders, Philadelphia, pp 269–283, 1978.
46. Skinner DG: Radical cystectomy. In: ED Crawford, TA Borden, eds, *Genitourinary Cancer Surgery*. Lea and Febiger, Philadelphia, pp 207–216, 1982.
47. Van der Werf-Messing B: Cancer of the urinary bladder treated by interstitial radium implant. *Int J Radiat Oncol Biol Physiol* 4: 373–378, 1978.
48. Miller LS: Bladder cancer: Superiority of preoperative irradiation and cystectomy in clinical stages B2 and C. *Cancer* 39:973–980, 1977.
49. Whitmore WF Jr, Batata MA, Oheneum MA, Grabstald H, Unal A: Radical cystectomy with or without prior irradiation in the treatment of bladder cancer. *J Urol* 108:184, 1977.
50. Prout GR Jr: The surgical management of bladder carcinoma. *Urol Clin North Am* 3:149–175, 1976.
51. Scardino PT, Skinner DG: Radical cystectomy, pelvic lymph node dissection, and urethrectomy. In: ED Whitehead, ed, *Current Operative Urology*, 2nd ed. Harper & Row, Hagerstown, MD, 1984.
52. Mathur VK, Krahn HP, Ramsey EW: Total cystectomy for bladder cancer.*J Urol* 125:784–786, 1981.
53. Schwartz S, Yagoda A, Natale RB, Watson RC, Whitmore WF Jr, Lesser M: Phase II trial of sequentially administered cisplatin, cyclophosphamide and doxorubicin for urothelial tract tumors. *J Urol* 130:681–684, 1983.
54. Sternberg CN, Yagoda A, Scher HI, Watson RC et al.: Preliminary results of M-VAC (methotrexate, vinblastine, doxorubicin, and cisplatin) for transitional cell carcinoma of the urothelium. *J Urol* 133:403–407, 1985.
55. Koch NG, Nilson AE, Nilson LO, Norlen LJ, Philipson BM: Urinary diversion via continent ileal reservoir: Clinical results in 12 patients. *J Urol* 128:469–475, 1982.
56. Richie JP: Techniques of ureterointestinal anastomoses and conduit construction. In: ED Crawford, TA Borden, eds, *Genitourinary Cancer Surgery*, Lea & Febiger, Philadelphia, pp 227–239, 1982.
57. Seidman H, Mushinski MH, Geib SK, Silverberg E: Probabilities of eventually developing or dying of cancer—United States, 1985, *CA* 35:36–56, 1985.
58. Frank LM: Latent carcinoma of the prostate. *J Path Bacteriol* 68:603, 1954.
59. McNeal JE: Origin and development of carcinoma in the prostate. *Cancer* 23:24, 1969.
60. Scardino PT: Early detection of prostate cancer. *Urol Clin N Am* 14:1170–1191, 1989.
61. Gleason DF, Mellinger GT, the VACRUG: Prediction of prognosis for prostatic adenocarcinoma by combined histological grading and clinical staging. *J Urol* 111:58–64, 1974.
62. Wheeler TM: Anatomical consideration in carcinoma of the prostate. *Urol Clin North Am* 16:623–634, 1989.
63. Whitmore WF: The natural history of prostatic cancer. *Cancer* 32:1104–1112, 1973.
64. Huggins C, Stevens RE, Hodges CV: Studies on prostatic cancer. II. The effect of castration on clinical patients with carcinoma of the prostate. *Arch Surg* 43:208–223, 1941.
65. Jobsis AC, DeVries GP, Anholt RRH, et al.: Demonstration of prostatic origin of metastases. An immunochemical method for formaline-fixed embedded tissue. *Cancer* 41:1788, 1978.
66. Guinan P, Bush I, Ray R, Veth R, Rao R, Bhatti R: The

accuracy of the rectal examination in the diagnosis of prostate carcinoma *N Engl J Med* 303:499–502, 1980.
67. Walsh PC, Lepor H: The role of radical prostatectomy in the management of prostatic cancer. *Cancer* 60 (Suppl 3):526–537, 1987.
68. Lee F, Torp-Pedersen ST, Siders DB, Littrup PJ, McLeary RD: Transrectal ultrasonography in the diagnosis and staging of prostatic carcinoma. *Radiology* 170:609–615, 1989.
69. Shinohara K, Wheeler T, Scardino PT: The appearance of prostate cancer on transrectal ultrasonography: Correlation of imaging and pathological examinations. *J Urol* 142:76–82, 1989.
70. Lee F, Littrup PJ, Torp-Pedersen ST, Mettlin C, McHugh TA, Gray JM, Kumasada GH, McLeary RD: Prostate cancer: Comparison of transrectal US and digital rectal examination for screening. *Radiology* 168:389–394, 1988.
71. Lee F, Torp-Pedersen S, Littrup PJ, McLeary RD, McHugh TA, Smid AP, Stella PJ, Borlaza GS: Hypoechoic lesions of the prostate: Clinical relevance of tumor size, digital rectal examination, and prostate-specific antigen. *Radiology* 170:29–32, 1989.
72. Gittes RF: Serum acid phosphatase and screening for carcinoma of the prostate. *N Engl J Med* 309:852–853, 1983.
73. Cooper JF: The radioimmunochemical measurement of prostatic acid phosphatase: Current state of art. *Urol Clin North Am* 7:653–665, 1980.
74. Bruce AW, Mahan DE, Belville WD: The role of the radioimmunoassay for prostatic acid phosphatase in prostatic carcinoma. *Urol Clin North Am* 7:645–652, 1980.
75. Andriole GL, Catalona W: Controversies in urologic oncology. *Urol Clin North Am* 14(4):657, 1987.
76. Wang MC, Papsidero LD, Kurtyama M, Valenzucla LA, Murphy GP, Chu FM: Prostatic antigen: A new potential marker for prostatic cancer. *Prostate* 2:89, 1981.
77. Papsidero LD, Wang MC, Valenzucla LA et al: A prostate specific antigen in SCRA of prostatic cancer patients. *Cancer Res* 40:2428, 1980.
78. Myrtle JF, Klimey PG, Iwor LP, Bruni JF: Clinical utility of prostate specific antigen (PSA) in the management of prostate cancer. *Adv Cancer Diagn*, 1986.
79. Kuriyama M, Wang MC, Lee CL, Kilian CS, Papsidero LD, Inaji H, Loor RM, Lin MF, Nishuria T, Slack NH, Murphy GP, Chu TM: Multiple marker evaluation in human prostate cancer with the use of tissue specific antigens. *J Natl Cancer Inst* 68: 99, 1982.
80. Killian CL, Yang N, Emirch LJ, Vargas FP, Kuriyama M, Wang MC, Slack NH, Papsidero LC, Murphy GP, Chu TM, the investigators of the National Prostatic Cancer Project: Prognostic significance of prostate specific antigen for monitoring patients with stages B2 to D1 prostate cancer. *Cancer Res* 45:886, 1985.
81. Ercole CJ, Lange PH, Mathisen M, Chiou RK, Reddy PK, Vessella RL: Prostatic specific antigen and prostatic acid phosphatase in the monitoring and staging of patients with prostatic cancer *J Urol* 138:1181, 1987.
82. Ferro PJB: Tumour markers in prostatic carcinoma: A comparison of prostate specific antigen with acid phosphatase. *Br J Urol* 60:69, 1987.
83. Stamey TA, Yang N, Hay AR, McNeal JE, Freiha FS, Redwine E: Prostate specific antigen as a serum marker for adenocarcinoma of the prostate. *N Engl J Med* 317:909, 1987.
84. Chan DW, Bruzek DJ, Oesterling JE, Rock RC, Walsh PC: Prostate specific antigen as a marker for prostatic cancer: A monoclonal and polyclonal immunoassay compared. *Clin Chem* 33:1916, 1987.
85. Stamey TA: Editorial comment. *J Urol* 139:764, 1988.
86. Lange PH, Ercole CJ, Lightner DJ, Fraley EE: The value of serum prostatic specific antigen determinations before and after radical prostatectomy. *J Urol* 141:873–879, 1989.
87. Wang TY, Kawaguichi TP: Preliminary evaluation of measurement of serum prostate specific antigen level in detection of prostate cancer. *Ann Clin Lab Sci* 16:461, 1986.
88. Oesterling JE, Chan DW, Epstein JI, Kimball AW Jr, Bruzek DJ, Rock RC, Brendler CB, Walsh PC: Prostate specific antigen in the preoperative and postoperative evaluation of localized prostatic cancer treated with radical prostatectomy. *J Urol* 139:766, 1988.
89. Cooner WH, Mosley BR, Rutherford CL Jr, Beard JH, Pond HS, Bass RB, Terry WJ: Clinical application of transrectal ultrasonography and prostate-specific antigen in the search for prostate cancer. *J Urol* 139:66–69, 1988.
90. Brawer MK, Lange PH: Prostate-specific antigen: Its role in early dectection, staging, and monitoring of patients with prostatic carcinoma. *J Endourol* 3:227–236, 1989.
91. Whitmore WF Jr: Hormone therapy in prostatic cancer. *Am J Med* 21:697, 1956.
92. Whitmore WF Jr, Catalona WJ, Grayhack JT, Hanks G, Peters PC, Shipley WV, Walsh PC: Organ systems program staging classification for prostate cancer. In: *A Multidisciplinary Analysis of Controversies in the Management of Prostate Cancer*. DS Coffey, MI Resnick, FA Dorr, JP Karr, eds, Plenum Press, New York, pp 295–297, 1988.
93. Neerhut GJ, Wheeler TM, Dunn JK et al.: Residual tumor after TUR: Pathologic features of stage A prostate cancer in the transurethral and radical prostatectomy specimens. *J Urol* 139:315A, 1988.
94. Schmidt JD, Mettlin CJ, Natarajan N, Peace BB, Beart Robert W Jr, Winchester DP, Murphy P: Trends in patterns of care for prostatic cancer, 1974–1983: Results of surveys by the American College of Surgeons. *J Urol* 136:416–421, 1986.
95. Newman AJ Jr, Graham MA, Carlton CE Jr, Lieman S: Incidental carcinoma of the prostate at the time of transurethral resection: Importance of evaluating every chip. *J Urol* 128:948–950, 1982.
96. Cantrell BB, DeKlerk DP, Eggleston JC, Boitnott SK, Walsh PC: Pathologic factors that influence prognosis in stage A prostatic cancer: The influence of extent versus grade. *J Urol* 125:516, 1981.
97. Donohue RE, Mani JH, Whitesel JA, Mohr S, Scanavino D, Augsburger RR, Biber RJ, Fauver EH, Wettlaufer JN, Pfister RR: Pelvic lymph node dissection: Guide to patient management in clinically locally confined adenocarcinoma of prostate. *Urology* 20:559–565, 1982.
98. Blute ML, Zincke H, Farrow GM: Long-term follow-up of young patients with stage A adenocarcinoma of the prostate. *J Urol* 136:840–843, 1986.
99. Carlton CE Jr, Scardino PT: Long-term results after combined radioactive gold seed implantation and external beam radiotherapy for localized prostatic cancer. In: *A Multidisciplinary Analysis of Controversies in the Management of Prostate Cancer*. DS Coffey, MI Resnick, FA Dorr, JP Karr, eds, Plenum, New York, pp 109–121, 1988.
100. Lin BP, Davies WE, Harmata PA: Prostatic aspiration cytology. *Pathology* 11:607–614, 1979.
101. Lee F, Littrup PJ, McLeary RD, Kumasaka GH, Borlaga GS, McHugh TA, Soideren MH, Roi LD: Needle aspiration and core biopsy of prostate cancer: Comparative evaluation with biplanar transrectal US guidance. *Radiology* 163:515–

520, 1987.
102. Shabsigh R, Carter S StC, Egawa S, Wright CD, Carlton CE Jr, Scardino PT: Transrectal ultrasound and/or digital guided biopsy of the prostate. *J Urol* 141:282A, 1989.
103. Scardino PT, Shinohara K, Carter S StC, Wheeler TM: Staging of prostate cancer: The value of ultrasonography. *Urol Clin North Am* 16:713–734, 1989.
104. Walsh PC, Donker PJ: Impotence following radical prostatectomy: Insight into etiology and prevention. *J Urol* 128:492–497, 1982.
105. Bagshaw MA: Radiation therapy of prostatic carcinoma. In: ED Crawford, TA Borden, eds, *Genitourinary Cancer Surgery*. Lea and Febiger, Philadelphia, pp 405–411, 1982.
106. Grossman HB, Batata M, Hilaris B, Whitmore WF Jr: ^{125}I implantation for carcinoma of the prostate. *Urology* 20:291, 1982.
107. The Leuprolide Study Group: Leuprolide versus DES in the initial therapy of advanced prostatic cancer: A randomized prospective trial. *N Engl J Med* 311:1281, 1984.
108. Crawford ED, McLeod D, Dorr H, et al.: A comparison of leuprolide with flutamide and leuprolide in previously untreated patients with clinical stage D2 cancer of the prostate. Phase III, Intergroup Study—0036. *N Engl J Med* 254:1989.
109. Scott WW, Menon M, Walsh PC: Hormonal therapy of prostatic cancer. *Cancer* 45:1929–1936, 1980.
110. Gibbons RP: Cooperative clinical trials of single and combined agent protocols: Adjuvant protocols. *Urology* 17 (Suppl):48–52, 1981.

CHAPTER 39

Toxic Nephropathies

JOHN F. MAHER

INTRODUCTION

Recently, toxic nephropathy has emerged as an important segment of clinical renal disease. The high prevealence of nephrotoxic lesions reflects increased human exposure to a wide variety of drugs, chemicals, and biologic products; improved diagnostic capability; and enhanced awareness.

The true incidence of toxic nephropathy is uncertain because of diagnostic inaccuracy. Since the structural and functional abnormalities caused by nephrotoxins are nonspecific, toxic causes are often overlooked. Conversely, an overinterpreted exposure history, without clinical, physiologic, and histologic evidence of compatible renal injury also misleads incidence data. Currently, the nephropahy of analgesic abuse accounts for about 3% of the worldwide population with end-stage renal failure (1) and as many as 30% of patients with chronic uremia in some geographic areas (2, 3). Lead nephropathy, mostly incorrectly diagnosed, may account for another 10% of chronic renal failure (4), and solvent exposure may be an underlying trigger for a high fraction of chronic glomerulopathies. Moverover, nephrotoxicity limits the use of some antibiotics (5), cancer chemotherapeutics (6), and diagnostic agents (7). Dectectable aminoglycoside nephrotoxicity may occur in as many as 50% of the several million patients so treated annually (8). Although overt acute renal failure represents a small fraction of aminoglycoside nephrotoxicity, the most severe end of the spectrum, it is one of the most frequent causes of acute renal failure encountered today.

DIAGNOSIS

The diagnosis of toxic nephropathy frequently depends on an exposure history. Often this history is occult. Special attention must be paid to the patients' occupation and hobbies (e.g., for lead exposure and hydrocarbon use). When the possibility of suicide or homicide is considered, heavy metals and other intoxicants should be suspected. The history may also reveal exposure to radiation; iodinated contrast media; prescribed drugs such as lithium or antibiotics; the use of nonprescription drugs including laxatives, analgesics, ointments, and antacids; or contact with fertilizers, paints, fumes, insecticides, or contaminated alcohol or food. Allergic patients should be suspected of hypersensitivity reactions involving the kidney. Abusers of drugs rarely offer the history and often deny their excesses, even to their family and themselves, especially when the query sounds punitive. Important environmental toxins causing acute renal failure include glycols, organic solvents, metals, pesticides, and herbicides, while exposure to hydrocarbons, cadmium, lead, silica, or radiation may underlie chronic renal failure (9). Occupational exposure can be monitored by measuring excretion of such urinary enzymes as N-acetyl-beta-D-glucosaminidase (10). Because the association of toxic exposure is more obvious with acute renal injury than with chronic nephropathy, the causative or contributory role of toxins in chronic lesions is more likely to be overlooked. The exposure history should be probed especially diligently when lesions that are particularly compatible with nephrotoxicity such as papillary necrosis are identified.

RENAL VULNERABILITY TO TOXINS

Explanations for the renal vulnerability to toxins have been reviewed elsewhere (11, 12). Both renal circulatory and renal tubular transport properties contribute to the high susceptibility to toxic injury, as outlined in Table 1.

Subsets of the population with increased susceptibility to nephrotoxic injury include the young and the elderly, in part because of pharmacokinetic differences, those with growing or hypertrophying kidneys, patients with impaired routes of elimination, those with vascular or hemodyamic abnormalities, and patients receiving more than one drug.

TREATMENT: GENERAL PRINCIPLES

General prinicples of treatment of toxic nephropathy are outlined in Table 2. Many types of toxic nephropathy remit spontaneously. Specific treatment depends on the type of renal injury, its clinical manifestations, and the

Table 1. Renal vulnerability to toxins

High blood flow rate
Neurogenic and hormonal effects on blood flow
Large endothelial surface area
High metabolic rate
Numerous renal enzymes
Uncoupling of toxins from plasma proteins
Transtubular cell transport
Medullary interstitial concentration
Urinary concentration
Urinary acidity

Table 2. Treatment of toxic nephropathy: General principles

1. Treat the syndrome as for nontoxic lesions
    Replete solute and water losses
    Modify diet as appropriate
    Control blood pressure
    Maintain renal perfusion, urinary drainage
    Chemotherapy
2. Discontinue or diminish exposure
3. Augment elimination
    Diuretics
    Increase solubility
    Chelates
    Induce (or inhibit) microsomes
    Dialysis, hemoperfusion
4. Limit renal exposure
    Block tubular secretion
    Decrease tubular reabsorption
    Chelate
5. Pharmacologic antagonists (needed)
6. Prevention is more important than all of the above

Table 3. Renal lesions caused by nephrotoxins

Ischemia without structural changes	Acute interstitial nephritis
Acute renal vasculitis	Chronic interstitial nephritis
Glomerulonephritis	Nephrocalcinosis
Glomerulosclerosis	Urinary crystallization
Lipoid nephrosis	Periureteral fibrosis
Membranous nephropathy	Papillary necrosis
Tubular necrosis	Renal cysts
Renal cortical necrosis	Uroepithelial carcinoma

Table 4. Toxic renal physiologic abnormalities and clinical syndromes

Hypertension	Sterile pyuria
Acute glomerulonephritis	Fanconi syndrome
Nephrotic syndrome	Renal glycosuria
Acute renal failure	Renal tubular acidosis
Chronic renal failure	Nephrogenic salt losing
Renal colic	Nephrogenic diabetes insipidus
Isolated hematuria	Water retention
Isolated proteinuria	Potassium retention

particular intoxicant, just as specific treatment of infectious or of immunologic renal disease depends on more detailed characterization of the illness. Some drugs and chemicals are bioactivated in the kidney into nephrotoxins. Experimental inhibition of the cytochrome P-450 enzyme system can protect against certain nephrotoxins (13, 14), while other toxins are biotransformed by this system into safer compunds and should be eliminated faster by enzyme induction. Interest in toxic nephropathy is heightened, however, because many of the lesions are treatable or, better yet, are preventable, and many can be reproduced readily in experimental animals, serving as models for many of the clinical syndromes in nephrology.

NEPHROTOXIC LESIONS AND SYNDROMES

Nephrotoxin exposure can produce a variety of pathologic changes, physiologic aberrations, and clinical abnormalities. These are outlined in Tables 3 and 4. The most frequently observed abnormalities are acute renal failure, usually related to tubular necrosis, acute interstitial nephritis, chronic renal failure associated with papillary necrosis, or chronic damage to the tubules resulting in interstitial nephritis and nephrotic syndrome, either due to lipoid nephrosis or membranous nephropathy.

Renal ischemia

A wide variety of toxins can cause hypotension with resultant acute ischemic injury to the kidney. Agents that cause hypersenitivity anaphylactoid reactions, depletion of blood or other body fluid volumes, or increase vascular capacitance and thereby cause shock can induce acute renal failure but are not usually categorized as nephrotoxins and will not be discussed here. Certain antihypertensive and other vasoactive drugs are particularly prone to cause renal ischemia, however. Although antihypertensive drugs can induce renal failure mediated by hypotension, a syndrome of normotensive renal ischemia characterized by reversible renal failure and severe hyperkalemia can occur with captopril therapy (15, 16). Susceptible patients typically have antecedent renal ischemia due to arterial disease or prior diuretic use.

Captopril can also cause tubular atrophy, possibly due to direct toxicity or to prolonged ischemia and membranous glomerulopathy. Monitoring renal function during captopril administration is advisable, and the drug should be discontinued when azotemia or hyperkalemia occur without another recognizable cause. Similar renal abnormalities have complicated enalapril therapy (17). Other vasoactive compounds that can induce renal ischemia include angiotensin, cimetidine, ergot, epinephrine, and norepinephrine (18–20). The severe vasospasm so induced should rapidly recede on discontinuing exposure, thereby restoring renal function. There is no clinicial precedent for the use of a vasodilator or other treatments for transient, spontaneously reversible renal ischemia.

PROSTAGLANDIN SYNTHETASE INHIBITORS

Recently, it has been recognized that nosteroidal antiinflammatory agents can induce reversible ischemic renal failure in certain patients, for example, those with congestive heart failure or systemic lupus erythematosus (21). The common denominator in susceptible patients is renal vasoconstriction mediated by increased activity of the renin-angiotensin system or other pressors such as catecholamines. Increased activity of vasodilator prostaglandins compensates for such vasoconstriction, thereby maintaining renal blood flow.

Blockade of prostaglandin synthetase by the nonsteroidal antiinflammatory drugs results in unopposed vasoconstriction with acute renal ischemia. Acute renal failure may occur early in the course of therapy without morphologic changes in the kidney. Indomethacin has caused this abnormality most frequently, but many other agents have been implicated (22, 23). Nonsteroidal antiinflammatory drugs that may cause such renal ischemia are listed in Table 5. Recognition of the problem and withdrawal of the culprit drug should lead to prompt reversal of renal failure, thereby sparing the patient from other diagnostic investigations that may be hazardous. When an antiinflammatory drug is needed but toxicity has occurred, an agent of a different class may be attempted under observation. Risk factors for acute ischemic renal failure secondary to nonsteroidal drugs are outlined in Table 6 (24, 25). The elderly, who are more likely to be given these drugs and are more susceptible to dehydration and diseases causing hypovolemia, should be monitored carefully when initiating therapy with these drugs (22).

Nonsteroidal antiinflammatory drugs cause a variety of other renal lesions (Table 7), some of which also relate directly to prostaglandin synthetase inhibition (23–28).

Severe bilateral flank pain with transient azotemia of unknown mechanisms after only a few doses of suprofen has recently been reported (29). Patients undergoing cancer chemotherapy may be at increased risk for uric acid precipitation when these agents are concurrently given, and patients with pyelonephritis or sepsis are more likely to manifest decreased glomerular filtration rates when these nonsteroidal drugs are administered. Severe hyperkalemia may complicate therapy, especially with indomethacin, mandating drug withdrawal. Although only a few cases of papillary necrosis and chronic interstitial nephritis have been reported, it is likely that long-term use of these new drugs will lead to an increased incidence of these chronic lesions.

Table 5. Nonsteroidal antiinflammatory drugs that can cause renal ischemia by inhibiting prostaglandin synthetase

Carboxylic acids
  Propionic acids
    ibuprofen, naproxen, fenoprofen
  Salicylates
    aspirin, diflunisal
  Indoleacetic acids
    indomethacin, sulindac
  Pyrrolacetic acids
    tolmetin, zomepirac
  Anthranilic acids
    meclofenamate
    mefanamic acid

Oxicams
  Piroxicam

Pyrazoles
  Phenylbutazone

Table 6. Risk factors for nonsteroidal drug-induced ischemic acute renal failure

Shock
Plasma volume depletion
Antecedent diuretics
Postoperative third spacing of fluids
Congestive heart failure
Nephrotic syndrome
Cirrhosis with ascites
Systemic lupus erythematosus
Atherosclerosis
Advanced age
Underlying renal disease
Gouty arthritis

Table 7. Adverse renal effects of nonsteroidal antiinflammatory drugs

Reversible ischemic acute renal failure
Acute hypersensitivity interstitial nephritis
Nephrotic syndrome usually with interstitial nephritis
Vasculitis
Chronic interstitial nephritis
Papillary necrosis
Hyperkalemia
Sodium retention, impaired diuretic action
Interference with antihypertensive therapy
Decreased water excretion
Uric acid precipitation
Circulatory shock, anaphylaxis
Hyporeninemic hypoaldosteronism

Acute renal vasculitis

Sporadic reports associate systemic vasculitis, often involving the renal arteries, with drug exposure. The lesions may present as hypersensitivity vasculitis, anaphylactoid purpura, or polyarteritis with focal proliferative and necrotizing glomerulonephritis. The drugs most frequently incriminated are the sulfonamides, penicillins, allopurinol, iodides, propylthiouracil, thiazides, quinine, tetracycline, phenylbutazone, and intravenous amphetamines (30, 31). Treatment consists of discontinuing the offending antigen and, where necessary, removing it by dialysis; the use of prednisone, rapidly tapering a high initial dosage, often in comination with an immunosuppressive drug such as cyclophosphamide; and control of blood pressure and uremia by standard methods (30).

Glomerulonephritis

In patients with glomerulonephritis, the history of an exposure to hydrocarbons in the form of engine fuels, paints, thinners, degreasing agents, solvents, hair sprays, or pesticides is elicited more often than occurs with other forms of chronic renal failure (32). The clinical course of such patients does not differ from other patients with glomerulonephritis and there is no specific treatment known to abort or ameliorate the glomerular lesions. The usual management, consisting of control of blood pressure and other supportive treatment, remains appropriate. The association with inhalation of petroleum fuel fumes is most striking in relation to the Goodpasture syndrome (33). The high incidence of circulating anti-glomerular basement membrane (GBM) antibody in those patients suggests a therapeutic benefit for plasmapheresis and immunosuppression. Usually the hydrocarbon exposure has been remote and already discontinued. Goodpasture's syndrome with circulating anti-GBM antibody has also been associated with penicillamine therapy, responding to plasmapheresis, immunosuppression, and hemodialysis after discontinuation of the drug (34).

Exposure to volatile hydrocarbons can also precede immune-complex-mediated glomerulonephritis. This can present as membranous nephropathy, when low-dose exposure is prolonged, or more acutely as crescentic glomerulonephritis (35, 36). Massive doses of hydrocarbons cause tubular necrosis with acute renal failure (37).

Glomerulosclerosis

Prolonged exposure of rats to carbon tetrachloride causes glomerular sclerosis with accumulation of fibrinogen in the glomerular tuft (38). Such an association has been postulated but not proved in humans.

Focal and segmental glomerulosclerosis, usually presenting as nephrotic syndrome and often progressing to chronic renal failure, has been associated with heroin abuse (39). The mesangium is expanded and focal deposition of IgM and complement occur, and a variety of other renal lesions are seen less frequently in drug abusers. The mechanism by which heroin or its adulterants induce the lesions is unkown. There is no specific treatment for glomerular sclerosis and the need for prevention of heroin use is already obvious.

Drug-induced lupus nephritis

Nephrotoxicity may also present as drug-induced systemic lupus erythematosus (40). While the incidence of renal involvment is much lower than in spontaneous disease, lesions indistinguishable from lupus nephritis may occur, and rarely fatal renal failure may ensue. Renal impairment, when present, is usually reversible, however. Drug-induced lupus is associated with (usually high doses of) hydralazine, isoniazid, penicillamine, propylthiouracil, procainamide, nitrofurantoin, or the anticonvulsants, phentoin, mesantoin, primidone, and trimethadione. Treatment consists of removal of the drug and use of adrenal corticosteroids. Rapid taper of the steroids should be possible in most cases.

Table 8. Nephrotoxic antecedents of nephrotic syndrome

Aminonucleoside of puromycin	Captopril
Vaccines and desensitization antigens	Tolbutamide
Oxazoladine anticonvulsants, e.g., trimethadione	Perchlorate
Prostaglandin inhibitors, e.g., indomethacin	Polyvinyl alcohol
Heavy metals, e.g., gold	Polycations
Beta-adrenergic blockers, e.g., propranolol	EDTA
Penicillamine	Trichlorethylene
Probenecid	Snake venom
Pheninedione	Heroin abuse

Nephrotic syndrome

Among the many factors that precipitate the nephrotic syndrome, nephrotoxin exposure is one of the most clearly defined and easily preventable. A variety of toxin exposures can be followed by the nephrotic syndrome, as outlined in Table 8. Evidence that a hypersensitivity glomerulopathy mediates a drug-related nephrotic syndrome includes the occurrence during desensitization procedures and after gamma globulin administration, remission on cessation of exposure with recurrence after rechallenge, and demonstration of specific antibodies in the glomerulus.

TRIMETHADIONE HYPERSENSITIVITY

When hypersensitivity occurs to such oxazoladine anticonvulsants as trimethadione or its congeners, ethadione and paramethadione, the nephrotic syndrome can be a prominent manifestation. Although this is a potentially fatal complication, remission usually occurs on withdrawal of the drug. Adrenal corticosteroids or immunosusppresive drugs may hasten remission, but such observations are uncontrolled (41). Unless the drugs are readministered, the nephrotic syndrome does not recur. Usually the glomerular changes are minimal, without detectable immune deposits in the glomeruli, but occasionally there are intramembranous deposits with eosinophilia and intraglomerular collections of eosinophils (42). Despite demonstrable dose-related toxicity in rats, these observations in patients are in accord with a hypersensitivity lesion that remits either spontaneously or with a short course of corticosteroids. Standard management of nephrotic syndrome, i.e., salt restriction, judicious use of diuretics, a high protein intake, and treatment of such complications as infection, hypertension, and thromboembolic disease, is warranted until remission occurs.

PENICILLAMINE TOXICITY

In 5–20% of patients with rheumatoid arthritis, cystinuria, or Wilson's disease treated with penicillamine, toxicity occurs, causing membranous nephropathy with nephrotic syndrome, which accounts for 10% of neprotic patients in some series (43). Subepithelial dense deposits containing IgG and complement are found in the glomeruli, sometimes with IgM deposition, and it is postulated that penicillamine itself or a haptene may be antigenic (44, 45). The onset is usually insidious, may occur after the drug has been stopped, and is usually preceded by treatment of about a year's duration, typically at a daily dose of 1 g of penicillamine (45). Proteinuria is maximal about 2 months later and then recedes gradually over several months with or without adrenal corticosteroid therapy. Immune deposits in glomeruli and proteinuria can persist for more than a year, however (46). Patients who manifest penicillamine hypersensitivity can benefit from desensitization. Once remission occurs, about 40% of patients will exacerbate within 3 months of reinstituting the drug. Proteinuria can remit despite continuation of the drug, however (47). Patients with penicillamine nephropathy should have a good prognosis when provided the usual management for the nephrotic syndrome, but a severe potentially fatal nephropathy with renal failure can occur, mandating aggressive treatment with immunosuppression and dialysis (34, 45).

GOLD NEPHROSIS

The toxicity of gold salts, used therapeutically for systemic lupus erythematosus and rheumatoid arthritis, includes cutaneous hypersensitivity, bone marrow depression, and renal injury. Nephrotoxicity, which occurs in 5–10% of patients receiving prolonged gold therapy, correlates poorly with the duration and dose of gold, is usually heralded by proteinuria with or without hematuria, and may progress to the nephrotic syndrome and renal failure (48). Most administered gold is not excreted rapidly but rather is retained and deposited in tissues, including the kidney. Gold may be recognized in glomeruli but is usually deposited to a greater extent in tubules, especially distal. Such deposition correlates with exposure to gold, rather than with nephrotoxicity (48). Glomerular abnormalities, typically epimembranous deposits of immunoglobulins and complement that do not contain gold, most likely result from autosensitization to renal tubular epithelial antigens released by cellular injury caused by the gold (48, 49). Such a pathogenetic mechanism has been demonstrated for other forms of chronic renal tubular injury (50). Prior gold nephropathy also increases the likelihood of penicillamine nephropathy, suggesting a similar pathogenesis (51). Moreover, enzymuria, an indicator of tubular injury, is a frequent early abnormality (52). Finally, ubiquitous tissue antigen has been recognized in the circulation weeks before the occurrence of proteinuria, and circulating immune complexes and tissue antibodies appear later (49). On withdrawal of gold, spontaneous recovery should be anticipated over a period of months or years (48, 49). Efficacy of adrenal corticosteroids has not been proved for the treatment of this lesion. Hypersensitivity to gold may occur, however, causing acute renal failure (53), for which steroids could be therapeutically useful.

MERCURY-INDUCED NEPHROTIC SYNDROME

Mercury also can induce nephrotic syndrome by causing autosensitization, preceded by chronic renal tubular injury, which evokes antibodies to renal tubular epithelial antigen and their deposition along with IgG and complement on the glomerular basement membrane (54). Usually, exposure to mercury, industrially (55) or as an ointment, diuretic, or teething powder (37), has preceded the onset of the nephrotic syndrome for several months or years. Increased renal excretion of mercury correlates with enzymuria and documents the exposure but not the nephrotoxicity, which may manifest overt proximal tubular injury with features of the Fanconi syndrome and usually focal glomerular basement membrane thickening without proliferation (56). Several reported cases have died, some with progressive renal failure. Cessation of exposure to mercury is usually followed, however, by spontaneous gradual remission. Adrenal corticosteroids occasionally have a salutary effect on the clinical course, and chelation of mercury with dimercaprol seems to induce remissions more often than occur spontaneously (55). The usual supportive treatments for the nephrotic syndrome are also appropriate.

NEPHROTIC SYNDROME WITH OTHER HEAVY METALS

Although chronic injury from other heavy metallotoxins should be capable of causing the nephrotic syndrome by the mechanism described above, only bismuth has been recognized clinically to cause this problem (57). In animals, saccharated iron oxide has induced the nephrotic syndrome, glomerular capillary occlusion, and proliferation (58); and nickel carbonyl inhalation has led to proteinuria and aminoaciduria (59). Awareness of such potential injury, for example, after industrial exposure, may be useful in preventing more severe damage.

NEPHROTIC SYNDROME WITH ANTIINFLAMMATORY AGENTS

The nonsteroidal antiinflammatory drugs can induced a reversible nephrotic syndrome occasionally (60, 61). Fenoprofen has been incriminated most frequently (23, 26). The glomeruli show only fusion of the podocytes, while an interstitial nephritis is usually the more obvious renal lesion. The interstitial infiltrate consists predominantly of cytotoxic/suppressor T lymphocytes, but includes some IgE-bearing B cells, suggesting a cell-mediated immune reaction (62). Whether inhibition of cyclooxygenase and consequent prostaglandin depletion also plays a pathogenetic role in such lesions has not been established. The nephrotic syndrome complicating the nonsteroidal drugs typically occurs after weeks or months of exposure, and may be accompanied by severe eosinophilia, hypertension, and acute renal failure. In addition to withdrawal of the drugs, the usual management of the nephrotic syndrome, hypertension, and renal failure are advised pending remission of the lesions. Adrenal corticosteroids probably accelerate remission.

OTHER TOXIC CAUSES OF THE NEPHROTIC SYNDROME

Recurrent episodes of the nephrotic syndrome have complicated probenecid use (63). Glomerular changes have been minimal and may represent a hypersensitivity reaction. Progressive renal failure with epimembranous deposits can occur, but the lesion usually reverses on withdrawal of the drug.

A variety of other drugs have caused the nephrotic syndrome (64), as outlined in Table 8. For most of these there has only been a single case reported, and neither the pathogenic mechanism nor appropriate therapy are known. Spontaneous remission is frequent, and it should not be assumed that all such reactions have a hypersensitivity or immunologic basis on which immunosuppressive drugs or corticosteroids can be justified. The nephrotic syndrome induced by the aminouncleoside of puromycin is unrelated to immunologic mechanisms, both in its genesis and progression (65). Moreover, glomerular podocyte fusion can be produced by perfusion of the kidney with polycations, so affecting the ionic charge of the glomerular basement membrane (66). This lesion also does not relate to immunologic mechanisms and can be reversed by reperfusion of the kidney with heparin, thereby neutralizing the polycation.

Acute renal failure

Acute renal failure with underlying tubular necrosis often results from nephrotoxin exposure. These toxins may injure the tubule directly, often with localization to the site of toxin transport or concentration, or may induce renal ischemia by any of several mechanisms, often with concurrent hemoglobinuria. Such acute renal failure often does not follow the course typical of that complicating hemorrhagic hypotension or a transfusion reaction. Rather, the renal failure may be polyuric and subtle in onset. Recognition may follow the unexpected discovery of azotemia or uremic symptoms. Continued toxin exposure may increase the severity of acute renal failure until progression to total, even irreversible, anuria occurs. The many causes of toxic acute renal failure are outlined in Table 9.

Table 9. Nephrotoxic causes of acute renal failure

Heavy metals, e.g., Hg, As, Bi, Pt
Glycols, e.g., ethylene glycol
Halogenated hydrocarbons, e.g., CCl$_4$
Iodides, i.e., radiographic contrast media
Antibiotics, e.g., aminoglycosides
Hemolysins, e.g., quinine
Drugs causing rhabdomyolysis
Drugs causing hypotension, e.g., by anaphylaxis
Drugs causing interstitial nephritis
Drugs causing acute urinary crystallization

HEAVY METAL INTOXICATION

In soluble inorganic forms, heavy metals are highly nephrotoxic, binding to cellular proteins and causing necrosis. Organic salts are less toxic, but their relative safety depends on rapid elimination.

Mercurial nephrotoxicity

Soluble salts of mercury cause granular or vacuolar degeneration, necrosis, and fragmentation of proximal tubular epithelium, spreading to involve the entire nephron as the dose increases. By combining with sulfhydryl groups of mitochondrial membrane protein, mercury causes mitochondrial disintegration, necrosis of nuclei, and subsequent loss of enzyme activity (67). The lethal dose can be as low as 1.0 g (two tablets), often ingested suicidally, but sometimes accidentally. Inhalation of mercury vapors, dermal absorption, or delayed elimination of organic mercurial drugs can also induce acute renal failure.

Clinical features of mercury intoxication include a bitter metallic taste, a sense of throat constriction and suffocation, gastritis, substernal burning, nausea, vomiting, abdominal pain, diarrhea, circulatory collapse, and anuric acute renal failure (68). Before anuria, the urine should show glycosuria, proteinuria, enzymuria, casts, erythrocytes, desquamated tubular epithelium, and a high mercury content. Recognition of these features can lead to early treatment, aborting the full-blow lesion. Once it occurs, anuria may persist for 3 weeks or more and the associated high catabolic rate often makes uremia severe. An interval between exposure to organic mercurials and the onset of renal injury suggests metabolism to more toxic compounds (69).

The best therapy for mercury intoxication is prevention. Depsite its overt labeling as poison, mercury is still ingested. Its availability should be discouraged. Industrial and agricultural use mandate saftey precautions. Should mercurial diuretics or ointments be used, they should be restricted to those with normal excretory mechanisms and the dose should be monitored carefully. Reduction of functional renal mass increases susceptibility to the nephrotoxicity of mercury, hence it should be avoided in all forms when renal insufficiency preexists.

After ingestion, emesis should be induced and the stomach lavaged and rinsed with egg white or medicinal charcoal. Dimercaprol (BAL), a highly effective antidote, binds absorbed mercuric ions competitively (70). Injections of 3.0 mg BAL/kg should be given every 4 hours, for up to six injections, depending on the severity of the intoxication. The BAL-mercury complex is eliminated by the kidney, and excess BAL causes such toxic symptoms and signs as vomiting, convulsions, and hypoglycemia. After anuria develops, subsequent doses of BAL can be removed by dialysis (71).

Hemodialysis systems employing chelates, such as N-acetyl cysteine and dimercaptosuccinic acid, can remove absorbed mercury from plasma and tissue depots (72), but dialysis ordinarily achieves little removal as clearances are below 5.0 ml/min (73). Nevertheless, such low rates can add significantly to the total removal rate in the anuric patient. Provided dialysis is initiated early and incorporates a chelation technique, it may lower the mortality rate (37). Salt depletion should be avoided since it aggravates the deleterious functional response to the tubular injury. Salt loading, furosemide, diethyl maleate, sodium maleate, and dimercaprol reduce renal toxicity by lowering the renal content of mercury (74). The metal chelator and sulfhydryl-reducing agent, dithiothreitol, lessens nephrotoxicity without decreasing renal mercury levels, presumably by an intrarenal effect, and cadmium-stimulated metallothionine decreases toxicity by shifting mercury from particulate to supernatant cellular fractions, a change also induced by spironolactone and sucrose (74). After acute renal failure is well established, the treatment outlined in Table 10 should continue, as for other causes of nephrotoxic acute renal failure, since the usual course and complications can be anticipated (75). Infusion of low doses of dopamine may hasten recovery from acute renal failure.

Platinum nephrotoxicity

Cis-dichlorodiammine-platinum has gained popularity as a potent cancer chemotherapeutic agent. Nephrotoxicity is the major impediment to the use of cisplatinum (6). In plasma, cisplatinum is mostly bound to proteins and is normally rapidly eliminated. Toxicity affects predominantly the S_3 segment of the proximal tubule, where platinum is most concentrated. It is dose dependent and complicates as many as 50% of therapeutic courses of the drug (76).

The first toxic effect of platinum is decreased renal blood flow. Often toxicity is heralded by enzymuria (77) and renal wasting of magnesium (78), following by acute renal failure with proximal tubular necrosis. Some newer analogues of platinum have comparable toxicity. Slow infusions and saline prehydration combined with mannitol and furosemide diuresis appear to lower the incidence of platinum-induced aucte renal failure (79), while probenecid increases platinum clearance and the mortality rate (80). Low molecular weight platinum compounds interact with essential cellular macromolecules, such as proteins, lipids, and nucleic acids. causing injury. By stimulating metallothionine production, zinc reduces platinum accumulation in the kidney (81). Once renal failure is established, it is not clear that the course is ameliorated by these or any other measures, except for discontinuing the drug and renal replacement therapy. The platinum half-life in plasma of intoxicated patients is 10 days and is not abbreviated by hemodialysis, which removes little platinum (82). The renal tissue half-life is several days, and platinum can be detected in tubular epithelium for as long as a month (83). On recovery, renal function may not return fully to normal, and with repeated courses of platinum, progressive loss of renal function can occur, especially if the patient is exposed to other nephrotoxins concurrently (84). Residual renal damage correlates better with the total dose than with the severity of a single episode of acute renal failure. Obviously, careful monitoring of platinum dosage is mandatory.

Other nephrotoxic heavy metals

Arsenic, a component of pigments, fertilizers, and insecticides; a potential contaminant of moonshine whiskey; and a notorious culprint in toxic homicides causes primarily gastrointestinal and neural lesions. By virtue of its concentration in the kidney, it may cause tubular necrosis with renal failure (85). Exposure to arsine gas, a hazard of the petroleum industry, can cause hemolysis with hemoglobinuric acute renal failure (86). Treatment consists of dimercaprol, as used for mercury poisoning, dialysis, and other supportive measures for acute renal failure. Established renal failure limits the use of dimercaprol, however. Although the BAL-arsenic complex can be removed by hemodialysis, it only eliminates a small fraction of the body burden, and its therapeutic value has not been established (87). Arsenical poisoning can also induce bilateral renal cortical necrosis with only partial recovery from acute renal failure and progression to renal atrophy, hypertension, and chronic renal failure (88).

Acute renal failure due to bismuth intoxication now most often occurs as an industrial hazard, whereas it was once a frequent complication of antisyphilitic therapy. After as little as 1.0 mg/kg of bismuth parenterally, patients can manifest signs of proximal tubular injury and oliguria, reflecting tubular necrosis (89), which results from selective concentration of the metal in tubules during its elimination. Management of bismuth-induced acute renal failure is the same as for that arising from other causes. Beneficial effects of early treatment with BAL have not been demonstrated unequivocally.

Other heavy metals that can cause acute renal failure include uranium, a classical model for experimental acute renal failure (90). Clinically toxicity is not a problem, however, reflecting inaccessibility rather than safety of the metal. Acute renal failure also may complicate copper-induced hemolysis, sulfhemoglobinuria, hypotension, and dehydration (91). Early recognition, hydration, and diuretics may ameliorate the lesion. Barium intoxication causes marked hypokalemia, with subsequent acute renal failure (92). Treatment with sulfate salts orally may precipitate barium in the gastrointestinal tract, augmenting elimina-

Table 10. Treatment of heavy-metal-induced acute renal failure

Prevention by labeling, restricting availability, monitoring exposure
Augment removal by emesis, chelates, extracorporeal techniques

Avoid salt depletion, other stimuli of the renin-angiotension system
Manage acute renal failure by diet, fluid and electrolyte control, dialysis
Treat extrarenal manifestations e.g., gastrointestinal bleeding
Manage complications of renal failure, e.g., hemorrhage, infection

tion. Acute renal failure in photographic film developers has been attributed to silver (93), a demonstrated cause of tubular degeneration in animals.

Chromium, which is also eliminated by the kidney, can cause acute renal failure (94), as can excessive doses of antimony, a treatment for kala-azar (95). Experimentally the intraperitoneal administration of aluminum nitrolotriacetate causes dose-dependent tubular degeneration and necrosis, with prior renal dysfunction increasing susceptibility (96), raising concern that the interaction of chelates and aluminum could accelerate the progression of chronic renal failure. Acute ferrous sulfate poisoning can also be accompanied by acute renal failure (97). Although hemodynamic abnormalities may be severe, iron deposition in the tubules occurs and a similar lesion is caused by deferrioxamine (98). Chelates may have direct toxicity or may induce renal injury by mobilization of tissue stores of metals (99). Nevertheless, in acute heavy-metal intoxication, chelate therapy is strongly indicated to prevent or lessen renal injury.

GLYCOL NEPHROTOXICITY

A variety of glycols can cause nephrotoxicity through several different mechanisms, including intrarenal oxalate crystallization, methemoglogin formation, hemolysis, and shock (100). Ethelyne glycol is highly toxic, readily available in antifreeze preparations, and rapidly metabolized to oxalate. Extensive precipitation of calcium oxalate in renal tubular lumens erodes the epithelium, causing tubular necrosis and oxalate nephrocalcinosis, and results in total anuria. Intoxicated patients present with central nervous system findings resembling acute ethanolism, followed by severe acute cardiopulmonary distress, after which anuria can develop abruptly. Proteinuria, oxalate crystalluria, flank pain and tenderness, severe metabolic acidosis, and acute renal failure develop within 48 hours of ingestion of as little as 30 ml. Ultrasonography may reveal increased renal echogenicity and sonic scattering.

Treatment consists of infusion of sodium bicarbonate and immediate hemodialysis to correct acidosis and to remove circulating ethylene glycol and oxalate (101). After the initial phase, the usual management of acute renal failure is appropriate, although total anuria may be prolonged, requiring careful attention to water balance, and the metabolic acidosis may be severe, accentuating hyperkalemia and requiring supplemental alkali therapy. As with other intoxication, prevention is better than treatment. Ethylene glycol solutions should only be stored in containers labeled as poison. Accidental intoxication has proved fatal.

Ethylene glycol dinitrate has caused methemoglobinuria with resultant acute renal failure. Propylene glycol, which is less toxic, has been used as a medicinal vehicle but can cause hemoglobinuric acute renal failure. Early management of these intoxications should include hydration and forced diuresis, as for other causes of pigment nephropathy. Diethylene glycol can cause tubular necrosis or cortical necrosis along with hepatic injury, while ingestion of ethylene dichloride causes circulatory collapse with resultant tubular necrosis. Management of these poisonings is supportive. They should be prevented by appropriated warnings on container labels.

HALOGENATED HYDROCARBONS

Various solvents cause acute renal tubular injury. Because these compounds are biotransformed to nephrotoxic metabolites, inhibitors of the cytochrome P-450 system reduce experimental injury (13). Carbon tetrachloride is widely used as an industrial solvent, household cleaning agent, fire extinguisher constituent, antihelminthic, and vermifuge. Inhaled, ingested, or absorbed through the skin, carbon tetrachloride can cause acute hepatic and renal failure (102). The initial symptom, irritation at the site of exposure, may be overlooked, central and peripheral nervous system abnormalities are easily misinterpreted, and gastrointestinal symptoms are nonspecific. Infrared analysis of characteristically odorous expired air may lead to an early diagnosis (103). Frequently, the insidious onset of acute renal failure, with or without oliguria, but usually with hepatic failure and jaundice, precedes the retrospective history of exposure. The prognosis often depends on the extent of hepatic injury, since the renal failure can be controlled adequately by dialysis. Impaired urea synthesis, however, can deceptively lead to underestimation of the severity of uremia. The mortality rate may approach 30%. Oliguria persists a mean of 9 days and reflects necrosis in the proximal tubule and the limbs of Henle's loop (37).

Proper recognition of the toxicity of carbon tetrachloride, adequate ventilation, with cognizance that it is heavier than air, and avoidance of ethanol during exposure are preventive measures. Therapy is less effective than prevention. It consists of terminating the exposure, cleansing the skin or gastric lavage, where appropriate, and managing the hepatic and renal failure and the hemorrhagic phenomena. When dialysis is used early after exposure, removal of carbon tetrachloride can be documented. Whether such removal is sufficient to affect the body burden appreciably or alter the clinical course remains to be demonstrated.

Tetrachloroethylene, a colorless organic solvent used mostly as a degreasing agent and spot remover, causes renal tubular necrosis and hepatic necrosis and a clinical course similar to that of carbon tetrachloride poisoning (37). Prevention and treatment should be as outlined for carbon tetrachloride intoxication.

Trichloroethylene, used as an anesthetic and also as a spot remover, induces toxicity after abusive sniffing of spot removers (104). The pathology and clinical picture resemble those of carbon tetrachloride intoxication, and the same prophylactic and therapeutic measures apply. Often severe central nervous system damage is lethal before acute uremia develops fully (105).

Other nephrotoxic hydrocarbons include chloroform, trichloroethane, and methylene chloride.

Toluene sniffing also frequently induces acute renal injury (106). Clinical abnormalities include hyperchloremic acidosis, proteinuria, rhabdomyolysis, hematuria, pyuria, magnesium and calcium loss, and, less frequently, renal failure. Repletion of electrolyte deficits along with cessation of exposure should promote recovery.

As discussed above, chronic exposure to organic solvents may be an important antecedent factor in several forms of glomerulonephritis.

IODINATED RADIOGRAPHIC CONTRAST MEDIA

Iodide, a component of contrast media for radiography of the vasculature, gall bladder, and kidney, and for computerized axial tomography, occasionally causes acute tubular necrosis (7). Iodide-induced nephrotoxicity occurs in 0.3% to as many as 40% of patients so exposed, depending on the associated risk factors outlined in Table 11 and on diagnostic criteria (7, 107–110). Arteriography carries the highest risk, especially if the dose exceeds 100 g of iodine, but the most important risk factor is preexisting renal insufficiency. Lower toxicity is observed with some newer agents that are less ionic, achieving radiographic visualization at lower osmolal concentrations and presumably inducing less vascular injury (109).

When possible, laxatives and diuretics should be avoided before contrast studies, volume depletion should be corrected, and adequate diuresis should be established. Because iodide nephrotoxicity has complicated diagnostic studies during the acute phase of pigment nephropathy, contrast medium exposure should be avoided or delayed when this problem coexists (111, 112). Typically, iodide-induced oliguric renal failure persists for 2–4 days, but nonoliguric renal failure or irreversible oliguria can occur. About 1% of patients undergoing angiography have severe nephrotoxicity requiring hemodialysis, usually permanently (108). An early clue to the diagnosis is the increasing density and persistence of the nephrogram during the culprit radiographic procedure (113).

Early diagnosis allows avoidance of exposure to further iodinated contrast procedures and other potential nephrotoxins. The pathogenesis of iodide nephrotoxicity is uncertain. It may involve vascular injury, hypersensitivity, iodide-induced uricosuria with obstructive crystalluria, interaction with Tamm–Horsfall protein, or, less likely, direct cellular toxicity (114). Tamm–Horsfall proteinuria does not increase with iodinated contrast medium exposure, but intrarenal gel formation or precipitation may

Table 11. Risk factors for iodide nephrotoxicity

Prior renal insufficiency	Congestive heart failure
Diabetes mellitus	Diuretic therapy
Multiple myeloma	Advanced age
Iodide dose	Vascular disease
Agent used	Hepatic insufficiency
Type of procedure	Hypoproteinemia
Injection site	Dehydration
Multiple contrast studies	Hyperuricemia

occur. A direct depression of renal blood flow and the glomerular filtration rate may be the result of the osmotic effects of the drugs (115). Less frequently, hypersensitivity acute interstitial nephritis has been documented (116).

Although intravenous pyelography is usually a safe procedure, the frequency of renal injury is high when patients are dehydrated, high doses are used, or renal failure preexists, notably that due to diabetes mellitus or multiple myeloma (108, 117). In the presence of such abnormalities, alternative diagnostic procedures such as sonography or radioisotope scanning should be used.

Cholecystography is more likely to cause nephrotoxicity when the iodide content of the contrast agent is increased, absorption of the agent is high, doses are doubled or repeated, or biliary elimination is impaired, as occurs with jaundice or hepatic failure (118). The clinical picture varies from mild nonoliguric renal failure to severe unrelenting anuria, and the mortality rate may be as high as 40%. Nephrotoxicity has been attributed to enhanced dissociation to inorganic iodide at low urinary pH (119). Renal failure is observed only rarely with the use of iopanoic acid but was frequent with bunamiodyl (120).

Iodide nephrotoxicity is best prevented by monitoring the dosage carefully, especially if the usual route of elimination is impaired; by maintaining adequate hydration before and diuresis during these radiographic examinations; and by testing for hypersensitivity. Hydration does not ensure protection against iodide nephrotoxicity, however. Organic iodides are normally eliminated rapidly but persist in the plasma of patients with acute renal failure, from where they can be efficiently removed by hemodialysis (121). Whether such removal of organic iodides after renal failure has occurred ameliorates the clinical course or affects the prognosis has not been established. The usual management for acute renal failure is appropriate once it has occurred.

ANTIBIOTIC NEPHROTOXICITY

The major problem complicating antibiotic therapy, especially of patients with underlying renal disease, is nephrotoxicity. The frequency and severity of nephrotoxicity varies substantially among the different antibiotics, some of which have a narrow margin of safety (5). Many antibiotics are excreted predominantly by the kidney. Such antibiotics are retained in patients with renal failure who require careful adjustment of their dosage according to published guidelines (122, 123). The diagnosis of antibiotic nephrotoxicity can be difficult amidst the hemodynamic effects of sepsis or the renal functional changes of acute pyelonephritis, so the problem can be either overdiagnosed or understimated. Specific functional abnormalities and toxin accumulation should be demonstrated. Predictors of nephrotoxicity of a given drug include such physical properties as aqueous and lipid solubility, molecular weight and protein binding, the type of metabolic transformation, the intrarenal localization and concentration, the extent and mode of renal excretion, and the behavior of subcellular elements in the presence of the drug.

Aminoglycoside nephrotoxicity

The aminoglycoside antibiotics are noted for their ototoxicity and nephrotoxicity. Neomycin and paromoycin are so toxic as to preclude their parenteral use. All of the aminoglycosides are poorly absorbed from the gastrointestial tract, however, so this route is relatively safe to use for enteric sterilization. Streptomycin is virtually not nephrotoxic. Although gentamicin was heralded as less toxic than kanamycin, it has been used more liberally, and today the aminoglycosides are the most frequent cause of acute renal failure in hospitalized patients.

Aminoglycoside nephrotoxicity is manifested functionally by lysosomal enzymuria, tubular proteinuria, mild glucosuria, impaired urinary concentration, saluresis, decreased ammonium excretion, and eventually depression of the glomerular filtration rate (124, 125). Histopathologic lesions are prominent in proximal tubules and include increased lysosomes and cytosegrosomes containing whorled myeloid bodies, disruption of the brush border, mitochondrial swelling, and overt tubular necrosis (124).

Toxicity relates to the dose and duration of treatment. It may be anticipated with persistently high trough plasma concentrations and correlates best, but imperfectly, with renal cortical concentrations of the aminoglycoside (125–128). Differences in affinity for the renal cortex, which relate to the number of cationic amino groups in the molecule, correlate with the likelihood of nephrotoxicity, neomycin binding most avidly, streptomycin least avidly, and gentamicin, kanamicin, and tobramycin achieving intermediate values. Other factors also relate to the lower intrinsic toxic potential of tobramycin, amikacin, and netilimicin (129, 130); toxicity correlates with the 2-deoxystreptamine component of aminoglycosides. With preexisting risk factors, as outlined in Table 12, expecially with prior renal dysfunction or extracellular volume depletion, nephrotoxicity is more likely (125–128). Individual risk factors predict toxicity imperfectly, however, and several cases have developed overt renal failure in the absence of such coexistent abnormalities (131).

Aminoglycosides are organic bases that are filtered across the glomerular capillaries and are reabsorbed to a modest extent by the proximal tubules by pinocytosis (124). The aminoglycosides then accumulate in proximal tubule lysosomes, binding phospholipids thereby inhibiting phospholipases, disrupting lysosomal membranes, interfering with mitochondrial respiration (132, 133), and causing necrosis with consequent acute renal failure and a decrease in the number and diameter of glomerular endothelial fenestrae.

At therapeutic doses for 10–14 days, as many as half of the patients will have a demonstrable renal functional abnormality, 20% will develop measurable renal failure, and a smaller fraction will acquire overt renal failure. The incidence of such abnormalities depends on the particular aminoglycoside (134). Altered pharmacokinetics can influence the likelihood of toxicity, and to reduce the probability doses must be adjusted carefully when renal insufficiency preexists (122, 123, 135). It has been demonstrated that prolonging the dosage interval, thereby decreasing the trough concentration, despite a high peak level, is safer than maintaining higher more constant levels by reducing the individual doses, when the total dosage remains constant (136).

The aminoglycosides are highly effective antibacterial agents, but must be used cautiously. There is little danger to their use for a few hours when sepsis is suspected. Continued use should be restricted to those instances where there is a clear-cut indication. Under these circumstances, renal function should be assessed and serum concentrations of the aminoglycoside should be assayed. The normal half-life of most aminoglycosides is 3 hours or less. After 2 or 3 days, therefore, equilibrium concentrations should be well established. The dosing interval should be prolonged as a multiple of the serum creatinine concentration, recalling, however, that there are many circumstances where a reduced glomerular filtration rate is not reflected by a quantitatively proportional accumulation of serum creatinine.

Aminoglycoside accumulation in the renal cortex is much more prominent during the second week of therapy, and characteristically nephrotoxicity begins after about 12 days of treatment. Prolonged aminglycoside treatment is thus ill advised. The half-life of aminoglycosides in renal tissue exceeds 100 hours. Accordingly, the lesion is not expected to reverse rapidly. With the onset of renal insufficiency, the aminoglycoside should accumulate in plasma, which should augment renal cortical accumulation. It is imperative, therefore that the drug be discontinued or the dose reduced drastically when presumptive evidence of renal insufficiency appears.

Experimental animals can recover from aminoglycoside nephrotoxicity despite continued exposure. The scenario in humans typically is progression from nonoliguric renal failure to oliguria to persistent anuria when the drugs are continued, but partial recovery has occurred despite continued drug exposure. Vigilance throughout the course of aminoglycoside therapy is mandatory. Although enzymuria may herald overt renal failure (137), this is not always a reliable predictor of impending azotemia. The appearance of urinary casts also predicts or accompanies the onset of renal failure (138). When possible, aminoglycosides with less nephrotoxic potential should used.

Comparative studies of nephrotoxicity indicate that tob-

Table 12. Risk factors for aminoglycoside toxicity

High dose	High renal cortical level
Prolonged drug use	High plasma trough level
Total dose	Impaired renal function
Advanced age	Concurrent nephrotoxin use
More toxic congener	Recent prior aminoglycoside
Female sex	Volume depletion
Shock	Potassium depletion
Bacteremia	Magnesium depletion
Obesity	Furosemide pretreatment
Liver disease	Hyperparathyroidism

Table 13. Comparative nephrotoxicity of aminoglycosides

Neomycin,* paromomycin*	Most
Gentamicin, kanamycin	
Sisomycin, dibekacin	
Tobramycin	
Netilmicin, Amikacin	
Streptomycin	Least

* Restricted to oral use.

ramycin, amikacin, and netilmicin cause less injury than the other broad-spectrum aminoglycosides (129, 130, 132, 134, 139–141), as outlined in Table 13. The lower toxic potential of these drugs can be offset, however, by only a modest increase in the dose. Although the roles of any single pathogenetic factor can be difficult to discern in so complicated a clinical setting as occurs in septic patients, concurrent cephalosporin use potentiates the risk of aminoglycoside nephrotoxicity (42).

Aminoglycoside dosage and renal function must be monitored especially carefully when cephalosporins are also used. Induction of extracellular volume depletion by furosemide or other potent diuretics often precedes overt gentamicin toxicity. The inappropriate practice of focusing on urine volume, rather than on body fluid volumes, can lead to such depletion, with consequent stimulation of the renin-angiotensin system aggrating the deleterious functional response to the tubular injury.

Once renal failure occurs, it is preferable to attempt to expand body fluid volumes toward normal than to artificially augment urinary volume. Sodium chloride loading lowers toxicity by decreasing aminoglycoside uptake by the kidney (143). Sometimes aminoglycoside toxicity manifests predominantly renal losses of potassium, magnesium, calcium, and glucose (144). Repletion of these solutes can prevent the pertinent deficiency syndromes. Calcium loading reduces aminoglycoside nephrotoxicity by competing with binding to tubular brush borders; lowering the renal cortical content. Independently of calcium effects, parathyroid hormone increases the renal uptake of aminoglycosides (145, 146). Thyroxine also protects against aminoglycoside-induced acute renal failure by maintaining Na-K-ATPase activity (47).

Occasionally, massive overdosage of an aminoglycoside has been encountered and treated by hemodialysis with clinical recovery (148, 149). Although removal of the aminoglycoside is demonstrable, total elimination is increased by dialysis by only a small percentage when renal function is normal, and there are no control observations to indicate that the favorable clinical outcome was not spontaneous. After renal failure has become established, the usual therapeutic management of this problem should be undertaken.

Cephalosporin nephrotoxicity

The cephalosporins are a family of antibiotics numbering about 30 congeners that chemically relate to the penicillins (150). Excreted predominantly by the kidney by filtration and secretion, the cephalosporins can cause dose-related renal toxicity as well as hypersensitivity interstitial nephritis (151). Cephalosporins interfere will cell-wall synthetic functions and cause mitochondrial injury, interfering with cell respiration (152). Dose-related toxicity occurs frequently with cephaloridine, which contains several toxic polymers that cause renal injury by polymerization from high intrarenal concentrations and covalent bonding in tubular epithelium, damaging first the brush border and leading to coagulative necrosis (153). This drug should be avoided.

Cephalothin and the other cephalosporin analogues recently introduced are less nephrotoxic (150), but with excessive dosage, preexisting renal impairment, advanced age, hypersensitivity, or concurrent use of other potential nephrotoxins, qualitatively similar renal changes occur (154, 155). Toxicity is usually manifested by proteinuria, cylindruria, hematuria, enzymuria, and acute renal failure, which may be nonoliguric (156) and should reverse as high plasma cephalosporin levels recede.

Although nephrotoxicity is infrequent, cephalosporins cannot be administered without precautions, at least in highly susceptible patients. By blocking tubular secretion of these drugs through the organic acid pathway, e.g., with probenecid, their accumulation in tubular epithelium should be prevented, so reducing toxicity (157). Accumulation of cephalosporins in plasma, however, can cause neurotoxicity comparable to that seen with penicillins. It is also preferable to use one of the less toxic cephalosporins (158). Because furosemide potentiates cephalosporin toxicity (151), the combination should be avoided and, when possible, saline diuresis should be achieved.

The management does not differ from that of acute renal failure of other causes, once it occurs. Should there be evidence of hypersensitivity, corticosteroids can be considered, but they are not proved to be efficacious. Although dialysis eliminates cephalosporins, it is not clear that such removal alters the clinical course or prognosis.

Polymyxin nephropathy

The polymyxins are a closely related group of polypeptide antibiotics with nephrotoxic properties of varying severity. Toxicity is likely to occur should the dose exceed 3.0 mg/kg/day or at lower doses when there is underlying renal dysfunction. Patients intoxicated with polymyxin B develop renal tubular degeneration and manifest cylindruria, proteinuria, abnormalities of tubular transport, and a decreased glomerular filtration rate (159). Similar nephrotoxic lesions occur in about 20% of patients treated with a therapeutic course of colistimethate (polymyxin E) and in a higher percentage of those with predisposing risk factors comparable to those for aminoglycoside-induced nephrotoxicity (160).

Prophylaxis and treatment of polymyxin nephrotoxicity follow the same guidelines as for aminoglycoside-induced renal injury. Polymyxins can cause irreversible acute renal failure and should be used only when other less toxic

Renal effect of tetracyclines

The most frequent disturbance caused by tetracyclines is the aggravation of azotemia caused by their impairment of amino acid incorporation into protein (161). Patients depleted of extracellular fluid or with antecedent renal insufficiency or both are at greater risk for tetracycline toxicity and may sustain irreversible renal failure from this antibiotic (162). Although doxycycline is less hazardous, even this congener has aggravated renal failure (163). Tetracyclines should be avoided in such patients. Outdated tetracycline has caused a reversible Fanconi syndrome mediated by its degradation products (164). No treatment is required, except for discontinuation of the drug.

Demeclocycline causes nephrogenic diabetes insipidus, inhibiting both the generation and action of cyclic AMP (165). Management of this problem involves rehydration and cessation of the antibiotic. This property of demeclocycline has been exploited for treatment of inappropriate antidiuretic hormone secretion and of dilutional hyponatremia complicating cirrhosis, but can lead to acute renal failure in these circumstances (166).

Sulfonamide nephrotoxicity

The nephrotoxic potential of sulfonamides has long been recognized. Sulfonamides of low solubility, when given in large doses or to dehydrated or acidotic patients, will readily obstruct the urinary tract, thereby injuring the kidney (167). Tubular necrosis with hematuria and acute renal failure also may occur without demonstrable sulfonamide crystallization. Sulfonamide mixtures and more soluble congeners decrease the frequency of nephrotoxicity but do not eliminate it. The likelihood of this complication is also reduced by maintaining a diuresis and by rendering the urine alkaline, usually with bicarbonate. Acetazolamide, a sulfonamide derivative, has rarely caused crystalline lesions resembling sulfonamide nephropathy. Renal failure has also complicated treatment with cotrimoxazole, a trimethoprim-sulfonamide combination, when large doses are given or some renal impairment preexists (168). Sulfonamides can also precipitate acute vasculitis, focal granulomatous interstitial nephritis, and an acute hypersenstivity interstitial nephritis.

Treatment of acute nephrotoxicity due to sulfonamides involves the usual management of acute renal failure, and if hypersensitivity is involved, corticosteroids may be indicated. Acute crystalline obstruction may require hydration, alkalinization, and even alkaline lavage of the ureters or dialysis. The removal of sulfonamides by dialysis (169) is augmented by the decreased protein binding (170) that occurs in uremic patients, but the contribution to clinical recovery has not been quantified.

Amphotericin B nephropathy

Antifungal therapy with the insoluble polyene antibiotic, amphotericin B, is often limited by dose-dependent, potentially reversible nephrotoxicity characterized by cylindruria, decreased renal blood flow and glomerular filtration rates, renal tubular acidosis, tubular necrosis, and interstitial calcification (171). Increased renal vascular resistance with a reduced glomerular filtration pressure precedes the increase in tubule permeability (172). Sodium depletion aggravates and sodium loading attenuates the decrements in renal blood flow and glomerular filtration rates, and concurrent use of furosemide also ameliorates these abnormalities in the dog, apparently by altering tubuloglomerular feedback (173). Maintenance of diuresis and alkali administration seem advisable during amphotericin B therapy.

Preexisting renal insufficiency does not mandate a reduction in dosage because elimination does not depend on the kidney (123). The appearance of azotemia, often preceded by hyperchloremic acidosis, is a warning to discontinue the drug or to reduce the dosage, however. Sometimes this efficacious fungicide must be continued nevertheless, but it can cause irreversible acute renal failure when high doses are prolonged (174). Usually, moderation of the dose, hydration, and electrolyte repletion improve renal function in these patients (175).

Other nephrotoxic antibiotics

Bacitracin is too nephrotoxic for systemic use (159). It may cause necrotizing changes in glomeruli as well as in tubules. Although early lots of vancomycin frequently caused renal damage, this was attributed to impurities, and the incidence of renal failure caused by vancomycin itself is low despite its accumulation in the kidney (176). Both viomycin and capreomycin are potentially nephrotoxic (5). There are no specific therapeutic recommendations for these forms of antibiotic nephrotoxicity; general measures for managing acute renal failure are appropriate.

PIGMENT NEPHROPATHY

Several drugs and chemicals can cause nontraumatic rhabdomyolysis. Although muscle injury can complicate deep coma of any cause, myoglobinuric renal failure is more often seen complicating abuse of heroin or other narcotics including codeine and methadone; sedative intoxication, particularly with barbiturates; massive ingestion of ethanol; amphetamine intoxication; and diazepam, amoxapine, propoxyphene, pentamadine, and amphotericin B toxicity (177–180). Prolonged coma with immobilization is not a necessary prerequisite for muscle and renal injury.

Such patients may manifest rapid increments in serum creatinine, potassium, phosphate, and uric acid concentrations and may require dialysis more frequently than those with acute renal failure due to other causes. When rhabdomyolysis occurs, forced hydration and solute diuresis are recommended to prevent or ameliorate the severity of acute renal failure, which is usually proportional to the extent of muscle injury. Hypercalcemia, a distinctive feature of this lesion, may appear late in the course. It usually subsides spontaneously. Occasionally, severe muscle swelling requires fasciotomy to prevent neural compression injury. Otherwise, conservative management, as used for acute renal failure of other causes, is appropriate.

Many drugs can cause severe hemolysis with the potential risk of hemoglobinuric acute renal failure. Table 14 lists some of the toxins that have caused hemoglobinuric renal failure (12, 181–183). Many other drugs cause hemolysis, but usually not so severely as to induce acute renal failure. For example, primaquin spares young erythrocytes, so hemolysis on the basis of 6-GPD deficiency may be insufficient to result in acute renal failure. Nevertheless, when hemoglobinuria occurs, any suspected hemolysins should be discontinued. It has been recommended to render the urine alkaline when hemoglobinuria occurs to avoid precipitation of acid hematin. Yet the pathogenetic role of obstruction by hemoglobin casts in acute renal failure has been questioned. The hemodynamic consequences of severe hemolysis seem more pertinent to the pathogenesis. Accordingly, repletion of blood volume, adequate hydration, and mannitol diuresis are generally preferred for the acute phase, followed by the usual management of acute renal failure. With massive hemolysis, special care may be required to control hyperkalemia.

Phenazopyridine can cause skin pigmentation, degenerative changes in collecting duct epithelium, pigmented urinary casts, and crystals and acute renal insufficiency, especially in patients with antecedent renal insufficiency or after overdose (184). The usual management of pigment nephropathy, cessation of toxin exposure, and avoidance of other nephrotoxins are recommended (111).

OTHER CAUSES OF ACUTE RENAL FAILURE

A variety of other drugs can cause acute renal failure with tubular necrosis (181, 185). Notable among such causes are certain insecticides; streptozoticin, a cancer chemo-

Table 14. Toxic causes of hemoglobinuric acute renal failure

Drugs
  Quinine sulfate, quinidine sulfate, sulfonamides, hydralazine, triamterene, mesantoin, nitrofuration nomifensine
Glycols
  Propylene glycol, ethylene glycol dinitrate
Metals
  Copper, arsine
Venoms
  Snake, spider
Miscellaneous toxins
  Aniline, benzene, cresol, phenol, glycerol, tribromoethanol, hydroquinine-pyrogallic acid, sodium chlorate, methyl chloride, djenkol beans, fava beans, coal-tar derivatives

therapeutic that first causes Fanconi syndrome (186); carbamazepine, a drug used for trigeminal neuralgia (187); the anticoagulant, hexadimethrine bromide (188); the cancer chemotherapeutic, mithromycin; and quinolones, a new type of urinary antiseptic. No special therapy is advised for these intoxications, however, except for withdrawal of the offending agent and the usual management of acute renal failure.

Cyclosporin A

Controlled trials of cyclosporin A indicate its value for the treatment of transplant rejection and other immunologically mediated diseases. Cyclosporins suppress T-lymphocyte production but not the bone marrow. The major limiting adverse effect of the drugs is dose-dependent nephrotoxicity, often reflected by only a transient mild increase in the serum creatinine concentration, but sometimes by protracted acute renal failure or even ischemic chronic renal failure (189). Acute vascular injury, sometimes with thromboses at the glomerular hilus and capillary tufts, correlates with the severity of functional impairment, while tubular vacuolization, inclusion bodies, microcalcification, and necrosis are distinctive features unrelated to the physiologic derangements (189, 190). Ischemically damaged kidneys are more vulnerable to cyclosporin injury. Enzymuria and distal renal tubular acidosis may accompany the clinical syndrome of ischemic acute renal failure. Cyclosporin itself appears to be the toxin, so induction of P-450 cytochrome oxidase-mediated elimination reduces toxicity, as do vasodilator prostaglandins and verapamil (190). Toxicity is best prevented by careful restriction of the total dose administered.

Mitomycin C

The cancer chemotherapeutic drug, mitomycin C, causes a clinical picure resembling hemolytic uremic syndrome with hemolysis, fibrin thrombi in glomeruli, and a hemorrhagic necrotizing glomerulonephritis, resulting in renal failure after a mean interval of 10 months (191). Early detection and withdrawl of the drug may stablize renal function, which should be monitored for several months after therapy. Plasmapheresis can reverse the microangiopathy but not the renal failure. This complication is dose dependent and occurs in 8–10% of patients treated with mitomycin.

TREATMENT OF TOXIC ACUTE RENAL FAILURE

From the foregoing, it is apparent that many cases of acute nephrotoxicity should undergo the same management as for acute renal failure of other causes. Early treatment consists of cessation of toxin exposure and restoration of body fluid volumes. Calcium-channel blockers and other vasodilators may reverse early ischemic lesions. Should oliguria persist, a trial of low-dose dopamine infusion can be justified (192). When oliguria does not respond, a short-term trial of agents that increase urine flow such as mannitol or furosemide should be considered, especially when hemoglobinuria or myoglobinuria is present.

In special circumstances, agents such as probenecid can be used to decrease secretion of potential toxins (e.g., of cephalosporins), agents that increase the solubility of drugs or metabolites can be employed (e.g., bicarbonate for sulfonamides), agents that chelate may be helpful (e.g., BAL for metals), or agents that decrease urate production (e.g., allopurinol) may be indicated (193). The increased catabolic response to certain intoxications may require more frequent use of dialysis and more diligent attention to hyperkalemia. Prevention of nephrotoxic acute renal failure calls for judicious use of toxic drugs but does not warrant withholding a needed drug because of inordinate concern about its potential toxicity.

Acute interstitial nephritis

Hypersensitivity to a variety of drugs can cause acute interstitial nephritis (194–196). A similar lesion can complicate certain infections, such as brucellosis or syphilis. Mild cases can easily go unrecognized and may manifest only evidence of tubular injury or transport abnormalities. Conversely, marked impairment of renal function can develop rapidly, causing uremia requiring dialysis treatment. The swollen kidneys show diffuse interstitial infiltration by plasma cells, lymphocytes, and frequently by eosinophils, often with little evidence of nephron destruction. Haptene formation sometimes incites immunologic injury to the tubular basement membrane, inducing the interstitial reaction.

Acute interstitial nephritis should be suspected in any case of unexplained acute renal failure, but especially when the kidneys are enlarged to palpation or radiographically or are tender, and when there are dermal or other signs of hypersensitivity such as features of serum sickness. Eosinophilia is frequent and eosinophiluria is considered a pathognomonic sign found in over half of the cases of hypersensitivity acute interstitial nephritis. In doubtful cases, a positive radiogallium scan of the kidney suggests the diagnosis (195).

Most frequently, acute interstitial nephritis has been associated with the penicillins, especially methicillin and ampicillin, but there are many causes as listed in Table 15 (12, 23, 60, 144, 194–199). In addition to the synthetic penicillins, the drugs most frequently causing hypersensitivity-mediated acute interstitial nephritis are sulfonamides, rifampin, pheninedione, and nonsteroidal antiinflammatory drugs such as fenoprofen. Often interrupted high-dose therapy precedes the sensitivity reaction. The signs of hypersensitivity are sometimes subtle. Hematuria, pyuria, and evidence of tubular dysfunction may predominate in less severe cases, but usually oliguric or nonoliguric acute renal failure dominates the clinical picture.

The syndrome is important to recognize because removal of the offending agent should be followed by spontaneous recovery, albeit slowly. Persistent drug exposure can be associated with prolonged oliguria and significant residual renal functional impairment (200). Clinical observations suggest that corticosteroids abbreviate the duration of oliguria compared to that of untreated patients (200, 201). It seems advisable to treat severely ill patients and those who do not show signs of early spontaneous recovery. Acute interstitial nephritis is another reason to avoid the pertinent drugs in patients with preexisting hypersensitivity, since recurrent episodes have been described.

A progressive form of irreversible acute interstitial nephritis may begin after treatment of malignancy with methyl CCNU (202–205). The pathogenesis of these nitrosourea-induced lesions is unknown, but among the few cases observed, nephrotoxicity bears a relation to the total drug dose. These drugs bind to intercellular amino acids, inhibiting protein synthesis. Symptoms often begin several weeks or months after a course of treatment. There is no therapy for this fibrotic lesion, and prevention can only be achieved by restricting the total dose.

Doxorubicin, structurally similar to daunorubicin, causes chronic renal failure with tubular atrophy, interstitial fibrosis, and glomerular proliferation, somewhat like the lesion of puromycin (206). The tumor response dose is close to that inducing nephrotoxicity. There is no specific treatment for this lesion either, but symptomatic and supportive care for the ensuing chronic renal failure is appropriate. Cytosine arabinoside also interferes with tubular epithelial DNA synthesis (205), and adriamycin causes tubular atrophy, interstitial fibrosis, and glomerular sclerosis (207).

Table 15. Drugs causing acute interstitial nephritis

Penicillins
 Methicillin, ampicillin, carbenicillin, penicillin, nafcillin, oxacillin, amoxicillin
Other antibiotics
 Sulfonamides, polymyxins, cephalosporins, rifampin, erythromycin, cotrimoxazole lincomycin, p-aminosalicylate
Nonsteroidal antiinflammatory agents
 Fenoprofen, benoxaprofen, glafenine, ibuprofen, indomethacin, ketoprofen, mefanamic acid, neproxen, phenylbutazone, sulfinpyrazone, tolmetin, zomepirac
Metals
 Gold, bismuth
Diuretics
 Thiazides, furosemide
Miscellaneous
 Allopurinol, amphetamine, antipyrine, azathioprine, captopril, cimetidine, clofibrate, phenazone, pheninedione, phenobarbital, phenytoin, propranolol

Chronic interstitial nephritis

Most chronic nephropathies cause interstitial inflammation and fibrosis, so the reaction is nonspecific. When a chronic interstitial inflammatory infiltrate and fibrosis are the predominant findings, however, nephrotoxicity is the likely cause. Preoccupation with the interstitial reaction, however, often focuses attention away from the primary site of injury, which can be the vasculature, glomeruli, collecting system, papillae, or tubular epithelial cells or their basement membranes. The difficulty in identifying the primary site of injury has been demonstrated by the progression of experimental crystal nephropathy from intraluminal crystallization to tubular cell injury to interstitial crystalline deposits, evoking an inflammatory reaction to disappearance of the crystals, with persistence of nonspecific interstitial abnormalities (208). Indeed, the only true form of interstitial nephritis may be infectious, i.e., pyelonephritis. The other causes usually affect the tubule primarily and may be recognized by abnormalities in tubular transport. The most important causes of such chronic tubulointerstitial nephritis are the nephropathy of analgesic abuse, chronic tubular injury due to heavy-metal intoxication, radiation nephritis, and nephrocalcinosis.

ANALGESIC NEPHROPATHY

A high incidence of renal papillary necrosis and consequent chronic interstitial nephritis complicates prolonged ingestion of large doses of mixed analgesic compounds, which are usually readily available without prescription (2, 209-213). Analgesic nephropathy varies geographically, accounting for 1-30% of end-stage renal failure in different localities (2, 211, 212). The 5-year mortality can exceed 50%.

Analgesic abuse causes chronic interstitial fibrosis and mononuclear infiltration with tubular atrophy and loss of nephrons. The earliest lesion is medullary fibrosis, a characteristic finding, accompanied by radiographically demonstrable papillary necrosis in about 25% of patients. Interstitial nephritis occurs in areas above affected papillae and is frequently complicated by pyelonephritis, which may accelerate renal functional deterioration. Urinary tract carcinoma is a late complication (214).

The most frequently used analgesic mixtures contain salicylate and phenacetin or its metabolite, acetaminophen, along with any of a number of unrelated drugs such as caffeine, codeine, sedatives, muscle relaxants, and tranquilizers. The newer nonsteroidal analgesics can also cause papillary necrosis, however (23). Nephrotoxicity should be suspected after ingestion of about 2 kg (of salicylate or phenacetin), is likely after 7 kg, and may not be recognized until after 20-50 kg are consumed. The pathogenesis is attributed to oxidant damage by arylating metabolites of acetaminophen, which accumulate in the papilla, by other metabolites, or by extraneous oxidants in patients rendered susceptible by the uncoupling of oxidative phosphorylation by salicylates (215). Coexistent laxative abuse or dehydration from any cause may contribute to the susceptibility to renal damage (216). Inhibition of prostaglandin synthetase by salicylates or other antiinflammatory drugs presumably contributes to the medullary ischemia, and indeed these drugs alone can induce papillary necrosis (2).

The syndrome of analgesic abuse is characterized by chronic headache, or backache in a neurotic patient, usually in a middle-aged female. Gastrointestinal distress, often including hematemesis and peptic ulcer, may have led to gastrectomy and iron-deficiency anemia, before hypertension, uremia, urinary infection, hematuria, or renal colic focus attention on the kidney (209-213). The earliest manifestation of renal dysfunction is usually impaired urinary concentration (217). Renal failure occurs late in the course and correlates with the quantity of analgesics ingested. Most patients have moderate proteinuria, cylindruria, slight or moderate hematuria, and leukocyturia, which are nonspecific findings. Indeed, today analgesic nephropathy is the most frequent cause of sterile pyuria. About half the patients develop bacilluria, which can be misleading. Renal tubular acidosis is frequent and sonography can detect calcified papillae. As many as one third of the patients are incorrectly diagnosed early in their course. Glomerular filtration decreases and with continued analgesic abuse the course progresses downhill with death in renal failure.

When analgesic intake is discontinued, acetaminophen excretion should cease (217) and renal function should improve in about half of the patients (2, 211). Once severe renal failure has occurred, appropriate management, including discontinuation of analgesics, should improve function in about one sixth of the patients, more than half should stabilize, and about one fourth will deteriorate, nevertheless (209). Appropriate management should also include control of hypertension, renal infection, sodium depletion, and intermittent obstruction from sloughed papillae. If analgesic abuse continues, attacks of papillary necrosis continue. Evaluation for uroepithelial carcinoma must continue as renal failure is treated, since tumors may occur as long as two decades after the nephropathy begins (214). Painless gross hematuria or colic must be evaluated urologically and by urinary cytology to identify and treat resectable lesions (218). Other complications such as cardiovascular disease, anemia, and osteodystrophy are especially frequent in these patients. Analgesic nephropathy represents a classical example of a preventable and a treatable form of chronic renal disease.

CHRONIC INTERSTITIAL NEPHRITIS DUE TO METALLOTOXINS

Extrarenal findings such as colic, encephalopathy, anemia, and peripheral neuritis may overshadow the nephropathy of chronic lead intoxication, but the diagnosis often is not so obvious (219). Lead persists in body stores for decades with only minimal blood levels. Chronic lead nephropathy may account for more than 5% of chronic renal failure, mostly undiagnosed (4). The renal manifestations are predominantly tubular and include proteinuria, casts, glycosuria, and aminociduria. Low renin hypertension and hyperuricemia are frequent. The urine may show increased excretion of lead, delta aminolevulinic acid, coproporphyrin, and urobilinogen. A history of illegally distilled alcohol use, childhood pica or industrial exposure may suggest the diagnosis, which can be confirmed by measuring increased urinary excretion of lead, particularly after chelation with disodium calcium ethylenediaminetetraacetate (EDTA) (220, 221). Childhood lead intoxication does not necessarily forbode nephropathy, however.

Recognition of characteristic eosinophilic intranuclear inclusion bodies in renal tubular cells on renal biopsy or in the urinary sediment can also establish the diagnosis (222). Tubular degeneration, interstitial fibrosis, and calcification progress slowly to renal failure, often with nonspecific vascular damage contributing to hypertension. Treatment consists of cessation of exposure to the metal; augmentation of lead excretion by chelates such as EDTA, sodium citrate, or BAL; control of hypertension; and symptomatic management of gout and uremia. Acute lead poisoning has been treated by a combination of EDTA infusion and hemodialysis, which achieves much more rapid elimination of lead than EDTA alone (223). Whether this combination can reverse chronic renal lesions more rapidly is uncertain.

Chronic exposure to cadmium, an inessential trace element that uncouples oxidative phosphorylation, can cause proximal tubular injury, leading to chronic interstitial nephritis (224–226). The characteristic abnormality, low molecular weight proteinuria, e.g., beta$_2$ microglobulinuria, occurs when food, water, or air are contaminated with cadmium (227, 228). Dose-dependent heavy exposure stimulates metallothioneion production which complexes with cadmium and accumulates in the kidney, where ionic cadmium may be released, leading to renal tubular acidosis with painful osteomalacia and nephrolithiasis, impaired urinary concentration, the Fanconi syndrome, and chronic renal failure, typically with low serum urate concentrations (224–226). Experimentally, pretreatment with zinc decreases cadmium nephrotoxicity. Cadmium nephropathy is treated by termination of exposure, the use of dimercaprol (which is not very effective), supportive therapy for the painful osteomalacia, and the usual management of renal tubular acidosis and nephrotlithiasis.

Beryllium toxicity can occur from inhalation of fumes derived from fluorescent lights or alloys. It causes chronic granulomatous interstitial nephritis with deposits of beryllium in the kidney and passage of small urinary calculi containing beryllium or calcium oxalate (229). Therapy should include discontinuation of exposure and hydration.

The chronic interstitial nephritis that complicates lithium therapy is discussed below.

RADIATION NEPHROPATHY

Chronic interstitial nephritis follows exposure of the kidney to excessive doses of radiation, usually more than 2500 rads. Irradiation nephritis is most likely after radiation of testicular, ovarian, or Wilm's tumors; retroperitoneal lymphoma; osteogenic sarcoma; neuroblastoma; or intraabdominal metastases. The young; those with kidneys undergoing hypertrophy, e.g., after nephrectomy; and patients with ectopic kidneys are especially susceptible to radiation injury.

Acute radiation nephritis becomes apparent several months after exposure. Clinically it resembles acute glomerulonephritis and is characterized by edema, hypertension, exertional dyspnea, anemia, headache, proteinuria, cylindruria, and uremia (230). The kidneys show degenerative changes in glomeruli and tubules and interstital edema and hemorrhage. The mortality approaches 50% and is determined primarily by the severity of hypertension. Treatment of acute radiation nephritis includes control of hypertension, management of congestive heart failure, and therapy of acute uremia.

Chronic radiation nephritis appears after an interval of up to 10 years following excessive radiation, either de novo or after recovery from acute radiation injury. Chronic radiation nephritis clinically resembles chronic glomerulonephritis, manifesting proteinuria, hyposthenuria, anemia, hypertension, and slowly progressive uremia (230, 231). Salt wasting may be prominent. Malignant hypertension may supervene at any time during the course. The kidneys show severe vascular sclerosis, decreased glomerular size, mesangial sclerosis, tubular atrophy, interstitial fibrosis with little inflammatory reaction, marked capsular fibrosis, and sometimes superimposed necrotizing vascular changes of malignant hypertension (230, 232, 233). Retroperitoneal fibrosis may contribute to renal failure and salt losing by obstructing one or both ureters (12). Coexisting radiation enteritis complicates management of renal failure by virtue of protein and electrolyte losses secondary to chronic diarrhea.

The treatment of radiation nephritis is symptomatic and supportive since the lesion cannot be reversed. The best therapy is prevention, which consists primarily of shielding the kidneys and carefully monitoring and restricting dosage. Spacing the exposure decreases the toxicity. Epinephrine infusion also limits toxicity by vasoconstricting normal tissue. Tumor vessels respond poorly to epinephrine, so the therapeutic effect is not decreased by the drug. Inhibitors of cell proliferation protect the skin but not the kidney from radiation injury.

It is important to manage the hypertension, particularly in the acute stage or when malignant. The usual vasodilators and diuretics are recommended, but the hypertension may resist treatment. Evaluation for unilateral nephritis and renal ischemia (often without increased plasma renin activity) should be undertaken. When the evidence supports unilateral disease, nephrectomy should be considered because it can cure such hypertension.

Otherwise, therapy includes management of heart failure, judicious repletion of water and electrolytes, improved nutrition, correction of superimposed obstruction by residual tumor or fibrosis when identified, antibiotic treatment of associated urinary tract infection when present, and the usual management of chronic renal failure.

NEPHROCALCINOSIS

An interstitial reaction to crystalline precipitates, nephrocalcinosis, can abruptly or gradually cause renal failure. In some diseases, nephrocalcinosis appears to be largely responsible for the observed functional disturbances, whereas in other it seems to be a relatively insignificant feature of the disease process. Many instances of nephrocalcinosis relate directly to toxin exposure.

Toxin crystallization is best exemplified by sulfonamide

intoxication, in which nephropathy correlates with the heterocyclic ring substitution, of the sulfonamide, its solubility, and the dose used and duration of treatment (167). Prevention and treatment depend on maintaining or restoring solubility, as discussed above.

Oxalate nephrocalcinosis can occur from ethylene glycol intoxication (101) or from the metabolism of fluoridated anesthetics to oxalate (234). These problems are prevented by avoiding and limiting exposure to these particular toxins. Discontinuation of exposure and control of acute renal failure are the most important treatments. With preexisting renal failure, excessive doses of ascorbic acid are not eliminated rapidly, allowing increased metabolism to oxalate, which may accelerate the deterioration of renal function (235, 236). Massive doses of ascorbic acid may induce acute failure of normal kidneys (237). Appropriate moderation of the intake will prevent this problem, for which there is no established therapy. Xylitol administration can also precipitate oxalosis, and high doses of this agent should be avoided (238).

Acute precipitation of uric acid throughout the urinary tract can complicate the chemotherapy of lymphoma or leukemia (205, 239); the use of uricosuric agents such as the diuretic, ticrynafin (240); or nonsteroidal antiinflammatory drugs (28), especially sulfinpyrazone (241). Prevention of acute renal injury depends on limiting the filtered load of uric acid by lowering the serum concentration with the use of allopurinol and by inducing aklaline diuresis. Extracellular-volume-depleted patients with hyperuricemia are at increased risk. After crystalline-induced anuria occurs, diuresis may be reinstituted by hydration and mannitol. If unsuccessful, alkaline lavage of the lower urinary tract may restore diuresis, or it may be necessary to remove uric acid by dialysis (239).

Toxic calcium precipitation in the renal interstitium can be a feature of the milk-alkali syndrome (242) and of vitamin-D intoxication (243). Prevention of these intoxications depends on avoiding excessive intakes and treatment consists of discontinuing exposure. Use of the active metabolites of vitamin D should not induce hypercalcemic complications, provided patients are monitored carefully and the dosage is not excessive. Should renal failure be aggravated by hypercalcemia (244), it is more likely to result from a metabolic effect than from nephrocalcinosis and should reverse rapidly because of the faster onset and offset of action of hydroxylated vitamin D than of the parent compound.

Obstructive uropathy

Ureteral obstruction can result from urate, calcium oxalate, or phosphate stones resulting from the toxins and mechanisms discussed under nephrocalcinosis. When such problems occur, the usual management of acute obstructive uropathy is appropriate. Prevention of recurrences depends on limiting toxic exposure, adequate hydration, and ensuring the appropriate urinary pH to maintain solubility. Ureteral obstruction can also result from passage of necrotic papillae. Cessation of analgesic abuse should terminate such episodes (2).

Methotrexate overdosage can cause acute renal failure by precipitation of the drug in the renal tubules (205, 245). Hydration and urinary alkalization may prevent methotrexate precipitation (204, 246), and leukovorin rescue can lower plasma levels and lessen toxicity. Nonsteroidal drugs may increase susceptibility to methotrexate precipation. Once it occurs, uremia is likely to persist. Neither forced diuresis nor dialysis are effective in removing methotrexate, but hemoperfusion may provide some benefit (245).

Reversible nonoliguric acute renal failure following acyclovir therapy has also been attributed to intratubular obstruction by the drug or a metabolite (247).

Gross hematuria complicating anticoagulant therapy also may induce obstructive nephropathy through intraluminal hemorrhage and clot formation, or by extrinsic compression secondary to retroperitoneal hemorrhage (248). After restoring coagulation to normal and rehydration, this problem should subside, but surgical intervention may be necessary. Epsilonaminocaproic acid can also induce clotting in the urinary tract, with obstruction that impairs renal function, so it should be used with caution.

Ureteral obstruction can occur from retroperitoneal fibrosis. It is typically painless because the obstruction is extrinsic. The presenting findings may be polyuria, recognition of desquamated tubular or ureteral epithelium in the urinary sediment, or unexplained uremia. Radiographically there is medial displacement of the ureters, and a long segment of obstructed ureter is identified. Rarely, the fibrosis encircles the vasculature. Table 16 lists toxins that can cause retroperitoneal fibrosis (249–251). Drug-induced retroperitoneal fibrosis has been most clearly recognized with prolonged ingestion of methysergide (250). It is a rare complication of beta-adrenergic blocker therapy, occurring most often with pindolol. In addition to discontinuation of toxic exposure, the ureters often must be released surgically. Corticosteroids may obviate the need for surgical lysis, however.

Renal tubular functional abnormalities

The Fanconi syndrome, reflecting proximal tubular injury, can follow exposure to a variety of toxins, notably heavy metals and streptozoticin. Management consists of removal from the toxin and repletion of electrolyte and nutrient losses.

Gradient limited or classical renal tubular acidosis can be a manifestation of vitamin-D overdosage, toluene

Table 16. Toxic causes of retroperitoneal fibrosis

Methysergide
Ergotamine
Dihydroergotamine
Hydralazine
Dextroamphetamine
Methyl dopa
Atenolol
Pindolol
Radiation

sniffing, cadmium poisoning, or amphotericin-B toxicity. Treatment with bicarbonate is usually required to offset urinary losses.

Nephrogenic diabetes insipidus can result from methoxyflurane anesthesia, prolonged use of demecylocycline, or chronic lithium therapy.

Methoxyflurane is an effective anesthetic, the major adverse effect of which is dose-dependent nephrotoxicity, characterized by vasopressin-resistant polyuria that subsides after several days or weeks (252, 253). Methoxyflurane is metabolized to both oxalate and fluoride, each of which contributes to renal tubular necrosis. Fluoride toxicity decreases free water reabsorption, and the hypovolemia resulting from such polyuria can cause ischemia, aggravating renal injury. Other fluoride anesthetics, such as fluorexene and enflurane, can cause similar toxic renal injury (254), but acute renal failure very rarely complicates halothane or isoflurane anesthesia (255). In addition to restricting the concentration of and limiting the duration of exposure to fluoride anesthestics, maintaining plasma concentrations below 50 µM/l, it is important to ensure adequate hydration of patients after fluoride anesthetic use. When renal failure occurs, the usual management is appropriate.

Renal toxicity of the chronic use of lithium salts, recognized for many years (256), has received increased attention recently (257). Nephrogenic diabetes insipidus, which is often reversible, occurs in as many as half of patients receiving chronic lithium therapy, when serum lithium concentrations exceed 1.5 mEq/l. Lithium inhibits vasopressin-stimulated water transport at a site biochemically proximal to that of cyclic AMP (258). Chronic excess of lithium results in chronic interstitial nephritis, which correlates with the severity of renal tubular dysfunction and can cause renal failure (259, 260). Often glomerular filtration remains normal, however, despite persistent collecting duct dysfunction (260).

The functional changes can reverse, but often only partially, when serum lithium concentrations are reduced by lowering the dose. Chronic progressive renal lesions consisting of cytoplasmic vacuoles, glycogen accumulation in distal tubular and collecting duct epithelium, interstitial fibrosis, tubular atrophy, casts, and glomerular sclerosis can be induced in animals by lithium (261). It should be recalled that patients who have enhanced sodium reabsorption also retain lithium, so the dose may have to be reduced. While nephrogenic diabetes insipidus exists, a high intake of solute-free water is mandatory. Chronic renal failure is not a frequent problem and usually needs no attention, except for maintaing serum lithium concentrations in the subtoxic level. Hypercalcemia, hypermagnesemia, and increased serum levels of parathyroid hormone occasionally occur in lithium-intoxicated patients (262). Because hypercalcemia and polyuria causing dehydration can aggravate lithium retention and renal failure, these problems should be treated by standard techniques as the lithium dosage is decreased or discontinued.

Numerous drugs impair free water elimination, either by stimulating the release of antidiuretic hormone or by augmenting its effect. Such drugs include barbiturates, chlorpropamide, clofibrate, cyclophosphamide, indomethacin, morphine, and vincristine. When such reactions occur, water restriction is necessary. It is also important to remember that diuretics that block sodium reabsorption in the ascending limb of Henle's loop inhibit free water clearance, also rendering the patient susceptible to water intoxication. Although these can be considered pharmacologic rather than toxic effects, considerable morbidity can ensue.

PREVENTION

The causes of toxic nephropathy may be considered as two groups, poisons and drugs. Although avoidance of the toxin is pertinent prophylactically for both types of compounds, specific recommendations differ.

Industrial hazards such as mercury vapors, cadmium wastes, and chlorinated hydrocarbons should be rendered less perilous by improved working conditions, such as better ventilation and safer waste disposal. Warnings on labels and safety education can reduce the number of accidents. Limiting accessibility to highly toxic substances may decrease the incidence of accidental and intentional self-poisoning. The development of safer chemicals is a long-term solution.

The incidence of nephrotoxicity due to drugs can be reduced by awareness of factors that increase the risk of injury on exposure, taking care to decrease these risk factors when possible, and, when vulnerability cannot be lessened, to lower dosages or to avoid pertinent drugs.

Because of the diversity of renal lesions resulting from drug toxicity, no recommendation except (inappropriate) therapeutic nihilism will be universally successful. Although some instances of nephrotoxicity appear without warning, many can be anticipated. To decrease the likelihood of nephrotoxicity some specific recommendations can be made. Avoid culprit drugs when susceptibility is high, e.g., nonsteroidals when dependent on vasodilator prostaglandins, and nephroallergens when there is a history of hypersensitivity. Be wary when resuming interrupted therapy with such allergens. Locate and shield kidneys before radiating. Limit and space radiation doses when possible. Use alternative imaging techniques in patients with risk facors for iodide nephrotoxicity, especially those with diabetic nephropathy. Monitor chronic exposure to toxins such as gold, lithium, and mixed analgesics. Educate those prescribing and taking medications about the potential dangers and early warning signs. Follow pharmacokinetic principles when treating patients with impaired elimination rates. Be wary of nephrotoxic antibiotics, especially in those having risk factors, undergoing prolonged therapy, or manifesting early signs of toxicity. Whenever possible use the least toxic congener. Maintain hydration, replete, and diurese patients receiving nephrotoxins. Maintain urinary solubility of drugs and metabolites.

In general, restricting the use of potentially nephrotoxic

drugs to definite indications, following dosing guidelines, monitoring plasma levels, seeking evidence of toxicity, and responding to early warning signs will lower the incidence of adverse reactions.

Prevention should involve education, both of physicians and other health profressionals, and of the pbulic. Most cases of nephrotoxicity could be avoided by anticipation and precautions.

In the long run, prevention can be greatly enhanced by research. The development of new analogues of effective drugs that have lower toxic potential can reduce or even eliminate the problem. Greater understanding of the mechanisms by which the kidney is injured and develops adverse reactions to injury, such as atrophy and interstitial fibrosis, should lead to methods to improve tolerance to toxic drugs for those instances when they are required. Identifying the cause and pathogenesis of the diseases for which toxic drugs are given could lead to more specific, less toxic treatments.

It is utopian, however, to anticipate that in the near future the judicious use of drugs, careful clinical observations, education, and research will relegate toxic nephropathy to historic interest.

NOTE

The opinions and assertions contained herein are the private views of the author and should not be considered as official or as necessarily representing those of the Uniformed Services University or the Department of Defense. There is no objection to publication.

REFERENCES

1. Wing AJ, Brunner FP, Brynger H, Chantler C, Donckerwolke RA, Jacobs C, Kramer P, Selwood NH: Combined report on regular dialysis and transplantation in Europe 1X, 1978. *Proc Eur Dial Transpl Assoc* 16:3–87, 1979.
2. Kincaid-Smith P: Analgesic abuse and the kidney. *Kidney Int* 17:250–260, 1980.
3. Gonwa TA, Hamilton RW, Buckalew VM Jr: Chronic renal failure and end-stage renal disease in northwest North Carolina. Importance of analgesic-associated nephropathy. *Arch Intern Med* 141:462–465, 1981.
4. Weeden RP, D'Haese P, Ven de Vyver FL, Verpooten GA, DeBroe MA: Lead nephropathy. *Am J Kidney Dis* 8:380–386, 1986.
5. Appel GB, Neu HC: The nephrotoxicity of antimicrobial agents. *N Engl J Med* 296:663–670; 722–728; 784–787, 1977.
6. Madias NE, Harrington JT: Platinum nephrotoxicity. *Am J Med* 65:307–314, 1978.
7. Byrd L, Sherman RL: Radiocontrast-induced acute renal failure: A clinical and pathophysiologic review. *Medicine* 58:270–279, 1979.
8. Kumin GD: Clinical nephrotoxicity of tobramycin and gentamicin. A prospective study. *JAMA* 244:1808–1810, 1980.
9. Finn WF: Environmental toxins and renal disease. *J Clin Pharmacol* 23:461–472, 1983.
10. Meyer BR, Fischbein A, Rosenman K, Lerman Y, Drayer DE, Reidenberg MM: Increased urinary enzyme excretion in workers exposed to nephrotoxic chemicals. *Am J Med* 76:989–998, 1984.
11. Maher JF: Clinicopathologic spectrum of drug nephrotoxicity. *Adv Intern Med* 30:295–316, 1984.
12. Maher JF: Toxic and irradiation nephropathies. In: LE Earley, CW Gottschalk, eds, *Strauss and Welt's Diseases of the Kidney*. Little, Brown, Boston, pp 1431–1474, 1979.
13. Masuda Y, Nakayama N, Yamaguchi A, Murohashi M: Effects of diethylthiocarbonate and carbon disulfide on acute nephrotoxicity induced by furan, bromobenzene and cephaloridine in mice. *Jpn J Pharmacol* 34:221–229, 1984.
14. Rush GF, Smith JH, Newton JF, Hook JB: Chemically induced nephrotoxicity: Role of metabolic activation. *CRC Crit Rev Toxicol* 13:99–160, 1984.
15. Hricik DE, Browning PJ, Kopelman R, Goorno WE, Madias NE, Dzau VJ: Captopril-induced functional renal insufficiency in patients with bilateral renal-artery stenosis or renal-artery stenosis in a solitary kidney. *N Engl J Med* 308:373–376, 1983.
16. Coulie P, DePlaen JF, van Ypersele de Strihou C: Captopril-induced acute reversible renal failure. *Nephron* 35:108–111, 1983.
17. Funck-Brentano C, Chatellier G, Alexandre JM: Reversible renal failure after combined treatment with enalapril and furosemide in a patient with congestive heart failure. *Br Heart J* 55:596–598, 1986.
18. Seidelin R: Cimetidine and renal failure. *Postgrad Med J* 56:440–441, 1980.
19. Webb J: Renal failure associated with ergot poisoning. *Br Med J* 2:1355, 1977.
20. Cronin RE, Erickson AM, de Torrente A, McDonald KM, Schrier RW: Norepinephrine-induced acute renal failure: A reversible ischemic model of aucte renal failure. *Kidney Int* 14:187–190, 1978.
21. Kimberly RP, Bowden RE, Keiser HR, Plotz PH: Reduction of renal function by newer nonsteroidal antiinflammatory drugs. *Am J Med* 64:804–807, 1978.
22. Lamp PP: Renal effects of nonsteroidal antiinflammatory drugs. Heightened risk to the elderly. *J Am Geriatric Soc* 34:361–367, 1986.
23. Carmichael J, Shankel SW: Effects of nonsteroidal antiinflammatory drugs on prostaglandins and renal function. *Am J Med* 78:992–1000, 1985.
24. Henrich WL: Nephrotoxicity of nonsteroidal antiinflammatory agents. *Am J Kidney Dis* 2:478–484, 1983.
25. Blackshear JL, Napier JS, Davidman M, Stillman MT: Renal complications of nonsteroidal antiinflammatory drugs: Identification and monitoring of those at risk. *Semin Arthritis Rheum* 14:163–175, 1985.
26. Garella S, Matarese RA: Renal effects of prostaglandins and clinical adverse effects of nonsteroidal antiinflammatory agents. *Medicine* 61:165–181, 1985.
27. Adams DH, Howie AJ, Michael J, McConkey B, Bacon PA, Adu D: Nonsteroidal antiinflammatory drugs and renal failure. *Lancet* 1:57–59, 1986.
28. Clive DM, Staff JS: Renal syndromes associated with nonsteroidal antiinflammatory drugs. *N Engl J Med* 310:563–572, 1984.
29. Hart D, Ward M, Lifschitz MD: Suprofen-related nephrotoxicity. A distinct clinical syndrome. *Ann Intern Med* 106:235–238, 1987.
30. Fauci AS, Haynes BF, Katz P: The spectrum of vasculitis: Clinicial, pathologic, immunologic and therapeutic considerations. *Ann Intern Med* 89:660–676, 1978.
31. Antonovych TT: Drug-induced nephropathies. *Pathol Annu*

19 (Pt 2):165–196, 1984.
32. Zimmerman SW, Groehler K, Beirne GJ: Hydrocarbon exposure and chronic glomerulonephritis. *Lancet* 2:199–201, 1975.
33. Beirne GL, Brennan JT: Glomerulonephritis associated with hydrocarbon solvents. *Arch Environ Health* 25:365–369, 1972.
34. Gavaghan TE, McNaught PJ, Ralston M, Hayes JM: Penicillamine-induced "Goodpasture's syndrome": Successful treatment of a fulminant case. *Aust NZ J Med* 11:261–265, 1981.
35. Ehrenreich T, Yunis SL, Chrug J: Membranous nephropathy following exposure to volatile hydrocarbons. *Environmental Res* 14:35–45, 1977.
36. von Scheele C, Althoff P, Kempi U, Schelin U: Nephrotic syndrome due to subacute glomerulonephritis—association with hydrocarbon exposure? *Acta Med Scand* 200:427–429, 1976.
37. Schreiner GE, Maher JF: Toxic nephropathy. *Am J Med* 38:408–449, 1965.
38. Zimmerman SW, Norbach DH: Nephrotoxic effects of long-term carbon tetrachloride administration in rats. *Arch Pathol Lab Med* 104:94–99, 1980.
39. Rao TKS, Nicastri AD, Friedman EA: Natural history of heroin-associated nephropathy. *N Engl J Med* 290:19–23, 1974.
40. Alarcon Segovia D: Drug induced lupus syndromes. *Mayo Clin Proc* 44:664–681, 1969.
41. Northway JD, West CD: Successful therapy of trimethadione nephrosis with prednisone and cyclophosphamide. *J Pediat* 71:259–263, 1967.
42. Bergstrand A, Bergstrand CG, Engstrom N, Herrlin KM: Renal histology during treatment with oxazolidine-diones (tremethadione, ethadione and paramethadione). *Pediatrics* 30:601–607, 1962.
43. Lange K: Nephropathy induced by D-penicillamine. *Contrib Nephrol* 10:63–74, 1978.
44. Jaffe IA, Treser G, Suzuki Y, Ehrenreich T: Nephropathy induced by D-penicillamine. *Ann Intern Med* 69:549–556, 1968.
45. Sternlieb I: Penicillamine and the nephrotic syndrome. *JAMA* 198:1311–1312, 1966.
46. Bacon PA, Tribe CR, MacKenzie JC, Verrier Jones J, Cuming RH, Amer B: Penicillamine nephropathy in rheumatoid arthritis: A clinicial pathological and immunological study. *Q J Med* 45:661–684, 1976.
47. Luke RG: Proteinuria during penicillamine therapy for cystinuria. *Postgrad Med J* 44 (Suppl 6):21–23, 1968.
48. Silverberg DS, Kidd EG, Shnitka TK, Ulan RA: Gold nephropathy: A clinical and pathologic study. *Arthritis Rheum* 13:812–825, 1970.
49. Palosuo T, Provost TT, Milgram F: Gold nephropathy: Serologic data suggesting an immune complex disease. *Clin Exp Immunol* 25:311–318, 1976.
50. Strauss J, Pardo V, Koss MN, Griswold W, McIntosh RM: Nephropathy associated with sickle cell anemia: An autologous immune complex nephritis. I. Studies on nature of glomerular-bound antibody and antigen identification in a patient with sickle cell disease and immune deposit glomerulonephritis. *Am J Med* 58:382–387, 1975.
51. Billingsley LM, Stevens MB: The relationship between D-penicillamine induced proteinuria and prior gold nephropathy. *Johns Hopkins Med J* 148:64–67, 1981.
52. Merle LJ, Reidenberg MM, Camacho MT, Jones BR, Drayer DE: Renal injury in patients with rheumatoid arthritis treated with gold. *Clin Pharmacol Ther* 28:216–222, 1980.
53. Robbins G, McIllmurray MB: Acute renal failure due to gold. *Postgrad Med J* 56:366–367, 1980.
54. Kelchner J, McIntosh JR, Boedecker E, Guggenheim S, McIntosh RM: Experimental autologous immune deposit nephritis in rats associated with mercuric chloride administration. *Experientia* 32:1204–1208, 1976.
55. Kazantzis G, Schiller KFR, Asscher AW, Drew RG: Albuminuria and the nephrotic syndrome following exposure to mercury and its compounds. *Q J Med* 31:403–418, 1962.
56. Cameron JS, Trounce FR: Membranous glomerulonephritis and the nephrotic syndrome appearing during mersalyl therapy. *Guy's Hosp Rep* 114:101–107, 1965.
57. Beattie JW: Nephrotic syndrome following sodium bismuth tartrate therapy in rheumatoid arthritis. *Ann Rheum Dis* 12:144–146, 1953.
58. Ellis JT: Glomerular lesions and the nephrotic syndrome in rabbits given iron oxide intravenously. *J Exp Med* 103:127–144, 1956.
59. Horak E, Sunderman FW Jr: Nephrotoxicity of nickel carbonyl in rats. *Ann Clin Lab Sci* 10:425–431, 1980.
60. Brezin JH, Katz SM, Schwartz AB, Chinitz JL: Reversible renal failure and nephrotic syndrome associated with nonsteroidal antiinflammatory drugs. *N Engl J Med* 301:1271–1273, 1979.
61. Gary NE, Dodelson R, Eisinger RP: Indomethacin-associated acute renal failure. *Am J Med* 69:135–136, 1980.
62. Stachura I, Joyakumar S, Bourke E: T and B lymphocyte subsets in fenoprofen nephropathy. *Am J Med* 75:9–16, 1963.
63. Ferris TF, Morgan WS, Levitin H: Nephrotic syndrome caused by probenicid. *N Engl J Med* 265:381–383, 1961.
64. Maher JF: Toxic disorders of the glomerulus. In: J Zabriskie, H Villaroel Jr, EL Becker, eds, *Perspectives in Clinical Immunology II: Kidney. Clinical Immunology of the Kidney*. John Wiley, New York, pp 293–306, 1982.
65. Alexander CS, Hunt VR: Evidence against immune mechanism in aminucleoside nephrosis in rats. *J Lab Clin Med* 62:103–108, 1963.
66. Seiler MW, Rennke HG, Venkstachalam MA, Cotran RS: Pathogenesis of polycation-induced alterations ("fusion") of glomerular epithelium. *Lab Invest* 36:48–61, 1977.
67. Robin AE, Crowson CN: Mercury nephrotoxicity in the rat. II. Investigation of intracellular site of mercury nephrotoxicity by correlated serial time histologic and histoenzymatic studies. *Am J Path* 41:485–499, 1962.
68. Peters JP, Eisenham AJ, Kydd DM: Mercury poisoning. *Am J Med Sci* 185:149–171, 1933.
69. Burgat–Sacaze V, Braun JP, Rico A, Benard P, Eghbali B: Methoxyethyl-mercury nephrotoxicity: Effects on enzymuria and kidney function. *Arch Toxicol* 43:277–231, 1980.
70. Longcope WT, Leutscher JA Jr, Calkins E, Grob D, Bush SW, Eisenberg H: Clinical uses of 2,3-dimercaptopropanol (BAL). XI. The treatment of acute mercury poisoning by BAL. *J Clin Invest* 25:557–567, 1946.
71. Doolan PD, Hess WC, Kyle LH: Acute renal insufficiency due to bichloride of mercury. Observations on gastrointestinal hemorrhage and BAL therapy. *N Engl J Med* 249:273–276, 1953.
72. Kostyniak PJ, Clarkson TW, Abbasi AH: An extracorporeal complexing hemodialysis system for the treatment of methylmercury poisoning II. In vivo applications in the dog. *J Pharmacol Exp Ther* 203:253–263, 1977.
73. Leumann EP, Brandenberger H: Hemodialysis in a patient

73. with acute mercuric cyanide intoxication. Concentrations of mercury in blood dialysate, urine, vomitus and feces. *Clin Toxicol* 11:301–308, 1977.
74. Klonne DR, Johnson DR: Amelioration of mercuric chloride-induced acute renal failure by dithiothreitol. *Toxicol Appl Pharmacol* 70:459–466, 1983.
75. Maher JF: Acute renal failure complicating intoxication. In: LH Haddad, JF Winchester, eds, *Clinical Management of Poisoning*. WB Saunders, Philadelphia, pp 170–184, 1983.
76. Blachley JD, Hill JB: Renal and electrolyte disturbances associated with cisplatin. *Ann Intern Med* 95:628–632, 1981.
77. Jones BR, Bhalla RB, Mladek J, Kaleya RN, Gralla RJ, Alcock NW, Schwartz MK, Young CW, Reidenberg MM: Comparison of methods of evaluating nephrotoxicity of cisplatinum. *Clin Pharmacol Ther* 27:557–562, 1980.
78. Schilsky RL, Anderson T: Hypomagnesemia and renal magnesium wasting in patients receiving cisplatin. *Ann Intern Med* 90:929–931, 1979.
79. Vogl SE, Zaravinos T, Kaplan BH: Toxicity of cis-diamminedichloroplatinum II given in a two hour regimen of diuresis and hydration. *Cancer* 45:11–15, 1980.
80. Daley-Yates PT, McBrien DCH: Enhancement of cisplatin nephrotoxicity by probenecid. *Cancer Treat Rep* 68:445–446, 1984.
81. Sharma RP: Cisplatinum: Effect of zinc acetate pretreatment on cellular uptake and interactions with cytosolic ligands. *Toxicology* 32:75–84, 1984.
82. Prestayko AW, Luft FC, Einhorn L, Crooke ST: Cisplatin pharmacokinetics in a patient with renal dysfunction. *Med Pediat Oncol* 5:183–188, 1978.
83. Goldstein RS, Mayor GH: Minireview: The nephrotoxicity of cisplatin. *Life Sci* 32:685–690, 1983.
84. Dentino M, Luft FC, Yum MN, Williams SD, Einhorn LH: Long term effect of cis-diamminedichloride platinum (CDDP) on renal function and structure in man. *Cancer* 41:1274–1281, 1978.
85. Vallee BL, Ulmer DD, Wacker WEC: Arsenic toxicology and biochemistry. *Arch Indust Health* 21:132–151, 1960.
86. Teitelbaum DT, Kier LC: Arsine poisoning. Report of five cases in the petroleum industry and a discussion of the indications for exchange transfusion and hemodialysis. *Arch Environ Hlth* 19:133–143, 1969.
87. Giberson A, Vaziri ND, Mirahadami K, Rosen SM: Hemodialysis of acute arsenic intoxication with transient renal failure. *Arch Intern Med* 136:1303–1304, 1976.
88. Gerhardt RE, Hudson JB, Rao RN, Sobel RE: Chronic renal insufficiency from cortical necrosis induced by arsenic poisoning. *Arch Intern Med* 138:1267–1269, 1978.
89. Burr RE, Botto AM, Beaver DL: Isolation and analysis of renal bismuth inclusions. *Toxicol Appl Pharmacol* 7:588–591, 1965.
90. Ryan R, McNeil JS, Flamenbaum W, Nagle R: Uranyl nitrate induced acute renal failure in the rat. Effect of varying doses and saline loading. *Proc Soc Exp Biol Med* 143:289–296, 1973.
91. Sanghvi LM, Sharma R, Misra SN, Samuel KC: Sulfhemoglobinemia and acute renal failure after copper sulfate poisoning; report or two fatal cases. *Arch Path* 63:172–175, 1975.
92. Wetherill SF, Guarino MJ, Cox RW: Acute renal failure associated with barium chloride poisoning. *Ann Intern Med* 95:187–188, 1981.
93. Lucke B: Lower nephron nephrosis. The renal lesions of crush syndrome, of burns, transfusions and other conditions affecting the lower segment of the nephrons. *Milit Surg* 99:371–396, 1946.
94. Franchini I, Mutti A, Cavatorta A, Corradi A, Cosi A, Olivetti G, Borghetti A: Nephrotoxicity of chromium. *Contrib Nephrol* 10:98–110, 1978.
95. Charlas R, Benabadji A: Nephrite azotemique au cours du traitement par l'antimoine d'un case de leishmanoise viscerale infantil. *Maroc Med* 41:1180–1182,1962.
96. Ebina Y, Okada S, Hamazaki S, Midorikawa O: Liver, kidney and central nervous toxicity of aluminum given intraperitoneally to rats: A multiple-dose subchronic study using aluminum nitrolotriacetate. *Toxicol Appl Pharmacol* 75:211–218, 1984.
97. Thompson J: Ferrous sulfate poisoning. Its incidence, symptomatology, treatment and prevention. *Br Med J* 1:645–646, 1950.
98. Batey R, Scott J, Jain S, Sherlock S: Acute renal insufficiency occurring during intravenous desferrioxamine therapy. *Scand J Haematol* 22:277–279, 1979.
99. Oliver LD, Mehta R, Sarles HE: Acute renal failure following administration of ethylenediaminetetraacetic acid (EDTA). *Tex Med* 80(2):40–42, 1984.
100. Laug EP, Calvery HP, Morris HJ, Woodard G: The toxicity of some glycols and derviatives. *J Indust Hyg Toxicol* 21:173–201, 1939.
101. Schreiner GE, Maher JF, Marc-Aurele J, Knowlan D, Alvo M: Ethylene glycol—two indications for hemodialysis. *Trans Am Soc Artif Intern Organs* 5:81–85, 1959.
102. Guild WR, Young JV, Merrill JP: Anuria due to carbon tetrachloride intoxication. *Ann Intern Med* 48:1221–1227, 1958.
103. Stewart RD, Boettner EA, Southwerth RR, Cerny JC: Acute carbon tetrachloride intoxication. *JAMA* 183:994–997, 1963.
104. Baerg RD, Kimberg DV: Centrilobular hepatic necrosis and acute renal failure in solvent sniffers. *Ann Intern Med* 73:713–720, 1970.
105. Halevy J, Pitlik S, Rosenfeld J, Eitan B: 1,1,1,-trichloroethane intoxication: A case report with transient liver and renal damage. Review of the literature. *Clin Toxicol* 16:467–472, 1980.
106. Streicher HZ, Gabow PA, Moss AH, Kono D, Kaehny WD: Syndromes of toluene sniffing in adults. *Ann Intern Med* 94:758–762, 1981.
107. Lang EK, Foreman J, Schlegel JU, Leslie C, List A, McCormick P: The incidence of contrast medium acute tubular necrosis following arteriography. *Radiology* 138:203206, 1981.
108. Gomes AS, Baker JD, Martin-Paredo V, Dixon SM, Takiff H, Machleder HI, Moore WS: Acute renal dysfunction after major angiography. *Am J Roentgenol* 145:1249–1253, 1985.
109. Tornquist C, Almén T, Golman K, Hotås S: Renal function following nephroangiography with metrizarnide and iohexal. Effects on renal blood flow, glomerular permeability and filtration rate and diuresis in dogs. *Acta Radio (Stockholm)* 26:483–489, 1985.
110. Taliercio CP, Vlietstra RE, Fisher LD, Burnett JC: Risks for renal dysfunction with cardiac angiography. *Ann Intern Med* 104:501–504, 1986.
111. Engle JE, Schoolwerth AC: Additive neprotoxicity from roentgenographic contrast media; its occurrence in phenazopyridine-induced acute renal failure. *Arch Intern Med* 141:784–785, 1981.
112. Winearls CG, Ledingham JGG, Dixon AJ: Acute renal failure precipitated by radiographic contrast medium in a patient with rhabdomyolysis. *Br Med J* 2:1603, 1980.

113. Older RA, Korobkin M, Cleeve DM, Schaaf R, Thompson W: Contrast-induced acute renal failure: Persistent nephrogram as clue to early detection. *Am J Roentgenol* 134:339–342, 1980.
114. Mudge GH: Nephrotoxicity of urographic radiocontrast drugs. *Kidney Int* 18:540–552, 1980.
115. Forrest JB, Howards SS, Gillenwater JY: Osmotic effects of intravenous contrast agents on renal function. *J Urol* 125:147–150, 1981.
116. Ihle BU, Byrnes CA, Simenhoff ML: Acute renal failure due to interstitial nephritis resulting from radio-contrast agents. *Aust NZ J Med* 12:630–632, 1982.
117. Healy JK: Acute oliguric renal failure associated with multiple myeloma. *Br Med J* 1:1126–1130, 1963.
118. Setter JG, Maher JF, Schreiner GE: Acute renal failure following cholecystography. *JAMA* 184:102–110, 1963.
119. Malt RA, Olken HG, Goade WJ Jr: Renal tubular necrosis after oral cholecystography. *Arch Surg* 87:743–746, 1963.
120. Canales CO, Smith GH, Robinson JC, Remmers AR Jr, Sarles HE: Acute renal failure after the adminstration of iopanoic acid as a cholecystographic agent. *N Engl J Med* 281:89–91, 1969.
121. Hansson R, Lindholm T: Elimination of hypaque (sodium-3,5 diacetamido -2,4,6 triiodobenzoate) and the effect of hemodialysis in anuria. A clinical study and experimental investigation on rabbits. *Acta Med Scand* 174:611–620, 1963.
122. Bennett WM, Aronoff GR, Morrison G, Golper TA, Pulliam J, Wolfson M, Singer I: Drug prescribing in renal failure: Dosing guidelines for adults. *Am J Kidney Dis* 3:155–193, 1983.
123. Maher JF: Pharmacologic aspects of regular dialysis treatment. In:W Drukker, FM Parsons, JF Maher, eds, *Replacement of Renal Function by Dialysis*. Martinus Nijhoff, The Hague, pp 749–797, 1982.
124. Kaloyanides GJ, Pastoriza-Munoz E: Aminoglycoside nephrotoxicity. *Kidney Int* 185:571–582, 1980.
125. Cronin RE: Aminoglycoside nephrotoxicity: Pathogenesis and prevention *Clin Nephrol* 11:251–256, 1979.
126. Humes HD, Weinberg JM, Knauss TC: Clinical and pathophysiologic aspects of aminoglycoside nephrotoxicity. *Am J Kidney Dis* 2:5–29, 1982.
127. Whelton A: Therapeutic initiatives for the avoidance of aminoglycoside toxicity. *J Clin Pharmacol* 25:67–81, 1985.
128. Smith CR, Moor RD, Leitman RD: Studies of risk factors for aminoglycoside nephrotoxicity. *Am J Kidney Dis* 8:308–313, 1986.
129. Luft FC, Block R, Sloan RS, Yum MN, Costello R, Maxwell DR: Comparative nephrotoxicity of aminoglycoside antibiotics in rats. *J Infect Dis* 138:541–545, 1978.
130. DeBroe ME, Paulus GJ, Veropooten GA, Roels F, Buyssens N, Weeden R, Van Hoof F, Tulkens PM: Early effects of gentamicin, tobramycin and amikacin on the human kidney. *Kidney Int* 25:643–652, 1984.
131. Gary NE, Buzzeo L, Salaki J, Eisinger RP: Gentamicin-associated acute renal failure. *Arch Intern Med* 136:1101–1104, 1976.
132. Tulkens PM: Experimental study of nephrotoxicity of aminoglycoside at low doses. Mechanisms and perspectives. *Am J Med* 80 (Suppl 6B):105–114, 1986.
133. Fillastre JP, Henet J, Tulkens P, Morin JP, Viotte G, Oiler B, Godin M: Comparative nephrotoxicity of four aminoglycosides: Biochemical and ultrastructural modifications of lysosomes. *Adv Nephrol* 2:253–275, 1982.
134. Brion B, Barge J, Godefroy I, Dromer F, Dobois C, Contrepois A, Carbon C: Gentamicin, netilmicin, dibekacin and amikacin nephrotoxicity and its relation to tubular reabsorption in rabbits. *Antimicrob Agents Chemother* 25:168–172, 1984.
135. Brogard JM, Comte F, Spach MO: Nephrotoxicity of aminoglycoside. Effects on pharmacokinetics and prevention. *Contrib Nephrol* 42:182–195, 1984.
136. Bennett WM, Plamp CE, Gilbert DN, Parker RA, Porter GA: The influences of dosage regimen on experimental gentamicin nephrotoxicity: Dissociation of peak serum levels from renal failure. *J Infect Dis* 140:576–580, 1979.
137. Sethi K, Diamond LH: Aminoglycoside nephrotoxicity and its predictability. *Nephron* 27:265–270, 1981.
138. Schentag JJ, Gengo FM, Plaut ME, Danner D, Mangione A, Jusko WJ: Urinary casts as an indicator of renal tubular damage in patients receiving aminoglycosides. *Antimicrob Agents Chemother* 16:468–474, 1979.
139. Sobern L, Bowman RL, Pastoriza-Munoz E, Kaloyanides GJ: Comparative nephrotoxicities of gentamicin, netilmicin and tobramycin in the rat. *J Pharmacol Exp Ther* 210:334–343, 1979.
140. Daschner FD, Just HM, Jansen W, Lorber R: Netilmicin versus tobramycin in multicentre studies. *J Antimicrob Chemother* 13 (Suppl A):37–42, 1984.
141. Engle JE, Abt AB, Schneck DW, Scohoolwerth AC: Netilmicin and tobramycin. Comparison of nephrotoxicity in dogs. *Invest Urol* 17:98–102, 1979.
142. Wade JC, Smith CR, Petty BG, Lipsky JJ, Conrad G, Ellner J, Lietman PS: Cephalothin plus an aminoglycoside is more nephrotoxic than methicillin plus an aminoglycoside. *Lancet* 2:604–606, 1978.
143. Bennett WM, Wood CA, Houghton DC, Gilbert DN: Modification of experimental aminoglycoside nephrotoxicity. *Am J Kidney Dis* 8:292–296, 1986.
144. Roxe DM: Toxic nephropathy from diagnostic and therapeutic agents. Review and commentary.*Am J Med* 69:759–766, 1980.
145. Bennett WM, Pulliam JP, Porter GA, Houghton DC: Modification of experimental gentamicin nephrotoxicity by selective parathyroidectomy. *Am J Physiol* 249:F832–F835, 1985.
146. Elliott WC, Patchin DS, Jones DB: Effect of parathyroid hormone activity on gentamicin nephrotoxicity. *J Lab Clin Med* 109:48–54, 1987.
147. Cronin RE, Newman JA: Protective effect of thyroxine but not parathyroidectomy on gentaimicin nephrotoxicity. *Am J Physiol* 248:F332–F339, 1985.
148. Ho PWL, Pien FD, Kominami N: Massive amikacin "overdose." *Ann Intern Med* 91:227–228, 1979.
149. Maher JF: The prognosis of toxic renal lesions. *Proc 8th Int Congr Nephrol* 8:761–767, 1981.
150. Moellering RC Jr, Swartz MN: The newer cephalosporins. *N Engl J Med* 294:24–28, 1976.
151. Barza M: The nephrotoxicity of cephalosporins: An overview. *J Infect Dis* 137:S60–S73, 1978.
152. Silverblatt F: Pathogenesis of nephrotoxicity of cephalosporins and aminoglycosides: A review of current concepts. *Rev Infect Dis* 4 (Suppl 5):S60–S65, 1982.
153. Boyd JF, Butcher BT, Stewart GT: The nephrotoxicity and histology of cephaloridine and its polymers in rats. *Br J Exp Pathol* 52:503–516, 1971.
154. Linton AL, Bailey R, Turnbull DI: Relative nephrotoxicity of cephalosporin antibiotics in an animal model. *Can Med Assoc J* 107:414–416, 1972.
155. Carling PC, Idelson BA, Casano A, Alexander EA,

McCabe WR: Nephrotoxicity associated with cephalothin adminstration. *Arch Intern Med* 135:797–801, 1975.
156. Fung–Herrere CG, Mulvaney WP: Cephalexin nephrotoxicity. Reversible nonoliguric acute renal failure and hepatotoxicity associated with cephalexin therapy. *JAMA* 299:318–319, 1974.
157. Tune B, Fravert D: Cephalosporin nephrotoxicity. Transport, cytotoxicity and mitochondrial toxicity of cephaloglycin. *J Pharmacol Exp Ther* 215:186–190, 1980.
158. Tune BM, Fravert D: Mechanisms of cephalosporin nephrotoxicity: A comparison of cephaloridine and cephaloglycine. *Kidney Int* 18:591–600, 1980.
159. Jawetz E: Polymyxin, colistin and bacitracin. *Pediatr Clin North Am* 8:1057–1071, 1961.
160. Kock–Weser J, Sidel VW, Federman EB, Kanarek P, Finer DC, Eaton AE: Adverse effects of sodium colistimethate. Manifestations and specific reaction rates during 317 courses of therapy. *Ann Intern Med* 72:857–868, 1970.
161. Shils ME: Renal disease and the metabolic effects of tetracycline. *Ann Intern Med* 58:389–408, 1963.
162. Philips ME, Eastwood JB, Curtis JR, Gower PE, de Wardener HE: Tetracycline poisoning in renal failure. *Br Med J* 2:149–151, 1974.
163. Orr LH Jr, Rudisill E Jr, Brodkin R, Hamilton RW: Exacerbation of renal failure associated with doxycycline. *Arch Intern Med* 138:793–794, 1978.
164. Frimpter GW, Timpanelli AE, Eisenmenger WJ, Stein HS, Ehrlich LI: Reversible Fanconi syndrome caused by degraded tetracycline. *JAMA* 184:111–113, 1963.
165. Singer I, Rotenberg D: Decmeclocycline-induced nephrogenic diabetes insipidus. In vivo and in vitro studies. *Ann Intern Med* 79:679–683, 1973.
166. Oster JR, Epstein M, Ulano HB: Deterioration of renal function with demeclocycline adminstration. *Curr Ther Res* 20:794–801, 1976.
167. Lehr D: Clinical toxicity of sulfonamides. *Ann NY Acad Sci* 69:417–447, 1957.
168. Kalowski S, Nanra RS, Mathew TH, Kincaid–Smith P: Deterioration in renal function in association with cotrimoxazole therapy. *Prog Biochem Parmacol* 9:129–140, 1974.
169. Skimming LH, Knies PT, Anthony MA, Melerango ES: Hemolytic anemia caused by sulfamethoxypridazine. Report of a case successfully treated by hemodialysis. *Ohio Med J* 57:280–281, 1961.
170. Kawamura T, Yagi N, Sugawara H, Yamahata K, Takada M: Efficacy of hemodialysis and the effects of certain displacing agents on plasma protein binding of sulfamethoxazole and sulfaphenazole in patients with chronic renal failure. *Chem Parmacol Bull (Tokyo)* 28:268–276, 1980.
171. Burgess JL, Birchall R: Nephrotoxicity of amphotericin B with emphasis on changes in tubular function. *Am J Med* 53:77–84, 1972.
172. Cheng JT, Witty RT, Robinson RR, Yarger WE: Amphotericin B nephrotoxicity: Increased renal resistance and tubule permeability. *Kidney Int* 22:626–633, 1982.
173. Gerkens JF, Branch RA: The influence of sodium status and furosemide on canine acute amphotericin B nephrotoxicity. *J Pharmacol Exp Ther* 214:306–311, 1980.
174. Takacs FJ, Tomkiewicz AM, Merrill JP: Amphotericin B toxicity with irreversible renal failure. *Ann Intern Med* 59:716–724, 1963.
175. Heidemann HT, Gerkens JF, Spickard WA, Jackson EK, Branch RA: Amphotericin B nephrotoxocity in humans decreased by salt repletion. *Am J Med* 75:476–481, 1983.
176. Appel GB, Given DB, Levine LR, Copper GL: Vancomycin and the kidney. *Am J Kidney Dis* 8:75–80, 1986.
177. Koffler A, Friedler RM, Massry SG: Acute renal failure due to nontraumatic rhabdomolysis. *Ann Intern Med* 85:23–28, 1976.
178. Cadnapaphornchai P, Taher S, McDonald FD: Acute drug-associated rhabdomolysis: An examination of its diverse renal manifestations and complications. *Am J Med Sci* 280:66–72, 1980.
179. Knochel JP: Rhabdomyolysis and myoglobinuria. *Semin Nephrol* 1:75–86, 1981.
180. Jennings AE, Levey AS, Harrington JT: Amoxapine-associated acute renal failure. *Arch Intern Med* 143:1525–1527, 1983.
181. Muehrcke RC: *Acute Renal Failure: Diagnosis and Management*. CV Mosby, Louis MO, 1969.
182. Takahashi H, Tsukada T: Triamterene-induced immune haemolytic anaemia with acute intravascular haemolysis and acute renal failure. *Scand J Hameatol* 23:169–176, 1979.
183. Prescott LF, Illingworth RN, Critchley JAJH, Frazer I, Stirling ML: Acute haemolysis and renal failure after nomifensine overdosage. *Br Med J* 2:1392–1393. 1980.
184. Alano F, Webster GD: Acute renal failure due to phenazopyridine (Pyridium). *Ann Intern Med* 72:89–91, 1970.
185. Maher JF: Effect of toxins on the kidney. *Contrib Nephrol* 7:42–68, 1977.
186. Sadoff L: Nephrotoxicity of streptozotocin (NSC 85998). *Cancer Chemother Rep* 54:457–459, 1970.
187. Nicholls DP, Yasin M: Acute renal failure from carbamazepine. *Br Med J* 4:490, 1972.
188. Haller JA, Randell HT, Stowens D, Rubel WF: Renal toxicity of polybrene in open heart surgery. *J Thorac Cardiovasc Surg* 44:486–493, 1962.
189. Myers BD: Cyclosporine nephrotoxicity. *Kidney Int* 30:964–974, 1986.
190. Thiel G: Experimental cyclosporine A nephrotoxicity: A summary of the International Workshop (Basle, April 24–26, 1985). *Clin Nephrol* 25 (Suppl 1):S205–210, 1986.
191. Hammer RW, Verani R, Weinman EJ: Mitomycin-associated renal failure; case report and review. *Arch Intern Med* 143:803–807, 1983.
192. Henderson IS, Beattie TJ, Kennedy AC: Dopamine hydrochloride in oliguric states. *Lancet* 2:827–828, 1980.
193. Tiller DJ, Mudge GH: Pharmacologic agents used in the management of acute renal failure. *Kidney Int* 18:700–711, 1980.
194. Heptinstall RH: Interstitial nephritis: A brief review. *Am J Path* 83:214–236, 1976.
195. Linton AL, Clark WF, Driedger AA, Turnbull DI, Lindsay RM: Acute interstitial nephritis due to drugs. Review of the literature with a report of nine cases. *Ann Intern Med* 93:735–741, 1980.
196. Mery J, Morel-Maroger L: Acute interstitial nephritis. A hypersensitivity reaction to drugs. *Proc 6th Int Congr Nephrol* 6:524–529, 1976.
197. Kleinhencht D, Kanfer A, Morel-Maroger L, Mery JP: Immunologically mediated drug-induced acute renal failure. *Contr Nephrol* 10:42–52, 1978.
198. Adler SG, Cohen AH, Border WA: Hypersensitivity phenomena and the kidney: Role of drugs and environmental agents. *Am J Kidney Dis* 5:75–96, 1985.
199. Hande KR, Noone RM, Stone WJ: Severe allopurinol toxicity. Description and guidelines for prevention in patients with renal insufficiency. *Am J Med* 76:47–56, 1984.
200. Woodroffe AJ, Thomson NM, Meadows R, Lawrence JR: Nephropathy associated with methicillin administration.

Aust NZ J Med 1:256–261, 1974.
201. Galpin JE, Shinaberger JH, Stanley TM, Blumenkrantz MJ, Bayer AS, Friedman GS, Montogmerie JZ, Guze LB, Coburn JW, Glassock RJ: Acute interstitial nephritis due to methicillin. Am J Med 65:756–765, 1978.
202. Harmon WE, Cohen HJ, Schneeberger EE, Grupe WE: Chronic renal failure in children treated with methyl CCNU. N Engl J Med 300:1200–1203, 1979.
203. Schacht RG, Feiner HD, Gallo GR, Lieberman A, Baldwin DS: Nephrotoxicity of nitrosureas. Cancer 48:1328–1334, 1981.
204. Raymond JR: Nephrotoxicities of antineoplastic and immunosuppressive agents. Curr Probl Cancer 8:1–32, 1984.
205. Healy HG, Clarkson AR: Renal complications of cytotoxic therapy. Aust NZ J Med 13:431–539, 1983.
206. Burke JF, Laucius F, Brodovsky HS, Soriano RZ: Doxorubicin hydrochloride-associated renal failure. Arch Intern Med 137:385–388, 1977.
207. Giroux L, Smeesters C, Boury F, Faure MP, Jean G: Adriamycin and adriamycin-DNA nephrotoxicity in rats. Lab Invest 50:190–196, 1984.
208. Farebrother DA, Hatfield P, Simmonds HA, Cameron JS, Jones AS, Cadenhead A: Experimental crystal nephropathy (one year study in the pig). Clin Nephrol 4:243–250, 1975.
209. Nanra RS: Clinical and pathological aspects of analgesic nephropathy. Br J Clin Pharmacol 10:359S–363S, 1980.
210. Gault MH, Wilson DR: Analgesic nephropathy in Canada. Clinical syndrome, management, and outcome. Kidney Int 13:58–63, 1978.
211. Buckalew VM, Schey HM: Analgesic nephropathy: A significant cause of morbidity in the United States. Am J Kidney Dis 7:164–168, 1986.
212. Maher JF: Renal failure in America is infrequently due to analgesic abuse. Am J Kidney Dis 7:169–173, 1986.
213. Cove–Smith JR, Knapp MS: Analgesic nephropathy: An important cause of chronic renal failure. Q J Med 47:49–69, 1978.
214. Bengtsson U: Prevention of renal disease. Proc Eur Dial Transpl Assoc 16:466–471, 1979.
215. Bluemle LW, Goldberg M: Renal accumulation of salicylate and phenacetin: Possible mechanisms in the nephropathy of analgesic abuse. J Clin Invest 47:2507–2513, 1968.
216. Wainscoat JS, Finn R: Possible role of laxatives in analgesic nephropathy. Br Med J 4:697–698, 1974.
217. Dubach VC, Levy PS, Rosner B, Baumeler HR, Mueller A, Peier A, Ehrensperger T: Relation between regular intake of phenacetin-containing analgesics and laboratory evidence for urorenal disorders in a female working population of Switzerland. Lancet 1:539–543, 1975.
218. Lornoy W, Morelle V, Becaus I, Fonteyne E, Mestdagh J, Thienpont L, Rollier A, Van Steenberge R, D'Haenens P: Malignant uroepithelial tumors of the upper urinary tract in sixteen patients with analgesic nephropathy. Acta Clin Belg 35:140–147, 1980.
219. Emmerson BT: Chronic lead nephropathy. Kidney Int 4:15, 1973.
220. Morgan JM, Hartley MW, Miller RE: Nephropathy in chronic lead poisoning. Arch Intern Med 118:17–29, 1966.
221. Emmerson BT: Chronic lead nephropathy. the diagnostic use of calcium EDTA and the association with gout. Aust Ann Med 12:310–324, 1963.
222. Goyer RA, May P, Cates MM, Krigman MR: Lead and protein content of isolated intranuclear inclusion bodies from kidneys of lead-poisoned rats. Lab Invest 22:245–251, 1970.
223. Smith Pederson R: Lead poisoning treated with haemodialysis. Scand J Urol Nephrol 12:189–190, 1978.
224. Kazantzis G: Cadmium nephropathy. Contr Nephrol 16:161–166, 1979.
225. Adams RG, Harrison JF, Scott P: The development of cadmium-induced proteinuria, impaired renal function and osteomalacia in alkaline battery workers. Q J Med 38:425–443, 1969.
226. Friberg L: Cadmium and the kidney. Environ Health Persp 54:1–11, 1984.
227. Roles HA, Lauverys RR, Bucket JP, Bernard A: Environmental exposure to cadmium and renal function of aged women in three areas of Belgium. Environ Res 24:117–130, 1981.
228. Smith TJ, Anderson RJ, Reading JC: Chronic cadmium exposures associated with kidney function effects. Am J Indust Med 1:319–337, 1980.
229. Barnett RN, Broun DS, Cadorna CB, Baker GP: Beryllium disease with death from renal failure. Conn Med 25:142–147, 1961.
230. Luxton RW: Radiation nephritis: A long-term study of 54 patients. Lancet 2:1221–1224, 1961.
231. Keane WF, Crosson JT, Staley NA, Anderson WR, Shapiro FL: Radiation-induced renal disease. Am J Med 60:127–137, 1976.
232. Churg J, Madrazo A: Radiation nephritis. Perspect Nephrol Hypertens 6:83–96, 1977.
233. Rosen S, Swerdlow MA, Muehrcke RC, Pirani CL: Radiation nephritis. Light and electron microscopic observations. Am J Clin path 41:487–502, 1964.
234. Frascino JA, Vanamee P, Rosen PP: Renal oxalosis and azotemia after methoxyflurane anesthesia. N Engl J Med 283:673–679, 1970.
235. Maher JF, Schreiner GE: Metabolic problems related to prolonged maintenance of life in oliguria. JAMA 176:393–403, 1961.
236. Schwartz RD, Wesley JR, Somermeyer MG, Lau K: Hyperoxaluria and renal insufficiency due to ascorbic acid administration during total parenteral nutrition. Ann Intern Med 100:530–531, 1984.
237. Lawton JM, Conway LT, Crosson JT, Smith CL, Abraham PA: Acute oxalate nephropathy after massive ascorbic acid administration. Arch Intern Med 148:950–951, 1985.
238. Ludwig B, Schindler E, Bohl J, Pfeiffer J, Kremer G: Reno-cerebral oxalosis induced by xylitol. Neuroradiology 26:517–521, 1984.
239. Maher JF, Rath CE, Schreiner GE: Hyperuricemia complicating leukemia: Treatment with allopurinol and dialysis. Arch Intern Med 123:198–200, 1969.
240. Paddack GL, Wahl RC, Holman RE, Schorr WJ, Lacher JW: Acute renal failure associated with ticrynafen. JAMA 243:764–765, 1980.
241. Orlandini G, Brognoli M: Acute renal failure and treatment with sulfinpyrazone. Clin Nephrol 20:161–162, 1983.
242. Randall RE, Strauss MB, McNeely WF: The milk-alkali syndrome. Arch Intern Med 107:163–181, 1961.
243. Chaplin H Jr, Clark LD, Ropes MW: Vitamin D intoxication. Am J Med Sci 221:369–378, 1951.
244. Christansen C, Rodbro P, Christensen MS, Hartnack B, Transbol I: Deterioration of renal function during treatment of chronic renal failure with 1,25 dihydroxycholecalciferol. Lancet 2:700–703, 1978.
245. Pitman SW, Frei E III: Weekly methotrexate-calcium leucovorin rescue: Effects of alkalinization on nephrotoxicity; pharmacokinetics in the CNS; and use in non-Hodgkin's

lymphoma. *Cancer Treatment Rep* 61:695–701, 1977.
246. Abelson HT, Fosberg MT, Beardsley GP, Goorin AM, Gorka C, Link M, Link D: Methotrexate-induced renal impairment: Clinical studies and rescue from systemic toxicity with high dose lecovorin and thymidine. *J Clin Oncol* 1:208–16, 1983.
247. Spiegel DM, Lau K: Acute renal failure and coma secondary to acyclovir therapy. *JAMA* 255:1882–1883, 1986.
248. Kaufman SA, McLellan P: Urinary tract complications of anticoagulation therapy; Pseudotumour of the kidney. *Br J Radiol* 41:180:185, 1968.
249. Curtis JR: Drug-induced renal disease. *Drugs* 18:377–391, 1979.
250. Graham JR, Suby HI, LeCompte PR, Sadowski NL: Fibrotic disorders associated with methysergide therapy for headache. *N Engl J Med* 274:359–368, 1966.
251. McCluskey DR, Donaldson RA, McGeown MG: Oxyprenol and retroperitoneal fibrosis. *Br Med J* 2:1459–1460, 1980.
252. Mazze RI, Trudell JR, Cousins MJ: Methoxyflurane metabolism and renal dysfunction: Clinical correlation in man. *Anesthesiology* 35:247–252, 1971.
253. Merkle RB, McDonald FD, Murray WJ: Human renal function following methoxyflurane anesthesia. *JAMA* 218:841–844, 1971.
254. Eichorn JH, Hedley–White J, Steinman TI, Kaufmann JM, Laasberg LH: Renal failure following enflurane anesthesia. *Anesthesiology* 45:557–560, 1976.
255. Cotton JR, Schwartz MM, Lindley JD, Hunsicker LG: Acute renal failure following halothane anesthesia. *Arch Pathol Lab Med* 100: 628–629, 1976.
256. Schou M: Litium studies I. Toxicity. *Acta Pharmacol* 15:70–84, 1958.
257. Singer I: Lithium and the Kidney. *Kidney Int* 19:374–387, 1981.
258. Singer I, Rotenberg D, Puschett JB: Lithium-induced nephrogenic diabetes insipidus. In vivo and in vitro studies. *J Clin Invest* 51:1081–1091, 1972.
259. Hansen HE, Hestbech J, Srensen JL, Norgaard K, Heilskov J, Amdisen A: Chronic interstitial nephropathy in patients on long-term lithium treatment. *Q J Med* 48:577–591, 1979.
260. Vestergaard P, Amidsen A: Lithium treatment and kidney function. A follow-up study of 237 patients in long-term treatment. *Acta Psychiat Scand* 63:333-343, 1981.
261. Walker RG, Escott M, Birchall I, Dowling JP, Kincaid-Smith P: Chronic progressive renal lesions induced by lithium. *Kidney Int* 29:875–881.
262. Christiansen C, Baastrup PC, Lindgreen P, Transbl I: Endocrine effects of lithium: II primary hyperparathyroidism. *Acta Endocrinol* 88:528–534, 1978.

CHAPTER 40

Acute Drug Intoxications

JAMES F. WINCHESTER

INTRODUCTION

The nephrologist is often called upon to aid in the treatment of poisoning in several ways: for guidance in the use of forced diuresis, for dialysis, and for expertise in sorbent hemoperfusion. Frequently consultation is sought for patients known to have ingested drugs with known rates of removal by dialysis and hemoperfusion. Advice may also be sought for substance removal where the exposure may be to a recently marketed drug or chemical for which there is scanty information on active drug removal with artificial organs. It is the purpose of this chapter to outline the factors governing active drug removal, to suggest areas in which drug removal may be invaluable or worthless, and to give guidelines for the employment of drug removal techniques.

In 1978 the National Center for Health Statistics (1) reported 12,171 deaths (mostly adults) attributable to poisoning. Of this number, 2452 were due to carbon monoxide, a situation almost identical to that in the United Kingdom (2), where the leading cause of death from poisoning, as in the United States, is carbon monoxide. In children over the last 20 years, a steady decline in accidental poison deaths has occurred, with only 100 deaths reported for 1980, in part due to safety closures on drug containers, improved medical training, consumer awareness, and voluntary industrial efforts limiting the toxic content of commercial products.

The number of deaths, however, does little to emphasize the amount of manpower expended in the treatment of poisoned subjects. For instance, for one drug, acetaminophen, the statistics are enlightening. In 1984, 35,074 cases of acetaminophen overdose were reported to the American Association of Poison Control Centers, National Data Collection System (AAPPC) (3), whereas, in 1983, 11,179 cases were reported to the AAPCC, with an additional 3332 reported exposures to other analgesics combined with acetaminophen. Acetaminophen accounted for 43% of all reported analgesic exposures in 1984, with the majority of patients being treated at home, only 38.8% being treated in a health care facility. The low mortality (0.07% or 23 deaths, from acute hepatic necrosis) is due to modern therapy, while 9.5% of patients developed major symptoms, 23.1% minor symptoms, and 383 "major outcomes" (1.1%).

There should be no complacency in the assessment and management of drug and chemical poisoning. The prevalence of poisoning remains high, with acute self-poisoning accounting for between 10% and 15% of medical emergencies presenting at hospitals both in the United Kingdom and in the U.S. (1, 2). Mortality in poisoned patients admitted to hospitals has been less than 1% since the adoption of the "Scandinavian method" of intensive supportive care as the mainstay of treatment (4).

DIAGNOSIS

The diagnosis of poisoning may or may not be straightforward, and it is necessary to ascertain from all sources any possibility of toxic ingestion, particularly in psychiatric patients, trauma victims, comatose patients, patients rescued from fires, or patients with an unexplained metabolic acidosis. If poisoning is suspected, simple qualitative chromatographic urinary drug screening methods are widely available and take less than 3 hours to make a tentative diagnosis. Following diagnosis, the approach to the poisoned patient can be divided into several phases (Table 1) (5).

In emergency stabilization of patients, the physician should direct his or her attention to cardiac and respiratory care, resuscitation, and fluid balance before any attempt at diagnosis is made. Intravenous fluids (saline) should be set up, and comatose patients may be given naloxone hydrochloride, followed by 50 g glucose as an IV bolus after blood and urine samples have been obtained for toxic screen, treating the common problems of opiate poisoning and hypoglycemia (6). In the comatose patient, particular attention should be paid to respiratory and cardiovascular systems, pupils, the body surfaces, the breath, and abdomen, since all may give clues to the etiology of poisoning. For example, in the comatose patient, pinpoint pupils suggest poisoning with organophosphate insecticides, opiates, or phenothiazines; whereas dilated pupils suggest tricyclic antidepressants, anticholinergic drugs, and sedatives such as glutethimide. Metabolic

Table 1. General approach to the management of poisoning

1. Emergency management
2. History and physical examination
3. Evaluation of major toxic signs
4. Laboratory evaluation
5. Elimination of poison
6. Administration of antidote
7. Elimination of absorbed substance
8. Supportive therapy
9. Observation and disposition

acidosis can be caused by several poisons. The following specifically contribute to acidosis: salicylates (7–10), methanol, ethylene glycol (11), and paraldehyde.

TREATMENT

Elimination of the poison from the gastrointestinal tract, skin, and eyes is the first major therapeutic goal. For organophosphates, it is imperative that the skin, eyes, and other body surfaces are thoroughly cleansed with soap and water initially, followed by alcohol rinses on exposed surfaces. Absorption of poisons from the gastrointestinal tract can be reduced by dilution with milk or water, gastric emptying (lavage or emesis), administration of activated charcoal, and administration of neutralizers (Bentonite, Fuller's earth or activated charcoal in paraquat poisoning), or cathartics. Contraindications to gastric lavage include the comatose patient prior to endotracheal intubation, kerosene ingestion, and lye ingestion. Drugs that have been reported to produce drug concretions in the stomach include meprobamate, carbromal, glutethimide, and carbamazepine (12). In this circumstance, warm saline lavage with abdominal massage, endoscopy, and endoscopic gastric removal of drug masses have been recommended (13).

Activated charcoal is the carbonaceous residue from destructive distillation of wood pulp, bone, coconut shells, peat, starch, lactose, or sucrose. Charcoal is "activated" by chemical or physical processes to form numerous surface pores; the small pores (micropores) determine the surface area and binding efficiency. Charcoal is administered frequently by mouth (or gastric/duodenal tube in the patient with active vomiting) in the form of a water-based slurry (along with a cathartic); the adult dose of activated charcoal is 50–100 g in 8 ounces of water, and the pediatric dose is 30–50 g in 4 ounces of water. Activated charcoal will adsorb many drugs, alcohols, and toxic compounds. There are very few contraindications to charcoal; charcoal will absorb ipecac and n-acetyl-cysteine, the antidote for acetaminophen poisoning (although in the latter it has been shown that the amount of n-acetylcysteine adsorbed is unimportant compared to the amount absorbed from the gastrointestinal tract (14)). Activated charcoal may also have a role in the management of poisoning from drugs that enter the enterohepatic circulation, such as barbiturates, digoxin, glutethimide, theophylline, and tricyclic antidepressants (15).

In certain situations such as poisoning with mercury, iron, iodine, strychnine, nicotine, and quinine, there are specific neutralizing agents that can be used instead of activated charcoal (5). Although cathartics are usually used in poisoning, there is no direct evidence of benefit, except for intestinal lavage with an osmotic agent in paraquat poisoning (16).

Very few antidotes are available for the treatment of drug poisoning. The following is a partial listing, the drug being followed in parentheses by its antidote: acetaminophen (n-acetyl-cysteine); cyanide (amyl nitrite, sodium nitrite); methanol and ethylene glycol (ethanol); iron, lead, mercury, gold, arsenic (chelating agents such as deferoxamine, calcium disodium versenate, and British anti-Lewisite [BAL or dimercaprol]); opiates, propoxyphene, and Lomotil (naloxone); organophosphates (atropine, pralidoxime); and atropine (physostigmine) (17).

Supportive therapy is the time-tested and proven therapeutic intervention for poisoning. This entails intensive care and a multidisciplinary approach to the management of respiration, circulation, and other vital functions. Only when intensive supportive care fails and the patient is deteriorating should recourse be made to other techniques such as dialysis or hemoperfusion. It must be remembered that certain poisons such as iron, acetaminophen, paraquat, amanita phalloides, carbon tetrachloride, mercury, and tricyclic antidepressants produce delayed effects and require prolonged periods of observation.

ACTIVE DRUG ELIMINATION TECHNIQUES

Forced diuresis

Most drugs are weak acids or bases that exist in the nonionized or ionized form. The nonionized molecules are lipid soluble and diffuse across cell membranes by nonionic diffusion. In contrast, the ionized form is unable to penetrate lipid membranes. In the kidney, drug excretion involves three main processes: glomerular filtration, where weakly protein-bound substances are ultrafiltered; tubular secretion at the proximal convoluted tubule with transport systems for acidic or basic drugs; and passive tubular reabsorption. The latter involves bidirectional movements of drugs across tubular epithelium, and a concentration gradient is created for reabsorption of the soluble drug back into the blood, limited to lipid-soluble drugs in the nonionized form. Increasing the pH of the tubular fluid increases the degree of ionization of weak acids and reduces tubular reabsorption. The reverse applies to weak bases. The dissociation of a weak acid or base is determined by both its dissociation constant (pKa) and the pH gradient across the tubular membrane. Elimination of weak acids by the kidney is increased in alkaline urine if the pKa of the drug lies between 3.0 and

7.5. For weak bases elimination is increased if the pKa of the drug is 7.5–10.5.

Drugs amenable to forced diuresis must be predominantly eliminated in the unchanged form via the kidney, be weak electrolytes with a pKa in the appropriate acidic or basic pKa range, and be distributed, with minimal protein binding, in the extracellular fluid compartment. Forced diuresis involves the administration of fluid in large quantities, alkaline and acidic agent, and mandates vigilance on urine pH (hourly) and plasma pH and electrolytes (every 1–2 hours). Changes in blood pH shifts potassium into and out of cells, requiring monitoring and replacement of potassium during the diuresis. Since urine flow rates should be accurately assessed, a catheter is placed in the bladder and, when appropriate, a Swan-Ganz line should be used to assess the fluid balance.

Alkaline diuresis is attained by using 1 l of 5% dextrose containing 25 mEq of bicarbonate and 75% mEq of sodium (18). Appropriate levels of potassium are given along with mannitol or furosemide every 1–2 hours until a urine flow of 300–500 ml/hr is reached. Alkaline diuresis is suitable for phenobarbital poisoning when the plasma level exceeds 10 mg/dl, barbital poisoning when the plasma level exceeds 10 mg/dl, salicylate poisoning when the plasma levels exceed 50 mg/dl, and also for 2, 4-dichlorophenoxyacetic acid (2, 4-D) poisoning. On the other hand, acid diuresis is attained by using 5% dextrose with added arginine or lysine, or with ammonium chloride 4 g every 2 hours given by mouth or intravenously. The dose should be adjusted to maintain a urinary pH near 6.5. Plasma potassium should be measured frequently. Forced acid diuresis increases excretion of amphetamines, fenfluramine, phencyclidine, and also quinine. Ascorbic acid, 1 g every 6 hours, can also be given orally to acidify the urine. A water and chloride diuresis increases the excretion of bromides, whereas lithium excretion is not enhanced further with saline (except in volume depletion), alkaline, or acid diuresis (19).

It has been shown that alkali alone may be associated with the same quantity of salicylate removal obtained with "forced" diuresis (20), avoiding the inherent dangers of high-volume fluid administration. In the latter study (20), however, the degree of salicylate poisoning was moderate (serum salicylate, 40 mg/dl) and the effect of alkali alone in more serious poisoning is unknown.

Dialysis techniques

In 1854 Graham predicted that "dialysis," would be used in the treatment of medical conditions (21). However, it was not until 1913 that Abel, Rowntree, and Turner (22) constructed the first hemodialyzer and demonstrated that salicylate could be removed. In 1951 Doolan et al. (23) demonstrated in a patient that aspirin was more rapidly removed with hemodialysis than occurred spontaneously, and in 1955 Schreiner et al. (24) reported the first successful use of hemodialysis in a patient intoxicated with aspirin.

Peritoneal dialysis and hemodialysis have now been used many times in the management of poisons (25–35). It has been appreciated that peritoneal dialysis is the least effective method for removing drugs compared with hemodialysis and hemoperfusion, in view of the slow mass transfer of drugs [for example, the maximal urea (60 daltons) clearance in humans is approximately 30 ml/min, and most drugs are much less rapidly removed than is urea]. It has, however, been shown that certain drugs that increase vascular permeability may increase peritoneal clearances of various solutes (36), but this has not yet been used extensively in the treatment of poisoning. Peritoneal dialysis has a particular role in the management of hypothermia complicating drug overdose (37).

Water-soluble drugs are more readily removed with hemodialysis, while lipid-soluble drugs are more readily removed with hemoperfusion. *Dialysance* or *clearance* describes removal of drugs similar to removal of uremic solutes. Clearance of drugs equals blood flow rate multiplied by A-V/A, where A is the arterial (or inlet) concentration, and V is the venous (or outlet) concentration of the drug. The A-V/A is equivalent to the extraction ratio across the dialyzer.

Not only are the volume of distribution, the lipid/water solubility, and the tissue binding of drugs relevant, but also the intercompartmental transfer rate of drugs from tissue into the plasma is important in the removal of drugs with devices (38). The intercompartmental transfer rate of drugs is largely unknown, except for a few specific drugs such as digoxin (39, 40). Plasma protein binding is also an important factor. Drugs such as salicylates, which in poisoning have very high ultrafilterable fractions, are ideal dialyzable drugs. Although lipid-soluble drugs were in the past removed with soybean oil hemodialysis at rates greater than with aqueous hemodialysis, this technique was abandoned when modern high-surface-area dialyzers were introduced and shown to be of equivalent or greater efficiency than "lipid dialysis." It has also been shown that hemofiltration (which utilizes more porous membranes than standard hemodialysis membranes) allows the transfer of larger molecules, up to approximately 1500 daltons, and has been suggested for removal of certain poisons (41).

A list of drugs and chemicals removed with various dialysis techniques is shown in Table 2. Many of the reports of clinical benefit from drug removal in humans are anecdotal, and the choice of dialysis for removal of a particular drug should take this into account. Information for agents not enclosed in brackets is indicative of efficient removal.

Sorbent hemoperfusion

The process of hemoperfusion (the passage of blood over sorbent particles) was introduced by Muirhead and Reid in 1948 for the removal of uremic toxins (42). In 1958 Schreiner (25) employed a lactated anion exchange resin column for the removal of pentobarbital in a uremic patient. While pentobarbital removal was achieved, the study was complicated by pyrogenic reactions, electrolyte

Table 2. Drugs and chemicals removed with dialysis

Barbiturates	Antimicrobials/anticancer	Cardiovascular
amobarbital	amikacin	acebutolol
aprobarbital	dibekacin	atenolol
barbital	fosfomycin	bretylium
butabarbital	gentamicin	captopril
cyclobarbital	kanamycin	(diazoxide)
pentobarbital	neomycin	(digoxin)
	netilmicin	(lidocaine)
phenobarbital	sisomicin	metoprolol
quinalbital	streptomycin	methyldopa
(secobarbital)	tobramycin	(ouabain)
	(vancomycin)	n-acetylprocainamide
		nadolol
Nonbarbiturate hypnotics, sedatives, tranquilizers, anticonvulsants	bacitracin	propranolol
	colistin	practolol
		procainamide
	ampicillin	(quinidine)
	amoxicillin	sotalol
carbamazepine	azlocillin	tocainide
carbromal	carbenicillin	
chloral hydrate	clavulinic acid	
(chlordiazepoxide)	(cloxacillin)	
(diazepam)	(floxacillin)	**Metals, inorganics**
(diphenylhydantoin)	mecillinam	
(diphenylhydramine)	mezlocillin	(aluminum)*
ethiamate	(nafcillin)	arsenic
ethchlorvynol	penicillin	(copper)*
ethosuximide	piperacillin	(iron)*
gallamine	temocillin	lead
glutethimide	ticarcillin	lithium
(heroin)		(magnesium)
meprobamate	(cefaclor)	(mercury)*
(methaqualone)	cefadroxil	potassium
methsuximide	cefamandole	phosphate
methyprylon	cefezolin	sodium
paraldehyde	cefixime	strontium
primidone	cefmenoxime	(tin)
valproic acid	(cefonicid)	(zinc)
	(cefoperazone)	
Antidepressants	ceforanide	bromide
	(cefotaxime)	chloride
(amitryptiline)	(cefotetan)	iodide
amphetamines	cefotiam	fluoride
(imipramine)	cefoxitin	
isocarboxazid	cefroxadine	**Miscellaneous**
MAO inhibitors	cefsulodin	
(pargyline)	ceftazidime	acipimox
(phenelzine)	(ceftriaxone)	aminophylline
tranylcypromine	cefuroxime	aniline
(tricyclics)	cephacetrile	borates
	cephalexin	boric acid
	cephaloridine	(chlorpropamide)
	cephalothin	chromic acid
	(cephapirin)	cimetidine
	cephradine	dinitro-o-cresol
		folic acid
	aztreonam	mannitol
Alcohols	cilastin	methylprednisolone
	imipinem	potassium dichromate
ethanol	moxalactam	sodium citrate
ethylene glycol		theophylline

Table 2. Drugs and chemicals removed with dialysis

Barbiturates	Antimicrobials/ anticancer	Cardiovascular
isopropanol	(chloramphenicol)	thiocyanate
methanol	ciprofloxacin	ranitidine
	(clindamycin)	
	(erythromycin)	**Solvents, gases**
	metronidazole	
Analgesics, antirheumatics	nitrofurantoin	acetone
	ornidazole	camphor
	sulfonamides	carbon monoxide
acetaminophen	tetracycline	(carbon tetrachloride)
acetophenetidin	tinidazole	(eucalyptus oil)
acetylsalicylic acid		thiols
colchicine	isoniazid	toluene
methylsalicylate	cycloserine	trichloroethylene
(d-propoxyphene)	ethambutol	
salicylic acid	5-fluorocytosine	**Plants, animals, herbicides, insecticides**
	(chloroquine)	
	quinine	
	amantadine	alkyl phosphate
	acyclovir	amanitin
		demeton sulfoxide
	(azathioprine)	dimethoate
	bredinin	diquat
	cyclophosphamide	methylmercury complex
	5-fluorouracil	(organophosphates)
	(methotrexate)	paraquat
		snake bite
		sodium chlorate
		potassium chlorate

( ) not well removed; ( )* removed with chelating agent.

disturbances, thrombocytopenia, and hemolysis. In 1964 Yatzidis (43) introduced the first usable activated charcoal device for removal of poisons and other solutes.

Yatzidis (43) demonstrated in vitro that barbital, phenobarbital, pentobarbital, salicylic acid, and glutethimide could be removed by hemoperfusion. The first clinical study in 1965 (44) demonstrated that in severe intoxication with barbiturates, three to five hemoperfusion episodes of 1 hour each were associated with clinical recovery. Largely through the work of Chang, polymer-coated charcoal devices were introduced (45). Clinical experiences with such devices (46) demonstrated safety and relief from many of the side effects of earlier devices. Nonionic resin hemoperfusion was introduced by Rosenbaum, showing that the nonionic polystyrene resin (XAD 4) was particularly useful in intoxication with lipid-soluble poisons such as glutethimide, methyprylon, and short-acting barbiturates (47). We demonstrated that coated charcoal hemoperfusion was useful in patients poisoned with various drugs and gave clearance values exceeding those with hemodialysis (48). Many reports of the successful treatment of severe poisoning with hemoperfusion has been published (49–52).

The side effects of hemoperfusion, which were of some concern with the early devices, since patients showed flushing, pyrogenic reactions, and platelet depletion, occurred especially with uncoated-charcoal-containing devices (43). Chang (45, 46) demonstrated that albumin-collodion-coated charcoal was not associated with severe platelet depletion. In general, coated charcoal has superceded all other forms of charcoal sorbent devices. A list of some drugs and chemicals that can be removed with hemoperfusion is shown in Table 3. Again, information on agents not enclosed in brackets indicates efficient removal with hemoperfusion.

Available hemoperfusion devices are described in Table 4. Hemoperfusion devices are generally cylindrical or biconcave columns containing activated charcoal particles or nonionic resin (XAD-4), through which anticoagulated blood is perfused. Heparin requirements are slightly higher than for hemodialysis and are slightly greater for resin than for charcoal hemoperfusion (approximately 6000 units for charcoal and 10,000 units for resin per hemoperfusion session). The devices are held in a vertical position to allow laminar blood flow without "channeling," and a pump is required to achieve blood flow rates of 200–300 ml/min with venovenous access.

Prolonged hemoperfusion is not usually necessary, since the prime aim of treatment is to reduce blood concentra-

Table 3. Drugs and chemicals removed with hemoperfusion

Barbiturates	Antimicrobials/anticancer	Cardiovascular
amobarbital	(adriamycin)	digoxin
butabarbital	ampicillin	(disopyramide)
hexabarbital	carmustine	n-acetylprocainamide
pentobarbital	chloramphenicol	procainamide
phenobarbital	chloroquine	quinidine
quinalbital	clindamycin	
secobarbital	dapsone	
thiopental	doxorubicin	**Metals, inorganics**
vinalbital	gentamicin	
	isoniazid	(aluminum)*
	(methotrexate)	(iron)*
	thiabendazole	
Nonbarbiturate hypnotics, sedatives, tranquilizers	**Antidepressants**	
	(amitryptiline)	**Miscellaneous**
	(imipramine)	
	(tricyclics)	aminophylline
carbromal		cimetidine
chloral hydrate		(fluoroacetamide)
chlorpromazine	**Plants, animals, herbicides, insecticides**	(phencyclidine)
(diazepam)		phenols
diphenhydramine		(podophyllin)
ethchlorvynol		theophylline
glutethimide	amanitin	
meprobamate	chlordane	
methaqualone	demeton sulfoxide	**Solvents, gases**
methsuximide	dimethoate	
methyprylon	diquat	carbon tetrachloride
promazine	methylparathion	ethylene oxide
promethazine	nitrostigmine	trichloroethanol
	organophosphates	
Analgesics, antirheumatic	phalloidin	
	polychlorinate biphenyls	
acetaminophen	paraquat	
acetylsalicylic acid	parathion	
colchicine		
d-propoxyphene		
methylsalicylate		
phenylbutazone		
salicylic acid		

( ) not well removed; ( )* removed with chelating agent.

tions of drug sufficiently to induce central nervous system recovery. Intermittent hemoperfusion has two major advantages: reduction in blood concentrations (often associated with saturation of devices for drug uptake when small quantities ($< 100\,g$) of charcoal are used) and reduction of the hematologic side effects of prolonged hemoperfusion (platelet loss and perhaps hemolysis). Replacement of saturated devices with fresh devices is not usually necessary in the usual clinical situation, but is another positive aspect of short intermittent hemoperfusion. Any rebound in plasma drug concentrations due to release from tissue can be advantageously reduced with further hemoperfusion (e.g., paraquat, glutethimide).

Hemoperfusion circuitry is similar to hemodialysis, except that no blood-warming apparatus is necessary, unless in the severely hypothermic patient. Blood access is best achieved through femoral or subclavian venous catheters or arteriovenous shunts. Blood flow is usually maintained by a pump unless an arteriovenous shunt is used.

Efficiency of dialysis or hemoperfusion for drug removal

Hemoperfusion relies on physical adsorption for its efficiency and in most cases is shown to give a higher solute clearance for drugs than occurs with hemodialysis, peritoneal dialysis, or forced diuresis. Activated charcoal tightly binds water-and lipid-soluble substances, in the molecular weight range between 113 and 40,000 daltons (at the latter level adsorption is less efficient when a polymer coating is used). Calculation of plasma or whole-blood (since red-cell drug removal has been demonstrated) extraction ratios gives an approximate guide to the efficiency of the devices for drug removal (15, 53). Table 4 shows that highly lipid-soluble drugs are more efficiently removed with the XAD-4 resin hemoperfusion than with hemodialysis. Drugs or chemicals that produce an acidosis or other metabolic complications are not generally highly lipid soluble, nor is the acidosis treatable with hemoperfusion alone (15). In this case dialysis is the preferred method of choice, particularly for methanol, ethylene glycol, and salicylates. Dialysis is also more efficient for small water-soluble drugs such as lithium and bromide (15).

In animal experiments, procedures such as hemodialysis and sorbent hemoperfusion reduce coma time and enhance elimination rates for certain drugs (53, 54). Mortality from intoxication with drugs such as barbiturates, salicylate, and paraquat has been reduced in animals, while increased drug elimination rates have been achieved with hemoperfusion in animals intoxicated with acetaminophen (54), barbital, ethchlorvynol, adriamycin (55), digoxin (38, 39), and digitoxin. In humans, however, it has not been conclusively demonstrated that a reduction in coma time or overall mortality is achieved, since controlled clinical trials have been difficult to perform (56). The severity of poisoning varies greatly depending on the geographic area (57), adding to differences of opinion on the efficacy of hemodialysis (58) or hemoperfusion (59) for poisoning. Adherence to the criteria for dialysis as iterated by Schreiner in 1958 (25) is of primary importance, since any procedure used in poisoning therapy should have a greater effect on drug elimination than occurs spontaneously. In conservatively managed barbiturate poisoning, the elimination half-life in humans ranges from 37 to 96 hours, whereas with hemodialysis the range is between 3.6 and 9.7 hours (60). In digoxin poisoning the elimination half-life in anephric patients can be substantially reduced with the addition of hemoperfusion (40).

Table 4. Hemoperfusion devices available in the US

Manufacturer	Device	Sorbent type	Amount of sorbent	Polymer coating
Chang	ACAC	Merck charcoal	300 g	Albumin-collodion
Clark	Biocompatible system	Charcoal	50, 100, 250 cc	Heparinized polymer
Gambro	Adsorba	Norit	100 or 300 g	Cellulose acetate
NMC	Hemocart	Petroleum-based charcoal	140 g	Albumin-collodion
Smith and Nephew	Hemocol or Haemocol	Sutcliffe Speakman charcoal	100 or 300 g	Hydrogel
Extracorporeal	XR-004	XAD-4 resin	350 g	None

Plasmapheresis and exchange blood transfusion

These techniques are useful for the removal of highly protein-bound substances that are not well removed with dialysis or hemoperfusion (e.g., chromic acid and chromate poisoning). Exchange blood transfusion is useful when hemolysis or methemoglobinemia complicate poisoning, e.g., sodium chlorate poisoning (61).

Criteria for hemodialysis and hemoperfusion

The criteria originally suggested by Schreiner (25) were expanded and further divided into clinical criteria and physical criteria for judging the applicability of dialysis or hemoperfusion in drug removal (15, 26–35, 53). These are given in condensed form in Tables 5 (15) and 6. In modern toxicology, mixed poisoning is common (approximately 30% of cases), and blood concentrations of a single drug may not necessarily reflect the clinical condition of the patient. Active treatment should only be used after due consideration of the severity. Intensive supportive therapy alone is associated with a reduction in mortality in barbiturate poisoning if central stimulants are avoided. Hemodialysis and hemoperfusion should be considered only if the severity of poisoning merits their use. Consideration might also be paid to cost reductions brought about by hemoperfusion, since rapid awakening from coma with barbiturates or nonbarbiturate hypnotics is likely to reduce hospitalization costs.

Table 5. Plasma drug extraction ratios with different devices*

Drug	Hemodialysis	Hemoperfusion Charcoal	Resin
Acetylsalicylic acid	0.5	0.5	—
Digoxin	0.2	0.3–0.6	0.4
Ethchlorvynol	0.2	0.7	1.0
Glutethimide	0.2	0.65	0.8
Paraquat	0.5	0.6	—
Theophylline	0.5	0.7	0.75

* Calculated for blood flow rate of 200 ml/min.

Table 6. Clinical and serum concentration criteria for dialysis or hemoperfusion in poisoning

Clinical
1. Progressive deterioration despite intensive care
2. Severe intoxication with midbrain dysfunction
3. Development of complications of coma
4. Impairment of normal drug excretory function
5. Intoxication with agents producing metabolic and/or delayed effects
6. Intoxication with an extractable drug that can be removed at a greater rate than endogenous elimination

Selected serum concentrations*

Drug	Serum conc (mg/dl)	Method of choice
Phenobarbital	10	HP > HD
Other barbiturates	5	HP
Glutethimide	4	HP
Methaqualone	4	HP
Salicylates	80	HD
Theophylline	40	HP > HD

* Suggested concentrations only, since clinical condition may warrant intervention at lower concentrations especially in mixed intoxications.
HP = hemoperfusion; HD = hemodialysis.

FUTURE TRENDS IN THERAPY OF POISONING

Fab fragments of antibodies contain binding sites for antibodies and have a molecular weight around 50,000 daltons. Using drug-hapten compounds, antibodies are generated and subjected to papain digestion, to yield Fac and Fab fragments. The latter, when injected combine with specific drug antigens with a high degree of specificity and thereby neutralize drug toxicity. Potentially fatal cases of digoxin poisoning have been treated successfully by this means (62, 63). In the future, drugs with a high toxicity ratio and poor removal with hemodialysis or hemoperfusion (e.g., tricyclic antidepressants) or drugs with delayed effects (e.g., paraquat) may be treated by such methods (64).

Recently administration of anticancer drugs into the carotid artery for unilateral cerebral tumors, with removal of the drugs from the systemic circulation by regional hemoperfusion, has been associated with successful tumor shrinkage and lower systemic toxicity (65).

POISON REMOVAL IN THE HEMODIALYSIS PATIENT

Since renal function is the primary determinant of the excretion of water-soluble drugs, renal insufficiency or failure is associated with a high prevalence of drug side effects. Dialysis or hemoperfusion may be useful where an excessive dosage of drugs is administered, such as antibiotics aminoglycosides, chloramphenicol, digitalis glycosides, and possibly in the distribution phase after anticancer drug administration. Digoxin intoxication is commonly encountered and may require a judgement as to whether to use hemoperfusion or immunopharmacology in dialysis patients. In addition, drug dosage adjustments are required for drugs that are removed with hemodialysis (e.g., antibiotics, etc.).

In cases of aluminum overload syndromes associated with refractory bone disease (osteomalacia) or dialysis dementia deferroxamine in conjunction with dialysis [continuous ambulatory peritoneal dialysis (66), hemodialysis (67)], or hemoperfusion (68, 69) is used for the removal of the deferroxamine-aluminum complex. Clinical improvement in the osteomalacic component of renal osteodystrophy (67, 70) and in encephalopathy (71) have been reported.

Iron overload in chronic dialysis patients, particularly if they possess the hemachromatosis alleles (HLA A_3, B_7, B_{14}) (72) is also fairly common. Dialysis (68, 74), hemofiltration (75), or hemoperfusion (68, 69), also in conjunction with deferroxamine, may be useful in these iron overload syndromes as well, since in hemoglobinopathy subjects the long-term iron deposition responsible for cardiomyopathy, diabetes, and other complications may improve with chelation treatment (76, 77).

REFERENCES

1. National Center for Health Statistics: DHEW, Public Health Service (HRA), 1977.
2. Jones DIR: Self poisoning with drugs: The last 20 years in Sheffield. *Br Med J* 1:28–20, 1977.
3. Litovitz T, Veltri J: 1984 Annual report of the American Association of Poison Control Centers. *Am J Emergency Med* 3:423, 1985.
4. Clemmesen C, Nilsson E: Therapeutic trends in the treatment of barbiturate poisoning: The Scandinavian method. *Clin Pharmacol Ther* 2:220–229, 1961.
5. Haddad LM: A general approach to the emergency management of poisoning. In: LM Haddad, JF Winchester, eds, *Clinical Management of Poisoning and Drug Overdose*. WB Saunders, Philadelphia, pp 4–17, 1983.
6. Haddad LM: A general approach to poisoning. In: JF Winchester, ed, *Office Procedures: Office Management of Poisoning*. Hanley and Belfus, Philadelphia, pp 325–342, 1986.
7. Proudfoot AT: Salicylates and salicylamides. In: LM Haddad, JF Winchester, eds, *Clinical Management of Poisoning and Drug Overdose*. WB Saunders, Philadelphia, pp 575–586, 1983.
8. Winters RW, White JS, Hughes MC, Ordway NC: Disturbances of acid-base equilibrium in salicylate intoxication. *Pediatrics* 23:260, 1959.
9. Gabow PA, Anderson RJ, Potts DE, Schrier RW: Acid-base disturbances in the salicylate-intoxicated adult. *Arch Intern Med* 138:1481, 1978.
10. Anderson RJ, Potts DE, Gabow PA, Rumack BH, Schrier RW: Unrecognized adult salicylate intoxication. *Ann Intern Med* 85:745, 1976.
11. Winchester JF: Methanol, isopropyl alcohol, higher alcohols, ethylene glycol, cellosolves, acetone and oxalate. In: LM Haddad, JF Winchester, eds, *Clinical Management of Poisoning and Drug Overdose*. WB Saunders, Philadelphia, pp 393–409, 1983.
12. Seyffart G: Meprobamate and related drugs. In: LM Haddad, JF Winchester, eds, *Clinical Management of Poisoning and Drug Overdose*. WB Saunders, Philadelphia, pp 520–526, 1983.
13. Schwartz HS: Acute meprobamate poisoning with gastrostomy and removal of a drug containing mass. *N Engl J Med* 295:1177, 1976.
14. Renzi FP, Donovan JW, Martin TG, Morgan L, Harrison EF: Concomitant use of activated charcoal and n-acetyl cysteine. *Ann Emerg Med* 14:568–572, 1985.
15. Winchester JF: Active methods for detoxification: Oral sorbents, forced diuresis, hemoperfusion, and hemodialysis. In: LM Haddad, JF Winchester, eds, *Clinical Management of Poisoning and Drug Overdose*. WB Saunders, Philadelphia, pp 154–169, 1983.
16. Okonek S, Hofman A, Hennigsen B: Efficacy of gut lavage, haemodialysis, and haemoperfusion in the therapy of paraquat and diquat intoxication. *Arch Toxicol* 36:43, 1974.
17. Shepherd SM, Litovitz TL: Antidotes. In: JF Winchester, ed, *Office Procedures: Office Management of Poisoning*. Hanley and Belfus, Philadelphia, pp 425–440, 1986.
18. Prowse K, Pain M, Marston AD, Cummings G: The treatment of salicylate poisoning using mannitol and forced alkaline diuresis. *Clin Sci* 38:327, 1970.
19. Winchester JF: Lithium. In: LM Haddad, JF Winchester, eds, *Clinical Management of Poisoning and Drug Overdose*. WB Saunders, Philadelphia, pp 372–379, 1983.
20. Prescott LF, Balali-Mood M, Critchley JA, Johnstone AF, Proudfoot AT: Diuresis or urinary alkalinization in salicylate poisoning? *Br Med J* 285:1383–1386, 1982.
21. Graham T: Bakerian lecture on osmotic force. *Philos Trans R Soc London*, p 177, 1854.
22. Abel JJ, Rowntree LG, Turner BB: On the removal of diffusible substances from the circulating blood of living animals by dialysis. *Clin Pharmacol ther* 5:275–316, 1913.
23. Doolan PD, Walsh WP, Kyle LH, Wishinsky H: Acetylsalicylic acid intoxication: A proposed method of treatment. *JAMA* 146:105–106, 1951.

24. Schreiner GE, Berman LB, Griffin J, Feys J: Specific therapy for salicylism. *N Engl J Med* 253:213–217, 1955.
25. Schreiner GE: The role of hemodialysis (artificial kidney) in acute poisoning. *Arch Intern Med* 102:896–913, 1958.
26. Maher JF, Schreiner GE: Editorial review: The dialysis of poisons. *Trans Am Soc Artif Intern Organs* 9:385–394, 1963.
27. Maher JF, Schreiner GE: Editorial review: The clinical dialysis of poisons. *Trans Am Soc Artif Intern Organs* 11:349–365, 1965.
28. Maher JF, Schreiner GE: The dialysis of poisons and drugs. *Trans Am Soc Artif Intern Organs* 13:369–393, 1967.
29. Maher JF, Schreiner GE: The dialysis of poisons and drugs. *Trans Am Soc Artif Intern Organs* 14:440–453, 1968.
30. Maher JF, Schreiner GE: Current status of dialysis of poisons and drugs. *Trans Am Soc Artif Intern Organs* 15:461–477, 1969.
31. Schreiner GE: Dialysis of poisons and drugs — annual review. *Trans Am Soc Artif Intern Organs* 16:544–568, 1970.
32. Schreiner GE, Teehan BP: Dialysis of poisons and drugs — annual review. *Trans Am Soc Artif Intern Organs* 17:513–544, 1971.
33. Schreiner GE, Teehan BP: Dialysis of poisons and drugs — annual review. *Trans Am Soc Artif Intern Organs* 18:563–599, 1972.
34. Knepshield JH, Schreiner Ge, Lowenthal DT, Gelfand MC: Dialysis of poisons and drugs — annual review. *Trans Am Soc Artif Intern Organs* 19:590–631, 1973.
35. Winchester JF, Gelfand MC, Knepshield JH, Schreiner GE: Dialysis and hemoperfusion of poisons and drugs — update. *Trans Am Soc Artif Intern Organs* 23:762–842, 1972.
36. Maher JF, Hirszel, P, Galen MA, Chamberlin M, Hohnadel DC: Enhanced peritoneal transport with dipyridamole. *Trans Am Soc Artif Intern Organs* 23:219–223, 1977.
37. Reuler JB, Parker RA: Peritoneal dialysis in the management of hypothermia. *JAMA* 240:2289, 1978.
38. Gibson TP, Atkinson AJ: Effect of changes in intercompartmental rate constants on drug removal during hemoperfusion. *J Pharm Sci* 67:1178–1179, 1978.
39. Gibson TP, Lucas SV, Nelson HA, Atkinson AJ, Okita GT, Ivanovich P: Hemoperfusion removal of digoxin from dogs. *J Lab Clin Med* 91:673–682, 1978.
40. Hoy WE, Gibson TP, Rivero AJ, Jain JK, Talley TT, Bayer RM, Montondo DF, Freeman RB: XAD-4 resin hemoperfusion for digitoxic patients with renal failure. *Kidney Int* 23:79–82, 1983.
41. Fairshter RD, Rosen SM, Smith WR, Glauser FL, McRae DM, Wilson AF: Paraquat poisoning. New aspects of therapy. *Q J Med* 45:180, 1976.
42. Muirhead EE, Reid AF: Resin artificial kidney. *J Lab Clin Med* 33:841–844, 1948.
43. Yatzidis H: A convenient haemoperfusion micro-apparatus over charcoal for the treatment of endogenous and exogenous intoxications. Its use as an artificial kidney. *Proc Eur Dial Transplant Assoc* 1:83–86, 1964.
44. Yatzidis H, Voudiclari S, Oreopoulos D, Tsaparas D, Triantaphyllidis D, Gavras C, Stavroulaki A: Treatment of severe barbiturate poisoning. *Lancet* 2:216–217, 1965.
45. Chang TMS: *Artificial Cells*. CC Thomas, Springfield, IL, 1972.
46. Chang TMS, Coffey JF, Lister C, Taroy E, Stark A: Methaqualone and glutethimide clearance by the ACAC microcapsule artificial kidney: In vitro and in patients with acute intoxication. *Trans Am Soc Artif Intern Organs* 19:87–91, 1973.
47. Rosenbaum JL, Winsten S, Kramer MS, Moros J, Raja R: Resin hemoperfusion in the treatment of drug intoxication. *Trans Am Soc Artif Intern Organs* 16:134–140, 1970.
48. Gelfand MC, Winchester JF, Knepshield JH, Hanson KM, Cohan SL, Strauch BS, Geoly KL, Kennedy AC, Schreiner GE: Charcoal hemoperfusion in the treatment of severe drug overdosage. *Trans Am Soc Artif Intern Organs* 23:599–604, 1977.
49. Ehlers SM, Zaske DE, Sawchuk RJ: Massive theophylline overdose. Rapid elimination by charcoal hemoperfusion. *JAMA* 240:474, 1978.
50. Trafford JAP, Jones RH, Evans R, Sharp P, Sharpstone P, Cook J: Haemoperfusion with R-004 amberlite resin for treating acute poisoning. *Br Med J* 2:1453, 1977.
51. Rosenbaum JL, Kramer MS, Raja R: Resin hemoperfusion for acute drug intoxication. *Arch Intern Med* 136:263, 1976.
52. Vale JA, Rees AJ, Widdop B, Goulding R: Use of charcoal haemoperfusion in the management of severely poisoned patients. *Br Med J* 1:5–9, 1975.
53. Winchester JF, Gelfand MC, Tilstone WJ: Hemoperfusion in drug intoxication: Clinical and laboratory aspects. *Drug Metab Rev* 8:69–104, 1978.
54. Winchester JF, Tilstone WJ, Edwards RO, Gilchrist T, Kennedy AC: Hemoperfusion for enhanced drug elimination — a kinetic analysis in paracetamol poisoning. *Trans Am Soc Artif Intern Organs* 20:358–363, 1974.
55. Winchester JF, Rhaman A, Tilstone WJ, Kessler A, Mortensen L, Schreiner GE, Schein PS: Sorbent removal of adriamycin in vitro and in vivo. *Cancer Treat Rep* 63:1787–1793, 1979.
56. Uldall PR: Controlled trial of resin hemoperfusion for the treatment of drug overdose at Toronto Western Hospital (TWH). *Trans Am Soc Artif Intern Organs* 28:676–677, 1982.
57. Maher JF: In discussion on hemoperfusion for poisoning — Is it really necessary? In: GE Schreiner, JF Winchester, eds, *Controversies in Nephrology*, Vol 2. Georgetown Nephrology Press, Washington DC, p 228, 1980.
58. Chazan JA, Garella S: Glutethimide intoxication: A prospective study of 70 patients treated conservatively without hemodialysis. *Arch Intern Med* 128:215, 1971.
59. Lorch JA, Garella S: Hemoperfusion to treat intoxications. *Ann Intern Med* 91:301, 1979.
60. Hadden J, Johnson K, Smith S, Price L, Giardana E: Acute barbiturate intoxication: Concepts in management. *JAMA* 209:893–901, 1969.
61. Seyffart G: Plasmapheresis in treatment of acute intoxication. *Trans Am Soc Artif Intern Organs* 28:673–676, 1982.
62. Marbury T, Mahoney J, Juncos L, Conti R, Cade R: Advanced digoxin toxicity in renal failure — Treatment with charcoal hemoperfusion. *South Med J* 72:279, 1979.
63. Tobin M, Cerra F, Steinvach J, Mookerjee B: hemoperfusion in digitalis intoxication: A comparative study of coated versus uncoated charcoal. *Trans Am Soc Artif Intern Organs* 23:730, 1977.
64. Colburn WA: Specific antibodies and Fab fragments to alter the pharmacokinetics and reverse the pharmacologic/toxicologic effects of drugs. *Drug Metab Rev* 11:233, 1980.
65. Oldfield EH, Dedrick RL, Yeager RL, Clark WC, DeVroom HL, Chatterji DC, Doppman JL: Reducd systemic drug exposure by continuous intrarterial chemotherapy with hemoperfusion of regional venous drainage. *J Neurosurg* 163:726–732, 1985.
66. Schwartz RD: Deferoxamine and aluminum removal. *Am J Kid Dis* 6:358–364, 1985.
67. Brown DJ, Dawborn JK, Ham KN, Xipell JM: Treatment of dialysis osteomalacia with desferrioxamine. *Lancet* 2:343–

347, 1982.
68. Chang TMS, Barre P: Effect of desferrioxamine on removal of aluminium and iron by coated charcoal haemoperfusion and haemodialysis. *Lancet* 2:1051–1054, 1983.
69. Hakim RM, Schulman JM, Lazarus JM: Hemoperfusion in the treatment of aluminum (Al) and iron (Fe) induced bone disease. *Abstr Am Soc Nephrol* 18:65a, 1985.
70. Andress DL, Maloney NA, Endres DB, Sherrard DJ: Aluminum-associated bone disease in chronic renal failure: High prevalence in a long term dialysis population. *J Bone Miner Res* 1:391–398, 1986.
71. Arieff AI: Aluminum and the pathogenesis of dialysis encephalopathy. *Am J Kid Dis* 6:317–321, 1985.
72. Bregman H, Gelfand MC, Winchester JF, Manz HJ, Knepshield JH, Schreiner GE: Iron overload-associated myopathy in patients on maintenance haemodialysis. A histocompatibility linked disorder. *Lancet* 2:882–885, 1980.
73. Winchester JF: Management of iron overload. *Seminars Nephrol* 4 (Suppl 1):22–26, 1986.
74. Falk RJ, Mattern WD, Lamanna RW, et al.: Iron removal during continuous ambulatory peritoneal dialysis using deferoxamine. *Kidney Int* 24:110–112, 1983.
75. McCarthy JT, Libertin CR, Mitchell JC III, et al.: Hemosiderosis in a dialysis patient. Treatment with hemofiltration and deferoxamine chelation therapy. *Mayo Clin Proc* 57:439–441, 1982.
76. Marcus RE, Davies SC, Bantock HM, et al.: Desferrioxamine to improve cardiac function in iron overloaded patients with thalassemia major. *Lancet* 1:392–393, 1984.
77. Wolfe L, Olivieri N, Sallan D, et al.: Prevention of cardiac disease by subcutaneous deferoxamine in patients with thalassemia major. *N Engl J Med* 312:1600–1603, 1985.

CHAPTER 41

Prevention of Progression of Renal Insufficiency

GIUSEPPE MASCHIO, LAMBERTO OLDRIZZI & CARLO RUGIU

DIETARY INTERVENTION

The optimum dietary composition for patients with chronic renal failure

Many factors that may explain the progressive nature of chronic renal disease have been so far identified or suggested. They include *hemodynamic adaptations* (increased glomerular pressures and flows), *metabolic abnormalities* (deposition of calcium and phosphate salts in renal parenchyma, deposition of urate salts in renal interstitium, and perhaps abnormalities of lipid and prostaglandin metabolism), *immunologic alterations* (immune response against renal antigens), and *coagulative disorders* (thrombosis of glomerular capillaries) (1).

In humans, nutritional and therapeutic maneuvers have been mainly directed at limiting the potentially harmful effects of elevated glomerular capillary pressures and flows and at preventing severe abnormalities of phosphate and parathyroid hormone metabolism early in the course of chronic renal disease. Dietary protein and phosphate restriction, for example, has been shown to slow the progression of chronic renal failure (CRF) in patients with a variety of chronic renal disease and to prevent, or even reverse, hyperphosphatemia and secondary hyperparathyroidism (2).

Two distinct clinical approaches using low-protein diets have been developed. In patients with advanced renal failure the administration of very low-nitrogen, low-phosphate diets — supplemented with essential amino acids or ketoanalogues — has been effective in delaying the end-stage phase of the disease and in postponing dialysis for a limited time (3).

In patients with early renal failure, based on the assumption that the degree of functional deterioration is critical in mediating the effects of dietary intervention, since 1972 we have been following a large number of patients in whom dietary protein and phosphate restriction was prescribed early in the course of their renal failure.

Basically, our diet contains about 40 kcal/kg, 0.6 g/kg of protein (mostly of high biologic value) and 700 mg of phosphate; 1000–1500 mg/day of calcium are given as a supplement. This diet overcomes the major causes of noncompliance, such as the absence of milk and meat, the small quantities of vegetables and fruit ingested, and the difficulty in preparing high-calorie, low-protein diets (the only non-natural food is the low-protein biscuit) (Table 1).

In 1980 we reported the results of a retrospective study in two groups of patients treated with dietary protein and phosphorus restriction. In group 1, the serum creatinine concentration increased from a mean value of 3.10 to 6.35 mg/100 ml over 4 years. In group 2, consisting of 20 patients with early renal failure, there was practically no change in the serum creatinine over 18 months (4).

In 1981 Giordano (5) reported two groups of patients with early renal failure whose survival time with dialysis treatment was very different, and he attributed this to a low-protein, low-phosphorus diet; the survival was 91.2 months in patients adhering to the diet, but only 16 months in those eating a free diet.

In the same year we reported (6) the changes in serum creatinine and glomerular filtration rate (GFR), evaluated by means of the renal clearance of iothalamate, of 20 patients with early renal failure. After 2 years of the low-protein diet, their serum creatinine had increased from 2.25 to 2.63 mg/100 ml, and their GFR had decreased from 40.06 to 32.56 ml/min.

In 1982 we presented (2) the results obtained in three groups of patients whose initial serum creatinine levels differed. Group 1 consisted of 25 patients with a mean serum creatinine of 2.18 mg/100 ml and group 2 of 20 patients with a mean serum creatinine of 4.24 mg/100 ml. All these patients were treated by restricting their dietary protein and phosphorus intake for 18–76 months. The 30 patients in group 3 had a mean serum creatinine of 2.28 mg/100 ml but followed no specific dietary regimen for 3–72 months. For most of the patients, a plot of the reciprocal creatinine against time gave a straight regression line, so that the data on changes in the reciprocal serum creatinine were analyzed by linear regression. We obtained slopes of -0.0008 and -0.0010 dl/mg/month in groups 1 and 2, and a slope of 0.020 dl/mg/month in the group 3 patients. The slopes for both the group 1 and group 2 patients were statistically different (analysis of variance and F test, $p < 0.01$) from that of group 3. Similar results were also obtained by other groups (7–9).

Table 1. Protein-restricted diet for patients with early renal failure

Milk (low cream)	200 ml	Calories	2600
Rice or pasta	70 g	Protein	40 g (cal 160)
Meat* or	100 g	Carbohydrate	270 g (cal 1080)
fish or	70 g	Lipid	120 g (cal 1080)
cheese	40 g		
Bread		Phosphate	670 mg
Marmalade	5 g	Calcium	710 mg
Biscuits (low protein)	100 g	Sodium	568 mg
Vegetables	300 g	Potassium	670 mg
Fruit	400 g		
Oil	80 g		
Butter	20 g		
Sugar	40 g		
Wine	250 ml		

* As alternative foods (40 g of cheese = 50 g of meat).

The effects of dietary protein and phosphorus restriction were also analyzed in patients who started the diet at a later stage of renal failure, when their serum creatinine averaged 6 mg/100 ml. The average rate of decrease in the reciprocal creatinine was significantly lower in patients treated at an earlier stage than in those treated after the serum creatinine reached 6 mg/100 ml. We have concluded, therefore, that dietary protein restriction is especially effective for patients with early renal failure (2).

In 1985 we reported (10) the clinical results obtained in 349 patients with early CRF of diverse etiology. The average followup was 35.4 months (6–156 months). At the end of followup, 213 patients (61%) presented stability of renal function (arbitrarily defined as no change in initial serum creatinine or an increase in serum creatinine ≤ 0.01 mg/dl/month), whereas 136 patients (39%) had progressive deterioration of renal function (defined as an increase in serum creatinine > 0.01 mg/dl/month). The two groups did not differ significantly as far as age, frequency of hypertension, known duration of hypertension, and serum calcium values on entry are concerned, whereas serum phosphate levels were significantly higher in patients with declining, than in those with stable, renal function (Table 2).

These data show that when a moderate dietary protein and phosphate restriction is started in the early phases of CRF, the progression of functional deterioration can be reduced or even halted for substantial periods of time in the large majority of patients. In addition, we have

Table 2. Clinical and biochemical data in 349 patients on protein-restricted diet (followup: 6–156 months, mean 35, 4)

	Stability of renal function	Deterioration of renal function
No. of patients	213 (61%)	136 (39%)
Age (years)	50 ± 4	47 ± 20
"Entry" serum creatinine	2.2 ± 1.2[2]	2.9 ± 1.4 mg/dl
"Entry" serum phosphate	3.2 ± 0.7[2]	3.7 ± 0.9 mg/dl
"Entry" serum calcium	9.3 ± 0.7	9.1 ± 0.6 mg/dl
DBP > 100 mmHg[1]	62%	61%
Known duration of hypertension (months)	49 ± 65	59 ± 63

[1] DBP = diastolic blood pressure.
[2] Significantly different ($p < 0.001$) from patients with stable renal funtion.

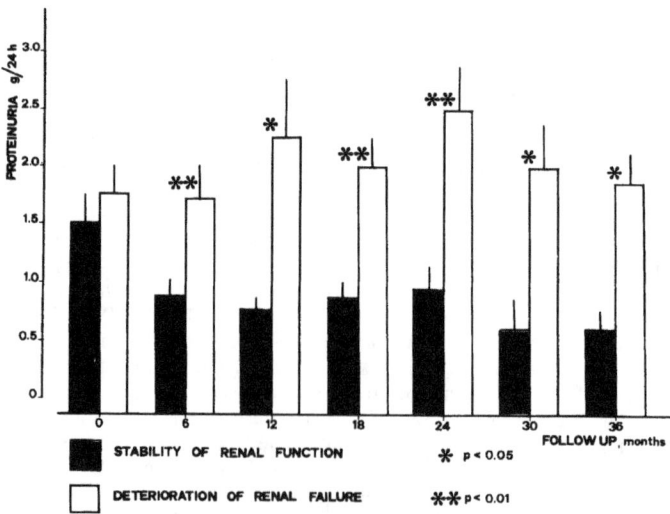

Figure 1. Changes in proteinuria (g/24 hr) during followup in two subgroups of patients on long-term dietary protein restriction with either stability (gray columns) or progressive deterioration (white columns) of renal function. Values are expressed as mean ± SD.

obtained evidence to support the assumption that dietary protein restriction is especially effective when prescribed at the early stages of CRF. Yet, proteinuria is generally believed to be an important negative factor in accelerating the progression of CRF, and a diet-induced decrease in proteinuria indicates an improved prognosis in patients with chronic glomerulonephritis, and even in those with nephrotic syndrome and early renal failure. In our patients, the two subgroups with either stability or deterioration of renal function had comparable levels of proteinuria on entry. During a 3-year followup, the subgroups of patients who started an earlier treatment (serum creatinine, 2.2 ± 1.2 mg/100 ml) had a progressive decrease in the magnitude of proteinuria and no deterioration of renal function. On the contrary, the subgroup of patients who started the diet later (serum creatinine, 2.9 ± 1.4 mg/100 ml) showed no change in proteinuria and continued loss of renal function (Figure 1).

A major point of criticism is the lack of controlled study protocols in our experience as well as in that of others. In a small number of patients we have performed a two-treatment self-controlled study to compare the progression of renal failure on two different protein and phosphate intakes. Ten patients with early CRF were studied after 18–42 months on dietary protein restriction (0.6 g/kg of protein and 700 mg of phosphate). During the study period, which was extended from 6 to 10 months, all patients were switched to a diet containing 0.9 g/kg of protein and 800 mg of phosphate. During the two study periods, changes in the serum creatinine/creatinine ratio plotted against time, GFR (iothalamate clearance), proteinuria, and mean arterial pressure were recorded. As shown in Table 3, progression of renal failure was significantly accelerated by the "normal protein diet" as compared to baseline values. In the meantime, urine protein excretion rose significantly during the normal protein diet.

Although limited, this study (11) demonstrates that dietary protein and phosphate intakes exceeding 0.6 g/kg and 700 mg/day, respectively, are harmful to renal function in patients with early-to-moderate CRF.

Factors affecting progression in patients on dietary protein restriction

Important differences in the progression of renal failure may be observed when patients are divided according to their *basic renal disease* (12). We evaluated the course of CRF in five groups of patients. Ninety-five patients (59 males and 36 females, mean age 48 ± 14 years) had CRF of unknown etiology (UE). Twenty-eight patients had proteinuria ranging from 1.5 to 3.0 g/24 hr, and 67 had minimal or no proteinuria. The mean initial serum creatinine values were 2.57 ± 1.50 mg/100 ml. The mean arterial pressure was 108 mmHg (63% of the patients had diastolic blood pressure ≥ 100 mmHg). Ninety-two patients (64 males and 28 females, mean age 41 ± 13 years) presented with chronic glomerulonephritis (CG), proven with biopsy in most of them. Twenty-five patients had clinical and biochemical evidence of nephrotic syndrome with proteinuria > 3.5 g/24 hr; 67 patients had minimal proteinuria (< 1.5 g/24 hr). The mean initial serum creatinine values were 2.34 ± 1.27 mg/dl. The mean arterial pressure was 110 mmHg (52% of the patients had diastolic blood pressure ≥ 100 mmHg). Eighty-six patients (52 females and 34 males, mean age 46 ± 14 years) had primary chronic pyelonephritis (PCP).

The diagnosis was made by history, clinical and radiologic data, and ultrasonography. Proteinuria ranging from 1.0 to 3.0 g/24 hr was present in 33 patients, whereas 53 patients had minimal or no proteinuria. The mean initial serum creatinine values were 2.54 ± 1.15 mg/100 ml. The mean arterial pressure was 111 mmHg (47% of the patients had diastolic blood pressure ≥ 100 mmHg). Forty patients (21 males and 19 females, mean age 46 ± 10 years) exhibited bilateral polycystic kidney disease (PKD), diagnosed by history and clinical and radiologic investigations. Proteinuria was absent or minimal (< 1 g/24 hr) in all patients. The mean initial serum creatinine values were 2.66 ± 1.42 mg/100 ml. The mean arterial pressure was 113 mmHg (70% of the patients had diastolic blood pressure ≥ 100 mmHg). Thirty-six patients (29 males and 7 females, mean age 55 ± 11 years) had hypertensive nephrosclerosis (HN), established by history and clinical and radiologic investigations. Proteinuria ranging from 1.0 to 3.5 g/24 hr was present in nine patients, whereas the remaining 27 had minimal or no proteinuria. The mean initial serum creatinine values were 2.16 ± 0.91 mg/100 ml. The mean arterial pressure was 105 mmHg (83% of the patients had diastolic blood pressure ≥ 100 mmHg).

All patients were kept on a diet containing about 40 cal/kg, 0.6 g/kg of protein, and 700 mg of phosphate. The diet for patients with the nephrotic syndrome was supplemented with an additional protein content of 0.5 g for each gram of proteinuria. Patients with high blood pressure received antihypertensive drugs (alphamethyldopa, clonidine, propranolol, and prazosin).

Deterioration of renal function was observed in 55% of

Table 3. Clinical course of patients on low- and normal-protein diets

	Low-protein diet	Normal protein diet
Monthly increase in SCr (mg/dl/mo)	−0.0062 ± 0.0084	0.0498 ± 0.024[2]
Percent increase in SCr	−13.4 ± 13.9	25.1 ± 10.4[2]
Starting GFR (ml/min)	43.6 ± 14.0	51.4 ± 14.8
Final GFR (ml/min)	45.3 ± 13.6	42.0 ± 0.15
Slope of 1/SCr (dl/mg/mo)	0.0022 ± 0.0032	−0.0193 ± 0.0138[1]
Proteinuria (g/24 hr)	0.68 ± 0.71	1.34 ± 0.82[1]
MAP (mmHg)	114.7 ± 7.8	115.4 ± 10.8 (ns)

SCr = serum creatinine; MAP = mean arterial pressure; ns = not significant.
[1] $p < 0.001$; [2] $p < 0.0001$.

patients with PKD, in 47% of those with CG, in 42% with PCP, in 30% with UE, and in 20% with HN. Accordingly, the actuarial survival probability at 72 months — assuming as "renal death" a serum creatinine level of 10 mg/100 ml — was 57% in patients with CG, 59% in those with PKD, 77% in those with UE, 78% in those with PCP, and 90% in those with HN.

Regular dialysis treatment was initiated in 18.5% of patients with CG, 17.5% of those with PKD, 11.5% of those with PCP, 10.5% of those with UE, and 8% of those with HN. We believe that the persistent immunologically mediated renal damage in glomerulonephritis and the constant growth of the cysts in polycystic kidney disease are the major, but not the only, determinants of "accelerated" progression in these patient groups.

In addition to the basic renal disease, *hypertension* has long been regarded as a potential damage to the kidney. Systolic blood pressure levels on entry were significantly higher in PCP patients who eventually had declining renal function than in those with stability of renal failure, and both systolic and diastolic blood pressure levels were significantly higher in PKD patients with continued loss than in those with stability of renal function. No significant difference was observed in the remaining groups of patients. However, in a previous study (2) we have shown that progressive functional deterioration was faster in hypertensive than in normotensive patients, regardless of their basic renal disease. Hypertension probably plays an important role in worsening the prognosis of patients with renal parenchymal disease and early CRF. However, its role in human pathology is not as clearly defined as in experimental animals (13).

The magnitude of *proteinuria* has been regarded as risk factor affecting the progression of renal disease. Admittedly, proteinuria reflects, to some extent, the degree of glomerular sclerosis that follows the progressive reduction of renal parenchyma in any chronic renal disease, and, therefore, it cannot be considered as a specific index of deterioration. Indirect evidence of the importance of proteinuria is supported by its significant reduction after the restriction of dietary protein in a variety of chronic renal diseases (10).

Among patients with proteinuria, apparently the worst prognosis is borne by those with the *nephrotic syndrome* (10). In the CG patients, this subgroup had faster deterioration than those with proteinuria in the non-nephrotic range. In the first subgroup, serum creatinine rose from 2.31 ± 1.36 to 4.16 ± 3.08 mg/100 ml in 40.8 months. The difference, however, is not statistically significant. The monthly increase in serum creatinine was 0.096 mg/dl/mo in patients with the nephrotic syndrome, and 0.053 mg/dl/mo in those without the nephrotic syndrome. In addition, 60% of patients with the nephrotic syndrome, in comparison with 42% of those without the nephrotic syndrome, had continued loss of renal function during followup. It seems likely that the constellation of endocrine and metabolic abnormalities that are usually associated with the nephrotic syndrome, rather than proteinuria per se, may have adversely affected the rate of progression in these patients (14).

Finally, the *degree of functional deterioration* at which dietary treatment is prescribed may be regarded as a discriminating factor in patients with CRF (10). In our large population of patients, serum creatinine and phosphate values on entry were significantly higher in patients who eventually had declining renal function than in those with stability of renal failure, and the best results were obtained in patients who started the diet at serum creatinine levels between 1.5 and 2.0 mg/100 ml. Conversely, the highest percentage of patients having continued loss of renal function was observed when the diet was prescribed at serum creatinine levels exceeding 4.0 mg/100 ml.

Compliance with the diet and nutritional problems in patients on protein-restricted diets

The extent to which our patients followed their prescribed diet was carefully monitored by members of our staff using the following procedures every two months: a) dietary interviews with each patient and with members of the family who prepared the patient's food and written diaries at 2-month intervals from each patient; b) measurement of the serum phosphate concentration and serum urea/serum creatinine ratios; and c) measurement of the urine phosphate and urea excretions.

The serum phosphate concentration was found to reflect the dietary intake of phosphate. In fact, mean values for the serum phosphate were within normal limits, even after years of the phosphate-restricted diet. In contrast, a significant increase in serum phosphorus was observed in

Table 4. Dietary intakes and urinary excretions of phosphate in patients with chronic renal failure (CRF) and in controls

	Patients with CRF on diet (n = 90)	Patients with CRF on free diet (n = 30)	Controls (n = 41)
Dietary intake of phosphate (mg/day)	683 ± 45	900 ± 135	900 ± 230
GFR (ml/min)	28.16 ± 13.00	30.00 ± 14.00	120.00 ± 15.00
Urine phosphate (mg/24 hr)	$410 \pm 90^*$	558 ± 160	594 ± 201
Urine phosphate (mg/100 ml GFR)	$1456 \pm 360^*$	1992 ± 440	495 ± 179

* Significantly different ($p < 0.01$) from values obtained both in controls and in patients with CRF on free diet.

patients eating a free diet. The serum urea concentrations generally reflected the prescribed protein intake at all levels of renal function. The serum urea/serum creatinine ratio, an index of dietary protein intake (15), showed little change in patients on dietary treatment, regardless of their degree of renal failure. The urinary urea and phosphate excretion of 90 patients with early renal failure undergoing dietary treatment were compared to those of patients with renal failure and of normal subjects eating a self-selected diet (Table 4).

In patients with CRF treated with our regimen, the daily or fractional renal phosphate excretion was decreased nearly 30% compared to that of patients on a free diet. There was a good correlation between the dietary intake and the urinary excretion of phosphate (averaging 58% of ingested phosphate). The mean values for urinary urea excretion were 7598 ± 2361 mg/day in patients on the protein-restricted diet and $10,878 \pm 2780$ mg/day in normal subjects. Individual variation in the daily urea excretion, however, limited its usefulness as a method of evaluating compliance with the diet. These results indicate that patients with early renal failure adhere well to a diet that daily provides at least 0.6 g/kg of primarily high-biologic-value protein.

The nutritional status of our patients was assessed by anthropometric measurements, including the relative body weight, ideal body weight, midarm circumference, subscapular and triceps skinfold thickness, and body fat. The mean values of these parameters before and after 24–72 months of a protein-restricted diet were not different from those obtained in normal individuals of similar age, height, and sex. Additionally, the mean values for the total serum protein, albumin, transferrin, complement, cholesterol, and triglycerides were within normal limits in patients on long-term dietary protein restriction (from 12 to 72 months) (Table 5). Furthermore, skeletal muscle biopsies, obtained from 40 unselected patients on dietary treatment after 24–68 months, showed normal values of phosphate and alkali-soluble protein nitrogen, in spite of long-term dietary protein and phosphate restriction. The muscle potassium content was slightly subnormal.

A recent investigation by Guarnieri et al. (16) of 12 unselected patients taken from our population showed that the RNA/DNA ratio (an index of the ribosomal capacity for protein synthesis) and alkali–soluble protein nitrogen/DNA ratio (an index of the cytoplasmatic protein synthesized by each nucleus) were not different from the values obtained in 15 controls matched for age, height, and sex. Therefore, our diet does not lead to progressive protein depletion or malnutrition.

Concluding remarks

Most reported clinical studies on the effects of dietary protein restriction in CRF may be open to some criticism for being retrospective and/or uncontrolled. However, they have one thing in common: all of them show a positive effect of dietary protein restriction in CRF. Admittedly, the dietary approach is only one of the many aspects of medical therapy in patients with CRF, and there is no controlled study to show whether protein restriction is superior to the control of blood pressure, for example. On the other hand, there is considerable evidence that a high protein and phosphorus intake is harmful to renal function, and, conversely, there is no clinical evidence that moderate dietary protein and phosphorus restriction is harmful to the patient.

NONDIETARY INTERVENTION

Management of arterial hypertension

Hypertension has long been regarded as potentially dangerous to the kidney, mainly through vasoconstriction and vascular sclerosis, eventually leading to ischemic glomerular sclerosis. In recent years, however, experimental evidence has indicated that hypertension may be transmitted directly to glomeruli, thus increasing glomerular capillary pressures and flows, and hence resulting in mesangial injury and glomerulosclerosis (17). These hemodynamic effects of systemic hypertension are magnified either when the nephron mass is reduced or in the presence of an experimentally induced glomerular disease.

Several studies have been performed in animals affected with different models of glomerular diseases (nephrotoxic serum nephritis, autologous and heterologous immune complex nephritis, ferritin/antiferritin immune complex nephritis, diabetes). In all of these experimental conditions, the superimposed hypertension resulted in deterioration of biochemical and functional parameters (increased proteinuria, reduced GFR) and in worsening of the structural damage (increased mesangial proliferation and sclerosis, crescentic formation, increased basement membrane thickness, vascular sclerosis) (17).

Indirect evidence of the harmful role of hypertension is provided by the observation that renal damage can be greatly improved by antihypertensive treatment. However, some antihypertensive agents (the combination of hydralazine, reserpine, and hydrochlorothiazide or that of clonidine, dihydralazine, and furosemide) were shown to induce undesired hemodynamic changes: they effectively lowered systemic blood pressure, but maintained an

Table 5. Serum proteins and lipid components in patients with chronic renal failure (CRF) on long-term dietary protein restriction

	Controls (n = 30)	Patients with CRF (n = 95)
Total protein (g/100 ml)	6.00–8.00	7.11 ± 0.60
Albumin (g/100 ml)	3.20–5.50	4.07 ± 0.40
Transferrin (mg/100 ml)	0.25–0.42	0.31 ± 0.05
Complement (units)	100.00–120.00	108.00 ± 3.50
C_3 (mg/100 ml)	55.00–120.00	82.00 ± 9.90
Cholesterol (mg/100 ml)	150.00–270.00	194.00 ± 49.00
Triglycerides (mg/100 ml)	54.00–177.00	157.00 ± 92.00

increased intraglomerular capillary pressure, probably due to predominant afferent arteriolar dilatation. As a result, the glomerular pathology was unchanged, or even worsened, after their use (18).

On the contrary, the administration of enalapril, whose vasodilator effect is predominantly exerted on the efferent arteriole, was followed by a concomitant reduction of systemic blood pressure, glomerular hydraulic pressure, proteinuria, and glomerular pathology in animals affected with different glomerular or systemic diseases and superimposed hypertension (13).

Although most reported clinical studies suggest that significant renal failure is uncommon in patients with essential hypertension, being observed in less than 10% of these patients, hypertension is believed to adversely affect the course of renal parenchymal disease. This assumption is based on the high incidence of vascular sclerosis during the intermediate phases of several forms of glomerulonephritis in which hypertension often precedes the onset of CRF. However, high blood pressure is not invariably associated with progressive functional deterioration in chronic renal disease of diverse etiology (19, 20), in which hypertension and dietary intakes of protein and phosphate appear to be independent, but complementary, risk factors.

We have examined (21) the role of hypertension on the progression of primary renal disease in 233 patients with CRF of diverse etiology (71 with CRF of unknown etiology, 61 with CG, 51 with PCP, 26 with PKD, and 24 with HN). On entry, 174 patients (74.6%) were hypertensive, i.e., with diastolic blood pressure $\geq$ 100 mmHg, and 59 (25.4%) were normotensive.

The mean initial serum creatinine ranged from 2.12 to 2.79 mg/100 ml in the various subgroups. The average followup was 51.4 ± 26.8 months (range 12–166). All patients were kept on a protein-and phosphate-restricted diet. Patients with high blood pressure were advised to regularly take antihypertensive drugs (alphamethyldopa, clonidine, propranolol, and prazosin). At the end of the followup, once again the progression of renal failure was much faster in patients with CG or with PKD than in the remaining groups. In the overall population, deterioration of renal function was more evident in hypertensive (112.8% increase in serum creatinine; monthly increase, 0.053 mg/100 ml) than in normotensive patients (70.9% increase; monthly increase, 0.032 mg/100 ml). This difference, however, was not statistically significant. The actuarial survival probability at 72 months (assuming as "renal death" a serum creatinine level of 10 mg/100 ml) was 77% in normotensive and 47% in hypertensive patients. At the end of the followup, 149 patients from the overall population (63.9%) had stability of renal function or slow deterioration of renal failure (arbitrarily defined as no change in serum creatinine or an increase in serum creatinine of less than 0.04 mg/100 ml/mo), whereas 84 patients (36.1%) had a faster deterioration of renal function, the increase in their serum creatinine exceeding 0.04 mg/100 ml/mo. In this latter subgroup of patients with "accelerated" renal functional deterioration, 71 (84.5%) were hypertensive and only 13 (15.5%) were normotensive (Table 6).

This study was performed on a larger population and supports our preliminary data showing that hypertension is associated with a more evident loss of renal function in patients with early CRF (20). Our patients with high blood pressure had been advised to regularly take "traditional" antihypertensive agents (Table 7). The compliance with these prescriptions was checked with frequent measurements of blood pressure, as well as with controls of fundoscopy and ECG, and was found to be rather poor. Admittedly, the role of antihypertensive therapy on the rate of progression of renal functional deterioration, both in essential hypertension and in primary renal parenchymal disease complicated by hypertension, is difficult to establish. The poor compliance with antihypertensive drug prescriptions is only one of the factors explaining this lack of information. It should be reminded that in human pathology it may prove quite difficult, and sometimes perhaps impossible, to establish the exact role of hypertension (and hence that of antihypertensive drugs) in the

Table 6. Progression of renal failure in 233 patients on protein-restricted diet (mean followup 51.3 months)

	Number of pts	Hypertensive	Normotensive
Stability or slow deterioration of renal function	149 (63.9%)	103 (69.1%)	46 (30.9%)
"Accelerated" deterioration of renal function	84 (36.1%)	71 (84.5%)	13 (15.5%)*

Stability or slow deterioration of renal function = SCr $\gtreqless$ < 0.04 mg/dl/mo.
"Accelerated" deterioration of renal function = > SCr > 0.04 mg/dl/mo.
* Chi-square = 6.29; p < 0.001.

Table 7. Antihypertensive drugs used in our clinical experience

Alphamethyldopa	500–1000 mg/day
Clonidine	0.150–0.600 mg/day
Prazosin	1–6 mg/day
Propranolol	40–80 mg/day
Atenolol	50 mg/day
Labetalol	100–600 mg/day
Furosemide	25–75 mg/day

Table 8. Antihypertensive drugs that might be potentially useful in patients with chronic renal failure

Nifedipine	20–60 mg/day
Verapamil	80–160 mg/day
Diltiazem	30–150 mg/day
Captopril	25–50 mg/day
Enalapril	5–20 mg/day

progression of functional deterioration. This puzzling topic is now made even more complicated by the recent experimental evidence showing opposite effects of the "traditional", as opposed to the "specific" antihypertensive agents (Table 8).

Only future studies aimed at comparing in a prospective, randomized manner the effects of these two categories of antihypertensive agents might be of value to elucidate the role of good pharmacologic control of hypertension in the progression of renal failure.

Treatment of disorders in mineral metabolism

Several experimental studies suggest a harmful role of increased phosphate intake on renal function. The proposed pathways leading to renal damage may be summarized as follows: a) hyperphosphatemia b) increased calcium x phosphate product, c) increased phosphate excretion per nephron, and d) calcium and phosphate deposition in renal parenchyma (22).

In animals this deposition has been found to be an early event that worsens the course of chronic renal disease. In humans, hyperphosphatemia may occur early in CRF before a significant decline in GFR can be detected. This hyperphosphatemia has been shown to be transient and postprandial (4) and results from renal failure in the excretion of the dietary phosphate load by the kidney.

Recently, evidence has been provided that the elevated serum phosphate is the most important factor in the sequence of events that leads to calcium and phosphate deposition in the kidney. In a large population of patients with renal disease of diverse etiology, increased calcium deposition in kidney biopsy specimens was directly correlated with renal impairment and was evident at the early stages of chronic renal disease even before significant renal failure was observed (23). In experimental animals, dietary phosphate restriction has been shown to prevent the development of secondary hyperparathyroidism, and even to reverse established hyperparathyroidism and, hence, to prevent calcium and phosphate deposition and progressive renal impairment.

In patients with early CRF, a moderate dietary restriction in phosphate (Table 9) has been effective in maintaining normal serum phosphate levels for years, in limiting the rise in serum parathyroid hormone concentration, and in preventing severe osteoclastic bone lesions (24).

A state of vitamin D deficiency probably exists, even in patients with early CRF (25). For this reason, the administration of vitamin D metabolites has been suggested,

Table 9. Suggested dietary phosphate and calcium intakes and vitamin-D dosage in patients with early chronic renal failure

Patients with GFR 70–30 ml/min	
Dietary phosphate	600–700 mg/day
Dietary calcium	1000–1500 mg/day
1,25-(OH)$_2$D3	0.25–1.00 µg/day
1 alpha (OH)$_2$D3	0.50–1.00 µg/day

either alone or associated with dietary phosphate restriction, in patients with GFR ranging from 30 to 60 ml/min. The results indicate that long-term treatment with 1,25-dihydroxycholecalciferol started early in the course of CRF could prevent the progression of renal osteodystrophy. The administration of 1,25-dihydroxycholecalciferol, however, has been claimed to have a deleterious effect on renal function (26). These data have not been confirmed (25) and it seems now established that a long-term treatment with low-dose 1.25-dihydroxycholecalciferol or 1-alpha-dihydroxycholecalciferol is an acceptable method for preventing the catabolic effect of secondary hyperparathyroidism without any significant impairment of renal function.

Treatment of disordered uric acid metabolism

As a common finding in patients with chronic renal failure, serum uric acid is increased and its total excretion is reduced. Since the major route of uric acid elimination is renal excretion, theoretically, when the renal function is reduced there should be a straight correlation between serum creatinine and serum uric acid values during the course of chronic renal failure. However, whatever the renal damage, the increase in serum uric acid is usually moderate and cannot be predicted from the fall in GFR.

Evidently there is a functional adaptation of renal uric acid handling; in fact, the net tubular reabsorption of urate falls from 90% (in healthy subjects) to 20% in end-stage renal failure. At the same time, the fractional excretion increases, changing from 10% to 80% of the filtered amount. The reduction of total uric acid excretion, on the other hand, could be due to a decreased production or to extrarenal clearance. The results of studies using labeled urate (C^{14}) showed, in patients with CRF, a quite normal production; accordingly, the same studies gave evidence that 10–30% of total urate production is excreted in gout and is degraded by uricase-bearing bacteria (27). Hypothetically, the hyperuricemic state is harmful for CRF patients because of interstitial deposits of urate salts, leading in turn to a further fibrosis.

Despite this logic, the clinical findings of renal damage due to uric acid deposition are uncommon in patients with chronic renal diseases. In 1965 Richet identified renal deposition of urate salts in only 17 of 1600 patients with CRF; Fessel in 1979 compared the clinical course of patients with mild hyperuricemia and of patients with gout; he observed that hyperuricemia per se apparently does not influence renal function. The studies of Berger and Yu (1975–1982) showed, once again, that hyperuricemia, even over a long-term followup, is not associated with a decline in renal function (28). These conclusions have been supported by the complementary observations that uric-acid-lowering agents, in particular allopurinol, did not play any role in preventing the progression of chronic renal failure.

In our experience, hyperuricemia is not a harmful condition for patients with CRF on long-term dietary protein restriction. We found no statistically significant difference in serum uric acid values between patients with a stable renal function and those with deterioration of renal function. Moreover, the percentage of patients treated with allopurinol in the two groups was not different.

Our results are in agreement with the study by Rosenfeld (29). Based on a controlled study design in patients with mild CRF, this study compared the effects on renal function of allopurinol and of placebo; no differences in creatinine clearance changes were found when comparing the treatments. Eventually, it was clearly demonstrated that hyperuricemia does not play any role in deteriorating renal function; in addition, the use of uric-acid-lowering agents has no benefit for the patients with chronic renal diseases and hyperuricemia.

Concerning our clinical experience, we believe that, besides the use of a low-protein diet (theoretically capable of lowering the uric acid load), allopurinol therapy is advisable when the serum uric acid value exceeds 9 mg/100 ml. We give patients 100 mg/day, further reducing the dosage to 50 mg/day when the GFR is very low (< 10 ml/min). In this way, the potential side effects of allopurinol (i.e., marrow failure, exfoliative dermatitis) can be minimized or even avoided (30).

REFERENCES

1. Mitch WE, Brenner BM, Stein JH eds: *The Progressive Nature of Renal Disease*. Churchill & Livingstone, New York, Chapters 1-8, 1986.
2. Maschio G, Oldrizzi L, Tessitore N, D'Angelo A, Valvo E, Lupo A, Loschiavo C, Fabris A, Gammaro L, Rugiu C, Panzetta G: Effects of dietary protein and phosphorus restriction on the progression of early renal failure. *Kidney Int* 22:371-376, 1982.
3. Alvestrand A, Ahlberg M, Bergstrom J: Retardation of the progression of renal insufficiency in patients treated with low-protein diets. *Kidney Int* 24 (Suppl 16):S268-S272, 1983.
4. Maschio G, Tessitore N, D'Angelo A, Bonucci E, Lupo A, Valvo E, Loschiavo C, Fabris A, Moracchiello P, Previato G, Fiaschi E: Early dietary phosphorus restriction and calcium supplementation in the prevention of renal osteodystrophy. *Am J Clin Nutr* 33:1546-1554, 1980.
5. Giordano C: Early diet to slow the course of chronic renal failure. In: *Proceedings of the 8th International Congress on Nephrology, Athens, 1981*. Plenum, New York, pp 71-81, 1981.
6. Maschio G, Tessitore N, Lund B, Bonucci E, Sorensen OH, D'Angelo A, Lund B, Loschiavo C, Lupo A, Valvo E, Chiaramonte S, Oldrizzi L, Fabris A, Previato G: Long-term effects of dietary phosphate restriction in chronic renal failure. In: C Giordano, EA Friedman, eds, *Uremia: Pathobiology of Patients Treated for 10 years or More*. Wichtig, Milan, pp 17-22, 1981.
7. Barsotti G, Morelli E, Giannoni A, Guiducci A, Lupetti S, Giovannetti S: Restricted phosphorus and nitrogen intake to slow the progression of chronic renal failure: A controlled trial. *Kidney Int* 24 (Suppl 16):S278-S284, 1983.
8. El Nahas AM, Masters-Thomas A, Brady SA, Farrington K, Wilkinson V, Hilson AJW, Varghese Z, Moorhead JF: Selective effect of low proteins diets in chronic renal diseases. *Br Med J* 289:1337-1341, 1984.

9. Rosman JB, Meijer S, Sluiter WJ, ter Wee PM, Piers-Becht TPM, Donker AJM:Prospective randomised trial of early dietary protein restriction in chronic renal failure. *Lancet* 2: 1291-1296, 1984.
10. Maschio G, Oldrizzi L, Rugiu C, Valvo E, Lupo A, Loschiavo C, Tessitore N, Fabris A, Gammaro L, Panzetta G: Factors affecting progression of renal failure in patients on long-term dietary protein restriction. *Kidney Int* 32, S22:S49-S52, 1987.
11. Oldrizzi L, Rugiu C, Maschio G: Different protein diets in renal failure: A self-controlled study. *Am J Nephrology* 85:344-348, 1988.
12. Oldrizzi L, Rugiu C, Valvo E, Lupo A, Loschiavo C, Gammaro L, Tessitore N, Fabris A, Panzetta G, Maschio G: Progression of renal failure in patients with renal disease of diverse etiology on protein-restricted diet. *Kidney Int* 27: 553-557, 1985.
13. Anderson S, Meyer T, Rennke HG, Brenner BM: Control of glomerular hypertension limits glomerular injury in rats with reduced renal mass. *J Clin Invest* 76:612-619, 1985.
14. Moorhead JF, Chan MK, Varghese Z: The role of abnormalities of lipid metabolism in the progression of renal disease. In: WE Mitch, BM Brenner, JH Stein, eds, *The Progressive Nature of Renal Disease*. Churchill & Livingstone, New York, pp 133-149, 1986.
15. Kopple JD, Coburn JW: Evaluation of chronic uremia. Importance of serum urea nitrogen, serum creatinine, and their ratio. *JAMA* 227:41-45, 1974.
16. Guarnieri G, Toigo G, Situlin R, Crapesi L, Del Bianco MA, Zanettovich A, Faccini L, Lucchesi A, Oldrizzi L, Rugiu C, Maschio G: Nutritional assessment in patients with early renal insufficiency on long-term low-protein diet. *Contrib Nephrol* 53:40-50, 1986.
17. Baldwin DS, Neugarten J: Role of hypertension in the evolution of renal disease. *Contrib Nephrol* 54:63-76, 1987.
18. Raij L: Role of hypertension in progressive glomerular injury in glomerulonephritis. *Hypertension* 8 (Suppl 1):30-31, 1986.
19. Arze RS, Ramos JM, Owen JP, Morely AR, Elliott RW, Wilkinson R, Ward MK, Kerr DNS: The natural history of chronic pyelonephritis in the adult. *Q Med* 204:396-41, 1982.
20. Oldrizzi L, Rugiu C, Maschio G: Hypertension and progression of renal failure in patients on protein-restricted diet. *Contrib Nephrol* 54:133-143, 1987.
21. Maschio G, Oldrizzi L, Rugiu C: The role of hypertension on the progression of renal disease in man. *Blood Purif* 6:250-257, 1988.
22. Klahr S: Metabolic adaptations of the nephron in renal disease. *Kidney Int* 29:80-89, 1986.
23. Lumlertgul D, Burke TJ, Gillum DM, Alfrey AC, Harris DC, Hammond WS, Schrier RW: Phosphate depletion arrests progression of chronic renal failure independent of protein intake. *Kidney Int* 29:658-666, 1986.
24. Maschio G, Bonucci E, D'Angelo A, Tessitore N, Fabris A, Lupo A, Valvo E, Loschiavo C, Oldrizzi L, Rugiu C, Panzetta G: Dietary management and the natural history of renal osteodystrophy. In: G D'Amico, G Colasanti, eds, *Nephrology 83*. Wichting, Milan, pp 57-60, 1983.
25. Massry S: Current status of the use of 1,25 (OH)2 D3 in the management of renal osteodystrophy. *Kidney Int* 18:409-418, 1980.
26. Christiansen C, Rodbro P, Christensen MS, Hartnack B, Trasbol I: Deterioration of renal function during treatment of chronic renal failure with 1,25 dihydroxycholecalciferol. *Lancet* 2:700-703, 1978.
27. Cameron JS, Simmonds HA: Uric acid, gout and the kidney.

J Clin Pathol 34:1245–1254, 1981.
28. Beck LH: Requiem for gouty nephropathy. *Kidney Int* 30:280–287, 1986.
29. Rosenfeld JB: Effect of long-term allopurinol administration on serial GFR in normotensive and hypertensive hyperuricemic subjects. *Adv Exp Med Biol* 41B:581–596, 1974.
30. Simmonds HA, Cameron JS, Morris GS, Davies PM: Allopurinol and the tumor lysis syndrome. *Clin Chim Acta* 160:189–195, 1986.

CHAPTER 42

Renal Insufficiency

EBERHARD F. RITZ

INTRODUCTION

This chapter will discuss the therapeutic approach in patients with chronic renal insufficiency (serum creatinine concentration ~2–10 mg/dl, GFR ~10–50% of normal), not yet requiring dialysis treatment. A number of conservative measures are indicated to maintain the patients in a state of well-being. To understand the rationale for these interventions it should be realized that chronically diseased kidneys often have a limited capacity to appropriately regulate body fluids and electrolytes (1), and this may be uncovered during stress (excessive potassium load, excessive fluid intake, or dehydration, etc.). In these circumstances, inadequate renal adaptation to the needs of the body may result in pernicious hyperkalemia, pulmonary edema, hyponatremia, or volume depletion. Furthermore, the long-term consequences of several abnormalities, such as malnutrition and disturbed calcium metabolism, require an early correction to prevent later complications at the time of dialysis. We shall discuss the prophylaxis of acute and chronic sequelae of chronic renal insufficiency, measures to slow the progression of functional renal deterioration, as well as the psychological handling of these patients.

COMPONENTS OF CHRONIC RENAL FAILURE THAT REQUIRE MANAGEMENT

The components of chronic renal failure that require management are:
Hypertension
Fluid and electrolyte overload or deprivation
Urinary tract infection
Urinary tract obstruction
Congestive heart failure

DIAGNOSIS AND TREATMENT OF REVERSIBLE CAUSES CONTRIBUTING TO RENAL FAILURE (2)

It is imperative that reversible factors causing or worsening renal failure be meticulously excluded (Table 1). The same applies to patients with an unexplained rapid progression of chronic renal insufficiency. The course of renal failure is expected to be slow in polycystic kidney disease, nephrocalcinosis, partial obstruction, and IgA nephropathy; intermediate in glomerulonephritis, and Alport's disease; or fulminant in end-stage juvenile diabetes, extracapillary glomerulonephritis, vasculitis, etc.

Dehydration (3)

Reversible prerenal azotemia from fluid or electrolyte depletion may occur as a consequence of vomiting, overzealous use of diuretics (including concealed diuretic abuse), sweating in hot climates, diarrhea, or inadequate fluid intake, particularly in patients with impaired mentation, nausea, etc. Some renal diseases predispose to renal electrolyte loss, e.g., analgesic nephropathy, polycystic kidney disease, renal tubular acidosis.

Remediable causes of vomiting (digitalis intoxication, coexisting intraabdominal disease, alcoholism, etc.) or renal electrolyte loss (concealed diuretic abuse, acute metabolic alkalosis of vomiting, uncontrolled hyperglycemia, diabetic ketoacidosis, administration of nonreabsorbable osmotic agents, e.g., mannitol, etc.) must be carefully investigated and corrected.

The diagnosis of volume depletion in the presence of renal insufficiency must be made clinically. The presence of the following signs should be sought:
Reduced skin turgor
Softness of the eyeballs
Absence of sweat from the axillae, dryness of mucous membranes
Orthostatic circulatory dysregulation (blood pressure and pulse-rate change in excess of 15% upon standing after lying supine)
Decreased central venous filling pressure (invisibility of pulse wave from internal jugular vein at the level of the clavicle when patient's head is flat or slightly raised)
Low central venous pressure, if available (< 5 mmHg)
Low pulmonary wedge pressure, if available (< 7 mmHg)
Laboratory findings in prerenal azotemia include:
Recent increase of hematocrit and total protein concentration

Table 1. Potentially reversible abnormalities contributing to chronic renal failure or azotemia

1. Dehydration (diarrhea, vomiting, excessive effect of diuretics, sweating, excessive salt restriction, fever)
2. Urinary tract infection
3. Obstructive uropathy (urinary tract obstruction, papillary necrosis, intratubular crystal precipitation)
4. Low cardiac output (congestive cardiac failure, cardiac arrhythmias, sequestration of fluid in "third spaces")
5. uncontrolled hypertension (including malignant hypertension)
6. Catabolism
7. Nephrotoxicity of drugs
8. Nephrotoxicity of contrast media
9. Renal vein thrombosis
10. Hypercalcemia
11. Complications of pregnancy

Serum urea increased disporportionally to serum creatinine concentration (ratio in excess of 10:1)
Relatively concentrated urine (U_{OSM} > 500 mOsm/kg H_2O, unless GFR is very low)

Management consists of treatment of underlying etiology and adequate fluid or electrolyte intake. If necessary, fluid must be administered intravenously until adequate urine output (> 40 ml/hr) is restored or a total of 3000 ml has been given. At this time, reevaluation of serum electrolyte parameters and exclusion of fluid overload are indicated before additional volume replacement is pursued. Monitoring of volume status and electrolyte concentrations is important because of the limited renal ability to excrete excess free water and electrolytes. Water intoxication is a hazard if > 3000 ml/24 hr of free water are given (particularly in patients treated with diuretics or a low-sodium diet).

Urinary tract infection (UTI)

An uncomplicated urinary tract infection is not a common cause for progression of renal failure. However, UTI may cause renal damage and require vigorous therapy when urodynamic abnormalities, renal stones, postrenal obstruction, or neurogenic bladder are present. Their recognition requires clinical examination, sonography, and plain films of the abdomen. In some cases, computerized tomography or gallium scans may be required. If excretory urography is used, the risk of worsening renal function must be considered.

Renal failure from UTI is usually associated with bacteremia, intrarenal microabscesses or papillary necrosis. Management includes recognition and, if possible, correction of coexisting urological problems, particularly obstruction, and judicious administration of antibiotics. Since patients often have a history of urinary tract instrumentation, bacteria that are resistant to multiple antibiotics are frequently encountered. Consequently, antibiotics should be selected on the basis of the in-vitro sensitivity test. In the absence of such information, or in emergency situations, gentamycin (in a dose adjusted for the degree of renal impairment) and/or broad-spectrum penicillins/ cephalosporins should be administered. Serum creatinine concentrations during treatment must be followed.

Urinary tract obstruction

Subvesical and supravesical obstruction frequently occur in the following clinical settings: diabetic papillary necrosis, papillary necrosis of phenacetin abusers, history of renal stone disease, prostatic hyperplasia, urethral narrowing (in patients with a history of indwelling bladder catheter, etc.). Bladder retention is also a common cause of deterioration of renal function in patients with mental obtundation and patients on tricyclic antidepressants. Recognition of obstruction requires sonography of the bladder and the upper urinary tract. Sonography should be repeated after 24 or 48 hours since evidence of distension may be absent in the first hours of obstruction. On plain abdominal x-rays, stones or necrotic papillae of phenacetin abusers cannot be regularly recognized since they are not always calcified. The usual clinical symptoms of obstruction, particularly colic, cannot be relied upon since they are frequently absent.

Congestive heart failure

Congestive heart failure is an important cause of deterioration of kidney function in renal failure patients. As in nonuremic patients, heart failure causes a reduction of GFR that is related to the decrease in cardiac output.

If symptoms and signs of congestion are present, i.e., dyspnea of exertion, orthopnea, pleural effusion, distended neck veins, hepatomegaly with hepatojugular reflux, dependent edema, pulmonary congestion, etc., one must consider different causes of congestion: extracardiac circulatory congestion, intrinsic myocardial insufficiency, or a combination of both. Measurement of cardiac output or circulation times are helpful for distinction but are rarely performed. Today, the preferred method is echocardiography (4, 5). Ejection fraction and other indices of contractibility are normal or high in cases in which pure volume overload causes extracardiac circulatory congestion and are depressed in cases with impaired pumping function of the heart, e.g., intrinsic myocardial disease. Coronary artery disease is the most common cause of myocardial insufficiency in patients with renal failure, and the above measurements, unfortunately, are unreliable if ischemic heart disease and segmental abnormalities of myocardial contraction are present.

Painless myocardial infarction is an important consideration, particularly in diabetics, when left heart failure or circulatory congestion supervene. Associated cardiomyopathy secondary to hypertension, ischemic heart disease, alcoholism, or amyloidosis must also be considered and adequately treated.

Finally, in patients with end-stage renal failure, pericarditis may supervene. It may be missed if the patient does not complain of precordial pain. Recognition requires careful auscultation and echocardiography. The sudden appearance of cardiomegaly in the absence of pulmonary congestion is suggestive of pericardial effusion.

Treatment of extracardiac circulatory congestion consists of the administration of high ceiling diuretics and negative fluid balance. Arterial blood pressure in supine and upright positions, serum creatinine, and BUN and serum electrolytes must be closely monitored. If a clear distinction between extracardiac congestion and intrinsic myocardial disease is not possible and patients remain symptomatic after administration of diuretics and control of blood pressure, a trial with digitalis is indicated. Afterload reduction with ACE inhibitors may be useful for the combined treatment of hypertension and cardiac insufficiency, e.g., with captopril or enalapril. Dose reduction is necessary because the drugs are excreted via the kidneys. Anemia rarely contributes to heart failure if hemoglobin levels are above 7–8 g/dl, except in elderly patients or in patients with symptomatic coronary disease.

Renal failure is not a contraindication for coronary bypass surgery. Coronary angiography should be performed in symptomatic patients to evaluate the indications for surgery, giving due consideration to the potential of contrast media to induce renal failure.

Uncontrolled hypertension (including malignant hypertension) (6, 7)

The prevalence of hypertension increases with progressive impairment of renal function. In preterminal renal failure, hypertension is observed in no less than 85% of patients. Hypertension is then only absent in renal diseases with renal wasting of sodium. Of note is the high proportion of patients with renal disease who go into the malignant phase of hypertension e.g., up to 10% of patients with mesangial IgA glomerulonephritis develp malignant hypertension. It was recently shown that at any given level of blood pressure, the incidence of malignant hypertension, i.e., grade III or IV retinopathy, is higher in patients with renal disease than in patients with essential hypertension (7). Malignant hypertension is an important cause for deterioration of renal function.

When treating hypertension, it is of note that renal autoregulation may be impaired so that a further increase of azotemia, usually transient in nature, is observed. It is imperative to normalize blood pressure despite such possible worsening of azotemia, because in the age of dialysis and transplantation, the long-term hazards of uncontrolled hypertension by far exceed those of uremia.

If hypertension is refractory to treatment, the possibility of unilateral or bilateral obstruction of renal arteries must be considered, particularly in elderly patients with diabetes mellitus. Abdominal auscultation, Doppler sonography, and renal angiography should then be considered, but the hazard of contrast media for renal function must be appreciated.

Catabolism

On the one hand, increased azotemia may result from massive dietary protein intake, parenteral hyperalimentation with infusion of amino acids, tube feeding in unconscious patients, etc. These conditions cause a rise of urea without a proportionate rise in serum creatinine. On the other hand, both urea and creatinine concentrations rise in patients who are catabolic from wasting or after administration of steroids, even in the absence of a change in GFR.

Nephrotoxicity of drugs (8)

Potentially reversible azotemia may result from unwanted side effects of several drugs. Diuretics may cause volume contraction. Cyclooxygenase inhibitors (indomethacin, aspirin) may cause a reduction of GFR (9, 10), particularly in patients with the nephrotic syndrome, SLE, glomerulonephritis, and hepatic insufficiency. Nephrotoxic antibiotics (e.g., aminoglycosides, amphotericin, etc.) cause reversible or irreversible renal impairment if given in the usual doses to patients with renal failure. Another important consideration is drug-induced interstitial nephritis, e.g., from diuretics, allopurinol, etc. Finally, an important indirect cause of drug-induced renal failure is digoxin intoxication with vomiting or arrhythmia.

Nephrotoxicity of contrast media

Administration of contrast media to patients with renal failure, especially to diabetics or patients with Bence Jones nephropathy, is particularly hazardous because of the risk of intratubular obstruction with acute renal insufficiency. Renal failure after contrast media is not always reversible. Renal impairment may follow excretory urography, cholecystography, angiography, or computed tomography with enhancement. Sonography should be chosen whenever possible. If contrast studies are necessary, the patient should be well hydrated before the examination is done. Recent studies showed that the renal risk is diminished with prophylactic administration of furosemide. Renal function must be closely monitored. Because polyuric renal failure is common, measuring fluid output is not sufficient and serum chemistry must be monitored.

Renal vein thrombosis

Sudden deterioration of renal function in patients with the nephrotic syndrome may result from renal vein thrombosis, which frequently does not cause any clinical signs and symptoms. The diagnosis should be suspected when sudden asymmetry of renal size is noted. The diagnosis can be substantiated by vena cavography and renal vein phlebography. Successful lysis of thrombi with streptokinase or urokinase has been reported. Anticoagulation is indicated in patients with documented renal vein thrombosis.

Hypercalcemia

Impairment of renal function occurs in hypercalcemia from any cause (tumors, especially multiple myeloma; hyperparathyroidism; vitamin D intoxication, particularly in patients with immobilization or fluid deprivation; oral administration of calcium salts, e.g., calcium carbonate; calcium-containing citrate salts for management of acidosis, etc.).

The main goal of therapy is to achieve and maintain intense natriuresis. This requires administration of large volumes of fluid (depending on the severity of hypercalcemia, 5–10 l/day with monitoring of central venous pressures and intensive care surveillance) and high doses of furosemide, unless oliguric renal failure is present.

If hypercalcemia results partially from intestinal hyperabsorption, low-calcium diets and oral administration of cellulose phosphate (3 × 20 g) are indicated. In vitamin D intoxication, administration of steroids may be indicated. Tumor hypercalcemia is best managed by administration of 10–20 μg/kg mithramycin in a single injection. Although nephrotoxicity after mithramycin has been noted, it can be given to patients with impaired renal function at the above low dose. Biphosphonates are currently under clinical evaluation; preliminary experience is so encouraging that they may become the drug of choice in this indication.

Complications of pregnancy

Although many patients with renal failure are infertile, conception may occur so that contraceptive advise should routinely be given to female patients with renal failure. If conception occurs, the main threat to renal function is hypertension. This risk is heralded by the failure of blood pressure to decrease in the first trimester, as expected during normal pregnancy. Recent studies showed that, in contrast to previous opinion, an adverse effect of pregnancy on renal function is by no means common in female patients with nonhypertensive renal disease, except in SLE. Consequently, pregnancy should be carefully monitored but not interrupted. On the other hand, the risk of preeclampsia is very high in pregnant women with hypertensive renal disease, and interruption of pregnancy may become necessary if the blood pressure is not normalized by bed rest, left lateral decubitus, and antihypertensive medication.

SPECIFIC APPROACHES TO THE CONSERVATIVE MANAGEMENT OF UREMIA

Fluid intake

An obligatory daily osmotic load of around 600 mOsm must be excreted when the patient is on a normal diet. Because of reduced renal concentrating ability (commonly not above 300–500 mOsm/kg H_2O) and an oral fluid intake of 1.5–2.5 l, it is necessary to maintain the external fluid balance. This is crucial for two reasons: a) With deficient fluid intake dehydration, volume contraction and a further decline of renal function are likely to follow; b) with excessive fluid intake (> 3 l/24 hr), dilution of body fluids and symptomatic hyponatremia will occur in cases of very low GFR (< 10 ml/min) due to the patient's impaired ability to excrete large quantities of free water, particularly if patients are on diuretics. If additional fluid loss (sweating, diarrhea, vomiting, fever) is present, the fluid intake must be higher; and if the patient is unable to ingest fluids, intravenous administration of fluids becomes necessary. One half of fluids should be given as normal saline and one half as 5% glucose. Body weight and urine output must be monitored during IV fluid administration.

Even as outpatients, renal failure patients should be advised to monitor their body weight every morning to avoid a gross fluid imbalance.

Dietary sodium restriction (3)

Dietary sodium should be restricted only when severe hypertension, pulmonary congestion, or massive peripheral edema are present. Concealed sources of sodium (penicillin and penicillin derivatives, etc.) should be considered. Because of the latent sodium wasting tendency of many uremic patients, it is wise to leave some residual peripheral edema as a buffer of safety.

Dietary restriction of protein (11–14)

This is an area of considerable controversy. It is not doubted that the end products of protein metabolism are responsible for, or at least contribute to, "uremic toxicity." Thus, in patients with end-stage renal failure the symptoms of uremia may be provoked by administration of protein, and conversely such symptoms are ameliorated by protein restriction. It remains controversial, however, to what extent the dietary restriction of protein can be safely implementated without the risk of malnutrition and protein depletion in patients with end-stage renal failure. Uremia is a hypercatabolic state. Furthermore, unless patients are properly instructed and supervised, energy (calorie) and protein intakes become easily inadequate, and the risk is aggravated by anorexia of renal insufficiency. As a rule, low-protein diets in end-stage renal failure cannot be safely implemented without the expert help of a dietician and without weighing food. Although the fraction of dietary protein that must consist of essential amino acids has not been established, it is recommended that protein consumed by uremic patients on a low-protein diet should be of high biologic value.

For the control of uremic symptoms, dietary protein restriction should be advised only in patients with slowly progressive renal disease, since instruction and habituation of patients to low-protein diets usually require considerable time.

One of the more exciting aspects of contemporary nephrology is the rediscovery that dietary protein restriction affects evolution of renal failure in experimental models of renal disease, particularly glomerular disease. It could be demonstrated that glomerular hyperperfusion induced by proteins (and possibly other nutrients) contributed to self-perpetuating renal damage and deterioration of renal function. Dietary protein restriction (and less certainly, dietary phosphate restriction) prevented or attenuated progression of renal failure in various models of renal damage. One controlled study showed a slower rise in serum creatinine levels in patients with modest renal failure with moderate protein restriction (60 g/day) and advanced renal failure with severe protein restriction (40 g/day). A 3-year followup (Rosman, personal communication) showed attenuated loss of C_{cr} on a low-protein diet for patients with glomerulonephritis, but not for other categories of renal disease. In preliminary communications, similar observations have been made in patients with other renal disease and specifically in those with diabetic nephropathy. It is currently unresolved by which mechanism protein restriction works and whether the action of protein restriction can be reproduced by drugs and antihypertensive therapy. It is furthermore unresolved whether this modality of treatment is only efficacious in glomerular diseases or is also useful in other renal diseases, specifically diseases involving renal ischemia. There is a curious discrepancy between the prominence that dietary intervention plays in the published literature and the infrequency with which it is prescribed in clinical practice. It is certainly prudent to assess the dietary protein intake in patients with known renal disease and early renal failure, measuring urinary urea excretion (protein intake = 3 × urinary urea (g/24 hr) + 15 ≃ g protein intake/24 hr). The usual protein intakes on Western diets of 1.3–1.5 g/kg/24 hr are neither necessary nor desirable. A reduction of protein intake to ~60 g/day (0.8 g/kg body weight/day) will not expose the patient to any nutritional risks and is feasible in daily practice. Nephrotic-range proteinuria is not necessarily a contraindication, since, paradoxically, protein balance may improve after protein restriction secondary to diminished proteinuria, but such patients clearly require careful anthropometric monitoring. The "success" of treatment should be monitored by sequential measurements of urinary protein (and albumin) excretion. Patients should also be monitored for compliance (serum urea/creatinine ratio; urinary urea excretion) and signs of protein malnutrition (total protein, transferrin, C_3 levels). At the current stage of knowledge, more severe dietary protein restriction, e.g., 0.4 g/kg body weight/day should not be undertaken outside controlled clinical trials without the possibility of regular followup and instructions by dietitians.

Hypertension (15–18)

Treatment of hypertension and maintenance of normal blood pressure is mandatory in patients with renal insufficiency. In several retrospective studies, a correlation has been noted between the degree of hypertension and the rate of deterioration of renal function. At least in patients with diabetic nephropathy, it could be clearly shown that lowering blood pressure by antihypertensive medication attenuates the rate of progression of renal failure. There is no logical reason why the same should not hold true for other renal, and specifically glomerular, diseases. The level to which blood pressure should be lowered has not been established. Studies in diabetics showed that the risk of retinal hemorrhage is related to the level of systolic blood pressure, even within the normotensive range; furthermore, studies in diabetics with "microproteinuria," i.e., urinary albumin excretion of 20–300 mg/day, showed that lowering of blood pressure within the normotensive range, e.g., from 140 mmHg systolic to 120 mmHg systolic, using beta blockers or ACE inhibitors reduces the level of albuminuria. This may indicate that the upper normal range of blood pressure, i.e., 140 mmHg systolic, may not be optimal for glomerular microcirculations with pre-existing damage, but no specific guidelines can currently be given in this respect other than that at least strict normotension must be achieved.

Based on experimental studies with renal ablation or models of glomerular injury, it has been argued that ACE inhibitors are superior to other antihypertensive agents with respect to their action on glomerular hydraulic pressure and attentuating glomerular injury. No definite clinical experience is available to date, but one controlled retrospective study showed less rise in serum creatinine in hypertensive patients with renal failure on ACE inhibitors compared to equally efficacious treatment with other antihypertensive agents. Following administration of ACE inhibitors, a rise in serum creatinine is commonly observed. This is the reason why these agents were considered to be contraindicated in renal failure. Such a rise of the serum creatinine concentration is the predictable consequence of the fall in glomerular capillary pressure. In our experience it never exceeded 70%. If greater increments of serum creatinine are noted, hypovolemia secondary to the use of diuretics should be excluded, and a careful search for renovascular disease is appropriate. In patients with bilateral renal artery stenosis or arterial stenosis of a single kidney, ACE inhibitors may cause an acute, mostly reversible, shutdown of renal function. Unsuspected atherosclerotic renovascular stenosis is particularly common in the elderly patient with renal failure.

Low-ceiling diuretics, i.e., thiazides, become usually, but not invariably, ineffective at GFR ~30 ml/min. More potent loop diuretics (e.g., furosemide 2 × 40 mg or more) must be given. In addition, potassium-sparing diuretics are contraindicated.

Some antihypertensive drugs, e.g., alpha methyldopa, atenolol, pindolol, captopril, and enalapril, accumulate in renal failure. An overdose of these drugs is generally rare because one usually measures blood pressure and selects the dosage according to the drug action; however, cardiac complications may arise from the accumulation of beta blockers, and adverse effects, e.g., exanthema, leukopenia, and pancytopenia, occur more frequently in patients with renal failure in whom the dosage of ACE inhibitors has not been reduced.

In patients with severe hypertension, a combination of high-ceiling diuretics (furosemide) or converting-enzyme inhibitors (captopril, enalapril) and calcium antagonists, beta blockers, or vasodilating drugs (prazosin, minoxidil) usually permits conservative control of blood pressure. In cases of excessive fluid retention, particularly in diabetics, it is often wise to start dialysis earlier to facilitate control of volume and management of hypertension.

Calcium and phosphorus metabolism (19, 20)

Three major interrelated mechanisms are operative in the genesis of renal osteodystrophy:
Hypocalcemia and secondary hyperparathyroidism
Renal retention of phosphorus and hyperphosphatemia
Impaired renal generation of the active vitamin D metabolite $1,25\text{-}(OH)_2D_3$

In renal failure, the intestine is unable to adapt to a low-calcium diet. On the other hand, such diets are commonly self-selected by anorectic uremic patients. Consequently hypocalcemia, secondary hyperparathyroidism, and negative calcium balance may ensue. If low serum calcium is found in the presence of normal total protein, oral calcium salts should be administered (e.g., 1 g elemental calcium as calcium carbonate per day), but this requires regular monitoring of serum and urinary calcium and of serum phosphorus.

Hyperphosphatemia is usually observed when the GFR has fallen to approximately 30 ml/min. Hyperphosphatemia must be avoided because of its role in the genesis of secondary hyperparathyroidism and in the genesis of extraosseous calcifications. In general, low-phosphorus diets are nutritionally inadequate because of their low protein content, but at least dairy products should be discouraged. Administration of calcium carbonate has the double advantage of simultaneously normalizing serum calcium and reducing the intestinal absorption of phosphate. If calcium carbonate alone is ineffective, one has to resort, in addition, to oral phosphate binders $[Al(OH)_3]$ or other Al compounds. Because of the recently recognized hazard of aluminum toxicity, we advise regular measurements of serum Al in such patients. Oral phosphate binders must be discontinued if Al serum levels exceed approximately 100–150 mg/l (or ppm). Noncompliance with oral phosphate binders is a common problem. It is often advisable to find the most accepted preparation (tablets, gels, cookies, etc.) by trial and error. Recently, oral administration of magnesium salts, e.g., magnesium carbonate, has been recommended for the control of serum phosphate. This medication is moderately effective but may cause hypermagnesemia and diarrhea.

Because of impaired renal generation of $1,25\text{-}(OH)_2D_3$, it appears logical to substitute for the failing kidney's role by administering $1,25\text{-}(HO)_2D_3$. The dose that maintains normocalcemia and normocalciuria in asymptomatic patients is usually $0.25\,\mu g/day$. However, the efficacy of such prophylaxis in preventing bone disease must still be evaluated in prospective studies. Despite some recent controversy, there is no solid evidence that vitamin D metabolites are nephrotoxic in the absence of hypercalcemia and hypercalciuria.

If patients have biochemical evidence of severe bone disease, i.e., elevated serum alkaline phosphatase (with elevated bone alkaline phosphatase); modest hypercalcemia; or normocalcemia with excessive hyperphosphatemia, higher doses of $1,25\text{-}(OH)_2D_3$ ($0.5-1.5\,\mu g/day$) or the parent vitamin D substances ($50-200\,\mu g$ $25\text{-}OH\text{-}D_3$ or 20,000–40,000 IU vitamin D_3 daily) are usually required. Because of the risk of soft-tissue calcifications, vitamin D metabolites should not be administered before hyperphosphatemia is under control. Such higher doses of vitamin D metabolites require regular monitoring of serum and urinary calcium and — at greater intervals — of serum alkaline phosphatase. Usually, the risk of vitamin D toxicity increases when the serum alkaline phosphatase levels start to decrease. The risk of hypercalcemia under vitamin D therapy is also considerably increased by immobilization, fluid deprivation, and concomitant therapy with $CaCo_3$. Success of therapy can usually be adequately followed by monitoring (bone) alkaline phosphatase and skeletal x-ray findings (hand skeleton in mammography technique or magnification technique) at 8-weekly intervals.

In patients with severe hypercalcemia ($\geq 12\,mg/dl$) or hyperphosphatemia resistant to oral phosphate binders, administration of vitamin D metabolites is contraindicated. In such cases one should resort to surgical reduction of the parathyroid mass. Today, the most widely used procedure is total parathyroidectomy with autotransplantation of parathyroid tissue into the forearm musculature.

Although, low $25\text{-}(OH)$ D levels are not a feature of uremia itself, low $25\text{-}(OH)$ D levels in patients with renal failure may occur for a variety of reasons: impaired actinic generation of vitamin D in the skin, possibly because of melanosis; reduced sun exposure because of a changed lifestyle; ingestion of drugs (e.g., phenobarbital) that stimulate the hepatic microsomal enzymes; and renal loss of vitamin D-binding protein and vitamin D metabolites in the nephrotic syndrome. It is therefore wise to monitor serum $25\text{-}(OH)$ D levels and to correct vitamin D deficiency if present.

Anemia (21–23)

Anemia of renal failure is multifactorial in origin. Obligatory gastrointestinal blood loss, reduced erythrocyte lifespan, normal or low plasma erythropoietin levels that are inappropriate for the prevailing hemoglobin concentration, and possibly accumulation of other inhibitors of erythropoiesis play a role in its genesis. Because adaptive mechanisms such as resetting the oxygen affinity of hemoglobin occur, patients usually tolerate anemia without major symptoms. Furthermore, even in terminal renal failure, hemoglobin levels usually do not fall below 7 g/dl.

If anemia is present in early renal failure (GFR > 30–50 ml/min) or if it is excessive (Hb < 7 g/dl), other problems are usually present: iron deficiency (this can be recognized by measuring serum ferritin levels, except in the presence of hepatic disease or infection, or by iron stains of bone marrow); folic acid deficiency (rare);

gastrointestinal blood loss (common); and malnutrition (common) or associated disease, e.g., myeloma, SLE, microangiopathic hemolytic anemia (HUS or malignant hypertension).

If no such remediable form of anemia is found, no therapy should be given, as long as the patient is asymptomatic. Anabolic steroids have little efficacy, cause adverse effects (priapism, painful gynecomastia), and pose potential long-term hazards (peliosis hepatis and hepatic tumors) that cannot be adequately assessed at present. Blood transfusions suppress erythropoiesis and carry the long-term hazards of hemosiderosis, hepatitis B, and generation of cytotoxic antibodies against HLA antigens. On the other hand, blood transfusions are today an obligatory part of patient preparation for renal homotransplantation.

Because of their associated risks and short-lived benefits, blood transfusions should be restricted to either patients with symptomatic cardiac failure, to those with symptomatic coronary artery disease whose symptoms improve with transfusion, or to elderly patients who do not tolerate anemia.

Recombinant human erythropoietin (rhEPO) has recently been introduced for the treatment of anemia in dialyzed patients. Such treatment is highly efficacious but is not devoid of side effects, particularly hypertension and thrombotic episodes. Its use in preterminal renal failure is currently under investigation; preliminary data show that it is effective, but more specific recommendations cannot currently be made.

Hyperkalemia (24)

For clinical purposes, two different forms of hyperkalemia should be distinguished: steady-state hyperkalemia and transient hyperkalemia due to diminished tolerance of potassium loads.

Because of the high capacity of tubules to secrete potassium, hyperkalemia is uncommon before patients are in the terminal oliguric stage of renal failure. However, hyperkalemia is observed in patients with moderate renal insufficiency when hyporeninemic hypoaldosteronism (RTA Type IV) is present; such patients have low circulating renin and aldosterone levels and/or an impaired tubular response to mineralocorticoids. This condition is mostly observed in patients with diabetes mellitus.

Because of the cardiac hazards (AV block), hyperkalemia should be treated with dietary K restriction, oral K exchange salts ($3 \times 10-20$ g polystyrene sulfonate with an equal amount of sorbitol), loop diuretics (furosemide 100–500 mg/day); in cases of hyporeninemic hypoaldosteronism 9-flurohydrocortisone (0.1–0.3 mg/day) or a combination of these procedures. Since patients are frequently hypertensive to begin with, mineralocorticoids are often not well tolerated and the blood pressure must be monitored.

Because of the reduced tolerance of potassium loads and the attendant risk of hyperkalemia, potassium supplements, potassium-sparing diuretics (triamterene, amiloride, spironolactone), potassium-containing salt substitutes, potassium-containing tonics, and transfusion of aged blood should be avoided in all patients with advanced renal failure.

Metabolic acidosis

The characteristic metabolic acidosis of renal failure is due to impaired renal generation of ammonia so that acid equivalents generated in protein metabolism, and to a lesser extent in phospholipid metabolism, can no longer be excreted by the kidneys. One additional factor is renal wasting of bicarbonate. A positive balance of acid equivalents and/or extrarenal disposal of acid equivalents must inevitably occur in the steady state.

Metabolic acidosis causes a decrease of bone carbonate content and of renal generation of $1,25\text{-}(OH)_2D_3$, but whether this is relevant in the genesis of uremic osteodystrophy remains undecided. Other long-term hazards of metabolic acidosis have not been clearly documented, but in experimental studies metabolic acidosis has been recognized as an important factor in the genesis of catabolism.

Metabolic acidosis of renal failure is usually quite well tolerated unless plasma bicarbonate levels fall below 15–17 mM/l. At this point, dyspnea occurs and circulatory disturbances resulting from catecholamine unresponsiveness may be observed.

Reduced dietary protein intake reduces the generation of acid equivalents but carries the risk of protein malnutrition unless properly supervised. In symptomatic patients, sodium bicarbonate po should be administered in amounts sufficient to raise the bicarbonate level until patients are asymptomatic. Higher bicarbonate levels usually necessitate the administration of excessive amounts of sodium bicarbonate because of renal bicarbonate wasting. Acid-base chemistry and plasma calcium levels should be monitored, and the patient should be watched for signs of tetany if acidosis is rapidly corrected. During long-term administration of sodium bicarbonate, patients must be examined to detect signs of overload (hypertension, dilutional anemia, edema); should these develop, sodium restriction or administration of loop diuretics (furosemide) become necessary. The risk of sodium retention is considerably less with sodium bicarbonate than with sodium chloride.

Hyperlipidemia (25–28)

The long-term atherogenic hazards of hyperlipidemia associated with renal failure (usually Type IV) and the nephrotic syndrome (usually Type II) are currently difficult to assess. There is growing consensus that, despite hyperlipidemia, uremia per se is not associated with a major acceleration of atherosclerosis. In experimental studies, the coexistence of hyperlipidemia in uremic animals accelerated progression of renal failure, but to what extent this holds true for humans has not been proven. Although hyperlipidemia of renal failure can successfully be corrected by dietary manipulation (high poly-unsaturated/saturated fatty acid ratio, carbohydrate restriction) or drug therapy (fibrates, cholestyramine), it is uncertain whether a therapeutic benefit is gained by such procedures. In particular, any dietary restrictions carry the risk of inadequate nutrition. Furthermore, in renal failure, clofibrate therapy requires careful supervision for toxicity (skeletal and heart muscle), since clofibrinic acid accumulates. Potential long-term hazards of clofibrate still remain to be defined. It is therefore our policy to treat hyperlipidemia, unless extreme, with benign neglect.

Hyperuricemia

In renal failure, hyperuricemia is common. Fractional excretion of urate increases to a variable extent, so that no constant relationship is observed between GFR (or serum creatinine), on the one hand, and serum uric acid levels, on the other hand. Gout undoubtedly may cause renal damage and kidney failure. However, there is little evidence that in the absence of gout hyperuricemia per se accelerates the development of renal failure. In several long-term studies over decades, no significant impairment of renal function was observed with serum uric acid levels up to 10 mg/dl. We would advise, however, to administer allopurinol (100–300 mg/day) when serum uric acid levels constantly exceed 10 mg/dl or if a history of gout can be obtained. If patients develop gout in the course of renal failure, lead intoxcation should be suspected and, if proven, it should be treated with chelating agents (Na_2, Ca-EDTA).

Principles of drug dosage in renal failure (8)

In renal failure, the handling of drugs (pharmacokinetics) may be altered because of impaired renal elimination, altered protein binding, or altered drug metabolism; in addition, the drug-response relationship (pharmacodynamics) may be altered. As a general rule, administration of any drug to patients with renal failure requires careful observation of the patient for potential side effects. In particular, for any given medication precise information should be obtained about drug elimination in renal failure. Common side effects include peripheral neuropathy from nitrofurantoin, hyperkalemia from potassium-sparing diuretics (triamterene, amiloride, spironolactone), deterioration of renal function, impaired vestibular function or hearing loss from aminoglycosides (gentamycin, tobramycin, sisomycin, kanamycin), severe hypoglycemia from sulfonylurea compounds or insulin, disturbed mentation from cimetidine, digoxin toxicity, impaired platelet function due to penicillin and penicillin derivatives, etc. For some medications, e.g., digoxin and gentamycin, measurement of serum levels is helpful. In any case, for maintenance therapy, an adjustment of the dosage should be made (using mathematical formulae or nomograms) for all drugs that are excreted via the kidneys.

Preservation of forearm veins

For every patient who is considered for maintenance hemodialysis, it is imperative to preserve future vascular access. Forearm veins should not be used for diagnostic venipuncture, infusions, or transfusions. If possible, veins of the dorsum of the hand or a central vascular access should be preferred.

Prophylactic surgical creation of an arteriovenous forearm fistula (Cimino fistula) should be considered when serum creatinine reaches 6–9 mg/dl, depending on the rate of progression of the underlying renal disease. This is particularly important in patients with poor forearm veins, e.g., diabetics, or elderly females, who usually require considerable time before venous walls have been arterialized and remodeled.

Psychological preparation and social adjustment for dialysis or transplantation (29)

Few diseases require such dramatic changes of life-style as terminal renal failure. Thus, it is not surprising that maladaptation to the dialysis procedure is quite common. Therefore, it is eminently important to accurately and promptly inform the patient, his or her partner, and his and her family of the need for dialysis without causing undue emotional upset. The procedures and options should be explained, and a discussion of all relevant problems should be offered. Group therapy and patient self-help groups may be quite beneficial. Of special importance is the evaluation of whether, when the patient is on dialysis in the future, the patient will be able to continue his or her present job and social activities.

Symptomatic therapy of neuromuscular symptoms

Neuromuscular changes include the syndrome of "restless legs," muscle cramps, and polyneuropathy. Severe neuromuscular symptoms should be treated by hemodialysis or transplantation, since polyneuropathy is potentially reversible if such treatment is initiated in time. It is advisable to ensure an adequate supply of vitamins (particularly water-soluble vitamins), protein (particularly in elderly patients), and to avoid drug neurotoxicity (especially nitrofurantoin, INH, hydralazine).

Clonazepam has been recommended for the treatment of restless legs, although we have not been particularly impressed by its efficacy. If muscle cramps are not due to sodium depletion, quinidine may be helpful. The drug does not accumulate in renal failure.

Pruritus and prurigo may become incapacitating in patients with renal failure. Recognized causes include: xerosis of the skin (which responds to emollients) and advanced secondary hyperparathyroidism (which responds to treatment with 1,25-$(OH)_2$ vitamin D_3 or parathyroidectomy). In most cases the cause remains unknown and symptomatic therapy must be chosen, e.g., cold showers, sedatives, or antihistaminics in low dosage.

In cases refractory to therapy, UV phototherapy (3 x/week for 6–8 weeks), oral administration of charcoal, or cholestyramine have been advocated.

Special problems in diabetics

Successful medical rehabilitation of diabetics on maintenance hemodialysis or transplantation is limited by the sequelae of retinopathy, hypertension, and atherosclerotic macroangiopathy. Visual impairment, nearly ubiquitous in the past, becomes quite manageable after prophylactic laser therapy of proliferative and preproliferative retinopathy; rigorous blood pressure control, and early dialysis have become the therapeutic standard.

Metabolic control usually becomes easier in uremic diabetics because of reduced dietary intake and increased sensitivity to insulin secondary to a prolonged insulin half-life. As a consequence, hypoglycemia from oral hypoglycemic agents (sulfonylurea) or insulin is common and should be carefully investigated. Malnutrition poses a particular problem in diabetics because of the dual influences of anorexia and habituation to dietary restriction.

Prospective studies suggest that rigorous control of arterial blood pressure retards the development of renal failure in established Kimmelstiel–Wilson's disease. Therefore, control of hypertension in the diabetic assumes even greater importance that in nondiabetic uremic patients. Control is difficult due to the general tendency for sodium retention and orthostatic hypotension in diabetic patients. It has been almost universely accepted that one should aim for earlier dialysis (at a serum creatinine concentration of approximately 7 mg/dl) when treating diabetic patients.

Anaesthesia in uremic patients (30)

Although morbidity and mortality during anaesthesia is clearly higher in uremic patients, renal failure in itself is not a contraindication against elective or emergency surgery. Patients should be well hydrated prior to surgery, because anaesthesia may interfere with renal function. If a major blood loss must be anticipated, the hematocrit should be raised to approximately 30% prior to surgery, because emergency intraoperative transfusions carry the risk of hyperkalemia. In patients with preterminal renal failure (serum creatinine approximately 6–10 mg/dl), it may be wise to dialyze patients prior to elective surgery to reduce the risks of hemorrhagic diatheses of renal failure and hyperkalemia.

Spinal or epidural anaesthesia carries less risk, but even with these modalities a fall in blood pressure and a further reduction in renal function may be observed. All depolarizing muscle relaxants may release potassium so that the serum potassium concentration may increase by up to 2 mM/l. Curare and pancuronium are preferable as relaxants, because gallamin and decamethonium are excreted virtually exclusively via the kidneys. All relaxants, however, carry the risk of postoperative redistribution with secondary relaxation and respiratory insufficiency after extubation. It must also be taken into account that the action of gallamine is potentiated by hypokalemia and after administration of morphine and aminoglycosides.

WHEN SHOULD CONSERVATIVE TREATMENT BE STOPPED?

Temporary dialysis is required in patients with preterminal renal failure when they become hypercatabolic from intercurrent illness and/or surgery (particularly abdominal surgery), or severely symptomatic from fluid overload and uncontrolled hypertension. One particular indication is presented by pregnant patients with renal failure, who almost invariably abort unless dialyzed daily or at least every other day.

Maintenance dialysis or transplantation is indicated when the patient's uremic symptoms can no longer be controlled with conservative management. In the past, nephrologists tended to go to extreme lengths with conservative therapy and to place patients on dialysis only when serum creatinine levels of 15–20 ml/dl had been reached. At present, it has become customary to put patients on dialysis at a GFR of 5–10 ml/min (corresponding to a serum creatinine of approximately 10 mg/dl). One should not however, stick, to narrow rules and should avoid treating biochemistry rather than patients. It appears desirable to start dialysis when a person is unable to continue his or her usual work, social activities, or school activities. Special problems are presented by patients who present with circulatory overload, congestive heart failure, hypertension, progressive peripheral neuropathy, uremic pericarditis, or severe microangiopathy or diabetes mellitus. In such patients, it may be necessary to start dialysis earlier and at higher levels of the GFR.

REFERENCES

1. Bricker NS: Adaptation in chronic uremia. Pathophysiologic "tradeoffs." *Hosp Pract* 9:119–126, 1976.
2. Blythe WB: The management of intercurrent medical and surgical problems in the patient with chronic renal failure. In: LE Early, CW Gottschalk, eds, *Strauss and Welt's Diseases of the Kidney*, 3rd ed, Little, Brown, Boston, 1979.
3. Levin DM, Cade R: Influence of dietary sodium on renal function in patients with chronic renal disease. *Ann Intern Med* 62:213–245, 1965.
4. Cohen MV, Diaz P, Scheuer J: Echocardiographic assessment of left ventricular function in patients with chronic uremia. *Clin Nephrol* 12:156, 1979.
5. D'Cruz IA, Bhatt GR, Cohen HC, Glick G: Echocardiographic detection of cardiac involvment in patients with chronic renal failure. *Arch Int Med* 138:720, 1978.
6. Rostand SG, Gretes JC, Kirk KA, Rutsky EA, Andreoli TE: Ischemic heart disease in patients with uremia undergoing maintenance hemodialysis. *Kidney Int* 16:600, 1979.
7. Vertes V, Cangiano JL, Berman LB, Gould A: Hypertension in end stage renal disease. *N Engl J Med* 280:978, 1969.
8. Bennett WM, Singer I, Golper T, Ferg P, Coggins CJ: Guidelines for drug therapy in renal failure. *Ann Intern Med* 86:764, 1977.
9. Kimberly RP, Plotz PH: Aspirin-induced depression of renal function. *N Engl J Med* 196:418, 1977.
10. Kimberly RP, Bowden RE, Keiser HR, Plotz PH: Reduction of renal function by newer non-steroidal antiflammatory drugs. *Am J Med* 64:804, 1978.
11. Brenner BM, Meyer TW, Hostetter TH: Dietary protein intake and the progressive nature of kidney disease: The role of hemodynamically mediated glomerular injury in the pathogenesis of progressive glomerular sclerosis in aging, renal ablation, and intrinsic renal disease. *N Engl J Med* 307:652–659, 1982.

12. Maschio G, Oldrizzi L, Tessitore N, D'Angelo A, Valvo E, Lupo A, Loschiavo C, Fabris A, Gammaro L, Rugiu C, Panzetta G: Effects of dietary protein and phosphorus restriction of the progression of early renal failure. *Kidney Int* 22:371–376, 1982.
13. Mitch WE: The influence of diet on the progression of renal insufficiency. *Ann Rev Med* 35:249–264, 1984.
14. Rosman JB, Meijer S, Sluiter WJ, Terwee PM, Piers–Bech TPM, Donker AJM: Prospective randomized trial of early dietary protein restriction in chronic renal failure. *Lancet* 2:1291, 1984.
15. Anderson S, Meyer TW, Rennke HG, Brenner BM: Control of glomerular hypertension limits glomerular injury in rats with reduced renal mass. *J Clin Invest* 76:612–619, 1985.
16. Anderson S, Rennke HG, Brenner BM: Therapeutic advantage of converting enzyme inhibitors in arresting progressive renal disease associated with systemic hypertension in the rat. *J Clin Invest* 77:1993, 1986.
17. Reisch CR, Mann J, Ritz E: Konversionsenzymhemmer in der antihypertensiven Behandlung niereninsuffizienter Patienten. *Dtsch Med Wschr* 112:1249, 1987.
18. Hrcik DE, Browning PJ, Kopelman R, Goorno WE, Madias NE, Dzau VJ: Captopril-induced functional renal insufficiency in patients with bilateral renal artery stenosis or renal artery stenosis in a solitary kidney. *K Engl J Med* 308:373, 1983.
19. Massry SG, Goldstein DA, Malluche HH: Current status of the use of $1,25(OH)_2D_3$ in the management of renal osteodystrophy. *Kidney Int* 18:409–418, 1980.
20. Ritz E, Drueke T, Merke J, Lucas PA: Genesis of bone disease in uremia. In: WA Peck, ed, *Bone and Mineral Research/5. A Yearly Survey of Developments in The Field of Bone and mineral metabolism.* Elsevier.
21. Naets JP: Hematologic disorders in renal failure. *Nephron* 14:181–194, 1975.
22. Winearls CG, Oliver DO, Pippard MJ, Reid C, Downing MR, Cotes PM: Effects of human erythropoeitin derived from recombinant DNA on the anaemia of patients maintained by chronic haemodialysis. *Lancet* 2:1175–1177, 1986.
23. Eschbach JW, Egrie JC, Downing MR, Browne JK, Adamson JW: Correction of the anemia of end-stage renal disease with recombinant human erythropoietin. *N Engl J Med* 316:73–78, 1987.
24. Ypersele De Strihou CVY: Potassium homeostasis in renal failure. *Kidney Int* 11:491–504, 1977.
25. Lindner A, Charra B, Sherrard DJ, Scribner BH: Accelerated artherosclerosis and survival in maintenance hemodialysis. *N Engl J Med* 290:697, 1974.
26. Mordasini R, Frey F, Flury W, Kloze G, Greten H: Selective deficiency of hepatic triglyceride lipase in uremic patients. *N Engl Med* 297:1362–1366, 1977.
27. Sanfelippo ML, Swenson RS, Reaven GM: Reduction of plasma triglyceride by diet in subjects with chronic renal failure. *Kidney Int* 11:54–61, 1977.
28. Ritz E, Augustin J, Bommer J, Gnasso A, Haberbosch W: Should hyperlipemia of renal failure be treated? *Kidney Int* 28 (Suppl):S84–S87, 1985.
29. Reichsman F, McKegney FP: Psychosocial aspects of maintenance hemodialysis. In: *Strategy in Renal Failure.* EA Friedman, ed, John Wiley & Sons, New York, Toronto, 1980.
30. Kountz SL, Villanua R: Operating on the uremic patient. In: EA Friedman, ed, *Strategy in Renal Failure.* John Wiley & Sons, New York, Toronto, 198.

CHAPTER 43

Anesthesia and Surgery in the Patient with Renal Failure

DAVID R. BEVAN

INTRODUCTION

Most patients with chronic renal failure(CRF) will receive an anesthetic, either for vascular access before hemodialysis or at the time of renal transplantation. Many have disseminated systemic disease, which increases the problems of anesthesia. The purpose of the present chapter is to review the major obstacles to safe anesthesia, to describe the modification in the activity of anesthetic drugs induced by renal failure, and to recommend safe approaches to anesthesia in the functionally anephric patient. Most patients are now dialyzed within 48 hours of transplantation so that severe cardiovascular and biochemical disturbances are seldom observed at the time of surgery.

SYSTEMIC DISEASE

Cardiovascular disturbances

ANEMIA

The commonest abnormality affecting the cardiovascular system is severe anemia. The causes are discussed elsewhere but include decreased erythropoiesis, hemolysis, bleeding, and iatrogenic blood sampling. In most studies (1–7) the mean hemoglobin concentration at the time of renal transplantation is 6–8 g/100 ml. Despite the more frequent use of preoperative transfusion (8), the hemoglobin concentration before surgery seldom exceeds 10 g/100 ml, a level below which most anesthesiologists often would advise the postponement of surgery (9, 10). The chronic anemia is compensated for by an increase in cardiac output and a shift to the right of the oxyhemoglobin dissociation curve by the stimulation of 2:3 DPG synthesis. Thus the offloading of oxygen at the tissues is increased. Nevertheless oxygen delivery (O_2 delivery = cardiac output × arterial oxygen content) is threatened and may be severely reduced in the presence of cardiac or respiratory disease. In addition, the increase in cardiac output predisposes to the development of congestive failure. Consequently, particular care is taken during and after anesthesia to preserve oxygen delivery with respect to blood loss replacement, oxygen therapy, and cardiovascular support. Most anesthetic agents are associated with some myocardial depression and impairment of pulmonary oxygen transfer, which exacerbate the problem.

HYPERTENSION

The majority of CRF patients are hypertensive. Arrhythmias and myocardial ischemia during anesthesia are common in the untreated hypertensive patient, particularly at the time of laryngoscopy and tracheal intubation (11). If time allows, attempts should be made to gain control of the blood pressure before anesthesia, but if impractical, deliberate hypotensive therapy may be necessary during and after surgery (12). Antihypertensive therapy should continue up to the time of surgery. It appears that the risk of uncontrolled hypertension far exceeds that of impaired cardiovascular responsiveness during surgery.

CONGESTIVE FAILURE

Preoperative fluid volume status will be determined by local hemodialysis practices. Nevertheless, a tendency to fluid overload persists. Some authors have found surprisingly high right- and left-sided filling pressures at the time of transplantation, even in the apparently well-controlled patient (13, 14). Thus, the theoretical advantages of "loading" the transplanted kidney to encourage early function (14, 15) may be hazardous. Uremic pericarditis is a rare complication of CRF but may, theoretically, contribute to hemodynamic complications.

Respiratory disturbances

Good hemodialysis treatment ensures that pulmonary edema is uncommon. Nevertheless the CRF patient usually has a PaO_2 that is lower than expected for his or her age. Several predisposing factors may be involved, particularly infection and, rarely, uremic lung disease. Consequently, attention should be paid to oxygen therapy in the perioperative period, particularly since O_2 delivery is already compromised. Hypoxemia during hemodialysis is common, although the cause is not understood clearly (16).

Electrolytes and hydrogen ion

Severe disturbances are uncommon, but mild hyponatremia and metabolic acidosis are not. The latter may induce hyperventilation and a compensatory respiratory alkalosis, and unless this is appreciated, positive-pressure ventilation without hyperventilation will encourage hyperkalemia (17).

Hyperkalemia is unusual, but if above 6 mEq/l should be treated with glucose, insulin, and calcium. There is a particular danger during anesthesia, because the muscle relaxant succinylcholine usually increases serum potassium concentration by a further 0.5 mEq/l (18), again predisposing to arrhythmias after, the induction of anesthesia. However, it seems that this risk has been exaggerated and a much greater increase in potassium concentration during transplantation occurs if the preserving fluid, with its high K^+ concentration, is not drained from the kidney before anastamotic connections are made (19).

Disordered calcium metabolism and the risk of pathologic fractures necessitate that the unconscious patient be moved carefully.

Alimentary tract

Renal transplantation is performed as an emergency procedure, so it must be assumed that recipients will have full stomachs and be prone to the dangers of regurgitation and pulmonary aspiration if adequate precautions are not taken. In addition, the CRF patient is at greater risk because of delayed gastric emptying (20). However, the routine precautions of preoxygenation, cricoid pressure, and rapid intubation will usually prevent this hazard. The routine use of magnesium trisilicate (4) as an antacid is not advised, as it may lead to hypermagnesemia.

Associated disease

In addition to hypertension, many CRF patients have widespread disease. Diabetes mellitus is common and may add particular vascular and neurologic complications. This will introduce further fluid imbalance if glucose levels are uncontrolled. Autonomic failure might predispose to hemodynamic instability and peripheral neuropathy encourages abnormal responses to neuromuscular blocking drugs (21).

Concomitant drug therapy is common. Those receiving corticosteroids for immunologic control may require additional steroids to maintain hemodynamic stability. However, this is not always necessary and should be administered as required (22). Immunologic suppression increases the risk of infection, and the associated antibiotic therapy may interact with drugs given during surgery, particularly the nondepolarizing muscle relaxants (23).

ANESTHETIC PROBLEMS

Anesthetic agents are fat-soluble compounds and consequently are normally reabsorbed by the kidney. Their termination of action depends upon redistribution, metabolism, and, for inhalational agents, excretion by the lungs. Thus, their action is unaffected in patients with renal disease unless the disease modifies organ sensitivity or unless cardiovascular effects are produced in the CRF patient.

The CRF patient must be handled gently to prevent damage to bone and to shunts and fistulae. For example IV and arterial cannulae and BP cuffs should be avoided on limbs used for hemodialysis access. The danger of sepsis exists so that all anesthetic instruments, laryngoscopes, suction apparatus, tracheal tubes, etc. should be sterilized before use. The immunologically impaired CRF patient may also be a carrier of viral diseases, so that medical staff should take appropriate precautions for their own safety.

The requirements for patient monitoring depend both on the severity and control of the renal failure, and the extent of surgery. In the well-controlled patient, hemodynamic monitoring may be restricted to blood pressure and ECG. However, the unstable patient, in whom considerable fluid and blood shifts are anticipated, will require central venous and probably pulmonary and systemic artery monitoring. The latter should be embarked upon judiciously because of the possible need for peripheral vessels for future hemodialysis.

The aim of anesthesia in the CRF patient is to provide comfort for the patient, access for the surgeon, and to avoid further compromise to the kidney by the direct or indirect effects of anesthesia. It should be remembered that these goals can be achieved by several techniques and that the success of transplantation depends upon immunologic techniques, ischemic time, and operative technique.

Fluid therapy

The principles of fluid therapy in the CRF patient are no different from normal. Fluid will be required for maintenance and to replace losses. Maintenance fluids, approximately 20 ml/kg/day, can be provided by 5% dextrose solution. The composition of other fluid will depend upon the composition of the fluid lost. Blood should be replaced with blood and, if the preoperative hemoglobin concentration is less than 10 g/100 ml, attempts should be made to ensure that it does not decrease during surgery. Third-space losses for intraabdominal operations can be replaced with either 0.9% saline or Ringer's lactate at the rate of approximately 5–10 ml/kg/hr during surgery. In this regard, the risks of fluid and sodium overload have been exaggerated to the detriment of the maintenance of hemodynamic integrity. There is no evidence that fluid loading or the addition of mannitol or loop diuretics improves postperative function in the CRF patient (5, 24).

Premedication

Several years of hemodialysis do not make repeated injections any more comfortable. CRF patients also realize that a successful transplant will have a profound effect on their lives. Understandably, the patients will be anxious before surgery and will require premedication to control their psychologic and cardiovascular states. Opiates, benzodiazapines, and droperidol have all been used successfully. Although these fat-soluble compounds are not excreted via the kidney, large doses of opiates seem to have a prolonged effect in renal failure (25), so that doses are reduced somewhat. Particular care should be taken with repeated narcotic administration after surgery.

Induction of anesthesia

Induction of general anesthesia is usually achieved with an intravenous barbiturate, thiopental. Its duration of action may be prolonged in the uremic patient as a result of decreased plasma protein binding (26), altered cerebral metabolism (27), or increased blood-brain barrier permeability (28). However, the duration of action in the recently dialyzed patient is not altered. Other induction agents, such as methohexital (11) or ketamine (29), produce more problems in the hypertensive patient.

Maintenance of anesthesia

In CRF patients anesthesia is maintained with O_2/N_2O, together with small concentrations of an inhalation agent and/or small doses of narcotics, either alone or as part of a neuroleptanalgesic sequence.

INHALATION ANESTHESIA

The choice of inhalation anesthetic vapors has changed considerably in the last decade. Ether and cyclopropane are avoided because they are flammable; methoxyflurane has been superceded because of a dose-related fluoride-induced, polyuric nephropathy (30, 31); and halothane has become a social outcast from exaggerated fears of the hepatotoxicity. These agents have been replaced by enflurane and isoflurane. Enflurane, like methoxyflurane, is metabolized to inorganic fluoride, but toxic concentrations are only approached in patients with augmented metabolism, isoniazid treatment(32), or who take up large quantities of the drug, such as the obese (33, 34). No untoward effects were observed after its use in 375 renal transplant recipients (35), and there is no evidence that it produces impairment in the restoration of function of the ischemic kidney (36). Thus, former advice to avoid enflurane seems to have been premature (37). Isoflurane, an isomer of enflurane, has been introduced more recently. Isoflurane undergoes less metabolism and is a reasonable, if somewhat expensive, alternative. It appears that anesthetic inhalation agents have little, if any, effect on renal function as long as hypovolemia is avoided.

NEUROLEPTANALGESIA

The combination of narcotics and tranquilizers is know as *neuroleptanalgesia* (NLA). A mixture of fentanyl and droperidol has been shown to maintain cardiovascular stability (38), and it has been suggested that the alpha-

Table 1. Complications associated with succinylcholine

Common	Rare
Hyperkalemia	Malignant hyperpyrexia
Fasciculations	Anaphylaxis
Muscle pains	Prolonged apnea
Myoglobinemia	Pulmonary edema
Cardiac bradyarrhythmias	Severe hyperkalemia
Catecholamine release	
Increased intraocular pressure	
Increased intragastric pressure	

blocking actions of droperidol may protect the kidney from catecholamines (5). Others have commented that a fluid load may be tolerated better with NLA than under halothane anesthesia (39). However, these observations have not been confirmed, so repeated doses of fentanyl (50–100 µg/hr) are often complemented with enflurane or isoflurane.

Muscle relaxation

Neuromuscular blocking drugs are necessary to facilitate tracheal intubation and to allow relaxation for intra-abdominal procedures. Abnormal effects can be anticipated with almost all muscle relaxants in the CRF patient.

DEPOLARIZING RELAXANTS

Succinylcholine is associated with many complications (Table 1), yet it remains the only relaxant with a rapid-onset (1 minute) and brief duration (5–8 minutes), and thus it maintains its place in the anesthetic armamentarium. In renal failure the most severe complication is *hyperkalemia* (19), so that succinylcholine is contraindicated if the serum potassium concentration exceeds 6 mEq/l, although the increase in renal failure is no greater than in normal patients.

Prolonged action of succinylcholine has been observed in renal failure because plasma cholinesterase concentrations are decreased by hemodialysis (40) and after transplantation (41). The latter is accentuated because the immunosuppressant azathioprine potentiates succinylcholine by phosphodiesterase inhibition, leading to increased acetylcholine release (42). Despite these problems, succinylcholine is normally used for rapid sequence induction of anesthesia and tracheal intubation in the emergency patient (1). Others have recommended its use by infusion to maintain neuromuscular blockade, although this function is usually obtained with the nondepolarizing relaxants.

NONDEPOLARIZING RELAXANTS

The kidney is the predominant route of excretion for most of the nondepolarizing relaxants that are ionized, water-soluble compounds. The kidney appears to be the only route of excretion for gallamine (43). Large doses produce plasma concentrations, even after redistribution of the drug, which are associated with a persistent paralysis that

Table 2. Median values for volume distribution (V_{ds}), plasma clearance (Cp), and terminal half-lives (t½ B) from several pharmacokinetic studies in normal patients and patients with renal failure (57)

	Normal			Renal failure		
	V_{ds} (l/kg)	Cp (ml/kg/min)	t½ B (min)	V_{ds} (l/kg)	Cp (ml/kg/min)	t½ B (min)
Atracurium	0.16	5.5	20	0.17	6.3	24
Gallamine	0.26	1.3	163	0.29	0.24	752
Metocurine	0.35	1.3	280	0.30	0.38	684
Pancuronium	0.23	1.9	145	0.25	0.67	534
Tubocurarine	0.39	1.9	239	—	—	330
Vecuronium	0.26	4.6	62	0.24	2.5	97

is overcome only by hemodialysis (45). The kidney is of graded importance for the excretion of other drugs: gallamine > metocurine > d-tubocurarine, pancuronium > vecuronium >> atracurium.

The liver forms an alternative route of excretion that is particularly important for vecuronium. The only nondepolarizing relaxant whose pharmacokinetic (47) and pharmacodynamic (48) activities are not altered in renal failure is atracurium, which undergoes spontaneous breakdown (49) and metabolism by nonspecific plasma esterases (50).

The sensitivity of the neuromuscular junction to the relaxants is not altered in renal failure (51) and neither is their volume of distribution (52, 53). Several pharmacokinetic studies have quantified the extent of the impaired clearances among the relaxants (Table 2). Similar doses, on a milligram per kilogram basis, are required to produce neuromuscular blockade, but the duration of block (54), with all except atracurium, will be prolonged, and repeated doses produce an increasing effect, cumulation, particularly with pancuronium.

It has been suggested that atracurium is the relaxant of choice in CRF. However, its short duration of action and possible hemodynamic effects from histamine release suggest its imperfections.

REVERSAL OF NEUROMUSCULAR BLOCKADE

The drugs used to antagonize muscle relaxants — anticholinergics and anticholinesterases — are also water-soluble, ionized compounds excreted by the kidney (57, 58). Indeed, the reduction of plasma clearance of the anticholinesterases is greater than can be explained by a decrease in GFR, so they are probably secreted actively into the tubular lumen (59). The reversal agents are given in normal doses in CRF. The fear of recurarization, reparalysis after initial antagonism as a result of differential rates of excretion of the relaxant and antagonist, is unlikely. Once adequate recovery has been established, reparalysis will not occur (60).

Regional analgesia

Several surgical procedures in the CRF patient are suitable for performance under regional analgesia. Brachial plexus block, axillary or interscalene, is ideal to allow the creation of shunts and fistulae in the arm. Some (61) but not all (62) investigators have noticed that the duration of action of the local anesthetic agents may be reduced in CRF. Regional analgesia becomes more difficult when several sites are required. Bilateral axillary blockade is inadvisable because of the risk of bilateral pneumothoraces.

Spinal or epidural analgesia has been recommended for renal transplantation (1, 63). They have the possible advantage of blockade of the autonomic stress responses to surgery. However, most patients prefer to sleep. Some consider epidural analgesia to be contraindicated in the patient with a hemorrhagic tendency (64), but there are no reports of epidural hematoma formation in the CRF patient.

PROTECTING THE KIDNEY

Major surgery in the CRF patient is often followed by deterioration in renal function. Several regimens have been recommended in an attempt to preserve function. Fluid loading, either in an arbitrary fashion or to predetermined indices of left atrial pressure, has been performed both for general surgical procedures (15) and renal transplantation (15, 65, 66). Unfortunately, most studies have been poorly controlled retrospective reviews, and the evidence has not been convincing. Such fluid administration is not without risk unless accompanied by CVP and pulmonary artery pressure measurement, because of the ease with which these patients can be induced into pulmonary edema (13, 14).

Similarly, routine diuretic administration with either mannitol or loop diuretics is of no proven benefit (24). Renal vasodilatation with low-dose dopamine 2–5 µg/kg/min has been attempted in the transplant donor (67) or the nontransplant patient (68). Again, the therapy is logical but has not proved to be effective.

At the present state of our knowledge, renal function seems to be preserved best by ensuring hemodynamic stability, by correcting preexisting fluid losses, and by replacing all fluid lost. Cardiovascular stimulant agents have a place in the compromised patient, but specific "renal" therapy needs to be justified.

REFERENCES

1. Vandam LD, Harrison JH, Murray JE, Merrill JP: Anesthetic aspects of renal homotransplantation in man. *Anesthesiology* 23:783–789, 1962.
2. Strunin L: Some aspects of anaesthesia for renal homotransplantation. *Br J Anaesth* 38:812–822, 1966.
3. Bastron RD, Bailey G, Deutsch S, Vandam LD: Anesthesia for patients with chronic renal failure for renal homotransplantation. *Anesthesiology* 30:335–336, 1969.
4. Samuel JR, Powell D: Renal transplantation. Anaesthetic experience of 100 cases. *Anaesthesia* 25:165–176, 1970.
5. Monks PS, Lumley H: Anaesthetic aspects of renal transplantation. *Ann Coll Surg Engl* 50:354–366, 1972.
6. Slawson KB: Anaesthesia for the patient in renal failure. *Br J Anaesth* 44:277–282, 1972.
7. Logan DA, Howie HB, Crawford J: Anaestheia for renal transplantation: An analysis of fifty-six cases. *Br J Anaesth* 46:69–72, 1974.
8. Uldall PR, Wilkinson R, Dewar PJ, et al.: Factors affecting the outcome of cadaver renal transplantation in Newcastle upon Tyne. *Lancet* 2:316–319, 1977.
9. Kowalyshyn TJ, Prager D, Young J: A review of the present status of preoperative hemoglobin requirements. *Anesth Analg* 51:75–80, 1972.
10. Gillies IDS: Anaemia and anaesthesia. *Br J Anaesth* 46:589–602, 1974.
11. Prys-Roberts C, Meloche R, Foex P: Studies of anaesthesia in relation to hypertension. I. Cardiovascular responses of treated and untreated patients. *Anesthesiology* 50:285–292, 1979.
12. Goldman L, Caldera DL: Risks of general anesthesia and elective operation in the hypertensive patient. *Anesthesiology* 50:285–292, 1979.
13. Cronnelly R, Kremer PF, Beaupre P, Cahalan MK, Salvatierra O, Feduska N: Hemodynamic response to fluid challenge in anesthetized patients with end-tidal renal disease. *Anesthesiology* 59:A49, 1983.
14. Carlier M, Squifflet J-P, Pirson Y, Gribomont B, Alexandre GPJ: Maximal hydration during anesthesia increases pulmonary arterial pressures and improves early function of human renal transplants. *Transplantation* 34:201–204, 1982.
15. Tasker PRW, MacGregor GA, de Wardener HE: Prophylactic use of intravenous saline in patients with chronic renal failure undergoing major surgery. *Lancet* 2:911–912, 1974.
16. Eiser AR: Pulmonary gas exchange during hemodialysis and peritoneal dialysis: Interaction between respiration and metabolism. *Am J Kidney Dis* 6:131–142, 1985.
17. Goggin MJ, Joekes AM: Gas exchange in renal failure. I. Dangers of hyperkalaemia during anaesthesia. *Br Med J* 2:244–247, 1971.
18. Koide M, Waud BE: Serum potassium concentrations after succinylcholine in patients with renal failure. *Anesthesiology* 36:142–144, 1972.
19. Soulillou JP, Fillaudeau F, Keribin JP, Guenel J: Acute hyperkalemia risks in recipients of kidney graft cooled with Collins' solution. *Nephron* 19:301–304, 1977.
20. McNamee PT, Moore GW, McGeown MG, Doherty CC, Collins BJ: Gastric emptying in chronic renal failure. *Br Med J* 291:310–311, 1985.
21. Azar I: The response of patients with neuromuscular disorders to muscle relaxants: A review. *Anesthesiology* 61:173–187, 1984.
22. Symreng T, Karlberg BR, Kagedal B, Schildt B: Physiological cortisol substitution of long-term steroid-treated patients undergoing major surgery. *Br J Anaesth* 53:949–954, 1981.
23. Sokoll MD, Gergis SD: Antibiotics and neuromuscular function. *Anesthesiology* 55:148–159, 1981.
24. Salaman JR, Calne RY, Pena J, Sells RA, White HJO, Yoffa D: Surgical aspects of clinical renal transplantation. *Br J Surg* 56:413–417, 1969.
25. Don HF, Dieppa RA, Taylor P: Narcotic analgesics in anuric patients. *Anesthesiology* 42:745–747, 1975.
26. Ghoneim MM, Pandya H: Plasma protein binding of thiopental in patients with impared renal or hepatic function. *Anesthesiology* 42:545–549, 1975.
27. Richet G, de Novales EL, Verroust P: Drug intoxication and neurological episodes in chronic renal failure. *Br Med J* 2:394–395, 1970.
28. Freeman RB, Sheff MF, Maher JF, Schreiner GE: The blood cerebrospinal fluid barrier in uremia. *Ann Intern Med* 56:233–240, 1962.
29. Hobika GH, Evers JL, Mostert JW, Trudnowski RJ, Moore RH, Murphy GP: Comparison of hemodynamic effects of glucagon and ketamine in patients with chronic renal failure. *Anesthesiology* 37:654–658, 1972.
30. Crandell WB, Pappas SG, Macdonald A: Nephrotoxicity associated with methoxyflurane anesthesia. *Anesthesiology* 27:591–595, 1966.
31. Cousins MJ, Mazze RI: Methoxyflurane nephrotoxicity. A study of dose response in man. *JAMA* 225:1611–1614, 1973.
32. Mazze RI, Woodruff RE, Heerdt ME: Isoniazid-induced enflurane defluorination in humans. *Anesthesiology* 57:5–8, 1982.
33. Miller MS, Gandolfi AJ, Vaughan RW, Bentley JB: Disposition of enflurane in obese patients. *J Pharmacol Exp Ther* 215:292–296, 1980.
34. Rice SA, Fish KJ: Anesthetic metabolism and renal function in obese and nonobese Fischer 344 rats following enflurane or isoflurane anesthesia. *Anesthesiology* 65:28–34, 1986.
35. de Temmerman P, Gribomont B: Enflurane in renal transplantation: Report of 375 cases. *Acta Anaesthesiol Scand* 71 (Suppl):24–31, 1979.
36. Wickstrom I: Effects of enflurane anesthesia on the function of ischemically damaged kidneys. *Acta Anaesthesiol Scand* 71 (Suppl):15–19, 1979.
37. Bastron RD: Anesthetic considerations in patients with renal disease. *ASA Refresher Courses* 128:1–4, 1981.
38. Mostert JW, Evers JL, Hobika GH, Moore RD, Murphy GP: Circulatory effects of analgesic and neuroleptic drugs in patients with chronic renal failure undergoing maintenance dialysis. *Br J Anaesth* 42:501–505, 1970.
39. Kay B: Antidiuretic effects of anaesthesia and neuroleptanaesthesia (NLA). In WF Henschel, ed, *International Bremer NLA Symposium*. Schattaner Verlag, Stuttgart, p 135, 1975.
40. Holmes JH, Makamoto S, Sawyer KC: Changes in blood composition before and after dialysis with the Kalff twin coil kidney. *Trans Am Soc Artif Intern Organs* 4:16–18, 1958.
41. Ryan DW: Postoperative serum cholinesterase activity following successful renal transplantation. *Br J Anaesth* 51:881–884, 1979.
42. Dretchen KL, Morgenroth VH, Standaert FG, Walts LF: Azathioprine: Effects on neuromuscular transmission. *Anesthesiology* 45:604–609, 1976.
43. Ramzan MI, Shanks CA, Triggs EJ: Gallamine disposition in surgical patients with chronic renal failure. *Br J Clin Pharmacol* 12:141–147, 1981.
44. Feldman SA, Levi JA: Prolonged paresis following gallamine: A case report. *Br J Anaesth* 35:804–806, 1963.

45. Singer MM, Dutton R, Way WL: Untoward results of gallamine administered during bilateral nephrectomy: Treatment with haemodialysis. *Br J Anaesth* 43:404–407, 1971.
46. Lebrault C, Berger JL, D'Hollander AA, Gomeni R, Henzel D, Duvaldestin P: Pharmacokinetics and pharmacodynamics of vecuronium (ORG NC 45) in patients with cirrhosis. *Anesthesiology* 62:601–605, 1985.
47. Fahey MR, Rupp SM, Fisher DM: The pharmacokinetics and pharmacodynamics of atracurium in patients with and without renal failure. *Anesthesiology* 61:699–702, 1984.
48. Hunter JM, Jones RS, Utting JE: Use of atracurium in patients with no renal function. *Br J Anaesth* 54:1251–1258, 1982.
49. Stenlake JB, Waugh RD, Dewar GH, Hughes R, Chappel DJ, Coker GG: Biodegradable neuromuscular blocking agents. Part 4. Atracurium besylate and related polyalkylene di-esters. *Eur J Med Chem* 16:515–524, 1981.
50. Nigrovic V, Pandya JB, Auen M, Wajskol A: Inactivation of atracurium in human and rat plasma. *Anesth Analg* 64:1047–1052, 1985.
51. Bevan DR, Donati F, Gyasi H, Williams A: Vecuronium in renal failure. *Can Anaesth Soc J* 31:491–496, 1984.
52. Somogyi AA, Shanks CA, Triggs EJ: The effect of renal failure on the disposition and neuromuscular blocking action of pancuronium bromide. *Eur J Clin Pharmacol* 12:23–29, 1977.
53. Fahey MR, Morris RB, Miller RD, Nguyen T-L, Upton RA: Pharmacokinetics of ORG NC45 (Norcuron) in patients with and without renal failure. *Br J Anaesth* 53:1049–1053, 1982.
54. Miller RD, Stevens WS, Way WL: The effect of renal failure on the duration of pancuronium neuromuscular blockade in man. *Anesth Analg* 52:661–665, 1973.
55. Fahey MR, Morris RB, Miller RD, Sohn YJ, Cronnelly R, Gencarelli P: Clinical pharmacology of ORG NC45 (Norcuron). *Anesthesiology* 55:6–11, 1981.
56. Shanks CA: Pharmacokinetics of the non-depolarizing neuromuscular relaxants applied to calculation of bolus and infusion dose regimens. *Anesthesiology* 64:72–86, 1986.
57. Cronnelly R, Stanski DR, Miller RD, Sheiner LB, Soh YJ: Renal function and the pharmacokinetics of neostigmine in anesthetized man. *Anesthesiology* 51:222–226, 1979.
58. Morris RB, Cronnelly R, Miller RD, Stanski DR, Fahey MR: Pharmacokinetics of edrophonium in anephric and renal transplant patients. *Br J Anaesth* 53:1311–1314, 1981.
59. Rennick BR: Renal tubule transport of organic cations. *Am J Physiol* 9:F83–F89, 1981.
60. Bevan DR, Archer DP, Donati F, Ferguson A, Higgs BD: Reversal of pancuronium in renal failure: No recurarisation. *Br J Anaesth* 54:63–68, 1982.
61. Bromage PR, Gertel M: Brachial plexus anesthesia in chronic renal failure. *Anesthesiology* 36:488–493, 1972.
62. Beauregard L, Martin R, Tetrault J-P: Brachial plexus block and chronic renal failure. *Can J Anaesth* 34:S118, 1987.
63. Wyant GM: The anaesthetist looks at tissue transplantation: Three years experience with kidney transplants. *Can Anaesth Soc J* 14:225–234, 1967.
64. Lofstrom B: Anaesthetic problems in renal transplantation. *J Urol Nephrol* 1:161–169, 1967.
65. Luciani J, Frantz P, Thibault P, Ghesquiere F, Conseiller C, Cousin M-T, Glaser P, LeGrain M, Viars P, Kuss R: Early anuria prevention in human kidney transplantation. Advantages of fluid load under pulmonary artery pressure monitoring during surgical period. *Transplantation* 28:308–312, 1979.
66. Tiggeler RGWL, Berden JHM, Hoitsma AJ, Koene RAP: Prevention of acute tubular necrosis in cadaveric kidney transplantation by the combined use of mannitol and moderate hydration. *Ann Surg* 201:246–251, 1985.
67. Raftery AT, Johnson RWG: Dopamine pretreatment in unstable kidney donors. *Br Med J* 1:522, 1979.
68. Parker S, Cardon GC, Isaacs M, Howlands WS, Kahn RC: Dopamine administration in oliguria and oliguric renal failure. *Crit Care Med* 9:630–632, 1981.

CHAPTER 44

Nutritional Management of the Uremic Patient

MARKUS TESCHNER & AUGUST HEIDLAND

INTRODUCTION

The dietary treatment of patients with chronic renal failure has many components. These include appropriate protein intake, sufficient adequate calories, and vitamins and trace element supplements (1). The clinical importance of the adequate dietary management of uremic patients is evident since uremia is characterized by a state of wasting and malnutrition (2–7).

The fact that many studies dealing with a low-protein diet and its effect on the progression of renal disease report a stable nutritional status of patients (8–10) seems surprising. However, these reports substantiate the crucial role of nutritional management in the prevention of wasting, since the nutritional intake of patients participating in these studies was carefully monitored.

REASONS FOR WASTING IN CONSERVATIVELY TREATED CHRONIC RENAL FAILURE (Table 1)

The pathogenesis of malnutrition in chronic uremia is probably multifactorial (11). Protein-energy undernutrition, however, has frequently been suggested as an important mediator of wasting in chronically uremic patients as well as in those on regular dialysis therapy (2,4,5,12). Poor dietary intake is due to anorexia, which is related to uremic toxicity, medicinal intake, emotional depression, or intercurrent illness (13). Furthermore, patients with renal failure are sometimes prescribed diets that are too low in protein intake or are inadequately supplemented by ketoacids or essential amino acids (14) and, in addition, are difficult to prepare and unpalatable to eat (15). Patients with chronic renal failure also develop an aversion to sweet products (16), as their taste recognition, especially for sweet and bitter foods, is impaired in uremia (17), and thus these patients may have difficulties in obtaining sufficient amounts of energy.

An overt clinical symptom of malnutrition is skeletal muscle wasting, which provides, as the main reservoir for body proteins, an increased supply of amino acids for the enhanced metabolic activity of the liver. Animal studies suggest that chronic uremia per se may promote mild catabolism and protein wasting (18). Up to now, it has not been completely determined whether decreased protein synthesis or enhanced protein degradation is responsible for muscle wasting. It has been suggested that muscle protein synthesis is reduced in fed rats with chronic renal failure (19) and enhanced protein degradation has also been demonstrated in experimental chronic uremia (20).

The multitude of endocrine disorders in clinically stable patients with chronic renal failure may also promote protein wasting (21). The resistance of target organs towards the anabolic action of insulin (22), as well as the enhanced levels of catabolic hormones such as glucagon (23) or PTH (24), might play a key role in uremic catabolism. Since 1949, glucocorticoids, as the classic catabolic hormones, have been suggested to play a considerable role in the protein catabolism of acute uremia (25), and this has recently been substantiated by Schaefer et al. (26). As far as the role of glucocorticoids in chronic renal failure is concerned, they might indirectly promote catabolism via insulin resistance, which leaves the catabolic effects of glucocorticoids on skeletal muscle unopposed (27).

Finally, metabolic acidosis of uremia represents a strong stimulus for protein breakdown (28) and may be an important mediator of catabolism in chronic renal failure.

Intercurrent illnesses such as infections and septicemia further increases protein catabolism in chronic renal failure, as it is the major catabolic factor in acute renal failure (29). The principal metabolic event in septicemia involves massive and apparently irreversible skeletal muscle proteolysis, called septic autocannibalism (30). A circulating peptide in patients suffering from septicemia was identified by Clowes et al. as playing a role in the pathogenesis of muscle proteolysis (31). Baracos et al. (32) suggested this peptide might be leukocyte pyrogen (interleukin 1). This peptide was assumed to stimulate muscle to produce prostaglandin E_2, thereby inducing enhanced proteolysis (33). Interleukin 1 is secreted during infections by monocytes and macrophages (34). It is interesting that the effect of interleukin 1 on protein breakdown is considerably enhanced during fever. Using incubated epitrochleares muscles from rats, a given dose

Table 1. Potential reasons for uremic malnutrition

Inadequate dietary intake
Enhanced protein breakdown due to
  Insulin resistance
  Catabolic hormone
    Glucocorticoids
    Glucagon
    PTH
  Metabolic acidosis
  Enhanced protease activity
  Intercurrent illness
    Septicemia
    Fever
    Congestive heart failure
Renal replacement therapy
  Regular hemodialysis treatment
    Losses of peptides, amino acids, glucose
    Blood losses
    Catabolic stimulus of the procedure
  Peritoneal dialysis
    Losses of proteins, peptides, amino acids (cave peritonitis!)
    Enhanced risk of reduced nutritional intake

Table 2. Diagnostic parameters for routine nutritional assessment in patients with chronic uremia

Nutritional intake
  Dietary interviews
  Dietary diaries
Protein intake
  Urinary urea excretion
  Plasma urea/creatinine ratio
  UNA
Anthropometric measurements
  Relative body weight
  Skinfold thickness
  Mid-arm-muscle circumference (MAMC)
Biochemical measurements
  Pseudocholinesterase
  Visceral proteins
    Albumin
    C_3, Clq
    Transferrin

of interleukin 1 at 39°C causes two or three times more rapid proteolysis than incubation at 36°C (35).

Hence, in conservatively treated patients with renal failure, there are many reasons for developing wasting. However, the degree of wasting is usually mild or moderate; only in a small percentage of patients, especially in those suffering from infectious complication, is it severe (36). The incidence of overt malnutrition increases in patients on renal replacement therapy who have to face the additional catabolic stress of hemodialysis or peritoneal dialysis treatment.

GUIDELINES FOR ASSESSING A PATIENT'S COMPLIANCE TO PROTEIN INTAKE AND NUTRITIONAL STATUS IN UREMIA (Table 2)

The assessment of nutritional status in chronic renal failure is complicated by the fact that many of today's traditional parameters, originally established to monitor the body composition of nonuremic individuals, have been shown to be markedly influenced by uremia (2). However, nutritional assessment guidelines are important in allowing early detection and categorization of the nutritional deficiency in order to start and control therapeutic interventions (37). In general, nutritional assessment is not a static diagnostic procedure. Accurate and reliable information about the patient's situation is based on serial (longitudinal) data. There are three cornerstones to evaluating a patient's adherence to dietary prescription and his nutritional status: assessment of dietary intake and anthropometric and biochemical measurements (2).

Assessment of dietary intake

Since a reduced dietary intake represents a leading factor in malnutrition, its assessment with the aid of dietary interviews and diaries (38, 39) is useful. According to El Nahas (40), a 4-day dietary history is usually adequate and correlates well with the true dietary intake. Apart from its diagnostic value, the interviews give the chance to engage the cooperation of the patient in the nutritional management of his or her disease (41).

In order to assess protein intake, apart from measuring the urinary urea excretion, the plasma urea/creatinine ratio has also been used (42). In a metabolically stable state, however, the relationship between the serum urea/creatinine ratio and protein intake may be influenced by the muscle mass, as well as by urine flow, as urea clearance may fall disproportionally compared with that of creatinine when the urine flow is low (16). The assessment of net urea generation or urea nitrogen appearance (UNA) (43), respectively, should avoid this disadvantage. UNA, which closely correlates with nitrogen intake as well as output, as long as the patient is in neutral nitrogen balance, is measured as the sum of urinary excretion plus accumulation (positive or negative) in the body pool of urea nitrogen (2). The calculation of the latter is based on the assumption that the concentration of urea is equal throughout the whole body fluids (44). That means that the urea space represents approximately 60% of the body weight. Changes in body weight during the 1 to 3-day period of assessing UNA have to be considered. They are supposed to be due to the gain or loss of body water. Thus, UNA can be calculated from the following equation,

$$\text{UNA (gN/day)} = \text{Urinary urea N (g/day)} + (SUN_f - SUN_i) \times 0.6\,BW + (BW_f - BW_i) \times SUN_f,$$

where i and f are the initial and final values for the period of measurement (15).

In patients undergoing hemodialysis treatment, UNA is usually calculated during the interdialytic interval, because the urea concentration in dialysate is low and is difficult to measure accurately (15). The same problem exists in peritoneal dialysate. In patients on CAPD, measurements of UNA are not very useful. Furthermore, in these patients, UNA is low due to protein, amino acid, and peptide loss in the dialysate and do not accurately reflect nitrogen intake (45).

If a patient is severely catabolic, nitrogen balance (the relationship of protein synthesis and degradation) is of special interest. It might roughly be estimated as the difference between nitrogen intake and UNA minus the average nonurea nitrogen excretion (44), which is approximately 31 mg N/kg BW/day (46).

In conclusion, the results of nitrogen balance studies have to be critically interpreted (11). They are influenced by previous dietary intake and the nutritional status of the patient (47). Malnourished patients may attain nitrogen equilibrium with less protein intake than well-nourished subjects (47). Therefore, attainment of nitrogen equilibrium is an uncertain parameter of nutritional adequacy if malnourished patients are studied. Furthermore, the results of short-term studies inadequately reflect disturbances of long-term conditions (48). Thus, the evaluation of the nutritional state has to be performed using additional parameters.

Body composition in uremic patients

Standard tests of nutritional assessments are largely quantitative measurements of body composition (49) and are markedly influenced by renal failure itself (2). As far as body weight and related indices are concerned, fluid retention or loss may influence these measurements (4). Up to now, there has been no agreement as to which index of body weight should be used as a basis for setting nutritional goals. The relative body weight (defined as the patient's weight, compared with the weight of normal persons of the same age, sex, and height) or premorbid weight might be the clue to nutritional goals in uremic patients (50). Blumenkrantz et al. attempt to maintain a patient at no less than 100% of his or her relative body weight.

Evaluation of somatic protein and fat components

Body weight indices, of course, do not indicate the proportion of body weight that is composed of fat, muscle, or body water (51). This is important in order to differenciate between the two types of protein and caloric malnutrition, which are kwashiorkor (depletion of somatic and visceral protein; increase in fat stores) and marasmus (depletion of proteins and fats) (2). Furthermore, restoration of lost weight does not necessarily mean successful nutritional care. For instance, it may derive from an increase in fat stores, a common event in patients on CAPD treatment. Replenishment of protein losses without weight gain may be a better goal (50).

With the neutron-activation and whole-body counting techniques presently available, the proportions of body composition can now be differentiated by direct measurements of the body cell mass via the total body potassium (TBK) and protein stores via the total body nitrogen (52).

Measurements of TBK with the aid of very sensitive detectors are based on the concept that potassium contains a natural radioactive tracer K^{40}, which emits a high-energy gamma ray (53). In chronic renal failure, however, potassium homeostasis is severely disturbed (54–56), rendering TBK less useful for the assessment of nutritional status in uremia (57). Isotopes of nitrogen do not occur naturally. They can be made radioactive, however, by neutron irradiation of the subject. Their measurement with very sensitive detectors is thought to very accurately reflect the body protein content ($+3\%$) (58) and has been successfully employed to study protein stores in patients on hemodialysis treatment (52).

However, these measurements do not fulfill the fundamental prerequisites for routine use in the assessment of the nutritional status of uremic patients: ease of use and low cost.

Since body fat closely correlates with subcutaneous fat, anthropometric measurements of skinfold thickness obtained from three different locations are thought to give inexpensive and reproducible information on body fat (2). The accuracy of this measurement is quite good in lean individuals but is poor in very obese patients (53). Skeletal muscle mass forms a major store for protein (57) and is commonly estimated from measurements of mid-upper-arm circumference. In order to estimate mid-arm-muscle circumference (MAMC) one has to calculate the mid-arm circumference from subcutaneous tissue (MAMC = mid-arm circumference (cm) $- 0.314 \times$ triceps skinfold thickness) (2). However, the data from such measurements have to be interpreted with caution. According to several studies, these anthropometric parameters have such a wide range of variance that only gross changes can be distinguished (59, 60). Thus, it is not surprising that MAMC correlated poorly with TBN in malnourished nonuremic patients as reported by Jeejeehoy et al. (58). Buzby et al. (61) did not find a correlation between nutritional risk factors and MAMC.

The basic requirement for anthropometric measurements is to get serial data on the same patient (50). In the patients on renal replacement therapy, anthropometric measurements should only be recorded when the patients are at dry body weight, since measurements of skinfold thickness and MAMC are influenced by a state of overhydration (37).

Evaluation of the visceral protein compartment by measuring serum proteins

Transport proteins have been used extensively to assess protein malnutrition in both uremic and nonuremic patients (62–65). However, the reliability of plasma proteins as an indicator of protein status is somewhat suspect, despite the widespread acceptance of serum albumin, prealbumin, retinol-binding protein, and transferrin as such indicators (50). To be reliable indices of protein status, the parameters must not respond to any other commonly encountered noxious influence (66). Apart from dietary factors, albumin concentration in plasma is lowered by pneumonia, trauma (67), and hepatic disease (66). Hypoalbuminemia in uremic patients has been corrected by renal transplantation, suggesting that it is related to uremia rather than to malnutrition (4).

Serum transferrin levels are supposed to react more sensitively to protein deficiency and to be less influenced by the state of hydration (68, 69). Because of the shorter half-life of transferrin (8-9 days) in comparison with albumin (20 days), the former might respond more rapidely to alterations in the diet (2). However, serum transferrin levels increase when iron stores are depleted, and they are diminished in iron overload and in patients with chronic diseases such as malignant tumors or rheumatoid arthritis (44). Particularly questionable is the validity of albumin and transferrin as nutritional indicators in patients on hemodialysis treatment. Periodic infusions of salt-poor albumin, given during hemodialysis to facilitate fluid removal, or multiple blood transfusions increasing the iron load, (70) rendering albumin and transferrin levels less useful as indicators of protein stores (37). Thus, it is not surprising that in the assessment of nutritional status in the National Cooperative Dialysis Study population, anthropometric measurements, together with dietary intake analyses, gave more appropriate data to determine the adequacy of nutritional therapy than the assessment of serum proteins, which had low sensitivity and specifity for the detection of nutritional abnormalities (71).

Many other serum proteins have been evaluated in uremia as nutritional indices, including prealbumin and retinol-binding protein (2). However, several reports demonstrate increased concentrations of both of these proteins, which have a rapid turnover, in chronic renal failure (72, 73), emphasizing the role of the kidney in the degradation of low molecular weight proteins (74).

In summary, there are many methods available for estimating the nutritional status of uremic patients. Single measurements, for example, of serum proteins, are appropriate to alert the clinician of the need to conduct a detailed evaluation of the patient's nutritional status. Combined serial anthropometric and biochemical measurements, together with dietary interviews, probably offer the best approach to routine assessment of the nutritional status.

PROTEIN RESTRICTION IN RENAL DISEASE

The fact that a protein-poor diet results in the amelioration of many uremic symptoms in patients with severe chronic renal failure was established as early as 1918 (75). With a decrease in functional renal mass, the waste products of protein metabolism accumulate in proportion to the loss of renal function; protein-poor diets thereby not only decrease urea levels, but also reduce the accumulation of phosphate, sulfate and numerous organic acids and amines, all of which are substances that may contribute to uremic toxicity (76). However, as early as 1961 it was recognized that it is difficult to bring a uremic patient into positive nitrogen balance during protein restriction (77).

The maintenance of protein stores in uremic patients is the primary aim of dietary treatment designed to prevent malnutrition. The preservation of nitrogen balance in a steady state requires an equilibrium between dietary protein, endogenous stores of amino acids, rates of protein breakdown, protein synthesis, and amino acid oxidation (78).

A proper balance of this complex protein metabolism can only be achieved if the concentrations of essential and nonessential amino acids are held stable. However, this is not assured if the protein intake is low, which causes a decrease in serum concentrations of essential amino acids but no change in those of nonessential amino acids. The relative decrease in plasma essential amino acid levels compared to nonessential amino acid levels is supposed to be a very sensitive indicator of protein malnutrition (79). An abnormal plasma amino acid composition contributes to amino acid imbalance, with the consequence of impaired protein synthesis (80, 81), since protein synthesis is thought to depend primarily on the availability of sufficient amounts of both the essential and nonessential amino acids, in the proper proportions and concentrations, in the intracellular pool (82, 83). In 1964, Giovanetti and Maggiore (84) pointed out that, despite substantially lower daily intakes of protein (20-25 g), nitrogen balance may be achieved if the proportion of essential amino acids (EAAs) in the selected protein is high. They supplemented a low-protein diet containing 1-1.5 g N (6-10 g protein) per day with proteins of high biologic value (egg protein), so-called high-quality proteins, corresponding to 1.5-2.2 g of N/day or the recomended daily intake of EAAs according to Rose (85). This clinical study was based on the data of Giordano (86), which proved that uremic patients on protein-free diets can be brought into a positive nitrogen balance when given EAAs.

These findings led to the development of a variety of diets with the common principle of supplying uremic patients with low quantities of high-quality proteins (approximately 0.3 g/kg BW/day). A beneficial effect on uremic toxicity was commonly observed (87-92). However, uremic patients on this diet usually were in a negative nitrogen balance (93-95). In time, these patients often died without uremic symptoms but had a progressive loss of body protein nitrogen (1). According to Giovanetti (96), however, these reports wrongly brought discredit upon dietary treatment for chronic uremia, since the negative results were often obtained in the presence of contraindications to dietary treatment such as poor compliance and concomitant illness (97).

Low protein diets supplemented with essential amino acids (EAA)

The very rigid restriction of using only proteins that are of high biologic value led to a monotonous and unpalatable diet. It is very fortunate that Bergström and coworkers created an alternative protein-restricted diet that is much more palatable and variable, and hence is easier for patients to accept. This diet contains 15-20 g of mixed-quality protein in conjunction with amino acid supplementation, which fulfills the demand for EAAs, so that there is no need for prescribing dietary protein of only high biologic value (98). The amino acids are supplemented in an amount that provides a nitrogen intake comparable to a diet containing 0.6 g protein/kg BW/day (1).

According to Mitch and Walser (44), EAA mixtures are the most efficiently used sources of nitrogen, i.e., they lead to the lowest rates of urea nitrogen appearance. Originally EAAs were supplemented in an amount that is two or three times the minimum requirements, but in the proportion recommended by Rose for normal humans (85), with the addition of histidine (98). Initially, this regimen sucessfully achieved a positive nitrogen balance in combination with a low-protein diet (16–20 g protein/day). Long-term treatment, however, failed to have this beneficial effect. It has been proposed that this is due to providing EAAs according to the regimen of Rose (85), which does not reflect the disturbed amino acid pattern in chronic renal failure. Although this pattern is similar to that seen in patients with protein malnutrition (99), it cannot be explained solely on this basis, since the abnormalities also occur in the presence of an adequate protein intake (44). Until now, several defects in amino acid metabolism have been identified in renal failure, including impaired conversion of citrulline to arginine (100); impaired hydroxylation of phenylalanine (101, 102), with resulting high phenylalanine and low thyrosine concentrations, accelerated destruction of valine (103), and altered protein binding of tryptophan (104). Finally, in uremia, there are high glycine levels (105) and low or normal levels of serine, perhaps due to diminished production of serine from glycine by the diseased kidney (106). Furthermore, it must be emphasized that in uremia the amino acid pattern is not an accurate reflection of the pattern within tissues such as muscle. Fürst et al., for example, found reduced plasma and intracellular levels of valine but normal muscle and low plasma concentrations of leucine (80) and isoleucine (107).

Based on the assumption that deficient intracellular amino acid pools may impair protein synthesis in patients with severe uremia, Alvestrand et al. (108) applied a low-protein diet (16–20 g/day) supplemented by a new amino acid formula with the addition of thyrosine, an amino acid that has been shown to be critically deficient in uremic patients treated with an EAA preparation, according to Rose (85) a higher proportion of valine and a lower proportion of phenylalanine. Improved nitrogen utilization was achieved by means of this amino acid formulation indicating that amino acid formulas reflecting the specific amino acid abnormalities of uremia might improve the problem of maintaining protein stores in severely uremic patients despite a protein-deficient diet.

Low-protein diet supplemented with ketoacids

For uremic subjects, it is especially important to ensure that the total intake of amino acids is sufficient to maintain nitrogen equilibrium but is not excessive, which would lead to the unnecessary accumulation of waste nitrogen. One means of achieving this goal is to supply a portion of the daily EAA requirements as nitrogen-free amino-acid analogues (109, 110), since as early as 1966 it was demonstrated that alpha-keto analogues of EAAs might spare nitrogen more efficiently than EAAs themselves in patients with chronic renal failure. These compounds are converted into amino acids by transamination reactions (111). Keto analogues administered as calcium salts were shown to be adequate substitutes for several EAAs [all but lysine and threonine (109)]. Later, the hydroxy analogues of methionine (112) and phenylalanine (113) were introduced as adequate dietary substitutes for the corresponding amino acids in uremia. Clinical results with a mixture of five l-analogues (i.e., the calcium salts of analogues of valine, leucine, isoleucine, methionine, and phenylalanine) and four EAAs, including l-histidine, were first reported by Walser et al. in patients on a mixed low-protein diet (109). He demonstrated a beneficial effect of such mixtures on nitrogen balance in comparison to EAA supplementation alone. These results have been confirmed by several other authors (114–116).

In 1982, Mitch et al. (117) reported on the long-term effects of a low-protein diet (20–25 g/day) supplemented with a combination of mixed salts formed from basic amino acids and keto analogues of EAAs in patients with severe chronic renal failure (mean GFR = 4.8 ml/min). The supplement was designed to minimize or reverse the amino acid abnormalities of chronic renal failure. In fact, as chronic renal failure is characterized by subnormal plasma concentrations of branched-chain amino acids (118) and branched-chain keto acids (119), the combination applied by Mitch et al. contained a high proportion of branched-chain keto acids but no phenylalanine and tryptophan and very little methionine. This analogue supplement regimen was able to forestall the need for dialysis therapy in those patients with end-stage kidney disease by an average of about 7 months, while maintaining protein stores. In addition, their nutritional status improved.

In addition to the advantage of a diminished nitrogen intake, a beneficial effect of the analogues on nutritional status — as measured by anthropometry, plasma protein levels, or nitrogen balance (120–124) — must be explained by a protein-sparing effect (76). The keto analogue of leucine has been shown, in contrast to leucine itself, to exert such a nitrogen-sparing effect (125). In a clinical study, a reduction of nitrogen wasting in postoperative patients following infusions of keto leucine was observed, although leucine did not have this beneficial effect (126). Mitch assumes this to be one important factor modulating the improvement of protein nutrition observed in these patients (117). Interestingly, no benefit was seen on a negative nitrogen balance from the supplementation of keto analogues when the level of nitrogen intake was greater than 20–30 g protein/day (127, 128). Presumably the more rapid oxidation of ketoacid that occurs when protein intake is increased (129) explains the different response (76).

Originally, nutritional studies of keto analogues always faced the problem of gastric distress. The high calcium content of the mixture of analogues and amino acids might have contributed to the gastrointestinal distress, apart from hypercalcemia (130, 131). Additionally, the calcium salts of branched-chain keto acids and of phenylpyruvate have a very unpleasant taste and must be taken as coated granules or tablets. In recent studies, the calcium salts of analogues (except for the calcium salt of the hydroxy analogue of methionine) have been replaced by mixed salts, which are formed from branched-chain keto acids and basic amino acids. Such mixtures are more soluble and less unpalatable than the calcium salts and can therefore be taken as powders dissolved in water or fruit juice (76).

Hence, in patients with severe uremia, a keto acid supplemented very-low-protein diet (20–30 g/day) might represent a realistic possibility for preserving protein stores while ameliorating uremic toxicity. However, careful assessment of nutrition is mandatory, since it has recently been demonstrated that some patients develop severe protein depletion when maintained on a very-low-protein diet supplemented by essential amino acids and keto acids (132).

When should protein restriction be started and how should it be adapted to renal function?

Patients with early renal failure are subjectively symptom free and, with the exception of anemia and hypertension, they do not have objective symptomatology. Low-protein diet (0.6 g protein/kg BW/day) at this stage of renal failure (serum creatinine <3 mg/dl), as advised by Giovanetti (97), may only have the benefit of slowing the progression of renal disease. It is doubtful, however, whether nitrogen equilibrium can be maintained in all patients with a diet that provides so small an amount of protein, despite a high proportion of high-quality proteins, since a recent review by the FAO/WHO/UNU Special Committee on Studies in Third World Countries has recommended 0.76 g/kg/day to ensure a sustaining nitrogen balance in most of the population (133). This is an increase when compared with the previous recommendation of 0.6 g/kg/day (134), which has been shown to be inadequate for some healthy subjects.

Furthermore, there is no reason to assume that patients with chronic renal failure, who are supposed to be in a catabolic stress, have a reduced protein requirement. This was recently confirmed by Guarnieri et al., who stated that patients with early renal insufficiency (mean serum creatinine 2.1 mg/dl) maintained on a long-term low-protein diet (0.6 g/kg BW/day 2/3 of high biologic value) and phosphate restriction (700 mg/day) have to be carefully monitored with regard to their nutritional and metabolic status since some of these patients have developed mild nutritional abnormalities such as a low serum protein content (11). Therefore, it is certainly useful that Alvestrand and Bergström (16) advise supplementing a diet providing 0.6 g protein/kg/day with a small amount of EAAs (5–10 g/day) in order to avoid malnutrition in all patients.

Uremic symptoms do not occur until the SUN is greater than 90 mg/dl. Thus, when focusing only on the prevention of uremic intoxication rather than the progression of renal disease, protein restriction is not necessary until the GFR is below 25 ml/min (15). According to Kopple, protein intake may be restricted progressively as the GFR falls according to the following guideline: a) GFR = 20–25 ml/min — protein intake=60–90 g/day; b) GFR = 15–20 ml/min — protein intake=50–70 g/day; c) GFR = 10–15 ml/min — protein intake=40–55 g/day (15).

When renal failure deteriorates with the appearance of uremic toxicity, a further restriction of protein intake becomes necessary. In patients with a GFR > 10 ml/min, a diet providing about 40 g protein/day containing a high proportion of high-quality protein might be adequate (95). However, in severe uremia (GFR < 5 ml/min) one has to switch to the very-low-protein diet (0.3 g protein/kg BW/day) supplemented by EAAs or KAs in order to avoid uremic toxicity.

Severe uremia certainly represents the most dangerous situation of developing malnutrition and wasting, since dietary prescription, especially at this stage of renal disease, critically faces the contradictory problem of limiting uremic toxicity while maintaining a good nutritional profile. There are several studies providing evidence that in patients with end-stage renal disease held on 20–30 g protein/day supplemented by EAAs or KAs, protein depletion does not occur (108, 117). However, there is a striking difference in nutritional status between non-dialyzed patients with a GFR of 5 ml/min and patients starting maintenance dialysis treatment, suggesting that some events during this brief period between these two stages of advanced renal failure produce wasting or malnutrition (21). Despite the beneficial effects of new formulas of EAA or KA supplementation (108, 117) on nutritional status in severe uremia, if the renal function is irreversibly reduced to less than 5% of normal, nutritional therapy should only be used until an adequate excess for dialysis is available (i.e., during maturation of an arteriovenous fistula) (44). Since it seems very difficult to improve nutritional status after hemodialysis therapy has started, nutritional therapy at this stage of renal disease should not primarily focus on postponing hemodialysis treatment rather than maintaining a good nutritional profile. The clinical relevance of this problem is indeed demonstrated by the fact that malnutrition prior to the initiation of dialysis is associated with a higher morbidity and mortality rate after the initiation of dialysis (2, 135). Very recently, El Nahas (40) warned not to exchange the benefits from postponing dialysis therapy by protein restriction for the loss of physical fitness at the time dialysis is started.

ADDITIONAL CATABOLIC FACTORS OF THE HEMODIALYSIS PROCEDURE

When dialysis is commenced, theoretically, the patient's nutritional status should improve, since the described wasting factors due to uremia should be alleviated by renal replacement therapy and since the patient's originally strictly reduced protein intake can be liberalized, rendering the diet more palatable. However, patients on regular hemodialysis treatment are particularly at risk of developing malnutrition (135, 137). Apart from the fact that uremia is only partially corrected (137), hemodialysis per se induces additional factors that may induce malnutrition. During dialysis and in the 24 hours after each dialysis, the patient may experience a number of symptoms, e.g., headache and vomiting, that lead to a reduction of food intake (137). According to Levine, the incidence and extent of depressed nutritional intake is especially pronounced in the population of diabetic patients on hemodialysis (138). Gastroparesis diabeticorum, a neuropathy associated with diabetes mellitus, is thought to be one major cause of the poor nutritional state of diabetic patients on regular hemodialysis treatment, as has recently been described by Miller et al. (70). Its symptoms include epigastric pain, early satiety, nausea, and vomiting (139).

The picture of malnutrition in hemodialysis patients does not suggest a simple caloric deficiency (140). Despite seemingly adequate protein intake, many patients display subclinical signs of protein deficiency (63). There are several reasons why the nitrogen requirements of hemodialysis patients are much greater than those of normal individuals or conservatively treated patients with chronic renal failure (141).

The amino acid and peptide losses into the dialysate are about 1–2 g of amino acids/dialysis/hr (142–144). This is dependent on the amino acid concentration in the blood, the type of membrane, the surface of the dialyzer, the transmembraneous pressure gradient, the blood flow rate, and the duration of dialysis (142, 143, 145). The total losses of amino acids could amount to 10–13 g/dialysis (146).

Wasting is further intensified by blood losses related to blood drawing, occult and profound gastrointestinal bleeding, and sequestration of blood in dialyzers (147). According to Kluthe, the total amount of blood loss per year is 6–8 l in a patient on regular hemodialysis treatment (148). These losses, however, do not solely account for the increased protein requirements of those patients (140). The blood membrane interaction during hemodialysis treatment is supposed to be an additional catabolic stimulus (141). The extensive protease release from leukocytes during the hemodialysis procedure has thereby been thought to represent a catabolic stimulus (149). Recently, Henderson (150) suggested that the negative side effects of hemodialysis might be due to a periodic release of interleukin at each hemodialysis, a known stimulator of protein breakdown, via enhanced prostaglandin E_2 liberation in skeletal muscle. In keeping to this hypothesis, Alvestrand et al. (151) demonstrated the strong catabolic stimulus of sham dialysis in healthy subjects to be prevented by indomethacin, suggesting that the enhanced protein breakdown due to the blood-membrane interaction is mediated by prostaglandins.

Finally, treatment regimens for hemodialysis patients aimed at the prevention of wasting have to reflect additional disorders currently present in this population. This includes effective chemotherapy in infectious disease, prevention of congestive heart failure, and fluid overload. Furthermore, Feinstein recommends the careful control of hyperparathyroidism, which may also cause severe debility and promote protein wasting (152).

Malnutrition as a mortality factor in patients on maintenence hemodialysis

Up to now, there exists no single study of uremic patients demonstrating, in a prospective and controlled fashion, that malnutrition or wasting, in itself, is associated with increased morbidity or mortality (152). In a noncontrolled prospective French study (Diaphane Registry), however, malnutrition was found to play a key role in the survival of those patients maintained on regular hemodialysis treatment (135). Low levels of body mass index, cholesterol, and triglyceride, as well as low urea predialysis blood levels, were associated with increased overall as well as cardiovascular mortality. Similarly, Acchiardo et al. (12) demonstrated that morbid events occurred more commonly in dialysis patients with an inadequate protein intake. In contrast to experiments with the general population, hypercholesteremia and hypertriglyceridemia do not seem to represent mortality risk factors in hemodialysis patients (153–155), although one could expect that a high cardiovascular mortality rate in RDT patients is related to the rapid progression of coronary artery disease due to the high atherogenic potential of their chronic uremic hyperlipemia.

Thus, these data indicate that, in addition to elevated blood pressure, adequate nutrient intake strikingly influences the prognosis of hemodialysis patients. In addition to cardiovascular mortality, infection and septicemia are important morbid events for malnourished hemodialysis patients (156). A causal relationship with malnutrition could be assumed, since in many studies a close correlation between nutritional status and reduced immunocompetence has been established (157, 158). Hobbs et al. reported that dialysis patients with albumin levels < 4 g/dl display a fivefold increase in the incidence of septicemia compared with patients whose serum albumin levels are > 4 g/dl (159). More recently, Wolfson has suggested a poor nutritional status of hemodialysis patients to be a cause of impaired lymphocyte function, thereby promoting the danger for a higher mortality rate (7).

Protein intake in patients on maintenance hemodialysis

Because of the prognostic importance of malnutrition, close attention should be paid to dietary prescription during maintenance dialysis treatment. The adequacy of hemodialysis therapy, however, may directly influence the nutrient intake of hemodialysis patients, since those who are suboptimally dialysed often develop anorexia and therefore decrease their caloric intake (71). Lowry et al. reported that the occurrence of morbid events in hemodialysis patients is associated with high BUN levels (160), which, in this case, do not reflect a high protein intake but instead reflect reduced urea clearance due to inadequate hemodialysis treatment. The patients of the National Cooperative Dialysis Study (160) with high BUN levels and a poor outcome suffered from malnutrition, since underdialysis seems to trigger a feedback mechanism, decreasing their dietary intake of nutrients and thereby reducing the level of metabolic waste products. Hence, an important prerequisite for successful nutritional therapy in patients on maintenance hemodialysis is adequate blood purification, thereby improving appetite with a subsequent increase of protein and caloric intake.

As already pointed out, patients on maintenance hemodialysis display many factors to develop malnutrition and wasting. Dialysis treatment further adds to catabolism of uremia by its effects on food intake, by blood loss, and by direct amino acid loss through dialysis itself. Despite careful instructions and considerable efforts, it is often difficult to achieve an optimal nutritional status in dialysis patients. This is demonstrated by the fact that, according to several reports (62, 63, 161), malnutrition exists even in dialysis patients who are on apparently adequate diets. Up to now, there has been no agreement as to whether in these patients low-caloric (162–164) or low-protein intake (62) predominates. There is no doubt, however, that as a consequence of malnutrition protein depletion is a common finding in these patients (62, 63, 162, 163, 165, 166), regardless of whether intake of proteins or calories is inadequate. This is not surprising, since the importance of energy intake for normal protein metabolism is well known (167, 168).

In the 1960s, when dialysis treatment was performed once or twice weekly, the patient's malnutrition worsened with a recommended daily dietary protein intake of 0.7–0.8 g of mixed dietary protein per kilogram of body weight (169). In the 1970s, however, when dietary treatment could be liberalized due to an improved dialysis procedure, protein malnutrition was even demonstrated in patients with seemingly adequate dietary adherence, including in those with a protein intake of 1 g/kg BW/day (62, 63, 161), indicating that the protein requirements of hemodialysis patients probably exceed those of normals and, in particular, of conservatively treated uremic patients. This was convincingly demonstrated by Borah et al., who showed that, despite a daily protein intake of 1.4 g protein/kg BW, the nitrogen balance of patients was still negative on dialysis days (170).

The problem of inducing uremic symptomatology due to a protein intake of 1.25 g/kg BW/day, as described by Kopple (171), will certainly not occur with the dialysis regimen currently used (148). The tolerance of protein intake with respect to uremic toxicity, however, is not unlimited in hemodialysis patients. Furthermore, even by using the most effective current hemodialyzers, correction of severe hyperphosphatemia is difficult if the protein intake is high (172).

Heidland and Kult (63) tried to overcome this problem by supplementing a diet containing 1.0 g/kg BW/day protein by 16.75 g EAAs and histidine intravenously at the end of each dialysis treatment, when protein synthesis is supposed to be accelerated (173). The concept of this trial was to equalize the amino acid losses during hemodialysis as one main factor of protein depletion in these patients. Furthermore, low plasma levels, of EAAs are frequently present in patients on maintenance hemodialysis, even when the diet contains theoretically adequate amounts of protein (137), substantiating the notion that EAA supplementation in these patients might be useful in maintaining nutritional status. In fact, the authors demonstrated that within 16 weeks of such treatment, a substantial reversal of protein malnutrition could be achieved. Similar results were obtained by Wolfson et al. (146), who, however, favored intravenous infusions of amino acids throughout the whole dialysis procedure. According to their results, this leads only to a marginal increase of free amino acid losses into the dialysate but avoids fluid overload, which could occur when nutrients are given at the end of hemodialysis. More recently, Acchiardo et al. indicated that oral supplementation of EAAs on a long-term basis is also an effective nutritional support for hemodialysis patients maintained on a diet of 1 g protein/kg BW/day (174). Rather than supplementing EAAs, Kluthe (148) recommends protein intake of 1.2 g/kg BW/day (0.8–0.9 g of high biologic value protein), since hemodialysis patients maintained on a diet of 1 g protein/kg Bw/day display subclinical signs of protein malnutrition. Alternatively, however, he also advises the intake of 1 g protein + 0.2 g/kg BW of amino acid supplementation or 1 g + 0.2 g/kg BW of high biologic value protein supplementation.

Up to now, there has been no agreement on the exact amount of recommended daily protein intake in patients on hemodialysis treatment. The current tendency is to raise the originally recommended daily protein intake of 1 g (171) slightly to 1.2 g protein/kg BW/day in order to maintain an optimal nutritional status in stable hemodialysis patients. Instead of supplementing EAAs intravenously or orally, losses of amino acids may be compensated to a certain extent by allowing a normal food intake during hemodialysis, although this has been questioned, since Grodstein et al. have demonstrated that gastric emptying is impaired even during uneventful hemodialysis in relatively healthy patients (175). To the wasted and malnourished patient who eats poorly, has gastrointestinal malfunction, or has catabolic stress due to intercurrent illness, the infusions of amino acids and glucose offer an opportunity to supplement dietary protein and energy intake as well as to replace the loss of amino acids during dialysis (146).

Another possibility of providing nutrients during dialysis treatment is through their addition to the dialysate, which was proposed as early as 1966 as a possibility for avoiding amino acid losses due to dialysis therapy (176). Recently, Feinstein et al. reintroduced this principle, proposing that the addition of glucose and amino acids to the dialysate fluid might be an important route to nutritional therapy in malnourished patients on regular hemodialysis treatment, thereby obviating the need for fluid administration (177). According to their results, however, efficient uptake of adequate amounts of nutrients requires that the dialysate flow rate is reduced markedly, thereby prolonging the treatment time. Thus, at least in a regular hemodialysis treatment, this strategy of nutritional treatment increases the workload of the medical staff and reduces the utilization of the dialysis facilities.

A more realistic idea for preventing the catabolic stress of hemodialysis treatment by manipulating the composition of the dialysate represents the proposition of adding glucose to the dialysate, therby theoretically reducing amino acid losses by as much as 50% (144). Kopple suggested that the use of glucose-containing dialysate facilitates glucose absorption through the dialysis membrane, leading to enhanced cellular uptake and decreased plasma levels of amino acids, making them less available for loss during dialysis. However, despite a similar study design, recently Ono et al. could not confirm these results (135).

ADDITIONAL FACTORS PROMOTING WASTING IN CAPD PATIENTS

Because of the growing importance of peritoneal dialyses, especially of CAPD, as dialysis therapy for patients with end-stage renal disease (178–180), the metabolic and nutritional effects reveal potentially critical limitations of this treatment (181). The metabolic effects consist of hypertriglyceridemia, probably in part induced by glucose uptake from the peritoneal dialysate (182). The absorption of large quantities of glucose may also contribute to obesity (183) and the initial weight gains in CAPD patients (182) without signs of fluid overload. As far as the nutritional effects are concerned, many patients undergoing long-term treatment with CAPD suffer from subclinical protein malnutrition and aggravation of muscle and plasma-free amino acid abnormalities (185, 186). It is well established that after 1 year of treatment CAPD patients may develop a significant decrease in their total body nitrogen, accompanied by lowered serum levels of albumin and transferrin (57, 187). Similar to hemodialysis treatment, it is thought that the dialytic procedure of CAPD per se also stimulates protein catabolism. Mediating substances could be microbial products (endotoxins), acetate, silicon, or other products from the system that elute into the peritoneal cavity (141). These compounds could stimulate peritoneal macrophages to produce interleukin 1 and other mediators, which in turn could induce protein catabolism (141). A CAPD-related production of peritoneal interleukin 1 has recently been reported (188). Furthermore, malnutrition appears to be brought about by a combination of decreased appetite and increased nutrient loss in the dialysate. Initially daily protein losses in patients on acute or chronic intermittent peritoneal dialysis were demonstrated to vary from 25 g to more than 200 g per dialysis (189–191). On CAPD, protein losses between 5 and 15 g/day have been described (179, 192, 196). This includes a considerable variety of proteins representing several functional classes such as albumin (192), immunglobulis (197), transferrin, and complement factors (192, 199). Differences in dietary protein intake, ultrafiltration volume (78), frequency and duration of dialysis (193, 194), and body surface area (137) may influence the quantity of protein losses. Furthermore, dialysate protein losses increase dramatically with peritonitis.

As far as the losses of free amino acids in clinically stable CAPD patients are concerned, they also vary in different studies; in fact, losses between 1.7 and 3.5 g/day have been described (198, 200–202). According to Dulaney (199) and Kopple (202), losses of proteins and amino acids should easily be replaced by an adequate intake of nitrogen.

Lack of appetite, however, often hinders the patient's compliance to a protein-rich diet (57). Abdominal distention because of the presence of dialysate in the peritoneal cavity may cause anorexia. Nausea, vomiting, and abdominal fullness often accompany CAPD (50); all of these interfere with food consumption. Similarly, hyperglycemia, caused by absorbed glucose, especially when hypertonic solutions are used as an osmotic agent, may also decrease appetite (203). Physicians and dietitions often face the problem that, despite careful and repeated consultation and supervision, patients spontaneously decrease the recommended level of nutrient intake (57, 203). Because of increased gastrointestinal symptoms, patients further reduce their nutrient intake when they suffer from peritonitis (204), which is especially deleterious to their nutritional status, since protein losses into the dialysate increase and, of course, the infection per se represents a strong catabolic stress. The adverse effect of recurrent peritonitis on nutritional status has recently been described by Rubin et al. (205).

Protein requirements in CAPD patients

The prognostic importance of nutritional status in CAPD patients is underlined by the data of Mackow et al. (206) demonstrating that patients with a low BUN or low nitrogen intake studied retrospectively have an increased incidence of morbidity and mortality early in the course of CAPD.

Current recommendations are that patients on CAPD consume 1.2–1.5 g protein/kg BW/day and that at least 50% be of high biologic value (45, 50, 206, 207) in order to compensate for the protein and amino acid losses into the dialysate and to ensure an equilibrated or even positive nitrogen balance (57). Clinically stable CAPD patients maintained on diets containing 0.96–1.44 g protein/kg BW/day have been shown to achieve a neutral or even a positive nitrogen balance (45, 206, 207).

Recently Schilling et al. indicated that long-term CAPD patients on a daily protein intake of 0.9 g/kg BW for women and 1.0 g/kg BW for men will lose body nitrogen (57). The great variability in protein needs depends on the amount of energy intake (50) or the varying quantities of nutrient losses into the dialysate. Since patients' adherence to a recommended anabolism-promoting daily intake of 1.5 g protein/kg BW has been shown to be poor (203), the recommended daily protein intake should probably be nearer to 1.2–1.3 g/kg BW (45). This recommendation slightly exceeds the recently demonstrated daily protein requirements for clinically stable patients undergoing CAPD (1.1 g/kg BW/day), based on the consideration that there will be variability among subjects in the calculations of recommended dietary allowances (208).

Malnourished patients on CAPD or those with intercurrent illnesses such as peritonitis might have greater protein needs. Since food intake is limited, alternative methods of treatment have been suggested.

In the case of these patients, Oreopoulus (209), recommended the replacement of glucose dialysate with a mixed amino acid solution. Following this procedure, one would hope to minimize the undesirable effects attributed to glucose absorption and to provide enough nitrogen to replace protein losses and to compensate for inadequate protein intake (181). Khanna et al. have demonstrated that a dialysate solution containing 2% amino acids produced similar amounts of ultrafiltration in comparison with a 4.25% dextrose solution (203). Furthermore, by the sixth hour of dialysis, 85–95% of the amino acids present in the dialysate have been shown to be absorbed (203). Oren studied the long-term effects, of alternating 2 l of 1% amino acid solutions with dialysate containing glucose in CAPD patients. He found an improved nutritional status from this therapy, as indicated by an increase in total body nitrogen and serum transferrin after 4 weeks of treatment (181).

In CAPD patients with peritonitis, however, nutritional supplementation with amino-acid-containing solutions failed to induce beneficial effects on a negative nitrogen balance (210).

ENERGY REQUIREMENTS IN CHRONIC RENAL FAILURE

Although the nephrologist's interest primarily concerns nitrogen homeostasis in uremic patients, energy is the body's first demand for maintenance of overall body balance. Metabolic and functional aspects of living are driven by energy (50). According to anthropometric data on malnourished chronically uremic patients and on patients on maintenance hemodialysis treatment, caloric malnutrition is a major aspect of their wasting (2–7, 163, 164, 182, 202). According to several studies (2, 148, 163), the energy intake of chronically uremic nondialyzed patients, as well as that of dialyzed patients, is below normal, i.e., 20–30% below 35 kcal/kg BW/day, which is the amount recommended by the Committee on Dietary Allowances, Food and Nutrition Board for Normal Adults (212). The energy expenditure of normals, of nondialyzed patients with chronic renal failure, and of patients on regular hemodialysis treatment was recently evaluated (36). According to Monteon et al. (36), the energy expenditure for a given physical activity in uremic patients — regardless of whether they are dialyzed or not — is not different from that of normals.

Since the amount of physical work carried out each day by uremic patients is estimated to not be different from normal, their reported low energy intake may be inadequate for their needs. Hence, their low energy intake does not seem to be an adaptive response to their low energy requirements, and this may be one factor causing wasting and malnutrition (36). A uremic patient is thus not able to reduce his or her basal energy expenditure as soon as energy intake decreases, as normals are (213). In conclusion, it seems suitable to gear recommendations of energy intake in uremic patients, regardless of whether or not they are on renal replacement therapy, to those of normal individuals. In contrast to the approximately doubled protein requirements of chronically stable patients on hemodialysis or CAPD in comparison to normal subjects or nondialyzed uremic patients, the energy requirements do not differ among these groups. In fact, energy recommendations for uremic patients, as for nonuremic individuals, should be based on their relative body weights. Severely underweight patients should receive extra calories, and patients who are more than 3% overweight should receive a restricted caloric intake (44).

An adequate caloric intake in the form of carbohydrate and fat will spare amino acids for use in synthesis and maintenance rather than for gluconeogenesis (50). The importance of energy intake for nitrogen balance has recently been demonstrated by Kopple et al. (214), who fed a low-protein diet (0.5 g/kg BW/day) to six clinically stable nondialyzed patients with chronic renal failure yet their energy intake varied between 45 and 15 kcal/kg BW/day. A daily energy intake of 35 kcal/kg BW was adequate to achieve neutral or positive nitrogen balance; low energy intakes were accompanied by a negative nitrogen balance, although the protein intake remained constant.

If energy requirements are not fulfilled by patients on renal replacement therapy, or are increased due to intercurrent illness and cannot be provided by dietary intake, energy supplementation such as amino acids, should be considered during the dialysis procedure. In stress states, the demand for glucose as a major cellular energy substrate increases. Liver and muscle glycogen stores are rapidly depleted. A subsequent release of gluconeogenic amino acids from skeletal muscle provides for the maintenance of adequate glucose concentrations (215). In order to interrupt this process, Wolfson et al. suggest providing for the enhanced energy demands of those patients by infusing hypertonic glucose throughout the hemodialysis procedure (146), in addition to amino acids. Due to a high blood flow, hypertonic glucose solutions can be infused into the venous line without causing damage to the peripheral vessels. Wolfson et al. advise that if glucose infusions are used, it is important to administer a carbohydrate source, such as bread, during the last 20–30 minutes of infusion to avoid reactive hypoglycemia (146). Although the addition of glucose to the dialysate makes it theoretically possible to supply energy in hemodialysis patients, it should not be used as a routine procedure because of the risk of bacterial growth in the glucose-containing dialysate.

In patients on CAPD, however, glucose absorption from the peritoneal cavity may provide a valuable source of energy to uremic patients. According to Gahl et al., 75% of dialysate glucose is absorbed, independent of what has been eaten, providing 20–30% of total calories (207). These additional calories from the peritoneal cavity certainly play an important role when patients on CAPD become anabolic due to a protein intake of 1.4 g/kg BW/day (45); however, patients on hemodialysis treatment do not become anabolic at a similar level of protein intake (170).

Taking into account the amounts of calories lost from the peritoneal cavity, Blumenkrantz (216) and Kopple (15) recommend the intake of 25–30 kcal/kg BW/day in CAPD patients, depending on the patient's mobility and state of health. Schilling proposes an intake of at least 23–24 kcal/kg BW/day to be compatible with long-term treatment on CAPD (57). Recently, however, Lindholm et al. suggested that a patient's spontaneous decrease in caloric intake within 1 year on CAPD from 34.6 to 28.7 kcal/kg BW/day was an important factor in the impairment of nitrogen balance that was commonly seen in his patients within the study period (217). Thus, energy recommendations should exceed 25–30 kcal/kg BW/day in patients on CAPD so that minimal energy requirements are met. In malnourished CAPD patients, it may be advisable to increase the number of exchanges with hypertonic glucose-containing dialysate (4.25%) to enhance their energy intake (218).

THERAPEUTIC APPROACHES TO LIPID ABNORMALITIES IN CHRONIC RENAL FAILURE

Dietary prescription in chronic uremia also faces the problem of hypertriglyceridemia. The characteristic uremic lipid abnormalities are reminiscent of those of Type IV hyperlipoproteinemia i.e., a moderate increase in serum triglycerides with essentially normal serum cholesterol (219). High-density lipoprotein (HDL) cholesterol concentrations tend to be somewhat reduced (220). In some cases, hypertriglyceridemia may be further accentuated by increased hepatic production of triglyceride-rich very-low-density lipoproteins (VLDL), partically mediated by increased levels of circulating insulin (221).

The major defect leading to hyperlipidemia in uremia is thought to be impaired lipoprotein catabolism due to diminished post heparin lipolytic activity (PHLA), particularly hepatic triglyceride lipase (222). Furthermore, reduced activities of lecithin cholesterol acyl transferase (LCAT) have been described (223). Recently Gnasso et al. (224) demonstrated that abnormalities in lipoprotein metabolism are not limited to end-stage renal failure. In addition to abnormalities in the composition of lipoprotein subclasses, they found diminished activities of hepatic triglyceride lipase activity in patients prior to end-stage renal failure. The total cholesterol and triglycerides were unchanged.

The nature of the lipid abnormalities in patients with end-stage kidney disease is compatible with those established as risk factors for coronary heart disease (225). However, the association between cardiovascular mortality and lipid abnormalities is not a cause and effect relationship. On the contrary, according to epidemiologic studies of patients on hemodialysis, hypertriglyceridemia cannot be demonstrated to play a role in the pathogenesis of accelerated atherogenesis (12). However, the more pronounced lipid abnormalities of white hemodialysis patients in comparison with black patients have been suggested to explain the higher cardiovascular mortality rates of whites (226). Thus, even though prospective controlled studies do not convincingly exclude uremic lipid abnormalities from being involved in the enhanced cardiovascular mortality rate of these patients, the improvement of such lipid abnormalities might be considered to be one of the major objectives of dietary therapy in patients with chronic renal failure.

A pharmacologic approach may be useful in the treatment of the lipid abnormalities. Clofibrate has been shown to increase the lipoprotein lipase activity of hemodialysis patients to normal, thereby correcting hypertriglyceridemia and decreasing HDL cholesterol (227). The active metabolites of clofibrate, however, accumulate in uremia and may cause toxicity (228). Hence, dietary intervention should be preferred. If this is not successful, extremely low doses of clofibrate may be suitable.

According to several clinical studies, uremic hyperlipemia can be beneficially influenced by dietary manipulations (229–231). A low-carbohydrate diet, for example, can lower high levels of serum triglycerides in nondialyzed patients with chronic renal failure (232). Over the last decades, many studies have shown that large amounts of polyunsaturated fat in the diet have a pronounced hypolipemic effect (233). This is also true in patients with chronic renal failure (234). Psukamato et al. demonstrated a significant decrease in serum triglycerides of 28% and an increase of HDL cholesterol levels due to consumption of a diet high in polyunsaturated fats (P/S ratio 4.2) (234). The high content of polyunsaturated fatty acids was obtained using highly polyunsaturated vegetable oils, such as safflower salad oil, which contains large amounts of the omega-6 fatty acid, linoleic acid.

However, according to Ritz (235), despite the efficacy of dietary interventions it is uncertain whether one should exchange the possible benefit of ameliorating lipid abnormalities for the disadvantage of an additional dietary impact on patients who are frequently anorexic and may easily become malnourished when put on restricted diets.

Carnitine supplementation may also reduce hyperlipidemia (236). This amino acid is required for the transport of fatty acids across the mitochondrial membrane, and seems to be deficient in hemodialysis patients (140). However, this has not been convincingly proved.

Another newly recognized aspect of the treatment of hyperlipidemia is the beneficial effect of fish oil on lipid abnormalities. It has been suggested that the low death rate from coronary heart disease among the eskimos of Greenland may be explained by their high consumption of fish (237). The fat of marine animals contains large quantities of long-chain highly polyunsaturated omega-3 fatty acids (238). According to Phillipson (233), the Eskimo diet differs from the typical American diet in at least two ways: a) It is somewhat low in saturated fatty acids and 2) more importantly, the primary polyunsaturated fatty acids in the Eskimo diet are of the omega-3-family, consisting largely of eicosapentaenoic (20:5 omega-3) and docosahexaenoic (22:6 omega-3) acids, rather than linoleic acid (18:2 omega-6), which is the predominant polyunsaturated fatty acid in the American diet. Very recently, it has been shown in a prospective study that an average daily intake of 30 g of fish had a substantial protective effect on the mortality from coronary heart disease (239). Phillipson demonstrated that a 4-week diet containing fish oil caused a marked reduction in the concentration of triglyceride-rich lipoproteins in the plasma of patients with hypertriglyceridemia. In contrast, a diet containing vegetable oil, i.e., a lot of linoleic acid, was less effective (233).

The beneficial effect of fish oil on lipid abnormalities has also been demonstrated in hemodialysis patients (240, 241), using fish oil capsules, which contain primarily eicosapentaenoic and docosahexaenoic acids. In fact, a significant decrease in triglycerides (240) and an increase in HDL cholesterol (240, 241) have been described.

Hypertriglyceridemia is especially pronounced in patients on CAPD. Both the absorption of large quantities of glucose (218) as well as the reduction of the catabolic clearance of very low density lipoprotein (VLDL) might contribute to this condition (50). Recently fish oil capsules were successfully used to lower hypertriglyceridemia in CAPD patients. Similarly, HDL cholesterol levels were shown to increase due to the intake of these capsulas (242).

Another potentially beneficial effect of omega-3 polyunsaturated fatty acids in atherogenesis is, in addition to besides their interference with the normal metabolism and function of platelets (241, 243), the blood pressure lowering effect of fish oil intake, which has been demonstrated in hemodialysis patients (240, 241). This effect is suggested to be induced by vasodilator prostaglandins from eicosapentaenoic acid modifying vascular reactivity (241).

Hence, fish oil consumption might provide a possible therapeutic approach that could diminish the mortality rates from cardiovascular or cerebral insult in hemodialysis patients by ameliorating important and proved risk factors of atherogenesis, such as hypertension, as well as possible risk factors, such as lipid abnormalities. However, up to now prospective controlled studies are lacking in this population.

VITAMINS

Inadequate dietary supply of vitamins in patients with chronic renal failure is due in part to anorexia and dietary restrictions of protein and phosphorus (41), since protein- and phosphorus-rich nutrients such as meat and milk are often valuable vitamin sources. As far as patients on hemodialysis who particularly have to restrict their potassium intake are concerned, their dietary supply of water-soluble vitamins is deficients, since foods high in these vitamins are also high in potassium (15). Cooking methods recommended for potassium leaching, such as extended soaking and boiling, may destroy the water-soluble vitamins (41). For example, cooking, canning, and refining destroys between 50% and 95% of the folate content of foods (244). An additional mechanism for developing deficiencies in water-soluble vitamins is the dialysis procedure, regardless of whether hemodialysis or CAPD is used (245, 246). Special attention should be given to the following water-soluble vitamins, whose deficiencies should be corrected by vitamin supplementation.

Pyridoxine

Assessment of vitamin B_6 status by enzyme functional tests of many patients with chronic renal failure, regardless of whether dialyzed or not, indicates a deficiency of this vitamin (246–248), although neither extreme dialysate losses (249) nor, with respect to the recommended intake for normals [2.2–2.9 mg/day (250)], markedly reduced intakes of this vitamin have been found. Therefore it is not surprising that normal vitamin B_6 serum levels were demonstrated in patients on hemodialysis (251, 253). The fact that enzyme functional tests (like the glutamic pyruvic transaminase test) indicate a vitamin B_6 deficiency, despite a normal plasma level suggests that uremics have higher requirements for this vitamin than normal individuals (251). Thus, the supplementation of pyridoxine hydrochloride is still advisable. An inadequate pyridoxine intake may contribute to central nervous system depression, anemia, peripheral neuropathy, and oxalosis in uremia (253, 254). Hemodialysis patients should receive 10 mg/day and patients on CAPD and conservatively treated should receive 5 mg/day. The need for pyridoxine increases when vitamin B_6 antagonists, such as hydralacine (255), are taken or when septicemia intervenes (248).

Ascorbic acid

Patients maintained on hemodialysis or CAPD have been shown to be vitamin-C deficient due to the restriction of potassium-rich fruits and vegetables, and losses of ascorbic acid during hemodialysis (245) or peritoneal dialysis (256). Usually a daily supplement of 100 mg ascorbic acid has been suggested for these patients (152). Recently Pru et al. (257) warned not to exceed this amount. This commonly happens due to vitamin C being added to the dialysate in some centers in order to neutralize chloramine and prevent hemolytic anemia (258, 259) and because the multivitamin tablets that are presently available often contain large amounts of vitamin C. In addition to interference with white-cell chemiluminescence, with resulting depressed phagocytic activity (260, 261), vitamin C, as a metabolic precursor of oxalic acid, when supplemented excessively, could aggravate uremic secondary hyperoxalemia (257).

Patients suffering from chronic renal failure and those on hemodialysis are known to show deposits of oxalate in the heart, kidneys, and blood vessels (257, 262, 263). According to Pru et al. (257), it is possible that vitamin C, by being shunted into the oxalic acid metabolic pathway, increases the level of oxalic acid and contributes to the vascular damage in patients on hemodialysis. Hence, vitamin C supplementation should be restricted to the minimal dosage necessary to correct the vitamin-C deficiency (100 mg).

Folic acid

Low plasma levels of folic acid have been reported in conservatively treated uremic patients, as well as in those on renal replacement therapy (264). In patients on hemodialysis treatment, this deficiency is supposed to be caused by inadequate dietary intake and by dialysis losses [9–32 µg/dialysis session (265)]. Red blood cell folate levels, however, have commonly been shown to be normal in thes patients (267). This is probably the reason why folic acid supplementation failed to improve erythropoesis in uremic patients (268). If a clinician, nevertheless, tends to maintain normal serum levels, a supplementation of 1 mg of folate is supposed to be adequate (269).

As far as the other water-soluble vitamins such as thiamin (vitamin B_1), riboflavin (vitamin B_2), bitotin, nicotinate, and panthotenate are concerned, no general supplementation seems to be necessary as long as the nutritional intake is adequate. Only in patients on CAPD, supplementation with 30 mg of thiamin has recently been recommended (246).

Fat-soluble vitamins

VITAMIN A

Plasma concentrations are quite divergent for fat- and for water-soluble vitamins. As far as vitamin A is concerned, it is well established that patients with chronic renal failure have significantly elevated plasma concentrations of both retinol (vitamin A) and retinol-binding protein (270). Hence, they are prone to develop hypervitaminosis A (271). Increased levels of vitamin A have been demonstrated in the liver (272) and skin (273). In general, supplementation of vitamin A should be avoided, especially since enhanced plasma levels of vitamin A are reported to be correlated with hypercalcemia (274) and hyperlipidemia (275) in chronically uremic patients. Hypercalcemia is thus thought to be related to enhanced parathyroid hormone secretion (276). Thus, hypervitaminosis A has been suggested to take part in the pathogenesis of renal osteodystrophy (277). Recently, however, Rylance et al. could not demonstrate a correlation of vitamin-A status and the severity of bone disease in chronic renal failure (278).

VITAMIN E

With respect to vitamin E, its supplementation cannot be recommended in patients with chronic renal failure, although there are data showing that high doses of vitamin E may ameliorate anemia in hemodialysis patients by reducing the susceptibility of red blood cells to osmotic hemolysis (279). Other authors, however, could not confirm these results (280, 281).

TRACE ELEMENTS

Toxicities as well as deficiencies of several trace elements have been described in patients with chronic renal failure (282), regardless of whether the patients are dialyzed or not. Toxicity particularly occurs in patients on renal replacement therapy due to contaminated dialysis fluid (283), blood contact with the dialyzer (284) or the tube system (285), or the intake of aluminium-containing phosphate binders. A deficiency might occur due to inadequate dietary intake (282), impaired gastrointestinal absorption (286), and losses in dialysate in CAPD patients (283). In patients on hemodialysis, the procedure per se is an unlikely cause of trace element deficiencies, because the trace elements in blood are complexed with proteins and cellular elements (282).

It is very difficult to ascertain what role, if any, these elemental disturbances play in the symptoms of uremic patients (287). However, deficiencies of some trace elements have been thought to be involved in the pathogenesis of the uremic syndrome, hence these elements deserve special consideration.

Zinc

Zinc deficiency, seems to mediate some of the uremic symptoms, since in humans the zinc-responsive defects include impaired gustatory and olfactory acuity, anorexia, delayed wound healing, and impaired leukocyte chemotaxis (288). Reports concerning the zinc status of chronic renal failure are, however, somewhat conflicting. Although, low plasma concentrations of zinc are common in uremic patients (289–291), this is not a reliable indicator of the total body zinc content, since plasma zinc levels represent only 0.5% of total body zinc (288). Smythe reported enhanced tissue zinc levels in uremic patients, although plasma levels and the levels in muscle were decreased, indicating an altered distribution of body zinc in chronic renal failure (287).

Hence, there is no specific laboratory finding of zinc deficiency. If a clinician believes certain symptoms of a uremic patient to be related to a zinc deficiency, he or she may try zinc supplementation. If the symptoms are reversed, the diagnosis could be correct. Zinc supplementation might be achieved by the intake of zinc-rich animal protein in the diet or by the use of oral zinc acetate or, in patients on hemodialysis, via dialysate enrichment (292). Up to now, beneficial effects on taste acuity (289) and sexual function (293) have been demonstrated, although other authors could not confirm these results (294). Recently, Antonio et al. demonstrated that zinc therapy improved lymphocyte function and viability in uremia, thereby improving cellular immunity (295).

SELENIUM

Another trace element, that is of pathophysiologic importance in uremia is selenium. In normals, a dietary selenium deficiency is an important risk factor for cardiovascular disease (296). Recently, Leung et al. suggested that a selenium-deficient status may be an additional factor in the pathogenesis of uremic cardiomyopathy and myopathy (297). The therapeutic consequences, however, have yet to be drawn from these results.

Iron

Iron deficiency in preterminal renal failure might be due to occult gastrointestinal bleeding or reduced iron intake due to protein restriction (298). Patients on hemodialysis should be particularly prone to develop an iron deficiency because of blood losses related to the dialysis procedure (299). However, iron stores are generally not depleted in chronic hemodialysis patients; features of iron deficiency anemia, such as hypochromic microcytic anemia, are rarely seen in these patients (300). Their iron stores are, on the contrary, commonly filled up by blood transfusions, often to an extent that iron overload and hemosiderosis develop (301). Moreover, the shortened half-lives of erythrocytes in uremia contribute to the iron overload.

In order to find the minority of patients on hemodialysis whose anemia would be ameliorated by iron supplementation, an accurate assessment of depleted iron stores is necessary (299). Serum iron and transferrin levels have been shown to be unreliable markers of iron status in patients with chronic renal failure. Serum ferritin levels, however, are a useful means of monitoring body iron stores (298).

Hence, if serum ferritin levels are below the normal limit of the assay used, iron supplementation may be considered (300). The oral route should be chosen, since gastrointestinal iron absorption has been shown to be normal in patients on hemodialysis (299).

However, since artificial erythropoietin is commonly available, iron supplementation must be considered because erythropoietin-treated patients often develop iron deficiency.

REFERENCES

1. Holliday MA: Nutrition therapy in renal disease. *Kidney Int* 30:3–6, 1986.
2. Blumenkrantz MJ, Kopple JD, Gutman RA, Chan YK, Barbour GL, Roberts C, Shen FH, Gandhi VC, Tucker CT, Curtis FK, Coburn JW: Methods for assessing nutritional status in patients with renal failure. *Am J Clin Nutr* 33:1567–1585, 1980.
3. Bansal VK, Popli S, Pickering J, Ing TS, Vertuno LL, Hano JE: Protein-caloric malnutrition and cutaneous anergy in hemodialysis maintained patients. *Am J Clin Nutr* 33:1608–1611, 1980.
4. Thunberg BJ, Swamy AP, Cestero RV: Cross-sectional and longitudinal nutritional measurements in maintenance hemodialysis patients. *Am J Clin Nutr* 34:2005–2012, 1981.
5. Young GA, Swanepoel CR, Croft MR, Hobson SM: Anthropometry and plasma valine, amino acids and proteins in the nutritional assessment of hemodialysis patients. *Kidney Int* 21:492–499, 1982.
6. Heide B, Pierratos A, Jhanna R, Pettit J, Ogilvje R, Harrison J, McNeil K, Siccion Z, Oreopoulos DG: Nutritional status of patients undergoing CAPD. *Peritoneal Dial Bull* 3:138–141, 1983.
7. Wolfson J, Strong CJ, Minturn D, Gray DK, Kopple JD: Nutritional status and lymphocyte function in maintenance hemodialysis patients. *Am J Clin Nutr* 37:547–555, 1984.
8. Alvestrand A, Ahlberg M, Bergstrom J: Retardation of the progression of renal insufficiency in patients treated with low protein diets. *Kidney Int* 24 (Suppl 16):268–272, 1983.
9. Mashio G, Oldrizzi L, Tessitore N, D'Angelo A, Valvo E, Lupo A, Loschiavo C, Fabris A, Gammaro L, Rugio C, Panzetta G: Early dietary protein and phosphorous restriction is effective in delaying progression of chronic renal failure. *Kid Int* 124 (Suppl 16): 273–277, 1983.
10. Rosman JB, Meijer S, Slinter WJ, ter Wee PM, Piers—Becht TPhM, Donker AJM: Prospective randomised trial of early dietary protein restriction in chronic renal failure. *Lancet* 2:1291–1295, 1984.
11. Guarnieri G, Toigo G, Situlin R, Crapesi L, Del Bianco MA, Zanettovich A, Faccini L, Lucchesi A, Oldrizzi L, Rugiu C, Maschio G: Nutritional assessment in patients with early renal insufficiency on long-term low protein diet. *Contr Nephrol* 53:40–50, 1986.
12. Acchiardo SR, Moore LW, Latour PA: Malnutrition as the main factor in morbidity and mortality of hemodialysis patients. *Kidney Int* 24 (Suppl 16):199–203, 1983.
13. Kopple JD, Jones M, Fukuda S, Swendseid ME: Amino acid and protein metabolism in renal failure. *Am J Clin Nutr* 31:1532–1535, 1978.
14. Bergström J: Discovery and rediscovery of low protein diet. *Clin Nephrol* 21:29–35, 1984.
15. Kopple JD: Nutritional therapy in kidney failure. *Nutr Rev* 39:193–206, 1981.
16. Alvestrand A, Bergström J: Nutritional management. In: WN Suki, SG Massry, eds, Therapy of Renal Diseases and Related Disorders. *Martinus Nijhoff, Boston*, pp 459–480, 1984.
17. Burge JC, Park HS, Whitlock CP, Schemmel RA: Taste acuity in patients undergoing long-term hemodialysis. *Kidney Int* 15:49–53, 1979.
18. LI J, Wassner S: Protein synthesis and degradation in skeletal muscle of chronically uremic rats. *Kidney Int* 29:1136–1143, 1986.
19. Garber A: Skeletal muscle protein and amino acid metabolism in experimental chronic uremia in the rat: Accelerated alanine and glutamine formation and release. *J Clin Invest* 62:623–632, 1978.
20. Garber A: The regulation of skeletal muscle alanine and glutamine formation and release in experimental chronic uremia in the rat. *J Clin Invest* 62:633–641, 1978.
21. Kopple JD: Nutrition in renal failure. In: RR Robinson, ed, *Nephrology*, Vol 2. Springer-Verlag, New York, pp 1498–1515, 1984.
22. De Fronzo RA, Alvestrand A, Smith D, Hendler R, Hend-

ler E, Wahren J: Insulin resistance in uremia. *J Clin Invest* 67:563–568, 1981.
23. Sherwin RS, Bastl C, Finkelstein FO, Fisher M, Black H, Hendler R, Felig P: Influence of uremia and hemodialysis on the turnover and metabolic effects of glucagon. *J Clin Invest* 57:722–731, 1976.
24. Kopple JD, Cianciaruso B, Massry SG: Does parathyroid hormone cause protein wasting? *Contr Nephrol* 20:138–148, 1980.
25. Bondy PK, Engel FL, Farrar B: The metabolism of amino acids and protein in the adrenalectomized nephrectomized rat. *Endocrinology* 44:476–483, 1949.
26. Schaefer RM, Teschner M, Kulzer P, Leipold J, Peter G, Heidland A: Evidence for reduced catabolism by the antiglucocorticoid RU 38486 in acutely uremic rats. *Am J Nephrol* 7:127–131, 1987.
28. May R, Kelly R, Mitch W: Metabolic acidosis stimulates protein degradation in rat muscle by glucocorticoid dependent mechanism. *J Clin Invest* 77:614–621, 1986.
29. Teschner M, Heidland A: Nutrition in acute renal failure *Blood Purif* 3:170–178, 1985.
30. Cerra FB, Siegel JH, Coleman B, Border JR, McMenamy RR: Septic autocannibalism: Failure of exogenous nutritional support. *Ann Surg* 192:570–580, 1980.
31. Clowes GHA, George BC, Villee CA, Saravis CA: Muscle proteolysis induced by a circulating peptide in patients with sepsis or trauma. *N Engl J Med* 308:545–552, 1983.
32. Baracos V, Rodemann P, Dinarello CA, Goldberg AL: Stimulation of muscle protein degradation and prostaglandin E_2 release by leukocytic pyrogen (Interleukin 1). *N Engl J Med* 308:553–558, 1983.
33. Goldberg AL, Baracos VE, Rodemann P, Waxmann L, Dinarello CA: Control of protein degradation in muscle by prostaglandins, Ca^{2+}, and leukocytic pyrogen (interleukin 1). *Fed Proc* 1301–1306, 1984.
34. Dinarello CA, Wolff SM: Molecular basis of fever in humans. *Am J Med* 72:799–819, 1982.
35. Baracos VE, Wilson JE, Goldberg AL: Effects of temperature on protein turnover in isolated rat skeletal muscle. *Am J Physiol* 246:125–130, 1984.
36. Monteon FJ, Laidlaw SA, Shaib JK, Kopple JD: Energy expenditure in patients with chronic renal failure. *Kidney Int* 30:741–747, 1986.
37. Levine SE, Madnnis MA: Pitfalls of nutritional assessment in end-stage renal disease: A case approach. *Dial Transpl* 14:610–617, 1985.
38. Madden JP, Goodman SJ, Guthrie HA: Validity of the 24-hr recall. *J Am Diet Assoc* 68:143–147, 1976.
39. Gersovitz M, Madden JP, Smiciklas-Wright H: Validity of the 24-hr dietary recall and seven-day recall for group comparisons. *J Am Diet Assoc* 73:48–55, 1978.
40. El Nahas AM, Coles GA: Dietary treatment of chronic renal failure: Ten unanswered questions. *Lancet* 2:597–600, 1986.
41. Holliday MA, McHenry-Richardson K, Portale A: Nutritional management of chronic renal disease. *Med Clin North Am* 63:945–963, 1979.
42. Kopple JD, Colwin JW: Evaluation of chronic uremia. Importance of serum urea nitrogen, serum creatinine and their ratio. *JAMA* 277:41–44, 1974.
43. Grodstein G, Kopple JD: Urea nitrogen appearance, a simple and practical indicator of total nitrogen output (abstract). *Kidney Int* 16:953, 1979.
44. Mitch WE, Walser M: Nutritional therapy of the uremic patients. In: BM Brenner, FC Rector, eds, *The Kidney*, Vol 2. WB Saunders, Philadelphia, pp 1759–1790, 1986.
45. Blumenkrantz MJ, Kopple JD, Moran JK, Coburn JW: Metabolic balance studies and dietary protein requirements in patients undergoing continuous ambulatory peritoneal dialysis. *Kidney Int* 21:849–861, 1982.
46. Maroni BJ, Steinman TI, Mitch WE: A method for estimating nitrogen intake of patients with chronic renal failure. *Kidney Int* 27:58–65, 1985.
47. Kopple JD, Swenseid ME: Amino acid and keto acid diet for therapy in renal failure. *Nephron* 18:1–12, 1977.
48. Ritz E, Mehls O, Gilli G, Heuck CC: Protein restriction in the conservative management of uremia. *Am J Clin Nutr* 31:1703–1711, 1978.
49. Berkelhammer CH, Leiler LA, Jeejeebhoy KN, Detsky AS, Oreopoulos DG, Uldall PR, Baker JP: Skeletal muscle function in chronic renal failure: An index of nutritional status. *Am J Clin Nutr* 42:845–854, 1985.
50. Flynn MA: Nutritional problems in continous ambulatory peritoneal dialysis. *Perit Dial Bull* 4 (Suppl):142–146, 1984.
51. Goldsmith GA: *Nutritional Diagnosis*. Charles C Thomas, Springfield, 1L, 1959.
52. Cohn S, Brennan BL, Yasamara S, Vartsky D, Vaswani AN, Ellis KJ: Evaluation of body composition and nitrogen content of renal patients on chronic dialysis as determined by total body nitrogen activation. *Am J Clin Nutr* 38:52–58, 1983.
53. Garrow JS: New approaches to body composition. *Am J Clin Nutr* 35:1152–1158, 1982.
54. Seedat YK: Exchangeable potassium study in patients undergoing chronic hemodialysis. *Brit Med J* 2:344–347, 1969.
55. Bilbrey GLNW, Carter MG, White J, Schilling F, Knochel JP: Potassium deficiency in chronic renal failure. *Kidney Int* 4:423–428, 1973.
56. Letteri JM, Ellis KJ, Asad SN, Cohn SH: Serial measurement of total body potassium in chronic renal disease. *Am J Clin Nutr* 31:1937–1944, 1978.
57. Schilling H, Wu G, Pettit J, Harrison J, McNeil K, Siccion Z, Oreopoulus DG: Nutritional status of patients on long-term CAPD. *Perit Dial Bull* 5:12–18, 1985.
58. Jeejeebhoy K, Baker JP, Wolman SL, Wesson DE, Langer B, Harrison JE, McNeill KG: Critical evaluation on the role of clinical assessment and body compositon studies in patients with malnutrition and after total parenteral nutrition. *Am J Clin Nutr* 35:1117–1127, 1982.
59. Collins JP, McCarthy ID, Hill GL: Assessment of protein nutrition in surgical patients — the value of anthropometrics. *Am J Clin Nutr* 32:1527–1530, 1979.
60. Forse RA, Shizgal HM: The assessment of malnutritions. *Surgery* 88:17–24, 1980.
61. Buzby GP, Mullen JL, Matthews DC, Hobbs CI, Rosate EF: Prognostic nutritional index in gastrointestinal surgery. *Am J Surg* 139:160–167, 1980.
62. Schaefer G, Heinze V, Jontofsohn R, Katz N, Rippich Th, Schäfer B, Südhoff A, Zimmermann W, Kluthe R: Amino acid and protein intake in RDT patients — a nutritional and biochemical analysis. *Clin Nephrol* 3:228–233, 1975.
63. Heidland A, Kult J: Long-term effects of essential amino acids supplementation in patients on regular dialysis treatment. *Clin Nephrol* 3:234–239, 1975.
64. Jensen TG, Englert AM, Dudrick SJ: Interpretation assessment data. *Nutr Suppl Serv* 1:14–20, 1981.
65. Shetty PS, Jung RT, Watrasiewicz KE, James WPT: Rapid turnover transport proteins: An index of subclinical protein-energy malnutrition. *Lancet* 2:230–232, 1979.

66. Golden M: Transport proteins as indices of protein status. *Am J Clin Nutr* 35:1159–1165, 1982.
67. Peters JP: Malnutrition and edema. *Nutr Rev* 8:33–36, 1950.
68. McFarlane H, Ogbeide MJ, Reddy S, Adcock JK, Adishina H, Gurney JM, Cooke A, Taylor GO, Mordie JA: Biochemical assessment of protein-calorie malnutrition. *Lancet* 1:392–396, 1969.
69. Kluthe R, Baumann G, Beschoff V, Quirin H: Serum transferrin und Eiweißernährung bei chronisch intermittierender Hämodialyse. *Med Ernährung* 12:73–77, 1971.
70. Miller DG, Levine S, Bistrian B: Diagnosis of protein calorie malnutrition in diabetic patients on hemodialysis and peritoneal dialysis. *Nephron* 33:127–132, 1983.
71. Schoenfeld PY, Henry RR, Laird NM, Roxe DM: Assessment of nutritional status of the national cooperative dialysis study population. *Kidney Int* 23 (Suppl 13):80–88, 1983.
72. Peterson PA: Demonstration in serum of two physiological forms of the human retinol binding. *J Clin Invest* 1:437–444, 1971.
73. Young GA, Keogh JB, Parson FM: Plasma amino acids and protein levels in chronic renal failure and changes caused by oral supplements of essential amino acids. *Clin Chim Acta* 61:205–213, 1975.
74. Mogielnicki RP, Waldmann TA, Strober W: Renal handling of low molecular weight proteins. 1. L-chain metabolism in experimental renal disease. *J Clin Invest* 50:901–909, 1971.
75. Volhard F: Die doppelseitigen hämatogenen Nierenerkrankungen (Bright'sche krankheit). In: *Mohr, Stachelin, Handbuch der Inneren Medizin.* Springer, Berlin, pp 1149–1722, special page 1400, 1918.
76. Walser M, Mitch WE, Abras E: Supplements containing amino acids and keto acids in the treatment of chronic uremia. *Kidney Int* 24 (Suppl 16):285–289, 1983.
77. Schreiner GE, Maher JF: In: IN Kugelmass, ed, *Uremia, Biochemistry, Pathogenesis and Treatment.* Charles C Thomas, Springfield, IL. p 81, 1961.
78. Walser M: Determinants of ureogenesis with particular reference to renal failure. *Kidney Int* 17:709–721, 1980.
79. Simmons WK: The plasma amino acid ratio as an indicator of the protein nutrition status: A review of recent work. *Bull World Health Org* 42:480–482, 1970.
80. Fürst P, Alvestrand A, Bergström J: Effects of nutrition and catabolic stress on intracellular amino acid pools in uremia. *Am J Clin Nutr* 33:1387–1395, 1980.
81. Giordano CC, de Pascale C, Pluvio M, De Santo NG, Fella A, Esposito R, Capasso G, Pota A: Adverse effects among amino acids in uremia. *Kidney Int* 7:306–310, 1975.
82. Harper AE, Benevenga NJ, Wolhuetin RM: Effects of ingestion of disproportionate amounts of amino acids. *Physiol Rev* 50:428–435, 1970.
83. Waterlow JC, Garlick PJ, Millward DJ: *Protein Turnover In Mammalian Tissues and in Whole Body.* North-Holland, Amsterdam, New York, 1978.
84. Giovannetti S, Maggiore Q: A low-nitrogen diet with proteins of high biological value for severe chronic uremia. *Lancet* 1:1000–1005, 1964.
85. Rose WC: The amino acid requirements of adult man. *Nutr Abstr Rev* 27:631–647, 1957.
86. Giordano C: Use of exogenous and endogenous urea for protein synthesis in normal and uremic subjects. *J Lab Clin Med* 62:231–246, 1963.
87. Berlyne GM, Shaw AB, Nilwarangkur S: Dietary treatment of chronic renal failure. Experiences with modified Giovanetti diet. *Nephron* 2:129–134, 1965.
88. Boström H, Edgren B, Engelke B: Experiences with the Giovanetti diet in chronic uremia. *Scand J Urol Nephrol* 1:171–176, 1967.
89. Kluthe R, Oechslen D, Quirin H, Jesdinsky HJ: Six years' experience with a special low-protein diet. In: R Kluthe, G Berlyne, B Burton, eds, *Uremia. Thieme, Stuttgart,* p 250, 1972.
90. Hodd CEA, Beale DJ, Housley J, Hardwicke J: Dialysed egg as nitrogen source in dietary control of chronic renal failure. *Lancet* 1:8–14, 1969.
91. Lonergan ET, Lange K: Use of special protein-restricted diet in uremia. *Am J Clin Nutr* 21:595–605, 1968.
92. Carmena R, Shapiro FL: Dietary management of chronic renal failure. *Geriatrics* 79:95–102, 1972.
93. Ford J, Phillips ME, Toye FE, Luck VA, de Wardener HE: Nitrogen balance in patients with chronic renal failure on diets containing varying quantities of protein. *Br Med J* 1:735–737, 1969.
94. Kopple JD, Sörensen MK, Coburn JW, Gordon S, Rubini ME: Controlled comparison of 20 g and 40 g protein diets in the treatment of chronic uremia. *Am J Clin Nutr* 21:553–564, 1968.
95. Kopple JD, Coburn JW: Metabolic studies of low protein diets in uremia. I. Nitrogen and potassium. *Medicine* 52:583–595, 1973.
96. Giovanetti S: Low protein diet in chronic uremia: A historical survey. *Contr Nephrol* 3:1–6, 1986.
97. Giovanetti S: Dietary treatment of chronic renal failure. Why is it not used more frequently? *Nephron* 40:1–12, 1985.
98. Bergström J, Fürst P, Noree LO: Treatment of chronic uremic patients with protein-poor diet and oral supply of essential amino acids. I. Nitrogen balance studies. *Clin Nephrol* 3:187–194, 1975.
99. Edozien JC: The free amino acids of plasma and urine in Kwashiorkor. *Clin Sci* 31:153–161, 1966.
100. Chan W, Wang M, Kopple JD, Swendseid ME: Citrulline levels and urea cycle enzymes in uremic rats. *J Nutr* 104:678–683, 1974.
101. Young GA, Parsons FM: Impairment of phenylalanine hydroxylation in chronic renal insufficiency. *Clin Sci* 45:89–97, 1973.
102. Wang M, Vyhmeister I, Swendseid ME, Kopple JD: Phenylalanine hydroxylase and tyrosine aminotransferase activity in chronically uremic rats. *J Nutr* 105:122–127, 1975.
103. Jones MR, Kopple JD: Valine metabolism in normal and chronically uremic man. *Am J Clin Nutr* 31:1660–1664, 1978.
104. Saito A, Niwa T, Maeda K, Kobayashi K, Yamamoto Y, Ohata K: Tryptophan and indolic tryptophan metabolites in chronic renal failure. *Am J Clin Nutr* 33:1402–1406, 1980.
105. Ahlmen J: Incidence of chronic renal insufficiency. A study of the incidence and pattern of renal insufficiency in adults during 1966–1971 in Gothenberg. *Acta Med Scand Suppl* 582:S3, 1975.
106. Tizianello A, DeFerrari G, Garibotto G, Gurneri G, Robando C: Renal metabolism of amino acids and amonia in subjects with normal renal function and in patients with chronic renal insufficiency. *J Clin Invest* 65:1162–1173, 1980.
107. Alvestrand A, Fürst P, Bergström J: Plasma and muscle free amino acids in uremia: Influence of nutrition with amino acids. *Clin Nephrol* 18:297–305, 1982.
108. Alvestrand A, Ahlberg M, Fürst P, Bergström J: Clinical results of long-term treatment with a low protein diet and a new amino acid preparation in patients with chronic uremia. *Clin Nephrol* 19:67–73, 1983.

109. Walser M, Coulter AW, Dighe S, Crantz FR: The effect of keto-analogues of essential amino acids in severe chronic uremia. *J Clin Invest* 52:678–690, 1973.
110. Mitch WE, Collier VU, Walser M: Treatment of chronic renal failure with branched chain keto acids plus the other essential amino acids or their nitrogen free analogues. In: M Walser, JR Williamson, eds, *Metabolic and Clinical Implications of Branched Chain Amino and Keto Acids.* Elsevier/North-Holland, New York, p 587, 1981.
111. Schloerb RR: Essential L-amino acid administration in uremia. *Am J Med Sci* 252:650–657, 1966.
112. Mitch WE, Walser M: Nitrogen balance of uremic patients receiving branched-chain keto acids and the hydroxyanalogue of methionine as substitutes for the respective amino acids. *Clin Nephrol* 8:341–344, 1977.
113. Mitch WE, Walser M: Utilization of calcium L-phenylacetate as a substitute for phenylalanine by uremic subjects. *Metabolism* 26:1041–1046, 1977.
114. Walser M: Keto acids in the treatment of uremia. *Clin Nephrol* 3:180–186, 1975.
115. Heidland A, Kult J, Röckel A, Heidbreder E: Evaluation of essential amino acids and keto acids in uremic patients on low-protein diet. *Am J Clin Nutr* 31:1784–1792, 1978.
116. Schmicker R, Vetter K, Kaschube I, Goetz KH, Fröhling P: Comparison between essential amino acid and keto acid substituted diet in patients with chronic renal failure (abstract). *Kidney Int* 24 (Suppl 16):350, 1983.
117. Mitch WE, Abras E, Walser M: Long-term effects of a new keto acid supplement in patients with chronic renal failure. *Kidney Int* 22:48–53, 1982.
118. Walser M: Conservative management of the uremic patient. In: B Brenner, FC Rector, eds, *The Kidney.* WB Saunders, Philadelphia, pp 383–2424, 1981.
119. Jones R, Dalton N, Turner C, Start K, Haycock G, Chantler C: Oral essential amino acid and keto acid supplements in children with chronic renal failure. *Kidney Int* 24:95–103, 1983.
120. Barsotti G, Guiducci A, Ciardella F, Giovannetti S: Effects on renal function of a low-nitrogen diet supplemented with essential amino acids and keto analogues and of hemodialysis and free protein supply in patients with chronic renal failure. *Nephron* 27:113–117, 1981.
121. Mitch WE, Walser M, Steinman TI, Hill S, Zeger S, Tungasanga K: The effect of a ketoacid/amino acid supplement to a restricted diet on the progression of chronic renal failure. *N Engl J Med* 311:623–629, 1984.
122. Broyer M, Guillor M, Niaudet P, Kleinknecht C, Dartois AM, Jean G: Comparison of three low-protein diets containing essential amino acids and their alpha analogues for severely uremic children. *Kidney Int* 24 (Suppl 16):290–294, 1983.
123. Barsotti G, Morelli E, Guiducci A, Ciardella F, Giannoni A, Luppatti S, Giovannetti S: Reversal of hyperparathyroidism in severe uremics following very low-protein and low-phosphorus diet. *Nephron* 30:310–313, 1982.
124. Barsotti G, Morelli E, Giannoni A, Guiducci A, Lupetti S, Giovannetti S: Restricted phosphorus and nitrogen intake to slow the progression of chronic renal failure. A controlled trial. *Kidney Int* 16:278–284, 1983.
125. Mitch WE, Walser M, Sapir DG: Nitrogen-sparing induced by leucine compared with that induced by its keto-analogue, α-ketoisoaproate in fasting obese man. *J Clin Invest* 67:553–562, 1981.
126. Sapir DG, Steward PM, Walser M: Effects of α-ketoisocaproate and of leucine on nitrogen metabolism in postoperative patients. *Lancet* 1:1010–1013, 1983.
127. Burns J, Cresswell E, Ell S, Fynn M, Jackson MA, Lee HA, Richards P, Rowlands A, Talbot S: Comparison of the effects of keto acid analogues and essential amino acids on nitrogen homeostasis in uremic patients on moderately protein-restricted diets. *Am J Clin Nutr* 31:1767–1775, 1978.
128. Hecking E, Andrzejewski L, Prellwitz W, Opferkuch W, Müller D: Double-blind cross-over study with oral alpha-ketoacids in patients with chronic renal failure. *Am J Clin Nutr* 33:1678–1681, 1980.
129. Epstein CM, Chawla RK, Waldsworth A, Rudman D: Decarboxylation of alpha-ketoisovaleric acid after oral administration in man. *Am J Clin Nutr* 33:1968–1974, 1980.
130. Jackson MA, Lee HA: Changes in serum calcium caused by supplementation of low protein diets with keto-acid analogues in patients with chronic renal failure. *J Parenter Enter Nutr* 5:52–56, 1981.
131. Walser M: Keto-analogues of essential amino acids in the treatment of chronic renal failure. *Kidney Int* 13 (Suppl 8):180–184, 1978.
132. Lucas PA, Meadows JH, Roberts DE, Coles GA: The risks and benefits of a low protein-essential amino acid-keto acid diet. *Kidney Int*, in press.
133. Rand WM, Uauy R, Scrimshaw NW (eds): *Protein Energy Requirement in Developing Countries: Results of International Research.* FAO/WHO/UNU, United National Bulletin, Supplement 10, p 327, 1984.
134. FAO/WHO: *Joint FAO/WHO Ad Hoc Committee on Energy and Protein Requirements.* Technical Report Series # 522, World Health Organization, Geneva, 1973.
135. Degoulet P, Legrain M, Reach I, Aime F, Devries C, Rojas P, Jacobs C: Mortality risk factors in patients treated by chronic hemodialysis. *Nephron* 31:103–110, 1982.
136. Ono K, Sasaki T, Waki Y: Glucose in the dialysate does not reduce the free amino acid loss during routine hemodialysis of non-fasting patients. *Clin Nephrol* 21:106–109, 1984.
137. Phillips ME, Havard J, Hovard JP: Oral essential amino acid supplementation in patients on maintenance hemodialysis. *Clin Nephrol* 9:241–248, 1978.
138. Levine SE: Nutritional care of patients with renal failure and diabetics. *J Am Diet Assoc* 81:261–265, 1982.
139. Braverman D, Bogoch A: Metoclopramide for gastroparesis diabeticorum. *Diabetis Care* 1:356–361, 1978.
140. Walser M: Nutritional support in renal failure: Future directions. *Lancet* 1:340–341, 1983.
141. Bergström J: Protein catabolic factors in patients on renal replacement therapy. *Blood Purif* 3:215–236, 1985.
142. Hecking E, Distler A, Dörr R, Mader H, Port FK, Zobel R: Losses of amino acids into the dialysate, Benefits of intravenous or oral substitution of amino acids in patients on chronic intermittent hemodialysis. *Akt Ernährungsemd* 2:15–20, 1977.
143. Klinkmann H, Holtz M: The permeating of essential amino acids through different dialysis membranes. *Proc EDTA* 9:402–408, 1972.
144. Kopple JD, Swendseid ME, Shinaberger JH, Umezava ChY: The free and bound amino acids removed by hemodialysis. *Trans Am Soc Artif Intern Org* 19:309–316, 1973.
145. Aviram A, Peters JH, Gulyassy PF: Dialysance of amino acids and related substances. *Nephron* 8:440–454, 1971.
146. Wofson M, Jones MR, Kopple JD: Amino acid losses during hemodialysis with infusion of amino acids and glucose. *Kidney Int* 21:500–506, 1982.
147. Möhring K, Sinn H, Schüler HW, Horsch R, Krüger H, Asbach HW: Comparison evaluation of iatrogenic sources

of blood loss during maintenance dialysis. *Proc EDTA* 13:233–238, 1976.
148. Kluthe R, Lüttgen FM, Capetianu T, Heinze U, Katz N, Südhoff A: Protein requirements in maintenance hemodialysis. *Am J Clin Nutr* 31:1812–1820, 1978.
149. Heidland A, Hörl WH, Heller N, Heine H, Neumann S, Schaefer RM, Heidbreder E: Granulocyte lysosomal factors and plasma elastase in uremia: A potential factor of catabolism. *Klin Wschr* 62:218–224, 1984.
150. Hendersen LW, Koch KM, Dinarello CA, Shaldon S: Hemodialysis hypotension: The interleukin hypothesis. *Blood Purif* 1:3–8, 1983.
151. Alvestrand A, Gutierrez A, Wahren J, Bergström J: Blood-membrane interaction without dialysis induces increased protein catabolism in normal man (abstract). In: *Fourth International Congress on Nutrition and Metabolism in Renal Disease*, Williamsburg, VA, USA, 1985.
152. Feinstein EI: Parenteral nutrition in acute renal failure. *Am J Nephrol* 5:145–149, 1985.
153. Vincenti F, Amend WJ, Abele J, Feduska NJ, Salvatierra O: The role of hypertension in hemodialysis-associated atherosclerosis. *Am J Med* 68:363–369, 1980.
154. Frank W, Rao TKS, Manis T: Uremic hyperlipoproteinemia: Correlation with residual renal function and duration of maintenance hemodialysis. *Trans Am Soc Artif Intern Org* 23:59–63, 1977.
155. Lundin AP, Adler AJ, Feinroth MV, Berlyne GM, Friedman EA: Maintenance hemodialysis: Survival beyond the first decade. *JAMA* 244:38–40, 1980.
156. Neff MS, Eiser AR, Seifkin RF, Baum M, Baez A, Gupta S, Amarga E: Patients surviving: 10 years of hemodialysis. *Am J Med* 74:996–1004, 1983.
157. Gross RL, Newberne PM: Role of nutrition in immunologic function. *Phyiol Rev* 60:188–302, 1980.
158. Law DK, Dudrick SV, Abdon NI: Immunoincompetence of patients with protein-calorie malnutrition. *Ann Intern Med* 79:545–550, 1973.
159. Hobbs CL, Murray TG, Mullen JL: Implications of malnutrition in chronic renal hemodialysis patients. *J Parenter Enter Nutr* 3:1, 1979.
160. Lowrie EG, Laird NM, Parker TF, Sargent JA: Effect of the hemodialysis prescription on patient morbidity: Report from the National Cooperative Dialysis Study. *N Engl J Med* 305:1176–1181, 1981.
161. Held E, Winkelmann W, Finke K, von Dohn H, Seyffart G, Gurland HJ: Plasma amino acids in chronic renal failure. *Klin Wschr* 52:974–978, 1974.
162. Kopple JD, Swendseid ME: Protein and amino acid metabolism in uremic patients undergoing maintenance hemodialysis. *Kidney Int* 7:64–72, 1975.
163. Kopple JD: Abnormal amino acid and protein metabolism in uremia. *Kidney Int* 14:340–348, 1978.
164. Guarnieri G, Faccini L, Lipartiti T, Ranieri F, Spangaro F, Giuntini D, Toigo G, Dardi F, Raimondi A: Simple methods for nutritional assessment in hemodialysis patients. *Am J Clin Nutr* 33:1598–1607, 1980.
165. Swendseid ME, Wang M, Schutz I, Kopple JD: Metabolism of urea cycle intermediates in chronic renal failure. *Am J Clin Nutr* 31:1581–1587, 1978.
166. Richards V, Hobbs C, Murray T, Mullen J: Incidence and sequelae of malnutrition (MNUT) in chronic hemodialysis (HD) patients (abstract). *Kidney Int* 14:683, 1978.
167. Munro HN: Energy and protein intakes as determinants of nitrogen balance. *Kidney Int* 14:313–316, 1978.
168. Garza CN, Scrimshaw NS, Young VR: Human protein requirements: The effect of variations in energy intake within the maintenance range. *Am J Clin Nutr* 29:280–286, 1976.
169. Comty CM, Shapiro FL: Hemodialysis. In: RJ Classock, ed, *Current Therapy in Nephrology and Hypertension 1984–1985*. BC Decker, New York, pp 261–268, 1984.
170. Borah MF, Schoenfeld PY, Gotch FA, Sargent FJA, Wolfson M, Humphreys MH: Nitrogen balance during intermittent dialysis therapy of uremia. *Kidney Int* 14:491–500, 1978.
171. Kopple JD, Shinaberger JH, Coburn JW, Sorensen M, Rubini ME: Optimal dietary protein treatment during chronic hemodialysis. *Trans Am Soc Artif Intern Org* 15:302–307, 1969.
172. Massry SG, Coburn JW, Peacock M, Kleeman CR: Turnover of endogenous parathyroid hormone in uremic patients and those undergoing hemodialysis. *Trans Am Soc Artif Intern Org* 18:416–422, 1972.
173. Fürst P, Bergström J, Josephson B, Norée LO: The effect of dialysis and administration of essential amino acids on plasma and muscle protein synthesis, studied with 15 N in uremic patients. *EDTA* 7:175–180, 1970.
174. Acchiardo S, Moore L, Cockrell S: Long term effect of essential amino acids on chronic hemodialysis patients (abstract). *Kidney Int* (Suppl 16):345, 1983.
175. Grodstein G, Harrison A, Roberts C, Ippoliti A, Kopple J: Impaired gastric emptying in hemodialysis patients (abstract). *Kidney Int* 16:952, 1979.
176. Young GA, Parson FM: Amino nitrogen loss during hemodialysis, its dietary significance and replacement. *Clin Sci* 31:299–307, 1966.
177. Feinstein EI, Collins JF, Blumenkrantz MJ, Roberts M, Kopple JD, Massary SG: Nutritional Hemodialysis. In: K Atsami, M Maekawa, K Ota, eds, *Progress in Artificial Organs*. SAO Press, Cleveland, p 421, 1984.
178. Oreopoulos DG, Robson M, Faller B, Ogilvie R, Rapoport A, DeVeber GA: continuous ambulatory peritoneal dialysis: A new era in the treatment of chronic renal failure. *Clin Nephrol* 11:125–128, 1979.
179. Popovich RP, Moncrief JW, Nolph KD, Ghods AJ, Twardowski ZJ, Pyle WK: Continuous ambulatory peritoneal dialysis. *Ann Intern Med* 88:449–456, 1978.
180. Nolph KD, Sorkin M, Rubin J: Continuous ambulatory peritoneal dialysis: Three-year experience at one center. *Ann Intern Med* 92:609–613, 1980.
181. Oren A, Wu G, Anderson GH, Marliss E, Khanna R, Pettit J, Mupas L, rodella R, Brandes L, Roncari DA, Kakis G, Harrison J, McNeil K, Oreopoulos DG: Effective use of amino acid dialysate over four weeks in CAPD patients. *Perit Dial Bull* 3:66–73, 1983.
182. Salusky IB, Fine AN, nelson B, Blumenkrantz MJ, Kopple JD: Nutritional status of children undergoing continuous ambulatory peritoneal dialysis. *Am J Clin Nutr* 38:599–611, 1983.
183. Moncrief JW, Popovich RO, Nolph KD, Rubin J, Robson M, Dombros N, De Veber GA, Oreopoulos DG: Clinical experience with the continuous ambulatory peritoneal dialysis. *Am Soc Artif Intern Organs* 2:114–118, 1979.
184. Kurtz SB, Wong VH, Andersson CF, vogel JP, McCarthy JT, Mitchell JC: Continuous ambulatory peritoneal dialysis. Three-years experience at the Mayo Clinic. *Mayo Clin Proc* 58:633–639, 1983.
185. Lindholm B, Bergström J: Nutritional aspects of CAPD. In: gokal R, ed. Continuous ambulatory peritoneal dialysis. Churchill Livingstone, London, in press.

186. Lindholm B, Bergström J, Alvestrand A: Muscle free amino acids in patients treated with CAPD, In: *Proceedings of the III International Symposium on Peritoneal Dialysis, 1984*, Washington DC, in press.
187. Williams P, Kay R, Harrison J: Nutritional and anthropometric assessment of patients on CAPD over one year: Contrasting changes in total body nitrogen and potassium. *Perit Dial Bull* 1:82–87, 1981.
188. Shaldon S, Koch KM, Quellhorst E, Dinarello CA: Pathogenesis of sclerosing peritonitis in CAPD. *Trans Am Soc Artif Organs* 30:193–194, 1984.
189. Burns RO, henderson LW: Peritoneal dialysis, clinical experience. *N Engl J Med* 267:1060–1066, 1962.
190. Berlyne GM, Jones JH: Protein loss in peritoneal dialysis. *Lancet* 1:738–741, 1964.
191. Gordon S, Rubini ME: Protein losses during peritoneal dialysis. *Am J Med Sci* 253:283–291, 1967.
192. Blumenkrantz MJ, Gahl GM, Kopple JD, Kamdar AV, Jones MR, Kessel M, Coburn JW: Protein losses during peritoneal dialysis. *Kidney Int* 19:593–602, 1981.
193. Giangrande A, Limido A, Cantu P, Allaria P: SDS-polyacrylamide electrophoresis of protein loss during continuous ambulatory peritoneal dialysis. *Ric Clin Lab* 10:117–120, 1980.
194. Katirtzoglou A, Oreopoulos DG, Husdan H, Leung M, Ogilvie R, Dombros N: Reappraisal of protein losses in patients undergoing continuous ambulatory peritoneal dialysis. *Nephron* 26:230–233, 1980.
195. Diaz–buxo JA, Walker PJ, Farmer CD, Chandler JT, Holt KL, Cox P: Continuous cyclic peritoneal dialysis. *Trans Am Soc Artif Intern Organs* 27:51–53, 1981.
196. Rubin J, Nolph KD, Arfania D, Prowant B, Fruto L, Brown P, Moore H: Protein losses in continuous ambulatory peritoneal dialysis. *Nephron* 28:218–221, 1981.
197. Twardowski Z, Ksiazek A, Majdan M, Janicka L, Bochenska–Nowacka E, Sokolowska G, Gutka A, Zbikowska A: Kinetics of continuous ambulatory peritoneal dialysis (CAPD) with four exchanges per day. *Clin Nephrol* 15:119–130, 1981.
198. Randerson DH, Chapman GV, Farrell PC: Amino acid and dietary status in CAPD patients. In: RC Atkins, NM Thomson, PC Farrell, eds, *Peritoneal Dialysis*. Churchill Livingstone, London, pp 179–191, 1981.
199. Dulaney JT, Hatch FE: Peritoneal dialysis and loss of proteins: A review. *Kidney Int* 26:253–262, 1984.
200. Fürst P, Bergström J, Lindholm B: Studies of amino acid metabolism in continuous ambulatory peritoneal dialysis patients — preliminary results. In: M Legrain, ed, *Continuous Ambulatory Peritoneal Dialysis*. Excerpta Medica, Amsterdam, pp 292–297, 1980.
201. Giordano C, DeSanto NG, Capodicasa G: Amino acid losses during CAPD. *Clin Nephrol* 14:230–232, 1980.
202. Kopple JD, Blumenkrantz MJ, Jones MR, Moran JK, coburn JW: Plasma amino acid levels and amino acid losses during continuous ambulatory peritoneal dialysis. *Am J Clin Nutr* 36:395–402, 1982.
203. Khanna R, Wu G, Rodella H, Oreopoulos DG: Use of amino acid containing solutions in CAPD patients. *Perit Dial Bull* 4:121–124, 1984.
204. Baeyer H von, Gahl GM, Riedinger H, Borowzak R, Averdunk R, Schurig R, Kessel M: Adaption of CAPD patients to the continuous peritoneal energy uptake. *Kidney Int* 23:29–34, 1983.
205. Rubin J, Kirchner K, Barnes T, Teal N, Ray R, Bower J: Evaluation of continuous ambulatory peritoneal dialysis. *Am J Kidney Dis* 3:199–204, 1983.
206. Giordano C, DeSanto NG, Pluvio M: Protein requirements of patients on CAPD: A study of nitrogen balance. *Int J Art Organs* 3:11–16, 1980.
207. Gahl GM, Bayer HV, Averdunk R: Outpatient evaluation of dietary intake and nitrogen removal in continuous ambulatory peritoneal dialysis. *Ann Intern Med* 94:643–646, 1981.
208. Committee On Dietary Allowances: Recommended Dietary Allowances. National Academy of Sciences, Washington DC, pp 1–15, 1980.
209. Oreopoulos DG, Crassweller P, Katirtzoglou A: Amino acids as an osmotic agent (instead of glucose) in continuous ambulatory peritoneal dialysis. In: M Legrain, ed, *First International Symposium on CAPD, Paris 1979*. Excerpta Medica, Amsterdam, pp 335–340, 1979.
210. Schilling H, Wu G, Pettit J, Mitwalli A, Anderson HG, Ogilve R, Oreopoulos DG: Use of amino acid containing solutions in continuous ambulatory peritoenal dialysis patients after peritonitis: Results of a prospective controlled trial. *Proc Eur Dial Transpl Assoc-ER ERA* 22:421–425, 1985.
211. Kopple JD: Abnormal amino acid and protein metabolism in uremia. *Kidney Int* 14:340–348, 1978.
212. Committee on Dietary Allowances, Food and Nutrition Board: Recommended Dietary Allowances, 9th ed. National Academy of Sciences, Washington DC, pp 16–30, 1980.
213. Keys A, Brozek J, Hanschel A, Mielson O, Taylor HL: *The Biology of Human Starvation*. University of Minnesota Press, Minneapolis, p 1385, 1950.
214. Kopple JD, Monteon FJ, Shaib JK: Effect of energy intake on nitrogen metabolism in non-dialyzed patients with chronic renal failure. *Kidney Int* 29:734–742, 1986.
215. Steefee WP: Nutritional support in renal failure. *Surg Clin North Am* 61:661–669, 1981.
216. Blumenkrantz MJ: Nutritional management of the adult patient undergoing peritoneal dialysis. *J Am Diet Assoc* 73:251–255, 1978.
217. Lindholm B, Ahlberg M, Alvestrand A, Fürst P, Tranaeus A, Bergström J: Nitrogen balance and protein and energy intake during CAPD (abstract). In: *Fourth Int. Congress on Nutrition and Metabolism in Renal Disease*, 1985.
218. Grodstein GP, Blumenkrantz MJ, Kopple JD, Moran JK, Coburn JW: Glucose absorption during continuous ambulatory peritoneal dialysis. *Kidney Int* 19:564–567, 1981.
219. Attman PO, Gustafson A: Lipid and carbohydrate metabolism in uremia. *Eur J Clin Invest* 9:285–291, 1979.
220. Attman PO: Long-term treatment with low protein diet in uremia. *Contr Nephrol* 53:128–136, 1986.
221. Bagdade JD, Yee E, Wilson DE, Shafrir E: Hyperlipidemia in renal failure. Studies of plasma lipoproteins, hepatic triglyceride production, and tissue lipoprotein lipase in a chronically uremic rat model. *J Lab Clin Med* 91:176–186, 1978.
222. Modasini R, Frey F, Flury W, Klose G, Greten H: Selective deficiency of hepatic triglyceride lipase in uremic patients. *N Engl J Med* 297:1362–1366, 1977.
223. Klose G, Ritz E, Weizel A, Greten H: Plasma lecithin-cholesterol acyltransferase (LCAT) activity and its relation to lipoprotein compositon in chronic hemodialysis (abstract). *Eur J Clin Invest* 10:111, 1980.
224. Gnasso A, haberbosch W, Augustin J, Ritz E: Abnormal lipoprotein metabolism in incipient renal failure. *Proc Eur Dial Transpl Assoc-ERA* 22:1129–1133, 1985.
225. Gofman JW, Young W, Tandy R: Ischemic heart disease,

atherosclerosis, and longevity. *Circulation* 34:679–697, 1966.
226. Goldberg AP, Harter MR, Patsch W, Schechtman KB, Province M, Weerts C, Kuisk I, McCrute MM, Schonfeld G: Racial differences in plasma high-density lipoproteins in patients receiving hemodialysis. *N Engl J Med* 308:1245–1252, 1983.
227. Goldberg AP, Applebaum–Bowden DM, Bierman EL, Hazzard WR, Haas LB, Sherrad DJ, Brunzell JD, Huttunen JK, Ehnholm C, Nikkila EA: Increase in lipoprotein-lipase during clofibrate treatment of hypertriglyceridemia in patients on hemodialysis. *N Engl J Med* 301:1073–1076, 1979.
228. Goldberg A, Hurrad D, Haas L, Brunzell J: Control of clofibrate toxicity in the treatment of uremic hyperlipemia. *Clin Pharm Ther* 21:314–319, 1977.
229. Sanfelippo ML, Swenson RS, Reaven GM, Reduction of plasma triglycerides by diet in subjects with chronic renal failure. *Kidney Int* 11:54–61, 1977.
230. Sanfelippo ML, Swenson RS, Reaven GM: Response of plasma triglycerides to dietary change in patients on hemodialysis. *Kidney Int* 14:180–186, 1978.
231. Cattran DC, Steiner G, Fenton SSA, Ampil M: Dialysis hyperlipemia: Response to dietary manipulations. *Clin Nephrol* 13:177–182, 1980.
232. Okubo M, Tsukamoto Y, Yoneda T, Homma Y, Nakamura H, Marumo F: Deranged fat metabolism and the lowering effect of carbohydrate-poor diet on serum triglycerides in patients with chronic renal failure. *Nephron* 25:8–14, 1980.
233. Phillipson BE, Rothrock DW, Connor WE, Harris WS, Illingworth DR: Reduction of plasma lipids, lipoproteins, and apoproteins by dietary fish oils in patients with hypertriglyceridemia. *N Engl J Med* 3 (12):1210–1216, 1985.
234. Tsukamoto Y, Okubo M, Yoneda T, Marumo F, Nakamura H: Effects of a polyunsaturated fatty acid-rich diet on serum lipids in patients with chronic renal failure. *Nephron* 31:236–241, 1982.
235. Ritz E, Augustin J, Bommer J, Gnasso A, Haberbosch W: Should hyperlipemia of renal failure be treated. *Kidney Int* 28 (Suppl 17):84–87, 1985.
236. Guarnieri GF, Ranieri F, Toigo G: Lipid-lowering effect of carnitine in chronically uremic patients treated with maintenance hemodialysis. *Am J Clin Nutr* 33:1489–1492, 1980.
237. Bang HO, Dyerberg J, Sinclair HM: The composition of the Eskimo food in north western Greenland. *Am J Clin Nutr* 33:2657–2661, 1980.
238. Bang HO, Byerberg J, Hjorne N: The composition of food consumed by Greenland Eskimos. *Acta Med Scand* 200:69–73, 1976.
239. Kromhout D, Bosschieter EB, Coulander C de L: The inverse relation between fish consumption and 20-year mortality from coronary heart disease. *N Engl J Med* 312:1205–1209, 1985.
240. Hamazaki T, Nakazawa R, Tateno S, Shishido H, Isoda K, Hattori Y, Yoshida T, Fujita T, Yano S, Kumagai A: Effects of fish oil rich in eicosapentaenoic acid on serum lipid in hyperlipidemic hemodialysis patients. *Kidney Int* 26:81–84, 1984.
241. Rylance PB, Gordge MP, Saynor R, Parsons V, Weston MJ: Fish oil modifies lipids and reduced platelet aggregability in hemodialysis patients. *Nephron* 43:196–202, 1986.
242. Acker BAC van, Gilo HJG, Popp–Snijders C, van Bronswijk H, Rustemeijer C, Oe PL, Donker AJM: Free University Hospital, Amsterdam, The Netherlands. *Kidney Int* 31:255, 1987.
243. Glomset JA: Fish, fatty acids and human health. *N Engl J Med* 312:1253–1254, 1985.
244. Herbert V: The vitamins: Folic acid and vitamin B_{12}. In: RS Goodhart, ME Shils, eds, *Modern Nutrition in Health and Disease*, Lea and Febiger, Philadelphia, 1973.
245. Sullivan JF, Eisenstun AB: Ascorbic acid depletion during hemodialysis. *JAMA* 220:1697–1699, 1972.
246. Blumberg A, Hauck A, Sander G: Vitamin nutrition in patients on continuous ambulatory peritoneal dialysis (CAPD). *Clin Nephrol* 20:244–250, 1983.
247. Stone WJ, Warnock LG, Wagner C: Vitamin B_6 deficiency in uremia. *Am J Clin Nutr* 28:950–957, 1975.
248. Kopple JD, Mercurio K, Blumenkrantz MJ, Jones MR, Roberts C, Card B, Saltzman R, Casciato DA, Swenseid MA: Daily requirement for pyridoxine supplement in chronic renal failure. *Kidney Int* 19:694–704, 1981.
249. Ito T, Niwa T, Matsui E: Plasma flavin levels of patients receiving long-term hemodialysis. *Clinica Chim Acta* 39:125–129, 1972.
250. Food and Nutritional Board, National Academy of Sciences: Recommended dietary allowances. National Academy of Sciences, Washington DC, 1980.
251. Ramirez G, Chen M, boyce HW, Fuller SM, Butcher DE, Brueggemeyer CD, Newton JL: The plasma and red cell vitamin B levels of chronic hemodialysis patients: A longitudinal study. *Nephron* 42:41–46, 1986.
252. DeBari VA, Frank O, Baker H: Water-soluble vitamins in granulocytes, erythrocytes, and plasma obtained from chronic hemodialysis patients. *Am J Clin Nutr* 39:410–415, 1984.
253. Dobblestein HW, Korner WF, Mempel W, Grosse–Wilde H, Edel HH: Vitamin B_6 deficiency in uremia and its implications for the depression of immune responses. *Kidney Int* 5:233–237, 1974.
254. Blacke P, Schmidt P, Zazgornik J, Kopsa H: Reduction of elevated plasma oxalic acid levels by pyridoxine therapy in patients on regular dialysis therapy (abstract). *Kidney Int* 24 (Suppl 16): 346, 1983.
255. Raskin NH, Fishman RA: Pyridoxine-deficiency neuropathy due to hydralazine. *N Engl J Med* 273:1182–1185, 1965.
256. Tsopas G, Magoula I, Paletas K, Concouris L: Effect of peritoneal dialysis on plasma levels of ascorbic acid. *Nephron* 33:34–37, 1983.
257. Pru C, Eaton J, Kjellstrand C: Vitamin C intoxication and hyperoxalemia in chronic hemodialysis patients. *Nephron* 39:112–116, 1985.
258. Day BR, Williams DR, Marsh CA: A rapid manual method for routine assay of ascorbic acid in serum and plasma. *Clin Biochem* 12:22–26, 1979.
259. Eswara Dutt VVS, Mottola HA: Detection and initial rate determination of oxalic acid at the microgram level. Application to the analysis of humans blood serum and urine. *Biochem Med* 9:148–157, 1974.
260. Dziubinski JE: The effects of mega doses of ascorbic acid on bacterial activity and chemiluminescence production by human polymorphonuclear leukocytes. Thesis. University of Minnesota, Minneapolis, MN, 1979.
261. Ritchey EE, Wallin JD, Shah SV: Chemiluminescence and superoxide anion production by leukocytes from chronic hemodialysis patients. *Kidney Int* 19:341–358, 1981.
262. Bennett B, Rosenblum BS: Identification of calcium oxalate crystals in the myocardium in patients with uremia. *Lab Invest* 10:947–955, 1961.
263. Macaluso MP, Berg NO: Calcium oxalate crystals in kidneys in acute tubular nephrosis and other renal diseases with functional failure. Institute of Pathology, University of Lund, Sweden, pp 197–205, 1959.

264. Hampers CL, Streiff R, Nathan DG, Snyder D, Merrill JP: Megaloplastic hematopoiesis in uremia and in patients on long-term hemodialysis. *N Engl J Med* 276:551–554, 1967.
265. Hemmeloff Andersen KE: Folic acid status of patient with chronic renal failure maintained by dialysis. *Clin Nephrol* 8:510–513, 1977.
266. Minar E, Zazgornik J, Bayer PM, Landschützer H, Mengele K, Marosi : Hämatologische Veränderungen bei Patienten mit chronicher Hämodialyse — und Hämofiltrationsbehandlung unter besonderer Berücksichtigung der Folsaure- und Vitamin B_{12}- Serumkonzentrationen. *Schweiz Med Wschr* 114:48–53, 1984.
267. Swainson CP: Do dialysis patients need extrafolate? *Lancet* 1:239, 1983.
268. Schmücher H, Franz HE: Zur Frage der Behandlung einer hyperchromen Anämie mit Folsäure bei Patienten mit chronischer, dialysepflichtiger Niereninsuffizienz. In: *Fortschritte in der Inneren Medizin*. Springer, Berlin/Heidelberg/New York, 1982.
269. Kopple JD, Swendseid ME: Vitamin nutrition in patients undergoing maintenance hemodialysis. *Kidney Int* 7 (Suppl 2):79, 1975.
270. Smith FR, Goodman DS, The effects of diseases of the liver, thyroid and kidneys on the transport of vitamin A in human plasma. *J Clin Invest* 50:2426–2436, 1971.
271. Vahlquist A, Berne B, Danielson BG, Grefberg N, Berne C: Vitamin A losses during continuous ambulatory peritoneal dialysis. *Nephron* 41:179–183, 1985.
272. Yatzidis H, Digenis P, Fountas P: Hypervitaminosis — a accompanying advanced renal failure. *Br Med J* 1:352–353, 1975.
273. Vahlquist A, Berne B, Berne C: Skin content and plasma transport of vitamin A and ß-carotene in chronic renal failure. *Eur J Clin Invest* 12:63–67, 1982.
274. Wieland RG, Hendricks FH, Amat Y, Leon F, Gutierrez L, Jones JC: Hypervitaminosis A with hypercalcemia. *Lancet* 1:698–701, 1971.
275. Werb R, Clarke WF, Lindsay RM, Jones EOP, Linton AL: Serum vitamin A levels and associated abnormalities in patients on regular dialysis treatment. *Clin Nephrol* 12:63–68, 1979.
276. Chertow BS, Williams GA, Norris RM, Baker GR, Hargis GK: Vitamin A stimulation of parathyroid hormone. Interactions with calcium, hydrocortisone and vitamin E in bovine parathyroid tissues and effects of Vitamin A in man. *Eur J Clin Invest* 7:307–314, 1977.
277. Farrington K, Miller P, Varghese Z, Baillod RA, Moorhead JF: Vitamin A toxicity and hypercalcemia in chronic renal failure. *Br Med J* 282:1999–2002, 1981.
278. Rylance PB: Brown IRF, Howells DW, Nisbet JA, Stone AN, Eastwood JB: Relationship between vitamin A and bone disease in chronic renal failure. *Nephron* 36:131–135, 1984.
279. Ono K: Effects of large dose vitamin E supplementation on anemia in hemodialysis patients. *Nephron* 40:440–445, 1985.
280. Sinsakal V, Drake JR, Leavitt JM, Harrison BR, Fitch CD: Lack of effect of vitamin E therapy on the anemia of patients receiving hemodialysis. *Am J Clin Nutr* 39:223–226, 1984.
281. Lillo-Ferez M, Dopommereulle C, Prieur P, Petrover M: Inefficacy of vitamin E supplementation on anemia in hemodialysis patients. *Nephron* 45:79–80, 1987.
282. Sandstead HH: Trace elements in uremia and hemodialysis. *Am J Clin Nutr* 33:1501–1508, 1980.
283. Wallaeys B, Cornelis R, Mees L, Lameire N: Trace elements in serum, packed cells and dialysate of CAPD patients. *Kidney Int* 30:599–604, 1986.
284. Bodgen JD, Zadzielski E, Weiner B, Oleske JM, Aviv A: Release of some trace methods from disponsible couils during hemodialysis. *Am J Clin Nutr* 36:403–409, 1982.
285. Bommer J: Deposits of silicone particles in organs of dialysis patients. *Nieren- und Hochdruckkrankheiten* 12:250–254, 1983.
286. Zumkley H, Bertram HP, Knok O, Graefe V, Lison A: Zinc and copper in chronic renal insufficiency. *Nieren- und Hochdruckkrankheiten* 12:221–224, 1983.
287. Smythe WR, Alfrey AL, Craswell PW, Ibels LS, Kubo H, Nunnelley LL: Trace elements abnormalities in chronic uremia. *Ann Int Med* 96:302–310, 1982.
288. Aggett PJ: Zinc metabolism in chronic renal insufficiency without dialysis therapy. *Contr Nephrol* 83:95–102, 1984.
289. Atkin-Thor E, Goddard B, O'Nion J, Stephen RL, Kolff WJ: Hypogeusia and zinc depletion in chronic dialysis patients. *Am J Clin Nutr* 31:1948–1951, 1978.
290. Condon CJ, freeman RM: Zinc metabolism in renal failure. *Ann Int Med* 73:531–536, 1970.
291. Leung A, Henderson I, Halls D, Fell G, Kennedy AG: Trace element abnormalities in CAPD. *Proc Eur Dial Transpl Assoc-ERA* 22:410–414, 1985.
292. sprenger KBG, Bundschuh D, Schmitz J, Franz HE: Therapy for zinc deficiency in dialysis patients. *Nieren- und Hochdruckkrankheiten* 12:230–234, 1983.
293. Mahajan SK, Prasad AS, McDonald FD: Sexual dysfunction in uremic man: Improvement following oral zinc supplementation. *Contr Nephrol* 38:103–111, 1984.
294. Brook AC, Johnston DG, Ward MK, Watson JM, Cook DB, Kerr DNS: Absence of a therapeutic effect of zinc in the sexual dysfunction of hemodialysed patients. *Lancet* 2:618–619, 1980.
295. Antoniou LD, Shalhoup RJ: Zinc-induced enhancement of lymphocyte function and viability in chronic uremia. *Nephron* 40:13–21, 1985.
296. Salonen JT, Alfthen F, Hattunen JK, Puska P: Association between cardiovascular death and myocardial function and serum selenium in a matched-pair longitudinal study. *Lancet* 1:175–177, 1982.
297. Leung A, Henderson I, Fell G, Hall D, Kennedy AC: Selenium deficiency in chronic uremia and dialysis. *Proc Eur Dial Transpl Assoc-ERA* 22:1134–1138, 1985.
298. Koch K-M, Bechstein PB, Fassbender W, Kaltwasser P, Schoeppe W, Werner E: Occult blood loss and iron balance in chronic renal failure. *Proc Eur Dial Transpl Assoc* 12:362–369, 1975.
299. Blumberg A, Marti HR, Graber Ch: Parameters for the assessment of iron metabolism in chronic renal insufficiency. *Contr Nephrol* 38:135–140, 1984.
300. Van de Vyrer FL, Vanheule AO, Verbueken AH, Haese PD, Visser WJ, Bekaert AB, van Grieken RE, Buyssens N, de Broe ME: Pattern of iron storage in patients with severe renal failure. *Contr Nephrol* 38:153–166, 1984.
301. Kothari T, Swamy AP, Lee JCK, Mangla JC, Cestero RVM: Hepatic hemosiderosis in maintenance hemodialysis patients. *Dig Dis Sci* 25:363–368, 1980.

CHAPTER 45

Cardiovascular Complications of Uremia and Dialysis

J. CARLOS AYUS & R. K. KROTHAPALLI

INTRODUCTION

Cardiovascular complications occur frequently in patients with renal disease. Furthermore, cardiovascular derangements constitute the leading cause of death in the population with end-stage renal failure on chronic dialysis (1, 2). Prevention and treatment of cardiovascular disorders is therefore of major importance in these patients.

Factors that contribute to the high cardiovascular morbidity and mortality in uremic patients are summarized in Table 1. Hypertension, either as a primary event or secondary to renal failure, is a major risk factor for the development and progression of atherosclerotic cardiovascular disease and has been found in approximately 80% of patients developing end-stage renal failure (3). The high frequency of hypertension in the uremic population suggests that it plays a major role in the development of cardiovascular pathology in this group. Two recent studies underscore the importance of arterial blood pressure control. The first found a significant correlation between the presence of atherosclerosis in iliac artery samples taken from chronic dialysis patients about to undergo renal transplantation and a previous history of hypertension (4). Studies done in our hospital have additionally shown a significant correlation between control of arterial blood pressure and improvement of left ventricular systolic function in uremic patients on chronic dialysis (5).

Other factors are felt to contribute to cardiovascular disease in uremic patients. Anemia and the presence of an arteriovenous fistula in hemodialyzed patients generate high cardiac output states that may eventually lead to myocardial failure. Chronic volume overload increases cardiac work requirements, which lead ultimately to myocardial dysfunction. Pericarditis and infective endocarditis, when present, further compromise the cardiovascular system. Alterations in lipid and carbohydrate metabolism can acclerate atherosclerosis, and secondary hyperparathyroidism with chronic increases in the blood calcium-phosphorus product can lead to vascular and cardiac calcification (6). Indeed, parathyroid hormone itself is thought to be cardiotoxic (7–9). The abrupt acid-base and electrolyte changes that can occur during hemodialysis may lead to arrhythmias with secondary cardiac malfunction. Last, but not least, hemodialysis per se has been postulated as an atherogenic factor in patients with end-stage failure (10). This last consideration is a much debated issue that will be addressed in more detail.

PERICARDITIS

Incidence

As shown in Table 2, the incidence of symptomatic uremic pericarditis prior to the initiation of dialysis has decreased in recent years. Availability and earlier initiation of dialysis have accounted for this, and it is likely that the incidence will decrease further in the future. The likelihood of symptomatic uremic pericarditis appearing in patients being chronically dialyzed is similar in most reported series (approximately 15%). In our study, however, none of the patients developed symptomatic pericarditis after being on dialysis for 10 months (17). The incidence of asymptomatic pericardial effusion in uremic patients who are about to initiate dialysis is between 15% and 40% (17, 18), while in chronically dialyzed patients it is approximately 30% (17–19).

Pathology

Table 3 depicts the pathologic findings of pericarditis associated with renal failure. There is some difference between the pathology of acute uremic pericarditis occurring prior to the initiation of dialysis and that occurring in

Table 1. Factors contributing to the increased incidence of cardiovascular disease in uremia

Hypertension	Alterations of lipid metabolism
Anemia	Alterations of carbohydrate metabolism
Arteriovenous fistula	Secondary hyperparathyroidism
Chronic volume overload	Electrolyte and acid-based alterations
Pericarditis	Dialysis
Endocarditis	

Table 2. Incidence of uremic pericarditis

Symptomatic pericarditis incidence		Asymptomatic pericarditis incidence	
Study (Ref.)	%	Study (Ref.)	%
Prior to initiation of dialysis			
11	51	16	15
12	41	17	39
13	13		
14	2		
15	9		
16	17		
17	6		
During chronic dialysis			
12	13	18	32
14	17	19	27
15	16	17	30

Table 3. Pathologic findings in uremic pericarditis

Type of pericarditis	Findings
1. Acute pericarditis	a. Fibrin formation
	b. Thickening of the pericardial walls
	c. Pericardial effusion
	— serous
	— serosanguinous
	— hemorrhagic
	d. Acute inflammation
2. Subacute constrictive pericarditis	a. Active inflammation
	b. Fibrin formation
	c. Vascularization of pericardial walls
	d. Fibrosis
3. Chronic pericarditis	a. Fibrosis and adhesions of both underlying epicardium

Table 4. Clinical features of pericarditis in patients with end-stage renal failure

Timing	Features
1. Prior to the initiation of dialysis	a. Chest pain
	b. Pericardial friction rub
	c. Fever
	d. Mental confusion
	e. Cardiomegaly
	f. Unexplained deterioration in renal function
2. During chronic dialysis	a. Chest pain
	b. Cough
	c. Dyspnea
	d. Mental confusion
	e. Fever
	f. Hypotension on dialysis
	g. Jugular venous distention
	h. Rapid weight gain
	i. Intolerance to ultrafiltration
	j. Cardiomegaly
	k. Cardiac arrhythmias

the chronically dialyzed patient. Generally, the pericardial fluid tends to be hemorrhagic in the dialyzed patients, while those with uremic pericarditis usually have serious effusions. As the disease becomes more chronic, the acute inflammatory features are replaced by fibrosis, which can eventually lead to constrictive pericarditis (20).

Clinical presentation

Table 4 depicts the clinical features of pericarditis associated with renal failure. Differences in presentation exist between the nondialyzed and the chronically dialyzed uremic patients. Symptoms of pericarditis in nondialyzed patients tend to be less severe, and pericardial tamponade is less frequent than in chronically dialyzed patients (21, 22). In both populations, chest pain is a presenting complaint in 60–70% of the cases, and pericardial friction rub is present in over 90% of the cases (13, 14).

Fever is most frequent in chronically dialyzed patients who develop pericarditis, occurring in 79–95% of cases (13, 14). Hypotension during dialysis and intolerance to ultrafiltration can be the result of hemodynamic compromise due to pericardial disease. Mental confusion, lethargy, and disorientation have been reported in patients with large pericardial effusions and probably reflect the low cardiac output syndrome that develops. (14).

Unexplained increases in heart size, especially in the absence of pulmonary congestion, should alert the physician to the presence of a progressively enlarging pericardial effusion. Cardiac arrhythmias, particularly refractory atrial tachyarrhythmias (atrial flutter, atrial fibrillation, and paroxysmal atrial tachycardia) can be the presenting manifestation of pericarditis in uremic patients (19–28%) (13, 14).

The most expedient method for diagnosing pericardial effusions in uremic patients is the echocardiogram. It is important to remember, though, that not all patients with pericarditis will have an effusion. This lack of correlation between clinical symptoms and signs suggesting pericarditis and the presence of a pericardial effusion has previously been documented (23). In fact, none of the three patients with symptomatic pericarditis in our series had a pericardial effusion on the echocardiogram (17). On the other hand, the use of routine echocardiography in patients with end-stage renal disease has revealed that a significant number of uremic patients have pericardial effusions that go clinically undetected (Table 5).

Etiology

The etiology of symptomatic pericarditis in the uremic nondialyzed patient seems to be related to the biochemical abnormalities found in renal failure, since restoration of biochemical control by dialysis or renal transplantation results in the resolution of the symptomatology in approximately 90% of the patients (20).

The etiology of pericarditis in the chronically dialyzed

Table 5. Incidence of pericardial effusion versus incidence of symptomatic pericarditis in patients with end-stage renal disease

Number of patients	Pericardial effusion (%) on echocardiogram (%)	Symptomatic pericarditis (%)	Study (Ref.)
46	30	17.4	16
150	62	7.3	24
49	39	6.0	17

Table 6. Complications of pericarditis in patients with end-stage renal failure

Timing	Complications
Acute	Pericardial tamponade
	Cardiac arrhythmias
	Myocarditis
Chronic	Constriction

patient is probably multifactorial. Uremia is likely to play a role in some patients, although blood urea nitrogen levels are frequently not different from those of the dialyzed population without pericarditis (13, 25). The pericarditis in most of these patients fails to respond when dialysis is intensified (20). Intensification of dialysis is more likely to help the hypercatabolic patient or those patients with poor biochemical control. The incidence of pericarditis is lower in patients on intermittent peritoneal dialysis than in those in hemodialysis, although the blood urea concentration is generally higher in the former (26). These facts tend to negate, in some respects, the role of uremia in the pathogenesis of pericarditis in the dialyzed patient.

The frequent presence of hemorrhagic peicardial fluid in dialysis-associated pericarditis has prompted some investigators to suggest that heparin administration plays a role in the initiation of this derangement (27, 28). There is little direct evidence that this is so; however, heparin administration during hemodialysis may perpetuate or aggravate the effusion by encouring bleeding from the inflamed pericardium (28–30). Infection must always be kept in mind when evaluating uremic patients with pericarditis, especially if they are diabetic. Fever in excess of 38.5 Cv, leukocyte counts greater than 15,000v, or concomitant systemic infections should alert the physician to the possibility of a purulent pericarditis.

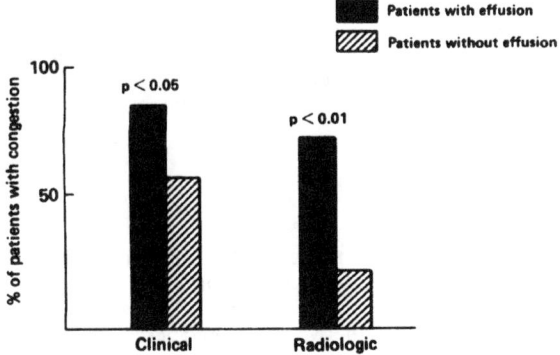

Figure 1. Clinical and radiologic evidence for fluid overload in renal disease patients with and without pericardial effusion.

Studies by our group and others suggest that volume overload plays an important role in the etiology of asymptomatic pericardial effusions in patients with endstage renal failure (16, 17, 24). Our study demonstrates that end-stage renal failure patients with pericardial effusions are less uremic and are more likely to have clinical and radiologic evidence of volume overload than those patients without an effusion (Figure 1). These findings are further supported by the study of Yoshida et al., who demonstrated that left atrial dimension, an indect measure of central hypervolemia, is significantly greater in patients with end-stage renal disease who have a pericardial effusion (24). Also, Wray and Stone found that most of their patients with pericardial effusion had clinical signs of volume overload (16).

Complications

Table 6 depicts the complications that might occur in a uremic patient with pericarditis. Acute pericardial tamponade resulting from rapid accumulation of pericardial fluid is a life-threatening emergency. In general, the slower the fluid accumulates in the pericardium, the larger the effusion will be before it causes hemodynamic compromise. The state of the pericardium itself also can determine the amount of fluid that can accumulate before tamponade occurs. A stiff, fibrotic, noncompliant pericardium with chronic pericarditis will accommodate far less fluid. The diagnosis of tamponade is not always easily made. Signs of right heart failure, with rapid increases in heart size, in the presence of clear lung fields on the chest roentgenogram, are suggestive of acute pericardial tamponade. Frequently, pulsus paradoxus will be present, although its absence by no means excludes cardiac tamponade. When congestive heart failure coexists with tamponade, the clinical diagnosis of tamponade can be very difficult, particularly in the presence of relative hypotension. In this case, the echocardiogram is very helpful when significant pericardial effusion is detected; right heart catheterization showing equalization of intracardiac diastolic pressure will provide the definitive diagnosis and should be employed any time a question remains concerning the differential possibilities. If the patient is volume depleted, this study may be falsely negative. In this case a fluid challenge may be necessary at any time of catheterization.

Myocarditis may accompany uremic pericarditis (13, 20). The functional contribution of this derangement is not well defined; however, it is likely to play a role in the hypotension and cardiac arrhythmias occurring in patients with pericarditis. Cardiac arrhythmias occur frequently in any patient with pericarditis, and uremic pericarditis is not an exception. Abrupt changes in the electrolyte composition occurring during hemodialysis can further contribute to the genesis of these arrhythmias. The arrhythmias that are most commonly seen in these patients are atrial in origin, including atrial fibrillation, atrial flutter, and paroxysmal atrial tachycardia (13, 14).

Now that patients with end-stage renal disease live longer, a long-term complication of uremic pericarditis has been observed: chronic constrictive pericarditis. Comty et al. reported an incidence of 4% (13). Chronic constrictive pericarditis is suggested in patients who seem particularly volume dependent during dialysis or in those with severe, refractory right heart failure. Cardiac catheterization may be required to differentiate between constrictive pericarditis, restrictive cardiomyopathy, and tamponade, and one should never hesitate to perform this diagnostic procedure.

Management

SYMPTOMATIC PERICARDITIS (MEDICAL)

Some aspects of the management of uremic pericarditis are agreed upon by all investigators. Most individuals will state that the appearance of symptomatic uremic pericarditis in a nondialyzed patient constitutes an indication for the initiation of dialysis (31). These patients generally show an excellent response to dialytic therapy, with approximately 90% having regression of their symptoms. The recurrence rate, however, is around 15% (20). Patients who do not respond to dialysis should be assessed carefully for other causes of pericarditis, such an infectious or immunologic processes. In these instances, uremia may mask the appropriate diagnosis.

Figure 2 depicts the therapeutic approach to symptomatic pericarditis in chronically dialyzed patients. Initially, the adequacy of dialysis should be assessed. If the patient has not achieved adequate biochemical control, intensification of dialysis is likely to be helpful. The response rate of these patients to intensification of dialysis, though, is low (40%), with only one third of the patients eventually recovering (20). A more effective method of managing these patients might be switching them to peritoneal dialysis until all signs and symptoms of pericarditis have subsided. This modality of dialysis avoids the use of heparin and appears to decrease the degree of pericardial fluid accumulation, and thus the incidence of tamponade (26, 27). Other investigators recommend that this group of patients be hemodialyzed with either regional or "tight" heparinization (25). These procedures lessen the systemic effect of heparin by either neutralizing it with protamine before it reaches the patient's veins in the former, or by decreasing the amount of heparin given to the patient in the latter.

None of these measures preclude simultaneous use of antiinflammatory agents. Indomethacin has been used in the treatment of uremic pericarditis (25 mg orally four times a day). Some authors have noted an excellent response, with an improvement in symptomatology (32). Others, in double-blind studies, have been unable to demonstrate a significant benefit of indomethacin on the course of uremic pericarditis (33). Indomethacin side effects, such as nausea, vomiting, headaches, and peptic ulceration, have required discontinuation of the drug in approximately 20% of the patients (33). Indomethacin, by blocking prostaglandin synthesis, may also cause a state of hyporeninemic hypoaldosteronism and thus may impair the uremic patient's defense against hyperkalemia (34).

The preferential use of systemic corticosteroids in the treatment of uremic pericarditis is a matter of debate. Comty et al. found a dramatic improvement in the symptoms and signs of pericarditis within 1 week in 72% of their patients after systemic administration of steroids. No complications occurred with short-term administration. They, therefore, recommend giving 40 mg of prednisone daily for 1 week, with subsequent dose tapering and discontinuation over 3–4 weeks (13). Serious complications, however, do occur with the use of systemic corticosteroids, and at least 1 of the 8 patients treated by Comty et al. died from complications following long-term corticosteroid administration. We believe that these antiinflammatory agents should be employed only in those patients with severe symptomatology. The use of corticosteroid agents may be dangerous if the etiology of the pericarditis is unknown, since they may either mask or disseminate an infection (35).

SYMPTOMATIC PERICARDITIS (SURGICAL)

Although the use of pericardiocentesis has a limited role in the management of uremic pericarditis, there is no doubt that it is the procedure of choice for acute pericardial tamponade. Pericardiocentesis may also be necessary for diagnostic purposes. Otherwise, repeated pericardiocentesis to treat uremic pericarditis carries a high morbidity and mortality risk. Although Silverberg et al. report that needle pericardiocentesis can be effective as a therapeutic

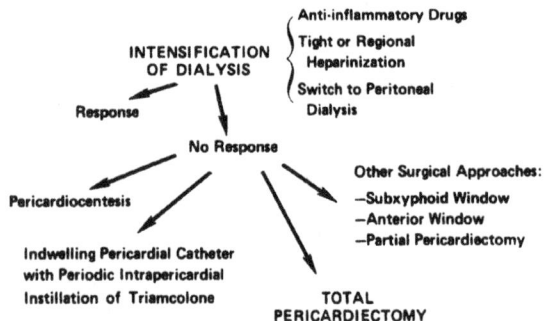

Figure 2. A schematic representation of the therapeutic approach to symptomatic pericarditis in the chronically dialyzed patient.

measure in pericardial tamponade from uremia, 1 of their 15 patients had a cardiac arrest during the procedure (26). Furthermore, most series show a high percentage of fluid reaccumulation when pericardiocentesis has been used as a mode of therapy (20). Thus, most authors now recommend alternative surgical approaches. We believe that pericardiocentesis should be employed only in the presence of acute hemodynamic impairment secondary to pericardial tamponade.

Busselmeier et al. report reasonable results in treating recurrent pericardial effusion by combining indwelling pericardial catheter drainage with periodic intrapericardial instillation of nonabsorbable corticosteroids. They report a 97% success rate in 45 patients, with only one recurrence and no deaths (36). It is possible, however, that some of the beneficial effects could have been due to a systemic steroid effect, since absorption of the steroids may have occurred across the inflamed pericardial membranes.

Other surgical drainage procedures have been used by different investigators. Formation of a pleural/pericardial window will drain the pericardium, however, window closure is frequent, and the rate of effusion recurrence is high. Partial pericardiectomy or a large anterior pericardial window have been advocated by some as the treatment of choice for acute pericardial tamponade and intractable effusions in these uremic patients (25, 37–41). However, we recommend total pericardiectomy as the standard treatment for patients with pericardial effusions that are hemodynamically significant or intractable. This latter procedure has a high success rate with a very low morbidity (3%) and mortality (1%) (42, 43). Recurrences are most likely to be a result of incomplete removal of the pericardium.

ASYMPTOMATIC PERICARDIAL EFFUSION

The therapeutic approach to asymptomatic pericardial effusion in the uremic patient has not been delineated, since this entity has only been recently appreciated. Indeed, it may be that no specific therapeutic measures need to be taken. Several authors have indicated that the natural history of these effusions is benign and that these patients rarely develop tamponade (19, 44). There is growing evidence, however, that the presence of these effusions in uremic patients may be a sign of chronic volume overload (16, 17, 24). Since chronic volume overload may, over time, be detrimental to myocardial function, volume reduction, either with diuretics or dialysis, appears to be indicated in these cases.

ACUTE PERICARDIAL TAMPONADE (TABLE 7)

Cardiac tamponade is a life-threatening emergency. When the patient is on dialysis, it should be discontinued and fluid should be administered in sufficient quantities to maintain venous return and cardiac output at an adequate level until tamponade has been alleviated. It is crucial to remember that further removal of intravascular volume in these patients may precipitate severe hypotension, which

Table 7. Management of acute pericardial tamponade in the uremic patient

1. Discontinue dialysis
2. Administer intravenous fluid to maintain adequate venous return
3. Never attempt to decrease extracellular volume since it may critically decrease venous return and lead to fatal hypotensive shock
4. Pericardiocentesis as soon as possible
5. Total pericardiectomy

can be fatal. Pericardiocentesis should be performed immediately in order to drain the pericardial fluid. This procedure allows for immediate improvement of the hemodynamic parameters. Subsequently, one must proceed total pericardiectomy as a definitive therapy, since, otherwise, the effusion is very likely to recur and further complicate the situation.

LEFT VENTRICULAR DYSFUNCTION

Incidence (Table 8)

The true incidence of left ventricular dysfunction in patients with renal failure is unknown since few studies have specifically addressed this point. It seems to vary from 25% to 39% in the series that have evaluated this parameter echocardiographically (5, 45, 46).

Etiology

Figure 3 depicts the factors that are commonly present in uremic patients that may be detrimental to cardiac function. Severe anemia can lead to high-output cardiac failure, even in subjects with initially normal cardiac and renal function. Although most patients with uremia are anemic, this problem can be particularly severe in anephric patients. The presence of an arteriovenous (AV) fistula in the hemodialysis patient is another potential source of high-output myocardial failure. Most authors, however, estimate that the AV fistula does not contribute significantly to increased cardiac output in the majority of these patients. This will obviously depend on the fistula size and the blood flow through it. There are, however, a few studies demonstrating that heart failure can result from the presence of an AV fistula in hemodialysis patients with poor myocardial function (47–49).

Table 8. Incidence of left ventricular dysfunction (ejection fraction < 50%) in patients with end-stage renal disease determined by echocardiography

Incidence (%)	Study (Ref.)
25	45
32	46
39	5

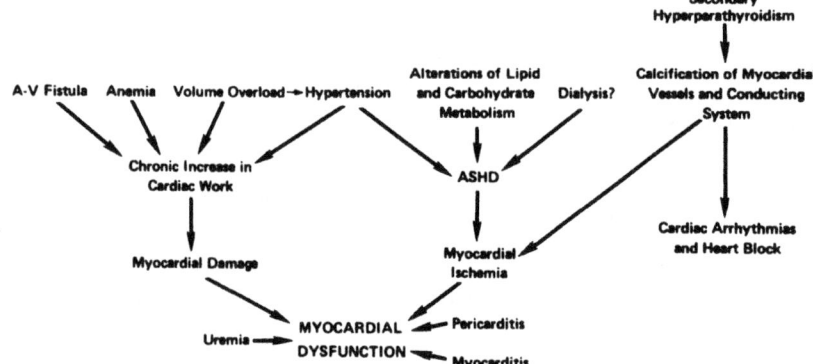

Figure 3. A schematic representation of factors in uremic patients that may be detrimental to cardiac function.

Secondary hyperparathyroidism, poor control of serum phosphorus, and administration of vitamin D in the uremic patient may result in a large increase of the serum calcium-solidus phosphorus ratio. This elevation can lead to calcification of myocardial vessels and of the conducting system of the heart, resulting in myocardial ischemia, intractable myocardial failure, heart block, and cardiac arrhythmias (6, 25). Pericarditis can affect myocardial function both by the restrictive effect of the inflamed pericardium and by the myocarditis, which is associated with uremic pericarditis (22).

The metabolic alterations that contribute to the progression of atherosclerotic heart disease (ASHD) will also be detrimental to myocardial function, since ASHD leads to myocardial ischemia and infarction, with a resultant decrease in ventricular function. Some authors have postulated that dialysis per se can accelerate the progression of atherosclerosis and thus contribute to the cardiovascular dysfunction of uremia (10). This view has been disputed by several investigators, and atherosclerosis in the uremic patient appears to relate more to underlying diseases and the presence of hypertension than to dialysis per se (4, 5, 50).

Uremia has also been postulated by some authors to exert a cardiodepressant effect. These hypotheses have been based on studies in which uremic patients who had a cardiomyopathy that was not due to other obvious causes promptly improved after initiation of dialysis or renal transplantation (51, 52). Experimental studies on the effects of uremia on cardiac muscle are contraindicatory and do not help to clarify this issue (53–58). In our studies, we have been unable to find a correlation between cardiac dysfunction and the degree of uremia (5). Still, the possibility exists that either uremia or other retained and unidentified compounds may contribute to the left ventricular dysfunction of patients with end-stage renal disease. The list of candidates for this toxin now includes middle molecules (59), phenols (60), trace elements (61), and PTH (7–9).

Obviously, other causes of heart failure in the population with normal renal function are also operative in patients with renal failure. However, pulmonary embolism as a cause for heart failure in uremia is probably rare. On the other hand, cardiac arrhythmias caused by abrupt acid-base and electrolyte changes in patients on dialysis may be more frequent.

Certainly, one of the most important etiologic factors in the myocardial failure of uremic patients is hypertension. The importance of arterial blood pressure control in patients with end-stage renal disease is underscored by results from our series that indicate a significant correlation between a reduction in arterial blood pressure and improvement in left ventricular systolic function in patients on long-term dialysis (5). Additionally, the most common cause of hypertension in the patient with end-stage renal failure is volume overload.

Management (Table 9)

The cornerstone of congestive heart failure management in the majority of patients with renal failure is the removal of fluid excess. This is especially true in the patient with no renal function who is on chronic dialysis. Patients with renal failure are unable to regulate their body fluid composition appropriately and are very vulnerable to volume overload. Thus, the most important principle, both in acute and chronic heart failure in these patients, consists of prompt removal of excessive fluid. Patients with some renal function (creatinine clearance > 10 ml/min) may respond to high doses of potent diuretics with a diuresis that may dispose of the excess fluid. To augment this effect, some authors have recommended the use of oral sorbitol, which removes fluid by causing an osmotic diarrhea. If the patient does not respond, or has no renal function and is on dialysis, removal of fluid by sequential ultrafiltration becomes the procedure of choice. Peritoneal dialysis with hypertonic solutions (4.5% dianel) and no dwelling time can remove several liters of fluid in a few hours. Unfortunately, patients with pulmonary edema may have further compromise of an already tenuous

Table 9. Management of left ventricular dysfunction in patients with chronic renal failure

Principle	Method of attainment
1. Adequate control of extracellular volume	a. Low-sodium diet b. Potent loop diuretics, dialysis
2. Adequate control of hypertension	a. Reduction of extracellular volume excess b. Antihypertensive medication c. Bilateral nephrectomy for refractory cases (very rare at the present time)
3. Correction of anemia	a. Anabolic steroids b. Transfusions when indicated
4. Decrease high-output state	a. Reduction or closure of the arteriovenous fistula in selected cases
5. Correction of calcium-phosphorus product	a. Oral use of phosphate binders b. Parathyroidectomy when indicated
6. Increase inotropy	a. Digitalization

Table 10. The acute effect of hemodialysis on left ventricular ejection fraction (LVEF) in chronic renal failure patients

Study (Ref.)	LVEF before acute dialysis		LVEF after acute dialysis	p
62		0.47	0.54	<0.001
63		0.59	0.67	ns
64	Group A	0.63	0.62	ns
	Group B	0.32	0.62	<0.01

Table 11. Effect of long-term dialysis on left ventricular ejection fraction in chronic renal failure patients

	LVEF before Chronic dialysis	LVEF after chronic dialysis	p
Entire group	0.51	0.57	<0.005
Patients with initially low LVEF	0.37	0.50	<0.001
Patients with initially normal LVEF	0.63	0.62	ns

respiratory function caused by the dialysis fluid pushing the diaphragm cephalad. A severely hypotensive patient might not tolerate the acute hemodynamic changes that occur during hemodialysis, and peritoneal dialysis then becomes the only therapeutic alternative.

The hemodynamic effects of acute hemodialysis have been studied by several investigators and are depicted in Table 10 (62–64). Acute hemodialysis will improve the left ventricular ejection fraction (LVEF) in patients who have a depressed LVEF (0.50) immediately prior to dialysis, while those who are normal remain unchanged. This enhancement of cardiac performance may be related to the increase in serum calcium achieved by hemodialysis. Recent work (65) has been done in which the effect of hemodialysis on ionized calcium was selectively controlled. Myocardial contractily improvement was related only to an increase in ionized calcium. Thus, changes induced by dialysis therapy are multifactorial depending on the baseline cardiac function (64) and the type of dialysis bath composition (acetate versus bicarbonate). In this regard, a recent study concluded that hemodialysis with bicarbonate produces a comparatively greater improvement in left ventricular systolic function than hemodialysis with acetate (66). Furthermore, the type of treatment utilized (hemodialysis vs. ultrafiltration vs. hemofiltration) could also play a role (67, 68). We have studied the effects of long-term dialysis on cardiac function in uremic patients (5). As seen in Table 11, the patients who had an abnormal LVEF (Group A; EF < 0.50) normalized this parameter after approximately 10 months on dialysis. LVEF in the group in which it was initially normal (Group B; EF=0.50) remained unchanged. Since we have shown the importance of arterial blood pressure reduction in the improvement of LVEF in these patients, the control of hypertension becomes of paramount importance (5). It is important to emphasize that the removal of volume excess and the control of hypertension constitute the main therapies for congestive heart failure in the patient with renal failure.

When congestive heart failure is secondary to acute myocardial infarction in the patient on hemodialysis, we recommend the insertion of a Tenckhoff catheter and institution of peritoneal dialysis until the patient has recovered completely and is hemodynamically stable. If this cannot be accomplished, it is advisable to postpone hemodialysis for at least 24 hours.

Other measures are also important for the correction of cardiac failure in uremia. Attenuation of the anemia by the administration of iron supplements, vitamins, folic acid, and anabolic steroids may decrease the cardiac work load. Patients who are anephric or have severe symptomatic ASHD may require periodic blood transfusions to maintain their blood hemoglobin concentration at a level of 7 g/dl or above. Correction of the serum calcium-phosphorus product by appropriate diet control, administration of phosphate binders, and parathyroidectomy, where indicted, may prevent calcification of the myocardium. If heart failure persists in spite of the above measures, it is important to consider unusual cases of cardiac failure, such as hyperthyroidism or bacterial endocarditis.

Digitalis is sometimes overused in patients with uremia and congestive heart failure, since the basic problem generally lies with lack of volume control. There are, however, circumstances in which digitalis is clearly indicated, such as the presence of supraventricular arrhythmias with a rapid ventricular response or the persistence of congestive heart failure in the presence of an adequate control of volume, anemia, and uremia. In such cases, we recommend that the patient be given the usual loading dose (0.25 mg q 6 h, up to a total of 0.75 mg or 0.25 mg per day for 10 days), but the maintenance dose needs to be adjusted according to the creatinine clearance. Patients with end-stage renal failure on dialysis usually require 0.125 mg of digoxin every other day. The use of appropriate serum drug levels is helpful in monitoring the adequacy of drug administration. Drugs such as prazosin and hydralazine may also improve myocardial performance by lowering the cardiac workload in the uremic patient and may be employed in appropriate doses. These drugs will improve cardiac output by causing arteriolar dilatation, thus reducing preload and afterload.

INFECTIVE ENDOCARDITIS IN END-STAGE RENAL DISEASE

Incidence

Excluding deaths from cardiovascular complications, infection is the most frequent cause of demise in patients with end-stage renal disease undergoing chronic hemodialysis (69–71). Estimates of mortality due to infections in chronically dialyzed patients range from 14% (46) to 33% (72).

Infective bacterial endarteritis with subsequent endocarditis has been observed in patients with arterial venous fistulae (73–75). Brecia et al. reported the first case of bacterial endocarditis complicating hemodialysis using venipuncture and a surgically created arteriovenous fistula (75). In this initial report of chronic hemodialysis being performed via surgically created fistulae, the only death occurred from acute infective endocarditis in a patient with rheumatic valvulitis.

In end-stage renal disease patients undergoing chronic hemodialysis, the incidence of infective endocarditis seems to be approximately 5%. Table 12 summarizes four studies in which the incidence of infective endocarditis was reviewed. Though the frequency of this complication is seemingly low, its potentially devastating effect forces us to pursue the problem aggressively.

Pathophysiology

Patients with end-stage renal disease on hemodialysis are particularly predisposed to developing infective endocarditis. Not only is their resistance to infection diminished,

Table 12. Incidence of infective endocarditis during hemodialysis for end-stage renal disease

Study (Ref.)	% of patients	Number of patients
71	2.7	9/330
76	6.6	7/106
77	4.4	
78	5.0	

but they have added risk factors in the form of arteriovenous fistulae and conduits. Indeed, chronic renal failure patients have been shown to have blunted immunologic responses, as well as malfunctioning lymphocytes and polymorphonuclear leukocytes (79).

The mere presence of an arteriovenous fistula seems to predispose patients to infective endocarditis. Lillehei et al. demonstrated that simple surgical creation of a fistulae produced infective endocarditis in dogs, even without the introduction of bacteria (80). The predisposition may be secondary to decreased clearance of pathogenic organisms from the bloodstream and the vascular intimal damage that is created by the turbulent flow associated with the fistula (81). The damaged vascular intima seemingly creates a nidus for infection to occur, ultimately developing from chronic bacteremia. Pathophysiologically, the creation of chronic bacteremia accounts for the predisposition of an individual under these circumstances to develop infections of the heart valve.

Clinical presentation

Cross and Steigbigel reviewed 35 episodes of infective endocarditis occurring in patients on chronic hemodialysis (82). They noted that the majority of infections were in males and that patients older than 46 were more likely to die. They also noted a wide range in duration of prior dialysis, with endocarditis occurring as early as 2 weeks as late as 106 months after the initiation of chronic hemodialysis. Death rates were not significantly different when patients with early endocarditis were compared to those with late infections. Additionally, infective endocarditis seemed as likely to occur in patients with arteriovenous fistulae as arteriovenous cannulae, and there was no difference in mortality of patients with fistulae compared with those with cannulae. Predisposing factors to the development of endocarditis included obvious access-site infection, steroid therapy, and prior dental manipulation.

Though clinical presentation of patients with end-stage renal disease and infective endocarditis is, for the most part, similar to the presentation of any individual with this affliction, one must be attuned to several atypical features that might occur. Firstly, these patients may not be febrile. Indeed, it is known that patients with chronic renal failure are occasionally unable to mount appropriate leukocyte responses and have attenuated febrile reactions to systemic infections. This is particularly the case when patients are receiving corticosteroids. Additionally, murmurs may be extraordinarily difficult to evaluate in this population. Generally, the anemic patient with renal disease tends to have multiple flow murmurs, which may or may not be of pathologic significance. Additionally, patients with septic thrombophlebitis tend to develop septic pulmonary emboli. Therefore, in any patient with pleuritic chest discomfort and pulmonary infiltrates suggesting cavitary lung lesions, endocarditis should be strongly considered.

Peripheral embolization will tend to occur, as in any patient with endocarditis, as well as pericardial effusion and congestive heart failure. Again, because end-stage renal disease patients are likely to have heart failure and pericardial effusion on the basis of their renal disease or intrinsic cardiac problems, it may at times be difficult to differentiate between infective endocarditis and intrinsic renal or cardiac pathology.

Echocardiography is a valuable tool for the evaluation of patients with possible infective endocarditis, as it may help to specifically identify valvular lesions and vegetations. Additionally, echocardiography in the face of infective endocarditis provides valuable prognostic information, as well as assisting in the overall care and planning for these patients.

Table 13 presents clinical findings frequently associated with infective endocarditis in the general population and the percent of patients in whom they can be appreciated. Patients with end-stage renal disease and endocarditis will also demonstrate these features, with the caveats noted above.

Etiology

Bacteriologic data reveals that the most frequent infecting organism in patients with infective endocarditis and end-stage renal disease is *Staphylococcus aureus*, followed by *Streptococcus viridans* and *Enterococcus*. *Listeria monocytogenes* is occasionally reported and its presence in these patients is interesting because this is an unusual organism to be causing endocarditis, seen usually only in those individuals who are immunologically compromised (83). In evaluating only arteriovenous fistulae and cannulae infections, *Staphylococcus aureus* again is the most frequent, accounting for 50–70% of these infections (84, 85).

Unlike end-stage renal failure patients with endocarditis, gram-negative bacillary infections are the second most frequent cause of arteriovenous fistulae infections, accounting for almost one third of these cases (78), with *Pseudomonas aeruginosa* causing approximately 10% of these afflications (84). There probably is no significant difference between the bacteriology of arteriovenous cannulae and arteriovenous fistulae infections. (86).

Another consideration, although frequent, is the possibility of fungal infection, especially in uremic patients with systemic septic emboli. *Candida* antibody levels and blood and thrombus cultures specifically for fungi may be helpful in identifying these organisms.

Complications

Patients with end-stage renal disease and infective endocarditis are likely to develop the same cardiovascular complications of endocarditis as the general population with this form of infection. Thus, the most common difficulty is valvular deterioration with resultant insufficiency. Additionally, sinus of Valsalva rupture with subsequent left-to-right shunts may be seen. Abscess formations in the perivalvular region, as well as multiple myocardial abscesses, may be noted. Myocardial infarction due to emboli coronary-artery occlusion has been observed, as well as ventricular septal defects, ventriculoatrial fistulae, aortopulmonary fistulae, and a diffuse myocarditis. Conduction disturbances are frequently noted when perivalvular or myocardial abscess formation is present. Pericarditis is also a frequent complication of this form of infection and may produce either a sterile, reactive, exudative inflammation of the pericardium or a pericardial effusion frankly contaminated with pus.

Additional difficulties that might develop in these patients include peripheral emboli events leading to infarction of vital organs, including the brain, spleen, mesenteric tract, and limbs. Pneumonia and pulmonary infarction may be present when right-sided endocarditis has developed.

Mortality in this group of patients seems to be much higher than that for the general population with endocarditis. Of 30 cases reviewed by Cross et al., where the clinical outcome was noted, 16 patients died (53%), clearly a higher death rate than the 20–30% usually reported during episodes of infective endocarditis in nonrenal disease patients (82, 87). Factors associated with a significant mortality in this group of patients (Table 14) seem to include: multivalvular involvement, enterococcal infections, steroid therapy, and patient age greater than 46. Additionally, patients with congestive heart failure not undergoing valve replacement tended to die. Not resecting the abscess site may also contribute to death, as it provides a source for continuing bacteremia.

Management

The ultimate management of patients with end-stage renal disease at risk for developing infective endocarditis is to prevent the occurrence of this infection. This might best be done by prevention of risk factors for endocarditis development (Table 15), particularly prevention of arteriovenous conduit or fistula infection. Prevention of these forms of infection should eliminate one of the more significant risk factors for the development of infective en-

Table 13. Presenting clinical features of infective endocarditis in the general population

Clinical feature	% present
CHF	25–65
Malaise, myalgias	95–100
Arthralgias	25
Fever	90–100
Roth spots	2–10
Heart murmurs	60
Neurologic deficits	33
Clubbing	10
Petechiae	33–60
Osler nodes	0–10
Janeway lesions	0–5
Splinter hemorrhages	2–10
Splenomegaly	33
Anemia	40–50
Leukocytosis	25–50
Hematuria	25–78

Table 14. Factors predisposing to mortality in patients with infective endocarditis and end-stage renal disease

Predisposing factor

1. Double valve infection
2. Enterococcal infections
3. Steroid therapy
4. Age over 46
5. Infection first year post-access insertion

Table 15. Factors predisposing to infective endocarditis in patients with end-stage renal disease

Predisposing factors

1. Antecedent infections
2. Access-site infections
3. Access-site manipulation
4. Steroid therapy
5. Immunosuppression
6. Dental work

Table 16. Management of infective endocarditis in patients with end-stage renal disease on hemodialysis

1. Switch to peritoneal dialysis
2. Remove access
3. Antibiotic therapy as outlined in Table 17
4. Valvular replacement
   a. Severe valvular destruction
   b. Class III or IV heart failure
   c. Recurrent systemic emboli
   d. Persistent infection

docarditis. Prophylactic antibiotics given routinely prior to hemodialysis, however, do not seem to prevent shunt infections (88). Furthermore, routine antibiotic administration in these patients may actually increase the incidence of gram-negative infections (88) or may induce infections with more resistant strains (88). Since bacteremia from post-dental manipulation also creates a risk for the development of shung-site infections, these patients should receive appropriate antibiotic prophylaxis for infective endocarditis prior to their dental mainpulation. Other procedures requiring prophylaxis include surgical manipulation of the genitourinary and gastrointestinal tracts. Still, it seems that the most important factors to be considered in the prevention of shunt infections are adequate antisepsis prior to needle insertion or dialysis hookup, and maintenance of appropriate aseptic techniques in the institution of the hemodialysis regimen. Table 16 depicts the general guidelines for the management of infective endocarditis in patients with end-stage renal failure on hemodialysis.

Removal of access

Abscess-site infection needs to be appropriately addressed and managed during infective endocarditis in these patients. Data that have been presented in the literature would suggest that, in addition to the usual indication for shunt removal — such as mycotic aneurysm of the arterial vessel, systemic septic emboli, and inadequate blood flow to keep the conduit open — it is also mandatory to remove an access site in any patient with infective endocarditis, particularly if the site is obviously infected. Indeed, experience with trauma-associated fistula formation indicates that antimicrobials alone will not cure an infected fistula in the presence of infective endocarditis. In one review, all cases of shunt-site infections were cured when surgical excision of the shunt was combined with medical therapy (89). When antimicrobials alone were used, the infection was not ameliorated. Thus, patients with obviously infected shunts, as well as those patients with infected shunts and endocarditis, should have their shunts removed. Additionally, patients with endocarditis and a vascular access shunt, though not obviously infected, should be considered for surgical excision of their shunt when the usual medical therapeutic programs are not controlling the infection.

Antibiotic therapy

After confirmation of the specific infecting organism, appropriate antimicrobial agents must be chosen. It is also important to administer the medication in a fashion that allows serum antibiotic levels to exceed the minimal bactericidal concentration for the particular etiologic agent. The monitoring of antibiotic therapy adequacy is, additionally, essential in any patient with endocarditis, but is particularly important in those with the added dimension of chronic renal failure, since the host immune and inflammatory systems may be compromised. Serum bactericidal titers of 1:8 or greater are thus desirable.

Table 17 lists the primary drugs of choice, dosages, administration route, and treatment duration as recommended by the Ad Hoc Subcommittee on Treatment of Bacterial Endocarditis of the American Heart Association's Council on Cardiovascular Disease in the Young (90), modified for patients with end-stage renal failure (91).

It should be obvious that patients with renal insufficiency or renal failure present added problematic dimensions to the therapy of infective endocarditis. Both the disease itself and its treatment may contribute to worsening of renal function. Many pharmacotherapeutic regimens in themselves are nephrotoxic (92). In particular, nafcillin, methicillin, and penicillin G may cause interstitial nephritis with hematuria, eosinophilia, eosinophiluria, and fever. Renal tubular damage may result from aminoglycosides, especially when combined with cephalosporins. Vancomycin and rifampin are also known nephrotoxic agents (87, 93).

Specific caution must also be taken when using other antibiotics in patients with renal failure. Complications

Table 17. Antibiotic therapy in patients with end-stage renal disease

Primary program of choice	Dose and route	Effect of dialysis	Treatment duration
a. Recommended antibiotic regimens in *Staphylococcus aureus* endocarditis (91, 92)			
Staphylococcus aureux (PCN sensitive)			
Aq. Penicillin G	Loading dose: 750 000 to 1.2 million units IV then 500 000 units IV every 8 hr	Need to supplement maintenance dose after hemodialysis. No loss in peritoneal dialysis	4–6 weeks
Staphylococcus (PCN resistant)			
Nafcillin	8–12 g/IV/q/day	Negligible dialysance by hemodialysis	4–6 weeks
Oxacillin	8–12 g/IV/q/day	Negligible dialysance by hemodialysis and peritoneal dialysis	4–6 weeks
Vancomycin	1 g/IV/q/week	Negligible dialysance by hemodialysis and peritoneal dialysis	4–6 weeks
Staphylococcus aureus (PCN allergy)			
Vancomycin	1 g/IV/q/week		4–6 weeks
Staphylococcus aureus (addition of aminoglycoside for synergy (93)			
Gentamycin	Give loading dose of 1.7 mg/kg/IV then 0.5–1 mg/kg after each dialysis	Readily removed by hemodialysis and peritoneal	5 days
Tobramycin		Readily removed by hemodialysis and peritoneal	5 days
b. Recommended antibiotic regimens in *Viridans* streptococcal and enterococcal endocarditis (91, 92)			
Viridans streptococci (PCN sensitive)			
Aq Penicillin G	Loading dose: 750 000 to 1.2 million U IV every 8 hr		4–6 weeks
Streptomycin	1 g loading dose followed by 0.5–1 g every 72–96 hr	Dialyzed: replace 250–500 mg after each dialysis	2 weeks
Viridans streptococci (PCN allergy)			
Vancomycin	1 g/IV/q/week		4 weeks
Enterococci			
Ampicillin	4–6 g/IV/q/day	Need supplemental maintenance dose after hemodialysis; poorly removed by peritoneal dialysis	4–6 weeks
Gentamycin	Give loading dose of 1.7 mg/kg/IV then 0.5–1 mg/kg/IV after each dialysis		4–6 weeks
Enterococci (PCN allergy)			
Vancomycin	1 g/IV/q/week		4–6 weeks
plus			
Gentamycin	Give loading dose of 1.7 mg/kg/IV then 0.5–1 mg/kg/IV after each dialysis		4–6 weeks

seen with penicillin G include cation overload and neurotoxicity (seizures) and are usually noted when blood levels exceed 100 µg/ml or when dosages reach 20 million U daily. In patients with chronic renal failure, the maximum predicted dosage (based on achieving a serum level of 20 µ/ml) can be estimated by employing the formula (94):

24 hr dose in million units = 3.2 + creatinine clearance/7.

When considering the use of nafcillin, oxacillin, or cloxacillin in the renal failure patient, one should use nafcillin, since 10% is cleared via the bile ducts and 60% is degraded primarily in the liver. No dosage adjustment, therefore, is necessary when using this antibiotic.

The dose of ampicillin needs to be reduced by approximately 50% in patients with severe renal impairment, since the half-life in anuric patients is approximately 8.5 hours. If the dosage is not diminished, these patients will almost certainly have an adverse response to the medication (mainly maculopapular rashes).

Aminoglycoside clearance is by glomerular filtration and therefore an adjustment of the dosage needs to be made. There is controversy regarding whether the dosage adjustment should be placed on variable dosages or variable dosing intervals (95, 96). In either event, drug levels, when available, should allow the most precise method of clinically adjusting the dosage. If regular intervals are chosen for gentamycin administration, the dose should be calculated by dividing the predicted dosage by the serum creatinine level. Alternatively, one can give the full calculated dose at an interval predicted by multiplying the usual dosage interval and the serum creatinine. In patients being dialyzed, a loading dose of 1.5 mg/kg of gentamycin should be given with subsequent dosing after each 4 hours of hemodialysis or 8 hours of peritoneal dialysis.

Most of the serum vancomycin (90%) is cleared unchanged by the kidney. It is not removed by either hemodialysis or peritoneal dialysis. This drug is being used increasingly in patients with end-stage renal failure because of its effectiveness and convenience of dosing (88). Patients with end-stage renal failure require initial dose of 1 g intravenously and then 1 g every 7 days (97–99). The drug should be administered over 1 hour in order to avoid side effects. Ototoxicity may occur at serum levles of 80–100 ng/ml, and severe tissue destruction occurs if the medication infiltrates locally.

Cephaloridine should be avoided in patients with renal failure since it is known to aggravate preexisting renal failure and to cause acute renal failure in patients concomitantly receiving aminoglycosides. Mild renal insufficiency does not require significant changes in the cephalosporin dosage. After the creatinine clearance has fallen to less than 30 ml/min a 50% reduction is needed. When it falls to 10 ml/min, a 75% reduction is required.

Still, the important point to remember is that each patient with infective endocarditis and chronic renal failure is an individual. Therefore, each therapeutic package must be carefully and thoughtfully designed in a tailor-made fashion, keeping in mind the severity of the renal failure, the infecting organism, and the general status of the host.

Surgical therapy

Acute surgical intervention can be lifesaving in any individual with infective endocarditis. The presence of chronic renal failure should not preclude the consideration of cardiovascular surgery. The major indications for surgery in the face of infective endocarditis remain valvular destruction severe enough to cause acute valvular insufficiency, the presence of New York Heart Association Class III or IV heart failure, repeated systemic emboli, and continued infection unresponsive to antibiotic administration. A decision for surgical intervention should be prompt and should not be based upon the duration of prior antimicrobial therapy (100).

REFERENCES

1. Bryan F Jr: National Registry Report. Proc 6th Ann Contractors Conference. Artificial Kidney Program. NIAMDD. *DHEW Publ No (NIH)* 74-248:201–207, 1973.
2. Parsons FM, Brunner FP, et al.: Combined report regular dialysis and transplantation in Europe II, Dialysis and renal transplantation. *Proceedings of the Eight Conference, Berline*, Vol 8. Pitman Medical, London, pp3–27, 1971.
3. Lazarus JM, Hampers CL, Merrill JP: Hypertension in chronic renal failure. Treatment with hemodialysis and nephrectomy. *Arch Intern Med* 133:1059–1066, 1974.
4. Vincenti F, Amend JW, Abele J, et al.: The role of hypertension in hemodialysis-associated atherosclerosis. *Am J Med* 68:363–369, 1980.
5. Ayus JC, Frommer P, Olivero JJ, et al.: Effect of long-term dialysis on left ventricular ejection fraction in end-stage renal disease. *Kidney Int* 19:142A, 1981.
6. Terman DS, Alfrey AC, Hammond WS, et al.: Cardiac calcification in uremia: A clinical, biochemical and pathologic study. *Am J Med* 50:744, 1971.
7. Drueke T, Fauchet M, Fleury J, et al.: Effect of parathyroidectomy on left ventricular function in haemodialysis patients. *Lancet* 1:112–114, 1980.
8. Bogin E, Massry SG, Harary I: Effect of parathyroid hormone on heart cells. *J Clin Invest* 67:1215–1227, 1981.
9. London GM, Fabiani F, Marchais SJ, et al.: Uremic cardiomyopathy: An inadequate left ventricular hypertrophy. *Kidney Int* 31:973–980, 1987.
10. Lindner A, Charra B, Sherrard DJ, et al.: Accelerated atherosclerosis in prolonged maintenance hemodialysis. *N Engl J Med* 290:697–701, 1974.
11. Wacker W, Merrill JP: Uremic pericarditis in acute and chronic renal failure. *JAMA* 156:764–765, 1954.
12. Bailey GL, Hampers CL, Hager EB, Merrill JP: Uremic pericarditis: Clinical features and management. *Circulation* 38:582–591, 1968.
13. Comty CM, Cohen SL, Shapiro FL: Pericarditis in chronic uremia and its sequels. *An Intern Med* 75:173–183, 1971.
14. Ribot S, Frankel JH, Gielchincky I, et al.: Treatment of uremic pericarditis. *Clin Nephrol* 2:127–130, 1974.
15. Comty CM, Wathen R, Shapiro FL: Incidence, mortality and effects of treatment on uremic pericarditis. *Am Soc Nephrol* 8:28, 1975.
16. Wray TM, Stone WJ: Uremic pericarditis: A prospective echocardiographic and clinical study. *Clin Nephrol* 6:295–302, 1976.
17. Frommer JP, Young JB, Ayus JC: Asymptomatic pericardial effusion in uremic patients: Effect of long-term dialysis. *Nephron* 39:296–301, 1985.
18. Lazarus JM, Gottlieb MN, Lowrie EG, et al.: Echocardiographic findings in stable hemodialysis patients. *Proc Dialysis Transplant Forum* 6:53–57, 1976.
19. Horton JD, Gelfand MC, Sherber HS. Natural history of asymptomatic pericardial effusions in patients on maintenance hemodialysis. *Proc Dialysis Transplant Forum* 7:76–78, 1977.
20. Renfrew RM Busselmeier TJ, Kjellstrand CM: Pericarditis and renal failure. *Ann Rev Med* 31:345–360, 1980.
21. Ayus JC, Frommer JP, Young JB: Cardiac and circulatory abnormalities in chronic renal failure. *Semin Nephrol* 1:112–123, 1981.
22. Comty CM, Shapiro FL: Cardiac complications of regular dialysis treatment. In: W Drukker, FM Parsons, JF Maher, eds, *Replacement of Renal Function by Dialysis*. Martinus Nihjoff The Hague, pp 519–537, 1978.
23. Markiewicz W, Brik A, Brook G, et al.: Pericardial rub in pericardial effusion: Lack of correlation with with amount of fluid. *Chest* 77:643–646, 1980.
24. Yoshida K, Shiina A, Asano Y, et al.: Uremic pericardial effusion: Detection and evaluation of pericardial effusion by echocardiography. *Clin Nephrol* 13:260–268, 1980.
25. Marini PV, Hull AR: Uremic pericarditis: A review of incidence and management. *Kidney Int* 7(1)11:163–166, 1975.
26. Silverberg S, Oreopoulos DG, Wise DJ, et al.: Pericarditis in patients undergoing long-term hemodialysis and peri-

toneal dialysis. Incidence, complications and management. *Am J Med* 63:874–880, 1977.
27. Cohen GF, Burgess JH, Kaye M: Peritoneal dialysis for the treatment of pericarditis in patients on chronic hemodialysis. *Can Med Assoc J* 102:1365–1368, 1970.
28. Alfrey AC, Goss JE, Ogden DA, et al.: Uremic hemopericardium. *Am J Med* 45:391–400, 1970.
29. Skov PE, Hansen HE, Spencer ES: Uremic pericarditis. *Acta Med Scand* 186:421–428, 1969.
30. Mitchell AG: Pericarditis during chronic hemodialysis therapy. *Postgrad Med J* 50:741–745, 1974.
31. Gulyassy PF, Yamauchi H, Depner TA: Conservative management of renal failure. In: LE Early, CW Gottschalk, eds, *Diseases of the Kidney, Strauss and Welt*. Little, Brown, Boston, Chapter 11, 1979.
32. Minuth ANW, Nottebohm GA, Eknoyan G, et al.: Indomethacin treatment of pericarditis in chronic hemodialysis patients. *Arch Intern Med* 135:807–810, 1975.
33. Spector D, Alfred H, Siedlecki M, et al.: A controlled study of the effect of indomethacin in uremic pericarditis. *Kidney Int* 24:663, 1983.
34. Tan SY, Shapiro R, Franco R, et al.: Indomethacin-induced prostaglandin inhibition with hyperkalemia. A reversible cause of hyporeninemic hypoaldosteronism. *Ann Int Med* 90:783–785, 1979.
35. Feinroth MV, Goldstein EJC, Josephson A, et al.: Infection complicating intrapericardial steroid instillation in uremic pericarditis. *Clin Nephrol* 15:331, 1981.
36. Buselmeier TJ, Davin TD, Simmons RL, et al.: Treatment of intractable uremic pericardial effusion. Avoidance of pericardiectomy with local steroid instillation. *JAMA* 240:1358–1359, 1978.
37. Ghavamian M, Gutch CF, Hughes RK, et al.: Pericardial tamponade in chronic hemodialysis patients. Treatment by pericardiectomy. *Arch Intern Med* 131:249–253, 1973.
38. Ali-Regiaba S, Gay WA, Sullivan JF, et al.: Treatment of uraemic pericarditis by anterior pericardiectomy. *Lancet* 2:12–14, 1974.
39. Singh S, Newmark K, Ishikawa I, et al.: Pericardiectomy in uremia. The treatment of choice for cardiac tamponade in chronic renal failure. *JAMA* 228:1132–1135, 1974.
40. Morin JE, Mulder DS, Long R: Pericardiectomy for uremic tamponade. *Can J Surg* 19:109–112, 1976.
41. Connors JP, Kleiger RE, Shaw RC, et al.: The indications for pericardiectomy in the uremic pericardial effusion. *Surgery* 80:689–694, 1976.
42. Engelman RM, Levitsky S, Konchigeri HN, et al.: Total pericardiectomy for uremic pericarditis. *World J Surg* 1:769–776, 1977.
43. Morin JE, Hollomby D, Gonda A, et al.: Management of uremic pericarditis: A report of 11 patients with cardiac tamponade and a review of the literature. *Ann Thorac Surg* 22:588–592, 1976.
44. Goldstein DH, Nagar C, Srivastava N, et al.: Clinically silent pericardial effusion in patients on long-term hemodialysis. Pericardial effusions in hemodialysis. *Chest* 72:744–747, 1977.
45. Cruz IA, Bhatt GR, Cohen HC, et al.: Echocardiographic detection of cardiac involvement in patients with chronic renal failure. *Arch Intern Med* 138:720–724, 1978.
46. Schott CR, LeSar JF, Kotler MN, et al.: The spectrum of echocardiographic findings in chronic renal failure. *Cardiovasc Med* 3(2):217–227, 1978.
47. Payne RM, Soderblom RE, Lobstein PH, et al.: Exercise-induced hemodynamic effects of arterio-venous fistulas used for hemodialysis. *Kidney Int* 2:344–348, 1972.
48. Anderson CB, Cod JR, Graff GM, et al.: Cardiac failure and upper extremity arterio-venous dialysis fistulas. *Arch Intern Med* 136:292–297, 1976.
49. Ahearn DH, Maher JF: Heart failure as a complication of a hemodialysis arteriovenous fistula. *Ann Intern Med* 77:201–204, 1972.
50. Burke JF, Francos GC, Moore LL, et al.: Accelerated atherosclerosis in chronic dialysis patients: Another look. *Nephron* 21:181–185, 1978.
51. Bailey GL, Hampers CL, Merrill JP: Reversible cardiomyopathy in uremia. *Trans Am Soc Artif Intern Organs* 13:263–272, 1967.
52. Ianhez LE, Lowen J, Sabbaga E: Uremic myocardiopathy. *Nephron* 15:17–28, 1975.
53. Nivatpumin T, Yipintsoi T, Penpargkul S, et al.: Increased cardiac contractility in acute uremia. Interrelationships with hypertension. *Am J Physiol* 229:501–505, 1975.
54. Scheuer J, Sterzoski SW: The effects of uremic compounds on cardiac function and metabolism. *J Mol Cell Cardiol* 5:287–300, 1973.
55. Kersting F, Brass H, Heintz R: Uremic cardiomyopathy: Studies on cardiac function in the guinea pig. *Clin Nephrol* 10:109–113, 1978.
56. Penpargukul S, Scheuer J: Effect of uraemia upon the performance of the rat heart. *Cardiovasc Res* 6:702–708, 1972.
57. Raab W: Cardiotoxic substances in the blood and heart muscle in uremia (their nature and action). *J Lab Clin Med* 29:725–734, 1944.
58. Knowlan DM, Piatnek DA, Olson RE: Myocardial metabolism and cardiac output in acute uremia. *Clin Res* 9:141, 1961.
59. Bernard P, Crest M, Rianado J, et al.: A study of the cardiotoxicity of uremic middle molecules on embryonic chick hearts. *Nephron* 31:135, 1982.
60. Lee JC, Downing SE: Negative inotropic effects of phenol on isolated cardiac muscle. *Am J Path* 102:367, 1981.
61. Pehrsson SK, Lins LE: The role of trace elements in uremic heart failure. *Nephron* 34:93, 1983.
62. Fernando HA, Friedman HS, Zaman Q, et al.: Echocardiographic assessment of cardiac performance in patients in maintenance hemodialysis. *Cardiovasc Med* 4:459–471, 1979.
63. Vaziri ND, Prakash R: Echocardiographic evaluation of the effect of hemodialysis on cardiac size and function in patients with end-stage renal disease. *Am J Med Sci* 278:201–206, 1979.
64. Hung J, Harris PJ, Uren RF, et al.: Uremic cardiomyopathy: Effect of hemodialysis on left ventricular function in end-stage renal failure. *N Engl J Med* 302:547–551, 1980.
65. Henrich WL, Hung J, Nixon JV: Increased ionized calcium and left ventricular contractitity during hemodialysis. *N Engl J Med* 310, 1984.
66. Ruder MA, Alpert MA, Van Stone J: Comparative effects of acetate and bicarbonate hemodialysis on left ventricular function. *Kidney Int* 27:768–773, 1985.
67. Aljama P, Martin-Malo A, Sanz R, et al.: Left ventricular function during haemofiltration and haemodialysis: A comparative study. *Proc Eur Dial Travpl Assoc* 19:281, 1982.
68. Cini G, Camici M, Pentimone F, Palla R: Echocardiographic hemodynamic study during ultrafiltration sequential dialysis. *Nephron* 30:124, 1982.
69. Brunner FP, Gurland HJ, Harlen H, Schafer K, Parsons

RM: Combined report on regular dialysis and transplantation in Europe, II, 1971. *Proc Eur Dial Transpl Assoc* 9:34, 1972.
70. Siddiqui JY, Fitz AE, Lawton RL, Kirkendall WN: Causes of death in patients receiving long-term hemodialysis. *JAMA* 212:1350–1354, 1970.
71. Vereerstraeten P: La survie du Brightique traite par l'hemodialyse. *S Sc Med Lille*, 88:49, 1970.
72. Cutler SS, Wolf J: Acquired arteriovenous fistula with coexistant subacute bacterial endocarditis and endoarteritis. *Ann Int Med* 25:972–981, 1946.
73. Hook EW, Wainer HS, McGee TJ, Sellers TF: Acquired arteriovenous fistula with bacterial endoarteritis and endocarditis. *JAMA* 164:1450–1454, 1957.
74. Lee SH, Fisher B, Fisher ER, Little A: Arteriovenous fistula and bacterial endocarditis. *Surgery* 52:463–467, 1982.
75. Brecia MJ, Cimino JE, Appel K, Hurwitz BJ: Chronic hemodialysis using venipuncture and a surgically created arteriovenous fistula. *N Engl J Med* 275:1089–1092, 1966.
76. Leonard A, Raij L, Shapiro FL: Bacterial endocarditis in regularly dialyzed patients. *Kidney Int* 4:407–422, 1973.
77. King LH, Bradley KP, Shires DL, Donohue JP, Glover JL: Bacterial endocarditis in chronic hemodialysis patients: A complication more common than previously suspected. *Surgery* 69:554–556, 1971.
78. Kuruvila KC, Beven EG: Arteriovenous shunts and fistulas for hemodialysis. *Surg Clin North Am* 51:1219–1234, 1971.
79. Wilson WEC, Kirkpatrick CH, Talmage DW: Suppression of immunologic responsiveness in uremia. *Ann Intern Med* 62:1–13, 1965.
80. Lillehei CW, Bobb JRR, Visscher MB: Occurrence of endocarditis with valvular deformities in dogs with arteriovenous fistulae. *Proc Soc Exp Biol Med* 75:9–16, 1950.
81. Rodbard S: Blood velocity and endocarditis. *Circulation* 27:18, 1963.
82. Cross AS, Steigbigel RT: Infective endocarditis and access site infections in paitents on hemodialysis. *Medicine* 55:453–466, 1976.
83. Gantz NM, Myerwitz RL, Medoiros AA, Camera GF, Wilson RE, O'Brien TF: Listeriosis in immunosuppressed patients: A cluster of eight cases. *Am J Med* 58:637–643, 1975.
84. Pendras JP, Smith MP: The silastic-Teflon arteriovenous cannula. *Trans Am Soc Artif Intern Organs* 12:222–228, 1966.
85. Ralston AJ, Harlow GR, Jones DM, Davis P: Infections of Scribner and Brescia arterio-venous shunts. *Br Med J* 3:408–409, 1971.

86. Levi J, Robson M, Rosenfeld JB: Septicemia and pulmonary embolism complicating use of arteriovenous fistula in maintenance haemodialysis. *Lancet* 2:288–290, 1970.
87. Garvey GJ, Neu HC: Infective endocarditis — an evolving disease. *Medicine* 57:105–127, 1978.
88. Morris AJ, Bilinsky RT: Prevention of staphylococcal shunt infections by continuous vancomycin prophylaxis. *Am J Med Sci* 262:87–91, 1971.
89. Martin AM, Clunie GJA, Tonkin RW, Robson JS: The aetiology and management of shunt infections in patients in intermittent hemodialysis, dialysis, and renal transplantation. *Proc Eur Dial Transplant Assoc* 4:67, 1967.
90. Bisno AL, Dismukes WE, Durack DT, et al.: Treatment of infective endocarditis due to *Viridans streptococci*. Council on Cardiovascular Disease in the Young. Ad Hoc Subcommittee on Treatment of Bacterial Endocarditis. *Circulation* 63:733A, 1981.
91. Bennett W, Muther RS, Parker R, et al.: A guide to drug therapy in renal failure. *Ann Int Med* 93:62–99, 1980.
92. Calderwood SB, Moellering RC: Common adverse effects of antimicrobial agents on major organ systems. *Surg Clin North Am* 60:65–81, 1980.
93. Watanakunakorn C, Glotzbecker C: Enhancement of the effects of anti-staphylococcal antibiotics by aminoglycosides. *Antimicrob Agents Chemother* 6:802–806, 1974.
94. Bryan CS, Stone WJ: "Comparably massive" penicillin G therapy in renal failure. *Ann Int Med* 82:189–195, 1975.
95. Cutler RE, Gyselynck AM, Fleet WP, Forrey AW: Correlation of serum creatinine concentration and gentamycin shelf life. *JAMA* 219:1037–1041, 1972.
96. Chan RA, Benner EJ, Hoeprich PD: Gentamycin therapy in renal failure: A nomogram for dosage. *Ann Int Med* 76:773–778, 1972.
97. Ayus JC, Eneas FJ, Tong TG, et al.: Peritoneal clearance and total body elimination of vancomycin during chronic intermittent peritoneal dialysis. *Clin Nephrol* 11(3):129–132, 1979.
98. Lindholm DD, Murray JS: Persistence of vancomycin in the blood during renal failure and its treatment of hemodialysis. *N Engl J Med* 274:1047–1051, 1966.
99. Krothapalli PK, Senekjian HO, Ayus JC: Efficacy of intravenous vancomycin in the treatment of grampositive peritonitis in long-term peritoneal dialysis. *Am J Med* 75:345–348, 1983.
100. Dtinson EB: Surgical treatment of infective endocarditis. *Progr Cardiovasc Dis* 22:145–168, 1979.

CHAPTER 46

Renal Osteodystrophy

SHAUL G. MASSRY

INTRODUCTION

Patients with end-stage renal failue display a multitude of signs and symptoms produced by derangements in the metabolism of divalent ions, vitamin D, parathyroid hormone, and bone (1). These abnormalities are collectively called "*renal osteodystrophy*". The biochemical, clinical, and pathologic features of renal osteodystrophy are listed in Table 1.

The objectives of the overall therapy of renal osteodystrophy are to prevent and/or manage its various components. Therefore the therapeutic approach is geared to: a) maintain the blood concentrations of calcium and phosphorus as near normal as possible; b) prevent the development of secondary hyperparathyroidism, and, if the latter already exists, to reduce the activity of the parathyroid glands; c) heal bone disease; d) prevent and reverse soft-tissue calcification; e) ameliorate or reverse the proximal myopathy, bone pain, pruritus, and soft-tissue necrosis; and f) prevent and treat aluminum bone disease.

Despite the advances in the understanding of the pathogenesis of renal osteodystrophy in patients with renal failure, there is still no unified approach to optimal therapy. The various therapeutic modalities currently in use are neither perfect nor without hazards. The overall management include the use of one or more of the following therapeutic approaches: a) control of phosphate retention and hyperphosphatemia, b) supplementation of calcium, c) treatment with vitamin D or one or more of its metabolites, d) parathyroidectomy, and e) appropriate dialysate composition in dialysis patients.

CONTROL OF PHOSPHATE RETENTION AND HYPERPHOSPHATEMIA

Phosphate retention and hyperphosphatemia play an important role in the pathogenesis of the disorders of divalent ion metabolism of renal failure (2–4). The prevention of phosphate retention in patients with mild or moderate renal insufficiency and the control of hyperphosphatemia in those with advanced renal failure represent important parts in the management of these patients.

The hyperphosphatemia of uremia may be reduced by dietary restriction of phosphate, the use of phosphate-binding antacids, an increased frequency of hemodialysis, and by the inhibition of PTH-mediated bone resorption.

The dietary intake of phosphate is a function of the meat and dairy products ingested by the patients. The usual phosphate intake of phosphate by a normal adult in the United States ranges between 1.0 and 1.8 g/day. One can reduce the dietary intake of phosphate by 40% (600–900 g/day) by the elimination of dairy products and the restriction of protein intake. Further reduction may be difficult to achieve without jeopardizing adequate protein intake or compromising the palatability of the food. Thus, restriction of dietary phosphate intake in proportion to the decrease in GFR as the sole measure for the prevention of phosphate retention is only feasible in patients with moderate renal failure (GFR, 60–30 ml/min). Indeed, this approach has been successful in reversing many of the abnormalities in divalent ion metabolism in such patients.

In patients with advanced renal failure, dietary phosphate restriction alone is not adequate to control the hyperphosphatemia. In a group of patients with creatinine clearance of 2–10 ml/min who were treated with rigid protein restriction (20 or 40 g/day) for 30–60 days, serum phosphorus levels remained elevated, with mean levels of 7.2 ± 0.86 and 7.3 ± 0.72 mg/dl, respectively, despite a continued negative phosphorus balance in some of the patients (5). It is evident that in patients with advanced renal failure other measures are needed to maintain serum phosphorus within the normal range. This could be achieved with the use of phosphate-binding antacids, which would render the ingested phosphate and the phosphate contained in the saliva (12 mM/l), bile (5 mM/l), and intestinal juices (1 mM/l) unabsorbable.

Several compounds that bind phosphate in the intestinal tract are available in liquid, tablet, and capsule forms (Table 2). The capsules are less effective than liquid gels in binding phosphate, but patient compliance is easier to achieve with capsules than with either the liquid or the tablets. The most frequently used compounds are Alu-Caps®, Amphojel®, and Basaljel® concentrate. The latter is tasteless and only a small volume is necessary per dose, and hence, the patients more readily follow the prescribed

Table 1. Biochemical, clinical and pathologic features of renal osteodystrophy

Hypocalcemia and occasionally hypercalcemia
Hyperphosphatemia
Elevated blood levels of parathyroid hormone
Elevated blood levels of alkaline phosphatase and hydroxyproline
Hyperplasia of the parathyroid glands
Defective intestinal absorption of calcium
Deficiency of $1,25\text{-}(OH)_2D_3$
Bone disease
    Defective mineralization (osteomalacias or rickets)
    Aluminum bone disease (low-turnover osteomalacia)
    Hyperparathyroid bone disease (enhanced bone resorption and endosteal fibrosis)
Soft-tissue calcification
Pruritus
Proximal myopathy
Spontaneous tendon rupture
Soft-tissue necrosis

regimen. The goal of the treatment is to reduce the level of serum phosphorus to near normal. Care should be exercised to avoid a fall in serum phosphorus to very low levels and the production of phosphate depletion with these agents. Phosphate depletion per se may aggravate bone disease and may even cause osteomalacia (6). Therapy may be started with two to three tablets of Amphojel or capsules or Alu-Caps or 5–10 ml of Basaljel with each meal. The levels of serum phosphorus should be monitored at least twice per month, and the dose of the phosphate binders should be adjusted accordingly. Continued coaxing and emphasis on the importance of this treatment are essential to obtain adherence to this therapy by the patients. These compounds are ineffective in controlling the concentration of serum phosphorus if the dietary phosphate intake exceeds 2.0 g/day.

The fall in serum phosphorus concentrations during therapy with dietary phosphate restriction and the use of phosphate binding antacids is usually associated with a rise in the level of serum calcium; if the magnitude of the latter is adequate, a fall in the blood levels of PTH may occur, and this, in turn, will contribute to the maintenance of the concentration of serum phosphorus at lower levels.

The aluminum in the phosphate-binding antacids is absorbed by the intestine and may accumulate in various tissues of the body such as the brain and bones. An increased aluminum burden of the brain has been incriminated in the pathogenesis of dialysis encephalopathy, and accumulation of aluminum in bone may be responsible for low-turnover osteomalacia, which is refractory to therapy. Despite these potential hazards, these compounds are still recommended for use in the control of hyperphosphatemia in patients with advanced renal failure and in dialysis patients. One approach that may minimize the hazards of aluminum toxicity is to begin therapy with aluminum compounds and then to replace these compounds with calcium carbonate once the serum phosphorus returns to normal. The use of magnesium-containing compounds should be avoided because of the risks of hypermagnesemia. If these compounds are given the patients should be dialyzed with a magnesium-free dialyzate.

CALCIUM SUPPLEMENTATION

The low dietary intake of calcium and the defect in intestinal calcium absorption, which is more evident at a low calcium intake (7, 8), put patients with renal failure in double jeopardy with regard to their calcium balance. Evidence exists indicating that normal amounts of calcium could be absorbed by the gut of these patients when the calcium intake is high (9). Indeed, long-term calcium supplementation has been associated with beneficial effects such as a rise in the concentration of serum calcium, a fall in the serum levels of alkaline phosphatase and PTH, and a reduction in bone resorption and the number and incidence of fractures; such therapy, however, did not achieve normal mineralization of osteoid. Thus, there is a good rational for calcium supplementation, but the time in the course of renal insufficiency at which such therapy should be initiated is not evident. It is reasonable to suggest that patients with a GFR between 40 and 10 ml/min should receive 1.2–1.5 g of calcium/day. Calcium supplements may be given to these patients to bring their total daily intake to this level. Patients with advanced renal failure (GFR < 10 ml/min) may need a supplement of 1.0–2.0 g of calcium/day.

Treatment with calcium salts is not without hazards. It is dangerous to administer large quantities of oral calcium compounds in the face of marked hyperphosphatemia

Table 2. Partial list of available phosphate-binding compounds

Generic name	Proprietary name	Manufacturer	Form available
Aluminum hydroxide gel	Amphojel	Wyeth	Tablets (0.3 and 0.6 g)
Aluminum hydroxide gel	Alu-Cap	Riker	Capsules (0.6 g)
Aluminum carbonate	Basaljel	Wyeth	Solution (3.6 g/30 ml) Tablets (0.5 g) Capsules (0.5 g)
Aluminum hydroxide and magnesium hydroxide	Aludrox	Wyeth	Tablets
Aluminum hydroxide and magnesium hydroxide	Maalox	Rorer	Tablets
Aluminum hydroxide, magnesium hydroxide, and simethicone	Gelusil	Parke–Davis	Tablets
Aluminum hydroxide, magnesium hydroxide, and simethicone	Mylanta	Stuart	Tablets

because of the danger of an elevation in the calcium-phosphorus product, predisposing to soft-tissue calcification. Thus, it is imperative that hyperphosphatemia is controlled and that the level of serum phosphorus is less than 5.5 mg/dl prior to treatment with calcium salts. Also, hypercalcemia may appear during therapy with large doses of oral calcium, especially in patients with advanced renal failure (10); this is particularly true when there has been a concomitant reduction in the levels of serum phosphorus to less than 2.0 mg/dl. A variety of symptoms may accompany even mild hypercalcemia in uremic patients. Nausea, vomiting, mental confusion, lethargy, pruritus, dysethesias, and severe hypertension have been encountered. Therefore, weekly or bimonthly monitoring of the concentration of serum calcium and phosphorus is advisable. If the serum concentration of calcium exceeds 10.5 mg/dl, calcium supplements may be cut in half or may even be discontinued temporarily.

Elemental calcium constitutes 40% of calcium carbonate, 12% of calcium lactate, and 8% of calcium gluconate. Calcium chloride should be avoided in uremic patients because of its acidifying properties. Calcium carbonate is inexpensive, tasteless, and relatively well tolerated. Calcium carbonate is available in several proprietary preparations such as Titralac®. Tums®, or Os-Cal®. Titralac provides 0.42 g of calcium carbonate and 0.18 g of glycine per tablet (160 mg of elemental calcium/tablet). Neo-Calglucon® syrup is another preparation that is well accepted by patients but it is costly; each 4 ml contains 92 mg of calcium ion. To maximize calcium absorption, the amount prescribed should be ingested in several small doses divided throughout the day rather than in one or two large doses.

USE OF VITAMIN-D COMPOUNDS

Since many of the features of abnormal calcium metabolism in uremia resemble those of vitamin-D deficiency, this compound and its related steroids have been used in the management of renal osteodystrophy. The currently available forms of vitamin-D metabolites for clinical use in the United States are vitamin D_2 (ergocalciferol); vitamin D_3 (cholecalciferol), which is the naturally occurring form of the steroid in mammals; dihydrotachysterol; 25-(OH)D_3; and 1,25-(OH)$_2D_3$. Another vitamin D analogue, 1α(OH)D_3, is available for clinical use outside the United States.

Because of its low cost, vitamin D_2, a steroid obtained from plant sources, has been most widely used in medicine. Vitamin D_3 can now be prepared inexpensively but it does not enjoy widespread use. Moreover, there is little evidence to indicate that vitamin D_2 differs in activity from vitamin D_3 in humans.

Vitamins D_2 and D_3

There is a great variability in the required amount of vitamin D by patients with advanced renal failure. Doses as high as 50,000 to 200,000 IU/day (1.25–5.0 mg) may be needed to achieve beneficial effects. The long-term therapy with large doses of vitamin D causes a rise in the serum calcium levels and may be followed by a fall in the serum levels of alkaline phosphatase and PTH, reduced bone resorption, and amelioration or healing of rickets in uremic children, or of osteomalacia in uremic adults. Because of the need for large doses of vitamin D, hypercalcemia is a real and frequent hazard. Such hypercalcemia may persist for weeks after the discontinuation of therapy. In addition to the clinical side effects of hypercalcemia, the elevation in the serum levels of calcium in a hyperphosphatemic patient would cause a marked rise in the calcium-phosphorus product, predisposing to soft-tissue calcification. Therapy with vitamin D should not be started prior to the normalization of the serum levels of phosphorus. Frequent monitoring of the levels of serum calcium and phosphorus during such therapy is advisable.

25-hydroxyvitamin D_3

Despite the block in the conversion of 25-(OH)D to 1,25-(OH)$_2$D, therapy with 50–100 µg of 25-(OH)D_3/day has been shown to be beneficial. Treatment with this metabolite was associated with amelioration of bone pain and proximal myopathy, a rise in serum calcium concentration, and a fall in serum levels of alkaline phosphatase and PTH. A decrease in the degree of osteitis fibrosa, and even improvement in bone mineralization, have been noted.

1,25-dihydroxyvitamin D_3

A relative deficiency of this active metabolite is present in patients with mild and moderate renal failure (4, 11, 12), and an absolute deficiency exists in those with advanced renal failure (13). Furthermore, the kidney is required to convert the parent vitamin D to this active metabolite. Therefore, it is rational to treat renal failure patients with this metabolite to correct the vitamin-D-deficient state. Indeed, such therapy has proven to be beneficial. It is important to emphasize at this point that some or most of the beneficial effects of 1,25-(OH)$_2D_3$ in the management of renal osteodystrophy could be produced by other vitamin-D compounds. The smaller dose of 1,25-(OH)$_2D_3$ that is needed to achieve beneficial effects and its shorter half-life make it, however, a better and safer agent than other vitamin-D compounds. On the other hand, the high biologic potency of 1,25-(OH)$_2D_3$ causes the early appearance of hazardous side effects (hypercalcemia and elevation in the calcium-phosphorus product) with even a very small dose. Thus, close monitoring of patients receiving 1,25-(OH)$_2D_3$ is mandatory.

The suggested initial dose of oral therapy is 0.5 µg/day, although it may be safer to begin therapy with 0.25 µg/day. The changes in the concentrations of serum calcium provide the best clinical guide for modification of the dose. Failure of the level of serum calcium to rise by at least 0.5 mg/dl with any particular dosage given for 4–6 weeks justifies increasing the dose by 0.25–0.5 µg/day. Such an approach may be used until the serum calcium reaches the upper normal range (10.0–10.5 mg/dl). When this is achieved, frequent monitoring of the serum calcium is needed, and if the latter approaches the hypercalcemic range, a reduction of the dose or temporary discontinuation of therapy should be considered. It is our experience and that of others that the requirement of and the tolerance for 1,25-$(OH)_2D_3$ may decrease progressively during treatment in many patients; therefore, reduction of the maintenance dosage after a prolonged period of therapy may be needed.

Among the most disturbing clinical symptoms of renal osteodystrophy are muscle weakness and bone pain. The muscle weakness is a clinical manifestation of uremic myopathy that is at least partly due to vitamin-D deficiency. The exact cause of bone pain is not known but may be related to the presence of osteomalacia and/or osteitis fibrosa or to a potential *algesic effect* of excess blood levels of PTH. These disturbances may interfere seriously with the daily activity of patients and may even render them totally disabled. Improvement in these symptoms appears rapidly after initiation of therapy with 1,25-$(OH)_2D_3$. The improvement in muscle strength may become noticeable within 2–5 weeks of treatment. A significant amelioration or complete disappearance of bone pain may also occur in some patients within 1–3 weeks of treatment, while in others it may take 6–28 weeks before a decrease in bone pain becomes evident. This clinical improvement produces a remarkable change in the physical disability of patients; many of them become symptom free and are able to perform their daily activity without limitation. Similar observations have been encountered in children. For example, three children who had ceased to walk for several months prior to therapy began walking within 1 month and were running after 4 months of treatment. Treatment of uremic children with 1,25-$(OH)_2D_3$ may also increase growth velocity; this effect is extremely important since retarded growth in uremic children is a very common and serious problem.

The most consistent effect of 1,25-$(OH)_2D_3$ in uremic and dialysis patients is the elevation in the serum concentration of calcium. Although it is reasonable to assume that the higher the dose of the metabolite, the greater this rise in the serum calcium concentration, many variables in addition to the dose may modify the calcemic response to therapy with 1,25-$(OH)_2D_3$. These may include the duration of treatment, dietary calcium intake, changes in the intestinal absorption of calcium, the type of bone disease and its response to treatment, and the severity of the state of secondary hyperparathyroidism. Occasionally, the serum calcium concentration may fall during the first 1–2 weeks of therapy, probably due to rapid remineralization of the skeleton.

Hypercalcemia is a frequent complication of treatment with 1,25-$(OH)_2D_3$. It has been reported that 30–67% of the patients treated with this metabolite developed one or more hypercalcemic episodes during the course of their therapy. The overall incidence of one episode was 42%. Hypercalcemia occurred with a dosage of 0.5–3.0 µg/day of 1,25-$(OH)_2D_3$ and was more frequent with a dosage of 1.0–3.0 µg/day. Two groups of patients are more prone to develop hypercalcemia; they are a) patients with osteitis fibrosa and a pretreatment serum calcium concentration greater than 10.5 mg/day and b) patients with low-turnover osteomalacia, a low serum concentration of PTH, and absent bone marrow fibrosis. Hypercalcemia may appear at any time during therapy with 1,25-$(OH)_2D_3$. It usually occurs after 2–3 months of therapy but has been encountered as early as 5 days and as late as 6–18 months after treatment. A high starting dose may be the cause for the early appearance of hypercalcemia. Early hypercalcemia within 1–4 weeks of therapy may also occur in patients with severe osteitis fibrosa and a pretreatment serum calcium concentration of 10.5 mg/dl. Extreme caution should be exercised in the management of such patients with 1,25-$(OH)_2D_3$. It has been noted that the incidence of hypercalcemia increases as serum alkaline phosphates activity returns to normal, and it is recommended to reduce the dosage of 1,25-$(OH)_2D_3$ when serum levels of alkaline phosphatase normalize. The hypercalcemia is usually mild and asymptomatic, but serum calcium concentrations is greater than 13.0 mg/dl, and occasionally even higher than 15.0 mg/dl, have been encountered during therapy with 1,25-$(OH)_2D_3$. The elevated levels of serum calcium usually return to normal shortly after reduction of the dose or discontinuation of the therapy. Occasionally, the hypercalcemia may persist for several weeks. It is advisable to stop treatment completely rather than to reduce the dose when hypercalcemia appears and to reinstitue therapy with a small dose as the serum calcium concentrations return to normal.

The effect of 1,25-$(OH)_2D_3$ treatment on the concentration of serum phosphorus in uremic or dialysis patients is not consistent. An increase, a decrease, and no change have been reported. This variability in the various patient populations may be related to differences in dietary intake of phosphate and/or the ingestion of phosphate-binding antacids, the dosage of 1,25-$(Oh)_2D_3$, the effect of the metabolite on intestinal absorption of phosphate, the degree of suppression of parathyroid gland activity, and the status of remineralization of bone. Monitoring of serum phosphorus concentrations during therapy with 1,25-$(OH)_2D_3$ is mandatory because the development of hyperphosphatemia, especially in the face of a rising serum calcium concentration, would result in elevation of the calcium-phosphorus product and would augment the hazards of soft-tissue calcification. If hyperphosphatemia occurs and the calcium-phosphorus product approaches 55, every effort should be made to control the levels of serum phosphorus with phosphate-binding antacids. If this procedure is not successful, the dose of 1,25-$(OH)_2D_3$ should be reduced or temporary cessation of therapy should be considered. It is recommended that the calcium-phosphorus product be maintained below 55.

Serum alkaline phosphatase activity usually decreases during therapy with 1,25-$(OH)_2D_3$, but several months elapse before levels return to normal. Occasionally, serum alkaline phosphatase may rise during the initial phase of therapy. Monitoring the serum alkaline phosphatase could provide an additional guide for the adjustment of the dosage of $1,25\text{-}(OH)_2D_3$ for two reasons. First, normalization of serum levels of alkaline phosphatase reflects an improvement in bone disease, and second, the occurrence of hypercalcemia increases as serum alkaline phosphatase returns to normal.

Long-term therapy with $1,25\text{-}(OH)_2D_3$ may be associated with a marked fall in or even normalization of serum levels of PTH. No change or even an increase in serum levels of the hormone has also been encountered during therapy with this metabolite. On the average, the blood levels of PTH fall by 50–60% with 1–2 years of oral therapy with $1,25\text{-}(OH)_2D_3$. The reduction in the serum levels of PTH during oral therapy with $1,25\text{-}(OH)_2D_3$ is probably due to the rise in the concentration of serum calcium (14), but a direct effect of $1,25\text{-}(OH)_2D_3$ on the activity of the parathyroid glands may also play a role (15). We have found an inverse correlation between the percentage change in serum calcium concentrations and PTH levels (14).

Intestinal absorption of calcium is usually increased in most uremic patients during therapy with $1,25\text{-}(OH)_2D_3$. The increment in calcium absorption is most evident during the first 2 hours after the ingestion of the ^{47}Ca, suggesting that the metabolite exerts its effect in the duodenum and the proximal part of the small intestine. This metabolite may also affect calcium absorption in the jejunum, since this segment of the intestine has receptors for $1,25\text{-}(OH)_2D_3$. There is a dose-response relationship between $1,25\text{-}(OH)_2D_3$ and intestinal absorption of calcium. Finally, the quantity of the sterol required to elicit an increase in intestinal calcium absorption in the uremic patient is greater than in normal subjects, suggesting that uremia per se may interfere with the action of the sterol on the gut. $1,25\text{-}(OH)_2D_3$ also augments intestinal absorption of phosphate. The metabolite may produce a modest rise in urinary calcium in uremic patients.

Therapy with oral $1,25\text{-}(OH)_2D_3$ for several months could be associated with a decrease in bone resorption, and treatment for 2–3 years may result in complete healing of bone resorption. The effect on bone resorption reflects the degree of success in suppressing the activity of the parathyroid glands. Endosteal fibrosis is either markedly reduced or completely reversed after several months of treatment, irrespective of whether serum levels of PTH are decreased or not. This observation raises the possibility that endosteal fibrosis is not entirely the result of excess PTH but could also be related to vitamin-D deficiency as well. The osteomalacia in patients with mixed bone disease (osteomalacia and osteitis fibrosa) responds well to therapy with $1,25\text{-}(OH)_2D_3$. Long-term treatment usually results in marked improvement or healing of the osteomalacia. In patients with pure low-turnover osteomalacia, the response to $1,25\text{-}(OH)_2D_3$ is poor; these patients may respond better to long-term therapy (4–6 months) with both $1,25\text{-}(OH)_2D_3$ and $24,25\text{-}(OH)_2D_3$ (2.5–10 µg/dl/day). The healing of the bone lesions during treatment with $1,25\text{-}(OH)_2D_3$ may also be evidenced by improvement in the radiographic findings of the skeleton.

Failure of therapy with $1,25\text{-}(OH)_2D_3$ to improve the clinical signs and symptoms has been reported. The treatment failure group appears to be heterogeneous and does not display a specific biochemical pattern of bone disease. Although patients had higher serum calcium concentrations than those who responded to treatment, the serum levels of PTH were normal, moderately elevated, or very high, and the bone lesions varied from pure osteomalacia in some to marked osteitis fibrosa in others. Further analysis of the data, however, indicates that there are two distinct subgroups among these patients. The first group consists of patients with severe osteitis fibrosa and marked elevation of serum PTH. In the second group, the patients had normal serum levels of PTH and pure osteomalacia without evidence of hyperparathyroid bone disease. Both of these groups rapidly develop hypercalcemia. As this complication requires cessation of treatment, it would preclude long-term therapy and, hence, failure to improve the clinical and histologic abnormalities of renal osteodystrophy.

Intravenous prepartion of $1,25\text{-}(OH)_2D_3$ in available for use in dialysis patients. This metabolite given in doses of 1.0–1.5 µg three times per weeks almost normalized blood levels of PTH within 2–3 months (16). It appears that intravenous administration of $1,25\text{-}(OH)_2D_3$ exerts a direct inhibitory effect on the parathyroid gland activity. Indeed, the blood levels of PTH began to fall before a significant rise in the concentration of serum calcium became evident. Data on the effect of this therapy on bone disease are as yet not available.

$1,25\text{-}(OH)_2D_3$ could also be used for the prevention of secondary hyperparathyroidism and of other derangements of divalent ion metabolism in patients with early-to-moderate renal failure. In a double-blind control study, it was found that 0.5–2.0 µg of $1,25\text{-}(OH)_2D_3$/day given for 1 year to patients with GFR ranging between 15 and 55 ml/min was associated with a rise in blood concentrations of calcium, a fall in those of alkaline phosphatase, a marked reduction in blood levels of PTH (50–60%), and healing of hyperparathyroid bone disease and osteomalacia. Blood levels of serum calcium should be monitored carefully during the therapy and hypercalcemia should be avoided.

It has been claimed that the administration of $1,25\text{-}(OH)_2D_3$ to patients with moderate renal failure produced a significant reduction in GFR due to a direct adverse effect. Analysis of all available and pertinent data does not support the contention that $1,25\text{-}(OH)_2D_3$ has a direct deleterious effect on renal function. The metabolite could produce a reversible or permanent fall in GFR, however, if sustained hypercalcemia develops during its administration. The use of the proper dosage, the frequent monitoring of serum calcium and creatinine concentrations, and the discontinuation of therapy as hypercalcemia develops are the precautionary measures that should be followed to reduce the likelihood of a harmful effect on renal function.

DIALYSATE AND ITS COMPOSITION

There is evidence for considerable geographic variations in the incidence of skeletal disease in patients undergoing hemodialysis. Various impurities and trace elements such as fluoride or aluminum may be responsible for these geographic variations. It is now accepted that water treatment and purification should be employed prior to the preparation of the dialysate.

Variations in the concentration of calcium in dialysate may affect the course of renal osteodystrophy. It should be emphasized that all the calcium present in dialysate is ionized and diffuses freely across the membrane of the dialyzer. This contrasts with calcium in the blood; only 60% of the total amount is not bound to protein and is able to move across the membrane. Depending upon the gradient, the dialysate calcium level, and the concentration of diffusible calcium in blood, there will be either a loss or a gain of this ion by the patient. The use of dialysate containing 5.0–5.5 mg of calcium/dl was associated with a high incidence of radiographic evidence of bone disease, progressively rising serum levels of alkaline phosphatase, loss of calcium from bone, and persistently elevated serum levels of PTH. For these reasons, dialysate containing such a low concentration of calcium should be abandoned. The use of dialysate containing 8.0 mg of calcium/dl may be hazardous in that it may cause hypercalcemia and may enhance soft-tissue calcification. Most authorities recommend a calcium concentration of 7.0 mg/dl. Occasionally, the use of this dialysate calcium in patients treated with 1,25-$(OH)_2D_3$ may be associated with hypercalcemia. If this occurs, either the dose of 1,25-$(OH)_2D_3$ is reduced or the dialysate calcium is decreased.

Most centers have used dialysate containing magnesium in a concentration varying between 0.6 and 1.8 mg/dl (0.5–1.5 mEq/l). With the lower magnesium dialysate, predialysis levels of magnesium are usually normal and are slightly below normal immediately after dialysis. Patients treated with dialysate containing the higher concentration of magnesium have moderate hypermagnesemia all the time. There is no evidence that variations in dialysate magnesium within this range have an effect on the incidence, course, or severity of skeletal disease, soft-tissue calcification, or symptoms related to altered divalent ion metabolism.

PARATHYROIDECTOMY

The various medical therapeutic modalities detailed earlier can result in suppression of the hyperplastic parathyroid glands in uremic patients. However, these measures may not be successful, and parathyroidectomy may be the only way to treat the clinical, biochemical, and skeletal manifestations of secondary hyperparathyroidism. Subtotal parathyroidectomy should be considered: a) when persistent hypercalcemia develops; b) when severe intractable pruritus that is unresponsive to dialysis is present, especially when the blood levels of PTH are markedly elevated; c) when marked soft-tissue calcification (especially vascular) and radiographic evidence of marked osteitis fibrosa are present, and they cannot be adequately controlled with conservative therapy; and d) when ischemic lesions of soft tissue with ulcerations and necrosis develop.

The amount of parathyroid tissue to be removed at surgery depends on the size of the parathyroid glands in any particular patient. We recommend that all four glands be first identified; three glands are then removed and weighed. By comparing the size of the fourth gland with those removed, one can roughly estimate the weight of the fourth gland. The surgeon should leave only 150–200 mg of this remaining gland. Since the residual parathyroid tissue may undergo further hyperplasia and a second operation may be required, it is recommended that the residual tissue be marked by a metal clip and a long black silk suture. An alternative approach is to remove all four glands and transplant part of a gland in the forearm. Occasionally, this has been associated with recurrent hyperparathyroidism due to development of sheets of parathyroid tissue along the entire arm, a situation that is not amenable to surgical correction. If fewer than four glands are identified in the neck, they should all be removed. Rarely, removal of three identified glands will result in a state of permanent hypoparathyroidism. Total parathyroidectomy may be considered in patients who will be maintained with hemodialysis and are not suitable for renal transplantation. The medical and/or surgical treatment of uremic secondary hyperparathyroidism assumes greater significance, with the accumulation of evidence indicating that excess PTH in blood may play a major role in uremic toxicity (17).

The technical problems during the surgical procedure are few. The glands are grossly enlarged and are easily identifiable. In the hands of an experienced surgeon, the operation is not hazardous, and the patient leaves the hospital within a week. The patients should be treated with dialysis 1 day prior to surgery.

A major problems during the postoperative period is the control of the serum calcium concentration. Its level invariably falls after the removal of three or more parathyroid glands. The magnitude and the duration of the hypocalcemia vary from one patient to another. Those with marked periarticular calcification usually maintain serum levels of calcium between 8.0 and 9.0 mg/dl until the ectopic calcifications disappear. Also, the use of dialysate containing 7.0 mg of calcium/dl causes a rise in the serum calcium concentration during dialysis and may alleviate the hypocalcemia during the interdialytic intervals. Profound hypocalcemia may develop in certain patients, especially in those with radiographic evidenced of bone resorption; treatment of such patients with 1,25-$(OH)_2D_3$ may reduce the severity of the postoperative hypocalcemia. Tetany may occur in those who develop severe hypocalcemia. When the level of serum calcium falls below 7.5 mg/dl, oral calcium supplementation may prevent a further decrease. The amount of oral calcium needed is usually quite large. The initial treatment should provide at least 2.0 g of calcium, and the dose can be increased at intervals of 3–7 days until an adequate rise in the serum calcium concentration is achieved. If the concentration of serum calcium falls to lower levels and if tetany appears, intravenous calcium should be given in addition to the oral supplements of calcium. In patients with profound and sustained hypocalcemia, 1,25-$(OH)_2D_3$ may be needed; careful monitoring of serum calcium and phosphorus should be undertaken with this therapy. Serum levels of phosphorus almost always fall after parathyroidectomy. Therefore, phosphate-binding antacids should be withheld if serum levels of phosphorus decrease to less than 3.0 mg/dl. Also, serum levels of phosphorus should not be allowed to rise above 4.0 mg/dl, because the hyperphosphatemia may aggravate the hypocalcemia in the parathyroidectomized patients.

ALUMINUM BONE DISEASE

Aluminum bone disease is a low-turnover osteomalacia. This type of osteomalacia does not usually respond to therapy with vitamin D. Treatment with 1,25-$(OH)_2D_3$ often causes hypercalcemia in these patients.

Aluminum can be removed from soft tissues and bone by the chelating agent deferoxamine. The intravenous infusion of this compound in patients treated with hemodialysis or the intraperitoneal instillation of deferoxamine in patients managed with continuous ambulatory pertioneal dialysis has been successful in removing large amounts of aluminum and in ameliorating aluminum bone disease.

Side effects of therapy with deferoxamine include hypotension, cataract formation, and increased sensitivity to infection, especially those due to *Yersinia*, *Salmonella*, and *Rhizopus* (*Mucromycosis*).

OTHER THERAPEUTIC MEASURES

The use of beta-adrenergic blocking agents (propranolol) may cause a decrease in the serum levels of PTH, but this action is variable and is not successful in the complete reversal of secondary hyperparathyroidism. Claims that cimetidine may be effective in controlling secondary hyperparathyroidism in uremic patients have not been convincingly substantiated. Occasionally, treatment with diphosphonate (disodium ethane-1-hydroxy-1, 1-diphosphonate (disodium ethane-1-hydroxy-1, 1-diphosphonate) may cause regression of ectopic calcification that is resistant to the usual therapy (control of the hyperphosphatemia, suppression of parathyroid gland activity, or parathyroidectomy. Treatment with disodium ethane-1-hydroxy-1, 1-diphosphonate, by itself, may produce osteomalacia.

REFERENCES

1. Massry SG: Divalent ion metabolism and renal osteodystrophy. In: SG Massry, RJ Glassock, eds, *Textbook of Nephrology*, 2nd ed. Williams and Wilkins, Baltimore, pp 1278–1311, 1989.
2. Slatopolsky E, Caglar S, Pennell JP, Taggart DD, Canterbury JM, Reiss E, Bricker NS: On the pathogenesis of hyperparathyroidism in chronic and experimental renal insufficiency in the dog. *J Clin Invest* 50:492–499, 1971.
3. Slatopolsky E, Caglar S, Gradowska L, Canterbury J, Reiss E, Bricker NS: On the prevention of secondary hyperparathyroidism in experimental chronic renal disease using "proportional reduction" of dietary phosphorus intake. *Kidney Int* 2:147–151, 1972.
4. Llach F, Massry SG: On the mechanisms of secondary hyperparathyroidism in moderate renal insufficiency. *J Clin Endocrinol Metab* 61:601–606, 1985.
5. Kopple JD, Coburn JW: Metabolic studies of low protein diets in uremia: II. Calcium, phosphorus and magnesium. *Medicine* 52:597–607, 1973.
6. Abrams DE, Silcot RB, Terry R, Berne TV, Barbour BH: Antacid induction of phosphate depletion syndrome in renal failure. *Western J Med* 120:157, 1974.
7. Coburn JW, Koppel MH, Brickman AS, Massry SG: Studies on intestinal absorption of calcium in patients with renal failure. *Kidney Int* 3:264–272, 1973.
8. Coburn JW, Hartenbower DL, Massry SG: Intestinal absorption of calcium and the effect of renal insufficiency. *Kidney Int* 4:96–104, 1973.
9. McDonald SJ, Clarkson EM, DeWardener HE: The effect of a large intake of calcium in normal subjects and patients with chronic renal failure. *Clin Sci* 26:27, 1964.
10. Ginsburg DS, Kaplan EL, Katz AI: Hypercalcemia after oral calcium carbonate therapy in patients on chronic hemodialysis. *Lancet* 1:1271, 1973.
11. Slatopolsky E. Gray R, Adams ND, Lewis J, Hruska K, Martin K, Klahr S, DeLuca H, Lemann J: Low serum levels of 1,25 $(OH)_2D_3$ are not responsible for the development of secondary hyperparathyroidism in early renal failure. *Kidney Int* 14:733A, 1978.
12. Cheung AK, Manolagas, Catherwood BD, Mosely CA Jr, Mitas JAB, Blantz RC, Deftos LJ: Determination of serum 1,25$(OH)_2D_3$ levels in renal disease. *Kidney Int* 24:104–109, 1983.
13. Haussler MR, Brumbaugh PF, Ogden DA: Radioreceptor assay of plasma 1 25-dihydroxy-vitamin D_3 in patients with chronic renal failure. *Clin Res* 22:531A, 1974.
14. Goldstein DA, Malluche HH, Massry SG: Management of renal osteodystrophy with 1,25$(OH)_2D_3$. I. Effects on clinical, radiographic and biochemical parameters. *Miner Electrolyte Metab* 2:35–47, 1979.
15. Chan W, McKay C, Dye E, Slatopolsky E: The effects of 1,25$(OH)_2D_3$ on PTH secretion by monolayer cultures of bovine parathyroid (PT) cells. *Proc Am Soc Nephrol* 17:13A, 1984.
16. Slatopolsky E, Weerts C. Thielan J, Horst R, Harter H, Martin KJ: Marked suppression of secondary hyperparathyroidism by intravenous administration of 1,25-dihydroxycholecalciferol in uremic patients. *J Clin Invest* 74:2136–2143, 1984.
17. Massry SG: The toxic effect of parathyroid hormone in uremia. *Semin Nephrol* 3:306–328, 1983.

CHAPTER 47

Neurologic and Psychiatric Disorders in Renal Failure

SUHAIL AHMAD & CHRISTOPHER R. BLAGG

While some of the effects of renal failure on the nervous system have been recognized for many years, it is only since the development of dialysis and kidney transplantation that these conditions have become important topics for study by neurologists and nephrologists. Neurologic problems are no longer regarded only as late or terminal events in the course of uremia; the importance of this recognition is the potential for reversibility with early and adequate treatment.

The pathophysiology of uremia is extremely complex, and patients with either acute or chronic renal failure may develop a complex of symptoms broadly described as *uremic encephalopathy*, frequently associated with involvement of the peripheral nervous system. Dialysis or a successful renal transplant can relieve many of these effects, but these treatments themselves may be associated with other neurologic complications. In dialysis patients the disequilibrium syndrome and dialysis dementia may occur, as well as other neurologic problems, which, while not specific to dialysis, are more common in these patients. Patients who receive a kidney transplant are prone to develop various tumors and infections of the central nervous system, primarily as a complication of immunosuppression. In addition, all patients with renal failure, however treated, are subject to a wide variety of psychological problems.

BRAIN ABNORMALITIES IN UREMIA

Uremic encephalopathy

Uremic encephalopathy is an organic brain syndrome occurring in patients with severely impaired renal function resulting from both acute or chronic renal failure (1). Clinically, the effects resemble those of other metabolic or toxic encephalopathies, and may be modified by the presence of acidosis, hypoxia, hypoosmolality and hyperosmolality, and other biochemical changes that can occur with renal failure.

The clinical manifestations of uremic encephalopathy are nonspecific, the symptom complex ranging from mild slurring of speech and tremors to coma and death. Affected patients differ in their presentation and, as with all metabolic encephalopathies, signs and symptoms can vary unpredictably in the same patient. The clinical features do not correlate well with the biochemical abnormalities or the degree of uremia, but correlate better with the rate of progression of renal failure. Consequently, encephalopathy may be more pronounced in pateints with acute renal failure and least obvious in patients with slowly progressive chronic renal failure. The signs and symptoms are relieved to a great degree by dialysis and are usually resolved completely by a successful kidney transplant. Thus it is important to recognize the development of uremic encephalopathy because it can be treated so readily, yet if untreated it may be fatal.

SYMPTOMS AND SIGNS

The earliest symptoms include disturbances of mental functions, malaise, irritability, difficulty in concentration, tiredness, insomnia, and apathy (2). These changes, which may be subtle, occur to some degree in most uremic patients prior to treatment and may be a sensitive index of early neurologic involvement. Signs and symptoms may be episodic or continuous and at first may be difficult to distinguish from the effects of nausea, anxiety, and depression, which are common in uremic patients who are aware of their disease and its implications. Similar symptoms result from the anemia associated with renal failure, and with recent development of recombinant human erythropoietin (3) it will be interesting to see how the early symptoms associated with uremia may be changed in patients who no longer develop anemia.

As uremia worsens, the symptoms progress and become continuous, and there may be a decreased attention span, further difficulty in concentration, inability to perform tasks such as subtraction of serial sevens, and worsening fatigue (4). Generally, patients are started on dialysis before these symptoms become marked. However, if untreated, the symptoms increase, and the patients becomes progressively drowsier or, in some cases, more nervous and restless.

Several specific neurologic disturbances also may develop. Dysarthria is a common early sign, with slow, slurred, and thickened speech because of difficulty with fine tongue movements, although palatal and lip movements are unaffected. Rapid irregular tremors may be an early sign of uremic encephalopathy (5), occurring during active movement and on extension of the hands, and these may become more obvious while eliciting asterixis. Asterixis usually develops simultaneously with the onset of clouding of consciousness, and the typical flapping tremor may be demonstrated in the hands, lower limbs, and face. These are not involuntary movements, but result from failure to maintain a sustained posture. Electromyography shows brief silent periods without muscular activity in extensors and flexors during the downward phase, followed by compensatory contraction of the extensors; there are no characteristic EEG changes. The cause is unknown, but asterixis is probably related to central nervous system dysfunction. Myoclonus is a sudden, asymmetrical, arrhythmical gross twitching, involving muscles in various parts of the body, particularly facial and proximal limb muscles, and is often preceded by muscular fasciculation. It is generally a late manifestation of uremic encephalopathy, often associated with stupor or coma. "Uremic twitching" is a combination of asterixis, tremors, and myoclonus (5), possibly representing cortical irritability resulting from metabolic changes. Movements may be so severe as to resemble multifocal seizures or an involuntary movement disorder, but chorea and athetosis have also been described in uremia.

Tetany is common and may occur with carpopedal spasm or may be latent and demonstrated by a positive Trousseau's sign. It results from abnormal peripheral nerve discharges, but in uremic patients may not respond to the administration of calcium and occurs despite the presence of metabolic acidosis, which normally would reduce the likelihood of tetany due to hypocalcemia. Tetany is usually associated with myoclonus and other manifestations of uremic encephalopathy.

Other motor abnormalities associated with early uremic encephalopathy include clumsiness, unsteady gait, and difficulty in performing fine movements. As uremia progresses, grasp and similar reflexes may be seen, resulting from depression of frontal lobe inhibitory mechanisms. Muscle tone is usually increased, especially in extensors, sometimes asymmetrically, and decorticate attitudes with lower limb extension and upper limb flexion may occur; diffuse muscle weakness is common, as are focal motor signs such as stretch reflex, asymmetry, and hemiparesis. These changes may be associated with severe acidosis and electrolyte abnormalities; for example, hyperkalemia may result in a flaccid quadriparesis resembling acute peripheral neuropathy.

Seizures generally are a late manifestation of uremia, and sudden death sometimes occurs during a convulsion. Usually these are generalized multiple motor seizures, although focal motor seizures may occur, often associated with local hemorrhage or other changes in the brain. The cause of the lowered seizure threshold in uremia is not known. Seizures in patients with renal failure can result from causes other than uremia, including the dialysis disequilibrium syndrome, hypertensive encephalopathy, and other toxic encephalopathies, but it is usually possible to distinguish these on clinical grounds. Hypertensive encephalopathy is generally associated with retinopathy and may be accompanied by focal signs and cerebral dysfunction such as aphasia or cortical blindness. Seizures may occur as a result of large doses of penicillins and are accompanied by an encephalopathy similar to uremic encephalopathy, with delirium, asterixis, myoclonus, and fasciculations. Penicillin encephalopathy is more common in uremic patients because penicillin is excreted by the kidney, and perhaps because of an increased intracerebral concentration of organic acids due to competitive inhibition of endogenous weak carboxylic acid transport from the ventricular fluid by the choroid plexus. The EEG in penicillin encephalopathy shows diffuse multifocal paroxysmal changes, unlike the smoother, slower records seen with metabolic encephalopathies.

Further progression of uremic encephalopathy leads to increasing clouding of consciousness, errors of perception, disorientation, confusion, agitation, delirium, and hallucinations, and some patients develop paranoid traits and/or depression (4). If not treated by dialysis, the patient becomes stuporous, then comatose, responding only to major stimuli, and eventually dies.

ENCEPHALOPATHY IN PATIENTS WITH ACUTE RENAL FAILURE

In patients with acute renal failure, the onset of lassitude and lethargy may be an early indication of uremic encephalopathy, followed by confusion and disorientation, which progress unless dialysis is begun. Nystagmus may be seen, dysarthria is common, and muscle weakness and fasciculation may occur, with marked variation in deep tendon reflexes (6). Untreated, progression can lead to coma and death.

THE ELECTROENCEPHALOGRAM IN RENAL FAILURE (7)

The EEG becomes abnormal early in the course of acute renal failure (6). Changes include increased abnormal delta slow-wave activity, an increase in the percentage of EEG power less than 5 Hz and 7 Hz, and reductions in the percentage of EEG frequencies above 9 Hz and below 5 Hz. Usually these changes are not significantly affected by dialysis, but return to normal only following recovery of renal function.

In patients with chronic renal failure the EEG shows slow background activity, loss of activity, and more frequent theta and delta waves. There is a good correlation between the percentage of EEG frequencies and power below 7 Hz and elevation of the serum creatinine level (8). After starting dialysis these changes improve gradually, but may not return completely to normal (9). Further improvement is usually seen following a successful kidney transplant.

There are many potential causes for the EEG abnormalities seen with uremic encephalopathy. In experimental animals and humans the degree of abnormality may be related to an increased blood level of parathyroid hormone. Studies in experimental animals have suggested the hormone exerts this effect by augmenting the accumulation of calcium in the brain (10). In patients with acute renal failure, EEG abnormalities develop rapidly and persist, generally unaffected by dialysis, gradually recovering some time after the return of normal renal function. This roughly corresponds with the duration of elevated parathyroid hormone levels in these patients (6). As a result of these and other findings, it has been suggested that parathyroid hormone may be a major uremic neurotoxin (11), although others disagree. A more recent suggestion is that uremic encephalopathy is caused by amino acid derangement resulting in an imbalance of neurotransmitters such as gamma-aminobutryic acid (GABA), dopamine, and serotonin (1, 12).

TREATMENT

In the patient with chronic renal disease the onset of uremic encephalopathy may be postponed by dietary protein restriction and control of hypertension. Once developed, the treatment is dialysis or kidney transplantation. Seizures may be related to encephalopathy or may result from the dialysis disequilibrium syndrome. The prevention of uremic encephalopathy is best achieved by starting dialysis before the patient becomes severely uremic.

Psychological complications of uremia

Patients with renal failure, particularly those with chronic renal failure, may develop a wide variety of psychological complications that affect intellectual functioning (13, 14), perception, consciousness, motor behavior, affective status, interpersonal relationships, and social functioning, but there is no specific psychological problem associated with uremia. Psychological disturbances may be associated with organic changes related to the uremia and, in addition, may be due to the patient's response to the chronic illness and its treatment.

ORGANIC BRAIN SYNDROME

As already noted, uremic encephalopathy can be associated with changes in mentation, apathy, fatigue, memory changes, disorientation, and difficulty with various intellectual functions. With more advanced encephalopathy, psychotic features may develop, including alterations in consciousness, hallucinations, delusions, and agitation.

REACTION TO ILLNESS AND ITS TREATMENT

Depression is a common problem in uremic patients, and particularly in dialysis patients. This is no different than the depression seen with other chronic illnesses. Symptoms include mood changes, psychomotor retardation, reduced libido, insomnia, loss of appetite, and weight loss. While these typical symptoms of depression occur in some patients, other may show behavioral changes such as irritability, anger, and headaches. Some patients develop symptoms of anxiety, including palpitations and hyperventilation. Both anxiety and depression are common in the later stages of chronic renal failure prior to beginning dialysis. The general improvement in well-being with the start of maintenance dialysis is often followed by a period of relative euphoria, a so-called honeymoon phase. In turn, this is often followed by a further period of depression some months after the commencement of treatment as the patient begins to understand the long-term nature of their illness. Nevertheless, most patients adjust with time. Successful transplantation is not generally associated with depression, but anxiety about long-term survival of the graft is common. Some patients may develop psychotic episodes, particularly if large doses of steroids are used. A study of dialysis and transplant patients showed that both subjective and objective measures of the quality of their life were somewhat lower than those of the general public (15). Nevertheless, these differences were slight, especially in patients with a successful transplant or treated by home hemodialysis.

NONCOMPLIANCE

Noncompliance with one or more aspects of their treatment is not uncommon in dialysis patients. Most patients have occasional episodes of dietary indiscretion, but some consistently fail to adhere to their dietary regimen. Excessive salt intake and fluid overload can result in increased weight gain between dialyses. On occasion, life-threatening hyperkalemia also may occur as a result of the ingestion of potassium-rich foods. A few patients are much more noncompliant, becoming abusive to staff and demanding shortening of their dialysis time or failing to attend for dialysis. Such patients can be a major management problem for the staff of a dialysis facility.

Suicide in dialysis patients does occur, and the rate is more frequent than in the general population, particularly if one includes deaths related to noncompliance. However, it would be more appropriate to compare the suicide rate in dialysis patients with that in patients with other life-threatening chronic diseases. In addition, an increasing number of dialysis patients, particularly the elderly and diabetics, may elect to discontinue dialysis when the complications of their disease become too burdensome (16).

PSYCHOLOGICAL TESTING

Several different tests have been used to study central nervous system dysfunction, many of which are related to measurement of cognition-dependent performance (17). Uremia is associated with impairment of such functions as sustained attention span, selective attention, speed of decision making, and short-term memory. Among the tests that can be used are the Choice Reaction Time (CRT) test, which measures sustained attention, as well as the speed of decision making, the Trailmaking Test, the Continuous Memory Test, and the Continuous Performance Test. Choice Reaction Time, discussed elsewhere in this chapter, correlates well with renal function, shows clear improvement with dialysis or transplantation, and is probably the best measure for clinical use.

Parathyroid hormone levels also have been shown to relate to psychological function, particularly measures of general cognitive function, nonverbal problem solving, and visual motor or visual spatial skills. Parathyroidectomy is associated with improvement in the results of the Trailmaking Test (18).

TREATMENT

For uremic patients in whom psychological symptoms appear to be associated with an organic brain syndrome, institution of dialysis usually results in improvement. When psychotic symptoms such as delusions or hallucinations occur in association with an organic brain syndrome, treatment with a phenothiazine or similar drug can help. Usually no dosage reduction is required because phenothiazines are metabolized by the liver. Haloperidol, 0.5 mg–2.0 mg twice or three times daily, may be preferred because it produces fewer anticholinergic side effects and little orthostatic hypotension.

For treatment of depression, an antidepressant such as one of the tricyclic compounds should be used. These, too, are primarily metabolized in the liver, and little dosage reduction is required. For anxiety, minor tranquilizers such as one of the benzodiazapines may be helpful.

Severly noncompliant patients can cause considerable stress for dialysis staff, who themselves may be assisted by a conference with a psychologist or psychiatrist. The possibility of a behavioral contract with the patient or transfer of the patient to another unit should be considered.

For the long-term support of dialysis patients and their families, social work intervention, vocational counseling, marital counseling, and individual and group psychotherapeutic management are helpful.

NEUROPATHY IN UREMIA

The occurrence of peripheral neuropathy in patients with chronic renal failure has been known for at least 100 years. As many as 65% of patients with end-stage renal disease have evidence of neuropathy at the time they start dialysis (5), and this appears to be more common and more severe in males, older patients, and in those with renal failure of long duration. Unless a systemic disease involving the nervous system is present, the underlying renal disease does not seem to play a role in the development of neuropathy, although this may be more common in patients with polycystic kidney disease or hereditary interstitial nephritis (19).

Clinical features

The clinical manifestions of uremic neuropathy are similar to those of the neuropathies associated with other metabolic diseases such as diabetes mellitus, alcoholism, and nutritional disorders. Usually it is a distal, symmetrical, mixed polyneuropathy involving both motor and sensory systems; generally, the legs are more severely involved, and ankle jerks are affected before knee jerks (20).

Symptoms related to neuropathy are unusual until the glomerular filtration rate declines below 15 ml/min (21). Initial symptoms are generally felt in the lower extremities, particularly the calves, and consist of paresthesiae, pruritus, and dull aches. These sensations are often worse at night and when the patient is at rest, and may be partially relieved by rapid movement of the legs. The patients had an irresistable compulsion to move the legs, hence the term *restless leg syndrome*. This occurs in 40% of patients with chronic renal failure (22) and is usually an early manifestation of neuropathy (23). It pathogenesis is obscure as there are no abnormalities of nerves or muscles (24). Restlessness causes insomnia and may be associated with nocturnal myoclonus. The syndrome can cause embarrassment and affect job performance, yet patients may not volunteer information on this problem except on direct questioning. Relief may occur with dialysis or the use of mild tranquilizers (25), and recently it has been suggested that levodopa may be effective (26).

Some uremic patients, particularly those with poor nutritional status, develop sensations of swelling, redness, tenderness, and constriction of the lower leg and soles and dorsa of the feet (22). This so-called burning foot syndrome may be relieved with improvement in the patient's nutritional status and may relate to vitamin deficiency, probably pantothenic acid and pyridoxine.

Muscle cramps are common in patients with uremia, tend to occur at night, and particularly affect the gastrocnemius and the intrinsic muscles of the arch of the feet. Cramping episodes last up to 10 minutes and usually are relieved by walking or other methods of stretching of the affected muscles. Cramps are often associated with increased fatiguability of muscles, muscle atrophy, and increased muscle irritability.

Loss of deep tendon reflexes, usually the ankle jerk and later the knee reflex, are early physical signs of uremic neuropathy and may be followed by development of hypoactive arm reflexes. At the same time, sensory changes occur. The vibration sense is impaired early in the course of neuropathy, again initially in the feet and legs. Varying degress of muscle weakness, sensory loss, and atrophic changes in the skin may be seen with advancing neuropathy. Loss of pain, tactile pressure, and the vibration sense are usually in the glove-stocking distribution. Loss of secondary skin appendages, dry skin with an unusual shine, and scaling and flakiness are common atrophic changes, and nail growth may be abnormal, with a predisposition to fungal infection of the nail beds.

Pathogenesis

Uremic neuropathy is a central peripheral axonopathy similar to various other peripheral neuropathies, and involves a symmetrical axonal degeneration starting peripherally. The cause is not clear, but like other neuropathies, there may be a toxic cause. Some combination of uremic toxins and abnormalities in metabolism and nutrition may be responsible (27) by inhibiting the nerve fiber enzymes necessary for the supply of energy to the axons. Depletion of glycolytic enzymes in the distal portion of the nerves results in a blockade of axonal transport, which is energy-dependent, and this chain of events may result in pathologic changes, culminating in the degeneration of distal nerve fibers.

Numerous compounds have been suggested as the uremic toxin or toxins. These have included creatinine, urea, "middle molecules," parathyroid hormone, methylguanidine, transketolase deficiency, vitamin deficiency, myoinositol, and magnesium. Vitamin deficiency does not seem to be the major cause, since large doses of vitamins do not alleviate uremic neuropathy (28). Red-cell transketolase, a thiamine-dependent enzyme, appears to be inhibited in uremic serum; however, there is no evidence for this as the cause of uremic neuropathy (29). There is some correlation between serum urea and creatinine concentrations and nerve function (21, 30). However, these are unlikely to be neurotoxic, as infusion of urea does not produce neuropathy in animals, and serum urea and creatinine levels in dialysis patients may be elevated without development of peripheral neuropathy. The classical example of this is the infrequency of clinical neuropathy in peritoneal dialysis patients, and this observation was the origin of the middle molecule hypothesis. Magnesium, once thought to play a role since it can block neuromuscular transmission (31), probably is not responsible. Myoinositol, methylguanidine, and guanidinosuccinic acid accumulate in renal failure and also have been suggested as possible neurotoxins (32, 33).

Middle molecules, compounds ranging in molecular weight from 300 to 2000 daltons, which are cleared less well than urea and creatinine during dialysis, have been suggested as a possible cause of uremic neuropathy (34). In a set of controlled experiments it has been shown that a reduction in middle molecule clearance and residual renal function resulted in worsening of nerve conduction velocity, while an increase in middle molecule clearance resulted in slow improvement (35).

Recently, the possible role of parathyroid hormone in the pathogenesis of uremic neuropathy has received attention (36), but the finding of a correlation between the plasma parathyroid hormone level and nerve conduction velocity (37) has not been confirmed (38). Administration of parathyroid hormone decreased the motor nerve conduction velocity in dogs (39), but in patients with primary or secondary hyperparathyroidism motor nerve conduction velocity may be normal and is unaffected by either medical or surgical treatment of hyperparathyroidism (40, 41). Similar results have been reported in dialysis patients (6, 38). In addition, motor nerve conduction velocity usually improves with time on dialysis, whereas the parathyroid hormone level remains elevated. Consequently, uremic neuropathy appears to result from axonal damage caused by the cumulative effects of various neurotoxins, and its etiology is complex and perhaps multifactorial.

Laboratory findings

Both motor and sensory nerve conduction velocities are depressed in uremia. Motor nerve conduction velocity has been used to judge the severity of uremia, but there are problems with this test, including a large variation in the same individual from day to day, as well as a wide variation from one laboratory to another (42, 43). The test may be helpful in assessing severe disease, but its usefulness is limited in milder cases. A correlation between clinical neuropathy and the motor nerve conduction velocity is either weak or lacking (44). The sensory nerve conduction velocity may be more sensitive but is not commonly used as measurement is uncomfortable. Evoked potentials also have been found useful in the assessment of uremic neuropathy (46). A large number of uremic patients have decreased nerve conduction velocity, particularly involving the distal segments of the peroneal fibers, even without clinical evidence of neuropathy. These findings are more pronounced in dialyzed patients than in those who are not yet on dialysis.

Usually in uremic neuropathy the protein level in the cerebrospinal fluid is normal, although rarely it may exceed normal limits. The creatinine phosphokinase level is also normal unless the patient is being treated with androgens (47).

Nerve biopsy shows a decrease in the number of nerve fibers, more pronounced distally, with loss of only 4% of fibers at the knee and 50% at the ankle (48). There is axonal degeneration with macrophages around the degenerated area, but little sign of inflammation; myelin fragments are marginated, and demyelination usually is mild. These changes are more severe distally, and there is a degeneration of distal axons of all sizes. Segmental demyelination is probably secondary to axonal abnormality (49). Axonal degeneration and demyelination can afflict axons of all sizes, but longer fibers seem to be more vulnerable. Neuropathy involves a dying back of nerve fibers from the periphery. These changes are nonspecific and are seen in association with various metabolic neuropathies. Thus nerve biopsy usually is not helpful unless there is question whether neuropathy is due to a systemic disorder such as vasculitis.

Autonomic nervous system

The presence of autonomic dysfunction in uremic patients is well recognized (50–52). An abnormal Valsalva response, reduced baroceptor sensitivity, an abnormal heart rate response to atropine, abnormal RR variations in the ECG, an abnormal sympathetic responses have been reported. The abnormal Valsalva response is not due to cardiomyopathy, and sympathetic reflex regulation and the reflex arc are preserved. It is postulated that either the carotid receptors or the parasympathetic pathways are abnormal. An abnormality of the parasympathetic system has been confirmed by use of the diving test and its effect on heart rate. Evaluation of noradrenaline responsiveness by the tilt test and the cold pressor test has shown normal noradrenaline increases, but blood pressure in uremic patients decreased, while the normal response is an increase. Thus end-organ responsiveness appears to be reduced in uremia.

Patients with different types of glomerulonephritis, polycystic kidney disease, and pyelonephritis have similar manifestations of autonomic neuropathy (51). However, parasympathetic lesions are more extensive, and the sympathetic system is more severely involved in diabetic patients with renal failure.

Cranial nerve abnormalities

Transient and fluctuating cranial nerve abnormalities occur in some uremic patients, and facial asymmetry with subtle and minimal muscle weakness is often noted. Hearing loss may result from Alport's syndrome, but careful audiometric examination shows evidence of hearing loss in the majority of patients with chronic renal failure (53). In addition, auditory-evoked responses are also commonly found to be abnormal. Some patients have visual loss (uremic amaurosis), which can ocurr rapidly over minutes to hours; loss of vision is complete, and pupillary reactions and fundoscopic examination are normal. Recovery usually occurs within weeks (2). Diplopia, nystagmus, and unilateral sixth nerve palsy have also been reported, particularly in severely hypertensive patients. Visual evoked responses are frequently abnormal in dialysis patients, retinal hemorrhages and exudates are common, and pupils may be assymetrical and their size may fluctuate. Various taste abnormalities are common in patients with chronic renal failure.

If cranial nerve abnormalities are found, other pathologic conditions should always be excluded. Thus retinal detachment as a cause of visual problems, overdose of anticonvulsant drugs causing nystagmus or speech problems, and hearing loss from ototoxic drugs such as aminoglycosides, furosemide, or vancomycin should always be ruled out. Similarly, nutritional or vitamin deficiencies should be considered. Occasionally zinc deficiency can present as hypogeusia, and zinc supplementation can correct this. Initiating or increasing dialysis may help if other causes have been ruled out.

Dialysis and transplantation

Generally, uremic neuropathy improves to some degree with dialysis, particularly in nondiabetic patients. However, significant neuropathy persists in many patients. In diabetic patients, neuropathy may worsen with dialysis (54). Autonomic dysfunction also improves with hemodialysis, but improvement is less with continuous ambulatory peritoneal dialysis (50). Successful kidney transplantation results in an initial rapid progressive improvement in neuropathy, followed by slow continuing improvement over as long as a year, but patients with severe peripheral neuropathy may have residual weakness and atrophy of muscles. While peripheral neuropathy improves after successful renal transplantation, autonomic dysfunction dose not (55).

Uremic polyneuropathy is a diagnosis of exclusion, once other causes have been excluded. If the patient appears uremic or underdialyzed, increasing dialysis might help. Patients with the restless leg syndrome may benefit with benzodiazipine or levodopa, especially taken at bedtime. Vitamin and nutritional deficiencies should always be considered and ruled out.

NEUROMUSCULAR SYSTEM

Diffuse proximal polymyopathy is common in patients with uremia and in those on dialysis (2). Wasting of the thigh muscles and pain and tenderness of the muscles are sometimes seen. Electromyography, nerve conduction velocity measurements, and muscle biopsy are not helpful, as EMG may show polyphasic potentials and biopsy may show nonspecific sarcolemmal proliferation with patchy areas of necrosis. The etiology of these changes is unknown, although hyperparpathyroidism is a common accompaniment and so has been implicated (56).

Potassium and myopathy

Both severe hypokalemia and hyperkalemia may present with flaccid areflexic muscle weakness. Most such patients respond to correction of the underlying problem. With hyperkalemia, other abnormalities such as acidosis and hyponatremia are frequently present and may require correction.

Carnitine deficiency

Carnitine is essential for the transport of lipids across the mitochondria where these are oxidized, providing energy for the muscles. There is mounting evidence that dialysis patients may have a carnitine deficiency. This may cause some of the muscular weakness seen in these patients and can be corrected by repletion with l-carnitine (57). Use of d-carnitine in the oral form has caused a myasthenialike syndrome; this responds to discontinuation of d-carnitine and changing to l-carnitine.

Other muscular problems

Recently, oxalate overload in dialysis patients has been recognized as a cause of muscle weakness and vascular calcification, and this can be exacerbated by excessive intake of vitamin C (58). Thus it is important to avoid the use of high doses of vitamin C in patients with renal failure.

Prune-belly syndrome is a congenital abnormality associated with the lack of abdominal musculature, urinary tract anomalies, cryptorchidism, and chronic renal failure. Surgical reconstruction is sometimes helpful.

FLUID AND ELECTROLYTE DISTURBANCES IN DIALYSIS PATIENTS

Hypernatremia and hyponatremia

Serum osmolality changes, manifested as hypernatremia or hyponatremia, may occur in patients with severe renal failure and in dialysis patients. As a result, contraction or expansion of the cells, including brain cells, may occur, and either may result in seizures and coma.

Hypernatremia can result from the use of a dialysate with a sodium concentration greater than 140 mEq/l, most likely as a result of problems with the dialysate delivery system or water purification; for example, malfunction of the dialysate proportioning system together with inaccurate setting of conductivity limits. Signs and symptoms include thirst, irritability, increased interdialytic weight gain, elevated blood pressure, and possibly congestive heart failure. If acute, hypernatremia can result in seizures, coma, and death.

Hyponatremia may occur in patients with advanced renal failure and in dialysis patients who ingest large quantities of water. In dialysis patients it can also be caused by use of a dialysate with a low sodium concentration as a result of human and/or mechanical error. If acute, hyponatremia results in weakness, fatigue, seizures, and acute hemolysis developing early after the start of dialysis. This may progress to coma, and death can occur from hyperkalemia as a result of the release of potassium from hemolyzed red blood cells.

Prevention of hypernatremia and hyponatremia requires careful dietary management of fluid and sodium intake in patients with renal failure and careful maintenance and use of dialysis equipment. Treatment of hypernatremia or hyponatremia due to dialysis errors includes stopping dialysis and restarting with appropriate dialysate. If significant hemolysis occurs, the patient should be monitored for the possible occurrence of hyperkalemia both during and after dialysis.

Hypermagnesemia and hypomagnesemia

Mild asymptomatic hypermagnesemia is not uncommon in patients with chronic renal failure. In dialysis patients, acute hypermagnesemia may occur in association with hypercalcemia in the "hard water syndrome," which results from inadequate water treatment. This syndrome is characterized by nausea, vomiting, headache, hypertension, and symptoms resembling acute pancreatitis; central nervous system symptoms and hypotension are particularly associated with hypermagnesemia (59). Accidental dialysis using a high-magnesium dialysate causes flushing, muscular weakness, hyporeflexia, ataxia, and blurred vision (60).

Hypomagnesemia can follow prolonged dialysis with magnesium-free dialysate and may result in an increased frequency of muscle cramps during dialysis (60).

Hypoglycemia

Hypoglycemia is not uncommon in dialysis patients, but does not generally lead to coma. It may be due to impaired gluconeogenesis and glycogenolysis, hepatic dysfunction, starvation, an increased insulin effect, and glucose utilization. Use of beta-blocking agents such as propanolol in dialysis patients has been associated with hypoglycemia, presumably because of their effects on hepatic glycogenolysis, glucagon release, and lipolysis (62). Hypoglycemia has also been reported in dialysis patients undergoing hyperalimentation with solutions of high dextrose content due to the rapid passage of glucose from the blood to the dialysate (63).

Nonketotic hyperosmolar coma

Nonketotic hyperosmolar coma associated with hyperglycemia has been described in both hemodialysis and peritoneal dialysis patients (64). Characteristically, it occurs during dialysis of a diabetic patient using dialysate with a high glucose concentration. This results in hyperglycemia, intracellular water depletion, and hyperosmolality, but without ketosis (65). The extracellular volume may be increased or decreased, depending on the rapidity of the shift of sodium and water; the extracellular fluid becomes hyperosmolar; and the cell volume is contracted. Symptoms include headache, nausea and vomiting, profound thirst, convulsions, coma, and death.

Dialysis-induced deficiency syndrome

Wernicke's encephalopathy has been described in a small number of dialysis patients (66), presumably because of poor dietary intake and loss of thiamine, a water-soluble vitamin, through the dialysis membrane. The characteristic triad of symptoms is confusion, ophthalmoplegia, and ataxia; this may be associated with a Korsakoff psychosis in which the patient becomes confused, confabulates, and has loss of memory. Chronic malnutrition may be a factor in some patients, and thiamine deficiency is more likely in patients not taking vitamin supplements (67). Wernicke's encephalopathy should be suspected in any patient on dialysis with an unexplained neurologic problem (66).

Treatment is with large doses of thiamine, and uremic patients appear to require much larger doses than do alcoholic patients with Wernicke's encephalopathy. Giving intravenous thiamine improves the ophthalmoplegia within hours, but the other components of the disorder may take several weeks to improve. Early treatment is essential in order to avoid the occurrence of irreversible changes.

SYNDROMES SECONDARY TO HEMORRHAGE IN DIALYSIS PATIENTS

Complications secondary to hemorrhage are not uncommon in uremic patients, particularly dialysis patients, and can involve the nervous system. In dialysis patients several factors may contribute to bleeding in the nervous system, including the abnormalities of the clotting mechanism seen in uremia; the use of anticoagulants during dialysis, and sometimes between dialyses; and the fact the dialysis patients may be more prone to head injuries as a result of episodes of hypotension.

Subdural hematoma

Subdural hematoma is a well-recognized complication of hemodialysis, occurring in about 3% of patients (68). It should be suspected in any dialysis patient presenting with headache or other neurologic symptoms suggestive of the dialysis disequilibrium syndrome. Subdural hematoma can also occur coincidentally with uremic or hypertensive encephalopathy (69).

Symptoms and signs are often nonspecific but generally may be distinguished from those of the dialysis disequilibrum syndrome. The latter is unusual in maintenance hemodialysis patients after the initial dialyses; the symptoms of disequilibrium usually do not fluctuate as much as those of subdural hematoma, and headaches, while frequent with disequilibrium, usually disappear shortly after dialysis. With subdural hematoma, the headache usually is severe, persisting through subsequent dialyses, and may be associated with fluctuating or constant, focal or multifocal, neurologic signs. Generally, neurologic signs are of no value in localizing the site of the intracranial bleeding.

Lumber puncture and electroencephalography are of little help in diagnosis, as abnormalities of both can also occur with the disequilibrium syndrome; radioisotope studies result in an appreciable percentage of false-negative results. The most useful investigations are cerebral arteriography and computerized tomography. When subdural hematoma is being seriously considered, it is preferable to use peritoneal dialysis rather than hemodialysis until the diagnosis is confirmed or rejected. If hemodialysis must be used, this should be done without the use of heparin. Treatment is by surgical exploration and clot removal. Results are disappointing, with a patient survival of less than 50%, although this is comparable to the results of treatment of acute subdural hematoma in nonuremic patients.

Cerebral hemorrhage

Intracerebral bleeding is frequently a fatal complication in uremic patients, occuring five times as often in dialysis patients as in the general population (70). It usually presents as a massive hemorrhage into the brain substance. Symptoms occur acutely over a short period of time and include development of hemiparesis, nausea, vomiting, meningial signs, coma, and death. Surgery is unlikely to be beneficial unless the patient's condition stabilizes rapidly.

Subarachnoid hemorrhage associated with a leaking berry aneurysm may be associated with polycystic kidney disease and can be aggravated by hypertension and anticoagulation. Surgical treatment should be considered, provided the patient survives the acute episode.

Epidural spinal hematoma

Epidural spinal hematoma occasionally occurs in patients taking anticoagulants. Symptoms of cord compression develop, with rapid onset of bilateral leg weakness and sensory loss, resulting in paraparesis and paraplegia. The occurrence of spinal cord signs in a dialysis patient is an indication for urgent treatment, as permanent paraplegia may result unless there is early surgical evacuation of the compressing hematoma.

INFECTIONS OF THE BRAIN AND MENINGES IN DIALYSIS PATIENTS

Dialysis patients have been reported to have an increased risk of infections of the central nervous system, perhaps because of the presence of some form of vascular access and more frequent episodes of local infection and septicemia. Development of meningeal signs and symptoms in a dialysis patient is always an indication for diagnostic lumbar puncture. Intracerebral infections are more common in patients following transplantation, frequently resulting from a systemic fungal infection with central nervous system involvement.

Cytomegalic inclusion disease is common in both dialysis and transplant patients, often without symptoms. Neurologic involvement with this disease usually is seen in conjuction with pulmonary disease. In transplanted patients in particular, active cytomegalic inclusion disease generally represents reactivation and dissemination of a preexisting latent infection.

DEGENERATIVE DISORDERS OF THE BRAIN IN DIALYSIS PATIENTS

Dialysis dementia

Dialysis dementia, or dialysis encephalopathy (71), a progressive frequently fatal neurologic disorder occurring in dialysis patients, was first described by Alfrey, who suggested that aluminum might be responsible for this disease (72, 73). It is characterized by the onset of dysarthria and dyspraxia, causing characteristic slurring, stuttering, and hesitancy of speech. This may be followed by difficulty in swallowing, the development of dementia, and the occurrence of psychoses, myoclonus, and seizures (74). At first, the symptoms may be intermittent and may be exacerbated by hemodialysis, but there is a gradual progression, with an increasing constancy of symptoms and eventual death following the development of full-blown dementia. Dialysis dementia tends to occur in patients who have been on dialysis for at least 2 years, and generally death occurs within 6 months of the onset (75). Electroencephalography shows paroxysmal high-voltage rhythmical and symmetrical delta activity, with spikes and sharp waves initially, and normal background alpha frequency. Eventually, the latter deteriorates into slow and disorganized activity (75).

No specific neuropathologic changes are seen in the brain on gross examination, but neurofibrillary material is found in the cortical neurons of patients dying with dialysis encephalopathy (76). This resembles that found in experimental aluminum toxicity, but differs from that seen in Alzheimer's disease.

An increased aluminum concentration in the gray matter of the brain of patients dying with dialysis dementia has been found (72), and epidemiologic studies appear to confirm aluminum as the cause. Some outbreaks have been epidemic in nature, frequently involving dialysis facilities using water with a high aluminum content for preparation of the dialysate. This may result from addition of aluminum salts to municipal water supplies to precipitate organic debris (77). Pretreatment of water for dialysis with a water softener dose not remove aluminum; deionization and/or reverse osmosis is necessary and can decrease the aluminum concentration in tap water to less than 1 µg/l (74). Institution of appropriate water treatment has been shown to halt epidemics of dialysis dementia in some dialysis units.

Aluminum is readily transferred across the dialysis membrane and can pass from the dialysate to blood or, if the dialysate is aluminum free, from blood to the dialysate. Transfer depends on the solubility of aluminum, which is dependent on the pH of the dialysate (78). Alfrey originally suggested that aluminum intoxication might be the result of the ingestion of aluminum-containing oral phosphate binders, but it was soon shown that most cases were associated with aluminum transferred from the dialysate. Nevertheless, a significant amount of aluminum can be absorbed from the gastrointestinal tract and is normally excreted by the kidneys. With the general use of effective water treatment, it is likely that most future cases of dialysis dementia will result from long-continued use of aluminum-containing antacids. For example, dialysis dementia has been a very unusual complication in dialysis patients in Seattle, Washington, because of water that does not contain significant amounts of aluminum, but now a number of patients have been found to have elevated bone aluminum levels, presumably acquired from long-continued antacid ingestion. Recently an acute and fatal aluminum-related encephalopathy has been reported in patients starting dialysis, apparently related to very high gut absorption of aluminum in patients also receiving a buffered citrate solution by mouth (79).

Some dialysis patients may show other manifestations of aluminum intoxication. These include osteomalacia with spontaneous bone fractures, proximal myopathy, normal serum calcium levels and low parathyroid hormone levels, and microcytic anemia. This aluminum bone disease is refractory to treatment with vitamin D metabolites and is associated with deposition of aluminum in bone, the amount of uncalcified osteoid correlating with the bone aluminum content.

The prevention of dialysis dementia is by the use of water treatment to ensure a dialysate aluminum level below 10 µg/l. Phosphate-binding aluminum antacids should be used with care in dialysis patients, and some have suggested the use of magnesium antacids in conjunction with a low-magnesium dialysate (61). Recently oral calcium carbonate has been used as a phosphate binder, but this must be used with caution, as hypercalcemia may develop in some patients. These alternatives should be considered in patients who show early signs of dialysis dementia. For the patient who develops seizures, diazapam or clonazepam are helpful in controlling these but have no effect on the eventual outcome of the disease. Established dialysis dementia, aluminum bone disease, and aluminum-related microcytic anemia should be treated with deferoxamine, up to 15 mg/kg/body weight administered intravenously over 2 hours at each dialysis, to chelate the aluminum (80). This treatment is discussed in more detail elsewhere in this book. One complication of deferoxamine treatment of aluminum bone disease may be the acute onset of dialysis dementia. Another potentially serious complication occurring in 1% of treated patients is mucomycosis, frequently with cerebral involvement. This and other bizarre infections that occur occasionally appear to be associated with siderophilic organisms. Yet another recently reported serious problem is the development of blindness and coma in patients treated with deferoxamine who are also receiving a benzodiazepine (81).

Other trace elements may be present in dialysate water and can be potential causes of central nervous system problems. These include boron, cadmium, copper, lead, manganese, mercury, nickel, thalium, tin, and vanadium (82). In addition, trace metals may be leached into dialysate water from plumbing beyond the deionizer. The best known example of problems related to other metals is copper intoxication. This has occurred when exhaustion of a deionizer used for water treatment produced acidic water that acted on the copper tubing used in some early dialysis equipment. Copper intoxication results in fever, nausea, vomiting, abdominal pain, headache, and diarrhea, and induces hemolytic anemia, metabolic acidosis, hyperkalemia, hepatitis, cirrhosis, pancreatitis, and myoglobinemia. The symptoms may be confused with dialysis disequilibrium, but are relieved by removing copper from the circuit.

Apart from dialysis dementia, a number of other degenerative disorders of the brain have occasionally been described in patients with end-stage renal disease. These include a progressive cerebellar syndrome resembling olivopontocerebellar disease, Creutzfeldt–Jakob disease, subacute spongiform degeneration of the white matter, and pontine myelinosis. The latter may be asymptomatic, may produce mild pyramidal and cerebellar signs, and occasionally may involve cranial nerves or the descending tracts to the medulla. This demyelinating disorder also occurs in alcoholism and other chronic diseases, and may be related to malnutrition.

Computerized tomography has revealed the presence of cerebral atrophy in some uremic patients (83). This is more marked in children, suggesting a possible inhibition of brain development by uremia, but also occurs to a lesser extent in adults. The cause is unknown. Because they appear to be particularly susceptible to the development of cerebral atrophy, it is important to treat uremia early in infants and small children (84).

DIALYSIS DISEQUILIBRIUM SYNDROME

The dialysis disequilibrium syndrome is now seen most commonly in patients beginning dialysis for acute renal failure, and occasionally in pateints with chronic renal failure commencing maintenance hemodialysis, particularly with the use of large surface-area dialyzers and short dialysis times.

In its mildest form, disequilibrium may present only as restlessness and headache during dialysis, sometimes associated with nasuea, vomiting, blurring of vision, and muscle twitching. Hypertension has been reported, and in more severe cases there may be disorientation, tremors, and seizures (85). Occasionally the latter may be accompanied by cardiac arrhythmias. Both grand mal and petit mal seizures may occur, but usually without focal signs unless there is preexisting neurologic damage. Most patients recover with appropriate treatment, but occasionally seizures are followed by coma and death. With current methods of dialysis, seizures, coma, and death are uncommon occurrences.

The major cause of the disequilibrium syndrome is thought to be cerebral edema, and this has been found at autopsy in patients dying with this disorder. Kennedy and associates (86) first noted that the urea concentration and osmolality in the cerebrospinal fluid fall more slowly than in the blood during rapid hemodialysis and that this is associated with an increase in the cerebrospinal fluid pressure. The rate of urea clearance from the brain more or less parallels that from the plasma, but there is some delay in the clearance of urea from the cerebrospinal fluid. Another possible cause may be the rapid correction of the metabolic acidosis, which results in worsening of the acidosis in the cerebrospinal fluid (87). The alteration in cerebrospinal fluid pH may impair mentation, and the intracellular acidosis in the brain contributes to brain edema by altering the osmotic activity of intracellular cations (88). In addition, brain edema may result from the generation of idiogenic osmoles in the brain during dialysis. These may be generated by changes in the intracellular binding of sodium and potassium caused by their displacement by ammonium ions from the equilibrium between glutamine and glutamic acid; and increased glutamic acid concentration in the brain could cause a fall in intracellular pH, loss of hydrogen ion to the cerebrospinal fluid, and a fall of cerebrospinal fluid pH and a rise in brain osmolality due to accumulation of acid osmoles.

Characteristically, the electroencephalogram in disequilibrium is said to show an increase of slow-wave activity, with increased spike-wave activity and bursts of delta waves, and with loss of normal alpha rhythm (89). However, others have shown that with the use of bicarbonate dialysate the EEG is normal and disequilibrium does not occur (9, 90). Cerebrospinal fluid pressure is normal in the nondialyzed uremic patient, but generally rises during dialysis, whether symptoms of disequilibrium occur or not. This increase does not necessarily indicate brain edema, but could result from an increase in the cerebrospinal fluid volume or an increase in the cerebral blood flow. However, autopsy of some patients who died during dialysis has shown brain swelling, often with tentorial herniation; and early studies on brain density using CT scan have shown that brain density falls significantly during and after hemodialysis, though not in patients on continuous ambulatory peritoneal dialysis. The changes are in keeping with a postdialysis gain in cerebral water, particularly marked in the region of the basal ganglia (91). More recent studies in stable hemodialysis patients, however, have shown on postdialysis change in brain density, ventricular size, or EEG deterioration (92).

The differential diagnosis of the dialysis disequilibrium syndrome includes hypotension, subdural hematoma, cerebrovascular accident, hypertensive encephalopathy, dialysis dementia, cardiac arrhythmias, hyponatremia, hypernatremia, hypoglycemia, uremia, copper intoxication, and other conditions.

Prevention of dialysis disequilibrium was originally achieved by adding osmotically active solute to the dialysate. Solutes used for this purpose have included urea, dextrose, fructose, mannitol, sodium chloride, and glycerol. Sequential ultrafiltration has also been used effectively. However, because disequilibrium occurs most commonly during rapid hemodialysis in a markedly uremic patient, the simplest preventive measure is to slow the rate of biochemical change during hemodialysis by using shorter and more frequent dialysis, with or without a reduction in the blood flow rate. Alternatively, peritoneal dialysis, which results in slower biochemical changes, is effective.

In addition to the use of shorter, more frequent hemodialyses, anticonvulsant drugs may be used in both the prevention and treatment of disequilibrium, although they have no effect on cerebral edema. In extremely uremic patients first starting dialysis, phenytoin may be useful, given as a loading dose of 100 mg at least one day before commencing dialysis, followed by a maintenance dose of 300–400 mg daily until the patient is stable and uremia is controlled. However, this is of little help during seizure activity since, although phenytoin enters the brain rapidly, the brain level declines very rapidly without continuous administration. Consequently, intravenous diazepam, which produces high brain levels within minutes, is one of the most effective agents for the suppression of acute seizure activity. The effect of an intravenous injection lasts $\frac{1}{2}$–1 hour, and respiratory depression is less than with barbiturates. Short-acting barbiturates, such as pentabarbital, are also effective within minutes, but are more dangerous because of the greater respiratory depression.

NERVE ENTRAPMENT

The carpal tunnel syndrome has been reported with increasing frequency in patients who have been on hemodialysis for more than 5 years. Originally it was suggested that this might relate to vascular access surgery and resultant ischemia or venous hypertension (93). More recently, the role of the deposition of amyloid derived from beta$_2$ microglobulin in causing the carpal tunnel syndrome in uremic patients has been suggested. Beta$_2$ microglobulin, a protein with a molecular weight of 11,818 daltons, is normally excreted by the kidneys and accumulates in maintenance dialysis patients (94). Deposition in the form of amyloid occurs in various tissues, resulting in asymptomatic lytic bone lesions, carpal tunnel syndrome, tenosynositis, arthropathies, and fractures. In addition to the carpal tunnel syndrome, this amyloid deposition may be responsible for many of the pains and discomforts around the shoulder and hip girdle in dialysis patients.

Higher serum beta$_2$ microglobulin levels are seen in patients dialyzed with cellulose membranes than in those dialyzed using polyacrylonitrile or polysulfone membranes. Thus it may be possible to prevent or delay the onset of the carpal tunnel syndrome by the use of these more biocompatible membranes (95–97). The recent development of high-efficiency dialysis using polysulfone hemodialyzers decreases serum beta$_2$ microglobulin levels by 30%–50%, and relief of symptoms occurs within a month or so (94). Nevertheless, when mechanical symptoms of nerve entrapment develop, surgery is required for prompt relief (98).

ADEQUACY OF DIALYSIS

As renal failure progresses and nephrons are destroyed, the internal hemostasis of the body changes, resulting in the uremic syndrome, which affects all bodily systems including the nervous system (99). This may influence posture, mood, activities, and verbal and nonverbal attitudes.

These abnormalities can be detected by several objective tests such as asking patients to perform complex tasks, looking for EEG abnormalities, and measurements of peripheral and autonomic nerve evoked potentials. As uremia progresses, the tests become progressively more abnormal. With the start of dialysis, these abnormalities improve, although they may or may not become completely normal. When dialysis becomes inadequate for any reason, one or several of these abnormalties may again become abnormal. Abnormalities of the EEG and of psychometric measurements occur with underdialysis (9, 100) and can be assessed quantitively (8, 101), as can changes in evoked potentials (46, 102). In particular, Scribner and colleagues have used nerve conduction velocity in assessing underdialysis of middle molecules (34, 35).

A simple task performance test, the Choice Reaction Time (CRT), has proved to be a relatively sensitive, albeit nonspecific, test for underdialysis. The patient is asked to respond to a flashing color of light by pressing the appropriate button, the response time is measured, and the average of 24 such responses is used in assessing the result of the test. Patients who are underdialyzed have the slowest CRT, and the score is significantly better in patients deemed to be well dialyzed, but the fastest score is achieved by normal subjects and transplanted patients. There is a relative improvement in the score after switching patients treated by intermittent peritoneal dialysis to hemodialysis. Similarly, when dialysis patients are transplanted, their score improves. Thus CRT appears to be a simple and useful clinical tool to assess the adequacy of dialysis.

COMPLICATIONS OF TRANSPLANTATION

Uremic encephalopathy, disequilibrium, EEG changes, and peripheral neuropathy in dialysis patients all tend to improve with a successful kidney transplant. Nevertheless, transplanted patients are subject to other neurologic complications, particularly the development of brain tumors and infections.

Tumors

Reticulum cell sarcoma and lymphoma are frequent in patients who have received a renal transplant (5). Typically these develop some months to years after transplantation, and generally present either with signs and symptoms of increased intracranial pressure or with focal signs. These tumors are usually radiosensitive.

The pathogenesis of these tumors is most likely related in some way to a drug-induced immune deficiency following transplantation, but similar tumors do not occur with increased frequency in patients on immunosuppressive therapy for other conditions. Consequently, their development may also relate to depression of the normal immunologic surveillance mechanisms in the brain and/or the proliferation of viruses. Lymphomas in other parts of the body are not more common in transplanted patients, and this may reflect a lessened capacity for an immune response by cerebral tissues.

Infections

Immunosuppression following transplantation is known to be associated with an increased risk of central nervous system infection, particularly in elderly patients (103).

Systemic fungal infections are common in transplanted patients at autopsy, and the central nervous system is frequently involved, usually from a primary source in the lung. Most fungal brain abscesses are associated with *Aspergillus* infection, although *Candida*, *Nocardia*, and *Histoplasma* infections also may occur. Intracerebral fungal infection usually presents with delirium and seizures, although focal neurologic signs may also be seen. Diagnosis can be difficult, and brain biopsy may be required.

Cytomegalic inclusion disease is frequent in transplanted patients, almost always in association with evidence of cytomegalic virus infection of the lungs. Most adults have complement-fixing antibodies to cytomegalovirus (5), and it seems likely that immunosuppression allows activation and dissemination of this preexisting cytomegalic virus infection. No specific clinical findings have been related to brain involvement in cytomegalic virus infection.

Toxoplasmosis is also not uncommon in transplanted patients and may result in encephalopathy, characterized by delirium, seizures, and coma. Meningoencephalitis with headache, stiff neck, seizures, and coma, or intracerebral focal lesions producing focal neurologic symptoms are also seen.

REFERENCES

1. Biasoli S, D'Andrea G, Feriani M, Chiaramonte S, Fabris A, Ronco C, LaGreca G: Uremic encephalopathy: An updating. *Clin Nephrol* 25:57–63, 1986.
2. Tyler HR, Tyler KL: Neurologic complications. In: G Eknoyan, JP Knochel, eds, *The Systemic Consequences of Renal Failure*. Grune and Stratton, Orlando, FL, pp 311–330, 1984.
3. Eschbach JW, Egrie JL, Downing MR, Browne JK, Adamson JW: Correction of the anemia of end-stage renal disease with recombinant erythropoietin. Results of a combined phase I and II clinical trial. *N Engl J Med* 8:73–78, 1987.
4. Ginn HE: Neurobehavioral dysfunction in uremia. *Kidney Int* 2 (Suppl):217–225, 1975.
5. Raskin NH, Fishman RA: Neurologic disorders in renal failure. *N Engl J Med* 294:143–148, 1976.
6. Cooper JD, Lazarowitz VC, Arieff AI: Neurodiagnostic abnormalities in patients with acute renal failure. *J Clin Invest* 61:1448–1455, 1978.
7. Bourne JR, Teschan PE: Computer methods: Uremic encephalopathy, and adequacy of dialysis. *Kidney Int* 24:496–506, 1983.
8. Teschan PE, Ginn HE, Bourne JR, Ward JW, Hamel B, Nunnally JC, Musso M, Vaughn WK: Quantitative indices of clinical uremia. *Kidney Int* 15:676–697, 1979.
9. Kiley JE, Woodruff MW, Pratt KL: Evaluation of encephalopathy by EEG frequency in chronic dialysis patients. *Clin Nephrol* 5:245–250, 1976.
10. Akmal M, Goldstein DA, Multani S, Massry SG: Role of uremia, brain calcium, and parathyroid hormone on changes in electroencephalogram in chronic renal failure. *Am J Physiol* 246:F575–F579, 1984.
11. Mahoney CA, Arieff AI: Central and peripheral nervous system effects of chronic renal failure. *Kidney Int* 24:170–177, 1983.
12. Perry TL, Yong VW, Kish SJ, Ito M, Foulks JG, Godolphin WJ, Sweeney VP: Neurochemical abnormalities in brains of renal failure patients treated by repeated hemodialysis. *J Neurochem* 45:1043–1048, 1985.
13. Arieff AI: Neurological complications of uremia. In: BM Brenner, FJ Rector Jr, eds, *The Kidney*, 2nd ed. WB Saunders, Philadelphia, pp 2306–2343, 1981.
14. English A, Savage RD, Britton PG, Ward MK, Kerr DN: Intellectual impairment in chronic renal failure. *Br Med J* 1:888–890, 1978.
15. Evans RW, Manninen DL, Garrison LP Jr, Hart LG, Blagg CR, Gutman RA, Hull AR, Lowrie EG: The quality of life of patients with end-stage renal disease. *N Engl J Med* 312:553–558, 1985.
16. Kjellstrand CM, Neu S: Stoppiong long-term dialysis, an empirical study of withdrawal of life-supporting treatment. *N Engl J Med* 314:14–20, 1986.
17. Ratner DP, Adams KM, Levin MW, Rourke BP: Effect of hemodialysis on the cognitive-motor functioning of the adult chronic hemodialysis patients. *J Behav Med* 6:291–311, 1983.
18. Cogan MG, Covey CM, Arieff AI: Wisniewski A, Clark OH, Lazarowitz VC, Leach W: Central nervous system manifestations of hyperparathyroidism. *Am J Med* 65:963–970, 1978.
19. Marin OS, Tyler HR: Hereditary interstitial nephritis associated with polyneuropathy. *Neurology* 11:999–1105, 1961.
20. Hollinrake K, Thomas PK: Electrical and morphological observations on uremic neuropathy. *Electroencephalogr Clin Neurophysiol* 25:398–399, 1968.
21. Nielsen VK: The peripheral nerve function in chronic renal failure. VI. The relationship between sensory and motor nerve conduction and kidney function, azotemia, age, sex, and clinical neuropathy. *Acta Med Scand* 194:455–462, 1973.
22. Nielsen VK: The peripheral nerve function in chronic renal failure: A survey. *Acta Med Scand* 573 (Suppl):1–32, 1974.
23. Asbury AK: Uremic neuropathy. In: PJ Dyck, PK Thomas, EH Lambert, eds, *Peripheral Neuropathy*. WB Saunders, New York, pp 982–992, 1975.
24. Harriman DGF, Taverner D, Woolfal AL: Ekbom's syndrome and burning paraesthesiae. *Brain* 93:393–406, 1970.
25. Telstad W, Sorensen O, Larsen S, Lillevold PE, Nyberg–Hansen R, Stensrud P: Treatment of the restless legs syndrome with carbamazepine: A double blind study. *Br Med J* 288:444–446, 1984.
26. Von Scheele C: Levodopa in restless legs. *Lancet* 2:426–427, 1986.
27. Spencer PS, Sabri MI, Shaumburg HH, Moore CL: Does a defect of energy metabolism in the nerve fiber underlie axonal degeneration in polyneuropathies? *Ann Neurol* 5:501–507, 1979.
28. Patten BM: Neuromuscular complications. In: G Eknoyan, JP Knochel, eds, *The Systemic Consequences of Renal Failure*. Grune and Stratton, Orlando, FL, pp 281–310, 1984.
29. Sterzel RB: Semar M, Lonergan ET, Treser G, Lange K: Relationship of nervous tissue transketolase to the neuropathy in chronic uremia. *J Clin Invest* 50:2295–2304, 1971.
30. Blagg CR, Kemble F, Taverner D: Nerve conduction velocity in relationship to the severity of renal disease. *Nephron* 5:290–299, 1968.
31. Fleming LW, Lenman JA, Stewart WK: Effect of magnesium on nerve conduction during regular dialysis treatment. *J Neurol Neurosurg Psychiatry* 35:342–355, 1972.
32. Clements RS, DeJesus PV Jr, Winegrad AI: Raised plasma myoinositol levels in uremia and experimental neuropathy. *Lancet* 1:1137–1141, 1973.
33. DeJesus PV Jr, Clements RS Jr, Winegrad AI: Hypermyoinositolemic polyneuropathy in rats. A possible mechanism for uremic polyneuropathy. *J Neurol Sci* 21:237–249, 1974.
34. Babb AL, Ahmad S, Bergstrom J, Scribner BH: The middle molecule hypothesis in perspective. *Am J Kid Dis* 1:46–50,

1981.
35. Ahmad S, Babb AL, Milutinovic J, Scribner BH: Effects of residual renal function on minimum dialysis requirements. *Proc Eur Dialys Transpl Assoc* 16:197–213, 1979.
36. Massry SG: Is parathyroid hormone a uremic toxin? *Nephron* 19:125–130, 1977.
37. Avram MM, Feinfeld DA, Huatuco AH: Search for the uremic toxin: Decreased motor-nerve conduction velocity and elevated parathyroid hormone in uremia. *N Engl J Med* 298:1000–1003, 1978.
38. DiGiulio SD, Chkoff N, Lhoste F, Zingraff J, Drueke T: Parathormone as a nerve poison in uremia. *N Engl J Med* 299:1134–1135, 1978.
39. Goldstein DA, Chui LA, Massry SG: Effect of parathyroid hormone and uremia on peripheral nerve calcium and motor nerve conduction velocity. *J Clin Invest* 62:89–93, 1978.
40. Aurbach GD, Patten BM, Bilezikian JP, Mallette LE, Prince A, Engel WK: Neuromuscular disease in primary hyperparathyroidism. *Ann Intern Med* 80:182–193, 1974.
41. Mallette LE, Patten BM, Engle WK: Neuromuscular disease in secondary hyperparathyroidism. *Ann Intern Med* 82;474–483, 1975.
42. McQuillen MP, Gorin FJ: Serial ulnar nerve conduction velocity measurements in normal subjects. *J Neurol Neurosurg Psychiatry* 32:144–148, 1969.
43. Kominami N, Tyler HR, Hampers CL, Merrill JP: Variations in motor nerve conduction velocity in normal and uremic patients. *Arch Intern Med* 128:235–239, 1971.
44. Preswick G, Jeremy D: Subclinical polyneuropathy in renal insufficiency. *Lancet* 2:731–732, 1964.
45. Versacci AA, Olsen KJ, McBain PB, Nakamoto S, Kolft WJ: Uremic polyneuropathy and nerve conduction velocity. *Trans Am Soc Artif Intern Organs* 10:328–330, 1964.
46. Albertazzi A, DiPaolo B, Capelli P, Spisni C, Del Rosso G: Evoked potentials in uremia. *Contr Nephrol* 45:60–68, 1985.
47. Ahmad S, Goodman W, Pagel M, Shen F: Accelerated creatinine generation and elevated CPK due to androgens. *Proc Clin Dial Transpl Forum* 10:174–176, 1980.
48. Thomas PK, Hollinrake K, Lascella RG, O'Sullivan DJ, Baillod RA, Moorhead JF, Mackenzie JC: The polyneuropathy of chronic renal failure. *Brain* 94:761–780, 1971.
49. Savazzi GM, Marbini A, Gemignani F, Cavatorta A, Govoni E, Bragaglia MM: The peripheral nervous system in dialyzed uremic patients: Regressive motor unit changes. *Contr Nephrol* 45:42–59, 1985.
50. Zucchelli P, Sturani A, Zucallà A, Santoro A, Degli Esposito E, Chiarini C: Dysfunction of the autonomic nervous system in patients with end-stage renal failure. *Contr Neurol* 45:69–81, 1985.
51. Solders G, Persson A, Gutierrez A: Autonomic dysfunction in non-diabetic terminal uremia. *Acta Nephrol Scand* 71:321–327, 1985.
52. Campese VM, Romoff MS, Levitan D, Lane K, Massry SG: Mechanisms of autonomic nervous system dysfunction in uremia. *Kidney Int* 20:246–253, 1981.
53. Charachon R, Moreno-Ribes V, Cordonnier D: Deafness due to renal failure. Clinicopathological study. *Ann Otolaryngol Chir Cervicofac* 95:179–203, 1978.
54. Heidbreder E, Schafferhaus K, Heidland H: Autonomic neuropathy in chronic renal insufficiency. Comparative analysis of diabetic and nondiabetic patients. *Nephron* 41:50–56, 1985.
55. Solders G, Persson A, Wilczek H: Autonomic system dysfunction and polyneuropathy in nondiabetic uremia: A one-year study after renal transplantation. *Transplantation* 41:616–619, 1986.
56. Lazaro RP, Kirshner HS: Proximal muscle weakness in uremia. Case reports and review of the literature. *Arch Neurol* 37:555–558, 1980.
57. Ahmad S, Golper T, Hirschberg R, Kopple J, Katz L, Kirtin P, Ashbrook D: Efficacy of l-carnitine in hemodialysis: A multi-center controlled clinical trial (abstract). *Am Soc Nephrol*:69A, 1986.
58. Ahmad S, Hatch M: Hyperoxalemia in renal failure and the role of hemoperfusion and hemodialysis in primary oxalosis. *Nephron* 41:235–240, 1985.
59. Freeman RM, Lawton RL, Chamberlain MA: Hard-water syndrome. *N Engl J Med* 276:1113–1118, 1967.
60. Govan JR, Porter CA, Cook JG, Dixon B, Traffor JA: Acute magnesium poisoning as a complication of chronic intermittent haemodialysis. *Br Med J* 2:278–279, 1968.
61. Kenny MA, Casillas E, Ahmad S: Magnesium, calcium, and PTH relationships in dialysis patients after magnesium repletion. *Nephron* 46:199–205, 1987.
62. Zarate A, Gelfand M, Novello A, Knepshield J, Preuss HG: Propanolol-asociated hypoglycemia in patients on maintenance hemodialysis. *Int J Artif Organs* 4:130–134, 1981.
63. Miller JD, Broom J, Smith G: Severe hypoglycaemia due to combined use of parenteral nutrition and renal dialysis. *Br Med J* 285:9–10, 1982.
64. Fernandez JP, McGinn JT, Hoffman RS: Cerebral edema from blood-brain glucose differences complicating peritoneal dialysis. Second membrane syndrome. *NY State J Med* 68:677–680, 1968.
65. Chazan BI: Rees SB: Balodimos MC, Younger D, Ferguson BD: Dialysis in diabetics. *JAMA* 209:2026–2030, 1969.
66. Jagadha V, Deck JH, Halliday WC, Smyth HS: Wernicke's encephalopathy in patients on peritoneal dialysis or hemodialysis. *Ann Neurol* 21:78–84, 1987.
67. Faris AA: Wernicke's encephalopathy in uremia. *Neurology* 22:1293–1297, 1972.
68. Leonard A, Shapiro FL: Subdural hematoma in regularly hemodialyzed patients. *Ann Intern Med* 82:650–658, 1975.
69. Nix WA: Coincidence of uremic and hypertensive encephalopathy with chronic subdural hematoma under hemodialysis. Case Report. *J Neurosurg Sci* 4:257–260, 1983.
70. Onoyama K, Kumagai H, Miishima T, Tsuruda H, Tommoka S, Motomura K, Fujishima M: Incidence of strokes and its prognosis in patients on maintenance hemodialysis. *Jpn Heart J* 27:685–691, 1986.
71. Alfrey AC: Dialysis encephalopathy. *Clin Nephrol* 24 (Suppl):S15–S19, 1985.
72. Alfrey AC, LeGendre GR, Kaehny WD: The dialysis encephalopathy syndrome: Possible aluminum intoxication. *N Engl J Med* 294:184–188, 1976.
73. Mayor GH, Burnatowska-Hledin M: The metabolism of aluminum and aluminum-related encephalopathy. *Semin Nephrol* 6:1–4, 1986.
74. Mahoney CA, Arieff AI: Uremic encephalopathies: Clinical, biochemical and experimental features. *Am J Kidney Dis* 2:324–336, 1982.
75. Dunea G, Mahurkar SD, Mamdami B, Smith EC: Role of aluminum in dialysis dementia. *Ann Intern Med* 88:502–504, 1978.
76. Scholtz CL, Swash M, Gray A, Kogeorgos J, Marsh F: Neurofibrillary neuronal degeneration in dialysis dementia: A feature of aluminum toxicity. *Clin Neuro Pathol* 6:93–97, 1987.
77. Wills MR, Savory J: Water content of aluminum, dialysis

dementia, and osteomalacia. *Environ Health Perspect* 63:141–147, 1985.
78. Gasek EM, Babb AL, Uvelli DA, Fry DL, Scribner BH: Dialysis dementia: The role of dialysate pH in altering the dialyzability of aluminum. *Trans Am Soc Artif Intern Organs* 25:409–415, 1979.
79. Bakir AA, Hryhorczuk DO, Berman E, Dunea G: Acute fatal hyperaluminemic encephalopathy in undialyzed and recently dialyzed uremic patients. *Trans Am Soc Artif Intern Organs* 32:171–176, 1986.
80. Ackrill P, Day JP: Deferoxamine in the treatment of aluminum overload. *Clin Nephrol 24* (Suppl 1):S94–S97, 1985.
81. Blake DR, Winyard P, Lunee J, Williams A, Good PA, Crewes SJ, Gutteridge JMC, Rowley D, Halliwell B, Cornish A, Hicker RC: Cerebral and ocular toxicity induced by desferoxamine. *Q J Med* 56:345–355, 1985.
82. Weiss B: The behavioral toxicology of metals. *Feder Proc* 37:22–27, 1978.
83. Savazzi GM, Cusmano F, Degasperi T: Cerebral atrophy in patients on long-term regular hemodialysis treatment. *Clin Nephrol* 23:89–95, 1985.
84. McGraw ME, Haka–Ikse K: Neurologic-developmental sequelae of chronic renal failure in infancy. *J Pediatr* 106:579–583, 1985.
85. Arieff AI: Dialysis disequilibrium syndrome: Current concepts on pathogenesis. In: GE Schreiner, JF Winchester, eds, *Controversies in Nephrology*, Georgetown University Press, Washington DC, pp 367–376, 1982.
86. Kennedy AC, Linton AL, Eaton JC, Urea levels in cerebrospinal fluid after haemodialysis. *Lancet* 1:410–411, 1962.
87. Arieff AI, Massry SG, Barrientos A, Kleeman CR: Brain water and electrolyte metabolism in uremia: Effects of slow and rapid hemodialysis. *Kidney Int* 4:177–187, 1973.
88. Posner JB, Plum F: Spinal fluid pH and neurologic symptoms in systemic acidosis. *N Engl J Med* 277:605, 1977.
89. Arieff AI: Massry SG: Dialysis disequilibrium syndrome. In: SG Massry, AL Sellers, eds, *Clinical Aspects of Uremia and Dialysis*. Charles C Thomas, Springfield, IL, pp 34–52, 1976.
90. Hampl H, Klopp HW, Michels N, Mahiout A, Schilling H, Wolfgruber M, Schiller R, Handfeld F, Kessel M: Electroencephalographic investigations of the disequilibrium syndrome during bicarbonate and acetate dialysis. *Proc Eur Dialys Transpl Assoc* 19:351–359, 1982.
91. LaGreca G, Biasioli S, Chiaramonte S, DeHor P, Dettori P, Fabris A, Feriana M, Pinna V, Pisani E, Ronco C: Studies on brain density in hemodialysis and peritoneal dialysis. *Nephron* 31:146–150, 1982.
92. Basil EC, Miller JD, Koles ZJ, Grace M, Ulan RA: The effects of dialysis on brain water and EEG in stable chronic uremia. *Am J Kidney Dis* 9:462–469, 1987.
93. Holtmann B, Anderson CB: Carpal tunnel syndrome following vascular shunts for hemodialysis. *Arch Surg* 112:65–66, 1977.
94. Di Raimondo CR, Stone WJ: A beta$_2$m amyloidosis. *Int J Artif Organs* 10:281–283, 1987.
95. Chanard J, Lavand S, Toupance O, Melin JP, Gillery P, Revillard JP: Beta$_2$-microglobulin-associated amyloidosis in chronic haemodialysis patients. *Lancet* 1:1212, 1986
96. Vandenbroucke JM, Jadoul M, Maldague B, Huaux JP, Noel H, vanYpersele de Strihou C: Possible role of dialysis membrane characteristics in amyloid osteoarthropahy. *Lancet* 1:1210–1211, 1986.
97. Haugelstaine D, Waer M, Michielsen P, Goebols J, Vandeputte M: Haemodialysis membranes, serum beta$_2$-microglobulin, and dialysis amyloidosis. *Lancet* 1:1211–1212, 1986.
98. Delmez JA, Holtmann B, Sicard GA, Goldberg AP, Harter R: Peripheral nerve entrapment syndromes in chronic hemodialysis patients. *Nephron* 30:118–123, 1982.
99. Teschan PE: Central and peripheral nervous system in uremia: An overview. *Contr Nephrol* 45:1–8, 1985.
100. Kiley JE, Hines O: Electroencephalographic evaluation of uremia. *Arch Intern Med* 116:67–73, 1965.
101. Teschan PE: Measurement of neurobehavioral responses to renal failure, dialysis and transplantation. In: Levy N, ed, *Psychonephrology I. Psychological Factors in Hemodialysis and Transplantation*. Plenum Press, New York, pp 13–18, 1981.
102. Rossini PM, Pirchio M, Treviso M, Gambi D, DiPaolo B, Albertazzi A: Checkerboard reversal pattern and flash VEPs in dialyzed and non-dialyzed subjects. *Electroencephalogr Clin Neurophysiol* 52:435–444, 1981.
103. Anderson RJ, Schafer LA, Olin DB, Eickhoff TC: Infectious risk factors in the immunosuppressed host. *Am J Med* 54:453–460, 1973.

CHAPTER 48

Hematologic Disorders in Renal Failure

K.M. KOCH

INTRODUCTION

Even though renal failure also affects the function of white blood cells and thrombocytes (1), renal anemia is the only hematologic disturbance of uremia for which well-founded possibilities of therapeutic intervention exist today. The basis for this exceptional and fortunate situation is our advanced understanding of the pathogenesis of renal anemia as well as recent progress in molecular biology. As this book is devoted to therapy, this chapter will restrict itself to renal anemia and its management.

CLINICAL FEATURES AND CONSEQUENCES

Anemia is one of main clinical symptoms of renal failure. It becomes manifest when creatinine clearance has dropped to 40–30 ml/min/1.73 m^2, and its severity increases with further deterioriation of excretory renal function. Renal anemia is normochronic and normocytic when no other aggravating factors such as iron deficiency or aluminum overload are coexisting with renal insufficiency. Renal anemia is hyporegenerative. The reticulocyte count, when corrected for normal hematocrit values, is inadequate.

The impact of renal anemia on physical and mental abilities is considerable and represents a major obstacle for the rehabilitation of patients in terminal renal failure. This applies even though the effect of anemia on tissue oxygenation may be partly balanced in uremic patients by a shift of the oxyhemoglobin dissociation curve to the right. This shift, which is attributed to acidosis and increased intraerythrocytotic levels of 2,3-diphosphoglycerate and other phosphates, reduces the peripheral affinity of hemoglobin for oxygen and thereby improves oxygen delivery to the tissues. A further compensating mechanism is an increase in cardiac output (2). However, many of the uremic patients have hypertension and myocardiopathy; therefore, their ability to compensate for the reduced hemoglobin level by an increase in cardiac output may be compromised. Also many of the patients have advanced coronary artery disease, and even renal anemia of a modrate degree may be accompanied by myocardial ischemia and angina.

PATHOGENESIS

The primary mechanisms involved in the pathogenesis of the anemia of renal failure are hemolysis, inadequate production of erythropoietin, and possibly also an inhibition of the response of erythroid precuror cells to erythropoietin (3). In addition, secondary mechanisms such as iron deficiency or aluminum intoxication may be operative.

Hemolysis

Hemolysis in terminal renal failure is of moderate degree, as red-cell survival in general is reduced by 25–30%. The cause for hemolysis appears to be extracellular and related to the effects of factors contained in the uremic plasma on membrane ATPase, as well as on the enzymes of the pentose phosphate shunt of erythrocytes. The malfunction of the pentose phosphate shunt renders erythrocytes vulnerable to hemoglobin oxidation with subsequent hemolysis. This defect may become especially critical when exogenous oxidants are introduced via the dialysate or as medication. Thus the use of chloramine-containing tap water for the production of dialysate can cause significant hemolysis in hemodialysis patients. Secondary hyperparathyroidism may also contribute to the reduction of red-cell survival in uremia, as intact PTH or its 1–34 fragment increase the osmotic fragility of human red blood cells, probably by increasing cellular rigidity (4). Also, chronic uremic dogs have a shortened red-cell survival, which is normalized by parathyroidectomy (5). These experimental findings are complemented by clinical reports of a rise of hemoglobin after parathyroidectomy in uremic patients. Another mechanism causing an increase of erythroyte rigidity with subsequent hemolysis in renal failure is intracellular phosphate depletion due to overtreatment with oral phosphate binders (6).

There are a number of additional less common mechanisms that occasionally may cause significant hemolysis such as accidental exposure of blood to excess copper, zinc, and formaldehyde, or to a overheated or very hypotonic dialysate in hemodialysis patients. Aggravation of hemolysis in renal failure may also be a consequence of additional pathologic processes such as hypersplenism or microangiopathy associated with periarteriitis nodosa, lupus erythematosus, and malignant hypertension.

Erythropoietin deficiency

The mild hemolysis caused by renal failure alone, without the action of additional aggravating factors, should not result in anemia if the response of erythropoiesis is sufficient. However, erythropoiesis is impaired. The major reason for this phenomenon is reduced production of erythropoietin in patients with advanced renal failure.

The inadequate production of erthropoietin is a consequence of progressive destruction of renal production sites of erythropoietin by the underlying renal disease. The important role erythropoietin deficiency in the pathogenesis of renal anemia is underscored by the more severe degree of anemia observed in bilateral nephrectomized hemodialysis patients. Furthermore, recent investigations applying reliable radioimmunoassays showed that, in comparison to anemic patients without renal disease, patients with anemia of renal failure display an inadequate rise of the serum erythropoietin concentration (7, 8).

Inhibition of erythropoiesis

In addition to the reduced availability of erythropoietin, inhibition of the response of erythroid precursor cells to erythropoietin has to be considered as a cause for the inadequate erythropoiesis in uremic patients.

The accumulation of inhibitors within the uremic organism is suggested by a number of clinical observations. One argument in favor of a role of inhibitors in the pathogenesis of the anemia of renal failure is the demonstration of elevated plasma levels of erythropoietin in some anemic patients with end-stage renal disease (9, 10), suggesting that the response of the bone marrow of these patients to erythropoietin is suppressed. Further support for the existence of "uremic" toxins suppressing erythropoiesis are the hematologic changes seen in patients with terminal renal failure after the induction of regular dialysis treatment. Hematocrit and red-cell production as measured by erythrocyte iron turnover usually rise (11) in spite of a parallel decline of serum erythropoietin levels (12).

Attempts to identify endogenous "uremic" inhibitors of erythropoiesis have led to conflicting results. Amongst the many substances implicated, the most intensively investigated were the ployamines spermin and spermidine (13) and parathyroid hormone (14). In spite of many observations supporting their involvement, the discussion is still controversial. This especially concerns the question of whether polyamines and parathyroid hormone are specific inhibitors of erythropoiesis (14, 15).

An additional inhibiting mechanism not directly linked to renal insufficiency can be aluminum intoxication due to exposure to high dialysate alumimum concentrations and/or extensive ingestion of aluminum-containing phosphate binders. Aluminum induces a microcytic anemia, which, when observed in the presence of normal or elevated serum ferritin levels, signals that the patient's renal anemia may be aggravated by aluminum intoxication. The exact pathogenesis of aluminum-associated anemia is not yet fully understood, but the available evidence strongly suggests that the toxic effects of aluminum on erythropoiesis involve inhibition of synthesis and ferrochelation of hemoglobin (16, 17).

MANAGEMENT

The principles of treatment of renal anemia range from the more symptomatic measure of transfusion of red cells to complete cure by renal transplantation. Blood transfusions are only of temporary benefit and carry inherent risks such as exposure to the viruses of hepatitis and human immune deficiency, as well as the development of secondary hemochromatosis. Renal transplantation in most cases is not available before a waiting period of variable length has passed, and not every regular dialysis patient, expecially amongst the steadily growing population of older patients, is eligible for transplantation. As shown in Table 1, there exist a variety of therapeutic approaches between the two poles of blood transfusion and transplantation that either interfere with the pathogenesis of renal anemia itself or prevent or correct the effects of secondary aggravating mechanisms.

Erythropoietin supplementation

As a treatment focused on the primary pathogenesis, a very effective and promising therapy has become available in that recombinant human erythropoietin (rh-Epo) has been produced for therapeutic application. When given intravenously to regular hemodialysis patients, rh-Epo caused a dramatic improvement of erythropoiesis (18, 19). It was even possible to keep hemoglobin levels normal after stopping blood transfusions in bilateral nephrectomized patients who had been in need for regular transfusions before. As shown in Figure 1, taken from a multicenter trial performed in regular hemodialysis patients, hematocrit increases within a few weeks when varying amounts of rh-Epo are given intravenously thrice a week

Table 1. Principles of treatment of renal anemia

Erthropoietin supplementation
Removal of endogenous inhibitors of erythropoiesis and endogenous hemolytic toxins by extracorporeal renal replacement therapy or peritoneal dialysis
Removal of excess aluminum by deferoxamine
Correction of hyperparathyroidism
Androgen therapy
Reduction of iatrogenic blood loss
Iron supplementation
Folate supplementation
Exclusion of physical and chemical hazards within the extracorporeal blood circuit

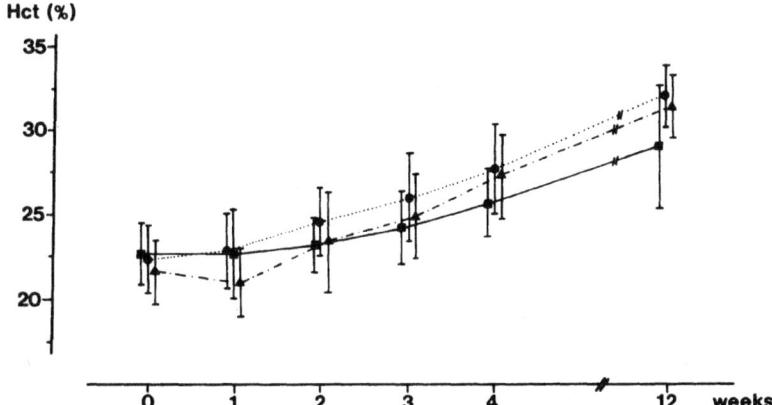

Figure 1. Hematocrit (median and interquartile range) of regular hemodialysis patients during treatment with human recombinant erythropoietin (■—■ = 40 IU kg/3 × week, n = 29; ●·····● = 80 IU kg/3 × week, n = 28; ▲-.-.-.-.▲ = 120 IU kg/3 × week, n = 28).

after dialysis. With higher doses of rh-Epo, the increase of hematocrit was faster and higher levels were achieved. In this trial the mean maintenance dose necessary to keep the hematocrit between 30–90 and 35% was found to be 3 × 36 IU/kg intravenously thrice weekly after dialysis (range 3 × 20 to 3 × 80 IU/kg/weekly). When erythropoiesis of regular hemodialysis patients improves under rh-Epo, iron deficiency may develop, necessitating oral or even intravenous iron supplementation.

The rise of hematocrit is accompanied by an immediate feeling of well-being and an improvement of exercise tolerance that can be quantitated by ergometry. Figure 2 shows the results we obtained in 15 regular hemodialysis patients with a mean age of 42.4 years (range 22–57) when we determined the physical work capacity at a heart rate of 130 beats/min (PWC 130) by bicycle ergometry. When the mean hematocrit had risen from $23 \pm 4\%$ (SD) to $35 \pm 6\%$ in approximately 12 weeks after starting rh-Epo therapy, the mean PWC 130 rose significantly ($p < 0.05$) from 73 ± 28 watts to 98 ± 38 watts, a value just reaching the lower limit of the range obtained in healthy volunteers of comparable age. Reports on long-term cardiovascular effects of rh-Epo therapy from the various study groups are still outstanding.

Up to now initial trials showed that antibodies against the recombinant material and resistance to its effect have not developed. The major side effects reported so far (Table 2) were increases in blood pressure and in some patients thrombosis of the vascular access site and other thrombotic events, together with a need for higher heparin doses to prevent clotting in the extracorporeal circulation (18, 19). There also were reports of increase of predialysis serum concentrations of creatinine, urea, and phosphate,

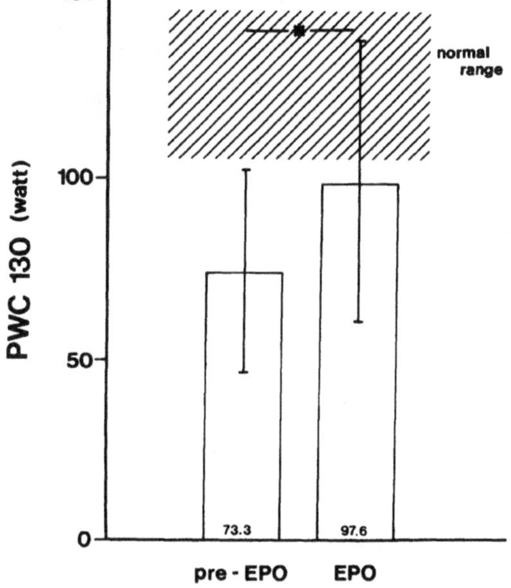

Figure 2. Physical work capacity at a heart rate of 130 beats/min. (PWC 130) in 15 regular hemodialysis patients before (pre-Epo) and during treatment (Epo) with human recombinant erythropoietin. Mean hematocrit pre-Epo: $23 \pm 4\%$; under Epo: $35 \pm 6\%$ (mean $\pm$ SD; * = $p < 0.05$, paired t-test).

Table 2. Treatment of anemia of regular hemodialysis patients by human recombinant erythropoietin: Side effects

Hypertension
Shunt thrombosis
Clotting within extracorporeal blood circuit
Increase of thrombocyte count
Increase of serum concentrations of phosphate, urea, creatinine, and potassium

and in individual patients severe hyperkalemia developed (18, 19).

In our multicenter trial, out of 92 regular hemodialysis patients finally evaluated 6 originally normotensive patients became hypertensive, and in 21 out of 43 initially hypertensive patients the doses of antihypertensive drugs had to be increased during treatment with rh-Epo. In three of the patients rh-Epo treatment had to be stopped because of severe hypertension. The rise of blood pressure following correction of anemia by rh-Epo is due to an increase peripheral resistance, which might be a consequence of two mechanisms. First, higher blood viscosity due to an increase of red-cell mass causes a rise of total peripheral resistance. Second, improvement of tissue oxygenation due to higher oxygen transport capacity increases arteriolar vascular tone (20) and thereby vascular resistance. Presently available data does not permit quantitation of the individual contributions of the two mechanisms towards a rise of peripheral resistance. As an example for the hemodynamic effects of the correction of renal anemia, Figure 3 shows calf blood flow measured by venous occlusion plethysmography and calculated regional peripheral resistance in seven regular hemodialysis patients before and 10–12 weeks after the start of rh-Epo treatment. Whereas calf blood flow decreased significantly ($p < 0.05$, paired t-test), the calculated peripheral resistance increased significantly ($p < 0.05$). None of the patients received antihypertensive drugs, hematocrit increased from 21% to 33%, and mean arterial blood pressure increased from 90 to 95 mmHg.

The reported thrombotic complications may also be related to higher blood viscosity. However, an increase of thrombocyte count — within the normal range — that was observed by us and by at least one other group of investigators (21) may also have contributed to the observed hypercoagulability. Higher predialysis serum concentrations of urea, creatinine, and phosphate, as well as reported incidences of hyperkalemia may be a consequence of both reduced dialyzer efficiency because of higher hematocrits and improved appetite because of increased general well-being.

All these observations indicate that therapy with rh-Epo should be used with caution. It is also possible that most of these side effects could be minimized if the hematocrit levels are not raised to normal but to levels between 30% and 35%. The production of rh-Epo and its clinical use represent a major breakthrough in the management of patients with uremia. Further experience will make the therapy safer. The results of the clincial trials support the concept that erthropoietin deficiency is the primary mechanism in the pathogenesis of renal anemia. However, the involvement of other factors, such as inhibitors of erythropoiesis, is not excluded, as their effect may have been overridden by the pharmacologic doses of erythropoietin applied.

Removal of inhibitors and toxins

All extracorporeal renal replacement therapies and peritoneal dialysis, in principle, could also interfere with the pathogenesis of anemia of renal failure, as they may remove toxins responsible for hemolysis and inhibition of erythropoiesis. Indeed, the clincial experience with all treatment modalities shows that a partial correction of the anemia is achieved. The improvement, however, falls significantly behind the results obtained with erythropoietin treatment. This also applies to the speed of improvement, which is much faster with erythropoietin therapy. The relative ineffectiveness of renal replacement therapies is a consequence of our limited knowledge of the toxins involved and the best way to remove them.

The simple approach to improve detoxification therapy of uremia by raising the upper limit of the molecular size

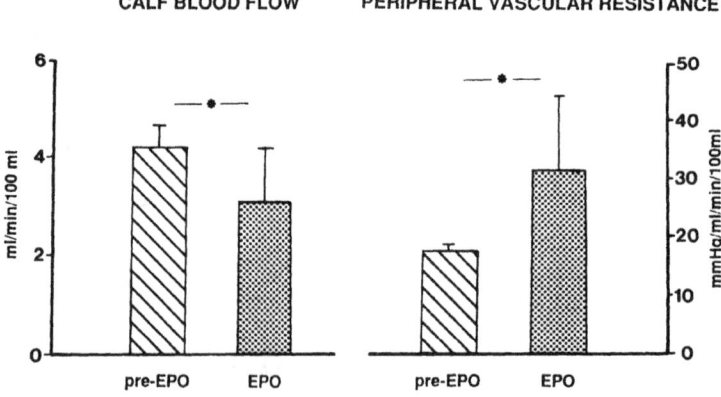

Figure 3. Calf blood flow and peripheral vascular resistance in seven regular hemodialysis patients before (pre-Epo) and during treatment (Epo) with human recombinant erythropoietin. Mean hematocrit pre-Epo: 21 ± 3%; under Epo: 33 ± 4%. Mean ± SD; * = $p < 0.05$, paired t-test.

removed by diffusive and/or convective transport did not produce unequivocal results. There exists, for instance, no data proving that hemofiltration or hemodiafiltration, which cover a larger molecular range of removal than hemodialysis with tight cellulosic membranes, are superior in correcting the anemia of renal failure. On the other hand, patients on continuous ambulatory peritoneal dialysis (CAPD), also a treatment with a larger molecular range of removal display better hematocrits than patients on standard hemodialysis with tight cellulosic membranes. It is still unclear whether this advantage of CAPD is really only due to better removal of inhibitors of erythropoiesis. As an alternative explanation, some observations indicate that CAPD by an unknown mechanism increases erythropoietin production, probably also at extrarenal sites, and therapy improves erythropoiesis (22, 23).

Removal of excess aluminum

When the inhibitor of erythropoiesis is known, as in the case of aluminum, intoxication treatment can be selective and effective. An aggravating effect of aluminum on the anemia of renal failure should always be assumed when in a regular hemodialysis patient microcytotic anemia coincides with normal or elevated serum ferritin levels. The diagnosis will be confirmed by elevated serum aluminum levels; by a history of aluminum exposure, orally or via dialysate; by further manifestations of aluminum intoxication, such as encephalopathy and aluminum bone disease; and by a successful therapeutic trial. The treatment of choice is the use of the chelator deferoxamine (DFO) intravenously during the last 1–2 hours of hemodialysis or hemofiltration, or intraperitoneally overnight in CAPD patients. The doses range from 0.5–2.0 g thrice weekly, depending on the side effects. DFO mobilizes aluminum as a soluable complex, which then is removed by the therapeutic dialytic or filtration procedure. The major side effects are hypotension, ocular toxicity, and neurologic complications such as seizures. These side effects respond to temporary interruption of therapy, reduction of dose, or termination of therapy.

Correction of hyperparathyroidism

Despite a potential role for secondary hyperparathyroidism in the pathogenesis of the anemia of renal failure, parathyroidectomy is not indicated for the sole purpose of treating severe renal anemia. When other complications, however, necessitate subtotal removal of the parathyroids, an improvement of anemia may be a welcome side effect. Medical suppression of parathyroid gland activity with $1,25\text{-}(OH)_2D_3$ in patients with end-stage renal disease very often is associated with an improvement of anemia.

Androgen therapy

Since the early 1970s a variety of androgens have been used in the treatment of the anemia of renal failure (24). Their positive effect is assumed to be mediated via increased erythropoietin production and increased proliferation of erythropoietin-sensitive stem-cell populations.

Testosterone esters (testosterone propionate), fluoxymesterone (17-methyl androstane), and 19-nortestosterone compounds (nandrolone decanoate) have been used successfully in the treatment of the anemia of renal failure. The response is slow and the effects of these drugs may become evident within 4 weeks of therapy. Nandrolone decanoate in doses of 100–200 mg given once a week is adequate. The 19-nortestosterone compounds have the highest anabolic/androgenic ratio of 6.0. Thus, they are the least hirsutizing and, therefore, they are tolerated by the female patient. Fluoxymesterone may cause priapism in the male patient. Cholestatic hepatocellular disease may complicate the use of these agents and is more common with the 17-methylated steroids. A progressive increase in blood transaminases or a rise in serum bilirubin levels requires the discontinuation of therapy. The hepatocellular changes are usually reversible following the cessation of treatment. Therapy with androgens may potentially aggravate the symptoms of prostatism or accelerate the growth of prostate carcinoma. Skin rashes, hoarseness of voice, and psychic disturbances are other side effects of this therapy.

In view of the side effects, androgens should be used with restraint. This point of view is supported by findings (25) that suggest due to simultaneous effects on red-cell metabolism, the positive effect of androgens on erythropoiesis and red-cell mass may not necessarily realize improved peripheral oxygenation. It is predictable that treatment of renal anemia by androgens will be stopped once recombinant human erythropoietin becomes available for general use.

Reduction of iatrogenic blood loss, iron supplementation, and other measures

Or course, the management of anemia in terminal renal failure also includes the prevention and correction of iatrogenic aggravating factors. Excessive loss of blood for laboratory investigation, into the extracorporeal blood circuit and from punctured access sites should be kept as low as possible. Monitoring of body iron stores by serum ferritin determination once or twice a year is indicated. When under treatment with human recombinant erythropoietin erythropoiesis is improving and iron demands are increasing, serum ferritin should be controlled more frequently.

As intestinal iron absorption is not affected by uremia, oral iron supplementation is preferable when iron deficiency is present. One should be aware, however, of the possibility that phosphate binders interfere with the intestinal absorption of iron. If oral therapy fails to correct iron deficiency, parenteral replacement of iron should be considered. This is done with iron dextran (inferon). The intravenous administration is safer and more comfortable than the intramuscular injection. Anaphylactic shock may occur in 1% of patients receiving parenteral iron. To reduce the incidence of this dangerous complication, the patient should be tested with a small dose 5 minutes prior to the administration of the total dose. The amount needed to replenish iron stores could be given in divided doses of 500 mg injected over 5–10 minutes every several days or in a single dose diluted in normal saline to give 5% iron dextran and infused slowly over a period of several hours.

Folate is lost into the dialysate from the blood. Therefore folate deficiency and macrocytotic anemia may develop in patients with a low protein intake. As the diet of regular dialysis patients is liberal and usually contains sufficient amounts of folate, folate deficiency and the need for oral folic acid supplementation is not common. Finally, the nephrologist should be aware that extracorporeal blood treatment carries many potential risks, predominantly in the form of contaminants of the blood and dialysate compartment such as metals and chemicals that could cause red-cell damage and hemolysis.

REFERENCES

1. Eschbach JW: Hematologic problems of dialysis patients. In: Drukker, Parsons, Maher, eds, *Replacement of Renal Function by Dialysis*. Martinus Nijhoff, Boston, pp 630–645, 1983.
2. Neff MS, Kim KE, Persoff M, Onesti G, Swartz C: Hemodynamics of uremic anemia. *Circulation* 43:876–883, 1971.
3. Eschbach JW, Adamson JW: Anemia of end-stage renal disease. *Kidney Int* 28:1–5, 1985.
4. Bogin E, Massry SG, Levi J, Mdaldeti M, Bristol G, Smith J: Effect of parathyroid hormone on osmotic fragility of human erythrocytes. *J Clin Invest* 69:1017–1025, 1982.
5. Akmal M, Telfer N, Ansari AN, Massry SG: Red blood cell survival in chronic renal failure: Role of secondary hyperparathyroidism. *J Clin Invest* 76:1695–1698, 1985.
6. Jacob HS, Amsden T: Acute hemolytic anemia with rigid red cells in hypophosphatemia. *N Engl J Med* 285:1146–1450, 1071.
7. Garcia JF, Ebbe SN, Hollander L, Cutting HO, Miller ME, Cronkite EP: Radioimmunoassay of erythropoietin: Circulating levels in normal and polycythemic human beings. *J Lab Clin Med* 99:624–635, 1982.
8. McGonigle RJS, Wallin JD, Shadduck RK, Fisher JW: Erythropoietin deficiency and inhibition of erythropoiesis in renal insufficiency. *Kidney Int* 25:437–444, 1984.
9. Caro J, Brown S, Miller O, Murray T, Erslev AJ: Erythropoietin levels in uremic nephric and anephric patients. *J Lab Clin Med* 93:449–458, 1979.
10. Radtke HW, Claussner A, Erbes PM, Scheuermann EH, Schoeppe W, Koch KM: Serum erythropoietin concentration in chronic renl failure: Relationship to degree of anemia and excretory renal function. *Blood* 54:877–884, 1979.
11. Eschbach JW, Adamson JW, Cook JD: Disorders of red blood cell production in uremia. *Arch Intern Med* 126:812–815, 1970.
12. Radtke HW, Frei U, Erbes PM, Schoeppe W, Koch KM: Improving anemia by hemodialysis: Effect on serum erythropoietin. *Kidney Int* 17:382–387, 1980.
13. Radtke HW, Rege AB, LaMarche MB, Bartos D, Bartos F, Campbell RA, Fisher JW: Identification of spermine as an inhibitor of erythropoiesis in patients with chronic renal failure. *J Clin Invest* 67:1623–1629, 1981.
14. Meytes D, Bogin E, Ma A, Dukes PP, Massry SG: Effect of parathyroid hormone on erythropoiesis. *J Clin Invest* 67:1263–1269, 1981.
15. Segal GM, Stueve T, Adamson JW: Spermine and spermidine are non-specific inhibitors of in vitro hematopoiesis. *Kidney Int* 31:72–76, 1987.
16. Kaiser L, Schwartz KA: Aluminum-induced anemia. *Am J Kidney Dis* 6:348–352, 1985.
17. Swartz R, Dombrouski J, Burnatowska — Hledin M, Mayor G: Microcytic anemia in dialysis patients: Reversible marker of aluminium toxicity. *Am J Kidney Dis* 9:217–223, 1987.
18. Eschbach JW, Egrie JC, Downing MR, Browne JK, Adamson JW: Correction of the anemia of end-stage renal disease with recombinant human erythropoietin. Results of a combined phase I and II clinical trial. *N Engl J Med* 316:73–78, 1987.
19. Winearls CG, Oliver DO, Pippard MJ, Reid C, Downing MR, Cotes PM: Effect of human erythropoietin derived from recombinant DNA on the anaemia of patients maintained by chronic haemodialysis. *Lancet* 2:1175–1177, 1986.
20. Duling BR, Pittman RN: Oxygen tension: Dependent or independent variable in local control of blood flow? *Fed Proc* 34(11):2012–2019, 1975.
21. Bommer J, Müller–Bühl E, Ritz E, Eifert J: Recombinant human erythropoietin in anaemic patients on haemodialysis (letter). *Lancet* 1:392, 1987.
22. Wideröe TE, Sanengen T, Halvorsen S: Erythropoietin and uremic toxicity during continuous ambulatory peritoneal dialysis. *Kidney Int* 24:208–217, 1983.
23. Chandra M, McVicar M, Clemons G, Mossey RT, Wilkes BM: Role of erythropoietin in the reversal of anemia of renal failure with continuous ambulatory peritoneal dialysis. *Nephron* 46:312–315, 1987.
24. Neff MS, Goldberg J, Slifkin RF, Eiser AR, Calamia V, Kaplan M, Baez A, Gupta S, Mattoo N: A comparison of androgens for anemia in patients on hemodialysis. *N Engl J Med* 304:871–875, 1981.
25. Hendler ED, Solomon L: Androgen therapy in hemodialysis patients: I. Effects on red cell oxygen transport. *Kidney Int* 31:100–106, 1987.

CHAPTER 49

Acute, Intermittent, and Cycled Peritoneal Dialysis

JOSE A. DIAZ-BUXO

INTRODUCTION

Peritoneal dialysis represents the first successful effort in replacing the funtion of a vital internal organ. Ever since 1923, when Ganter applied the concept of peritoneal lavage to treat renal insufficiency (1), we have been modifying the technique of peritoneal dialysis in our goal of providing renal substitution in the most physiologic manner. The inability to obtain an adequate peritoneal access greatly hindered the progress of peritoneal dialysis for several decades. The development of a permanent peritoneal dialysis catheter by Tenckhoff in the late 1960s marked the beginning of the golden age of peritoneal dialysis (2). Within the next 15 years dialysate delivery systems were developed, the novel concept of equilibration dialysis was proposed, and the mechanisms of peritoneal solute and fluid transfer were better characterized.

Peritoneal dialysis has enjoyed a prominent position in the treatment of acute renal failure. Prior to the advent of hemodialysis, peritoneal dialysis was reserved for patients with a reasonable chance of recovery of renal function. However, despite the advances and availability of hemodialysis, peritoneal dialysis has played an important role in the treatment of the acute patient. Among the advantages of peritoneal dialysis figure its simplicity, the ability to obtain a peritoneal access without complicated surgical techniques, and the provision of dialysis without specialized equipment.

This chapter will focus on the therapeutics of peritoneal dialysis while providing a limited background of the rationale for the dialysis prescription and a means of calculating the magnitude of fluid and solute removal for specific schedules of dialysis.

ACUTE PERITONEAL DIALYSIS

Peritoneal dialysis is an attractive option for the treatment of acute renal failure (3, 4). It can be performed in practically any hospital and does not require specialized equipment or surgical skills. It is the preferred modality of dialysis for small children (5, 6) due to the difficulties in obtaining adequate circulatory access for hemodialysis and the technical difficulties in matching the size of the hemodialyzer to the child's surface area. Although acute peritoneal dialysis is a relatively simple procedure, the clinician should be knowledgeable of its limitations and potential complications and must always pay strict attention to sterile technique.

Indications and contraindications

The most frequent indications for acute peritoneal dialysis are: acute renal failure and its common manifestations — uremic syndrome, hyperkalemia, extracellular fluid overload, and metabolic acidosis; isolated electrolytic disorders, where conservative therapy is ineffective; and, intractable congestive heart failure. Peritoneal dialysis is the preferred method of renal replacement in patients with bleeding disorders and those in whom heparinization is contraindicated, in those with unstable cardiovascular systems, and in patients with poor or abused peripheral and central veins that are not suitable as a vascular access for hemodialysis.

The indications for dialysis in acute renal failure are usually relative, and the decision to start therapy is often made in the setting of progressive azotemia long before life-threatening complications present. Since acute renal failure frequently occurs as a consequence, or concomitantly, with sepsis, surgery, and malnutrition, the patient may be hypercatabolic (7). Because of the limitations of peritoneal dialysis in achieving solute removal (vide infra), it is recommended that peritoneal dialysis be started early in order to facilitate adequate nutrition and to prevent further catabolism. Although a specific BUN level is seldom the indication for peritoneal dialysis, levels in excess of 120 mg/dl should be monitored closely and should be considered in the decision to commence therapy.

Severe hyperkalemia (potassium ≥ 6 mEq/l) that cannot be treated or has not responded to conservative management (sodium polysterene sulfonate, bicarbonate, glucose/insulin infusions) is an indication for acute dialysis. Evidence of myocardial toxicity should immediately trigger the initiation of therapy; however, an occasional patient may have severe hyperkalemia in the absence of clinical cardiovascular manifestations or electrocardiographic abnormalities such as tall T waves, prolonged PR intervals, QRS widening, or cardiac arrhythmias.

Acute peritoneal dialysis may also correct electrolyte aberrations that are less frequent and are usually controlled with pharmacologic therapy. Severe hyponatremia typically responds to the administration of hypertonic saline or to water intake restriction. Conversely, hypernatremia is treated by the administration of free water. However, in the presence of overhydration and advanced renal insufficiency, dialysis may be indicated. Acute peritoneal dialysis can correct hypercalcemia (8, 9), but the slow rate of calcium removal warrants the use of hemodialysis with a low-calcium bath whenever possible.

Overhydration manifested by peripheral edema (or sacral edema in bedridden patients), elevations in central venous pressure, pulmonary rales, cardiac gallops, pleural effusions, and ascites is a common indication for peritoneal dialysis. Acute peritoneal dialysis has proven to be of benefit in the temporary treatment of patients with cardiomyopathy and life-threatening congestive failure in the absence of renal failure (10-14). It may also benefit nephrotic patients with cardiopulmonary compromise while awaiting the benefits of specific therapy for parenchymal renal disease.

Peritoneal dialysis has been successfully used in the treatment of acute drug intoxication (15, 16). Certain substances can enhance drug removal when added to the dialysate. Examples of accepted practices to augment drug removal by peritoneal dialysis are: a) alteration of the dialysate pH to enhance anion diffusion (17); b) addition of albumin to the dialysate to increase protein binding and to prevent reabsorption of the toxin (18, 19); and c) intraperitoneal administration of vasocative agents to augment peritoneal clearances (16). Despite the proven benefit of peritoneal dialysis in the treatment of acute intoxication, it is known that its effetiveness is only a fraction of that of hemodialysis or hemoperfusion. Peritoneal dialysis should be reserved for the treatment of drug overdoses when hemoperfusion or hemodialysis are unavailable or contraindicated.

Miscellaneous indications for acute peritoneal dialysis include profound hypothermia, which can be reversed by slowly increasing core temperature (20-22); acute pancreatitis (23, 24), often associated with oliguric renal failure; prolonged hypoglycemia associated with the use of oral hypoglycemic agents (25); hepatic coma (26); psoriasis (27).

Although there are no absolute contraindications for acute peritoneal dialysis, several conditions may interfere with adequate dialysate flow or peritoneal access. In the immediate postoperative period, peritoneal dialysis may prove impossible due to the presence of drains or profuse leakage around the surgical wound. The presence of adhesions from previous inflammatory processess or surgery could make peritoneal access impossible and may limit the peritoneal surface area. Similarly, intraabdominal masses, large polycystic kidneys, or extreme obesity may impair the fluid dynamics. Finally, conditions such as severe pulmonary disease and diaphragmatic, abdominal, or inguinal hernias may be aggravated by the increased abdominal pressure generated by dialysate infusion.

Acute peritoneal access

Peritoneal access for acute dialysis can be readily obtained by insertion of a semirigid catheter under local anesthesia. Strict sterile precautions should be observed, and the operator and assistants must wear masks and sterile gloves. The abdomen is prepared in the usual manner by shaving the area between the umbilicus and symphysis pubis, and cleansing the area with povidone-iodine. A local anesthetic is injected in the midline 2-3 cm under the umbilicus. A small stab wound is made and extended to the fascial plane. If the patient is conscious, his or her cooperation is requested by performing a Valsalva maneuver in order to stiffen the anterior abdominal wall. The catheter, with the stylet in place, is inserted into the stab wound and directed slightly caudad into the peritoneum. In order to avoid bowel perforation, it is recommended that the operator uses one hand to thrust the catheter into the abdominal cavity, while the other hand holds the catheter 2-3 cm from its distal end. As the catheter and stylet are pushed through the fibrous tissues of the anterior abdominal wall and peritoneum, resistance increases. Once the peritoneum is pierced a sudden "pop" is felt, signaling entrance into the peritoneal cavity. At this point, the stylet can be withdrawn and the catheter advanced towards the left lower quadrant or other dependent area in the pelvis. The advance of the catheter should be smooth. Whenever resistance is encountered, rotary or back-and-forth motion should be used to facilitate placement and to prevent visceral perforation. The system can then be tested by infusing dialysate and obtaining adequate return.

Some clinicians prefer to fill up the abdominal cavity with 2 or 3 of dialysate, prior to insertion of the catheter, in order to obtain abdominal distention, which both approximates the peritoneum against the abdominal wall and allows the bowel to float in the solution, making the procedure safer. This maneuver has been criticized by others, who contend that the risk of visceral perforation is greater with the use of a sharp needle for the infusion of dialysate than with a blunt stylet.

Once the semirigid catheter is in place, a small metal ring is fitted around the external shaft of the catheter to limit the path of the cathether into the abdominal wall. This same disk can be used to properly anchor the catheter to the abdominal wall with adhesive tape.

Semirigid catheters can be used for several days; however, it is recommended that the catheter be removed between sessions of acute peritoneal dialysis. Because of the inconvenience of multiple punctures and the potential risks involved in catheter insertion, some centers have elected to insert one-cuff acute Tenckhoff catheters if repeated procedures are anticipated. The technique for insertion is similar to that described for the chronic Tenckhoff catheter in a subsequent section.

Table 1. Peritoneal dialysis solutions

		IPD concentrate[1]	Standard dialysate[2]
Volume	(l)	2	0.25, 0.5, 1, 1.5, 2, 2.5, 3, 6
Glucose	(%)	1.5, 2.5	1.5, 2.5, 4.25
Sodium	(mEq/l)	118–132	131–141
Potassium	(mEq/l)	0	0
Calcium	(mEq/l)	3.5	3.4–4.0
Magnesium	(mEq/l)	1.0	0.5–1.5
Acetate	(mEq/l)	35	35–45
Lactate	(mEq/l)	—	35–40

[1] Concentration resulting after 1:19 dilution.
[2] Dialysate used for acute and chronic IPD, CAPD, CCPD, and NPD.

Peritoneal dialysis solutions

Commercial dialysate is available from several manufacturers in containers varying in size from 0.25 l for pediatric use to 6 l. Table 1 provides the formulation for different dialysate solutions. Standard commercial dialysate is usually utilized during acute peritoneal dialysis.

Reverse osmosis systems use a dialysate concentrate that is diluted 19 times to produce the final dialysate. A 2-l bottle of concentrate is diluted to make 40 l of dialysate. The concentration of solutes in the final solution is similar to commercially available dialysate. When rapid cycling with extremely short dwell times (<30 minutes) is performed in combination with hypertonic glucose solutions, greater removal of extracellular water is accomplished, leading to hypernatremia (28, 29). This can be prevented with the use of a low-sodium dialysate.

Technique and schedules for acute peritoneal dialysis

INTERMITTENT PERITONEAL DIALYSIS (IPD)

The oldest and simplest technique for the provision of IPD consists of the periodic manual infusion of commercial dialysate from crystal or plastic containers into the peritoneal cavity and its drainage into a calibrated collecting device with the use of a closed tubing set. The initial exchange volume for adults can be set at 1 l and gradually increased to 2 l if comfortably tolerated by the patient and if no pericatheter leaks are oberved. Variable dwell times and dialysate flow rates can be utilized. For practical purposes, dialysate flow of 2–3 l/h of dialysate can be obtained using infusion and dwell times of 20–30 minutes and drain times of 15–20 minutes. Manual IPD is usually carried on for approximately 24–48 hours and repeated whenever necessary.

IPD can be more conveniently performed with the use of an automated reverse osmosis delivery system or a dialysate cycler (see Chronic IPD). These devices allow provision of automated peritoneal dialysis with excellent control of flow, dwell time and drainage time. Modern equipment is also available that can determine ultrafiltration.

CLINICAL EXPERIENCE WITH IPD IN THE TREATMENT OF ACUTE RENAL FAILURE

IPD is considered an acceptable alternative to hemodialysis for the treatment of patients with acute renal failure (4, 30). The mortality rate in various series has been comparable to that of hemodialysis (3, 30). Control of biochemical parameters has been acceptable, except in cases of extreme hypercatabolism. Fluid removal can be easily manipulated by altering the dialysate flow and the osmolality of the solution. Although heparin is usually recommended in order to avoid catheter obstruction from fibrin strands, the use of intraperitoneal heparin does not result in systemic heparinization (31, 32).

IPD, being a high-flow peritoneal system, provides a relatively high small-molecule removal. The following sample prescription for IPD using an automated delivery system demonstrates its efficiency for urea clearance:

Length of session — 24 hours
Dialysate flow — 24, 2-l exchanges/session (48 l/session)
  Exchange duration — 1 hour (inflow time, 5 minutes; dwell time, 40 minutes; drainage time, 15 minutes)
Dialysate — 1.5% dextrose; sodium, 132 mEq/l; chloride, 101 mEq/l; calcium, 3.5 mEq/l; magnesium, 1.5 mEq/l; acetate, 37 mEq/l
Dialysate/plasma urea ratio — 0.5
Drainage volume — 48 l + 2 l ultrafiltrate = 50 l
Urea clearance — 50 l × 0.5 = 25 l/day.

The net ultrafiltration accomplished with IPD can be easily altered by either increasing the dextrose concentration of the solution or by reducing the dwell time.

CONTINUOUS EQUILIBRATION PERITONEAL DIALYSIS (CEPD)

CEPD is a low-flow, continuous system that maintains stable levels of nitrogenous waste products and a steady hydration status, thus making parenteral alimentation and the regular infusion of intravenous medications feasible (33–35). The kinetics of CEPD are similar to continuous ambulatory peritoneal dialysis (CAPD). The use of a cycler to administer dialysate exchanges ensures precise scheduling and reduces nursing labor.

A typical dialysis schedule for adults consists of a 2-l dialysate/exchange using standard solutions for a total length of exchange of 2–4 hours. Variable ultrafiltration is achieved by adjusting the dialysate dextrose concentration. The following sample prescription illustrates the efficiency of the system:

Dialysate flow — 6, 2-l exchanges/day (12 l/day)
Exchange duration — 4 hours (inflow, 10 minutes; dwell time, 210 minutes; drainage time, 20 minutes)
Dialysate — 2.5% dextrose standard solution
Dialysate/plasma urea ratio — 0.88
Drainage volume — 12 l dialysate + 3 l ultrafiltrate = 15 l
Urea clearance — 15 l × 0.88 = 13 l/day

The reduced urea removal of CEPD compared to IPD is readily compensated by the fact that it is carried continuously. The steady state attained with this technique

Table 2. Complications of acute peritoneal dialysis

Infectious complications
  Peritonitis
  Catheter exit-site infections
Catheter-related complications
  Laceration of internal organs
  Dialysate leaks
  Catheter obstruction
    One-way
    Complete
Mechanical complications
  Abdominal pain
  Shoulder pain
  Hernia
Medical complications
  Cardiovascular
    Dehydration
    Overhydration
    Arrhythmias
  Pulmonary
    Effusion
    Atelectasis
    Aspiration
    Pneumonia
  Neurologic
    Disequilibrium syndrome
    Hyponatremia
  Metabolic
    Hyperglycemia

makes it particularly valuable for critical care patients in need of parenteral alimentation and those with unstable cardiovascular systems.

Complications of acute peritoneal dialysis (Table 2)

INFECTIOUS COMPLICATIONS

Peritonitis

Although peritonitis is a relatively common complication of acute peritoneal dialysis, it is much less frequent than in chronic peritoneal dialysis. The rate of peritonitis is dependent on the length of the procedure, its frequency, maintenance of sterile control, and the presence of concomitant infection of the skin in proximity to the catheter exit site. Immunocompromised patients, and those with abdominal stomas and poorly healed wounds are more susceptible to this complication.

The incidence of peritonitis in recent series ranges between 1.2% and 2.5% of all procedures (3). The first signs of peritonitis are a cloudy outflow, abdominal pain or tenderness, and fever. Prompt diagnosis and treatment usually results in complete eradication of the infection without significant sequela. The therapy of peritonitis is discussed in Chapter 50.

Catheter exit-site infections are infrequent when acute semirigid catheters are used, due to their short length of implantation. The presence of a catheter exit-site infection is an indication for immediate removal of the semirigid catheter and replacement in a different location. When exit-site infections are diagnosed with permanent catheters, immediate antibotic therapy should be initiated, and the area should be cleansed on a regular basis with peroxide and povidone-iodine. If there is tenderness, erythema, or extrusion of purulent material from the subcutaneous tunnel, the catheter should be removed and antibiotics continued for at least 1 week following clinical healing of the infection.

CATHETER-RELATED COMPLICATIONS

Laceration of internal organs

Perforation of a viscus or laceration of a blood vessel may occur during catheter implantation. Laceration of a blood vessel is immediately manifested by a bloody peritoneal outflow. If the initial peritoneal outflow is clear but turns progressively darker, it suggests minor bleeding from the anterior abdominal wall. The addition of heparin, 500–1000 U/l of dialysate, is recommended to prevent occlusion of the catheter from blood clots or fibrin. Rapid dialysate exchanges are used to clear intraperitoneal blood and to assess the severity and activity of the bleeder. In most cases, bleeding is self-limited and does not interfere with the procedure. However, it is imperative to monitor the patient's vital signs, dialysate outflow, and hemoglobin concentration at frequent intervals while bleeding persists.

The perforation of an internal viscus may be more difficult to diagnose. A whistling sound through the peritoneal catheter during the initial entrance into the peritoneal cavity suggests perforation of the large bowel and extrusion of colonic gas. The catheter should be removed and a new catheter inserted at a different site. If puncture of the large bowel is suspected, the patient should be treated with prophylactic antibiotics. If intestinal content is suspected in the outflow, the sample should be immediately inspected under the microscope to verify the diagnosis. Intestinal or bladder perforation not recognized at the time of catheter insertion is usually manifested by either diarrhea or profuse urination after infusion of dialysate. In those circumstances dialysate cultures should be obtained, the catheter should be removed and replaced in an adequate location, and the patient should be treated with antibiotics. Cloudy fluid shortly after insertion of the catheter and confirmation of polymicrobial peritonitis are suggestive of bowel perforation.

Dialysate leaks

Extravasation of dialysate around the catheter is a common complication of acute dialysis and is encountered in approximately 20% of patients (37–39). This complication can be partially prevented by controlling the size of the initial incision and avoiding frequent manipulation of the catheter. When leaks occur, the exchange volume should be reduced in order to lower the intraabdominal pressure. The presence of a dialysate leak may be a source of discomfort to the patient and to the paramedical personnel caring for the patients, but it is seldom of any significant consequence. A large leak may interfere with proper determination of fluid balance.

Preperitoneal leaks may cause dissection of the peritoneum into the scrotum or vulva, resulting in significant edema. Action should be taken depending on the severity and rate of fluid accumulation. The first step in managing this complication is to reduce the volume of the exchange. Progressive edema may dictate removal of the catheter and temporary discontinuation of peritoneal dialysis.

Catheter obstruction

One-way or ball-valve obstruction is more commonly seen with intermittent than with continuous peritoneal dialysis (40). This complication is characterized by easy dialysate inflow but poor or no outflow. The most common causes of one-way obstruction are wrapping of the omentum around the catheter, introduction of the catheter into a small compartment created by adhesions, or a catheter resting against the pelvic or abdominal wall. The use of enemas to stimulate the bowel and omentum, changing the position of the paient in bed, or manipulation of the catheter often correct the problem.

Complete catheter obstruction to inflow and outflow suggests an intraluminal blood or fibrin clot, or kinking of the catheter. If a clot is suspected, brisk infusion of 20–30 ml of dialysate or saline usually corrects the problem. A sharp kink in the catheter is best corrected by manipulation or replacement of the catheter.

OTHER MECHANICAL COMPLICATIONS

Abdominal pain

Many patients complain of diffuse abdominal pain or shoulder pain shortly after initiation of acute peritoneal dialysis. The pain is most severe during inflow and subsides during dwell. Inflow pain is more frequently seen with high-flow acute peritoneal dialysis using automated equipment. This type of pain is often relieved by adjustment of the dialysate pH to 6.5–7 with sodium hydroxide (41). In some instances, abdominal pain is not due to the acidity of the dialysate but to the hypertonicity of the dialysate. A 1% or 2% xylocaine solution added to the dialysate (5 ml/l) may relieve the pain. Severe pain on inflow that increases in proportion to dialysate infusion suggests that the catheter tip may be located inside a peritoneal compartment. An air-contrast study or Tenckhoff cannulography should help diagnose this condition (42).

Shoulder pain can result from introduction of air into the peritoneal cavity during insertion of the catheter. This type of pain usually subsides spontaneously. However, if the pain persists, the air bubble can be displaced by filling the peritoneal cavity with dialysate and manipulating the patient's position into Trendelenburg while letting the air escape through the catheter.

Hernias

A hernia may manifest shortly after initiation of acute peritoneal dialysis in patients who already have a weak anterior abdominal wall or weak inguinal rings. Nevertheless, it is relatively rare when compared to chronic peritoneal dialysis.

MEDICAL COMPLICATIONS

Cardiovascular complications

Acute peritoneal dialysis can result in dehydration or overhydration of the patient if careful monitoring of the hydration status is not maintained. Dehydration can always be corrected by infusion of intravenous fluids, reduction of the dialysate osmolality, or both. Overhydration can be corrected by reducing the dialysate dwell time and/or increasing the dialysate glucose concentration. Cardiac arrhythmias may be the consequence of fluctuations in hydration status, hyperkalemia, or hypokalemia.

Pulmonary complications

Pleural effusions manifesting immediately after initiation of peritoneal dialysis suggest a pleuroperitoneal communication. The diagnosis can be readily made by draining the peritoneal cavity and obtaining a chest x-ray. If the level of a pleural effusion fluctuates with the volume of the intraperitoneal dialysate, the complication is confirmed. If this relationship is not so clear, infusion of a small amount of radioactive material into the peritoneal cavity with appearance of the radioisotope in the pleural cavity is diagnostic (43). In such circumstances, the peritoneal cavity should be drained and dialysis discontinued.

Basal atelectasis, pneumonia, and aspiration are occasional complicaions of acute peritoneal dialysis (44).

Neurologic complications

The disequilibrium syndrome is seldom seen with acute peritoneal dialysis. It is usually manifested by headaches, nausea, vomiting, hypertension, seizures, and coma. This syndrome is the consequence of cerebral edema, which may occur when a rapid osmotic gradient is created between the brain and the extracellular compartment due to the lag in removal of urea across the blood-brain barrier (45).

Confusion, irritability, generalized weakness, and cloudy sensorium can be a complication of hyponatremia when very short dwell times and standard solutions are used. This complication can be prevented by adjusting the dialysate sodium concentration (28).

Metabolic complications

Severe hyperglycemia and a hyperosmolar state can occur in diabetic patients during acute peritoneal dialysis, particularly when hypertonic solutions are used. Careful monitoring of blood sugar, intraperitoneal or intravenous infusion of insulin, and reduction of the dialysate glucose concentration usually correct this complication.

CHRONIC PERITONEAL DIALYSIS

Chronic peritoneal dialysis can be used in the treatment of most patients with end-stage renal disease (ESRD). The development of safe and permanent peritoneal dialysis catheters, dialysate in plastic containers of variable volume, and dialysis techniques, which offer improved and continuous solute removal, have been responsible for the increased proportion of ESRD patients treated with chronic peritoneal dialysis. Peritoneal dialysis is the most common form of renal replacement therapy used by patients at home. According to the NIH USA CAPD Registry, 16,400 patients are being treated with CAPD/CCPD, or approximately 20% of all patients undergoing dialysis in the USA (46). In some European countries the proportion of patients on peritoneal dialysis is even higher (47).

The explosive growth of chronic peritoneal dialysis in general, and CAPD in particular, together with a relatively high rate of abandonment of therapy, frequent episodes of peritonitis, and failure of the peritoneal membrane to provide adequate ultrafiltration and solute removal has generated serious concern about the future of chronic peritoneal dialysis as chronic therapy. Although peritonitis and loss of peritoneal ultrafiltration remain the two principal deterrents of peritoneal dialysis growth, significant progress has been made in the prevention, diagnosis, and treatment of these complications and reaffirms the important role of peritoneal dialysis in the chronic treatment of uremia.

In 1968 Tenckhoff and Schechter (2) introduced a silastic peritoneal catheter with Dacron cuffs that has proven effective in providing adequate dialysate flow, and is safe, longlasting, and easy to insert. A four-part trocar was also designed to allow entrance into the peritoneal cavity and insertion of the flexible catheter at the bedside. A single-cuff Tenckhoff catheter, designed for acute use, became available shortly afterwards and remains in demand for acute use when dialysis is necessary for a short period of time.

The Tenckhoff peritoneal catheter can be inserted in the traditional manner using the special trocar, surgically (48), under peritoneoscopy (49), or using the Seldinger technique (50). However, the original technique described by Tenckhoff remains the most common method of insertion and probably is the simplest to perform. Several modifications of the Tenckhoff catheter have been introduced, including the curled catheter and those with disks, ballons and other devices in the distal end, designed to avoid omental wrapping and to improve dialysate drainage. Other catheters have been designed to improve flow dynamics. Nonetheless, the traditional double-cuff catheter remains the most popular catheter for chronic peritoneal dialysis use.

IMPLANTATION OF THE TENCKHOFF CATHETER

The abdomen is shaved and cleansed with povidone-iodine. One percent xylocaine is used for local anesthesia. A 14- or 16-gauge plastic needle with stylet is used to enter the peritoneal cavity while the patient exerts a Valsalva maneuver, and 2–3 l of dialysate are injected into the peritoneal cavity. Following this, the needle is removed. A 3–4 cm midline incision is created approximately 3 cm below the umbilicus and extended into the fascial plane (linea alba). The fully assembled trocar is now used to penetrate the peritoneal cavity while the patient again stiffens the anterior abdominal muscles. Penetration into the peritoneal cavity is verified by removing the central stylet and obtaining free flow of dialysate through the lumen of the trocar. The Tenckhoff catheter with a blunt flexible wire in place is then introduced into the lumen of the trocar and gently directed towards the left lower quadrant. Proper location is often associated with perirectal discomfort. The guidewire is removed and the dialysate outflow is checked. If clear and brisk outflow is observed, the trocar is disassembled into its parts and removed. The inner catheter cuff is placed over the rectus fascia and a purse-string suture is tied around the cuff, assuring proper anchoring, but avoiding collapse of the catheter lumen by excessive tension.

A straight or curled subcutaneous tunnel is created with a straight or semiflexible probe, and the outer end of the catheter is pulled through a small skin puncture. The catheter is pulled through the incision, leaving the outer cuff 2–3 cm from the skin exit site. The midline incision is now closed and the abdominal cavity is drained.

BREAK-IN TECHNIQUE

Many protocols have been suggested for the care and use of a new peritoneal catheter. Some centers recommend a period of rest of 24 hours to 1 week before using the catheter. Although this practice allows proper time for healing and avoidance of pericatheter or incisional dialysate leaks, it has the disadvantage of preventing an early diagnosis of catheter dysfunction. Whether the catheter is used immediately or a healing period is allowed, the use of 500–1000 U heparin/l of dialysate is recommended to avoid clotting of the catheter lumen with fibrin strands. Most centers use the catheter immediately after implantation. The volume of dialysate during the first few days of use should be limited to 1 l in normal-size adults in order to minimize intraabdominal pressure and consequent discomfort and pericatheter leaks. The dialysate volume can be gradually increased to 2 or 3 l/exchange as tolerated by the patient. The sutures should be removed within 1 week or whenever proper healing is noted.

Peritoneal dialysis delivery systems

REVERSE OSMOSIS PROPORTIONING SYSTEMS

The reverse osmosis (RO) proportioning system combines an RO water treatment device with a product water-dialysate concentrate proportioning unit (51). Tap water is filtered to remove sediment or particulate matter prior to entering the RO pump. The water is then forced through an RO membrane, where pyrogens and trace elements are removed to form the product water. The product water is then mixed with dialysate concentrate at a 19:1 ratio to produce dialysate. These systems allow automated delivery of dialysate to the patient and can be preprogrammed to provide specific rates of inflow, dwell times, and variable drain periods. Although the RO proportioning systems provide the convenience of automated dialysis delivery in a reliable and safe manner, the complexity of the systems, their large size, the high initial purchase price, the high cost of maintenance, the relatively long training period, and the complex sterilization procedure required hindered their popularity. These systems are only used for acute therapy in the hospital or for IPD.

PERITONEAL DIALYSIS CYCLERS

All cyclers are designed following Lasker's original design using the principles of gravity infusion and drainage (52). Peritoneal cyclers automatically deliver a prescribed volume of commercial dialysate and allow variable dwell and drain times. Their simplicity and short procedural requirements have made them readily acceptable for home use for IPD, CCPD, and nocturnal IPD (NPD). A cycler consists of three main parts: the stand/base, heater cabinet, and control unit. Dialysate flow from the bags or bottles takes place by gravity. Surgical-grade polyvinyl chloride tubing and bags are used. The dialysate originates at the highest point of the system and flows into the heating cabinet, where it is premeasured, heated, and delivered to the patient. After the prescribed volume of dialysate is allowed to dwell for the predetermined time, the abdominal cavity is drained by gravity and the effluent dialysate is collected in a drainage bag, where it is weighed and stored.

Newer cyclers are capable of precisely monitoring ultrafiltration, and some models can keep record of the number of exchanges, length of exchanges, and ultrafiltration.

Intermittent peritoneal dialysis

Chronic IPD was mostly used in the 1970s before the introduction of CAPD and CCPD. IPD represented the first automated modality of peritoneal dialysis capable of providing long-term renal replacement. Some of the factors that influenced the selection of IPD included: its relative simplicity, no need for venipunctures or blood access, avoidance of systemic heparinization, and gradual removal of nitrogenous products and water. The rate of peritonitis was generally low, at approximately 0.3% of all dialyses (53, 54). Although the initial clinical experience claimed control of biochemical parameters and mortality rates similar to chronic hemodialysis for the first years of therapy (54), the long-term experience was very disappointing. The mortality rate after 2 years exceeded

Table 3. Comparative clearances of selected solutes obtained with various modalities of peritoneal dialysis in liters/day

	C_{urea}	$C_{creatinine}$	Dialysate flow
Acute PD	25	16	24, 2 l exchanges/24 hrs
CAPD	8.1	6.2	4, 2 l exchanges/24 hrs
CCPD	8.0	6.0	Nocturnal:
			4, 2 l exchanges (10 hrs)
			Diurnal:
			1, 2 l exchange (14 hrs)
NPD	7.5	4.5	12, 1.9 l exchanges or 23 l/8 hrs
TPD	8.4	5.0	TV 1.7 l
			RV 0.9 l or 23 l/8 hrs

50%, and the mortality among diabetic patients was significantly higher (55).

The typical IPD prescription is a 10-hour session every other night or three times per week, using dialysate flow rates of 2–4 l/hr delivered via an RO proportioning unit or a peritoneal dialysis cycler. Although adequate ultrafiltration can usually be accomplished, total solute removal is less than desirable, as note in Table 3. Patients with residual renal function (GFR 3–5 ml/min) can benefit from supplementary IPD and often remain healthy; however, anuric patients and those with minimal renal function eventually develop uremic complications and malnutrition (55–57).

The use of chronic IPD has plummeted due to the inadequate dialysis it provides, the high cost of dialysate, other disposables and equipment, and the introduction of simpler and more effective forms of peritoneal dialysis. IPD is now reserved for patients with residual renal function, those who refuse continuous peritoneal dialysis, and the few that require hospital dialysis due to their unstable medical condition and unfavorable socioeconomic environment.

Continuous cyclic peritoneal dialysis (CCPD)

The introduction of continuous equlibration peritoneal dialysis by Popovich et al. in 1976 offered a potential solution to the problem of inadequate dialysis (58). Although the clearances offered by CAPD are rather limited, the continuous nature of the treatment overcomes this problem, achieving total weekly clearances that are definitely superior to those of IPD for small molecules and greater than those of hemodialysis for middle-size molecules (Table 3). Notwithstanding CAPD's simplicity, ability to maintain a steady physiologic state, and adequate ultrafiltration, multiple drawbacks, such as the long and interrupted procedural time and high rate of peritonitis, stimulated development of CCPD (59, 60).

TECHNIQUE

CCPD provides continuous peritoneal dialysis and is a virtual reversal of CAPD. The scheldule consists of a long diurnal dwell exchange and multiple shorter nocturnal exchanges delivered by a peritoneal cycler. Before retiring at night, the patient prepares the peritoneal cycler with the necessary dialysate and sets the cycler controls that determine the volume of each exchange, the duration of dwell, and drainage. The connection between the cycler's patient line and the peritoneal catheter takes place under sterile control. During the night the patient receives three to five exchanges of variable volumes (2–3 l/exchange). Standard dialysis solution containing 1.5–4.25% dextrose is used for the noctural exchanges (Table 2). The last exchange consists of hypertonic (4.25%) solution. The nocturnal cycles last approximately 10 hours. In the morning the patient disconnects the cycler line from the catheter after infusing 1500–2000 ml of hypertonic solution. The disconnection can be achieved by traditional methodology or with the newly developed external occlusion technique, which is much simpler and faster to perform (61). The diurnal exchange lasts approximately 14 hours.

CLINICAL EXPERIENCE

The clinical experience with CCPD has been similar to that reported with CAPD. Improvement in hematocrit levels, normalization of acid-base balance, adequate control of nitrogenous waste products, and modest reductions in blood albumin concentrations have been reported (55, 59–64). Although a small percentage of patients have developed frank hypertriglyceridemia and/or obesity, the proportion of patients with these complications seems to be less than in those undergoing CAPD. A possible explanation for this phenomenon lies in the increased ultrafiltration per gram of absorbed glucose observed with shorter peritoneal cycles (65). The shorter nocturnal cycles of CCPD accomplish ultrafiltration earlier in the cycle, while dialysate glucose concentrations are higher. Therefore, the same or higher ultrafiltration is attained with lower glucose absorption.

Peritoneal protein losses in uninfected patients average 6–9 g/day, which is similar to that reported for noninfected CAPD patients (65, 66).

Peritonitis rates have been reported to be significantly lower than with CAPD in most adult series (61). In our series, the rate of peritonitis has been one episode every 2 years. This experience is not exclusive to our institution and has been corroborated or surpassed by other centers primarily caring for adult patients (61). The most recent update from the NIH USA CAPD Registry reports a significant difference in the rate of peritonitis between CAPD and CCPD patients (46). Conversely, several large pediatric centers have failed to show a significant difference in the rate of peritonitis between these two therapies (61, 63).

Several factors that may explain the lower rate of peritonitis among CCPD patients should be mentioned. The fact that all connections for CCPD take place only once daily in the home environment may allow better aseptic control, greater concentration, the possible use of a partner, and less stress on the patient and his or her relatives. The number of actual connections can be reduced by utilizing large volume dialysate containers. The dialysate outflow following a connection conceivably reduces the bacterial concentration at the connecting site in case of contamination. This last possibility should be further scrutinized in view of the extremely low rates of peritonitis reported by several investigators with the double-bag CAPD systems, which share the common feature with CCPD of an initial dialysate outflow following a connection. Finally, it is possible that the long diurnal dwell of CCPD allows repopulation of the peritoneal resident macrophages and provides a better host immune defense. We have reported elevated peritoneal fluid cell counts in noninfected patients following the diurnal cycle of CCPD (67). This observation requires further investigation.

CCPD is capable of providing adequate dialysis for patients with normal peritoneal permeability. CCPD provides solute clearances similar to CAPD (Table 3). The minor differences observed may not be of clinical importance and could be corrected by increasing dialysate flow during the nocturnal cycles. The cumulative patient and technique survival for nondiabetic patients on CCPD exceeds 80% at 3 years for patient survival and 60% for technique survival (55). In our program, these figures are comparable to those of CAPD and hemodialysis.

INDICATIONS AND CONTRAINDICATIONS

The major indications for CCPD are summarized in Table 4. Most patients select CCPD due to the daytime freedom that it allows, the improved self-image provided by the freedom from bags and procedural exchanges during the day, and the reduced fatigue from the procedure.

CCPD has become the most common form of therapy for pediatric use in many large centers. The main reasons for this preference is that this procedure allows the participation of a parent in performing connections and disconnections, and daytime freedom for school and recreational activities, while retaining all the other advantages inherent in continuous peritoneal dialysis.

Additional advantages of CCPD relate to the physical effects of a reduced intraabdominal volume. Aside from the direct correlation between intraabdominal volume and pressure, it has been shown that position further influences

Table 4. Indications for CCPD

Patient preference
   Employed, active patients
   Unwilling or unable to perform exchanges
   Poor eye-hand coordination
   Need for partner
   Psychological (self-image)
Children
Poor compliance with number of exchanges
Frequent peritonitis
Hernias
Chronic low-back pain
Severe cardiopulmonary compromise
Recurrent catheter exit-site leakage

intraabdominal pressure (64, 68). The same volume of dialysate increases the intraabdominal pressure when the patient changes from the supine to the standing or sitting position. An increase in intraabdominal pressure can lead to a higher incidence of abdominal discomfort, lumbosacral strain, pericatheter leaks, and hernias. Many patients with these complications benefit from a reduced diurnal intraabdominal volume.

Nocturnal peritoneal dialysis (NPD)

Nightly peritoneal dialysis is similar to IPD but is performed nightly (65). The total exchange time is 8–10 hours, using cycle times of 20–60 minutes. Although NPD has the disadvantages of not being able to provide a steady physiologic state, is expensive due to the high dialysate flow, and requires a delivery system capable of infusing large amounts of dialysate during every session, it has some specific indications. The indications fall into two main categories: a high peritoneal membrane permeability and mechanical indications.

Patients with high peritoneal permeability accomplish osmotic equilibration within a relative short dwell period. Consequently, ultrafiltration becomes inadequate and absorption of dialysate takes place. The use of short dwell times leads to drainage of the fluid while the peritoneal osmotic gradient is still effective. Solute equilibration also takes place faster than in normal permeability states, thus allowing adequate solute removal with shorter dwell times. Therefore, a patient with high peritoneal permeability can achieve adequate ultrafiltration and solute removal with a high flow, short dwell schedule, while the long dwell periods of CAPD and CCPD may prove detrimental.

Patients suffering from abdominal leaks and hernias, bladder prolapse, low back pain, and restrictive lung disease may be intolerant of the increased intraabdominal pressure associated with the infusion of 1 or 2 l of dialysate during the day while the patient is sitting or standing. These patients may tolerate equal volumes of dialysate in the supine position, as provided by NPD.

Table 3 provides the average clearances obtained with NPD in patients with normal permeability using 14 l of dialysate over an 8-hour period for 7 days. The weekly clearances for urea and creatinine are lower than those obtained with CAPD or CCPD.

The clinical experience with NPD is limited, preventing any firm conclusions regarding the long-term safety and efficiency of this technique. However, there are preliminary data to suggest that patients with increased peritoneal permeability who remain on peritoneal dialysis may develop further deterioration of peritoneal membrane function. It has also been speculated that this group of patients may eventually develop peritoneal sclerosis.

Tidal peritoneal dialysis (TPD)

A technique referred to as TPD has been recently introduced that consists of maintaining a constant reserve volume of dialysis solution in the peritoneal cavity at all times and an additional tidal volume of dialysate that is intermittently cycled in and out of the peritoneal cavity (69, 70). The rationale behind this technique is that a sufficent reserve volume in contact with the peritoneal membrane at all times, and the additional tidal volume, which assures adequate mixing of the dialysate and frequent restoration of the dialysate/plasma gradient, will enhance peitoneal clearance.

The preliminary results (Table 3) using high dialysate flows (23 l over 8 hours) show urea and potassium clearances superior to CAPD or CCPD, with creatinine clearances being slightly lower (70). The main disadvantages of this procedure are the need for a specially modified cycler, which is regulated by volume rather than time, and the extremely high dialysate flows, both of which result in additional cost. The procedure remains experimental and no long-term clinical experience has been reported.

Complications of chronic peritoneal dialysis (Table 5)

PERITONITIS

Peritonitis remains the most common complication of chronic peritoneal dialysis. However, significant differ-

Table 5. Complications of chronic peritoneal dialysis

Infectious compliations
    Peritonitis
    Exit-site and tunnel infections
Catheter-related complications
    Abdominal pain
    Bloody outflow
    Pericatheter leaks
    Perforations or lacerations of blood vessels and internal organs
    Catheter obstruction
        one-way
        complete
Peritoneal membrane dysfunction
    Ultrafiltration failure
    Peritoneal sclerosis
Complications due to increased intraabdominal pressure
    Dialysate leaks
    Hernias
    Low-back pain
    Gastroesophageal reflux
    Hemorrhoids
    Pulmonary compromise
    Cardiac compromise
Medical complications
    Metabolic
        Protein malnutrition
        Obesity
        Hyperlipoproteinemia
        Renal osteodystrophy
    Neurologic
        Disequilibrium syndrome
        Peripheral neuropathy
        Dialysis dementia
    Hematologic
        Anemia

ences in the incidence of this complication have been reported for IPD, CCPD, and CAPD. The peritonitis rate for IPD is approximately 0.3% of all procedures, or one episode of peritonitis every 2–3 years (53, 54). The peritonitis rate for CCPD in most large adult series has been in the range of one episode every 1.5–2 years (61). The NIH USA CAPD Registry reports a combined rate for adults and children of one episode/year (46). Peritonitis rates for CAPD remain higher and approximate one episode every 9 months. Peritonitis and peritoneal dialysis infectious complications are discussed in detail in Chapter 52.

CATHETER-RELATED COMPLICATIONS

Abdominal pain can present immediately after insertion of the peritoneal catheter or late during treatment of the chronic peritoneal dialysis patient. The pain can be related to pressure of the catheter against the abdominal or pelvic wall and usually subsides after a few days or weeks on peritoneal dialysis. Introduction of the catheter into a small peritoneal compartment formed by previous adhesions can also cause pain on inflow. These complications should always be suspected when the pain increases as a function of the volume of peritoneal dialysate infused. The problem should be corrected by removal and replacement of the catheter. Abdominal pain associated with the use of acetate-containing dialysate concentrate or commercial dialysate is very uncommon at present, since these solutions are seldom used. The problem can be remedied by the addition of sodium hydroxide to increase the pH to between 6 and 7 (41). Abdominal pain and peritoneal eosinophilia have been noted to occur shortly after insertion of a new peritoneal dialysis catheter. Daugirdas et al. have demonstrated a direct relationship between the infusion of intraperitoneal air and this syndrome (71). The symptoms usually subside spontaneously and do not require specific therapy.

Bloody peritoneal outflow occurring immediately after insertion of a peritoneal catheter suggests laceration of a major blood vessel or continous oozing from the anterior abdominal wall at the site of the peritoneal catheter entrance. Therapy will depend on the severity and persistence of the bleeding. Close monitoring of the dialysate outflow and the hemoglobin concentration should be maintained and exploratory laparotomy considered if the bleeding persists or results in a significant hemoglobin drop. The late presentation of peritoneal bleeding should be viewed in a different manner. The possibility of erosion of the peritoneal catheter into a blood vessel or spleen is rare but possible. Displacement of the Tenckhoff catheter to the left upper quadrant associated with severe intraperitoneal bleeding due to rupture of the spleen has been reported (72). Hemoperitoneum during continuous peritoneal dialysis has also been ascribed to postradiation peritoneal injury (73). Recurrent bloody peritoneal outflow, with or without associated vaginal bleeding, is not uncommon among women of menstruating age undergoing continuous peritoneal dialysis. This phenomenon is often referred to as *retrograde menstruation* and does not require specific therapy.

Dialysate leaks around the catheter exit site are common complications of peritoneal dialysis. Patients who suffer from malnutrition, debilitating diseases, or who are under the effects of corticosteroid therapy are at high risk. Internal dialysate leaks manifested by infiltration of dialysate into the anterior abdominal wall, scrotum, and vulva usually occur shortly after catheter implantation and suggest leakage around the catheter entrance into the peritoneum. Reduction in the volume of dialysate or temporary discontinuation of peritoneal dialysis usually correct the problem. Persistence of leakage after these maneuvers suggests a larger tear in the peritoneal entrance or a pinhole in the catheter itself, resulting in continuous leakage. In such instances, the catheter must be removed and replaced with a new device, preferably after allowing a 10- to 14-day rest to assure proper healing of the original incision. The use of technetium-99 m scintigraphy or CT scanning of the abdomen have been proposed for the diagnosis of dialysate leakage (74, 75). Although this procedure has a high diagnostic yield in cases of pleuroperitoneal communications and open processus vaginalis, it is seldom diagnostic in cases of small cracks or pinholes in the Tenckhoff catheter itself (76).

Late dialysate leaks are less common and probably are due to increased intraabdominal pressure (vide infra). The complication can be adequately treated in most cases by either decreasing the dialysate volume, interrupting peritioneal dialysis with temporary transfer to hemodialysis, or use of IPD or NPD. Removal and reimplantation of the catheter is seldom necessary. Vaginal leakage of dialysate by way of the Fallopian tubes and uterus has been observed both in asymptomatic women and associated with peritonitis (77). Although women have the potential anatomic vaginoperitoneal communication, this complication has been rare.

Early perforation or laceration of an internal organ is relatively rare with the use of a Tenckhoff trocar. The criteria for diagnosis are similar to those already introduced under complications of acute peritoneal access. The organs most frequently injured are the bowel, bladder, liver, renal cysts, and blood vessels. Perforation of the bowel and mesenteric vessels is most likely to occur in patients who have undergone previous abdominal surgery and have developed adhesions and fixation of the organ to the anterior abdominal wall. Also at higher risks are patients with bowel distention due to paralytic ileus, toxic magacolon, or bowel obstruction. Recognition of visceral perforation requires prompt removal of the catheter, with or without reinsertion, appropriate peritoneal cultures, prophylactic antibiotic therapy, and close observation. If symptoms of peritoneal inflammation manifest within the first 48 hours, suggesting continuous leakage of visceral content and peritoneal contamination, consideration should be given to exploratory laparotomy.

Perforation or laceration of internal organs as a late complication of the peritoneal catheter is uncommon. However, erosion of the catheter into the colon has been reported as late as 9 months after insertion of the catheter (78). Erosion of the catheter into the pelvic wall with eventual vaginal penetration has also been reported after

17 months of successful chronic peritoneal dialysis (79). The causative factors offered to explain these complications include pressure necrosis due to the continuous pressure of the catheter against tissue and chemical irritation caused by the jet current during dialysate infusion. Malnutrition and peritonitis may serve as predisposing factors.

Catheter obstruction can be partial or complete. The most common type of catheter dysfunction is the one-way or ball-valve type. The diagnosis and correct therapy for these complications are similar to those described for acute peritoneal access. One-way obstruction has been reported to be the cause of catheter failure in 14–23% of the cases (40, 80, 81). However, this complication is more frequent in patients undergoing IPD than in those on continuous peritoneal dialysis (40). The likely explanation for this difference is that the fluid is always present during continuous peritoneal dialysis and reduces the concentration of fibrin strands and prevents omental wrapping around the peritoneal catheter.

PERITONEAL MEMBRANE DYSFUNCTION

Although some patients can remain on peritoneal dialysis for as long as 8 or 10 years, many others have developed evidence of peritoneal membrane dysfunction (82, 83). With the increased use of peritoneal dialysis as a chronic means of renal replacement, the incidence of this type of complication has increased. The earliest and most frequently recognized form of peritoneal dysfunction is the syndrome of ultrafiltration failure. This condition has been characterized as an increase in peritoneal permeability, which results in rapid absorption of dialysate glucose with prompt blunting of the osomtic gradient between dialysate and plasma. The transport of solutes remains intact but failure to achieve ultrafiltration of water precludes adequate peritoneal dialysis. Many investigators have suggested that the use of acetate in dialysate solutions is a causative factor for this condition (83–85). Although the data are not conclusive, there is enough circumstantial evidence to implicate acetate as a possible etiology. This syndrome has been much more frequently seen in France than in North America, but has been diagnosed in isolated patients throughout the world. Whether this condition progresses to the more serious complication of peritoneal membrane thickening and sclerosis is uncertain. The wealth of data today suggest that the etiology of peritoneal ultrafiltration failure may be multifactorial, that it may be present at the initiation of peritoneal dialysis in some patients or may gradually develop in others, that a temporary transfer to hemodialysis or the use of IPD or NPD may restore normal permeability in some patients, and that a few patients may progress to peritoneal sclerosis if peritoneal dialysis is continued (86, 87). Proper evaluation of peritoneal permeability is indicated in any patient who fails to achieve adequate water ultrafiltration with CAPD or CCPD and in those who progressively require a higher proportion of hypertonic exchanges in order to accomplish the same ultrafiltration. If peritoneal hyperpermeability is diagnosed, a transfer to higher flow dialysis using shorter dwell times and elimination of the long diurnal dwells of CCPD or long nocturnal dwells of CAPD are indicated.

A more dreadful complication of peritoneal dialysis is peritoneal sclerosis. In this condition the peritoneal membrane becomes thickened and eventually leads to strangulation of the bowel by the formation of a leathery cocoon that envelopes all intra-abdominal organs. The condition has been reported in patients on IPD, CAPD, and CCPD (88). Peritoneal sclerosis eventually leads to decreased solute and water movement across the peritoneal membrane due to loss of peritoneal permeability or surface area. Repeated episodes of peritonitis, the use of acetate solutions, regular use of hyperosmolar dialysate, chlorhexidine, plasticizers, and particulate matter in the dialysate have all been implicated as etiologic factors. Peritoneal sclerosis has also been associated with the use of other pharmacologic agents such as propranolol and oxprenolol. There is no specific therapy for this condition, which may prove fatal in its most advanced forms.

COMPLICATIONS DUE TO INCREASED INTRAABDOMINAL PRESSURE (IAP)

IAP is directly proportional to the volume of dialysate infused intraperitoneally (89). Changes in position further affect IAP (64, 68). The highest IAP is observed with the patient in the sitting position, followed by the standing and supine positions. This phenomenon probably explains the higher incidence of certain complications in patients undergoing CAPD and those on CCPD using high diurnal volumes, as compared to those undergoing IPD or NPD. Additional factors that influence the rate of development of these complications include intraabdominal masses such as large polycystic kidneys, previous abdominal surgery, weak abdominal walls from malnutrition, and multiparity.

Late dialysate leaks are often a product of these circumstances. Similarly hernias, which may include incisional, umbilical, inguinal, abdominal, and diaphragmatic, can be observed with relatively high frequency. Although the incidence of abdominal hernias with CAPD and CCPD using exchanges of 2 or more liters has been reported to be 9–12% (90, 91), the incidence is 2–3% among patients on IPD and those on CCPD with reduced diurnal volumes (40).

Low back pain can present de novo or may become aggravated with the infusion of large volumes of intra-abdominal fluid. High IAP increases the lordotic curvature, which is associated with lumbosacral strain and pain (92). The use of exercise to strengthen the paravertebral and the anterior abdominal wall muscles may help prevent or ameliorate these symptoms. However, if symptomatology persists, a reduction in the exchange volume is indicated.

Increased IAP can affect changes in cardiac and pulmonary function. Gotloib et al. have demonstrated a significant decrease in cardiac output and stroke volume in response to increase in IAP. Mean arterial blood pressure increased as a consequence of a significant increase in peripheral resistance (89). More recently, Alpert et al. have shown that in CAPD patients with left ventricular hypertrophy, intraperitoneal volumes exceeding 2 l produce a significant decrease in left ventricular systolic function due to preload reduction, probably from increasing IAP (93). Nevertheless, for practical purpose the infusion of 2 l of dialysate intraperitoneally does not adversely affect hemodynamics in most patients.

Increases in intraabdominal volume and IAP may also result in pulmonary compromise. Marked deterioration of vital capacity, forced vital capacity, and forced expiratory volume at 1 second have been reported in some patients with intraperitoneal volumes in excess of 2 l (68, 94). In our experience very few patients with chronic obstructive pulmonary disease tolerate dialysate volumes in excess of 2 l in the sitting position.

Other symptoms that are occasionally associated with increased IAP include gastroesophageal reflux and hemorrhoidal discomfort.

Medical complications

METABOLIC COMPLICATIONS

Protein malnutrition develops in some patients undergoing chronic peritoneal dialysis. Dialysate protein losses vary widely among patients and average 6–10 g/day (66). It is of interest that the total weekly dialysate losses are relatively constant for the same patient, regardless of the dialysate schedule. This is probably due to the fact that during long dwell cycles or periods of interruption of dialysis, higher concentrations of protein accumulate in the dialysate, which are removed during the next exchange. Conversely, patients undergoing regular exchanges have much lower concentrations of protein. The majority of patients can maintain total protein and seurm albumin levels that are either slightly low or in the lower range of normal. Close monitoring of plasma protein concentration is recommended. Evidence of progressive protein malnutrition should alert the physician to intervene with either dietary supplementation or temporary discontinuation of dialysis. Although the use of intraperitoneal administration of amino acids has been explored, no long-term studies have been published. Amino acid solutions have been shown to provide adequate ultrafiltration, comparable to glucose, and transient improvement in plasma amino acid concentrations (95). However, they also result in an increased metabolic acid load and azotemia. Predisposing factors to protein malnutrition include peritonitis, which can dramatically increase protein losses in the dialysate; surgery, infection, and other hypercatabolic states; poor protein intake; and inadequate caloric intake with impaired utilization of amino acids.

The caloric load of patients undergoing chronic peritoneal dialysis can be markedly increased in patients using high dextrose concentrations in their dialysate. Patients undergoing chronic peritoneal dialysis receive 20–35% of their daily caloric intake from intraperitoneal glucose absorption (96). This can result in obesity or uncontrolled hyperglycemia in diabetics. The constant infusion of glucose can also lead to lipid abnormalities such as hypertriglyceridemia. This problem is best approached by controlling dietary salt intake and thus reducing the need for high ultrafiltration; the use of shorter dwell times, which increases the ultrafiltration/glucose absorption ratio; and dietary restriction of carbohydrates.

There has been concern about the possibility of a depletion syndrome in patients undergoing chronic peritoneal dialysis due to peritoneal losses of important nutrients such as vitamin B_{12}. Although the equilibration and losses of certain vitamins through dialysate outflow have been studied, the lack of exhaustive studies in this area preclude firm recommendations for vitamin supplementation. The same general guidelines recommended for vitamin supplementation among hemodialysis patients have been temporarily used in the treatment of the chronic peritoneal dialysis patient.

Renal osteodystrophy is one of the most frequent and crippling complications of uremia. This complication usually develops long before the patient reaches end-stage renal disease and starts dialysis. The particular influences of chronic peritoneal dialysis on renal osteodystrophy have not been well characterized. Multiple studies have provided conflicting results (97–100). However, it is apparent that both osteitis fibrosa and osteomalacia are prevalent among patients undergoing chronic peritoneal dialysis. The management of this complication is similar for both hemodialysis and peritoneal dialysis patients (see Chapter 48).

Specific neurologic, psychiatric, and hematologic complications are discussed in Chapters 47 and 48.

REFERENCES

1. Ganter G: Ueber die beseitigung giftiger stoffe aus dem blute durch dialyse. *Munch Med Wochschr* 70-II:1478–1480, 1923.
2. Tenckhoff H, Schechter H: A bacteriologically safe peritoneal access device. *Trans Am Soc Artif Intern Organs* 14:181–186, 1968.
3. Firmat J, Zucchini A: Peritoneal dialysis in acute renal failure. *Contrib Nephrol* 17:33–38, 1979.
4. Mathew TH: Comparison of peritoneal dialysis and haemodialysis in acute renal failure. In: RC Atkins, NM Thomson, PC Farrell, eds, *Peritoneal Dialysis*. Churchill Livingstone, Edinburgh, pp 80–86, 1981.
5. Segar WE, Gibson RK, Rhamy R: Peritoneal dialysis in infants and small children. *Pediatrics* 27:603–613, 1961.
6. Chan JCM, Campbell RA: Peritoneal dialysis in children, a survey of its indications and applications, *Clin Pediatr* 12:131–139, 1973.
7. Camerson JS, Ogg C, Trounce JR: Peritoneal dialysis in hypercatabolic acute renal failure. *Lancet* 1:1188–1191, 1967.
8. Stolz ML, Nolph KD, Maher JF: Factors affecting calcium removal with calcium-free peritoneal dialysate. *J Lab Clin Med* 78:389–398, 1971.
9. Counts SJ, Baylink DJ, Shen FH, Sherrard DJ, Hickman RO: Vitamin D intoxication in an anephric child. *Ann Intern Med* 82:196–200, 1975.
10. Mailloux LU, Swartz CD, Onesti GO, Heider C, Ramirez

O, Brest A: Peritoneal dialysis for refractory congestive heart failure. *JAMA* 199:873–878, 1967.
11. Cairns KB, Porter GA, Kloster FE, Bristow JD, Griswold HE: Clinical and hemodynamic results of peritoneal dialysis for severe cardiac failure. *Am Heart J* 76:227–234, 1968.
12. Raja RM, Krasnoff SO, Moros JG, Kramer MS, Robenbaum JL: Repeated peritoneal dialysis in treatment of heart failure. *JAMA* 213:2268–2269, 1970.
13. Shapira J, Lang R, Jutrin I, Robson M, Ravid M: Peritoneal dislysis in refractory congestive heart failure, Part I: Intermittent peritoneal dialysis. *Perit Dial Bull* 3:130–132, 1983.
14. Robson M, Biro A, Knobel B, Schai G, Ravid M: Peritoneal dialysis in refractory congestive heart failure, Part II: Continuous ambulatory peritoneal dialysis. *Perit Dial Bull* 3:133–134, 1983.
15. Winchester JF, Gelfand MC, Knepshield JH, Schreiner GE: Dialysis and hemoperfusion of poisons and drugs — update. *Trans Am Soc Artif Intern Organs* 23:762–842, 1977.
16. Maher JF: Principles of dialysis and dialysis of drugs. *Am J Med* 62:475–481, 1977.
17. Knochel JP, Mason AD: Effect of alkalinization on peritoneal diffusion of uric acid. *Am J Physiol* 210:1160–1162, 1966.
18. Campion DS, North JDK: Effect of protein binding of barbituates on their rate of removal during peritoneal dialysis. *J Lab Clin Med* 66:549–563, 1965.
19. Etteldorf JN, Dobbins WT, Summitt RL, Rainwater WT, Fischer RL: Intermittent peritoneal dialysis using 5% albumin in the treatment of salicylate intoxication in children. *J Pediatr* 58:226–236, 1961.
20. Reuler JB, Parker RA: Peritoneal dialysis in the management of hypothermia. *JAMA* 240:2289–2290, 1978.
21. Zawada ET Jr: Treatment of profound hypothermia with peritoneal dialysis. *Dial Transpl* 9:255–256, 1980.
22. O'Connor J: The treatment of profound hypothermia with peritoneal dialysis. *Perit Dial Bull* 2:171–173, 1982.
23. Wall AJ: Peritoneal dialysis in the treatment of severe acute pancreatitis. *Med J Aust* 52:281–283, 1965.
24. Glenn LD, Nolph KD: Treatment of pancreatitis with peritoneal dialysis. *Perit Dial Bull* 2:63–68, 1982.
25. Skoutakis VA, Black WD, Acchiardo SR, Wood GC: Peritoneal dialysis in the treatment of acetohexamide induced hypoglycemia. *Am J Hosp Pharm* 34:68–70, 1977.
26. Sidek M, Sieberth HG, Schmitz G, Redlich A: Extrarenal indications for peritoneal dialysis. *Proc Eur Dial Transpl Assoc* 3:335, 1966.
27. Twardowski ZJ, Nolph KD, Rubin J, Anderson PC: Peritoneal dialysis for psorasis, an uncontrolled study. *Ann Intern Med* 88:349–351, 1978.
28. Shen FH, Sherrard DJ, Scollard D, Merritt A, Curtis FK: Thirst, relative hypernatremia, and excessive weight gain in maintenance peritoneal dialysis. *Trans Am Soc Artif Intern Organs* 24:142–149, 1978
29. Nolph KD, Sorkin ML, Moore H: Autoregulation of sodium and potassium removed during continuous ambulatory peritoneal dialysis. *Trans Am Soc Artif Intern Organ* 26:334–338, 1980.
30. Stewart JH, Tuckwell LA, Sinnett PF, Edwards KDG, Whyte HM: Peritoneal and haemodialysis: A comparison of their morbidity and of their mortality suffered by dialysed patients. *J Med* 35:406–420, 1966.
31. Furman KL, Gomperts ED, Hockley J: Activity of intraperitoneal heparin during peritoneal dialysis. *Clin Nephrol* 9:15–18. 1978.
32. Thayssen P, Pindborg T: Peritoneal dialysis and heparin. *Scand J Urol Nephrol* 12:73–74, 1978.
33. Posen GA, Luisello J: Continuous equilibration peritoneal dialysis in the treatment of acute renal failure. *Perit Dial Bull* 1:6–7, 1980.
34. Katirzoglou A, Digenis G, Mayopoulou–Symvoulidis D, Zervaris D, Symvoulidis A, Komninos Z: Continuous equilibration peritoneal dialysis versus acute peritoneal dialysis. In: *GM Gahl, M Kessel, KD Nolph, eds, Advances in Peritoneal Dialysis.* Excerpta Medica, Amsterdam pp 122–125, 1981.
35. Katirtzoglou A, Kontesis P, Maopoulou–Symvoulidis D, Digenis GE, Symvoulidis A, Komninos Z: Continuous equilibration peritoneal dialysis in hypercatobolic renal failure. *Perit Dial Dull* 3:178–180, 1983.
36. Oreopoulos DJ: Report of a symposium: Pan Pacific Symposium on Peritoneal Dialysis, Melborne, Australia 1980. *Perit Dial Bull* 3:18–19, 1980.
37. Maher JF, Schreiner GE: Hazards and complications of dialysis. *N Eng J Med* 273:370–377, 1965.
38. Vaamonde CA, Michael VF, Metzger RA, Carrd KE: Complications of acute peritoneal dialysis. *J Chron Dis* 28:637–659, 1975.
39. Valk TW, Swartz RD, Hsu CH: Peritoneal dialysis in acute renal failure: Analysis of outcome and complications. *Dial Transpl* 9:64–68, 1980.
40. Diaz-Buxo JA, Geissinger WT: Single cuff versus double cuff Tenckhoff catheter. *Perit Dial Bull* 4:S100–S102, 1984.
41. Gutman RA: Automated peritoneal dialysis for home use. *Q J Med* 47:261–280, 1978.
42. Tucker CT, Cunningham JT, Nichols AM, Greer CF, Bailey CT: Cannulography with peritoneal air contrast study. *Contemp Dial* 3:9–16, 1982.
43. O'Conner J, Rutland M: Demonstration of a pleuroperitoneal communication with radionuclide imaging in a CAPD patients. *Perit Dial Bull* 1:153, 1981.
44. Berlyne GM, Lee HA, Ralston AJ, Woodlock JA: Pulmonary complications of peritoneal dialysis. *Lancet* 2:75–78, 1966.
45. Port F, Johnson WJ, Klass DW: Prevention of dialysis disequilibrium syndrome by use of high sodium concentration in the dialysate. *Kidney Int* 3:327–333, 1973.
46. Nolph KD, Cutler SJ, Steinberg SM, Novak JW: Special studies from the NIH USA CAPD registry. *Perit Dial Bull* 6:28–34, 1986.
47. Kramer P, Broyer M, Brunner FP, Brynger H, Challah S, Oules R, Rizzoni G, Selwood NH, Wing AJ, Balas EA: Combined report on regular dialysis and transplantation in Europe, XIV, 1983. *Proc Eur Dial Transpl Assoc* 21:5–68, 1984.
48. Scott DF, Marshall VC: Insertion and complications of Tenckhoff catheters — surgical aspects. In RC Atkins, NM Thomson, PC, Farrell, eds, *Peritoneal Dialysis.* burg. Churchill Livingstone, Edinburg, pp 61–72, 1981.
49. Ash SR, Handt AE, Bloch R: Peritoneosopic placement of the Tenckhoff catheter: Further clinical experience. *Perit Dial Bull* 3:8–12, 1983.
50. Zappacosta AR, Perras ST: Seldinger technique for Tenckhoff catheter placement. *Perit Dial Bull* 6–S24, 1986.
51. Diaz–Buxo JA: Peritoneal dialysis reverse osmosis machines and cylers. In: AR Nissenson, RN Fine, eds, *Dialysis Therapy.* Hanley & Belfus, Philadelphia, pp 41–47, 1986.
52. Lasker N, McCawley EP, Passarotti CT: Chronic peritoneal dialysis. *Trans Am Soc Artif Intern Organs* 12:94–96, 1966.
53. Boen ST: Overview and history of peritoneal dialysis. *Dial*

Transpl 6:12–18, 1977.
54. Diaz-Buxo JA, Chandler JT, Farmer CD, Smith DL: Chronic peritoneal dialysis at home — A comparison with hemodialysis. *Trans Am Soc Artif Intern Organs* 23:191–193, 1977.
55. Diaz-Buxo JA, Walker PJ, Chandler JT, Burgess WP, Farmer CD: Experience with intermittent peritoneal dialysis and continuous cyclic peritoneal dialysis. *Am J Kidney Dis* 4:242–248, 1984.
56. Schmidt RW, Blumenkrantz MJ: IPD, CAPD, CCPD, CRPD — Peritoneal dialysis: Past, present and future. *Int J Artif Organs* 4:124–129, 1981.
57. Ghantous WN, Salkin MS, Adelson BN, Ghantous S, McGinnis K, Valenziano A, Cronin M: Limitations of peritoneal dialysis in the treatment of ESRD patients. *Trans Am Soc Artif Intern Organs* 25:100–103, 1979.
58. Popovich RP, Moncrief JW, Decherd JF, Bomar JB, Pyle WK: The definition of a novel portable/reusable equilibrium peritonel dialysis technique (abstract). *Am Soc Artif Intern Organs* 5:64, 1976.
59. Diaz-Buxo JA, Walker PJ, Farmer CD, Chandler JT, Holt KL: Continuous cyclic peritoneal dialysis — a preliminary report. *Artif Organs* 5:157–161, 1981.
60. Price CG, Suki WN: Newer modifications of peritoneal dialysis: Options in the treatment of patients with renal failure. *AmJ Nephrol* 1:97–104, 1081.
61. Diaz-Buxo JA, Walker PJ, Burgess WP, Chandler JT, Farmer CD, Holt KL: Current status of CCPD in the prevention of peritonitis. In: R Khanna, et al. eds, *Advances in Continuous Ambulatory Peritoneal dialysis*. Perit Dial Bull, University of Toronto Press, pp 145–148, 1986.
62. Walls J, Smith BA, Feehally J, Tavernel D, Turgan C: CCPD — an improvement on CAPD. In: GM Gahl, M Keisel, KD Nolph, eds, *Advances in Peritoneal Dialysis*. Excerpta Medica, Amsterdam, pp 141–143, 1981.
63. Fine RN, Salusky IB: CAPD/CCPD in children: Four years' experience. *Kidney Int* 30:S7–10, 1986.
64. Diaz-Buxo JA: CCPD is even better than CAPD. *Kidney Int* 28:S26–28, 1985.
65. Twardowski ZJ, Nolph KD, Khanna R, Gluck Z, Prowant BF, Ryan LP: Dialy clearances with continuous ambulatory peritoneal dialysis and nightly peritoneal dialysis. *Trans Am Soc Artif Intern Organs* 32:575–580, 1986.
66. Blumenkrantz MJ, Gahl GM, Kopple JD, Kamdar AV, Jones MR, Kessel M, Coburn JW: Protein losses during peritoneal dialysis. *Kidney Int* 19:593–602, 1981.
67. Diaz-Buxo JA: Continuous ambulatory and continuous cycling peritoneal dialysis. In: G La Greca, et al. eds, *Peritoneal Dialysis*. Wiching Editore, Milano, pp 257–264, 1986.
68. Twardowski ZJ, Prowant BF, Nolph KD, Martinez AJ, Lampton RN: High volume, low frequency continuous ambulatory peritoneal dialysis. *Kidney Int* 23:64–70, 1983.
69. Di Paolo N: Semicontinuous peritoneal dialysis with a subcutaneous peritoneal catheter. *Dial Transpl* 7:834–838, 1978.
70. Frock J, Twardowski Z, Nolph K, Khanna R, Prowant B, Dobbie J, Serkes K, Kennley R, Witsoe D, Garber J: Tidal peritoneal dialysis (abstract). *Kidney Int* 31:250, 1987.
71. Daugirdas JT, Leehey DJ, Popli S, Gandhi VC, Zayas I, Hoffman W, Ing TS: Induction of peritoneal fluid eosinophilia by intraperitoneal air in patients on continuous ambulatory peritoneal dialysis. *N Engl J Med* 313:1481, 1985.
72. Abaete de los Santos C, Von Eye O, d'Avila D, Mottin CC: Rupture of the spleen: A complication of continuous ambulatory peritoneal dialysis. *Perit Dial Bull* 6:203–204, 1986.
73. Hassell LH, Moore J, Conklin JJ: Hemoperitoneum during continuous ambulatory peritoneal dialysis: A possible complication of radiation induced peritoneal injury. *Clinical Nephrol* 21:241–243, 1984.
74. Orfei R, Seybold K, Blumberg A: Genital edema in patients undergoing continuous ambulatory peritoneal dialysis. *Perit Dial Bull* 4:251–252, 1984.
75. Twardowski ZJ, Tully RJ, Nichols WK, Sunderrajan S: Computerized tomography CT in the diagnosis of subcutaneous leak sites during continuous ambulatory peritoneal dialysis. *Perit Dial Bull* 4:163–166, 1984.
76. Schleifer CR, Smink RD, Baum SF: Dialysate leakage with a negative Technetium scan — a diagnostic dilemma. *Perit Dial Bull* 5:255–256, 1985.
77. Coward RA, Gokal R, Wise M, Mallick NP, Warrell D: Peritonitis associated with vaginal leakage of dialysis fluid in continuous ambulatory peritoneal dialysis. *Br Med J* 284:1529, 1982.
78. Watson LC, Thompson JC: Erosion of the colon by a long-dwelling peritoneal dialysis catheter. *JAMA* 243:2156–2157, 1980.
79. Diaz-Buxo JA, Burgess WP, Walker PJ. Peritoneovaginal fistula — unusual complication of peritoneal dialysis. *Perit Dial Bull* 3:142–143, 1983.
80. Bierman MH, Kasperbauer J, Kusek A, Hammeke MD, Fitzgibbons RJ, Egan: Peritoneal catheter survival and complications in end-stage renal disease. *Perit Dial Bull* 5:229–233, 1985.
81. Odor A, Alessio-Robles LP, Leuchter J, Mendoza A, Bordes J, Wadgymar A, Gonzalez RF, Peon FC: Experience with 150 consecutive permanent peritoneal catheters in patients on CAPD. *Perit Dial Bull* 5:226–229, 1985.
82. Diaz-Buxo JA, Chandler JT, Farmer CD, Walker PJ, Holt KL, Burgess WP, Orr SL: Long-term observations of peritoneal clearances in patients undergoing peritoneal dialysis. *Am Soc Artific Intern Organs* 5:21–25, 1983.
83. International Cooperative Study Group: A survey of ultrafiltration in continuous ambulatory peritoneal dialysis. *Perit Dial Bull* 4:137–142, 1984.
84. Faller B, Marichal JF: Loss of ultrafiltration in continuous ambulatory peritoneal dialysis: A role for acetate. *Perit Dial Bull* 4:10–13, 1984.
85. Nielsen LH, Nolph KD, Khanna R, Moore H: Sclerosing peritonitis on CAPD; the acetate-lactate controversy (abstract). *Am J Nephrol* 17:82A, 1984.
86. Manuel MA: Failure of ultrafiltration in patients on CAPD. *Perit Dial Bull* S38–40, 1983.
87. Hasbargen JA, Smith BJ, Rodgers DJ: Ultrafiltration failure at the initation of CAPD. *Perit Dial Bull* 6:46–47, 1986.
88. Junor BJR, Briggs JD, Forwell MA, Dobbie JW, Henderson I: Sclerosing peritonitis — The contribution of chlorhexidine in alcohol. *Perit Dial Bull* 5:101–104, 1985.
89. Gotloib L, Mines M, Garmizo L, Varka I: Hemodynamic effects of increasing intra-abdominal pressure in peritoneal dialysis. *Perit Dial Bull* 1:41–43, 1981.
90. Wetherington GM, Leapman SB, Robison RJ, Filo RS: Abdominal wall and inguinal hernias in continuous ambulatory peritoneal dialysis patients. *Am J Surg* 150:357–360, 1985.
91. Rocco MV, Stone WJ: Abdominal hernias in chronic peritoneal dialysis patients: A review. *Perit Dial Bull* 5:171–174, 1985.
92. Goodman CD, Husserl FE: Etiology, prevention and treat-

ment of back pain in patients undergoing continuous ambulatory peritoneal dialysis. *Perit Dial Bull* 1:119–122, 1981.
93. Alpert MA, Franklin JO, Twardowski ZJ, Khanna R: Effect of increasing intra-abdominal pressure and posture on left ventricular function in patients on CAPD. *Kidney Int* 31:248, 1987.
94. Gotloib LA, Garmizo L, Varak T, Mines M: Reduction of vital capacity due to increased intra-abdominal pressure during peritoneal dialysis. *Perit Dial Bull* 1:63–64, 1981.
95. Williams PF, Marliss EB, Anderson GH, et al.: Amino acid absorption following intraperitoneal administration in CAPD patients. *Perit Dial Bull* 2:124–130, 1982.
96. Grodstein GP, Blumenkrantz MJ, Kopple JD, Moran JK, Coburn JW: Glucose absorption during continuous ambulatory peritoneal dialysis. *Kidney Int* 19:564–567, 1981.
97. Delmez JA, Fallon MD, Bergfeld MA, Gearing BK, Dougan CS, Teitelbaum SL: Continuous ambulatory peritoneal dialysis and bone. *Kidney Int* 30:379–384, 1986.
98. Buccianti G, Bianchi ML, Valenti G: Progress of renal osteodystrophy during continuous ambulatory peritoneal dialysis. *Clinical Nephrol* 22:279–283, 1984.
99. Renal osteodystrophy and the status of albumin and other trace metals in CAPD: A panel review. *Perit Dial Bull* 4:129–135, 1984.
100. Taber T, Hageman T, York S, Miller R: Removal of aluminum with intraperitoneal deferoxamine. *Perit Dial Bull* 6:213–216, 1986.

CHAPTER 50

Continuous Ambulatory Peritoneal Dialysis

ROBERT A. MACTIER & KARL D. NOLPH

INTRODUCTION

The potential use of the peritoneum as a dialyzing membrane was recognized as early as 1923 (1, 2). Nevertheless, not until a permanent indwelling peritoneal catheter was developed in 1964 by Palmer et al. (3) and later modified by Tenckhoff (4), did long-term intermittent peritoneal dialysis (IPD) become a practical alternative to hemodialysis. However, due to inadequate dialysis and repeated episodes of peritonitis, the cumulative technique survival on IPD was low (5) and hemodialysis remained the predominant form of dialysis therapy.

The concept of portable/wearable equilibrium peritoneal dialysis was introduced by Popovich and Moncrief in 1976 (6). Initial clinical studies with four or five 2-1 exchanges per day showed that adequate steady-state control of uremia, sodium and water balance, hyperkalemia, and acidosis could be achieved in patients with end-stage renal failure, and this technique was retermed *continuous ambulatory peritoneal dialysis* (CAPD) (7). Oreopoulos replaced the use of glass bottles containing dialysis solution with a polyvinylchloride (PVC) bag, which could be rolled up when empty and carried under the clothing without being disconnected from the transfer set (8). After equilibrating for the selected dwell time (4–10 hours), the dialysate was drained into the PVC bag and the connection-disconnection procedure was repeated using an aseptic, nontouch technique. This development markedly reduced the peritonitis rate and, apart from further minor modifications, this basic CAPD system (peritoneal catheter, transfer set, PVC bag containing dialysis solution, four exchanges per day) remains unchanged today.

During the past decade the number of patients on CAPD has increased annually (9, 10), and CAPD now has an established role in renal replacement therapy (11). Factors identified as being of paramount importance in a successful CAPD program include:
1. Patient selection
2. Peritoneal access
3. Patient training and education
4. Individualized dialysis
5. Avoidance of complications

PATIENT SELECTION

Advantages of CAPD

CAPD offers the patient with end-stage renal disease a relatively simple home dialysis therapy that does not require routine vascular access, a machine, a supervising partner, limitation of activity during dialysis, or rigid dietary restriction. CAPD provides steady-state control of serum biochemistry and fluid balance, thus avoiding the problems of transcellular disequilibrium, interdialysis weight gain, and hemodynamic instability that are observed with intermittent dialysis therapies. Comparison of solute clearances with CAPD (four exchanges and 10-1 dialysate drain volume per day), IPD (40 hours per week), and hemodialysis with cellulose membranes (12 hours per week) are shown in Table 1. The low solute clearance rates in CAPD are due to the very low dialysate flow rate (7 ml/min) and are compensated for by dialysis being performed continuously (12). Weekly removal of solutes of molecular weight greater than 100 daltons (creatinine = 113) is higher with CAPD, since the peritoneum has a greater permeability to larger solutes than standard hemodialysis membranes and serum solute concentrations decrease markedly during hemodialysis, reducing solute mass transfer at a given clearance rate. Consequently it has been proposed that great removal of uremic toxins, such as middle molecules, with CAPD (13) may improve well-being and reduce the severity of anemia, the incidence of pericarditis, and the progression of peripheral neuropathy (14–18). A further benefit for the community in this modern age of finanical restraint in health care is that CAPD has lower initial capital expenditure and annual maintenance costs than hemodialysis (19) and has enabled the number of patients receiving dialysis to be expanded in some countries (20, 21).

Indications and contraindications

The aforementioned medical advantages make CAPD a more appropriate initial therapy than hemodialysis for children (22) and patients with cardiac failure (23) or

Table 1. Comparison of solute clearances in IPD, CAPD, and hemodialysis

Solute (molecular weight)	IPD ml/min	l/wk	CAPD ml/min	l/wk	HD ml/min	l/wk
Urea (60)	25	60	7	70	150	108
Creatinine (113)	17	41	6	60	120	86
Vitamin B_{12} (1355)	8	19	4	42	17	12
Inulin (5200)	5	12	2.6	26	5.5	4

Table 2. Indications for CAPD

1. Age of patient	children elderly
2. Medical complications	diabetes cardiac failure anephric/severe anemia recurrent hemorrhage
3. Psychosocial factors	*patient choice* self-motivated long distance from in-center dialysis freedom to travel
4. Transfer from hemodialysis	no vascular access uncontrolled hypertension hemodynamic instability high interdialysis weight gain postdialysis dysequilibration syndrome dialysis-associated ascites
5. Awaiting transplantation	

Table 3. Contraindications to CAPD

Major	Minor
1. *Extensive peritoneal fibrosis*	Chronic obstructive pulmonary disease
2. Recent major abdominal surgery	Peripheral vascular disease
3. Inflammatory bowel disease	Diverticulosis
4. Colostomy, ileal conduit	Hernias
5. Immunosuppressed	Polycystic kidney disease
6. Poor motivation	Hepatitis B antigenemia
7. Psychosis*	Systemic vasculitis
8. Impaired intellect*	Hyperlipidemia
9. Neurologic deficit*	Obesity
10. Grippling arthritis of hands*	Lumbar backache
11. Blindness*	Protein malnutrition

* For Self-therapy only.

diabetes (24). Moreover, intraperitoneal administration of insulin in diabetic CAPD patients can the improve control of blood glucose, and CAPD avoids the need for systemic heparinization, which may increase the risk of retinal or vitreous hemorrhage (24–26). Social factors and complications encountered with hemodialysis may also influence the decision in favor of beginning or transferring to CAPD (Table 2). It was feared that CAPD immediately prior to renal transplantation would predispose the patient to peritonitis, but this has not been verified (27, 28), and indeed CAPD has been advocated as the preferred dialysis therapy for patients who are likely to receive an allograft in the near future (11). However, as with home hemodialysis, patient motivation for self-treatment is essential in CAPD, and the patient has to be able to perform the dialysis schedule correctly and safely. The latter need not apply if a partner is willing to be trained to perform the exchanges for the patient every day. The major and minor contraindications to CAPD are summarized in Table 3. The only absolute contraindication to CAPD is extensive peritoneal fibrosis. An assessment of the advantages and disadvantages of each mode of dialysis will help determine the dialysis therapy best suited for the individual patient. Since CAPD is self-dialysis, it is emphasized that "patient selection" should refer to the dialysis choice of the patient as well as the physician.

PERITONEAL ACCESS

Swan Neck catheters

A durable indwelling peritoneal catheter providing reliable and safe access to the peritoneal cavity is a prerequisite for long-term peritoneal dialysis. The Tenckhoff catheter (3, 4) and implantation technique (29) has been the most widely used for peritoneal access in CAPD but has been associated with an unacceptably high incidence of complications (30, 31). Modifications in catheter design and implanation technique have been introduced in recent years in an attempt to reduce the frequency of catheter-related complications (32). These developments have been directed mainly at reducing the incidence of intraperitoneal catheter-tip migration, outflow (one-way) obstruction, dialysate leakage, external cuff extrusion, exit-site and tunnel infection, and incisional hernias. The Swan Neck catheters now available incorporate features designed to prevent most of these complications (Table 4) (33, 34). Catheters with the advantage of an intraperitoneal disc or balloon to prevent catheter displacement (Toronto Western, Lifecath, Valli catheter) also have the disadvantage of requiring open surgery through a relatively large incision in the peritoneum and fasica for both implantation and removal. However, peritoneal catheter survival with surgical placement is higher than with bedside (medical) insertion (35), and open surgical implantation through the belly of the rectus abdominis muscle results in fewer dialysate leaks and incisional hernias than midline insertion (36, 37). Accordingly, we now advocate open insertion of a Swan Neck catheter through a lateral approach in the rectus muscle for patients beginning CAPD (38).

Table 4. Features of Swan Neck catheter design and implantation technique that prevent complications

Complication	Catheter design	Catheter implantation
1. a. Catheter tip migration	Internal segment of tunnel anchored in caudal direction by the slanted internal cuff (Toronto and Missouri catheters)	At open insertion, catheter tip placed in true pelvis under direct visualization
b. Outflow obstruction	Discs in Toronto catheter impede displacement and wrapping by omentum	
2. Pericatheter dialysate leak	Flange sutured to posterior rectus sheath and purse-string suture on peritoneum, transversalis fascia, and posterior rectus sheath between flange and bead (Missouri and Toronto catheters)	Lateral insertion through the belly of rectus abdominis muscle Avoid scars
3. Tunnel infection	External cuff	Caudal direction of external segment of turnnel may aid drainage
4. a. External cuff extrusion	Permanent bend (Swan Neck) in subcutaneous segment	Cuff implanted 2 cm from skin exit site
b. Exit-site infection		Avoid skin folds or beltline
5. Incisional hernia		Lateral approach

Surgical insertion of the Swan Neck catheter

The preferred catheter site should be marked on the skin prior to surgery. The use of a stencil of the catheter helps ensure correct creation of the arcuate tunnel and positioning of the external cuff (Figure 1). Care should be taken to keep the exit site out of skinfolds, distant from scars, and a least 2 cm above or below the patient's beltline. Preoperatively the patient should be given an enema and asked to empty the bladder. Vancomycin 1 g should be infused intravenously over 1 hour immediately before surgery.

Best results are achieved if implantation is performed by a single surgical team that is fully acquainted with the technique. Local anesthesia is preferred. After surgical preparation a 3 cm transverse incision is made in the skin over the rectus muscle. Rectus muscle fibers are dissected bluntly as far as the posterior rectus sheath. A purse-string suture is placed through the posterior rectus sheath, transversalis fascia, and peritoneum, and then a small incision is made in the peritoneum. The sterilized catheter is threaded over a stylet until the tip is in the true pelvis. At this point the patient may be aware of rectal or bladder discomfort, which should resolve if the catheter is withdraw slightly. After ensuring free inflow of dialysis solution through the catheter into the peritoneal cavity, the purse string is tightened, placing the bead of the catheter in the peritoneal cavity and sewing the flange to the posterior rectus sheath (Figure 1). A small stab wound in the anterior rectus sheath and a subcutaneous pocket are then created above the transverse incision to accommodate the intercuff segment of the catheter. Using a trocar, the catheter is passed anteriorly and superiorly through the stab incision in the anterior rectus sheath, and the arcuate portion of the catheter is then positioned carefully in the subcutaneous pocket. Finally the trocar is directed inferiorly through the marked exit site, and the external cuff is placed 2 cm from the skin surface. Care is taken to ensure that the exit site and tunnel lateral to the external cuff are of similar diameter to the catheter and that the radiopaque stripe of the catheter always lies anteriorly. A 1-l bag of dialysis solution containing 1000 U heparin is connected to the catheter via an extension tubing and titanium adaptor (39), and inflow and outflow

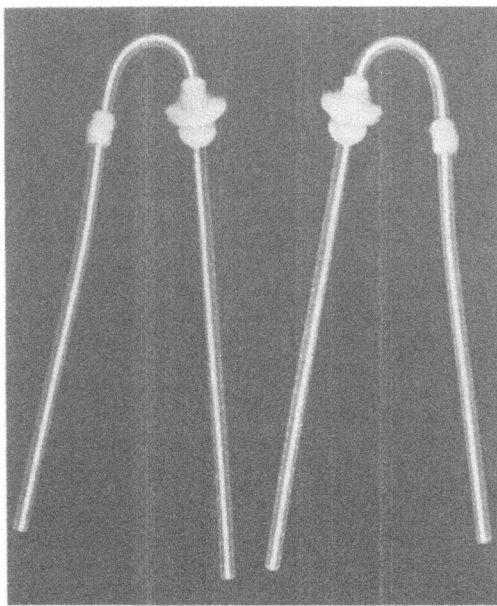

Figure 1. Swan Neck Missouri catheters with two cuffs and slanted flange and bead. The radiopaque stripe always lies anteriorly and identifies the right and left catheters. Reproduced with permission from Twardowski et al. (38).

through the catheter is evaluated. At least 200 ml of dialysate should drain within the first minute. In-and-out exchanges are continued until the solution is free of blood. If good inflow and drainage are obtained, the incision is closed with absorbable subcuticular sutures and covered with a gauze dressing. Finally, the extension tubing is taped to the abdomen to prevent inadvertent tugging on the newly inserted catheter. This surgical approach can be easily modified for implantation of the other types of catheters currently available (32).

Catheter break-in

Early postoperative management aims to maintain catheter patency, to minimize the risk of pericatheter dialysate leak, and, if needed, to control uremia. Malnutrition and uremia are associated with poor wound healing and delayed tissue ingrowth into the external cuff, and thus predispose to dialysate leaks. In the immediate postoperative period, three in-and-out exchanges are performed using 0.5–1.0 l of 1.5% dextrose dialysis solution containing 1000 U/l heparin to assess catheter patency. Further exchanges may be necessary if the dialysate remains bloodstained. An abdominal film is obtained to determine the catheter position. If the tip of the catheter is outside the true pelvis but the catheter is functioning, no correction of the catheter malposition is attempted, since it may translocate into the pelvis spontaneously. For the patient who does not need immediate peritoneal dialysis (elective placement of peritoneal catheter, temporary or chronic vascular access available), the catheter lumen is filled with 3 ml undiluted heparin solution (5000 U/ml) and the external tip is covered with a sterile cap. The incision is kept clean with hydrogen peroxide, the surrounding skin is painted with betadine and air dried, and the incision is covered with a nonadhesive dressing. CAPD training is commenced in 10–14 days unless the patient is diabetic, multiparous, on corticosteroids, or had a wound infection, in which case further delay may be required until the wound is healed. If the patient requires earlier peritoneal dialysis, rapid exchanges (1–2 hourly) with small volumes of dialysis solution can be performed either manually or using a cycler machine (IPD) with the patient supine. This approach will minimize the risk of dialysate leak since, for any given dialysate volume, the intraabdominal pressure is lowest in the supine position (40).

A dialysate leak will usually resolve if peritoneal dialysis is discontinued temporarily. Dialysis solution may not infuse in the postoperative period if the catheter is occluded by blood, fibrin, a kink (seen on x-ray), or omentum. Clot or fibrin in the catheter can often be dislodged by flushing the catheter with heparinized saline or streptokinase and recurrence can usually be prevented with irrigation with dialysis solution containing 1000 U/l heparin. Partial omental wrapping is usually associated with outflow (one-way) obstruction and migration of the catheter tip out of the pelvis. If this does not resolve after correction of constipation and several days of one-way irrigation of the catheter, replacement of the catheter will be required and the need for concurrent partial omentectomy should be evaluated at operation.

PATIENT TRAINING AND EDUCATION

The success of a CAPD program depends on proper patient training and education (41). A well-trained and dedicated nursing team with a special interest in peritoneal dialysis facilitates achieving these objectives (42). Training is best conducted as an outpatient and on a one-to-one basis by the nurse who will later follow up the patient at home. As well as systematic training in aseptic technique, patients require a basic knowledge of the CAPD system and education in early recognition of complications and simple problem solving. These teaching goals are aided by providing patients with a training manual containing protocols for unit procedures dealing with CAPD techniques and complications. The time taken to train a CAPD patient varies, but averages 10 days and is dependent on many factors, including age, mental alertness (state of uremia), presence of physical handicaps, and level of family support. After completion of training, the patient's progress is assessed at regular clinic visits. Home visits and telephone calls by the patient's nurse and social worker provide further patient support during intervals between clinic attendances (43).

INDIVIDUALIZED DIALYSIS

Mass transfer of urea and creatinine

In peritoneal dialysis the rate of equilibration of dialysate solutes with plasma depends on the solute molecular weight (7). Accordingly in CAPD, small molecular weight solutes, such as urea, almost completely equilibrate with the plasma within 4 hours (dialysate/plasma urea = 1), whereas larger solutes continue to equilibrate until the end of the dwell time (Figure 2) (44). The mass transfer of solutes not present in the infused dialysis solution is equal to the drained dialysate solute concentration × daily drain volume product. Thus the daily net removal of small solutes in CAPD is primarily determined by the daily drain volume (dialysate flow rate), while the mass transfer rates of larger solutes are predominantly influenced by the patient's peritoneal permeability-area product (45). If the exchange dwell time is reduced below 3 hours (Figure 2), the mass transfer of small solutes is also influenced by peritoneal permeability times area.

The peritoneum is a composite biologic "membrane" (capillary endothelium and endothelial basement membrane, interstitium, and mesothelium) that is subjected to chronic reuse during CAPD. Consequently, not only is there interindividual variation in the peritoneal permeability-area product, but the peritoneal membrane transport kinetics of each patient may also change with time. Moreover, the dialysis requirements of CAPD patients also vary and depend on several factors, including body

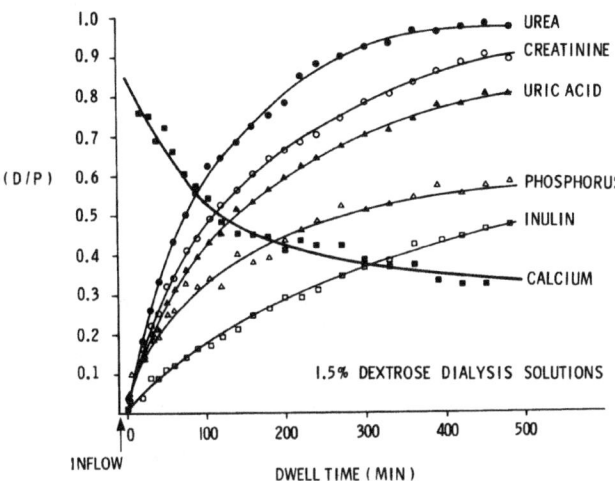

Figure 2. Equilibration of dialysate and plasma solute concentrations during long-dwell exchanges using 2 l of 1.5% dextrose dialysis solution. Reproduced with permission from Nolph et al. (44).

weight, dietary protein intake, catabolic rate, and residual renal clearance. Thus individualized dialysis schedules are recommended to ensure that CAPD patients with differing peritoneal transport and dialysis requirements all receive adequate dialysis (46).

After the peritoneal catheter break-in period, most adult patients on CAPD are initially prescribed four 2-l exchanges per day, which commonly results in dialysate drain volumes and urea clearances of around 10 l/day. Dialysis solution tonicity and/or volume can be increased until there are no symptoms attributable to uremia and the desired biochemical values are achieved. Hypertonic exchanges increase solute clearances by increasing both the drain volume and the peritoneal permeability-area product (47). Furthermore, the peritoneal permeability-area product remains increased for several exchanges after the dialysate osmolality is reduced (48). Large adult patients can usually tolerate 2.5 or 3.0-l exchanges, provided that there are no contraindications to a further increase in intraabdominal pressure (49). Alternatively, solute clearances on CAPD can be augmented by increasing the number of exchanges per day. However, the inconvenience of the extra exchange procedures each day negates its therapeutic application for most CAPD patients.

CAPD creatinine clearance rates average 6 ml/min, and so an endogenous creatinine clearance at the beginning of dialysis of only a milliliters per minute makes a significant contribution to the total clearance. Moreover, for each decrease in residual renal urea clearance of 1 ml/min, the CAPD urea clearance (drain volume) must be increased by 1.43 l/day to maintain the same total urea clearance. Consequently residual renal function should be conserved for as long as possible, and nephrotoxic drugs, such as aminoglycosides and nonsteroidal antiinflammatory drugs, should be prescribed with caution. If the dialysis schedule remains unchanged during progressive loss of residual renal function, underdialysis may occur. Furthermore, inadequate dialysis may not be recognized early unless the nutritional intake and status are routinely assessed, since the concomitant anorexia result in failure to adhere to recommended protein and calorie intakes, reduced urea nitrogen appearance rate, and muscle wasting, and thus relatively stable or low serum urea nitrogen and creatinine levels. Nevertheless, underdialysis usually manifests as a rise in serum urea nitrogen and creatinine, especially if there is an acute decline in total daily clearances.

Studies of transperitoneal solute and fluid transport during standardized exchanges (2 l, 2.5% dextrose dialysis solution with a 4-hour dwell time) are a clinically useful index of the peritoneal permeability-area and are helpful in selecting the patient's individualized dialysis schedule (50, 51). Equilibration curves relating the dialysate/plasma urea nitrogen, creatinine, and protein, and sequential/initial dialysate glucose, concentration ratios to dwell time show wide interindividual variation, but reference values are available (Figure 3). Baseline equilibration studies, performed soon after beginning CAPD, can predict the adequacy of dialysis on standard CAPD after the loss of residual renal function. Patients with high peritoneal solute transport (more than 1 SD above the mean in Figure 3) usually require four or more short dwell exchanges during the day (daytime ambulatory peritoneal dialysis) in order to capture maximum ultrafiltration and solute clearances. Patients with low peritoneal solute transport (more than 1 SD below the mean) are at risk of underdialysis on

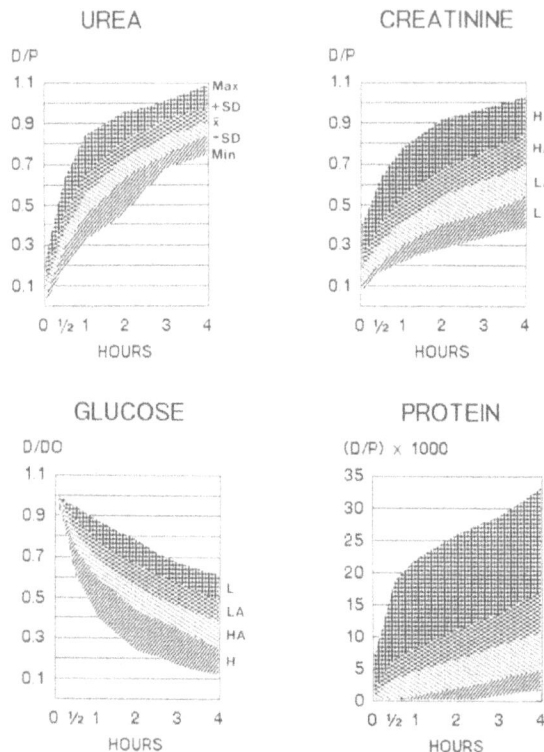

Figure 3. Equilibration curves during standardized 4 hour exchanges using 2 l of 2.5% dextrose dialysis solution (n = 103). The mean and mean + 1 SD solute ratios categorize patients with high (H), high average (HA), low average (LA), and low (L) peritoneal transport. Reproduced with permission from Twardowski et al. (51).

standard CAPD after the loss of residual function, especially if they are of high body weight. These patients often require dialysis solution inflow volumes of at least 10 l per day. Patients with average peritoneal transport rates (within 1 SD of the mean in Figure 3) can usually be maintained on standard CAPD unless they have a very high body weight, are catabolic, or have a significant change in the peritoneal permeability-area product. The latter can be confirmed by repeating the standardized equilibration test, and the dialysis schedule should be modified appropriately. These alterations in peritoneal transport have been observed infrequently in North America but may reflect underlying pathologic changes in the peritoneum and may forewarn of the future development of sclerosing peritonitis (52).

Ultrafiltration

In peritoneal dialysis ultrafiltration is induced by the transperitoneal osmotic gradient of the hypertonic (glucose) dialysis solution (53). The ultrafiltration rate decreases exponentially from the beginning of the exchange due to dissipation of the osmotic gradient by absorption of dialysate glucose and dilution of dialysate glucose by the ultrafiltrate (53). The peritoneal cavity lymphatics, in contrast, absorb intraperitoneal fluid at a constant rate during the long dwell exchanges of CAPD (54). Consequently, the maximum net ultrafiltration volume is observed before osmotic equilibrium is reached, when the transperitoneal ultrafiltration and lymphatic absorption rates are equal (55). Thereafter the lymphatic flow rate exceeds the transperitoneal ultrafiltration rate and intraperitoneal fluid volume decreases (55). For any given patient, increasing the tonicity and volume of the dialysis solution increases the maximum intraperitoneal volume, increases the absorbed glucose load, and prolongs the exchange dwell time until net fluid absorption occurs (Figure 4) (56).

Fluid balance is achieved when the daily net ultrafiltration and residual urine volumes balance fluid intake. Excessive fluid intake, necessitating extra hypertonic exchanges and an increased obligatory glucose load from the dialysis solution, should be discouraged. High-dose furosemide may be prescribed to try to preserve residual urine volumes for as long as possible after the onset of dialysis (57) and so minimize the need for hypertonic exchanges. However, as residual renal function decreases, the increased number of hypertonic exchanges needed

Ultrafiltration (UF) Related to Dwell Time With 2 and 3L Volumes, 1.5, 2.5, and 4.25% Glucose Concentrations

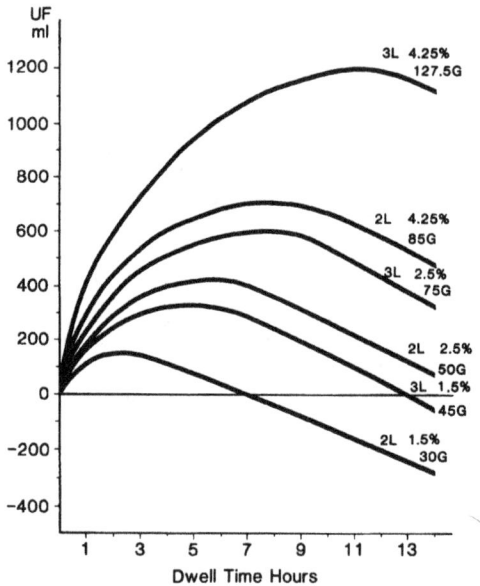

Figure 4. Effect of volume and tonicity of dextrose dialysis solutions on net ultrafiltration during the dwell time. Reproduced with permission for Twardowski et al. (56).

Table 5. Diagnostic value of repeat standardized equilibration studies in CAPD patients with apparent and actual loss of ultrafiltration

Drain volume	Peritoneal solute transport[1]		Residual volume (51)	Diagnosis	Diagnostic test	Recommended therapy
	Baseline study	Repeat study				
L	H	H	N	Loss of residual urine volume[2]	—	4 or more short dwell exchanges during daytime (DAPD)
L	N	H	N	Peritoneal hyperpermeality change	Equilbration study	Temporary hemodialysis (52)
L	N	L	N	Massive adhesions or sclerosing peritonitis	Laparotomy	Permanent hemodialysis (52)
L	N	N	N	High lymphatic absorption or	Intraperitoneal albumin removal (62)	DAPD or hemodialysis
L	N	N	N	Dialysate leak	Abdominal CT with intraperitoneal contrast (60)	Temporary hemodialysis or supine IPD
L	N	N	H	Catheter malposition	Abdominal x-ray	Reposition catheter
N	N	N	N	High fluid intake[2]	—	Dietary counseling

[1] Patients with high transperitoneal solute transport (H) have high dialysate/plasma nonglucose solute ratios and low dwell/initial dialysate glucose ratios. Patients with low peritoneal transport (L) demonstrate the reverse pattern of solute ratios during the standardized equilibration study (Figure 3).
[2] Apparent loss of ultrafiltration occurs when patients with high peritoneal transport lose residual renal function or when patients with normal (N) peritoneal transport have excessive fluid intake.

to ensure fluid balance augment peritoneal small-solute clearances as well as drain volumes and thus help prevent underdialysis. Nevertheless, with the loss of residual urine volume some patients continue to have insufficient ultrafiltration despite extra hypertonic exchanges (58, 59). Standardized peritoneal equilibrium studies (Figure 3) can often delineate the cause of loss of ultrafiltration, especially if a baseline study is available for comparison (50, 51). The diagnosis and recommended therapy for each causes of failure of ultrafiltration is summarized in Table 5. Apparent loss of ultrafiltration is observed in patients with a high peritoneal permeability-area product when they lose residual urine volume or in patients with an injudiciously high fluid intake. Actual loss of ultrafiltration occurs when the daily cumulative peritoneal cavity lymphatic absorption (55) and/or dialysate leakage (60) equals or exceeds the daily net transperitoneal ultrafiltration. Extraperitoneal dialysate leaks may occur with abdominal wall edema and hernias, as well as overtly with a pericatheter leak. Consequently, in the absence of a dialysate leak, true failure of ultrafiltration is observed when transperitoneal water transport is relatively low (61) and/or peritoneal cavity lymphatic drainage is relatively high (62). Leaving the peritoneal cavity empty overnight and resting the peritoneum may reverse, at least in part, peritoneal hyperpermeability changes and so increase transperitoneal ultrafiltration (50), but at present there is no therapy to reduce lymphatic absorption during CAPD.

Alternatively excessive ultrafiltration may lead to a sudden weight loss and orthostatic tachycardia and hypotension. This is most likely to occur when the patient with a reduced fluid intake or increased gastrointestinal fluid losses continues to use several hypertonic exchanges each day. Since extraperitoneal fluid is absorbed at around 50 ml per hour after osmotic equilibrium is approached (63, 64), minor dehydration can be corrected by using 1.5% glucose exchanges with a prolonged dwell time (8–12 hours). Chronic orthostatic hypotension unrelated to a recent negative fluid balance may indicate sodium depletion (65).

Control of blood pressure and sodium balance

The improvement in blood pressure control on CAPD is attributed to daily controlled ultrafiltration, which can maintain patients at their dry body weight (14, 66). A reduction in blood pressure is most marked in the first weeks of CAPD (66) and emphasizes the importance of volume status in the pathogenesis of hypertension in end-stage renal disease. Indeed, hypertension can often be controlled without antihypertensive therapy despite an increase in plasma renin and aldosterone levels (67). CAPD results in daily net removal of sodium as well as water. Peritoneal mass transfer of sodium can be readily calculated as the sum of (drain volume × drained dialysate sodium concentration) − (infusion volume × infused dialysate sodium concentration) for each exchange. The dialysate sodium concentration decreases during the first 2–3 hours of each exchange due to solute sieving with ultrafiltration (68) and thereafter equilibrates with serum sodium by diffusion (69). Thus net ultrafiltration of 1.0–1.5 l/day of dialysate at the standard infused dialysate sodium concentration (132 mEq/l) will result in sodium losses of 132–198 mEq/day. Consequently, CAPD patients with high daily ultrafiltration volumes require a liberal dietary sodium intake to avoid sodium depletion. However, as serum sodium decreases, the equilibration of serum and dialysate sodium concentrations during long dwell exchanges tends to autoregulate net sodium removal (69). Nevertheless symptomatic hypotension in nondiabetic CAPD patients has been attributed to sodium depletion (70) and, in a small series of such patients, symptoms improved and exchangeable sodium increased with sodium supplementation (65).

Acid-base balance

Commercial peritoneal dialysis solutions for CAPD contain lactate as a buffer base. A dialysis solution lactate concentration of 40 mEq/l can maintain the serum concentration of total CO_2 at 28 mEq/l in most patients using four 2-l exchanges per day (71), whereas with solutions containing 35 mEq/l of lactate, serum total CO_2 averages 22 mEq/l (14). There is interindividual variation, however, and the dialysate lactate concentration for CAPD patients needs to be individualized. It has been reported that acidosis is better controlled by CAPD than by other forms of dialysis (72).

Dialysis solutions containing acetate are no longer commercially available. Acetate solutions were withdrawn, since their long-term use has been associated with increased absorption of dialysate glucose and loss of ultrafiltration (59, 73). The development of sclerosing peritonitis in some patients has been linked with exposure to acetate-containing dialysis solutions, but a causative role remains unproven (74, 75). Bicarbonate has not been used routinely in CAPD, since insoluble calcium and magnesium salts form in the dialysis solution during storage. This problem can be avoided if sodium bicarbonate and buffer-free dialysis solution are stored in separate compartments in the dialysis bag and are not mixed until immediately prior to infusion (76). However, the clinical application of this formulation remains to be evaluated.

Prevention of hyperkalemia

In CAPD patients serum potassium is maintained at the level where dietary intake is balanced by dialysate, fecal, and urinary losses. Hyperkalemia is observed infrequently, even though potassium intake is usually 70–80 mEq/day and dialysate losses average only 35 mEq/day (69). This discrepancy has been explained by an increase in fecal potassium losses during CAPD and by a concurrent increase in dialysate potassium losses as serum potassium rises (69). Indeed, metabolic balance studies in CAPD patients have shown that a positive potassium balance was not observed until the potassium intake exceeded 67 mEq/day (77).

Mineral metabolism

Transperitoneal transport of calcium depends on the direction of the concentration gradient between the dialysate and serum ionized calcium. In normocalcemic patients, peritoneal dialysis solutions containing 3.5 mEq/l of calcium result in a positive calcium balance during 1.5% dextrose exchanges (78, 79) but net removal of calcium during more hypertonic exchanges due to hypotonic ultrafiltration. Thus daily peritoneal mass transfer of calcium depends on the tonicity of the exchanges used each day as well as the serum ionized calcium concentration. Most normocalcemic CAPD patients using three 1.5% dextrose and one 4.25% dextrose exchanges/day have a daily net uptake of calcium from the dialysate (77, 78).

The rate of diffusion of phosphate into the dialysate is slower than predicted from its molecular weight (MW = 98) and is attributed to its hydration shell and anionic charge (Figure 2). Nevertheless, with the long dwell exchanges of CAPD 250–350 mg of phosphorus are removed in the dialysate each day (78). Most patients on an adequate protein diet will ingest 800–1200 mg of phosphorous per day, and, assuming 50% phosphorus absorption and no residual renal function, will need to use phosphate binders to remove 150–250 mg phosphorus each day. After serum phosphorus has been lowered below 6.0 mg/dl with dialysis and aluminium-containing phosphate binders, calcium carbonate can be prescribed with food in increasing dosages until serum ionized or total calcium is in the upper-normal range (80). Only after calcium carbonate has been given in a maximum dosage should aluminium-containing phosphate binders be added to control serum phosphorus levels. This therapeutic approach helps ensure adequate calcium supplementation, while the use of calcium carbonate as a phosphate binder (81) lessens the requirement for aluminum-containing antacids. The latter is important since cumulative aluminum intake from aluminum-containing phosphate binders is the major determinant of serum aluminum levels in CAPD patients maintained on dialysis solutions containing less than 15 µg/l aluminum (82, 83). Net removal of aluminum has been observed with the currently available dialysis solutions (84, 85) and may explain the infrequent reports of overt aluminum toxicity in adult CAPD patients (86) unless exposed to dialysate contaminated with aluminum (87). Reducing the dialysate magnesium concentration from 1.5 to 0.5 mEq/l prevents magnesium uptake from the dialysate during 1.5% dextrose exchanges (79) and corrects hypermagnesemia in CAPD patients (71). This lower magnesium dialysate concentration may enable magnesium hydroxide to be use as a phosphate bind for patients on CAPD (88)

1.25-dihydroxycholecalciferol levels are often reduced at the beginning of CAPD (89) and 25-hydroxycholecalciferol levels may fall during CAPD due to losses in the dialysate (90, 91). However, therapy with vitamin D analogues has the potential hazards of worsening hyperphosphatemia, hypercalcemia, and metastatic calcification, and has usually been reserved for CAPD patients with worsening secondary hyperparathyrodism despite optimum existing therapy or osteomalacia unrelated to aluminum toxicity. With this overall management strategy, most patients on CAPD show an improvement in radiologic and histologic features of renal bone diseae (80, 90).

Daily dietary requirements of CAPD patients

The nutritional requirements of patients on CAPD are significantly influenced by losses of proteins, amino acids, and water-soluble vitamins into the dialysate and by absorption of glucose from the dialysate (92). Protein losses in the dialysis solution range from 6 to 12 g/day and are unrelated to dietary protein intake or ultrafiltration volume (93–95). Dialysate protein losses remain relatively constant in the same patient but markedly increase during episodes of peritonitis (96, 97). Amino acid losses in the dialysate reflect the plasma amino-acid profile and range from 2.0 to 3.5 g/day (98–100). Serum levels of vitamin C, vitamin B_1, vitamin B_6, and folic acid decrease in CAPD patients not receiving vitamin supplementation to the diet (101, 102). Absorption of intraperitoneal glucose varies from 100 to 200 g/day depending on the number, volume, and tonicity of dextrose dialysis solutions used each day (103, 104). This obligatory glucose load promotes insulin secretion and anabolism in CAPD patients (104) but has the disadvantages of also predisposing the patients to obesity, impaired glucose tolerance, and hypertriglyceridemia (105–107).

CAPD patients without peritonitis are in a neutral to positive nitrogen balance while on a diet providing at least 1.2 g protein/kg/day (77, 108). Fifty percent of the daily protein intake should be of high biologic value to replace the dialysate losses of essential amino acids (98, 100). Several other dietary manipulations have been proposed to lessen the risk of metabolic complications (105–107) and at the same time to maintain adequate nutrition: Only 35% of ingested calories should be in the form of carbohydrate, fat intake should be mainly polyunsaturated fatty acids, and daily total calorie (diet and dialysate) and protein intakes should reflect the patient's normalized rather than actual weight. Trace element supplements are not recommended unless there is both biochemical and clinical evidence of a deficiency state (109). These considerations rationalize the daily dietary allowances currently advocated for CAPD patients (Table 6).

COMPLICATIONS

Peritonitis

Peritonitis is the most common acute complication of CAPD (Table 7) and is the major cause of technique

Table 6. Daily dietary allowances for CAPD patients

Energy (diet and dialysate)	35–42 kcal/kg normalized body weight
Protein	1.2–1.3 g/kg normalized body weight
Carbohydrate (diet)	35% of ingested calories
Fat	Remainder of nonprotein ingested calories
Polyunsaturated : saturated fatty acid ratio	1.5 : 1
Minerals	
Calcium	At least 1000–1400 mg
Phosphorus	800–1200 mg
Magnesium	200–300 mg
Potassium	70–80 mEq
Sodium and water	As tolerated by fluid balance
Aluminum hydroxide	Minimum intake required to control serum phosphorus
Ferrous sulphate	200 mg
Supplemental vitamins	
Ascorbic acid	100 mg
Pyridoxine HCL	10 mg
Thiamine HCL	2 mg
Folic acid	1 mg
Other water-soluble vitamins	Recommended daily allowances for normal adults
Fat-soluble vitamins (A, D, E, K)	None routinely

Table 7. Complications of CAPD

1. *Peritonitis*
   Bacterial
   Culture negative
   Fungal
   Eosinophilic
2. *Catheter-related*
   Exit-site and/or tunnel infection
   External cuff extrusion
   Inflow and/or outflow obstruction
   Dialysis solution infusion pain
3. *Related to increased intraabdominal pressure*
   Abdominal hernia
   Pericatheter dialysate leak
   Abdominal wall or genital edema
   Massive hydrothorax
   Cardiorespiratory compromise
   Hiatus hernia
4. *Membrane failure*
   Inadequate ultrafiltration and/or inadequate dialysis
   Sclerosing peritonitis
5. *Metabolic*
   Protein depletion
   Hyperlipidemia and obesity
6. *Medical*
   Cardiovascular disease
   Progression of renal osteodystrophy

failure (10). More than half of all patients using standard manual exchange procedures experience at least one episode of peritonitis during the first year of CAPD. The host defenses of the peritoneal cavity are compromised by CAPD and thus predispose patients to develop peritonitis (110):
1. The peritoneal catheter provides a ready route for recurrent intraperitoneal contamination with skin comensals and opportunistic organisms.
2. The dialysate concentrations of opsonins (IgG and C3) and resident peritoneal macrophanges are diluted by the daily exchange of large volumes of dialysis solution (111, 112).
3. The intraperitoneal volume of dialysis solution impairs the localization of infection within the peritoneal cavity by the omentum.
4. The phagocytic and bactericidal activity of the influx of polymorphonuclear leukocytes is suppressed by the acidic pH and hypertonicity of freshly infused dialysate (113).

Passive immunization with intraperitoneal IgG may reduce the incidence of peritonitis (114), especially in patients with very low opsonic activity in the dialysate, but this needs further evaluation. Existing improvements in connector technology and aseptic technique may have contributed to the gradual decrease in peritonitis rates of patients in the USA to one episode every 12 patient months (115).

DIAGNOSIS OF PERITONITIS

The diagnosis of peritonitis requires two of the following criteria:
1. Abdominal pain or tenderness
2. Absolute WBC count $> 100/mm^3$ and differential count $> 50\%$ polymorphs (cloudy dialysate)
3. Microorganisms in the dialysate (gram stain, positive culture)

Other symptoms of peritonitis include nausea and vomiting, fever, chills, diarrhea, and dialysate drainage problems. Some patients may notice cloudy dialysate before the onset of abdominal pain. However, turbid dialysate alone is not diagnostic of peritonitis, since it may be caused by fibrin, lymph leakage, or minor bleeding into the dialysate. Similarly, the differential diagnosis of abdominal pain in CAPD patients should also include pancreatitis, cholecystitis, appendicitis, diverticulitis, and underlying bowel perforation.

For the laboratory diagnosis of peritonitis, it is best to send all of the first cloudy drainage bag for examination. This simple approach ensures an adequate dialysate sample volume for microbiologic concentrating techniques and avoids potential sample contamination. Gram stain of the sediment from the dialysate establishes the presence of microorganisms in only 20–30% of cases of peritonitis. Culture for identification and antimicrobial sensitivities of the causative organism(s) has the highest yield if bacterial concentrating techniques such as centrifugation and microfiltration are performed (116). Cloudy dialysate can be stored overnight at 4°C without reducing the accuracy of bacteriologic diagnosis (117). However, even in the presence of fever or severe systemic symptoms, blood cultures in patients with CAPD-associated peritonitis are seldom positive.

Gram-positive cocci are isolated in 60–70%, gram-negative bacilli in 20–25%, anaerobes in 3–5%, and fungi in 3–5% of culture-positive episodes of peritonitis. *Staphylococcus epidermidis* is by far the most frequent isolate (35–40% of peritonitis episodes), but many unusual bacteria and fungi can occasionally cause peritonitis in CAPD patients (118). *Tuberculous peritonitis* should be considered in patients with predominantly mononuclear cells in the dialysate and culture-negative results by standard methods (119). Isolates of more than one organism should raise suspicion of visceral perforation. Peritoneal eosinophilia (cloudy dialysate; differential WBC count $>15\%$ eosinophils) is always culture negative and is usually asymptomatic (120). Dialysate eosinophilia is most frequently observed within the first weeks of beginning chronic peritoneal dialysis (121); has been attributed to peritoneal reaction to intraperitoneal air, the catheter, or other irritants (122, 123); and usually resolves spontaneously without altering the dialysis schedule or solutions used (120, 124).

TREATMENT OF PERITONITIS

Two or three rapid exchanges can be performed to alleviate symptoms while the diagnosis is being confirmed. If peritoneal fluid cytology and the gram stain indicate peritonitis, empirical antibiotic therapy should be initiated immediately. Many different routes of administration and combinations of antibiotics have been sucessfully used to treat CAPD-associated peritonitis (124). However, intraperitoneal antibiotic therapy is usually preferred; the antibiotic has a direct effect at the site of infection, adequate systemic absorption is readily achieved due to increased peritoneal permeability during peritonitis, and treatment can be commenced by the patient at home. Our protocol for selecting first-line antibiotic treatment, pending the results of dialysate effluent culture, is summarized in Figure 5. Most commonly no organisms are seen in the gram stain of the peritoneal fluid, and both cephalothin and tobramycin are commenced. This combination of a cephalosporin and an aminoglycoside is active against most isolates from peritoneal effluent (116). Admixtures of these two antibiotics are stable in the dialysate, but should be injected into the dialysis solution using different syringes (126, 127). In patients with hypersensitivity to beta-lactam antibiotics, the cephalosporin can be replaced by vancomycin (Figure 5) (128). CAPD, rather than rapid exchange peritoneal lavage, should be continued during intraperitoneal antibiotic treatment since long dwell exchanges maintain higher white blood cell counts and better leukocyte function in the dialysate (129, 130). Modifications in antibotic therapy may be required when the culture results and antimicrobial sensitivities become available after 24–36 hours or if symptoms and serial dialysate white

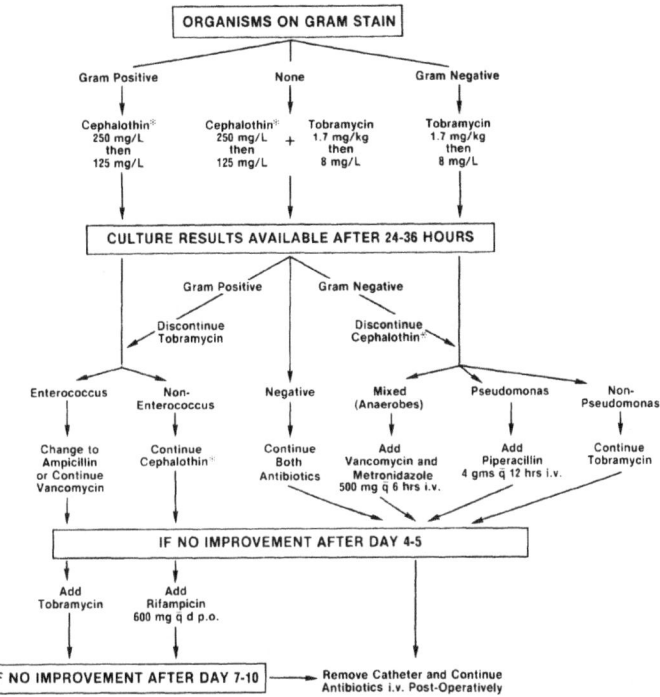

Figure 5. Decision analysis for antibiotic treatment of CAPD peritonitis. Recommended intraperitoneal dose of antibiotics is in mg/l dialysis solution for CAPD exchanges unless stated otherwise; i.v. = intravenous; p.o. = oral.
* For patients with betalactam antibiotic hypersensitivity, cephalothin can be replaced by intraperitoneal vancomycin at a 1000 mg/l loading dose and a 10 mg/l maintenance dose.

blood cell counts do not decrease despite "appropriate" therapy. To lessen the risk of loss of residual renal function, tobramycin should be discontinued if dialysate culture yields gram-positive isolates. The optimum duration of antibiotic therapy is not established, but many centers continue antibiotics for 7 days after either the dialysate effluent becomes clear (less than 100 WBC/mm^3) or the last positive culture (116).

The addition of heparin to the dialysis solution (250–500 U/l) during the acute phase of peritonitis reduces the formation of fibrin and may prevent subsequent adhesion formation (131). Increased peritoneal permeability during peritonitis results in increased protein losses in the dialysate, more rapid glucose absorption, and reduced ultrafiltration volume (97). Moreover, patients are catabolic and often anorexic. Consequently, adequate protein intake during peritonitis (1.2–1.6 g/kg/day) needs to be actively encouraged, and short dwell exchanges may be required to maintain fluid balance or to reduce dialysate turbidity. Glycemic control in diabetics requires careful monitoring during episodes of peritonitis, since insulin requirements often increase.

With early diagnosis and appropriate antibiotic and adjuvant therapy, around 80% of patients have clear peritoneal fluid and negative cultures within 7 days without detectable sequelae. If peritonitis fails to improve despite several days of appropriate antibiotic therapy, catheter removal and intravenous antibiotic therapy are recommended (Figure 5) (134). This approach usually results in prompt resolution of symptoms, avoids the protracted negative nitrogen balance that is associated with refractory peritonitis, and may reduce the risk of intraperitoneal sequelae. *Staphylococcus aureus*, *Pseudomonas*, multiple organism, and fungal peritonitis account for a high proportion of refractory peritonitis that leads to catheter removal and/or intraperitoneal adhesion formation. Peritonitis due to mixed organisms, especially anerobes, is also frequently associated with bowel perforation or diverticulitis, and early surgical intervention may be required. There is no generally accepted therapy for fungal peritonitis. However, the morbidity and mortality rates are relatively high when peritoneal dialysis is continued during antifungal therapy, and peritonitis often persists until the catheter is eventually removed (135–137). Consequently many centers now advocate removal of the catheter as soon as the diagnosis is confirmed, administration of intravenous amphotericin B, and temporary hemodialysis (137–139). Catheter replacement in patients with refractory peritonitis should be delayed for at least 2 weeks.

Relapsing peritonitis, defined as peritonitis caused by the same organism within 2 weeks of stopping antibiotic treatment (140), occurs in over 10% of peritonitis episodes (132, 141). If the recurrent organism is either gram-negative or can be isolated from a concurrent catheter exit-site or tunnel infection, long-term resolution of peritonitis is uncommon and catheter removal will be required.

PREVENTION OF PERITONITIS

Strict aseptic technique is the single most important factor in preventing intraluminal contamination of the transfer set and catheter. However, only the most motivated patients can maintain high aseptic standards indefinitely, and many different connecting devices have been developed to further reduce the risk of intraluminal contamination:

1. Beta-cap system (142)
2. Oreopoulos–Zellerman connector (143)
3. Bazzato double-bag system (144)
4. Italian Y connector (145, 146) and its modification, the O set
5. Ultraviolet germicidal system (147)
6. Sterile connection device (148)
7. In-line bacterial filters (149)

Encouraging preliminary results have been reported with most of these connectors, but only the Y connector has been prospectively evaluated in controlled trials and been shown to reduce the peritonitis rate significantly (146). Moreover this bagless system may also improve patient freedom and reduce body image problems associated with the attached collapsible bag in standard CAPD. However, with the combined use of antiseptic solutions and connectors (142, 146), there is the potential danger that resistant organisms may emerge in the connector (150) or that repeated intraperitoneal injection of the antiseptic may induce peritoneal sclerosis (151). These risks may be avoidable, since a Y connector system that does not use an antiseptic has been reported recently to reduce peritonitis rates significantly during a 2-year prospective study (152). If the benefits of the Y connector are confirmed, variants of this system could become the connectors of the future.

An alternative approach has been to reduce the number of connection-disconnections per day by using a cycler machine to perform continuous cyclic peritoneal dialysis (CCPD). However, the USA National CAPD Registry has failed to demonstrate any major difference in peritonitis rates between CAPD and CCPD (10). Conversely, intraperitoneal insulin administration may theoretically increase the risk of intraluminal contamination, but no difference has been observed in peritonitis rates between diabetic and non-diabetic patients (10). For episodes of potential contamination of the CAPD system, such as accidental disconnection or transfer set leak, oral or intraperitoneal cephalothin should be prescribed prophylactically for 2 days. However, long-term prophylactic oral antibiotics are not recommended, since they do not reduce the incidence of CAPD peritonitis (153) and indeed may increase the risk of fungal peritonitis (136).

Catheter exit-site and tunnel infections can lead to periluminal contamination and peritonitis. Recent innovations in catheter design and implantation technique include features intended to prevent these complications (Table 4). Exit-site skin care is not standardized, but leaving the exit site uncovered after healing is complete and daily gentle cleansing with soap and water are as effective as more active wound care in preventing exit-site infections. The diagnosis of exit-site infection is dependent on the presence of erythema and/or purulent drainage and not culture results, which are usually positive, even in the absence of signs of inflammation. Oral antibiotic therapy should be commenced without delay and, if no improvement, deroofing of the exit site with or without shaving of the external cuff may be attempted. If exit-site infection persists or if the tunnel is infected, the catheter is best removed because of the risk of developing peritonitis.

Diverticulosis and severe constipation may increase the risk of transmural migration of fecal organisms and many cause peritonitis in CAPD patients. Accordingly, all patients should be encouraged to increase the fiber content of their diet and to take bulk laxatives as required to prevent constipation. Rarely, peritonitis is associated with vaginal leakage of dialysate, and tubal ligation is then necessary to prevent recurrence of retrograde infection (154).

Catheter-related complications

The prevention and treatment of catheter-related complications (Table 7) is described in detail in Chapter 51.

Complications related to increased intraabdominal pressure

ABDOMINAL HERNIAS

Increased intraabdominal pressure with CAPD may predispose the patient to develop an abdominal hernia. Alternatively, the initiation of peritoneal dialysis may facilitate the clinical presentation of a previously unrecognized hernia. More than 10% of CAPD patients develop a hernia, and all forms of abdominal hernia have been reported (155, 157). The elderly, multiparous women, patients on steroids appear to be more prone to develop hernias on CAPD (156). Incisional hernias are more common with midline insertion of the peritoneal catheter (36) and paramedian placement is now preferred (Table 4) (36, 37).

Abdominal hernias should be carefully looked for and repaired before peritoneal dialysis is begun. If patients develop hernias after starting CAPD, temporary transfer to hemodialysis or low-volume supine IPD is required until the surgical repair is healed. Thereafter most patients are able to resume CAPD.

DIALYSATE LEAKAGE

Pericatheter external dialysate leaks most commonly occur during the first weeks after catheter insertion. The incidence of these dialysate leaks is reduced if peritoneal dialysis can be delayed for 7-10 days, if low dialysate volumes are used in the break-in period, and if a paramedian rather than a midline approach is used for catheter insertion (36, 37). Patients with internal dialysate leaks usually present with a combination of abdominal wall or genital edema, a sudden decrease in dialysate drain volume, and a rapid weight gain. The most common sites of leakage are around the peritoneal entrance of the catheter, through previous scars, or through an open processus vaginalis and, if not evident clinically, can be localized using computerized tomography with contrast added to the dialysis solution (60). External dialysate leaks usually resolve after the patient has been changed temporarily to hemodialysis or supine IPD. Internal dialysate leaks are much more likely to persist when CAPD is resumed and to then require surgical intervention. Genital edema usually indicates a patent processus vaginalis and merits surgical correction. Occasionally genital edema without a cough impulse may be the initial presentation of an inguinal hernia (158).

MASSIVE HYDROTHORAX

Transdiaphragmatic leakage of dialysate is an uncommon but serious complication that usually requires that CAPD be discontinued. Acute hydrothorax almost always occurs on the right side and usually presents within hours to a few weeks of beginning peritoneal dialysis (159, 160). The pleural fluid glucose concentration is high and the protein concentration is low (160). The presence of a pleuroperitoneal communication can often be confirmed by radionuclide scanning using technetium-99 m-labeled macroaggregated albumin added to the dialysis solution (159, 161). However, anatomic evidence of either an acquired or congenital pleuro-peritoneal connection can be found at autopsy in only some of the patients (160, 161). Thoracocentesis may be required for acute respiratory distress or, if less acute, the effusion may be allowed to resolve spontaneously once peritoneal dialysis is discontinued. The patient should be transferred from CAPD permanently, since hydrothorax is likely to reoccur if peritoneal dialysis is reinstituted at a later date (161). Alternatively, sclerosing agents can be instilled into the pleural cavity in an attempt to close the leak (162), but the long-term success of this approach needs confirmation.

CARDIORESPIRATORY COMPROMISE

Increased intraabdominal pressure and intraperitoneal fluid volume during CAPD may compromise pulmonary and cardiac function. Nevertheless, in adult CAPD patients at stable dry weight, vital capacity (40), maximum expiratory flow rate (163), and left ventricular function (164) are not significantly changed with standard volumes of dialysis solution (2.0-2.5 l). These parameters are not adversely influenced in most patients until infusion volumes of dialysis solution are at least 3 l (40, 164). However, in the supine position, some patients may experience dyspnea and a reduction in vital capacity at lower infusion volumes (40, 49). Patients with a low body surface area or a poor cardiopulmonary reserve (chronic obstructive pulmonary disease, pulmonary edema) are unlikely to tolerate infusion volumes greater than 2 l and, indeed, may require lower dialysate volumes, especially when supine overnight.

Membrane failure

INADEQUATE ULTRAFILTRATION AND/OR INADEQUATE DIALYSIS

The ability of the peritoneum to function as a long-term dialysis membrane is not well established. The durability of the peritoneum in CAPD may be adversely influenced by continuous exposure to unphysiologic dialysis solutions, intercurrent episodes of peritonitis, and/or coincident drug therapy. Nevertheless, at least in North America and Australasia, peritoneal solute transport has rarely been reported to change significantly with time on CAPD (51, 132, 165, 166). Loss of ultrafiltration (true and apparent) is more common (73). However, a change in peritoneal membrane transport is only one of the potential mechanisms of ultrafiltration failure in CAPD patients (Table 5). A persistent increase in the peritoneal permeability-area product, resulting in rapid glucose absorption from the dialysate, early dissipation of the osmotic gradient, and decreased ultrafiltration volume, has been observed most frequently in Europe (52) and is termed *Type I membrane failure* (138). Almost complete equilibration of solutes during the dwell time compensates in part for the reduction in the dialysate drain volume and helps maintain adequate solute removal. This pattern of peritoneal transport is simulated transiently during peritonitis (96, 97). Hypertonic dialysis solutions containing acetate or lactate induce vasodilatation, and their long-term use may predispose to increased peritoneal permeability (167). Several clinical studies from Europe have implicated acetate-containing dialysis solutions as a risk factor for gradual loss of ultrafiltration (58, 59), and this has been supported by an international survey of ultrafiltration in CAPD patients (73). However, the ultrafiltration volume did not correlate with the number of prior episodes of peritonitis (73).

The formation of fibrous adhesions or peritoneal sclerosis following most episodes of peritonitis is probably limited, since peritoneal transport is usually unchanged and there is no interference with dialysate inflow or outflow. However, massive adhesion formation may occasionally complicate refractory peritonitis, especially if due to *Staphylococcus aureus* or fungi, and prevent reinstitution of peritoneal dialysis (132). In addition to mechanical complications (loculation of intraperitoneal fluid, abdominal pain during dialysate infusion, bowel obstruction), extensive adhesions can lead to an acute reduction in the peritoneal permeability-area product and initially a greater reduction in solute transport than ultrafiltration (Type II membrane failure). It is emphasized that, in the absence of laparotomy, intraperitoneal adhesions are only diagnosed early after peritonitis if complications develop, but remain unassessed in patients who are initially asymptomatic on peritoneal dialysis.

SCLEROSING PERITONITIS

Sclerosing peritonitis is characterized by the development of progressive peritoneal sclerosis and may be unrelated to an episode of acute infectious peritonitis (168, 169). Clinical features include Type II membrane failure, relapsing culture-negative peritonitis, and/or acute bowel obstruction. At laparotomy dense laminated fibrous tissue may be found around the viscera (encapsulating peritonitis), in the peritoneum, or even within the bowel wall (168, 170). Peritoneal fibrosis may progress despite cessation of CAPD, and patients may first develop symptoms while on chronic hemodialysis. The etiology remains unknown but is most likely to be multifactorial. The clustering of cases within some centers suggests that local exogenous factors may be important, but an international survey has failed to identify a common etiology (171). Factors associated with the occurrence of sclerosing peritonitis include: severe or recurrent episodes of peritonitis leading to the cessation of CAPD, increased past incidence of *Staphylococcus aureus* peritonitis, potential dialysate contamination with antiseptics, beta-blocker therapy, and exposure to acetate-containing dialysis solutions (151, 168, 171). An increase in peritoneal permeability (Type I membrane failure) has been claimed to precede symptomatic sclerosing peritonitis (52, 172). If peritoneal dialysis is discontinued and the catheter is removed at this stage or before acute complications develop, progression of peritoneal sclerosis may be halted. For patients presenting with acute or subacute bowel obstruction, mortality exceeds 50% despite surgical intervention and cessation of peritoneal dialysis (168, 169).

Metabolic complications

PROTEIN DEPLETION

Persistent anorexia, nausea, and early satiety are not uncommon symptoms in CAPD patients and may lead to chronic protein and/or calorie malnutrition. Dietary assessment, serial anthropometric measurements, and biochemical monitoring (serum albumin and transferrin) are invaluable for the early detection of undernutrition in patients on CAPD. With progressive loss of residual renal function, underdialysis on CAPD and undernutrition are often interrelated (72). Dietary protein intake in stable CAPD patients can be estimated from the measurement of urea nitrogen appearance (UNA) (173, 174), where:

UNA (g/day) = Blood urea nitrogen (mg/dl) × total urea clearance (l/day) and
Total urea clearance (l/day) = drain volume + residual renal urea clearance.

These results help verify the dietary history and establish whether an increase in dietary protein intake and/or dialysis clearance is required. If, despite adequate dialysis, the daily nutritional intake remains poor (Table 7), temporary enteral or parenteral nutritional supplementation may be required. Alternatively, in the future amino acids may be administered in the dialysis solution (175, 176).

HYPERLIPIDEMIA AND OBESITY

Hyperlipidemia is common in uremic patients and is due, at least in part, to reduced activity of serum lipoprotein lipase and hepatic lipase (177). Dyslipoproteinemia would be expected to worsen during CAPD because of the additional glucose load from the dialysate (103) and hyperinsulinemia (178). Indeed, the prevalence of hypertriglyceridemia and de-novo hypercholesterolemia in patients during their first year of CAPD is reported to be 60–80% and 20–30%, respectively (89, 107). However, except in a small subgroup of patients (107), hyperlipidemia reaches a peak after 3–12 months of CAPD and thereafter falls to pretreatment levels (89, 107).

Patients also frequently gain more than 5 kg in weight during the first year on CAPD (14, 105). Despite evidence of net anabolism and an increase in lean body mass after beginning CAPD (179, 180), the major proportion of this weight gain appears to be increased body fat (105, 181). Nevertheless, most patients do not become obese during CAPD, but rather tend to return to their premorbid nonuremic weight (181).

For CAPD patients who require treatment for hyperlipidemia and/or obesity, the oral carbohydrate intake can be restricted and exercise can be increased (106, 182). Decreasing oral fluid intake will reduce the number of hypertonic exchanges required and will limit the dialysate glucose load, but the reduced dialysate drain volume will also decrease the small-solute clearances (45). An alternative osmotic agent would be invaluable for such patients (56, 183). Lipid-lowering drugs, such as clofibrate, should be prescribed with caution to uremic patients since side effects are not uncommon.

Medical complications

CARDIOVASCULAR DISEASE

Cardiovascular disease is by far the major cause of death in CAPD patients (184). This may be related to the high proportion of "at risk" patients selected for CAPD (diabetic, known cardiac disease, elderly) and/or the acceleration of atherogenesis by metabolic sequelae of CAPD (hyperlipidemia, hyperinsulinemia). Indeed, more than 25% of patients now beginning CAPD in the USA are diabetic (10). However, when standardized dialysis populations (15–55 years, nondiabetic, normotensive, no malignancy) are compared, no difference in actuarial patient survival is observed between CAPD and hemodialysis (185, 186). Therefore, it is unlikely that the choice of the dialysis modality per se significantly alters the risk of cardiovascular disease in patients with end-stage renal failure. Primary and secondary prevention of cardiovascular risk factors before and after beginning dialysis is much

Table 8. Life table analysis of CAPD patients*

Duration of analysis (years)	1	2	3
% patient survival	84	72	60
% technique survival	80	66	57
% survival of first catheter	79	70	70
% peritonitis free	43	32	27
% without prior exit-site or tunnel infection	67	55	37

* Extrapolated from Steinberg et al. (10).

more likely to lessen cardiovascular morbidity and mortality.

CONCLUSION

During the first 10 years of CAPD, improvements in patient selection, modifications in catheter design and implantation, an increased range of dialysis solutions and schedules, and a reduction in complications (especially peritonitis) have all contributed to increased patient and technique survival. Patients beginning CAPD at present can expect results at least equal to historical cohorts (Table 8). CAPD now has a well-established role in the short-to medium-term management of patients with end-stage renal failure and in the provision of an integrated renal replacement program.

REFERENCES

1. Putnam J: The living peritoneum as a dialyzing membrane *Am J Physiol* 63:548–565, 1923.
2. Ganter G: Uber die beseitigung gigtiger stoffe dein blute durch dialyse. *Munch Med Wochenschr* 70:1478–1480, 1923.
3. Palmer RA, Quinton WE, Gray JF: Prolonged peritoneal dialysis for renal failure. *Lancet* 1:700–702, 1964.
4. Tenckhoff H, Schechter H: A bacteriologically safe peritoneal access device. *Trans Am Soc Artif Int Organs* 14:181–186, 1968.
5. Ahmad S, Gallagher N, Shen F: Intermittent peritoneal dialysis: Status reassessed. *Trans Am Soc Artif Intern Organs* 25:86–88, 1979.
6. Popovich RP, Moncrief JW, Decherd JF, et al.: The definition of a novel portable/wearable equilibrium dialysis technique. *Trans Am Soc Artif Intern Organs* 5:64A, 1976.
7. Popovich RP, Moncrief JW, Nolph KD, et al.: Continuous ambulatory peritoneal dialysis. *Ann Intern Med* 88:449–456, 1978.
8. Oreopoulos DG, Robson M, Izatt S, et al.: A simple and safe technique for continuous ambulatory peritoneal dialysis. *Trans Am Soc Artif Intern Organs* 24:484–489, 1978.
9. Wing AJ, Broyer M, Brunner FP, et al.: Combined report on regular dialysis and transplantation in Europe, XV, 1984. *Proc Eur Dialys Tranpl Assoc* 22:3–54, 1985.
10. Steinberg SM, Cutler SJ, Novak JW, et al.: Report of the National CAPD registry of the National Institutes of Health. *NIH, Washington DC*, 1986.
11. Gokal R: World-wide experience, cost effectiveness and future of CAPD — its role in renal replacement therapy. In: R Gokal, ed, *Continuous Ambulatory Peritoneal Dialysis*. Churchill Livingstone, Edinburgh, pp 349–369, 1986.
12. Nolph KD, Popovich RP, Moncrief JW: Theoretical and practical implications of continuous ambulatory peritoneal dialysis. *Nephron* 21:117–122, 1978.
13. Bergstrom J, Asaba H, Furst P, et al.: Middle molecules in chronic uremic patients treated with continuous ambulatory peritoneal dialysis. *Perit Dial Bull* 3:S7–S9, 1983.
14. Nolph KD, Sorkin M, Rubin J, et al.: Continuous ambulatory peritoneal dialysis: Three-year experience at one center. *Ann Intern Med* 92:609–613, 1980.
15. Zappacosta AR, Caro J, Erslev A: Normalization of hematocrit in patients with end-stage renal disease on continuous ambulatory peritoneal dialysis. The role of erythropoietin. *Am J Med* 72:53–57, 1982.
16. De Paepe MBJ, Schelstraete KGH, Ringoir SMG, et al.: Influence of continuous ambulatory peritoneal dialysis on the anemia of end-stage renal disease. *Kidney Int* 27:744–748, 1983.
17. Sunderrajan S, Nolph KD: Longitudinal study of nerve conduction velocities during continuous ambulatory peritoneal dialysis. *Perit Dial Bull* 5:48–50, 1985.
18. Kim D, Blair G, Wu G, et al.: Electrophysiological studies of nerve function in patients on CAPD over long periods. *Perit Dial Bull* 5:45–48, 1985.
19. Levery AS, Harrington JT: Continuous peritoneal dialysis for chronic renal failure. *Medicine* 61:330–339, 1982.
20. Gokal R, Marsh F: Survey of CAPD in UK — 1982. *Perit Dial Bull* 4:240–243, 1984.
21. Nichols AJ, Waldek S, Platts MM, et al.: Impact of CAPD on treatment of renal failure in patients over 60. *Br Med J* 288:18–19, 1984.
22. Fine RN: Peritoneal dialysis update. *J Pediatrics* 100:1–7, 1982.
23. Rubin J, Bell R: Continuous ambulatory peritoneal dialysis as treatment of severe congestive heart failure in the face of chronic renal failure. *Arch Int Med* 146:1533–1538, 1986.
24. Amair P, Khanna R, Leibel B, et al.: Continuous ambulatory peritoneal dialysis in diabetics with end-stage renal disease. *N Engl J Med* 306:625–630, 1982.
25. Flynn CT, Nanson JA: Intraperitoneal insulin with CAPD — an artificial pancreas. *Trans Am Soc Artif Int Organs* 25:114–117, 1979.
26. Madden MA, Zimmerman SW, Simpson DP: CAPD in diabetes mellitus — the risks and benefits of intraperitoneal insulin. *Am J Nephrol* 2:133–139, 1982.
27. Gokal R, Ramos JM, Veitch P, et al.: Renal transplantation in patients on continuous ambulatory peritoneal dialysis. *Proc Eur Dialys Tranpl Assoc* 18:222–227, 1981.
28. Stephanidis CJ, Balfe JW, Arbus GS, et al.: Renal transplantation in children treated with continuous ambulatory peritoneal dialysis. *Perit Dial Bull* 3:5–8, 1983.
29. Tenckhoff H: Home peritoneal dialysis. In: SG Massry, AL Sellars, eds, *Clinical Aspects of Uremia and dialysis*. CC Thomas, Springfield, 1976.
30. Rubin J, Adair C: Peritoneal access using the Tenckhoff catheter. *Perspect Perit Dial* 1:2–3, 1983.
31. Gloor HJ, Nichols WK, Sorkin MI, et al.: Peritoneal access and related complications in continuous ambulatory peritoneal dialysis. *Am J Med* 74:593–598, 1983.
32. Khanna R, Oreopoulos DG: Peritoneal access for chronic peritoneal dialysis. *Int J Artif Organs* 8:1–6, 1985.
33. Twardowski ZJ, Nolph KD, Khanna R, et al.: The need for a "swan neck" permanently bent, arcuate peritoneal dialysis

catheter. *Perit Dial Bull* 5:219–223, 1985.
34. Khanna R, Izatt S, Burke D, et al.: Experience with the Toronto Western Hospital permanent peritoneal catheter. *Perit Dial Bull* 4:95–97, 1984.
35. Ponse SP, Pierratos A, Izatt S, et al.: Comparison of the survival and complications of three permanent peritoneal dialysis catheters. *Perit Dial Bull* 2:82–86, 1982.
36. Helfrich GB, Pechan BW, Alijani MR, et al.: Reduced catheter complications with lateral placement. *Perit Dial Bull* 3:S2–S4, 1983.
37. Khanna R, Oreopoulos DG: Peritoneal access using the Toronto Western Hospital permanent catheter. *Perspect Perit Dial* 1:4–6, 1983.
38. Twardowski ZJ, Khanna R, Nolph KD, et al.: Preliminary experience with the Swan Neck peritoneal dialysis catheters. *Trans Am Soc Artif Intern Organs* 32:64–67, 1986.
39. Nolph KD: Continuous anbulatory peritoneal dialysis. *Am J Nephrol* 1:1–10, 1981.
40. Twardowski ZJ, Khanna R, Nolph KD, et al.: Intraabdominal pressures during natural activities in patients treated with continuous ambulatory peritoneal dialysis. *Nephron* 44:129–135, 1986.
41. Moncrief JW, Sorrels PAJ, Druger VG, et al.: Development of training programs for continuous ambulatory peritoneal dialysis — historical review. In: M Legrain, ed, *Continuous Ambulatory Peritoneal Dialysis*. Excerpta Medica, Amsterdam, pp 149–151, 1980.
42. Oreopoulos DG: Requirements for the organisation of a CAPD Program. *Nephron* 24:261–263, 1979.
43. Moon J, Uttley L, Manos J, et al.: Home CAPD nurse, an asset to a CAPD programme? In: JF Maher, JF Winchester, eds, *Frontiers in peritoneal Dialysis*. Field Rich and Associates, New York, pp 360–363, 1986.
44. Nolph KD, Twardowski ZJ, Popovich RP, et al.: Equilibration of peritoneal dialysis solutions during long dwell exchanges. *J Lab Clin Med* 93:246–256, 1979.
45. Nolph KD, Popovich RP, Ghods AJ, et al.: Determinants of low clearances of small solutes during peritoneal dialysis. *Kidney Int* 13:117–123, 1978.
46. Twardowski ZJ: Individualized dialysis for CAPD patients. *Uremia Invest* 8:35–43, 1984.
47. Henderson LW: Peritoneal ultrafiltration dialysis: Enhanced urea transfer using hypertonic peritoneal dialysis fluid. *J Clin Invest* 45:950–955, 1966.
48. Henderson LW, Nolph KD: Altered permeability of the peritoneal membrane after using hypertonic peritoneal dialysis fluid. *J Clin Invest* 48:992–1001, 1969.
49. Twardowski ZJ, Prowant B, Nolph KD, et al.: High volume, low frequency continuous ambulatory peritoneal dialysis. *Kidnet Int* 23:64–70, 1983.
50. Khanna R, Nolph KD: Ultrafiltration failure and sclerosing peritonitis in peritoneal dialysis patients. In: AR Nissenson, RN Fine, eds, *Dialysis Therapy*. Hanley and Belfus Philadelphia, pp 122–125, 1968.
51. Twardowski ZJ, Nolph KD, Khanna R, et al.: Peritoneal equilibration test. *Perit Dial Bull*, in press.
52. Verger C, Larpent L, Dumontet M: Prognostic value of peritoneal equilibration curves in CAPD patients. In: *Frontiers in Peritoneal Dialysis*. JF Maher, JF Winchester eds, Field, Rich and Associates, New York, pp 88–93, 1986.
53. Nolph KD, Miller FN, Pyle WK, et al.: An hypothesis to explain the ultrafiltration characteristics of peritoneal dialysis. *Kidney Int* 20:543–548, 1981.
54. Mactier RA, Khanna R, Twardowski Z, et al.: Role of peritoneal cavity lymphatic absorption in peritoneal dialysis. *Kidney Int*, in press.
55. Mactier RA, Khanna R, Twardowski Z, et al.: Lymphatic absorption in CAPD. *Kidney Int* 31:252A, 1987.
56. Twardowski ZJ, Khanna R, Nolph KD: Osmotic agents and ultrafiltration in peritoneal dialysis. *Nephron* 42:93–101, 1986.
57. Rottembourg J, El Shahat Y, Agrafiotis A, et al.: Continuous ambulatory peritoneal dialysis in insulin-dependent diabetic patients. A 40-month experience. *Kidney Int* 23:40–45, 1983.
58. Slingeneyer A, Canaud B, Mion C: Permanent loss of ultrafiltration capacity of the peritoneum in long-term peritoneal dialysis: An epidemiological study. *Nephron* 33:133–138, 1983.
59. Faller B, Marichal JF: Loss of ultrafiltration in continuous ambulatory peritoneal dialysis: A role for acetate. *Perit Dial Bull* 4:10–13, 1984.
60. Twardowski ZJ, Tully RJ, Nichols WK, et al.: Computerized tomography in the diagnosis of subcutaneous leak sites during CAPD. *Perit Dial Bull* 4:163–166, 1984.
61. Wideroe TE, Smeby LC, Mjaaland S, et al.: Long-term changes in transperitoneal water transport during continuous ambulatory peritoneal dialysis. *Nephron* 38:238–247, 1984.
62. Mactier RA, Khanna R, Twardowski Z, et al.: Ultrafiltration failure in CAPD due to excessive peritoneal cavity lymphatic absorption. *Am J Kidney Dis* in press.
63. Pyle WK, Popovich RP, Moncrief JW: Mass transfer evaluation in peritoneal dialysis. In: JW Moncrief, RP Popovich, eds, *CAPD Update*. Masson, New York, pp 35–52, 1981.
64. Twardowski Z, Ksiazek A, Majdan M, et al.: Kinetics of continuous ambulatory peritoneal dialysis (CAPD) with four exchanges per day. *Clin Nephrol* 15:119–130, 1981.
65. Leenen FHH, Shah P, Boer WH, et al.: Hypotension in CAPD: An approach to treatment. *Perit Dial Bull* 3:S33–35, 1983.
66. Young MA, Nolph KD, Dutton S, et al.: Anti-hypertensive drug requirements in continuous ambulatory peritoneal dialysis. *Perit Dial Bull* 4:85–88, 1984.
67. Glasson PH, Favre H, Valloton MB: Response of blood pressure and the renin-angiotensin-aldosterone system to chronic ambulatory peritoneal dialysis in hypertensive end-stage renal failure. *Clin Sci* 63:S207–209, 1982.
68. Nolph KD, Hano JE, Teschan PE: Peritoneal sodium transport during hypertonic peritoneal dialysis: Physiologic mechanisms and clinical implications. *Ann Intern Med* 70:931–941, 1969.
69. Nolph KD, Sorkin MI, Moore H: Autoregulation of sodium and potassium removal during continuous ambulatory peritoneal dialysis. *Trans Am Soc Artif Intern Organs* 6:334–337, 1980.
70. Marquez-Julio A, Dombros N, Osmond D, et al.: Hypotension in patients on continuous ambulatory peritoneal dialysis. In: M Legrain, ed, *Proc First Int Symp CAPD*. Excerpta Medica, Amsterdam, pp 263–267, 1979.
71. Nolph KD, Prowant B, Serkes KD, et al.: Multicenter evaluation of a new peritoneal dialysis solution with a high lactate and a low magnesium concentration. *Perit Dial Bull* 3:63–65, 1983.
72. Nissenson AR: Acid-base homeostasis in peritoneal dialysis patients. *Int J Artif Organs* 7:175–176, 1984.
73. An International Cooperative study (Third Report): A survey of ultrafiltration in CAPD. In: R Khanna, KD Nolph, B Prowant, ZJ Twardowski, DG Oreopoulos, eds, *Advances in Continuous Ambulatory Peritoneal Dialysis*. University of

Toronto Press, pp 79–86, 1985.
74. Gandhi VC, Humayun HM, Ing TS, et al.: Sclerotic thickening of the peritoneal membrane in maintenance peritoneal dialysis patients. *Arch Intern Med* 140:1201–1203, 1980.
75. Novello AC, Port FK: Sclerosing encapsulating peritonitis. *Int J Artif Organs* 9:393–396, 1986.
76. Feriani M, Biasioli S, Borin D, et al.: Bicarbonate buffer for CAPD solutions. *Trans Am Soc Artif Organs* 31:668–672, 1985.
77. Blumenkrantz MJ, Kopple JD, Moran JK, et al.: Metabolic balance studies and dietary protein requirements in patients undergoing continuous ambulatory peritoneal dialysis. *Kidney Int* 21:849–861, 1982.
78. Delmez JA, Slatopolsky E, Martin KJ, et al.: Minerals, vitamin D, and parathyroid hormone in CAPD. *Kidney Int* 21:862–867, 1982.
79. Parker A, Nolph KD: Magnesium and calcium transfer during CAPD. *Trans Am Soc Artif Int Organs* 26:194–196, 1980.
80. Cassidy MJD, Owen JP, Ellis HA, et al.: Renal osteodystrophy and metastatic calcification in long-term CAPD. *Q J Med* 213:29–48, 1985.
81. Slatopolsky E, Weerts C, Lopez-Hilker S, et al.: Calcium carbonate as a phosphate binder in patients with chronic renal failure undergoing dialysis. *N Engl J Med* 315:157–161, 1986.
82. Mactier RA, Nolph KD, Khanna R, et al.: Risk factors for hyperaluminemia in continuous ambulatory peritoneal dialysis. *Perit Dial Bull* 6:188–193, 1986.
83. Salusky IB, Coburn JB, Paunier L, et al.: Role of aluminum hydroxide in raising serum aluminum levels in children undergoing CAPD. *J Pediatrics* 105:717–720, 1984.
84. Rottembourg J, Gallego JL, Jaudon M, et al.: Serum concentration and peritoneal mass transfer of aluminum during treatment by continuous ambulatory peritoneal dialysis. *Kidney Int* 24:919–924, 1984.
85. Sorkin MI, Nolph KD, Anderson HO, et al.: Aluminum mass transfer during continuous ambulatory peritoneal dialysis. *Perit Dial Bull* 1:91–94, 1981.
86. Bertholf RL, Roman, Brown S, et al.: Aluminum hydroxide induced osteomalacia, encephalopathy and hyperaluminemia in CAPD, treatment with desferrioxamine *Perit Dial Bull* 4:30–32, 1984.
87. Cumming AD, Simpson G, Bell D, et al.: Acute aluminum intoxication in patients on continuous ambulatory peritoneal dialysis. *Lancet* 1:103–104, 1982.
88. Guillot AP, Hood BL, Runge CF, et al.: Use of magnesium containing phosphate binders in patients with end-stage renal disease on maintenance hemodialysis. *Nephron* 30:114–117, 1982.
89. Nolph KD, Ryan L, Prowant B, et al.: A cross-sectional assessment of serum vitamin D and triglyceride concentration in a CAPD population. *Perit Dial Bull* 4:232–237, 1984.
90. Gokal R, Ramos JM, Ellis HA, et al.: Histological renal osteodystrophy, and 25 hydroxycholecalciferol and aluminum levels in patients on continuous ambulatory peritoneal dialysis. *Kidney Int* 23:15–21, 1983.
91. Aloni Y, Shany S, Chaimovitz C: Losses of 25-hydroxy vitamin D in peritoneal fluid: Possible mechanisms for bone disease in uremic patients treated with CAPD. *Miner Electrolyte Metab* 9:82–86, 1983.
92. Kopple JD, Blumenkrnatz MJ: Nutritional requirements for patients undergoing continuous ambulatory peritoneal dialysis. *Kidney Int* 24:S295–S302, 1983.
93. Dulaney JT, Hatch FE: Peritoneal dialysis and loss of proteins: A review. *Kidney Int* 26:253–262, 1984.
94. Rubin J, Nolph KD, Arfania D, et al.: Protein losses in continuous ambulatory peritoneal dialysis. *Nephron* 28:218–221, 1981.
95. Blumenkrantz MJ, Gahl GM, Kopple JD, et al.: Protein losses during peritoneal dialysis. *Kidney Int* 19:593–602, 1981.
96. Rubin J, Ray R, Barnes T, et al.: Peritoneal abnormalities during infectious episodes of continuous ambulatory peritoneal dialysis. *Nephron* 29:124–127, 1981.
97. Krediet RT, Zuyderhoudt FMJ, Boeschoten EW, et al.: Alterations in peritoneal transport of water and solutes during peritonitis in continuous ambulatory peritoneal dialysis patients. *Eur J Clin Invest*, in press.
98. Dombros N, Oren A, Marliss EB, et al.: Plasma amino acid profiles and amino acid losses in patients undergoing CAPD. *Perit Dial Bull* 2:27–32, 1982.
99. Giordano C, De Santo NG, Capodicasa G, et al.: Amino acid losses during CAPD. *Clin Nephrol* 14:230–232, 1980.
100. Kopple JD, Blumenkrantz MJ, Jones MR, et al.: Plasma amino acid levels and amino acid losses during continuous ambulatory peritoneal dialysis. *Am J Clin Nutr* 36:395–402, 1982.
101. Blumberg A, Hanck A, Sander G: Vitamin nutrition in patients on continuous ambulatory peritoneal dialysis. *Clin Nephrol* 20:244–250, 1983.
102. Henderson IS, Leung ACT, Shenkin A: Vitamin status in continuous ambulatory peritoneal dialysis. *Perit Dial Bull* 4:143–145, 1984.
103. Grodstein GP, Blumenkrantz MJ, Kopple JD, et al.: Glucose absorption during continuous ambulatory peritoneal dialysis. *Kidney Int* 19:564–567, 1981.
104. Von Baeyer H, Gahl GM, Riedinger H. et al.: Adaptation of CAPD patients to the continuous peritoneal energy uptake. *Kidney Int* 23:29–34, 1983.
105. Young GA, Hobson SM, Young SM, et al.: Adverse effects of hypertonic dialysis fluid during CAPD. *Lancet* 2:1421, 1983.
106. Cattran DC, Steiner GS, Fenton SSA, et al.: Dialysis hyperlipemia: Response to dietary manipulations. *Clin Nephrol* 13:177–182, 1980.
107. Ramos JM, Heaton A, Mc Gurk JC, et al.: Sequential changes in serum lipids and their subfractions in patients receiving continuous ambulatory peritoneal dialysis. *Nephron* 35:20–23, 1983.
108. Giordano C, De Santo NG, Pluvio M, et al.: Protein requirement of patients on CAPD: A study of nitrogen balance. *Int J Artif Organs* 3:11–14, 1980.
109. Thomson NM, Stenens BJ, Humphery TJ, et al.: Comparison of trace elements in peritoneal dialysis, hemodialysis and uremia. *Kidney Int* 23:9–14, 1983.
110. Keane WF, Peterson PK: Host defense mechanisms of the peritoneal cavity and continuous ambulatory peritoneal dialysis. *Perit Dial Bull* 4:122–127, 1984.
111. Keane WF, Comty CM, Verbrugh HA, et al.: Opsonic deficiency of peritoneal dialysis effluent in continuous ambulatory peritoneal dialysis. *Kidney Int* 25:539–543, 1984.
112. Verbrugh HA, Keane WF, Hoidal JR, et al.: Peritoneal macrophage and opsonins: Antibacterial defense in patients on chronic peritoneal dialysis. *J Infect Dis* 147:1018–1029, 1983.
113. Duwe AK, Vas SI, Weatherhead JW: Effect of the composition of peritoneal dialysis fluid on chemiluminescence, phagocytosis and bactericidal activity in vitro. Infection and

Immunity 33:130–135, 1981.
114. Lamperi S, Carozzi S: Defective opsonic activity of peritoneal effluent during continuous ambulatory peritoneal dialysis. *Perit Dial Bull* 6:87–92, 1986.
115. Steinberg SM, Culter SJ, Novak JW, et al.: Report of the National CAPD Registry of the National Institutes of Health. NIH, Washington DC, 1987.
116. Vas SI: Microbiologic aspects of chronic ambulatory peritoneal dialysis. *Kidney Int* 23:83–92, 1983.
117. Vas SI: Peritoneal fluid cultures remain positive for days. *Perit Dial Bull* 2:144, 1982.
118. Arfania D, Everett ED, Nolph KD, et al.: Uncommon causes of peritonitis in patients undergoing peritoneal dialysis. *Arch Int Med* 141:61–64, 1981.
119. Morford DW: High index of suspicion for tuberculous peritonitis in patients on CAPD. *Perit Dial Bull* 2:189–190, 1982.
120. Nolph KD, Sorkin MI, Prowant BF, et al.: Asymptomatic eosinophilic peritonitis in continuous ambulatory peritoneal dialysis. *Dial Transpl* 11:309–313, 1982.
121. Digenis GE, Khanna R, Pantalony D: Eosinophilia after implantation of the peritoneal catheter. *Perit Dial Bull* 2:98–99, 1982.
122. Steiner R, Clinical observations on the pathogenesis of peritoneal dialysate eosinophilia. *Perit Dial Bull* 2:118–119, 19
123. Daugirdas JT, Leehey DJ, Popli S, et al.: Induction of peritoneal fluid eosinophilia by intraperitoneal air in patients on continuous ambulatory peritoneal dialysis. *N Engl J Med* 313:1481, 1985.
124. Gokal R, Ramos JM, Ward MK, et al.: Eosinophilic peritonitis in continuous ambulatory peritoneal dialysis. *Clin Nephrol* 15:328–330, 1981.
125. Nolph KD: Peritoneal dialysis. In: BM Brenner, FC Rector Jr, eds, *The kidney,* 3rd ed. WB Saunders, Philadelphia, pp 1875–1877, 1986.
126. Sewell DL, Golper TA, Brown SD, et al.: Stability of single and combination antimicrobial agents in various peritoneal dialysates in the presence of insulin and heparin. *Am J Kidney Dis* 3:209–212, 1983.
127. Loeppky C, Tarka E, Everett ED: Compatibility of cephalosporins and aminoglycosides in peritoneal dialysis fluid. *Perit Dial Bull* 3:128–129, 1983.
128. Krothapalli RK, Senekjain HD, Ayus JC: Efficacy of intravenous vancomycin in the treatment of gram-positive peritonitis in long-term peritoneal dialysis. *Am J Med* 75:345–348, 1983.
129. Williams P, Khanna R, Vas SI, et al.: The treatment of peritonitis in patients on CAPD: To lavage or not. *Perit Dial Bull* 1:12–14, 1980.
130. Digenis GE, Khanna R, Pierratos A, et al.: Morbidity and mortality after treatment of peritonitis with prolonged exchanges and intraperitoneal antibiotics. *Perit Dial Bull* 2:45–46, 1982.
131. O'Leary JP, Malik FS, Donahue RR, et al.: The effects of a minidose of heparin on peritonitis in rats. *Surg Gynecol Obst* 148:51–55, 1979.
132. Gokal R, Ramos JM, Francis DMA, et al.: Peritonitis in continuous ambulatory peritoneal dialysis. *Lancet* 2:1388–1391, 1982.
133. Rubin J, Nolph K, Arfania D, et al.: Follow-up of peritoneal clearances in patients undergoing continuous ambulatory peritoneal dialysis. *Kidney Int* 16:619–623, 1979.
134. Vas SI: Indications for removal of the peritoneal catheter. *Perit Dial Bull* 1:149, 1981.
135. Rault R: Candida peritonitis complicating peritoneal dialysis: A report of five cases and review of the literature. *Am J Kidney Dis* 2:544–547, 1983.
136. Johnson RJ, Ramsey PJ, Gallagher N, et al.: Fungal peritonitis in patients on peritoneal dialysis: Incidence, clinical features and prognosis. *Am J Nephrol* 5:169–175, 1985.
137. Rubin J: Management of fungal peritonitis. *Perspect Perit Dial* 4:10–11, 1986.
138. Khanna R, McNeely DJ, Oreopoulos DG, et al.: Treating fungal infections: Fungal peritonitis in CAPD. *Br Med J* 280:1147–1148, 1980.
139. Kerr CM, Perfect JR, Craven PC, et al.: Fungal peritonitis in patients on continuous ambulatory peritoneal dialysis. *Ann Intern Med* 99:334–337, 1983.
140. Pierratos A: Peritoneal dialysis glossary. *Perit Dial Bull* 4:2–3, 1984.
141. Rubin J, Rogers WA, Taylor HM, et al.: Peritonitis during continuous ambulatory peritoneal dialysis. *Ann Intern Med* 92:7–13, 1980.
142. Mabichak V, Moriarty MV, Cameron EC, et al.: Three and a half year experience with CAPD using the Beta-Cap technique. *Trans Am Soc Artif Organs* 28:253–257, 1982.
143. Fenton SSA, Wu G, Bowman C, et al.: The reduction in peritonitis rate among high risk CAPD patients with the use of the Oreopoulos–Zellerman connector. *Trans Am Soc Artif Intern Organs* 31:560–563, 1985.
144. Bazzato G, Coli U, Landini S, et al.: Continuous ambulatory peritoneal dialysis method without wearing a bag: Complete freedom of patients and significant reduction in peritonitis. *Proc Eur Dial Transpl Assoc* 17:266–274, 1980.
145. Buoncristiani U, Bianchi P, Cozzari M, et al.: A new simple safe connection system for CAPD. *Int J Nephrol Urol Androl* 1:50–53, 1980.
146. Maiorca R, Cantaluppi A, Cancarini GC, et al.: Prospective controlled trial of a Y-connector and disinfectant to prevent peritonitis in continuous ambulatory peritoneal dialysis. *Lancet* 2:642–644, 1983.
147. Nolph KD, Prowant B, Serkes KD, et al.: A randomized multicentric clinical trial to evaluate the effects of an ultraviolet germicidal system on peritonitis rate in continuous ambulatory peritoneal dialysis. *Perit Dial Bull* 5:19–24, 1985.
148. Hamilton RW, Disher BA, Dillingham GA, et al.: The sterile weld, a new method for connection in continuous ambulatory peritoneal dialysis. *Perit Dial Bull* 3:S8–S10, 1983.
149. Ash SR, Hoswell R, Heefer EM, et al.: Effect of the Peridex filter on peritonitis rates in a CAPD population. *Perit Dial Bull* 3:89–93, 1983.
150. Parrott PL, Terry PM, Whitworth EN, et al.: *Pseudomonas aeruginosa* peritonitis associated with contaminated poloxamer-iodine solution. *Lancet* 2:683–685, 1982.
151. Junor BJR, Briggs JD, Forwell MA, et al.: Sclerosing peritonitis: Role of chlorhexidine in alcohol. *Perit Dial Bull* 5:101–104, 1985.
152. Rottenbourg J, Brouard R, Issad B, et al.: Prospective randomized study about Y connectors in CAPD patients. *Perit Dial Bull* 6:S17, 1986.
153. Low DE, Vas SI, Oreopoulos DG, et al.: Randomized clinical trial of prophylactic cephalexin in CAPD. *Lancet* 2:753–754, 1980.
154. Coward RA, Gokal R, Wise M, et al.: Peritonitis associated with vaginal leakage of dialysis fluid in continuous ambulatory peritoneal dialysis. *Br Med J* 284:1529, 1982.
155. Chan MK, Biallod RA, Tanner A, et al.: Abdominal her-

155. nias in patients receiving continuous ambulatory peritoneal dialysis. *Br Med J* 283:826. 1981.
156. Digenis GE, Khanna R, Mathews R, et al.: Abdominal hernias in patients undergoing CAPD. *Perit Dial Bull* 2:115–118, 1982.
157. Rubin J, Raju S, Teal N, et al.: Abdominal hernia in patients undergoing continuous ambulatory peritoneal dialysis. *Arch Int Med* 142:1453–1455, 1982.
158. Cooper JC, Nicholls AJ, Simms AG, et al.: Genital edema in patients treated by continuous ambulatory peritoneal dialysis: An unusual presentation of inguinal hernia. *Br Med J* 286:1923–1924, 1983.
159. Singh S, Vaidya P, Dale A, et al.: Massive hydrothorax complicating continuous ambulatory peritoneal dialysis. *Nephron* 34:168–172, 1983.
160. Grefberg N, Danielson BG, Benson L, et al.: Right-sided hydrothorax complicating peritoneal dialysis. *Nephron* 34:130–134. 1983.
161. Spadaro JJ, Thakur V, Nolph KD: Technetium-99m-labelled macroaggregated albumin in demonstration of transdiaphragmatic leakage of dialysate in peritoneal dialysis. *Am J Nephrol* 2:36–38, 1982.
162. Rudnick MR, Coyle JF, Beck LH, et al.: Acute massive hydrothorax complicating peritoneal dialysis, report of 2 cases and review of the literature. *Clin Nephrol* 12:38–44, 1979.
163. Epstein SW, Inouye T, Robson M, et al.: Effect of peritoneal dialysis fluid on ventilatory function. *Perit Dial Bull* 2:120–122, 1982.
164. Franklin JO, Alpert MA, Twardowski ZJ, et al.: Effect of intraperitoneal infusion volume and posture on left ventricular systolic function in patients on continuous ambulatory peritoneal dialysis. *J Am Soc Artif Intern Organs* 15:49A, 1986.
165. Spencer PC, Farrell PC: Solute and water kinetics in CAPD. In: R Gokal, ed, *Continuous Ambulatory Peritoneal Dialysis*. Churchill Livingstone, Edinburgh, pp 38–55, 1986.
166. Gilmour J, Wu G, Khanna R, et al.: Long-term continuous ambulatory peritoneal dialysis. *Perit Dial Bull* 5:112–118, 1985.
167. Miller FN, Nolph KD, Joshua IG, Weigman DL, Harris PD, Anderson DB: Hyperosmolality, acetate and lactate: Dilatory factors during peritoneal dialysis. *Kidney Int* 20:397–402, 1981.
168. Slingeneyer A, Faller B, Beraud JT: Progressive sclerosing peritonitis: Late and severe complication of maintenance peritoneal dialysis. *Trans Am Soc Artif Intern Organs* 29:633–638, 1983.
169. Rottembourg J, Gahl GM, Piognet JL, et al.: Severe abdominal complications in patients undergoing continuous ambulatory peritoneal dialysis. *Proc Eur Dial Transpl Assoc* 20:236–241, 1983.
170. Bradley JA, McWhinnie DL, Hamiton DNH, et al.: Sclerosing obstructive peritonitis after continuous ambulatory peritoneal dialysis. *Lancet* 2:113–114, 1983.
171. Slingeneyer A, Elie M: Co-operative international study on sclerosing encapsulating peritonitis: Preliminary report. In: R Khanna, KD Nolph, B Prowant et al., eds, *Advances in Continuous Ambulatory Peritoneal Dialysis*. University of Toronto Press, pp 118–123, 1985.
172. Verger C, Brunschvicg O, Le Carpentier Y, et al.: Structural and ultrastructural peritoneal membrane changes and permeability alterations during CAPD. *Proc Eur Dial Transpl Assoc* 18:199–203, 1981.
173. Gahl GM, Von Baeyer H, Averdunk R, et al.: Outpatient evaluation of dietary intake and nitrogen removal in continuous ambulatory peritoneal dialysis. *Ann Intern Med* 94:643–646, 1981.
174. Blumenkrantz MJ, Kopple JD, Moran JK, et al.: Nitrogen and urea metabolism during continuous ambulatory peritoneal dialysis. *Kidney Int* 20:78–82, 1981.
175. Williams P, Marliss E, Anderson GH, et al.: Amino acid absorption following intraperitoneal administration in CAPD patients. *Perit Dial Bull* 2:124–129, 1982.
176. Oren A, Wu G, Anderson GH, et al.: Effective use of amino acid dialysate over 4 weeks in CAPD patients. *Perit Dial Bull* 3:66–73, 1983.
177. Chan MK, Varghese Z, Moorhead JF: Lipid abnormalities in uremia, dialysis and transplantation. *Kidney Int* 19:625–637, 1981.
178. Heaton A, Johnston DG, Burrin JM, et al.: Carbohydrate and lipid metabolism during continuous ambulatory peritoneal dialysis (CAPD): The effect of a single cycle. *Clin Sci* 65:539–545, 1983.
179. Williams P, Kay R, Harrison J, et al.: Nutritional and anthropometric assessment of patients on CAPD over 1 year: Contrasting changes in total body nitrogen and potassium. *Perit Dial Bull* 1:82–87, 1981.
180. Rubin J, Flynn MA, Nolph KD: Total body potassium — a guide to nutritional health in patients undergoing continuous ambulatory peritoneal dialysis. *Am J Clin Nutr* 34:94–98, 1981.
181. Rubin J, Kirchner K, Barnes T, et al.: Evaluation of continuous ambulatory peritoneal dialysis. *Am J Kidney Dis* 3:199–204, 1983.
182. Turgan C, Feehally J, Bennett S, et al.: Accelerated hypertriglyceridemia in patients on continuous ambulatory peritoneal dialysis — a preventable abnormality. *Int J Artif Organs* 4:158–160, 1981
183. Wu G: Osmotic agents for peritoneal dialysis solutions. *Perit Dial Bull* 2:151–154, 1982.
184. Canadian Renal Failure Register: *Kidney Foundation of Canada — 1986 report*, 1987.
185. Wing AJ, Broyer M, Brunner FP, et al.: Combined report on regular dialysis and transplantation in Europe. *Proc Eur Dial Transpl Assoc* 20:2–75, 1983.
186. Hutchison TA, Thomas DC, MacGibbon B: Predicting survival in adults with end-stage renal disease: An age equivalent index. *Ann Intern Med* 96:417–423, 1982.

CHAPTER 51

Dialysis Access Surgery

GEORGE P. NOON & H. DAVID SHORT

INTRODUCTION

To a great degree, the increase in utilization of dialysis has paralleled the development of technically feasible access devices that may be used on a short-term or long-term basis. In this chapter we will summarize the surgical techniques for inserting and maintaining access devices currently available for hemodialysis and peritoneal dialysis. While we will not dwell on the indications for one type of access over another, we will indicate our preferences whenever technical factors bear upon the choice.

From the outset it should be emphasized that renal failure patients on dialysis do not merely require dialysis for their lifetime; they may live only so long as dialysis is available. Efforts should begin with insertion of the first dialysis access device to conserve dialysis access sites. With proper care and foresight, in most patients, dialysis can be provided for many years.

HEMODIALYSIS

Considerable progress has been made in providing devices for angioaccess since the demonstration by Kolff of the clinical feasibility of hemodialysis (1). Early efforts were restricted to cannulation of peripheral vessels with metal or glass cannulas under direct vision. Because the cannulas thrombosed after use and the vessels had to be ligated when the cannulas were removed, dialysis was limited by the number of peripheral vessels available. This in effect meant that only temporary renal failure could be treated.

The introduction in 1960 of the indwelling arteriovenous cannula by Scribner and associates represented the first real long-term device for chronic dialysis (2). At present, angioaccess devices can be roughly divided into those for immediate use and those for delayed use. For the most part, angioaccess devices for immediate use are for patients with acute renal failure where return of renal function may reasonably be expected or for patients with chronic renal failure as a temporary measure until a delayed-use device is available for chronic dialysis. Delayed-use devices make up the majority of access devices used for chronic dialysis.

Acute use

Effective dialysis can be accomplished utilizing cannulas inserted percutaneously into peripheral or central vessels. Early clinical use involved outflow catheters introduced into brachial or femoral arteries, with inflow provided by other catheters introduced into the femoral vein or peripheral arm vein. It later became evident that inflow and outflow could both be provided by percutaneous vein cannulation, avoiding the problems inherent in arterial cannulation.

Percutaneous catheters

Separate cannulas may be used in two different veins for outflow and inflow, or a single, large-bore catheter may be used for both. The large catheters can be inserted directly into the subclavian, internal juglar, or femoral vein over a guidewire using the Seldinger technique (3). Single-lumen catheters provide outflow and inflow alternately with recycle. Double-lumen catheters have one lumen for outflow, with another separate lumen that supplies inflow simultaneously. In our experience, double-lumen catheters achieve superior performance and are currently our access of choice for temporary, immediate hemodialysis (Figure 1).

In addition to short-term use percutaneous catheters for hemodialysis, double-lumen catheters placed through a subcutaneous tunnel are available for long-term or permanent use. These catheters have a subcutaneous cuff of Dacron that allows fibroblastic ingrowth, preventing ascending infection of the catheter tract. These catheters are inserted using a local anesthesia in the operating room under strict sterile conditions. They may be inserted into the central venous circulation either from the subclavian or internal juglar approach (Figure 2). Peel-apart introducer sheaths have greatly facilitated the insertion of these catheters. With increased use of large-bore central venous catheters for hemodialysis, the incidence of central venous stenosis or thrombosis has become more common (4). Problems with upper extremity edema are especially prominent when the obstruction occurs above a functioning arteriovenous fistula. For this reason, the internal

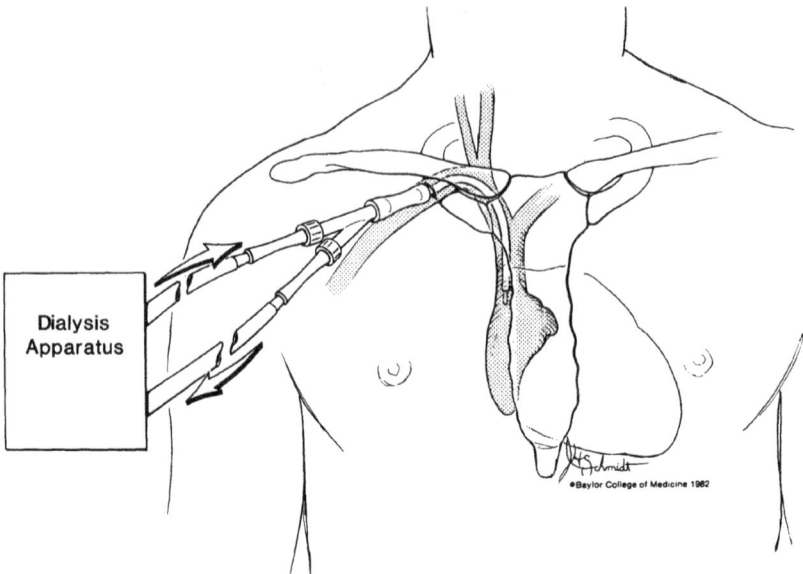

Figure 1. Double-lumen hemodialysis catheter introduced via the right subclavian vein.

jugular vein may theoretically be preferable to the subclavian vein for temporary catheter insertion. The surgical approach to correction of venous obstruction is dealt with later in this chapter.

Shunts

Until the introduction of effective percutaneous venovenous catheters, the silastic arteriovenous shunts were the angioaccess of choice for immediate use.

The most popular of the shunts is the silastic/Teflon shunt described by Scribner (2). This shunt is presently composed of standard-sized silastic tubing with Teflon connectors and Teflon vessels tips of varying sizes and lengths. The tubing is recurved so that peripheral vessles may be cannulated very distal in the extremity where they are more superficial, but the shunt will not interfere with motion in the wrist or ankle. The outflow of this shunt is provided by direct cannulation of a peripheral artery just proximal to be wrist or ankle, and inflow through another cannular in a suitable peripheral vein. These cannulas are connected externally by a Telfon connector, which may be easily disconnected for dialysis.

Because shunts with subcutaneous recurved portions are difficult to thrombectomize if they clot, some people prefer to use straight shunts. These have the disadvantage of encroaching more on the distal joint, so must be placed slightly more proximal (and deeper) in the extremity. In addition, dislodgement is easier with straight shunts. This problem was partially solved by the introduction of a "winged" shunt, such as that described by Ramirez (5).

Insertion of a temporary shunt at the wrist is more convenient for the mobile patient and has the advantage of better arterial flow in older patients with arteriosclerotic peripheral vascular disease. However, for patients who are immobilized or who may be candidates for chronic dialysis, some consideration should be given to shunts inserted at the ankle. This preserves arm vessels that may be needed later for chronic angioaccess sites. If the arm is used, the shunt is generally placed in the dominant arm so that the chronic device can be placed in the nondominant arm.

OPERATIVE TECHNIQUE (FIGURE 3)

Shunts are easily inserted using local anesthesia. Perioperative antibiotics are not used routinely, but meticulous care of wounds and exit sites is necessary to prevent shunt infection.

In the ankle, the saphenous vein and posterior tibial arteries are generally used for shunts. In the wrist, the radial artery and cephalic vein are usually used. They can often be exposed through the same incision, although it may be more convenient to use two separate incisions if a satisfactory vein is not close to the artery. Since the radial artery is ligated distally, it is essential to determine if ulnar flow alone will be adequate to maintain viability of the hand. The Allen test is useful to evaluate the adequacy of ulnar flow and the presence of an intact palmar arch.

The vein is usually opened first, using a longitudinal incision. It is ligated distally and dilators of up to 4 mm are passed proximally to determine the lumen size and patency. Finally, heparinized saline is flushed proximally, both to prevent thrombosis and to estimate the resistence to flow. Undue resistance to saline flushing indicates obstruction to venous outflow. This requires correction to prevent shunt thrombosis. The largest Teflo vessel tip that will easily fit in the vein is selected and inserted into the shunt.

The use of a blunt stilette while inserting the vessel tip into the shunt will help to avoid crimping the tip. The shunt is then flushed with heparinized saline and clamped. Then it is inserted into the vein and tied securely into place. One tie around the vein where the tip is inserted will prevent leaking around the tip. The other tie is placed around the vein and the shunt to prevent dislodgement. Chronic cat-gut ties are used because they dissolve in time, facilitating future shunt removal. This also prevents the

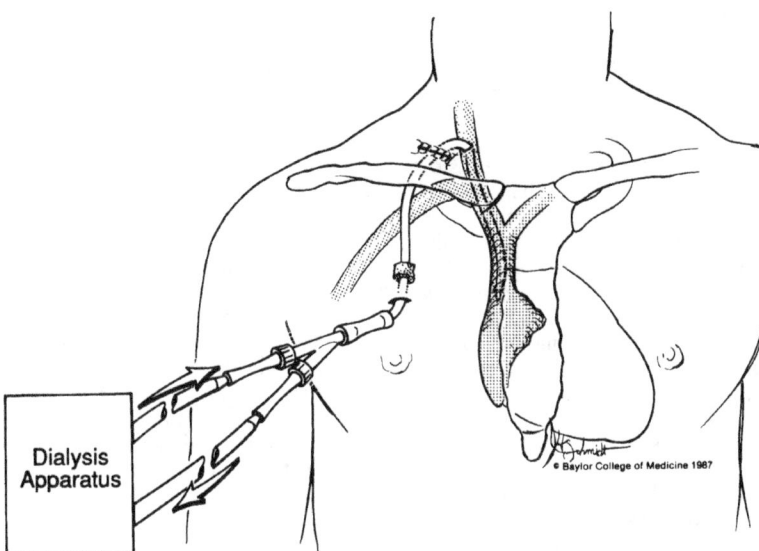

Figure 2. Surgical correction of venous obstruction.

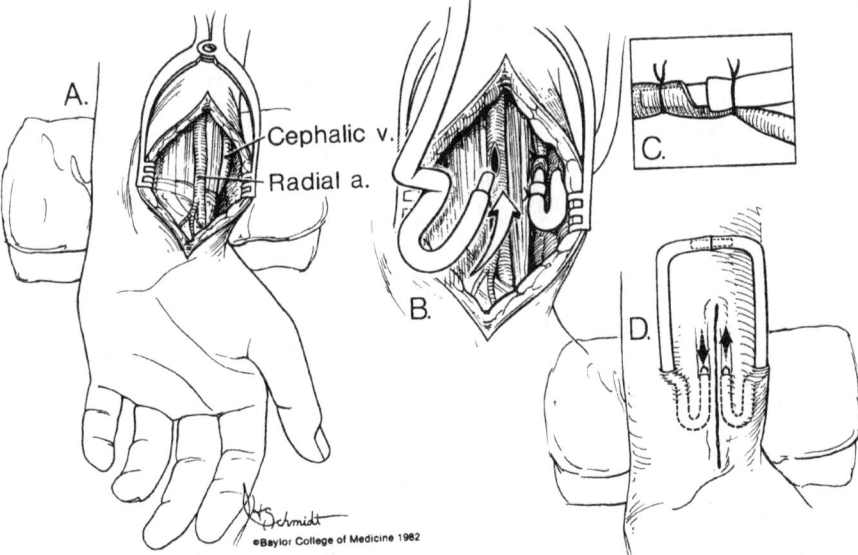

Figure 3. Technique of insertion of hemodialysis cannulas in the radial artery and cephalic vein. A: Artery and vein exposed. B: Cannulas inserted in the artery and vein. C: Cannuals fixed in place with suture ligature. D: Cannulas connected while not dialyzing.

formation of foreign-body granulomas from nonabsorbable sutures. A subcutaneous pocket is then made for the recurved portion of the shunt, and the shunt is brought out through a separate stab wound lateral to the incision. At this point the shunt should be inspected in the subcutaneous pouch to be sure that it is not kinked or twisted. It is flushed once again to ensure free flow and then it is clamped. The arterial limb of the shunt is inserted in an identical manner. Finally, when both limbs of the shunt are in place, they are cut to length such that they lie in a gentle external loop and connect with a Teflon connector. When the clamps are released, prompt flow from the arterial to the venous limb should occur. If hemostasis is adequate, the wounds are then closed in two layers.

Sometimes the vein will be found inadequate at the level at which the artery is exposed. For these cases, shunts of varying configurations (e.g., longer of U shaped) are available. Although they are inserted into the vein in the usual manner, the external portion may be routed differently to connect easily with the arterial limb of the shunt. When removal is required, the shunt is merely clamped for 24 hours to allow the artery and vein to thrombose, then the shunt is pulled out using local anesthesia. Shunts with interchangeable vessel tips should be inspected to ensure that the tip is removed with the tubing. If the vessel tip remains in the vessel, it should be removed, wither through the exit site or, if necessary, by reopening the wound.

Once superficial vessels have been exhausted, shunts may be placed in deeper vessels. Branches of the common femoral artery and vein, such as the superficial circumflex iliac vessels or the superficial eqigastric vessels, may be cannulated directly with straight shunts. If these vessels are too small, special shunts have been devised for use on larger deep vessels that cannot be sacrificed after use. Shunts composed of silastic tubing bonded to Dacron tube grafts may be sutured directly to vessels such as the common femoral artery by means of the graft. Ths silastic tubes exit the skin and are connected externally by means of a Teflon connector. Although insertion and removal of this type of shunt is more complicated, removal does not require sacrifice of the vessels. The grafts are merely reexposed, transected, and oversewn, leaving a short stump of graft attached to the side of the vessel.

COMPLICATIONS

Thrombosis is the most common complication of shunt use. In each case, efforts should be made to establish the exact cause of thrombosis in order to prevent recurrence. Sometimes, the cause is obvious, such as hypotension or inadvertent clamping of the shunt. In this circumstance, simple thrombectomy should be adequate to reestablish patency. Small-caliber (2F or 3F) Fogarty catheters may be used to remove the clot from each limb of the shunt. In recurved shunts, this is facilitated by pulling the recurved portion out of the skin exit site and straightening out the shunt tubing. Because the balloon catheter may not extract all of the clots, copious flushing is employed to remove the remaining clot. We have not encountered any problem from thromboenbolism due to flushing a clotted shunt. Undue resistance to flushing in the venous limb may demonstrate poor run-off to be the cause of shunt thrombosis. When this occurs, revision of the venous limb may be required to maintain a patent shunt. This may require insertion higher in the vein or selection of another vein for venous run-off.

If no obvious cause for shunt thrombosis is apparent, the vessels should be reexposed and the insertion sites examined. Early shunt occlusion may be caused by an intimal flap created by the vessel tip. Late shunt occlusion may be due to hyperplasia or fixed stenosis at the vessel tip. Revision by insertion more proximal in the vessel will then reestablish adequate shunt flow.

Dislodgment

Dislodgment of a shunt can present a serious problem. If the arterial cannula is removed, brisk arterial bleeding will ensue from the open end of the artery. This is easily controlled by direct pressure but necessitates reoperation for reinsertion. Usually, shunts are only partially dislodged, resulting in thrombosis. Passage of thrombectomy catheters will be difficult, and on exploration the reason is evident. Dislodgment is more likely with a straight shunt than a recurved one, and efforts to prevent it with the attachment of subcutaneous "wings" are only partially successful.

Infections

Infections of shunts occur at the skin exit site. Attention to local wound care can delay or prevent this complication. Purulent drainage or cellulitis may respond to local wound care and antibiotics, but in patients who manifest septicemia it is best to remove the shunt. Hemorrhage and shunt dislodgment is more common in the presence of infection.

Chronic use

Although historically shunts were used chronically for hemodialysis, at present most long-term dialysis is achieved by means of arteriovenous fistulas. In the parlance of angioaccess, fistulas differ from shunts in that fistulas are totally internal, where shunts are at least partially external. Fistulas may involve either a direct arteriovenous anastomosis or a conduit of tissue of prosthetic origin. Most require some delay before use is advisable, so immediate use devices are used simultaneously if immediate dialysis is required.

PRIMARY FISTULAS

Direct arteriovenous anastomosis between the radial artery and cephalic vein for dialysis access was first described by Brescia (6). Blood flowing from the radial artery distends the superficial venous system of the arm.

When the veins dilate, they may be used for hemodialysis outflow and inflow by means of needles inserted percutaneously. Since several weeks to months are required for the veins to dilate, they are generally not available for immediate use. An exception to this is when a previously constructed radial-cephalic shunt has been in place long enough for venous dilatation to occur. After direct arteriovenous anastromosis, the veins remain dilated, and immediate dialysis is possible.

Primary arteriovenous fistulas have several advantages over graft fistulas. First, no foreign material except suture is implanted, so infection is rare. Second, patency rates are higher with primary AV fistulas. Finally, primary AV fistulas require very little maintenance. These are such attractive features that we use primary fistulas whenever possible, but proper selection of suitable candidates requires considerable judgement.

If arterial flow into the fistula is inadequate, thrombosis usually occurs. If the flow is only marginal or limited by fixed obstruction, the veins may never dilate enough to be usable. Older patients with arteriosclerosis may not be good candidates for a radial-cephalic fistula for this reason. Likewise, if venous outflow is inadequate, thrombosis usually ensues. Patients who have small arm veins, or whose veins have been obliterated by frequent vein punctures or phlebitis, are not suitable candidates for primary AV fistulas. Also, patients with very fat arms and deep veins are not good candidates for primary fistulas.

Some patients may have inadequate veins in the distal portion of the arm, but adequate veins more proximally. Primary fistulas constructed using the brachial artery and vein have been recommended by some authors, although we would prefer to use a graft in this situation. The key to initial success with primary arteriovenous fistulas is selection of patients with adequate arteries and veins with which to construct satisfactory fistulas.

Operative technique (Figure 4)

Construction of a primary radial-cephalic fistula can be accomplished using local anesthesia supplemented with mild intravenous sedation. A single vertical incision placed between the course of the cephalic vein and radial artery is adequate to expose both vessels. Each vessel is mobilized for several centimeters so that it may be anastomosed without tension. Generally an end-artery to side-vein anastomosis is used, although side-to-side or end-to-end anastomoses may be preferable in some anatomic situations. Whenever contemplating interruption of the radial artery, the existence of an intact palmar arch with normal ulnar flow must be ascertained to prevent ischemia of the hand.

Systemic anticoagulation with 10,000 U of heparin given intravenously is used to prevent clot formation during the creation of the fistula. Topical papaverine is also sometimes employed to reduce vessel spasm, which may make the anastomosis more difficult.

The cephalic vein is clamped distally and opened with a

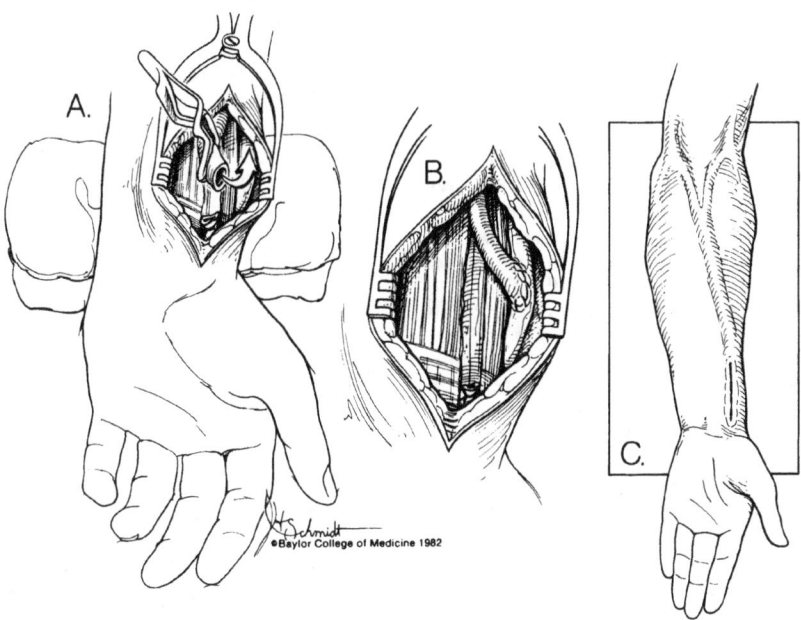

Figure 4. Construction of an arteriovenous fistula for hemodialysis utilizing the radial artery and cephalic vein. A: Radial artery isolated and transected. B: An end-artery to side-vein anastomosis. C: Cephalic vein distends and is used for dialysis.

longitudinal incision. It may not be necessary to clamp the vein proximally if valves prevent backflow. Dilators of up to 4 mm in diameter are gently passed proximally to ensure adequate lumen size and patency. Flushing the vein proximally with heparinized saline will allow estimation of venous resistance. The artery is then clamped proximally, ligated distally, and transected. The artery is splayed open and then anastomosed to the vein using a running 7–0 or 8–0 polypropylene suture and loop magnification. As the suture line is completed, before tying the dilator is again passed proximally in each vessel to ensure patency. The artery and vein are then flushed to remove any clot or debris, then the clamps are removed and the sutures tied. As this point there should be an easily palpable pulse in the vein proximal to the anastomosis, and often there is a palpable thrill. Each of the limbs is checked to be sure that it lies without kinking or undue tension. Protamine sulfate is given to reverse the heparin and then, if hemostasis is adequate, the wound is closed in two layers.

Complications

Complications with primary arteriovenous fistulas are uncommon. Because they are constructed with autogenous tissue, infections almost never occur. When they do, they are usually superficial wound infections and the fistulas continue to function.

Thrombosis. Thrombosis is the most common complication of primary arteriovenous fistulas. If it occurs early, either the vessels were inadequate to support flow or a technical error has been committed. If thrombosis occurs late, obstruction of flow by localized stenosis in the venous system or hyperplasia at the anastomosis should be suspected. Sometimes, in critically ill patients, an episode of hypotension may be enough to cause thrombosis in an adequately functioning fistula. Thrombosis should be corrected as soon as possible, because undue delay may make correction not only more difficult, but impossible. We generally employ systemic heparinization for thrombectomy. These cases may be prolonged and tedious, and this prevents rethrombosis in the limbs after the clot is removed and obviates the need for excessive flushing.

The anastomosis should be exposed and inspected. A twist or kink severe enough to cause thrombosis should be obvious on initial inspection. In any case, the anastomosis will have to be taken down to thrombectomize the afferent and efferent limbs. Since the radial artery has few branches below its origin at the brachial artery, it usually thromboses along its entire length. This thrombus is easily removed with a 3F or 4F Fogarty catheter. A 4F Fogarty catheter has a balloon diameter of 9 mm, generally larger than any radial artery. Care must be taken when using this catheter to not damage the radial artery. Inflow from the radial artery adequate enough to sustain a fistula is easily estimated by merely flushing this vessel.

Generally, thrombosis of a primary fistula is due to poor outflow with increasing venous resistance. After the venous limb has been thrombectomized, it may be checked for stenosis by passing dialtors or a Fogarty catheter proximally or by flushing heparinized saline into the venous limb. Resistance to the flow of saline is a clue to obstruction somewhere in the venous limb. If the exact location of stenosis is not easily determined at the time of surgery, intraoperative venography after thrombectomy may localize the area responsible for thrombosis. Localized areas of venous obstruction may be amenable to patch-graft angioplasty or segmental resection and repair by primary anastomosis or graft interposition. Fistulas that have functioned well for a while but thrombose later are worth strenuous attempts at repair, even if it requires graft interposition in the arterial of venous limbs. If flow can be reestablished in these cases, function can often be restored for prolonged periods. However, primary fistulas that fail very early and require elaborate reconstruction are probably best abandoned in favor of a graft fistula.

Aneurysms. Aneurysms may occur along the course of the venous limb of primary fistulas. These may rarely be true aneurysms due to dilatation of the vein by arterial pressure, or false aneurysms formed by frequent punctures for dialysis. in contrast to graft fistulas, aneurysms of primary fistulas rarely cause problems that require surgical correction.

Venous hypertension

The success of primary arteriovenous fistulas depends upon venous hypertension to dilate proximal veins enough to be used for dialysis. Sometimes, however, the venous dilatation occurs in the distal veins across the dorsum of the hand. Sometimes this may occur without apparent proximal obstruction in the cephalic vein. In these cases, less resistance exists in the distal cephalic vein than the proximal cephalic vein and blood flows preferentially, or at least equally across the hand. Edema of the hand may be quite severe and may produce nonhealing ulcers on the fingers. Ligation of the cephalic vein distal to the anastomosis may be required to relieve the venous hypertension causing the hand edema. Venous hypertension of later onset in a previously well-functioning fistula should alert one to the development of proximal venous stenosis. Palpation of the vein for a pressure differential may localize the area of obstruction. A "fistulogram" performed at this time should reveal the area of obstruction, and timely surgical intervention will not only relieve the obstruction, but also help avoid future thrombosis.

Graft fistula

Although primary fistulas may function satisfactorily for many years, ultimately they, like shunts, are doomed as distal vessels fail. The solution to the problem of inadequate distal peripheral vessels has been aided by the introduction of AV graft fistulas. These large-caliber conduits, placed between more proximal vessels, provide adequate flow for hemodialysis. They are placed subcutaneously, so puncture is easy, and repeated puncture causes no direct damage to the native circulation.

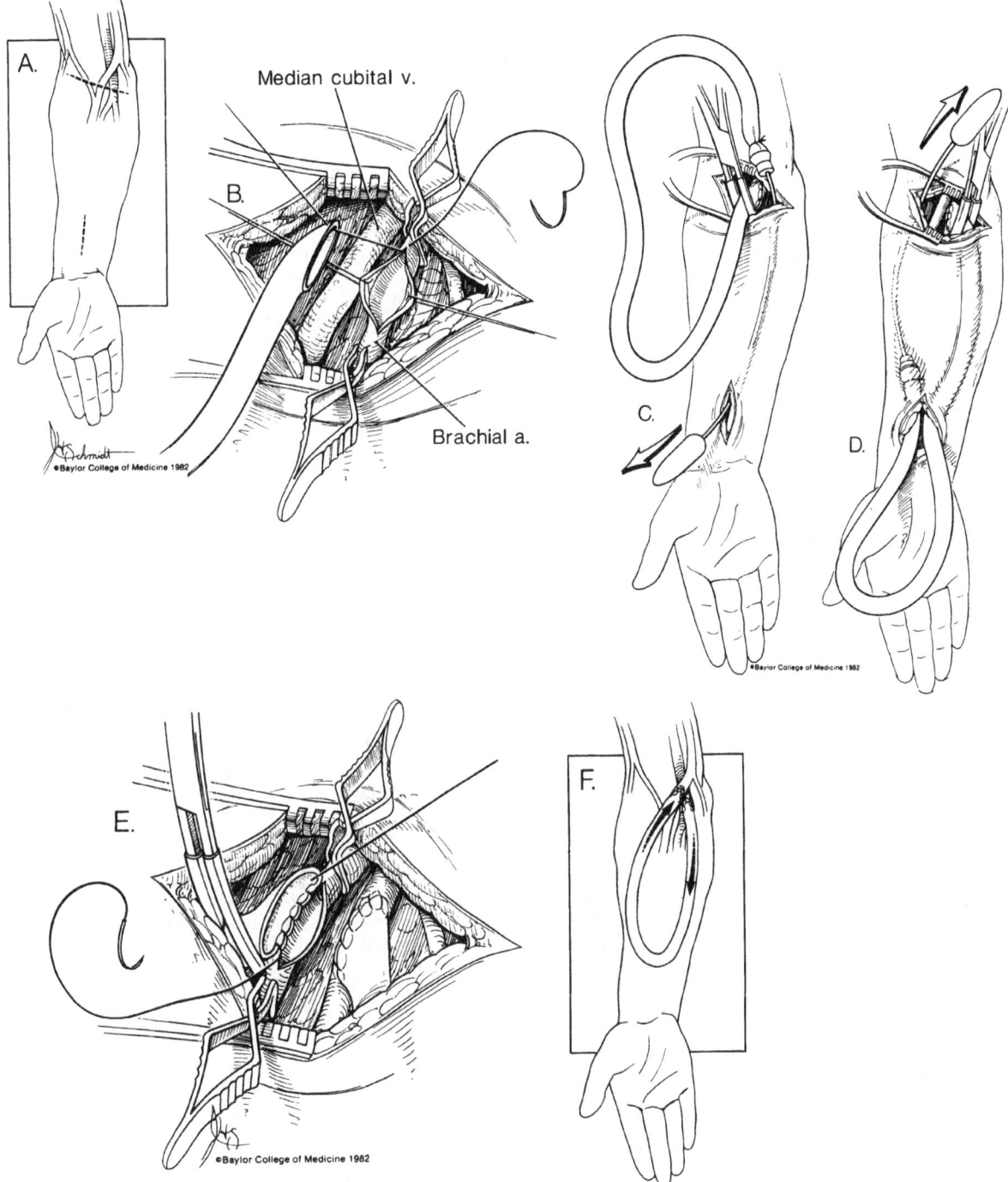

Figure 5. A: Incisions used for implantation of hemodialysis access graft. B: Anastomosis of the graft to the brachial artery. C, D: Graft is tunneled subcutaneously in the forearm. E: Graft is anastomosed to the median cubital vein. F: Functioning graft at completion of the procedure.

Because there is a tunnel through which the graft is placed, early puncture of the graft for dialysis can result in perigraft hematoma, especially if improper pressure after needle removal or poor needle technique is used. For this reason, a period of several weeks is required for graft "maturation." Healing around the graft then prevents dissecting hematomas, leading to graft compression by a false aneurysm. If immediate dialysis is required, it is best supplied by some other access.

Operative technique (Figure 5)

Graft fistulas are inserted in the operating room, using local anesthesia with intravenous sedation. Prophylactic antibiotics with activity against gram-positive organisms are begun before the procedure and continued for several days thereafter. In patients with some renal function, we generally use a cephalosporin antibiotic. They have cidal activity and a low incidence of toxicity or allergy. In patients with no renal function, vancomycin is a good alternative. This drug is nondialyzable, so only one dose is needed; in addition, its major toxicity (nephrotoxicity) is no factor in functionally anephric patients.

Historically, various conduits have been used for graft fistulas: antogenous or homograft veins, Dacron grafts, and bovine grafts (7). Our present choice of graft material is a Gore-Tex straight tube graft (8). This graft is easy to use, readily available, and has low porosity. This last feature is important whenever systemic heparinization is ued for graft insertion. Gore-Tex grafts have demonstrated good patency rates over long periods of time. Grafts allowed to mature show a low incidence of false aneurysm formation and true aneurysms are rare. In addition, graft infections, should they occur, are easier to control with less risk of hemorrhage compared with the other graft materials available. We generally prefer 8 mm grafts, because they are easier to puncture and maintain a larger lumen after neotintima has formed. In patients with very small vessels, the 6 mm graft may be preferable because of less disparity between the graft and vessel diameters.

Grafts are generally placed as loops on the volar aspect of the nondominant forearm. The vessels are exposed through a single transverse incision in the antecubital fossa distal to the flexion crease. Since finding an adequate vein is more often a problem than an adequate artery, this is sought first. The cephalic, basilic, or median cubital veins are used most commonly. If none of these is adequate, the deep brachial veins around the artery are usually adequate.

The brachial artery is exposed by incising the aponeurosis of the biceps muscle, and is mobilized proximally and distally for several centimeters. The arterial anastomosis is usually performed first. The brachial artery is clamped proximally and distally, and opened through a longitudinal arteriotomy. The graft is anastomosed with a running 7-0 Prolene suture. After the suture line is completed, the brachial artery is flushed through the graft to remove any clot of debris. Heparinized saline is then flushed back through the graft, which is then clamped just distal to the anastomosis with a rubber-shod hemostat. At this point, blood flow is reestablished through the brachial artery.

Some authors have recommended sewing the arterial anastomosis on the radial or ulnar artery. If the graft becomes infected, the entire graft can be removed and the vessel sacrificed, if necessary, to control the infection. In our experience, this is a rare circumstance, and cannot justify the decrease in flow caused by the narrow lumen of the radial or ulnar artery.

After infiltrating the path in the arm with xylocaine, the graft is then passed through a subcutaneous loop in the forearm. This is facilitated by making a second incision at the apex of the loop. The graft is first delivered from the incision in the antecubital fossa into the distal incision, then back into the incision in the antecubital fossa near the selected vein. This may be done using a special tunneler or a long, narrow clamp. Care should be taken to avoid kinking or twisting the graft.

With the arterial anastomosis completed first, it is possible at this point to fill the graft with heparinized saline and, compressing the graft distally, to remove the proximal clamp. The arterial pressure will distend the graft filled with heparinized saline. This will demonstrate how the graft will lie when completed, and any kinking or twisting will be obvious. The graft is then flushed again with heparinized saline and reclamped at the distal incision.

The vein is then clamped proximally and distally. It is opened through a longitudinal incision and dilators of up to 4 mm are passed proximally to check for any areas of unsuspected stenosis. Heparinized saline is flushed proximally in the vein. Any resistance to flow should alert one to significant proximal venous obstruction, which could lead to early graft thrombosis. If the vein is satisfactory, the graft is cut to length and sutured to the venotomy with a running 7-0 Prolene suture. When this suture line is completed, the clamps are removed, establishing flow from the brachial artery through the graft into the vein. There is often a palpable pulse or thrill in the vein at this time. The ourflow from the vein may be so good that the graft pulse is very weak. Momentary compression of the vein or graft will then produce an increased graft pulse, demonstrating adequate inflow with low resistance. Other cause of low graft pressure are poor arterial inflow, graft thrombosis, twisting or kinking, and hypotension.

There is generally very little bleeding from the suture line using 7-0 suture. If the hemostasis is adequate, the wounds are then closed over the graft in two layers, completing the procedure.

Complications

Some of the operative techniques for complications differ from those used with the original procedures and need special emphasis. The operative correction of complications of graft fistulas can usually be accomplished using local anesthesia with intravenous sedation. This is performed in the operating room using strict sterile technique. We routinely employ antibiotics directed against gram-positive organisms in the perioperative period. In cases of known infection, we use antibiotics with documented activity against the offending organism. Because the operation may be prolonged or complicated, systemic anticoagulation with heparin is often used. This allows the graft to be clamped at any level without fear of thrombosis and minimizes the blood loss due to flushing. Once reconstruction is accomplished, the heparin is reversed with protamine sulfate to decrease the risk of bleeding or hematoma formation.

Extensive dissection during graft revision may create dead spaces adjacent to the graft. To avoid hematoma formation or perigraft fluid collection, small closed-suction drains are sometimes inserted. These are fashioned from butterfly IV catheters by cutting off the hub and cutting several side holes in the tubing. These are brought out through the wound and the needles are inserted into sterile vacutainer tubes. The drains are removed from the wound whenever drainage ceases, usually about 2 or 3 days later.

Angiograms are employed frequently in the evaluation of graft complications. Edema or high graft resistence by venous obstruction may be diagnosed by angiography. This helps to plan elective revision to relieve edema, and high resistence and may help to prevent graft thrombosis. Intraoperatively, after thrombectomy of a grft, angiography may demonstrate mechanical causes for graft thrombosis that cannot be discerned by other methods. Unusual graft configurations or diffuse venous dilitation can be distinguished from an aneurysm of the graft or native vessels, thereby avoiding unnecessary exploration of what externally appears to be an aneurysm.

Streptokinase. Streptokinase may have a role in the treatment of thrombosis of grafts due to iatrogenic factors. The low porosity of Gore-Tex grafts makes bleeding a remote risk. However, if the graft has occluded spontaneously, streptokinase is contraindicated, because invariably a problem exists in the graft that requires surgical correction.

Noninvasive studies. Noninvasive vascular studies play a part in the differentiation of pain syndromes in the hand and arm, where grafts are implanted. Doppler studies at the wrist or digital pulse volume recordings may demonstrate markedly reduced flow, which augments to normal with temporary graft compression. In the absence of abnormal peripheral nerve studies, this is evidence for a steal syndrome contributing to the symptom of hand pain distal to a dialysis fistula.

Occlusion. Graft occlusion is a common complication of graft fistulas. Thrombosis is most easily dealt with as soon as possible, before the thrombus becomes organized and adherent to the graft. When occlusion occurs early after insertion, technical problems, poor run-off, or hypotension should be suspected. The graft must be examined, and if an obvious technical problem exists, it must be corrected. After thrombectomy, the adequacy of arterial inflow and venous outflow should be reassessed. Poor inflow from the brachial artery should be a rare cause of early graft occulsion. It is easily evaluated by flushing the brachial artery, and it should have been obvious at the time of initial graft insertion. Inflow that was initially brisk but diminished after graft insertion should alert one to the possibility of iatrogenic stenosis or dissection of the brachial artery. Efforts should then be directed toward the detection and correction of these technical errors.

Poor venous outflow may be due to venous narrowing near the anastomosis or more proximal in the vein. Passing dilators proximally in the vein will give an estimation of the lumen of the vein, and flushing heparinized saline proximally can give an appreciation of the impedence to flow. Stenosis of the vein may be correctable with patch angioplasty or may require graft interposition proximally to the same vein or a different vein to establish adequate outflow.

If no obvious cause of early graft occlusion is found, intraoperative angiography of the graft may be performed after thrombectomy renders the graft functional. This may demonstrate areas of stenosis that were not demonstratable by any other means.

Late graft occlusion may be precipitated by obvious causes. Occlusion may result from a period of hypotension in a critically ill patient. Once the cause of hypotension is corrected and the patient is stable, reestablishment of graft patency is easily accomplished by simple thrombectomy.

Thrombosis of a graft can also result from placement of a compression dressing or blood pressure cuff above the graft. Should this occur, simple thrombectomy will again reestablish graft patency.

Early puncture of a Gore-Tex graft can result in perigraft hematoma formation with compression the thrombosis. Before "maturation" of the graft has occurred due to fibroblastic ingrowth, this is a real hazard. We generally allow 2–4 weeks of healing around a graft before use. If hematoma formation with occlusion does occur, the hematoma must be evacuated the thrombectomy of the graft performed.

Prevention of compression occlusion of the graft by bandages or hematoma should be possible by proper education of the medical staff who deal with chronic renal failure patients.

Most late graft occlusions occur without an obvious precipitating event. Reexploration of the graft is necessary, generally exposing the venous anastomosis first (Figure 6). The most common etiology in this circumstance is pseudo-intimal build-up, especially at the venous anastomosis. After the patient is systemically anticoagulated with heparin, the graft is opened just proximal to be venous anastomosis using a longitudinal incision, which may be extended through the anastomosis. The thrombectomy is accomplished with a 5F or 7F Fogarty catheter. Use of a large catheter with only partial balloon inflation is helpful, because the ballon will not be as easily disrupted by the rough inner surface of the graft. Care must be taken to avoid overdistention and injury to native vessels. Dilators may then be passed through the anastomosis and up into the vein to identify any areas of narrowing. Narrowing of the anastomosis due to psuedo-intimal build-up is corrected by patch-graft angioplasty. The incision is extended through the anastomosis and onto the vein past the pseudo-intimal build-up. The Fogarty catherter is passed proximally into the graft to remove the thrombus back to the arterial anastomosis. The graft is flushed to remove any clot or debris and can be clamped, since the patient is systemically heparinized. Finally, the incision is closed using a Gore-Tex patch and running 5-0, 6-0, or 7-0 Prolene suture. Occasionally it will be difficult to pass the Fogarty catheter back to the arterial anastomosis and to adequately thrombectomize the graft. In this case, a second incision is made in the graft, near the arterial anastomosis, and the catheter is then passed in both directions to remove the thrombus material. Control of bleeding from the brachial artery during thrombectomy is easy with simple manual compression. The incision on the arterial limb of the graft, however, should be placed far enough from the arterial anastomosis so that after thrombectomy the graft can be clamped for proximal control. This obviates any need for direct exposure or clamping of the native artery.

If the venous anastomosis and outflow appear adequate, the arterial anastomosis and inflow should be evaluated. Although uncommon, pseudo-intimal build-up at the arterial anastomosis can produce sufficient narrowing to precipitate occlusion. This is corrected by extending the graft incision through the arterial anastomosis and performing a patch-graft angioplasty. Proximal control of the brachial artery in these cases must be established by either exposing the vessel and clamping it directly, or by inserting balloon catheters to occulde the lumen while sewing on the patch.

Whenever a patch-graft angioplasty is performed on the arterial or venous anastomosis, the running suture of the previous anastomosis is obviously divided. This is not a problem in a healing graft, because separation of the graft from the native vessel with false aneurysm formation usually does not occur. However, if possible, the new suture can be tied to the old or interrupted sutures can be placed on either side of the incision and this will secure it. Venous obstruction more proximal in the arm may lead to graft occlusion. Localized areas can sometimes be dilated, or, once identified, be exposed directly and treated with local patch angioplasty. Serial obstructions of long narrow segments in the upper arm vein are best treated by bypass. A Gore-Tex interposition from the venous limb of the dialysis graft to the vein above the obstruction or to another vein in the upper arm will reestablish the outflow. We have experienced no difficulty with graft occlusions due to the interposition grafts extended across the flexion crease of the antecubital fossa.

Infection. Dialysis graft infections may be localized or may involve the entire graft. Before graft maturation occurs, infections often involve the entire length of the graft. These infections may require total graft removal for control, but because fibroblastic ingrowth has not occurred, it may be accomplished relatively easily. After healing around the graft has occurred, infections are often local-

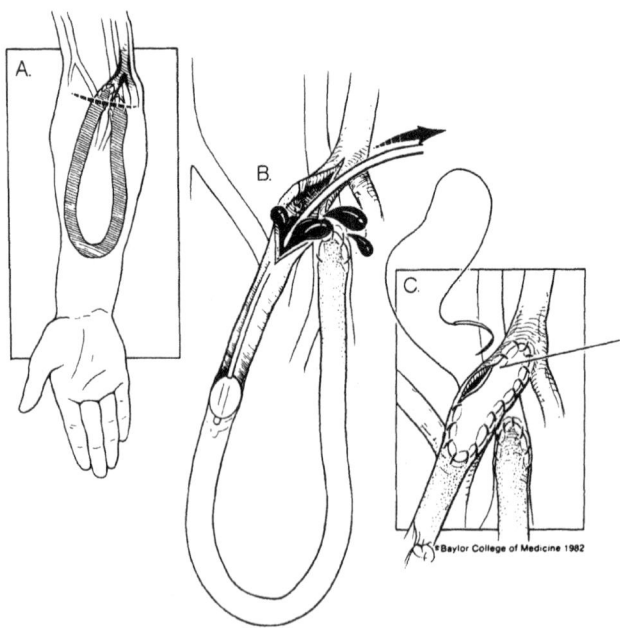

Figure 6. A: Thrombosis of a hemodialysis access graft secondary to intimal hyperplasia at the venous anastomosis. B: Thrombectomy performed. C: Patch-graft angioplasty of the venous anastomosis.

ized by the firm adherence of surrounding tissue to the graft. Thse infections are often at a puncture site or an area of skin breakdown over the graft. If the infection can be controlled by the administration of appropriate antibiotics, the wound may heal over the exposed graft. If healing does not occur, a cure may be accomplished by bypassing the graft through uninfected tissue, then later removing the detached infected piece of graft. This conservative approach to graft infection is really only applicable to polytetrafluroethylene grafts, because biologic grafts have a much greater risk of rupture or hemorrhage. Ultimately, even some Gore-Tex grafts have to be ligated and removed because of bleeding or uncontrollable sepsis.

Aneurysms (Figure 7). Aneurysms are much more common with bovine grafts and vein conduits. False aneurysms can occur with equal frequency, however, in Gore-Tex grafts, especially if used before graft healing has occurred. Aneurysms cause problems of bleeding or graft thrombosis, and are best repaired before complications arise. Segmental resection and graft interposition are usually employed. Proximal and distal control may be gained by direct exposure of the graft on both sides of the aneurysm. An alternative is temporary compression of the graft while the aneurysm is opened directly. Balloon catheters may then be inserted into the graft for proximal and distal control. After gaining control, the aneurysm is resected and a segment of Gore-Tex is interposed using 4-0 Prolene for the anastomosis. Drains may be employed around the graft to avoid fluid collection in the space created by the aneurysm resection.

Steal. When resistance is a very low in an AV graft fistula, diminished flow in the hand may occur. This will be manifested by a cool, pale hand, with diminished or absent radial pulse. Momentary compression of the graft will restore a normal radial pulse, demonstrating the existence of a steal syndrome. Patients may complain of numbness or parathesias in the hand, which must be distinguished from neuropathy or carpal tunnel syndrome. When symptoms occur immediately after graft insertion, they usually improve with time, and expectant treatment is warranted. In a few cases, the graft has to be ligated to relieve the neurologic symptoms or, rarely, reverse ischemic changes in the hand.

Congestive failure. On very rare occasions, flow through a graft fistula will comprise so much of the cardiac output that congestive failure occurs. This is usually in patients with limited cardiac reserve from intrinsic cardiac disease. It may be possible to limit flow through the graft by narrowing the graft or interposing a smaller segment of graft. If this does not suffice, the graft will require ligation and dialysis must be supplied by other means.

Edema. Edema, along with erythema and tenderness, around a newly inserted Gore-Tex graft fistula is common. The swelling may extend into the upper arm and down to

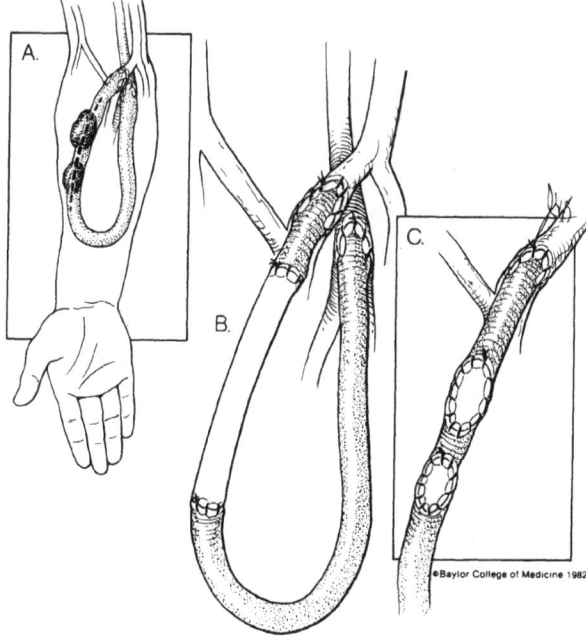

Figure 7. A: Aneurysms of a hemodialysis access graft. B: Resection of aneurysms and graft replacement. C: Resection of aneurysm and patch-graft angioplasty.

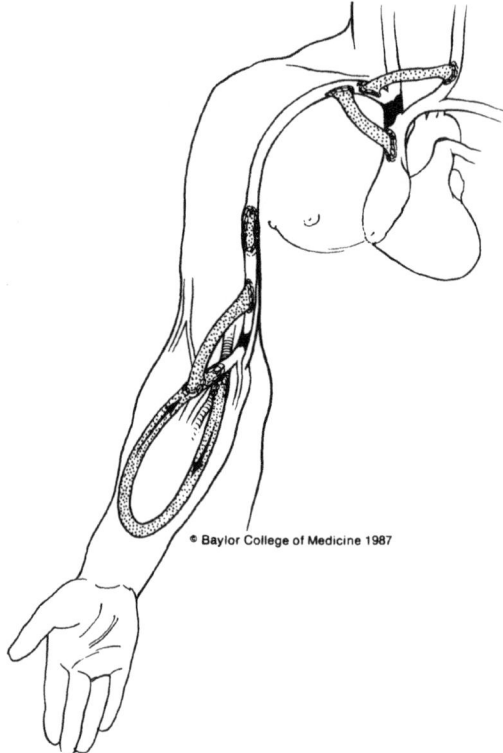

Figure 8. Perm Cath® introduced via the internal jugular.

the hand, and may be accompanied by low-grade fever. This inflammatory reaction usually resolves spontaneously in several weeks, but is aided by elevation of the extremity. Edema that is persistent or appears late is abnormal. Persistent inflammation, high fevers, or purulent drainage may signify infection. A gram stain and cultures should be taken and appropriate antibiotic coverage instituted. Edema without inflammation is rarely due to lymphatic obstruction and may be the first clue to venous outflow obstruction. If allowed to go untreated, severe skin changes, including brawny edema and ulceration, can occur. Graft angiography should be employed to localize areas of venous obstruction.

SURGICAL CORRECTION OF VENOUS OBSTRUCTION

Obstruction to the venous outflow at any level above a functioning arteriovenous fistula can result in severe edema of the extremity below the level of obstruction. The higher the level of venous obstruction, the more of the arm that will be invoved in the edema process. Localized area of stenosis in the arm vein may be treated with patch angioplasty or localized bypasses. Stenosis in the central circulation at the level of the subclavian or innominate vein may require bypasses to other veins in the central venous circulation to correct upper extremity edema. Occasionally a functioning graft will have to be ligated in order to allow the resolution of upper-extremity edema. In spite of the persistent obstruction of the central venous circulation, ligation of the functioning graft normally will provide adequate resolution of edema in the extremity. Edema that has been allowed to progress to severe degrees may be slow to resolve, even after the obstruction has been relieved (Figure 8).

Increased resistance

Increased graft resistance on dialysis may also be an early clue to venous outflow obstruction. If relieved early, graft thrombosis may be averted. Graft angiography is very useful to demonstrate areas of obstruction that may be amenable to correction, either by dilitation or surgery.

Pain

Persistent pain or late development of pain in the hand below a graft fistula is an occasional complaint. Since some of the causes are remediable, it is important to establish the etiology in each specific case. Angiography, noninvasive vascular studies, and nerve conduction studies are helpful to distinguish the various syndrome that may cause pain.

Generalized neuropathy in renal failure patients may cause hand pain. Nerve conduction studies should show decreased nerve conduction in all the nerves in the arm and in the other extremities as well. This type of pain is difficult to treat, and surgery has no role in the therapy.

Accumulating case reports in the literature indicate that carpal tunnel syndrome associated with functioning dialysis fistulas may be more common than is generally appreciated. Hand pain is in the median nerve distribution, and nerve conduction studies show decreased conduction across the wrist. Frequently, the transverse carpel ligament is very thick and densely calcified, but open carpal tunnel release will relieve the pain. It is important to distinguish this syndrome from neuropathy, because proper surgical treatment can provide a lasting cure.

The steal syndrome may produce hand pain that is difficult to distinguish from neuropathic pain. Normal nerve conduction testing along with noninvasive vascular studies that show diminished perfusion identify steal as the probable cause of pain. The pathophysiology and approach to relief of the steal syndrome is described elsewhere in this chapter.

PERITONEAL DIALYSIS

As with hemodialysis, the possibility of dialysis by means of the peritoneal cavity has been known for many years (9), but the popularization of this technique has awaited the development of reliable hardware. Peritoneal dialysis has an advantage over chronic methods of hemodialysis in that it may be used immediately, and also can be used as a chronic dialysis access. Because the dialysate is left in the peritoneal cavity while equilibrium is taking place, the patient is not inseparably linked to the dialysis machine. Finally, because no direct access to the bloodstream is involved, it does not represent as much of a hazard or require quite as rigid supervision.

The device we presently use for peritoneal dialysis is a Tenckhoff catheter with two Dacron cuffs (10). The peritoneal end of the catheter has numerous small holes to facilitate inflow and drainage. The two cuffs are designed to receive fibrobastic ingrowth: one at the fascial level to establish a watertight seal and the other subjacent to the skin to prevent infection along the catheter.

Operative technique (Figure 9)

The catheters are placed with local anesthesia using mild intravenous sedation, but in the operating room, using strict sterile technique. Antibiotic prophylaxis for gram-positive organisms is used routinely. In patients with no prior abdominal surgery, the catheter is placed subumbilically, through a midline incision. If previous surgery has been performed through a lower abdominal midline incision, a paramedian muscle splitting incision or a supraumbilical midline incision may be used. The peritoneal cavity should be opened under direct vision and digital palpation ensures that an adequate free peritoneal cavity exists for catheter insertion. The peritoneal end of the catheter is gently introduced and positioned in the pelvis. This is facilitated by a stilette that is temporarily inserted into the catheter. Once the catheter is positioned, it is irrigated and aspirated to ascertain free flow. Meticulous watertight fascial closure is accomplished using vicryl sutures, catching a stitch or two in the fascial cuff of the catheter to prevent migration. The external end is then brought out a separate stab wound lateral to the incision. This exit site should be placed such that the catheter is not kinked in the subcutaneous tissue, and the superficial cuff is far enough beneath the skin that it will not later erode through the skin. At this point, the catheter is again irrigated to enusre adequate flow, and if it is satisfactory the catheter is capped. The wound is then closed in two layers, completing the procedure.

Local care of the exit site, including daily dressing changes and the use of povidone-iodine ointment, is important to prevent the development of infection of the exit site. This is usually continued at least until healing around the site has occurred (about 7–10 days). Meticulous sterile technique is also important at the connector to prevent the development of peritonitis.

Complications

INFECTION

Infection is one of the most common complications of peritoneal dialysis. This may be a localized infection of the exit site or generalized peritonitis. Because the catheter is a foreign body, infections are frequently difficult to eradicate and are the most common indication for catheter removal. Infections may be caused by gram-positive cocci, gram-negative rods, or fungi. Knowledge of specific pathogens and their antibiotic sensitivities is important in treating the infections if any hope of cure without catheter removal is to be expected.

Patients with peritonitis frequently have high fevers and marked abdominal tenderness. Dialysis may be continued during the episode of peritonitis, and indeed antibiotics may be delivered along with the dialysate. Patients who do not respond to appropriate antibiotics in several days or who have recurrent infections may need to have their catheter removed to control the infection. In our experience, infections due to *Psuedomonas* or *Candida* species usually will not resolve without removing the catheter.

Patients with exit-site infections usually do not manifest systemic symptoms, but if the infection spreads, generalized peritonitis may ensue. Attempts to suppress exit-site

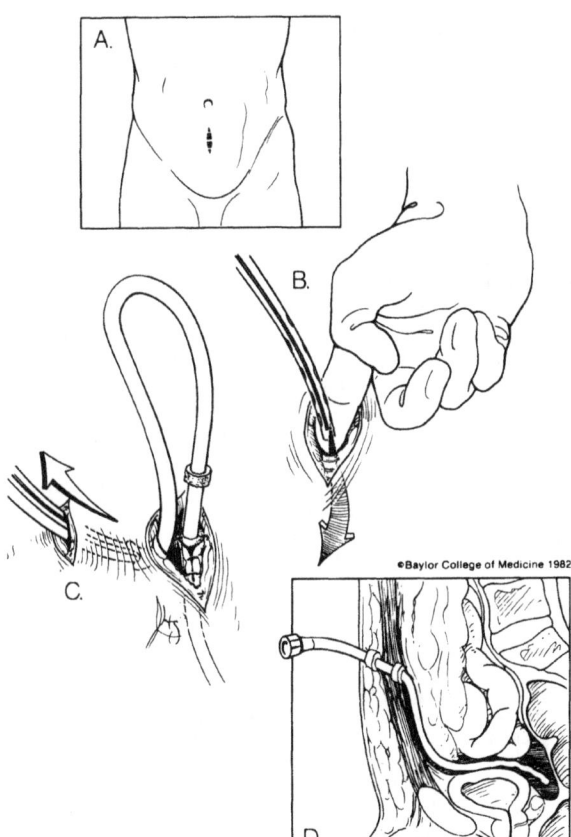

Figure 9. Technique of insertion of a double-cuff peritoneal dialysis catheter. A: Lower abdominal incision. B: Peritoneum entered and digitally explored and catheter inserted into pelvis using a stilette. C: The deep cuff is incorporated in the abdominal closure. The catheter is pulled through a separate stab-wound exit site. D: Position of catheter after completion of the procedure.

infections are worthwhile, but frequently catheter removal is required.

The previous incision is reopened under local anesthesia and the fascia is exposed. The fascial cuff has to be dissected free from the fascia to get the catheter out. The wound is irrigated with povidine-iodine, then closed. We generally prefer to wait several weeks before reinsertion of another peritoneal dialysis catheter after infection has precipitated removal and avoid using the previous incision, regardless of how well healed it appears. If dialysis is required during the waiting period, a subclavian vein catheter for dialysis is inserted.

LEAKING

Secure fascial closure around the catheter is important to prevent leaking during dialysis. Waiting several days before using the catheter is helpful to allow some healing to occur, although this is not always necessary. New catheters that leak may be revised by exploring the incision and placing more fascial sutures to establish a watertight closure. Recurrent leaking or leaking in a chronic catheter is often the first clue to the presence of infection.

POOR OUTFLOW

Poor outflow is a common problem with chronic peritoneal dialysis. Usually the dialysis will flow easily into the peritoneal cavity, but returns slowly or not at all. This can be due to a poor position of the catheter. The catheter position can be checked with a plain x-ray of the abdomen. Sometimes a previously well-placed catheter will be seen to have moved or kinked, presumably as a result of intestinal motility. Contrast injected through the catheter using x-ray or image intensification may demonstrate the cause of poor outflow in catheters that appear well positioned on plain film. In cases where the position of the catheter appears to be acceptable, the holes in the catheter may be occluded by omental fat or by fibrin or protein. Streptokinase infusion may improve the outflow in the later cases, but in the former case repositioning is usually necessary. When repositioning a catheter, it is helpful to go through a separate incision that is lateral to the previous incision used for insertion. In this way, the fascial closure around the catheter and the previously healed wound are not disrupted.

POOR DIALYSIS

Finally, there are some patients who either initially, or later as a result of recurrent peritonitis, have obliteration of their free peritoneal cavity. They do not have enough absorptive surface to dialyze adequately. These patients should be recognized as poor candidates for peritoneal dialysis so that provisions for hemodialysis may be made.

INTESTINAL PERFORATION

Intestinal perforation is fortunately a rare complication of peritoneal dialysis. The use of temporary dialysis catheters with sharp stilettes designed for blind insertion through the fascia make this complication more frequent. However, insertion under direct vision into the peritoneal cavity should not result in this complication. Overzealous attempts to free up the peritoneal cavity by blunt dissection could cause intestinal perforation at the time of insertion, but the soft Teflon catheter used for chronic peritoneal dialysis will not erode into the bowel lumen.

BLEEDING

Bleeding from various sources may be encountered after Tenckhoff catheter insertion. Bleeding at the exit site is usually from small subcutaneous blood vessels and, if clotting studies are normal, is of little significance. Significant bleeding, however, may occur in the peritoneal cavity. Early after surgery it is usually from the incision or from adhesions disrupted during catheter insertion. Later, spontaneous intraperitoneal bleeding can occur, presumably due to the disruption of omental vessels by the catheter. Peritoneal bleeding from any of these cause almost always resolves spontaneously, and reexploration to control hemorrhage is rare.

PAIN

Some patients experience pain during the inflow or outflow of the peritoneal dialysate. For the most part, pain on inflow is the discomfort of distention of the peritoneal cavity. Patients gradually become accustomed to this sensation, and it becomes subjectively tolerable. Pain on outflow is due to catheter impingement upon an intraabdominal viscus or entrapment of omentum in the holes of the catheter. Blind maneuvers to reposition the catheter, such as changing the patient's position, rapid flushing of the catheter, or enemas, may resolve the problem. Contrast material injected through the catheter may show the position of the catheter and the organ involved. Conservative measures are usually successful in resolving this complication, but ultimately, in some patients, surgical repositioning of the catheter may be necessary.

REFERENCES

1. Kolff WJ, Berk HTJ, ter-Welle M, van der Leg JW, van Dijk EC, van Nordwijk J: The artificial kidney: A dialyser with a great area. *Acta Med Scand* 117:121, 1944.
2. Scribner BH, Caner JEZ, Buri R, Quinton W: The technique of continuous hemodialysis. *Trans Am Soc Artif Intern Organs* 12:220, 1966.
3. Uldall PR, Dyck RF, Woods F: A subclavian cannula for temporary vascular access for hemodialysis or plasmapheresis. *Dial Transplant* 8(10):963, 1979.
4. Scheinin, S, Short, HD, Noon, GP: Surgical management of venous complications of dialysis access graft. In preparation.
5. Ramirez O, Swartz C, Onesti G, Mailloux L, Brest AN: The winged in-line shunt. *Trans Am Soc Artif Intern Organs* 12:220, 1966.
6. Brescia MJ, Cimino JE, Appel K, Hurwich BJ: Chronic

hemodialysis using vein puncture and a surgically created arteriovenous fistula. *N Engl J Med* 275:1089, 1966.
7. Lefrak EA, Noon GP: Surgical technique for creation of an arteriovenous fistula using a looped bovine graft. *Ann Surg* 182:782, 1975.
8. Rapaport A, Noon GP, McCollum CH: Ploytetrafluoroethylene (PTEE) grafts for haemodialysis in chronic renal failure. *Aust NZ J Surg* 51:562, 1981.
9. Frank HA, Seligman AM, Fine J: Treatment of uremia after acute renal failure by peritoneal irrigation. *JAMA* 130:703–1946.
10. Striker GE, Tenckhoff H: A transcutaneous prosthesis for prolonged access to the peritoneal cavity. *Surgery* 69:71, 1971.

CHAPTER 52

Dialyzers, Dialysates, and Water Treatment

N.K. MAN & J.L. FUNCK-BRENTANO

INTRODUCTION

The principles underlying hemodialysis are the physical and chemical laws governing mass transfer across semipermeable membranes (1–3). Semipermeable membranes used in hemodialysis allow the passage of low molecular weight (MW) solutes but prohibit transfer of blood proteins and blood cells (4). Solutes are removed from the bloodstream by making appropriate adjustments in the composition of the dialysate (5). Excess water is removed by ultrafiltration resulting from increasing the hydrostatic pressure differences between the blood and the dialysate compartments (6).

Dialyzers are characterized both by their design parameters and by their performance with regard to solute and water removal.

Solute removal

Schematically, a hemodialyzer is composed of a semipermeable membrane separating two compartments in which blood and dialysate flow (Figure 1).

Blood and dialysate flow rates are respectively designated as Q_B and Q_D (cm^3/min), with index i (inlet) and o (outlet), and blood and dialysate solute concentrations as C_B and C_D (g/cm^3) with the same indices.

Mass solute removal from the bloodstream per unit time (N, g/min) may be expressed as the difference between solutes present in the inflowing blood and those in the outflowing blood:

$$N = (Q_{Bi} \cdot C_{Bi}) - (Q_{Bo} \cdot C_{Bo}). \quad (1)$$

If ultrafiltration is negligible, Q_{Bi} and Q_{Bo} may be assumed to be equal, and equation (1) may be simplified as follows:

$$N = Q_B(C_{Bi} - C_{Bo}).$$

Taking into account ultrafiltration (Q_F), which is the difference in volumetric flow rate (cm^3/min) between both streams entering and leaving the dialyzer,

$$Q_F = Q_{Bi} - Q_{Bo} = Q_{Do} - Q_{Di},$$

the solute mass removal can be written

$$N = Q_{Bi}(C_{Bi} - C_{Bo}) - Q_F C_{Bo}.$$

In steady state, the solute mass balance across the dialyzer will be

$$N = Q_{Bi}(C_{Bi} - C_{Bo}) + Q_F C_{Bo} = Q_{Di}(C_{Do} - C_{Di}) - Q_F C_{Do}.$$

It is clear that solute mass transfer can be calculated by two independent sets of measurements, based on either the blood or dialysate concentrations and flow rates.

Clearance (cm^3/min) is defined as the amount of solute removed from the bloodstream per unit of time divided by the inflowing blood concentration:

$$C = \frac{N}{C_{Bi}} \text{ or } C = Q_{Bi}\frac{C_{Bi} - C_{Bo}}{C_{Bi}} + Q_F\frac{C_{Bo}}{C_{Bi}}$$

In terms of dialysance (cm^3/min):

$$D = \frac{N}{C_{Bi} - C_{Di}} \text{ or } D = Q_{Bi}\frac{C_{Bi} - C_{Bo}}{C_{Bi} - C_{Di}} + Q_F\frac{C_{Bo}}{C_{Bi} - C_{Di}}$$

Clearance and dialysance are related as follows:

$$C = D\left(1 - \frac{C_{Di}}{C_{Bi}}\right)$$

For single-pass dialysis, C_{Di} is zero and clearance equals dialysance. In analogy with the natural kidneys (7), clearance is the most meaningful quantity, since it describes the dialyzer as part of the circulatory system.

Mass transfer across a semipermeable membrane is based on two mechanisms, diffusion and convection. Diffusion transport (D_d, g/min) depends on three factors: overall mass transfer of the dialyzer (K_o, cm/min), effective membrane surface area (A, cm^2), and mean concentration difference (c, g/cm^2) for a given solute:

$$N_d = K_o \cdot A \cdot \overline{\Delta C}$$

The overall mass transfer coefficient depends on the resistance to solute transfers (8), not only of the membrane (R_M), but also of the blood film (R_B) and the dialysate (R_D).

The overall mass tranfer resistance (R_o) is equal to the sum of the above resistances:

$$R_o = R_B + R_M + R_D.$$

The average overall mass tranfer resistance, R_o, is the reciprocal of K_o:

In order to improve diffusion mass transfer, individual resistances must be reduced.

R may be reduced by dialyzer design (9), R_D by a high

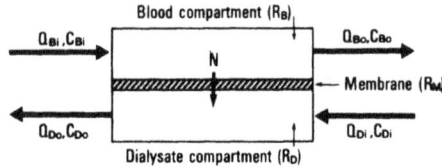

Figure 1. Schematic representation of flows, concentrations, and resistances to solute transport during countercurrent dialysis.

$$R_o = \frac{1}{K_o} = \frac{1}{K_B} + \frac{1}{K_M} + \frac{1}{K_D}$$

dialysate flow rate (10), and R_M by diminishing membrane thickness for a given membrane (11).

Newer membranes, such as polyacrylonitrile (12), polycarbonate (13), and polymethylmethacrylate (14), have low R_M compared to the standard cuprophan membrane (Table 1).

The respective influences of R_B, R_M, and R_D on mass transfer varies greatly according to the molecular weight. For low molecular weight solutes such as urea (60 daltons), R_B and R_D contribute greatly to overall resistance, while the influence of R_M is negligible. On the contrary, for high molecular weight solutes between 1000 and 10,000 daltons, R_M represents nearly the entire overall resistance to diffusion (15).

Fluid removal

Reproducible and controllable removal of excess body water by ultrafiltration is an important function of the dialyzer. The ultrafiltration rate is governed by the following equation:

$$Q_F = K_h \cdot A(\Delta P - \Delta \pi)$$

where Q_F: ultrafiltration rate (cm^3/min)
  K_h: membrane hydraulic permeability (cm^3/min.cm^2.mm Hg)
  A : effective membrane area (cm^2)
  ΔP: hydrostatic transmembrane pressure (mm Hg)
  $\Delta \pi$: effective osmotic pressure difference, essentially oncotic pressure of plasma proteins (25–30 mm Hg)

Mean hydrostatic transmembrane pressure is given by:

$$\Delta P = \frac{P_{Bi} + P_{Bo}}{2} - \frac{P_{Di} + P_{Do}}{2}$$

where P_{Bi} and P_{Bo} are the inlet and outlet blood pressure and P_{Di} and P_{Do} are the inlet and outlet dialysate pressure.

Generally, the desired ultrafiltration rate is achieved by control of the mean transmembrane pressure. In most devices, pressure is monitored at the outlet of the blood and dialysate compartments. Such limited pressure monitoring is accurate, provided the presssure drop in both compartments is low and predictable.

Table 1. Membrane resistance (min/cm) to solute diffusion and hydraulic permeability of standard cuprophan (cellulose), gambrane (polycarbonate), cuprophan F 1 (modified cuprophan) and AN 69 N (acrylonitrile and sodium methallyl sulfonate copolymer) membranes

Solute	MW	Cuprophan st Enka	Gambrane Gambro	Cuprophan F 1 Enka	AN 69 S Hospal
Urea	60	15	14	14	11
Creatinine	113	30	24	16	16
Glucose	180	30	35	—	24
Vitamin B_{12}	1355	256	128	152	71
Inulin	5200	2500	830	286	196
Myoglobin	17,800	—	1111	—	570
Hydraulic permeability (cm^3/H.M^2.mmHg)		1.8	4.1	5.5	29

Table 2. Transmittance coefficient (filtrate/filtrand) for various solutes and hydraulic permeability of the glomerular basement membrane and dialysis membranes

Solute (MW)	Molecular Radius (A)	PMMA Toray	Hemophan HP Enka	AN 69 S Hospal	Polysulfon fresenius	Glomerular basement membrane
Urea (60)	1.6	1.0	1.0	1.0	1.0	1.0
Vitamin B_{12} (1355)	8.6	0.95	0.95	1.0	1.0	1.0
Inulin (5200)	14.8	0.75	0.76	0.95	0.99	0.98
Hydraulic permeability (cm^3/H.M^2.mmHg)		10	22	50	210	190

PMMA = polymethylmethacrylate; Hemophan HP = modified cellulose; AN 69 S = acrylonitrile and sodium methallyl sulfonate copolymer.

The ultrafiltration rate may vary among dialyzers. It reflects the variability in the fabrication of the support structures and of the membrane permeability. The ultrafiltration rate may be nonlinear with increasing pressure because the effective membrane area may change with pressure (16).

In order to eliminate the variables associated with inaccurate ultrafiltration rates, a growing number of dialysate monitors measure the actual ultrafiltration flow rate or remove a predetermined amount of fluid from the patient's blood (17–19).

Ultrafiltration would be expected to increase clearance (20) due to the additional convective component, according to:

$$N_c = Q_h \cdot \bar{C} \cdot T$$

where N_c: convective mass transfer rate (g/min)
  Q_h: ultrafiltration rate (cm^3/min)
  $\bar{C}$: average solute concentration (g/cm^3)
  T : transmittance coefficient (filtrate to filtrand ratio)

The degree of clearance increase depends on the diffusive mass transfer rate to the solute, the ultrafiltration rate, and the transmittance coefficient (Table 2). As the diffusive mass transfer rate decreases at a greater rate than the transmittance coefficient with an increased molecular size, the influence of convection is more significant for larger molecules (21).

For plate dialyzers, there is significant membrane stretching with increasing transmembrane pressure. This results in increased membrane diffusive permeability (22). But membrane stretching may result in more significant membrane masking by the support structure, which reduces the effective membrane area. If the reduction of the effective membrane area is more significant than the increase of the membrane diffuse permeability, the net effect could be a reduction, rather than the expected increase in clearance with increasing ultrafiltration (23).

For hollow-fiber dialyzers, where no support masking can occur, clearance increases with increased ultrafiltration (24).

DIALYZERS

Three types of dialyzers, plate, coil and hollow fiber, are currently in clinical use (Table 3).

Plate dialyzers (Figure 2 and 3)

Plate dialyzers are composed of a variable number of rectangular compartments in a parallel structure separated by rigid support structures. This arrangement provides low compliance of the blood compartment. As blood flow resistance is low, ultrafiltration is predictable and easily controlled.

Early plate dialyzers (Kill type) consisted of three heavy polypropylene boards with longitudinal grooves (25, 26) or with crossing grooves (9, 27) covered by a membrane that formed two large blood compartments. These dialyzers were manually assembled before each dialysis session.

Multilayer plate dialyzers have more recently been introduced. They are supplied ready for use, are sterilized by gamma rays or ethylene oxide, and are intended to be fully disposable (28–30).

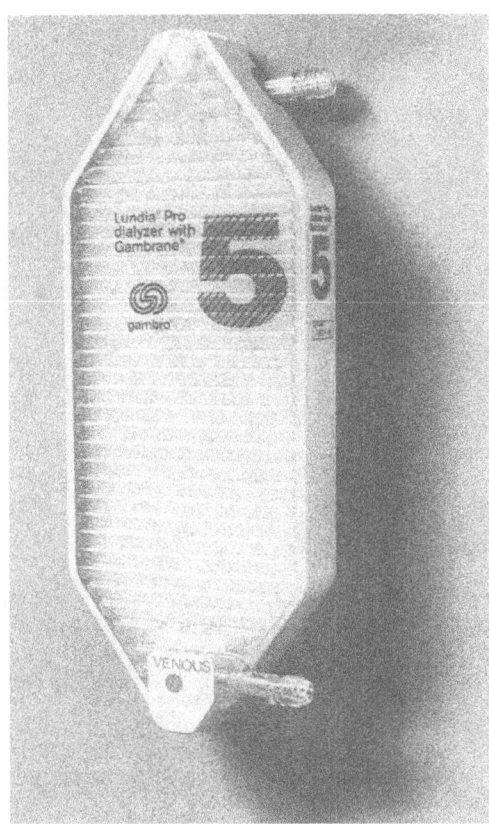

Figure 2. The Gambro Lundia Pro 5 plate dialyzer: 1.1 m^2 Gambrane (polycarbonate), ethylene oxide gas sterilization. Weight: 916 g.

Table 3. In-vito ultrafiltration flow rate and clearance characteristics of typical coil-pate and hollow-fiber dialyzers (effective membrane area = 1 m^2 cuprophran).

Dialyzer	Ultrafiltration flow rate (ml/h.mmHg)	Clearance (ml/min)	
		Urea (60)	Vit. B$_{12}$ (1355)
Coil	5.0	160	35
Plate	4.0	150	35
Hollow fiber	4.0	160	40

Clearance measurements at $Q_D = 500$ ml/min, $Q_B = 200$ ml/min and $Q_F = 10$ ml/min.

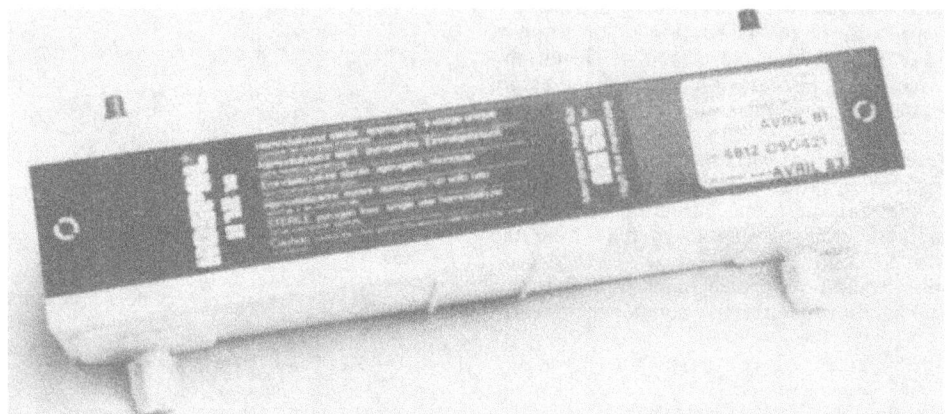

Figure 3. The Hospal H 12–10 plate dialyzer: $1.0\,m^2$ AN 69 (acrylonitrile and sodium methallylsulfonate copolymer), ethylene oxide gas sterilization. Weight: 1300 g.

Coil dialyzers (Figure 4)

The coil dialyzer is made of one or two single-piece lengths of membrane tubing wound concentrically with a mesh supporting screen around a central core. Blood flows through the tubing while dialysate is pumped at a high flow rate (25–30 l/min) perpendicular to the blood flow through the supporting screen, thereby coming into contact with the outside of the blood membrane (31).

Coil dialyzers have a high flow resistance, which necessarily results in a high ultrafiltration rate (32). The blood compartment volume is larger (200–250 ml) than that of either the plate or hollow-fiber dialyzers and is more compliant.

This type of dialyzer has several advantages: high solute dialysance, easy set-up, and easy use.

Hollow-fiber dialyzers (Figures 5–14)

Hollow-fiber dialyzers consist of 10,000–15,000 hollow fibers in a bundle. They have an internal diameter of 200–300 µm and a wall thickness of 10–30 µm. The bundle is encased in a plastic jacket. Due to its high surface area to priming volume ratio, its stable dimensions, and virtual lack of compliance, this design is theoretically the best among the three types of dialyzers (33).

Within the bundle of fibers, blood flows through each fiber, while a countercurrent of dialysate flows around the fibers. This system results in a high mass transfer capacity, low blood flow resistance, and easily controlled ultrafiltration. The dialyzer is also compact and easy to handle. All these advantages combine to make it the most popular dialyzer to date (34).

Large surface area dialyzers and high permeability membrane dialyzers

Large surface area dialyzers and high permeability membrane dialyzers were developed to reduce the weekly

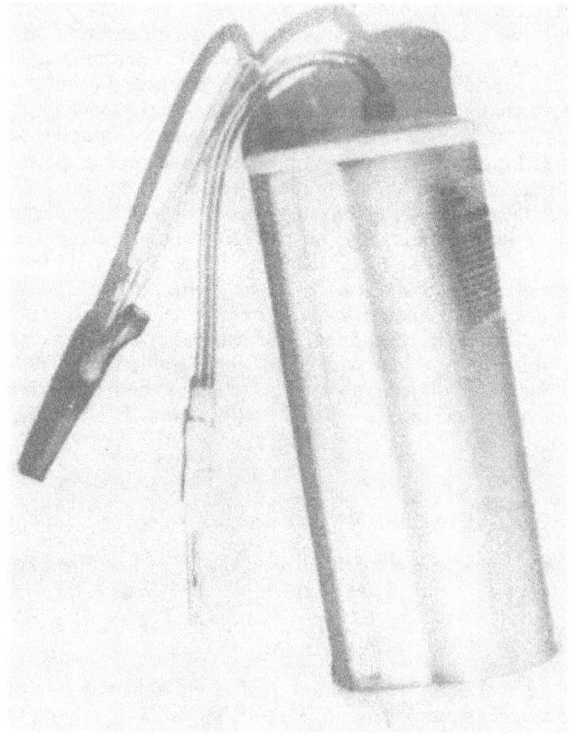

Figure 4. The Travenol 1000 coil dialyzer: $1.0\,m^2$ cuprophan (cellulose), ethylene oxide gas sterilization.

dialysis duration without diminishing the adequacy of dialysis, according to the middle molecule hypothesis (35, 36).

Improved design has allowed the use of a standard

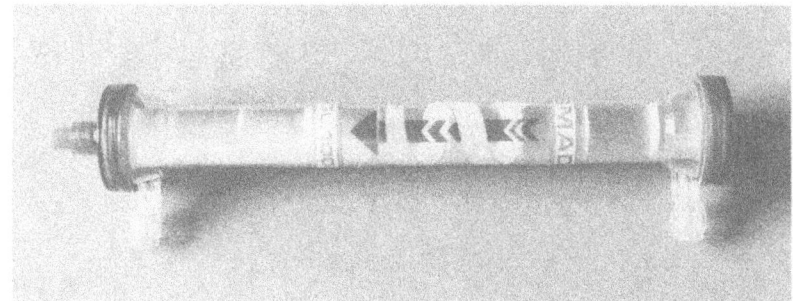

Figure 5. The Smad GL 100 hollow-fiber dialyzer: $1.0\,m^2$ cuprophan $9\,\mu m$ (cellulose), ethylene oxide gas sterilization. Weight: 111 g.

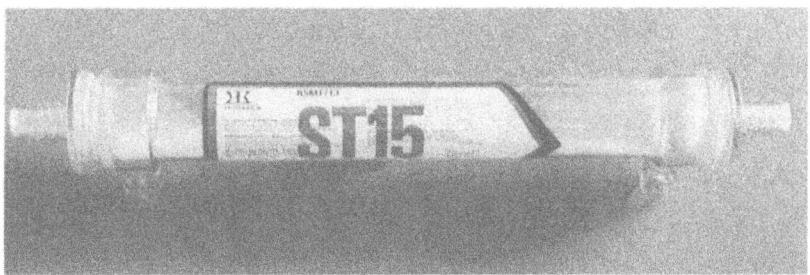

Figure 6. The Travenol ST 15 hollow-fiber dialyzer: $0.9\,m^2$ Cuprophan $8\,\mu m$ (cellulose), ethylene oxide gas sterilization. Weight: 66 g.

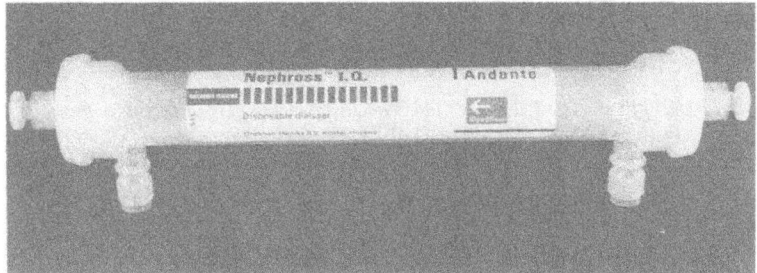

Figure 7. The Organon Teknika Nephross I.Q. Andante hollow-fiber dialyzer: $0.7\,m^2$ cuprophan $8\,\mu m$ (cellulose), ethylene oxide gas sterilization. Weight: 83 g.

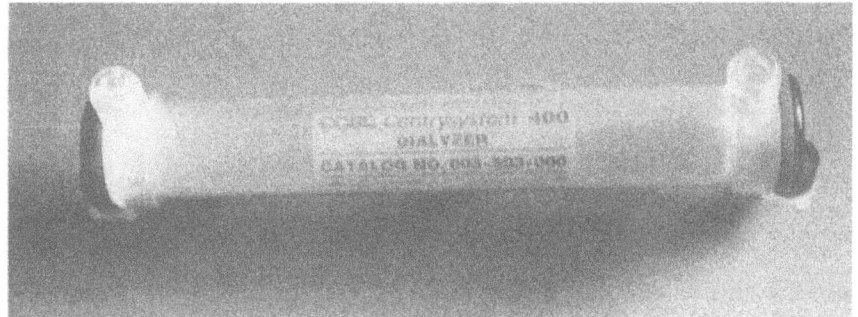

Figure 8. The Cobe Centry System 400 hollow-fiber dialyzer: $1.0\,m^2$ cuprophan $6.5\,\mu m$ (cellulose), ethylene oxide gas sterilization. Weight: 63 g.

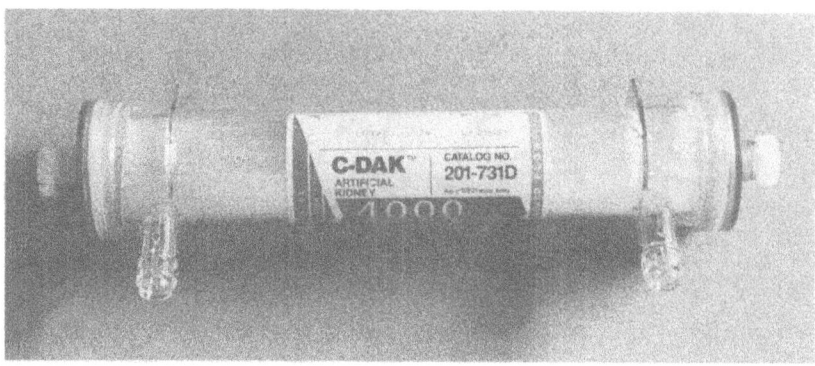

Figure 9. The CD medical CDAK 4000 hollow-fiber dialyzer: 1.4 m² cellulate (cellulose acetate), ethylene oxide gas sterilization. Weight: 206 g.

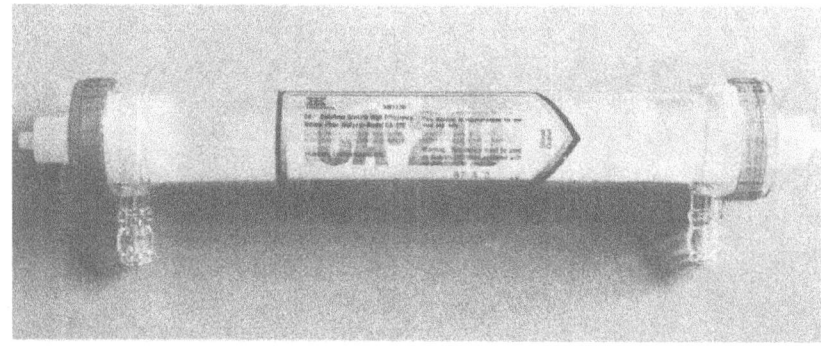

Figure 10. The Travenol CA 210 hollow-fibre dialyzer: 2.1 m² cellulose acetate, ethylene oxide gas and gamma ray sterilization. Weight: 197 g.

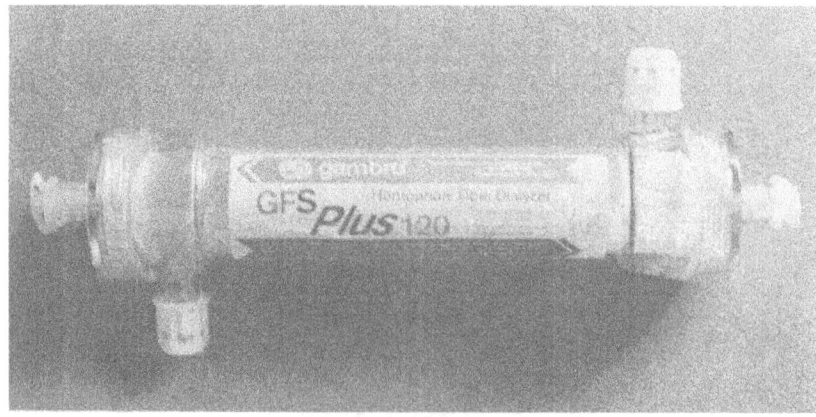

Figure 11. The Gambro GFS Plus 120 hollow-fiber dialyzer: 1.3 m² hemophan (modified cuprophan), steam sterilization. Weight: 204 g.

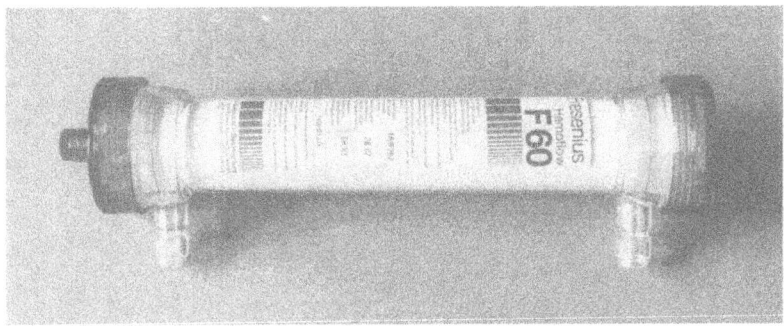

Figure 12. The Fresenius F 60 hollow-fiber dialyzer: 1.3 m² Polysulfon, ethylene oxide gas sterilization. Weight: 232 g.

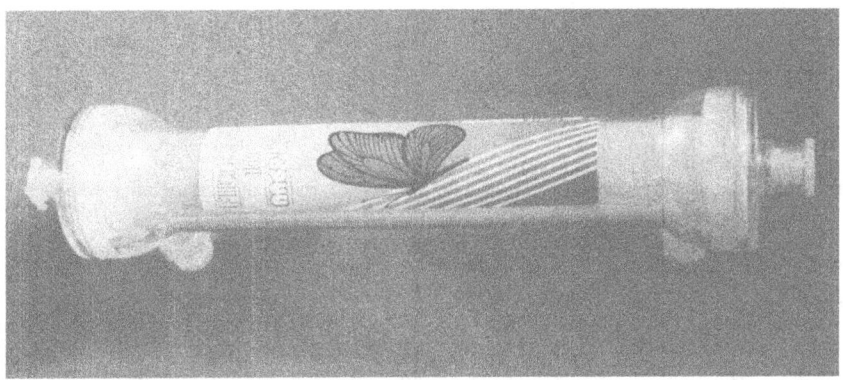

Figure 13. The Hospal Filtral 10 hollow-fiber dialyzer: 1.0 m² AN 69 HF (acrylonitrile and sodium methallylsulfonate copolymer), ethylene oxide gas sterilization. Weight: 206 g.

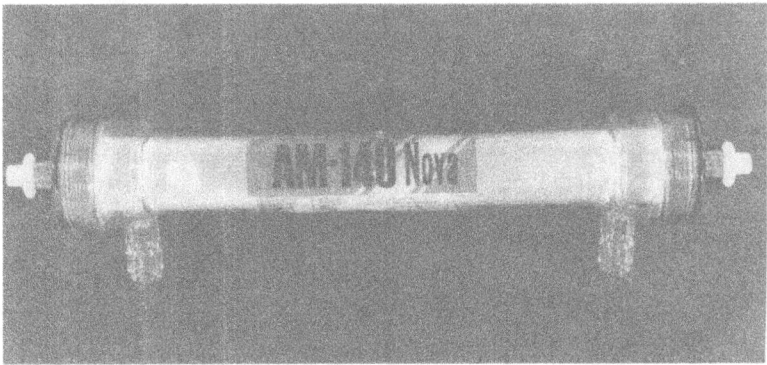

Figure 14. The Asahi AM-140 Nova hollow-fiber dialyzer: 0.9 m² cuproammonium rayonne (cellulose), steam sterilization. Weight: 150 g.

Table 4. Characteristics and performances of high flux dialyzers

Dialyzer model manufacturer	Membrane material	Surface area (m^2)	Priming volume (ml)	Ultra filtration rate (ml/H.mmHg)	Clearance	
					Urea (ml/min)	Vit. B_{12} (ml/min)
Pan 250 Asahi	PAN	1.8	120	27	184	132
Duo flux HP CD Medical	CA	1.8	120	15	171	88
Lundia IC-6 HF Gambro	CU	1.4	169	21	177	88
Filtral 10 Hospal	ANMS	0.9	60	32	165	68
F-60 Fresenius	PS	1.3	75	40	190	125
FB-210 H Nipro	CA	2.1	130	15	197	100
Filtryzer B-l-L Toray	PMMA	2.1	150	20	185	104
CA-210 Travenol	CA	2.1	133	10	198	77

Clearance measurements at QS = 200 ml/min, QD = 500 ml/min, and QF = 10 ml/min.
PAN = polyacrylonitrile; CA = cellulose acetate; CU = cuprophan; ANMS = acrylonitrile and sodium methallyl sulfonate copolymer; PS = polysulfone; PMMA = polymethylmethacrylate.

dialysis membrane with a large surface area and an acceptably low priming volume. This can best be achieved with hollow-fiber dialyzers, which have the lowest priming volume/surface area ratio (37).

Several highly permeable membranes have been manufactured such as acrylonitrile and sodium methallyl sulfonate copolymer (Hospal, France), polymethylmethacrylate (Toray, Japan), high-flux cuprophan (Enka, W. Germany), polyacrylonitrile (Asahi, Japan), polycarbonate (Gambro, Sweden), and polysulfone (Amicon, USA and Fresenium, Germany) membrane. Table 4 gives the characteristics and performances of high flux dialyzers equipped with these membranes that are currently in clinical use. The high hydraulic permeability of these dialyzers necessitates their use in association with monitoring devices that allow the control of the ultrafiltration rate (17–19).

Residual blood volume

Patient blood loss due to residual blood in the extracorporeal circuit should be minimal (38). The residual blood volume depends upon the flow-path geometry of the dialyzer, provided adequate heparinization is achieved, and upon the backwash technique (39, 40).

Considerable progress in blood flow-path geometry has been achieved, and losses are now relatively small (about 1 ml) compared with other sources of blood loss such as bleeding from fistula sites and sampling for biochemical analysis (41, 42).

Dialyzer thrombogenicity

Dialyzers and blood tubings are thrombogenic and require anticoagulation, either of the patient or of the extracorporeal blood circuit (43, 44). Systemic anticoagulation is achieved with heparin, and regional anticoagulation is also achieved with heparin, which is inactivated by protamine prior to blood return to the patient (45). The materials and flow geometry of the dialyzer are the most significant parameters that affect the clotting system. Thrombus formation could be fibrin deposits and/or red-cell inclusions (46). Inadequate heparinization may result in significant thrombus formation, which reduces the membrane surface area and consequently decreases the clearance and ultrafiltration characteristics of the dialyzer (47).

Numerous coagulation tests are used to monitor heparin therapy during hemodialysis (48), such as Lee–White clotting time, plasma-activated partial thromboplastin time, activated whole blood clotting time, and plasma thrombin time (49, 50). A modified coagulation test, the whole-blood-activated partial thromboplastin time, has been found to be a fast and accurate method for monitoring heparin therapy during hemodialysis (51, 52).

Complement activation

Hemodialysis with cellulosic membranes is known to induce transient and marked leukopenia and to activate complement (81–83). Activation of human complement is mainly through the alternative pathway (83). Synthetic membranes, such as polyacrylonitrile, polycarbonate, polysulfone, or modified cellulosic membranes, have appeared to show less effect on leukopenia an complement activation (84–87). It is of interest that cellulosic dialyzers reused after a saline rinse and formalin sterilization protocol have a striking reduction in their tendency to activate complement (88, 89). Complement activation during exposure of plasma to cellulosic dialysis membranes has been postulated to cause leukocyte-mediated hypoxemia in hemodialysis patients through release of the anaphylotoxin C5a, which provokes pulmonary lekuoagglutination (83). In spite of variable degrees of leukopenia, all the patients treated with an acetate-containing dialysis showed, with any type of membrane, a similar and significant hypoxemia, which was progressive throughout the dialysis run (85). The fact that hypoxemia was also found in patients treated with noncellulosic membranes, whether neither leukopenia nor complement activation occurred, does not entirely support this mechanism (90). Moreover, virtual elimination of hypoxemia in patients treated with cellulose dialyzers was demonstrated when using a bicarbonate-containing dialysate (91).

The clinical implications of the transient complement activation found with cellulosic dialysis membranes are not well established. Continuous exposure to these membranes may potentially deplete complement proteins, which in turn may predispose chronic hemodialysis patients to bacterial infections (92). However, there is no drop in titer of any complement component before dialysis, and complement abnormalities are an unlikely explanation for the predisposition of dialysis patients to bacterial infections (85). With the long survival of patients on hemodialysis, repeated release of anaphylatoxins may result, via interleukin-1 overproduction, in long-term complications such as destructive lesions in joints and bones, generation and deposition of abnormal proteins in tissues, and disorders of the immunosuppressive system (93). This could be a factor that influences membrane choice for some patients (94).

First-use syndrome and hypersensitivity during hemodialysis

The first-use syndrome can be defined as a subset of symptoms that occurs during hemodialysis when a dialyzer is used for the first time (95, 96). These reactions are significantly diminished with reuse of the dialyzer (97). Reactions can range from mild to life threatening, and include both hyperesensitivity-related reactions and nonspecific reactions (98).

The hypersensitivity reaction presents as an anaphylacticlike reaction, which starts immediately on the initiation of hemodialysis. Symptoms include nausea, pruritus, urticaria, a sensation of burning or heat throughout the body, flushing, dyspnea, and, in some rare cases, vascular collapse and cardiopulmonary arrest (98, 99). Most of these symptoms can be explained by the release of chemical mediators from circulating basophilic leukocytes and tissue mast cells (101, 102). These reactions are often severe, requiring immediate termination of dialysis and/or administration of antihistamines, epinephrine, or steroids (103).

The nonspecific reactions, commonly chest and back pain, take place during the first hour of dialysis. They are typically mild, and it is usually not necessary to discontinue dialysis (103).

These adverse reactions may be the result of a variety of factors, including the dialyzer manufacturing process and characteristics of the patient. For example, leachable derivatives from cellulosic membrane (104); residues from the manufacturing process for fiber, such as isopropylmyristate and organic solvent; ethylene oxide used for dialyzer sterilization (105–107); endotoxins from contaimined dialysate (108); etc. have been identified as contributive factors.

Changes in the manufacturing process and intensive dialyzer rinsing procedures have been associated with a reduced incidence and/or severity of these adverse reactions (96).

Reuse of dialyzers

Economic considerations have made the reuse of dialyzers desireable, particularly with the introduction of expensive devices, such as large surface area or highly permeable membrane dialyzers (81–83). However, the safety and efficacy of reuse is the subject of some controversy.

There are a great variety of reuse procedures, and analysis of the risks and hazards reported in the literature suggest that the adverse effects observed are specific to a given reuse procedure rather than inherent to reuse per se (84).

The reuse procedure is simple. At the completion of dialysis, the dialyzer and blood tubings are both rinsed with water and/or sodium hypochlorite and sterilized with formaldehyde. The dialyzer and blood tubings, full of sterilant, are then stored at room temperature. Before reuse, the sterilant is drained off of the dialyzer and blood tubings. Then the dialysate compartment is rinsed thoroughly with water. During this sequence the remaining sterilant in the blood compartment is dialyzed. Finally, the blood compartment, including the tubings, are rinsed with 1 l of sterile isotonic saline, and the absence of formaldehyde is verified with a very sensitive reagent such as Schiff's reagent, rather than with a Clinistix® (85). These procedures can be performed either automatically or manually (86, 87).

Among the risks and hazards is the reinfusion into the patient of the residual sterilant and/or the blood products that have reacted with the chemicals used to clean and sterilize the dialyzer, thereby producing undesirable toxic and immunologic reactions in the patient. The immunologic reactions have been demonstrated by the detection of anti-N-like antibodies in the sera of patients who have been on hemodialysis with reused dialyzers sterilized with formaldehyde (88). The incidence of this antibody in

Table 5. Maximum contaminant levels allowed in water used for dialysate preparation

Contaminant	Max. level allowable (mg/l)	
	Ass. for the Advancement of Medical Instr. Proposed standard, 1981	French Pharmacopea 11 ed., 1981
Calcium	2	2
Magnesium	4	1.2
Sodium	70	50
Potassium	8	2
Fluoride	0.2	0.5
Chlorine	0.5	0.1
Nitrate	2	0.2
Sulfate	100	50
Chloramine	0.1	—
Chloride	—	50
Ammonia	—	0.2
Phosphate	—	5
Copper, barium (each)	0.1	—
Zinc	0.1	0.05
Arsenic, lead, silver (each)	0.005	—
Heavy metals	—	0.1
Cadmium	0.001	—
Chromium	0.014	—
Selenium	0.09	—
Tin	—	0.1
Aluminum	0.01	0.03
Mercury	0.0002	0.004

dialysis patients has been implicated in renal allograft failure (89), a shortened red-cell lifespan (90), and clotting of extra-corporeal devices, leading to increased transfusion requirements (91).

WATER FOR HEMODIALYSIS

In most cases, tap water is unsuitable for use in preparing the dialysate (92). Its organic solute and mineral content is both variable and excessive, which may be detrimental for the patient (Table 5).

During dialysis, an excessive concentration of calcium may induce acute hypercalcemia ("hard water syndrome") (93), nitrates and nitrites may induce methemoglobinemia (94), chloramines (95, 96) or copper (97) may provoke hemolysis, excess iron may lead to hemosiderosis (98), excess aluminum to "dialysis encephalopathy" (99, 100), and the presence of pyrogens may provoke febrile reactions (101, 102).

The most complete water treatment system (Figure 15) is composed of a filter to remove particulate material in suspension, an exchange softener to remove calcium and magnesium, an activated charcoal filter to absorb chlorine and organic matter, reverse osmosis to remove most ions, and finally a deionizer to remove residual ions. The final product is pure water.

One of three filters is commonly used for mechanical filtration: a sand filter, a wound cartridge filter, or a membrane filter. Mechanical filtration does not remove dissolved material. While the water flows through the filter, the insoluble particles it contains are collected on the media.

Insoluble particles between 25 and 100 µm can be efficiently collected by sand filters, those in the 5 µm range by cartridge filters, and particles down to 0.2 µm by membrane filters.

Sand filters can be regenerated by backwashing the collected particles. Cartridge filters and membrane filters, however, must be discarded when they become saturated.

Activated charcoal will absorb organic matter, chloramines, chlorine, pyrogens, and odor-producing material from water. However, because of its porosity and its attraction for organic matter, an activated charcoal bed can become the source of bacterial growth and pyrogens.

In ion-exchange softeners, the cation exchange resin is in the sodium ion (Na^+) form. When hard water containing calcium and magnesium salt enters the resin bed, the sodium absorbed to the ion-exchange bed exchanges with the calcium and magnesium on an ion equivalent-weight basis.

In a deionizer, the cation-exchange resin is in the hydrogen ion (H^+) form and the anion-exchange resin is in the hyroxide ion (OH^-) form. As the water enters the resin bed, the N^+, K^+, Ca^{2+}, and Mg^{2+} cations exchange with the H^+ cation on the exchange resins; the Cl^-, HCO_3^-, SO_4^{2-}, and NO_3^- anions exchange with the OH^- anion on the exchange resin; subsequently, the hydrogen and hyroxyl ions combine to form pure water.

The two resin beds can be combined in a mixed resin bed or can be maintained in separate tanks and serve in a series pattern. It is recommended that water for dialysate preparation achieve a resistivity of 1 Mohm-cm after deionization treatment.

Like activated charcoal beds, ion-exchange resin beds introduce the risk of bacterial growth and subsequent pyrogen generation.

Reverse osmosis is a semipermeable membrane and pressure process that repels ions and screens out organic particles while water is fed across the membrane. Pressure forces pure water through the pores of the membrane.

Salt ions are rejected by the reverse osmosis membrane according to their valence. Ninety to 95% of monovalent ions are removed as well as more than 95% of divalent ions. Consequently, when reverse osmosis treatment is used, it should be remembered that up to 10% of these ions will remain in the purified water. To obtain water having a very low salt content for use in dialysate preparation, water treated by reverse osmosis must be polished with deionization.

Organic particles are rejected by the reverse osmosis membrane through another mechanisms, a physical sieving or screening action. Amost all particles of a molecular weight over 200 daltons are rejected by most commercially

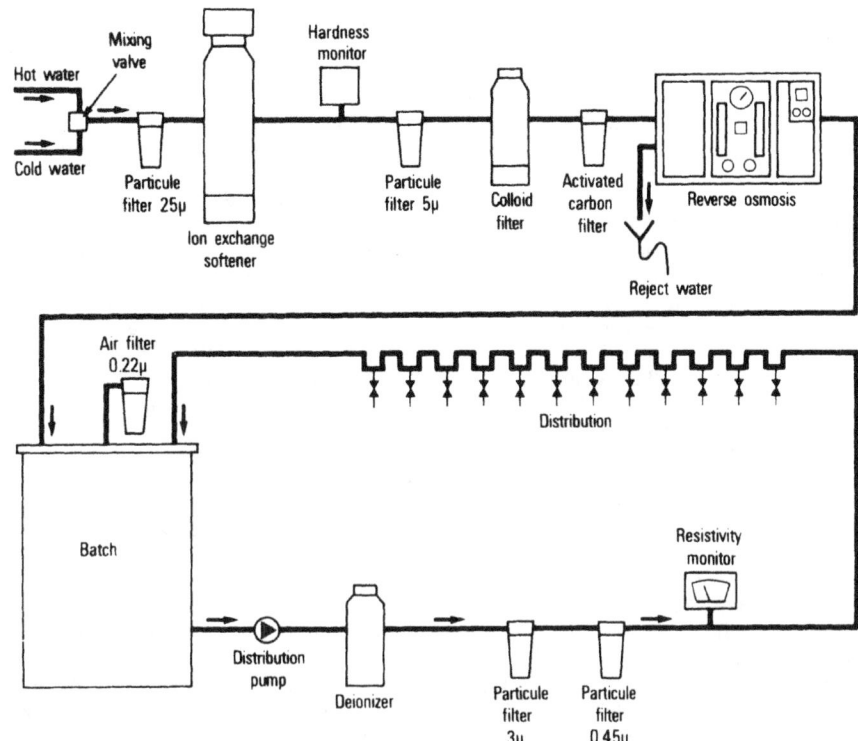

Figure 15. Schematic representation of a typical hemodialysis water treatment system.

available reverse osmosis membranes. This, therefore, includes bacteria, viruses, and pyrogens (103).

Composition of the dialysate

The dialysis fluid or dialysate is essentially an electrolyte solution with a composition similar to that of extracellular fluid. Considerable variation has been advocated in both cation and anion composition in order to correct the abnormalities that develop between dialyses. Table 6 shows the dialysate composition generally used in France with its range variations. The concentration of each electrolyte will be discussed below (104, 105).

Dialysate is prepared from pharmaceutical grade salts and treated water. Salt concentrates are provided in powdered or liquid form. According to their solubility in water, the concentration may be 1:35–1:40 (acetate concentrate or 1:20 (bicarbonate concentrate). A variety of formulas, with and without glucose, are available, according to individuals requirements and the mode of therapy.

A dialysate delivery system delivers dialysate to the hemodialyzer in appropriate conditions of concentration, temperature, pressure, and flow. Monitors and alarms incorporated in the system monitor, in addition to these parameters, fluid removal, blood leak into the dialysate, and air entering the blood line. Dialysate may be prepared as a batch or may be continuously proportioned on line (112).

SODIUM

Sodium is the major component of dialysate and the major determinant of its osmolality. In the early artificial kidney, no membrane support was present, prohibiting ultrafiltration. For this reason, dialysate contains a high concentration of glucose (15 g/l) for fluid removal and a low sodium concentration (130 mM/l) for sodium removal by diffusive

Table 6. A survey of dialysate composition from commercially available dialysate concentrates (France, 1987)

	Dialysate concentration range (mM/l)	
Solute	Acetate dialysis	Bicarbonate dialysis
Sodium	135–145	137–147
Potassium	1–3	0–3
Calcium	1.5–1.75	1.5–2
Magnesium	0.75	0.35–1.5
Chloride	103–118	103–120
Acetate	35–42	2–10
Bicarbonate	0	26–36

processes (5). In current hemodialyzers, fluid is extracted by ultrafiltration, which concomitantly removes water and sodium, as well as other permeable solutes (106, 107). Therefore, the dialysate sodium concentration should be at least similar to the plasma concentration in order to prevent an additive loss of sodium by the diffusive process (108). Since ultrafiltrate is isonatric to plasma, removal of sodium by ultrafiltration may be in excess of sodium intake, which is usually hyponatric to plasma. For example, ultrafiltration of 3 l of fluid will remove about 400 mM of sodium, for a mean sodium concentration in plasma of 137 mM/l. If the patient's sodium intake is 100 mM/day for 3 days, 100 mM of excess sodium is removed. With hyponatric dialysate, essentially all the fluid removed during dialysis comes from the extracellular compartment. This could result in an overreduction of plasma volume with subsequent symptomatic hypotension. Furthermore, fluid shifts from the extracellular compartment to the intracellular compartment, and therefore the total water loss from the extracellular compartment, exceeds the total water loss from the body by ultrafiltration (109). Therefore, hyponatric dialysate is associated with increased symptomatic hypotension. Moreover, a decrease in serum sodium and serum osmolality provokes a disequilibrium syndrome, which is commonly characterized by headaches, muscle cramps, nausea, and vomiting (110–112). With hypernatric dialysate, water is removed from both the intracellular and extracellular compartments and a correction of fluid overload is better achieved (113–121).

Usually, a sodium dialysate concentration of ~ 140 mM/l is sufficient for the removal of 3 l of fluid with minimal dialysis-associated symptoms in almost all dialysis patients.

Actually, the sodium concentration of dialysate should be adapted to each individual in order to match the sodium removal during dialysis to the sodium intake during the interdialytic period. In contrast to fluid intake, which is easily assessed by body weight gain, sodium intake is not readily available. Therefore, it is difficult to determine the dialysate sodium concentration required for each patient. The modeling of sodium and water kinetics during dialysis led to a sodium dialysate concentration that allows adequate sodium and water removal (122–125). Based on this model, the monitoring of the sodium dialysate concentration during dialysis was proposed to achieve this goal. (126, 127).

Careful manipulation of the sodium dialysate concentration is critical for the prevention of dialysis-induced symptoms. This does not exclude other factors such as acetate intolerance, blood-material interactions, or endotoxin transfer from contaminated dialysate (128).

POTASSIUM

Hyperpotassemia occurs often in renal insufficiency. The extracellular concentration of potassium may be a poor reflection of total body stores of this cation, but it is usually the only data available (129, 130).

Potassium accumulation in chronic renal failure is influenced by the rate of endogenous catabolism of protein, the maintenance of cell gradients, and exogenous intake of the cation (131, 132). Potassium is derived from the intake of animal or vegetable cells in food or drink. The average potassium ingestion is 35–100 mEq daily and is subject to random variations. An increase in the serum potassium concentration may be a consequence of a decreased cellular uptake of potassium and/or an increased transfer of potassium from the intracellular to the extracellular compartment, which could be due to hyponatremia, metabolic acidosis, anoxia, and uremic toxicity (133).

Excessive hyperpotassemia should be investigated, not only because it indicates a possible excessive potassium intake, but also to determine the adequacy of dialysis. Insufficient dialysis could influence the acid-base status of the patient and the maintenance of Na-K cell gradients. Therefore, the potassium concentration in the dialysate depends not only on the dietary intake, and the duration and frequency of dialysis, but also on the patient's clinical status.

In the steady state and assuming that daily endogenous potassium is 0.5 mEq/l TBW and exogenous potassium is 1 mEq/kg, 15–20 g of an orally administered cation exchange resin (sodium or calcium polystyrene sulfonate) should be sufficient to maintain potassium balance for a subject of 70 kg body weight (134).

Changes in predialysis and postdialysis plasma concentrations of potassium should be in the range of 4 ± 1 mEq/l to prevent symptomatic hyperpotassemia before dialysis and hypopotassemia after dialysis (135, 136). This could be achieved with a potassium dialysate concentration of 2 mEq/l for a dialysis of 4–5 hours duration. However, a dialysate concentration of potassium up to 3 mEq/l, and even 4 mEq/l, may be necessary when potassium depletion at the end of a dialysis session provokes cardiac arrythmia. This is particularly true in elderly patients with cardiac instability and in those undergoing glycoside treatment for cardiac disorders (137).

CALCIUM

The concentration of calcium in the plasma of patients with chronic renal failure is often reduced, primarily due to diminished absorption of calcium from the intestines (138–140). The impairment of intestinal calcium absorption results from a deficiency in the active vitamin-D metabolite, 1,25-$(OH)_2$ vitamin D_3, and probably also from a relative insensitivity to vitamin D (141, 142). The elevated concentration of plasma phosphate that results from failure of renal excretion is considered to be partly responsible for the lowered serum calcium concentration (143, 144). Finally, systemic acidosis with an increased proportion of plasma ionized calcium may partially counteract the tendency to hypocalcemia but may, on the other hand, unfavorably influence vitamin-D metabolism (145).

Patients on a normal diet have a negative balance because of fecal calcium losses in the range of 1.5 g per week.

Dialysis with a high calcium dialysate concentration

relative to the serum concentration or prescription of oral calcium salt could balance this net loss of calcium. The use of calcium carbonate is of particular interest, since the administration of this compound may be an effective way to control serum phosphorus levels and elicits a steady improvement in the serum concentration of calcium and bicarbonate (146–148). However, attaining a positive calcium balance alone may not be sufficient for the achievement of a normal calcium homeostasis. The addition of the active vitamin-D metabolite, $1,25\text{-}(OH)_2D_3$, which enhances intestinal calcium absorption and modulates the synthesis and secretion of parathyroid hormone, is beneficial in that it leads to better bone mineralization (149–154). Thus, administration of active vitamin D and calcium carbonate seems to be adequate for the treatment of calcium disorders and renal osteodystrophy in dialysis patients. The combined treatment requires close followup, however, because of the risk of hypercalcemia (155–157). The calcium concentration in the dialysate fluid should be high enough to achieve a zero or slightly positive balance during dialysis. Since the diffusible fraction of calcium is approximately 60% of total, and since it is slightly higher in uremic than in healthy subjects, no significant diffusive transfer occurs with a dialysate calcium of 3 mEq/l (1.5 mM/l) (158–161). Moreover, the calcium balance during dialysis may be negative due to calcium loss in the ultrafiltrate. Actually, ultrafiltration for body weight loss causes significant calcium losses, which can be estimated as the ultrafiltrate volume multiplied by the diffusible calcium concentration. For example, ultrafiltration of 3 l of fluid will remove about 8–9 mEq (4–4.5 mM) of calcium for a calcium concentration in serum of 4.5 mM to 5 mEq/l (2.25–2.50 mM/l). Therefore, dialysate calcium concentrations of 3.25–2.5 mEq/l (1.63–1.75 mM/l) are recommended to yield an adequately positive calcium balance (162–165). Raising the dialysate calcium concentration from 3.5 to 4.0 mEq/l (1.75–2.0 mM/l) was not associated with a further benefit in terms of bone disease, and it could induce inappropriate hypercalcemia at the end of dialysis and subsequent complications (166, 167).

ACETATE

Historically, bicarbonate was used in dialysis fluid to correct metabolic acidosis in patients with renal failure (5). Because of the high pH of the solution, which affects the solubility of calcium and magnesium salts, bubbling of CO_2 into the dialysis fluid was necessary to decrease the inital pH of 8.1–8.6 to 7.1–7.6 (168, 169). Furthermore, in the on-line proportioning dialysate delivery system, an extra proportioning pump for bicarbonate is needed, since concentrated bicarbonate solution cannot be mixed with other concentrated salts. To avoid these disadvantages, the substitution of sodium acetate for sodium bicarbonate was proposed as an alternative (170).

After cellular conversion into acetyl-CoA, acetate can be metabolized to carbon dioxide and water, entering the fatty acid synthesis or organic acid production pathways (171, 172). In substituting sodium acetate for sodium bicarbonate, it is presumed that rapid peripheral utilization of acetate results in an equimolar oxidative generation to sodium bicarbonate. According to kinetic studies of serum bicarbonate levels during dialysis with a modified Kiil dialyzer, the concentration of 35 mEq/l was recommended and is still in use at the present time (170).

Acetate metabolism takes place in the liver and in peripheral tissues, predominantly in skeletal muscles. Healthy subjects can metabolize up to 300 mM/hr of acetate (173). The maximum acetate utilization rate in dialysis patients has been estimated to be 3.0–3.5 mM/kg/hr (174). Thus, hyperacetemia develops whenever the transfer rate of acetate from the dialysate exceeds the maximum utilization rate of exogenous acetate. This could be the case in high-efficiency dialysis and/or in patients with a low, lean body mass (175–178). Actually, during hemodialysis, the plasma acetate concentration increase from a normal level of < 1 mM/l to 3–7 mM/l and is normalized within 1 hour after termination of hemodialysis (179). On the contrary, plasma bicarbonate and pCO_2 decrease during dialysis and increase after termination of dialysis. These changes are due to a) the simultaneous transfer of bicarbonate and CO_2 from the blood to the dialysate and the transfer of acetate from dialysate to blood and b) the fact that bicarbonate generation is less rapid than bicarbonate loss, particularly in the case of a high ultrafiltration rate (179–182).

The hypoxemia occurring in the first hour of dialysis could also result from the loss of CO_2 and bicarbonate, which ultimately depresses ventilation (183–186).

A high acetate load has been implicated as a factor in the increase of dialysis-associated signs and symptoms with the use of high-efficiency dialyzers. Acetate itself has a depressant effect upon the cardiovascular system. Vasodilation with a reduction in systemic vascular resistance and diminished myocardial contractility with a reduction in cardiac output can contribute to hypotensive episodes during acetate dialysis (187, 188). Muscle cramps could be triggered by local tissue hypoxemia induced by acetate metabolism (189). However, manipulation of the dialysate sodium concentration has shown that hypotensive episodes and muscle cramps can be prevented, even with an acetate-containing dialysate, provided that the dialysate sodium concentration is adequate (108). Headache, nausea and vomiting are more related to the increased cerebral acidosis resulting from bicarbonate loss and/or production of organic acids in the cerebral tissue during acetate dialysis (190–192). Finally, it has been suggested that hypertriglyceridemia could result from the de-novo synthesis of triglycerides from acetate transferred to the patient from dialysate (193–195). However, other reports indicate that acetate does not play an important role in the genesis of hypertriglyceridemia and that its presence in the dialysate does not significantly affect cholesterol levels (196, 197).

The possible contribution of acetate to acute and long-term complications leads to a renewed interest in bicarbonate as a base replacement in dialysis fluid. Some of this interest is generated by refinement of techniques in the bicarbonate dialysate delivery system. However, standard acetate dialysis still remains popular because it has the advantage of simpler proportioning devices, and a large proportion of ambulatory chronic dialysis patients seem to do well with acetate dialysis.

BICARBONATE

Bicarbonate, as a base repletion agent in dialysis fluid, provides a more physiologic correction of metabolic acidosis than does acetate. In contrast to acetate dialysis, the blood bicarbonate concentration and pH rise gradually during dialysis and an abrupt postdialysis increase is avoided. This results in less dialysis-associated symptomatology and improved patient well-being (198–200).

Dialysis fluid is prepared from two dialysate concentrates, one containing sodium bicarbonate with or without sodium chloride, the other containing all other dialysate constituents and acetic acid. Acetic acid is used to maintain the pH of the final dialysis fluid at about 7.1–7.6 to prevent formation and precipitation of calcium and magnesium carbonate. This precipitation not only changes the dialysate composition, but also impairs proper machine function. This results in complicated hardware and a need for frequent troubleshooting, which in turn decreases the reliability and increases the cost of maintenance.

Usually, liquid bicarbonate concentrate is supplied to give a final concentration in dialysate of 26–36 mM/l, taking into account the amount of sodium bicarbonate consumed by acetic acid for the generation of carbon dioxide. In fact, the bicarbonate concentration in dialysis fluid should be adjusted to the patient's needs. Therefore, careful monitoring of the predialysis serum bicarbonate concentration over weeks or months is important to determine the optimal bicarbonate concentration in dialysate and to prevent acute metabolic alkalosis (201–203).

It is likely that, in long-term acetate dialysis, a chronic base deficit may occur, as bone buffers are used to correct acidosis in the interdialytic period. Furthermore, phosphate release from bone as a buffering agent could participate in increasing the plasma phosphate level. Thus, replacement of bicarbonate dialysis not only corrects the base deficit, but also diminishes phosphate production of endogenous origin. Consequently, bicarbonate dialysis should reduce osteodystrophy, and lower doses of phosphate binder will be needed to control the plasma phosphate concentration (203–205).

Notwithstanding the potential problems encountered with bicarbonate dialysis, which are easily preventable, it is advisable to use bicarbonate-containing dialysate in critically ill patients and in those with adverse reactions related to acetate. In high-efficiency dialysis, bicarbonate dialysis becomes mandatory (204, 205).

MAGNESIUM

Magnesium is concentrated in the intracellular space. The usual magnesium concentration range in plasma is 0.75–1.0 mM/l (1.5–2.0 mEq/l). In the physiologic pH range, about 20% of plasma magnesium is protein bound (206). Although the great majority of ingested magnesium is excreted in the feces, the absorbed magnesium is mainly excreted by the kidneys (207, 208). Absorption of magnesium is reduced in renal failure. However, normal dietary intake results in magnesium retention. An extra source of magnesium, which must be taken into account, is the use of magnesium-containing drugs, such as laxatives or antacids (209). Magnesium excess has been associated with atrioventricular and intraventricular condition abnormalities and nervous system depression, and chronic hypermagnesemia may play a role in renal bone disease and soft-tissue calcification (210). Therefore, it appears desirable to avoid hypermagnesemia, even when it is asymptomatic. Clinical manifestations are generally present for plasma concentration > 2 mM/l (4 mEq/l) (77). Dialysis attempts to reduce hypermagnesemia in renal failure. The magnesium content in dialysate varies, but the effects of various magnesium concentrations in the dialysate have not been clearly elucidated. For example, a low magnesium concentration in the dialysate in the range of 0–0.2 mM/l was used for the improvement of motor nerve conduction velocity, pruritus, and renal osteodystrophy, and a high magnesium concentration of up to 1.25 mM/l was suggested for the suppression of PTH production (211–218). However, the results obtained from the manipulation of the magnesium dialysate concentration were controversal (219). Finally, the concentration commonly used for the majority of patients remains in the range of 0.5–0.75 mM/l (1–1.5 mEq/l), which is the range of the diffusible plasma magnesium concentration in normal adults (220–223).

CHLORIDE

When the concentrations of sodium, potassium, magnesium, and acetate or bicarbonate are chosen, the concentration of chloride in the dialysate is determined according to the electrochemical neutrality of aqueous solutions, where the concentration of chloride anions is equal to the total concentration of cations minus the concentration of acetate of bicarbonate anions. Since the sum of the potassium, calcium, and magnesium concentrations is small (2.5–5.5 mEq/l), the concentration of sodium (135–145 mEq/l) becomes the determinant factor. The chloride concentration in dialysate in current use varies between 105 and 120 mEq/l, and clinical manifestations specifically related to different chloride concentrations in dialysate have not been reported.

GLUCOSE

Hemodialysis is usually performed with a glucose-free dialysate (224, 225). The amount of glucose transferred from blood to the dialysate has been estimated to be 25–30 g for each dialysis (226). The loss of glucose during dialysis may alter plasma glucose, insulin, and several steps of intermediary metabolism (227–230). This could be responsible for dialysis-associated symptoms such as headache, nausea, and postdialysis fatigue (231). Formerly, with devices where hydrostatic pressure could not be applied, glucose was added to the dialysis fluid to provide osmotic pressure for the removal of water. The rationale for the addition of glucose to the dialysis fluid then shifted to the metabolic changes induced by the loss of glucose during dialysis (226). For example, in response to the loss of glucose, hepatic glucogenesis will be enhanced (236). To meet the energy demand of glucogenesis, catabolism of protein and lipid body stores will occur. The loss of amino acids could be as high as 10 g per dialysis session performed without a glucose-containing dialysate, whereas the presence of glucose in dialysis fluid could reduce this loss to 1–3 g. Loss of amino acids into the dialysate and the increased protein catabolism stimulated by the loss of glucose into dialysate could lead to a negative nitrogen balance (232–235). Thus, with glucose-free dialysis, the patient runs the risk of critical hypoglycemia if the catabolism of protein and lipid is impaired in order to meet the glucogenesis demand (237). A diabetic patient undergoing chronic dialysis might be considered particularly susceptible to the glycogenic demands of glucose-free dialysis in that such patients have inadequate endogenous insulin and hyperglycemia (226).

The use of a dialysate containing glucose close to that of normal plasma glucose prevents the hypoglycemia and related symptoms commonly observed in dialysis performed with a glucose-free dialysate (238). Furthermore, dialysis without glucose would adversely affect protein and lipid metabolism (239). However, the major disadvantage of adding glucose is the enhancement of bacteria growth and endotoxin generation, which could provoke adverse reactions, particularly with the use of a highly permeable membrane dialyzer (108).

For patients without glucogenesis disorders and/or with food intake available during dialysis, glucose-free dialysate seems to be well tolerated.

REFERENCES

1. Graham T: Liquid diffusion applied to analysis. *Phil Trans R Soc London* 151:183, 1961.
2. Wolf AV, Remp DG, Kiley JE, Currie GD: Artificial kidney function: Kinetics of hemodialysis. *J Clin Invest* 30:1062, 1951
3. Michaels AS: Operating parameters and performance criteria for hemodialysers and other membrane-separation devices. *Trans Am Soc Artif Intern Organs* 12:387, 1966.
4. Abel JJ, Rowntree LG, Turner BB: On the removal of diffusible substances from the circulating blood of living animals by dialysis. *J Pharmacol Exp Ther* 5:275, 1914.
5. Kolff WJ, Berk HThJ, ter Well M, van der Ley AJW, van Dijk EC, van Noordwijk J: The artifical kidney, a dialyzer with a great area. *Acta Med Scand* 117:121, 1944.
6. Alwall N: On the artificial kidney. I: Apparatus for dialysis of blood in vivo. *Acta Med Scand* 128:317, 1947.
7. Smith HW: *Principles of Renal Physiology*. Oxford University Press, New York, 1956.
8. Leonard EF, Bluemle LW, JR: The permeability concept as applied to dialysis. *Trans Am Soc Artif Intern Organs* 6:33, 1960.
9. Edson HB, Keen ML, Gotch FA: Comparative solute transport and therapeutic effectiveness of multiple point support and standard Kiil hemodialyzers. *Trans Am Soc Artif Organs* 18:113, 1972.
10. Babb AL, Mauer CJ, Fry DL, Popovich RP, McKee RE: The determination of membrane permeabilities with applications to hemodialysis. *Chemical Engineering Progress Symposium Series* 64:59, 1968.
11. Leonard EF, Bluemle LW: Evaluation of dialysis membranes. *Trans Am Soc Artif Intern Organs* 8:182, 1962.
12. Man NK, Granger A, Rondon-Nucete M, Zingraff J, Jungers P, Sausse A, Funck-Brentano JL: One year follow up of short dialysis with a membrane highly permeable to middle molecules. *Proc Eur Dial Trans Assoc* 10:236, 1973.
13. Fisher BS, Highley WS, Cantor PA, Stone W: Modified polycarbonate membranes for hemodialysis. *Trans Am Soc Artif Intern Organs* 19:420, 1973.
14. Ota K. Okazawa J, Kumagaya E, Agishi T, Sugino N, Mitani N, Fugii Y, Kimura M, Nagao Y, Tsukamoto H, Tanzawa H, Sakai Y: Polymethylmethacrylate capillary kidney highly permeable to middle molecules. *Proc Eur Dial Transplant Assoc* 12:559, 1975.
15. Babb AL, Farrell PC, Uvelli DA, Scribner BH: Hemodialyzer evaluation by examinatio of solute molecular spectra. *Trans Am Soc Artif Intern Organs* 18:98, 1972.
16. Mrava G, Weber DC, Malchesky PS, Masuda K, Nose Y: Computerized data analysis of hemodialyzers by a standard protocol shows true effective membrane area. *Trans Am Soc Artif Intern Organs* 16:155, 1970.
17. Funck-Brentano JL, Sausse A, Man NK, Granger A, Rondon-Nucette M, Zingraff J, Jungers P: Une nouvelle methode d'hemodialyse associant une membrane a haute permeabilite pour les movennes molecules et un bain de dialyse en circuit ferme. *Proc Eur Dial Transplant Assoc* 9:55 ff, 1972.
18. Kunitomo T, Lowrie EG, Kumazawa S, O'Brien M, Lazarus JM, Gottlieb MN, Merrill JP: Controlled ultrafiltration with hemodialysis: Analysis of compling between convective and diffusive mass transfer in a new HD-UF System. *Trans Am Soc Artif Intern Organs* 23:234 ff, 1977.
19. Gentile DE: Clinical evaluation of a computerized dialysate-delivery system. *Kidney Int* 18 (Suppl 10):S44 ff, 1980.
20. Klein E (chairman): *Evaluation of Hemodialyzers and Dialysis Membranes*. Artificial kidney chronic uremia program of the National Institute of Arthritis, Metabolism and Digestive Diseases. DHEW Publication (NIH) #77–1294, 1977.
21. Villarrroel F, Klein E, Holland F: Solute flux in hemodialysis and hemofiltration membranes. *Trans Am Soc Artif Intern Organs* 23:225, 1977.
22. Frost TH, Jolly D, Kerr DNS: Effect of membrane grain orientation on in vitro performance of a Kiil dialyzer. *Kidney Int* 3:186, 1973.
23. Nolph KD, Hopkins CA, van Stone JL: Decreases in small solute clearance with ultrafiltration in parallel plate dialyzers. *Clin Nephrol* 8:443, 1977.
24. Gotch FA, Sargent JA, Teisinger CL, Jones PO, Lipps BJ: The hollow fibre artifical kidney (Cordis Dow) 1968–1971. *Proc Eur Dial Transplant Assoc* 8:568, 1971.
25. Kiil F: Development of a parallel flow artifical kidney in plastics. *Acta Chir Scand* 253:143, 1960.
26. Scribner BH, Caner JEZ, Buri R, Quinton W: The technique of continuous hemodialysis. *Trans Am Soc Artif Intern Organs* 6:88, 1960.

27. von Hartitzsch B, Hoenich NA: Meltec multipoint haemodialyzer. *Br Med J* 1:237, 1972.
28. Alwall N: A new disposable artifical kidney: Experimental and clinical experience. *Proc Eur Dial Transplant Assoc* 5:18, 1968.
29. Funck-Brentano J, Sausse A, Vantelon J, Granger A, Zingraff J, Man NK: A new disposable plate-kidney. *Trans Am Soc Artif Intern Organs* 15:127 ff, 1969.
30. Hoeltzenbein J: Efficient and inexpensive no prime, no blood loss haemodialysis system. *Proc Eur Dial Transplant Assoc* 5:316, 1969.
31. Kolff WJ, Watschinger B: Further development of a coil kidney. Disposable artificial kidney. *J Lab Clin Med* 47:969, 1956.
32. Lowrie EG, Hampers CI, Merrill JP; Twin coil: Performance and predictasbility. *Trans Am Soc Artif Intern Organs* 15:60, 1969.
33. Stewart RD, Lipps BJ, Baretta ED, Piering WR, Roth DA, Sargent JA: Short term hemodialysis with the capillary kidney. *Trans Am Soc Artif Intern Organs* 14:121 ff, 1968.
34. Brynger H, Brunner FP, Chantler C, Donckerwolcke RA, Jacobs C, Kramer P, Selwood NH, Wing AJ: Combined report on regular dialysis and transplantation in Europe, X, 1979. *Proc Eur Dial Transpl Assoc* 17:4 ff, 1980.
35. Babb AL, Popovich RP, Christopher TG, Scribner BH: The genesis of the square meter hour hypothesis. *Trans Soc Artif Intern Organs* 17:81 ff, 1971.
36. Man NK, Terlain B, Paris J, Werner G, Sausse A, Funck-brentano JL: An approach to "middle molecules" identification in artificial kidney dialysate, with reference to neuropathy prevention. *Trans Am Soc Artif Intern Organs* 19:320, 1973.
37. Gotch F, Lipps B, Weaver J, Brandes J, Rosin J, Sargent J, Oja P: Chronic hemodialysis with the hollow fiber artificial kidney (HFAK). *Trans Am Soc Artif Intern Organs* 15:87, 1969.
38. Lindsay RM, Burton JA, Edward N, Dargie HJ, Prentice CFM, Kennedy AC: Dialyzer blood loss. *Clin Nephrol* 1:29, 1973.
39. Evans DB, Clarkson Em, Curtiss JR: Blood loss using the modified two layer Kiil dialyser. *Br Med J* 4:651, 1967.
40. Lindsay RM, Burton JA, King P, Davidson JF, Boddy K, Kennedy AC: The measurement of dialyser blood loss. *Clin Nephrol* 2:25, 1973.
41. von Hartitzsch B, Hoenich NA, Samson P, Erickson J, Ashcroft RA, Kerr DNS: A clinical evaluation of the new dialysers. *Kidney Int* 3:35, 1973.
42. Hoenich NA, Kerr DNS: Dialysers. In: JP Maher, (eds): *Replacement of Renal Function by Dialysis*, 2nd ed. Martinus Nihoff, Boston, pp 106–141, 1983.
43. Salzman EW, Deykin D, Shapiro RM, Rosenberg R: Management of heparin therapy. Controlled prospective trial. *N Engl J Med* 292:1046, 1975.
44. Glazier RL, Crowell EB: Randomized prospective trial of continuous vs. intermittent heparin therapy. *JAMA* 236:1365, 1976.
45. Maher JF, Lapierre L, Schreiner GE, Geiger M, Westervelt FB: Regional heparinization for hemodialysis. *N Engl J Med* 268:451, 1963.
46. Mason RG, Wolf RH, Zucker WH, Shinoda WH, Shinoda BA: Dynamics of thrombus formation upon an artificial surface in vivo: Effects of antithrombotic agents. *Am J Path* 82:187, 1976.
47. Farrell PC, Eschbach JW, Vizzo JE, Babb AL; Hemodialyzer reuse: Estimation of area loss from clearance data. *Kidney Int* 5:446, 1974.
48. Congdon JE, Kardinal CG, Wallin JD: Monitoring heparin therapy in hemodialysis. *JAMA* 226:1529, 1973.
49. Zucker S, Cathey MH: Control of heaprin therapy: Sensitivity of the activated partial thromboplastin time for monitoring the antithrombotic effects of heparin. *J Lab Clin Med* 73:320, 1969.
50. Basu D, Gallus A, Hirsh J, Cade J: A prospective study of the value of monitoring heparin treatment with the activated partial thromboplastin time. *N Engl J Med* 287:324, 1972.
51. Blakely JA: A rapid bedside method for the control of heparin therapy. *Can Med Ass J* 99:1072, 1968.
52. Gotch FA, Keen ML: Precise control of minimal heparinization for high bleeding risk hemodialysis. *Trans Am Soc Artif Intern Organs* 23:168 ff, 1977.
53. Kaplow LS, Goffinet JA: Profound neurtropenia during the early phase of hemodialysis. *JAMA* 203:133, 1968.
54. Henderson LW, Miller ME, Hamilton RW, Norman ME: Hemodialysis leukopenia and polymorph random mobility. A possible correlation. *J Lab Clin Med* 85:191, 1975.
55. Craddock PR, Fehr J, Dalmasso AP, Brigham KL, Jacob HS: Hemodialysis leukopenia. Pulmonary vascular leukostasis resulting from complement activation by dialyzer cellophane membrane. *J Clin Invest* 58:879, 1977.
56. Aljama P, Bird PAE, Ward MK, Feest TG, Walker W, Tanboga H, Sussman M, Kerr DNS: Haemodialysis-induced leucopenia and activation of complement. Effects of different membranes. *Proc Eur Dial Transpl Assoc* 15:144, 1978.
57. Jacob AI, Gavellos G, Zarco R, Perez G, Bourgoignie JJ: Leukopenia, hypoxia and complement function with different hemodialysis membranes. *Kidney Int* 18:505, 1980.
58. Chenoweth DE, Cheung AK, Henderson LW: Anaphylatoxin formation during hemodialysis: Effects of different dialyzer membranes. *Kidney Int* 24:764–769, 1983.
59. Man NK, Tien NQ, Lesavre P, Funck-Brentano JL: Leukopenia and complement activation induced by different dialysis membranes. *Contr Nephrol* 37:142–148, 1984.
60. Hakim RM, Lowrie EG: Effect of dialyzer reuse on leukopenia, hypoxemia and total hemolytic complement system. *Trans Am Soc Artif Intern Organs* 26:159, 1980.
61. Chenoweth DE, Cheung AK, Ward DM, Henderson LW: Anaphylatoxin formation during demodialysis: Comparison of new and reused dialysers. *Kidney Int* 24:770–774, 1983.
62. Man NK, Fournier G, Thireau P, Gaillard J, Funck-Brentano, JL: Effect of bicarbonate-containing dialysate on chronic hemodialysis patients. A comparative study. *Artif Organs* 6:421, 1982.
63. Raja R, Kramer MS, Rosenbaum JL, Bolisay CG, Krug MJ: Hemodialysis associated hypoxemia. Role of acetate and pH in etiology. *Trans Am Soc Artif Intern Organs* 27:180, 1981.
64. Hakim RM, Fearon DT, Lazarus JM: Biocompatibility of dialysis membranes: Effects of chronic complement activation. *Kidney Int* 26:194–200, 1984.
65. Dinarello CA: The biology of interleukin-1 and its relevance to hemodialysis. *Blood Purif* 1: 197–224, 1983.
66. Henderson LW, Cheung AK, Chenoweth DE: Choosing a membrane. *Am J Kidney Dis* 3:5–20, 1983.
67. Ogden DA: New dialyzer syndrome. *N Engl J Med* 302:1262–1263, 1980.
68. Villaroel F, Ciarkowski AA: A survey on hypersensitivity reactions in hemodialysis. *Artif Organs* 9:231–238, 1985.
69. Robson MD, Charoenpanich R, Kant KS, Peterson DW, Flynn J, Cathey M, Pollak VE: Effect of first and subsequent use of hemodialyzers on patient well-being. *Am J*

Nephrol 6:101–106, 1986.
70. Daugirdas JT, Ing TS: Classification of first-use reactions. *Int J Artif Organs* 9:194, 1986.
71. Ing TS, Daugirdas JT, Popli S, Gandhi VC: First-use syndrome with cuprammonium cellulose dialyzers. *Int J Artif Organs* 6:235–239, 1983.
72. Foret M, Kuentz F, Meftahi H, Milongo R, Hachache T, Elsener M, Dechelette E, Cordonnier D: Acute anaphylactoid reactions during hemodialysis in France. *Artif Organs* 11:168–172, 1982.
73. Hamilton RG, Adkinson NF: Mechanisms of acute allergic reactions. *Artif Organs* 8:311–317, 1984.
74. Hakim RM, Breillat J, Lazarus M, Port FK: Complement activation and hypersensitivity reactions to dialysis membranes. *N Engl J Med* 311:878–882, 1984.
75. Ing TS, Ivanovich PT, Daugirdas JT: First-use syndrome and hypersensitivity during hemodialysis: Some pieces of the puzzle are falling into place. *Artif Organs* 11:79–81, 1987.
76. Pearson FC, Bohon J, Lee W, Bruszer G, Sagona M, Jakubowski G, Dawe R, Morrison D, Dinarello C: Characterization of limulus amoebocyte lysate-reactive material from hollow fiber dialyzers. *Appl Environ Microbiol* 48:1189–1196, 1984.
77. Dolovich J, Marshall CP, Smith EKM, Shimizu A, Pearson FC, Sugona MA, Lee W: Allergy to ethylene oxide in chronic hemodialysis patients. *Artif Organs* 8:334–337, 1984.
78. Bommer J, Barth HP, Wilhelms OH, Schindele H: Anaphylactoid reactions in dialysis patients: Role of ethylene oxide. *Lancet* 2:1382, 1985.
79. Ciancioni C, Naret C, Picot A, Poignet JL, Delons S, Man NK: Cutaneous hypersenitivity reactions to dialyzer extract and ethylene oxide in hemodialyzed patients. *Proc Eur Dial Transpl Assoc* 22:187–191, 1985.
80. Man NK, Ciancioni C, Guyomard S, Blasis D, Delons S, Funck-Bretano JL: Risks and hazards of contaminated dialysate associated with high flux membrane. In: G Buccianti, *Prevention in Nephrology*, Masson Italia, Milano, pp 227–234, 1987.
81. Shaldon S, Silva H, Rosen SM: Technique of refrigerated coil preservation hemodialysis with fermoral catheterization. *Br Med J* 2:411, 1964.
82. Poliard TL, Barnett BMS, Eschbach HW, Scribner BH: A technique for storage and multiple reuse of the Kiil dialyzer and blood tubing. *Trans Am Soc Artif Intern Organs* 13:24 ff, 1967.
83. Wing AJ, Brunner FP, Brynger HOA, Chantler C, Donckerwolcke RA, Gurland HJ, Jacob C, Selwood NH: Mortality and morbidity of reusing dialysers. *Br Med J* 2:853 ff, 1978.
84. Keshaviah P: Investigation of the risks and hazards associated with hemodialysis devices. US Department of Health Education and Welfare. Public Health Service. *FDA Bureau of Medical Device*. Silver Spring, MD, p 338, 1980.
85. Orringer EP, Mattern WD: Formaldehyde induced hemolysis during chronic hemodialysis. *N Engl J Med* 294:1416, 1976.
86. De Palme JR, Mason B, Abukurah AR: New artificial kidney reuse machine. *Trans Am Soc Artif Intern Organs* 20:584–588, 1974.
87. Man NK, Glace M, Becker A, Di Giulio S, Zingraff J, Funck-Brentano J: A new dialyzer re-use machine. In: Frost TH, ed, *Technical Aspects of Renal Dialysis*. Pitman Medical, London, 1:256, 1978.
88. Kaehny WD, Miller GE, White WL: Relationship between dialyzer re-use and the presence of anti-N-like antibodies in chronic hemodialysis patients. *Kidney Int* 12:59, 1977.
89. Belzer FO, Kountz SL, Perkins HA: Red cell cold autoagglytinins as a cause of failure of renal allotransplantation. *Transplantation* 11:422, 1971.
90. Fassbinder W, Pilar J, Schuermann E, Koch ML: Formaldehyde and occurrence of anti-N-like cold agglutinins in RDT patients. *Proc Eur Dial Trans Assoc* 13:333, 1976.
91. Harrison PB, Jansson K, Kronenberg H, Mahony FJ, Tiller D: Cold agglutinins formation in patients undergoing haemodialysis: A possible relationship to dialysis re-use. *Aust NZ J Med* 5:195, 1975.
92. Comty C, Luchmann D, Wathen R, Shapiro F: Prescription water for chronic hemodialysis. *Trams Am Soc Artif Intern Organs* 20:189, 1974.
93. Freeman RM, Lawton RL, Chamberlain MA: Hard water syndrome. *N Engl J Med* 276:1113, 1967.
94. Carlson DJ, Shapiro GL: Methemoglobinemia from well water nitrates, a complication of home dialysis. *Ann Intern Med* 73:757, 1970.
95. Eaton JW, Koplin CF, Swofford HS, Kjellstrand CM, Jacobs HS: Chlorinated urban water — of dialysis-induced hemolytic anemia. *Science* 181:463, 1973.
96. Kjellstrand CM, Eaton JW, Yawata Y, Swofford H, Koplin CF, Buselmeier TJ, Hartiszsch B, Jacob AS: Hemolysis in dialyzed patients caused by chloramines. *Nephron* 13:427, 1974.
97. Lyle WH: Chronic dialysis and copper poisoning. *N Engl J Med* 276:1209, 1967.
98. Lawson DH, Boddy K, King PC, Linton AL, Will G: Iron metabolism in patients with chronic renal failure on regular dialysis treatment. *Clin Sci Mol Med* 41:345, 1971.
99. Alfrey AC, Legendre GR, Kaehny ND: The dialysis encephalopathy syndrome possible aluminum intoxication. *N Engl J Med* 294:184, 1976.
100. Flendrig JF, Kruis H, Das HA: Aluminum intoxication: The cause of dialysis dementia? *Proc Europ Dial Trans Assoc* 13:355, 1976.
101. Kidd E: Bacterial contamination of dialysing fluid of artificial kidney. *Br Med J* 1:880, 1964.
102. Biangini M, Rindi P. Rizzo G, Giovannetti S: Removal of pyrogens from dialysate of artificial kidney. *Proc Europ Dial Trans Assoc* 7:467, 1970.
103. Madsen RF, Nielsen B, Olsen OJ, Raaschou F: Reverse osmosis as a method of preparing dialysis water. *Nephrorn* 7:545, 1970.
104. Parsons FM, Steward WK: The composition of dialysis fluid. In: W Drukker, FM Parsons, JF Maher, eds, *Replacement of Renal Function by Dialysis*, 2nd ed. Martinus Nijoff Publishers, Boston, pp 148–170, 1983.
105. Port FK: Fluid and electrolyte disorders in dialysis. In: JH Kokko, Tannen, eds, *Fluid and electrolytes*. WB Philadelphia, Saunders, pp 593–618, 1986.
106. Sargent JA, Gotch FA: Principles and biophysics of dialysis. In: M Drukker, F Parsons, eds, *Replacement of Renal Function by Dialysis*, 2nd ed. Martinus Nijhoff, Boston, pp 242–264, 1983.
107. Henderson LW: Biophysics of ultrafiltration and hemofiltration. In: W Drukker, FM Parsons, eds, *Replacement of Renal Function by Dialysis*, 2nd ed. Martinus Nijhoff, Boston, pp 242–264, 1983.
108. Man NK, Sausse A, Di Giulio S, Zingraff J, Drueke T, Jungers P, Funck-Brentano JL. Relationship between Na-free water clearance and asymptomatic high body water clearance and asymptomatic high body weight changes in

hemodialyzed patients. *Artif Organs* 3(Suppl):54, 1979.
109. Van Stone JC, Bauer J, Carey J: The effects of dialysate sodium concentration on body fluid distribution during hemodialysis. *Trans Am Soc Artif Intern Organs* 26:383–386, 1980.
110. Kennedy AC, Linton AL, Luke RG, Renfrew S: Electroencephalographic changes during haemodialysis. *Lancet* 1:408, 1963.
111. Arieff AI, Guisado R, Massry SG, Lazarowitz VC: Central nervous system pH in uremia and the effects of hemodialysis. *J Clin Invest* 58:306, 1976.
112. Port FK, Johnson WJ, Klass DW: Prevention of dialysis disequilibrium syndrome by use of high sodium concentration in the dialysate. *Kidney Int* 3:327, 1973.
113. Steward WK, Fleming LW, Manuel MA: Benefits obtained by the use of high sodium dialysate during maintenance haemodialysis. *Proc Eur Dial Transpl Assoc* 9:111, 1972.
114. Locatelli F, Costanzo R, Di Filippo S, Pedrini L, Marai P, Pozzi C, Ponti R, Sforzini S, Redaelli B: Ultrafiltration and high sodium concentration dialysis: Pathophysiological correlation. *Proc Eur Dial Transpl Assoc* 15:253, 1978.
115. Wehle B, Asaba H, Castenfors J, Furst O, Grahn A, Gunarsson B, Shaldon S, Bergstrom J: The influence of dialysis fluid composition on the blood pressure response during dialysis. *Clin Nephrol* 10:62, 1978.
116. Man NK, Pils P, Di Guilio D, Zingraff J, Drueke T, Jungers P, Funck-Brentano JL: Tolerance to high ultrafiltration rates during closed batch hemodialysis. *Artif Organs* 2:154, 1978.
117. Maeda KS, Kawaguchi S, Kobayashi T, Niwa T, Kobayashi K, Saito A, Iyoda S, Ohta K: Cell wash dialysis. *Trans Am Soc Artif Intern Organs* 26:213–218, 1980.
118. Man NK, Di Giulio S, Zingraff J, Sausse A, Funck-Brentano JL: The role of sodium in the prevention of vascular instability during haemodialysis. *Proc Eur Dial Transpl Assoc* 18:255–261, 1981.
119. Shaldon S, Baldamus CA, Beau MC, Koch KM, Mion CM, Lysaght MJ: Acute and chronic studies of the relationship between sodium flux in hemodialysis and hemofiltration. *Trans Am Soc Artif Intern Organs* 29:641–644, 1983.
120. Murisasco A, France G, Leblond G, Stroumza P, Durand C, Reynier JP, Crevat A, Elsen R: Separation of Na$^+$ and H$_2$O transport during hemodialysis and quantification of high-low NaDi levels during sequential sodium therapy. *Trans Am Soc Artif Intern Organs* 29:645–648, 1983.
121. Raja A, Kramer M, Barber B, Chen S: Sequential changes in dialysate sodium during hemodialysis. *Trans Am Soc Artif Intern Organs* 29:649–651, 1983.
122. Gotch FA: Sodium-volume modeling of hemodialysis therapy. *Proc Clin Dial Transpl Forum* 10:12, 1980.
123. Kimura G, Van Stone JC, Bauer JH, Keshaviah P: A stimulation of transcellular fluid shifts induced by hemodialysis. *Kidney Int* 24:542–548, 1983.
124. Petitclerc T, Man NK, Funck-Brentano JL: Sodium modeling during hemodialysis: A new approach. *Artif Organs* 8:418–422, 1984.
125. Man NK, Petitclerc T, Jehenne G, Funck-Brentano JL: Clinical validation of a predictive modeling equation for sodium. *Artif Organs* 9:150–154, 1985.
126. Man NK, Tien NQ, Petitclerc T, Jehenne G, Funck-Brentano JL: On-line monitoring of sodium dialysate concentration during hemodialysis. In: K Atsumi, M Maekawa, K Ota, eds, *Progress in Artificial Organs* — 1983. ISAO Press, Cleveland, pp 487–490, 1984.
127. Petitcler T, Man NK, Goureau Y, Jehenne G, Funck-Brentano NL: Optimization of sodium dialysate concentration by plasma water conductivity monitoring. In: Y Nose, C Kjellstrand, P Ivanovich, eds, *Progress in Artificial Organs* — 1985. ISAO Press, Cleveland, pp 234–236, 1986.
128. Henderson LW, Koch KM, Dinarello CA, Shaldon S: Hemodialysis hypotension: The interleukin hypothesis. *Blood Purif* 1:197–224, 1983.
129. Johny KV, Lawrence JR, O'Halloran MW, Welby ML, Worthy BW: Studies on total body, serum and erythrocyte potassium in patients on maintenance haemodialysis. The value of erythrocyte potassium as a measure of body potassium. *Nephron* 7:230, 1970.
130. Seedat YK: Total body potassium and chronic renal failure. *Br Med J* 2:405, 1972.
131. Boddy K, King PC, Lindsay RM, Briggs JD, Winchester JF, Kennedy AC: Total body potassium in non-dialysed and dialysed patients with chronic renal failure. *Br Med J* 1:771, 1972.
132. Butkus DE, Alfrey AC, Miller NL: Tissue potassium in chronic dialysis patients. *Nephron* 13:314, 1974.
133. Morgan AG, Burkinshaw L, Robinson PJA, Rosen SM: Potassium balance and acid-base changes in patients undergoing regular haemodialysis therapy. *Br Med J* 00:779, 1970.
134. Berlyne GM, Janabi K, Shaw AB, Hocken AG: Treatment of hyperkalemia with a calcium-resin. *Lancet* 1:169, 1966.
135. Feig PU, Shook A, Sterns RH: Effect of potassium removal during hemodialysis on the plasma potassium concentration. *Nephron* 27:25–30, 1981.
136. Ward RA, Williams TE, Wathen RL: Factors affecting potassium removal during hemodialysis. *Kidney Int* 23:164, 1983.
137. Morrison G, Michelson EL, Brown S, morganroth J: Mechanism and prevention of cardiac arrhythmias in chronic hemodialysis patients. *Kidney Int* 17:811–819, 1980.
138. Stanbury SW: Azotemic renal osteodystrophy. *Clin Endocrinol Metab* 1:267–304, 1972.
139. Coburn JW, Hartenbower DL, Massry SG: Intestinal absorption of calcium and the effect of renal insufficiency. *Kidney Int* 4:96–104, 1973.
140. Malluche HH. Werner E, Ritz E: Intestinal absorption of calcium and whole body calcium retention in incipient and advanced renal failure. *Miner Electrolyte Metab* 1:263–270, 1978.
141. Massry SG, Lee DBN, Kleeman CR: Skeletal resistance to parathyroid hormone in renal failure. Studies in 105 human subjects. *Ann Intern Med* 78:357–364, 1973.
142. Coburn JW, Slatopolsky E: Vitamin D parathyroid hormone and renal osteodystrophy. In: BM Brenner, FC Rector Jr, eds, *The Kidney*, 2nd ed, WB Saunders, Philadelphia, pp 1657–1729, 1985.
143. Bricker NS: On the pathogenesis of the uremic state. An exposition of the "trade-off hypothesis." *N Engl J Med* 268:1093–1100, 1972.
144. Massry SG, Ritz E, Verberckmoes R: Role of phosphate in the genesis of secondary hyperparathyroidism of renal failure. *Nephron* 18:77–81, 1977.
145. Lee SW, Russell J, Avioli LV: 25-hydroxycholecalciferol to 1,25-dihyroxycholecalciferol: Conversion impaired by systemic metabolic acidosis. *Science* 195:994–996, 1977.
146. Meyrier A. Marsac J, Richet G: The influence of a high calcium carbonate intake on bone disease in patients undergoing hemodialysis. *Kidney Int* 4:146–153, 1973.
147. Fournier A, Moriniere PH, Coevoet B. Prevention and medical treatment of hyperparathyroidism secondary to renal failure. *Adv Nephrol* 11:241, 1982.

148. Slatopolski E, Weerts C, Lopez-Hilker S, Norwood K, Zink M, Windus D, Delmez J: Calcium carbonate as a phosphate binder in patients with chronic renal failure undergoing dialysis. *N Engl J Med* 315:157-161, 1986.
149. Pierides AM, Ward MK, Alvarez-Ude F, Ellis HA, Peart KM, Simpson W, Kerr DNS, Norman A: Long term therapy with 1,25 (OH)$_2$D$_3$ in dialysis bone disease. *Proc Eur Dial Transpl Assoc* 12:237, 1975.
150. McIntosh CHS, Fuch C, Dorn D, Quelhorst E, Henning HV, Hesch RD, Scheler F: Effect of dialysate calcium concentration on plasma parathyroid hormone during hemodialysis. *Nephron* 19:88, 1977.
151. Winney RJ, Tothill P, Robson JS, Abbot SR, Lidgard GP, Cameron EHD, Smith MA, Macpherson JN, Strong JA: The effect of dialysate calcium concentration and 1-hydroxyvitamin D$_1$ on skeletal calcium loss and hyperparathyroidism in haemodialysis patients. *Clin Endocrinol (Oxford)* (Suppl):151s, 1977.
152. Goldstein DA, Malluche HH, Massry SG: Management of renal osteodystrophy with 1,25 (OH)$_2$D$_3$ 1. Effect on clinical, radiographic and biochemical parameters. *Miner Electrolyte Metab* 2:35, 1979.
153. Malluche HH, Goldstein DA, Massry SG: Management of renal osteodystrophy with 1,25 (OH)$_2$D$_3$ II. Effects on histopathology of bone, evidence for healing of osteomalacia. *Miner Electrolyte Metab* 2:48-55, 1979.
154. Slatopolsky E, Weerts C, Thielan J, Horst R, Harter H, Martin KJ: Marked suppression of secondary hyperparathyroidism by intravenous administration of 1,25-dihydroxycholecalciferol in uremic patients. *J Clin Invest* 74:2136-2143, 1984.
155. Ginsburg DS, Kaplan EL, Katz AI: Hypercalcemia after oral calcium-carbonate therapy in patients on chronic haemodialysis. *Lancet* 00:1271-1274, 1973.
156. Parfitt AM: Soft-tissue calcification in uremia. *Arch Intern Med* 00:544-556, 1969.
157. Haque AK, Rubin SA, Leveque CM. Pulmonary calcification in long-term hemodialysis: A mimic of pulmonary thromboembolism. *Am J Nephrol* 4:109-113, 1984.
158. Ogden DA, Holmes JH: Changes in total and ultrafilterable plasma calcium and magnesium during hemodialysis. *Trans Am Soc Artif Intern Organs* 12:200, 1966.
159. Moore EW: Ionized calcium in normal serum, ultrafiltrates and whole blood determined by ion-exchange electrodes. *J Clin Invest* 49:318-334, 1970.
160. Conceicao S, Hoenich NA, Ward MK, White T, Aljama P, Dewar J, Kerr DNS: Ionised calcium during haemodialysis. *Proc Eur Dial Transpl Assoc* 14:229, 1977.
161. Goldsmith RS, Furszyfer J, Johnson WJ, Beeler GW, Jr, Taylor WF: Calcium flux during hemodialysis. *Nephron* 20:132, 1978.
162. Wing AJ: Optimum calcium concentration of dialysis fluid for maintenance hemodialysis. *Br Med J* 4:145-149, 1968.
163. Soyannwo MAO, Oreopoulos DG, Mustafo G, McGeown MG: Studies on dialysate calcium requirements on maintenance haemodialysis: With observations on phosphate and magnesium. *Proc Eur Dial Transpl Assoc* 5:288, 1969.
164. Bouillon R, Verberckmoes R, de Moor P: Influence of dialysate calcium concentration and vitamin D on serum parathyroid hormone during repetitive dialysis. *Kidney Int* 7:422, 1975.
165. Regan RJ, Peacock M, Rosen SM, Robinson PJ, Horsman A: Effect of dialysate calcium concentration on bone disease in patients on hemodialysis. *Kidney Int* 10:246, 1976.
166. Drueke T, Bordier PJ, Man NK, Jungers P, Marie P: Effects of high dialysate calcium concentration on bone remodeling, serum biochemistry, and parathyroid hormone in patients with renal osteodystrophy. *Kidney Int* 11:267, 1977.
167. Asad SN, Ellis KJ, Cohn SH, Letteri JM: Changes in total body calcium on prolonged maintenance hemodialysis with high and low dialysate calcium. *Nephron* 23:223, 1979.
168. Merrill JP, Thorn JW, Walter CW, Callahan EJ, Smith LH: The use of an artifical kidney. I. Technique. *J Clin Invest* 29:412-424, 1950.
169. Hamburger J, Richet G: Le rein artificiel Compute-rendu de l'Academie Nationale de Medecine Seance du 8 Janvier 1957, 12-25, 1957.
170. Mion CM, Hegstrom RM, Boen ST, Scribner BH. Substitution of sodium acetate for sodium bicarbonate in the bath fluid for hemodialysis. *Trans Am Soc Artif Intern Organs* 10:110, 1964.
171. Kveim M, Nesbakken R: Utilization of exogenous acetate during hemodialysis. *Trans Am Artif Intern Organs* 21:138, 1975.
172. Rorke SJ, Davidson WD, Guo SS, Morin RJ: Metabolic fate of ^{14}C-acetate during dialysis. *Proc Eur Dial Transpl Assoc* 13:394, 1976.
173. Lundquist F, Tygstrup N, Winkler K, Mellemgaard K, Munck-Petersen S: Ethanol metabolism and production of free acetate in the human liver. *J Clin Invest* 41:955, 1962.
174. Tolchin N, Roberts JL, Hayashi J, Lewis EJ: Metabolic consequences of high mass-transfer hemodialysis. *Kidney Int* 11:366, 1977.
175. Port FK, Easterling RE: Metabolism of acetate during hemodialysis and I.V. infusion. *Kidney Int* 8:432, 1975.
176. Novello A, Kelsch R, Easterling R: Acetate intolerance during hemodialysis. *Clin Nephrol* 5:29-32, 1976.
177. Kaiser BA, Potter DE, Bryant RE, Vreman JH, Weiner MW: Acid-base changes and acetate metabolism during routine and high-efficiency hemodialysis in children. *Kidney Int* 19:70, 1981.
178. Weiner MW: Acetate metabolism during hemodialysis. *Artif Organs* 6:370-377, 1982.
179. Graefe U, Milutinovich J, Follette WC, Vizzo JE, Babb AL, Scribner BH: Less dialysis-induced morbidity and vascular instability with bicarbonate in dialysate. *Ann Intern Med* 88:332, 1978.
180. Tolchin N, Roberts JL, Lewis EJ: Respiratory gas exchange by high-efficiency hemodialyzers. *Nephron* 21:137-145, 1978.
181. Vreman HJ, Assomull VM, Kaiser BA, Blaschke TF, Weiner MW: Acetate metabolism and acid-base homeostasis during hemodialysis, influence of dialyzer efficiency and rate of acetate metabolism. *Kidney Int* 18:S62, 1980.
182. Raja RM, Kramer MS, Rosenbaum JL, Bolisay CG, Krug MJ: Hemodialysis associated hypoxemia. Role of acetate and pH in etiology. *Trans Am Soc Artif Intern Organs* 27:180, 1981.
183. Sherlock J, Ledwith J, Letteri J: Hypoventilation and hypoxemia during hemodialysis: Reflex response to removal of CO$_2$ across the dialyzer. *Trans Am Soc Artif Intern Organs* 23:406, 1977.
184. Aurigemma MM, Feldman NT, Gottlieb M, Ingram RH, Lazarus JM, Lowrie EG: Arterial oxygenation during hemodialysis. *N Engl J Med* 297:871, 1977.
185. Nissenson AR: Prevention of dialysis induced hypoxemia by bicarbonate dialysate. *Trans Am Soc Artif Intern Organs* 26:339, 1980.
186. Dolan MJ, Whipp EJ, Davidson WD, Weitzman RE, Wasserman K: Hypopnea associated with acetate hemodialysis:

Carbonate dioxide-flow-dependent ventilation. *N Engl J Med* 305:72, 1981.
187. Kirkendol PL, Devia CJ, Bower JD, Holbert RD: A comparsion of the cardiovascular effects of sodium acetate, sodium bicarbonate and other potential sources of fixed base in hemodialysate solutions. *Trans Am Soc Artif Intern Organs* 23:399, 1977.
188. Aizawa Y, Ohmori T, Imai K, Nara Y, Matsuoka M, Hirikawa Y: Depressant action of acetate upon the human cardiovascular system. *Clin Nephrol* 8:477, 1977.
189. Liang CS, Lowenstein JM: Metabolic control of the circulation. Effects of acetate and pyruvate. *J Clin Invest* 62:1029, 1978.
190. Richet GE, Lopez–DeNovales E, Verroust P: Drug intoxication and neurological episodes in chronic renal failure. *Br Med J* 1:394–395, 1970.
191. Posner JB, Plum F: Spinal-fluid pH and neurological symptoms in systemic acidosis. *N Engl J Med* 277:605–613, 1967.
192. Hampel H, Klopp H, Wolfgruber M, Pustelnik A, Schiller R, Hanefeld F, Kessel M: Advantages of bicarbonate hemodialysis. *Artif Organs* 6(4):410, 1982.
193. Gonzalez FM, Pearson JE, Garbus SE, Holbert RD: On the effects of acetate during hemodialysis. *Trans Am Soc Artif Intern Organs* 20:169, 1974.
194. Giorcelli G, Dalmasso F, Bruno M, Pellegrino S, Tondolom M, Sirkka M, Vacha G: Regular dialysis treatment with acetate-free bicarbonate buffered dialysis fluid: Long-term effects on lipid pattern, acid-base balance and oxygen delivery. *Proc Eur Dial Transplant Assoc* 16:115, 1979.
195. Man NK, Fournier G, Thireau P, Gaillard JL, Funck–Brentano JL: Effect of bicarbonate-containing dialysate on chronic dialysis patients: A comparative study. *Artif Organs* 6:421–425, 1982.
196. Savdie E, Mahoney J, Stewart J: Effect of acetate on serum lipids in maintenance hemodialysis. *Trans Am Soc Artif Intern Organs* 23:385–392, 1977.
197. Sanfelippo ML, Swenson RS, Reaven GM: Reduction of plasma triglyceride by diet in subjects with chronic renal failure. *Kidney Int* 11:54, 1977.
198. Ahmad S, Pagel M, Vizzo J, Scribner BH: Effect of the normalization of acid-base balance on post-dialysis plasma bicarbonate. *Trans Am Soc Artif Intern Organs* 26:318, 1980.
199. Ward RA, Wathen RL: Utilization of bicarbonate for base repletion in hemodialysis. *Artif Organs* 6:396–403, 1982.
200. Ward RA, Wathen RL: Effects of long-term bicarbonate hemodialysis on acid-base statue. *Trans Am Soc Artif Intern Organs* 28:295–298.
201. Sargent JA, Gotch FA: Bicarbonate and carbon dioxide transport during hemodialysis. *Am Soc Artif Intern Organs* 2:61, 1979.
202. Gotch FA, Sargent JA, Keen ML: Hydrogen ion balance in dialysis therapy. *Artif Organs* 6:388–395, 1982.
203. Fournier G, Gaillard JL, Man NK: Control of acid-base status and phosphatemia with bicarbonate-containing dialysate. A long term study. In: K Atsumi, M Maekawa, K Ota, eds, *Progress in Artificial Organs — 1983*. ISAO Press, Cleveland, pp 470–473, 1984.
204. Ward RA, Wathen RL, Williams TE, Harding GB: Hemodialysate composition and intradialytic metabolic, acid-base and potassium changes. *Kidney Int* 32:129–135, 1987.
205. Vinay P, Prud'Homme M, Vinet B, Cournoyer G, Degoulet P, Leville M, Gougoux A, St-Louis G, Lapierre L, Piette Y: Acetate metabolism and bicarbonate generation during hemodialysis: 10 years of observation. *Kidney Int* 31:1194–1204, 1987.
206. Gunther T: Biochemistry and pathobiochemistry of magnesium. *Artery* 9:167–181, 1981.
207. Massry SG: The clinical pathophysiology of magnesium. *Contrib Nephrol* 14:64, 1978.
208. Silver L, Robertson JS, Dahl LK: Magnesium turnover in humans studied with 28 Mg. *J Clin Invest* 39:420–425, 1960.
209. Paymaster NJ: Magnesium metabolism: A brief review. *Ann R Coll Surg (England)* 58:309, 1976.
210. Ferdinandus J, Pederson JA, Whang R: Hypermagnesemia as a cause of refractory hypotension, respiratory depression and coma. *Arch Intern Med* 141:669–670, 1981.
211. Fleming LW, Lenman JAR, Stewart WK: Effect of magnesium on nerve conduction velocity during regular dialysis treatment. *J Neurol Neurosurg Psychiatry* 35:342, 1972.
212. Hollinrake K, Thomas PK, Wills MR, Baillod RA: Observations on plasma magnesium levels in patients with uremic neuropathy under treatment by periodic hemodialysis. *Neurology* 20:939, 1970.
213. Alfrey AC, Miller NL: Bone magnesium pools in uremia. *J Clin Invest* 52:3019, 1973.
214. Brautbar N, Kleeman CR: Disordered divalent ion metabolism in kidney disease: Comments on pathogenesis and treatment. *Adv Nephrol* 8:179, 1979.
215. Graf H, Kovarik J, Stummvol HK, Wolf A: Disappearance of uraemic pruritus after lowering dialysate magnesium concentration. *Br Med J* 2:1478, 1979.
216. Parsons V, Papapoulos SE, Weston MJ, Tomlinson S, O'Riordan JLH: The long term effect of lowering dialysate magnesium on circulating parathyroid hormone in patients on regular haemodialysis therapy. *Acta Endocrinol (Copenh)* 93:455, 1980.
217. Pletka P, Bernstein DS, Hampers CL, Merrill JP, Sherwood LM: Effects of magnesium on parathyroid hormone secretion during chronic haemodialysis. *Lancet* 2:462, 1971.
218. Burnell JM, Teubner E: Effects of decreasing dialysate magnesium in patients with chronic renal failure. *Proc Clin Dial Transpl Forum* 5: 191, 1976.
219. Gonella M, Bonaguidi F, Buzzigoli G, Bartolini V, Mariani G: On the effect of magnesium on the PTH secretion in uremic patients on maintenance hemodialysis. *Nephron* 27:40, 1981.
220. Johny KV, Lawrence JR, O'Halloren MW, Wellby ML: Effect of haemodialysis on erythrocyte and plasma potassium, magnesium, sodium and calcium. *Nephron* 8:81, 1971.
221. Heierli C, Hill AVL: The relationship between the magnesium concentration in the dialysis fluid used and in the plasma and erythrocytes of patients with chronic renal failure being treated by regular haemodialysis. *Clin Sci* 43:779, 1972.
222. Stewart WK, Fleming LW: The effect of dialysate magnesium on plasma and erythrolyte magnesium and potassium concentrations during maintenance haemodialysis. *Nephron* 10:222, 1973.
223. Catto GRF, Reid IW, MacLeod M: The effect of low magnesium dialysate on plasma, ultrafiltrable, erythrocyte and bone magnesium concetrations from patients on maintenance haemodialysis. *Nephron* 13:372, 1974.
224. Alwall N, Hagstam KE, Lingergard B, Lindholm T: A clinical trial with a glucose-free dialysate. *Proc Eur Dial Transpl Assoc* 7:55, 1970.
225. Hubner W, Sieberth UG, Diemer A, Finke K, Prange E. Effect of regular hemodialysis with glucose and glucose free dialysate on hyperlipidemia. *Proc Eur Dial Transplant Assoc* 8:174–181, 1971.

226. Wathen RL, Keshaviah P, Hommeyer P, Cadwell K, Comty CM: The metabolic effects of hemodialysis with and without glucose in the dialysate. *Am J Clin Nutr* 31:1870–1875, 1978.
227. Alfrey AC, Sussman KE, Holmes JH: Changes in glucose and insulin metabolism induced by dialysis in patients with chronic uremia. *Metab Clin Exp* 733–740, 1967.
228. Bilbrey GL, Faloona GR, White MG, Atkins C, Hull AR, Knochel: Hyperglycagonemia in uremia: Reversal by renal transplantation. *Ann Intern Med* 82:525–528, 1985.
229. Feldman HA, Singer I: Endocrinology and metabolism in uremia and dialysis: A clinical review. *Medicine* (Baltimore) 54:345–376, 1975.
230. Sherwin RS, Basti C, Finkelstein FO, Fisher M, Black H, Hendler R, Felig P: Influence of uremia and hemodialysis on the turnover and metabolic effect of glucagon. *J Clin Invest* 57:722–730, 1976.
231. Leski M, Niethammer T, Wyss T: Glucose enriched dialysate and tolerance to maintenance hemodialysis. *Nephron* 24:271–273, 1979.
232. Ginn HE, Frost A, Lacey WW: Nitrogen balance in hemodialysis patients. *Am J Clin Nutr* 21:385, 1968.
233. Young GA, Parsons FM: Amino nitrogen loss during haemodialysis, its dietary significance and replacement. *Clin Sci* 31:299, 1966.
234. Ganda OP, Aoki TT, Soeldner JS, Morrison RS, Cahill GF Jr: Hormone-fuel concentrations in anephrie subjects. *J Clin Invest* 57:1403, 1976.
235. Borah MF, Schoenfeld PY, Gotch FA, Sargent JA, Wolfson M, Hymphreys MH: Nitrogen balance during intermittent dialysis therapy of uremia. *Kidney Int* 14:491–500, 1978.
236. Wathen R, Keshaviah P, Hommeyer P, Cadwell K, Comty C: Role of dialysate glucose in preventing gluconeogenesis during hemodialysis. *Trans Am Soc Artif Intern Organs* 23:393, 1977.
237. Ward RA, Shirlow MJ, Hayes JM, Chapman GV, Farrell PC: Protein catabolism during hemodialysis. *Am J Clin Nutr* 32:2443, 1979.
238. Fournier G, Joseph O, Crochon B, Palluel AM, Man NK: Metabolic, hormonal and solute mass transfer removal changes during hemodialysis with and without glucose in dialysate. In: Y Nose, C Kjellstrand, P Ivanovich, eds, *Progress in Artifical Organs — 1985*. ISAO Press, Cleveland, pp 161–164, 1986.
239. Swamy AP, Cestero RVM, Campbell RG, Freeman RB: Long-term effect of dialysate glucose on the lipid levels of maintenance hemodialysis patients. *Trans Am Soc Artif Intern Organs* 22:54, 1976.

CHAPTER 53

Membrane Biocompatibility

ALFRED K. CHEUNG

INTRODUCTION

The primary purpose of the hemodialysis and hemofiltration membranes in the extracorporeal circuits is to act as a barrier to retain cellular elements and larger solutes, while allowing removal of water and solutes of smaller sizes. However, these artificial surfaces behave differently from the vascular endothelial cells in that they are more likely to alter the blood elements with which they come in contact. The exact clinical effects of these alterations may not be apparent. They are, however, not the purpose of the extracorporeal circulation and are usually considered to be undesirable. There is not any unanimous definition of the term *membrane incompatibility*. However, many bioengineers and nephrologists would agree that a biocompatible membrane is one that causes no perturbation from normal anatomy, compositions, or functions of the body, except for the changes that are specifically targeted by the treatment. To achieve this goal, if possible, we have to recognize the different aspects that are bioincompatible, and then try to correct them (1). Klinkmann et al. suggested several issues that should be considered for the biocompatibility of biomaterials. These include: thrombosis, toxicity, allergy, inflammatory reactions, destruction of formed elements, changes in plasma proteins and enzymes, immunologic reactions, carcinogenicity, and deterioration of adjacent tissues (2). The mechanisms by which the extracorporeal circuits cause changes usually can be classified into one of the following four categories: a) cell adhesion, aggregation, and activation; b) protein transformation at the membrane interface; c) mechanical shear effects; and d) leaching of materials into the fluid phase and spallation of particulate matters (1).

It should be emphasized from the beginning that biocompatibility of an artificial kidney does not depend on the membrane structure alone. Many other factors such as potting materials, casing materials, sterilizing agents, and the geometry of the blood paths are all important considerations. Besides the artificial kidney itself, the blood lines and cannulae are also in direct contact with the blood. In fact, the cannulae probably provide the greatest shear in the hemodialysis circuits (3) and are therefore important sources of trauma to cells. The blood pump may have an indirect influence by causing spallation of particles from the pump segment of the blood tubing. The dialysate, in some instances, could have profound impacts on the patient. Not only does the dialysate determine the net exchange of ions such as calcium, which has hemodynamic implications (4) it may also be a potential source of bacterial and endotoxin contamination, as well as a potential factor in the generation of interleukins. Finally, comparison of the long-term sequelae of treatments with different types of membranes has to take into account not only the biocompatibility, but also the differences in the solute clearance profiles. This chapter will concentrate primarily on the effects of biocompatibility of hemodialyzer membranes. Discussions on the other types of membranes and the many other components of the extracorporeal circuits will be brief.

COMPOSITIONS OF MEMBRANES

A brief introduction of the materials for commonly used artificial kidney membranes is in order before we discuss their biocompatibility. Cellulosic membranes, which encompass all membranes generated from cellulose (5), have been the most commonly employed types for many years. Cellulose is part of the matrix of plant cell walls. The form of cellulose used to manufacture dialysis membranes is a polysaccharide composed of linear chains of glucosan rings containing free hydroxyl groups. The membranes are prepared from cellulose by two different processes of regeneration. One involves a solution of cellulose in sodium hydroxide, the product of which is known as *cellophane*. The second involves solubilization of cellulose in an ammonium solution of cupric oxide, the product of which is known as *cuprophan* (or cuprophane). Cuprophan has largely replaced cellophane as a hemodialyzer membrane material.

Cellulose acetate is another form of cellulosic membrane. In this membrane, however, 5 out of 6 hydroxyl groups on the glucose rings are acetylated. As a result of this acetylation, the properties of the membrane are changed. This has particular interesting ramifications in terms of biocompatibility that will be discussed later.

Recently, a new cellulose-based membrane (Hemophan®) has been manufactured by Akzo (FRG), which has only 1 out of 150 free hydroxyl groups substituted by a tertiary amino group. This minor change in structure, however, leads to significant effects on its biocompatibility (6, 7).

Other materials used to manufacture artificial kidney membranes include polyacrylonitrile (PAN), polysulfone, polymethylmethacrylate (PMMA), polycarbonate, and polyamide. Many of these noncellulosic membranes possess high ultrafiltration coefficients and are used for high-flux hemodialysis, heomfiltration, or hemodiafiltration.

Membranes of different materials are fabricated primarily into one of three formats (coils, flat plates, and hollow fibers) with different surface areas, casing designs, and sterilization methods. The use of coil dialyzers is proportionately diminishing compared to the other two formats. Some examples of hemodialyzers and hemofilters made from various materials are listed in Table 1.

ERYTHROCYTES

Hemolysis

Blood loss during hemodialysis contributes to the many causes of anemia in dialysis patients. Besides the obvious causes such as bleeding, blood loss can also be due to hemolysis and thrombus formation inside the dialyzer. The latter may lead to gross clotting of the dialyzer or high blood residual left in the dialyzer after treatment. The loss from hemolysis is usually minor. It may stem from mechanical trauma by shearing during the flow of blood through the dialyzer (8) or blood pump. Hemolysis of a serious nature occurs rarely; it can result from overheating or incorrect composition of the dialysate.

Rarely, hemolysis may result from the formation of anti-N antibodies (9, 10). The MN blood group system consists of two alleles, M and N. Anti-N is a cold agglutinin directed against the N antigen on the red cells. The emergence of this rare antibody has been proposed to result from exposure of red cells to formaldehyde during processing for dialyzer reuse (9, 11, 12). Presumably, the formaldehyde alters the antigenicity on the cell surface and elicits an antibody response. Reports from the earlier literature suggest that this antibody is of clinical significance. One such report described a dialysis patient who had an increased transfusion requirement resulting from blood exposure to lower temperature in the extracorporeal circuit. This problem was corrected by minimizing heat loss from the blood (10). Another report attributed the acute failure of a transplanted kidney to this antibody, which presumably caused erythrocyte agglutination in the chilled transplanted organ (13). Subsequent studies (11, 12), however, showed that despite a documented increase in the incidence of anti-N antibody in patients practicing dialyzer reuse, there was no apparent clinical sequela. No clinical or laboratory evidence of hemolysis in these patients was observed. No renal graft loss could be attributed to the presence of the antibody. However, cautions should be taken during transplantation surgery for patients who are known to have this antibody.

The incidence of anti-N antibody is significantly increased in patients practicing dialyzer reuse. Its occurrence is related to the amounts of residual formaldehyde in the dialyzer effluent after reprocessing, i.e., the amounts of formaldehyde to which the patients are exposed. In patients whose dialyzer residual formaldehyde concentrations were 3–13 µg/ml, the prevalence of this antibody was as high as 31% (12). This was in contrast to the absence of anti-N in patients whose dialyzer effluent formaldehyde concentrations were < 1 µg/ml. It should be noted that the Clinitest® tablets only detect formaldehyde concentrations over 3 µg/ml. The anti-N antibodies can disappear with time after the exposure to formaldehyde has been eliminated (12).

Adherence

Erythrocytes usually adhere to the dialyzer membrane surfaces less readily than leukocytes and platelets (14).

Table 1. Examples of artificial kidneys*

	Name	Format	Manufacturer
Cuprophan	CF 1511	Hollow fiber	Baxter, USA
	PPD 1.6	Plate	Cobe Lab, USA
	CD	Coil	Baxter, USA
Cellulose acetate	CA 90	Hollow fiber	Cobe Lab, USA
	Hemofresh	Plate	Daicel, Japan
Hemophan	APF	Hollow fiber	National Medical Care, USA
Polyacrylonitrile	Filtral	Hollow fiber	Hospal, USA
	1210 H	Plate	Hospal, USA
Polymethymethacrylate	Filtryzer B1	Hollow fiber	Toray, Japan
Polysulfone	Diafilter 20	Hollow fiber	Amicon, USA
Polycarbonate	Lundia Pro	Plate	Gambro, Sweden
Polyamide	FH 66	Hollow fiber	Gambro, Sweden

* Listed are examples of some of the artificial kidneys for hemodialysis and/or hemofiltration purposes. They are categorized by membrane materials.

However, inadequate anticoagulation can lead to microthrombi formation, increased residual blood, or overt clotting of the dialyzers. Under these circumstances, red cells are mixed inside the thrombi with the other types of cells and plasma proteins. Damaged erythrocytes can also contribute to the thrombolic process by releasing thromboplastic substances and adenosine diphosphate (ADP).

PLATELETS

Adhesion and activation of platelets

Clotting of the dialyzers was a major problem in the early days of hemodialysis. It continues to be a problem, especially in patients who have a hypercoagulable state or in those who have a high risk of bleeding which makes the use of anticoagulants hazardous. A number of factors influence the clotting tendency on hemodialysis. These include the structure of the membrane, surface free energy, surface roughness, configuration of the blood compartment, blood flow characteristics, and anticoagulation, as well as the composition of the patient's blood.

Absorption of plasma proteins onto the artificial membrane surface occurs immediately after blood contact. Adherence of platelets, leukocytes, and, to a lesser extent, erythrocytes (14, 15) to these proteins follows. Platelets seem to have a predilection for fibrinogen over gamma globulins; adsorption to albumin is minimal (16). Adhesion to cellulosic membrane surfaces stimulates the platelets to undergo morphologic changes characterized by pseudopod formation and spreading of the cells over the surfaces. Activation of platelets, either mechanically or by virtue of their involvement in coagulation, causes release of a variety of substances from the cells. The release of adenosine diphosphate (ADP), thromboxane A_2 (TXA_2), as well as platelet-activating factor (PAF) (17), and the binding of activated factor V (18) and X (19) leads to further aggregation of cells. Activation of platelets also leads to the release of platelet factor 4 (PF4) and β-thromboglobulin (βTG), which are stored inside these cells. An increase of these substances in the plasma usually denotes activation of platelets. PF4 is cleared by its binding to the endothelial cells; infusion of heparin can increase the plasma level of PF4 (20), a cationic protein, by releasing it from the endothelial cells. PF4 binds to heparin and neutralizes it instantaneously (21). βTG is cleared by the kidneys; renal failure, therefore, leads to elevation of its plasma concentration (22).

Once formed by activation of the coagulation pathway, thrombin also stimulates platelets to undergo the release reaction. The aggregation of platelets may lead to mural thrombi, which are then stabilized by fibrin. Microemboli can ensue. The importance of platelets in the clotting of dialyzers can be illustrated by the effectiveness of antiplatelet agents such as aspirin and dipyridamole in preventing these events (23, 24). Prostacyclin, another inhibitor of platelet aggregation with high potency, can be used as the sole anticoagulant in the absence of heparin for successful hemodialysis treatments (25, 26). Again, this underscores the importance of platelet activation in the generation of thrombosis in the extracorporeal circuit.

Assessment of platelet activation in hemodialysis

Platelet activation during hemodialysis has been assessed by different methods, including changes in peripheral platelet counts, morphologic alterations, and the increase in plasma concentrations of the released substances such as TXB_2, PF4 and βTG. Thrombocytopenia usually occurs in the initial 15–30 minutes of hemodialysis. The degree is usually mild, with only a 10–15% decrease in platelet counts (27–29). This decrease per se usually does not pose a problem in terms of systemic bleeding during or after the treatment. The most likely cause of the peripheral thrombocytopenia is adhesion of the platelets to the dialyzer membranes and the formation of mural thrombi (14). Peripheral thrombocytopenia, however, is a crude indicator of platelet activation.

As indicated above, because of the other factors that may affect their plasma concentrations, data on platelet activation by dialysis membranes using markers such as PF4 and βTG should be interpreted with caution. Although renal failure per se leads to the accumulation of βTG, acute changes in plasma levels may reflect activation of platelets during hemodialysis. Some investigators have demonstrated that successful prevention of dialyzer clotting is associated with effective suppression of the rise in plasma βTG levels (30). Others have shown that the increase in plasma βTG levels during hemodialysis is only partially inhibitable by the administration of dipyridamole, suggesting that the release of this protein is not totally dependent on the functional activity of the cells (31). Instead, it may result from the mechanical disruption of the platelets by the dialysis membranes or other components of the extracorporeal circuit that cannot be inhibited by antiplatelet agents. Since heparin is a potent stimulus to the dissociation of PF4 from endothelial cells, and it is also used extensively as an anticoagulant during hemodialysis, assessment of platelet activation by plasma PF4 concentrations alone is difficult.

Comparison between different membranes

Dialyzers differ in their abilities to sequester platelets, thereby affecting their thrombogenicity (32). Cuprophan membranes have been shown to activate platelets more than polyacrylonitrile membranes, as assessed by the rise in plasma βTG during dialysis with the former and the lack of rise with the latter (33). Platelet factor 4 rose with both membranes, because of the heparin effect mentioned above. Dialysis with cuprophan has also been shown to be associated with more severe thrombocytopenia than the thrombocytopenia seen with polymethylmethacrylate membranes (34).

In another study comparing cuprophan with polycarbonate, significant platelet adherence to the cuprophan membrane surfaces was found, accompanied by several lines of evidence of platelet activation (27). There were spreading of the cells with pseudopod formation and cytoplasmic bridging by scanning electron microscopy. The plasma βTG levels were increased and platelet counts were decreased by 13%. Furthermore, platelet aggregation to collagen decreased, and the template bleeding time at the end of dialysis was significantly prolonged. In comparison, the changes in platelet counts, morphology, and platelet functions were much milder with polycarbonate membranes, despite a comparable increase in plasma βTG. Although the blood lines may be partially responsible for the platelet activation, this study points out the different ways in which platelets are affected by different membranes. In addition, it points out the lack of precise correlation of the platelet release reaction (as measured by βTG) with morphologic and functional changes. It should be emphasized that, besides the polymers, flow characteristics and other factors may differ between the two types of dialyzers employed in this study.

The utility of these markers to compare platelet activation by different membranes can be improved with careful control of other conditions such as anticoagulants, blood flow rates, and patient variability. For example, in an in-vivo model utilizing human blood in a single-pass mode without heparin, Spencer et al. found that Hemophan membrane dialyzers were associated with a lower generation rate (assessed by the difference between arterial and venous lines) of PF4 than cuprophan dialyzers (6).

Dialyzer membranes may also affect platelet activation and aggregation by their abilities to activate complement and to degranulate leukocytes (34). As will be discussed later, both of these events have been shown to occur during hemodialysis. Complement activation product C_{3a} can stimulate thromboxane production (35, 36). Degranulation of basophils can lead to the release of platelet-activating factor (37). Both thromboxane and platelet-activating factor, to a lesser extent, can stimulate platelet. Membranes that differ in these properties may therefore influence platelets to different degrees.

CLOTTING FACTORS

Activation of coagulation cascades

Protein adsorption onto dialyzer membrane surfaces occurs immediately when blood is exposed to the membranes, followed by the adsorption of the cellular elements. The layering of proteins have important effects on the transport of molecules, which is beyond the scope of this chapter. Membrane-protein interactions can, however, also lead to activation of different cascades in the plasma. Activation of the Hageman factor (factor XII) results in activation of the intrinsic coagulation pathway that potentiates the effects of platelets in causing thrombosis (38). The fibrinolytic system is also activated as a result of membrane contact. Tissue thromboplastin on the plasma membranes of the adherent leukocytes may also activate the extrinsic pathway of coagulation. The thrombin formed as a result of activation of these cascades has a high tendency to bind to artificial surfaces, possibly through its binding to the adherent platelets (39). As indicated in the last section, thrombin can also stimulate the release reactions of platelets. Stagnation of blood in the dialyzers enhances thrombus formation, partly because the activated coagulaton components are not removed and are therefore concentrated on the membrane surfaces.

Assessment of activation of coagulation cascades

During clinical hemodialysis, heparinization is usually monitored by measurements of whole-blood clotting time, activated clotting time or activated partial thromboplastin time. Seemingly adequate heparinization, as assessed by these clotting studies, does not always prevent mural thrombus because of platelet activation.

Activation of the fibrinolytic system can be detected by an increase in serum fibrinogen degradation products (29). Activation of the coagulation cascades can be detected by various methods. Consumption of clotting factors during hemodialysis is reflected in a decrease in fibrinogen's half-life. A more commonly used method is the measurement of fibrinopeptides by radioimmunoassay. During activation of the coagulation system, fibrinogen is cleaved by thrombin into fibrin, releasing the fragments fibrinopeptides A and B (FPA and FPB). When heparin was given in sufficient amounts during hemodialysis to achieve a concentration $> 0.5 \, \text{IU/ml}$, plasma FPA levels did not rise, reflecting the absence of thrombin activity (40, 41). Plasma FPA should also be interpreted with caution. As in the case of βTG, FPA elimination is impaired in renal failure (42). Baseline plasma levels can therefore be higher than normal. Furthermore, this peptide carries a molecular weight of only 1527 daltons. As such, they are dialyzable to some extent. Indeed, dialyzer efferent concentrations of FPA have been shown to be lower than the afferent concentrations in some instances (40). Therefore, the efferent concentrations may not accurately reflect the generation of this peptide. However, if the cleavage of fibrinogen is very active in the presence of inadequate heparinization, the removal of FPA by the dialyzer membrane is unlikely to completely mask its production.

Thrombogenicity is definitely an important issue in the biocompatibility of hemodialysis membranes. Ongoing research is directed at developing thromboresistant membranes. One approach is to develop polymers that do not activate platelets or clotting factors. Alternatively, a more promising approach is to incorporate pharmacologically active anticoagulants such as heparin or prostaglandins onto the membranes. Detachment of these anticoagulant molecules from the membrane surfaces and the binding of these molecules by adsorbed proteins are problems that need further research.

KALLIKREIN AND KININ

As discussed in the last section, contact of blood with foreign surfaces leads to activation of the Hageman factor (factor XII) (38). A series of events can theoretically follow. Besides activating the intrinsic coagulation cascade, activated Hageman factor can also convert prekallikrein to kallikrein (43, 44). Kallikreins can a) provide a positive feedback for the activation of Hageman factor; b) convert kininogen to kinins, which can cause increased vascular permeability, vasodilatation, smooth muscle contraction, and chemotaxis; and c) activate plasmin and therefore fibrinolysis and C_3 conversion. To what extent the kallikrein and bradykinin systems are actually activated during clinical hemodialysis is uncertain (45, 46).

COMPLEMENT

Complement activation

The complement system has received a lot of attention in the area of extracorporeal circulation in recent years. This is probably so for a number of reasons: a) There have been significant advances in the past 10 years in the understanding of the basic mechanisms involved in the activation and control of the complement system. b) There has been increasing understanding of the interactions between the complement system and the other biologic systems. c) There has been increasing realization of the roles of complement in various pathologic states. d) Activation of the complement system is readily detectable with currently available techniques.

The complement system can be activated via the classical or alternative pathway (47, 48). Activation of the classical pathway is usually initiated by formation of antigen-antibody complexes or by antibody bound to cellular or particulate antigens. Although not exclusively so, the alternative pathway is usually activated in the absence of specific antibody. It can be viewed as a first-line defense mechanism by which the immune system can respond to foreign substances expeditiously. Many of the substances known to activate the alternative pathway contain carbohydrate moieties, such as zymosan (a derivative of yeast cell walls) and gram-negative bacterial lipopolysaccharide. Cuprophan membranes are also capable of activating the alternative pathway of complement, presumably because of its carbohydrate structure (49, 50).

The alternative pathway activation is initiated by spontaneous hydrolysis of circulating C_3 molecules, with subsequent generation of trace amount of C_{3b} in the serum (47, 48, 51–53). The C_{3b} attaches to neighboring surfaces. Covalent binding of the α chain of C_{3b} to the surface hydroxyl group of an "activating" biologic surface such as zymosan leads to amplification of the pathway. Under these circumstances, binding of factor B to the C_{3b} is favored over the binding of the regulatory protein factor H. The presence of Mg^{2+} is required for this binding. The factor B bound to C_{3b} can hence be activated by factor D, resulting in the formation of a $C_{3b}Bb$ complex, which is an active C_3 convertase. This pathway is further amplified when another C_3 molecule is cleaved by the C_3 convertase, resulting in another C_{3b} and the anaphylatoxin C_{3a}. The combination of two C_{3b} molecules with the active form of factor B (Bb) is a C_5 convertase, capable of converting C_5 to C_{5b} and another anaphylatoxin, C_{5a}. Although the free hydroxyl groups on the glucosan rings of the cuprophan membrane seem to be ideal moieties for covalent binding of C_{3b}, they may not be the actual sites on the membrane surfaces to which the C_{3b} molecules bind (54). The exact manner in which the activated C_3 is attached to the cuprophan membrane remains unknown at present. Nonetheless, the carbohydrate structure does seem to provide a favorable activating surface, leading to the formation of C_{3a} and C_{5a} (50).

Evidence supporting the hypothesis that activation of complement during hemodialysis is via the alternative pathway is convincing. C_3 activation products have been demonstrated on cuprophan membrane surfaces after clinical hemodialysis (54, 55), in concurrence with the manner in which alternative pathway activation has been described to occur. More evidence is the demonstration of the conversion of factor B, an alternative pathway activating protein, in the dialyzer efferent blood of patients (49). Finally, no increment in the plasma concentration of C_{4a} during hemodialysis is detectable (50), an observation against the activation of the classical pathway.

Figure 1 is a schematic diagram of the proposed mechanism by which the alternative pathway of complement is activated and anaphylatoxins are generated by the cuprophan membrane.

Anaphylatoxins

Some of the in-vitro biologic effects of C_{3a} and C_{5b} have been described for many years. They are termed *anaphylatoxins* because of their abilities to contract guinea-pig ileal smooth muscles (56), to increase vascular permeability (57), and to cause histamine release from mast cells (58). The spasmogenic property of human C_{3a} occurs at nanamolar concentrations, whereas that of C_{5a} occurs at subnanamolar concentrations. More recently, the anaphylatoxins have also been shown to stimulate the production of various arachidonic acid metabolites (35, 59–62), which has further ramifications. In addition, C_{5a} also has granulocyte-directed activities at nanamolar concentrations (63). They bind to C_{5a} receptors present on granulocyte surfaces (64). This ligand-receptor interaction is capable of stimulating the granulocytes to aggregate, to become adhesive to endothelial cells, and to release intracellular oxygen radicals capable of damaging the pulmonary endothelium (65–67). These granulocyte-directed effects of C_{5a} and $C_{5a_{desArg}}$ are probably the major causes of hemodialysis-induced leukopenia. Once released into the circulation, the carboxy-terminal arginine is removed from the anaphylatoxins by a serum carboxypeptidase, resulting in the formation of $C_{3a_{desArg}}$ and $C_{5a_{desArg}}$ (68). These desArginine derivatives are markedly less spasmogenic than their precursors (69). However, $C_{5a_{desArg}}$ retains significant chemotactic activities (63).

Assays for anaphylatoxins

The availability of the radioimmunoassays (RIA) for C_{3a} and C_{5a} antigens has facilitated the detection of complement activation by hemodialysis membranes. They are much more sensitive than hemolytic assays because the baseline concentrations of C_{3a} (76 ± 15 ng/ml) and C_{5a} (14 ± 4 ng/ml) antigens in human plasma are low (50) relative to the plasma levels of intact C_3 and C_5. Activation of a small fraction of the total plasma pool of C_3 and C_5 would be difficult to assess by conventional hemolytic assays. However, the same degree of C_3 and C_5 activation would result in relatively sizable increases in plasma C_{3a} and C_{5a} antigens. The RIA for C_{5a} is also preferable to the leukocyte aggregation bioassay because of its specificity. The bioassay detects any substances that would aggregate leukocytes, such as C_{5a}, leukotrienes, and neutrophil cationic proteins, whereas the RIA for C_{5a} detects C_{5a}-related peptides only.

Anaphylatoxin and hemodialysis membranes

The generation of C_{3a} and C_{5a} during hemodialysis with cuprophan membranes has been clearly demonstrated (50, 70, 71). As seen in Figure 2, the plasma concentrations of C_{3a} antigen in the venous (dialyzer to patient) blood increase abruptly during the initial 15 minutes to a mean value above 6000 ng/ml, which is 15 times above the mean baseline values (50). The plasma C_{3a} antigen concentrations bear a close temporal correlation with the degree of peripheral leukopenia. This, however, does not imply that C_{3a} or its desArg derivative is responsible for the leukopenia. Rather, the increase in its plasma concentration only serves as a marker for complement activation.

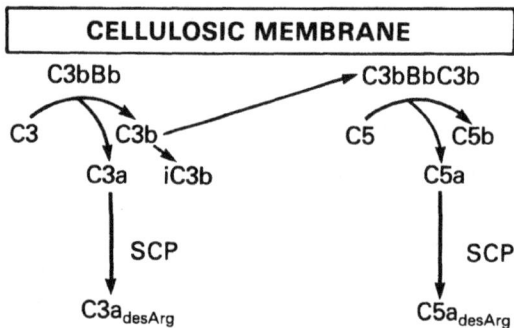

Figure 1. Schematic diagram of the proposed mechanism by which complement activation via the alternative pathway occurs on the cuprophan dialyzer membrane. C_{3b} spontaneously generated in the plasma binds to the membrane surface. Presumably the carbohydrate structure of the membrane favors the binding of factor B to the surface-bound C_{3b}. Factor B is then converted to the active form Bb by the action of factor D. The $C_{3b}Bb$ complex is a C_3 convertase, capable of converting intact C_3 to C_{3a} and C_{3b}. The latter can be converted to the inactive form (iC_{3b}) by factors H and I. The complex of two C_{3b} molecules and Bb is a C_5 convertase, capable of converting C_5 to C_{5a} and C_{5a}. Both C_{3a} and C_{5a} are anaphylatoxins. They are converted into $C_{3a_{desArg}}$ and $C_{5a_{desArg}}$ by a serum carboxypeptidase (SCP). $C_{3a_{desArg}}$ is biologically rather inactive, but $C_{5a_{desArg}}$ retains significant leukocyte-directed properties.

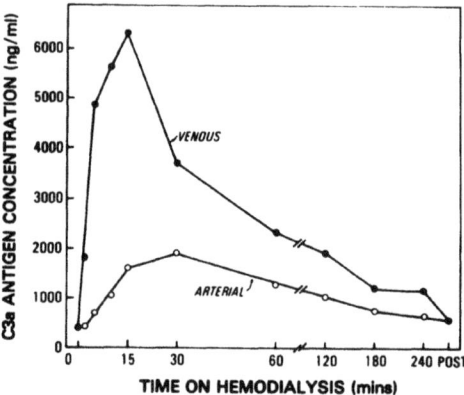

Figure 2. Concentrations of C_{3a} antigens in plasma obtained from patients during hemodialysis with new (unused) cuprophan membrane dialyzers. Each data point represents the mean of 12 observations. The rapid accumulation of C_{3a} antigens in the plasma during the initial 15 minutes coincides with the development of peripheral leukopenia. Clearance of these antigens by the patient's body leads to the decline in subsequent hours (see text). The arterial (patient to dialyzer) concentrations are consistently lower than the venous concentrations, suggesting the C_{3a} were formed during the passage of blood through the cuprophan dialyzers. Modified from Chenoweth et al. (50) with permission from *Kidney International*.

Other products of this activation further down the cascade (C_{5a} and $C_{5a_{desArg}}$) are likely to be the causative agents. The increase in C_{3a} antigen concentrations in the first 15 minutes is followed by a gradual decrease during the next few hours towards baseline values. This decrease is due to the decreased generation rate and increased clearance by the patients' body (70). Arterial (patient to dialyzer) plasma concentrations of C_{3a} antigen are consistently below those in the venous samples, indicating that the C_{3a} is generated during the passage of blood through the cuprophan dialyzers.

The maximum plasma C_{5a} antigen concentrations during cuprophan hemodialysis are usually around 200 ng/ml, which are significantly lower than those of C_{3a} antigens (50, 71). The difference between the peak plasma concentrations of C_{3a} and C_{5a} antigens is probably due to multiple factors. First, the predialysis baseline C_{3a} antigen concentrations are higher than those of C_{5a} antigens. Second, the efficiency of C_5 conversion is lower than that of C_3 conversion. Third, the clearance of C_{5a} antigens by the patient's body seems to be more efficient than that of C_{3a} (70). As mentioned above, C_{5a} binds to receptors on the surfaces of granulocytes. However, this binding to granulocytes does not seem to be the only clearance mechanism for C_{5a}. In fact, the body clearance of C_{5a} is maximal (almost 900 ml/min) at 15–30 minutes from the beginning of cuprophan hemodialysis, when the circulating leukocyte counts are at their nadir, suggesting that other tissues contribute significantly to its clearance. This concurs with animal studies demonstrating the uptake of injected C_{5a} by extravascular tissues independent of neutrophil attachment (72).

The transfer of these anaphylatoxins into the dialysate compartments from the blood compartments is small because of their relatively large sizes (9000–11,000 daltons) (73). Dialysis membranes, however, have the capabilities of adsorbing the anaphylatoxins onto their surfaces. In-vitro models show that different dialysis membranes adsorb anaphylatoxins to different extents. Polyacrylonitrile membranes adsorb a significant amount of $C_{5a_{desArg}}$ onto their surfaces. This concurs with the observation that granulocyte-aggregating activity generated in serum by zymosan activation can be removed by exposure to these membranes (74). Cuprophan membranes adsorb significantly less anaphylatoxins than polyacrylonitrile. Cellulose acetate membranes are intermediate between the two. The adsorption of anaphylatoxins in nonspecific, in that cytochrome C, a molecule with similar size and charge, is adsorbed onto the polyacrylonitrile surfaces almost as well (73) as anaphylatoxins.

Polyacrylonitrile membranes also possess other interesting properties that had previously generated controversy in the literature. The topic of hemodialysis-induced leukopenia will be further discussed in the section on granulocytes. Here, we shall only discuss some aspects related to complement activation.

It had previously been shown that polyacrylonitrile membranes produced minimal leukopenia, yet they were associated with a significant decrease in complement hemolytic titers (CH50) (75). If CH50 is an accurate indicator of complement activation, these two observations would superficially appear to be inconsistent with the notion that complement activation products are responsible for dialysis induced leukopenia. Subsequent studies provide plausible explanations for this apparent discrepancy. When cuprophan and polyacrylonitrile membranes were incubated with serum in vitro, more C3 activation was found to occur in the presence of polyacrylonitrile membranes (76). Most of the generated C3a, however, remained bound to the polyacrylonitrile membrane surface. The concentration of this anaphylatoxin in the serum was therefore low. Presumably, C5a behaves in a similar manner, resulting in less leukocyte-aggregating activity in the serum. Complement activation induced by polyacrylonitrile membranes causes consumption in complement proteins and therefore decrease in the CH50. In addition, because of the large capacity of polyacrylonitrile membranes to adsorb proteins, more C3 and C5 may be adsorbed onto their surfaces. This removal of unactivated complement from the plasma may also lead to a decrease in CH50. It is of further interest that, in addition to the adsorption of complement components, polyacrylonitrile membranes also seem to have significant capacities to absorb a variety of other substances such as fibrinogen, IgG, Cl_q (77), and interleukin-1 (78).

Attenuation of hemodialysis-induced complement activation

Complement activation via the alternative pathway by hemodialysis membranes can be attenuated by various means. A number of noncuprophan membranes have been shown to be associated with less complement activation. Among the family of cellulosic membranes, cellulose acetate membranes have been shown to be associated with less complement activation and perhaps less intradialytic symptoms than cuprophan membranes (79). Another cellulosic membrane manufactured by Akzo, Hemophan®, also activates less complement than cuprophan, as assessed by plasma C_{3a} concentrations (6,7). Likewise, noncellulosic membranes such as polysulfone and polymethylmethacrylate are also more biocompatible in this regard (34, 71, 73). Compared to cuprophan, membranes that

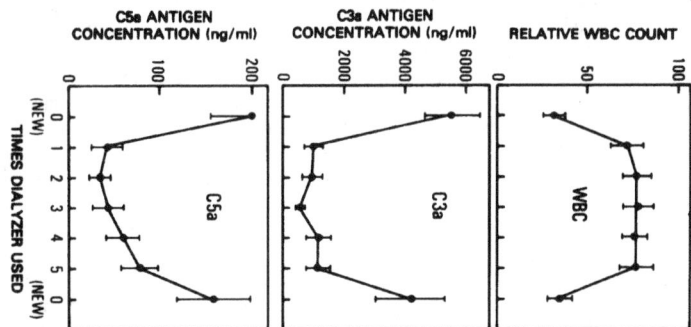

Figure 3. Effects of dialyzer reuse on leukopenia and complement activation. Depicted are peripheral leukocyte (WBC) counts (top panel), venous plasma C_{3a} antigen concentrations (middle panel), and C_{5a} antigen concentrations (bottom panel) at 15 minutes after starting hemodialysis with new cuprophan membranes and the same membranes during five subsequent reuses. Each data point represents the mean of 11 observations. Dialyzer reuse is associated with less complement activation and peripheral leukopenia. Most of the changes from new membranes occur during the first reuse. Modified from Chenoweth et al. (55) with permission from *Kidney International.*

activate less complement (generate less anaphylatoxins) are also associated with less leukopenia.

Of particular interest are reused cuprophan membranes sterilized with formaldehyde, which are associated with less complement activation and less leukopenia than their unused counterparts (55, 80). Figure 3 depicts the peripheral leukocyte counts, and plasma C_{3a} and C_{5a} antigen concentrations, at 15 minutes from the beginning of hemodialysis employing new and sequentially reused cuprophan membranes (55). As can be seen, the improvement in biocompatibility in terms of leukopenia and complement activation occurs after the first use and does not change significantly during susbsequent reuses. However, when the used cuprophan membranes were treated with sodium hypochlorite, the capabilities of the membranes to activate complement and to induce leukopenia are resumed (81–83). These correlations between the degrees of complement activation and the degrees of leukopenia by different types of membranes further support the causal relationship between the two phenomena.

The reasons for the relatively lower potentials of certain membranes to activate complement are not completely understood. Presumably, the noncellulosic membranes do not contain the carbohydrate moieties that make the membranes favorable for factor-B binding. In the case of cellulose acetate membranes, substitution of the hydroxyl groups on the glucose rings with acetyl groups apparently exerts a negative influence on complement activation. Nonetheless, the mechanism is unlikely to be a simple blockade of C_{3b} binding to the hydroxyl groups (54, 84), since Hemophan membranes are also associated with significantly less complement activation (6, 7). On the Hemophan membranes, only 1 out of 150 hydroxyl groups is substituted by a tertiary amino group. In the case of reused cuprophan membranes, attenuation of complement activation is not due to formaldehyde exposure per se, since treatment of new dialyzers with formaldehyde does not prevent activation (55). Using a polyclonal antibody, C_{3b} antigens have been demonstrated to be present on these used membranes after 4 hours of clinical hemodialysis. Presumably, the presence of some biologically inactive breakdown products of C_{3b} (iC_{3b}, C_{3c}, and/or C_{3dg}) prevents binding of active C_{3b} during subsequent reuses. Without the binding of C_{3b}, the active alternative pathway C_3 convertase cannot be formed. The cleansing agent sodium hypochlorite may resume the C_{3b} binding capacity of the used membranes by removing these inhibitory proteins (54, 85).

Modulation of complement activation during hemodialysis can also be achieved in other manners. For example, cooling of the dialysate has been used to diminish intradialytic hypotension (86, 87). Since complement activation is temperature dependent, such treatments are associated with less C_{3a} and C_{5a} generation, and correspondingly less leukopenia (88). Regional citrate anticoagulation has been used as an alternative to heparinization for hemodialysis in some centers. Since alternative pathway complement activation is dependent on the availability of divalent cations, chelation of these cations in the extracorporeal circuits also attenuates C_{3a} generation (89).

In-vivo effects of dialysis membrane biocompatibility and the effects of anaphylatoxins in animal models

The physiologic effects of blood or plasma exposure to dialysis membranes have been studied in several animal models. Craddock et al. initially examined the effects of cellophane-activated plasma in sheep (90). Infusion of autologous plasma previously incubated with cellophane membranes into the animals produced significant pulmonary leukose-questration, leukopenia, pulmonary hypertension, increased lymph outflow from the lungs, and arterial hypoxemia. These effects could be abolished by heat inactivation of plasma, depletion of complement with cobra-venom factor, or chelation of divalent cations with EDTA prior to incubation with cellophane, suggesting that complement activation products are the mediators of these physiologic disturbances.

The swine model has also been employed to study the physiologic effects of blood-membrane interactions (36, 91). This species provides certain advantages for studies in this particular area. a) It is a sensitive model. b) The structures and the in-vitro properties of porcine anaphylatoxins have been well characterized (69, 92–94). c) The physiologic responses of swine to exercise resemble those in human (95).

Bolus infusion of autologous plasma that has been previously recirculated through cuprophan hemodialyzers into the swine also produces peripheral leukopenia, pulmonary hypertension, hypoxemia, acute fluctuation in systemic arterial pressure, a decrease in cardiac output, and an increase in left ventricular end-diastolic pressure (91). Infusion of zymosan-activated plasma or purified $C_{5a_{desArg}}$ produce similar results, suggesting that these physiologic responses are mediated by anaphylatoxins. The pulmonary hypertension is inhibited by a specific thromboxane synthetase inhibitor (36), suggesting that the arachidonic acid metabolites, thromboxanes, are mediators of the vasoconstrictive response induced by anaphylatoxins in the pulmonary vascular bed. The sources of the thromboxanes in this setting are primarily the lungs, instead of the peripheral leukocytes and platelets. It has further been shown in experimental animals that the pulmonary hypertension induced by cuprophan-activated plasma precedes the development of pulmonary leukostasis (96) and peripheral leukopenia (36).

From the currently available data, the following sequence of events can be postulated. Exposure of the animals' plasma to cuprophan membranes in vitro or ex vivo stimulates alternative pathway complement activation and the production of anaphylatoxins, C_{3a} and C_{5a}. When this activated plasma is infused into the animals, the anaphylatoxins stimulate the release of thromboxanes, primarily from the lungs. These potent eicosanoids then act locally to contract vascular smooth muscles to produce pulmonary hypertension. The participation of the leukotrienes and other mediators cannot be excluded. In addition, anaphylatoxins C_{5a} and $C_{5a_{desArg}}$ also cause the granulocytes to aggregate in the pulmonary vasculature with subsequent peripheral leukopenia. Hypoxemia likely results from the deranged pulmonary physiology induced directly or indirectly by the anaphylatoxins, which probably includes bronchial constriction and interstitial fluid accumulation from increased vascular permeability. In such animal models, the anaphylatoxins are undoubtedly the initiating factors.

Animal models have also been employed to compare the effects of different types of dialysis membranes (97). In parallel to the plasma anaphylatoxin levels in humans, cuprophan-activated plasma induces a significant increase in pulmonary arterial pressure, whereas cellulose acetate, polyacrylonitrile (97), and reused cuprophan membranes sterilized with formaldehyde (98) are associated with lesser degrees of pulmonary hypertension. Exposure of blood or plasma to polyvinylchloride blood tubings per se does not produce these physiologic alterations. Thus, the dialysis membrane itself is the important factor (91, 97).

Such animal models using bolus infusion of membrane-activated plasma or blood tend to produce drastic responses. Nonetheless, they may be analogous to the clinical events in patients who might have defective inactivation of anaphylatoxins or abnormal end-organ responsiveness to various mediators. In addition, it is useful to employ models with exaggerated responses to bring out the more subtle changes that might be induced by continuous exposure of blood to dialysis membranes and allow for the study of their pathogenetic mechanisms. In this regard, it should be noted that mock dialysis of swine with cuprophan membranes in the absence of dialysate also produces pulmonary hypertension (91). Mock dialysis in human volunteers is also associated with hypoxemia (99).

LEUKOCYTES

Adherence of leukocytes to dialyzer membranes

Besides platelets and erythrocytes, leukocytes also adhere to artificial membrane surfaces (14, 100). Although the adherence is prominent on microscopic examination, it is not a major cause of the hemodialysis-induced leukopenia phenomenon. Polymorphonuclear cells are the predominant leukocyte associated with the membranes, although eosinophils are occasionally seen in clusters. The predilection of granulocytes to adhere to the dialyzer membranes may be due to their responsiveness to chemotactic factors generated during hemodialysis, such as C_{5a}, its desArginine derivative, C_3 activation products, neutrophil cationic proteins, and leukotriene B_4. Adhesion of leukocytes to the artificial membrane surfaces results in the exposure of tissue thromboplastin (101), which is an activator of the extrinsic coagulation pathway. In addition, the intragranular proteolytic enzymes released by the stimulated leukocytes can also activate clotting factors. Hence, the leukocytes may also have a role in thrombogenesis in the extracorporeal circuit.

Hemodialysis-induced leukopenia

Kaplow and Goffinet first described the phenomenon of transient leukopenia during hemodialysis with cellophane membranes almost 20 years ago (102). It typically occurs shortly after blood contact with dialyzer membranes. The leukocyte counts achieved their nadir at 10–15 minutes. Recovery from the leukopenia occurs during the next 30–45 minutes and is occasionally accompanied by rebound of the leukocyte counts to values above the baselines. The cells that disappear from the peripheral circulation are primarily the neutrophils, monocytes, and, occasionally, eosinophils (103, 104). Lymphocytes are usually not affected. After almost 20 years, debates on the pathogenesis of this phenomenon still continue. Although leukocytes have been found to adhere to the dialyzer membrane surfaces, this sequestration of cells is only a minor contributing factor, since changes in the leukocyte counts across the dialyzers are small (50, 102). Furthermore, limited studies using indium-labeled neutrophil did not show an increase in the radioactivity over the dialyzers when peripheral leukopenia occurred (105). Plasma seems to be an important factor for this phenomenon since infusion of saline previously exposed to cellophane did not produce this phenomenon (106).

Craddock et al. first demonstrated that complement activation occurred via the alternative pathway during cellophane hemodialysis (49, 90). They suggested that the complement activation product C_{5a} was responsible for the pulmonary leukosequestration, peripheral leukopenia, and hypoxemia in the dialysis patients. The granulocyte aggregation bioassay they employed was not specific for C_{5a}. Their hypothesis for the mechanism of hemodialysis-induced hypoxemia was probably inaccurate. Nonetheless, their series of elegant studies were innovative, informative, and stimulated exciting investigations in the areas of immunology, renal and pulmonary diseases, artificial organs, and several other fields.

As discussed previously, their studies strongly suggest that complement activation products can, and probably do, produce dialysis leukopenia. The specific complement activation product was proposed to be C_{5a}. They further suggested that the pulmonary leukosequestration was responsible for the hemodialysis-induced hypoxemia. Indeed, their studies (90) and those of others (91, 97) clearly demonstrated that infusion of cuprophan-activated plasma into experimental animals produced profound pulmonary hypertension and hypoxemia. In their clinical studies on hemodialysis patients, they demonstrated a fall in pulmonary diffusion capacity and an increase in closing volumes. In addition, they cited an increased alveolar-arterial oxygen tension gradient as evidence for the dialysis membrane effect on oxygenation (90). However, the oxygen gradient was calculated assuming that the respiratory quotient remained constant during hemodialysis. This assumption was later shown to be inaccurate, because the carbon dioxide excreted through the lungs did not reflect the total amount produced by the body during acetate hemodialysis (107–109). The issue of hypoxemia will be further explored in the Clinical section below.

Since these provocative, though not completely accurate, postulates of Craddock et al., many clinical and animal studies have emerged to support, expand, modify, or refute them. Complement activation via the alternative pathway during cuprophan hemodialysis has been clearly demonstrated, as indicated above. The pulmonary leukosequestration during hemodialysis has been demonstrated in patients using indium-labeled neutrophils (105). The production of anaphylatoxins C_{3a} and C_{5a} have also been confirmed by radioimmunoassays. The time course of complement activation correlates well with that of peripheral leukopenia (50, 71). Attenuation of complement activation by reuse of cuprophan membranes, employment of other types of membranes, citrate administration, or cooling of dialysate all lead to a corresponding decrease in leukopenia. This further adds support to the role of complement activation products in the pathogenesis of hemodialysis leukopenia. Pulmonary hypertension has been shown to occur during clinical hemodialysis (110, 111). Animal studies are also supportive of the role of anaphylatoxins in this phenomenon, although it is more likely to be caused by pulmonary vasoconstriction than by leukocyte plugging of the blood vessels (91).

The causal relationship between complement activation and leukopenia has, however, been disputed. Studies that have often been cited to dissociate these two phenomena are those that employed hemolytic assays to detect complement activation (75, 112). The pitfalls of using these assays are two-fold. First, these bioassays are rather insensitive because of the relatively small fractions of plasma complement components that are usually activated and consumed during hemodialysis. As such, there may be relatively small changes in C_3 or CH50 titers despite a substantial generation of C_{3a}, i.e., they are false negatives. Secondly, the decrease in CH50 titers may be caused by removal or adsorption of C_3 and C_5, rather than consumption by activation of complement, i.e., they are false-positives. Convincing data that refute the hypothesis that complement activation products cause dialysis induced peripheral leukopenia is still lacking.

Recovery of dialysis-induced leukopenia is rapid. Factors contributing to this recovery are multiple: a) The rate of complement activation abates after the initial 15 minutes (50). b) The granulocytes are released after only a brief period of sequestration in the pulmonary vasculature (103, 105). c) The bone marrow responds to the leukopenia by releasing more granulocytes (103). d) After the period of leukopenia, the peripheral granulocytes have been reported to become unresponsive to further chemotactic stimulation by C_{5a}. Presumably, this results from downregulation of the C_{5a} receptors on the granulocyte surfaces (113). To what extent this phenomenon of receptor downregulation actually occurs and contributes to the recovery of the leukopenia is uncertain (114).

More recently, other candidates, such as neutrophil cationic proteins (NCP) and platelet activating factor (PAF), have been proposed as alternative mediators of dialysis-induced leukopenia (115). In-vitro studies demonstrated the release of these substances when plasma-free human neutrophils were incubated with cuprophan membranes (116). These substances have also been shown to promote neutrophil aggregation. However, these observations do not refute the role of complement activation products in dialysis leukopenia, especially in view of the many potential interactions of these mediators with the complement system (37, 117). It is probable that the cuprophan membrane activates the neutrophils by C_{5a}-dependent and C_{5a}-independent mechanisms, resulting in the production of NCP and PAF. These neutrophil products then potentiate the action of C_{5a} (and $C_{5a_{desArg}}$) to induce neutrophil aggregation. In addition, NCP also activates C_5, probably by direct proteolysis. A simplified scheme of the proposed effects of the anaphylatoxins and some of their interactions with the neutrophils are presented in Figure 4. It should be pointed out that some of the events depicted in the diagram have only been demonstrated in vitro or in animal studies, and have not been documented in dialysis patients.

It is clear that anaphylatoxin C_{5a} (and probably some other mediators) possess the properties to aggregate granulocytes and cause them to attach to endothelial cells. Regardless of whether the granulocytes aggregate before they embolize to the lungs or they adhere to the pulmonary endothelium as individual cells, the net result is the formation of "leukocyte thrombi" in the pulmonary vasculature. The presence of these thrombi per se is unlikely to be the cause of hypoxemia, nor are they essential for the development of pulmonary hypertension (36, 96). However, the release of intracellular substances by the activated granulocytes may potentiate the anaphylatoxins to exert deleterious effects on the lungs.

Degranulation of granulocytes

Mature neutrophils contain two types of granules, azurophil (primary) and specific (secondary) (118). These granules contain a wide variety of enzymes, and many of them are proteinases that catalyze catabolic reactions. The azurophil granules contain myeloperoxidase, which potentiates the microbicidal and chemiluminescence activities of hydrogen peroxide; lysozyme and cationic proteins, which are involved in bacterial killing; and elastase, which has a broad substrate specificity and may be involved in collagen vascular diseases. The specific granules also contain lysozyme. In addition, they contain lactoferrin, which chelates iron and therefore has bacteriostatic properties. With the proper stimuli, such as phagocytosis, complement activation products, and endotoxins, neutrophils degranulate and extrude certain granular contents extracellu-

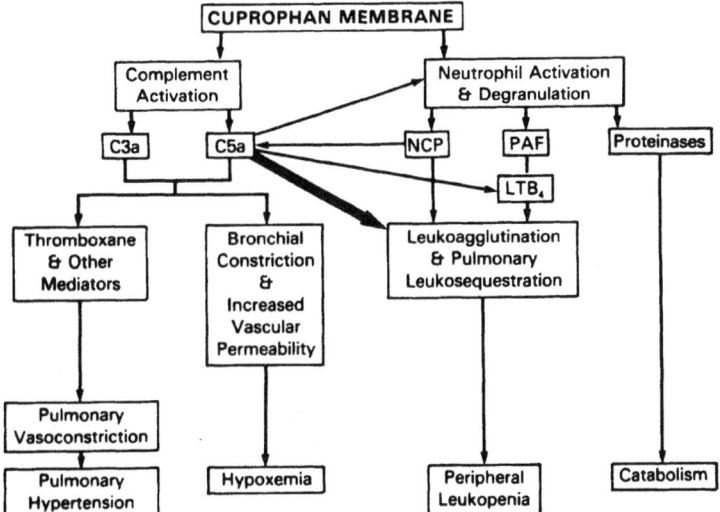

Figure 4. Proposed effects of anaphylatoxins and their interactions with the neutrophils. The dialyzer membrane triggers complement activation with the resultant formation of anaphylatoxins C_{3a} and C_{5a}. The dialyzer membrane, and probably C_{5a}, also activate the granulocytes and cause them to degranulate, releasing biologically active substances. Some of these are proteinases from intracellular granules, which may contributed to intradialytic catabolism. C_{5a} and its desArg derivative are largely responsible for the hemodialysis leukopenia. Platelet-activating factor (PAF), neutrophil cationic proteins (NCP), and leukotriene B_4 (LTB_4) from neutrophils are probably contributory. The interactions between the complement system and the granulocytes are complex; this diagram is a simplified view of some of their interactions as they may relate to dialyzer membranes. Note that the anaphylatoxins also stimulate thromboxane production to cause pulmonary hypertension, which is independent of the pulmonary leukosequestration. They probably also contribute to the pathogenesis of dialysis-induced hypoxemia.

larly. The released proteinases can result in tissue injury and the breakdown of plasma proteins. These proteolytic activities are controlled by plasma proteinase inhibitors such as α_2-macroglobulin and α_1-proteinase inhibitor (α_1-antitrypsin).

Degranulation of both azurophil and specific granules have been shown during hemodialysis, as evident by the increase in serum levels of myeloperoxidase, lactoferrin, and elastase (79, 119). Although in-vitro studies demonstrate that the release of lysozyme from specific granules can be enhanced by adherence to certain artificial surfaces and C_{5a} (120), clinical studies could not demonstrate an increase in plasma lysozyme levels during hemodialysis with a variety of membranes (49, 121). Instead, plasma lysozyme levels decrease during dialysis with polyacrylonitrile or polymethylmethacrylate membranes (121, 122). This decrease is probably due to the adsorption of lysozymes onto the polyacrylonitrile membranes. It is known that polyacrylonitrile membranes have a high propensity to adsorb a large variety of proteins and that lysozymes have a high tendency to bind to membranes (123).

It is well known that C_{5a} has granulocyte-directed activities. It causes granulocytes to aggregate and stimulates their release of intracellular proteins (124) and oxygen radicals (67). Plasma lactoferrin levels increase during hemodialysis with cellulosic membranes and seem to correlate with the degree of complement activation (79). It therefore seems logical to propose that the C_{5a} generated as a result of complement activation during hemodialysis is the cause of proteinase release from the granulocytes. However, recent studies suggest that this release may be independent of complement activation. Hörl et al. assessed the release of neutrophil elastase by measuring the elastase-α_1-proteinase inhibitor (E-α_1PI) complexes in the plasma of patients undergoing dialysis with different types of membranes (125). Cuprophan membranes induced higher E-α_1PI levels than polyacrylonitrile and polysulfone membranes. Of interest are polymethylmethacrylate membranes. Despite their minimal ability to activate complement and induce leukopenia, polymethylmethacrylate membranes were found to be associated with high plasma concentrations of myeloperoxidase, elastase, and lactoferrin, indicating release from both azurophil and specific granules (119). In fact, these membranes were associated with higher E-α_1PI levels than cuprophan, polysulfone, and polyacrylonitrile membranes after 5 hours of dialysis (125). These data suggest that degranulation may occur independent of complement stimulation and leukoagglutination. Mechanical shearing of the neutrophils per se can induce degranulation and release of enzymes (126). Shearing can also enhance the aggregation of leukocytes, which is another potential stimulus for enzyme release (3, 127). These observations do not, however, preclude the participation of C_{5a} in neutrophil degranulation.

There has been speculation about the significance of neutrophil degranulation during hemodialysis. Hemodialysis has been considered to be a catabolic event (128, 129). Potential causes of this catabolism proposed were gluconeogenesis and protein breakdown to replace the amino acid and glucose losses into the dialysate. However, replacement of amino acid losses by infusion of amino acids or prevention of glucose losses by increasing the dialysate glucose concentration does not prevent the catabolism. With the demonstration of the release of intracellular proteolytic enzymes from neutrophil granules, it has been postulated that this release phenomenon contributes to the catabolism during hemodialysis (130). Despite the differences in the intradialytic increases in plasma proteinases concentrations associated with different dialysis membranes, it is unclear at present how these differences translate into the degrees of intradialytic catabolism.

The proteolytic enzyme elastase can also degrade fibronectin (131). Indeed, the serum concentrations of fibronectin have been shown to decrease transiently at 10 minutes after starting dialysis with cellulosic membranes (132, 133). The time course coincides with pulmonary leukosequestration of neutrophils but does not coincide with the changes in plasma E-α_1PI concentrations (125). How this decrease in plasma levels translates into changes in tissue levels of fibronectin and what impact this has on the integrity of the pulmonary vascular endothelium are unknown.

Besides neutrophils, eosinophils also degranulate during hemodialysis with the release of eosinophil cationic proteins (123, 134, 135). The dialysis membranes per se seems to be an important factor in eosinophil degranulation independent of complement activation (135). The exact effects of these released cationic proteins on dialysis patients are unknown, although these proteins have been shown to be active in the coagulation and fibrinolytic systems (136, 137).

Intradialytic alterations in other neutrophil functions

It has been demonstrated that peripheral mature neutrophils consist of two populations. One that comprises 80% of the peripheral pool is able to form rosettes with IgG-sensitized erythrocytes. The other population, which does not form such rosettes, performs inferiorly in bioassays of adherence, phagocytosis of opsonized bacteria, bactericidal activities, and chemotaxis to stimuli such as $C_{5a_{desArg}}$ or endotoxin-activated serum (138). Neutrophils obtained from patients at 15–20 minutes after starting hemodialysis with cellulosic membranes when peripheral neutrophil counts are at their nadir showed a significant shift of the predominant population to the non-rosette-forming variety. In addition to their unresponsiveness to the chemotactic stimulus of $C_{5a_{desArg}}$, the cells remaining in the peripheral circulation also displayed an impairment in adherence (139). Furthermore, they have been shown to have defective oxidative metabolism, which is manifested by a decreased production of hydrogen peroxide and luminol-enhanced chemiluminescence (140).

Neutrophils obtained at 60 minutes from patients undergoing cuprophan hemodialysis also showed decreased chemiluminescence in response to zymosan stimulation (141). At this time point, however, the neutrophils sequestered in the pulmonary vasculature have already returned to the peripheral circulation. This decreased chemiluminescence is therefore unlikely to be due to a shift in neutrophil subsets. Potentially, the decrease is due to the degranulation of neutrophils and loss of myeloperoxide, which is essential for the phenomenon of chemiluminescence.

Hemodialysis with cuprophan membranes is also associated with an increase in the expression of C_{3b} receptors on neutrophils (142). C_{3b} receptors (also known as CR1) on neutrophils serve to enhance phagocytosis (143). The degree of this upregulation of C_{3b} receptors seems to correlate with the degree of complement activation. Since C_{5a} has also been shown to stimulate C_{3b} receptor expression in vitro, it is likely that this anaphylatoxin is responsible for the upregulation of neutrophil C_{3b} receptors during hemodialysis. Intravascular stimulation of the neutrophils in such a purposeless manner thrice weekly in the absence of infection has been proposed to be an undesirable event.

The functional abnormalities of neutrophils induced by membrane exposure depend on the nature of membrane materials. For example, neutrophils exposed to cellulose acetate membranes result in decreased chemotaxis, phagocytosis, and random motility, whereas only chemotaxis is abnormal in neutrophils exposed to polysulfone membranes (144).

Lymphocytes

Although peripheral lymphocytopenia does not usually occur during hemodialysis, changes in the characteristics of the peripheral lymphocytes have been reported. Using cell electrophoretic analysis, it has been shown that at 15 minutes after starting dialysis with regenerated cellulose membranes, there was a shift in the electrophoretic mobility histograms of the patients' peripheral lymphocytes (145). The relative number of low-mobility cells (primarily B cells) decreased. In contrast, there is not a noticeable alteration induced by polyacrylonitrile membranes. The etiology of such an alteration by cellulosic membranes and its effects are unknown at present.

Preliminary data showed that dialysis membranes also had an effect on natural killer cell function (146). Natural killer cells in the peripheral blood that were exposed to cuprophan membranes had decreased function compared to those exposed to polycarbonate membranes. This adverse effect on natural killer cell function can potentially impair the patients' defense against viral infection and tumors.

INTERLEUKIN-1

Properties of interleukin-1

The potential role of interleukin-1 (IL-1) in the pathogenesis of fever in the dialysis patient has stimulated significant interest among nephrologists. There has been a large volume of literature and several comprehensive reviews on IL-1 published in the past few years (147–149). Some of the aspects pertinent to hemodialysis will be discussed here. IL-1 represents a class of polypeptides that possess a wide variety of biologic activities coded by more than a single gene. The molecular weights of the various species of human IL-1 are between 15,000 and 35,000 daltons. The primary sources of IL-1 are blood monocytes, pulmonary macrophages, and phagocytic cells in the liver and spleen. They have recently been recognized as important mediators of acute responses to infection and inflammation. A prominent function of IL-1 is its ability to activate lymphocytes in the presence of antigens or mitogens. In fact, bioassays for IL-1, in general, exploit this particular property and involve enhancement of the murine thymocyte mitogenic responses to phytohemagglutinin by IL-1.

Many exogenous substances can stimulate the production IL-1. Most of them originate from microorganisms, including viruses, bacteria, mycobacteria, and fungi. Substances from other sources are also effective. One of the best known stimuli of IL-1 production is endotoxin lipopolysaccharide (LPS) from gram-negative bacteria. LPS is ubiquitous and is often resistant to autoclaving, organic solvents, acids, and ethanol. Endotoxin carries a molecular weight of 1×10^6 daltons and is therefore unable to cross intact dialysis membranes. However, a fragment of endotoxin that is also pyrogenic, lipid A, carries a molecular weight as small as 2000 daltons. Furthermore, muramyl dipeptides (400–1000 daltons) derived from bacterial cell walls that are not detected by the limulus amebocyte lysate assay are also potent stimuli of IL-1 production. Endogenous substances such as lymphokines are also inducers of IL-1. It should be noted that the production of IL-1 by phagocytic cells as the result of exogenous stimuli begins with transcription of new mRNA before protein synthesis. Therefore, it is unlikely that fever occurring in the early phase of hemodialysis is caused by dialysis-induced IL-1 production.

Stimulation of interleukin-1 production by the hemodialysis circuit

Recently, Bingel et al. studied the production of IL-1 by human blood monocytes after recirculation of the blood through regenerated cellulose hollow-fiber dialyzers in vitro (150). Increased production or IL-1 was demonstrated only when purified endotoxins were added to the dialysate. Although the intact endotoxins in the dialysate compartments cannot cross the intact dialysis membranes, they may be able to cross membranes with microruptures. In addition, as discussed above, the other smaller derivatives of the bacterial cell wall can cross the intact membranes. It has been proposed that lysozymes released from granulocytes as a result of degranulation at the dialysis membrane interphase may cleave off small muramyl dipeptides from the bacterial envelopes (contained in the endotoxin preparation), which can then cross the dialysis membranes and stimulate IL-1 production.

C_{5a} generated as a result of complement activation is known to promote the production of IL-1 (151). Preliminary in-vitro data suggested that dialysis membrane can induce IL-1 production in the absence of endotoxin and activated complement (78). In particular, polyacrylonitrile membrane sheets stimulated monocytes to generate IL-1 far more than regenerated cellulose membranes did. However, removal of IL-1 from PAN dialyzers were also greater, presumably because of greater membrane adsorption and transfer to the dialysate compartments.

Potential effects of interleukin-1 on dialysis patients

A prominent action of IL-1 is its ability to induce fever, presumably by increasing the prostaglandin E level in the brain, thereby raising the hypothalamic temperature setpoint (148). Because of this property, IL-1, or at least one form of this class of molecules, have been called *endogenous pyrogen*. It has been speculated that IL-1 participates in the pathogenesis of fever in dialysis patients. To what extent these peptides are actually produced in vivo during the 4 or 5 hours of clinical hemodialysis is currently unknown.

The spectrum of reported biologic activities of IL-1 is wide. Some of these activities that have potential effects on hemodialysis patients are depicted in Table 2. Although plasma IL-1 levels have been shown to be elevated in hemodialysis patients (152), direct evidence for IL-1 as the pathogenetic factor in causing these abnormal-

Table 2. Biologic activities of interleukin-l*

Fever
Lymphocyte stimulation
Muscle proteolysis and negative nitrogen balance
Hypozincemia
Effects on neutrophils
   Release of neutrophils from bone marrow
   Neutrophil degranulation*
   Chemotaxis
Bone resorption
Anorexia
Enhanced procoagulant activity
Changes in production of hepatic proteins
   Increase acute-phase reactants such as amyloid AA protein
   Decrease albumin synthesis

* The spectrum of biologic activities of interleukin-l is broad. Listed are some of the activities that potentially affect the hemodialysis patient. However, at present, there is no convincing data to support their actual participation in these phenomena in this population.

ities is lacking. As the methodology for assaying IL-1 becomes more widely available, more studies will evolve to delineate the possible roles of these substances with multiple biologic functions. For example, because of their muscle proteolytic properties, they may contribute to the catabolic effects of hemodialysis. IL-1 is also a potent inducer of synthesis of hepatic acute-phase reactants, including serum AA protein, which is a precursor of the amyloid fibril in patients with secondary amyloidosis. It is tempting to postulate that the IL-1-induced production of AA protein is the cause of the amyloidosis seen commonly in dialysis patients. However, in view of the recent identification of β_2 microglobulin in the tissues of localized amyloidosis in hemodialysis patients (see next section), the importance of AA in the pathogenesis of the amyloidosis seen in these patients is unclear.

β_2 MICROGLOBULIN

Arthropathy afflicts dialysis patients commonly. One form of arthropathy that seems to be much more prevalent in these patients compared to the general population is amyloid osteoarthropathy. It is manifested by periarticular bone erosions and cystic lesions in the bones (153, 154). Hemodialysis patients also have a higher incidence of carpal tunnel syndrome, some of which has been shown to be caused by localized amyloidosis (155–157). Recently, some of these amyloid deposits in dialysis patients have been identified as β_2 microglobulin (β_2MG) (158–162). β_2MG carries a molecular weight of 11,000 daltons. Similar to the AA proteins of the classical secondary amyloid, β_2MG also loses Congo-red staining when the tissues are treated with potassium permanganate. However, they can be distinguished from AA by specific immunochemical staining (158). Carpal tunnel syndromes and amyloid tumors in bones that lead to fractures have been reported to be associated with β_2MG (161).

In two studies, carpal tunnel syndrome caused by amyloidosis was primarily reported to be associated with long-term dialysis with cuprophan membranes. Dialysis with polyacrylonitrile membranes is either associated with no or a lower incidence of this disease (154, 157). Recently, the effects of dialysis membranes on β_2MG levels have been described in a number of preliminary reports. Serum β_2MG levels are higher in patients dialyzed with cuprophan than with polyacrylonitrile membranes (163). Plasma β_2MG levels are increased during the course of hemodialysis with a cellulose ester membrane.

It is unclear whether the production or release of these molecules actually increased in this setting and, if so, how they occurred. Interestingly, this increase may be attenuated with reuse (164). In addition, high-flux dialysis utilizing polysulfone, polymethylmethacrylate, or polyacrylonitrile membranes was associated with a decrease, rather than an increase, in β_2MG levels during hemodialysis (165). This decrease is probably due to lower generation as well as higher adsorption and removal to the dialysate compartment. It should be noted that, although the serum concentrations of β_2MG in dialysis patients with localized β_2MG amyloidosis are high, they are not different from those found in dialysis patients without the disease (around 20–100 mg/l) (166).

CLINICAL EFFECTS OF MEMBRANE BIOCOMPATIBILITY

Thrombogenicity

Some aspects of dialysis membrane biocompatibility have indisputable clinical impact. Clotting of the dialyzers is an obvious example. A tendency to thrombosis is innate to blood exposure to most foreign surfaces and involves activation of platelets as well as of the coagulation cascades. Prevention of activation of the coagulation cascades is usually achieved with systemic heparinization, although regional heparinization or regional citrate anticoagulation is occasionally used. A detailed discussion on anticoagulation is beyond the scope of this chapter. It should be kept in mind that the clotting cascade is only one facet of the problem; platelets and perhaps leukocytes are also important in the thrombogenesis of dialyzers. Heparin may actually promote the aggregation of platelets (167). Overzealous usage of this agent may lead to systemic complications without necessarily preventing dialyzer clotting.

We have already mentioned the effectiveness of antiplatelet agents in decreasing microthrombi formation in dialyzers. In rare instances, these agents are even necessary in order to perform successful hemodialysis. Besides aggregating to form thrombi, activated platelets also release platelet factor 4, which has heparin-neutralizing properties. In this regard, membranes that activate platelets to a less extent are probably more desirable. As noted above, polyacrylonitrile (33), polycarbonate (27), and polymethylmethacrylate (34) membranes seem to activate platelets less than cuprophan membranes; polymethylmethacrylate is also associated with less intradialytic thrombocytopenia. It should be emphasized that stagnant or turbulent blood flow is a major contributor to thrombogenesis. The importance of blood-flow characteristics can be illustrated by successful hemodialysis treatments with a high blood-flow rate and no anticoagulant.

Although activation of platelets during hemodialysis can be problematic, normal platelet function to promote necessary clotting in between dialysis treatments is desirable. It is well known that platelet function defects are common in uremic patients. The abnormality in platelet adhesiveness and bleeding time seen in patients dialyzed with cuprophan membranes could be improved by dialysis with polyacrylonitrile membranes (168). Whether this improvement is due to the difference in membrane biocompatibility or differences in solute removal profile is unknown.

Hypoxemia

Hypoxemia is common during hemodialysis. The magnitude of the hypoxemia is relatively mild with the drop of arterial tension of oxygen (p_{O_2}) usually around 8–12 mmHg. This degree of hypoxemia is of little clinical significance to most patients. However, in patients with cardiac or pulmonary diseases, it may have a significant impact. The use of acetate as dialysate is undoubtedly the major contributing factor to the pathogenesis of the hypoxemia (107–109, 169–170). There are at least two mechanisms proposed for the effects of acetate. First, carbon dioxide and bicarbonate are lost by diffusion from the blood into the dialysate (107, 108). Second, acetate diffuses from the dialysate into the blood. During the metabolism of acetate, two moles of oxygen are consumed for each mole of carbon dioxide produced (109). Either mechanism would explain the decrease in respiratory quotients seen in acetate hemodialysis. The decrease in the carbon dioxide burden decreases the respiratory drive. Hypoventilation and hypoxemia ensue, as documented in a number of reports (107, 108). Yet hypoxemia can still develop during hemodialysis in patients mechanically ventilated with constant minute volume and inspired oxygen concentrations (171). Thus, other mechanism are likely to be involved.

Much of the debate in the literature is focused on the relative contributions of membrane biocompatibility to the pathogenesis of hemodialysis-induced hypoxemia. Table 3 lists some of the studies supporting the notion that the dialysis membrane per se is a contributing factor. A decrease in pulmonary diffusion capacity ($D_L CO$) can be seen (90, 172–174), which is compatible with the concept of anaphylatoxin-induced interstitial fluid accumulation. Whether a decrease in $D_L CO$ would impair oxygenation in a particular patient depends on the degree of the decrease and on the transit time of blood through the pulmonary vessels available for gas exchange. Other observations including a decrease in transthoracal impedance (173), widening of the alveolar-arterial oxygen tension ($[(A-a)DO_2]$) (174–176), increase in the dead space/tidal volume ratio (V_D/V_T) (108), and an increase in closing volumes (90) also suggest a defect in intrapulmonary gas exchange, and not alveolar hypoventilation. The degree of hypoxemia has been shown to correlate with the degree of leukopenia (177). Replacement of cellulosic membranes with either polyacrylonitrile or polymethylmethacrylate (176, 178, 179) membranes without a change in the dialysate composition can also ameliorate, although not abolish, the hypoxemia. Furthermore, replacement of acetate with bicarbonate dialysate does not necessarily eliminate the hypoxemia (177).

Further support of the effects of membranes can be drawn from studies involving infusion of cuprophan-activated plasma into humans (173) and animals (90, 91, 97), which produces significant hypoxemia. In a recent study in which normal human subjects were subjected to sham hemodialysis with cuprophan membranes in the absence of dialysate, hypoxemia was also observed (99).

A few points need to be emphasized regarding the effects of the membranes and the possible mechanisms of their action: a) The effect is relatively small compared to that of the acetate dialysate. b) "Membrane-effects" are not synonymous with "complement effects" or "leukocyte effects." Dialysis membranes have effects independent of complement. Complement activation products may cause pulmonary dysfunction independent of its leukocyte-directed effects (see Figure 4). Potentially, the anaphylatoxins may cause hypoxemia by bronchial smooth-muscle contraction and increased vascular permeability, leading to an impedance in airflow and accumulation of interstitial fluid. On the other hand, the stimulated granulocytes that aggregate in the pulmonary vasculature may cause pulmonary injury by the release of intracellular enzymes and oxygen radicals. Conceivably, membrane effects may be attributed to neither the occurrence of leukoagglutination nor the formation of anaphylatoxins, which may only be coincidental events. c) The effects of membranes on hypoxemia are likely to be more important in the first 30 minutes (175, 176) when complement activation is intense than during the subsequent hours. However, the effects of complement activation potentially can last longer. For example, if the pulmonary vascular permeability is increased by the anaphylatoxins, the resultant interstitial fluid accumulation may not resolve immediately despite cessation of mediator production.

In summary, although the impact is rather mild and the mechanisms are not completely understood, certain membranes such as the potent complement activator

Table 3. Studies supporting the role of dialyzer membranes in the pathogenesis of dialysis-induced hypoxemia

Author	Reference	Observations
Craddock et al.	90	↓ $D_L CO$, ↑ closing volume
Mahajan et al.	172	↓ $D_L CO$ and ↓ pO_2 correlate with leukopenia
Graf et al.	173	↓ $D_L CO$, ↓ transthoracal impedence
Morrison et al.	174	↓ $D_L CO$, ↑ $(A-a)DO_2$, ↓ Q_c
Hakim et al.	178	More hypoxemia with cuprophan than polymethylmethacrylate
Dolan et al.	108	↑ V_D/V_T
Debacker et al.	175, 176	↓ pO_2 and ↑ $(A-a)DO_2$, which is abolished by prostacyclin
Vaziri et al.	179	More hypoxemia with cuprophan than polyacrylonitrile
Abu-Hamdan et al.	177	Hypoxemia not abolished by bicarbonate; hypoxemia is proportionate to leukopenia

$(A-a)DO_2$ = alveolar-arterial oxygen gradient; $D_L CO$ = diffusing capacity of lungs for carbon monoxide; Q_c = pulmonary capillary blood flow; V_D/V_T = dead space to tidal volume ratio.

The cause of hemodialysis-induced hypoxemia is primarily hypoventilation because of the acetate-containing dialysate. However, membrane biocompatibility is likely to contribute to this phenomenon.

cuprophan seem to induce more hypoxemia than other membranes. In patients with significant cardiac or pulmonary problems such as congestive heart failure and obstructive airway disease with or without pulmonary hypertension, the hemodialysis prescription should take into account the choice of the dialysis membrane.

Hemodynamic alterations

Severe pulmonary hypertension is readily seen when cuprophan-activated plasma is infused intravenously into experimental animals (36, 90, 91, 96, 97). An increase in pulmonary arterial pressure has also been observed in patients undergoing hemodialysis with cuprophan membranes (110). It is occasionally associated with cardiac decompensation (111). Although pulmonary hypertension per se is unlikely to be the cause of hypoxemia, it may very well contribute to the chest pain and dyspnea sometimes seen in clinical hemodialysis. It should be noted that pulmonary hypertension was not observed during mock hemodialysis in normal volunteers (99).

The systemic hemodynamics may also be affected by the blood-membrane interaction, which can be demonstrated in experimental animals (91, 97). In a clinical comparative study where acetate dialysate was used and ultrafiltration was controlled, hemodialysis with cuprophan membranes was associated with a larger decrement of peripheral vascular resistance than with cellulose acetate membranes (180). This fall of resistance could be further accentuated by the administration of indomethacin.

Dialyzer reuse

Dialyzer reuse is often a difficult issue encountered by dialysis unit directors. It has medical, ethical, economic, and social implications. The performance of the reused dialyzers in terms of ultrafiltration and solute removal are acceptable if proper guidelines are followed. Details on the processing techniques and performance are readily available elsewhere (181). This chapter will only deal with some aspects pertinent to membrane biocompatibility and clinical outcomes.

Sterilization and cleansing of the dialyzers between uses are usually accomplished with formaldehyde or sodium hypochlorite. A few newer agents are also available, but the information about their effects on membrane biocompatibility is relatively sparse. Infections and pyrogenic reactions are potential problems associated with dialyzer reuse. However, with careful handling of the used dialyzers, periodic microbiologic monitoring of the water source, and appropriate exclusions of certain patients (e.g., carriers of hepatitis B), infection should not be a major problem (182-184).

Despite the lack of consensus from all medical personnel and patients involved in hemodialysis, reuse of dialyzers seems to be potentially beneficial in certain aspects. Reuse of cuprophan membrane dialyzers with a formaldehyde rinse is associated with attenuation of complement activation and leukopenia (55, 80). Treatment with sodium hypochlorite, on the other hand, restores the potential of the cuprophan membranes to activate complement (54) and to induce leukopenia (81, 82). The intradialytic morbidity and long-term outcomes of dialyzer reuse will be discussed in the following sections.

First-use syndrome (FUS)

Many different terms have been used to describe this poorly-defined "syndrome," including *dialyzer hypersensitivity syndrome*, *cuprophan hypersensitivity*, *new dialyzer syndrome*, and *first-use syndrome*, reflecting the lack of understanding and confusion of this problem. Henderson et al. have coined the term *FUS-1*, which refers to the drastic onset of signs and symptoms within seconds to minutes from the beginning of a treatment with a previously unused (new) dialyzer (185). The manifestations include various combinations of hypertension or shock; respiratory symptoms such as dyspnea, coughing, sneezing, and wheezing; choking sensations, rhinorrhea, conjuctival injection, headache, muscle cramps, back, abdominal, and chest pain; nausea, vomiting, fever, chills, flushing, and urticaria; as well as pruritis. This effects can be severe and even fatal (186). The incidence of this phenomenon obviously depends on the definition. Although relatively rare, it seems to afflict some patients repeatedly. In other words, there seems to be a subset of the dialysis population who are susceptible to these reactions.

In the past few years, a number of anecdotal reports have appeared in the literature describing this syndrome (186-194). Villarroel and Ciarkowski reported the results of a survey conducted jointly by the Food and Drug Administration, the Center for Devices and Radiological Health, and seven dialyzer manufacturers (195). This survey covers primarily a 24-month period between January 1982 and December 1983. Several aspects of the report are interesting: a) A total of 363 cases were reported with a frequency of 4.3 per 100,000 for hollow-fiber and 0.2 per 100,000 for plate dialyzers sold in the United States. b) The severity of the reactions were classified into three types: Type I, mild reactions that allow the patients to continue dialysis without medication and comprised 9.9% of the reported cases; Type II, reactions requiring medications or discontinuation of dialysis, which comprised 87.3% of the cases; Type III, death, which occurred in 10 patients (2.8%). c) 25.2% of the afflicted patients had previous reactions to the same brand of dialyzers; 13.3% of the afflicted patients had previous reactions to other brands or models of dialyzers. These patients, therefore, seem to comprise the subset of population who are prone to these reactions. d) Cellulose acetate membranes were associated with the lowest rate among the membranes studied. e) Blacks and other minorities, as well as young patients, were afflicted more often. f) Interestingly, 1.4% of the reactions were associated with reused dialyzers.

One difficulty in interpreting the data from this large-scale survey is again the lack of a precise definition of the problem. Only 54.6% of these reactions were considered by the reporting dialysis units to be due to dialyzer hypersensitivity. Potentially, the remainder may stem from other factors such as rapid fluid removal or intercurrent illness. Likewise, the small number of cases (1.4%) reported with reused dialyzers may or may not have a hypersensitivity etiology. Their manifestations may be mild and may not fit into the definitions of hypersensitivity reactions employed by other investigators.

There has been considerable debate about the etiology of FUS-1, with complement activation products and ethylene oxide being the prime candidates. Most likely, this is a constellation of syndromes with different pathogenetic mechanisms rather than a single entity. Those occurring during the first 30 seconds, before the blood has passed through the dialyzer and returned to the patient (192), are probably not the result of complement activation. Residual noxious materials from the manufacturing process are much more likely to be the causative agents. On the other hand, symptoms developing after the first 10–15 minutes are more likely to be due to products of the blood-membrane interaction such as anaphylatoxins, since this is the time when the peak plasma C_{3a} antigen concentration occurs (193). The bulk of the noxious materials in the lumen of the blood compartment that are unbound to the membrane would have already been washed into the patient during the first few minutes.

Any hypothesis on the etiology of FUS-1 has to take into consideration the following clinical observations: a) Cuprophan membranes are primarily incriminated; however, it can also occur with other types of regenerated cellulose or noncellulosic membranes (196). b) In the United States, hollow-fiber dialyzers are associated with a much higher incidence of FUS-1 than plate dialyzers. Some patients who experience these symptoms when dialyzed with cuprophan hollow-fiber dialyzers can subsequently be dialyzed with cuprophan plate dialyzers without incidence. c) A patient may experience reactions with a particular cuprophan hollow-fiber dialyzer without even changing the brand. d) Intensifying and correcting the method of rinsing the blood compartments before dialysis diminish the problem in some units (197). e) There seems to be clustering of cases in certain dialysis units. Whether they indeed occur in this manner or there is underreporting from other units in unclear.

Ethylene oxide (ETO) is commonly used to sterilize dialyzers during the manufacturing process. Its toxicity to the workers exposed to this agent is well recognized. The potting material, polyurethane, seems to be the main "reservoir" of the ethylene oxide in the hollow-fiber dialyzers (198). The content decreases with the time of storage, presumably from slow continuous dissipation from the reservoir. To examine the possible role of ethylene oxide in the pathogenesis of these seemingly allergic phenomena, investigators have studied the sera of patients and have found that some of these patients with FUS-1 have specific IgE antibodies directed against ethylene oxide. The IgE is usually detected by using a radioadsorbant test (RAST), which utilizes albumin exposed to ethylene oxide (ETO-HSA) as the antigen. ETO-induced histamine release in vitro from peripheral leukocytes of an afflicted patient has been described (199).

Nicholls and Platts described some patients in Europe who suffered from anaphylactoid reactions to previously unused artificial kidneys sterilized with ethylene oxide (197). These reactions occurred within 1–2 minutes from the onset of the treatments. The manifestations were wheezing, urticaria, chest pain, sneezing, rhinorrhea, flushing, and watery eyes. These reactions were likely to be caused by eluted residues from the manufacturing process. The evidence suggests ethylene oxide to be the culprit. This report is interesting from a few standpoints. a) Many of these patients had high titers of IgE directed specifically against ETO-HSA. The total serum IgE was, however, not elevated. b) Most of these reactions occurred with hemodialyzers; however, hemofilters and plasma membrane separators were also incriminated. c) Most of the dialyzers used by these afflicted patients were plate dialyzers, in contrast to the United States experience in which reactions to plate dialyzers were much less frequent than those to hollow-fiber dialyzers.

The demonstration of specific IgE to ETO-HSA in patients is supportive, but not conclusive, evidence of ETO being the causative agent. Marshall et al. (200) found that about 12% of their hemodialysis population studied have IgE directed against ethylene oxide. This test was more sensitive than the skin-prick test using ETO-HSA as the antigen. All patients with a positive skin test also had the specific IgE antibodies. However, the presence of positive specific IgE and a positive skin test were not associated with FUS-1 in this study. Besides the development of hives on the fistula arm in one patient, only pruritis or an absence of symptoms was observed. Among their peritoneal dialysis population, only 1 out of 41 tested patients had specific IgE antibodies, and none developed positive skin tests. These data suggest that IgE against ETO develops in a substantial portion of the general hemodialysis population, probably as the result of recurrent exposure to ETO in the extracorporeal circuits. The presence of these antibodies, even in the presence of a positive skin test, is seldom associated with FUS-1. Nonetheless, ETO as the causative agent of FUS-1 in other patients cannot be ruled out by these data. These patients with specific IgE antibodies may also develop blocking IgG that are protective. Furthermore, these particular patients might not have been exposed to large enough amounts of ETO during a single hemodialysis session to trigger the clinical reactions.

Peripheral eosinophilia, even if present, is also nonspecific. This laboratory abnormality occurs in a substantial fraction of the general dialysis population (201–203). The incidence depends on the definition. Around 25% of hemodialysis patients may have peripheral eosinophil counts > 500 cells/mm^3. Some of these patients indeed develop peripheral eosinophilia as the result of allergy to certain components of the dialyzers. Similar to other forms of allergy, the clinical symptoms and eosinophilia abate with discontinuation of exposure to the allergenic agent (189).

Besides acting as a haptene to elicit the IgE response, ethylene oxide can also have other effects through the generation of metabolites. Reaction of ethylene oxide with chloride ions produces 2-chloroethanol, which is a toxic substance. This compound had been found in the effluent of the blood compartment of the dialyzer from a patient who suffered sudden severe back, chest, and head pain within the first 10 minutes of hemodialysis (194). Cuprophan was shown to support the in-vitro generation of 2-chloroethanol from ethylene oxide more readily than polyethylene and polyvinylchloride.

Another potential etiology of FUS-1 is complement activation by the dialysis membrane. Specifically, the anaphylatoxins C_{3a} and C_{5a} (and $C_{5a_{desArg}}$) are proposed to be the causative agents. Hakim et al. studied six patients who experienced recurrent reactions to new cuprophan membranes (193). Respiratory symptoms were present in all the patients. Chest and back pain, nausea, flushing, and angioedema were present in some. These symptoms were more severe during the initial 15–30 minutes of the treatments. The peak plasma C_{3a} antigen concentration during hemodialysis in these six patients, as well as in two additional patients who suffered cardiopulmonary collapse, were significantly higher than those in hemodialysis patients without these reactions. Furthermore, the production of C_{3a} antigens was exaggerated when the plasma from these patients was incubated in vitro with the alternative pathway complement activator zymosan. These data suggest that the anaphylatoxins or mediators of their biologic effects may cause these reactions. The reactors were more prone to activate complement, possibly because of abnormalities in their complement regulatory proteins. Alternatively, they might have defects in inactivating the anaphylatoxins or abnormal end-organ sensitivities to them. To what extent the anaphylatoxins might have contributed to the reactions of these six particular patients is uncertain. These reactions were, however, somewhat different from those labeled as *new dialyzer syndrome* by some other investigators, in that they occurred later in the course of the dialysis sessions and the manifestations were in some instances less drastic than those seen in other patients. These particular reactions described by Hakim et al. may very well be attributable to complement activation, which is usually maximal at the time when these symptoms occurred (15–20 minutes). They may fall into the gray area between FUS-1 and FUS-2, which will be described below. In the same context, it should be pointed out the patient described by Agar et al. (111), who experienced signs of pulmonary hypertension and cardiac decompensation, had the onset of symptoms at 10–40 minutes. The timing was more compatible with the complement hypothesis than the cases which occur within a minute that have been described by others.

If one chooses the terms *FUS* or *new dialyzer syndrome* instead of the others, then by definition it does not occur with reuse. During the course of the first use of a cuprophan dialyzer, the membrane becomes coated with inactive C_3 molecules, which probably inhibits further complement activation. Leachable noxious or allergenic substances, such as ethylene oxide, are also removed to a substantial extent during the first use. Thus, regardless of the etiologic agents of FUS-1, it is not surprising that the problem is less likely to occur during reuse.

Since the etiology of FUS-1 is unclear at present, the treatment is largely symptomatic (Table 4). In mild situations, such as sneezing and rhinorrhea, the dialysis treatment can be continued and the symptoms may abate after the first ½–1 hour with or without antihistamines. If the manifestations are severe, more aggressive measures may have to be taken. The dialysis treatment should be terminated immediately. The blood in the extracorporeal circuit should not be returned to the patient, since it is likely to carry the offending agents. Bronchodilators and other sympathomimetics are used to treat bronchospasm. Administration of corticosteroids and antihistamines are empirical but theoretically sensible if IgE, complement activation products, or even other noxious agents are considered to be the pathogens. Blood pressure support with fluids, sympathomimetics, and oxygen supplement are instituted as necessary.

For prevention of future episodes, the patients are usually switched to another type of dialyzer if the reactions are severe. Often a noncuprophan or noncellulosic membrane is used as a substitute. Occasionally, even switching from a cuprophan hollow-fiber to a cuprophan parallel-plate dialyzer may prevent further episodes. The blood compartments should be rinsed extensively with normal saline prior to use. Although rinsing with 1 l is frequently performed, some investigators recommend 2 l of normal saline in a single pass (196). The dialysate compartment should also be rinsed at the same time. Some recommend

Table 4. Prevention and treatment of first-use syndrome*

Prevention
    Extensive rinsing of the blood compartment (>1 liter) and dialysate compartment before dialysis
    Change the dialyzer to another brand if the syndrome occurs in a particular patient
    Employ membranes with low potentials to activate complement

Acute treatment
    Discontinue dialysis
    Do not return the blood in the extracorporeal circuit to the patient
    Antihistamine for "allergic" symptoms such as rhinorrhea and pruritis
    Oxygen supplement
    Bronchodilators and sympathomimetics for bronchospasm
    Corticosteroids
    Fluid and sympathomimetics for hypotension
    Resuscitation with usual measures if there is cardiopulmonary arrest

* Since the etiology of this "syndrome" is not well understood at present, the strategies for prevention and treatment are empirical. The aggressiveness depends on the severity of the manifestations. Listed are some suggestions that include the usual symptomatic and supportive measures, as well as medications counteracting the effects of anaphylatoxins and histamine.

10 l of dialysate at 500 ml/min with a negative pressure of 200 mmHg be maintained in the dialysate compartment. Pretreatment of new dialyzers with formaldehyde has been reported to prevent the occurrence of FUS-1. In these instances, the effectiveness is more likely to be due to the rinsing procedure, which removes the formaldehyde and the offending agents, than to any action of the formaldehyde per se.

The term *FUS-2* refers to the statistically significant increase in symptoms during dialysis treatment with new membranes compared to the symptoms occurring during reuse (185). These symptoms are usually not life threatening, and the time of onset is variable. It is possible that FUS-2 and FUS-1 are a continuum and that the only difference is the severity of the clinical manifestations. For example, the first use of the dialyzer may be associated with severe symptoms because a large amount of the offending agent (anaphylatoxins, allergenic or noxious substances) is transferred from the dialyzer to the patient. During the second use, the innoculum of these substances is substantially reduced, so that the onset of the symptoms is less abrupt and the manifestations are less severe. The causative agents may be identical in both the first and subsequent uses. If this hypothesis is correct, one should not be surprised that the reuse of dyalyzers is associated with less symptoms.

Indeed, in a double-blind study, the incidence of back pain and chest pain was found to be lower with reused cellulosic membrane dialyzers than with new dialyzers (204). In another study, Robson et al. reported their experience in Cincinnatti with dialyzer reuse in 147 patients over a 26-month period (205). In this study, all the dialyzers were made of cellulosic membranes. Symptoms that occurred more frequently during first use than during reuse included hypotension, cramps, nausea, vomiting, headache, itching, chest pain, back pain, dyspnea, chills, and tremor. In particular, chest pain occurred 2.6 times and back pain occurred six times more frequently with the first use. In contrast, there was no complication that occurred more frequently with reuse than with the first use.

Long-term effects of dialyzer reuse

The long-term safety of dialyzer reuse have also been reported in the United States and the United Kingdom. Wing et al. reported the data from the United Kingdom, which was part of a survey conducted by the European Dialysis and Transplantation Association in 1976 (206). To eliminate the bias of disparity in age distribution, only patients with ages between 15 and 34 years were included in the report. The results showed that, in both the hospital and the home dialysis setting, the reuse of dialyzers was associated with lower 1-year mortality rates than not reusing them. More recently, Pollak et al. reported their experience on 1318 patients from Cincinnati and Detroit with a followup of 2744 patient years. The data showed that the mortality rates in their patients practicing dialyzer reuse were no higher than the mortality rates reported by the other dialysis units in their geographic areas (183). There was also no increase in the hospitalization rates associated with reuse.

It, therefore, seems that dialyzer reuse conducted properly is safe and effective. It may be associated with less intradialytic complications. Hospitalization and mortality rates were at least not higher than in patients not practicing reuse. One of the frequently cited arguments against reuse pertains to the potential ill effects of the sterilizing agents. Formaldehyde, being the most commonly used sterilant for years, has been particularly criticized. Most people are familiar with the irritant effects of formaldehyde gas, which can cause itchy eyes, rhinorrhea, and coughing. Sensitivity dermatitis has also been recognized. The issue of anti-N against red cells has been discussed above. In addition, there seems to be an increased incidence of squamous cell carcinoma of the nasal turbinate in rats and mice exposed to formaldehyde fumes (207). All these problems are associated with high concentrations of the reagent, which should not be present in the reused dialyzers after proper rinsing and testing. Furthermore, formaldehyde is used widely in many industries, including the handling of biologic tissues by our pathologist colleagues. Studies linking these exposures to carcinogenesis in humans is lacking. Although the long-term effects of a patient's exposure to the trace amount of residual formaldehyde is unknown, it does not seem to adversely affect the longevity of the hemodialysis population. In the study of Pollak et al. mentioned above, where formaldehyde was used as sterilant for reuse, the followup on 14% of the study population exceeded 5 years and 3% exceeded 7 years (183). Although there are obviously other factors that contribute to the overall success of their dialysis programs, their data demonstrate that dialyzer reuse using formaldehyde is safe for a number of years. We expect that large centers that keep meticulous records on reuse will continue to be able to supply us with information regarding its long-term impacts on dialysis patients.

Although it is not the purpose of this chapter to discuss the financial, ethical, and other aspects of dialyzer reuse, it should be mentioned that unless the costs of new (especially high flux) dialyzers are substantially reduced, the financial savings of reuse is indisputable and should not be disregarded. This is especially important for countries where resources are more scarce for the treatment of patients with end-stage renal diseases. Newer sterilizing agents are now employed which would hopefully make reuse an even safer practice.

Comparisons between dialyzers of different polymers

Dialysis with cellulose acetate membranes has been reported to be associated with less fatigue, pruritis, and a better sense of well-being than with cuprophan (79). Plasma levels of anaphylatoxin C_{3a} antigens, CH50 titers, the granulocyte product lactoferrin, and granulocyte-aggregating activities (presumably reflective of $C_{5a_{desArg}}$) were correspondingly lower. These laboratory phenomena were potentially related to the mild clinical advantages of the cellulose acetate membranes. In another clinical study comparing patients dialyzed with cuprophan membranes versus patients dialyzed with polyacrylonitrile membranes, the polyacrylonitrile group was associated with a lower number of hospitalization days and a lower incidence of intradialytic complications such as vomiting, headache, cramps, and hypotension (208). When these two membranes were compared within the same patient group, there was no difference in the number of hospitalization days, but the incidence of intradialytic complications was still lower with polyacrylonitrile. To what extent the difference in the control of ultrafiltration accounted for the differences in the clinical outcome could not be ascertained.

Preliminary results of a retrospective study showed that patients dialyzed with polyacrylonitrile membranes were also associated with less thromboembolic complications and cardiovascular death than cuprophan membranes (209). These complications included clotting of arteriovenous fistulae, lower extremity thrombosis, and pulmonary embolism. Here again, if the results can be confirmed, we have to speculate whether the difference is due to differences in molecule clearance profiles or membrane biocompatibility, such as the degrees of platelet activation.

Fever

Besides intercurrent illness, febrile reactions during dialysis can also be caused by infectious agents or pyrogenic substances contaminating the extracorporeal circuits. Dialysis with reused membranes can be due to inadequate sterilization of the dialyzers. The dialysis unit water is occasionally contaminated with bacteria and mycobacteria that are resistant to even 2–4% formaldehyde (210, 211). Addition of ethanol and raising of the temperature to 40°C sometimes potentiates the killing of the organisms by formaldehyde. Patients exposed to the dialyzers processed with water that is not adequately sterilized with extra means can sometimes be infected by these organisms.

Pyrexial reactions may also occur with new dialyzers. Rinsing of new dialyzers with water in order to prevent the first-use syndrome may paradoxically result in contamination of the dialyzers with infectious agents. Pyrexial reactions associated with new dialyzers may also occur in the absence of intact live organisms. Vomiting, back pain, and hypotension sometimes accompany the fever (212). As discussed above in the Interleukin-1 section, endotoxins may cross dialysis membranes with microrupture. Alternatively, smaller fragments of the bacterial cell wall may traverse even the intact membranes.

The presence of bacterial endotoxins is often detected with the limulus amebocyte lysate (LAL) assay. Substances that react in the LAL assay have been found in the blood compartments of new dialyzers and in the venous blood of a patient (213). Subsequent investigations, however, demonstrated that these LAL-positive materials eluted from dialyzers might not be pyrogenic endotoxins (214–216). Instead, they were probably products derived from cellulose, the raw material from which the cellulosic dialysis membranes are manufactured. These products react in the LAL assay, presumably because of their high molecular weight polysaccharide structure. These observations, however, do not preclude the transfer of true endotoxins or smaller fragments of bacterial origin across the damaged dialyzer membranes from contaminated water in certain instances. Finally, the production of interleukin-1 from monocytes, regardless of the sources of stimuli, may induce fever in hemodialysis patients.

Pyrexial reactions and the so-called first-use syndrome share certain features in common. Both of them can be accompanied by other signs and symptoms such as nausea, vomiting, backache, and hypotension. Indeed, there may be an overlap between these two entities. For example, a pyrexial reaction occurring during hemodialysis with a new dialyzer accompanied by hypotension and chest pain may be caused by endotoxins. Depending on the definition one chooses, this reaction can also be classified as first-use syndrome. Until we have a better understanding of the pathogenesis and stricter definitions of these entities, it will be difficult, and may even be unreasonable, to dogmatically distinguish one from another.

Other sequelae of membrane bioincompatibility

Purposeless cyclic activation of complement and stimulation of leukocytes may predispose dialysis patients to infections. Indeed, chronic use of new cellulosic membranes can result in a decrease in predialysis leukocyte counts (71), impaired neutrophil chemotactic response (217), as well as defective adherence (218) and phagocytic capabilities of neutrophils (219).

Increased vascular permeability has been observed in hemodialysis patients for many years and predisposes patients to pulmonary edema (220). The etiology is unknown. Calcification of the lungs, especially along the alveolar septal walls, is also commonly seen in this population (221, 222). Anaphylatoxins are known to increase vascular permeability. The sequestered granulocytes in the pulmonary vasculature may also release intracellular enzymes and oxygen radicals. Serum fibronectin levels are decreased during hemodialysis. Whether these observed phenomena are related to the increased permeability and pulmonary calcification in dialysis patients remains speculative.

Leaching and spallation of materials

Not only do loosely associated substances such as ethylene oxide leach from dialyzers, spallation of materials from dialysis tubings can also occur. One substance that has attracted attention is silicone. As a result of mechanical damage to the tubings by blood roller pumps, fragments of silicone can be released into the bloodstream and enter the patient's body (223). Refractile materials in macrophages and foreign-body giant cells within the lungs, liver, spleen, bone marrow, skin, and lymph nodes have been reported. By energy-dispersive x-ray fluorescence microanalysis, this refractile material has been demonstrated to be the non-biodegradable element silicone. The exact mechanisms by which these activated macrophages and giant cells damage the visceral organs are unknown. However, human and animal studies indicate that these macrophages (or splenic cells) produce more arachidonic acid metabolites than normal macrophages under basal and stimulated conditions (224, 225). How these abnormal metabolisms translate to tissue injury is unclear at present.

These organ injuries can be manifested clinically (223, 225). Liver involvement includes hepatomegaly, granulomatous hepatitis, and transaminase elevations. Splenomegaly sometimes leads to pancytopenia, requiring splenectomy. Disturbance in macrophages may lead to impairment of immunity.

Silicone is not the only substance that is problematic. Other commonly used biomaterials, such as polyurethane and polyvinylchloride, also stimulate the abnormal production of arachidonic acid metabolites by splenic cells in vitro. They are, therefore, potentially capable of inducing organ damage. Improvement of the materials in the extracorporeal circuits and mechanical factors are needed to eliminate the problem of spallation. For example, reduction of the occlusion pressure in the blood pump segments can reduce spallation from silicone tubings (226).

Many other organic and inorganic substances are contained in the various components of dialyzers and are potentially capable of causing side effects. There is copper used in the cuprammonium process of cellulose regeneration, styrenes used as casing material, polyethylene used as supporting plates, isopropyl myristate used as bore fluid, and polyurethane used as potting compound. Polyvinylchloride from blood tubings had been associated with necrotizing dermatitis (227). The plasticizer di-2-ethylhexyl phthalate can be leached from plastics into patients and may cause liver abnormalities (228).

CONCLUSIONS

Despite all the documented and potential problems related to the bioincompatibility of the materials, artificial kidney treatments have been remarkably successful in maintaining the lives of many patients with end-stage renal disease. Exposure of blood to foreign surfaces in these treatments is inevitable. The job of bioengineers and physicians taking care of these patients is to further understand blood-foreign surface interactions and to improve the design of the biomaterials and structures of the extracorporeal circuits. Hopefully, then, treatments with extracorporeal circulations can attain removal of molecules with minimal side effects to the patients. The process of investigating the different aspects of biocompatibility of materials would also contribute to the understanding of body homeostasis and pathogenesis of diseases.

ACKNOWLEDGMENTS

The author acknowledges support from the Veterans Administration Research Service and the Department of Medicine, University of Utah School of Medicine. He also wishes to thank Drs. Lee Henderson and Kathleen McElligott for reviewing the manuscript, and Ms. Sharon Henn for preparation of the manuscript.

REFERENCES

1. Leonard EF: Dialysis membranes. *Proc Eur Dial Transplant Assoc* 21:99–109, 1984.
2. Klinkmann H, Wolf H, Schmit E: Haemodialysis and membrane biocompatibility. *Contr Nephrol* 37:70–77, 1984.
3. Leonard EF, Van Vooren C, Hauglustaine D, Haumont S: Shear-induced formation of aggregates during hemodialysis. *Contr Nephrol* 36:34–45, 1983.
4. Parsons FM, Stewart WK: The composition of dialysis fluid. In: W Drukker, FM Parsons, JF Maher, eds. *Replacement of Renal Function by Dialysis*. Martinus Nijhoff Publishers, Boston, pp 148–170, 1983.
5. Lyman DJ: Membranes. In: W Drukker, FM Parsons, JF Maher, eds, *Replacement of Renal Function by Dialysis*. Martinus Nijhoff, Boston, pp 97–105, 1983.
6. Spencer PC, Schmidt B, Samtleben W, Bosch T, Gurland HJ: *Trans Am Soc Artif Intern Organs* 31:495–498, 1985.
7. Falkenhagen D, Zinner G, Falkenhagen U, Ahrenholz P, Holtz M, Behm E, Klinkmann H: A modified cellulose membrane (MC) with reduced complement activation. *Kidney Int* 28:331, 1985.
8. Blackshear PL Jr, Droman FD, Steinbach JH: Some mechanical effects that influence hemolysis. *Trans Am Soc Artif Intern Organs* 11:112–117, 1965.
9. Fassbinder W, Pilar J, Scheuermann E, Koch M: Formaldehyde and the occurrence of anti-N-like cold agglutinins in RDT patients. *Proc Eur Dial Transpl Assoc* 13:333–338, 1976.
10. Harrison PB, Jansson K, Kronenberg H, Mahony JF, Tiller D: Cold agglutinin formation in patients undergoing hemodialysis. A possible relationship to dialyser re-use. *Aust NZ J Med* 5:195–197, 1975.
11. Kaehny WD, Miller GE, White WL: Relationship between dialyzer reuse and the presence of anti-N-like antibodies in chronic hemodialysis patients. *Kidney Int* 12:59–65, 1977.
12. Lewis KJ, Dewar PJ, Ward MK, Kerr DNS: Formation of anti-N-like antibodies in dialysis patients: Effect of different methods of dialyzer rinsing to remove formaldehyde. *Clin Nephrol* 15:39–43, 1981.
13. Belzer FO, Kountz SL, Perkins HA: Red cell cold autoagglutinins as a cause of failure of renal allotransplantation. *Transplantation* 11:422–424, 1971.
14. Marshall JW, Ahearn DJ, Nothum RJ, Estherly J, Nolph KD, Maher JF: Adherence of blood components to dialyzer membranes morphological studies, *Nephron* 12:157–170, 1974.
15. Salzman EW: Role of platelets in blood-surface interactions. *Fed Proc* 30:1503–1508, 1971.
16. Mason RG, Chuang HYL, Mohammed SF: Extracorporeal thrombogenesis: Mechanisms and prevention. In: W Drukker, FM Parsons, JF Maher, eds. *Replacement of Renal Function by Dialysis*. Martinus Nijhoff, Boston, pp 186–200, 1983.
17. Chap H, Mauco G, Simon MF, Benveniste J, Douste–Blazy L: Biosynthetic labelling of platelet activating factor from radioactive acetate by stimulated platelets. *Nature* 289:312–314, 1981.
18. Osterud B, Rapaport SI, Lavine KK: Factor V activity of

platelets: Evidence for an activated factor V molecule and for a platelet activator. *Blood* 49:819–834, 1977.
19. Miletich JP, Jackson CM, Majerus PW: Interaction of coagulation factor Xa with human platelets. *Proc Natl Acad Sci USA* 74:4033–4036, 1977.
20. Kaplan KL, Owen J: Plasma levels of β-thromboglobulin and platelet factor 4 as indices of platelet activation in vivo. *Blood* 57:199–202, 1981.
21. Nath N, Niewiarowski S, Joist JH: Platelet factor 4 — antiheparin protein releasable from platelets — purification and properities. *J Lab Clin Med* 82:754–768, 1973.
22. Dawes J, Smith RC, Pepper DS: The release, distributions, and clearance of human β-thromboglobulin and platelet factor 4. *Thromb Res* 12:851–861, 1978.
23. Lindsay RM, Prentice CRM, Ferguson D, Burton JA, McNicol G: Reduction of thrombus formation on dialyser membranes by aspirin and RA 233, *Lancet* 2:1278–1290, 1972.
24. Salter MCP, Crow MJ, Donaldson DR, Roberts TG, Rajah SM, Davison AM: Prevention of platelet deposition and thrombus formation on hemodialysis membranes: A double-blind randomized trial of aspirin and dipyridamole. *Artif Organs* 8:57–61, 1984.
25. Zusman RM, Rubin RH, Cato AE, Cocchetto DM, Crow JW, Tolkoff-Rubin N: Hemodialysis using prostacyclin instead of heparin as the sole antithrombotic agent. *N Engl J Med* 304:934–939, 1981.
26. Smith MC, Danviriyasup K, Crow JW, Cato AE, Park GD, Hassid A, Dunn MJ: Prostacyclin substitution for heparin in long-term hemodialysis. *Am J Med* 73:669–678, 1982.
27. Sreeharan N, Crow MJ, Salter MCP, Donaldson DR, Rajah SM, Davison AM: Membrane effect on platelet function during hemodialysis: A comparison of cuprophan and polycarbonate. *Artif Organs* 6:324–327, 1982.
28. Docci D, Turci F, Del Vecchio C, Bilancioni R, Cenciotti L, Pretolani E: Hemodialysis-associated platelet loss: Study of the relative contribution of dialyzer membrane composition and geometry. *Int J Artif Organs* 7:337–340, 1984.
29. Gasparotto ML, Bertoli M, Vertolli U, Ruffatti A, Stoppa ML, Di Landro D, Romagnoli GF: Biocompatibility of various dialysis membranes as assessed by coagulation assay. *Contr Nephrol* 37:96–100, 1984.
30. Ireland H, Lane DA, Curtis JR: Objective assessment of heparin requirements for hemodialysis in humans. *J Lab Clin Med* 103:643–652, 1984.
31. Green D, Santhanam S, Krumlovsky FA, del Greco F: Elevated β-thromboglobulin in patients with chronic renal failure: Effect of hemodialysis. *J Lab Clin Med* 95:679–685, 1980.
32. Lindsay RM, Rourke J, Reid B, Friesen M, Linton AL, Courtney J, Gilchrist T: Platelets, foreign surfaces, and heparin. *Trans Am Soc Artif Int Organs* 22:292–295, 1976.
33. Adler AJ, Berlyne GM: β-thromboglobulin and platelet factor-4 levels during hemodialysis with polyacrilonitrile. *Am Soc Artif Int Organs* 4:100–102, 1981.
34. Hakim RM, Schafer AI: hemodialysis-associated platelet activation and thrombocytopenia. *Am J Med* 78:575–580, 1985.
35. Hartung H-P, Bitter-Suermann D, Hadding U: Induction of thromboxane release from macrophages by anaphylatoxic peptide C_{3a} of complement and synthetic hexapeptide C_{3a} 72–77. *Immunol* 130:1345–1349, 1983.
36. Cheung AK, Baranowski RL, Wayman AL: The role of thromboxane in cuprophan-induced pulmonary hypertension. *Kidney Int* 31:1072–1079, 1987.
37. Camussi G, Mencia-Huerta JM, Benveniste J: Release of platelet-activating factor and histamine. *Immunology* 33:523–534, 1977.
38. Vroman L, Adams AL, Klings M: Interactions among human blood proteins at interfaces. *Fed Proc* 30:1494–1502, 1971.
39. Mohammed SF, Whitworth C, Chuang HYK, Lundblad RL, Mason RG: Multiple active forms of thrombin: Binding to platelets and effects on platelet function. *Proc Natl Acad Sci USA* 73:1660–1663, 1976.
40. Wilhelmsson S, Asaba H, Gunnarsson B, Kudryk B, Robinson D, Bergstrom J: Measurement of fibrinopeptide A in the evaluation of heparin activity and fibrin formation during hemodialysis. *Clin Nephrol* 15:252–258, 1981.
41. Wilhelmsson S, Ivemark CK, Kudryk B, Robinson D, Biberfeldt P: Thrombin activity during hemodialysis: Evaluation by the fibrinopeptide A assay. A comparison between a high and a low heparin dose regime. *Thromb Res* 31:685–693, 1983.
42. Lane DA, Ireland H, Knight I, Wolff S, Kyle P, Curtis JR: The significance of fibrinogen derivatives in plasma in human renal failure. *Br J Haematol* 56:251–261, 1984.
43. Murano G: The Hageman connection: Interrelationships of blood coagulation, fibrino(geno)lysis, kinin generation and complement activation. *Am J Hematol* 4:409–417, 1978.
44. Arias R, Schulman G, Kaplan AP, Silverberg M, Arbeit LA: Generation of activated Hageman factor (HF_a), kallikrein (KK) and bradykinin (BK) by cuprophane dialysis membranes (C). *Kidney Int* 29:44A, 1986.
45. Vaziri ND, Toohey J, Paule P, Alikhani S, Hung E: Effect of hemodialysis on contact group of coagulation factors, platelets, and leukocytes. *Am J Med* 77:437–442, 1984.
46. Stratta P, Canavese C, Mangiarotti G, Pacitti A, Tetta C, Coppo R, Ragni R, Vercellone A: Heparin is unable to prevent contact activation by three different membranes. *Proc Eur Dial Transpl Assoc* 18:269–274, 1981.
47. Muller-Eberhard HJ, Schreiber RD: Molecular biology and chemistry of the alternative pathway of complement. *Adv Immunol* 29:1–53, 1980.
48. Reid KBM, Porter RR: The proteolytic activation systems of complement. *A Rev Biochcm* 50:433–464, 1981.
49. Craddock PR, Fehr J, Dalmasso AP, Brigham KL, Jacob HS: Hemodialysis leukopenia: Pulmonary vascular leukostasis resulting from complement activation by dialyzer cellophane membranes. *J Clin Invest* 59:879–888, 1977.
50. Chenoweth DE, Cheung AK, Henderson LW: Anaphylatoxin formation during hemodialysis: Effects of different dialyzer membranes. *Kidney Int* 24:764–769, 1983.
51. Tack BF, Harrison RA, Janatova J, Thomas ML: Evidence for presence of an internal thiolester bond in third complement of human complement. *Proc Natl Acad Sci USA* 77:5764–5768, 1980.
52. Law SK, Lichtenberg NA, Levine RP: Covalent binding and hemolytic activity of complement proteins. *Proc Natl Acad Sci USA* 77:7194–7198, 1980.
53. Pangburn MK, Morrison DC, Schreiber RD, Muller-Eberhard HJ: Activation of the alternative complement pathway: Recognition of surface structures on activators by bound C_{3b}. *Immunol* 124:977–982, 1980.
54. Cheung AK, Parker CJ, Janatova J: Analysis of the complement C_3 fragments associated with hemodialysis membranes. *Kidney Int* 35:576–588, 1989.
55. Chenoweth DE, Cheung AK, Ward DM, Henderson LW: Anaphylatoxin formation during hemodialysis: Comparison of new and re-used dialyzers. *Kidney Int* 24:770–774, 1983.

56. Cochrane CG, Muller-Eberhard HJ: The derivation of two distinct anaphylatoxin activities from the third and fifth components of human complement. *J Exp Med* 127:371–386, 1968.
57. Lepow IH, Wilms-Kretschmer K, Patrick RA, Rosen FS: Gross and ultrastructural observations on lesions produced by intradermal injection of human C_{3a} in man. *Am J Path* 61:13–24, 1970.
58. Johnson AR, Hugli TE, Müller-Eberhard HJ: Release of histamine from mast cells by the complement peptides C_{3a} and C_{5a}. *Immunology* 28:1067–1080, 1975.
59. Stimler NP, Bloor CM, Hugli TE: C_{3a}-induced contraction of guinea pig lung parenchyma: Role of cyclooxygenase metabolites. *Immunopharmacology* 5:251–257, 1983.
60. Claesson H-E, Lundberg U, Malmsten C: Serum-coated zymosan stimulates the synthesis of leukotriene B_4 in human polymorphonuclear leukocytes. Inhibition by cyclic AMP. *Biochem Biophys Res Commun* 99:1230–1237, 1981.
61. Stimler NP, Bach MK, Bloor CM, Hugli TE: Release of leukotrienes from guinea pig lung stimulated by $C_{5a_{desArg}}$ anaphylatoxin. *J Immunol* 128:2247–2252, 1982.
62. Stimler NP, Brocklehurst WE, Bloor CM, Hugli TE: Complement anaphylatoxin C_{5a} stimulates release of SRS-A-like activity from guinea-pig lung fragments. *J Pharm Pharmacol* 32:804, 1980.
63. Fernandez HN, Henson PM, Otani A, Hugli TE: Chemotactic response to human C_{3a} and C_{5a} anaphylatoxins. *Immunol* 120:109–115, 1978.
64. Chenoweth DE, Hugli TE: Demonstration of specific C_{5a} receptor on intact human polymorphonuclear leucocytes. *Proc Natl Acad Sci USA* 75:3943–3947, 1978.
65. Craddock PR, Hammerschmidt D, White JG, Dalmasso AP, Jacob HS: Complement (C_{5a})-induced granulocyte aggregation in vitro. *J Clin Invest* 60:260–264, 1977.
66. Hammerschmidt DE, Harris PD, Wayland JH, Craddock PR, Jacob HS: Complement-induced granulocyte aggregation in vivo. *Am J Path* 102:146–150, 1981.
67. Sacks T, Moldow CF, Craddock PR, Bowers TK, Jacob HS: Oxygen radicals mediate endothelial cell damage by complement-stimulated granulocytes. *J Clin Invest* 61:1161–1167, 1978.
68. Bokisch VA, Müller-Eberhard HJ: Anaphylatoxin inactivator of human plasma: Its isolation and characterization as a carboxypeptidase. *J Clin Invest* 49:2427–2436, 1970.
69. Gerard C, Hugli TE: Identification of classical anaphylatoxin as the des-Arg form of the C_{5a} molecule: Evidence of a modulator role for the oligosaccharide unit in human des-Arg[74] C_{5a}. *Proc Natl Acad Sci USA* 78:1833–1837, 1981.
70. Smeby LC, Jørstad ST, Balstad T, Widerøe TE: Dialyzer generation and plasma clearance of activated complement during hemodialysis. In: LC Smeby, S Jorstad, T-E Wideroe, eds, *Immune and Metabolic Aspects of Therapeutic Blood Purification Systems*. Karger, Basel, pp 76–84, 1985.
71. Hakim RM, Fearon DT, Lazarus JM: Biocompatibility of dialysis membranes: Effects of chronic complement activation. *Kidney Int* 26:194–200, 1984.
72. Webster RO, Larsen GL, Henson M: In vivo clearance and tissue distribution of C_{5a} and C_{5a} des arginine complement fragments in rabbits. *J Clin Invest* 70:1117–1183, 1982.
73. Cheung AK, Chenoweth DE, Otsuka D, Henderson LW: Compartmental distribution of complement activation products in artifical kidneys. *Kidney Int* 30:74–80, 1986.
74. Amadori A, Candi P, Sasdelli M, Massai G, Favilla S, Passaleva A, Ricci M: Hemodialysis leukopenia and complement function with different dialyzers. *Kidney Int* 24:775–781, 1983.
75. Aljama P, Bird PAE, Ward MK, Feest TG, Walker W, Tanbago H, Skussman M, Kerr DNS: Haemodialysis-induced leucopenia and activation of complement: Effects of different membranes. *Proc Eur Dial Transplant Assoc* 15:144–153, 1979.
76. Cheung AK, Parker CJ, Wilcox L, Janatova J: Activation of complement by hemodialysis membranes: Polyacrylonitrile binds more C_3 than cuprophan. *Kidney Int* 37:1055–1059, 1990.
77. Chuang HYK, Sharpton TR, Mohammad SF: Adsorption and reactivity of human fibrinogen and immunoglobulin G on two types of hemodialysis membranes. *Int J Artif Organs* 6:199–206, 1983.
78. Lonnemann G, Koch KM, Shaldon S, Dinarello CA: Induction of interleukin-1 (IL-1) from human monocytes adhering to hemodialysis (HD) membranes. *Kidney Int* 31:238A, 1987.
79. Ivanovich P, Chenoweth DE, Schmidt R, Klinkmann H, Boxer LA, Jacob HS, Hammerschmidt DE: Symptoms and activation of granulocytes and complement with two dialysis membranes. *Kidney Int* 24:758–763, 1983.
80. Hakim RM, Lowrie EG: Effect of dialyzer reuse on leukopenia, hypoxemia and total hemolytic complement system. *Trans Am Soc Artif Intern Organs* 26:159–164, 1980.
81. Gagnon RF, Kaye M: Hemodialysis neutropenia and dialyzer reuse: Role of the cleansing agent. *Uremia Invest* 8:17–23, 1984.
82. Hoenich NA, Johnston SRD, Woffindin C, Kerr DNS: Haemodialysis leucopenia: The role of membrane type and re-use. *Contr Nephrol* 37:120–128, 1984.
83. Dumler F, Zasuwa G, Levin NW: Effect of dialyzer reprocessing methods on complement activation and hemodialyzer-related symptoms. *Int J Artif Organs*, in press.
84. Cheung AK, Parker CJ, Janatova J, Wayman AL: Acetylation does not affect C_3 deposition on cellulosic dialysis membranes. *Clin Res* 35:174A, 1987.
85. Cheung AK, Parker CJ, Wayman AL: Sodium hypochlorite (NaOCl) regenerates the complement(C)-activating potential of cuprophan membranes (CuM). *Kidney Int* 31:230A, 1987.
86. Sherman RA, Rubin VP, Cody RP, Eisinger RP: Amelioration of hemodialysis-associated hypotension by the use of cool dialysate. *Am J Kidney Dis* 5:124–127, 1985.
87. Sherman RA, Faustino EF, Bernhoic AS, Eisinger RP: Effect of variations in dialysate temperature on blood pressure during hemodialysis. *Am J Kidney Dis* 4:66–68, 1984.
88. Maggiore Q, Enia G, Catalano C, Misefari V, Mundo A, Creazzo G, Zaccuri F: Anaphylatoxin release and leukopenia during cool hemodialysis (HD). *Kidney Int* 27:167A, 1985.
89. MacDougall M, Diederich D, Wiegmann T: Dissociation of hemodialysis leukopenia and hypoxemia from complement changes during citrate anticoagulation. *Kidney Int* 27:166A, 1985.
90. Craddock PR, Fehr J, Brigham KL, Kronenberg RS, Jacob HS: Complement and leukocyte-mediated pulmonary dysfunction in hemodialysis. *N Engl J Med* 296:769–774, 1977.
91. Cheung AK, LeWinter M, Chenoweth DE, Lew YW, Henderson LW: Cardiopulmonary effects of cuprophane-activated plasma in the swine. *Kidney Int* 29:799–806, 1986.
92. Hugli TE, Vallota EH, Müller-Eberhard HJ: Purification and partial characterization of human and porcine C_{3a} anaphylatoxin. *J Biol Chem* 25:1472–1478, 1975.
93. Gerard C, Hugli TE: Anaphylatoxin from the fifth com-

ponent of porcine complement. Purification and partial chemical characterization. *J Biol Chem* 254:6346–6351, 1979.
94. Gerard C, Hugli TE: Amino acid sequence of the anaphylatoxin from the fifth component of porcine complement. *J Biol Chem* 255:4710–4713, 1980.
95. Hastings AB, White FC, Sanders TM, Bloor CM: Comparative physiological responses to exercise stress. *J Appl Physiol* 52:1077–1083, 1982.
96. Walker JF, Lindsay RM, Sibbald WJ, Linton AL: Acute pulmonary hypertension, leukopenia and hypoxia in early haemodialysis. *Proc Eur Dial Transplant Assoc* 21:135–142, 1984.
97. Walker JF, Lindsay RM, Peters SD, Sibbald WJ, Linton AL: A sheep model to examine the cardiopulmonary manifestations of blood-dialyzer interactions. *Am Soc Artif Intern Organs J* 6:123–130, 1983.
98. Lindsay RM, Walker JF, Sibbald WJ, Linton AL: The influence of sterilizing agents on the biocompatibility of reused dialysers. *Kidney Int* 27:166A, 1985.
99. Bergström J, Danielsson A, Freyschuss U: Dialysis, ultrafiltration and sham-dialysis in normal subjects. *Kidney Int* 27:157A, 1984.
100. Ahearn DJ, Marshall JW, Nothum RJ: Morphologic studies of dialysis membranes adherence of blood components to air rinsed coils. *Trans Am Soc Artif Intern Organs* 19:435–439, 1973.
101. Gary SK, Niemetz J: Tissue factor activity of normal and leukemic cells. *Blood* 42:729–735, 1973.
102. Kaplow LS, Goffinet JA: Profound neutropenia during the early phase of hemodialysis. *JAMA* 203:133–135, 1968.
103. Brubaker LH, Nolph KD: Mechanisms of recovery from neutropenia induced by hemodialysis. *Blood* 38:623–631, 1971.
104. Danielsson A, Bergstrom J, Freyschuss U, Hammarstrom L, Lantz B: Biocompatibility of hemodialysis membranes in normal man. In: LE Smeby, S Jørstad, T-E Widerøe, eds, *Immune and Metabolic Aspects of Therapeutic Blood Purification Systems*. Karger, Basel, pp 155–160, 1985.
105. Dodd NJ, Gordge MP, Tarrant J, Parsons V, Weston MJ: A demonstration of neutrophil accumulation in the pulmonary vasculature during haemodialysis. *Proc Eur Dial Transpl Assoc* 20:186–189, 1983.
106. Gral T, Schroth P, De Palma JR, Gordon A: Leukocyte dynamics with three types of hemodialyzers. *Trans Am Soc Artif Intern Organs* 15:45–49, 1969.
107. Aurigemma NM, Feldman NT, Gottlieb M, Ingram RH, Lazarus JM, Lowrie EG: Arterial oxygenation during hemodialysis. *N Engl J Med* 297:871–873, 1977.
108. Dolan MJ, Whipp BJ, Davidson WD, Weitzman RE, Wasserman K: Hypopnea associated with acetate hemodialysis: Carbon dioxide-flow-dependent ventilation. *N Engl J Med* 305:72–75, 1981.
109. Oh MS, Uribarri J, Del Monte ML, Heneghan F, Kee CS, Friedman EA, Carroll HJ: A mechanism of hypoxemia during hemodialysis. *Am J Nephrol* 5:366–371, 19 .
110. Walker JF, Lindsay RM, Driedger AA, Sibbald WJ, Linton AL: Hemodialysis commonly causes transient pulmonary hypertension. *Kidney Int* 25:195A, 1984.
111. Agar JW, Hull JD, Kaplan M, Pletka PG: Acute cardiopulmonary decompensation and complement activation during hemodialysis. *Ann Intern Med* 90:792–793, 1979.
112. Jacob AI, Gavellas G, Zarco R, Perez G, Bourgoignie JJ: Leukopenia, hypoxia, and complement function with different hemodialysis membranes. *Kidney Int* 18:505–509, 1980.
113. Skubitz KM, Craddock PR: Reversal of hemodialysis granulocytopenia and pulmonary leukostasis: A clinical manifestation of selective down-regulation of granulocyte responses to $C_{5a_{desArg}}$. *J Clin Invest* 67:1383–1391, 1981.
114. Lewis SL, Van Epps DE, Chenoweth DE: Leukocyte C_{5a} receptor modulation during hemodialysis. *Kidney Int* 31:112–120, 1987.
115. Camussi G, Pacitti A, Tetta C, Bellone G, Mangiarotti G, Canavese C, Segoloni G, Vercellone A: Mechanisms of neutropenia in hemodialysis (HD). *Trans Am Soc Artif Intern Organs* 30:364–367, 1984.
116. Camussi G, Segoloni G, Rotunno M, Vercellone A: Mechanisms involved in acute granulocytopenia in hemodialysis: Cell-membrane direct interactions. *Int J Artif Organs* 3:123–127, 1978.
117. Venge P, Olsson I: Cationic proteins of human granulocytes. Effects on the complement system and mediation of chemotactic activity. *J Immunol* 115:1505–1508, 1975.
118. Silber R, Moldow CF: Biochemistry and function of neutrophils. Composition of neutrophils. In: WJ Williams, E Brutler, A Erslev, M Lichtman, eds, *Hematology*, 3rd ed. McGraw Hill, New York, pp 726–734, 1983.
119. Hörl WH, Riegel W, Schollmeyer P, Rautenberg W, Neumann S: Different complement and granulocyte activation in patients dialyzed with PMMA dialyzers. *Clin Nephrol* 25:304–307, 1986.
120. Wright DG, Gallin JI: Secretory responses of human neutrophils: Exocytosis of specific (secondary) granules by human neutrophils during adherence in vitro and during exudation in vivo. *J Immunol* 123:285–294, 1979.
121. Hörl WH, Steinhauer HB, Schollmeyer P: Plasma levels of granulocyte elastase during hemodialysis: Effects of different dialyzer membranes. *Kidney Int* 28:791–796, 1985.
122. Buscaroli A, Stefoni S, Costa AN, Feliciangeli G, Coli L, Mosconi G, Borgnino LC, Iannelli S, Galanti S, Lucatello A, Boni P, Bonomini V: Evaluation of lysozyme kinetics in dialysis patients treated with different membranes. In: LE Smeby, S Jørstad, T-E Widerøe, eds, *Immune and Metabolid Aspects of Theraeutic Blood Purification Systems*. Karger, Basel, pp 39–43, 1985.
123. Hallgren R, Venge P, Danielson BG: Neutrophil and eosinophil degranulation during hemodialysis are mediated by the dialysis membrane. *Nephron* 32:329–334, 1982.
124. Goldstein IM, Brai M, Osler AG, Weissmann G: Lysosomal enzyme release from human leukocytes: Mediation by the alternative pathway of complement activation. *J Immunol* 111:33–37, 1973.
125. Hörl WH, Schaefer RM, Heidland A: Effect of different dialyzers on proteinases and proteinase inhibitors during hemodialysis. *Am J Nephrol* 5:320–326, 1985.
126. Dewitz TS, McIntire LV, Martin RR, Sybers HD: Enzyme release and morphological changes in leukocytes induced by mechanical trauma. *Blood Cells* 5:499–510, 1979.
127. Dewitz TS, Hung TC, Martin RR, McIntire LV: Mechanical trauma in leukocytes. *J Lab Clin Med* 90:728–736, 1977.
128. Gotch FA, Borah M, Keen M, Sargent J: The solute kinetics of intermittent dialysis therapy (IDT). *Proc Ann Contractors Conf Artif Kidney Program NIAMDD* 10:105–107b, 1977.
129. Farrell PC, Hone PW: Dialysis-induced catabolism. *Am J Clin Nutr* 33:1417–1422, 1980.
130. Heidland A, Horl WH, Heller N, Heine H, Neumann S, Heidbreder E: Proteolytic enzymes and catabolism: Enhanced release of granuloctye proteinases in uremic intoxication and during hemodialysis. *Kidney Int* 24 (Suppl 16):S27–S36, 1983.

131. McDonald JA, Kelly DG: Degradation of fibronectin by human leukocyte elastase. *J Biol Chem* 255:8848–8858, 1980.
132. Schwarz HP, Graf H, Luger A, Kovarik J, Stummvoll HK: Fibronectin during hemodialysis. *Nephron* 34:138–139, 1983.
133. Schwarz HP, Graf H, Luger A, Kovarik J, Stommvoll HK: Dialysis hypoxemia: The role of fibronectin and its pathophysiological implication. *Contr Nephrol* 37:107–110, 1984.
134. Hällgren R, Venge P, Wikström B: Hemodialysis-induced increase in serum lactoferrin and serum eosinophil cationic protein as signs of local neutrophil and eosinophil degranulation. *Nephron* 29:233–238, 1981.
135. Danielson BG, Hällgren R, Venge P: Neutrophil and eosinophil degranulation by hemodialysis membranes. *Contr Nephrol* 37:83–88, 1984.
136. Venge P, Dahl R, Hällgren R: Enhancement of factor XII dependent reactions by eosinophil cationic protein. *Thromb Res* 14:641–649, 1979.
137. Dahl R, Venge P: Enhancement of urokinase-induced plasminogen activation by the cationic protein of human eosinophil granulocytes. *Thromb Res* 14:599–608, 1979.
138. Klempner MS, Gallin JI: Separation and functional characterization of human neutrophil subpopulation. *Blood* 51:649–669, 1978.
139. Klempner MS, Gallin JI, Balow JE, Van Kammen DP: The effect of hemodialysis and $C_{5a_{des\ arg}}$ on neutrophil subpopulations. *Blood* 55:777–783, 1980.
140. Cohen MS, Elliott DM, Chaplinski T, Pike MM, Niedel JE: A defect in the oxidative metabolism of human polymorphonuclear leukocytes that remain in circulation early in hemodialysis. *Blood* 60:1283–1289, 1982.
141. Lucchi L, Acerbi MA, Cappelli G, Leonardi M, Lusvarghi E: The biocompatibility of Cuprophan®, cellulose acetate, polyacrylonitrile assessed by polymorphonuclear leukocyte chemiluminescence. In: LE Smeby, S Jørstad, T-E Widerøe, eds, *Immune and Metabolic Aspects of Therapeutic Blood Purification Systems*. Karger, Basel, pp 11–17, 1985.
142. Lee J, Hakim RM, Fearon DT: Increased expression of the C_{3b} receptor by neutrophils and complement activation during haemodialysis. *Clin Exp Immunol* 56:205–214, 1984.
143. Fearon DT, Wong WW: Complement ligand-receptor interactions that mediate biological responses. *Ann Rev Immunol* 1:243–271, 1983.
144. Henderson LW, Miller ME, Hamilton RW, Norman ME: Hemodialysis leukopenia and polymorph random mobility — a possible correlation. *J Lab Clin Med* 85:191–197, 1975.
145. Thomaneck U, Schutt W, Behrend D, Falkenhagen D, Klinkmann H: Cell electrophoretic investigations of lymphoid cells after contact with biomaterials. In: LE Smeby, S Jørstad, T-E Widerøe, eds, *Immune and Metabolic Aspects of Therapeutic Blood Purification Systems*. Karger, Basel, pp 161–167, 1985.
146. Kay NE, Raij, L: Differential effect of hemodialysis membranes on human lymphocyte natural killer function. *Artif Organs* 11:165–167, 1987.
147. Dinarello CA: An update on human interleukin-1: From molecular biology to clinical relevance. *J Clin Immunol* 5:287–297, 1985.
148. Dinarello CA: Interleukin-1. *Rev Infect Dis* 6:51–95, 1984.
149. Dinarello CA: Pathogenesis of fever during hemodialysis. *Contr Nephrol* 36:90–99, 1983.
150. Bingel M, Lonnemann G, Shaldon S, Koch KM, Dinarello CA: Human interleukin-1 production during hemodialysis. *Nephron* 43:161–163, 1986.
151. Goodman MG, Chenoweth DE, Weigle WO: Induction of interleukin 1 secretion and enhancement of humoral immunity by binding of human C_{5a} to macrophage surface C_{5a} receptors. *J Exp Med* 1156:912–917, 1982.
152. Koch KM, Shaldon S, Bingel M, Dinarello CA: Plasma interleukin-1 (IL-1) is elevated in ESRD patients on long-term hemodialysis (HD). *Kidney Int* 31:237A, 1987.
153. Fenves AZ, Emmett M, White MG, Greenway G, Michaels DB: Carpal tunnel syndrome with cystic bone lesions secondary to amyloidosis in chronic hemodialysis patients. *Am J Kidney Dis* 7:130–134, 1986.
154. Vanderbroucke JM, Jadoul M, Maldague B, Huaux JP, Noel H, Van Ypersele de Strihou C: Possible role of dialysis membrane characteristics in amyloid osteoarthropathy. *Lancet* 1:1210–1211, 1986.
155. Walts AE, Goodman MD, Matorin PA: Amyloid, carpal tunnel syndrome, and chronic hemodialysis. *Am J Nephrol* 5:225–226, 1985.
156. Cambi V, Nizzoli M, Paganelli E, David S, Bono F: Danger of an unnecessarily prolonged dialysis session: Carpal tunnel syndrome. *Artif Organs* 10:178–181, 1986.
157. Chanard J, Lavaud S, Toupance O, Roujouleh H, Melin J-P: Carpal tunnel syndrome and type of dialysis membrane used in patients undergoing long term hemodialysis. *Arthritis Rheum* 29:1170–1171, 1986.
158. Casey TT, Stone WJ, DiRaimondo CR, Page DL: Dialysis-related amyloid is amyloid of beta-2-microglobulin ($AM_{\beta 2M}$) origin. *Arthritis Rheum* 29:1170–1171, 1986.
159. Sethi D, Gower PE: Synovial-fluid β_2-microglobulin levels in dialysis arthropathy. *N Engl J Med* 315:1419–1420, 1986.
160. Gejyo F, Homma N, Suzuki Y, Arakawa M: Serum levels of β_2-microglobulin as a new form of amyloid protein in patients undergoing long-term hemodialysis. *N Engl J Med* 314:585–586, 1986.
161. Gorevic PD, Casey TT, Stone WJ, DiRaimondo CR, Prelli FC, Frangione B: Beta-2 microglobulin is an amyloidogenic protein in man. *J Clin Invest* 76:2425–2429, 1985.
162. Gejyo F, Yamada T, Odani S: A new form of amyloid protein associated with chronic hemodialysis was identified as β_2-microglobulin. *Biochem Biophys Res Commun* 129:701–706, 1985.
163. Kostic S, Djordjevic, Lecic N, Stefanovic V: Serum β_2-microglobulin in patients on maintenance hemodialysis: The effect of dialysis membrane. *Kidney Int* 28:338, 1985.
164. Levin NW, Dumler F: Effect of reprocessing dialyzers on serum β_2 microglobulin in hemodialysis patients. *Kidney Int* 31:238A, 1987.
165. Petersen J, Hyver S, Yeh I: Evaluation of new synthetic membranes for high-flux hemodialysis (HFD). *Kidney Int* 31:241A, 1987.
166. DiRaimondo CR, Casey TT, Gorevic PD, DiRaimondo CV, Stone WJ: Beta-2-microglobulin amyloidosis in chronic hemodialysis patients. *Clin Res* 34:82A, 1986.
167. Mohammad SF, Anderson WH, Smith JB, Chuang HYK, Mason RG: Effects of heparin on platelet aggregation, release reaction and thromboxane A_2 production. *Am J Pathol* 104:132–141, 1981.
168. Mingardi G, Vigano G, Massazza M, Remuzzi G, Mecca G: Polyacrylonitrile membranes for hemodialysis: Long-term effect on primary hemostasis. In: LE Smeby, S Jorstad, T-E Wideroe, eds, *Immune and Metabolic Aspects of Therapeutic Blood Purification Systems*. Karger, Basel, pp 310–314, 1985.
169. Garella S, Chang BS: Hemodialysis-associated hypoxemia. *Am J Nephrol* 4:273–279, 1984.

170. Kraut J, Garter U, Brautbar N, Miller J, Shinaberger J: Prevention of hypoxemia during dialysis by the use of sequential isolated ultrafiltration-diffusion dialysis with bicarbonate dialyzate. *Clin Nephrol* 15:181–184, 1981.
171. Jones RH, Broadfield JB, Parsons V: Arterial hypoxemia during hemodialysis for acute renal failure in mechanically ventilated patients: Observations and mechanisms. *Clin Nephrol* 14:18–22, 1980.
172. Mahjan S, Gardiner H, De Tar B, Desai S, Muller B, Johnson N, Briggs W, McDonald F: Relationship between pulmonary functions and hemodialysis induced leukopenia. *Trans Am Soc Artif Intern Organs* 23:411–415, 1977.
173. Graf H, Stummvoll HK, Haber P, Kovarik J: Pathophysiology of dialysis related hypoxaemia. *Proc Eur Dial Transplant Assoc* 17:155–161, 1980.
174. Morrison JT, Wilson AF, Vaziri ND, Brunsting L, Davis J: Determination of pulmonary tissue volume, pulmonary capillary blood flow and diffusing capacity of the lung before and after hemodialysis. *Int J Artif Organs* 3:259–262, 1980.
175. DeBacker WA, Verpooten GA, Borgonjon DJ, Van Waeleghem JP, Vermeire PA, DeBroe ME: Hypoxemia during hemodialysis: Effects of different membranes and dialysate compositions. *Contr Nephrol* 37:134–141, 1984.
176. De Backer WA, Vepooten GA, Borgonjon DJ, Vermeire PA, Lins RR, De Broe ME: Hypoxemia during hemodialysis: Effects of different membranes and dialysate compositions. *Kidney Int* 23:738–743, 1983.
177. Abu-Hamban DK, Desai SG, Mahajan SK, Muller BF, Briggs WA, Lynne-Davies P, McDonald FD: Hypoxemia during hemodialysis using acetate versus bicarbonate dialysate. *Am J Nephrol* 4:248–253, 1984.
178. Hakim RM, Lowrie EG: The relative effect of leukopenia and dialysate composition on the dialysis-associated hypoxemia. *Proc Clin Dial Transplant Forum* 10:190–195, 1980.
179. Vaziri ND, Barton CH, Warner A, Toohey J, Lintner C, Hung E, Mullin P, Samiminina B, O'Donnell M, Mallot K: Comparison of four dialyzer-dialysate combinations: Effects on blood gases, cell counts, complement contact factors and fibrinolytic system. *Contr Nephrol* 37:111–119, 1984.
180. Branger B, Deschodt G, Baudin G, Oules R, Granolleras C, Shaldon S: Improvement of hemodynamic tolerance during acetate short dialysis with biocompatible membranes: Mechanisms involved. In: LE Smeby, S Jorstad, T-E Wideroe, eds, *Immune and Metabolic Aspects of Therapeutic Blood Purification Systems*. Karger, Basel, pp 214–217, 1985.
181. Deane N, Bemis JA: Multiple use of hemodialyzers. In: W Drukker, FM Parsons, JF Maher, eds, *Replacement of Renal Function by Dialysis*. Martinus Nijhoff, Boston, pp 286–304, 1983.
182. Kant KS, Pollak VE, Cathey M, Goetz D, Berlin R: Multiple use of dialyzers: Safety and efficacy. *Kidney Int* 19:728–738, 1981.
183. Pollak VE, Kant KS, Parnell SL, Levin NW: Repeated use of dialyzers is safe: Long-term observations on morbidity and mortality in patients with end-stage renal disease. *Nephron* 42:217–223, 1986.
184. Favero MS, Deane N, Legev RT, Sosin AE: Effect of multiple use of dialyzers on hepatitis B incidence in patients and staff. *JAMA* 245:166–167, 1981.
185. Henderson LW, Cheung AK, Chenoweth DE: Choosing a membrane. *Am J Kidney Dis* 3:5–20, 1983.
186. Foley RJ, Reeves WB: Acute anaphylactoid reactions in hemodialysis. *Am J Kidney Dis* 5:132–135, 1985.
187. Ogden DA: New-dialyzer syndrome. *N Engl J Med* 302:1262–1263, 1980.
188. Rault R, Silver MR: Severe reactions during hemodialysis. *Am J Kidney Dis* 5:128–131, 1985.
189. Michelson EA, Cohen L, Dankner RE, Kulczycki A: Eosinophilia and pulmonary dysfunction during cuprophan hemodialysis. *Kidney Int* 24:246–249, 1983.
190. Caruana RJ, Hamilton RW, Pearson FC: Dialyzer hypersensitivity syndrome possible role of allergy to ethylene oxide. *Am J Nephrol* 5:271–274, 1985.
191. Key J, Nahmias M, Acchiardo S: Hypersensitivity reaction on first-time exposure to cuprophan hollow fiber dialyzer. *Am J Kidney Dis* 2:664–666, 1983.
192. Popli S, Ing TS, Daugirdas JT, Kheirbek AO, Wiol GW, Vilbar RM, Gandhi VC: Severe reactions to cuprophan capillary dialyzers. *Artif Organs* 6:312–315, 1982.
193. Hakim RM, Breillatt J, Lazarus JM, Port FK: Complement activation and hypersensitivity reactions to dialysis membranes. *N Engl J Med* 311:878–882, 1984.
194. Gutch CF, Eskelson CD, Ziegler E, Ogden DA: 2-chloroethanol as a toxic residue in dialysis supplies sterilized with ethylene oxide. *Dial Transplant* 5:21–25, 1976.
195. Villarroel F, Ciarkowski AA: A survey on hypersensitivity reactions in hemodialysis. *Artif Organs* 9:231–238, 1985.
196. Ing TS, Daugirdas JT, Popli S, Gandhi VC: First-use syndrome with cuprammonium cellulose dialyzers. *Int J Artif Organs* 6:235–239, 1983.
197. Nicholls AJ, Platts MM: Anaphylactoid reactions during haemodialysis are due to ethylene oxide hypersensitivity. *Proc Eur Dial Transpl Assoc* 121:173–177, 1984.
198. Lee FF, Durning CJ, Leonard EF: Urethanes as ethylene oxide reservoirs in hollow-fiber dialyzers. *Trans Am Soc Artif Intern Organs* 31:526–533, 1985.
199. Poothullil J, Shimizu A, Day RP, Dolovich J: Anaphylaxis from the product(s) of ethylene oxide gas. *Ann Intern Med* 82:58–60, 1975.
200. Marshall C, Shimizu A, Smith EKM, Dolovich J: Ethylene oxide allergy in a dialysis center: Prevalence in hemodialysis and peritoneal dialysis populations. *Clin Nephrol* 21:346–349, 1984.
201. Scheuermann EH, Fassbinder W, Frei U, Koch KM, Baldamus CA: Eosinophilia in hemodialysis. *Contr Nephrol* 36:133–138, 1983.
202. Spinowitz BS, Simpson M, Manu P, Charytan C: Dialysis eosinophilia. *Trans Am Soc Artif Intern Organs* 26:161–163, 1981.
203. Röckel A, Abdelhamid S, Fiegel P, Hertel J, Panitz N, Walb D: Clinical relevance of the ethylene-oxide-RAST in patients on RDT. In: LE Smeby, S Jorstad, T-E Wideroe, eds, *Immune and Metabolic Aspects of Therapeutic Blood Purification Systems*. Karger, Basel, pp 97–104, 1985.
204. Bok DV, Pascual L, Herberger C, Sawyer R, Levin NW: Effect of multiple use of dialyzers on intradialytic symptoms. *Proc Clin Dial Transpl Forum* 10:92–95, 1986.
205. Robson MD, Charoenpanich R, Kant KS, Peterson DW, Flynn J, Cathey M, Pollak VE: Effect of first and subsequent use of hemodialyzers on patient well-being. *Am J Nephrol* 6:101–106, 1986.
206. Wing AJ, Brunner FP, Brynger HOA, Chantler C, Donckerwolcke RA, Gurland HJ, Jacobs C, Selwood NH: Mortality and morbidity of reusing dialysers. *Br Med J* 2:853–855, 1979.
207. Swenberg JA, Kerns WD, Mitchell RI, Gralla EJ, Pavkov KL: Induction of squamous cell carcinomas of the rat nasal cavity by inhalation exposure to formaldehyde vapor. *Can-*

cer Res 40:3398–3402, 1980.
208. Chanard J, Brunois JP, Melin JP, Lavaud S, Toupance O: Long-term result of dialysis therapy with a highly permeable membrane. *Artif Organs* 6:261–266, 1982.
209. Simon P, Ang KS, Cam G: Influence of membrane biocompatibility on thrombosis and/or embolism in hemodialysis patients. *Kidney Int* 29:225A, 1986.
210. Hakim RM, Friedrich RA, Lowrie EG: Formaldehyde kinetics and bacteriology in dialyzers. *Kidney Int* 28:936–943, 1985.
211. MMWR-Centre for Disease Control: Nontuberculous mycobacterial infections in hemodialysis patients — Louisiana, 1982. 32:244–246, 1983.
212. Robinson PJA, Rosen SM: Pyrexial reactions during haemodialysis. *Br Med J* 1:528–530, 1971.
213. Petersen NJ, Carson JA, Favero MS: Bacterial endotoxin in new and reused hemodialyzers: A potential cause of endotoxemia. *Trans Am Soc Artif Intern Organs* 26:155–160, 1981.
214. Henne W, Schulze H, Pelger M, Tretzel J, Von Sengbusch G: Hollow-fiber dialyzers and their pyrogenicity testing by limulus amebocyte lysate. *Artif Organs* 8:299–305, 1984.
215. Butcher BT, Reed MA, O'Neil CE, Leech S, Pearson FC: Immunologic studies of hollow-fiber dialyzer extracts. *Artif Organs* 8:318–324, 1984.
216. Pearson FC, Bohon J, Lee W, Bruszer G, Sagona M, Dawe R, Jakubowski G, Morrison D, Dinarello C: Comparison of chemical analyses of hollow-fiber dialyzer extracts. *Artif Organs* 8:291–298, 1984.
217. Greene WH, Ray C, Mauer SM, Quie PG: The effect of hemodialysis on neutrophil chemotactic responsiveness. *J Lab Clin Med* 88:971–974, 1976.
218. Lespier-Dexter LE, Guerra C, Ojeda W, martinez-Maldonado M: Granulocyte adherence in uremia and hemodialysis. *Nephron* 24:64–68, 1979.
219. Ritchey EE, Wallin JD, Shah SV: Chemiluminescence and superoxide anion production by leukocytes from chronic hemodialysis patients. *Kidney Int* 19:349–358, 1981.
220. Crosbie WA, Snowden S, Parsons V: Changes in lung capillary permeability in real failure. *Br Med J* 4:338–390, 1972.
211. Conger JD, Hammond WS, Alfrey AC, Contiguglia SR, Stanford RE, Huffer WE: Pulmonary calcification in chronic dialysis patients. *Ann Intern Med* 83:330–336, 1975.
222. Haque AK, Rubin SA, Leveque CM: Pulmonary calcification in long-term hemodialysis: A mimic of pulmonary thromboembolism. *Am J Nephrol* 4:109–113, 1984.
223. Bommer J, Ritz E: Spallation of dialysis materials: Problems and perspectives. *Nephron* 39:285–289, 1985.
224. Bommer J, Gemsa D, Waldherr R, Kessler J, Ritz E: Plastic filing from dialysis tubing induces prostanoid release from macrophages. *Kidney Int* 26:331–337, 1984.
225. Bommer J, Gemsa D, Kessler J, Ritz E: Evidence for macrophage activation in dialysis patients exposed to silicone filing. *Nephron* 39:395–397, 1985.
226. Bommer J, Pernicka E, Kessler J, Ritz E: Reduction of silicone particle release during haemodialysis. *Proc Eur Dial Transpl Assoc* 21:287–290, 1984.
227. Bommer J, Ritz E, Andrassy K: Necrotizing dermatitis resulting from hemodialysis with polyvinylchloride tubing. *Ann Intern Med* 91:869–870, 1979.
228. Kevy S, Jacobson M: Hepatic effects of the leaching of phthalate ester plasticizer and silicon. *Contr Nephrol* 36:82–89, 1983.

CHAPTER 54

Dialysis, Ultrafiltration and Hemofiltration

RAYMOND C. VANHOLDER, NICOLAS H. HOENICH & SEVERIN M. RINGOIR

INTRODUCTION

The management of renal insufficiency by extracorporeal circulatory support is a well-recognized and widely practiced technique. Hemodialysis is the most widely used method of extracorporeal circulatory support, and it is in this technique that a number of improvements have been made over the past decade through the introduction of biocompatible membranes, bicarbonate buffering of the dialysis fluid, and the availability of ultrafiltration during therapy.

Despite the widespread use of hemodialysis techniques for both chronic and acute renal insufficiency, dialyzed patients continue to exhibit metabolic derangements, related to a mixture of deficiency syndromes, as well as to incomplete extraction of nitrogenous and other metabolites elevated as a consequence of renal insufficiency. These shortcomings of hemodialysis therapy have led to the development and clinical application of new concepts of extracorporeal therapy such as hemofiltration, hemodiafiltration, continuous arteriovenous hemofiltration (CAVH), as well as plasma separation and hemoperfusion.

The purpose of this chapter is to review the techniques of extracorporeal therapy available, to examine their relationship to each other, and to focus on specific aspects relating to the clinical use of these modes of therapy.

VASCULAR ACCESS FOR EXTRACORPOREAL THERAPY

The need for adequate and reliable vascular access remains one of the major problems in extracorporeal therapy, since contact with the bloodstream must be obtained and a substantial blood flow must be achieved to allow the therapeutic technique to be performed. Within this context a number of solutions have been proposed, some of which are suitable for short-term acute use, while others are intended for long-term chronic use.

Temporary access techniques

Acute vascular access was historically first obtained by the creation of external arteriovenous shunts (1). This technique necessitates surgical intervention, makes reintervention necessary in the case of thrombosis, and can be the cause of the loss of one or more veins that could be useful for subsequent creation of endogenous arteriovenous fistulae. Alternative temporary access procedures include the placement of catheters in the femoral (2-4), internal jugular (5), or subclavian (6-7) positions. In the latter technique a number of acute complications, such as hemothorax or pneumothorax (8-12), and long-term central venous thrombosis (13-14) have been described, although large population studies show that these techniques have a low complication rate when properly performed (15-16).

Central venous catheters are available either in a single- or double-lumen version, the latter sometimes characterized by a higher blood-flow resistance, thereby limiting the availability of blood flow (17).

Long-term access techniques

Within this context the Cimino Brescia fistula remains the most widely used method of vascular access (18). This type of fistula is established at the wrist between the cephalic vein and the radial artery. Long-term access can be achieved only if the fistula is established well before the patient needs to use it, in order to allow the vasculature to enlarge before the needles are inserted for extracorporeal therapy. Clearly, such access requires the availability of an adequate vascular system and, in the absence of such system, a number of artificial alternate solutions have been described, such as the implantation of exogenous polymeric materials (Gortex or PTFE) (19), bovine grafts (20), or specially prepared cadaveric or umbilical veins (21).

TECHNIQUES OF EXTRACORPOREAL THERAPY

Hemodialysis

Hemodialysis relies upon the use of a hemodialyzer containing a semipermeable membrane, on one side of which blood flows, while the other side is bathed by a fast-flowing electrolyte solution (dialysis fluid). The format of the

Table 1. Requirements of an ideal dialyzer

High clearance of small and middle molecular weight solutes
Negligible loss of vital solutes or uptake of impurities across the semipermeable membrane
Adequate range of ultrafiltration
Low blood volume contained within the device
Good washback characteristics
High reliability
Biocompatible construction
Reuse potential (if desired)

membrane may be a flat sheet, tube, or hollow fiber. Metabolites elevated as a consequence of renal insufficiency diffuse across the membrane and are carried to the waste. Formed elements are prevented from passing across the membrane by their size. Fluid retained as a consequence of oliguria is removed principally by the application of a hydrostatic pressure across the semipermeable membrane and also by osmosis.

A wide variety of hemodialysers, suitable for use for small children up to large adults, are available for clinical use. They offer a range of solute and water removal efficiencies depending upon their size and the type of membrane used. The choice is a complex decision, which is dependent not only upon its functional performance, but also on its biocompatibility and economic as well as other considerations. It is not proposed to discuss the criteria of choice in detail, but instead to state the requirements of an ideal hemodialysis (Table 1) in order that the reader may have a yardstick of comparison against which potential choices may be matched.

In common with other modes of extracorporeal therapy, safety precautions during the use are mandatory, and consequently both the blood and the dialysate circuits incorporate a variety of safety devices to enable the safe use of the technique to be undertaken. These include monitoring the pressure in the extracorporeal blood circuit and the composition and temperature of the dialysis fluid, which after passage through the hemodialyser is also monitored for the presence of hemoglobin, since there is a risk of rupture of these semipermeable membranes.

Blood flow through the extracorporeal circuit is maintained by the use of a blood pump, which is linked to the above safety and monitoring devices, and this ensures that the blood flow is stopped in the event of a malfunction. The use of a pump in the blood circuit increases the risk of an air embolism, and in consequence an air detector is an integral part of the blood circuit monitoring system.

DIALYSIS FLUID

Hemodialysis relies on the diffusion from the blood to the dialysis fluid of metabolites with an elevated concentration as a consequence of renal insufficiency. The dialysis fluid is obtained by the mixing of commercially available concentrate with treated tap water by a proportionating system designed for use either by a single patient or for batch production suitable for multiple patient use.

DIALYSIS FLUID COMPOSITION

In theory, the composition of dialysis fluid should probably be similar to that of interstitial fluid, with a suitable correction for the small protein fraction. In practice, considerable variations in both cation and anion composition may occur.

The electrolyte content of the dialysate can be important for clinical tolerance, and a dialysate containing low sodium level is, in general, less well supported, especially in hemodynamically labile patients (22)

A specific series of problems is related to the composition of the buffer. Dialysis was first performed with bicarbonate as a buffer, however, the advent of early single-patient proportionating systems meant that, for chemical reasons, bicarbonate-based dialysis fluid could not be produced in batch in the presence of calcium in the concentrate, which is essential for the attainment of a positive calcium balance and the prevention of bone decalcification. For these reasons, Mion proposed in 1964 to use acetate as an alternative buffer (23).

By the early 1970s it became possible to mix bicarbonate and calcium without precipitation, and this led to the more widespread use of bicarbonate-based dialysis fluids. A further interest in the return to bicarbonate buffering from the more commonly used acetate buffer came with the introduction of high-efficiency dialysers and shorter dialysis times, which resulted in the abnormalities of acid-base parameters of dialysis patients subject to such schedules (24).

CLINICAL PROBLEMS RELATED TO BUFFER COMPOSITION

A number of clinical studies have demonstrated that patients on acetate-based dialysis treatment are prone to hemodynamic problems (22, 25, 26). There is, however, no universal agreement on this observation, partly due to differences in the efficiency of the dialysers used in the studies and the patient's cardiovascular status (27, 28). Acetate hemodialysis is also associated with a marked hypoxia, resulting from the loss of CO_2 from the blood across the membrane into the dialysate (29, 30). In contrast, this aspect of dialysis therapy may be prevented, or at least ameliorated, by the use of bicarbonate buffering. There is also the possibility that acetate may be metabolized into lactate or be incorporated into lipids and be responsible for the hyperlipidemia observed in dialyzed patients (31), and be contributory to the cardiovascular problems of patients treated by long-term hemodialysis. The data presented in support of this hypothesis are not convincing.

Furthermore, Morin et al. (32) failed to demonstrate significant differences in the serum lipid profiles of patients on acetate-or bicarbonate-based dialysis fluids. Acetate may also interfere with the buffering mechanism, not only in the extracellular fluid, but also in the bone. This latter fact may be of importance in chronic acidosis when calcium phosphate and calcium carbonate crystals from the bone dissolve, releasing their respective ions, which then act as a buffering agent.

The use of bicarbonate as a buffer allows a quick correction of the acid-base disturbances in uremic patients. It would seem that bicarbonate is preferabe to acetate, but despite all the apparent theoretical and practical advantages of bicarbonate over acetate, many nephrologists continue to use acetate, possibly due to the fact that such systems are simpler and less expensive.

Sequential ultrafiltration and hemodialysis

In conventional hemodialysis, fluid removal is sustained during the period of treatment to rid the patient of excess of water and extracellular electrolytes. Bergström et al. (33) showed that by introducing a period of ultrafiltration without dialysate flow in the dialysis schedule, i.e., separating the process of ultrafiltration and dialysis, it was possible to remove up to 3 l/hour of fluid from an overhydrated patient without adverse affects. The absence of hypotension or muscle cramps during the period of ultrafiltration appeared to be related to the absence of osmolality changes.

Sequential ultrafiltration and dialysis may be performed in a number of different ways, the simplest is by the application of a positive pressure on the blood side or a vacuum on the dialysate side in the absence of rinsing fluid flowing through the dialyzer. With the availability of hemofilters or high-flux hemodialyzers, sequential ultrafiltration and hemodialysis remains of interest mainly to those with access only to conventional hemodialyzers. In spite of the relative simplicity of the procedure, the treatment time is prolonged because of the necessity to sequence ultrafiltration and hemodialysis. Furthermore, there is also a danger of imbalance in the electrolytes, e.g., hypercalcemia.

In the treatment of chronic renal failure, sequential ultrafiltration and dialysis should only be used on selected patients or in special situations. It may be considered for patients who develop symptomatic hypotension during hemodialysis, patients whose interdialytic weight gain is excessive, or patients with cardiovascular disease or myocardial insufficiency who are intolerant of conventional dialysis. In addition, it may also be useful in controlling volume-related hypertension in the early stage of dialysis treatment.

Hemofiltration

During conventional dialysis, the principal method of solute removal is by diffusion, which is augmented to a lesser extent by convective mass transport (ultrafiltration). In hemofiltration, the ultrafiltrate flow through highly permeable membranes is augmented with a substitution fluid, which is a modified Ringer lactate solution. The augmentation may take place either before (predilution) or after (postdilution) the hemofilter. Predilution requires about 30% more substition fluid than postdilution. This, coupled with the fact that postdilution corresponds to the filtration process in the human kidney, has meant that of the two, postdilution has become the more widely used technique.

The total volume of exchange ranges from 20 to 40 per treatment, which is typically carried out in three times weekly sessions, lasting 4–5 hours each.

The equipment for hemofiltration consists of the extracorporeal blood circuit, which is analogous to that used in hemodialysis. Ultrafiltration across the hemofilter is achieved by the exertion of a hydrostatic pressure gradient across the membrane, resulting in the transfer of plasma, water, and solutes. In contrast to the complex hydraulic system required for hemodialysis, the hydraulic circuit used to achieve this in hemofiltration is markedly simpler. In general, a roller pump creates the negative pressure in the dialysate compartment and carries the ultrafiltrate from the hemofilter through a disposable tubing set to a collection canister. A negative pressure monitor in the circuit prevents the pressure limits from being exceeded, and the circuit also contains a blood leak detector that stops the extracorporeal blood flow in the event of a membrane rupture. In a separate circuit, substitution fluid is delivered from its containers into the extracorporeal circuit by a separate roller pump.

Due to the large volume of fluid exchange during each treatment, an accurate balancing and monitoring system is used, which generally is microprocessor operated and balances the amount of fluid removed from the circuit with that infused. The removal of low molecular weight substances, such as urea and creatinine, with postdilution hemofiltration is less effective than with hemodialysis (Figure 1). In contrast, however, hemofiltration is considerably more effective in removing substances of a higher molecular weight.

Treatment of chronic renal failure by long-term hemofiltration was first described in 1974 (34); by 1984 statistical returns from the EDTA-ERA Registry (35) showed that 1740 patients, representing 2.4% of the European treatment group, used this method of treatment. No records are available for the USA regarding the number of hemofiltration procedures performed, but its clinical use has been described by several workers (36, 37).

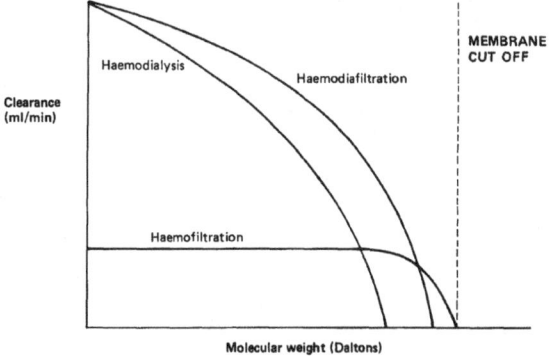

Figure 1. Comparative solute removal rate by hemodialysis, hemofiltration, and hemodiafiltration.

The need for special equipment to allow hemofiltration to be performed safely, together with the high cost of replacement fluid, unless it is manufactured on site, has limited the use of this technique to patients with vascular instability episodes, hypertension, or hypotension between treatments, as well as to those patients with autonomic insufficiency. In addition, it has also been used successfully in the treatment of acute renal failure (38).

Hemodiafiltration

Hemodiafiltration or biofiltration combines conventional hemodialysis with hemofiltration. The combination of the two methods allows an increased clearance rate for both middle and small molecules compared to the use of a single technique alone. Low molecular weight substances are removed predominantly by diffusion, whereas middle molecules are removed by convection.

In contrast to hemofiltration, during hemodiafiltration only 8–10 l of replacement solution is used, which is infused into the venous return of the extracorporeal circuit. In contrast with hemofiltration, during biofiltration a hypertonic substitution fluid containing bicarbonate is used (39).

Continuous arteriovenous hemofiltration (CAVH)

In continuous arteriovenous hemofiltration, fluid, electrolytes and small-and middle-molecular-sized solutes are removed from the patient by ultrafiltration for an extended period ranging from several hours to days. Simultaneously, the blood volume is reconstituted by the administration of a fluid with an electrolyte composition comparable to that of normal plasma. The process relies on a small filter containing a highly permeable membrane, and the patient's arterial to venous pressure gradient is usually sufficient to provide circulation through the extracorporeal circuit.

Continuous arteriovenous hemofiltration was originally intended as a form of therapy for renal failure, as opposed to the intermittent modes of therapy described above. However, it has seen a much wider acceptance as a mode of treatment in patients with acute renal failure.

CAVH is ideally suited for patients with acute renal failure who are hemodynamically unstable, or those who have a contraindication for the use of peritoneal dialysis. Patients with multiple organ failure or patients with traumatic injuries and acute renal failure are considered ideal candidates for CAVH.

It may also be used advantageously for the initial dehydration in the cases of diuretic-resistant cardiac insufficiency. Shock lung syndrome, a complication frequently accompanying acute renal failure, is considered another indication for the application of continuous hemofiltration, because oxygenation is improved only when dehydration of the patient is performed simultaneously with PEEP respiration. Although CAVH is a treatment that permits access to the extracellular fluid of patients with a variety of diseases, it should not be performed on patients who are severely hypotensive or catabolic despite hyperalimentation, nor in patients with systemic bleeding, since under these conditions the technique is difficult to sustain.

Plasma separation

The separation of plasma from cells may be achieved either by centrifugation or by filtration through membranes. There is little difference in the therapeutic effects of plasmafiltration through membranes and cell centrifugation, and the choice of technique is dictated by the facilities available.

When using plasma separators an extracorporeal circuit comparable to that used in hemodialysis or hemofiltration may be used. Plasma separation is used in the treatment of disorders that are provoked by plasma components such as immunoglobulins, immune complexes, and substances with a strong protein binding, which are eiiminated through the large pores of the plasma filter and are substituted by a protein-containing solution.

Hemoperfusion

In hemoperfusion direct contact between the blood and the sorbent system occurs. Most clinically available sorbent systems use activated carbons (charcoals), ion-exchange resins, or nonionic macroporous resins. The sorbents are generally contained within cartridges or columns. Such devices may be used not only in the treatment of uremia, but also in the treatment of drug intoxication and hepatic encephalopathy.

Hemoperfusion alone, however, is not sufficient for the control of symptoms or removal of water in uremic subjects, and, because of this, composite devices combining a charcoal column with a hemodialyzer have been developed.

SPECIFIC ASPECTS OF EXTRACORPOREAL THERAPY

Single-needle dialysis

As stated earlier, the current access method for extracorporeal therapy is by the use of two needles or catheters to gain access to the patient's circulation and to facilitate the return of blood from the extracorporeal circuit. Since 1972 the possibility has existed to perform extracorporeal procedures such as dialysis through the insertion of a single needle by a technique known as single-needle dialysis (40). Such a method of access is more comfortable and acceptable for the patient, but, despite this, it has not been as widespread a technique as might be expected.

The reluctance to adopt this technique routinely may be attributed to the belief that single-needle dialysis is inadequate. This prejudice is based on the poor clinical experience obtained with the older systems (41), which resulted in low blood flows, as high recirculation rates were achieved during clinical use (42). Furthermore, in the past such a technique of vascular access has been preferentially used in patients with poor fistulae when it was not possible to insert two needles.

Recent data obtained in a group of patients treated by a more recently developed single-needle technique operating on a pressure-pressure basis has demonstrated that the adequacy of dialysis when estimated by clearance measurements as well as urea kinetics is similar to conventional two-needle dialysis (43), with patient mortality and morbidity equivalent to that achieved by the more conventional method of access.

In addition to the benefits offered to patients when using this system, the newer systems also allow ultrafiltration control to be achieved in the absence of the newer proportioning systems offering this option, which results in a greater hemodynamic stability in patients in whom this technique is used (44).

Uremic toxin removal

The uremic syndrome has many characteristics in common with the clinical picture arising from the ingestion of an exogenous toxin (45). The mean difference is that a major part of the responsible toxins are formed in the body itself as a consequence of metabolic breakdown of food and other ingested substances. It has long been recognized that the uremic syndrome affects multiple organ systems, particularly the neurologic, cardiovascular, hematologic, and gastrointestinal systems (46).

On the other hand, it has also been demonstrated that uremic biologic fluids, such as serum or the ultrafiltrate of serum, may affect several biologic functions and that these disturbances may be dose related (47). The most important systems in this context are in immunologic systems, especially phagocytosis (48–50), the production and fragility of red blood cells (51–56), drug protein binding (62–65), and nerve conduction (66).

It is well recognized that, whereas substances are retained during uremia and many of these are partially removed by extracorporeal therapy, it is less clear what the link between the uremic symptoms and the inhibitory effects on biologic systems and the responsible retained solutes is. The possibility may well exist that a single substance is not toxic in isolation but becomes toxic only when it is mixed with other substances that are retained. One of the major problems in this identification has been incomplete recognition of metabolites retained, as well as technical difficulties in isolating substances responsible for biologic changes.

The most commonly used separation technique has been gel chromatography, one of the major pitfalls of this technique being an incomplete separation of uremic substances, as well as the presence of sugar and salt in the eluate, which may alter biologic functions (67, 68). Recently, HPLC has been used as an alternative technique of separation, and this allows a better separation with less chance for the presence of interfering factors (69, 70).

In light of these difficulties relating to the technique of separation and identification, only a few metabolites have been recognized as having a truly toxic effect. One such substance is urea, although it is accepted that most of its side effects only occur at high concentrations that are rarely seen today (71, 72). Methylguanidine has also been shown to have adverse effects, principally on nerve function (73, 74). Parathormone, which is oversecreted in the majority of renal failure patients due to an inappropriate homeostatic action of the parathyroids, also interferes with several biologic functions (53, 55, 57). Indoxylsulphate and hippuric acid decrease drug protein binding (64, 65). Beta$_2$-microglobulin has been shown to accumulate in uremic patients (75) and has recently been linked to the development of the amyloidosis that occurs after several years of dialysis therapy (76–78).

A wide range of molecular-weight metabolites are retained as a consequence of renal insufficiency and are inadequately removed by replacement renal therapy. A few years ago there was a tendency to attribute at least part of the uremic toxicity to the retention of so-called middle molecules whose molecular weight is between 500 and 10,000 daltons (68). A number of investigations were started in an attempt to identify the substances responsible and to define their toxicity. The resulting studies were conflicting: despite extensive evaluations, only two distinct substances were isolated, one a glucuronide, of orthohydroxy hippuric acid, and the other, an as yet unidentified compound (79–81). Both these substances have molecular weights below 600 daltons. It is therefore probable that some molecules behave during dialysis and chromatography like middle molecules, although their molecular weight is lower than could be expected from their intradialytic behavior. A further problem has been the fact that one of the two recognized products, the glucuronide of orthohydroxy hippuric acid, turned out to be a major metabolite of aspirin (82).

The middle molecular hypothesis thus remains unproven, and focus is shifting towards establishing the toxicity of smaller molecules, some of them behaving like middle molecules. It should, however, be stressed that beta$_2$-microglobulin and parathormone are two substances in the middle molecular weight range whose toxicity has been demonstrated.

The importance of small molecules and their removal during extracorporeal therapy has been further emphasized by the American National Cooperative Dialysis Study (NCDS), which showed urea to be an adequate parameter of dialysis efficiency and a predictor of dialytic morbidity (83).

Urea, however, can only be considered as an indirect indicator and, furthermore, it should be stressed that the data presented in the American National Cooperative Dialysis Study were obtained with hemodialyzers containing cellulose-based (cuprophan) membranes and not with the newer devices that have been recently introduced into clinical practice, which contain synthetic membranes that are not only more porous to middle molecules, but also offer an improved biocompatibility. It cannot be denied, therefore, that uremic toxicity is a multifactorial problem, and our knowledge of it, at present, is characterized by multiple blind spots. Until our knowledge becomes less scanty, one should pursue an overall solute elimination that encompasses as wide a molecular weight range as possible. The ideal situation would be to obtain postdialysis serum profiles in uremia that are comparable to normal serum profiles.

Reuse of hemodialyzers

The initial motivation for reuse of hemodialyzers was economy and convenience. Interest in dialyzer reuse has been rekindled in the last few years, principally for economic reasons, and due to the fact that improved biocompatibility may exist for reused dialysers when compared with new dialyzers. The technique of reuse, the practice in which hemodialysers are used for multiple dialyses of the same patient, may be subdivided into four distinct steps: rinsing of the dialyzer at the termination of dialysis, cleaning, and sterilization to allow its storage between uses. The preparation of the dialyzer prior to subsequent use is the final stage of the procedure. The technique may be carried out manually or automatically, using equipment designed specifically for this purpose. Several different sterilants are available for reuse; the most popular is formaldehyde (84). It is frequently used at a 2% concentration, although sterilization may be incomplete under these conditions and contamination by non-tuberculous microbacteria has been reported (84). A 4% concentration may be more appropriate.

The use of formaldehyde as a sterilant for hemodialyzers poses risks not only to the patients, but also to the staff. Occupational exposure to formaldehyde may be associated with respiratory tract and eye irritation. Prolonged handling of formaldehyde by the staff and patients is associated with contact dermatitis and asthma (85–87). A more serious concern is its carcinogenecity or cocarcinogenecity. Animals exposed to atmospheric levels of 6 and 15 ppm over an 18-month period developed nasal squamous-cell carcinomas. A spillage of 1 ml of 37% formalin in a $3 \times 4 \times 7$ meter room will, if completely volatile, produce vapors of about 3.6 ppm.

Additional potential hazards in patients receiving regular dialysis treatment in which the dialyzer has been exposed to formalin is the increased presence of anti-N-like antibodies (88); this, in turn, may result in hemolytic anemia (89, 90). The reduction of formaldehyde concentrations in the venous effluent of the dialyzer to below 3 ppm has been recommended to avoid this problem (89), although in our own experience target concentrations of below 1 ppm have still resulted in anti-N-like antibody development.

Alternative sterilants that may be more suitable than formalin are peracetic acid (91) and gluteraldehyde (92). Although with these sterilants no adverse reactions have been reported to date, their use has been limited in order to be cautious with regard to their long-term safety.

Peracetic acid, however, is degraded quickly when brought into contact with human blood, so it is possible that this reagent may turn out to be a safe alternative to formaldehyde.

Sodium hypochlorite has also been used as a sterilant (93); it breaks down the protein layer on the membrane surface instead of fixing it, so that there is no gain in biocompatibility when using this agent (94). It is especially suitable for the reuse of primarily biocompatible synthetic membranes such as polyacrylonitrile (95), since it does not structurally weaken such membranes, in contrast to cellulose-based membranes, where repeated exposure to sodium hypochlorite reduces the membrane strength and leads to blood leak during use.

The issues surrounding the reuse of hemodialyzers are complex and involve medical, ethical, social, and financial considerations. Despite these complex issues, the practice remains firmly established. At present, no national codes of practice exist relating to the reuse of devices intended for single use, although some centers have drawn up their own guidelines.

Biocompatibility

Biocompatibility may be defined as the absence of a reaction when the body or part of the body is brought in contact with a foreign chemical structure (96). Biocompatibility problems have been observed with all types of artificial organs. The biocompatibility of hemodialysis has been extensively studied, since patients receiving this type of therapy are exposed to foreign materials regularly over a period of several years. The exposure of blood to the membrane contained within the hemodialyzer may be associated with a rapid, transient fall in white cells, activation of the complement system, and a fall in arterial oxygenation. The fall in white cell counts occurs during the first hour of treatment. Its duration is short, with the nadir being reached between 10 and 20 minutes after the commencement of treatment. This is followed by a gradual return to pretreatment levels by the end of the first hour. Differential counts performed during the phenomenon indicate that the leukopenia is due to a fall in neutrophils and monocyte counts.

Activation of the complement system also occurs and may be demonstrated by a fall in the total complement activity of serum (CH50), or by falls in the concentration of complement components such as C_3 and factor B.

Craddock and coworkers (97, 98) demonstrated that this activation was a direct consequence of blood-membrane contact. They based their hypothesis on the fact that polysaccharides, which are similar in structure to cellulose, are capable of activating complement by the alternative pathway with depletion of both C_{3a} and factor B. In addition, they also showed that contact between plasma and the membrane releases a granulocyte aggregant (C_{5a}) that increases the stickiness of the leukocytes and cause them to adhere to the first vascular surface with which they come into contact after passing through the hemodialyzer, namely, the pulmonary capillaries. Patients receiving dialysis treatment experience a fall in arterial oxygen tension (Pa_{O_2}). This fall occurs over the same time span as leukopenia and ranges between 5% and 25%. The onset of hypoxia is rapid, but, unlike leukopenia, it may persist throughout treatment, with the arterial oxygen tension not returning to predialysis levels until the termination of dialysis. The study of this aspect of extracorporeal therapy has concentrated on three areas. First, the relationship between leukopenia, complement activation, and hypoxia; secondly, the role of the membrane materials; and third, clinical implications of these phenomena.

Craddock et al., demonstrated in their studies that leukopenia was associated with changes in pulmonary function manifested by a rise in the intrapulmonary arterial pressure and an increase in lymph effluent from the lungs, a consequence of endothelial leakage when cellophane incubated with plasma was injected into animals. Based on their findings, they concluded that the most probable sequence of events was complement activation, leading to neutrophil aggregation in the lungs, which resulted in impaired oxygen transport across the lungs, which led to hypoxia.

Several studies recently revealed a relationship between intradialytic leukopenia and complement activation, on one hand, and pulmonary function, more precisely, lung diffusion capacity, on the other (30, 99); although other studies state that the changes induced by complement-activating cellulosic membranes and by noncomplement-activating synthetic membranes are comparable (100, 101).

It can, however, not be denied that other mechanisms may also play a role in the development of intradialytic hypoxia (102, 103): firstly, the loss of CO_2 through the dialyzer and, secondly, the increased oxygen consumption and decreased CO_2 production resulting from the metabolism of acetate contained in the dialysis fluid.

The membranes used in hemodialyzers currently may be divided into two categories: those that are based on cellulose and those that are synthetic copolymers. Leukopenia induced by synthetic membranes is signifiantly lower than that induced by cellulose membranes, although a new generation of cellulose-based membranes in which the structure has been modified is being introduced into clinical use, and in such membranes, the magnitude of leukopenia induced is comparable with that for synthetic membranes (104, 105).

In common with the leukopenia, complement activation is also reduced for synthetic membranes when measurements using the recently developed radioimmunoassays for anaphylatoxins C_{3a} and C_{5a} and their desArg derivates are used. On the other hand, studies of complement activation using the more common CH50, factor B, and C_3 and C_4 assays have provided conflicting results between cellulose-based and synthetic membranes, which may be a consequence of their insensitivity in measuring complement levels. The clinical implications of these phenomena and their long-term consequences are far from clear.

Leukopenia may be associated with functional changes in neutrophils such as chemotaxis, phagocytability, decreased random mobility, and an increased adherence. Although phagocytic function is generally depressed in dialysis patients (48), Nguyen et al. demonstrated that phagocytic activity increased during cuprophan dialysis in contrast with dialysis with polyacrylonitrile membranes (49). It is not clear from the available data whether the currently observed predialysis depression of phagocytic systems can be attributed to exhaustion of the phagocytic system due to its repeated intradialytic stimulation. In any case, phagocytic function is more depressed in dialyzed than in nondialyzed renal patients (106). Furthermore, Henderson showed that a decrease in phagocytic mobility after contact of white blood cells with cellulose acetate occurred, whereas this reaction remained absent after contact with a more biocompatible membrane (107).

The clinical implications of repeated complement activation have received little attention. Hakim and colleagues investigated complement activation in patients with and without the first-use syndrome in cuprophan-containing hemodialyzers (108). They demonstrated an association between the level of complement activation, as measured by C_{3a}, and adverse allergic reactions experienced during treatment. Since such allergic reactions may result from other causes, such as an allergy to ethylene oxide (109), its dependance on a single cause is speculative.

The possibility exists that the difference between synthetic and cellulose-based membranes may exert an important influence on the pulmonary and cardiac functions of patients receiving regular dialysis therapy. Studies by Chanard et al. (110) and Kant et al. (111) have demonstrated markedly less intradialytic morbidity during dialysis when using membranes that are more biocompatible.

In patients who have experienced hypersensitivity or allergic reactions with cellulose-based membranes, especially in specific groups of patients such as the eldery, as well as in those with coexisting cardiovascular and pulmonary complications, the use of more biocompatible synthetic membranes in conjunction with bicarbonate-based dialysis appears to be preferable.

Coagulation

Contact of blood with surfaces other than the vascular wall triggers coagulation. This process is dependent upon the chemical characteristics of the contact surface, such as the charge and structure, but also on the geometrical structure and shear-generating capacity of the surface or material in contact with the blood (112, 113). Extracorporeal therapy may trigger coagulation not only by membrane contact, but also by blood contact with components of the extracorporeal circuit. In-vitro data on the degree of coagulability due to different materials is conflicting; in-vivo results, however, show no clearcut differences between membranes (114). Different polymers have been developed in an attempt to minimize coagulability, and polyurethane is probably one of the most widely used polymers that has the least pronounced coagulability.

During extracorporeal therapy, it is therefore necessary to administer an anticoagulant to prevent clotting in the extracorporeal circuit. Intravenously administered heparin is widely used for this purpose. If the level of anticoagulation is too low, clotting of the circuit can occur, while in excessive anticoagulation there is an increased risk of patient bleeding after therapy. The goal of heparinization is to achieve a uniform adequate level of anticoagulation, and the dose of heparin required may vary considerably from patient to patient. To overcome these difficulties, kinetic modeling techniques may be used for the calculation of heparin requirements for an individual patient.

In patients where there is adverse risk associated with the use of heparin, prostacyclin may be used (115, 116). Prostacyclin is expensive for routine use and may cause hemodynamic side effects. Low moleucular weight heparin is another alternative that has recently become available (117). The incorporation of heparin or other anticoagulants into the polymer structures and other contact surfaces is an appealing alternative to the routine administration of anticoagulants during therapy, but is only being used experimentally at present.

Elution of toxic substances

The elution of toxic substances from components of the extracorporeal circuit is a well-recognized complication of extracorporeal therapy. Substances released during extracorporeal therapy include the spallation of silicone from blood tubings (118); the degree of spallation has been shown to correlate with the duration of dialysis, with the weight of the reticuloendothelial system organs at autopsy, and with functional liver disturbances (119). The intravenous injection of silicone into rats caused an increase in prostaglandin E_2 and thromboxane release from the spleen into the blood (120). The magnitude of spallation may be modified by careful attention to the occlusion pressure of the peristaltic blood pumps used in the extracorporeal circulation (121–123). Other materials that has been shown to be released from extracorporeal circuits are plasticizers. The most commonly used plasticizer is DI-2-ethylplexyl phthalate (DEHP), which may represent up to 40% of the dry weight of polyvinylchloride (PVC). DEHP is released during extracorporeal therapy and may accumulate in the body and cause liver damage (124). Ethylene oxide is commonly used for sterilization of devices and may slowly release into the blood, especially after inadequate rinsing of the extracorporeal circuit (125). In capillary hemodialyzers, the polyurethane potting material has a specific affinity for ethylene oxide. An ethylene oxide allergy may develop in a substantial fraction of patients routinely subjected to extracorporeal therapy and is characterized by positive radioimmunoabsorbent tests (126).

WHEN SHOULD TREATMENT BE STARTED?

The most appropriate time to start renal replacement therapy depends upon the indication and the treatment modality. In acute renal failure, especially when the established phase has been reached, hemodialysis or related techniques should be started early and a serum BUN of 1 g/l or more is currently accepted as the lower limit at which to commence treatment (127). Dialysis should be started even earlier in the case of total anuria, fluid overload, hypercalcemia, and/or acidosis.

Hemodialysis for chronic renal failure without complications is generally started at a glomerular filtration rate of 5 ml/min (128), although some groups start earlier (129). Dialysis should be started earlier in diabetic patients or in those suffering from severe hypertension; in these cases, 10 ml/min glomerular filtration rate may be considered the minimum at which to initiate therapy (128). It should be stressed that if hemodialysis is planned in diabetics, fistula creation should be started early, e.g., at a glomerular fltration rate of 20 ml/min or a creatinine level of 4 mg% due to the risk of fistula thrombosis and other fistula problems in this group of patients.

Plasma separation or plasmapheresis remains a controversial issue in many aspects and should only be used in life-threatening situations, if its benefit is proven (130, 131).

WHICH TREATMENT MODALITY SHOULD BE USED?

The wide range of therapies currently available makes it difficult to reach a consensus regarding specific advantages and disadvantages.

Conventional diaysis with acetate remains the standard treatment for the majority of dialysis patients. Bicarbonate-based dialysis may be considered as the method of choice, however, in acute renal failure patients, as well as in those with cardiovascular instability and in the older age group. The question as to whether to use a more biocompatible membrane in these treatment groups remains partially unanswered at present.

Sequential ultrafiltration and dialysis may be useful in the case of patients with a high interdialytic weight gain, especially those who are hemodynamically labile.

Hemofiltration or hemodiafiltration may also be of help in patients with problematic hemodynamics, although the availability of bicarbonate or variable sodium during dialysis may also resolve these problems.

Continuous arteriovenous hemofiltration (CAVH) is a technique that may be useful for acute renal failure patients.

Accepted indications for the use of *plasma separation* include Goodpasture's syndrome, rapidly progressive glomerulonephritis, hyperviscosity syndrome, thyrotoxic crisis, thrombotic thrombocytopenic purpura, and intoxication with digitalis or amanita phalloides (130, 131). For other renal-related diseases such as lupus erythematodes disseminatus, other treatments must be first considered.

The use of *hemoperfusion* may be useful in the treatment of severely drug-intoxicated patients.

Single-needle dialysis is an accepted indication for bad fistulas or hemodialysis in children, and in our opinion the newer types of pressure-pressure single-needle dialysis, with their proven adequacy, should replace two-needle dialysis with time.

REFERENCES

1. Hegstrom RM, Quinton WE, Dillard DH, Cole JJ, Scribner BH: One year's experience with the use of indwelling teflon cannulas and bypass. *Trans Am Soc Artif Intern Organs* 7:47, 1961.
2. Shaldon S, Chiandussi L, Higgs B: Haemodialysis by percutaneous catheterisation of the femoral artery and vein with regional heparinisation. *Lancet* 2:857, 1961.
3. Shaldon S, Rae AI, Rosen SM, Silva H, Oakley J: Refrigerated femoral venous-venous haemodialysis with coil preservation for rehabilitation of terminal uraemic patients. *Lancet* 1:1716, 1963.
4. Fuchs HJ, Jenett G, Klehr V, Richter G, Wilbrandt R, Frotscher U: Die perkutane punktion der vena femoralis zur hämodialysebehandlung. *Dtsch Med Wschr* 102:1280, 1977.
5. Bambauer R, Jutzler GA: Jugularis-interna-punktion zur Shaldon-katheterisierung. Ein neuer Zugang für akute Hämodialysen, *Nieren Hochdruckkrankheiten* 3:109, 1980.
6. Uldall PR, Dyck RF, Woods F, Merchant N, Martin GS, Cardella CJ, Sutton D, Deveber GA: A subclavian cannula for temporary vascular access for hemodialysis or plasmapheresis. *Dial Transpl* 8:963, 1979.
7. De Cubber A, De Wolf C, Lameire N, Schurgers M, Ringoir S: Single needle hemodialysis with the double headpump via the subclavian vein. *Dial Transplant* 7:1261, 1978.
8. Fine A, Churchill D, Gault H, Mathieson G: Fatality due to subclavian dialysis catheter. *Nephron* 29:99, 1981.
9. Merrill RH, Raab SO: Dialysis catheter-induced pericardial tamponade. *Arch Int Med* 142:1751, 1982.
10. Barton BR, Hermann G, Weill R: Cardiothoracic emergencies associated with subclavian hemodialysis catheters. *JAMA* 250:2660, 1983.
11. Vaziri ND, Maksy M, Lewis M, Martin D, Edwards K: Massive mediastinal hematoma caused by a double-lumen subclavian catheter. *Artif Organs* 8:223, 1984.
12. Ducatman BS, Mac Michan JC, Edwards MD: Catheter-induced lesions of the right side of the heart. A one year prospective study of 142 autopsies. *JAMA* 253:791, 1985.
13. Ratcliffe PJ, Oliver DO: Massive thrombosis around subclavian cannulas used for hemodialysis. *Lancet* 1:1472, 1982.
14. Cheung AK, Gregory MC: Subclavian vein thrombosis in hemodialysis patients. *Trans Am Soc Artif Int Organs* 31:131, 1985.
15. Vanholder R, Lameire N, Verbanck J, Van Rattinghe R, Kunnen M, Ringoir S: Complications of subclavian hemodialysis: A 5 year prospective study in 257 consecutive patients. *Int J Artif Organs* 5:297, 1982.
16. Vanholder R, Hoenich N, Ringoir S: Morbidity and mortality of central venous catheter hemodialysis. *Nephron* 47:274, 1987.
17. Uldall PR, Joy C, Merchant N: Further experience with double lumen subclavian cannula for hemodialysis. *Trans Am Soc Artif Int Organs* 28:71, 1982.
18. Brescia MJ, Cimino JE, Appel K, Hurwich BJ: Chronic hemodialysis using venipuncture and a surgically created arteriovenous fistula. *N Engl J Med* 275:1089, 1966.
19. Tellis VA, Kohnberg WJ, Bhat DJ, Driscoll B, Veith FJ: Expanded polytetrafluoroethylene graft fistula for chronic hemodialysis. *Ann Surg* 189:101, 1979.
20. Knutson R, Wathen R, Comty CM, Shapiro FL: Bovine carotid artery grafts as blood access devices. *Proc Eur Dial Transpl Assoc* 10:229, 1973.
21. Zerbino VR, Tice DA: Successful use of preserved allograft vein for chronic hemodialysis. *Nephron* 10:61, 1973.
22. Wehle B, Asaba H, Castenfors J, Fürst P, Grahn A, Gunnarson B, Shaldon S, Bergström J: The influence of dialysis fluid composition on the blood pressure response during dialysis. *Clin Nephrol* 10:62, 1978.
23. Mion CM, Hegstrom RM, Boen ST, Scribner BH: Substitution of sodium acetate for sodium bicarbonate in the bath fluid for hemodialysis. *Trans Am Soc Artif Intern Organs* 10:110, 1964.
24. Graefe U, Milutinovich J, Follette WC, Vizzo JE, Babb AL, Scribner BH: Less dialysis-induced morbidity and vascular instability with bicarbonate in dialysate. *Ann Intern Med* 88:332, 1978.
25. Aizawa Y, Ohmori T, Imai K, Nara Y, Matsuoka M, Hirasawa Y: Depressant action of acetate upon the human cardiovascular system. *Clin Nephrol* 8:477, 1977.
26. Leenen FHH, Buda AJ, Smith DL, Farrel S, Levine DZ, Uldall PR: Hemodynamic changes during acetate and bicarbonate hemodialysis. *Artif Organs* 8:411, 1984.
27. Borges HF, Fryd DS, Rosa AA, Kjellstrand CM: Hypotension during acetate and bicarbonate dialysis in patient with acute renal failure. *Am J Nephrol* 1:24, 1981.
28. Vanholder R, Piron M, Ringoir S: Absence of a beneficial hemodynamic effect of bicarbonate versus acetate hemodialysis. *Proc Eur Dial Transpl Assoc* 21:195, 1984.
29. Dolan MJ, Whipp BJ, Davidson WD, Weitzman RE, Wasserman K: Hypopnea associated with acetate hemodialysis: Carbon dioxide-flow-dependent ventilation. *N Engl J Med* 305:72, 1981.
30. De Backer WA, Verpooten GA, Borgonjon DJ, Vermeire PA, Lins RR, De Broe ME: Hypoxemia during hemodialysis: Effects of different membranes and dialysate compositions. *Kidney Int* 23:738, 1983.
31. Novello AC, Kjellstrand CM: Is bicarbonate dialysis better than acetate dialysis? *J Am Soc Artif Intern Organs* 6:103, 1983.
32. Morin RJ, Srikantaiah MV, Woodley Z, Davidson WD: Effect of hemodialysis with acetate vs. bicarbonate on plasma lipid and lipoprotein levels in uremic patients. *J Dial* 4:9, 1980.
33. Bergström J, Asaba H, Fürst P, Oules R: Dialysis, ultrafiltration and blood pressure. *Proc Eur Dial Transpl Assoc* 13:293, 1976.
34. Quellhorst EA: Ultrafiltration and haemofiltration. Practical applications. In: W Drukker, FM Parsons, JF Maher, eds, *Replacement of Renal Function by Dialysis*, 2nd ed. Martinus Nijhoff, Boston, pp 265–274, 1983.
35. Brunner FP, Broyer M, Brynger H, Challah S, Fassbinder W, Oules R, Rizzoni G, Selwood NH, Wing AJ: Combined report on regular dialysis and transplantation in Europe, XV, 1984. *Proc Eur Dial Transpl Assoc* 22:5, 1985.
36. Bosch JP, Lauer A, Glabman S: Mortality and morbidity associated with hemofiltration. *J Am Soc Artif Intern Organs* 8:28, 1985.
37. Collins AJ, Keshaviah P, Ilstrup KM, Shapiro F: Clinical comparison of hemodialysis and hemofiltration. *Kidney Int* 28:S18, 1985.
38. Hakim M, Wheeldon D, Bethune DW, Milstein BB, English TAH, Wallwork J: Haemodialysis and haemofiltration on cardiopulmonary bypass. *Thorax* 40:101, 1985.

39. Meloni C, Taccone-Gallucci M, Morosetti M, Valentini G, Tozzo C, Mazzarella V, Elli M, Marciani MG, Rossini PM, Casciani CU: Clinical evaluation of biofiltration in uremic patients undergoing chronic hemodialysis. *Int J Artif Organs* 9 (Suppl 3):39, 1986.
40. Kopp KF, Gutch CF, Kolff WJ: Single needle dialysis. *Trans Soc Artif Intern Organs* 18:75, 1972.
41. Beretta-Piccoli C, Golder S, Weidmann P, Descoeudres C: Einnadelhämodialyse. *Scheiz Med Wschr* 105:289, 1975.
42. Luno J, Hoenich NA, Conceicao S, Feest TG, Lian F, Ward MK, Kerr DNS: In vivo evaluation of three single needle haemodialysis systems. In: TH Frost, ed, *Technical Aspects of Renal Dialysis*. Pitman Medical, Tunbridge Wells, UK, pp 174-183, 1978.
43. Vanholder R, Hoenich NA, Ringoir S: Adequacy studies of fistula single needle dialysis. *Am J Kidney Dis* 10:417, 1987.
44. Vanholder R, Hoenich N, Piron M, Billiouw JM, Ringoir S: Haemodialysis in a single and a two needle vascular access system: A comparative study. *Proc Eur Dial Transpl Assoc* 20:176, 1983.
45. Knochel JP: Pathogenesis of the uremic syndrome. *Postgrad Med* 64:88, 1978.
46. Teschan PE: The presentation of the patient with chronic renal failure. In: WJ Stone, PL Rabin, eds, *End-Stage Renal Disease*. Academic Press, New York, pp 31-56, 1983.
47. Vanholder R, Schoots A, Ringoir S: Uraemic toxicity. In: JF Maher, ed, *Replacement of Renal Function by Dialysis*. Martinus Nijhoff, Boston, pp 4-19, 1989.
48. Ritchey EE, Wallin JD, Sham SV: Chemiluminescence and superoxide anion production by leucocytes from chronic hemodialysis patients. *Kidney Int* 19:349, 1981.
49. Nguyen AT, Lethias C, Zingraff J, Herbelin A, Naret C, Descamps-Latscha B: Hemodialysis membrane-induced activation of phagocyte oxidative metabolism detected in vivo and in vitro within microamounts of whole blood. *Kidney Int* 28:158, 1985.
50. Ringoir S, Van Looy L, Van de Heyning P, Leroux-Roels G: Impairment of phagocytic activity of macrophages as studied by the skin window test in patients on regular hemodialysis treatment. *Clin Nephrol* 4:234, 1975.
51. Ota K, Sanaka T, Agishi T, Nakajima O: Influence of uremic middle molecules on blood cells. *Artif Organs* 4:113, 1980.
52. Wallner SF, Vautrin RM: The anemia of chronic renal failure: Studies of the effect of organic solvent extraction of serum. *J Lab Clin Med* 92:363, 1978.
53. Meytes D, Bogin E, Ma A, Dukes PP, Massry SG: Effect of parathyroid hormone on erythropoiesis. *J Clin Invest* 67:1263, 1981.
54. Delwiche F, Segal GM, Eschbach JW, Adamson JW: Hematopoietic inhibitors in chronic renal failure: Lack of in vitro specifity. *Kidney Int* 29:641, 1986.
55. Bogin E, Massry SG, Levi J, Djaldetti M, Bristol G, Smith J: Effect of parathyroid hormone on osmotic fragility of human erythrocytes. *J Clin Invest* 69, 1017, 1982.
56. Malachi T, Bogin E, Gafter U, Levi J: Parathyroid hormone effect on the fragility of human young and old red blood cells in uremia. *Nephron* 42:52, 1986.
57. Bogin E, Massry SG, Harary I: Effect of parathyroid hormone on rat heart cells. *J Clin Invest* 67:1215, 1981.
58. Mann JFE, Jakobs KH, Riedel J, Ritz E: Reduced chronotropic responsiveness of the heart in experimental uremia. *Am J Physiol* 250 (Heart Circ Physiol 19):H846, 1986.
59. Defronzo RA, Smith D, Alvestrand A: Insulin action in uremia. *Kidney Int* 24:S102, 1983.
60. Dzurik R, Spustova V, Gerykova M: Pathogenesis and consequences of the alteration of glucose metabolism in renal insufficiency. In: S Massry, R Vanholder, S Ringoir, eds, *Uremic Toxins*. Plenum, New York pp 105-110, 1987.
61. Lockwood DH: The insulin resistance inducing factor. In: S Massry, R Vanholder, S Ringoir, eds, *Uremic Toxins*. Plenum, New York pp 97-104, 1987.
62. Reidenberg MM, Odar-Cederlof I, Van Bahr C, Borga O, Sjoqvist F: Protein binding of diphenylhydantoin and desmethylimipramine in plasma from patients with poor renal function. *N Engl J Med* 285:264, 1971.
63. Depner TA, Gulyassy PF: Plasma protein binding in uremia: Extraction and characterisation of an inhibitor. *Kidney Int* 18:86, 1980.
64. Gulyassy PF, Bottini AT, Stanfel LA, Jarrard EA, Depner TA: Isolation and chemical identification of inhibitors of plasma ligand binding. *Kidney Int* 30:391, 1986.
65. Mac Namara PJ, Lalka D, Gibaldi M: Endogenous accumulation products and serum protein binding in uremia. *J Lab Clin Med*, 98:730, 1981.
66. Funck-Brentano JL, Boudet J, Sausse A, Cueille G, Man NK: In vitro sural nerve test for the evaluation of middle molecule neurotoxicity in uraemia. In: TH Frost, ed, *Technical Aspects of Renal Dialysis*. Pitman Medical, Tunbridge Wells, UK, pp 256-263, 1978.
67. Schoots AC, Mikkers FEP, Claessens HA, De Smet R, Van Landschoot N, Ringoir S: Characterization of uremic "middle molecular" fractions by gas chromatography, mass spectrometry, isotachophoresis and liquid chromatography. *Clin Chem* 28:45, 1982.
68. Schoots A, Mikkers F, Cramers C, De Smet R, Ringoir S: Uremic toxins and the elusive middle molecules. *Nephron* 38:1, 1984.
69. Schoots AC, Homan HR, Gladdines MM, Cramers C, De Smet R, Ringoir S: Screening of UV-absorbing solutes in uremic serum by reversed phase HPLC-change of blood levels in different therapies. *Clin Chim Acta* 146:37, 1985.
70. Schoots A, Vanholder R, De Smet R, Cramers C, Ringoir S: Hippurate and an unknown compound as indicators of residual renal function in dialysed patients. In: LC Smeby, S Jorstad, TE Wideroe, eds, *Immune and Metabolic Aspects of Therapeutic Blood Purification Systems*. Karger, Basel pp 240-245, 1986.
71. Sargent JA, Gotch FA: Mathematic modeling of dialysis therapy. *Kidney Int* 18:2, 1980.
72. Scheuer J, Stezoski SW: The effects of uremic compounds on cardiac function and metabolism. *J Mol Cell Cardiol* 5:287, 1973.
73. Giovannetti S, Balestri PL, Barsotti G: Methylguanidine in uremia. *Arch Int Med* 131:709, 1973.
74. Giovannetti S, Barsotti G: Uremic intoxication. *Nephron* 14:123, 1975.
75. Vincent C, Revillard JP, Galland M, Traeger J: Serum beta 2-microglobulin in hemodialyzed patients. *Nephron* 21:260, 1978.
76. Shirahama T, Skinner M, Cohen AS, Gejyo F, Arakawa M, Suzuki M, Hirasawa Y: Histochemical and immunohistochemical characterization of amyloid associated with chronic hemodialysis as beta 2-microglobulin. *Lab Invest* 53:705, 1985.
77. Gejyo F, Odani S, Yamada T, Honma N, Saito H, Suzuki Y, Nakagawa U, Kobayashi H, Maruyama Y, Hirasawa Y, Suzuki M, Arakawa M: Beta 2-microglobulin: A new form of amyloid protein associated with chronic hemodialysis. *Kidney Int* 30:385, 1986.

78. Vandenbroucke JM, Jadoul M, Maldague B, Huaux JP, Noël H, van Ypersele de Strihou C: Possible role of dialysis membrane characteristics in amyloid osteo-arthropathy. *Lancet* 1:1210, 1986.
79. Zimmerman L, Furst P, Bergström J, Jornvall H: A new glycine containing compound with a blocked amino group from uremic body fluids. *Clin Nephrol* 14:109, 1980.
80. Cueille G: Mise en évidence et évaluation des "moyennes molécules" de la taille de la vitamine B_{12} présents dans les liquides biologiques de sujets normaux et de patients urémiques. *J Chromatogr* 146:55, 1978.
81. Cueille G, Man NK, Farges JP, Funck-Brentano JL: Characterization of sub-peak b4.2 middle molecule. *Artif Organs* 4:28, 1980.
82. Asaba H, Zimmerman L, Bergström J: On drug artifacts in middle molecule analysis. *Nephron* 39:73, 1985.
83. Lowrie EG, Laird NM, Parker TF, Sargent JA: Effect of the hemodialysis prescription on patient morbidity. *N Engl J Med* 305:1176, 1980.
84. Bland L, Alter M, Favero M, Carson L, Cusick L: Hemodialyzer reuse: Practices in the United States and implication for infection control. *Trans Am Soc Artif Int Organs* 31:556, 1985.
85. Sakula A: Formalin asthma in hospital laboratory staff. *Lancet* 2:816, 1975.
86. Porter JAH: Acute respiratory distress following formalin inhalation. *Lancet* 2:603, 1975.
87. Hendrick DJ, Lane DJ: Formalin asthma in hospital staff. *Br Med J* 1:607, 1975.
88. Lewis KJ, Dewar PJ, Ward MK, Kerr DNS: Formation of anti-N-like antibodies in dialysis patients: Effects of different methods of dialyzer rinsing to remove formaldehyde. *Clin Nephrol* 15:39, 1981.
89. Koch KM, Frei U, Fassbinder W: Hemolysis and anemia in anti-N-like antibody positive hemodialysis patients. *Trans Am Soc Artif Intern Organs* 24:709, 1978.
90. Fassbinder W, Koch KM: A specific immunohaemolytic anaemia induced by formaldehyde sterilisation of dialyzers. *Contr Nephrol* 36:51, 1983.
91. Berkseth R, Luehmann D, Mac Micael C, Keshaviah P, Kjellstrand C: Peracetic acid for reuse of hemodialyzers: Clinical studies. *Trans Am Soc Artif Intern Organs* 30:270, 1984.
92. Petersen NJ, Carson LA, Doto IL, Aguero SM, Favero MS: Microbiologic evaluation of a new glutaraldehyde-based disinfectant for hemodialysis systems. *Trans Am Soc Artif Intern Organs* 28:287, 1982.
93. Rancourt M, Senger K, De Oreo P: Cellulosic membrane induced leukopenia after reprocessing with sodium hypochlorite. *Trans Am Soc Artif Intern Organs* 30:49, 1984.
94. Hoenich NA, Johnston SRD, Woffindin C, Kerr DNS: Haemodialysis leukopenia: The role of membrane type and reuse. *Contr Nephrol* 37:120, 1984.
95. Hoenich NA, Kerr DNS, Ward MK, Aljama P, Sussman M: Two special properties of polyamylonitrile membrane — suitability for reuse and biocompatibility. *Contemp Dialysis* 1:31, 1984.
96. Ringoir S, Vanholder R: An introduction to biocompatibility. *Artif Organs* 10:20, 1986.
97. Jacob HS, Craddock PR, Hammerschmidt DE, Moldow CF: Complement induced granulocyte aggregation. An unsuspected mechanism of disease. *N Engl J Med* 302:789, 1980.
98. Craddock PR, Fehr J, Dalmasso AP, Brigham KL, Jacob HS: Hemodialysis leukopenia. Pulmonary vascular leukostasis resulting from complement activation by dialyzer cellophane membranes. *J Clin Invest* 59:879, 1977.
99. Vanholder RC, Pauwels RA, Vandenbogaerde JF, Lamont HH, Van Der Straeten ME, Ringoir SM: Cuprophan reuse and intradialytic changes of lung diffusion capacity and blood gases. *Kidney Int* 32:117, 1987.
100. Fawcett S, Hoenich NA, Woffindin C, Ward MK: Influence of high permeability synthetic membranes on gas exchange and lung function during hemodialysis. *Contr Nephrol* 46:83, 1985.
101. Woffindin C, Hoenich NA, Wilkinson R: Biocompatibility studies on new synthetic membranes. (abstract). *Nephrol Dial Tranpl* 1:108, 1986.
102. Eiser AR: Pulmonary gas exchange during haemodialysis and peritoneal dialysis: Interaction between respiration and metabolism. *Am J Kidney Dis* 6(3):131, 1985.
103. Nissenson AR, Kraut JA, Shinaberger JA: Dialysis associated hypoxemia. Pathogenesis and prevention. *J Am Soc Artif Intern Organs* 7:1, 1984.
104. Mahiout A, Meinhold H, Kessel M, Schulze H, Baurmeister U: Dialyzer membranes: Effect of surface area and chemical modification of cellulose on complement and platelet activation. *Artif Organs* 11:149, 1987.
105. Akizawa T, Kitaoka T, Koshikawa S, Watanabe T, Imamura K, Tsurumi T, Suma Y, Eiga S: Development of a regenerated cellulose non-complement activating membrane for hemodialysis. *Trans Am Soc Artif Intern Organs* 32:76, 1986.
106. Hallgren R, Fjellstrom KE, Hakanson L, Venge P: Kinetic studies of phagocytosis II. The serum-independent uptake of IgG-coated particles by polymorphonuclear leukocytes from uremic patients on regular dialysis treatment. *J Lab Clin Med* 94:277, 1979.
107. Henderson LW, Miller ME, Hamilton RW, Norman ME: Hemodialysis leukopenia and polymorph random mobility — a possible correlation. *J Lab Clin Med* 85:191, 1975.
108. Hakim RM, Breilatt J, Lazarus JM, Port FK: Complement activation and hypersensitivity reactions to dialysis membranes. *N Engl J Med* 311:878, 1984.
109. Rumpf KW, Seubert A, Valentin R, Ippen H, Seubert S, Lowitz HD, Rippe H, Scheler F: Association of ethyleneoxide-induced IgE in dialysis patients. *Lancet* 2:1385, 1985.
110. Chanard J, Brunois JP, Melin JP, Lavaud S, Toupance O: Long-term results of dialysis therapy with a highly permeable membrane. *Artif Organs* 6:261, 1982.
111. Kant KS, Pollak VE, Cathey M, Goetz D, Berlin R: Multiple use of dialyzers: Safety and efficacy. *Kidney Int* 19:728, 1981.
112. Klinkmann H, Wolf H, Schmidt E: Definition of biocompatibility. *Contr Nephrol* 37:70, 1984.
113. Lyman DJ, Knutson K, Mc Neill B, Shibatani K: The effects of chemical structure and surface properties of synthetic polymers on the coagulation of blood. IV. The relation between polymer morphology and protein absorption. *Trans Am Soc Artif Intern Organs* 21:49, 1975.
114. Gasparotto ML, Bertoli M, Vertolli U, Ruffatti A, Stoppa ML, Di Landro D, Romagnoli GF: Biocompatibility of various dialysis membranes as assessed by coagulation assay. *Contr Nephrol* 37:96, 1984.
115. Rylance PB, Gordge MP, Ireland H, Lane DA, Weston MJ: Haemodialysis with prostacyclin (epoprostenol) alone. *Proc Eur Dial Transpl Assoc ERA* 21:281, 1984.
116. Camici M, Evangelisti L: Prostacyclin and heparin during haemodialysis. Comparative effects. *Life Support Systems* 4:205, 1986.

117. Renaud H, Morinière P, Dieval J, Abdull-Massin Z, Dkhissi H, Toutlemonde F, Delobel J, Fournier A: Low molecular weight heparin in haemodialysis and haemofiltration — comparison with unfractioned heparin. *Proc Eur Dial Transpl Assoc ERA* 21:276, 1984.
118. Leong ASY, Disney APS, Gove DW: Spallation and migration of silicone from blood-pump tubing in patients on hemodialysis. *N Engl J Med* 306:135, 1982.
119. Bommer J, Waldherr R, Ritz E: Silicone storage disease in long-term hemodialysis patients. *Contr Nephrol* 36:115, 1983.
120. Bommer J, Gemsa D, Waldherr R, Kessler J, Ritz E: Plastic filing from dialysis tubing induces prostanoid release from macrophages. *Kidney Int* 26:331, 1984.
121. Bommer J, Pernicka E, Kessler J, Ritz E: Reduction of silicone particle release during haemodialysis. *Proc Dur Dial Transpl Assoc ERA* 21:287.
122. Barron D, Harbottle S, Hoenich NA, Morley AR, Appleton D, McCabe JF: Particle spallation induced by blood pumps in hemodialysis tubing sets. *Artif Organs* 10:226, 1986.
123. Morley AR, Barron D, Thompson P, Hoenich NA, Harbottle S, Kerr DNS: Surface alterations in dialysis roller pump inserts: A scanning electron microscopy study. *J Biomed Eng* 8:255, 1986.
124. Kevy S, Jacobson M: Hepatic effects of the leaching of phthalate ester plasticizer and silicon. *Contr Nephrol* 36:82, 1983.
125. Dolovich J, Marshall CP, Smith EKM, Shimizu A, Pearson FC, Sugona MA, Lee W: Allergy to ethylene oxide in chronic hemodialysis patients. *Artif Organs* 8:334, 1984.
126. Marshall C, Shimizu A, Smith EKM, Dolovich J: Ethylene oxide allergy in a dialysis center: Prevalence in hemodialysis and peritoneal dialysis populations. *Clin Nephrol* 21:346, 1984.
127. Ng RCK, Suki WN: Treatment of acute renal failure. In: BM Brenner, JH Stein, eds, *Treatment of Acute Renal Failure*. Churchill Livingstone, New York, pp 229–273, 1980.
128. Delano BG: Regular dialysis treatment (RDT). In: W Drukker, FM Parsons, JF Maher, eds, *Replacement of Renal Function by Dialysis*. Martinus Nijhoff, Boston, pp 391–409, 1983.
129. Bonomini V, Albertazzi A, Vangelista A, Bartolotti GC, Stefoni S, Scolari MP: Residual renal function and effective rehabilitation in chronic dialysis. *Nephron* 16:89, 1976.
130. Kiprov DD: An overview of therapeutic apheresis. *Dial Transpl* 14:195, 1985.
131. Gurland HJ, Lysaght M, Samtleben W: Immunomodulation: Clinical aspects. *Artif Organs* 10:122, 1986.

CHAPTER 55

Use of Drugs in Uremia and Dialysis

D. CRAIG BRATER

INTRODUCTION

A host of drugs are eliminated by the kidney and thereby require dose adjustment in patients with renal insufficiency (1–5). In addition, some drugs that are not themselves dependent upon the kidney for excretion are converted in the liver to active metabolites, which accumulate in patients with diminished renal function (6–7). Examples include N-acetylprocainamide and normeperidine, the metabolites of procainamide and meperidine, respectively, which can accumulate in toxic concentrations in patients with renal insufficiency. To avoid toxicity from either parent drug or active metabolites, the doses of many drugs must be adjusted downward in patients with decreased renal function. The precision required in this dose adjustment is not always great and depends upon the therapeutic index of individual drugs. For example, penicillin and cephalosporin antibiotics have wide margins of safety. Many antibiotics in these classes are administered in smaller doses to patients with severe renal insufficiency, but doing so does not require the same degree of precision as dose adjustment with drugs having narrow therapeutic indices, such as aminoglycoside antibiotics. With the latter, more precise dosing guidelines are followed plus serum concentrations are measured to ensure the attainment of therapeutic and nontoxic levels (8).

In addition to drug accumulation because of compromised elimination pathways, the patient treated with hemodialysis or peritoneal dialysis presents an additional challenge. Drug may be removed by the dialysis procedure itself, thereby requiring compensatory dose supplementation, the extent of which is a function of the amount of drug removed (1). The ability of dialysis to remove drugs is influenced by factors such as the binding of drug to protein, which limits dialyzability, molecular size, etc. These factors are highly variable among drugs, even those in the same chemical class, rendering *a priori* predictions impossible. As a result, one must rely on experimental data in appropriate patient populations to guide therapy.

In this chapter the principles of drug dosing, which will serve as a framework for dosing regimen adjustments in patients with renal insufficiency, will first be discussed. Subsequently, dosing guidelines for patients with various degrees of renal dysfunction, including dialysis, will be offered. The objective of the chapter, then, is to provide both a conceptual framework and specific recommendations for treating such patients.

PRINCIPLES OF DOSE ADJUSTMENT IN PATIENTS WITH RENAL DISEASE

Loading dose

Use of some drugs entails a "loading dose strategy" in which an initial dose larger than the maintenance dose is administered to rapidly attain therapeutic drug concentrations (9–11). This approach is usually employed in therapeutic settings in which an effective drug concentration is needed quickly. As such, examples include the use of lidocaine, digoxin, and aminoglycoside antibiotics. The loading dose needed is a function of the volume of distribution (V_d) of the drug and the target blood concentration to initially be attained ($C_{initial}$):

$$\text{Loading dose} = (C_{initial})(V_d).$$

For example, if the V_d for an aminoglycoside antibiotic is 0.25 l/kg and the desired peak serum concentration is 8 µg/ml (= 8 mg/l), the necessary loading dose can be calculated as follows:

$$\begin{aligned}\text{Loading dose} &= (8\,\text{mg/l})(0.25\,\text{l/kg}) \\ &= 2\,\text{mg/kg}.\end{aligned}$$

It is customary for clinicians to think in terms of the loading dose itself, as opposed to calculating it from V_d and the desired concentration. So doing can be hazardous, particularly in settings where the patient's disease may influence V_d and thereby mandate a change in the loading dose. For example, if the V_d of a drug in a patient with renal insufficiency were one half that of a patient with normal renal function, and the patient with renal disease received a "standard" loading dose, the resulting initial concentration would be twice that expected, with a consequent risk of toxicity. In the previous example, if the "normal" loading dose of 2 mg/kg were administered to a patient whose V_d was 0.125 l/kg (i.e., half the usual value), then a concentration of 16 mg/l would result:

$$2\,\text{mg/kg} = (C_{initial})\,(0.125\,\text{l/kg})$$
$$C_{initial} = 2\,\text{mg/kg} \div 0.125\,\text{l/kg}$$
$$= 16\,\text{mg/l}.$$

If this scenario occurred with an aminoglycoside antibiotic, serious ototoxicity and/or nephrotoxicity could result.

It should be clear from this example that clinicians need to be alert to changes that occur in the V_d of drugs. Table 1 lists drugs in which a change in V_d has been documented in patients with renal disorders. If a loading-dose strategy is used in such patients, the dose to be administered can be calculated as shown previously if the desired concentration is known. Alternatively, if the clinician knows the usual loading dose, the data in the table can be used to calculate a modified dose:

$$\frac{\text{Usual loading dose}}{\text{Modified loading dose}} = \frac{\text{Normal } V_d}{\text{Patient's } V_d}, \text{ or}$$

$$\text{Modified loading dose} = \frac{\text{Patient's } V_d}{\text{Normal } V_d}\,(\text{usual loading dose}).$$

The direct proportionality between loading dose and V_d should make such dose adjustments easy and routine. Unfortunately, the need for altering the loading dose and the method for doing so is often ignored.

Another caution that needs emphasis concerning loading doses and V_d is the influence of changes in drug protein binding. When V_d is determined experimentally in pharmacokinetic studies, it is usually the total concentration of drug in serum that is used as a reference point. For drugs that are highly protein bound, assessing V_d (or other pharmacokinetic parameters) solely in terms of total drug concentrations can be misleading (12). For example, consider a drug that is 90% protein bound and has an initial total serum concentration of 10 mg/l. This value constitutes 9 mg/l of protein-bound drug but only 1 mg/l of unbound, free drug. It is the latter that is able to gain access to tissues and is active. If a loading dose of 100 mg was needed to attain this concentration of drug, one can calculate the V_d for both total and unbound drug:

$$V_d = \frac{\text{Loading dose}}{C_{initial}},$$

$$V_d\,(\text{total}) = \frac{100\,\text{mg}}{10\,\text{mg/l}} = 10\,\text{l},$$

$$V_d\,(\text{free}) = \frac{100\,\text{mg}}{1\,\text{mg/l}} = 100\,\text{l}.$$

In patients with renal insufficiency, many drugs manifest diminished protein binding (13). This is particularly true of acidic drugs bound to serum albumin in which accumulated endogenous organic acids (e.g., hippuric acid) can displace drug from binding sites (14). In the preceeding example, such a scenario could manifest in two different fashions.

For drugs like phenytoin, valproate, and warfarin, all of which are metabolized by the liver, a decrease in binding

Table 1. Drugs for which the volume of distribution is affected by renal disease

Drug	V_d(l/kg) Normal renal function	ESRD
Anesthetics and drugs used during anesthesia		
Thiopental	1.9 (12)	3.0 (12)
Analgesics		
Salicylate	0.15	Increase (no change)
Antiinflammatory agents		
Azapropazone	0.15–0.25	No change (decrease)
Antianxiety agents		
Oxazepam	1.0	Increase (no change)
Anticoagulants, antifibrinolytics and antiplatelet agents		
Sulfinpyrazone	0.06	Increase (no change)
Warfarin	0.14	Increase (no change)
Anticonvulsants		
Phenytoin	0.6	Increase (no change)
Valproate	0.19	Increase (no change)
Antimicrobial agents/ antibacterials		
Cephalosporins		
Cefazolin	0.14	Increase
Cefoxitin	0.27	Increase
Macrolide antibiotics		
Erythromycin	0.78	Increase
Penicillins		
Temocillin	0.15–0.24	Increase (no change)
Antifungals		
Miconazole	21	Decrease
Cardiovascular agents		
Antiarrhythmics		
Disopyramide	0.91	Decrease
Encainide	5.7	Decrease
Blood lipid-lowering agents		
Clofibrate	0.14	Increase (no change)
Cardiac inotropes		
Digitoxin	0.73	Increase (no change)
Digoxin	$V_d = 3.84 + 0.0446\,Cl_{Cr}$	

V_d = volume of distribution; ESRD = end-stage renal disease; Cl_{Cr} = creatinine clearance.
Values in parentheses indicate data for unbound drug.

to albumin might be expected to cause an increase in the unbound concentration and thereby to result in an increased effect. However, the increased free drug is also readily available for metabolism by the liver such that the unbound concentration is no different from patients with normal renal function (12, 13). In other words, using the example outlined above, in patients with normal renal function a total serum concentration of 10 mg/l may yield 1 mg/l of free drug; in contrast, in a patient with end-stage renal disease (ESRD), a total concentration of 5 mg/l may result in the same free concentration:

	Bound	+	Free	=	Total	% Bound
Normal renal function	9	+	1	=	10 mg/l	90%
ESRD	4	+	1	=	5 mg/l	80%

From this information, one can examine the various volumes of distribution that might be calculated:

Normal renal function

$$V_d \text{(total)} = \frac{100 \text{ mg}}{10 \text{ mg/l}} = 10 \text{ l} \qquad V_d \text{(free)} = \frac{100 \text{ mg}}{1 \text{ mg/l}} = 100 \text{ l}$$

ESRD

$$V_d \text{(total)} = \frac{100 \text{ mg}}{5 \text{ mg/l}} = 20 \text{ l} \qquad V_d \text{(free)} = \frac{100 \text{ mg}}{1 \text{ mg/l}} = 100 \text{ l}$$

If one calculated V_d in the patient with ESRD using total drug concentration, the conclusion would be that such patients had twice as great a V_d as subjects with normal renal function (20 l vs. 10 l). If one then used these data to calculate a loading dose in a patient with ESRD, a dose double that in patients with normal renal function would be recommended. However, since it is the free, unbound drug that is pharmacologically active, it is the V_d of this component of the total drug concentration that is therapeutically relevant. As should be apparent, in the example chosen this V_d was the same in both patients, 100 l. Thus, in terms of unbound drug concentration, if the V_d from the total drug concentration were used to guide therapy, and the loading dose were doubled to 200 mg, the free concentration would double to 2 mg/l and might lead to toxicity:

$$C_{\text{initial}} \text{(free)} = \frac{\text{Loading dose}}{V_d} = \frac{200 \text{ mg}}{100 \text{ l}} = 2 \text{ mg/l}.$$

Early studies with phenytoin reported an increase in the V_d in patients with renal insufficiency (13). As our knowledge in this area increased, it became clear that the scenario exemplified above was applicable to phenytoin; namely, decreased protein binding occurred and the free drug concentration, and therefore the V_d of the free drug, was unchanged. Until this was discovered, misleading data led to inappropriate dosing recommendations for phenytoin. Clinicians should be alert to this potential problem in reading the proliferating medical literature dealing with the disposition of drugs in patients with renal diseases. For acidic drugs that are highly protein bound (> 90%), V_d and other pharmacokinetic parameters expressed as total drug concentration may be misleading and the reader should search for data concerning unbound drug concentrations.

Another misleading scenario can also occur that is the converse of that discussed above. In the preceeding example, V_d calculated from total serum concentrations led to a misleading conclusion that a modification of the loading dose was needed. With some drugs (e.g., naproxen) the V_d for the total drug appears normal (implying no change in loading dose), whereas the V_d for the free drug is altered, mandating a change (15).

For example, this situation might occur if a drug is displaced from protein binding but the increased free drug concentration is not eliminated and remains elevated:

	Bound	+	Free	=	Total	% Bound
Normal renal function	9	+	1	=	10 mg/l	90%
ESRD	8	+	2	=	10 mg/l	80%

Note, that the percent binding in patients with ESRD is identical to that in the previous example, 80%. However, in this example the free drug concentration is doubled to 2 mg/l. Again, one can calculate the V_d's for both the total and unbound drug:

Normal renal function

$$V_d \text{(total)} = \frac{100 \text{ mg}}{10 \text{ mg/l}} = 10 \text{ l} \qquad V_d \text{(free)} = \frac{100 \text{ mg}}{1 \text{ mg/l}} = 100 \text{ l}$$

ESRD

$$V_d \text{(total)} = \frac{100 \text{ mg}}{10 \text{ mg/l}} = 10 \text{ l} \qquad V_d \text{(free)} = \frac{100 \text{ mg}}{2 \text{ mg/l}} = 50 \text{ l}$$

The misleading conclusion in this setting from values related to the total drug concentration would be that no change in the loading dose is indicated. In contrast, if assessed as free concentration, it is apparent that the V_d in patients with ESRD is half that in patients with normal renal function. If the loading dose given to the patient with ESRD were not decreased proportionally, then an elevated free drug concentration could result, with the possibility of toxicity.

These examples are meant to emphasize the importance of the assessment of V_d (and other pharmacokinetic parameters) in terms of the free drug concentration. It should be clear that basing conclusions as to the loading dose adjustment on the total drug concentration can be misleading, sometimes erroneously assuming no change is needed and, with other drugs, incorrectly assuming that a modified loading dose is needed. When pertinent data on free drug concentrations are available, they have been used in Table 1. Unfortunately for many drugs, the experimental design of studies has been flawed and free drug concentrations have not been measured. In this setting, the clinician must be aware of the potential pitfalls illustrated above. Realizing these problems inherent in the extant data should result in cautious dosing and close assessment of the patient.

Maintenance dose

As the name implies, a maintenance dose is administered to maintain the desired drug concentrations at steady state (9-11). It is determined by the desired average steady-state drug concentration, $C_{average}$, and the elimination rate of the drug from the body, clearance (Cl):

Maintenance dose = $(C_{average})$ (Cl).

Note the similarity between this relationship and that for loading dose. This relationship is easy to derive and is a function of the definition of steady state; namely, at steady state, the rate of drug entering the body must equal the rate of removal. In turn,

Rate in = Administration rate = maintenance dosing-rate,

and

Rate out = $(C_{average})$ (Cl).

Administration of drugs by different routes affects the above relationship. For example, if a drug is administered as a continuous intravenous infusion, the maintenance dosing rate is the infusion rate of the drug. If a drug is administered as separate, intermittent doses, the dosing rate is the individual dose divided by the dosing interval. Lastly, if a drug is administered by mouth, one must incorporate a term that accounts for incomplete bioavailability, the fraction of the dose absorbed (F). In this circumstance the maintenance dosing rate becomes:

(F) (individual dose)/Dosing interval.

Hence, depending on the route of administration, any of the following relationships may apply:

Infusion rate = $(C_{average})$ (Cl),
Dose/dosing interval = $(C_{average})$ (Cl),
F × dose/dosing interval = $(C_{average})$ (Cl).

It should be apparent from these relationships that a change in clearance mandates a proportional change in the rate of drug administration if the average drug concentration is to remain the same. In patients with renal insufficiency, the clearance of drugs is often diminished and, consequently, maintenance doses must be adjusted.

In a subsequent section, specific guidelines will be offered for maintenance doses of a variety of drugs; these recommendations derive from studies that quantify the effect of renal insufficiency on the clearance of these drugs.

When analyzing published literature concerning the clearance of a drug and whether or not a clinical condition mandates a change in the maintenance dose, the caveats discussed in detail previously concerning the influence of protein binding on V_d are also applicable to clearance (12, 13). Hence, if changes in binding occur, clearance calculations based on the total drug concentration can be misleading and one should seek data relevant to the unbound drug. The recommendations that follow are based on free drug concentrations when data are available; unfortunately, for many drugs this information does not exist.

Half-life

The half-life ($t_{1/2}$) of a drug refers to the time required for the serum concentration to decrease by one half. The rate of elimination of most drugs (the exceptions being phenytoin and salicylates) is independent of the drug serum concentration and is referred to as being *linear*. This also means that the $t_{1/2}$ is independent of the serum concentration, and as such the time for a drug's concentration to decrease from 100 to 50 units of concentration is the same as it takes to decrease from 10 to 5 units.

Many clinicians use $t_{1/2}$ synonymously with clearance of a drug. As such, they presume that an increase in $t_{1/2}$ indicates a decrease in clearance and thereby requires a compensatory decrease in the maintenance dose. This popular misconception can lead to errors in dose adjustment in patients with renal insufficiency. As opposed to being a reflection of the clearance of a drug $t_{1/2}$ is a function of both V_d and Cl (9-11):

$$t_{1/2} = 0.693 \, V_d/Cl.$$

Hence, a change in $t_{1/2}$ can reflect either a change in V_d, a change in Cl, or a change in both. The correct dosing regimen adjustment that must be made depends on whether an alteration in V_d or Cl is responsible for the change in $t_{1/2}$. If $t_{1/2}$ increases solely because of an increase in V_d, the loading dose should be increased while the maintenance dose should remain unchanged. In this example, if one incorrectly assumed that $t_{1/2}$ increased because Cl decreased, and therefore administered a "normal" loading dose and a diminished maintenance dose, the result would be that the too-small loading dose would not attain the desired initial concentration and the inappropriately diminished maintenance dose would maintain a lower drug concentration than desired. The result could be lack of efficacy.

A good example of this potential scenario is digoxin in patients with renal insufficiency. In patients with mild-to-moderate renal insufficiency, the V_d of digoxin is approximately the same as in patients with normal renal function, while Cl may be about one half to two thirds of normal (16). In such patients, the $t_{1/2}$ is prolonged inversely propor-

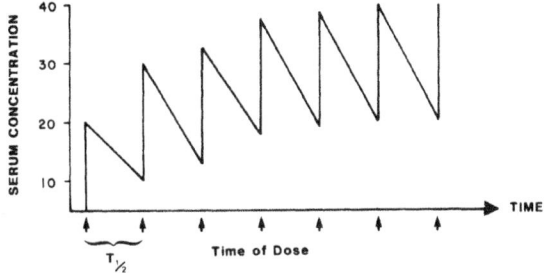

Figure 1. Schematic illustration that four to five times the half-life ($t_{1/2}$) are needed to reach steady state serum concentrations of a drug. Arrows represent the time of dosing, and the drug is administered every $t_{1/2}$.

tional to the diminished Cl. In patients with severe renal insufficiency, however, V_d is decreased to one-half to two-thirds normal and Cl is decreased even more, to about one-third normal (16, 17). In this setting, $t_{1/2}$ is influenced by both parameters, and, though it would be prolonged compared to patients with normal renal function, it may be little different than in the patient with mild-to-moderate renal insufficiency. In the patient with severe renal insufficiency, if the change in $t_{1/2}$ were erroneously presumed to quantitatively reflect the decrease in digoxin clearance and thereby the maintenance dose, a serious dosing error would occur. Since no downward adjustment in the loading dose would be made, the initial concentration would be higher than desired; in addition, the needed decrease in the maintenance dose would be underestimated so that the patient's steady state serum concentration would be maintained at a higher concentration. The hazards of such an error are obvious.

One must realize the limitations of using $t_{1/2}$ to predict needed dosing adjustments, and instead one must dissect it into its component parts of V_d and Cl. Of what use, then, is $t_{1/2}$? Knowing $t_{1/2}$ allows one to determine the time necessary for serum drug concentrations to reach steady state. As illustrated in Figure 1, steady state is reached after administering a drug for four to five times the $t_{1/2}$. If the clinician is starting drug therapy, this delay in attaining plateau drug concentrations can be avoided by giving a loading dose designed to attain the desired drug concentration quickly; this concentration can then be maintained. It is important to remember that the concept of attainment of steady state applies to any change in dose, not just starting therapy. For example, if a maintenance dose is doubled, four to five times the $t_{1/2}$ is required for the serum concentration to reach the new plateau. Similarly, if the maintenance dose is decreased, four to five times the $t_{1/2}$ must elapse for the new, lower steady state concentration to be reached. Lastly, if the drug is stopped altogether, four to five times the $t_{1/2}$ are needed for concentrations to become negligible.

In summary, the half-life should be used to predict the time necessary for a drug to reach steady state concentrations. It is a hybrid value influenced by both V_d and Cl, and as such provides no direct information about the loading or maintenance dose.

Dosing regimens

When renal dysfunction dictates a need to modify the dosing regimen, several options are available. Changes in the loading dose simply entail giving a larger or smaller dose, depending on whether V_d is increased or decreased. It must be emphasized that one is often uncertain as to the need to modify a loading dose. In such cases one should first decide whether or not a loading-dose strategy is actually necessary. If so, one should err on the side of caution and administer a smaller loading dose than usual. If monitoring of clinical end points and/or serum drug concentrations shows the dose to have been too low, a supplementary dose can be given. In contrast, if too large a dose is administered, the clinician may be faced with iatrogenic drug toxicity and the need for remedial measures until the drug concentration diminishes.

For adjusting maintenance doses of a drug, several strategies can be employed. The primary objective is to maintain the same average drug concentration as would occur if the patient did not have renal disease. Because the vast majority of drugs obey linear or first-order elimination kinetics, a change in clearance can be compensated by a proportional change in the dosing rate:

$$\frac{\text{Usual maintenance dose}}{\text{Modified maintenance dose}} = \frac{\text{Usual clearance}}{\text{Patient's clearance}},$$

or

$$\text{Modified maintenance dose} = \frac{\text{Patient's clearance}}{\text{Usual clearance}} (\text{usual maintenance dose}).$$

Hence, if the clearance of a drug in a patient with renal insufficiency is one-half the "normal" value, then the patient's maintenance dose should be one-half that usually administered. Such dose modifications will maintain average steady state drug concentration of the same level in patients with renal disease as in those with normal renal function.

If a patient is receiving a drug by continuous intravenous infusion, a maintenance dose modification simply requires a modified infusion rate. If, however, the patient is receiving intermittent doses, reduction of the total dose being administered can be accomplished in three different fashions:

1. Decreasing each individual dose and maintaining the same dosing frequency, which is often referred to as the *variable dose method*.
2. Maintaining the same individual dose but administering each dose less frequently, which is called the *variable frequency* (or *interval*) *method*.
3. Modifying both individual doses and the frequency of their administration, which is a *combination method*.

All three methods attain the same average drug concentration. For example, if a drug is administered to a patient with normal renal function as 500 mg every 12 hours and

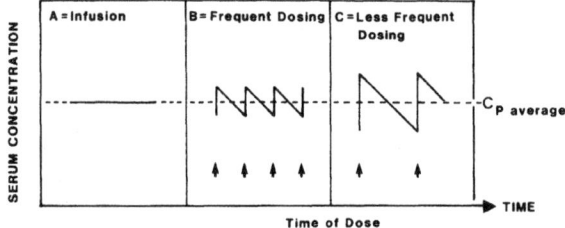

Figure 2. Illustration of three different dosing regimens in all of which the total amount of drug administered is the same so that the average drug concentration, C_p average, is identical. The regimen with the least frequent administration of large doses results in the greatest difference between the peak and trough concentrations.

one wished to administer half as much drug to a patient with renal insufficiency, viable options according to the above include:
1. 250 mg every 12 hours
2. 500 mg every 24 hours
3. 375 mg every 18 hours

Over a course of therapy, the total amount of drug administered with each of these regimens is the same, and it is half that in the patient with normal renal function. These regimens differ, however, in the profile of the serum drug concentrations. Regimens with closer dosing frequencies and smaller individual doses result in less difference between peak and trough drug concentrations (Figure 2).

Which of these options is best to employ is unclear. For aminoglycoside antibiotics, an extensive literature has evolved with derivation of numerous dosing nomograms employing all three options (18, 19). As is apparent from Figure 2, modifying only the individual dose and maintaining the same frequency results in lower peak and higher trough concentrations than alternative methods. With aminoglycosides, in particular, the elevated trough concentration may increase the risk of toxicity, while in some patients the peak may be so low as to be subtherapeutic. In contrast, regimens that diminish the total dose of a drug solely by decreasing the frequency of administration (increasing the dosing interval) may result in long periods of time with subtherapeutic serum drug concentrations. For these reasons, I recommend a combination approach to dose adjustment. For aminoglycosides, for example, the method of Hull and Sarubbi seems best (20). They suggest that a variable frequency method be used with these antibiotics, with the limitation that the dosing interval never be longer than 24 hours. When this point is reached, they suggest switching to a variable dose method; hence, in patients with severe renal insufficiency the dosing interval would be 24 hours and individual doses would also be smaller than usual.

There is no general rule that can be applied in terms of the maximum length of a dosing interval. Twenty-four hours seems a reasonable rule of thumb. Clinicians should realize the different options available and try to collate these options with individual therapeutic settings. For example, if a patient is not responding to a drug, the clinician should realize that a possible explanation is an inappropriate dosing regimen. Similarly, signs of toxicity shortly after administration of an individual dose may indicate the need to give a drug more frequently in smaller doses. Simply realizing the possibilities can help tailor therapy to individual patients, whereas their ignorance can lead to inadequate therapeutics.

Dialysis

Patients with end-stage renal disease treated with hemodialysis or chronic ambulatory peritoneal dialysis (CAPD) have a unique additional mechanism by which drugs can be eliminated from the body (21, 22). If substantial elimination by these routes occurs, the dosing regimen must be modified. In patients maintained on hemodialysis, this is most easily accomplished by administering a supplemental dose of drug at the completion of the dialysis session. The dose given is the amount of drug removed during the hemodialysis procedure. With CAPD there is a more or less continual process of drug removal. In this setting the patient's total clearance of a drug equals clearance relative to the patient's residual level of renal function plus clearance via CAPD. One simply adjusts the dosing regimen (either individual dose, dosing interval, or both) upwards in proportion to the added increment in clearance from CAPD.

It is not infrequent for clinicians to encounter a setting where they are administering a drug to a patient receiving dialysis and are unable to find any information about dialytic removal of the agent. In this setting, one can often gain insight into the dialyzability of a drug by examining some of its pharmacokinetic parameters. One limitation to removal by dialysis is molecular size. If a drug is too large to pass across the dialysis membrane (including the peritoneum), it will not be removed by dialysis. This consideration, for example, applies to vancomycin and amphotericin. Drugs that are highly bound to serum proteins have restricted access to the dialysis membrane, since only free, unbound drug can cross this barrier. Hence if a drug is bound in excess of 90%, it is unlikely that dialysis will contribute appreciably to its elimination. Drugs that are water soluble are more readily dialyzed; in turn, a clue that a drug is water soluble is the fact that these drugs are usually eliminated predominantly by the kidneys as unchanged drug. Lastly, drugs with large volumes of distribution have minimal dialyzability. Conceptually, one can think of such drugs in terms of having only a small portion in the vascular space and a predominant portion in peripheral tissues. The drug in the vascular space can be removed, but once dialysis ends, the large amount of drug in the tissues can refill the vascular compartment and the dialysis procedure thereby removes only an insignificant quantity of the total amount of drug in the body.

Specific examples can be used to illustrate these principles. Aminoglycoside antibiotics are water soluble and are eliminated primarily by the kidney (fraction of dose excreted unchanged is approximately 100%), they have negligible protein binding, and they have small volumes of distribution (0.25 l/kg). These drugs are removed by dialysis procedures in sufficient quantities to require dose supplementation. In contrast, cefonicid has a small V_d (0.10 l/kg) but is highly bound to serum proteins (98%) and thereby is not removed by hemodialysis or CAPD. Cefadroxil, on the other hand, though having a somewhat larger V_d than cefonicid (0.30 l/kg), is only 16% bound to serum proteins. Hemodialysis is sufficient with this cephalosporin to require a supplemental dose. Lastly, drugs such as phenothiazines and tricyclic antidepressants that have very large V_d's (> 10 l/kg) are not eliminated by dialysis, even if they are negligibly bound to serum proteins.

Gwilt and Perrier have examined the relationship between dialyzability, protein binding, and V_d in detail (23) and have quantified the general relationships discussed above. If the percent of free drug in serum divided by V_d (expressed in l/kg) is greater than 80, 6 hours of hemodialysis will in general remove 20–50% of the body burden of the drug and thereby will require a supplemental dose at the end of the procedure. In contrast, if this ratio is less than 20, in general less than 10% of a drug will be removed and no supplemental dosing would be necessary. As with any generalization, there are exceptions to the above concepts; however, when specific information concerning removal by dialysis is lacking, these guidelines can be used as a starting point for therapeutic decisions, with further refinements based on clinical end points and/or measured serum drug concentrations.

Table 2 lists the amount of a drug removed by dialysis (as percent of a "normal" dose in a patient with normal renal function). This value allows calculation of the increment in dosing that must be given to compensate for removal by dialysis. The table does not include removal of drugs by hemoperfusion, hemofiltration, or hemodiafiltration. Hemoperfusion is applicable to toxicologic settings and is outside the scope of this chapter. Insufficient data are available for newer dialysis techniques to offer guidelines for dose adjustment.

Active metabolites

As noted in the introductory comments, even though many drugs are not themselves eliminated by renal routes, they are converted by the liver to active metabolites that depend on the kidney for excretion. Hence, in patients with renal disease, the metabolite can accumulate, causing its own pharmacologic effect(s) (6, 7). For example, meperidine is converted to normeperidine, which is not an analgesic like the parent drug, but rather is a central nervous system stimulant. It is excreted by the kidney and accumulates in patients with renal insufficiency. Even in elderly patients with mild decrements in renal function, this metabolite can reach sufficient concentrations to cause seizures. It use in patients with renal compromise requires lower doses of meperidine (which may limit its efficacy). A better alternative is to use another analgesic, such as morphine, for which the parent drug does not depend on the kidney for elimination and the metabolite is not active.

Procainamide is another good example of the difficulties engendered in constructing dosing regimens when an active metabolite is formed. Procainamide itself is metabolized by the liver to N-acetylprocainamide (NAPA), a drug with a different spectrum of antiarrhythmic effect than procainamide. In patients with normal renal function, procainamide concentrations exceed those of NAPA, and the latter has negligible pharmacologic effects. As such, dosing regimens are aimed at maintaining therapeutic concentrations of the parent drug. In patients with renal insufficiency, NAPA accumulates and patients often have NAPA concentrations exceeding those of procainamide. In this circumstance, the patient essentially has circulating pharmacologic (and perhaps toxic) concentrations of two different antiarrhythmics. Designing a dosing regimen that will precisely maintain desired concentrations of each is virtually impossible. Hence, therapy can be hazardous and alternative drugs should be sought.

Table 3 lists drugs that are converted to active metabolites, which in turn are eliminated by the kidney. It is important to emphasize that numerous other drugs are metabolized to active compounds that are eliminated by other routes (e.g., many benzodiazepines), and thus there is no need for dose adjustment of these drugs in patients with renal disease. For those drugs listed in Table 3, the degree of accumulation of the active metabolite is difficult to predict, and therefore precise dosing guidelines are not possible. If these drugs are used in patients with renal insufficiency, caution is mandatory and the clinical end points of the drug and metabolite effect must be monitored closely. Whenever possible, it would seem prudent to use alternative therapeutic agents.

DOSING RECOMMENDATIONS IN PATIENTS WITH VARIOUS DEGREES OF RENAL INSUFFICIENCY

When renal insufficiency affects the volume of distribution of a drug (as previously listed in Table 1 and discussed above), the loading dose must be modified. More commonly, one needs to compensate for decreased clearance of drugs by adjusting the maintenance dose. Principles for doing so have been discussed previously, the single most important of which is the proportionality that exists between the clearance, dose, and steady state serum drug concentration. Hence, a clearance that is half normal can be compensated for by decreasing the dose by one half. Different strategies for dose adjustment have also been discussed, and the clinician can change each individual dose, the interval between them, or both. Which strategy to use depends on the drug and the individual patient, but a reasonable starting point for most drugs is to first lengthen the interval until a maximum of 24 hours is reached, after which further modification of the individual dose is appropriate.

Table 4 offers recommendations for modification of the maintenance dose in patients with various degrees of renal

Table 2. Dialyzability of drugs: Percent of a normal dose removed by one session of hemodialysis or 24 hours of CAPD

Drug	Hemodialysis	CAPD
Anesthetics and drugs used during anesthesia		
Gallamine	Considerable	Considerable
Analgesics		
Meperidine	Negligible	Negligible
Methadone	Negligible (< 1%)	Negligible (< 1%)
Propoxyphene	Negligible	Negligible
Salicylates	Negligible Considerable in overdose settings	Negligible
Antiinflammatory agents		
Azapropazone	Negligible	Negligible
Oxaprozin	Negligible	Negligible
Antianxiety agents, sedatives, and hypnotics		
Buspirone	Negligible	
Chloral hydrate	Negligible	
Ethchlorvynol	Negligible	
Glutethimide	Negligible	
Meprobamate	Negligible	
Methaqualone	Negligible	
Oxazepam	Negligible	
Phenobarbital	Negligible	
Zopiclone	Negligible	
Anticholinergics and cholinergics		
Metoclopramide	Negligible	
Pirenzipine	11–15%	
Anticoagulants, antifibrinolytics and antiplatelet agents		
Warfarin	Negligible	Negligible
Anticonvulsants		
Phenytoin	Negligible	Negligible
Primidone	30%	
Valproic acid	4%	Negligible
Antideoressants, antipsychotics, and antimaniacals		
Lithium	Considerable	Considerable
Antihistamines		
Cimetidine	10–20%	Negligible
Famotidine	Negligible	
Ranitidine	50–60%	
Antimicrobial agents/ antibacterials		
Aminoglycosides	50%	20–25%
Spectinomycin	50%	
Carbapenems		
Imipenem	80–90%	
Cephalosporins		
Cefaclor	33%	
Cefadroxil	> 50%	
Cefamandole	> 50%	5%
Cefazolin	50%	20%
Cefixime	Negligible (1.6%)	Negligible
Cefmenoxime		Negligible (< 10%)

Table 2. (Con't)

Drug	Hemodialysis	CAPD
Cefonicid	Negligible	Negligible (6.5%)
Cefoperazone	Negligible	Negligible
Ceforanide	20%	
Cefotaxime	60%	Negligible (5%)
Cefotetan	Negligible (5–9%)	
Cefoxitin	> 50%	Negligible
Cefroxadine	> 50%	
Cefsulodin	60%	
Ceftazidime	50%	Negligible
Ceftizoxime	50%	Negligible
Ceftriaxone		Negligible (4–5%)
Cefuroxime		20%
Cephacetrile	> 50%	
Cephalexin	> 50%	Negligible
Cephaloridine	> 50%	
Cephalothin	50%	
Cephapirin	20%	
Macrolide antibiotics		
Clindamycin	Negligible	Negligible
Lincomycin	Negligible	Negligible
Monobactams		
Aztreonam	40%	Negligible
Moxalactam	30–50%	Negligible (15–20%)
Penicillins		
Amdinocillin	32–70%	Negligible (< 4%)
Amoxicillin	30%	
Ampicillin	40%	
Azlocillin	30–45%	
Carbenicillin	50%	
Cloxacillin	Negligible	
Dicloxacillin	Negligible	
Mecillinam	50%	
Methicillin	Negligible	
Mezlocillin	20–25%	Negligible
Nafcillin	Negligible	
Oxacillin	Negligible	
Penicillin	> 50%	
Piperacillin	50%	
Temocillin	50%	
Ticarcillin	50%	Negligible
Polymyxins		
Colistin	Negligible	Negligible
Quinolones		
Ciprofloxacin	Negligible (2%)	Negligible (0.4–1.6%)
Norfloxacin	Negligible	
Sulfonamides		
Sulfamethoxazole	50%	Negligible (8%)
Trimethoprim	50%	Negligible (7%)
Tetracyclines		
Doxycycline	Negligible	
Vancomycin	Negligible	Negligible (15–20%)
Antifungals		
Amphotericin B	Negligible	
Flucytosine	50%	
Ketoconazole		Negligible
Miconazole	Negligible	Negligible
Antimalarials		
Chloroquine	Negligible	
Quinine	Negligible	

Table 2. (Con't)

Drug	Hemodialysis	CAPD
Antiparasitics and antihelmintics		
Metronidazole	25–50%	Negligible
Ornidazole	50%	Negligible
Tinidazole	40%	
Antituberculous agents		
Paraaminosalicylic acid	>50%	
Ethambutol	33–50%	
Isoniazid	75%	
Antiviral agents		
Acyclovir	60%	
Amantadine	Negligible	
Antineoplastics and antimetabolites		
Cyclophosphamide	30–60%	
Etoposide	Negligible	
Methotrexate	Negligible	
Antiulcer agents and antacids		
Omeprazole	Negligible	
Bronchodilators		
Dyphylline	28%	
Theophylline	40%	
Cardiovascular agents		
Antianginal agents		
Nifedipine	Negligible (<1%)	Negligible
Antiarrhythmics		
N-acetylprocainamide	50%	Negligible
Amiodarone	Negligible	
Bretylium	Negligible	
Disopyramide	Negligible (2–4%)	
Flecainide	Negligible (1%)	
Lorcainide	Negligible (8–12%)	
Mexiletine	Negligible	Negligible
Procainamide	Negligible	Negligible
Tocainide	25%	
Antihypertensives		
Acebutolol	Negligible	
Atenolol	50%	
Captopril	35–40%	
Clonidine	Negligible	
Diazoxide	Negligible	
Doxazosin	Negligible	
Enalapril	50%	
Guanfacine	Negligible	
Labetalol	Negligible (2.5%)	Negligible (0.14%)
Metoprolol	Negligible	
Minoxidil	24–43%	
Nadolol	50%	
Sotalol	40%	
Cardiac inotropes		
Digoxin	Negligible	Negligible
Hypouricemic agents		
Allopurinol	40%	
Steroids		
Prednisone	Negligible	
Miscellaneous		
Cyclosporine	Negligible	

Table 3. Drugs with active metabolites dependent on the kidney for elimination

Drug	Active metabolite	Drug	Active metabolite
Anesthetics and drugs used during anesthesia		Antineoplastics and antimetabolites	
Pancuronium	3-OH pancuronium	Cyclophosphamide	4-Hydroxycyclophosphamide Aldophosphamide
Analgesics		Antispasticity agents	
Meperidine	Normeperidine	Dantrolene	Hydroxy and amino metabolites
Propoxyphene	Norpropoxyphene	Cardiovascular agents	
Anticoagulants, antifibrinolytics and antiplatelet agents		Antiarrhythmics	
		Disopyramide	Mono-N-desisopropyl-disopyramide (MND)
Sulfinpyrazone	Thioether metabolite	Encainide	O-desmethylencainide (ODE) 3-methoxy-ODE (MODE)
Anticonvulsants		Flecainide	Meta-O-dealkylflecainide
Primidone	Phenylethylmalonamide	Procainamide	N-acetylprocainamide (NAPA)
Antihistamines		Antihypertensives	
		Acebutolol	N-acetalacebutolol (diacetolol)
Climetidine	Cimetidine sulfoxide	Captopril	Mixed disulfides with endogenous thiols
Antimicrobial agents/antibacterials		Enalapril	Enalaprilat
		Methyldopa	Methyldopamine
Cephalosporins		Metoprolol	α-hydroxymetoprolol
Cefotaxime	Desacetylcefotaxime	Nitroprusside	Thiocyanate
Cefoxitin	Decarbamoylcefoxitin	Blood-lipid lowering agents	
Cephalothin	Desacetylcephalothin	Clofibrate	Parachlorophenoxyisobutyric acid (CPIB)
Cephapirin	Desacetylcephapirin		
Quinolones		Cardiac inotropes	
Ciprofloxacin	Three different metabolites	Digitoxin	Digoxin
Enoxacin	Oxoenoxacin	Diuretics	
Norfloxacin	Six different metabolites	Triamterene	Sulfuric ester of hydroxytriamterene
Pefloxacin	N-desmethylpefloxacin		
Sulfonamides		Hypoglycemic agents	
Sulfamethoxazole	Acetyl metabolite	Acetohexamide	Hydroxyhexamide
Sulfisoxazole	Acetyl metabolite	Tolbutamide	Hydroxytolbutamide Carboxytolbutamide
Antiparasitics and antihelmintics		Hypouricemic agents	
Metronidazole	Hydroxymetabolite	Allopurinol	Oxipurinol

Table 4. Dosing recommendations in patients with renal insufficiency (relative to normal dose)

Drug	Creatinine Clearance (ml/min)			Drug	Creatinine Clearance (ml/min)		
	>50	20–50	<20		>50	20–5	<20
Antesthetics and drugs used during anesthesia				Anticoagulants, antifibrinolytics, and antiplatelet agents			
Alcuronium			1/3	Tranexamic acid	1/2	1/4	1/8
Gallamine			1/8				
Metocurine			1/2	Antihistamines			
Pancuronium			1/5	Cimetidine		1/2	1/6
D-tubocurarine			1/2	Famotidine			1/3
				Ranitidine	1/2	1/3	1/4
Antiinflammatory agents							
Azapropazone	1/2	1/5	1/10	Antimicrobial agents/antibacterials			
Anticholinergics and cholinergics							
Metoclopramide		1/2	1/4	Aminoglycosides	1/3	1/2	1/4
Neostigmine		1/2	1/3	Carbapenems			
Pyridostigmine	1/2	1/3	1/5	Imipenem		1/2	1/4

Table 4. (Con't)

Drug	Creatinine Clearance (ml/min) > 50	20–50	< 20	Drug	Creatinine Clearance (ml/min) > 50	20–5	< 20
Cephalosporins				Sulfisoxazole	3/4	1/2	1/4
Cefaclor		1/2	1/4	Trimethoprim			1/2
Cefadroxil	1/2	1/4	1/8	Tetracyclines			
Cefamandole	1/2	1/3	1/4	Tetracycline		1/3	1/10
Cefazolin	1/2	1/4	1/6	Vancomycin	2/3	1/2	1/10
Cefixime		1/2	1/3	Antifungals			
Cefmenoxime	1/2	1/4	1/6	Flucytosine	1/2	1/3	1/4
Cefonicid	1/2	1/5	1/10	Miconazole			1/3
Ceforanide	1/2	1/3	1/5	Antituberculous agents			
Cefotaxime		1/2	1/4	Ethambutol		1/2	1/3
Cefotetan	1/2	1/4	1/10	Isoniazid			1/2
Cefoxitin	1/2	1/4	1/6	Antiviral agents			
Cefroxadine		1/2	1/4	Acyclovir		1/2	1/5
Cefsulodin	1/2	1/4	1/10	Amantadine	1/2	1/5	1/10
Ceftazidime	1/2	1/5	1/10	Cardiovascular agents			
Ceftizoxime	1/2	1/4	1/10	Antiarrhythmics			
Cefuroxime		1/2	1/4	N-acetylprocainamide (NAPA)		1/2	1/4
Cephacetrile	1/2	1/4	1/10	Bretylium			1/5
Cephalexin		1/3	1/10	Cibenzoline		1/2	1/3
Cephalothin	2/3	1/2	1/6	Disopyramide		1/2	1/5
Cephapirin		1/2	1/3	Encainide		1/2	1/4
Cephradine		1/3	1/10	Flecainide			1/3
Chloramphenicol and thiamphenicol				Procainamide		(see NAPA)	
Thiamphenicol	1/2	1/3	1/10	Tocainide		3/4	1/2
Macrolide antibiotics				Antihypertensives			
Lincomycin		1/2	1/3	Acebutolol		1/2	1/3
Monobactams				Atenolol		1/2	1/4
Aztreonam	1/2	1/3	1/4	Betaxolol			1/2
Carumonam	2/3	1/3	1/6	Captopril	1/2	1/6	1/12
Moxalactam	1/2	1/3	1/10	Carteolol		1/2	1/4
Penicillins				Clonidine		1/2	1/3
Amdinocillin		1/2	1/4	Diazoxide		2/3	1/2
Amoxicillin		1/2	1/6	Enalapril		1/3	1/5
Ampicillin	1/2	1/4	1/10	Methyldopa			1/2
Azlocillin		1/2	1/4	Metoprolol			1/2
Carbenicillin	1/3	1/5	1/10	Nadolol	3/4	1/2	1/4
Mecillinam		1/2	1/4	Sotalol		1/3	1/8
Methicilin		1/2	1/4	Blood lipid-lowering agents			
Mezlocillin	1/2	1/4	1/8	Bezafibrate	2/3	1/3	1/6
Penicillin		1/5	1/8	Clofibrate	1/2	1/4	1/10
Piperacillin		1/2	1/3	Cardiac inotropes			
Temocillin		1/2	1/4	Digoxin	1/2	1/3	1/5
Ticarcillin	1/2	1/3	1/4	Hypouricemic agents			
Polymyxins				Allopurinol	2/3	1/3	1/6
Colistin	1/2	1/3	1/6	Colchicine			1/2
Quinolones				Miscellaneous			
Ciprofloxacin			1/2	Dextran 40			1/4
Enoxacin	1/2	1/3	1/4	EDTA		1/2	1/4
Norfloxacin			1/2				
Ofloxacin			1/2				
Sulfonamides							
Sulfamethoxazole			1/2				

insufficiency. It must be emphasized that these guidelines should serve only as starting points of therapy. Subsequent dosing requires tailoring the regimen to each individual patient, which in turn must be based on the clinical end points for all drugs and measurement of serum concentrations for drugs with narrow therapeutic indices.

REFERENCES

1. Brater DC: *Pocket Manual of Drug Use in Clinical Medicine*, 4th ed. BC Decker, Toronto, 1990.
2. Brater DC: The pharmacological role of the kidney. *Drugs* 19:31–48, 1980.
3. Bjornsson TD: Nomogram for drug dosage adjustment in patients with renal failure. *Clin Pharmacokinet* 11:164–170, 1986.
4. Bennett WM, Muther RS, Parker RA, Feig P, Morrison G, Golper TA, Singer I: Drug therapy in renal failure: Dosing guidelines for adults, Part I: Antimicrobial agents, analgesics. *Ann Intern Med* 93:62–89, 1980.
5. Bennett WM, Muther RS, Parker RA, Feig P, Morrison G, Golper TA, Winger I: Drug therapy in renal failure: Dosing guidelines for adults. Part II: Sedatives, hypnotics, and tranquilizers; cardiovascular, antihypertensive, and diuretic agents; miscellaneous agents. *Ann Intern Med* 93:286–325, 1980.
6. Drayer DE: Pharmacologically active drug metabolites: Therapeutic and toxic activities, plasma and urine data in man, accumulation in renal failure. *Clin Pharmacokinet* 1:426–443, 1976.
7. Verbeeck RK, Branch RA, Wilkinson GR: Drug metabolites in renal failure: Pharmacokinetic and clinical implications. *Clin Pharmacokinet* 6:329–345, 1981.
8. Koch-Weser J: Serum drug concentrations as therapeutic guides. *N Engl J Med* 287:227–231, 1972.
9. Grenblatt DJ, Koch-Weser J: Clinical pharmacokinetics. *N Engl J Med* 293:702–705, 964–970, 1975.
10. Gibaldi M, Levy G: Pharmacokinetics in clinical practice. I. Concepts. *JAMA* 235:1864–1867, 1976.
11. Gibaldi M, Levy G: Pharmacokinetics in clinical practice. 2. Applications. *JAMA* 235:1867–1872, 1976.
12. Oie S: Drug distribution and binding. *J Clin Pharmacol* 26:583–586, 1986.
13. Reidenberg MM, Drayer DE: Alteration of drug-protein binding in renal disease. *Clin Pharmacokinet* 9 (Suppl l):18–26, 1984.
14. Gulyassy PF, Bottini AT, Stanfel LA, Jarrard EA, Depner TA: Isolation and chemical identification of inhibitors of plasma ligand binding. *Kidney Int* 30:391–398, 1986.
15. Anttila M, Haataja M, Kasanen A: Pharmacokinetics of naproxen in subjects with normal and impaired renal function. *Eur J Clin Pharmacol* 18:263–268, 1980.
16. Sheiner LB, Rosenberg BG, Marathe VV: Estimation of population characteristics of pharmacokinetic parameters from routine clinical data. *J Pharmacokinet Biopharm* 5:445–479, 1977.
17. Gault MH, Churchill DN, Kalra J: Loading dose of digoxin in renal failure. *Br J Clin Pharmacol* 9:593–597, 1980.
18. Burton ME, Vasko MR, Brater DC: Comparison of drug dosing methods. *Clin Pharmacokinet* 10:1–37, 1985.
19. Chennavasin P, Brater DC: Nomograms for drug use in renal disease. *Clin Pharmacokinet* 6:193–214, 1981.
20. Hull JH, Sarubbi FA: Gentamicin serum concentrations: Pharmacokinetic predictions. *Ann Intern Med* 85:183–189, 1976.
21. Gibson TP, Nelson HA: Drug kinetics and artificial kidneys. *Clin Pharmacokinet* 2:403–426, 1977.
22. Christopher TG, Blair AD, Forrey AW, Cutler RE: Hemodialyzer clearances of gentamicin, kanamycin, tobramycin, amikacin, ethambutol, procainamide, and flucytosine, with a technique for planning therapy. *J Pharmacokinet Biopharm* 4:427–441, 1976.
23. Gwilt PR, Perrier D: Plasma protein binding and distribution characteristics of drugs as indices of their hemodialyzability. *Clin Pharmacol Ther* 24:154–161, 1978.

CHAPTER 56

Donor and Recipient Selection

STUART M. FLECHNER

INTRODUCTION

Kidney transplantation has become well established as an acceptable and perhaps the preferred form of replacement therapy for patients with end-stage renal disease (ESRD) (1-3). While the number of transplants performed has usually risen each year in the United States, the total represents less than 10% of the dialysis-dependent population. As reported to the Health Care Financing Administration at the end of the fourth quarter of 1989, there were over 116,000 ESRD patients receiving dialysis therapy. During this same interval 8882 patients received renal transplants, 6982 of which came from cadaveric donors and 1900 from living donors (4). In addition, about 14,000 patients remained on waiting lists, unable to secure a cadaveric organ. It has been estimated that an additional 10,000 patients would seek the option of transplantation if they received further education and if more plentiful donor sources existed.

The increasing demand for transplantation is a natural trend that parallels the ever-diminishing recipient mortality and the increasing graft survival enjoyed by renal transplant patients (5). At the same time, previous obstacles and impediments to transplantation have been steadily lifted. Absolute criteria that render a patient too old, too young, too small, too weak, or diabetic have been liberalized or eventually eliminated by many transplant teams. In recent years the predominant indication for transplantation has been the patient-driven desire to return to preillness levels of activity, well-being, employment status, self-image, and sexual performance. While not a cure for renal failure, a well-functioning renal allograft can best provide the means to these goals (6, 7). Nevertheless, transplantation must be tailored for each individual patient. The proper evaluation of every potential recipient and donor is of critical importance to ensure the best clinical outcome and the best utilization of a limited resource.

INDICATIONS FOR TRANSPLANTATION

The option of renal transplantation should be entertained by any patient with permanent renal failure. Of course, transplantation may not be medically suitable for every patient, nor would every individual want to inherit the unique responsibilities imposed on immunosuppressed recipients. Nevertheless, a complete discussion of treatment options at the onset of renal failure permits maximal patient involvement in treatment planning. Transplantation and dialysis are truly complementary forms of renal replacement therapy, rather than alternatives. The majority of recipients have been chronically dialyzed for months or years prior to transplantation, and many patients return to dialysis after a failed transplant, while awaiting another kidney. A candid presentation of treatment options may also relieve anxiety in certain patients who fear the loss of control over their own destiny (8).

The timing of renal transplantation may also have a significant impact on the outcome. Some renal physicians advocate a period of mandatory dialysis prior to transplantation so patients can "get used to" renal failure. Clearly, transplantation should not be done as an emergency, and patients who first present with florid uremia require acute dialysis and stabilization. However, for those with slowly progressive renal insufficiency, an increasing number want to be transplanted without prior chronic dialysis (9). Many of these individuals see elective transplantation as less disruptive to their lives, and they can avoid additional surgery to create vascular access. Such an approach is possible in highly motivated patients, especially those who have a willing and healthy family donor. Ultimately, though, the majority of transplant recipients will come from the pool of patients on chronic dialysis (Figure 1). They will usually be awaiting a cadaveric kidney. They will seek the option of transplantation because they want to "feel better."

Controversy exists as to the impact of transplantation on patient survival among various ESRD populations. As yet, no prospective analysis has been forthcoming in which the treatment option is randomized. Patient survival comparisons between dialysis and transplantation are usually plagued by a poor case mix, in which younger patients are transplanted and older patients with multiorgan system disease are placed on maintenance dialysis (10). A general consensus today would be that over a 5-year period, patient survival after living related transplantation (Figure 2) is about 10% better than survival after either a

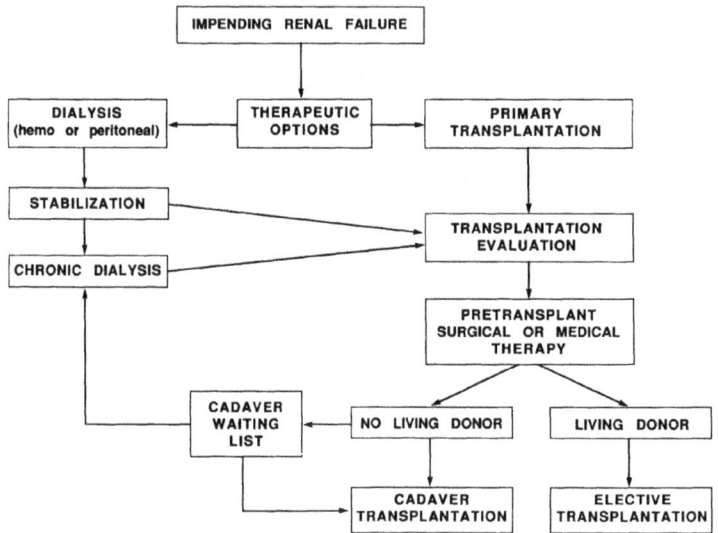

Figure 1. Patient options in end-stage renal disease.

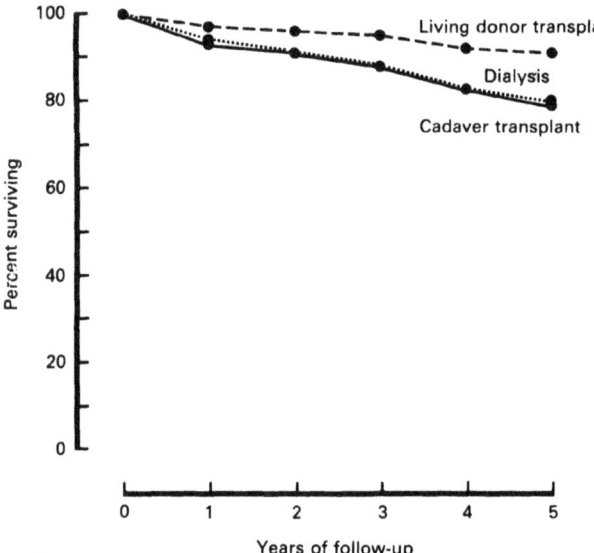

Figure 2. Percent survival of renal failure patients treated by cadaveric or living, related transplantation or dialysis. Results corrected for adverse pretreatment prognosis. From Hutchinson TA, Thomas DC, Lemieux JC, et al: Prognostically controlled comparison of dialysis and renal transplantation. Kidney Int 26:44, 1984, with permission.

cadaveric renal transplant or maintenance dialysis (11–13). However, it is important to caution that this issue is evolving rapidly. The use of cyclosporine-based immunosuppressive protocols and the transplantation of the older age patient (over 55 years) during the last few years may have a significant impact on the analysis of long-term patient survival by the end of this decade.

The predominant indication to proceed with transplantation for patients with renal failure is their ability to return to a more normal life style. There is little controversy that patients with a functioning renal allograft have increased exercise tolerance and are able to increase their physical activity and participation in sporting activities and travel (14, 15). For many, increased libido, sexual performance, and the ability to have children are major contributors to an improved sense of well-being. In addition, individual patients who were plagued by certain uremic symptoms, such as chronic nausea, vomiting, hiccups, headaches, itching, leg cramps, belching, weakness, lassitude, poor appetite, etc., which were not relieved by the artificial kidney, experience dramatic relief from a functioning kidney transplant. Other uncontrollable uremic complications, such as anemia, peripheral neuropathy, hyperparathyroidism, pericarditis, pleuritis, and enteropathy, are rapidly reversed in most instances. These changes permit the majority of motivated recipients to return to the work force and to pursue educational goals that were sharply curtailed when the diagnosis of renal failure was made.

CONTRAINDICATIONS TO TRANSPLANTATION

The shortage of donor organs worldwide creates inevitable judgements about how best to distribute such a resource (16). While it is beyond the scope of this chapter to debate the socioeconomic, moral, psychosocial, ethical, and ultimately political ramifications of organ distribution, it remains an inherent responsibility of all transplant practitioners to ensure that the "gift" of organ donation is allocated wisely. The continued altruism of donor families is ever dependent on the doctrine that needy recipients will have equitable access to organs and that recipient selection will be based on sound medical criteria. It is therefore prudent to consider who will not benefit from renal transplantation.

Simply put, the option of renal transplantation should not be entertained when the risks of the surgical procedure and the attendant life-long immunosuppression outweigh the benefits of a functioning kidney. Each individual must be evaluated for any coexistent medical or psychosocial problem that would lead to a poor outcome if not corrected. The following considerations should be part of the process of patient evaluation.

Chronologic age has often been a barrier to transplantation, with arbitrary cut-offs established for upper and lower age ranges at many centers. While a decade ago, the ideal candidate may have been between 15 and 45 years of age (17), improved transplant practice and delivery of immunosuppression has permitted the transplantation of small children of less than 10 kg in weight and older patients in their 60s and 70s (18–20). The physiologic age of the patient is a more significant determinant of outcome. Such older candidates should be aggressively screened for active cardiovascular disease. Posttransplant myocardial infarction, stroke, and peripheral vascular disease remain the most common cause of morbidity and mortality in these patients, whether they are transplanted or remain on dialysis (21). Therefore, careful history and physical examination, and the liberal use of noninvasive and invasive (angiography) studies, when indicated, best determine their suitability for transplantation. The older age patient with atherosclerotic disease should have realistic goals regarding rehabilitation and physical activity. Those patients with severe, noncorrectable atherosclerotic disease and little expectation for physical rehabilitation are probably best served by chronic dialysis, regardless of their chronologic age. On the other hand, those patients with identifiable atherosclerotic lesions should have them repaired by surgery and/or angioplasty prior to transplant.

Small children of less than 20 kg in size have been considered high-risk patients because of technical difficulties associated with dialysis and surgery in this group (22). In addition, many small babies with progressive uremia are severely malnourished, and have somatic and neurologic growth retardation. The wisdom of replacement therapy for uremic infants with severe cerebral impairment, and possibly other nonrenal organ system anomalies, has been questioned (23). Clearly, such decisions should be carefully individualized, and require the input of the parents and other social, ethical, religious, and legal support services where appropriate. Refinements in pediatric anesthesia, intensive care practice, and surgical technique have substantially improved transplant outcome, and size per se should no longer be considered a contraindication (24). While some have advocated the transplantation of small infants on an urgent basis, such a practice is rarely if ever indicated (25). Small uremic children can be safely stablized with peritoneal dialysis (26). During this period of time, they can be nutritionally repleted. The use of small nasogastric tubes for enteral hyperalimentation during continuous peritoneal dialysis has been a major advance. Since many such children have willing parental donors, the once high-risk endeavor of transplanting small children can now procede in an orderly, elective fashion.

Patients with metastatic malignancy should not be transplanted, regardless of which organ system is involved. The use of continuous immunosuppressive therapy may exacerbate tumor growth and prevent the possibility of cure (27). A more formidable dilemma concerns the suitability for transplantation of patients who have been considered cured of a primary malignancy. It would appear that the incidence of tumor recurrence posttransplant is inversely proportional to the length of time after tumor excision (28). This point is best illustrated by the post-transplant recurrence rate after the excision of a renal cell carcinoma. If patients are transplanted within 12 months of nephrectomy, the recurrence rate is 48%; between 13 and 24 months, the rate drops to 20%; after 24 months, 14%; and no recurrences were reported if the interval was greater than 4 years. It would therefore appear prudent to wait at least 18–24 months after tumor excision to ensure that a potential recipient remains NED (no evidence of disease). A thorough repeat metastatic evaluation should be performed prior to transplantation in these select cases. Transplantation can probably proceed more quickly in patients who have been successfully treated for tumors with a very slow growth potential such as superficial skin tumors (basal and squamous cell carcinoma), bladder papillomas, and stage A-1 prostate adenocarcinoma (29).

Renal transplantation should be delayed or even avoided in patients with active infectious disease. Patients should be carefully screened to rule out bacterial, viral, fungal, and/or parasitic infections that can have life-threatening consequences under immunosuppressive therapy (30). All infectious illnesses should be properly diagnosed, treated with full courses of antibiotics and/or surgical drainage, and adequately monitored after therapy is complete. This includes a number of occult (31), and at times asymptomatic, infections, such as sinus infections, dental abscesses, perirectal abscesses, vaginal discharges, nonhealing bone or osteomyelitis, chronic epididimitis or prostatitis, and infected vascular access grafts or peritoneal dialysis catheters. Chronic leukocytosis or eosinophilia should not be overlooked in the dialysis-dependent population. Newly uncovered cardiac murmurs should be throughly evaluated as well.

Patients with active tuberculosis (TB) should complete a full course of therapy prior to transplantation (32, 33). This usually entails two-drug therapy for pulmonary TB and three-drug therapy for extrapulmonary TB. Patients with well-documented renal tuberculosis should have the affected renal unit removed, as drug delivery will be inadequate in tubercular nonfunctioning kidneys (34). Potential recipients with a well-documented but remote history of TB, or those with a strong likelihood of recent exposure, create a special problem. Skin testing may not be useful due to the high frequency of anergy in uremic patients. Such patients are probably best treated with prophylactic isoniazid posttransplant. However, possible hepatotoxicity and drug interactions with isoniazid may complicate posttransplant management.

Patients who develop end-stage renal disease and become infected with hepatitis B comprise a high-risk group for renal transplantation. It appears that dialysis patients who remain HB_s Ag positive at the time of or become positive after transplantation have a diminished chance of clearing the virus and are at an increased risk of developing chronic liver disease (35). The use of chronic immunosuppression in HB_s Ag-positive patients may predispose to the development of chronic active hepatitis, cirrhosis, hepatoma, and increased mortality related to liver failure. Much of this information emerges from longitudinal studies done (36, 37) on a group of recipients who were immunosuppressed with azathioprine and prednisone. Some have implicated azathioprine in liver disease progression, and, therefore, the impact of newer immunosuppressive protocols remains unknown (38). As yet there has been no matched prospective study demonstrating that HB_s Ag-positive patients have a greater life expectancy on dialysis *vis à vis* transplantation. Until such data is forthcoming, it is prudent to alert potential recipients to the real risk of progressive liver disease and presumably increased mortality post-transplant if they are HB_s Ag positive. It is advisable to monitor serial liver function tests and to avoid transplantation in those patients with rising transaminases. In certain cases it may be best to wait 3–6 months, in order to observe the clinical course of a patient with fluctuating liver function. Liver biopsy may be helpful in identifying chronic active hepatitis and/or cirrhosis. These patients would not be well served by life-long immunosuppressive therapy.

CAUSES OF RENAL FAILURE

The pathologic entities listed in Table 1 represent the leading causes of kidney disease that eventuate in the diagnosis of end-stage renal disease. This large spectrum includes both congenital and acquired renal disease, and those isolated to the kidney or part of a systemic process. With few exceptions, patients with any of these primary diagnoses have been successfully transplanted with either a living related or a cadaveric organ.

The spectrum of glomerulonephritis represents the most common form of renal failure and the most common etiology leading to renal transplantation. If patients are biopsied early in the course of their disease, a more precise histopathologic diagnosis can be made. Unfortunately, many patients present uremic, with small contracted and

Table 1. Most common forms of chronic renal failure leading to renal transplantation

Glomerular disease
   Membranoproliferative glomerulonephritis
   Rapidly progressive glomerulonephritis
   Antiglomerular basement membrane disease
   Membranous nephropathy
   IgA nephropathy (Berger's)
   Focal segmental glomerulosclerosis

Diabetic nephropathy

Arteriolar nephrosclerosis
   Essential hypertension
   Malignant hypertension
   Bilateral renovascular disease

Interstitial disease
   Chronic pyelonephritis
   Analgesic nephropathy
   Toxic nephropathy

Congenital disorders
   Renal agenesis
   Renal dysplasia
   Posterior urethral valves
   Vesico-ureteral reflux
   Prune-belly syndrome
   Ureteropelvic junction obstruction

Neurogenic bladder
   Congenital (meningomyelocele)
   Acquired

Hereditary diseases
   Polycystic kidney disease
   Medullary cystic disease
   Alport's syndrome

Nephrolithiases
   Infection stones
   Hyperoxaluria
   Cystinuria

Systemic diseases
   Lupus erythematosis
   Hemolytic uremic
     syndrome
   Amyloidosis
   Scleroderma
   Polyarteritis nodosa
   Fabry's disease
   Henoch-Schonlein
     purpura

Infections
   Tuberculosis
   Schistosomiasis

Surgical nephrectomy
   Trauma
   Renal malignancy

scarred kidneys that have nonspecific changes. As might be predicted, patients with primary glomerular diseases may develop recurrent disease in the transplant kidney. The rates of recurrence of membranoproliferative glomerulonephritis (38, 40), focal sclerosis (41, 42), IgA nephropathy (43, 44), and antiglomerular basement membrane (anti-GBM) disease (45, 46) have been reported to be as high as 50% on posttransplant biopsies. However, the continuous use of immunosuppressive drugs may significantly retard the progression of recurrent disease, and actual graft loss from recurrent disease occurs in only a few percent of patients. "De-novo" glomerular disease, such as membranous nephropathy, has also been reported (47, 48). While the fear of recurrent disease should not alter the decision to proceed with transplantation, the timing of the transplant should be considered carefully. Patients with a very rapid and aggressive course to renal failure, such as those with focal segmental sclerosis, rapidly progressive crescentic glomerulonephritis, or those with high titers of anti-GBM or circulating immune complexes, should probably wait 6–12 months on dialysis until the disease is quiescent.

Insulin-dependent diabetics comprise a steadily increasing percentage of the ESRD population. They now represent up to 25–30% of transplant recipients in many centers (49). While not a cure for diabetes, uremic diabetics often experience dramatic improvement in exercise tolerance, mobility, and well-being after renal transplantation. Much of this improvement is due to a reversal of uremic neuropathy, which often compounds the peripheral neuropathy of diabetes (50). Diabetics with severely compromised vision often experience a similar degree of rehabilitation as sighted patients and should not be excluded from transplantation (51). Unfortunately progressive vasculopathy post-transplant continues, which leads to a higher frequency of myocardial infarction, stroke, and amputation than in the nondiabetic transplant population (52). For this reason, it is very important to screen diabetics for correctable coronary artery, carotid, and peripheral vascular lesions prior to transplantation.

Arteriolar nephrosclerosis, often associated with malignant hypertension, is another frequent cause of renal failure. This represents the most common etiology leading to renal transplantation in young black males. While some patients have dramatic improvement in blood pressure control with the onset of dialysis, others may require nephrectomy to prevent cardiovascular and cerebrovascular accidents. It should be noted that control of blood pressure with medications may significantly improve renal function in previously untreated patients (53). Such patients should not be transplanted until irreversible renal failure has been established.

The transplantation of patients with metabolic, hereditary, and systemic diseases will be discussed in another chapter. Each group has some unique considerations in recipient preparation and posttransplant management. The transplantation of patients with a previous history of self-destructive behavior leading to renal failure, such as those with analgesic-abuse nephropathy, intravenous-drug-use nephropathy, etc., must be carefully individualized. This often requires the input of various family, community, social service, and religious support systems.

PRETRANSPLANT EVALUATION OF THE POTENTIAL RECIPIENT

It is imperative that each potential recipient undergo a complete evaluation prior to transplantation by the team responsible for his or her surgery and immunosuppression. The relative physiologic age and health of the patient, as well as social circumstances and distance from the transplant center, may dictate whether such an evaluation can be done on an inpatient or outpatient basis. The main purposes of such an evaluation are twofold. Firstly, every effort should be made to uncover any existing medical or psychosocial conditions that would increase the risk for morbidity or mortality after transplantation. Any such condition, if identified, should be corrected prior to surgery and the administration of immunosuppression. Secondly, such information serves as a database to use as a baseline for possible organ system complications posttransplant and/or the comparison of different treatment plans.

The precise evaluation for transplantation varies from center to center, depending on practice philosophies and patient populations. In recent years there has been a trend to streamline transplant practice and to eliminate studies when a particular complication has not been observed in recent months. One reason for this has been pressure to contract medical services by financing agencies. Another has been competitive marketing practices between centers in close proximity to a fixed dialysis-dependent population. Whatever the circumstance, it is incumbent on all transplant practitioners to ensure that patients are thoroughly prepared and can therefore maximize their opportunity for a successful outcome. These considerations may become more important in the future, as a broader ESRD population seeks the option of transplantation. The following evaluation is used by the Division of Transplantation, Department of Surgery at Stanford University Medical Center (Table 2).

History

The initial history should address the onset of renal failure and its presentation. Hypertension, proteinuria, edema, fever, weight gain, etc. may have resolved or remain active. The cause of the disease and any available biopsy material should be reviewed. Associated problems such as recurrent urinary tract infections or pyelonephritis, stone disease, or gross hematuria should be explored. If the patient still produces urine, the voiding pattern should be ascertained, in an effort to diagnose bladder outlet obstruction. Symptoms related to vascular disease should be elicited, specifically looking for coronary or carotid artery

Table 2. Pretransplant evaluation for potential recipients

1. General studies
   a. History and physical exam
   b. Pelvic exam with PAP smear
   c. Stool for occcult blood
   d. CXR, EKG
2. Blood chemistry
   a. BUN, creatinine, electrolytes
   b. Total protein, albumin, transferrin
   c. Ca, PO_4, Mg, alkaline phosphatase
   d. SGOT, SGPT, bilirubin, LDH
   e. Cholesterol, triglycerides, FBS
   f. Amylase, uric acid, PTH
3. Hematologic studies
   a. cbc and differential
   b. PT, PTT, platelets
   c. Direct Combs
   d. Cold agglutinins
4. Serology
   a. CMV, herpes, VDRL
   b. HIV
   c. HB_sAg, HB_sAb, HB_cAg
5. Immunologic studies
   a. FANA, rheumatoid factor
   b. Serum complement
   c. T-cell subsets
   d. Panel MLC
   e. Spontaneous blastogenesis
   f. Skin testing — recall antigens
6. Tissue typing
   a. ABO type
   b. HLA A, B, C
   c. Anti-HLA cytotoxic antibody screen
   d. Donor-specific MLC
7. Infectious work-up
   a. Blood cultures
   b. Urine cultures
   c. Nasal cultures
8. Urologic studies
   a. Urinalysis
   b. 24-hour creatinine clearance
   c. Voiding cystourethrogram
9. Radiologic studies
   a. Upper GI series
   b. Barium enema (age over 50)
   c. Ultrasound kidneys, gallbladder
   d. Bone x-rays, sinus films
   e. Panarex — teeth, mandible
10. Selected studies
    a. Plumonary function tests
    b. Arterial blood gases
    c. Cystoscopy
    d. Cystometrogram
    e. Echocardiogram
    f. Coronary angiography

disease and peripheral vascular disease. A careful GI history is important to uncover gallbladder, pancreatic, liver, or peptic ulcer disease symptoms. The family history may uncover a pattern of cancer, bleeding diatheses, or inherited renal disease. Previous use of immunosuppressive drugs and any complications should be noted. The quantity and time of administration of blood products should be recorded.

Physical exam

The initial physical examination may reflect patient compliance with dialysis or with medical therapy. Fluid overload and edema may represent intentional noncompliance. The eyes may reveal lipid abnormalities or cataracts. The fundi can demonstrate the degree of diabetic retinopathy or nephrosclerosis with hypertension. The cardiac exam may reveal new murmurs that have an infectious origin. All major blood vessels from the carotids to the dorsalis pedis should be palpated and/or auscultated. Diminished pulses or bruits should be evaluated further. Sources of occult infections, such as otitis, cervical, axillary, and inguinal lymph nodes; dental abscesses; genital or perirectal abscesses; and the lower extremities of diabetics, should be carefully inspected. A pelvic exam in females should include a PAP smear if one has not been done in the past year. A rectal exam should include a stool sample for occult blood.

Laboratory tests

The purpose of these studies is to identify metabolic or physiologic derangements that will complicate transplant surgery and immunosuppression. Ideally, recipients should be well nourished and in metabolic balance. Vitamin-deficiency anemia should be corrected. Serologic studies will identify previous exposure to common pathogens encountered by transplant recipients. Patients with a positive VDRL, which has been confirmed by specific treponemal antibody studies, should have documented evidence of treatment with a long-acting penicillin prior to transplant. Patients who have no antibody to the CMV virus should receive a CMV-negative donor kidney, if possible (54). All potential recipients should be tested for antibody to HIV (55). Positive tests should be reconfirmed by western blot analysis. Hepatitis B status should be identified.

Screening immunologic studies test for persistent immune activity. This is especially important in patients with autoimmune disease such as systemic lupus erythematosis (SLE), rapidly progressive glomerulonephritis, antiglomerular basement membrane (anti-GBM) antibody disease, and focal sclerosis. Patients with low serum complement, high titers of anti-GBM, or immune complexes should not be transplanted for 6–12 months, until quiescence has been documented. Baseline studies, such as T-cell subsets, panel MLC, and spontaneous blastogenesis, are useful predictors of weak versus strong immune responders (56). Skin testing to microbial recall antigens and PPD will identify anergic patients and those at risk for certain infections post-transplant (57).

Patients with positive blood or urine cultures should be treated after the source of the infection is identified. Recently, nasal cultures have been added to identify recipients who are colonized with methicillin-resistant *Staphylococcus aureus* (MRSA). This virulent organism can cause serious problems if introduced on a ward with immunosuppressed transplant recipients. Every effort is made to clear patients who are chronic MRSA carriers prior to transplant (58).

Urologic studies

Routine urologic studies include a urine culture, urinalysis, 24-hour urine collection for volume, protein excretion, and creatinine clearance, and a voiding cystourethrogram. Patients with hematuria, a history of prostatism (males over 55), filling defects, incontinence, or a history of previous lower urinary tract pathology should be cystoscoped. Retrograde pyelograms may be useful in selected cases. Cystometrograms may be useful in patients with incontinence, diabetics with a sensory neuropathy, or if there is any question of neurogenic bladder disease. It should be noted that virtually all dialysis patients with defunctionalized bladders (< 200 cc per day) will have diminished flow rates and high voiding pressures. This is usually readily reversible after normal urine volumes are restored.

Radiographic studies

Routine radiographic studies include an upper GI series (endoscopy may be preferred) and a barium enema in patients over 50. Ultrasound exam of the gallbladder, bile ducts, and pancreas to rule out gallbladder disease, and the kidneys to rule out acquired cystic disease, tumors, stones, hydronephrosis, etc. are necessary. Plain films of the sinuses, mandible and teeth are done to rule out occult infections.

Selected studies

Patients with an extensive smoking history are instructed to stop prior to transplant. Such patients, and those with a history of frequent pulmonary infections, undergo pulmonary function tests with blood gases. Reversible bronchospasm should be corrected.

Coronary artery disease is a significant cause of morbidity and mortality for diabetic and elderly ESRD patients (21, 59, 60). It has therefore been our policy to perform coronary angiography on all diabetics, patients over 60 years, and any patient with symptomatic angina. Potential recipients with critical coronary artery lesions are referred for percutaneous transluminal angioplasty (PTCA) or aortocoronary bypass. Using such a policy, several centers have demonstrated a reduction in death from myocardial infarction in this high-risk group up to 3–4 years posttransplant (61–63).

PRETRANSPLANT SURGICAL PREPARATION

The use of continuous chemical immunosuppression posttransplant increases the risks of complications for elective or emergency surgical procedures. Wound healing is impaired, sutured anastomoses have a greater tendency to leak, and wound hematomas are more likely. In addition, postoperative pulmonary disease can become a major problem. For this reason, with few exceptions, it is recommended that all elective surgical procedures be performed and healed prior to transplantation. It should be cautioned, however, that many of the same pitfalls will occur with greater frequency in uremic individuals compared with otherwise normal patients. Examples of such procedures include inguinal or incisional hernias, hemorrhoids, cosmetic surgery, minor skin biopsies, orthopedic procedures, extensive dental work, etc. The following major surgical procedures may be required to enhance the chances of a successful kidney transplant and should be completed prior to transplantation as well.

Native nephrectomy

The indication for bilateral nephrectomy has become much more conservative during the last few years. The procedure was quite common in the 1960s, presumably to remove the stimulus of immune-mediated renal injury. Such practice was supported as recently as 1977, with data suggesting improved graft survival (64). This idea has been largely outweighed by the advantages of retained native kidney function. Even severely contracted kidneys contribute to red cell production, calcium homeostasis, and provide an additional source of fluid and potassium loss, which make life on dialysis more comfortable. Therefore, nephrectomy is required in only about 10% of recipients. Indications would include recurrent bacterial pyelonephritis, infected renal cysts, active stone passage, high-grade vesicoureteral reflux with residual urine, refractory hypertension, renal tumors, and patients with severe proteinuria causing malnutrition. Occasionally, patients may have massive polycystic kidneys that cause abdominal symptoms or gross hematuria, which require selective nephrectomy. In patients with reflux, tuberculosis, hydronephrosis, or other ureteral pathology, nephroureterectomy may be required.

Parathyroidectomy

Uremic patients with tertiary hyperparathyroidism should have a subtotal parathyroidectomy prior to transplant. This is usually reserved for symptomatic patients with either metastatic calcification, peptic ulcer disease, pancreatitis, itching, and/or severe bone mineral reabsorption. Many of these patients have serum calcium levels at the upper limit of normal, but radioimmunoassay parathormone levels are elevated to 10–100 times normal. This group represents a small percentage of the dialysis population, since the majority of patients have secondary hyperparathyroidism, which will reverse with a functioning renal allograft.

Gastrointestinal disease

Uremic patients with active peptic ulcer disease are at high risk for bleeding and/or perforation in the early posttransplant period, when steroid doses are highest (65, 66). Patients with a history of recurrent ulcers or hemorrhage requiring transfusion should have a prophylactic acid-reducing procedure. Selective vagotomy has been popularized in recent years (67). Endoscopic evidence of complete healing should be documented before proceeding with transplantation. Intensive antacid therapy should continue posttransplant. Unfortunately the H_2 blockers, cimetidine and ranitidine, exacerbate cyclosporine nephrotoxiciy and should be used cautiously with cyclosporine-based immunosuppressive protocols (68).

Patients with active gallbladder disease or those with gallstones or common bile-duct stones should be stone free prior to transplantation. Cholecystectomy with choledocograms is usually required.

The presence of colon diverticula (usually patients over 45) create a management dilemma. Those patients with a well-documented history of diverticulitis should have a prophylactic colectomy (usually left) if they are to be immunosuppressed. The mortality of posttransplant colon perforation has been reported to be as high as 50% (69, 70). Those patients with scattered diverticula and no history of bowel symptoms need to be appraised of the possibility of such a catastrophic complication. Although prophylactic colectomy in these patients seems hard to justify, the decision to proceed with transplantation should not be taken lightly.

Lower urinary tract dysfunction

As the number of older aged male recipients increases, bladder outlet obstruction will be seen with increasing frequency. Uremic patients who produce at least a liter of urine per day may describe typical symptoms of prostatism. Those who produce only a small volume of urine daily will be difficult to evaluate. Patients may have a large amount of postvoid residual urine (over 200 cc), a low flow rate, cellules, and diverticula on voiding cystogram. Obstructed patients, usually over 55 years of age, who produce over a liter of urine per day should undergo transurethral prostatectomy (TURP) prior to transplant. However, those patients who produce small urine volumes frequently develop bladder-neck contractures and urethral strictures after a resection (71). Therefore, TURP should be delayed until they receive a functioning kidney. Patients with urethral stricture disease should be treated with a direct-vision internal urethrotomy, if possible. If these patients produce small urine volumes pretransplant, then daily self-catheterizations of the urethra should be done to prevent recurrent strictures.

On occasion an ESRD patient may present with a small, contracted, severely fibrosed bladder. This is usually caused by either tuberculosis, schistosomiasis, or severe interstitial cystitis. In addition, some patients may have total urinary incontinence, not infrequently associated with a high-pressure neurogenic bladder. In these cases, the existing bladder is not suitable for transplantation, and an intestinal conduit is required. An ileal loop is preferred, which should be created at least 6 weeks prior to the anticipated transplantation (72). One may also encounter a patient in whom an ileal loop has been in place for many years. These patients may have developed chronic pyelonephritis as the cause of their ESRD, and their loops can be used for transplantation. It should be emphasized, however, that the creation of an intestinal loop is a last resort. Many small (< 50 cc) defunctionalized bladders will dilate nicely after urine volumes are restored from a functioning kidney. Patients with flaccid bladders that empty poorly (some diabetics) can be managed with intermittent clean catheterization with excellent results, as long as their continence mechanism is intact (73). Bladder filling, emptying, and the continence mechanism can be reliably tested pretransplant by the insertion of a small percutaneous suprapubic tube and saline irrigation (74).

Splenectomy

Surgical removal of the spleen for the purpose of augmenting immunosuppression was once an integral component of pretransplant preparation. Previous reports justified the procedure on the basis of improved graft survival (75, 76). Indeed, splenectomy would obviate persistent leukopenia and permit maximal doses of antiproliferative drugs such as azathioprine. Routine splenectomy has all but been abandoned due to an increased long-term risk of sepsis, the absence of persistent leukopenia in cyclosporine-based immunosuppressive regimens, and the associated morbidity of the procedure itself (77). On rare occasions, splenectomy may be indicated for massive hypersplenism causing pancytopenia.

BLOOD TRANSFUSIONS

In perhaps no other arena does the pendulum swing back and forth from consensus to controversy as in the use of intentional pretransplant blood transfusions. In the 1960s the administration of blood transfusions to dialysis patients was discouraged, due to the formation of anti-HLA cytotoxic antibodies. Patients who developed broadly reacting antibodies were too often unable to find a crossmatch negative kidney. However, in 1973 Opelz and Terasaki reported that cadaver allograft survival rose in proportion to the number of pretransplant third-party blood transfusions (78). This observation was corroborated in numerous retrospective studies worldwide over the next 10 years (79–82). Virtually all of the patients in those reports were immunosuppressed with azathioprine and prednisone.

Although the blood transfusion effect is cited as a major contributor to successful outcome, the mechanism of this effect is poorly understood. Some have attributed the effect to a "selecting out" of patients who develop broadly reacting cytotoxic antibodies due to the transfusions and subsequently are not transplanted. Others have reported the induction of nonspecific suppressor networks or enhancing antibodies (83, 84). During the past few years, several changes have taken place that have curtailed the enthusiasm for routine transfusions.

Firstly, there has been a steady improvement in the results of cadaver graft survival in untransfused patients, which was initially observed using azathioprine and prednisone immunosuppression. Opelz reported a 1-year graft survival under 40% in untransfused patients in 1973 (78), while Terasaki reported a jump to nearly 60% in 1984 (85). This observation may relate to the fact that transplant outcome is a multifactorial phenomena and is not based on a single determinant, such as transfusion history. It should be pointed out that, to this day, a truly prospective study, in which similar subsets of patients are randomized to receive intentional third-party transfusions or to remain untransfused, has not been accomplished.

Secondly, the use of cyclosporine has improved graft survival in virtually all donor-recipient combinations and may have obscured the blood-transfusion effect (86–89).

In one single-center report, there was no difference in graft survival, incidence of rejection, or renal function between transfused and untransfused cyclosporine-treated, cadaver recipients (90). A similar finding was originally reported in mismatched, living, related recipients treated with cyclosporine and prednisone (91).

Thirdly, a decrease in the requirement for pretransplant surgery, such as bilateral nephrectomy and splenectomy, has eliminated many tranfusions that were previously administered during these procedures. Such practices not only diminish the perioperative transfusion requirement, but also that of the anephric patient awaiting transplantation. During the coming years, blood transfusions required for dialysis patients with symptomatic anemia may be further reduced as recombinant human erythropoietin becomes available (92).

A fourth, and perhaps the most vexing, consideration is the increasing patient fear of disease transmission by blood products. The transmission of the human immunodeficiency virus by blood transfusion has been prominent in the lay and scientific media. The incidence of such transmission should be low in the dialysis population with the introduction of mandatory screening of blood donors for antibody to the virus (93). However, of far greater concern to ESRD patients is the transmission of viral hepatitis by blood products. Unfortunately, the screening of blood donors for hepatits B will not eliminate the problem, as the major disease vector is now non-A, non-B hepatitis (94). Post-transfusion hepatitis has been reported to occur in as high as 5-7% of patients. Blood transfusion is also a major vehicle for the transmission of cytomegalovirus.

Should all recipients be routinely transfused prior to transplantation? This question is perhaps best answered by individual centers. Since the majority of potential recipients will have had previous transfusions from either previous surgical procedures, failed transplants, symptomatic anemia, etc., the question primarily addresses new, first kidney-transplant patients. If ESRD patients are to receive pretransplant blood transfusions for no other reason than to improve graft survival, then each center should demonstrate this beneficial effect in its own particular environment. Since blood transfusion allegedly diminishes accelerated graft loss during the first month posttransplant (95), this can be assessed at repeated intervals as new immunosuppressive protocols are developed at various centers.

SELECTION OF RENAL DONORS

Human renal allografts come from one of four sources. The first kidneys used for transplantation were removed from patients who had suffered recent cardiac arrest and died. Due to an obligatory period of warm ischemia that such organs undergo, and the uncertainty surrounding such events, the use of these donors has all but been abandoned. Currently, the largest source of donor kidneys come from individuals who have suffered irreversible brain death and whose vital organs can be maintained for a limited period of time by artifical life-support systems. Donated organs and tissues from so-called heart-beating cadavers can usually be recovered with minimal warm ischemic injury. Healthy, willing, and highly motivated living relatives of the recipient, such as siblings, parents, or children, comprise another source of kidneys. More distant relatives such as aunts, uncles, grandparents, or cousins may also be suitable donors. The last and most controversial source of kidneys come from living nonrelated individuals. A healthy spouse is the most likely representative in the latter group, but unusually motivated "friends" of the recipient have been used. At the present time xenograft kidneys have not been successfully transplanted in humans. There are certain advantages and disadvantages to the recipient from each donor source. The selection of the best donor for each recipient should be an individualized process, which often highlights the art of transplantation medicine as well as the science.

Living related donors

The use of a living related donor (LRD) in human renal transplantation has created a unique ethical dilemma for those involved with the daily care of transplant patients. In no other area in medicine is an otherwise healthy individual asked to subject himself or herself to the potential morbidity and mortality of major surgery for no apparent physical benefit. There are two basic reasons why LRD transplants are done, and each presents a variable degree of significance for a given donor-recipient pair. Firstly, LRD kidneys work better and last longer. This fact has been continuously observed using virtually all combinations of nonspecific chemical immunosuppression during the past 25 years (5). Secondly, there is a global shortage of suitable cadaver kidneys (96). Therefore, LRD transplantation will expedite the process for some recipients and may permit transplantation to be done in some patients who have been unable to secure a cross-match negative cadaver kidney after waiting an extended period of time. These benefits, solely to the recipient, must be balanced against the potential short-term and long-term harm to the donor.

Living related renal transplantation has been the clinical laboratory that validates the role of the major histocompatibility complex (MHC), on chromosome 6, in allograft rejection. While the importance of tissue typing in cadaver transplantation is debated, there is little question as to the impact of immune responsiveness evoked by histoincompatibilities among family members. These differences appear to correlate directly with the eventual graft survival and clinical course (5). Assuming that medical and psychosocial parameters are equal, donors are selected based on their degree of histocompatibility. Table 3 provides, in descending order, the degree of tissue similarity among potential donors and suggests the order of preference for a specific recipient.

Tissue typing is done to identify the class I (HLA A, B) and class II (Dr) antigens present in each family member.

Table 3. Donor selection by immunologic similarity

Monozygotic twins
HLA identical siblings
Haploidentical siblings, parents, children, relatives
Less than haploidentical siblings, parents, children, relatives
Distant relatives

Unrelated living donors (spouse, etc.)

Cadaveric donors

Since each individual receives two alleles (one from each parent), a recipient has a 25% chance that a potential sibling donor is identical for each HLA antigen. In addition, there is a 50% chance that the potential sibling donor has inherited the same HLA antigens from one parent (called a haplotype). Since HLA antigens are inherited as a group on chromosome 6 within a family, a specific haplotype may be found on more distant relatives as well. The tissue type between parents and children are almost always haploidentical, but aunts, uncles, grandparents, and cousins may also share a haplotype. The reason that matching among family members has such a powerful effect on outcome is that matching for the known HLA determinants within a family virtually assures compatibility for all the gene products of the entire MHC region. Tissue typing among unrelated individuals does not carry the certainty of linkage with other (as yet undetermined) products of the MHC. An additional MHC region gene product that can be identified is the HLA-D antigen. This requires a lengthy 6 to 7-day assay, the mixed lymphocyte culture (MLC). HLA identical siblings will share HLA-D antigens and will have a nonproliferative MLC reaction. The MLC test can be used to further stratify potential donors who have similar serologic HLA typing to a specific recipient. Diminished MLC responses between two individuals may signify not only similarity at the D locus, but also at other as yet undetermined loci in the MHC region. Therefore, the strength of the MLC response should be coupled with tissue-typing information to select the most compatible potential donor (97).

The first successful human renal transplant was performed between monozygotic twins without immunosuppression (98). Thirty such isografts have been done at the Brigham Hospital in Boston, and none has experienced graft rejection (99), thus validating the role of the MHC in human organ transplantation. The most common cause of graft loss in these recipients has been recurrence of glomerulonephritis in the graft or death from unrelated causes (99). Recurrent nephritis can be prevented (in those recipients who developed ESRD from this etiology) by delaying transplantation until the disease process is quiescent, as is done for patients with lupus nephritis. Long-term graft survival in HLA identical and haploidentical LRD transplants, as compiled by Terasaki, appears in Figure 3. A clear difference between these groups and cadaveric recipients can be observed using azathioprine and prednisone immunosuppression. While these curves have been pushed upward and to the right with the use of cyclosporine and prednisone, a similar separation of these groups remains. As reported by Flechner et al., rejection episodes occur in less than 10% of cyclosporine-prednisone treated HLA-identical recipients, and graft loss is exceedingly rare (100). In fact, over half of these patients can be treated by cyclosporine alone and avoid the long-term consequences of steroid therapy. Several groups have reported over 90% 2 to 3-year graft survival in haploidentical recipients treated with this regimen (101–103).

Prior to the introduction of cyclosporine-based immunosuppression, a marked improvement in HLA nonidentical LRD transplants was observed if the recipient was given three pretransplant blood transfusions from the specific kidney donor (DST). As first reported by Cochrum et al., if such patients did not develop donor-specific cytotoxic

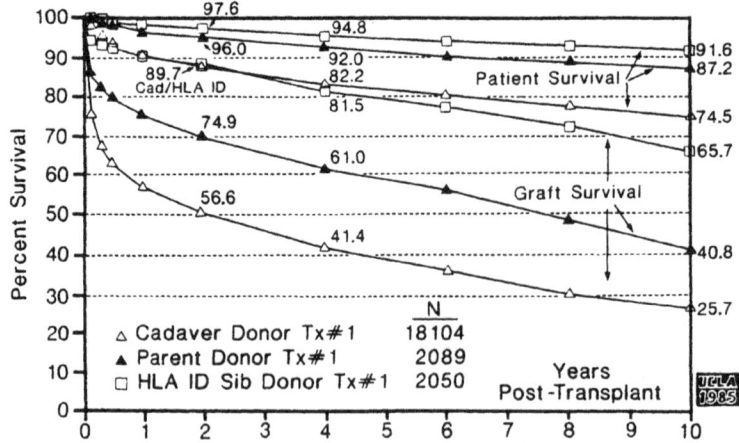

Figure 3. Ten-year patient and graft survival for transplant recipients according to donor source, from UCLA registry. From Terasaki PI: *Clinical Kidney Transplants. 1986.* University of California Press, Los Angeles, CA, p 5, 1986.

antibodies to recipient T cells after the transfusions, graft survival of 90% at 1 year could be achieved with azathioprine and prednisone immunosuppression (104). While some centers prefer this approach, up to 30% of recipients become sensitized from DSTs, and therefore cannot receive their potential donor's kidney (105). For those who remain unsensitized, they can be transplanted without cyclosporine, thereby avoiding the potential nephrotoxicity. However, the incidence of acute rejection episodes exceeds 60% in DST-prepared patients, which necessitates further courses of steroid therapy (105).

Despite the compelling arguments for the use of livng donors, such procedures should not be done if significant morbidity or mortality were to be experienced by the donor. The concept of self-sacrifice and organ donation has been extensively examined by the medical, ethical, and legal professions. Postdonation analyses have consistently found that the donor experience was an overwhelmingly positive one, regardless of the outcome of the kidney in the recipient (106, 107). The courts have found that donor altruism is an acceptable motivation to undergo nephrectomy. In fact some courts have found that the donor will not only benefit psychologically and spiritually from the act of charity, but might even be psychologically harmed if prevented from donating when the life and well-being of a loved one was at stake (108). This argument is the basis for use of potential donors who are legal minors. Life insurance companies have also considered the impact of renal donation. In a survey of over 60 major carriers by Santiago et al., 97% responded that they would accept renal donors, assuming that the remaining renal function was normal. Half of the companies felt that there is a minimal and temporary risk to the donor (relating to the surgical procedure), and the other half did not feel there was any increased risk (109).

Clearly, renal donation is not an innocuous procedure, as all donors experience some degree of anxiety, physical pain, and disruption of their employment schedule, schooling, and home life. In addition, a degree of pressure and coercion can be present among family members that is not readily apparent to health care professionals. For these reasons, each donor must b given the opportunity to give their independent, informed consent to this decision. We have found that it is very important to counsel the spouse of the potential donor and to permit his or her input into the process as well. It is also helpful to allow the potential donor to determine the pace of the evaluation. Some may truly be undecided and may require more time to evaluate their commitment, or want to opt out of the process. These complex social interactions make it very difficult to consider minors, uner age 18, as potential donors in all but the most unusual of circumstances.

What, then, is the risk to the potential renal donor? While the number of donor deaths worldwide is quite low, they have occurred. It has been reported that the 5-year life expectancy of a unilaterally nephrectomized 35-year-old healthy male donor will be 99.1%, as compared with 99.3% for a matched control with two kidneys (110). Another estimate is that the mortality for donor nephrectomy is less than 0.1% (111). The long-term risk by actuarial methods has been calculated to equal that of commuting in a car 16 miles each working day. Fortunately, major postoperative complications, such as life-threatening infections or cardiopulmonary events, are rare. Minor complications, such as atelectasis, urinary tract infection, phlebitis, urinary retention, etc., are reported to occur in 10–20% of cases (112). A flurry of concern has been generated from the findings of Brenner et al. that rats who underwent renal ablation were subject to glomerular hyperfiltration in the remnant kidney (113). This process led to glomerular sclerosis and deterioration in renal function, which was related to protein intake and time. However, several studies of renal donors with 15–20 years of follow-up failed to identify this problem in humans (112, 114, 115). Progressive renal deterioration is not observed, and the incidence of hypertension was consistent with that of the population at large. Some uninephrectomized donors did have an increased urinary protein excretion, the implications of which are presently unknown. Whether these findings will remain constant with 50 years of follow-up is open to conjecture. Similar findings were observed in patients who underwent unilateral nephrectomy in childhood for other reasons, after more than 23 years of observation (116).

Living unrelated donors

The utilization of kidneys from living unrelated individuals is a subject that raises the passions, both pro and con, of many in the transplant community. For some, it is a logical extension of the practice of transplantation; for others it is anathema to the principal of *primum non nocere* (doctor do no harm). The impetus behind the use of living nonrelated donors comes from patients and physicians. Firstly, there has been an undeniable increase in the number of dialysis-dependent patients every year, and a corresponding increase in the number of potential recipients awaiting a cadaveric transplant (Table 4). This trend, coupled with an insufficient quantity of available organ donors to meet the demand, creates pressure to explore all donor sources (117). Secondly, the bond between two individuals, such as husband and wife, is arguably as firm as that between blood relations. The same satisfaction in helping a loved

Table 4. Dialysis and transplantation in the united states

Year	New dialysis patients	CAD transplants	LRD transplants	Patients on dialysis at year end
1981	21,367	3427	1458	58,924
1982	22,797	3681	1677	65,765
1983	24,218	4333	1796	71,961
1984	27,113	5264	1704	78,479
1985	29,995	5819	1876	84,797
1986	33,451	7089	1887	90,880
1987	36,659	7060	1907	98,432
1988	40,545	7278	1845	106,009
1989	44,630	6982	1900	116,172

one that is attributed to living related donation can be conveyed by spousal donation. In fact, the improved health and well-being of the recipient may provide more tangible benefits within a household than that obtained by more distant family members. Thirdly, as the results of transplantation continue to improve, the expectation for success with living unrelated donors has never been better. There is little question that the net histoincompatibility in these donor-recipient pairs is as great as that of cadaveric transplant. However, the virtual elimination of donor warm ischemia, preservation injury, and the optimal condition of the recipient at the time of transplantation should potentiate the outcome. Indeed, 1-year patient and graft survival in excess of 90% has been reported by at least three centers using living unrelated donors (118–120).

While the arguments for the use of living unrelated donors may appear cogent, they bypass an important reality, namely, that the number of kidneys available for transplantation is far less than the predicted number of potential organ donors that exist. Bart et al. have estimated that between 50 and 100 donors per million population in the United States could be realized each year (121). Currently, only about 10–20% of this total are recovered. Therefore, some have argued, greater efforts in education and commitment to cadaver organ procurement should be undertaken, rather than a reliance on living unrelated donors (122). The latter are considered to be merely a solution of expedience and convenience, since the living unrelated donor would be subject to the same risk and uncertain long-term consequences of kidney donation as the living related donor. Perhaps the greatest concern raised over this type of medical intervention is the possibility for exploitation and commercialization of living organ procurement. Precisely these consideration have made the sale and trafficking of human organs and tissues illegal in the United States (Public Law 98–507) and have been decried by virtually every transplantation organization (123, 124).

In conclusion, the decision to use a living unrelated donor is not a trivial one and should be carefully individualized by any transplant unit considering this approach. While clearly not a panacea fo the global cadaver-organ shortage problem, it may have a role in highly selected circumstances. Those teams who wish to perform such procedures should make special efforts to ensure that proper informed consent has been obtained and that donor altruism is the predominant indication to proceed. Living unrelated transplantation will thus remain limited and should not interfere with the larger goal to expand cadaver organ procurement efforts.

PRETRANSPLANT EVALUATION OF THE POTENTIAL LIVING DONOR

The purpose of this evaluation is to uncover any prexisting renal disease or predilection for renal disease in the potential donor (Table 5). These patients are also screened for risk factors that would preclude a major surgical procedure such as donor nephrectomy. Not surprisingly, certain conditions may be identified that will not only lead to exclusion of the donor, but may require medical or surgical therapy for the donors' benefit. Therefore, prior to evaluation, every potential donor must be informed as to the nature of these studies and how the information will be used. It is important to maintain a strict doctor-patient relationship with donors and to accede to their requests for confidentiality. In addition, it is important to identify any diseases that could be transmitted from the donor to the recipient by the transplanted kidney.

Table 5. Pretransplant evaluation of potential living donor

1. General studies
  a. History and physical exam
  b. Pelvic exam with PAP smear
  c. Stool for occult blood
  d. CXR, EKG
2. Blood chemistry
  a. BUN, creatinine, electrolytes
  b. Total protein, albumin, uric acid
  c. SGOT, SGPT, bilirubin, LDH
  d. Cholesterol, triglycerides, FBS
  e. Ca, PO_4, alkaline phosphatase
3. Hematologic studies
  a. Cbc and differential
  b. PT, PTT, platelets
	4. Serology
	  a. CMV, VDRL
	  b. HIV
	  c. HB_s, Ag, HB_sAb, HB_cAg
	5. Tissue typing
	  a. ABO type
	  b. HLA A, B, C, Dr
	6. Urologic studies
	  a. Urinanalysis
	  b. Urine culture
	  c. 24-hour urine collection: creatinine clearance protein excretion
	7. Radiographic studies
	  a. Excretory urogram
	  b. Renal angiogram (standard or DSA)
	8. Special studies
	  Glucose tolerance test (diabetic families)

History and physical examination

Potential donors should be adults, age 18 or over, who are competent to give their own informed consent for renal donation. It is unusual that potential donors over age 65 would be suitable candidates (125). Donors should not have unexplained fevers, urinary tract infections, pyelonephritis, hematuria, or stone disease. Any history of urologic surgery should be documented. In general, donors with hypertension, diabetes, cardiovascular disease, or systemic illnesses involving the kidneys are excluded. Daily medications, nonprescription drug use, and allergy should be noted. The sexual history of the donor is recorded. They are reassured that renal donation will not alter present performance (126). Any abnormal physical findings should be explained.

Laboratory tests

Screening chemistry and hematologic studies should be consistent with a normal physiologic state. Abnormalities such as elevated liver transaminases or prolonged coagulation profiles should be further evaluated. Serologic studies and cultures are necessary to identify present and/or past exposure to transmissable diseases. Donors with a previously unknown history of exposure to venereal disease should be completely treated prior to consideration for renal donation. Potential donors who are infected with the hepatitis-B or human immunodeficiency virus should not donate organs or tissues (127). Donors with previous exposure to the CMV virus may place seronegative recipients at increased risk for primary CMV disease (128).

Renal function studies are essential and should be performed in triplicate. While no absolute criteria have been established, renal donors should have a creatinine clearance in excess of 80 cc/min. We have seen several donors, usually thin, middle-aged females, with a serum creatinine of 1.2–1.4 mg/dl, who have had a creatinine clearance under 60 cc/min. Such patients are excluded from donation. An inulin clearance or radionuclide determination of the glomerular filtration rate may be helpful in certain patients. The 24-hour urinary protein excretion should be less than 200 mg in adults. Patients with crystalluria on urinanlysis require metabolic stone evaluation.

Radiographic studies

The final piece to the donor evaluation confirms the anatomic integrity of the donor kidneys. An excretory urogram is performed initially to document two functioning renal units of generally normal size, shape, and position. Abnormalities, such as a solitary kidney, severe atrophy or scarring, stones, obstruction, a horse-shoe kidney, tumors, etc., would exclude renal donation. If the urogram is normal, an angiogram is done to identify the abdominal aorta, number, position, and patency of renal vessels and to further delineate the renal parenchyma. The introduction of digital subtraction angiography techniques has been reported to be a less-invasive alternative to standard catheter angiography in donor evaluation (129).

CADAVERIC DONORS

The majority of renal transplant recipients will not have a healthy, willing family donor and will therefore be candidates for a cadaveric kidney. A well-functioning cadaveric organ will provide the same opportunity for rehabilitation from ESRD as a live-donor organ. A major advantage of cadaveric transplantation is the absence of potential morbidity to a living donor. Complicating factors in cadaveric transplantation arise from the fact that organ availability is a random event, which makes this surgery nonelective in nature. Generally, kidneys can be preserved ex vivo for a maximum of 48–72 hours, but are preferably transplanted within 24 hours of removal. During this period of time, a previously evaluated and waiting recipient is identified and prepared for surgery. This may require transportation of the recipient or the organ across the country. An obligatory minimum period of 6–8 hours is required in order to tissue type the donor and perform specific cross-match tests to identify donor-directed cytotoxic antibody using sera from a number of waiting recipients of compatible ABO blood type.

In general, potential renal donors come from individuals who have suffered irreversible head trauma, cerebral vascular accidents, or anoxic brain injury. Preferably, they should be between 1 and 60 years of age. The continued shortage of cadaver kidneys has created a recent plea to consider the use of anencephalic fetuses as organ donors (130). Patients over age 60 usually have a degree of arteriolar nephrosclerosis, which can cause diminished renal function. However, in an otherwise healthy donor it would seem reasonable to use a kidney up to age 70 for potential recipients who are in the same age group.

One of the great uncertainties in cadaveric transplantation arises from an incomplete past medical history of the potential donor. This can be a special problem when the mortal injury has occurred far from the patient's home. It is always important to obtain a medical history, if possible, from an individual who has had recent contact with the donor. There should be no history of systemic diseases that involve the kidneys, such as hypertension, diabetes mellitus, autoimmune disease, etc. Patients with a history of malignant tumors other than localized brain or skin (not melanoma) tumors are not acceptable. There should be no history of transmissable infectious disease. It is probably best not to consider potential donors with a documented history of intravenous drug use, active homosexuals, or hemophiliacs requiring blood transfusions (131).

Organs for transplantation cannot be removed until the surviving family gives specific permission for this act and brain death has been declared. The act of donation is therefore completely dependent upon the good will and altruism of the public at large. The use of a signed donor card on the back of a driver license is not sufficient consent and has been of marginal value in increasing the donor supply. It is hoped that "required request" legislation, in which families of expired individuals must be informed of the possibility of organ donation by their attending physicians or his/her delegate, will expand the pool through greater public awareness (132). Such legislation has had a positive effect in the few states where it has already been enacted. In California the diagnosis of brain death requires strict medical criteria to be met and a signed declaration of death note by two physicians, neither of which can be a transplant team member. Brain death remains a clinical diagnosis (Table 6), but can be supported by other objective tests. Due to its ease of performance, we prefer an isotopic cerebral blood flow scan (133). Absence of flow is not compatible with a return of brain function.

Once declared brain dead and after family consent is obtained, the donor should be kept in a state as close to normal homeostasis as possible. Appropriate ventilatory support is required, and normothermia should be maintained. Blood transfusion is not routinely necessary, except in cases with ongoing hemorrhage. Quite often, donors are volume contracted and dehydrated (the appropriate management of brain injury), and must be resuscitated with fluids. Ringer's lactate is usually sufficient. In an effort to maintain systolic blood pressure over 100 mmHg, various

880 Therapy of Renal Diseases and Related Disorders

Table 6. Diagnosis of brain death

I. Clinical criteria
  a. Unresponsive to external stimuli:
     pain, sound, light, noxious, ice water calorics
  b. Absence of spontaneous breathing
  c. No cranial nerve function
  d. Above findings present with body temperature over 90°F
  e. Absence of CNS depressant drugs

II. Clinical criteria can be supported by
  a. Isoelectric electroencephalogram
  b. Lack of cerebral perfusion by angiogram or radioisotopic flow scan
  c. Absence of evoked potentials

pressors may be required. Dopamine, which maintains renal blood flow, is helpful. Urine output in adults should be maintained at over 1 ml/kg/hr. Frequently, donors may have massive urine output (> 500 ml/hr) due to diabetes insipidus, in which case vasopressin or similar agents can be used. The serum creatinine should be 1.5 mg/dl or less. A rising creatinine may be due to prolonged hypotension, which may cause irreversible renal ischemic injury. The maintenance of the donor prior to surgical nephrectomy is one of the most important factors that, contribute to immediate renal function after revascularization and minimizing ex-vivo preservation injury.

Cadaveric kidneys should be removed *enbloc* with the aorta and vena cava to prevent injury to kidneys with multiple renal vessels. Brain dead, heart-beating cadavers provide an excellent opportunity to procure organs with minimal warm ischemia in a good physiologic state. Once removed, kidneys are flushed with a hypothermic (4°C) electrolyte solution, which is hyperosmolar and mimics intracellular sodium and potassium concentrations (134), Ex-vivo renal preservation is hypothermic and is done by one of two methods. The majority of transplant centers in the United States now preserve kidneys using simple cold storage, with the organ immersed in the same flushing solution. An alternative preservation method utilizes continuous pulsatile perfusion with perfusates such as albumin or colloid solutions (135). The former method is simpler and cheaper, and is therefore preferred for preservation up to 48 hours. The latter method may be beneficial if extended preservation up to 72 hours is to be anticipated.

THE ROLE OF TISSUE TYPING

Histocompatibility has had an intimate relationship with transplantation since the elucidation of the ABO system by Landsteiner in the early 1900s (136). Today ABO compatibility is still important, as most renal transplants done across the ABO barrier result in early graft failure. Recent investigations have demonstrated that the A_2 subgroup, representing no more than 20% of blood group A patients, can be transplanted into recipients of blood group O (137). However, this remains an exception. In fact, most transplant centers group their patients awaiting cadaver transplantation according to their ABO type. The Rh antigen has no deleterious effect on renal allograft outcome and is not considered in determining donor suitability.

Unlike the strong impact of HLA on living related renal transplantation, tissue typing for the purpose of improving cadaver graft survival has produced variable results in different transplant centers. If possible, donor-recipient pairs should be identified in which there are no serologically defined mismatches at the HLA class I (A, B) and class II (Dr) loci. Prospective cadaver matching at the HLA D locus, which requires MLC testing, is of course not possible. However, due to the extreme polymorphism of the HLA alleles, it is very unlikely that two unrelated individuals will be identical for all six HLA antigens. During the past few years, zero mismatches have been uncommon in North America. Cicciarelli et al. report that among 15,000 first cadaver-kidney recipients accumulated by the UCLA Transplant Registry between 1982 and 1986, only 201 were zero HLA mismatches (138). They report that transfused, zero-mismatched recipients treated with cyclosporine had a 91% 1-year graft survival that was similar to LRD recipients. Comparable data has been reported by Gilks et al, using over 2200 kidney recipients from the United Kingdom Transplant Service (139). Both reports emphasize that there is little impact of typing when two to six HLA mismatches are present, therein creating a dilemma. Discrepancies among previous studies often involved differences in the number of mismatches, with very few zero-mismatched patients included.

A positive influence of tissue typing has been reported to be lasting, beyond 5 years after transplantation when azathioprine and prednisone immunosuppression was used (140–143). The majority of studies supporting the influence of tissue typing come from large multicenter data banks that represent several thousand patients. The advantages of such studies depend on large patient numbers, whereby small difference are statistically supported, and a sufficient number of very well-matched recipients can be included. The disadvantages of these reports are highlighted by multiple methods of patient selection, immunosuppression, and transplant practices (144). In addition, the use of univariate analysis for tissue typing has been questioned, considering the multifactorial influences on cadaver graft outcome. On the other hand, many single-center reports demonstrating little impact of tissue typing (86, 87, 145) cite consistent clinical management practices for all patients groups. However, these reports usually contain very few well-matched recipients, and small differences are usually statistically nonsignificant. Thus, many centers use HLA matching as a means to avoid the worst possible mismatches among recipients on their local waiting list.

The incorporation of cyclosporine into standard immunosuppressive regimens has added an additional variable to these considerations. The shipping of kidneys for the purpose of maximizing histocompatibility, which leads to prolonged preservation times, increased the likelihood of posttransplant acute tubular necrosis and cyclosporine nephrotoxicity (146). In fact, one study has reported that locally procured and utilized but poorly matched kidneys produce better results than well-matched but shipped kidneys when cyclosporine is utilized (147). These latter observations were usually made with very few zero-mismatched patients.

Thus, much of the controversy arises from comparisons between groups with a large number of HLA mismatches. Apparently even one class I or class II antigen mismatch will significantly diminish the matching effect (138, 139). This may be due to the ability of the immune system to recognize and target one antigen as effectively as several HLA antigens. If this is the case, then the goal of identifying zero-mismatched donor-recipient combinations will be very limited. It has been estimated that a given HLA-typed kidney (assuming six antigens can be identified) has a 19% probability of finding a zero-mismatched recipient if the recipient pool size is 10,000 (148). The probability falls to 6% for a pool size of 800 and 1.5% for a pool of 100 recipients. These figures emphasize the need for large recipient populations in order to maximize the opportunity to locate zero antigen mismatches.

The role of tissue typing then becomes one of regional and national policy. The previous arguments would favor a maximal effort to obtain zero-mismatched donor-recipient pairs. However, extensive transportation of organs with extended preservation times does not appear justified to offset the difference between two or four HLA mismatches. For a given transplant waiting list, tissue typing can then be incorporated into one of a number of factors that should be considered in cadaver kidney assignment. These would include, but are not limited to, the length of time on waiting list, number of transplants, level of cytotoxic antibody, blood group, unusual medical conditions, etc. An example of one such system was reported by the University of Pittsburg (149). At the present time, the sharing of zero-mismatched kidneys and the distribution of kidneys among transplant centers has been mandated by the United Network for Organ Sharing (UNOS), according to these principles.

VIRAL INFECTIONS

Viral illnesses represent the most common identifiable cause of infectious morbidity in renal transplant recipients. The spectrum of disease is broad, ranging from self-limited skin eruptions to life-threatening sepsis and multiorgan system failure. By far the most common offenders are the herpes viruses: cytomegalovirus (CMV), Epstein-Barr virus (EBV), herpes simplex virus (HSV), and varicella-zoster virus (VZV) (150). Each of these double-stranded DNA viruses share the property of latency, meaning they can exist in a dormant state within cells such as neural tissue, lymphocytes, and leukocytes. Recipients can experience primary infections due to new viral exposure or secondary infections due to reactivation of latent virus. Posttransplant immunosuppression and allograft rejection can lead to reactivation of latent virus. Primary infections are usually the more severe and are associated with overt clinical symptoms.

CMV is the most frequently encountered viral illness among renal transplant patients (54, 151). Primary infections can arise from viral transmission by blood products or more frequently from the allograft itself (152). In addition, recent evidence has been accumulated that a recipient previously infection with one CMV strain can acquire a second strain from the new allograft (153). The impact of CMV infection on patient and graft survival has been variable, but clearly represents a source of morbidity. Those centers that utilize higher doses of immunosuppression, especially polyclonal antilymphocyte preparations (ALG), experience a greater incidence of infection (154). Reports of newer protocols that utilize cyclosporine, lower steroid doses, and less ALG suggest a decrease in the incidence and severity of CMV disease (155).

These data suggest that a CMV-seronegative recipient should receive a CMV-seronegative kidney. This, however, is not possible in all circumstances, and it should be noted that a CMV-seropositive recipient at the time of transplant is not protected from post-transplant CMV disease. Any recipient receiving a CMV-seropositive donor kidney is at risk for some form of CMV disease, which should be considered in the differential diagnosis of any posttransplant febrile illness. The use of CMV immunoglobulin and the development of a specific CMV vaccine may diminish the impact of this agent in transplant recipients in the future (128). In addition, it has been demonstrated that the EBV can be transmitted by the donor kidney (157).

There has been little experience with human immunodeficiency virus (HIV) in transplant patients at the present time. The Center for Disease Control has established policy that no patient with evidence of antibody to HIV be used as an organ or tissue donor (127). Unfortunately, there may be a window of a few months in which a prospective donor has been infected with HIV but has no demonstrated antibody formation. For this reason we have elected not to use donors who have been documented to be in an established high-risk group for HIV infection. In addition, we have elected not to consider antibody-positive potential recipients for chronic immunosuppression. The natural history of asymptomatic antibody-positive uremic individuals on dialysis is presently not known (156).

REFERENCES

1. Levey AS, The improving prognosis after kidney transplantation: New strategies to overcome immunologic rejection. *Arch Intern Med* 144:2382–2387, 1984.
2. Terasaki PI, Perdue ST, Sasaki N, Mickey R, Whitley L: Improving success rates of kidney transplantation. *JAMA* 250:1065–1068, 1983.
3. Strom TB: The improving utility of renal transplantation in the management of end-stage renal disease. *Am J Med* 73:105–124, 1982.
4. End stage renal disease Network Coordinating Counsel, Program report. National Forum of End Stage Renal Disease Networks, 1989

5. Terasaki PI, Toyotome A, Mickey R, Iwaki Y, Cecka M, Tiwari J: Patient, graft, and functional survival rates. In: *Clinical Kidney Transplants*. University of California Press, Los Angeles, CA, pp 141–257, 1988
6. Flechner SM, Novick AC, Braun WE, Popowniak K, Steinmuller D: Functional capacity and rehabilitation of recipients with a functioning renal allograft 10 years or more. *Transplantation* 35:572–576, 1983.
7. Rosenbaum I, Atcherson E, Lorry, RJ: Rehabilitation and the transplant patient. *Dial Transplant* 10:136–140, 1981.
8. Devins GM, Binik YM, Hutchinson TA: The emotional impact of end-stage renal disease. Importance of patients perceptions of intrusiveness and control. *Int J. Psychiatry Med* 13:327–335, 1984.
9. Migliori RJ, Simmons R, Payne WD, Ascher N, Sutherland D, Najarian JS: Renal transplantation done safely without prior chronic dialysis therapy. *Transplantation* 43:51–55, 1987.
10. Hutchinson TA, Thomas DC, MacFibbon B: Predicting survival in adults with end-stage renal disease: An age equivalency index. *Ann Intern Med* 96:417–424, 1982.
11. Krakauer H, Grauman JS, McMullan MR, Creede CC: The recent U.S. experience in the treatment of end stage renal disease by dialysis and transplantation. *N Engl J Med* 308:1558–1562, 1983.
12. Vollmer WM, Wahl RW, Blagg CR: Survival with dialysis and transplantation in patients with end stage renal disease. *N Engl J Med* 308:1553–1557, 1983.
13. Hutchinson TA, Thomas DC, Lemieux JC, Harvey CE: Prognostically controlled comparison of dialysis and renal transplantation. *Kidney Int* 26:44–49, 1984.
14. Simmons RG, Kamstra-Hennen L, Thompson CR: Psychosocial adjustment 5–9 years post transplant. *Transplant Proc* 13:40–43, 1981.
15. Frisk B, Blohme I, Brynger H: The social rehabilitation and quality of life in patients living with kidney transplants for more than 10 years. *Scan J Urol Nephrol* 54:100–105, 1980.
16. Engelhardt HT: Allocating scarce medical resources and the availability of organ transplantation. *N Engl J Med* 311:66–71, 1984.
17. Jacobs C, Branner FP, Chantler C, Donckerwolcke RA, Gurland HJ, Hathaway R, Wing AJ: *Proc EDTA* 14:3–69, 1977.
18. Okiye SE, Engen DE, Sterioff S: Primary renal transplantation in patients 50 years of age and older. *Transplant Proc* 15:1046–1053, 1983.
19. Ost L, Lundgren G, Groth C: Renal transplantation in the older patient. In: P Morris, N Tilney, eds, *Progress in Transplantation*. Churchill-Livingstone, New York, pp 1–15, 1985.
20. Miller LC, Bock GH, Lum C, Najarian JS, Mauer SM: Transplantation of the adult kidney into the very small child. *J Pediatr* 100:675–680, 1982.
21. Helderman JH: The role of cardiovascular disease in renal transplantation. In: M Garovoy, R Guttmann, eds, *Renal Transplantation*. Churchill-Livingstone, New York, pp 209–232, 1986.
22. Moel DI, Butt K: Renal transplantation in children less than 2 years of age. *J Pediatr* 99:535–539, 1981.
23. Fletcher JC: Moral problems and ethical issues in the management of children with chronic renal failure. In: *Proceedings of Conference on Chronic Renal Disease: Unique problems of the child with renal failure*. National Institutes of Health, March 5–6, 1981.
24. Najarian SS, So K, Simmons R, Fryd D, Nevins T, Sutherland D, Payne W, Chavers B, Mauer S: The outcome of 304 primary renal transplants in children. *Ann Surg* 204:246–256, 1986.
25. So SK, Nevins T, Chang P, Mauer S, Ascher N, Fryd D, Simmons R, Najarian J: Preliminary results of renal transplantation in children under 1 year of age. *Transplant Proc* 17:182–183, 1985.
26. Fine R: Peritoneal dialysis in children. *J Pediatr* 100:1–4, 1982.
27. Penn I: Leukemias and lymphomas associated with the use of cytotoxic and immunosuppressive drugs. *Recent Results Cancer Res* 69:7–17, 1979.
28. Penn I: Renal transplantation in patients with pre-existing malignancies. *Transplant Proc* 15:1079–1082, 1983.
29. Matas AJ, Simmons R, Kjellstrand C, Buselmeier T, Johnson T, Najarian J: Successful renal transplantation in patients with prior history of malignancy. *Am J Med* 59:791–796, 1975.
30. Rubin RH, Wolfson JS, Cosimi AB, Rubin NT: Infection in the renal transplant patient. *Am J Med* 70:405–411, 1981.
31. Reyna J, Richardson J, Mattox D, Banowsky L, Lutton J: Head and neck infection after renal transplantation. *JAMA* 247:3337–3339, 1982.
32. Andrew OT, Schoenfeld P, Hopewell PC, Humphreys M: Tuberculosis in patients with end stage renal disease. *Am J Med* 68:59–65, 1980.
33. Jones RH, Weston M, Bewick M, Parsons V: Management of TB occurring in patients with chronic renal failure requiring dialysis or transplantation. In: *14th Congress Eur Dial Transplant Assoc*, Helsinki, p 241, 1977.
34. Flechner SM, Gow JG: Role of nephrectomy in treatment of nonfunctioning unilateral tuberculous kidney. *J Urol* 123:822–825, 1980.
35. Parfrey PS, Forbes R, Hutchinson TA, Beaudoin J, Hollomby D, Guttmann R: The clinical and pathological course of hepatitis B liver disease in renal transplant recipients. *Transplantation* 37:461–465, 1984.
36. Parfrey PS, Forbes R, Hutchinson T, Kenick S, Frarge D, Seely F, Guttman R: The impact of renal transplantation on the course of hepatitis B liver disease. *Transplantation* 38:610–615, 1985.
37. Pirson Y, Alexandre G, Ypersele de Strihou C: Longterm effect of HB_s antigenemia on patient survival after renal transplantation. *N Engl J Med* 296:194–198, 1977.
38. Weller IV, Bassendine M, Murray A, Crasi A, Thomas H, Sherlock S: Effects of prednisolone/azathioprine in chronic hepatitis B viral infection. *Gut* 23:650–656, 1982.
39. McLean RH, Geiger H, Burke B, Simmons R, Najarian J: Recurrence of membranoproliferative GN following kidney transplantation. *Am J Med* 60:60–65, 1976.
40. Droz D, Nabarra B, Noel L, Liebowitch J, Crosnier J: Recurrence of dense deposits in transplanted kidneys. *Kidney Int* 15:386–395, 1979.
41. Leumann EP, Briner J, Donckerwolke R, Kuijten R, Largiader F: Recurrence of FSGN in the transplanted kidney. *Nephron* 25:65–70, 1980.
42. Malekzadeh MH, Heuser E, Ettenger R, Pennisi A, Fine RB: Focal glomerulosclerosis and renal transplantation. *J Pediatr* 95:249–254, 1979.
43. Berger J, Yaneva H, Nabarra B, Barbanel C: Recurrence of mesangial deposition of IgA after renal transplantation. *Kidney Int* 7:232–241, 1975.
44. Hamburger J, Crosnier J, Noel L: Recurrent glomerulonephritis after renal transplantation. *Ann Rev Med* 29:67–72, 1978.

45. Cameron JS: Recurrent glomerulonephritis in allograft kidneys. *Clin Nephrol* 7:47, 1977.
46. Couser WG, Wallace A, Monaco AP, Lewis E: Successful renal transplantation in patients with circulating antibody to glomerular basement membrane. *Clin Nephrol* 1:381–388, 1973.
47. Briner J, Binswanger U, Largiader F: Recurrent and de novo membranous GN in renal cadaveric allografts. *Clin Nephrol* 13:189–196, 1980.
48. Steinmuller DR, Stilmant M, Idelson B, Monaco A, Lewis E, Davis R, Couser W: De novo development of membranous nephropathy in cadaver renal allografts. *Clin Nephrol* 9:210–218, 1978.
49. Friedman EA, L'Esperance F: *Diabetic Renal-Retinal Syndrome*. Grune and Stratton, New York, 1980.
50. Okiye S, Engen D, Steriolf S, Johnson W, Offord K, Zincke H: Primary and secondary renal transplantation in diabetics *JAMA* 249:492–495, 1983.
51. Haber W, Hoffken B, Frieling U, Ritz E: Professional training for the blind diabetic with nephropathy. *Diabetic Nephropathy* 4:88–92, 1985.
52. Najarian J, Sutherland D, Simmons R, Howard R, Kjellstrand C, Ramsay R, Goetz F, Sommer B: Ten year experience with renal transplantation in juvenile onset diabetics. *Ann Surg* 190:487–498, 1979.
53. Mamdani B: Recovery from prolonged renal failure in patients with accelerated hypertension. *N Engl J Med* 291:1343, 1974.
54. Peterson P, Balfour H, Marker S: CMV disease in renal allograft recipients: A prospective study of the clinical features, risk factors, and impact on renal transplantation. *Medicine* 59:283–300, 1980.
55. Kerman R, Flechner S, VanBuren C, Lorber M, Dawson G, Gutierrez R, Hollinger B, Kahan B: Investigation of HTLV-3 serology in a renal transplant population. *Transplantation* 43:24–248, 1987.
56. Kerman R, Kahan B: Immunological evaluation of transplant rejection. Pre and postoperative indices detecting immune responsiveness. *Ann Clin Res* 13:244–263, 1981.
57. Rolley RT, Widman D, Parks L, Steriolf S, Williams GM: Monitoring of responsiveness in dialysis-transplant patients by delayed cutaneous hypersensitivity tests. *Transplant Proc* 10:505–509, 1978.
58. Aldridge KE: Methicillin resistent staph aureus: Clinical and laboratory features. *Infection Control* 6:461–465, 1985.
59. Ibels LS, Mahony J, Sheil AGR: Deaths from occlusive arterial disease in renal allograft recipients. *Br Med J* 3:552–557, 1974.
60. Traeger J, Dubernard JM, Bosi E, Piatti P, Gelef A, Pozza G: Patient selection and risk factors in organ transplantation in diabetes. *Transplant Proc* 577–582, 1984.
61. Lorber MI, VanBuren C, Flechner S, Cameron L, Walker W, Smalling R, Kahan B: Pretransplant coronary arteriography for diabetic renal transplant recipients. *Transplant Proc* 19:1539–1541, 1987.
62. Braun W, Phillips D, Vidt D, Novick A: The course of coronary artery disease in diabetics with and without renal allografts. *Transplant Proc* 15:1114–1119, 1983.
63. Weinrauch L, D'Elia J, Healy R: Asymptomatic coronary artery disease: Angiography in diabetics before renal transplantation. *Ann Intern Med* 8:346–352, 1978.
64. Advisory Committee to the Renal Transplant Registry. The 13th Report of the Human Renal Transplant Registry. *Transplant Proc* 9:9–15, 1977.
65. Stuart FP, Reckard C, Schulak J, Ketel B: Gastroduodenal complications in kidney transplant recipients. *Ann Surg* 194:339–345, 1981.
66. Faro R, Corry R: Management of surgical GI complications in renal transplant recipients. *Arch Surg* 114:310–312, 1979.
67. Spanos PK: Peptic ulcer disease in the transplant recipient. *Arch Surg* 109:193, 1974.
68. Jarowenko MV, VanBuren C, Flechner S, Kramer W, Lorber M, Kahan B: Ranitidine, cimetidine, and the transplant kidney. *Transplantation* 42:311–312, 1986.
69. Demling R, Salvatierra O, Belzer F: Intestinal necrosis and perforation after renal transplantation. *Arch Surg* 110:251–253, 1975.
70. Guice K, Rattazi L., Marchioro J: Colon perforation in renal transplant patients. *Am J Surg* 138:43–48, 1979.
71. Bissada NK: Incidence of vesical neck contracture complicating prostatic resection in hemodialysis patients. *J. Urol* 00:192–193, 1977.
72. Peters PC: The management of renal transplant recipients with abnormal lower urinary tract — reconstruction vs. diversion. *Urol Clin North Am* 3:685–694, 1976.
73. Flechner S, Conley S, Brewer E, Benson G, Corriere J: Intermittent clean catheterizations. An alternative to diversion in continent transplant recipients. *J. Urol* 130:878–881, 1983.
74. Kogan S, Levitt S: Bladder evaluation in patients before undiversion in previously diverted urinary tracts. *J Urol* 118:443–446, 1977.
75. Stuart F, Reckard C, Ketel B, Schulak J: Effect of splenectomy on first cadaver kidney transplants. *Ann Surg* 192:553–560, 19 .
76. Fryd D, Sutherland D, Simmons R, Ferguson R, Kjellstrand C, Najarian J: Results of a prospective randomized study on the effect of splenectomy vs. no splenectomy in renal transplant patients. *Transplant Proc* 13:48–56, 1981.
77. Alexander JW, First M, Majeski J, Munda R, Fidler J, Suttman M: The late adverse effect of splenectomy on patient survival following cadaver renal transplantation. *Transplantation* 37:467–470, 1984.
78. Opelz G, Sengar D, Mickey R, Terasaki P: Effect of blood transfusions on subsequent kidney transplants. *Transplant Proc* 5:253–259, 1973.
79. Persijn G, Cohen B, Lansberger O, VanRood J: Retrospective and prospective studies on the effect of blood transfusions in renal transplantation in the Netherlands. *Transplantation* 28:396–401, 1979.
80. Fehrman I, Lundgren G, Moller E, Groth C: Cadaver graft survival: The bearing of the number of blood transfusions and of dialysis treatment. *Scand J Nephrol* 54:49–51, 1980.
81. Van Es A, Balner H: Effect of pretransplant transfusions and kidney transplantation. *Transplant Proc* 11:127–137, 1979.
82. Opelz G, Terasaki P: Improvement in kidney graft survival with increased numbers of blood transfusions. *N Engl J Med* 299:799–803, 1978.
83. Singal DP, Joseph S, Szewczuk M: Possible mechanisms of the beneficial effect of pretransplant blood transfusions on renal allograft survival in man. *Transplant Proc* 14:316–318, 1982.
84. Fagnilli L, Singal D: Blood transfusions may induce anti-T-cell receptor antibodies in renal patients. *Transplant Proc* 14:319–322, 1982.
85. Perdue S, Terasaki P: The transfusion effect in renal allograft recipients. *Proceedings of 11th International Congress of Nephrology*. 11:1674–1679, 1984.
86. Kahan B, VanBuren C, Flechner S, Payne W, Kerman P:

Cyclosporine immunosuppression mitigates immunological risk factors in renal allotransplant patients. *Transplant Proc* 15:2463–2477, 1983.
87. Lundgren G, Albrechtsen D, Flatmark A, et al.: HLA matching and pretransplant blood transfusion in cadaveric renal transplantation — changing picture with CSA. *Lancet* 1:66–69, 1986.
88. Opelz G: Improved kidney graft survival in nontransfused recipients. *Transplant Proc* 19:149–152, 1987.
89. Groth C: There is no need to give blood transfusions for renal transplantation in the CSA era. *Transplant Proc* 19:153–154, 1987.
90. Kerman R, VanBuren C, Lewis R, Kahan B: Successful transplantation of 100 untransfused cyclosporine treated primary recipients of cadaver renal allografts. *Transplantation* 45:37–40, 1988.
91. Flechner SM, Kerman R, VanBuren C, Kahan B: Successful transplantation of cyclosporine treated haploidentical living related recipients without blood transfusions. *Transplantation* 37:73–76, 1984.
92. Eschbach J, Egrie J, Downing M, Browne J, Adamson J: Correction of the anemia of ESRD with recombinant human erythropoietin. *N Engl J Med* 316:73–78, 1987.
93. The impact of routine HTLV-3 antibody testing of blood and plasma donors on Public Health. NIH Consensus Conference. *JAMA* 256:1778–1783, 1986.
94. Hoofnagle JH, Alter H: Chronic non A — non B hepatitis: In: RY Dodd, LF Barker, eds, *Progress in Clinical and Biomedical Research. Infection, Immunity, and Blood Transfusion.* Alan R Liss, New York, pp 63–69, 1985.
95. Terasaki P, Perdue S, Ayoub G: Reduction of accelerated failures by transfusions. *Transplant Proc* 14:251–259, 1982.
96. Koop CE: Increasing the supply of solid organs for transplantation. *Public Health Rep* 98:566–572, 1983.
97. Cochrum KC, Salvatierra O, Belzer F: Correlation between MLC stimulation and graft survival in living related and cadaver transplants. *Ann Surg* 1801:617–622, 1974.
98. Murray J, Merrill J, Harrison J: Renal homotransplantation in identical twins. *Surg Forum* 6:432–435, 1955.
99. Tilney NL: Renal transplantation between identical twins: A review. *World J Surg* 10:381–388, 1986.
100. Flechner SM, Kerman R, VanBuren C, Lorber M, Barker C, Kahan B: Does CSA improve the results of HLA-identical renal transplantation? *Transplant Proc* 19:1485–1488, 1987.
101. Flechner SM, Kerman R, Van Buren C, Epps L, Kahan BD: The use of CSA in living related renal transplantation. *Transplantation* 38:685–691, 1984.
102. Leivstad T, Albrechtsen D, Flatmark A, Thorsby E: Renal transplants from HLA haploidentical living related donors. *Transplantation* 42:35–38, 1986.
103. Sommer BG, Ferguson R: Mismatched living related renal transplantation: A prospective randomized study. *Surgery* 98:269–275, 1985.
104. Cochrum K, Hanes D, Potter D, Vincent F, Amend W, Perkins H, Salvatierra O: Donor specific blood transfusions in HLA-D disparate one haplotype related allografts. *Transplant Proc* 11:1903–1907, 1979.
105. Salvatierra O, Vicenti F, Amend W, Garovoy M, Iwaki Y, Terasaki P, Potter D, Duca R, Hopper S, Feduska N: 4 year experience with donor specific blood transfusions. *Transplant Proc* 15:924–931, 1983.
106. Simmons RG: Long term reactions of renal recipients and donors. In: NB Levey ed, *Psychonephrology 2: Psychological Problems in Kidney Failure and their Treatment.* Plenum Press, New York, pp 275–287, 1983.
107. Marshall J, Fellner C: Kidney donors revisited. *Am J Psychiatry* 134:575–576, 1977.
108. Madsen vs. Harrison (1957). Massachussetts Supreme Judicial Court Equity number 68651.
109. Santiago EA, Simmons R, Kjellstrand C, Buselmeier T, Najarian J: Life insurance prospective for the living kidney donor. *Transplantation* 14:131–133, 1972.
110. Merrill JP: Moral problems of artificial and transplanted organs letter. *Ann Intern Med* 61:355–364, 1964.
111. Leary F, DeWeerd J: Living donor nephrectomy *J Urol* 109:947–951, 1973.
112. Weiland D, Sutherland D, Chavers B, Simmons R, Ascher N, Najarian J: Information on 628 living related kidney donors at a single institution with longterm follow up on 472 cases. *Transplant Proc* 16:5–7, 1984.
113. Brenner B, Meyer T, Hostetter T: Dietary protein intake and the progressive nature of kidney disease. *N Engl J Med* 307: 652–659, 1982.
114. Vincenti F, Amend W, Kaysen G, Feduska N, Duca R, Salvatierra O: Longterm renal function in Kidney donors. *Transplantation* 36:626–659, 1984.
115. Dunn J, Nylander W, Richie R, Johnson K, Sawyers J: Living related kidney donors. *Ann Surg* 203:637–642, 1986.
116. Robitaille P, Lortie L, Mongean J, Sinnassamy P: Longterm followup of patients who underwent unilateral nephrectomy in childhood. *Lancet* 1:1297–1299, 1985.
117. Levey A, Hou S, Bash H: Sounding board: Kidney transplantation from unrelated living donors *N Engl J Med* 314:914–916, 1986.
118. Sodal G, Albrechtsen D, Berg K, Bondevik H, Brekke I, Talseth T, Thorsby E, Flatmark A: Renal transplantation from living donors mismatched for two HLA haplotypes. *Transplant Proc* 19:1509–1510, 1987.
119. Belzer F, Kalayoglu M, Sollinger H: Donor specific transfusion in living unrelated renal donor-recipient combinations. *Transplant Proc* 19:1514–1517, 1987.
120. Kumar M, White A, Samhan M, Abouna G: Nonrelated living donors for renal transplantation *Transplant Proc* 19:1515–1517, 1987.
121. Bart KJ, Macon E, Humphreys A: Increasing the supply of cadaveric kidneys for transplantation. *Transplantation* 31:383–387, 1981.
122. Kries H: Why living related donors should not be used whenever possible. *Transplant Proc* 17:1510–1514, 1985.
123. Council of the Transplantation Society: Commercialization in transplantation: The problems and some guidelines for practice. *Lancet* 2:715–716, 1985.
124. Carpenter C, Ettinger R, Strom T: "Free market" approach to organ donation. *N Engl J Med* 310:395–396, 1984.
125. Askari A, Novick A, Braun W, Steinmuller D: The older living related donor: Prognosis for the donor and recipient. *J Urol* 129:779–780, 1980.
126. Buszta C, Steinmuller D, Novick A, Schreiber M, Strum S, Steinhilber D, Braun W: Pregnancy after donor nephrectomy. *Transplantation* 40:651–654, 1985.
127. Testing donors of organs, tissues, and semen for antibody to HTLV-3. *MMWR* 34:294, 1985.
128. Snydman DR, Werner B, Lacey B, et al.: Use of CMV immune globulin to prevent CMV disease in renal transplant recipients. *N Engl J Med* 317:1049–1054, 1988.
129. Flechner, SM, Sandler C, Houston G, VanBuren C, Lorber M, Kahan B: 100 living related kidney donor evaluations using DSA. *Transplantation* 40:675–679, 1985.
130. Harrison M: Organ procurement for children: Anencephalic

fetus as donor. *Lancet* 2:1383–1385, 1986.
131. Feduska N, Perkins H, Melzer J, Amend W, Vincenti F, Garovoy M, Salvatierra O: Observations relating to the incidence of AIDS in a large population of renal transplant recipients. *Transplant Proc* 19:2161–2166, 1987.
132. Izenson S: Required request laws. A successful state approach to meet the increasing need for cadaver kidneys. *Contemp Dial Nephrol* 00:54–58, 1987.
133. Schwartz J, Baxter J, Bull D, Burns R: Radionuclide cerebral imaging confirming brain death. *JAMA* 249:246–247, 1983.
134. Collins G, Bravo-Sugarman M, Terasaki P: Kidney preservation for transplantation: Initial perfusion and 30 hour ice storage. *Lancet* 2:1219–1222, 1969.
135. Belzer F, Kountz S: Preservation and transplantation of human cadaver kidneys. A 2 year experience. *Ann Surg* 172:394–399, 1970.
136. Landsteiner R, Levine P: On the inheritance of agglutinogens of human blood demonstrable by immune agglutinins. *J Exp Med* 48:731–740, 1928.
137. Brynger H, Blohme I, Lindholm A, Rydberg L, Sandberg L: Transplantation of cadaver kidneys from blood group A_2 donors. *Transplant Proc* 14:195–000, 1982.
138. Cicciarelli J, Terasaki P, Mickey R: The effect of zero HLA class I and II mismatching in cyclosporine treated kidney transplant patients. *Transplantation* 43:636–640, 1987.
139. Gilks W, Bradley B, Gore S, Klouda P: Substantial benefits of tissue matching in renal transplantation. *Transplantation* 43:669–674, 1987.
140. Festenstein H, Doyle P, Holmes J: Longterm followup in London transplant group recipients of cadaver renal allografts. *N Engl J Med* 314:7–13, 1986.
141. Persijn G, Hendricks G, VanRood J: HLA matching, blood transfusions, and renal transplantation. *Clin Immunol Allergy* 4:535–565, 1984.
142. Sanfilippo F, Vaughn W, Spees E, Light J, Lefor W: Benefits of HLA A and B matching on graft and patient outcome after cadaver kidney transplantation. *N Engl J Med* 311:358–364, 1984.
143. Opelz G: Correlation of HLA matching with kidney graft survival in patients with or without cyclosporine. *Transplantation* 40:240–243, 1985.
144. Opelz G, Mickey M, Terasaki P: HLA matching and cadaver kidney transplant survival in North America: Influence on center variation and presensitization. *Transplantation* 23:490–497, 1977.
145. Harris K, Gosling D, Campbell M, Sharman V, Digard N, Tate G, Slapak M: Azathioprine and cyclosporine: Different tissue matching criteria needed. *Lancet* 2:802–804, 1985.
146. Salaman J, Ross W: Exchanging Kidney transplants — is it worth it? *Lancet* 1:1480–1481, 1987.
147. Alexander JW, Vaughn W, Pfaff W: Local use of kidneys with poor HLA matches is as good as shared use with good matches in the cyclosporine era. *Proc ASTS* 12:25, 1986.
148. Baur M, Neugebauer M, Albert E: Reference tables of two haplotype frequencies for all MHC marker loci. In: E Albert, M Baur, W Mayr, eds, *Histocompatibility Testing 1984*. Springer, New York, pp 677, 1984.
149. Starzl T, Hakala T, Tzakis A, Gordon R, Stieber A, Makowka L, Klimoski J, Bahnson H: A multifactorial system for equitable selection of cadaver kidney recipients. *JAMA* 257:3073–3075, 1987.
150. Rubin R, Tolkoff-Rubin N: Viral infection in the renal transplant patient. *Proc EDTA* 19:513–520, 1982.
151. Glenn G: CMV infection following renal transplantation. *Rev Inf Dis* 3:1151–1178, 1981.
152. Betts R, Freeman R, Douglas R: Transmission of CMV infection with the renal allograft. *Kidney Int* 8:385–390, 1975.
153. Chou S: Aquisition of donor strains of CMV by renal transplant recipients. *N Engl J Med* 314:1418–1422, 1986.
154. Simmons RL, Lopez C, Balfour H: CMV: Clinical, virological correlations in renal transplant recipients. *Ann Surg* 180:623–634, 1974.
155. Bia M, Andima W, Gaudio K: Effect of treatment with CSA vs. azathioprine on incidence and severity of CMV infection post transplant. *Transplantation* 40:610–614, 1985.
156. Peterman T, Lang G, Mikes N, Solomon S, Schable C, Britz J, Allen J: HTLV-3 infection in hemodialysis patients. *JAMA* 255:2324–2326, 1986.
157. Denning D, Weiss LM, Martinez K, Flechner, SM: Transmission of EBV by a transplanted kidney with activation by OKT3 antibody. *Transplantation* 48:141–144, 1989.

CHAPTER 57

Immunosuppression and Treatment of Rejection

YVES F.CH. VANRENTERGHEM

INTRODUCTION

When a kidney is transplanted in a recipient other than a monozygous twin, antigenic disparity between the donor and the recipient will elicit a cascade of immunologic reactions, resulting in progressive damage and ultimate loss of the grafted kidney unless some form of immunosuppression is given. New insights into the immunologic events involved in the recognition and response to the histocompatibility or transplantation antigens has led to a better understanding of the action of various immunosuppressive agents and constitute a basis for a more rational use of these agents in clinical transplantation.

In the first part of this chapter the mechanisms whereby an allograft is recognized and rejected, and how the immunosuppressive agents currently in use in clinical practice interfere with these mechanisms, will be briefly reviewed.

THE ALLOGRAFT RESPONSE

T lymphocytes play a pivotal role in the recognition and response to transplantation antigens, of which Class I and Class II HLA-antigens are the most important (Figure 1). Class I antigens can be found on the cell membrane of almost all nucleated cells, while Class II antigens have a more restricted tissue distribution and are present on B lymphocytes, monocytes, and dendritic cells (1). Recent studies have, however, shown that both Class I and Class II antigens have a dynamic tissue distribution and that their expression on the cell membrane can be upregulated or downregulated by various regulatory mechanisms (2).

Class II antigens, such as HLA-DR, are responsible for the initiation of the immune response and are recognized by T-helper lymphocytes (T4 cells, now called CD4 positive cells) (1). Upon activation these lymphocytes release lymphokines, including macrophage stimulating factor (identical to gamma-interferon?), which stimulates the production of interleukin 1 (IL1) by macrophages (3). Class I antigens are usually recognized by cytotoxic T lymphocytes (T8 cells, now called CD8 positive cells), which upon activation develop interleukin 2 (IL2) receptors (4).

IL1 stimulates the release of IL2 activated T-helper lymphocytes (5). This IL2 interacts with specific IL2 receptors on both activated CD4 and CD8 positive cells. The interaction between IL2 and these cells results in clonal proliferation of these cells. IL2 also stimulates the release of gamma interferon, which activates macrophages, and of B-cell growth factor, which stimulates the proliferation of B lymphocytes (6). Gamma interferon enhances the expression of Class II antigens on cells that constitutively express these antigens, and it induced de-novo expression in negative cells. In addition, the expression of Class I antigens is enhanced by gamma interferon (2). Parenchymal cells of the normal kidney, like those of most other organs, have little or no constitutional Class I expression. Lymphocyte-stimulated expression of these HLA antigens will make them more vulnerable to cytotoxic cells.

Both delayed-type hypersensitivity (mainly mediated by CD4 positive cells) and cytotoxic responses (mediated by CD8 positive cells), as well as antibody-mediated responses, play a role (7) in the destruction of the allogenic tissue. Direct cytolysis can occur either by CD4 positive cells, which attach to cells bearing Class II antigens, and CD8 positive cells, which attach to Class I antigen bearing targets (7). In normal tissue, the target for CD4 positive cells would be restricted to tissue macrophages, dendritic cells, B lymphocytes, and vascular endothelium. In rejecting tissue, somatic cells will gain a marked Class II expression, making them more vulnerable to cytolytic attack (2, 7).

In addition to direct and specific cytolysis by T lymphocytes, unspecific delayed hypersensitivity reactions also help in the destruction of the rejected tissue, as the release of lymphokines by the effector lymphocytes will recruit and activate monocytes and macrophages (7).

SITE OF INTERACTION OF THE CURRENTLY USED IMMUNOSUPPRESSIVE AGENTS

Corticosteroids

Since the early studies of Billingham and Medawar with skin grafts in rabbits (8), later confirmed by many other

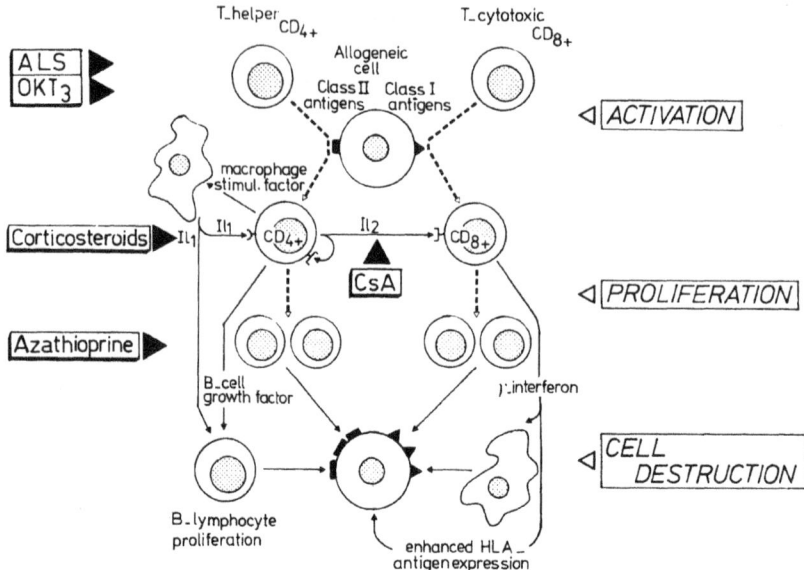

Figure 1. Schematic representation of the mechanisms whereby an allograft is recognized and rejected and how immunosuppressive agents interfere with these mechanisms.

studies, it is well known that, for maximal suppression, glucocorticosteriods should be present at the initiation of the immune response. Over the last years it has become clear that corticosteroids primarily act on IL1 production early in the induction phase of T-cell activation. Secondary to its effect on IL1 production, IL2 release will also be affected. In addition, corticosteroids will also affect the expression of Class II antigens on human lymphocytes, probably via their effect on gamma-interferon production (9, 10).

In addition to their inhibitory effect on lymphokine production early in the activation of the T lymphocyte, corticosteroids have a lot of other effects on the immune system. Corticosteroids induce a rapid sequestration of lymphocytes and monocytes in the extravascular pool, thereby protecting the graft against further invasion with cytotoxic T cells and macrophages (9). This effect on lymphocyte and moncyte circulation kinetics may also explain their beneficial effect on an ongoing rejection. Furthermore, much of their immunosuppressive properties are attributable to their antiinflammatory properties (11).

Cyclosporin

Cyclosporin appears to have a more restricted site of action on the immune system than corticosteroids. Like corticosteroids, cyclosporin interferes with the activation phase of lymphocytes, and its predominant effect is on the T-helper lymphocyte. Cyclosporin blocks the release of IL2 from activated T-helper cells, probably at the transcriptional level of IL2 production (12). In contrast to steroids, cyclosporin does not block the release of IL1 by macrophages. As the release of other lymphokines is IL2 dependent, cyclosporin will also affect the release of other lymphokines, such as gamma interferon, by activated T lymphocytes. Furthermore, it became rapidly obvious that cyclosporin does not interfere with the activation and the proliferation of suppressor T lymphocytes (13). Because of its selective effect on T lymphocytes, cyclosporin has no effect on bone marrow elements nor on T-cell-independent antibody synthesis.

Azathioprine

The immunosuppressive effect of azathioprine is mainly via its hepatic metabolite, 6-mercaptopurine. 6-mercaptopurine is a structural analogue of the purine base hypoxanthine and, therefore, interferes with purine biosynthesis, killing all dividing cells in the G_1 phase of the cell cycle (14, 15). As antigen recognition and stimulation of lymphocytes causes rapid cell division of helper and cytotoxic T lymphocytes, azathioprine will reduce the proliferation of these activated cells. On the other hand, as the antiproliferative effect of azathioprine is not restricted to lymphocytes, all other rapidly dividing cells will also be affected, often resulting in generalized bone marrow depression.

Antilymphocyte serum (ALS)

The immunosuppressive property of ALS lies in its gamma-globulin 7S-fraction, which is usually prepared by precipitation or chromatographic purification of heterologous serum from horses or rabbits immunized with human lymphocytes, thymocytes, or cultered lymphoblasts (16). The antibodies are directed against the surface antigens of the injected lymphoid cells. Although some of these antigens are unique for T lymphocytes, most of them are also present on other tissues. This explains why polyclonal ALS contains antibodies directed not only against T lymphocytes, but also directed against B lymphocytes and even nonlymphoid cells. The antibody-coated lymphocytes may bind complement, leading to complement activation and cell lysis. They also undergo opsonization and are removed from the circulation by the monocytic-phagocytic system.

Although depletion of recirculating long-living thymus-dependent lymphocytes may play an important role in the immunosuppressive effect of ALS (17), the peripheral lymphopenia is, however, transient, and there is no quantitative correlation between the immunosuppressive activity and the peripheral lymphocyte count (18). Evidence has been gained that the immunosuppressive effect of ALS is at least in part mediated by the induction of suppressor T lymphocytes (19, 20).

Monoclonal antibodies

The major disadvantages of polyclonal ALS (lack of specificity and variability in immunosuppressive activity) are avoided by using monoclonal antibodies. There antibodies are produced by a hybridoma cell line formed by fusion of the myeloma cell clone and the specific subclass of human lymphocytes against which the antibody should be directed. This technique alllows the production of antibodies with well-defined specificity against those subpopulations of lymphocytes responsible for graft rejection (helper or cytotoxic cells) while sparing suppressor cells. Up to now only antibodies directed against all T lymphocytes (pan-T-antibodies such as OKT3 and anti-T12) were available for clinical use. OKT3 antibodies react with the T3 antigen recognition structure of T lymphocytes (21). Administration of OKT3 results in an early and total disappearance of circulating T lymphocytes bearing the T3 antigen on their cell surface (both CD4 and CD8 positive lymphocytes bear the T3 antigen) (22). Binding of the OKT3 antibody to the T3 receptor results in the suppression of all T3 cell functions (22). This dramatic effect on T3 lymphocytes explains the potent effect of OKT3 on an acute allograft rejection. With cessation of the administration of OKT3, normally functioning T3 positive cells rapidly reappear in the circulation, explaining the high incidence of recurrent rejections after cessation of the therapy.

Total lymph node irradiation (TLI)

Lymphocytes, particularly the small T lymphocytes, are one of the most radiosensitive cells of the mammalian organism and are killed by only small doses of ionizing radiation (23). Total body irradiation used in the early years of transplantation has been abandoned because of its serious side effects. Local graft irradiation has been used in many centers to treat acute rejection crises. As the favorable effect of local graft irradiation could never be substantiated in a controlled trial, most centers have also abandoned this technique (24).

During the last few years there has been renewed interest in the use of ionizing radiation, since it became obvious from Hodgkin's patients that TLI has profound immunosuppressive effects in humans (25). Most experimental work performed today with regard of the mechanisms of action of TLI points at the pivotal role of suppressor-cell induction (26). TLI also induces a striking and long lasting inversion of the ratio between T helper/inducer (CD4 positive) cells over T suppressor/cytotoxic (CD8 positive) cells. This is due to a decrease of the number of CD4 positive cells after TLI and to a rapid and supranormal recovery of CD8 positive cells early after TLI (27).

From the foregoing it is obvious that several possible approaches to immunosuppression after kidney transplantation exist appart from the "conventional" therapy with corticosteroids and azathioprine, which has been the mainstay of clinical immunosuppression for more than 20 years. The possibility of switching from one approach to another or of combining different protocols in case of inefficiency or toxicity is a major step forward in clinical transplantation. In the next section some of the practical problems with the use of these protocols will be described.

THE "CONVENTIONAL" APPROACH: AZATHIOPRINE AND CORTICOSTEROIDS

High-versus low-dose corticosteroids

Up to 1980 almost all centers used high doses of corticosteroids during the first weeks after transplantation. These high doses of steroids often resulted in a high mortality and a significant morbidity such as steroid-induced diabetes, avascular bone necrosis, cushingoid appearance, and severe infectious complications. In 1980 McGeown from Belfast first showed that excellent results could be obtained with low doses of corticosteroids (20 mg prednisone daily for the first 6 months together with azathioprine 1.5 mg/kg/day) (28). The uncontrolled Belfast results were subsequently confirmed by a lot of controlled trials, but as reviewed by Gore and Oldhan (29), authoritative conclusions about the safety of the low-dose regime cannot yet been given. In several of these studies, higher doses of steroids (up to three times higher) were used, and in same groups additional pulses of intravenous steroids were given (30). Furthermore, not all authors were able to confirm the optimistic Belfast results. In some subgroups of patients a significantly higher graft loss was seen in the low-dose group (31). In the study of d'Apice, low-dose steroids were only safe in the subgroup of patients who received at least 1.75 mg/kg/day of azathioprine (31). It is also important to note that in most of these trials the 1-year graft survival was as low as 50–60%, a figure that is substantially lower than the 89% 1-year graft survival that is obtained with a high-dose prednisone protocol together with prophylactic ALG (32).

In determination of the corticosteroid dose, especially for long-term maintenance therapy, the concomitant administration of drugs that may influence the bioavailability of corticosteroids should be considered. Drugs causing induction of microsomal enzymes in the liver, such as phenytoin, barbiturates, and rifampicine, can shorten the half-life of prédnisolone (33–35). The increased prednisolone clearance shown in patients taking anticonvulsive drugs (36) may explain the lower graft survival described in these patients (37). It is therefore advisable to give slightly higher doses of maintenance corticosteroids to patients taking these drugs.

Time of administration

Little attention has been paid to the time of the day at which corticosteroids are taken. However, a significantly lower graft failure has been found in patients taking immunosuppressives twice daily than in those taking all immunosuppressive drugs in the evening (38). It is also of interest to note that McGeown's patients all took steroids once daily in the morning (28). Endogenous cortisol secretion is highest in the early morning, and adrenopituitary suppression is minimal when steroids are taken in the morning (39). It has also been shown that the immunosuppressive effect of methylprednisolone is prolonged when given close to the transition from sleep to activity (40, 41). We advise the administration of a single morning dose, especially when low daily maintenance doses of steroids are given.

Choice of steroids

For oral administration, prednisone, prednisolone, and methylprednisolone have been used. Prednisone and prednisolone are rapidly absorbed and reach a peak plasma concentration after 1–3 hours. Prednisone is converted to prednisolone in the liver (42). Although the bioavailability of prednisolone after oral prednisone is approximately 80% of that after prednisolone, in subjects with hepatic dysfunction the plasma levels will be more variable (43). This could be a reason for preferring prednisolone over prednisone, especially in patients with liver dysfunction. However, a wide intersubject variation in prednisolone concentration is still seen even after prednisolone (42). A prospective double-blind crossover study comparing oral prednisone and methylprednisolone could not demonstrate any difference in the immunosuppressive capability of both drugs (44). In an attempt to reduce the risk of peptic ulcerations, the use of enteric-coated tablets has been suggested. As the absorption of prednisolone from these tablets is very variable (45) and as peptic ulcerations can now easily be prevented by prophylactic use of H_2-receptor antagonists (46), the use of these enteric-coated tablets is not recommended. Dexamethasone does not appear to be suitable for maintenance immunosuppression (47).

Alternate-day steroid therapy

It has been shown in the past that alternate-day steroid therapy is as effective as daily therapy in controlling the activity of several diseases, such as asthma, rheumatoid arthritis, nephrotic syndrome, etc., and alternate-day therapy has a substantially lower incidence of side effects (48). A theoretic basis for at least one of the advantages of alternate-day therapy has been given by Dale et al., who showed that alternate-day prednisone administration reduced the neutrophil response to inflammation considerably less than daily administration (49). On the "on" day, both monocyte and neutrophil accumulation were decreased, whereas on the "off" day, monocyte but not neutrophil accumulation was decreased. Early uncontrolled studies on mostly living, related transplant recipients were enthusiastic, indicating a substantial reduction of several side effects, such as hypertension, Cushing, obesity, contaract, and growth retardation without a higher risk of rejection and renal function impairment (50–54). Two studies emphasized the potential risks of precipitating rejection (55, 56). This could not be confirmed by the controlled study of McDonald et al. in 1976 (57). These authors were not able to confirm the previously claimed benefits. Of these benefits only the lower incidence of hypertension reached statistically significance in the recently published controlled trial by De Vecchi et al. in 91 cadaver kidney recipients with a mean followup of 44 months (58). The most important benefit of alternate-day therapy seems to be an accelerated growth rate in children, where the risks of renewed rejection can outweigh the benefits of improved growth. Alternate-day therapy is not effective in reversing acute rejection (50).

Discontinuance of corticosteroid therapy

Anecdotal reports in the past have shown that, as in animals, kidney transplants in humans can survive following withdrawal of all immunosuppressive treatment (59, 60). However, a retrospective survey of 165 United States renal transplant units showed that of the 32 living, related grafts, 12 failed within a mean of 234 days after cessation of all immunosuppressants. Of the 16 cadaveric grafts, nine failed within a mean of 59 days (61). The data are consistent with the findings of other (62–64) and suggest that it is not prudent to stop both azathioprine and corticosteroids in kidney allograft recipients.

The question of whether corticosteroids can be stopped in patients under continued azathioprine therapy is also not yet resolved. Although this can be done more safely in recipients of HLA-identical sibling transplants (65), studies dealing with only cadaver kidney recipients have been less optimistic. Turcotte et al. found that a daily dose of < 17.5 mg/day is associated with an increasing number of rejections (66). Thaysen and Lokkegaard demonstrated that rejection occurred in 9 of 43 patients with a daily dose of prednisone of < 10 mg (67). These authors also found that when rejections occurred, they were more severe, leading to irreversible destruction of the graft.

It is not yet clear to what extent complications that are already present, such as cataracts and avascular necrosis, can be favorably influenced by a further reduction of a low maintenance steroid dose. In the study of Naik et al., antihypertensive therapy could be reduced after a reduction of the maintenance steroid dose (64) in only 3 of 8 patients receiving antihypertensive medication. Antihypertensive drugs could be stopped in 6 of the 9 patients in the study of Steinman (68).

Based on these data, we use prednisone at a dose at 12.5 mg/day until the end of the fifth post-transplant year. Afterwards prednisone is tapered to 10 mg/day but only in these patients who can tolerate a daily dose of at least 1.5 mg/kg of azathioprine.

Discontinuation of azathioprine therapy

Several patients have been described in whom azathioprine was omitted without subsequent deterioration of renal function. When rejection did occur afterwards, it could be easily controlled with methylprednisolone alone (69–73). Reports from other authors have warned that withdrawal of azathioprine might be dangerous for the survival of the allograft (62, 74–76). In view of these conflicting data, it should be emphasized that in most patients in which azathioprine was withdrawn (except in 15 of the 23 patients in Sheriff's study) (69), azathioprine was stopped because of leukopenia, hepatotoxicity, severe infections, or intercurrent malignancies.

Side effects of "conventional" immunosuppression

The side effects of the standard azathioprine-corticosteroid regimen are numerous and well known. Since the initial high doses of corticosteroids were abandoned, early mortality due to infectious and/or gastrointestinal complications has been significantly reduced. Even the short-term courses of high doses of corticosteroids used to treat acute rejection episodes can still result in the occurrence of avascular bone necrosis, while long-term administration of low doses of steroids is associated with a lot of side effects, such as diabetes, cataracts, and skin bruisability. As mentioned earlier, alternate-day prednisone therapy has been advocated to adminish these long-term side effects.

The main toxic effect of azathioprine is on the bone marrow, leading to leukopenia, thrombocytopenia, and anemia. Leukopenia is seen in almost 20% of kidney transplant recipients, most frequently during the first month of therapy (78). Renal function impairment, viral infections, and association with other drugs such as allopurinol (79) and trimethoprim-sulfamethoxazole (80, 81) may enhance bone marrow toxicity. Eosinophilia may precede granulocytopenia (82). Chronic administration of azathioprine can lead to progressive bone marrow depression with leukopenia, thrombopenia, and anemia. In these cases, conversion to cyclosporin can be tried (83).

Although azathioprine has been shown to be hepatotoxic in experimental animals (84), its pathogenic role in the hepatic dysfunction so often seen in human kidney allograft recipients is controversial (85). Apart from cholestatic liver injury, which is probably idiosyncratic and is rapidly reversible after azathioprine interruption (86–88), it is not at all certain how much of the other hepatic dysfunctions seen are due to azathioprine or to acute or chronic viral infections.

Long-term therapy with azathioprine in the doses used after kidney transplantation appears to not have adverse effects on fertility (89–91). In contrast to animal studies, which clearly demonstrated a teratogenic effect of azathioprine, it appears that the frequency of congenital malformations in humans is rather small (92–95). The problem of determining whether permanent genomal or gonadal damage will become manifest later in life in the children born from allograft recipients, or even in subsequent generations, is not yet resolved.

The adjunctive use of antilymphocyte serum

Since the pioneering work of Starzl in 1966 (96), several centers have used antilymphocyte (ALG) or antithymocyte (ATG) globulins in conjunction with corticosteroids and azathioprine during the first weeks after transplantation. Although the differences in graft survival did not usually reach statistical significance, the overall results of the available controlled studies show that the adjunctive use of ALG or ATG results in a 10–15% improvement of 1-year graft survival, with no alteration in patient survival (16, 97). The major advantage of the adjunctive use of ALG or ATG is certainly the reduction of the number and the severity of the acute rejection reactions, leading to reduce steroid requirements (16). It is interesting to note that, in most of the recent studies that could not show a further improvement of the 1-year graft survival with cyclosporin, conventional immunosuppression always included prophylactic antilymphocyte serum (32, 98–100).

The use of ALG or ATG may result in the occurrence of minor side effects, such as chills, skin rash, fever, and pruritus, in about 15% of patients. In these cases we always have stopped further administration. Leukopenia and thrombocytopenia is seen in 10% of patients. Anaphylactic reactions are seldom seen, but we advise performing a skin test before the first intravenous administration. Most authors have reported an increased incidence and severity of CMV infections, although this did not lead to an increased patient mortality (16).

MAINTENANCE IMMUNOSUPPRESSION WITH CYCLOSPORIN

The introduction of cyclosporin in clinical transplantation has set an end point after many of the still controversial problems of the conventional approach of immunosuppression, such as the issue of initial high-versus low-dose corticosteroids, and whether or not prophylactic antilymphocyte serum should be added. That cyclosporin is a powerful immunosuppressive drug became rapidly obvious from the pioneering studies of Calne's group (101) and from the European Multicenter Trial (102), which showed that, at least in some patients, transplantation with cadaveric kidneys was possible without the use of corticosteroids at all. In most centers with 1-year graft survivals between 50% and 60% under conventional immunosuppression, the use of cyclosporin resulted in a significant increase of graft survival of about 20%. In those centers with high survival rates under conventional immunosuppression, cyclosporin had a clear-cut steroid-sparing effect. In a retrospective analysis of 67 conventionally treated and 67 cyclosporin-treated cadaveric renal transplant recipients, we found that the mean number of rejections per patient during the first 6 post-transplant months was 1.49 ± 1.11 and 0.51 ± 0.82, respectively (mean ± SD; $p < 0.001$) (32).

Although the usefulness of cyclosporin in clinical transplantation is not of doubt, the introduction of cyclosporin has also created new problems. The diagnosis of rejection has become much more difficult, as the classic symptoms are often absent and a differential diagnosis with cyclosporin nephrotoxicity is not always easy. Much controversy also remains regarding the optimal clinical use of cyclosporin. Some of these problems will now be reviewed.

Cyclosporin alone or in combination with low-dose corticosteroids

In the initial studies of Calne, cyclosporin was used as the sole immunosuppressive drug and corticosteroids were only given to treat acute rejection episodes (101). The same protocol was also followed by the European Multicenter Trial and, according to the 3-year followup report of this study, 56% of the patients were still receiving cyclosporin as their sole immunosuppressive drug (102). In their report on 5 years' experience, Calne's group found that in 41% of the patients corticosteroids were completely avoided (103). The adjunctive use of corticosteroids was advocated by Starzl (104) and was subsequently followed by most transplant groups.

Only a few centers have conducted controlled studies on whether adjunctive administration of corticosteroids indeed has any advantage over cyclosporin alone (105–108). The conclusion of these studies was that low-dose steroids do not augment the immunosuppressive properties of cyclosporin but do diminish the cyclosporin-related nephrotoxicity. In the study of Johnson et al., the rate of conversion for nephrotoxicity was only 14% in the prednisone group versus 41% in the nonprednisone group (105). In the Cardiff study, 74% of the patients receiving cyclosporin alone experienced at least one episode of nephrotoxicity compared with 55% of the group that received steroids in addition ($p < 0.05$) (106). Furthermore, in the initial post-transplant period, steroids may have a cyclosporin-sparing effect, reducing indirectly the toxic side effects of cyclosporin. In our own patients, 50 mg of prednisolone is given intravenously during the first postoperative day. Thereafter 16 mg methylprednisolone is given orally in a single morning dose. Each month this daily dose is decreased by 2 mg to reach a maintenance dose of 8 mg/day.

Timing and dosage considerations

In their pilot studies in kidney graft recipients, Calne's group used initial doses of 25 mg/kg/day (101). This high dose was associated with serious nephrotoxicity. Later these authors recommended an initial dose of 17 mg/kg/day, gradually tapered to 8–10 mg/kg/day over 6–8 weeks. At present most centers start cyclosporin at a dose of 10–15 mg/kg/day. This dose is gradually tapered to a maintenance dose of 5–7 mg/kg/day after 3–6 months. Most centers also adjust the cyclosporin dose to the cyclosporin trough levels. In Kahan's group, the trough levels during the first post-transplant months are maintained between 100 and 250 ng/ml (109). Like most authors, we too have gradually diminished the dose of cyclosporin given during the first weeks after transplantation. In our patients transplanted between February 1983 and May 1984, cyclosporin serum trough levels during the first post-transplant month were maintained at 200–250 ng/ml, in the period between June 1984 and May 1985 they were maintained at 150–200 ng/ml, and since June 1985 at 100–150 ng/ml. In Table 1 is shown the effect of the lower cyclosporin level on the number of rejections during the first post-transplant month. These data suggest that reducing the cyclosporin levels to < 150 ng/ml during the first weeks after transplantation is not safe.

Because of the well-known nephrotoxicity of cyclosporin and the fear that an ischemically damaged kidney may be more vulnerable to the toxic side effects of cyclosporin, many authors have recommended withholding the

Table 1. Effect of cyclosporin trough level on the incidence of acute rejection episodes

	Evaluation at one month after transplantation		
	Cyclosporin trough level (ng/ml)	Number of rejections/patient	Serum creatinine (mg/dl)
February 1983–May 1984 (n = 50)	230 ± 7.8	0.3 ± 0.07	2.03 ± 0.10
June 1984–May 1985 (n = 49)	161 ± 3.7 ***	0.3 ± 0.07 **	1.81 ± 0.12
June 1985–March 1987 (n = 108)	129 ± 2.7 ***	0.6 ± 0.07 **	2.25 ± 0.24

Data are given as mean ± SE.
Comparaison by Student t-test. *$p < 0.05$; **$p < 0.01$; ***$p < 0.001$.

Table 2. Incidence of initial nonfunctioning (INF) in recently published controlled trials

Reference	Azathioprine	Cyclosporin	Significance
114	68.9	72.5	ns
115	27	33	ns
116	58	72	ns
117	23	20	ns
118	32	46	ns
119	32	50	$p < 0.05$
120	26	32	ns
	Mean 38.1	46.5	

drug until good graft function has occurred. The first question to be answered in this regard is whether the incidence of initial nonfunction (INF) is indeed higher in cyclosporin-treated than in conventionally treated allografts. Secondly, it should be determined whether initial nonfunctioning influences on short- and long-term graft survival differ with the type of immunosuppression used.

With regard to the incidence of INF, retrospective studies have given rather conflicting results. While some authors found a significant increase in the incidence of INF in their cyclosporin-treated patients compared to azathioprine-treated controls (100, 110), others could not confirm these finding (111–113). Table 2 summarizes the data from some recently published randomized controlled trials (114–120). It appears that in these studies the incidence of INF is slightly, but usually not significantly, higher in the cyclosprin-treated group than in the control group. In most of the published series, however, the incidence of INF is significantly higher in retransplants than in first transplants (115, 121, 122). Prolonged warm and cold ischemia times are also associated with an increased incidence of INF (123).

Only two of the controlled studies mentioned in Table 2 give a clear answer to the second question. Canafax et al. found a 1-year graft survival of 92% in the cyclosporin-treated group for kidneys with immediate function and a 1-year survival of 73% in kidneys with INF ($p = 0.008$) (115). In the azathioprine group, the difference of 14% was not significant. In the Canadian trial the risk of graft loss was increased twofold to fourfold ($p = 0.004$ in the cyclosporin group; $p = 0.06$ in the azathioprine group) (118). The same trend was also seen in several retrospective trials (110, 112, 121, 122), although this was not the case in all of the trials (111, 113, 123). At present we can conclude that under cyclosporin therapy the incidence of

Table 3. Effect of initial nonfunction (INF) on the 1-year graft survival

	Conventional immunosuppression		Cyclosporin	
	– INF	+ INF	– INF	+ INF
Total group	80%	79%	95%	84%[1]
First transplants	80%	82%	94%	94%
Retransplants	75%	67%	100%	44%[2]

[1] $p < 0.05$; [2] $p < 0.001$

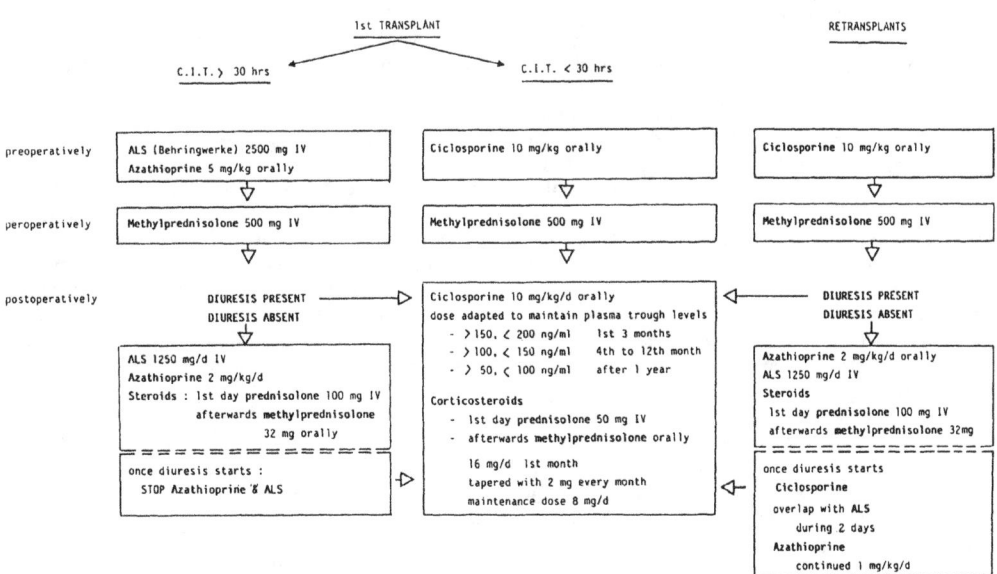

Figure 2. Immunosuppressive protocol presently in use by the Leuven Collaborative Group for Transplantation.

INF is slightly increased, as compared with noncyclosporin-treated patients and that under cyclosporin the deleterious effect of INF on graft survival is more pronounced than when azathioprine is used. This deleterious effect is especially marked in retransplants (121, 124) and in kidneys that have undergone prolonged preservation (113). In our own experience the incidence of INF when using cyclosporin was 34%. The effect on the 1-year graft survival is given in Table 3. The presence of INF had no deleterious effect on the outcome of our first transplants, but a marked negative effect was seen in retransplants.

Based on the data from the literature and on our own experience, the following policy has been adopted (Figure 2): For first transplants cyclosporin is started 4 hours before transplantation and is continued after transplantation, irrespective of whether or not the kidney is functioning. Only when the preservation is longer than 30 hours, is cyclosporin started once the kidney function begins. In the meantime, azathioprine, ALG, and steroids are given. ALG and azathioprine are stopped once therapeutic cyclosporin levels are reached. In retransplants, cyclosporin is also given before transplantation, but it is not continued when the kidney is not functioning immediately. In this case, azathioprine, prednisone, and ALS are given until the kidney starts functioning. Then ALS is stopped and azathioprine is continued.

There is also great concern regarding the potential chronic and permanent damage to the kidney when cyclosporin is given over several years after transplantation. For this reason several authors have advocated limiting cyclosporin administration to the first months after transplantation when the risk of graft loss due to rejection is the highest and converting to conventional immunosuppression afterwards (119, 125). The improved renal function after conversion must, however, be balanced against the possibility of acute rejection episodes, some of which may result in loss of the kidney. A preliminary question to be answered is whether long-term administration of cyclosporin results in progressive deterioration of renal function, as suggested by the findings of the Stanford group in heart-transplant recipients (126). Only a few groups have published their long-term results with patients chronically treated with cyclosporin. In the 5-year followup report of Calne's group, serum creatinine was $221 \pm 10\,\mu M/l$ at discharge and $213 \pm 13\,\mu M/l$ at the most recent followup visit (104). Stable serum creatinines levels were also seen as long as 3 years after transplantation in other large series, such as those from Boston, Houston, and Basel (127–129). In a group of 80 cadaveric kidney-graft recipients treated for a second year with cyclosporin, we also did not find a progressive deterioration of renal function — serum creatinine at 1 year = $1.52 \pm 0.07\,mg/dl$ and at 2 years = $1.61 \pm 0.07\,mg/dl$ (130). It can therefore be concluded that, in general, long-term cyclosporin administration in renal transplant recipients dose not result in progressive deterioration of renal function.

The outcome after conversion is largely dependent on the reason for conversion. Early conversion in the face of persistent nonfunction or rejection is in most cases not very useful, as a high percentage of the kidneys will be lost after conversion (119, 131–133). The experience with elective conversion (e.g., for reasons of cost) is more conflicting. Controlled studies comparing the outcome of a group of converted patients with a group of patients in which cycloporin was not stopped are lacking. The two recently published "controlled" studies (119, 125) compared the outcome of their converted groups with the outcome of groups of conventionally treated patients. Only Veitch et al., in a retrospective study, compared the outcome of their converted group with the outcome of their nonconverted group (134). In our experience an unacceptably high number of reversible rejections occurred after conversion-rejection was seen in 8 of the 9 patients converted after 1 month and in 7 of the 9 patients converted after 3 months (135). In most other series, a lower incidence of rejections is seen, ranging between 20% and 35% (119, 136–140). One group reported a very low incidence of only 3%, but in a followup study a substantial number of late-onset rejections was reported (141). A comparable high number of later-onset rejections was also reported by Maddux et al. (140). Because of the lack of clear-cut data indicating that long-term cyclosporin administration results in a progressive deterioration of kidney-graft function, and because of the considerable risk of acute rejection (and eventual graft loss), we cannot recommend elective conversion to cyclosporin versus conventional immunosuppression.

Conversion may, however, be necessary in the case of severe nephrotoxicity. If this is needed within the first year after transplantation, conversion to triple therapy with low doses of cyclosporin, azathioprine, and steroids is probably preferable (141–143). In the Houston experience, a significantly lower incidence of rejection and graft loss was seen after conversion to triple therapy with low doses of cyclosporin (2.5–3 mg/kg/day), azathioprine (2 mg/kg/day), and prednisone than after conversion to azathioprine and corticosteroids alone (142).

Triple and quadruple therapy

Three-drug therapy using cyclosporin, azathioprine, and prednisone has been used as initial immunosuppressive regimen in an attempt to reduce cyclosporin nephrotoxicity while preserving its unique immunosuppressive effect (144, 145). When used in rather high doses (8–10 mg/kg/day of cyclosporin, 2 mg/kg/day of azathioprine, and intermediate doses of corticosteroids), this regimen has proven its efficacy in immunologically high-risk patients (146), but can be associated with a high incidence of severe infectious complications (147). When used in low doses (2 mg/kg/day cyclosporin, 1 mg/kg/day azathioprine, and 16 mg prednisone), the regimen was not proven to be superior to cyclosporin and steroids alone in terms of efficacy as well as toxicity (148).

Some authors have also used so-called quadruple therapy, consisting of azathioprine, corticosteroids, and antilymphocyte serum started at the time of transplantation. Once the serum creatinine is below a given level (3–5 mg/

dl), cyclosporin is started, and antilymphocyte serum is stopped after 1 or 2 days of overlap (149–151). This aggressive immunosuppressive approach should, however, be used with severe caution, as overwhelming infection due to overimmunosuppression has been reported (138, 152).

Therapeutic drug monitoring

Although there may be a considerable overlap of blood concentrations between patients suffering nephrotoxicity and those with allograft rejection (due to insufficient dosage), we believe, like many others (153, 154), that therapeutic drug monitoring should be recommended for the rational use of cyclosporin after kidney transplantation. The interindividual variations in drug absorption, distribution, and clearance make regular monitoring of cyclosporin levels mandatory.

Until now, two types of methods have been used to measure cyclosporin. High-performance liquid chromatography (HPLC) measures the native compound but usually involves time-consuming and expensive extraction processes. Radioimmunoassay (RIA) has the advantage of rapidly processing large numbers of samples but, at least with the use of the polyclonal antibody, measures not only the native compound, but also several metabolites, and the immunosuppressive properties and toxic side effects of these measured metabolites are mostly unknown. This also explains why cyclosporin concentrations measured by RIA are systematically twofold to fourfold higher than HPLC results. Fortunately, monoclonal antibodies directed against the native compound alone will shortly become available for clinical use (155).

There has been considerable controversy regarding the appropriate matrix for cyclosporin measurement: serum or whole blood. Almost 60% of the blood cyclosporin is associated with erythrocytes. The distribution in the erythrocytes and plasma is temperature dependent. When the blood is allowed to stand and clot at room temperature, cyclosporin rapidly diffuses into the blood cells, reaching an equilibrium after 2 hours, thereby resulting in a ± 25% lower level in whole blood (153). Within the limits of the hematocrit seen in renal-graft recipients, blood concentrations are independent of variations in the hematocrit (156). Because of the general trend to use lower doses of cyclosporin, the drug levels in serum are often close to the limit of sensitivity of the method. This is one reason to use blood instead of serum or plasma as the matrix for drug monitoring.

Several authors have tried to define the upper and lower limits of the therapeutic window. Predose whole-blood trough levels above 800 ng/ml are often associated with nephrotoxicity (154). The lower limit for adequate immunosuppression is less firmly defined and should be reduced as a function of time after transplantation. During the first month after transplantation, we maintain the serum trough levels between 150 and 200 ng/ml, as levels lower than 150 ng/ml are associated with more rejection episodes (Table 1). Between 6 and 12 months, serum levels are maintained between 100 and 150 ng/ml. After 1 year, levels lower than 100 ng/ml seem to be safe (157).

Interactions of other drugs with cyclosporin

Cyclosporin is mainly metabolized by the hepatic monooxygenase system (cytochrome P-450). Drugs that induce cytochrome P-450 activity will thus accelerate cyclosporin elimination, while drugs that compete for cytochrome P-450 will decrease cyclosporin clearance. A third level of interaction is additive nephrotoxicity when other nephrotoxic drugs are associated. For a comprehensive review of the many drug interactions reported up to now, the reader is referred to the paper of Cockburn (158). In Table 4 we have summarized the most relevant clinical drug interactions.

Side effects of cyclosporin

Since its introduction into clinical practice, a wide array of more or less frequently occurring complications and side effects have been reported (Table 5). The data given in Table 5 are based on the third interim report of the ongoing long-term safety followup study being conducted by Sandoz in renal transplant recipients treated with cyclosporin. These data were kindly provided by Prof. Krupp of the Drug Monitoring Center of Sandoz in Basel, Switzerland. In this table, only the adverse effects reported in more than 2% of the patients are mentioned. For each of these events, the estimated incidence of experiencing these effects during the first, second, and third year of observation is given. It is obvious that several of the re-

Table 4. Drug interactions with cyclosporin

Induction of cytochrome P-450 (accelerated metabolism high doses of cyclosporine are needed)	Competition with cytochrome P-450 (reduced metabolism lower doses of cyclosporine are needed)	Additive nephrotoxicity
Rifamycin (159)	Erythromycin (163)	Amphotericin B (167) Trimethoprim with or without sulfamethoxazole (168)
Dilantin (160)	Ketoconazole (164)	
Phenobarbital (161)	Furosemide in high doses (165)	
Combination of trimethoprim and sulphadimidine (162) (mechanism unknown)	High doses of corticosteroids (166)	Aminoglycoside antibiotics (169)

Table 5. Adverse events reported under cyclosporin therapy

	Incidence in percent per year		
	First	Second	Third year
Renal dysfunction	57.6	7.6	11.1
Hypertension	46.4	7.8	12.6
Hypertrichosis	43.2	3.6	2.3
Tremor	25.4	3.1	1.1
Gum hypertrophy	20.0	4.5	2.6
Hepatic dysfunction	18.9	4.3	2.3
Infectious complications			
Unspecified	18.0	3.4	2.0
Bacterial	14.7	2.8	1.7
Viral	14.2	2.2	2.2
Disorders of the upper G.I. tract (dyspepsia, nausea...)	5.6	2.0	1.7
Cushing disease	5.5	0.3	0.9
Neuropathy	4.8	1.5	1.1
Hyperuricemia	3.8	1.5	1.0
Disorders of the lower G.I. tract	3.1	0.7	0.4
Lipid disturbances	2.9	0.3	0.1
Glucose disturbances	2.8	0.6	0.1
Hyperthermia	2.7	0.5	0
Acne	2.4	0.3	0.3
G.I. ulcer	2.3	0.5	0
Thromboembolic complications	2.1	0.5	0.1
Edema	2.0	0.5	0.4

ported adverse effects are primarily due to the concomitant corticosteroid therapy, e.g., acne, hyperglycemia, Cushing's disease, and gastrointestinal ulcer. This table indicates that most side effects occur during the first year of administration, suggesting that their occurrence is mainly dose dependent and that their manifestation can be minimized by given the lowest effective dose of cyclosporin.

The most disturbing side effect of cyclosporin after kidney transplantation is certainly its nephrotoxicity. The clinical picture of this nephrotoxicity is a reduced creatinine clearance with increased serum creatinine, hyperkalemia, hyperuricemia, and hyperkalemic, hyperchloremic renal tubular acidosis (Type IV). The frequently observed elevation of arterial blood pressure may also be related to its nephrotoxicity. The mechanisms of this acute and chronic nephrotoxicity are unknown but may be multifactorial (170). Several aspects of this nephrotoxicity and of the approaches to avoid it have already been mentioned earlier in this chapter. For a more through discussion of cyclosporin-associated nephrotoxicity, the reader is referred to the excellent review of Kahan (170).

Another side effect of cyclosporin, possibly related to its nephrotoxicity, is the vascular injury described by several authors in experimental animals as well as in humans. An illness that resembles the hemolytic uremic syndrome has been described in liver and bone-marrow transplant recipients treated with cyclosporin (171, 172), while glomerular capillary thrombosis has been seen in kidney biopsies of renal transplant recipients (173). In a retrospective survey, we also found a significant increase in thromboembolic complications in 90 cyclosporin-treated patients compared with 90 azathioprine-treated patients (174), a finding that could not be confirmed by others (175–177). The cause of this cyclosporin-related vasculopathy is unknown, but several mechanisms have been suggested, including a direct toxic effect of cyclosporin on endothelial cells (178), decreased synthesis of prostacyclin-stimulating factor (179), and increased factor-VIII-related antigen (180). Hypercoagulability could be mediated by the increased monocyte proagulant activity induced by cyclosporin (181) and/or by platelet hyperaggregability (173, 174).

TOTAL LYMPH NODE IRRADIATION (TLI)

TLI has been used during the past 5 years by several groups as an immunosuppressive protocol for kidney transplantation. Irradiation is mostly given in daily fractions of 1 Gy up to a cumulative dose of 10–40 Gy. The irradiation is delivered through two ports, the so-called mantle port, including the lymph nodes of the neck, the axilla, and the mediastinum, and the inverted Y port, including the aortic, iliac, and pelvic lymph nodes.

We have used TLI (between 20 and 30 Gy) in combination with a low dose of prednisone (15 mg/kg) in all our diabetic kidney-graft recipients transplanted between September 1981 and January 1987 (n = 23) (182, 183). The last nine patients were enrolled in a controlled study comparing TLI and cyclosporin, both with low-dose steroids (184). Although this experience confirmed the potent immunosuppressive effect of TLI, it appeared that this protocol is not optimal, certainly not with regard to the prevention of rejection, as 8 of the 9 TLI patients of the controlled trial had at least one rejection episode within the first 6 post-transplant months versus only 2 of the 9 in the cyclosporin group. Other groups have used TLI in conjunction with either conventional immunosuppression (Minneapolis) (185), post-transplant antithymocyte globulin (Standford and San Francisco) (186), or cyclosporin (Rome and Johannisburg) (187, 188). These combined immunosuppressive protocols seem to be much more efficient, resulting in a rejection-free course in almost half of the patients, although a higher incidence of infectious complications has been seen. More carefully planned trials comparing these high-efficiency TLI schedules with the better known cyclosporin regimens are needed before this technique can be more widely recommended.

TREATMENT OF ACUTE REJECTION

Corticosteroids

Increased doses of corticosteroids have been the mainstay of the treatment of acute cellular rejections since the early days of transplantation. Since the work of Bell et al. (189), most transplant centers have used pulses of high doses of methylprednisolone (20 mg/kg) in three to six daily doses. These high doses of intravenous steroids, especially when repeated courses are given, are associated with a significant mortality and morbidity. Nakajima et al. were among the first to compare intravenous pulses of methylprednisolone with lower doses of oral prednisone (300, 200, and 100 mg in 3 days) (190). They found that these oral doses were equally successful in reversing rejection and that although oral treatment tended to be associated with a greater morbidity, This difference was not statistically significant. Kauffman et al. compared the effect of bolus therapy of IV methylprednisolone at 30 mg/kg versus 3 mg/kg and could not find any therapeutic benefit in using higher doses (191). We normally use lower doses of intravenous prednisolone (200–200–150–150 mg) followed by oral methylprednisolone 72 mg, tapered daily with 8 mg until the maintenance dose of 16 mg is reached.

Because of the serious side effects of corticosteroids (even in the lower used by our group and others), and because steroids are not always effective in reversing rejection, there has been an intensive search for alternative antirejection therapies, such as antilymphocyte or antithymocyte globulin and monoclonal anti-T-cell antibodies.

Antilymphocyte and antithymocyte globulins

Shield et al. performed the first controlled trial comparing antithymocyte globulin with high doses of steroids in related-donor kidney recipients and noted a more rapid reversal of rejection, fewer further rejections, and better long-term survival (192). The same favorable results were also found in cadaver kidney recipients by Hoitsma et al., who compared rabbit antithymocyte globulin with high oral doses of prednisone (193), and by Broyer et al. in pediatric kidney-graft recipients (194). Several groups have also demonstrated that antilymphocyte or antithymocyte globulin used with a standard antirejection treatment are more effective than a standard antirejection therapy alone in reversing acute rejection episodes (195, 196). Antilymphocyte globulins have also been used with success to treat rejections that have failed to respond to large doses of steroids (197–199). In all of the aforementioned studies, maintenance immunosuppression consisted of azathioprine and steroids. Antilymphocyte globulins have also recently been used with success to treat rejections in patients under cyclosporin therapy, either as an alternative therapy to steroids or as rescue therapy in the case of steroid-resistant rejections (200–202).

Monoclonal antibodies

In recent years monoclonal antibodies against T3 positive lymphocytes (Orthoclone OKT3) have also been tested with success, either as first-line antirejection therapy (203, 204) or as rescue therapy in the case of steroid-resistant rejections (205–210), both in patients under conventional immunosuppression or under cyclosporin maintenance therapy. A very limited experience is also available with monoclonal antibodies against blast cells (211) and against T12 positive cells (212). It must be noted that the administration of Orthoclone OKT3 can be associated with severe adverse reactions. Almost all patients develop an acute symptom complex after the first injection. This typically commences 4–6 hours after the injection and can last several hours (213). It is manifested as fever, chills, frontal headache, chest lightness, nausea and diarrhea, and pulmonary edema. Pulmonary edema was especially disturbing during the first clinical trials and was the cause of death in two cases. In retrospective it appears that all cases of pulmonary edema were seen in patients with significant fluid retention during the immediate pretreatment period. A high percentage of rerejection has also been noted (214). This may in part be due to the mitogenic effect of OKT3 in vitro (215).

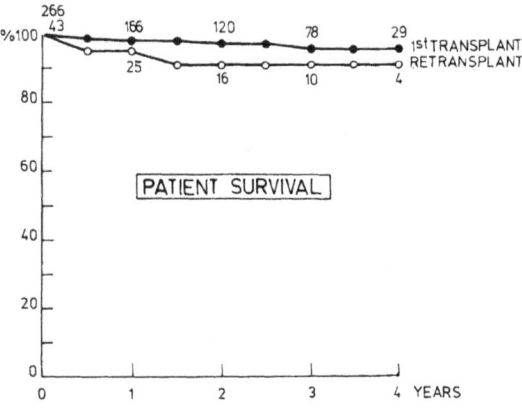

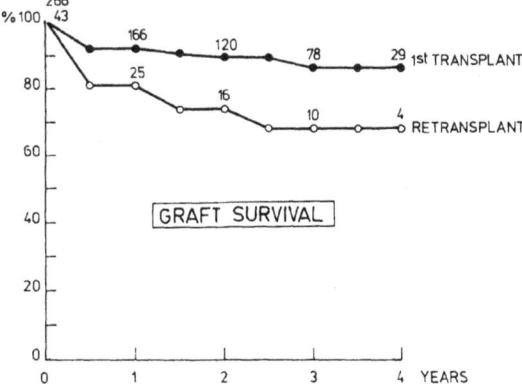

Figure 3. Patient and graft survival for first transplants and retransplants treated with cyclosporin sinc 1983.

IMMUNOSUPPRESSIVE PROTOCOL USED BY THE LEUVEN COLLABORATIVE GROUP FOR TRANSPLANTATION

In Figure 2 the immunosuppressive protocol presently in use by the Leuven Collaborative Group for Transplantation is shown. The patient and graft survival of the patients transplanted with this protocol since January 1983 are shown in Figure 3. All patients are cadaveric graft recipients.

REFERENCES

1. Thorsby E: Structure and function of HLA-molecules. *Transplant Proc* 19:29, 1987.
2. Fabre JW, Milton AD, Spencer S, Settaf A, Houssin D: Regulation of alloantigen expression in different tissues. *Transplant Proc* 19:45, 1987.
3. Moore RN, Oppenheim JJ, Farrar JJ, Carter CS, Waheed A, Shadduck RK: Production of LAF (IL$_1$) by macrophages activated with colony stimulating factors. *J Immunol* 125:1302, 1980.
4. Robb RJ, Munck A, Smith KA: T cell growth factor receptors quantitation, specificity and biological relevance. *J Exp Med* 154:1455, 1981.
5. Smith KA, Lachman LB, Oppenheim JJ, Favata MF: The functional relationship of the interleukins. *J Exp Med* 151:1551, 1980.
6. Farrar WL, Johnson HM, Farrar JJ: Regulation of the production of immune interferon and cytotoxic T lymphocytes by interleukin-2. *J Immunol* 126:1120, 1981.
7. Hall BM: Cellular infiltrates in allografts. *Transplant Proc* 19:50, 1987.
8. Billingham RE, Krohn PL, Medawar PB: Effects of cortisone on survival of skin homografts in rabbits. *Br Med J* 1:1157, 1951.
9. Dupont E, Wybran J, Toussaint C: Glucocorticosteroids and organ transplantation. *Transplantation* 37:331, 1984.
10. Cupps TR, Fauer AS: Corticosteroid-mediated immunoregulation in man. *Immunol Rev* 65:113, 1982.
11. Claman HN: How corticosteroids work. *J Allergy Clin Immunol* 55:145, 1975.
12. Bunjes D, Hardt C, Rollinghoff M, Wagner H: Cyclosporin A mediates immunosuppression of primary cytotoxic T cell responses by impairing the release of interleukin-1 and interleukin-2. *Eru J Immunol* 11:657, 1981.
13. Hutchinson IF, Shadur CA, Duarte AJS, Strom TB, Tilney NL: Cyclosporin A spares selectively lymphocytes with donor specific suppressor characteristics. *Transplantation* 32:210, 1981.
14. Elion GB: Biochemistry and pharmacology of purine analogues. *Fed Proc* 26:898, 1967.
15. Wheeler GP, Bowdon BJ, Adamson DJ, Wail MH: Comparison of the effects of several inhibitors of the synthesis of nucleic acids upon the viability and progression through the cell cycle of cultured H.Ep No-2 cells. *Cancer Res* 32:2661, 1972.
16. Monaco AP: antilymphocyte globulin: A clinical transplantation research opportunity. *Am J Kidney dis* 2:67, 1982.
17. Lance EM, Medawar PB, Taub RN: Antilymphocyte serum. *Advances Immunol* 17:1, 1973.
18. Tyler RW, Everett NB, Schwartz MR: Effect of antilymphocyte serum on rate lymphocytes. *J Immunol* 102:179–186, 1968.
19. Maki T, Simpson M, Monaco AP: Development of suppressor T cells by antilymphocyte serum treatment in mice. *Transplantation* 34:376, 1982.
20. Thomas JM, Carver FM, Haisch CE, Fahrenbruck G, Deepe RM, Thomas FT: Suppressor cells in Rhesus monkeys treated with antithymocyte globulin. *Transplantation* 34:83, 1982.
21. Reinherz EL, Meuer S, Fitzgerald KA, Mussey RE, Levine H, Schlossman SF: Antigen recognition by human T lymphocytes is linked to surface expression of the T3 molecular complex. *Cell* 30:735, 1982.
22. Bach JF, Chatenoud L: Immunologic monitoring of orthoclone OKT3 treated patients: The problem of antimonoclonal immune response. *Transplant Proc* 19 (suppl 1):17, 1987.
23. Trowell OA: The sensitivity of lymphocytes to ionizing radiation. *J Path Bact* 64:687, 1952.
24. Godfrey AM, Salaman JR: Is graft irradiation of value in renal transplant rejection? *Transplant Proc* 9:1005, 1977.
25. Fuks Z, Strober S, Bobrove AM, Sasazuki T, McMicheal A, Kaplan HS: Longterm effects of radiation on T and B lymphocytes in peripheral blood of patients with Hodgkin's disease. *J Clin Invest* 58:803, 1976.
26. Strober S: Natural suppressor (NS) cells, neonatal tolerance, and total lymphoid irradiation: Exploring obscure relationships. *Ann Rev Immunol* 2:97, 1984.
27. Waer M, Vanrenterghem Y, Roels L, Ang K, Bouillon R, Lerut T, Gruwez J, van der Schueren E, Vandeputte M, Michielsen P: Immunologic and clinical observations in diabetic kidney graft recipients pretreated with total lymphoid irradiation. *Transplantation* 43:371, 1987.
28. McGeown MG, Douglas JF, Brown WA, Donaldson RA, Kennedy JA, Loughridge WG, Mehta S, Nelson SD, Dohertry CC, Johnstone R, Todd G, Hill CM: Advantages of low dose steroid from the day after renal transplantation. *Transplantation* 29:287, 1980.
29. Gore SM, Oldham JA: Randomized trials of high-versus-low-dose steroids in renal transplantation. Does the evidence favor a consensus? *Transplantation* 41:319, 1986.
30. Morris PJ, French ME, Chan L, Ting A: Low dose oral prednisolone in renal transplantation. *Lancet* 1:525, 1982.
31. d'Apice AJF, Becker GJ, Kincaid-Smith P, Mathew TH, Ng J, Hardie IR, Petrie JJB, Rigby RJ, Dawborn J, Heale WF, Miach PJ: A prospective randomized trial of low-dose versus high-dose steroids in cadaveric renal transplantation. *Transplantation* 37:373, 1984.
32. Vanrenterghem Y, Roels L, Lerut T, Waer M, Gruwez J, Michielsen P: Evaluation of cyclosporine in a center with high survival rates using conventional immunosuppression. *Transplant Proc* 17:2666, 1985.
33. Stjernholm MR, Katz FH: Effects of diphenylhydantoin, phenobarbital and diazepam on the metabolism of methylprednisolone and its sodium succinate. *J Clin Endocr* 41:887–893, 1975.
34. Hendrickse W, McKierman J, Pickup M, Lowe J: Rifampicin-induced non-responsiveness to corticosteroid treatment in nephrotic syndrome. *Brit Med J* 1:306, 1979.
35. Buffington Ga, Comingues JH, Piering WF, Hebert LA, Kauffmen N, Lemann J Jr: Interaction of rifampicin and glucocorticoids. Adverse effects on renal function. *JAMA* 236:1958, 1976.
36. Gamberloglio JG, Holford NHG, Kapusnik JE, Nishikawa R, Saltiel M, Stanik-Lizak P, Birnbaum JL, Hau T, Amend WJC Jr: Disposition of total and unbound prednisolone in

36. renal transplant patients receiving anticonvulsants. *Kidney Int* 25:119, 1984.
37. Wassner SJ, Malekzadeh MH, Pennisi AJ, Ettenger RB, Uittenbogaart CH, Fine RN: Allograft survival in patients receiving anticonvulsant medication. *Clin Nephrol* 8:293, 1977.
38. Knapp MS, Byrom NP, Pownall R, Mayor P: Time of day of taking immunosuppressive agents after renal transplantation: A possible influence on graft survival. *Brit Med J* 281:1382, 1980.
39. Harter JG, Reddy WJ, Thorn GW: Studies on an intermittent corticosteroid dosage regimen. *N Engl J Med* 269:591, 1963.
40. Kabler TA, Knapp MS, Pownall R: The effects of corticosteroids given at various clock times on cell-mediated immunity to oxazolone. *Br J Pharmacol* 64:427P, 1978.
41. Pownall R, Knapp MS: A circadian study of corticosteroid suppression of delayed hypersensitivity. *Int J Immunopharmacol* 1:293, 1980.
42. Pickup ME: Clinical pharmacokinetics of prednisone and prednisolone. *Clin Pharmacokinet* 4:111, 1979.
43. Davis M, Williams R, Chakraborty J, English J, Marks V, Ideo G, Tempini S: Prednisone or prednisolone for the treatment of chronic active hepatitis? A comparison of plasma availability. *Br J Clin Pharmacol* 5:301, 1978.
44. Burleson RI, Marberger PD, Jermanovich N, Brennan AM, Scruggs BF: A prospective study of methylprednisolone and prednisone as immunosuppressive agents in clinical renal transplantation. *Transplant Proc* 13:339, 1981.
45. Henderson RC, Wheatly T, English J, Chakraborty J, Marks V: Variation in plasma prednisolone concentration in renal transplant recipients given enteric-coated prednisolone. *Br Med J* 1:1534, 1979.
46. Vanrenterghem Y, Roels L, Michielsen P: Prohylactic treatment with cimetidine after renal transplantation. In: *Further Experience with H₂-Receptor Antagonists in Peptic Ulcer Disease and Progress in Histamine Research*. Excerpta Medica, Amsterdam, Congress Series No 521, pp 159, 1980.
47. Bennett WM, Barry JM: Failure of dexamethasone to provide adequate chronic immunosuppression for renal transplantation. *Transplantation* 27:218, 1979.
48. Harter JG, Reddy WJ, Thorn GW: Studies on an intermittent corticosteroid dosage regimen. *N Engl J Med* 269:591, 1963.
49. Dale DC, Fauci AS, Wolff SM: Alternate-day prednisone: Leukocyte kinetics and susceptibility to infections. *N Engl J Med* 291:1154, 1974.
50. Reed WP, Lucus ZJ, Cohn R: Alternate-day prednisone therapy after renal transplantation. *Lancet* 1:747, 1970.
51. Siegel RR, Luke RG, Hellebusch AA: Reduction of toxicity of corticosteroid therapy after renal transplantation. *Am J Med* 53:159, 1972.
52. Wilson CJ, Kaye J, Belzer FO, Kountz SL, Potter DE: Growth following renal transplantation: Daily vs. alternate-day steroid therapy. *Pediat Res* 6:415, 1972.
53. Sampson D, Albert DJ: Alternate-day therapy with methylprednisolone after renal transplantation. *J Urol* 109:345, 1973.
54. McEnery PT, Gonzalez LL, Martin LW, West CD: Growth and development of children with renal transplantation. Use of alternate-day steroid therapy. *J Pediat* 83:806, 1973.
55. Potter D, Belzer FO, Rames L, Holliday NA, Kountz SL, Najarian JS: The treatment of chronic uremia in childhood. 1. Transplantation. *Pediatrics* 45:432, 1970.
56. Diethelm AG, Sterling WA, Hartley MW, Morgan JM: Alternate-day prednisone therapy in recipients of renal allografts. *Arch Surg* 111:867, 1976.
57. McDonald FD, Horenstein ML, Moyor GB, Turcotte JG, Selezinka W, Schork MA: Effect of alternate-day steroids on renal transplant function. A controlled study. *Nephron* 17:415, 1976.
58. DeVecchi A, Cantaluppi A, Montagnino G, Tarantino A, Maestri O, Ponticelli C: Long-term comparison between single-morning daily and alternate-day steroid treatment in cadaver kidney recipients. *Transplant Proc* 12:327, 1980.
59. Owens ML, Maxwell JG, Goodnight J, Wolcatt MW: Discontinuance of immunosuppression in renal transplant patients. *Arch Surg* 110:1450, 1975.
60. Di Padova F, Morandi E, Mazzei D: Is long-term immunosuppressive treatment necessary to maintain good kidney graft function? *Br Med J* 2:421, 1979.
61. Zoller KM, Cho SI, Cohen JJ, Harrington JT: Cessation of immunosuppressive therapy after successful transplantation: A national survey. *Kidney Int* 18:110, 1980.
62. Najarian JS: Editorial comment. *Arch Surg* 110:1451, 1975.
63. Ueling DT, Hussey JL, Weinstein AB, Wank R, Bach FH: Cessation of immunosuppression after renal transplantation. *Surgery* 79:278, 1976.
64. Naik RB, Abdeen H, English J, Chakraborty J, Slapak M, Lee HA: Prednisolone withdrawal after 3 years in renal transplant patients receiving only this form of immunosuppression. *Transplant Proc* 11:39, 1979.
65. First MR, Munda R, Kant KS, Fidler JP, Alexander JW: Steroid withdrawal following HLA-identical related donor transplantation. *Transplant Proc* 13:319, 1981.
66. Turcotte JG, Dickerman RM, Harper ML: Minimum steroid requirements in the late post-transplant period. *Transplant Proc* 7:83, 1975.
67. Thaysen JH, Lokkegaard H: Permanent withdrawal of prednisone in necro-kidney transplantation. *Scand J Urol Nephrol* 42:198, 1977.
68. Steinman TI, Zimmerman CE, Monaco AP, Brown RS, Yager HM, Clive DM, Ransil BJ: Steroids can be stopped in kidney transplant recipients. *Transplant Proc* 13:323, 1981.
69. Sheriff MHR, Yayha T, Lee HA: Is azathioprine necessary in renal transplantation? *Lancet* 1:118, 1978.
70. Pirson Y, van Ypersele de Strihou C, Alexandre GPJ: Is azathioprine necessary in renal transplantation (letter)? *Lancet* 1:506, 1978.
71. Schmidt P, Kapsa H, Zazgornik J, Pils P, Balcke P: Renal graft acceptance without azathioprine. *Lancet* 2:314, 1978.
72. Dandavino R, Trunet P, Descamps B, Kreis H: Prolonged withdrawal of azathioprine in kidney transplantation. *Transplant Proc* 10:655, 1978.
73. Ozaki A, Ywazaki Y, Miyaji T: Withdrawal of azathioprine after renal transplantation. *Transplant Proc* 12:513, 1980.
74. Haesslein HC, Pierce JC, Lee HM, Hume DM: Leukopenia and azathioprine management of renal homotransplantation. *Surgery* 71:598, 1972.
75. Woods JE, de Weerd JH, Johnson WJ, Anderson CF: Splenectomy in renal transplantation — Influence on azathioprine sensitivity. *JAMA* 218:1430, 1972.
76. Toussaint C, Kinnaert P, Vereerstraeten P, Dupont E, Van Geertruyen J: Azathioprine is necessary in kidney transplantation. *Transplantation* 27:145, 1979.
77. Parfrey PS, Hutchinson TA, Lowny RP, Knaack J, Guttmann RD: The role of azathioprine reduction in late renal allograft failure. *Transplantation* 39:147, 1985.
78. Pierce JC, Hume DM: Toxicity of azathioprine. *Laval Méd* 41:295, 1970.

79. Stockhausen G, Hopf U, Glogner P: Panzytopenie nach kombinations-behandlung mit allopurinol and azathioprin. *Med Welt* 28:198, 1977.
80. Hulme B, Reeves DS: Leukopenia associated with trimethoprim-sulphamethoxazole after renal transplantation. *Br Med J* 3:610, 1977.
81. Bradley PP, Warden GD, Maxwell JG, Rothstein G: Neutropenia and thrombocytopenia in renal allograft recipient treated with trimethoprim-sulfamethoxazole. *Ann Intern Med* 93:560.
82. Hamburger J, Crosnier J, Dormont J, Bach JF: *La Transplantation Rénale*. Flammarion Médecine-Sciences, Paris, p 213, 1971.
83. Ebel H, Lange H: Conversion from azathioprine and/or prednisolone to cyclosporine A in renal allograft recipients. *Transplant Proc* 19:2005, 1987.
84. Starzl TE, Marchioro TL, Porter KA, Taylor PD, Faris TD, Herrmann TH, Alad CJ, Waddell WR: Factors determining short- and long-term survival after orthotopic liver homotransplantation in the dog. *Surgery* 58:131, 1965.
85. Penn I, Hammond W, Bell P: Hepatic disorders in renal homograft recipients. *Curr Top Surg Res* 1:67, 1969.
86. Freise J, May B, Schmidt E: Cholestatischer ikterus nach azathioprin (cholestatic jaundice after azathioprine treatment). *Dtsch Med Wschr* 101:1223, 1976.
87. Haas J, Stamm T: Intrahepatische cholestase eine allergische reaktion bei azathioprine-therapie? (Intrahepatic cholestasis: an allergic reaction to azathioprin therapy?) *Dtsch Med Wschr* 103:1576, 1978.
88. Davis M, Eddeston AL, Williams R: Hypersensitivity and jaundice due to azathioprine. *Postgrad Med J* 56:274, 1980.
89. Golby M: Fertility after renal transplantation. *Transplantation* 10:201, 1970.
90. Penn I, Makowski E, Froegemueller W, Halgrimson C, Starzl TE: Parenthood in renal homograft recipients. *JAMA* 216:1755, 1971.
91. Phadke AG, Mac Kinnan KJ, Dossetor JB: Male fertility in uraemia: Restoration by renal allografts. *Can Med Ass J* 102:607, 1970.
92. Rudolph JE, Schweizer RT, Bartus SA: Pregnancy in renal transplant patients. A review. *Transplantation* 27:26, 1979.
93. Rifle G, Traeger J: Pregnancy after renal transplantation: An international survey. *Transplant Proc* 7:723, 1957.
94. Sciarra JJ, Toledo-Pereyra LH, Bendel RP, Simmons RL: Pregnancy following renal transplantation. *Am J Obstet Gynec* 125:141, 1975.
95. Penn I, Makowski EL, Harris P: Parenthood following renal transplantation. *Kidney Int* 18:221, 1980.
96. Startzl TE, Marchioro TL, Porter KA, Iwasaki Y, Cerilli GJ: The use of heterologous antilymphoid agents in canine renal and liver homotransplantation and in human renal transplantation. *Surg Gynecol Obstet* 124:301, 1967.
97. Hardy MA: Beneficial effects of heterologous antilymphoid globulins in renal transplantation: One "believer's" view. *Am J Kidney Dis* 2:79, 1982.
98. Squifflet JP, Pirson Y, Jamart J, Wallemacq K, Alexandre GPJ: Cyclosporine in cadaver renal transplantation at a center with good results using conventional treatment. *Transplant Proc* 17:1212, 1985.
99. Sutherland DER, Strand M, Fryd DS, Ferguson RM, Simmons RL, Ascher NL, Najarian JS: Comparison of azathioprine-antilymphocyte globulin versus cyclosporine in renal transplantation. *Am J Kidney Dis* 3:456, 1984.
100. Cho SI, Bradley JW, Monaco AP, Tilney NL: Comparison of kidney transplant survival between patients treated with cyclosporine and those treated with azathioprine and antithymocyte globulin. *Am J Surg* 147:518, 1984.
101. Calne RY, White DJG, Thiru S, Evans DB, McMaster P, Dunn DC, Craddock GN, Pentlow BD, Rolles K: Cyclosporin A in patients receiving renal allografts from cadaver donors. *Lancet* 2:1323, 1978.
102. European Multicentre Trial Group: Cyclosporin in cadaveric renal transplantation: One-year followup of a multicentre trial. *Lancet* 2:986, 1983.
103. Merion RM, White DJG, Thiru S, Evans DB, Calne RY: Cyclosporine: Five years' experience in cadaver renal transplantation. *N Engl J Med* 310:148, 1984.
104. Starzl TE, Weil III R, Iwatsuki S, Klintmalm G, Schröter GPJ, Koep LJ, Iwaki Y, Terasaki PI, Porter KA: The use of cyclosporin and prednisone in cadaver kidney transplantation. *Surg Gynec Obstet* 151:17, 1980.
105. Johnson RWG, Wise MH, Bakram A, Short C, Dyer P, Mallick NP, Gokal R: A four-year prospective study of cyclosporine in cadaver renal transplantation. *Transplant Proc* 17:1197, 1985.
106. Griffin PJA, Gomes Da Costa CA, Salaman JR: A controlled trial of cyclosporine-treated renal transplant recipients. *Transplantation* 43:505, 1987.
107. MacDonald AS, Daloze P, Dandavino R, Jindal S, Bear L, Dossetor JB, Klassen J, Stiller CR, Lockwood B, Reeve CE, and the Canadian Transplant Group: A randomized study of cyclosporine with and without prednisone in renal allograft recipients. *Transplant Proc* 19:1865, 1987.
108. Albert FW, Schmidt U: Cyclosporine therapy with or without steroids in cadaveric kidney transplantation — a prospective randomized one-center study. *Transplant Proc* 17:2669, 1985.
109. Kahan BD, Flechner SM, Lorber MI, Golden D, Conley S, Van Buren CT: Complications of cyclosporine-prednisone immunosuppression in 402 renal allograft recipients exclusively followed at a single center for from one to five years. *Transplantation* 43:197, 1987.
110. Gonwa TA, Nghiem DD, Schulak JA, Corry RJ: Cyclosporine use in early graft dysfunction. *Transplant Proc* 18:104, 1986.
111. Flechner SM, Payne WD, Van Buren C, Kerman R, Kahan BD: The effect of cyclosporine on early graft function in human renal transplantation. *Transplantation* 36:268, 1983.
112. Castro LA, Hillebrand G, Land W, Schneider B, Günther K, Gurland H: Cyclosporine in patients with oligoanuria after cadaveric kidney transplantation. *Transplant Proc* 15:2699, 1983.
113. Bradley JW, Cho SI, Cosimi AB, Monaco AP: Cyclosporine immunosuppression and perfusion preservation of cadaver kidneys. *Transplant Proc* 19:2104, 1987.
114. Hall BM, Tiller DJ, Duggin GG, Horvath JS, Farnsworth A, May J, Johnson JR, Sheil AGR: Post-transplant acute renal failure in cadaver renal recipients treated with cyclosporine. *Kidney Int* 28:178, 1985.
115. Canafax DM, Torres A, Fryd DS, Heil JE, Strand MH, Ascher NL, Payne WD, Sutherland DER, Simmons RL, Najarian JS: The effects of delayed function on recipients of cadaver renal allografts. *Transplantation* 41:177, 1986.
116. Novick AC, Ho-Hsieh H, Steinmuller D, Streem SB, Cunningham RJ, Steinhilber D, Goormastic M, Buszta C: Detrimental effect of cyclosporine on initial function of cadaver renal allografts following extended preservation. *Transplantation* 42:154, 1986.
117. Henny FC, Kootte AMM, Van Bockel JH, Baldwin WM, Hermans J, Bos B, van Es LA, Paul LC: A prospective

randomised comparative study on the influence of cyclosporin and azathioprine on renal allograft survival and function. *Nephrol Dial Transplant* 1:44, 1986.
118. The Canadian Multicentre Transplant Study Group: A randomized clinical trial of cyclosporine in cadaveric renal transplantation. Analysis at three years. *N Engl J Med* 314:1219, 1986.
119. Morris PJ, Allen RD, Thompson JF, Chapman JR, Ting A, Dunnill MS, Wood RFM: Cyclosporin conversion versus conventional immunosuppression: Long-term followup and histological evaluation. *Lancet* 1:586, 1987.
120. Gianello P, Squifflet JP, Pirson Y, Stoffel M, Dereme Th, Alexandre GPJ: Cyclosporine-steroids versus conventional therapy in cadaver kidney transplantation: Analysis of a randomized trial at two years. *Transplant Proc* 19:1867, 1987.
121. Taylor RJ, Landreneau MD, Makowka L, Rosenthal TJ, Gordon RD, Tzakis AG, Starzl TE, Hakala TR: Cyclosporine immunosuppression and delayed graft function in 455 cadaveric renal transplants. *Transplant Proc* 19:2100, 1987.
122. Rocher LL, Landis C, Dafoe DC, Keyserling C, Swartz RD, Campbell DA Jr: The long-term deleterious effect of delayed graft function in cyclosporine-treated renal allograft recipients. *Transplant Proc* 19:2093, 1987.
123. Kahan BD, Mickey R, Flechner SM, Lorber MI, Wideman CA, Kerman RH, Terasaki P, Van Buren CT: Risk factors for cadaveric donor allograft survival in cyclosporine-prednisone-treated recipients. *Transplant Proc* 19:1835, 1987.
124. Keown PA, Stiller CR, Wallace AC, McKenzie FN, Wall W: Cyclosporine nephrotoxicity: Exploration of the risk factors and prognosis of the renal injury. *Transplant Proc* 17:247, 1985.
125. Hoitsma AJ, Van Lier HJJ, Wetzels JFM, Berden JHM, Koene RAP: Cyclosporin treatment with conversion after three months versus conventional immunosuppression in renal allograft recipients. *Lancet* 1:584, 1987.
126. Myers BD, Ross J, Newton L, Luetscher J, Perlroth M: Cyclosporine-associated chronic nephropathy. *N Engl J Med* 311:699, 1984.
127. Tilney NL, Milford EL, Carpenter CB, Lazarus JM, Strom TB, Kirkman RL: Long-term results of cyclosporine treatment in renal transplantation. *Transplant Proc* 18:179, 1986.
128. Flechner SM, Van Buren CT, Kerman RH, Lorber MI, Barker CJ, Golden DL, Kahan BD: Long-term results of cyclosporine therapy in recipients of mismatched living related kidneys. *Transplant Proc* 18:44, 1986.
129. Thiel G, Mihatsch M, Landmann J, Hermle M, Brünner FP, Harder F: Is cyclosporin-A induced nephrotoxicity in recipients of renal allografts progressive? *Transplant Proc* 17 (Suppl 1):169, 1985.
130. Vanrenterghem Y, Waer M, Roels L, Lerut T, Michielsen P: Is cyclosporine associated nephrotoxicity progressive? *Transplant Proc* 1987, in press.
131. McDonald AS, Belitzky P, Gupta R, Bitter–Suermann H, Campbell R, Cohen A, Lannon SC: Conversion from cyclosporine to azathioprine in renal graft recipients. *Transplant Proc* 17:1940, 1985.
132. Land WS, Castro LA, Hillebrand G, Günther K, Gokel JM: Conversion rejection consequences by changing the immunosuppressive therapy from cyclosporine to azathioprine after kidney transplantation. *Transplant Proc* 15 (Suppl 1):2857, 1983.
133. Flechner SM, Lorber M, Van Buren C, Kerman R, Kahan BD: The case against conversion to azathioprine in cyclosporine-treated renal recipients. *Transplant Proc* 17 (Suppl 1):276, 1985.
134. Veitch PS, Taylor JD, Feehally J, Walls J, Bell PRF: Elective conversion from cyclosporine to azathioprine: Long-term follow-up. *Transplant Proc* 19:2017, 1987.
135. Vanrenterghem Y, Waer M, Michielsen P: A controlled trial of one versus three months' cyclosporine and conversion to azathioprine in renal transplantation. *Transplant Proc* 17:1162, 1985.
136. Rocher LL, Milford EL, Kirkman RL, Carpenter CB, Strom TB, Tilney NL: Conversion from cyclosporine to azathioprine in renal allograft recipients. *Transplantation* 38:669, 1984.
137. Ramos CP: Cyclosporin A or azathioprine combined with prednisone in renal allotransplantation with conversion from cyclosporin A to azathioprine at four months. *Proc Eur Dial Transpl Assoc-ERA* 22:571, 1985.
138. Simmons RL, Canafax DM, Strand M, Ascher NL, Payne WD, Sutherland DER, Najarian JS: Management and prevention of cyclosporine nephrotoxicity after renal transplantation: Use of low doses of cyclosporine, azathioprine and prednisone. *Transplant Proc* 17 (Suppl 1):266, 1985.
139. Weimar W, Versluis DJ, Wenting GJ, Derkx FHM, Schalekamp MADH, Jeekel J: Prolonged cyclosporine therapy to induce solid engraftment after renal transplantation. *Transplant Proc* 19:1998, 1987.
140. Maddux MS, Veremis SA, Pollak R, Mozes MF: Conversion from cyclosporine to azathioprine improves renal function without increased risk of graft failure. *Transplant Proc* 19:2007, 1987.
141. Canafax DM, Martel EJ, Asscher NL, Payne WD, Sutherland DER, Simmons RL, Najarian JS: Two methods of managing cyclosporine nephrotoxicity: Conversion to azathioprine, prednisone, or cyclosporin, azathioprine and prednisone. *Transplant Proc* 17:1176, 1985.
142. Lorber MI, Flechner SM, Van Buren CT, Sorensen K, Kerman RH, Kahan BD: Cyclosporine toxicity: The effect of combined therapy using cyclosporine, azathioprine and prednisone. *Am J Kidney Dis* 9:476, 1987.
143. Henry ML, Sommer BG, Ferguson RM: Triple drug therapy: An alternative regimen in renal transplantation. *Transplant Proc* 19:1920, 1987.
144. Fries D, Hiesse C, Charpentier B, Rieu P, Neyrat N, Cantarovich M, Ouziala, Bellamy J, Benoit G: Triple combination of low-dose cyclosporine, azathioprine and steroids in first cadaver donor renal allografts. *Transplant Proc* 19:1911, 1987.
145. Slapak M, Shell T, Digard N, Gosling DC, Qerchi della Rovera G, Crockett RC, Ahmed K: Triple and quadruple therapy after renal transplantation in patients from developing countries. *Transplant Proc* 19:1922, 1987.
146. Fries D, Kechrid C, Charpentier B, Hammouche M, Moulin B: A prospective study of a triple association: Cyclosporine, corticosteroids, and azathioprine in immunologically high-risk renal transplantation. *Transplant Proc* 17:1231, 1985.
147. Salaman JR, Griffin PJA, Ross WB, Williams JD: A controlled trial of triple therapy in renal transplantation. *Transplant Proc* 19:1935, 1987.
148. De Vecchi A, Tarantino A, Montagnino G, Egidi F, Vegeto A, Berardinelli L, Ponticelli C: A controlled prospective trial of triple therapy with low-dose azathioprine, cyclosporine and methylprednisolone in renal transplantation. *Transplant Proc* 19:1933, 1987.
149. Light JA, Aquino A, Ali A, Rodriguez R, Ali S: Quadruple drug therapy prevents graft loss from acute rejection without

increasing mortality. *Transplant Proc* 19:1927, 1987.
150. Deierhoi MH, Sollinger HW, Kalayoglu M, Belzer FO: Quadruple therapy for cadaver renal transplantation. *Transplant Proc* 19:1917, 1987.
151. Halloran P, Ludwin d, Bear R, Aprile M, McQuarrie B, Poole R, White N: Intermodal immunosuppression for cadaver renal transplantation: Results using antilymphocyte globulin, azathioprine, cyclosporine and prednisone. *Transplant Proc* 19:1931, 1987.
152. Halloran P, Ludwin D, Aprile M and the Canadian Multicentre Transplant Study Group: Comparison of antilymphocyte globulinimuran, cyclosporine, and antilymphocyte globulin-cyclosporine therapy for cadaver renal transplantation. *Transplant Proc* 17:1201, 1985.
153. Kahan BD: Individualization of cyclosporine therapy using pharmacokinetic and pharmacodynamic parameters. *Transplantation* 40:457, 1985.
154. Holt DW, Marsden JT, Johnston A, Bewick M, Taube DH: Blood cyclosporin concentrations and renal allograft dysfunction. *Br Med J* 293:1057, 1986.
155. Quesniaux V, Tees R, Schreier MH, Maurer G, van Regenmoortel MHV: Potential of monoclonal antibodies to improve therapeutic monitoring of cyclosporine. *Clin Chem* 33 (1):32, 1987.
156. Reid M, Gibbons S, Kwak D, Van Buren CT, Flechner S, Kahan BD: Cyclosporine levels in human tissues of patients treated for one week to one year. *Transplant Proc* 15:2434, 1983.
157. Kupin WL, Venkat KK, Norris C, Florence–Green Dollie, Dienst S, Oh HK, Feldkamp C, Levin NW: Effective long-term immunosuppression maintained by low cyclosporine levels in primary cadaveric renal transplant recipients. *Transplantation* 43:214, 1987.
158. Cockburn I: Cyclosporine A: A clinical evaluation of drug interactions. *Transplant Proc* 18 (Suppl 5):50, 1986.
159. Langhoff E, Madsen S: Rapid metabolism of cyclosporin and prednisone in kidney transplant patients on tuberculostatic treatment. *Lancet* 2:1303, 1983.
160. Freeman DJ, Laupacis A, Keown PA, Stiller CR, Carruthers SG: Evaluation of cyclosporin-phenytoin interaction with observations on cyclosporin metabolities. *Br J Clin Pharmacol* 18:887, 1984.
161. Carstensen H, Jacobsen N, Dieperink H: Interaction between cyclosporin A and phenobarbitone. *Br J Clin Pharmacol* 21:550, 1986.
162. Wallwork J, McGregor CGA, Wells FC, Cory–Pearce R, English TAH: Cyclosporin and intravenous sulphadimidine and trimethoprim therapy. *Lancet* 1:366, 1983.
163. Hourmant M, Le Bigot JF, Vernillet L, Sagniez G, Remi JP, Soulillou JP: Coadministration of erythromycin results in an increase of blood cyclosporine to toxic levels. *Transplant Proc* 17:2723, 1985.
164. Ferguson RM, Sutherland DER, Simmons RL, Najarian JS: Ketoconazole, cyclosporin metabolism, and renal transplantation. *Lancet* 2:882, 1982.
165. Whiting PH, Cunningham C, Thomson AW, Simpson JG: Enhancement of high dose cyclosporin A toxicity by furosemide. *Biochem Pharmacol* 33:1075, 1984.
166. Klintmalm G, Säwe J: High dose methylprednisolone increases plasma cyclosporin levels in renal transplant recipients. *Lancet* 1:731, 1984.
167. Kennedy MS, Deeg HJ, Siegel M, Crowley JJ, Storb R, Thomas ED: Acute renal toxicity with combined use of amphotericin B and cyclosporin after marrow transplantation. *Transplantation* 35:211, 1983.
168. Thompson JF, Chalmers DHK, Hunisett AGW, Wood RFM, Morris PJ: Nephrotoxicity of trimethoprim and cotrimoxazole in renal allograft recipients treated with cyclosporine. *Transplantation* 36:204, 1983.
169. Whiting PH, Simson JG, Davidson RJL, Thompson AW: The toxic effects of combined administration of cyclosporin A and gentamycin. *Br J Exp Pathol* 63:554, 1982.
170. Kahan BD: Cyclosporine nephrotoxicity: Pathogenesis, prosphylaxis, therapy, and prognosis. *Am J Kidney Dis* 8:323, 1986.
171. Shulman H, Striker G, Deeg HJ, Kennedy M, Strob R, Thomas ED: Nephrotoxicity of cyclosporin A after allogeneic marrow transplantation: Glomerular thromboses and tubular injury. *N Engl J Med* 305:1392, 1981.
172. Bonses RS, Adu D, Franklin I, McMaster P: Cyclosporin-induced hemolytic uremic syndrome in liver allograft recipient. *Lancet* 2:1337, 1984.
173. Neild GH, Reuben R, Hartley RB, Cameron JS: Glomerular thrombi in renal allografts associated with cyclosporin therapy. *J Clin Pathol* 38:253, 1985.
174. Vanrenterghem Y, Roels L, Lerut T, Gruwez J, Michielsen P, Gresele P, Deckmijn H, Colucci M, Arnout J, Vermylen J: Thromboembolic complications and haemostatic changes in cyclosporin-treated cadaveric kidney allograft recipients. *Lancet* 1:999, 1985.
175. Choudhury N, Neild GH, Brown Z, Cameron JS: Thromboembolic complications in cyclosporin-treated kidney allograft recipients. *Lancet* 2:606, 1985.
176. Allen RD, Michie CA, Morris PJ, Chapman JR: Venous thrombosis and cyclosporin. *Lancet* 2:1004, 1985.
177. Brunkwall J, Bergqvist D, Bergentz S-E, Bornmyr S, Husberg B: Postoperative deep venous thrombosis after renal transplantation. Effects of cyclosporine. *Transplantation* 43:647, 1987.
178. Zoja C, Furci L, Ghilardi F, Zilio P, Benigni A, Remuzzi G: Cyclosporin-induced endothelial cell injury. *Lab Invest* 55:455, 1986.
179. Neild GH, Rocchi G, Imberti L, Fumagalli F, Brown Z, Remuzzi G, Williams DG: Effect of cyclosporine on prostacyclin synthesis by vascular tissue in rabbits. *Transplant Proc* 15:2398, 1983.
180. Brown Z, Neild GH, Willoughby J, Somia NV, Cameron SJ: Increased factors VIII as an index of vascular injury in cyclosporine nephrotoxicity. *Transplantation*:42, 150, 1986.
181. Carlsen E, Mallet AC, Prydz H: Effect of cyclosporine A on procoagulant activity in mononuclear blood cells and monocytes in vitro. *Clin Exp Immunol* 60:407, 1985.
182. Vanrenterghem Y, Waer M, Kian Ang K, Lerut T, Bouillon R, Vandeputte I, Vandeputte M, van der Schueren E, Gruwez J, Michielsen P: Renal cadaveric transplantation after total lymphoid irradiation in patients with diabetes. *Kidney Int* 23 (Suppl 14):S-69, 1983.
183. Waer M, Vanrenterghem Y, Roels L, Kian Ang K, Bouillon R, Lerut T, Gruwez J, van der Schueren E, Vandeputte M, Michielsen P: Immunological and clinical observations in diabetic kidney graft recipients pretreated with total-lymphoid irradiation. *Transplantation* 43:371. 1987.
184. Vanrenterghem Y, Waer M, Roels L, Michielsen P: A controlled trial comparing pretransplant total lymphoid irradiation versus posttransplant cyclosporine in type I diabetic cadaveric kidney graft recipients: Short-term results. *Transplant Proc* 19:1542, 1987.
185. Najarian S, Sutherland DER, Ferguson RM, Simmons RL, Kersey J, Mauer SM, Slavin S, Kim TH: Total lymphoid

irradiation and kidney transplantation: A clinical experience.
186. Levin B, Hoppe RT, Collins G, Miller E, Waer M, Bieber C, Girinsky T, Strober S: Treatment of cadaveric renal transplant recipients with total lymphoid irradiation, antithymocyte globulin, and low-dose prednisone. *Lancet* 2:1321, 1985.
187. Cortesini R, Berloco P, Famulari A, Trovati A, Iapelli M, Molajoni ER, Bachetoni A, Pretagostini R, Marinucci G, Capua A, Rossi M, Alfani D: Influence of total lymphoid irradiation plus cyclosporine on kidney graft outcome in high-risk patients. *Transplant Proc* 19:1949, 1987.
188. Myburgh JA, Meyers AM, Botha JR, Thomson PD, Smit JA, Browde S, Lakier R: Wide field low-dose total lymphoid irradiation in clinical kidney transplantation. *Transplant Proc* 19:1974, 1987.
189. Bell PRF, Briggs JD, Calman KC, Paton AM, Wood RFM, McPherson SG, Kyle K: Reversal of acute clinical and experimental organ rejection using large doses of intravenous prednisolone. *Lancet* 1:876, 1971.
190. Nakajima N, Rao TKS, Sakai A, Butt KH, Kountz SL: Effects of intravenous bolus dosages of methylprednisolone and local irradiation on renal allograft rejection and patient mortality. *Surg Gyn Obstet* 144:63, 1977.
191. Kauffman HM Jr, Stromstad SA, Sampson D, Stawicki AT: Randomized steroid therapy of human kidney transplant rejection. *Transplant Proc* 9:36, 1979.
192. Shield CR, Cosimi AB, Tolkoff–Rubin N, Rubin RH, Herrin J, Russell PS: Use of antithymocyte globulin for reversal of acute allograft rejection. *Transplantation* 28:461, 1979.
193. Hoitsma AJ, Reekers P, Kreeftenberg JG, van Lier HJJ, Capel PJA, Koene RAP: Treatment of acute rejection of cadaveric renal allografts with rabbit antithymocyte globulin. *Transplantation* 33:12, 1982.
194. Broyer M, Niaudet P, Bijaoui, Gagnadoux MF: Treatment of acute rejection crisis by antilymphocyte globulins: A randomized prospective study in pediatric kidney transplantation. *Transplant Proc* 19:1886, 1987.
195. Filo RS, Smith EJ, Leapman SB: Therapy of acute cadaveric renal allograft rejection with adjunctive antithymocyte globulin. *Transplantation* 30:445, 1980.
196. Nowygrod R, Appel G, Hardy MA: Use of ATG for reversal of acute allograft rejection. *Transplant Proc* 13:469, 1981.
197. Light JA, Alijani MR, Biggers JA, Oddenino K, Reinmuth B: Antilymphocyte globulin (ALG) reverses irreversible allograft rejection. *Transplant Proc* 13:475, 1981.
198. Hardy MA, Nowygrod R, Erlberg A, Appel G: Use of ATG in treatment of steroid-resistant rejection. *Transplantation* 29:162, 1980.
199. Griffin PJA, Williams GT, Salaman JR: Antilymphocyte globulin for the treatment of steroid non-responsive acute renal allograft rejection. *Clin Nephrol* 21:115, 1984.
200. Veremis SA, Maddux MS, Pollak R, Kline SS, Mozes MF: Alternative antirejection treatment with steroids or antilymphoblast globulin in renal transplant patients receiving cyclosporine. *Transplant Proc* 19:1893, 1987.
201. Benvenisty AI, Tannenbaum GA, Cohen DJ, Appel G, Hardy MA: Use of antithymocyte globulin and cyclosporine to treat steroid-resistant rejection episodes in renal transplant recipients. *Transplant Proc* 19:1889, 1987.
202. Matas AJ, Tellis VA, Quinn T, Glichlick D, Soberman R, Weiss R, Karwa G, Veith FJ: ALG treatment of steroid-resistant rejection in patients receiving cyclosporine. *Transplantation* 41:579, 1986.
203. Ortho Multicenter Transplant Study Group: A randomized clinical trial of OKT3 monoclonal antibody for acute rejection of cadaveric renal transplants. *N Engl J Med* 313:337, 1985.
204. Ponticelli C, Rivolta E, Tarantino A, Egidi F, Banfi G, DeVecchi A, Montagnino G, Vegeto A: Clinical experience with Orthoclone OKT3 in renal transplantation. *Transplant Proc* 18:942, 1986.
205. Thistlethwaite JR Jr, Gaber AO, Haag BW, Aronson AJ, Broelsch CE, Stuart JK, Stuart FP: OKT3 treatment of steroid-resistant renal allograft rejection. *Transplantation* 43:176, 1987.
206. Ponticelli C, Rivolta E, Tarantino A, De Vecchi A, Vegeto A: Rescue of severe steroid-resistant rejection with OKT3.PAN. *Transplant Proc* 19:1908, 1987.
207. Norman DJ, Barry JM, Funnell B, Henell K, Goldstein G: OKT3 for treatment of acute and steroid- and ATG-resistant acute rejection in renal allograft transplantation. *Transplant Proc* 17:2744, 1985.
208. Flye W, Kashgarian M, Gaudio K, Siegel N, Smith D, Kliger A, Schiff M, Bia MJ: Cyclosporine and OKT3 salvage for steroid-and ATG-resistant renal transplant rejection.
209. Monaco A, Goldstein G, Bernes L: Use of Orthoclone OKT3 monoclonal antibody to reverse acute renal allograft rejection unresponsive to treatment with conventional immunosuppressive regimens. *Transplant Proc* 19 (Suppl 1):28, 1987.
210. Hirsch RL, Layton PC, Barnes LA, Kremer AB, Goldstein G: Orthoclone OKT3 treatment of acute renal allograft rejection in patients receiving maintenance cyclosporine therapy. *Transplant Proc* 19 (Suppl 1):32, 1987.
211. Takahashi H, Terasaki PI, Kinukawa T, Chia D, Miura K, Okazaki H, Iwaki Y, Taguchi Y, Hardiwidjaja S, Ishizaki M, Billing B: Reversal of transplant rejection by monoclonal antiblast antibody. *Lancet* 2:1155, 1983.
212. Kirkman RL, Araujjo JL, Busch GJ, Carpenter CB, Milford EL, Reinherz EL, Schlossman SF, Strom TB, Tilney NL: Treatment of acute renal allograft rejection with monoclonal anti-T12 antibody. *Transplantation* 36:620, 1983.
213. Cosimi AB: Treatment of rejection: Antithymocyte globulin versus monoclonal antibodies. *Transplant Proc* 17:1562, 1985.
214. Norman DJ, Shield III CF, Barry J, Henell K, Funnell MB, Lemon J: A U.S. clinical study of Orthoclone OKT3 in renal transplantation. *Transplant Proc* 19 (suppl 1):21, 1987.
215. Van Wauwe JP, De Mey JR, Goossens JG: OKT3: A monoclonal antihuman T lymphocyte antibody with potent mitogenic properties. *J Immunol* 124:2708, 1980.

CHAPTER 58

Tubular and Metabolic Dysfunction Following Kidney Transplantation

J. WINAVER, J. GREEN & O.S. BETTER

INTRODUCTION

The transplanted kidney is exposed to a wide range of injuries. These may afflict the kidney before, during, and after the surgical procedure. The trauma, shock, or morbidity that caused the death of the donor may affect the kidney even before the operation. In addition, the handling of the kidney, the extracorporeal perfusion, and the surgery itself may cause damage to the kidney during the operative and perioperative phase. After transplantation the kidney is also subjected to rejection and other deleterious conditions (summarized in Table 1). The resulting kidney damage is frequently associated with a generalized decrease in renal function characterized by oliguria or anuria of variable duration. Occasionally, however, despite this hostile environment, the glomerular filtration rate is relatively spared and the injury is predominantly tubulointerstitial (see Table 2). These tubular syndromes may cause profound changes in the acid-base balance and disturbances in electrolyte and mineral homeostasis, which may aggravate preexisting bone disease and lead to nephrocalcinosis or nephrolithiasis.

Alteration in renal tubular functions may appear in the early phase following kidney transplantation. Many of these early tubular syndromes are consequences of the acute tubular necrosis sustained by the transplanted kidney and therefore are potentially reversible. Disturbances in electrolyte and mineral metabolism in the early posttransplant period may also represent metabolic and hormonal derangements of chronic renal failure that persist into the setting of a "normally" functioning kidney. Finally, aberrations in tubular functions may occur as a late consequence, i.e., months and even years afer successful kidney transplantation. The appearance of such a disturbance in a patient with an allograft that was hitherto functioning normally may be the first sign of rejection.

It is therefore important to recognize the various forms of tubular syndromes and metabolic abberrations that have been reported following kidney transplantation. Understanding their pathogenetic mechanisms is not merely of academic interest, but may also have important prognostic and therapeutic implications. The present chapter will review the various tubular and metabolic defects that have been described following renal transplantation.

RENAL TUBULAR ACIDOSIS (RTA)

Hyperchloremic metabolic acidosis due to a tubular defect in the transplanted kidney was first reported in 1967 by Massry and associates (1). Subsequently, the occurrence of RTA following kidney transplantation was confirmed in many other studies (2–12). Most of the patients reported presented with a mild spontaneous hyperchloremic acidosis associated with an inappropriately high urinary pH. The latter finding is highly suggestive of an impairment in distal acidification, i.e., distal RTA (1–6). Proximal RTA, either as an isolated finding or more frequently as a part of generalized proximal tubular dysfunction (Fanconi syndrome), have been also reported (1, 6, 7–13).

Finally, an incomplete form of distal RTA, which may be uncovered only during a challenge with an acid load, has been described following kidney transplantation in patients who otherwise displayed a normal acid-base status (3, 6). Thus, a wide spectrum of tubular defects that result in impaired renal acid excretion may be encountered in the transplanted kidney.

RTA is not a rare finding following renal transplantation. In the study of Gyory et al. (2), evidence for impaired tubular acidification was obtained in 13 of 21 patients (61%) with a cadaver renal allograft. In three of these patients this defect resulted in moderate-to-severe hyperchloremic acidosis. In the study of Wilson and Siddiqui (6), 14 of 32 patients who were studied 3–6 weeks after renal transplantation displayed evidence of defective distal acidification (complete or incomplete forms). Six additional patients had signs compatible with proximal tubular acidosis. In the late phase, i.e., 1–3 years after kidney transplantation, 13 of 30 patients (43%) showed evidence of impaired distal acidification (6). Therefore, episodes of hyperchloremic renal tubular acidosis may be frequently encountered both in the early and the late phase following kidney transplantation.

In most studies the impairment in urinary acidification was observed in the first few months after transplantation

Table 1. Potential causes for tubular dysfunction following transplantation

1. Ischemic damage following acute tubular necrosis
2. Acute and chronic rejection
3. Unresolved hyperparathyroidism with or without hypercalcemia
4. Use of nephrotoxic agents
5. Lack of renal innervation
6. Urinary tract infection
7. Obstructive uropathy
8. Ischemia due to renal artery stenosis

Table 2. Tubular dysfunction following kidney transplantation

1. Renal tubular acidosis (RTA): proximal, distal and mixed type
2. Fanconi syndrome (generalized defect in proximal reabsoroption of bicarbonate, glucose, amino acid, phosphate, and uric acid)
3. Urinary phosphate leak (PTH dependent and PTH independent)
4. Defects in tubular calcium reabsorption, nephrolithiasis, and nephrocalcinosis
5. Impaired ability to excrete potassium resulting in hyperkalemia (nonazotemic hyperkalemia)
6. Hypoaldosteronism resulting in hyperkalemia and acidosis Type 4 RTA)
7. Impaired ability to maximally concentrate and dilute the urine
8. Any combination of disturbances described above

and in some cases appeared to be reversible (2, 5, 6). The defect was ascribed to several potential factors, such as acute rejection episodes, ischemic tubular damage, and proximal bicarbonate wasting due to secondary hyperparathyroidism (2–6).

Distal renal tubular acidosis

Renal tubular acidosis due to impaired distal acidification (DRTA) has been traditionally ascribed to the inability of the distal nephron to maintain a steep hydrogen gradient between tubular urine and peritubular blood (gradient limitation RTA) (14, 15). This view was challenged by Halperin, who suggested that DRTA may also result from impaired H^+ ion secretion (16). More recent data based on studies in human subjects, experimental animal models, and membrane analogues of mammalian collecting duct have clearly indicated that DRTA is a heterogeneous group of disorders originating from various pathophysiologic mechanisms (17–19). These include a primary defect in the proton pump (secretory defect), an inability to generate an appropriate electrical gradient for H^+ ion secretion (voltage defect) and increased permeability of the collecting duct to protons or carbonic acid (gradient or backleak defect) (17–19). In addition, the association of RTA with various forms of primary and secondary hypoaldosteronism has been increasingly recognized in recent years (18, 20–23). This syndrome (commonly referred to as Type IV RTA) is characterized by hyperchloremic metabolic acidosis, hyperkalemia, and a normal ability to lower urinary pH during systemic acidosis. Suppression of urinary ammonium secretion, probably secondary to the hyperkalemia, has been proposed as a major pathogenetic mechansim in this interesting clinical entity (24).

The various subtypes of DRTA may be distinguished by evaluating the following: a) urinary pH and net acid excretion in response to systemic acidosis and sodium sulfate administration, b) measurements of urine minus blood p_{CO_2} difference (U-Bp_{CO_2}) during bicarbonate and neutral phosphate infusion, and c) the plasma potassium level and urinary potassium excretion, as well as the renin-angiotensin-aldosterone axis (17, 19).

Because many of the descriptions of RTA following kidney transplantation were published before this newly developed classification became available, many cases were incompletely evaluated. However, based on data available in the literature, it appears that the syndrome of RTA in the transplanted kidney is not a unifying entity, and several pathophysiologic mechanisms may contribute to its development. Thus, the patient described by Massry et al. (1) failed to increase titratable acid excretion after an intravenous phosphate load, which suggests a tubular defect in proton secretion. In contrast, Better et al. (3) showed a considerable increase in titratable acid excretion during neutral phosphate infusion, indicating a different underlying mechanism in their patients. Batlle et al. (25) have recently evaluated six patients with persistent hyperchloremic metabolic acidosis developing in the first 2 months after kidneys transplantation. Five of these patients displayed a DRTA highly suggestive of a primary secretory defect (i.e., inability to lower urinary pH below 5.5, impaired acidification response to Na_2SO_4 administration, and failure to generate a steep U-Bp_{CO_2} gradient during $NaHCO_3$ and neutral phosphate infusions). The sixth patient manifested the characteristics of Type IV RTA associated with hypoaldosteronism and hyperkalemia. Urinary ammonium excretion was low during spontaneous systemic acidosis despite the fact that his urinary pH was below 5.5. Followup of these patients revealed in each patient, with the exception of one who lost his kidney due to accelerated early rejection, histologic features suggestive of chronic allograft rejection. The authors hypothesized that the impaired renal acidification in their patients resulted from immunologically mediated renal damage. The deposition of complement (C_3) along the tubular basement membrane and mononuclear cell infiltrates in the renal interstitium found in these patients are similar to those described in other autoimmune diseases complicated by RTA such as systemic lupus erythematosus (26) and Sjogrens syndrome (27). They further conclude that DRTA in the transplanted kidney is indicative of permanent tubular damage and should be considered as an ominous sign of graft survival.

Indeed, the association between renal allograft rejection and the appearance of renal tubular acidosis has also been emphasized by previous authors (4, 6). Mookerjee and coworkers (4) reported the occurrence of hyperchloremia and impaired urinary acidification in 33.6% of 122 rejection episodes. They claimed that the occurrence of hyperchloremic acidosis was a reliable early sign of rejection sufficient to warrant treatment, even when signs of rejection were not clearly present. Furthermore, reestablishment of normochloremia could be taken as a good prognostic guide to the efficacy of the treatment of the rejection episode (4). In a long-term followup of 32 patients whose allograft had been functioning for 1–3 years, Wilson and Siddiqui (6) found that persistent DRTA could be considered as a functional equivalent of chronic rejection. In contrast, proximal RTA and reduced ammonia secretion had a tendency to disappear. These data clearly indicate the possible association between distal tubular acidosis and rejection of the transplanted kidney.

On the other hand, defects in distal acidification have also been described as a consequence of acute tubular necrosis (14, 28–30). Therefore, the latter phenomenon could also be a sequel of the ischemic damage occurring in the early phase of cadaveric renal transplantation. The finding of spontaneous remissions of the acidification defect might indicate that the latter may be possible (2, 3, 6). Futhermore, we have recently demonstrated a defect in distal acidification in an experimental model of acute renal ischemia in the dog (31). This defect appears to be of a secretory type and is identical to the one described by Batlle et al. (25) as a characteristic sign of allograft rejection. It seems, therefore, that both acute tubular necrosis and allograft rejection may lead to similar acidification defects in the early phase following renal transplantation. Thus, we believe that the finding of DRTA in the early post-transplant period is not necessarily a poor prognostic sign. Certainly, the significance of the impaired renal acidification in patients with renal allograft has not been fully elucidated. Additional long-term studies with sequential assessments of the distal acidifying capacity will be required in order to determine the prognostic implications of DRTA following renal transplantation.

Recent studies (32, 33) have suggested that cyclosporin A (CSA), the recently introduced immunosuppressive agent, may impair urinary acid excretion and lead to the development of hyperchloremic metabolic acidosis. Although no detailed evaluation of the tubular defect had been performed in these patients, the finding of a preserved capacity to lower urinary pH is probably compatible with the diagnosis of Type IV RTA (32, 33). In two patients described by Stahl et al. (33), reversal of the acidosis and hyperchloremia was noticed upon cessation of (CSA) treatment. In view of the increasing use of the drug, this rare complication should be added to the differential diagnosis of post-transplant RTA.

Other factors such as nephrocalcinosis, interstitial nephritis, and obstructive uropathy may be associated with DRTA in patients with a kidney transplant (18, 34). Of particular interest in this respect is the association between obstructive uropathy and hyperkalemic distal tubular acidosis that has been described by Batlle and coworkers (34). This potentially curable complication should be considered as a possible cause of DRTA and the deterioration of renal function after kidney transplantation.

Proximal tubular dysfunction (Fanconi syndrome)

FOLLOWING RENAL TRANSPLANTATION

Alterations in proximal tubular functions have been reported in the original patient with post-transplant RTA described by Massry et al. (1). Since this initial study few other reports have described the association of proximal tubular dysfunction with kidney transplantation (6–13). In its full expression, proximal tubular dysfunction may present in the form of the Fanconi syndrome, (glycosuria, amino aciduria, phosphaturia, and bicarbonate wasting). Uric acid clearance may reach 30% or more of GFR under these circumstances. In our experience, however, excessive uricosuria or hypouricemia is not commonly seen following transplantation (3). The pathophysiology of the Fanconi syndrome in renal transplant patients remains obscure. Both primary and secondary hyperparathyroidism (35, 36) have been suggested as contributing to urinary bicarbonate wasting (proximal RTA) and could also account for the phosphaturia seen in many patients. Persistent secondary hyperparathyroidism could certainly be a factor in renal tubular acidosis after renal transplantation, since patients with chronic renal failure usually have excessive levels of this hormone circulating at the time of the transplantation and for several months thereafter (37). The losses of bicarbonate and phosphate in the urine may perpetuate the acidosis and aggravate the bone disease of these patients. Tubular dysfunction due to graft rejection or ischemic acute renal failure may be another cause for the development of the Fanconi syndrome after transplantation.

Since the report by Butler et al. (38) of Fanconi syndrome in an adult nephrotic patient receiving mercaptopurine, it has been claimed that immunosuppressive therapy caused tubular dysfunction. However, this has never been substantiated. Moreover, in the patient described by Vertuno et al. (11), some of the proximal tubular dysfunction remitted while the patient was receiving immunosuppressive drugs.

In summary, renal tubular acidosis is the most prevalent tubular syndrome following kidney transplantation. It may encompass the entire spectrum of RTA, namely, proximal, distal (both secretory and nonsecretory), Type 3 (mixed proximal and distal), and Type 4 RTA. Acidification disorders may vary as a function of time after transplantation. As a general rule, RTA that appears early following transplantation resolves spontaneously and is predominantly a sequel to acute renal failure (acute tubular necrosis). On the other hand, defects that exist in the late post-transplant period are due to chronic rejection. A contributory minor role in the pathogenesis of RTA may also be played by secondary hyperparathyroidism, reduced ammonium excretion (due to protein malnutrition or hyperkalemia), urinary tract infection, and obstructive uropathy. Chronic RTA following transplantation may interfere with bone metabolism and may rarely lead to nephrocalcinosis and nephrolithiasis. Therefore, if sustained and complicated by hypophosphatemia, phosphate and bicarbonate should be supplemented, at least to protect the skeleton. Fortunately, in most patients RTA remits spontaneously and no special treatment seems to be indicated.

DISORDERS OF POTASSIUM HOMEOSTASIS FOLLOWING KIDNEY TRANSPLANT

In the recovery phase after kidney transplantation, most patients have a tendency to develop hypokalemia. Among the causes contributing to this phenomenon are the osmotic diuresis and polyuria of the recovery phase from acute tubular necrosis, administration of large doses of steroids, and occasionally the occurrence of renal tubular acidosis. On the other hand, in our experience hyperkalemia is rare after successful kidney transplantation. Yet, the danger of hyperkalemia is always a potential threat to patients who undergo an emergency operation without endogenous kidney function. Such a patient should receive potassium-binding resins per rectum (Kayexalate®) before being operated, particularly if time has elapsed since the previous dialysis. Transfusion of old, stored blood or administration of the muscle relaxant, succinylcholine, should be avoided because of their tendency of cause hyperkalemia (39).

The defense against hyperkalemia depends on the normal uptake of potassium by cells (internal balance) as well as elimination of excess potassium by the kidneys (external balance) (40, 41). A brief summary of the various alterations in the internal and external potassium balance that may lead to the development of hyperkalemia is given in Tables 3 and 4.

Many reports expanding on the subject of nonazotemic hyperkalemia have appeared since the original study of Hudson et al. (42), namely, hyperkalemia that may occur in patients with only modest kidney failure. This type of hyperkalemia has been also described within the particular setting of kidney transplantation.

The first report of a cluster of patients with kidney grafts and hyperkalemia came from Australia (2). The second communication describing this complication appeared in the USA (43). DeFronzo et al. (43) observed hyperkalemia in 23 of 75 patients in the first 3 months following transplantation. The hyperkalemia was unrelated to rejection, renal failure, oliguria, or acidosis. Urinary potassium excretion was sufficient to achieve potassium balance, but was inappropriately low relative to the hyperkalemia. In all patients, the hyperkalemia resolved spontaneously. An unusual feature of this hyperkalemia was its refractoriness to furosemide. Few patients responded, however, to thiazides with an increase in urinary potassium excretion and a fall in serum potassium. When the renin-angiotensin-aldosterone axis was studied, it was found to be normal under basal conditions and responded adequately and appropriately to stimulation (43). However, the patients displayed refractoriness to the kaliuretic action of exogenous mineralocorticoids and to infusions of acetazolamide and bicarbonate. Based on the latter findings, the authors concluded that their hyperkalemic patients had an end-organ (distal tubular) defect of potassium excretion, the nature of which has not been elucidated (43).

The acquired transient distal tubular defect in the excretion (secretion) of potassium observed in these transplant patients (43) is reminiscent of a similar, but permanently impaired renal ability to secrete potassium seen in several other patients. The growing list of such patients includes single case reports with hyperkalemia and hypertension seen in Australia (44, 45), children with hyperkalemia and short stature (46, 47), patients with lupus erythematosus (48), patients with sickle cell disease (49), and patients with familial hypertension, hyperkalemia, and acidosis reported from Israel (50–52). After scanning the data of these familial cases, it appears that in at least one member of the family the hyperkalemia was resistant to furosemide (50). In contrast, in other members of the family (51, 52), thiazides corrected the hyperkalemia by increasing urinary excretion of potassium. This pattern of response to different diuretics is similar to that seen in the transplant patients of DeFronzo et al. (43).

A defect in potassium excretion has been induced experimentally in animals by selectively damaging the medullary portion of the kidney (53). Conceivably, therefore, medullary interstitial kidney damage, which is common after transplantation, in sickle cell anemia (49), and perhaps in lupus erythematosus (48), is the common denominator of the impaired renal handling of potassium.

Table 3. Factors producing nonazotemic hyperkalemia by influencing the internal balance of potassium

1. Hypoinsulinism or end-organ refractoriness to the action of insulin
2. Hypoaldosteronism
3. β-adrenergic blockade
4. Acidosis
5. Hyperglycemia in the presence of factors 1, 2, or 3

Table 4. Factors producing nonazotemic hyperkalemia by interfering with urinary excretion of potassium (external balance)

1. Primary tubular defect in potassium excretion
2. Factors related to mineralocorticoid hormone "deficiency"
   a. Primary mineralocorticold deficiency
   b. Syndrome of hyporeninemic hypoaldosteronism (SHHA)
   c. Heparin
   d. Pseudohypoaldosteronism (with high blood levels of aldosterone)
3. Use of potassium-sparing diuretics (spironolactone, amiloride, triamterene)
4. Use of cyclosporin A

In addition to a primary tubular defect in potassium secretion, other factors, in particular those associated with impaired function of the renin-angiotensin-aldosterone system, have been invoked as a possible cause of posttransplant hyperkalemia. The syndrome of hyporeninemic hypoaldosteronism (SHHA) (54, 55) should be sought as a potential cause of hyperkalemia, especially in patients with diabetes mellitus (55). It should be noted that patients with "primary renal hyperkalemia" may masquerade as having the syndrome of (SHHA). This is because hyperkalemia per se may suppress plasma renin activity. Although hyperkalemia should directly stimulate aldosterone secretion, the stimulation could be overridden by volume overload secondary to excessive salt reabsorption (56). In addition, it has been suggested that the direct stimulation of aldosterone secretion by potassium requires the presence of angiotensin II (57) and therefore may be diminished in cases of hyporeninemia.

Roll et al. (58) reported two patients in whom transient hyperkalemia appeared after kidney transplantation. The hypokalemia was excessive in relation to the graft function and urine output. Plasma renin and aldosterone were low and did not respond to standard stimulation. Administration of mineralocorticoids corrected the hyperkalemia by augmenting the urinary potassium excretion. This suggests that hyporeninemic hypoaldosteronism contributed to the hyperkalemia of these two patients. It is not known what caused the suppression of the renin-angiotensin-aldosterone axis in the patients of Roll et al. (58). Possible causes may be a prolonged pretransplant volume overload (56) and chronic exposure to heparin during hemodialysis, which is known to suppress adrenal function (59).

Hyperkalemia due to hypoaldosteronism has been also observed in 2 of the 6 patients reported by Batlle et al. (25) as suffering from distal RTA following renal transplantation. One of these patients also had a tubular defect in potassium secretion, as evidenced by the blunted kaliuretic response to sodium sulfate and fluorohydrocortisone administration. Finally, hyperkalemia has been also described as a manifestation of "pseudohypoaldosteronism," i.e., renal refractoriness to high circulating levels of aldosterone (60).

The spectrum of hyperkalemia following kidney transplantation has been broadened since the introduction of cyclosporin A (CSA) as an important immunosuppressive tool. Cyclosporin A is currently used in many centers as a useful agent for preventing the rejection of renal allografts. Nephrotoxicity is a well-documented side effect of this agent, usually manifested by a reduction in GFR and an increase in plasma creatinine and BUN levels (61, 62). Several studies have reported an increased incidence of hyperkalemia in patients with kidney transplant treated with (CSA) (32, 63–65). Thus, Adu and coworkers (32) found hyperkalemia in 7 of 43 cyclosporin-treated renal transplant recipients. In the renal transplant patients of the University of Minnesota, 25% of those receiving CSA developed hyperkalemia sufficient to warrant treatment, whereas only 6% of the patients receiving azathioprine needed such treatment (63, 65). The mechanism leading to the development of hyperkalemia in patients treated with CSA is not clear. It is obvious, however, that the reduction in GRF reported in these patients was not sufficient to decrease urinary potassium excretion. Bantle and coworkers (65) have recently demonstrated a decrease in plasma renin activity, as well as a reduction in the kaliuretic response to KCl loads in renal allograft recipients treated with CSA. The authors have suggested that CSA-induced hyperkalemia is the result of both the defect in tubular potassium secretion and the suppression of plasma renin activity. In contrast to the findings in humans (65), studies in experimental animals suggest that the renin-angiotensin system is actually stimulated by CSA (66). Whatever the mechanism, a higher incidence of hyperkalemia in transplant patients is expected in the future due to increasing use of the drug. Plasma potassium levels, therefore, should be carefully monitored, and the use of potassium-containing medications and potassium-sparing diuretics should be minimized in patients receiving CSA. Special care should be taken in patients with diabetes mellitus in whom potassium regulation is further compromised by the lack of insulin.

The instances of nonazotemic hyperkalemia described above were mainly due to impaired elimination of potassium by the kidneys (positive external balance). Potassium load from tissue catabolism, because of infection, hemolysis, massive blood transfusion, and acidosis are additional factors aggravating the hyperkalemia.

An important impairment in the internal balance of potassium has been described in a diabetic patient (67). In this patient, who was insulin dependent and had an adequately functioning kidney graft, hyperglycemia was associated with hyperkalemia. Interestingly, plasma and urinary aldosterone levels were normal. It was considered that insulinopenia resulted in impaired cellular uptake of both glucose and potassium, leading to hyperglycemia and hyperkalemia. Solvent drag from the intracellular to the extracellular compartment under the influence of the hyperosmolality of hyperglycemia probably contributed to the hyperkalemia as well.

The renal response to diuretics may give a clue to the cause of hyperkalemia in post-transplant patients. Correction of the hyperkalemia with furosemide or exogenous mineralocorticoids suggests hypoaldosteronism with normal end-organ function. Refractoriness of the hyperkalemia to furosemide or mineralocorticoids, but its correction with thiazides, suggests a primary defect in renal handling of potassium.

In summary, transient hyperkalemia may be seen occasionally following kidney transplantation, even when the graft function is otherwise normal. The mechanism of this hyperkalemia could be due to a) a primary tubular defect of potassium excretion, b) impaired function of the renin-angiotensin-aldosterone system with mineralocorticoid deficiency, or c) disturbances in internal potassium balance reflecting diminished translocation from the extracellular to the intracellular compartment. The clinical implication of these findings is that careful monitoring of serum potassium is mandatory following renal transplants.

This is especially true in diabetic patients and/or in those receiving CSA in whom administration of potassium-sparing diuretics and a potassium supplement may result in life-threatening hyperkalemia.

IMPAIRED ABILITY TO CONCENTRATE AND DILUTE THE URINE

Clinically, a normal state of hydration is well maintained following transplantation. However, when the body is subjected to fluid overload or prolonged thirst, the ability to maximally dilute or concentrate the urine is impaired (3, 68). In some of these patients defects in urinary dilution and concentration were found in the presence of normal GFR (68). In some reports, RTA was associated with either impaired concentration or dilution of urine (69, 70), suggesting an impaired tubulointerstitial function. Post-transplant hypercalcemia, which occurs in up to one third of these patients (71), may contribute to the defect in maximal urinary concentration.

OBSTRUCTIVE UROPATHY FOLLOWING RENAL TRANSPLANTATION

Ureteral obstruction following kidney transplantation may have several adverse effects on the graft. The main causes of post-transplant obstructive uropathy are surgical complications at the ureteral anastomosis and nephrolithiasis. There have also been reports of some rare causes such as periureteral fibrosis developing after transplantation, probably produced by retroperitoneal hemorrhage or retroperitonitis (72, 73).

Obstructive lesions in the transplanted kidney may lead to deterioration of the graft function, defects in urinary concentration resembling nephrogenous diabetes insipidus, and hypertension (73). All these defects may remit following relief of the obstruction.

Batlle et al. (34) showed that distal RTA and hyperkalemia may complicate obstructive uropathy of various etiologies. These disturbances were attributable either to tubular dysfunction or to hyporeninemic hypoaldosteronism. It is conceivable that obstructive uropathy following transplantation may cause similar defects.

The clinical implication of these potential complications requires that a pyelography or ultrasonography of the graft be performed as early as possible after transplantation in order to achieve baseline data for future reference.

DISORDERS OF DIVALENT ION METABOLISM FOLLOWING KIDNEY TRANSPLANTATION

Disturbances of divalent ions and mineral metabolism are common after successful renal transplantation. These include transient and persistent hypercalcemia due to hyperparathyroidism (37, 71, 74-83), a defect in tubular calcium reabsorption, and subnormal intestinal calcium absorption (84). Hypophosphatemia, secondary to either renal phosphate loss or impaired intestinal absorption, is also frequently encountered following kidney transplantation (37, 85).

The occurrence of hypercalcemia after kidney transplantation was first reported in 1964 (74) and subsequently has been described in a number of other studies (37, 71, 75-84). The onset of hypercalcemia may occur as early as 1 day, or as late as 1 year following kidney transplantation (71). The incidence of hypercalcemia in patients with kidney transplantation has varied from 9% to more than one third of the patients (71, 75, 78, 82, 83).

Although several mechanisms may contribute to the development of hypercalcemia in the post-transplant period, hyperfunction of the parathyroid glands is undoubtedly the predominant factor responsible for the latter phenomenon. The hyperparathyroidism of chronic uremia and dialysis usually persists into the post-transplant period despite resolution of uremic state. Persistence of hyperparathyroidism in the face of a normal functioning kidney is related to the fact that the hyperplastic parathyroid glands undergo hypoplasia at a very slow rate (86). As was pointed out recently by Parfitt (86), the normal human parathyroid gland has a low rate of cell turnover and poorly developed mechanisms for cell deletion. As a consequence, the involution of the enlarged parathyroid gland is an extremely slow process in comparison to other endocrine glands. Since the majority of the patients have enlarged parathyroid glands at the time of transplantation, it is reasonable to assume that hyperfunctioning of the gland will persist in the post-transplant period. Indeed, evidence for hyperparathyroidism can be found in approximately two thirds of transplant recipients when parathormone levels are measured (78, 87). On the other hand, the metabolism of vitamin D returns to normal in most patients (84, 85, 88). Restoration of metabolic conversion of 25-hydroxycholecalciferol to 1,25-dihydroxycholecalciferol, the active metabolite of vitamin D, enhances skeletal sensitivity to parathyroid hormone and increases intestinal absorption of calcium. Normalization of the uremic environment under these conditions may augment the tendency to hypercalcemia and unmask vitamin-D intoxication. Additional factors may aggravate the hyperparathyroidism and accentuate hypercalcemia. Hypophosphatemia can potentiate hypercalcemia when phosphate depletion is produced by overzealous use of phosphate-binding gels or by increased urinary loss due to corticosterioid therapy or tubular leak of phosphate (33, 85). Increased demand for phosphate by the skeleton due to improved mineralization following successful transplantation may also contribute to the hypophosphatemia. Finally, mobilization of soft-tissue "metastatic," calcifications is another possible cause of hypercalcemia after renal transplantation (89).

According to Parfitt (86) three stages can be discerned in the evolution of post-transplant hypercalcemia: early severe hypercalcemia, transient hypercalcemia, and persistent hypercalcemia. Severe hypercalcemia, probably reflecting the poor control of hyperparathyroidism during dialysis, was more frequent in early reports and often required emergency parathyroidectomy. This form has become rare because of improved control of hyperparathyroidism in patients on chronic dialysis. Transient hypercalcemia (duration of 1 year of less) is of more frequent occurrence, although its incidence has become relatively less common in recent years. Factors such as iatrogenic phosphate depletion, mobilization of soft-tissue calcifications, and a too rapid reduction in the dose of corticosteroids may play an important role in the pathogenesis of transient hypercalcemia, in addition to hyperparathyroidism. Of major importance, however, especially with regard to appropriate management, is the persistent form of post-transplant hypercalcemia. The latter form, arbitrarily assigned to cases where hypercalcemia persists for longer than 1 year, has become more common in the last decade (86). In the studies of David et al. (71), persistent hypercalcemia of more than 1 year's duration was reported in 5 of his 22 hypercalcemic patients. Chattergee et al. (79) found persistent hypercalcemic for 2–4 years in 7 of 16 hypercalcemic patients, and in two patients the hypercalcemia persisted for 7 years. Persistent hypercalcemia, however, is not synonymous with permanent hypercalcemia. Cases have been reported in which normocalcemia was eventually restored after 2–6 years (79–81).

David et al. (71) found a correlation between the time of onset of hypercalcemia and its severity and duration: Early onset (within the first 10 days after transplantation) was associated with a greater severity of hypercalcemia, frequently necessitating urgent parathyroidectomy. A negative correlation was also documented between kidney function in the early post-transplant period and the development of hypercalcemia. Hypercalcemia did not develop in any of the patients with a creatinine clearance of less than 30 ml/min (71). It is noteworthy that no correlation was found between the presence of renal osteodystrophy before transplantation and the occurrence of hypercalcemia following transplantation (37).

Several issues have been raised regarding the optimal management of persistent hypercalcemia following kidney transplantation. Although parathyroidectomy was advocated in several earlier studies, in particular if normocalcemia was not restored after some arbitrary time interval, more recent studies have questioned this policy (80, 81, 90, 91). Even if hypercalcemia persists for a long period, most cases are asymptomatic and the disease appears to be of a benign nature. Of particular interest is the fact that complications such as renal calculi and bone disease are rare in patients with post-transplant hypercalcemia. The recent large series in which hundreds of post-transplant patients have been followed for years confirm that impression (80, 81, 90). Thus in the study of Christensen et al. (80), post-transplant hypercalcemia was detected in 29 of 174 long-term allograft recipients, and parathyroidectomy was performed in five patients, of whom only one was symptomatic. In a series of 400 kidney transplants reported by Diethelm et al. (81), 113 patients developed hypercalcemia, but only 34 followed the criteria of persistent hypercalcemia. Six of these patients underwent parathyroidectomy, whereas 28 patients remained asymptomatic in a followup of 3 months to 9 years. In view of the favorable outcome and the benign sequelae of the disease, several recent studies recommended reserving surgical intervention only for cases with progressive clinical or roentgenographic findings (81, 90, 91). Parathyroidectomy is clearly indicated in patients with a rapid deterioration in renal function due to severe hypercalcemia, bone fractures, or those developing kidney stones. However, these complications are rare, in most patients with mild asymptomatic hypercalcemia nonsurgical management with careful observation is currently recommended (81, 91). The degree of hypercalcemia is of importance in this regard. It has been claimed that persistent elevation of serum calcium of < 12 mg/dl does not damage the function of the allograft (71). On the other hand, serum calcium levels > 13 mg/dl may produce a decrease in creatinine clearance, which improves after subtotal parathyroidectomy (71, 77, 79). Thus, it seems prudent to follow renal function carefully and frequently in renal transplant recipients. If renal function deteriorates in the absence of evidence for rejection, then parathyroidectomy should be seriously considered. Finally, since phosphate depletion might contribute to the development of post-transplant hypercalcemia, Alfrey et al. (37) recommended a trial of repletion with phosphate-containing agents. Phosphate supplementation is probably worth trying for a short period. However, long-term treatment with phosphate may actually stimulate the parathyroid gland and aggravate soft-tissue calcification (92). It is therefore recommended to try this treatment for a period of no longer than 3 months (77). If the hypercalcemia persists thereafter, or metastatic calcifications develop, phosphate supplementation should be stopped and parathyroidectomy considered.

NEPHROLITHIASIS AND NEPHROCALCINOSIS AFTER RENAL TRANSPLANTATION

Nephrolithiasis and nephrocalcinosis may occur following successful renal transplantation (93–99). Calcium deposition in transplanted kidneys has been noted as early as 5 days and as late as 16 months postoperatively. Although there are certain favorable metabolic conditions for the formation of kidney stones following transplantation, the actual incidence of post-transplant nephrolithiasis is surprisingly low.

Hypercalcemia, secondary to hyperparathyroidism, is an important factor in the pathogenesis of nephrolithiasis and nephrocalcinosis in the transplanted kidney. Nevertheless, most patients in whom hypercalcemia develops or is maintained after renal transplantation will not demonstrate calcium deposition or calculi in the kidney. This low incidence of calcium deposition in allografts is contrary to renal involvement in primary hyperparathyroidism, in which case 48–78% of patients clinically demonstrate stones or nephrocalcinosis (100). The low incidence of stone formation in transplanted kidneys may be reflected in the transient nature of the hypercalcemia and in the early medical or surgical treatment that this closely observed group of patients receives. Apart from hyperparathyroidism, urinary tract infection (by urea-splitting organisms) and distal RTA may have a contributory role in stone formation. Renal tubular acidosis, which is quite a common tubular defect after transplantation, predisposes to stone formation due to hypercalciuria, alkaline pH of the urine, and a low rate of urinary citrate excretion.

In order to prevent deterioration of graft function, parathyroidectomy should seriously be considered in all patients who manifest nephrolithiasis or nephrocalcinosis. In fact, all patients reported so far as suffering from these complications benefitted from such a procedure.

In addition to parathyroidectomy, control of urinary tract infection, correction of renal tubular acidosis if it exists, and institution of a high water-intake regimen are also necessary to ensure effective therapy. Stone removal may be required only if there is calyceal or ureteral obstruction. However, nonoperative management of stones is preferable because of the increased risk of infection and impairment of wound healing in the immunosuppressed patient.

HYPOPHOSPHATEMIA FOLLOWING KIDNEY TRANSPLANTATION

Hypophosphatemia is common following successful kidney transplantation, particularly in the early posttransplant period, and is frequently associated with hypercalcemia (37, 85). The introduction of a normal kidney into an environment with excessive circulating PTH levels may readily explain the hypophosphatemia encountered in this setting. However, hypophosphatemia is frequently also observed in the late post-transplant period (101–103). Several factors, in addition to persistent hyperparathyroidism, may play an important role in the pathogenesis of hypophosphatemia. These include extrarenal mechanisms such as decreased intestinal phosphate absorption due to overzealous use of phosphate-binding antacids (37), steroid treatment, reduced dietary phosphate intake or a relative deficiency of vitamin D (88, 104). Hypophosphatemia in renal allograft recipients may also be the result of an augmented urinary loss of phosphate. Indeed, several studies have documented a reduced rate of tubular

Table 5. Possible causes for hypophosphatemia following kidney transplantation

---

External causes
1. Use of phosphate-binding antacids
2. Post-transplant hyperparathyroidism
3. Use of steroids
4. "Hungry-bones syndrome" following resolution of hyperparathyroidism
5. Impaired intestinal phosphate reabsorption, secondary to inadequate vitamine-D levels

Renal causes
1. Intrinsic tubular defect in phosphate reabsorption
2. Increased tubular sensitivity to PTH

---

phosphate reabsorption (TRP) after kidney transplantation (12, 85, 105, 107). This diminished phosphate reabsorption by the kidney has been attributed to persistent hyperparathyroidism (77, 78) and increased tubular sensitivity to PTH (102, 105). In addition, it has been proposed that a PTH-independent tubular leak of phosphate may result in an augmented phosphaturia following transplantation. The latter could be a consequence of an immunologic injury (12), the action of immunosuppressive agents and steroids (102, 106), and a tubular adaptive response to nephron reduction (105, 107). The diminished intestinal phosphate absorption may act in concert with the increased urinary losses of phosphate, thus contributing to the development of hypophosphatemia. The various possible causes for hypophosphatemia following renal transplantation are summarized in Table 5.

Hypophosphatemia following kidney transplantation has several deleterious effects. These include increased osteolysis, unmasking of hypercalcemia associated with persistent secondary hyperparathyroidism, and a tendency to metabolic acidosis (108). It appears, therefore, that early recognition and treatment of post-transplant hypophosphatemia is essential in order to avoid severe bone disease.

RENAL TRANSPLANTATION AND AMYLOIDOSIS

In Europe, amyloidosis of diverse causes was diagnosed in approximately 0.6% of registered hemodialysis patients (109). On the other hand, patients suffering from amyloidosis undergoing hemodialysis in Israel constitute 6–10% of the total population on dialysis treatment. This high prevalence in Israel as compared with other countries is attributed mostly to the high incidence of familial Mediterranean fever (FMF). This genetic disorder is common among Sephardic Jews, Arabs, and Armenians. All afflicted patients may eventually develop amyloidosis that is of the AA type and therefore is believed to be secondary to hereditary, recurrent inflammatory disorder (110). The kidney is the organ most commonly infiltrated with amyloid in this disease, and thus the renal lesion is responsible for death or end-stage renal failure at an early of these patients (111, 112).

The extraordinarily high incidence of FMF and amyloidosis in Israel (the Sephardic Jews consitute at least half of Israel's population), has led to accumulated experience regarding the treatment of these patients either by chronic hemodialysis (113) of by kidney homotransplantation (114).

Hemodialysis is often fraught with difficulties in patients with amyloidosis. Intolerance to hemodynamic alterations and persistent hypotension (despite advanced kidney disease) are common. Diminished adrenal reserve due to amyloid involvement may play a role, not only in hemodynamic instability, but also in mortality (115). In fact, in their extensive survey of FMF, Sohar et al. (111) have clearly demonstrated that two vital organs, i.e., the kidneys and the adrenals, were mainly involved with amyloid in this type of systemic disease. It is likely that the longer the patients are maintained on hemodialysis, the greater will be the degree of adrenal infiltration by amyloid. In addition to adrenal insufficiency, many causes combine to lower blood pressure in these patients, including hypovolemia secondary to hypoproteinemia, malnutrition due to longstanding nephrotic syndrome and, occasionally, due also to intestinal malabsorption. Involvement of the autonomic ganglia and the wall of the arterioles with amyloid may also impair normal homeostasis of blood pressure. The hypotension promotes arteriovenous fistula clotting and failure. Therefore, patients suffering from amyloidosis and subjected to recurrent vascular operations, and eventually all possible sites for AV fistula construction may become exhausted. Thus, the average lifespan of AV fistulas in FMF patients is one third of that in nonamyloidotic renal disease.

In addition, because of the associated adrenal insufficiency and problematic vascular access, the survival of patients with amyloidosis is affected as well. In fact, European studies show that the life expectancy of patients suffering from renal amyloidosis who are maintained on long-term hemodialysis is 15–23% less than that of patients without amyloidosis (109). It appears, therefore, that these patients might benefit much more from kidney transplantation as compared with chronic hemodialysis. The severe problems associated with vascular access would thus be avoided. Furthermore, steroids that are routinely administered after transplantation as an antirejection treatment would automatically compensate for any reduction in endogenous glucocorticoid secretion.

Experience with renal transplantation in systemic amyloidosis has been limited by the relative rarity of the disease (114, 116–119). The first study that comprised a statistically significant series of patients (ten patients with FMF) was that of Jacob et al. (114). Three years later the same group reported their experience with 21 renal transplants in 20 amyloidotic recipients (120). The data accumulated thus far demonstrate that long survival with a well-functioning graft is attainable in this high-risk population. Moreover, these patients enjoyed a quality of life and rehabilitation comparable to nonamyloidotic transplant recipients. Although actuarial survival of amyloidotic recipients was still lower compared to other transplant recipients, their graft survival at 5 years was greater than in the nonamyloidotic group. The latter finding was attributed to the lower incidence fo treated rejection episodes in the amyloidotic recipients (120).

Continuing amyloid deposition is anticipated in the patient whose life has been prolonged by dialysis and transplantation, which would eventually lead to involvement of other organs by amyloid. Indeed, hepatic and cardiac involvement have been reported (111, 112, 120) and intestinal malabsorption has appeared in one FMF patient with a kidney transplant (118). Deposition of amyloid in renal allografts has been found to occur within $2\frac{1}{2}$–4 years (and sometimes as early as 6 months) after transplantation (116–119). However, in most of the cases reported, proteinuria was absent and graft function was adequate, suggesting that amyloidosis was at a preclinical stage. It is obvious, therefore, that amyloid deposits may exist in the kidney for long periods without causing overt organ dysfunction. Thus, the limiting factor in graft functions and survival remains the immunologic fate of the transplant.

The recent establishment of the effectiveness of colchicine in preventing amyloidosis of FMF is of vast importance in this regard (121, 122). In a followup of 1070 FMF patients, Zemer et al. (122) demonstrated that colchicine prevented the development of amyloid and the deterioration in renal function in patients with proteinuria. The drug was ineffective in patients who already developed the nephrotic syndrome (122). Protection of the transplanted kidney and other organs from continuing amyloid deposition appears to be an attainable goal in the future, extending life expectancy and graft survival in these patients.

HYPERTENSION FOLLOWING RENAL TRANSPLANTATION

Hypertension is commonly seen after kidney transplantation. It occurs in approximately 30–50% of the recipients and may be present even in patients with a normally functioning kidney (123–125). In patients who have not had a bilateral nephrectomy, the incidence of hypertension 6 months after grafting may appraoch 80% (12, 126). Furthermore, based on recent data, it is clear that the prevalence of post-transplant hypertension remains high, even up to 10 years after being operated (124). These patients, therefore, may face the long-term effects of hypertension on the cardiovascular system with the subsequent increased risks of complications such as cerebrovascular accidents and myocardial infarction.

The pathogenesis of hypertension following renal transplantation appears to be multifactorial. Several mechanisms related either to the donor, the recipient, or the post-transplantation course have been suggested:
1. Hypersecretion of renin by the native kidneys (126–130).
2. Acute and chronic transplant rejection (131–133).
3. Transplant renal artery stenosis (131, 133–136).
4. Corticosteroid therapy (137).
5. Hypercalcemia and hyperparathyroidism (138, 139)
6. Recurrence of the original disease in the transplanted kidney (140).

Among these potential causes, the first three mechanisms account for a major percentage of patients with post-transplant hypertension. Interestingly, these causes are also associated with activation of the renin-angiotensin-aldosterone axis.

Role of the renin-angiotensin system in post-transplant hypertension

Activation of the renin-angiotensin system in the post-transplantation period may be related to the presence of host diseased kidneys, acute or chronic rejection, and to the development of renal artery stenosis in the transplanted kidney.

In 1973, Cohen (126) pointed out the role of native kidneys in the pathogenesis of post-transplant hypertension. More recently, McHugh and coworkers (127) measured renin, aldosterone, and exchangeable sodium in hypertensive and normotensive renal transplant recipients with good renal function and without renal artery stenosis. They found that hypertension was uncommon and plasma renin activity (PRA) was low when bilateral nephrectomy was performed. PRA and urinary aldosterone were higher in the hypertensive patients, and angiotensin II blockade with saralasin produced a fall in blood pressure proportional to preinfusion PRA levels. The latter suggest that hypersecretion of renin is an etiologic factor in the hypertension following transplantation. Since renin levels were lower in patients subjected to bilateral nephrectomy, the source of the excess renin was probably the host's native kidneys. These observations support earlier findings of Linas et al. (128) suggesting a role of the native kidneys in post-transplant hypertension. They found that salt depletion and saralasin administration did not lower blood pressure in patients with one kidney (the homograft), whereas blood pressure was reduced by the latter combination in patients with more than one kidney. These findings suggest that post-transplant hypertension is more likely to be renin dependent in patients with more than one kidney. Interestingly, one of the patients who responded to saralasin had two transplanted kidneys but no original kidneys. It appears, therefore, that the absolute number of the kidneys available to release renin may determine the renin dependency of post-transplant hypertension.

The role of the native kidneys in the pathogenesis of post-transplant hypertension has been recently underscored by Curtis and coworkers (129, 130). These authors have demonstrated a substantial increase in renal (allograft) plasma flow and a decrease in the renal vascular resistance of the graft in six patients after removal of their native kidneys (130). Based on the response to salt loading and restriction, and to captopril administration, they suggested that the native kidneys seemed to exert their hypertensive effect via the renin-angiotensin system (129, 130).

A peculiar role of renin secretion by the graft in the pathogenesis of excessive hypertension has been demonstrated following transplantation of kidneys obtained from donors dying of "hepatorenal syndrome" in anephric recipients (141). This type of hypertension was probably due to a combination of high endogenous renin levels in the transplanted kidney and high circulating renin substrate in the recipients.

The association between hypertension and acute and/or chronic rejection is well recognized (131–133). A higher incidence of post-transplant hypertension was found in recipients of cadaver kidneys in which rejection episodes were more likely to occur (142). Measurements of PRA have shown a wide variation during the course of transplant rejection (132, 143). However, the response of some of these patients to angiotensin blockade indicates that this hypertension is renin dependent (144).

Renal artery stenosis is a well-recognized complication in patients with kidney transplantation. It has been reported to occur in 1–10% of patients undergoing kidney transplantation (133–136). The onset of hypertension secondary to renal artery stenosis usually occurs within 6 months after transplantation, with a range of 3 months to 2 years. In the series of Lacombe (134), a higher incidence of renal artery stenosis was found in cadaver transplants than in living-donor related transplants.

Characteristic features of patients with post-transplant hypertension secondary to renal artery stenosis are the refractoriness of the high blood pressure to conventional treatment, increased PRA (135, 136), the presence of transplant bruits, and erythrocytosis (145, 146). However, none of the above findings is an exclusive marker of post-transplant renal artery stenosis. In fact, transplant bruits are commonly found in patients with excellent renal function with no evidence of renal artery stenosis. In this situation disappearance of the bruit may indicate a reduction in blood flow and a worsening of renal function. Furthermore, in these patients, PRA has been found to be elevated, normal, or low, similar to patients with post-transplant hypertension without renal artery stenosis (124, 125).

It is important to recognize and diagnose renal artery stenosis in the transplanted kidney as early as possible, since it is a potentially curable cause of post-transplant hypertension. Failure to do so may ultimately lead to the deterioration of renal function and hypertensive crisis (145).

Pharmacologic blockade of the renin-angiotensin system, either by saralasin or the converting-enzyme inhibitor, captopril, has been used in the diagnosis and treatment of renal artery stenosis related hypertension in patients with kidney transplantation (144, 147, 148). Saralasin administration is an important screening test for the diagnosis of renovascular hypertension and may also be used as a therapeutic means to control severe renin-dependent hypertension that is refractory to sodium nitroprusside (144). The use of captopril is increasing due to its effectiveness as an antihypertensive drug. Of particular interest in that respect is the deterioration in renal function that has been observed in renal allograft recipients with renal artery stenosis (147, 148). The renal insufficiency induced by captopril in these patients is probably related to intrarenal hemodynamic changes and therefore is potentially reversible. The drug should be used with great caution, however, whenever the possibility of renal artery stenosis is raised.

Strict control of blood pressure is a desirable goal in the management of patients with hypertension after kidney transplantation. Medical treatment is effective in more than 75% of the resistant cases of hypertension (124). In addition to conventional treatment, the powerful vasodilator minoxidil and the converting-enzyme inhibitor captopril may be used to control blood pressure in resistant cases. Like captopril, minoxidil may also cause reversible renal failure. Among the major causes of post-transplant hypertension, graft artery stenosis and hypertension related to the native kidneys may be amenable to surgical treatment. Percutaneous transluminal angioplasty (149) has been recently introduced as an alternative method of treatment in selected cases of renal artery stenosis. This procedure will probably reduce the need for definitive surgery in the future. However, at present no reliable diagnostic procedure is available to predict which individual will benefit from surgery (124). Therefore, surgery should be considered in cases where medical treatment failed to adequately control hypertension.

ERYTHROCYTOSIS AFTER RENAL TRANSPLANTATION

Erythrocytosis has been described as a transient complication following renal transplantation (145, 146, 150–154) and its incidence may range between 5% and 17%, according to recent reports. Post-transplant erythrocytosis may occur as early as 3 months or as late as 7.5 years after transplantation (154). In many patients the elevated hematocrit is of a transient nature and is self-limited. However, persistence for more than 1.5 years is not an uncommon finding (154). The pathogensis of this complication appears to be multifactorial. Few cases have been reported in which a decrease in plasma volume was primarily responsible for the elevated hematocrit (155). However, in most cases, true erythrocytosis with a normal plasma volume and an elevated red blood cell mass has been found. Increased production of erythropoietin has been documented in many studies and could play a major role in the pathogenesis of post-transplant erythrocytosis (146, 151–153, 156, 157). The source of the elevated levels of erythropoietin could be the transplanted kidney, secondary to acute or chronic rejection (150, 151, 153) or renal artery stenosis (145, 146).

Overproduction of erythropoietin by the native kidneys (156, 157) and ectopic erythropoietin production (158) has also been suggested as a causative factor. Other mechanisms that have been proposed are the resolution of hypoparathyroidism with the associated bone marrow fibrosis and ureteral obstruction (159, 160). The association between a post-transplant erythropoiesis and acute or chronic allograft rejection has been underscored in earlier studies (150, 151, 153). However, in the large series of 53 patients with post-transplant erythrocytosis reported recently by Wickre et al. (154), erythrocytosis generally occurred in those with good kidney function and with no evidence of acute or chronic rejection. In the latter study, diabetes, smoking, and a rejection-free course were the most obvious risk factors for the development of erythrocytosis (154).

Renal artery stenosis should also be considered in patients developing erythrocytosis following renal transplantation (145, 146). It has been suggested that increased renin activity directly affects erythropoietin production by the kidney. However, in-vitro experiments failed to show such evidence (161).

The combination of erythrocytosis, hypertension, and deterioration in renal function is certainly compatible with either renal artery stenosis or transplant rejection. Yet, the absence of proteinuria and the preserved ability to concentrate the urine despite azotemia (prerenal azotemia) are highly suggestive of renal artery stenosis rather than a diffuse parenchymal lesion secondary to rejection (145). It is crucial to make the correct diagnosis in order to avoid erroneous treatment with immunosuppressive drugs.

Post-transplant erythrocytosis may be associated with a significant morbidity due to thromboembolic complications (151, 154). Therefore, it has been recommended that therapeutic phlebotomies should be consistently performed when the hematocrit reaches 51% (154). Such an approach seems entirely rational, although evidence for its efficacy awaits further controlled clinical trials.

REFERENCES

1. Massry SG, Preuss HG, Maher JF, Schreiner GE: Renal tubular acidosis after cadaver kidney homotransplantation. *Am J Med* 42:284–292, 1967.
2. Gyory AZ, Stewart JH, George CRP, Tiller DJ, Edwards KDG: Renal tubular acidosis, acidosis due to hyperkalemia hypercalcemia, disordered citrate metabolism and other tubular dysfunction following human renal transplantation. *Q J Med* 38:231–254, 1969.
3. Better OS, Chaimowitz C, Naveh Y, Stein A, Nahir AM, Barzilai A, Erlik D: Syndrome of incomplete renal tubular acidosis after cadaver kidney transplantation. *Ann Intern Med* 71:39–46, 1969.
4. Mookerjee B, Gault MH, Dossetor JB: Hypechloremic acidosis in early diagnosis of renal allograft rejection. *Ann Intern Med* 71:47–57, 1969.
5. Better OS, Chaimowitz C, Alroy GG, et al.: Spontaneous remission of the defect in urinary acidification after cadaver kidney homotransplantation. *Lancet* 1:110–112, 1970.
6. Wilson DR, Siddiqui AA: Renal tubular acidosis after kidney transplantation. Natural history and significance. *Ann Intern Med* 79:352–361, 1973.
7. Rubini ME, Agre KL, Mims MM, et al.: Curious tubular syndromes after homotransplantation (abstract). *Clin Res* 16:167, 1968.
8. Henderson LW, Nolph KD, Puschett JB, Goldberg M: Proximal tubular malfunction as a mechanism for diuresis after renal homotransplantation. *N Engl J Med* 278:467–473, 1968.
9. Liebau G, Muller R, Schad H, Edel HH: Proximale tubulare acidose bei nieretransplantierten patienten. *Klin Wochenschr* 48:624–629, 1970.
10. Briggs WA, Kominami N, Wilson RE, Merril JP: Kidney transplantation and Fanconi syndrome. *N Engl J Med* 286:25, 1972.
11. Vertuno LL, Preuss HG, Argy WP, Schreiner GE: Fanconi syndrome following homotransplantation. *Arch Intern Med* 133:302–305, 1974.
12. Vaziri ND, Nellands RE, Brueggmann RM, Barton CH, Martin DC: Renal tubular dysfunction in transplanted kidneys. *Southern Med J* 72:530–534, 1979.

13. Reubi FC, Montandon A: Renal glycosuria in renal homograft recipients. *Klin Wochenschr* 62:876–884, 1984.
14. Wrong O, Davies H: The excretion of acid in renal disease. *Q J Med* 28:259–313, 1959.
15. Morris RC Jr: Renal tubular acidosis: Mechanisms, classification and implications. *N Engl J Med* 281:1405–1413, 1968.
16. Halperin ML, Goldstein MB, Haig A, Johnson MD, Stinebaugh BJ: Studies on the pathogenesis of type I (distal) renal tubular acidosis as revealed by the urinary PCO_2 tensions. *J Clin Invest* 53:669–677, 1974.
17. Arruda JAL, Kurtzman NA: mechanisms and classification of deranged distal urinary acidification. *Am J Physiol* 239:F515–F523, 1980.
18. Batlle DC, Sehy JT, Roseman MK, Arruda JAL, Kurtzman NA: Clinical and pathophysiologic spectrum of acquired distal-tubular acidosis. *Kidney Int* 20:389–396, 1981.
19. Helperin ML, Goldstein MB, Richardson RMA, Stinebaugh BJ: Distal renal tubular acidosis syndromes: A pathophysiological approach. *Am J Nephrol* 15:1–8, 1985.
20. Schambelan M, Stockgit J, Bigliery E: Isolated hypoaldosteronism in adults: A renin-deficiency syndrome. *N Engl J Med* 287:573–578, 1972.
21. Perez GO, Oster JR, Vaamonde CA: Renal acidosis and renal potassium handling in selective hypoaldosteronism. *Am J Med* 57:809–816, 1974.
22. Hulter HW, Ilnicki LP, Harbottle JA, Sebastian A: Impaired renal H^+ secretion and NH_3 production in mineralocorticoid deficient glucocorticoid replete dogs. *Am J Physiol* 232:F136–F146, 1977.
23. Ditella P, Sodhi B, McCreary J, Arruda JAL, Kurtzman NA: The mechanism of the metabolic acidosis of selective mineralocorticoid deficiency. *Kidney Int* 14:466–477, 1978.
24. Szylman P, Better OS, Chaimowitz C, Rosler A: Role of hyperkalemia in the metabolic acidosis of isolated hypoaldosteronism. *N Engl J Med* 294:361–365, 1976.
25. Battle DC, Mozes DF, Manaligod J, Arruda JAL, Kurtzman NA: The pathogenesis of hyperchloremic metabolic acidosis associated with kidney transplantation. *Am J Med* 70:786–796, 1981.
26. Tu WH, Shearn MA: Systemic lupus erythematosus and latent renal tubular dysfunction. *Ann Intern Med* 67:100–109, 1967.
27. Shioji R, Furuyama T, Onodera S, et al.: Sjogren syndrome and renal tubular acidosis. *Am J Med* 48:456–463, 1970.
28. DeOliviera HL: Excretion of ammonium in cases of acute tubular necrosis with acidosis and alkaline urine. *Metabolism* 2:36–46, 1953.
29. De Luna MB, Metcalfe-Gibson A, Wrong O: Urinary excretion of hydrogen ion in acute oliguric renal failure. *Nephron* 1:3–15, 1964.
30. Briggs JD, Kennedy AD, Young LN, Luke RG, Gary M: Renal function after acute tubular necrosis. *Br Med J* 33:513–516, 1967.
31. Winaver J, Agmon D, Harari R, Better OS: Impaired renal acidification following acute renal ischemia in the dog. *Kidney Int* 30:906–913, 1986.
32. Adu D, Turney J, Michael J, McMaster P: Hyperkalemia in cyclosporine-treated renal allograft recipients. *Lancet* 2:370–372, 1983.
33. Stahl PAK, Kantz L, Maier B, Schollmeyer P: Hyperchloremic metabolic acidosis with high serum potassium in renal transplant recipients: A cyclosporine A associated side effect. *Clin Nephrol* 25:245–248, 1986.
34. Batlle DC, Arruda JAL, Kurtzman NA: Hyperkalemic distal renal tubular acidosis associated with obstructive uropathy. *N Engl J Med* 304:373–380, 1981.
35. Muldowney FP, Carrol D, Donohoe JF, Freaney RF: Correction of renal bicarbonate wastage by parathyroidectomy. *J Med* 40:487–498, 1971.
36. Muldowney F, Donohoe J, Carrol D, Powell D, Freaney RF: Parathyroid acidosis in uremia. *Q J Med* 41:321–342, 1972.
37. Alfrey AC, Jenkins D, Groth CG, Schorr WS, Gecelter L, Ogden DA: Resolution of hyperparathyroidism, renal osteodystrophy and metastic calcification after renal homotransplantation. *N Engl J Med* 279:1349–1356, 1968.
38. Butler HE Jr, Morgan JM, MacSmythe CM: Mercaptopurine and acquired tubular dysfunction in adult nephrosis. *Arch Intern Med* 116:853–856, 1965.
39. Gronert GA, Theye RA: Pathophysiology of hyperkalemia induced by succinylcholine. *Anaesthesiology* 43:89–99, 1975.
40. Cox M, Sterns RH, Singer I: The defense against hyperkalemia. The roles of insulin and aldosterone. *N Engl J Med* 299:525–532, 1978.
41. Field MJ, Giebisch GJ: Hormonal control of renal potassium excretion. *Kidney Int* 27:379–387, 1985.
42. Hudson JB, Chobanian AV, Relman AS: Hypoaldosteronism. A clinical study of a patient with an isolated adrenal mineralocorticoid deficiency, resulting in hyperkalemia and Stokes–Adams attacks. *N Engl J Med* 257:529–536, 1957.
43. DeFronzo RA, Goldberg M, Cook CR, Barker C, Grossman RA, Agus ZA: Investigations into the mechanisms of hyperkalemia following renal transplantation. *Kidney Int* 11:357–365, 1977.
44. Arnold JE, Healy JK: Hyperkalemia, hypertension and systemic acidosis without renal failure associated with a tubular defect in potassium excretion. *Am J Med* 47:461–472, 1969.
45. Gordon RD, Geddes RA, Pawsey CGK, O'Halloran MW: Hypertension and serve hyperkalemia associated with suppression of renin and aldosterone and completely reversed by dietary sodium restriction. *Aust Ann Med* 4:287–294, 1970.
46. Spitzer A, Edelman CM, Goldberg LD, Hanneman PH: Short stature, hyperkalemia and acidosis. A defect in renal transport of potassium. *Kidney Int* 3:251–257, 1973.
47. Weinstein SF, Allan DME, Mendosa SA: Hyperkalemia, acidosis and short stature associated with a defect in renal potassium secretion. *J Pediat* 85:355–358, 1974.
48. DeFronzo RA, Cooke CR, Goldberg M, Cow M, Myers AR, Agus ZS: Impaired renal tubular potassium secretion in systemic lupus erythematosus. *Ann Intern Med* 86:268–271, 1977.
49. DeFronzo RA, Taufield PA, Black H, McPhedran P, Cooke CR: Impaired tubular potassium secretion in sickle cell disease. *Ann Intern Med* 90:310–316, 1979.
50. Brautbar N, Levi J, Rosler A, Lietsdorf E, Djaldeti M, Epstein M, Kleeman CR: Familial hyperkalemia, hypertension and hyperreninemia with normal aldosterone levels. A tubular defect in potassium handling. *Arch Intern Med* 138:607–610, 1978.
51. Farfel Z, Iaina A, Rosenthal T, Waks U, Shibolet S, Gafni J: Familial hyperpotassemia and hypertension accompanied by normal plasma aldosterone levels. Possible hereditary cell membrane defect. *Arch Intern Med* 138:1828–1832, 1978.
52. Farfel Z, Iaina A, Levi J, Gafni J: Proximal tubular acidosis associated with familial normoaldosteronemic hyperpotassemia and hypertension. *Arch Intern Med* 138:1837–1840, 1978.

53. Finkelstein FO, Hayslett JP: Role of medullary structures in the functional adaptation of renal insufficiency. Kidney Int 6:419–425, 1974.
54. DeFronzo RA: Hyperkalemia and hyporeninemic hypoaldosteronism. Kidney Int 17:118–134, 1980.
55. Perez G, Lespier L, Knowles R, Oster J, Vaamonde C: Hyporeninemia and hypoaldosteronism in diabetes mellitus. Arch Intern Med 137:852–855, 1977.
56. Oh MS, Carrol HJ, Clemmons JE, Vagnucci A, Levinson S, Whang E: A mechanism for hyporeninemic hypoaldosteronism in chronic renal disease. Metabolism 23:1157–1166, 1974.
57. Pratt JH: Role of angiotensin II in potassium mediated stimulation of aldosterone secretion in the dog. J Clin Invest 70:667–672, 1982.
58. Roll D, Licht A, Rosler A, Durst AK, Kleeman CR, Czaczkes JW: Transient hypoaldosteronism after renal allotransplantation. Isr J Med Sci 15:29–34, 1979.
59. Wilson ID, Goetz FC: Selective hypoaldosteronism after prolonged heparin administration. Am J Med 36:635–640, 1964.
60. Uribarri J, Oh MS, Butt KMH, Carrol HJ: Pseudohypoaldosteronism following kidney transplantation. Nephron 31:368–370, 1982.
61. Hamilton DV, Evans DB, Henderson RG et al.: Nephrotoxicity and metabolic acidosis in transplant patients on cyclosporine A. Proc Eur Dial Transpl Assoc 18:400–409, 1981.
62. Myers BD: Cyclosporine nephrotoxicity. Kidney Int 30:964–974, 1986.
63. Najarian JS, Strand M, Fryd DS, et al.: Comparison of cyclosporine versus azathioprine-antilymphocyte globulin in renal transplantation. Transplant Proc 15:2463–2468, 1983.
64. Foley RJ, Van Buren CT, Hammer R, Weinmann EJ: Cyclosoporine-associated hyperkalemia. Transplant Proc 15:2726–2729, 1983.
65. Bantle JP, Nath KA, Sutherland DER, Najarian JS, Ferris TF: Effect of cyclosporine on the renin-angiotensin aldosterone system and potassium excretion in renal transplant recipients. Arch Intern med 145:505–508, 1985.
66. Siegel H, Ryffel B, Petric R, Shoemaker P, Miller A, Donatsch P, Mihatsch M: Cyclosporine, the renin-angiotensin-aldosterone system, and renal adverse reactions. Transplant Proc 15:2719–2725, 1983.
67. Rosenbaum R, Hoffsten PE, Cryer P, Klahr S: Hyperkalemia after renal transplantation. Arch Intern Med 138:1270–1272, 1978.
68. Ogden DA, Porter KA, Terasaki PI, et al.: Chronic renal homograft function. Correlation with histology and lymphocyte antigen matching. Am J Med 43:837–845, 1967.
69. Gyory AZ, Edwards KDG: Renal tubular acidosis. A family with an autosomal dominant genetic defect in renal hydrogen ion transport, with proximal tubular and collecting duct dysfunction and increased metabolism of citrate and ammonia. Am J Med 45:43–62, 1968.
70. Gill JR, Bell HN, Bartter FC: Impaired conservation of sodium and potassium in renal tubular acidosis and its correction by buffer anions. Clin Sci 33:577–592, 1967.
71. David DS, Sakai S, Brennan BL, Riggio RA, Cheigh J, Stenzel KH, Rubin AL, Sherwood LM: Hypercalcemia after renal transplantation. N Engl J Med 289:398–401, 1973.
72. Krane RJ, Sang IC, Olson CA, et al.: Renal transplant ureteral obstruction simulating retroperitoneal fibrosis. JAMA 225:607–609, 1973.
73. Nagar D, Ferris FZ, Schacht RA: Obstructive polyuric renal failure following renal transplantation. Am J Med 60:702–706, 1976.
74. McPhaul JJ Jr, McIntosh DA, Hammond WS, Park OK: Autonomous secondary (renal) parathyroid hyperplasia. N Engl J Med 271:1342–1345, 1964.
75. Hampers CL, Katz AI, Wilson RE, Merrill JP: Calcium metabolism and osteodystrophy after renal transplantation. Arch Intern Med 124:282–291, 1969.
76. Schwartz GH, David DS, Riggio RR, Saville PD, Whitsell JC, Stenzel KH, Rubin AL: Hypercalcemia after renal transplantation. Am J Med 49:42–51, 1970.
77. Geis WP, Popovtzer MM, Corman JL, Halgrimson CG, Groth CG, Starzl TE: Diagnosis and treatment of hyperparathyroidism after renal homotransplantation. Surg Gynecol Obstet 137:997–1010, 1973.
78. Pletka PG, Strom TB, Hampers CL, Griffiths H, Wilson RE, Bernstein DS, Sherwood LM, Merrill JP: Secondary hyperparathyroidism in human kidney transplant recipients. Nephron 17:371–381, 1976.
79. Chatterjee SN, Friedler RM, Berne TV, Oldham SB, Singer FR, Massry SG: Persistent hypercalcemia after successful renal transplantation. Nephron 17:1–7, 1976.
80. Christensen MS, Nielsen HE, Torring S: Hypercalcemia and parathyroid function after renal transplantation. Acta Med Scand 201:35–39, 1977.
81. Diethelm AG, Edwards RP, Whelchel JD: The natural history and surgical treatment of hypercalcemia before and after renal transplantation. Surg Gynecol Obst 154:481–490, 1982.
82. Conceicao SC, Wilkinson R, Feest TG, Owen JP, Dewar J, Kerr DNS: Hypercalcemia following renal transplantation: Causes and consequences. Clin Nephrol 16:235–244, 1981.
83. Cundy T, Kanis JA, Heynan G, Morris PJ, Oliver DO: Calcium metabolism and hyperparathyroidism after renal transplantation. Q J Med 52:67–78, 1983.
84. Sakhaee K, Brinker K, Helderman H, Bengfort JL, Nicar MJ, Hull AR, Pak CYC: Disturbances in mineral metabolism after successful renal transplantation. Miner Electrolyte Metab 11:167–172, 1985.
85. Ulmann A, Chkoff N, Lacour B: Disorders of calcium and phosphorus metabolism after successful kidney transplantation. In: J Hamburger, J Crosnier, JP Grunfeld, MH Maxwell, eds, Advances in Nephrology, Vol 12. Year Book Medical, Chicago, pp 331–340, 1983.
86. Parfitt AM: Hypercalcemic hyperparathyroidism following renal transplantation: Differential diagnosis, management and implications for cell population control in the parathyroid gland. Miner Electrolyte Metab 8:92–112, 1982.
87. Bernheim J, Touraine JL, David L, Faivre JM, Traeger J: Evolution of secondary hyperparathyroidism after renal transplantation. Nephron 16:381–387, 1976.
88. Garabedian M, Silve C, Bentolila DL, Bourdeau A, Ulmann A, Nguyen TM, Lieberherr M, Broyer M, Balsan S: Changes in plasma 1,25 and 24,25-dihydroxyvitamin D after renal transplantation in children. Kidney Int 20:403–410, 1981.
89. Hornum I: Post transplant hypercalcemia due to mobilisation of metastic calcifications. Acta Med Scand 189:199–205, 1971.
90. Blohme I, Eriksson A: parathyroidectomy after renal transplantation. Scand J Urol Nephrol 42 (Suppl):134–136, 1977.
91. Garvin PJ, Castaneda M, Linderer R Dickhans M: Management of hypercalcemic hyperparathyroidism after renal transplantation. Arch Surg 120:578–583, 1985.
92. Laflamme GH, Jowsey J: Bone and soft tissue changes with oral phosphate supplements. J Clin Invest 51:2834–2840, 1972.
93. Dominguez JM, Mautalen CA, Rodo JE, Barcat JA, Molins

ME: Tertiary hyperparathyroidism diagnosed after renal homotransplantation. *Am J Med* 49:423-428, 1970.
94. Rosenberg JC, Arnstein AR, Ing TS, et al.: Calculi complicating renal transplant. *Am J Surg* 129:326-330, 1975.
95. Lattimer RG, Renning J, Stevens LE, Northway JD, Reemtsma K: Tertiary hyperparathyroidism following successful renal allografting. *Am Surg* 172:137-141, 1970.
96. Starzl TE, Groth CG, Putnam CW, et al.: Urologic complications in 216 human recipients of renal transplants. *Ann Surg* 172:1-22, 1970.
97. Walsh A: Nephrocalcinose sur rein greffe. *J Urol Nephrol* 75 (Suppl) 75:244, 1969.
98. Leapman SB, Vidne BA, Butt KMH, et al.: Nephrolithiasis and nephrocalcinosis after renal transplantation: A case report and review of the literature. *J Urol* 115:129-132, 1976.
99. Caralps A, Lloveras J, Masramon J, et al.: Urinary calculi after renal transplantation (letter). *Lancet* 1:544, 1977.
100. Cope O: The study of hyperparathyroidism at the Massachusetts General Hospital. *N Engl J Med* 274:1174-1182, 1966.
101. Ward HN, pabico RC, McKenna BA, Freeman RB: The renal handling of phosphate by renal transplant patients: Correlation with serum parathyroid hormone, cycle 3'5' adenosine monophosphate urinary excretion, and allograft function. *Adv Exp Med Biol* 81:173-181, 1977.
102. Moorhead JF, Wills MR, Admed KY, Baillad RA, Varghese Z, Tatler GLV: Hypophosphataemic osteomalacia after cadaveric renal transplantation. *Lancet* 1:649-697, 1974.
103. Graf H, Kovarik J, Stummvol HK, Wolf A, Pinggera WF: Handling of phosphate by the transplanted kidney. *Proc Eur Dial Transpl Assoc* 16:624-629, 1979.
104. Olgaard K, Madsen S, Lund BJ, Sorensen OH: Pathogenesis of hypophosphatemia in kidney necrograft recipient: A controlled trial. *Adv Exp Med Biol* 128:255-261, 1980.
105. Rosenbaum RW, Hruska KA, Korkor A, Anderson C, Slatopolsky E: Decreased phosphate reabsorption after renal transplantation: Evidence for a mechanism independent of calcium and parathyroid hormone. *Kidney Int* 19:568-578, 1981.
106. Ingbar S, Kon E, Burnett C, Relman A, Burrows B, Sisson J: The effect of cortisone on the renal tubular transport of uric acid, phosphorus, and electrolytes in patients with normal renal and adrenal function. *J Lab Clin Med* 38:533-541, 1951.
107. Parfitt AM, Kleerekoper M, Cruz C: Reduced phosphate reabsorption unrelated to parathyroid hormone after renal transplantation: Implications for the pathogenesis of hyperparathyroidism in chronic renal failure. *Miner Electrolyte Metab* 12:356-362, 1986.
108. Gold LW, Massry SG, Arieff AL, Coburn JW: Renal bicarbonate wasting during phosphate depletion. A possible cause of altered acid-base homeostasis in hyperparathyroidism. *J Clin Invest* 52:2556-2562, 1973.
109. Gurland HJ, Brunner FP, Ghanther C, et al.: Combined report on regular dialysis and transplantation in Europe. VI 1975. In: BHB Robinson, P Vereerstraeten, JE Hawkins, eds, *Dialysis, Transplantation, Nephrology. Proceedings of the European Dialysis and Transplantation Association*, Hamburg, Germany. Pitman Press, Bath, England, pp 22-25, 1975.
110. Levin M, Franklin EC, Frangione B, Pras M: The amino acid sequence of a major nonimmunoglobulin component of some amyloid fibrils. *J Clin Invest* 51: 2773-2776, 1972.
111. Sohar E, Gafni J, Pras M, Heller H: Familial Mediterranean fever: A survey of 470 cases and review of the literature. *Am J Med* 43:227-253, 1967.
112. Gafni J, Ravid M, Sohar E: The role of amyloidosis in familial Mediterranean fever: A population study. *Isr J Med Sci* 4:995-999, 1968.
113. Ben Ari J, Zlotnik M, Oren A, Berlyne GM: Dialysis in renal failure caused by amyloidosis of familial Mediterranean fever. *Arch Intern Med* 136:449-451, 1976.
114. Jacob ET, Bar-Nathan N, Shapira Z, Gafni J: Renal transplantation in the amyloidosis of familial Mediterranean fever. *Arch Intern Med* 139:1135-1138, 1979.
115. Better OS, Tuma S, Barzilai D: Diminished adrenocortical function reserve in patients with familial Mediterranean fever and renal amyloidosis. In: *Frontiers in Internal Medicine*. Karger, Basel, p 339, 1974.
116. Jones NF: Renal amyloidosis: Pathogenesis and therapy. *Clin Nephrol* 6:459-464, 1976.
117. Kennedy CL, Castro LE: Transplantation for renal amyloidosise. *Transplantation* 24:382-385, 1977.
118. Jones MB, Adams JM, Passer JA: Amyloidosis in renal allograft in familial Mediterranean fever (letter). *Ann Intern Med* 87:579-580, 1977.
119. Benson MD, Skinner M, Cohen AS: Amyloid deposition in renal transplant in familial Mediterranean fever. *Ann Intern Med* 87:31-34, 1977.
120. Jacob ET, Siegal B, Bar-Nathan N, Gafni J: Improving outlook for renal transplantation in amyloid nephropathy. *Transplant Proc* 14:41-45, 1982.
121. Zemer D, Revach M, Pras M, et al. A controlled trial of colchicine in preventing attacks of familial Mediterranean fever. *N Engl J Med* 291:934-937, 1974.
122. Zemer D, Pras M, Sohar E, Modan M, Cabili S, Gafni J: Colchicine in the prevention and treatment of the amyloidosis of familial Mediterranean fever. *N Engl J Med* 314:1001-1005, 1986.
123. Pollini J, Guttmann RD, Beaudoin JB, Morehouse DD, Klassen J, Knacck J: Late hypertension following renal allotransplantation. *Clin Nephrol* 11:202-212, 1979.
124. Ypersele de Strihou CV, Vereestraeten P, Wauthier M, et al.: Prevalence, etiology and treatment of late post transplant hypertension. In: J Hamburger, J Corsnier, JP Grunfeld, MH Maxwell, eds, *Advances in Nephrology*, Vol 12. Yearbook Medical, Chicago, pp 41-60, 1983.
125. Waltzer WC, Turner S, Frohnert P, Rapaport FT: Etiology and pathogenesis of hypertension following renal transplantation. *Nephron* 42:102-109, 1986.
126. Cohen S: Hypertension in renal transplant recipients: Role of bilateral nephrectomy. *Br Med J* 3:78-81, 1973.
127. McHugh MI, Tanboga H, Marcen R, Liano F, Robson V, Wilkinson R: Hypertension following renal transplantation. The role of the host's kidneys. *Q J Med* 196:395-403, 1980.
128. Linas SL, Miller PD, McDonald KM, Stables DP, Katz P, Weil R, Schrier R: Role of the renin-angiotensin system in post transplantation hypertension in patients with multiple kidneys. *N Engl J Med* 298:1440-1444, 1978.
129. Curtis JJ, Luke RG, Jones P, Diethelm AG, Welchel JD: Hypertension after successful renal transplantation. *Am J Med* 79:193-200, 1985.
130. Curtis JJ, Luke RG, Diethelm AG, Whelchel JD, Jones P: Benefits of removal of native kidneys in hypertension after renal transplantation. *Lancet* 2:739-742, 1985.
131. Bennett WM, McDonald WJ, Lawson RK, Porter GA: Post tranplant hypertension: Studies of cortical blood flow and the renal pressor system. *Kidney Int* 6:99-108, 1974.
132. West TH, Turcotte JG, Vander A: Plasma renin activity,

sodium balance and hypertension in a group of renal transplant recipients. *J Lab Clin Med* 73:564–573, 1969.
133. Bachy C, Alexandre GPJ, Ypersele de Strihou CV: Hypertension after renal transplantation. *Br Med J* 2:1287–1289, 1976.
134. Lacombe M: Arterial stenosis complicating renal allotransplantation in man. *Ann Surg* 181:283–288, 1975.
135. Lindsey ES, Garbus SB, Golladay ES, et al.: Hypertension due to renal artery stenosis in transplanted kidneys. *Ann Surg* 181:604–610, 1975.
136. Lindfors O, Lassonon L, Fyhrquist F, Kock B, Lindstrom B: Renal artery stenosis in hypertensive renal transplant recipients. *J Urol* 118:240–243, 1977.
137. Popovtzer MM, Pinnggera W, Katz FH, Corman JL, Robinette J, Lonois B, Halgrimson CG, Starzel TE: Variations in arterial blood pressure after kidney transplantation. *Circulation* 47:1297–1305, 1973.
138. Weidmann P, Massry SG, Coburn JW, Maxwell MH, Atleson J, Kleeman CR: Blood pressure effects of acute hypercalcemia — studies in patients with chronic renal failure. *Ann Intern Med* 76:741–745, 1972.
139. Earll JM, Kurtzman NA, Moser RH: Hypercalcemia and hypertension. *Ann Intern Med* 64:378–381, 1966.
140. Posborg PV, Steen OT, Kessmeyer-Neilsen F: Late failure of human renal transplant. *Medicine* 54:45–71, 1975.
141. McDonald FD, Brennan LA, Turcotte JG: Severe hypertension and elevated plasma renin activity following transplantation of "hepatorenal donor" kidneys into anephric recipients. *Am J Med* 54:39–43, 1973.
142. Whelton PK, Russel RP, Harrington DP, Williams GM, Walker WG: Hypertension following renal transplantation: Causative factors and therapeutic implications. *JAMA* 241:1128–1131, 1979.
143. Beckerhoff R, Uhlschmid G, Vetter W, Armbuster H, Siegenthaler W: Plasma renin and aldosterone after renal transplantation. *Kidney Int* 5:39–46, 1974.
144. Zawada ET, Maxwell MH, Marks LS: The diagnostic and therapeutic uses of saralasin in renal transplant hypertension. *J Urol* 123:148–152, 1980.
145. Schramek A, Adler O, Hashmonai M, Better OS, Tuma S, Barzilai A: Hypertensive crisis, erythrocytosis and uremia due to renal-artery stenosis of kidney transplants. *Lancet* 1:70–71, 1975.
146. Bacon BR, Rothman SA, Ricanati ES, Rashad FA: Renal artery stenosis with erythrocytosis after renal transplantation. *Arch Intern Med* 140:1206–1211, 1980.
147. Curtis JJ, Luke RG, Whelchel JD, Diethelm AG, Jones P, Dustan HP: Inhibition of angiotensin converting enzyme in renal transplant recipients with hypertension. *N Engl J Med* 308:377–381, 1983.
148. Waltzer WC, Anaise D, Arbeit L, Weinstein S, Rapaport FT: Usefulness of captopril in the management of hypertension after renal transplantation. *Transplant Proc* 16:1372–1374, 1984.
149. Reilly OT, Wood RFM, Watkin EM: Attempted balloon catheter dilation of transplant renal artery stenosis and subsequent operative correction. *Transplantation* 32:444–445, 1981.
150. Nies BA, Cohn R, Schrier SL: Erythemia after renal transplantation. *N Engl J Med* 273:785–788, 1965.
151. Westerman MP, Jenkins JL, Dekker A, Kreutner A, Fisher B: Significance of erythrocytosis and increased erythropoietin secretion after renal transplantation. *Lancet* 2:755–757, 1967.
152. Wu KK, Gibson TP, Freeman RM, Bonney WW, Fried W, DeGowin RL: Erythrocytosis after renal transplantation. Its occurrence in two recipients of kidneys from the same cadaver donor. *Arch Intern Med* 132:898–902, 1973.
153. Nellans R, Otis P, Martin DC: Polycythemia following renal transplantation. *Urology* 6:158–163, 1975.
154. Wickre CG, Norman DJ, Bennison A, Barry JM, Bennett WM: Post renal transplant erythrocytosis: A review of 53 patients. *Kidney Int* 23:731–737, 1983.
155. Obermiller LE, Tzamaloukas AH, Avasthi PS, Halpern JA, Sterling WA: Decreased plasma volume in post transplant erythrocytosis. *Clin Nephrol* 23:213–217, 1985.
156. Dagher FJ, Ramos E, Erslev AJ, Alongi SV, Karmi SA, Caro J: Are the native kidneys responsible for erythrocytosis in renal allorecipients? *Transplantation* 28:496–498, 1979.
157. Thevenod F, Radke HW, Grutzmacher P, Vincent E, Koch KM, Schoeppe W, Fassbinder W: Deficient feedback regulation of erythropoiesis in kidney transplant patients with polycythemia. *Kidney Int* 24:227–232, 1983.
158. Meyrier A, Simon P, Boffa G, Brissot P: Uremia and the liver: The liver and erythropoiesis in chronic renal failure. *Nephron* 29:3–6, 1981.
159. Barbour GL: Effect of parathyroidectomy on anemia in chronic renal failure. *Arch Intern Med* 139:889–891, 1979.
160. Hammond D, Winnick S: Paraneoplastic erythrocytosis and ectopic erythropoietins. *Ann NY Acad Sci* 230:219–227, 1974.
161. Anagnostou A, Baranowski R, Pillary VK, Kurtzman N, Vercellotti G, Fried W: Effect of renin on extrarenal erythropoietin production. *J Lab Clin Med* 88:707–715, 1976.

CHAPTER 59

Renal Transplantation in Systemic Inherited and Metabolic Disease

ELEANOR D. LEDERER & WADI N. SUKI

INTRODUCTION

The ever-growing success of renal transplantation in the treatment of end-stage renal disease has encouraged nephrologists and transplant surgeons to broaden its application. Previously reserved for the young, healthy individual with chronic glomerulonephritis, renal transplantation is now available to less than ideal patients, high-risk patients, and those suffering from systemic disorders. In some clinical situations such as enzyme deficiency disorders, renal transplantation may offer an advantage over dialysis in that the transplanted organ may act as a source for a deficient cell product as well as a kidney. Experience has demonstrated that transplantation can be successfully accomplished in a variety of common and uncommon renal diseases. Thus patients with many causes of renal failure have benefitted from this form of therapy. In turn, the community of practicing and investigative nephrologists has gained considerable insight into the nature of these several renal diseases. This chapter is devoted to the experience with transplantation in systemic, hereditary, and metabolic disorders resulting in renal failure, with emphasis on unusual problems that have been encountered, patient selection, degree of success, and particular therapeutic considerations.

SYSTEMIC DISEASES

Paraproteinemias

A number of primary paraproteinemias and other systemic diseases complicated by the development of paraproteinemias may eventuate in renal insufficiency, the most common being idiopathic light-chain deposition disease, multiple myeloma, and amyloidosis.

LIGHT-CHAIN DISEASE

Light-chain nephropathy describes the chronic, slowly progressive tubulointerstitial disease associated with the excretion of immunoglobulin light chains. The toxicity of light chains appears to depend at least in part upon an alkaline isoelectric point and perhaps other factors, such as dehydration, excretion of a very concentrated acid urine, and the total load of light chains (1). Additionally, these patients may be prone to episodes of acute renal failure, hastening the decline in renal function (2). Pathologic findings include interstitial fibrosis and tubular casts surrounded by multinucleated giant cells (3). As chronic renal failure is a relatively common occurrence in both multiple myeloma and light-chain disease, a significant number of patients who are long-term survivors are eligible for renal replacement therapy.

There are now nine individually reported cases of renal transplantation in patients in whom chronic renal failure was secondary to ligh-chain disease (4–11). Survival after transplantation has ranged from 14 to 114 months. Four patients have died, three with evidence of recurrent nephropathy 20, 44, and 114 months after transplantation. Five were alive at the time of report, although three had suffered disease recurrence. Penn has also reported the accumulated experience from the Cincinnati Transplant Tumor Registry (12). As of 1986, he had a series of ten patients, six of whom were transplanted with active disease. Of the four patients who were disease free prior to transplantation, only one patient remained in remission, 51 months after transplantation. The other three patients developed tumor 11.5, 12, and 18 months after remission. (One tumor was a pulmonary immunoblastoma, felt possibly to have been a plasmacytoma).

The major concerns in transplanting these individuals are patient survival, recurrent paraprotein damage to the allograft, and the hazards of immunosuppression in a patient with a history of a prior malignancy. Where frank multiple myeloma has been the underlying disease and is in remission at the time of transplantation, excellent results have been obtained in a few cases. Even pathologic recurrence of light-chain disease within the allograft has still been accompanied by relatively normal kidney function for varying periods of time, thus offering the patient a better quality of life (6). Interestingly, the type of paraprotein has not seemed to have made a difference in patient survival or in the future development of recurrence, although the numbers are too small to be truly meaningful. With regard to the issue of immunosuppression following antineoplastic therapy, it is not clear, primarily because of the absence of an acceptable control population, whether or not immunosuppression accelerates tumor recurrence or spread (12). Myeloma follows a variable course, from very indolent with few extrarenal manifestations to a rapidly progressive course involving multiple organ systems. Thus the course after transplantation likely reflects the prior course of disease.

With proper criteria for patient selection, therefore renal transplantation should be considered an acceptable option for the treatment of chronic renal failure secondary to light-chain damage in certain circumstances. These criteria would include complete remission of multiple myeloma for a defined period of time, at least 2 years, and minimal extrarenal manifestation of their illness. For individuals with light-chain disease without bone marrow evidence of a plasma cell dyscrasia, the management is less clear. Frequently, these patients are not treated as myeloma patients, as they do not have frank plasmacytosis. The likelihood of recurrent nephropathy would seem to be quite high because of the persistence of the toxic paraprotein. If transplantation is attempted, maintenance of a high urine output and perhaps alkalinization of the urine may be beneficial (13, 14). Finally, because of the substantial possibility of recurrence of disease, living related donation should be discouraged.

AMYLOIDOSIS

The other clinically significant paraproteinemia that results in renal failure is amyloidosis. Amyloidosis is a disorder characterized by the extracellular deposition of a nonbranching fibrillar protein into a variety of different organs, including the kidneys (15). The disease has been classically divided into primary amyloidosis, in which there is no apparent underlying cause for the production and deposition of amyloid protein, and secondary amyloidosis, in which the development of the syndrome accompanies another systemic illness. Kidney involvement can occur with either form and is generally manifested as proteinuria, diabetes insipidus, renal tubular acidosis, or chronic renal failure (16). Although initially denied renal replacement therapy because of the concern about extrarenal organ involvement, over 100 patients have now received transplants. The first reported case was by Belzer et al. in 1968 (17). According to a later report (18), this patient died of a perforated gallbladder several months after the transplant without evidence of recurrent amyloid in the allograft. Numerous case reports have subsequently appeared documenting both successes and failures in this disease (18–21). Kennedy and Castro described two patients with secondary amyloidosis who received renal transplants (18). One died 2 years post-transplant of a myocardial infarction and sepsis. He had moderately severe renal insufficiency and demonstrated amyloid in the allograft on autopsy. The other patient had excellent renal function at 7 months. The authors also reviewed the literature on the subject, culling the experience of 24 transplants in 23 patients. Five patients who received living related transplants had excellent renal function 7–61 months posttransplant. Of the 16 remaining patients, only six were alive. Four had died within 1 month, three of sepsis and one of cardiac amyloid. Only three patients had survived over 1 year, two dying of infection and one of myocardial infarction. Three of the patients in that series had evidence of recurrent disease. Additionally, patient and graft survival were significantly worse in amyloid patients when compared with other transplant recipients: 40% versus 68% patient survival and 40% versus 50% graft survival at 1 year; 12% versus 50% patient survival and 12% versus 30% graft survival at 5 years. The authors felt that, although these patients fared worse than average, they should be offered transplantation.

Small series have tended to confirm the findings of the case reports. Jones reported ten patients who received cadaveric renal transplants (22). After the first 6 months, patient survival rates were clearly inferior to other transplant patients: 60% versus 73% at 12 months and 38% versus 66% at 24% months. Five of six deaths were secondary to infection. Pasternack et al. reported on their experience in Finland, initially in 1981 (23), then updated to 45 patients in 1986 (24). Three patients had primary amyloid; in the others it was secondary to some form of arthritis or chronic inflammatory condition. The mean age at the time of transplant was 45. These patients were compared with a control group of patients receiving renal transplants for chronic renal failure secondary to glomerulonephritis. Patient survival in the amyloid group was clearly inferior, with a high percentage of deaths in the amyloid group in the first 6 months. Twelve-month patient survival was 50% in the amyloid patients versus 78% in the control group. The causes of death were primarily infection and cardiovascular disease, although four patients died of generalized amyloid. Four patients demonstrated recurrent amyloid in the transplant, all of whom had been transplanted for greater than 1 year. On the other hand, 19 patients who had had their kidneys for less than a year and six who had had theirs for greater than a year showed no amyloid. Drawing on the experience in the literature, they felt that the incidence of recurrence was at least 20%. Interestingly, rejection as a cause of graft failure was less frequent in the amyloid than in the control patients, and there were fewer rejection episodes.

Amyloidosis associated with familial Mediterranean fever may account for as much as 10% of the end-stage renal disease in areas where the disease is endemic. One group has now documented their transplant experience in this population of patients, initially in 1979 (25), then again in 1982 (26). The authors compared 20 amyloid with 123 nonamyloid patients (21 and 143 transplants, respectively). In addition to the usual immunosuppression, amyloid patients received colchicine, 1 mg/day. Their experience confirmed the inferior patient survival but noted that there was a marked difference between their early experience, where 5 of 10 patients died very soon posttransplant, and their later experience, where only 1 of 10 had died, a difference they attributed to a less aggressive approach to immunosuppression. Interestingly, graft survival in their amyloid patients was superior to control. A recurrence of amyloid in the allograft was found pathologically without clinical manifestations.

The major concerns in transplanting individuals with amyloidosis are the effects of extrarenal organ involvement and the possibility of recurrence within the transplanted graft. In the small series and case reports available for evaluation, it is apparent that neither concern should preclude transplantation for the entire population of patients with this disease. These individuals have posed no unexpected difficulties in management or outcome. Patient survival appears to be inferior to nonamyloid patients. On the other hand, the mean age at transplant may be higher (27). Graft survival, if anything, may be better, suggesting that these individuals may be low immunologic responders. Causes of death are primarily cardiovascular and infectious, as is seen in nonamyloid patients. Progressive disseminated amyloid has been noted as a cause of death occasionally. The recurrence rate may be as high as 20% pathologically. Although many of these cases showed pathologic but not clinical recurrence, at least one case has demonstrated recurrence resulting in loss of the transplant (19). Several authors have noted early recurrence of disease in the patients with underlying familial Mediterranean fever and have advocated the routine use of prophylactic colchicine as a preventive measure (26, 28–29). The usual dose has been 1–1.5 mg/day. This practice is supported by experimental evidence of the usefulness of this agent in experimental amyloid (30). Additionally some investigators have commented on the apparent inability of many patients with familial Mediterranean fever to tolerate cyclosporin (29). A large number of patients develop recurrent abdominal pain and other gastrointestinal complaints, necessitating withdrawal or reduction of this immunosuppressive agent. On the other hand, they have noted excellent graft survival on low-dose or no cyclosporin in this group of transplant recipients.

The conclusions to be drawn in considering renal transplantation in this population of patients are as follows. It is reasonable to offer transplantation to these patients. They should be screened for significant involvement of other organs, particularly the heart and liver, prior to transplantation and discouraged from this modality of renal replacement therapy if widespread disease is present. Despite the fact that the disease may recur, the experience with living related donation would suggest that it is a reasonable and ethically defendable choice. It is not clear whether or not recurrence can be prevented, but some authors have recommended that colchicine, 1–1.5 mg/day, should be added to the regimen. Finally, there is some evidence that cyclosporin may be poorly tolerated in these patients. Clinical intolerance, therefore, should be looked for and substitution with azathioprine should be contemplated.

RHEUMATOLOGIC DISORDERS

Systemic lupus erythematosus

Despite innovative and aggressive therapy in this disease, renal involvement remains a major cause of morbidity and mortality. The unpredictable course and the immunologic nature of the disorder have been cause for hesitation in offering the option of transplantation to those individuals who develop renal failure. Lupus pathologically affects the kidneys in a variety of ways, all of which may eventuate in renal failure. Once the patient reaches end-stage renal disease, however, it has been noted that most of the clinical and serologic manifestations of the disease disappear (31–33).

Early reports of renal transplantation in patients with lupus noted that recurrence of the disease in the transplanted kidney was unusual. The first two cases were reported by Roenigk et al. in 1965 (34). Both patients died 1 and 2 months after transplantation of mechanical and infectious complications without evidence of recurrent lupus in their transplanted organs. The Renal Transplant Registry reported on 56 patients who received 60 transplants (35). Of the transplanted kidneys, 28 were from living related sources. Patient survival at the time of analysis (1973) was 66%. There was a 55% allograft survival: 80% living related and 32% cadaveric. No evidence of recurrent disease was found in biopsy or autopsy specimens of allograft material, but the number of specimens examined was not detailed. As these results were comparable with those obtained in non-lupus patients, the authors felt that transplantation was justifiable in these individuals. Amend et al. reported on their experience with transplantation in 11 patients with dialysis-dependent renal failure and clinically quiescent systemic lupus erythematosus (36). Five of 10 cadaver transplants were functioning, with a mean followup of 30 months. Five had failed, three in less than 3 months and two at 10 and 18 months. Three living related grafts were functioning well at a mean of 19 months post-transplant. Serologic parameters, including ANA, anti-DNA, and C3, were not found to be helpful in predicting disease activity or graft function, although there was a suggestion that profound hypocomplementemia may portend either rejection or extrarenal lupus flares. Pathologically, no evidence of disease recurrence was found, even by electron microscopy. These results served to confirm prior sanguine opinions. Mejia et al. confirmed these findings in 1983 with a report on their experience with 20 transplants in 18 patients between 1971 and 1982 (37). Eight kidneys were lost to acute rejection within the first month. One-year patient survival was 100%. One-year graft survival was 34% for cadaveric kidneys and 80% for living related kidneys. Ten patients had functioning allografts for greater than 1 year: seven living related, one living unrelated with donor-specific transfusions, and two cadaveric. The mean time on dialysis prior to transplantation was 10.6 months. The mean followup post-transplantation in this group was 4.5

years. Three developed symptoms of recurrent extrarenal active lupus, though none had had active disease at the time of transplantation. The only patient with clinically significant proteinuria and renal insufficiency had biopsy-proven chronic rejection. Low-titer ANA positivity was found in five and low complement levels in four patients. The authors concurred wholeheartedly with prior recommendations for transplantation.

Although apparently uncommon, recurrent disease in the kidney allograft has been reported. In 1970, Buda et al. found viruslike particles in a transplanted kidney 5 weeks after transplantation (38). At 10 months, however, the patient was reportedly clinically free of disease. Yakub et al. described three patients with lupus who received cadaveric transplants (39). Two with serologically active lupus lost their kidneys within 1 year, one with demonstrable anti-DNA antibody in the graft, although histologically the cause of the loss of function appeared to be rejection. Finally, Amend et al. reported two cases of recurrent lupus nephritis in kidney transplants (40). Both patients experienced significant extrarenal lupus activity prior to renal involvement. Additionally, both became hypocomplementemic just prior to transplant involvement. Interestingly, hypocomplementemia had preceded their original disease as well.

Several problems other than the recurrence of disease have emerged in these individuals. Because of autoantibodies, it may be difficult to cross-match these patients successfully for a transplant. The degree of presensitization as measured by panel reactive antibody screen may be quite high. Additionally, the development of isoantibodies against major blood group determinants has been reported (41). These patients may come to transplantation with a background of extensive immunosuppression and attendant side effects, rendering them less than optimal candidates for further immunosuppressive therapy. Finally, Terasaki and coworkers have noted that living related grafts demonstrate a decreased survival in lupus patients compared with patients with pyelonephritis, suggesting that these kidneys, by virtue of genetic predisposition, may be prone to immunologic damage (42). Despite this intriguing finding, the few reported series continue to support a superior graft survival in living related as opposed to cadaveric sources.

It would appear, on balance, that patients suffering from end-stage lupus nephritis are reasonable candidates for renal transplantation. Clinical experience would support the contention that those patients fare as well as other patients with renal transplants. Several idiosyncrasies peculiar to these patients warrant attention, however. Evidence exists that a significant number of patients who reach end-stage renal disease may be able to discontinue dialysis, at least temporarily. These tend to be individuals who very rapidly deteriorate to renal failure and who have other aggravating factors. However, no serologic features distinguish those who do from those who do not come off dialysis (43). Therefore, it would appear prudent to allow a period on dialysis prior to transplantation. In this regard, hemodialysis appears to be preferable to peritoneal dialysis in achieving disease remission (44, 45). Additionally, although serologic parameters are of indeterminant significance in patients on dialysis, a few cases would suggest that hypocomplementemia precedes either recurrent disease or acute rejection (46, 47). Thus it would also be safer to transplant when the patient is normocomplementemic, if possible. It is probably also advisable to monitor serologic status after transplantation periodically, on the assumption that the development of hypocomplementemia may alert the medical team to the potential for disease recurrence. Recurrent disease is rare, but even if it does occur this may not signify loss of the graft. Many of these patients exhibit high performed antibody titers. Absorption of serum or treatment with dithiotreitol to remove autoantibodies may be necessary to ensure that a false-positive cross-match does not occur. Finally, transplant candidates who have suffered the ravages of prior steroid therapy may benefit from immunosuppressive regimens employing minimal steroid usage, such as cyclosporine alone or in combination with azathioprine.

Progressive systemic sclerosis

Scleroderma is an uncommon but well documented cause of end-stage renal disease. This illness affects primarily young women in the second to fourth decades, affecting a number of different organ systems. The renal lesion is characterized most commonly by intensive arteriolar nephrosclerosis, often culminating in a malignant-hypertension-type picture and rapidly progressive renal failure (48). Even into this decade, patients were dying of the severe hypertensive crisis that characterizes the clinical course of these patients. Because of the relative rarity of the entity, the literature on the subject of renal transplantation in these patients is confined to case reports and very small clinical series. The picture that emerges, however, is more optimistic than may be expected. Multiple reports confirm that not only can these patients be successfully transplanted, but that in some cases extrarenal manifestations of the disease, such as the Raynaud's phenomenon and skin changes, may actually regress. The first reported case appeared in 1973, in which a man with longstanding scleroderma received a cadaveric renal transplant after bilateral nephrectomy for control of hypertension (49). Eighteen months later he had excellent renal function and had noted disappearance of arthralgias and Raynaud's as well as loosening of the skin. This report was followed by a mention by Cannon et al., in their 1974 review, of one patient who had excellent function 7 months after receiving a living related transplant (50). While other case reports have continued to document the possibility of successful transplantation in this condition (51–54), recurrent disease has been reported in at least two separate cases, resulting in loss of the allograft (55, 56). In one of the cases there was accelerated loss of the transplant, in which the pathology was indistinguishable from the native illness. It is well known, however, that the pathologic findings of acute accelerated rejection mimic those of malignant hypertension. Therefore, whether this report truly represents an example of recurrent disease is not clear.

Despite the paucity of clinical material, there would appear to be no reason to discourage transplantation in these patients. In some institutions these patients routinely undergo nephrectomy prior to transplant, primarily in an effort to control severe hypertension. However, transplantation has been accomplished successfully, even without nephrectomy. Therefore, in the opinion of the authors, the decision to nephrectomize the patient prior to transplantation should be based on blood pressure control or infection control, but is otherwise not necessary. The disease may recur, and some authors have suggested that this is more likely if the patient has sustained a very fulminant course that culminates in renal failure (56). Additionally, since progressive systemic sclerosis affects many other organ systems, these patients should be screened for significant pulmonary, cardiac, or esophageal involvement. While evidence of extrarenal disease does not necessarily preclude transplantation (especially in view of the reports of regression of some of the manifestations after transplantation), it may influence the decision on the form of renal replacement therapy or on the source of the transplant allograft.

Vasculitis

The experience in renal transplantation for vasculitic causes of end-stage renal disease is quite limited because of the infrequency of these disorders. Nonetheless, a literature review has uncovered case reports of individuals with Wegener's, Henoch Schonlein purpura, polyarteritis nodosa, and Goodpasture's syndrome having undergone renal transplantation.

WEGENER'S GRANULOMATOSIS

Wegener's granulomatosis is a disease of unknown etiology, manifesting clinically as recurrent respiratory disease, sinus inflammation, and renal insufficiency. Renal failure is a common sequela, even with aggressive therapy and, before the onset of chronic hemodialysis, was the major cause of death (57). Renal transplantation in this disease was first described by Lyons and Lindsay in 1972 (58). A 29-year-old patient received a living related transplant from his sister after control of his underlying disease, splenectomy, and nephrectomy. He was doing well 14 months later. This report was followed by several others documenting the long-term success in patients with different presentations and clinical courses (59–62). Recurrent disease has been reported, however, both in the allograft and extrarenally, despite continuous immunosuppression. One patient described by Steinman et al. had been disease free on azathioprine and prednisone for 4 years when he developed upper respiratory tract disease, sinus symptoms, and microscopic hematuria, but stable renal function (63). Recurrent Wegener was documented by sinus, turbinate, and nasopharyngeal biopsies, and his immunosuppression was changed from azathioprine to cyclophosphamide. Subsequently he experienced relief of his symptoms as well as his hematuria. Severe leukopenia necessitated discontinuation of cyclophosphamide after 3 months and reinstitution of azathioprine, but the patient remained disease free at 7 months after the switch. The authors suggested that cyclophosphamide may be preferable to azathioprine on a chronic basis. Another patient described by Curtis et al. developed recurrent disease on chronic azathioprine therapy, however, with evidence clinically and pathologically of renal involvement (64). This man received cyclophosphamide and high-dose prednisone but developed Listeria meningitis and lost his allograft. Kuross et al, reviewed the nine patients with this disorder who had been transplanted up to 1981 (65). Three had died of infection, and six were alive 7 months to 7 years posttransplant. Only one patient had experienced recurrent disease but had been successfully treated.

HENOCH SCHONLEIN PURPURA

Renal transplantation for other vasculitides is less well reported. Henoch Schonlein purpura is a rare cause of renal failure, but recurs commonly in the transplanted kidney. Single cases documenting pathologic recurrence have been reported since 1974 (66); graft loss secondary to recurrent disease, however, has been seen rarely (67–69). Levy et al. reported on transplantations in 11 children with Henoch Schonlein purpura (70). Biopsies of eight patients revealed mesangial IgA desposits in six, whereas only one had clinical evidence of disease, i.e., hematuria and proteinuria. Transplantation was delayed 21–99 months after the onset of clinical disease, a factor that the authors felt was significantly related to their low clinical recurrence rate. Cameron reported no IgA deposition in 7 of 10 kidneys transplanted into such patients (71). Bachman et al. also reported no recurrence in three patients with Henoch Schonlein purpura (72). Only one patient was biopsied, however, and this was quite soon after transplantation. Two patients had proteinuria, but no biopsy was performed. All three patients had good kidney function. On the whole, therefore, it seems reasonable to offer renal transplantation to this population of patients, delaying the transplant until the patient is free of clinical disease for at least 1 year. Pathologic recurrence would appear to be quite common, near 50%, but does not correlate with the clinical outcome. Cameron has suggested that measuring IgA levels and transplanting at a time when they are normal may be advisable, but this hypothesis has not been tested (71).

POLYARTERITIS NODOSA

Polyarteritis nodosa is even less well reported *vis à vis* renal transplantation. Montalbert et al. reviewed the subject in 1980 (73). Eight patients had been reported to the transplant registry. Fifty percent of the transplants were functioning 1–4 years posttransplantation. Their patient had done well and had experienced marked improvement in neuropathy posttransplant. No recurrence of disease was noted on biopsies performed 5 and 21 months postoperatively.

GOODPASTURE'S SYNDROME

Goodpasture's syndrome is another extremely unusual cause of renal failure. In its full form, it is characterized by the appearance of hemoptysis, anemia, and rapidly progressive renal failure. Histologically, there is extensive crescent formation and linear deposition of IgG along the glomerular basement membrane. Concomitantly anti-GBM antibodies can be detected in the serum. Wilson and Dixon reviewed the transplant experience in patients with anti-GBM-associated chronic renal failure, both with and without Goodpasture's syndrome, who underwent transplantation (74). At the time of report, seven patients with Goodpasture's were alive 2 months to 4–5 years posttransplant; three had died. All of these patients had received therapy for their underlying disease. Of those without Goodpasture's syndrome, 8 of 15 were alive and seven had died of sepsis and hemorrhage. Two of these patients had detectable circulating levels of antiglomerular basement membrane antibodies and eight had antibody detectable in kidney tissue. There is evidence that the active disease is self-limited, such that after a delay, transplantation could be successfully performed without disease recurrence (75). However, recurrent disease has been reported on several occasions, even years after clinical quiescence (76–79). In fact, successful transplantation has taken place in the face of detectable levels of anti-GBM in the serum (80). Therefore, serologic activity does not absolutely preclude transplantation; although, generally, recurrent nephritis has not occurred if transplantation is delayed until serum anti-GBM is undetectable (75). Additionally, it may be advisable to monitor anti-GBM levels periodically after transplantation.

THROMBOTIC MICROANGIOPATHIC DISORDERS

The term *thrombotic microangiopathy* covers a group of disorders affecting the small vessels of a variety of organs and producing a picture of a microangiopathic hemolytic anemia accompanied by derangement of the function of affected organs. The three major clinical entities include hemolytic uremic syndrome, thrombotic thrombocytopenic purpura, and postpartum renal failure.

Hemolytic uremic syndrome

The hemolytic uremic syndrome is a disease that primarily affects children under the age of 5, characterized clinically by hematuria, acute oliguric renal failure, and hemolytic anemia, and pathologically by endothelial cell swelling and hyaline thrombi of glomerular capillaries and extraglomerular arterioles and venules (81). Cerilli and coworkers in 1972 reported the first two cases of renal transplantation as the therapy for chronic renal failure secondary to hemolytic uremic syndrome (82). It is not clear from the reports whether or not the hematologic manifestations of the diseases had cleared prior to transplantation. The first patient underwent bilateral nephrectomy and splenectomy prior to transplantation and received conventional immunosuppression with azathioprine, rabbit antilymphocyte globulin, and steroids. She did well without evidence of rejection or recurrence of disease for 13 months posttransplantation at the time of the report. The other patient was treated similarly but experienced what appeared to be an acute exacerbation of the hemolytic uremic syndrome 12 hours posttransplant and recovered spontaneously. There was no evidence of cytotoxic antibody formation to the donated kidney. Since those two reports, several more case reports have documented the experience with transplantation in this disorder (83–85). It would appear that recurrence of the disease is common (86–88), although it does not necessarily result in failure of the graft. In uncontrolled trials, some patients have been treated prophylactically with heparinization or antiplatelet agents. Additionally, these agents plus fresh-frozen plasma have been used when a presumptive recurrence has happened.

Some of the major questions to be addressed in the determination of the role of renal transplantation in the hemolytic uremic syndrome include: Is the disease the same in adults as in children? Should the evidence of potential genetic predisposition to the illness be considered in the decision as to the source of the kidney, i.e., should living related transplantation be discouraged? Should any form of therapy specific for the hemolytic uremic syndrome be maintained prophylactically in these patients? Should pregnancy be discouraged? Should cyclosporine, which itself occasionally produces a similar picture (89, 90), be used as the immunosuppressive agent of choice? There are no clear-cut answers to any of these questions.

A major stumbling block in the evaluation of therapy in these diseases has been the lack of understanding of the pathogenesis. While the hemolytic uremic syndrome in adults may resemble that in children clinically at the onset, there are distinct differences. In children the outcome is, for the most part, good; on the other hand, in adults chronic renal failure is a more common situation (85). Additionally, a syndrome clearly resembling hemolytic uremic syndrome has been seen in adults in other situations such as postpartum, after the use of some chemotherapeutic agents such as mitomycin C or cyclosporine, and with the use of hormonal agents such as birth control pills or estrogens (81). It is not clear, therefore, that the disease in children and adults should be regarded or treated in a similar manner.

At this time it would appear from reports from most centers that there is no indication for prophylactic antiplatelet drugs, fresh-frozen plasma, or other forms of therapy that have been employed in the treatment of the thrombotic microangiopathies. Recurrences of disease have been reported to occur from 1 week and to as long as several months after transplantation. Recurrent disease has not correlated with the use of prophylactic therapy to prevent hemolytic uremic syndrome.

With regard to the third issue, that of potential genetic predisposition, both living related and cadaveric kidneys have been transplanted into victims of hemolytic uremic syndrome. In either circumstances there are reported cases of recurrence as well as nonrecurrence. The question, therefore, becomes more of a general philosophical question as to whether or not living related transplantation should be allowed in a disease that can recur. Most transplant centers have formulated their own policy on this issue. In the opinion of the authors, living related transplantation can be considered provided that all parties understand the potential risk of recurrence in the recipient and of de-novo disease in the donor (91).

The question of pregnancy in a renal transplant recipient in whom the original disease was idiopathic hemolytic uremic syndrome is again one that has no answer based on solid fact. Successful renal transplantation has been performed in at least four patients whose disease was initially postpartum renal failure (92, 93). However, none of these patients has become pregnant again, at least to the knowledge of the authors. Again it would seem reasonable to apprise the patient of the potential risk of pregnancy in this particular situation and to leave the final decision to her.

Although cyclosporine has been associated with the hemolytic uremic syndrome de novo in organ transplant recipients, the occurrence is quite rare (79, 80). At this time there can no firm recommendations made concerning the use of cyclosporine in this situation. Recurrent disease, however, should be a major consideration in the event of renal transplant dysfunction (94).

Thrombotic thrombocytopenic purpura

The reports on the use of renal transplantation in the therapy of chronic renal failure secondary to thrombotic thrombocytopenia purpura (TTP) are scant indeed. TTP is a syndrome characterized by fever, altered mental status, thrombocytopenia, microangiopathic hemolytic anemia, and renal dysfunction (81). The major disease manifestations are extrarenal, and chronic renal failure is a relatively infrequent sequela in survivors. The pathogenesis of this disorder is unknown, although there is evidence for endothelial cell damage, resulting in suboptimal production of the antiplatelet aggregatory prostaglandin, prostacyclin, thus culminating in diffuse intravascular thrombosis. These patients die of cardiac or central nervous system manifestations of this disease, although renal failure can be seen as well. The general therapy of TTP has undergone a significant advance in the last decade, resulting in a marked improvement in morbidity and mortality. Thus far there are three case reports of renal transplantation for TTP, one without and two with recurrence. One patient with frequently recurrent TTP responded well to repeated plasma infusions (95). In another patient a donor-specfiic antimonocyte antibody was identified in the recipient and postulated to be an initiating event in the recurrence of the thrombotic microangiopathy in this individual (93). The paucity of reports reflects the infrequency of the syndrome, as well as chronic renal failure resulting therefrom. From what is presented in the literature, it would appear that transplantation is feasible in these individuals.

Postpartum renal failure

Postpartum renal failure (PPRF) is another of this group of diseases characterized by acute renal failure and a microangiopathic hemolytic anemia (96). The onset of generally within a few days after delivery, but many occur up to months later. As above, the cause is unknown, but may also be a result of endothelial injury produced by some as yet uncharacterized insult resulting in intravascular platelet aggregation. In the past the mortality in this illness has ranged from 50% to 80%. Improved supportive measures have lessened this mortality, but chronic renal failure remains a significantly common sequela. There are now at least four case reports of successful renal transplantation in this disorder, again suggesting that these patients are suitable recipients for this form of therapy (92, 93). Although recurrent postpartum renal failure has not been reported in the renal transplant population, we have seen one case of de-novo occurrence (97).

In summary, the thrombotic microangiopathies are a group of disorders characterized by intravascular platelet coagulation producing dysfunction of a variety of organs, but commonly resulting in renal failure. Renal transplantation has been utilized in the therapy of all three clinical syndromes with success. There are several specific recommendations to be made regarding transplantation in these individuals. The possibility of recurrence of disease must be recognized, and aggressive measures to exclude disease recurrence must be performed in the evaluation if graft dysfunction should it occur. These individuals may respond to specific therapeutic modalities such as antiplatelet drugs, fresh-frozen plasma, or plasmapheresis in the case of a recurrence, whereas none of these therapies would be used in the treatment of acute rejection. Severe acute rejection and recurrent thrombotic microangiopathy may be difficult to distinguish histopathologically, and clinically these two processes may present similarly. Significant hematuria, however, is quite uncommon in acute rejection, whereas it is quite common in HUS or TTP. Additionally, on biopsy an intense inflammatory infiltrate in the interstitium is the hallmark of severe cell-mediated rejection, whereas this is not seen in the thrombotic microangiopathies. Finally, the time course may be of some diagnostic aid in that acute severe rejection tends to occur less frequently after the first month. Therefore, a fulminant episode of acute renal failure with a picture of severe glomerular thrombosis and fibrin deposition occurring several months posttransplantation would be more consistent with a recurrence of disease. Although recurrence does not appear to be the rule, the patient should be informed of the potential prior to transplantation. Additionally, any potential donor should be aware of the possibility of recurrence in the recipient and of potential de-novo disease in the case of a living related donor. Finally, careful counseling regarding the potential hazards of pregnancy and oral contraceptive agents should be a part of the posttransplantation agenda, bearing in mind that for many female patients the possibility of successful parenthood may have been a major consideration in the decision to choose transplantation as a therapeutic option.

DIABETES MELLITUS

Without a doubt, diabetes mellitus is the single most common systemic disease resulting in renal failure. Previously considered unsuitable candidates for end-stage renal disease therapy, diabetics now constitute nearly 25% of all patients entering renal failure programs (98). Clinically significant renal diseases strikes 30–50% of type 1 and 10% of type 2 diabetics, after 10–20 years of disease and, once apparent, relentlessly progresses to renal failure within 3–5 years (99). Clinically, these individuals exhibit a high glomerular filtration rate initially, followed by proteinuria, hypertension, nephrotic syndrome, and a progressive decline in renal function. The characteristic pathologic lesions are nodular and diffuse glomerulosclerosis. Early histologic changes can be seen as soon as 2 years after the onset of diabetes, literally decades before clinical disease is apparent. While theories abound, the precise pathophysiologic mechanisms for the initiation and progression of diabetic nephropathy remain unknown. What seems to be clear, however, is that diabetic renal disease is a result of the diabetic milieu and not a coexistent independent phenomenon. Several lines of evidence support this contention. Diabetic nephropathy complicates the course of type 1, type 2, and other forms of diabetes. Recurrent diabetic nephropathy has been well documented in the literature in cases where kidneys from nondiabetic donors are transplanted into diabetic recipients (100–102). Likewise, there has been a report of a kidney from a diabetic transplanted into a nondiabetic with subsequent loss of the pathologic lesions of diabetes from the transplanted kidney (103). All of these findings support the conclusion that diabetic nephropathy is a result of the metabolic derangements of the disease. The consequences of long-term diabetes manifest not only in the kidneys, but also in the nerves, heart, retina, and vasculature. Thus the diabetic with renal failure comes to dialysis or transplantation with significant multiorgan pathology. The survival of diabetic patients on dialysis is clearly inferior to nondiabetic patients. The major concerns, therefore, in the decision to transplant a diabetic patient with end-stage renal disease have been related to the systemic nature of the disease. Is the survival of diabetic patients who have been transplanted equivalent to nondiabetics? If not, how does it compare with the survival of diabetic patients on dialysis? Since diabetes recurs in the transplanted kidney, should they be transplanted? Should living related donors be used? What pretransplant evaluation should be done, and under what medical circumstances should a diabetic be denied a transplant? Does transplantation affect the natural history of the disease and its complications, and can we alter the natural history in any way? Finally, should we alter immunosuppression protocols for diabetic patients?

Even with favorable patient selection, diabetics exhibited a significantly inferior renal allograft survival in the precyclosporine era. The Transplant Registry in 1977 reported a significant difference in 1-year graft survival between diabetics and nondiabetics, particularly when the donor was cadaveric (104). These findings were echoed in a number of other series (105–108). Additionally, some investigators reported an excessive rate of complications, early and late (109–112). In one series of 77 transplanted diabetics, 10 of the 77 had urinary leakage, 5 had severe infection, and 10 died from cardiac complications in the early postoperative period (109). Eight of the 77 underwent amputation, six underwent surgical procedures for ischemic extremities, and two sustained cerebrovascular accidents in the later period of follow-up. Zincke and coworkers also reported a high rate of complications in 69 diabetics, including nine wound infections, seven of which were fatal; one wound dehiscence; four patients with ileofemoral thrombosis and pulmonary embolism; eight with fatal myocardial infarctions; one with a cerebrovascular accident; and 15 patients (25%) with amputation (110). On the other hand, Sutherland and coworkers have reported comparable graft and patient survival rates between diabetics and nondiabetics since 1979 (113). They attributed the improvement in their diabetic statistics to a policy of pretransplant splenectomy and transfusions, posttransplant intensive insulin therapy, and less aggressive rejection therapy. These investigators did not experience an increased incidence of surgical or urologic complications. Admittedly there was a 15% cardiovascular mortality in diabetics compared with 2% in nondiabetics and an equally high incidence of amputations, but these complications have tended to occur after the first 2 years. This center tends to perform a large number of living related transplants, approximately 60% of the total number. Other investigators have documented the superiority of living related as opposed to cadaveric graft survival especially in the diabetic (114–116).

Newer survival statistics in diabetics in the cyclosporine era have been reported from Minnesota and Pittsburg recently. Sutherland reported a 76% 2-year cadaveric graft and patient survival with the use of cyclosporine, representing a significant improvement in graft survival in this population (117). Rosenthal has reported from Pittsburgh a comparable cadaveric graft survival at 2 years, 70%, as well as a lower steroid dose, a decreased number of hospital days in the first year, a lesser increase in the insulin dose posttransplant, and a decreased incidence of septic complications in cyclosporine- as opposed to azathioprine-treated patients (118, 119). Importantly, there was also a marked decrease in patient mortality with cyclosporine. It would appear, therefore, that cyclosporine use has resulted in patient and graft survival rates that justify the role of transplantation in the diabetic patient.

The next issue is how transplantation compares with dialysis in the diabetic patient in terms of patient survival, quality of life, and rehabilitation potential. In 1978, Goldstein and Massry published their experience with diabetics who came to hemodialysis (120). One-year mortality was greater than 50%. On the whole, a large percentage of these patients had numerous diabetic complications, besides nephropathy, and a considerable problem with vascular access. More recent survival statistics have demonstrated substantial improvement in diabetic patient survival on dialysis with a 1-year survival rate of greater than 80% and 3-year rates of 50% (98, 121). Because of the high incidence of transplant complications in diabetics, it is pertinent to compare the modalities in determining the optimal mode of therapy for these patients. One of the earlier reviews disclosed that, despite a higher rate of complications in the diabetic posttransplant relative to the nondiabetic, survival and rehabilitation were superior in the transplanted versus the dialyzed diabetic (116). The authors recognized, however, that patient selection may have influenced the statistics, in that younger and healthier diabetics would be more likely to be accepted for renal transplantation. Other groups, however, also showed superior patient survival up to 5 years with either a living related or cadaveric transplant as opposed to any form of dialysis (122). One study that attempted to control for age disparity and other potentially confounding factors was published by Parfrey and coworkers (123). The groups were small and all but one of the transplants were cadaveric and were treated with azathioprine. They found that morbidity and mortality were comparable for both modalities, except for a higher rate of hospitalization in the transplanted patient.

It is clear, therefore, that patient selection is of paramount importance in the decision on therapeutic modality in the diabetic patient with end-stage renal disease. Diabetic complications that may confound rehabilitative potential include vision disturbances, neuropathy, peripheral vascular disease, and coronary artery disease. Regrettably, the initiation of end-stage renal disease therapy has little or no effect on progressive retinopathy. Many of the initial reports of maintenance hemodialysis commented on the acceleration of eye disease, felt to be, in part, secondary to the use of heparin. Although some studies have suggested that deterioration of vision slows after transplantation, most studies have documented progressive loss of vision (98). More recent statistics demonstrating improved visual prognosis for all modalities may be related to more timely intervention with laser therapy.

The evaluation of neuropathy is a more complex issue in that both uremia and diabetes result in neuropathic disease. Undoubtedly transplantation ameliorates uremic neuropathy far better than either form of dialysis (124). Diabetic neuropathy, on the other hand, progresses under the influence of both dialysis and transplantation (98). Interestingly, despite a higher incidence of bladder dysfunction secondary to autonomic neuropathy in the diabetic transplanted patient, there is not an increase in hospitalization days or allograft loss relative to the nondiabetic recipient.

Vascular disease is a more significant issue in the evaluation of long-term prognosis. Cardiovascular complications are the most frequent cause of death in the dialysis population and in transplanted patients alike, along with infection. A sizable number of patients, ranging from 15% to 35% of those transplanted, will undergo amputation after transplantation (105–112, 126–129). More importantly, preexisting vascular disease has been shown to adversely affect patient survival in a number of studies (128–131). Rimmer et al. compared ten diabetic patients with and 20 patients without vascular disease pretransplantation who subsequently underwent renal transplantation (128). One- and 2-year patient survival rates were 48% and 24% in those with vascular disease and 85% in those without. Braun et al. published their experience with 61 transplanted diabetics who had undergone coronary angiography prior to transplantation (131). Patients with greater than 70% occlusion of the coronary vessels had a 2-year survival of 40%, those with left ventricular dysfunction had a 60% 2-year survival, and those without coronary disease had an 81% survival. They recommended against transplantation in the high-risk cardiac group. They also recommended screening for cardiac disease in all diabetics contemplating transplantation.

In summary, therefore, renal transplantation is a reasonable mode of therapy in the diabetic end-stage renal failure patient. A living related completely matched graft offers the best opportunity for rehabilitation and survival of both the patient and graft. Cadaveric renal transplantation is associated with at least equivalent if not better patient survival and quality of life than either mode of dialysis. Additionally, high MLC, mismatched kidneys from related donors with donor specific transfusion and azathioprine (133), or cyclosporine without DSTs (134) have yielded excellent results. More data are emerging that allografts from unrelated living donors may also produce comparable results (135–137). Selection of recipients is, however, of paramount importance. Neither eye disease nor neuropathy should preclude transplantation. Progressive retinopathy has been described in all forms of therapy of renal failure in this population. Neuropathy is more likely to improve with a transplant than with dialysis therapy. Screening for coronary and peripheral vascular disease, however, is critical, both in establishing suitability for transplantation as well as prognosis. Because of the high incidence of silent coronary disease, evaluation based on symptoms alone is inadequate. Experience in other centers suggesting a lack of acceptable correlation between noninvasive testing and the results of coronary angiography in diabetic patients mandates screening coronary angiography on most if not all diabetics prior to transplantation. Studies by Morrow (138) and Philipson (139) demonstrated that only about 10% of diabetic patients were able to achieve 85% maximal heart rate on stress thallium testing. A negative stress thallium test was found to correspond well to the lack of significant coronary disease in Philipson's study. However, Morrow found that a negative stress thallium test pretransplantation did not predict a lack of coronary morbidity posttransplantation. It is not clear, however, if these were truly negative in the face of an 85% maximal heart rate, or whether many fell into a nondiagnostic category. If no significant disease is seen, angiography should be repeated every 18 months to verify the absence of new coronary disease. Critical coronary lesions should be addressed prior to transplantation. If percutaneous transluminal angioplasty is the selected procedure, then followup angiography should be performed on a semiannual basis to determine persistent patency of the coronary arteries. Surgically corrected coronary artery disease should be evaluated with yearly angiographic follow-up. Careful pretransplant evaluation of symptoms of potential peripheral vascular disease should be performed with particular attention to neurologic symptoms, claudication, and examination of the peripheral pulses. Doppler studies of the iliac vessels should be obtained as a screen to exclude significant atherosclerosis, which may complicate the vascular anastamosis of the transplant. Suspicious Doppler results may prompt full angiography for better anatomic definition of potential disease. Patients with untreated or untreatable coronary artery disease or significant left ventricular dysfunction should not be offered a transplant, not because transplant gives inferior results, but because of their overall poor prognosis.

Although in some institutions they are not considered high-risk patients, diabetics with renal failure are felt to be prone to an increased frequency of complications, particularly related to steroid use. They may experience significant deterioration of metabolic control, more frequent accelerated cataract and bone disease, and more infectious complications. Thus every attempt should be made to optimize their generally metabolic state and to minimize steroid dose. Ideally, a well-matched living related donor transplantation performed on an elective basis offers the best clinical situation. If cadaveric donation is contemplated, then the best match with the least ischemic time is optimal. What, if any, alteration in nonimmunosuppressive drugs is needed is unknown at this time. A brief induction course of steroids or initial elimination of steroids altogether may be feasible, using cyclosporine alone or in combination with azathioprine. Extra careful attention to potential sources of infection, such as indwelling urinary catheters, central intravenous lines, or Tenckhoff catheters, is crucial during the period of maximum immunosuppression. That diabetes can recur in the transplanted kidney is well documented. It is not known, however, if measures such as tight metabolic control, low protein diet, or the use of angiotensin-converting enzyme inhibitors are of benefit in eliminating or delaying this problem. In the final analysis, successful concomitant or sequential pancreas transplantation along with renal transplantation probably offers our best chance of alleviating the problem of the diabetic renal failure patient.

INHERITED AND METABOLIC DISORDERS

This group of disorders includes a wide variety of diseases of diverse pathogenesis, affecting either the kidney alone or a multitude of organs. As a combined cause of end-stage renal disease in this country, they account for only a small percentage of the total population of individuals with renal failure. Despite this, a significant experience with the use of renal transplantation has accrued in many of these diseases.

Hematologic Diseases

SICKLE CELL DISEASE

The S form of human hemoglobin is present in the black population of the United States in 1% as the homozygous disease, sickle cell disease, and in 8% as the heterozygous form of the illness, sickle cell trait (140). It has long been recognized that both forms of hemoglobinopathy produce renal disease, albeit much more severely in the homozygous form, and that chronic renal failure can result. The most common clinical manifestation of sickle cell involvement of the kidney is hematuria; however, a multitude of manifestations can occur, such as hyposthenuria, hyperkalemia, proteinuria ranging to the frank nephrotic range, papillary necrosis, and end-stage renal disease (141). Both interstitial and glomerular involvement have been reported. The mechanism of renal disease of the interstitial variety is felt to be secondary to recurrent ischemic episodes that are secondary to intravascular sickling within the hyperosmolar, relatively hypoxic medulla, resulting in progressive loss of medullary tissue. The mechanism of glomerular disease is not clear and indeed may be simply coincidental. The contribution of sickle cell disease and trait to the development of chronic renal failure is unknown, but has generally been felt to be small. However, in Jamaica and other Caribbean countries renal failure has been found to be responsible for up to 20% of deaths in individuals with sickle hemoglobin disease (142). Despite the frequency of this disorder, there is a relative paucity of data on the transplantation experience in this population. Chatterjee has accumulated, through a questionnaire, the experience of 110 centers, resulting in data concerning 45 transplants in 40 patients: 13 homozygous sicklers and 27 heterozygous (143). Thirty-four of the kidneys were from cadaveric sources and the remainder were from living related donors. Despite a high mortality in the first year (12%), graft survival at the first year was satisfactory: 82% in the living related population and 62% in the cadaveric group. Based on this experience, he recommended renal transplantation as a reasonable modality of therapy for end-stage renal disease in these patients.

Individual case reports have documented problems unique to the sickle cell patient. Chartterjee reported a patient with sickle trait who lost two cadaveric allografts by what clinically appeared to be rejection-induced intravascular sickling (144). He postulated that mild rejection may have rendered the kidney tissue more vulnerable to the extensive sickling process, thus exacerbating the underlying ischemia and contributing significantly to graft loss. Spector et al. reported the case of a patient with sickle cell anemia who developed frequent and severe painful crisis after successful renal transplantation following a 13-year pain-free hiatus (145). She responded to repeated and frequent transfusions with relief from painful crises. Interestingly, she also demonstrated relative hyposthenuria, with a maximum concentrating ability of 532 mOsm/l despite an otherwise well-functioning kidney. Not only crisis, but recurrent sickle cell nephropathy as well, has been reported in a living related kidney (146).

With this background in mind, it is recommended that all black patients awaiting renal transplantation undergo hemoglobin electrophoresis to determine the presence or absence of hemoglobinopathy, which may later have a bearing on transplant function. Additionally, it is recomemded by some authors that these patients remain well hydrated throughout the transplant procedure, with a low-dose dopamine drip (3–5 μg/kg/min) to ensure excellent renal vasodilation and supplemental oxygen administration to avoid tissue hypoxia. Some authors have also recommended repeated transfusions to maintain Hb S less than 20% (147), but the potential benefits of this therapy must be weighed very carefully against the very real and potential hazards of transfustion and iron overload. Certainly in the case of the individual such as the one reported who developed repeated severe episodes of painful crises, one is justified in such a therapeutic regimen. In summary, these patients can be considered good candidates for either living related or cadaveric renal transplantation with certain precautions being maintained. There may be a higher first-year mortality than in the general population of transplant recipients, but otherwise the results are satisfactory.

Inherited primary renal disorders

POLYCYSTIC KIDNEY DISEASE

Polycystic kidney disease is a disease of unknown etiology manifested as the relentless cystic enlargement of different portions of the renal tubule, resulting in the eventual destruction of normal renal parenchyma and chronic renal failure. It is second only to glomerulonephritis as a primary renal cause of end-stage renal disease in this country. Patients with this disorder as a rule tend to do well as chronic renal failure patients, but may have continuing problems with bleeding, pain in the kidneys, and cyst infections. Additionally, there are several extrarenal manifestations of the disease that may become problematic, including hypertension, diverticulosis, cerebral aneurysms, and possibly aortic aneurysms (148).

Several series now document the efficacy of renal transplantation in this disorder. In 1975 Mendez and coworkers reported 17 patients who received cadaveric renal transplants between 1969 and 1973 (149). Nine patients retained either one or both of their native kidneys, while eight had had bilateral nephrectomy for bleeding or infection. Those patients who retained at least one native kidney had a graft survival rate of 44%, 33%, and 18% at 6, 12, and 18 months. Four of these patients died of a variety of causes; however, of note, one patient who had been discovered to have a urinary tract infection prior to transplant died of pyelonephritis post-transplant. The transplant survival rate in the nephrectomized group was 86%, 68.6%, and 58.8% at 6, 12, and 18 months, in sharp contrast to the nonephrectomized group. Nonetheless, this group recommended a continued practice of selective nephrectomy, as they could implicate the retained kidney in only one of the patient deaths.

Salvatierra et al. reviewed the course of 31 patients who received 35 transplants in 1976 (150). Seven of these individuals had undergone bilateral nephrectomy specifically for bleeding or infection and two had undergone unilateral nephrectomy. With an average follow-up of over 3 years, there was 81% patient survival, with a 71% graft survival (virtually all were cadaveric recipients). There was no differentiation made between nephrectomized and nonnephrectomized individuals. Two patients who had had renal infections in the past and who had not undergone nephrectomy developed infection posttransplant, requiring emergency nephrectomy and considerable morbidity but not mortality. These authors addressed several issues concerning polycystic patients. They recommended nephrectomy for patients who had had a history of urinary tract infections or bleeding. They specifically commented that there wre no technical difficulties in placing the kidney in the iliac fossa, even when the kidneys were in place, and therefore there was no surgical indication for nephrectomy. Finally, they suggested that living related donation should be considered, but the potential donors should be carefully screened for the presence of this disease and the minimum age of donation should be 30 years.

De Bono ad Evans reviewed their experience with 65 patients who received renal transplants (151). One-year graft survival was 46% compared with a general 1-year graft survival of 53% at their institution. They also noted that in many of their patients the cause of death was something that could have been anticipated, such as diverticulitis, myocardial infarction, or urinary tract infection. They recommended adding barium enema examinations, evaluation of serum lipids, and evaluation of peripheral vascular disease to the usual pretransplant evaluation.

Sanfilippo et al. in 1983 reviewed their experience with 108 patients who had received renal transplants during the prior 4 years, 1977–1981 (152). Overall graft and patient survival were similar to a control group: 50% at 1 year and 45% at 2 years. Although there were no mortality rates quoted, more polycystic patients died of sepsis. The presence or absence of pretransplant nephrectomy made no difference in the rate of sepsis. However, the use of antilymphocyte serum was associated with a higher rate of sepsis in the polycystic patients than in the nonpolycystics. Additionally, if the individuals had undergo bilateral nephrectomy prior to transplantation and then returned to dialysis secondary to graft loss, there was a higher incidence of significant anemia and death. Based on their experience, they endorsed the use of renal transplantation for the treatment of end-stage polycystic kidney disease. They also recommended nephrectomy only for selected indications and advised caution in the use of antilymphocyte immunosuppressive products.

With the exception of one report (153), most of published literature would suggest an excellent outcome for transplanted polycystic patients (154–156). Based on a review of the combined reports in the literature, the authors recommend the use of renal transplantation in this population. Nephrectomy should be considered only for specific indications, either infection or bleeding. Whether all patients who have had a history of urinary tract infection should undergo nephrectomy is not clear, but the fact that the mere history of an infection does not ensure the development of infection or sepsis post-transplant suggests that nephrectomy under those circumstances should not be mandatory. Additionally it may be difficult to determine which kidney or kidneys are infected, resulting in prophylactic bilateral nephrectomy, a procedure that carries substantial postoperative morbidity (157). Also, these patients should be screened well for comorbid disease, such as cerebral aneurysm, diverticulitis, or peripheral vascular disease, including abdominal aortic aneurysm. Certainly not all patients should undergo cerebral arteriography or CAT scanning, but a careful neurologic history and physical examination should be performed and symptoms should be investigated. Finally, the possibility that antilympocyte immunosuppressive agents may be detrimental in these patients is intriguing and needs further investigation. In the meantime, the modality of immunosuppression at this institution is no different in polycystic patients than in nonpolycystics.

ALPORT'S SYNDROME

Alport's syndrome is a hereditary form of renal disease, generally manifesting within a family as progressive chronic renal failure and deafness (158). The clinically significant forms of renal disease are generally far more prevalent in the male members of the pedigree, resulting in renal failure generally within the second or third decade, and accompanied frequently by clinically significant hearing loss. Additional features include lenticonus and other ocular abnormalities. However, none of the extrarenal manifestations need to be present in order to make a diagnosis of familial nephritis. Pathologically one sees the presence of cells within the interstitium, and on electron microscopy the presence of splitting and thinning of the basement membrane without deposition of immunoglobulins or complement. Biochemical determination of basement membrane content has revealed in a large percentage of patients suffering from Alport's syndrome the absence of a normal constituent of renal basement membrane (159). In 1975 the ASC/NIH Renal Transplant Registry had recorded 73 patients with Alport's syndrome who had undergone renal transplantation with a very satisfactory 2-year graft survival of 53% and 2-year patient survival of 71% (35). Of 24 transplants lost, 80% were attributed to rejection and no mention of either de-novo glomerulonephritis or recurrent disease was made. In 1979, the EDTA recorded 127 patients who had been transplanted, but no survival data or indeed any patient detail was given (160).

Milliner et al. in 1987 reviewed their experience with 11 patients in more detail (161). All of their patients were male, with a mean age of 36.5 years at the time of their first transplant. Fourteen allografts were performed in these 11 patients, seven living related and seven cadaveric. With a mean follow-up of 6 years, 10 of 11 patients had functioning kidneys and nine of them had creatinine less than 2 mg/dl. The one patient on dialysis had lost two allografts very early. Seven had microscopic hematuria and six had proteinuria, although three of these patient had native kidneys in place. Three allografts were removed and studied histologically. Two of three had linear IgG along the glomerular basement membrane by immunofluorescence, one with a positive serum anti-GBM antibody titer and one with a negative titer. The authors hypothesized that in the patients with anti-GBM staining, the normally present GBM antigen in the transplanted kidney was triggering an immune response, resulting in the above finding. However, the clinical significance of this finding was unclear, as was the prevalence with which this would occur. Interestingly, one of the patients with positive anti-GBM staining had 75% crescents on light microscopy, suggesting the development of a true de-novo crescentic glomerulonephritis in this individual.

Carrying these observations further, Querin and coworkers studied the incidence of anti-GBM staining in renal transplant specimens of 767 allograft recipients (162). Twelve of these 767 developed linear IgG deposits along the glomerular basement membrane. Circulating anti-GBM antibody was not found. Anti-tubular basement membrane antibody was found in two individuals. Interestingly, 5 of the 12 patients had Alport's syndrome and the others had a variety of renal diseases. There were several patterns of occurrence of linear fixation. One patient had persistent anti-GBM fixation over time; in eight patients it occurred in only one biopsy, including two patients in whom the linear deposits actually disappeared over time. There was no correlation between the presence of linear deposits and clinical disease, and the authors concluded that generally there was no adverse effect of linear deposits. They agreed with the authors of the previously discussed paper that these deposits were very likely to be related to the presence of an antigenic determinant in the transplanted kidney, which is absent in the native kidneys, triggering an immune response.

On the basis of the foregoing discussion, it is clear that renal transplantation is a reasonable option for patients with end-stage renal disease secondary to Alport's syndrome. One group has reported the recurrence of disease in a transplanted kidney (163). This was the second cadaveric renal transplant for a 27-year-old man. The precise histology of the native and transplanted kidneys, however, was not presented in the paper, and with our current hypotheses concerning the nature of the disease, it would seem very unlikely that this case represented a true recurrence of disease. The likelihood of the development of linear deposition of IgG along the glomerular basement membrane is a consideration that must be recognized. By the data presented thus far it would appear that histologic evidence of anti-GBM disease may be present far more frequently than clinically significant sequelae of it. Therefore, there is no indication either for surveillance biopsy solely to determine the presence or absence of linear anti-GBM staining or for surveillance of the serum level of anti-GBM antibody. On the other hand, in the event of deterioration of graft function, it may be prudent to search for these two factors as an aid to the determination of the cause of transplant dysfunction, and possibly to the treatment of it.

Metabolic disorders involving the kidney

HEREDITARY HYPEROXALURIA

Primary hyperoxaluria is a rare disease resulting from the absence of crucial enzymes in oxalate metabolism. Types I and II have been characterized biochemically, but clinically their manifestations are very similar, and the transmission of both is thought to be autosomal recessive (164). The disease generally presents in early childhood as recurrent nephrolithiasis, progressing to end-stage renal disease secondary to chronic obstruction, nephrocalcinosis, and pyelonephritis resulting from deposition of oxalate in the kidney. Some individuals may respond to pharmacologic doses of pyridoxine, and other therapeutic modalities such as methylene blue have been tried (165). However, the disease generally results in renal failure by the third decade.
It has been recognized for many years that these individuals fare less well on either hemodialysis or peritoneal dialysis than patients suffering from other causes of renal failure; however, renal transplantation, especially in the early years, seemed to offer no benefit. The early reports documented rapid deposition of calcium oxalate in the transplanted kidney, with early failure of the allograft, leading to the initial impression that renal transplantation was contraindicated in these patients (166–169).

The first report of a long-term successful renal transplant was by Morgan in 1974 (170). Since then, multiple case reports have ensued, supporting the impression that renal transplantation may be a viable modality of end-stage renal disease therapy in these individuals (171–178). Toussaint reported a case of an individual who died 7 months posttransplant of miliary tuberculosis with normal renal function (171). Postmortem examination of the transplanted kidney revealed calcium oxalate crystals within the renal tubules as well as a few small stones in the renal pelvis. There was a small amount of interstitial edema, but no gross oxalate deposition in the kidneys, although there were oxalate deposits in the eye and heart. Leumann et al. also reported 3-year graft survival in a patient whose course had been complicated by an acute rejection (172). These authors reviewed previous cases and suggested that early failure of the transplants may have been related to complications that enhanced deposition of oxalate within the kidneys, such as acute tubular necrosis and acute rejection.

With the knowledge that the transplanted kidney did not supply sufficient enzyme to alleviate the underlying biochemical abnormality and that the allograft seemed to serve as a sink for accelerated oxalate deposition, the dilemma in transplantation for these individuals became not so much whether or not to transplant, but how to modify the standard protocols to meet the special needs of these patients. The largest series documenting consistent success in transplanting patients with primary hyperoxaluria was reported by Scheinman et al. in 1984 (173). Eleven patients of various ages received renal transplantations according to a specific protocol, which included aggressive dialysis in the peritransplant period, the use of a well-matched donor kidney, high-dose pyridoxine, neutral phosphate magnesium, and prolonged aggressive diuresis. Ten of the 11 received living related transplants, while one was cadaveric. The time on dialysis prior to transplant varied from a few months to 4 years, with a mean of about 1 year. Of the eight patients who received a transplant within 1 year of the development of end-stage renal disease, seven have good renal function, with a mean follow-up of 30.9 months. Two patients who received transplants after 3 or more years on dialysis developed rapidly recurrent oxalosis in the allografts. The one patient who received a cadaveric transplant developed multiple complications of progressive oxalosis and loss of renal function. Renal biopsies performed on well-functioning kidneys have revealed no oxalate deposits. On the other hand, biopsy specimens quantitated for oxalate did not correlate well with the clinical picture. At the conclusion of the report, these authors suggested that, far from a questionable therapy, early renal transplantation was the treatment of choice for patients with primary hyperoxaluria, provided that the above-mentioned protocol changes were made.

The results of the above study, long-term good renal function in 7 of 11 renal transplant recipients with primary hyperoxaluria, provide strong endorsement for the use of renal transplantation in this situation. Two facts, however, should be noted. Of the now 30 of more patients who have received renal transplants, long-term function has been seen in only 25–30%. Additionally, despite good renal function, these patients are still vulnerable to the late complications of primary hyperoxaluria that are seen on hemodialysis, that is, deposition in the bone and joints with disabling, crippling bone disease (179); deposition in the heart, resulting in cardiac conduction abnormalities; and deposition in the vasculature, resulting in localized ischemia (180, 181). With these facts in mind, one group has attempted combined liver and kidney transplantation in an individual with severe progressive oxalosis (182, 183). Despite the fact that the patient died of infection, measurements of the exchangeable oxalate pool suggested that the transplanted liver was providing sufficient enzyme to correct the underlying biochemical defect. The approach, however, remains entirely experimental at this time.

In summary, renal transplantation is a viable therapeutic option, perhaps even the treatment of choice, for the treatment of end-stage renal disease secondary to primary hyperoxaluria. The nature of the disease necessitates modifications of the standard transplant protocol (173). It is recommended that renal transplantation be performed at the early end-stage period, even predialysis. Because of the accelerated accumulation of oxalate with worsening renal function, intensive daily hemodialysis should be performed for 5–10 days prior to transplantation when a living related transplant is planned and during any period of decreased renal function, such as an acute rejection or acute tubular necrosis, to minimize the deposition of oxalate within the allograft. Dietary oxalate but not calcium should be restricted. Immediate therapy with magnesium, (5–10 mEq/1.73 m^2/day), neutral phosphate (2 g elemental P/1.73 m^2/day), and pyridoxine (500 mg 1.73 m$_2$/day), intravenously initially, then orally, should be institued and maintained indefinitely. A vigorous diuresis should be maintained with noncalciuretic diuretics (such as thiazides). In the case of a cadaveric transplant, the best match with the least ischemic time would be ideal additional maneuvers to minimize the chances of early allograft loss secondary to oxalate deposition. The justification of a living related transplant over a cadaveric one is substantiated by the larger series, which clearly demonstrates an enhanced survival, particularly when the transplant occurs early in renal failure. However, the well-documented occurrence of extrarenal manifestations of oxalosis, even with a well-functioning transplant, is cause for hesitation in risking a living related transplant. This issue is one that will have to be resolved at each individual institution.

HEREDITARY CYSTINOSIS

This disorder is characterized by the accumulation of cystine within lysosomes in several organs of the body, including the kidney (184). Transmitted in an autosomal recessive pattern, the renal manifestations become apparent within the first year of life, specifically polyuria, polydipsia, nausea, vomiting, failure to thrive, and growth retardation. Generally, end-stage renal disease occurs in the first decade. The other two organs that exhibit evidence of significant infiltration include the eye (retina and cornea) and thyroid, resulting in significant visual impairment in a high percentage of patients and clinical as well as biochemical hypothyroidism. There are, as well, some reports of hepatomegaly. Histologically, the kidneys demonstrates thinning and attenuation of the early proximal tubule, known as the swan-neck deformity. Clusters of cystine crystals can be seen within the proximal tubular cells, and in some cases have been seen in glomerular cells as well. The crystals appear to be free or localized within lysosomal structures. The cystine content of the kidney can attain tremendous values, being several times higher than normal.

Renal transplantation has been performed in over 90 patients with this metabolic defect (185–192). The specific questions addressed have been, first, does the implanted organ supply enough of the missing enzyme to rectify the defect in the rest of the body? Second, does the disease recur in the transplanted kidney histologically, clinically, or both? Third, can living related donor kidney be used safely? Overall, when compared with patients transplanted during the same time frame, individuals with cystinosis have fared at least as well if not better than individuals with other forms of primary renal diseases. Broyer et al. reported on 47 children who have been transplanted (185). Patient survival at 1 year was 89%, compared with 81% in patients with other renal disease; while 1-year graft survival was 82% compared with 67% in a control group of transplanted children. Langlois and coworkers reported in somewhat more detail on ten children who had received 13 transplants (186). Six of the ten patients were doing well 6–62 months posttransplant (4 of the 6 had been followed for at least 2 years). None of the patients with well-functioning transplants developed hypothroidism, and photophobia resolved in three of the transplanted individuals. Serial biopsies of the allografts revealed increasing cystine deposits with time. From a quality-of-life standpoint, these children were far better off after transplant than before, when examining factors such as growth and exercise tolerance. The authors suggested that renal transplantation, even before dialysis, may be the optimal mode of therapy. Obviously, however, the metabolic defect was not entirely remedied by the allograft, as cystine accumulation was demonstrable. The fact that cystine accumulation progresses in the nondonor organs and nondonor cells within the allograft, however, is not surprising in view of the underlying pathogensis.

A recent long-term follow-up study on patients with cystinosis was reported by Gahl and coworkers, who obtained data on 80 patients older than age 10 with the disease (187). Over 90% of the patients had received at least one renal transplant, all over the age of 7. Although not stated explicitly, the implication was that indeed 90% had functional transplants at the time of the report. The striking finding of this article was the high incidence of extrarenal complications of cystinosis. Almost 75% required thyroid replacement, 30% had splenomegaly, 42% had hepatomegaly, and 85% had photophobia. More severe ocular complications included impaired visual acuity in 32% and corneal ulcerations in 15%. Interestingly, central nervous system complications were uncommon and were confined to recipients of transplants. These included seizures, speech difficulties, tremor, transient ischemic attacks, and muscular weakness. The authors concluded that continued cystine depletion therapy should follow successful renal transplant to perhaps minimize the degree of posttransplant long-term complications.

In summary, therefore, renal transplantation is not only viable, but may be the preferred form of renal replacement therapy. These individuals tend to maintain a transplant more readily than other children receiving renal transplants (192–194). The allograft does not provide enzyme replacement to prevent extrarenal manifestations of hereditary cystinosis. This is well documented now in the relatively high incidence of hypothyroidism, and ocular complications, as well as the finding of increased cystine content in the allograft, even after successful transplant. Although higher than normal cystine levels have been found in the kidneys, histologically the characteristic swan-neck deformity of the early proximal tubule is not seen in the transplanted kidney (188). Additionally, in living related donor allografts, the increased cystine content may be attributable to a lower than normal level of enzyme activity in thses individuals, who are of necessity heterozygous for the cystinotic state. Despite this potential problem, living related allografts are well tolerated and function well for years, suggesting that the use of these donors is entirely justified.

FABRY'S DISEASE (ANGIOKERATOMA CORPORIS DIFFUSUM)

Fabry's disease, an X-linked recessive disorder of galactosidase deficiency, is a relatively uncommon cause of renal failure (195). The illness is characterized by the accumulation of ceramide trihexoside by all body tissues, resulting in a characteristic clinical picture of burning paresthesias, erythematous skin lesions, and renal failure by the third or fourth decade. Although renal failure is the most common cause of death in this population, hypertension and cardiac disease are seen as well. Only about 20 patients with this disorder have been tranplanted (196–202). Philippart et al. reported one of the earliest cases of renal transplantation in the treatment of this disease in 1972 (196). A 38-year-old man received a cadaveric kidney transplant, following which normal levels of galactosidase were measured in his urine, with subnormal but detectable levels in the plasma. Additionally, he sustained a remission of his pain and anhidrosis, which had characterized his pretransplant clinical condition. Kidney biopsy 14 months posttransplant revealed only evidence of early acute rejection, and a liver biopsy revealed evidence of some reversal of glycolipid storage in that organ. At the time of the case report, 31 months post-transplant, the patient was reportedly clinically doing well, with acceptable renal function of 60 ml/min creatinine clearance, absence of pain, presence of sweating for the first time in his life, and no mention of clinical cardiac disease. These authors suggested that renal transplantation had the potential for reversing the metabolic abnormality in these patients and should be seriously considered as a therapeutic modality.

These encouraging results were confirmed by a report of two patients by Desnick et al. at the University of Minnesota (198). The authors were also able to document low but detectable levels of the absent enzyme in the two transplant recipients and decreased levels of trihexosyl ceramide. Neither patient suffered typical Fabry's-type pain and both patients noted increased sweating posttransplant. Histologic and biochemical evaluation of one of the transplanted kidneys revealed no evidence of recurrent disease.

More recent studies, however, have failed to substantiate earlier claims of successful reversal of the disease process. Van den Bergh et al. reported the case of a 40-year-old man who received a cadaveric renal transplant for renal failyre secondary to documented Fabry's disease (199). In contrast to the above related cases, the authors were unable to document a significant rise in plasma enzyme activity. Further, the patient suffered arrhythmias and died several months posttransplant, presumably as a result of an arrhythmia. Autopsy revealed no evidence of Fabry's disease in the transplanted organ, as had been shown previously; however there was significant deposition in the heart, liver, spleen, and vasculature of trihexosyl ceramide. The authors felt that there was no suggested that the apparent normalization of plasma levels of abnormal lipid previously reported merely reflected changes in the uremic state and subsequent substrate availability. The largest single reported series from Maizel et al. recounted ten transplants in eight patients over a 10-year period of time from 1970 to 1980 (145). Six of the eight patients had died, four from sepsis. Patients survival was 57% at 12 months and 26% at 60 months, significantly inferior to a control group, whose survival was 92% and 78% for the same period of time. The two surviving patients had both had episodes of pain and had suffered cardiovascular complications 5 and 8 years posttransplant. The authors commented specifically on an unusually high incidence of death from sepsis and wound complications. Consequently, their recommendations for renal transplantation were considerably more conservative, advising a period of observation on hemodialysis to exclude the development of long-term complications of Fabry's disease; other authors have documented the development of progressive extrarenal manifestations of Fabry's disease with subsequent death, specifically intestinal and cardiac disease (202).

After consideration of the above limited experience, the following conclusions concerning renal transplantation for end-stage kidney disease secondary to Fabry's disease can be made. There is some evidence of inferior survival in patients transplanted with this disease, relative to other transplanted patients, with an increased incidence of sepsis and othe complications. Renal transplantation, however, is feasible and is not associated with a recurrence in the allograft. It is debatable whether the allograft kidney provides sufficient enzyme to ameliorate the underlying metabolic abnormality. Finally, while some patients may experience a lessening of some of the clinical manifestations of their disease after renal transplantation, there is ample evidence of persistent progressive extrarenal involvement by the disease. With this in mind, the authors suggest that renal transplantation be considered as a therapeutic option in these patients, with the understanding that the incidence of sepsis and wound complications may be higher than in other comparable patients. A trial on dialysis with careful evaluation for the presence of significant cardiac or hepatic involvement would seem prudent as well. At this time there is no information that would bias the choice of immunosuppressive therapy in this disease or would mandate any specific alteration in the management of these individuals.

REFERENCES

1. Fang LST: Light chain nephropathy. *Kidney Int* 27:582–592, 1985.
2. DeFronzo RA, Humphrey RL, Wright JR, Cook CR: Acute renal failure in multiple myeloma. *Medicine* 54:209–223, 1975.
3. Martinez-Maldonado M, Carayalde A: Renal involvement

in multiple myeloma, In: WN Suki, G Eknoyan: *The Kidney in Systemic Disease*, 2nd ed. Wiley Medical, New York: pp 197–209, 1981.
4. Cosio FT, Pence TV, Shapiro FL, Kjellstrand CM: Severe renal failure in multiple myeloma. *Clin Nephrol* 15(4):206–210, 1981.
5. Walker F, Bear RA: Renal transplantation in light chain multiple myeloma. *Am J Nephrol* 3:34–37, 1983.
6. Gerlag PGG, Koene RAP, Berden JHM: Renal transplantation in light chain nephropathy: Case report and review of the literature. *Clin Nephrol* 25(2):101–104, 1986.
7. Spence RK, Hill GS, Goldwein MI, Grossman RA, Barker CF, Perloff LJ: Renal transplantation for end-stage myeloma kidney. *Arch Surg* 114:950–952, 1979.
8. Humphrey RL, Wright JR, Zachary JB, Sterioff S, DeFronzo RA: Renal transplantation in multiple myeloma. *Ann Intern Med* 83:651–653, 1975.
9. De Lima JJG, Kourilsky O, Meyrier A, Morel–Maroger L, Sraer JD: Kidney transplantation in multiple myeloma. *Transplantation* 31(3):223–224, 1981.
10. Medical Staff Conference: The kidney in multiple myeloma. *Western J Med* 129:41–59, 1978.
11. Briefel GR, Spees EK, Humphrey RL, Hill GS, Saral R, Zachary JB: Renal transplantation in a patient with multiple myeloma and light chain nephropathy. *Surgery* 93:579–584, 1983.
12. Penn I: Kidney transplantation following treatment of tumors. *Transplant Proc* 18(4) (Suppl 3):16–20, 1986.
13. Bryan CW, McIntire KR, Princler GL: Effect of sustained diuresis on the renal lesions of mice with Bence–Jones protein-producing tumors. *J Lab Clin Med* 83(3):409–416, 1974.
14. Clyne DH, Pesce AJ, Thompson RE: Nephrotoxicity of Bence Jones proteins in the rat: Importance of protein isoelectric point. *Kidney Int* 16:345–352, 1979.
15. Kyle RA, Byrd ED: Amyloidosis: Review of 236 cases. *Medicine* 54:271–300, 1975.
16. McIntosh RM, Durante D, Gilboa N: Gammopathies: Glomerular and tubular diseases. In: WN Suki, G Eknoyan, *The Kidney in Systemic Disease*, 2nd ed. Wiley Medical, New York: pp 140–145, 1981.
17. Belzer FO, Ashby BS, Gulyassy PF, Powell M: Successful seventeen-hour preservation and transplantation of human-cadaver kidney. *N Engl J Med* 278(11):608–610, 1968.
18. Kennedy CL, Castro JE: Transplantation for renal amyloidosis. *Transplantation* 24(5):382–385, 1977.
19. Dorman SA, Gamelli RL, Benziger JR, Trainer TD, Foster RS: Systemic amyloidosis involving two renal transplants. *Human Patho* 12(8):735–738, 1981.
20. Cohen AS, Bricetti AB, Harrington JT, Mannick JA: Renal transplantation in two cases of amyloidosis. *Lancet* 1:513–516, 1971.
21. Kuhlback B, Falck H, Tornroth T, Wallenius M, Lindstrom BL, Pasternack A: Renal transplantation in amyloidosis. *Acta Med Scand* 205:169–172, 1979.
22. Jones NF: Renal amyloidosis: Pathogenesis and therapy. *Clin Nephrol* 6(5):459–464, 1976.
23. Helin H, Pasternack A, Falck H, Kuhlback B: Recurrence of renal amyloid and de novo membranous glomerulonephritis after transplantation. *Transplantation* 32(1):6–9, 1981.
24. Pasternack A, Ahonen J, Kuhlback B: Renal transplantation in 45 patients with amyloidosis. 42(6):598–601, 1986.
25. Jacob ET, Bar-Nathan N, Shapira Z, Gafni J, Renal transplantation in the amyloidosis of familial Mediterranean fever. *Arch Intern Med* 139:1135–1138, 1979.
26. Jacob ET, Siegal B, Bar-Nathan N, Gafni J: Improving outlook for renal transplantation in amyloid nephropathy. *Transplant Proc* 14(1):41–45, 1982.
27. Wilson RE: Transplantation in patients with unusual causes of renal failure. *Clin Nephrol* 5(2):51–53, 1976.
28. Benson MD, Skinner M, cohen AS: Amyloid deposition in a renal transplantation familial Mediterranean fever. *Ann Intern Med* 87:31–34, 1977.
29. Siegal B, Zemer D, Pras M: Cyclosporine and familial Mediterranean fever amyloidosis. *Transplantation* 41(6):793–794, 1986.
30. Skirahama T, Cohen AS: Blockage of amyloid induction by colchicine in an animal model. *J Exp Med* 140:1102, 1974.
31. Coplon NS, Diskin CJ, Petersen J, Swensen RS: The long term clinical course of systemic lupus erythematosus in end stage renal disease. *N Engl J Med* 308:186–190, 1983.
32. Cheigh JS, Stenzel KH, Rubin AL, Chami J, Sullivan JF: Systemic lupus erythematosus in patients with chronic renal failure. *Am J Med* 75:602–606, 1983.
33. Kimberly RP, Lockshin MD, Sherman RL, Beary JF, Mouradian J, Cheigh JS: "End stage" lupus nephritis: Clinical course to and outcome on dialysis. *Medicine* 60(4):277–287, 1981.
34. Roenigk HH, Haserich JR, Nakamoto S, McCormack LJ: Systemic lupus erythematosus and renal transplantation. *Arch Dermatol* 92:263–270, 1965.
35. Advisory Committee to the Renal Transplant Registry: Renal transplantation in cogenital and metabolic disease – A report from the ASC/NIH Renal Transplant Registry. *JAMA* 232:148–153, 1975.
36. Amend W, Vincenti F, Covey C, Epstein W, Feduska N, Salvatierra O: Renal transplantation in systemic lupus erythematosus. *Proc Dialysis Transpl Forum* 7:18–21, 1977.
37. Mejia G, Zimmerman SW, Glass NR, Miller DT, Sollinger HW, Belzer FO: Renal transplantation in patients with systemic lupus erythematosus. *Arch Intern Med* 143:2092–2098, 1983.
38. Buda JA, Lattes CG, Grant JP, Meltzer JI, Hsu KC, Tannenbaum M: Feasibility of renal transplantation in systemic lupus erythematosus. *Surg Forum* 21:252–254, 1970.
30. Yakub YN, Freeman RB, Pabico R: Renal transplantation in systemic lupus erythematosus. *Nephron* 27:197–201, 1981.
40. Amend WJC, Vincenti F, Feduska NJ, Salvatierra O, Johnston WH, Jackson J, Tilney N, Garovoy M, Burwell EL: Recurrent systemic lupus erythematosus involving renal allografts. *Ann Intern Med* 94:444–448, 1981.
41. Stevens J, Callendar CO, Jilly PN: Emergence of red blood cell agglutinins following renal transplantation in a patient with systemic lupus erythematosus. *Transplantation* 32(5):398–400, 1981.
42. Cats S, Terasaki PI, Perdue S, Mickey MR: Increased vulnerability of the poor donor organ in related kidney transplants for certain diseases. *Transplantation* 87(6):575–579, 1984.
43. Kimberly RP, Lockshin MD, Sherman RL, Mouradian J, Saal S: Reversible end stage lupus nephritis. *Am J Med* 74:361–368, 1983.
44. Nolph KD, Husted FC, Sharp GC, Siemsen AW: Antibodies to nuclear antigens in patients undergoing long-term hemodialysis. *Am J Med* 60:673–676, 1976.
45. Rodby RA, Korbet SM, Lewis EJ: Persistence of clinical and serologic activity in patients with systemic lupus erythematosus undergoing peritoneal dialysis. *Am J Med* 83:613–

618, 1987.
46. Steinman C, Achad A: Appearance of circulating DNA during hemodialysis. *Am J Med* 62:693–697, 1977.
47. Gladman DD, Urowitz MB, Keystone EC: Serologically active clinically quiescent systemic lupus erythematosus. *Am J Med* 66:210–215, 1979.
48. Traub YM, Shapiro AP, Rodnan GP, Medsger TA, McDonald RH, Steen VD, Osial TA, Tolchin SF: Hypertension and renal failure (scleroderma renal crisis) in progressive systemic sclerosis. *Medicine* 62(6):335–352, 1983.
49. Richardson JA: Hemodialysis and kidney transplantation for renal failure from scleroderma. *Arthritis Rheum* 16(2):265–271, 1973.
50. Cannon PJ, Hassar M, Case DB: Relationship of hypertension and renal failure in scleroderma to structural and functional abnormalities of the renal cortical circulation. *Medicine* 53:1–45, 1974.
51. Keane WF, Danielson B, Raij L: Successful renal transplantation in progressive systemic sclerosis. *Ann Intern Med* 85:199–202, 1976.
52. LeRoy EC, Fleishmann RM: The management of renal scleroderma. *Am J Med* 84:974–978, 1978.
53. Oliver JA, Cannon PJ: The Kidney in scleroderma. *Nephron* 18:141–150, 1977.
54. McKinney TD, McAllister CJ, Stone WJ, Johnson HK, Ginn HE: Hemodialysis and renal transplantation in progressive systemic sclerosis: Report of two cases. *Clin Nephrol* 12(4):178–185, 1979.
55. Woodhall PB, McCoy RC, Gunnell's JC, Seigler HF: Apparent recurrence of progressive systemic sclerosis in a renal allograft. *JAMA* 236(9):1032–1034, 1976.
56. Merino GE, Sutherland DER, Kjellstrand CM, Simmons RL, Najarian JJ: Renal transplantation for progressive systemic sclerosis with renal failure. *Am J Surg* 133:745–749, 1977.
57. Godman GC, Churg J: Wegener's granulomatosis: Pathology and review of the literature. *Arch Pathol* 58:533, 1954.
58. Lyons GW, Lindsay WG: Renal transplantation in a patient with Wegener's granulomatosis. *Am J Surg* 124:104–107, 1972.
59. Kjellstrand CM, Simmons RL, Uranga VM, Buselmeier TJ, Najarian JS: Acute fulminant Wegener granulomatosis. *Arch Intern Med* 134:40–43, 1974.
60. Fauci AS, Balow JE, Brown R, Chazan J, Steinman T, Sakyoun AI, Monaco AP, Wolff SM: Successful renal transplantation in Wegener's granulomatosis. *Am J Med* 60:437–440, 1976.
61. von Ypersele de Strihou C, Pirson Y, Vandenbroucke JM, Alexander OPJ: Hemodialysis and transplantation in Wegener's granulomatosis. *Br Med J* 2:93–94, 1979.
62. Chandran PKG, First MR, Weiss MA, Hess EV, Alexander JW, Pazmino P, Pollak VE: Wegener's granulomatosis: Prolonged patients survival after penumonectomy and renal transplantation. *Am J Nephrol* 2:325–329, 1982.
63. Steinman TI, Jaffe BF, Monaco AP, Wolff SM, Fauci AS: Recurrence of Wegener's granulomatosis after kidney transplantation. Successful reinduction of remission with cyclophosphamide. *Am J Med* 68:458–460, 1980.
64. Curtis JJ, Diethelm AG, Herrera GA, Crowell WT, Whelchel JD: Recurrence of Wegener's granulomatosis in a cadaver renal allograft. *Transplantation* 36(4):452–454, 1983.
65. Kuross S, Davis T, Kjellstrand CM: Wegener's granulomatosis with severe renal failure: Clinical course and results of dialysis and transplantation. *Clin Nephrol* 16(4):172–180, 1981.
66. Baliah T, Kim KH, Anthone S, Anthone R, Montes M, Andres CA: Recurrence of Henoch Schonlein purpura glomerulonephritis in transplanted kidneys. *Transplantation* 18(4):343–346, 1974.
67. Hamburger J, Crosnier J, Noel LH: Recurrent glomerulonephritis after renal transplantation. *Ann Rev Med* 29:67, 1978.
68. Weiss JH, Bhathma DB, Curtis JJ, Lucas BA, Luke RG: A possible relationship between Henoch–Schonlein syndrome and IgA nephropathy (Berger's disease) *Nephron* 22:582, 1978.
69. Sabai T, Tanaka T, Kasai N, Shinagawa I, Endo T: Recurrence of Henoch Schonlein purpura glomerulonephritis in transplant kidneys. *Sixth International Congress of Nephrology*, Florence, 1975, Abstract 1023.
70. Levy M, Moussa RA, Habib R, Gagnadoux MF, Broyer M: Anaphylactoid purpura nephritis and transplantation. *Kidney Int* 22:326, 1982.
71. Cameron JS: Glomerulonephritis in renal transplants. *Transplantation* 34:237–245, 1982.
72. Bachman U, Biava C, Amend W, Feduska N, Melzer J, Salvatierra O, Vincenti F: The clinical course of IgA nephropathy and Henoch Schonlein purpura following renal transplantation. *Transplantation* 42(5):511–515, 1986.
73. Montalbert C, Carvallo A, Broumand B, Noble D, Anstine LA, Currier CB: Successful renal transplantation in polyarteritis nodosa. *Clin Nephrol* 14(4):206–209, 1980.
74. Wilson CB, Dixon FJ: AntiGBM antibody induced glomerulonephritis. *Kidney Int* 3:74–89, 1973.
75. Cameron JS, Turner DR: Recurrent glomerulonephritis in allografted kidneys. *Clin Nephrol* 7:47–54, 1977.
76. Cove–Smith JR, McLeod AA, Blamey RW, Knapp MS, Reeves WG, Wilson CB: Transplantation, immunosuppression and plasmapheresis in Goodpasture's syndrome. *Clin Nephrol* 9(3):126–128, 1978.
77. Beleil OM, Coburn JW, Shinaberger JH, Glassrock RJ: Recurrent glomerulonephritis due to anti-glomerular basement membrane antibodies in two successive allografts. *Clin Nephrol* 1(6):377–380, 1973.
78. Hind CRK, Bowman C, Winearls CG, Lockwood CM: Recurrence of circulating anti-glomerular basement membrane antibody three years after immunosuppressive treatment and plasma exchange. *Clin Nephrol* 21(4):244–246, 1984.
79. Almkuist RD, Buckalew VM Jr, Hirszel P, Maher JF, James PM, Wilson CB: Recurrence of antiglomerular basement membrane antibody mediated glomerulonephritis in isograft. *Clin Immunol Immunopathol* 18:54, 1981.
80. Couser WG, Wallace A, Monaco AP, Lewis AP: Successful renal transplantation in patients with circulating antibody to glomerular basement membrane: Report of two cases. *Clin Nephrol* 1(6):381–387, 1973.
81. Byrnes JJ, Moake JL: Thrombotic thrombocytopenic purpura and the haemolytic uraemic syndrome: Evolving concepts of pathogenesis and therapy. *Clinics Haematol* 15(2):413–442, 1986.
82. Cerilli GJ, Nelson C, Dorfmann L: Renal homotransplantation in infants and children with the hemolytic uremic syndrome. *Surgery* 71(1):66–71, 1972.
83. Arias-Rodriguez M, Sraer JD, Kourilsky O, Smith MD, Verroust PJ, Meyrier A, Kuntziger HE, Kanfer A, Nessim V, Neuilly G, Morel-Maroger L, Richet G: Renal transplantation and immunological abnormalities in thrombotic microangiopathy of adults. *Transplantation* 23(4):360–365,

1977.

84. Folman R, Arbus GS, Churchill B, Gaum L, Huber J: Recurrence of the hemolytic uremic syndrome in a 3½ year old child, 4 months after second renal transplantation. *Clin Nephrol* 10(3):121–127, 1977.
85. Morel Maroger L, Kanfer A, Solez K, Sraer JD, Richet G: Prognostic importance of vascular lesions in acute renal failure with microangiopathic hemolytic anemia (hemolytic-uremic syndrome): Clinicopathologic study in 20 adults. *Kidney Int* 15:548–558, 1979.
86. Hebert D, Sibley RK, Mauer SM: Recurrence of hemolytic uremic syndrome in renal transplant recipients. *Kidney Int* 30:S51–S58, 1986.
87. Case Records of the Massachusetts General Hospital Case 15-1986: *N Engl J Med* 314(16):1032–1040, 1986.
88. Van Den Berg-Wolf M, Kootte AMM, Weening JJ, Paul LC: Recurrent hemolytic uremic syndrome in a renal transplant recipient and review of the Leiden experience. *Transplantation* 45(1):248–251, 1988.
89. Shulman H, Striker G, Deeg HJ, Kennedy M, Stork R, Thomas ED: Nephrotoxicity of cyclosporin A after allogeneic marrow transplantation: Glomerular thrombosis and tubular injury. *N Engl J Med* 305:1392–1394, 1981.
90. Bonser RS, Adur D, Fanklin I, McMaster P: Cyclosporin induced haemolytic-uraemic syndrome in liver allograft recipient. *Lancet* 2:1337, 1984.
91. Bergstein J, Michael A, Kellstrand C, Simmons R, Najarian J: Hemolytic-uremic syndrome in adult sisters. *Transplantation* 17(5):487–490, 1974.
92. Sun NCJ, Johnson WJ, Sung DTW, Woods JE: Idiopathic postpartum renal failure: Review and case report of a successful renal transplantation. *Mayo Clin Proc* 50:395–401, 1975.
93. Bonsib SM, Ercolani L, Ngheim D, Hamilton HE: Recurrent thrombotic microangiopathy in a renal allograft. Case report and review of the literature. *Am J Med* 79:520–527, 1985.
94. Leithner C, Sinzinger H, Pohanha E, Schwartz M, Kretschamer G, Syre G: Recurrence of hemolytic uremic syndrome triggered by cyclosporin A after renal transplantation. *Lancet* 2:1470, 1982.
95. Stevenson JA, Dumke A, Glassock RJ, Raifer J, Cohen AH: Thrombotic microangiopathy: Recurrence following renal transplant and response to plasma infusion. *Am J Nephrol* 2:227–231, 1982.
96. Robson JS, Martin AM, Puckley VA, MacDonald MK: Irreversible postpartum renal failure: A new syndrome. *Q J Med* 37:423–435, 1968.
97. Lederer ED, Truong L, Suki WN: Postpartum renal failure in a renal transplant recipient. *Transplantation* 47:717–719, 1989.
98. Skyh T-P, Beyer MM, Friedman EA: Treatment of the uremic diabetic. *Nephron* 40:129–138, 1985.
99. Tisher CC, McCoy RC: Diabetes mellitus and the kidney. In: WN Suki, G Eknoyan, eds, *The Kidney in Systemic Disease*, 2nd ed. Wiley Medical, New York: pp 479–507, 1981.
100. Maryniak RK, Mendoza, N, Clyne D, Balakrishnan K, Weiss MA: Recurrence of diabetic nodular glomerulosclerosis in a renal transplant. *Transplantation* 39(1):35–38, 1985.
101. Mauer SN, Barbosa J, Vernier RC: Development of diabetic vascular lesions in normal kidney transplanted into patients with diabetes mellitus. *N Engl J Med* 295:916, 1976.
102. Personal observation.
103. Abouna GM, Kremer GD, Daddah SK, Al-Adnani MS, Kumar SA, Kusma G: Reversal of diabetic nephropathy in human cadaveric kidneys after transplantation into nondiabetic recipients. *Lancet* 2:1274–1276, 1983.
104. Advisory Committee to the Renal Transplant Registry: The 13th report of the Human Renal Transplant Registry *Transplant Proc* 9:9–26, 1977.
105. Hoitsma A, Wetzels JFM, Berden JHM, Koene RAP: Kidney transplantation in patients with diabetic nephropathy. *Kidney Int* 28:700, 1985.
106. Kjellstrand CM, Goetz FC, Shideman JR, Simmons RL, Buselmeier TJ, Von Hartitzsch B, Najarian JS: Renal transplantation in patients with insulin dependent diabetes. *Lancet* 2:4–8, 1973.
107. Totten MA, Izenstein B, Glaeson RE, Kassissieh SD, Libertino JA, D'Elia JA: Chronic renal failure in diabetes survival with hemodialysis versus transplantation. *Kidney Int* 12:492, 1977.
108. Jones RH, Rudge CJ, Watkins PJ, Bewick M, Parsons V: Renal transplantation in insulin requiring diabetics. *Lancet* 1:153, 1979.
109. Konrad P, Husberg BS, Takolander R, Bergentz SE: Renal transplantation in patients with end-stage diabetic nephropathy. *Transplant Proc* 14(1):28–29, 1987.
110. Zincke H, Woods JE, Sterioff S, Johnson WJ, Palumbo PJ, Mitchell JC, Frohnert PP, Anderson CF, Service FJ, Leary FJ: Renal transplantation in patients with diabetes mellitus–Revisited. *Transplant Proc* 11(1):55–59, 1979.
111. Jervell J, Dahl BO, Jakobsen A, Lund PK, Thayssen P, Fjeldborg O, Hansen HE, Koch B, Lindstrom B, Larson O, Brynger H, Groth CG, Lundgren G, Husberg B, Wieslander J, Frodin L, Wickstrom B: Renal transplantation in insulin treated diabetics. *Transplant Proc* 11(1):60–62, 1979.
112. Larsson O, Attman PO, Blohme I, Brynger H: Transplantation in patients with diabetic nephropathy: A 10-year experience. *Transplant Proc* 14(1):30–32, 1981.
113. Sutherland DER, Morrow CE, Fryd DS, Ferguson R, Simmons RL, Najarian HS: Improved patient and primary renal allograft survival in uremic diabetic recipients. *Transplantation* 34(6):319–325, 1982.
114. Okiye SE, Engen DE, Sterioff SS, Frohnert PP, Johnson WJ, Offord KP, Zincke H: Primary and secondary renal transplantation in diabetic patients. *JAMA* 249(4):492–495, 1983.
115. Jervell J: Joint Scandinavian report: Renal transplantation in insulin dependent diabetics. *Lancet* 2:915–917, 1978.
116. Najarian JS, Sutherland DER, Simmons RL, Howard R, Kjellstrand C, Ramsay R, Goetz F, Fryd D, Sommer B: Ten year experience with renal transplantation in juvenile onset diabetics. *Ann Surg* 109:487–500, 1979.
117. Rosenthal JT: Transplantation in diabetics with end stage renal disease transplantation and immunology. *Letter* 1(3):1, 6–7, 1985.
118. Sutherland DER, Fryd DS, Morrow CE, et al.: Kidney transplantation in diabetics at the University of Minnesota: An analysis of results by era. *Transplantation Proc* 15:1110, 1983.
119. Sutherland DER, Fryd DS, Payne WD, Ascher N, Simmons RL, Najarian JS: Kidney transplantation in diabetics patients. *Transplant Proc* 19(Suppl 2):90–94, 1987.
120. Goldstein DA, Massry SG: Diabetic nephropathy. Clinical course and effect of hemodialysis. *Nephron* 20:286–296, 1978.
121. McCrary RF, Pitts TO, Puschett JB: Diabetics nephropathy:

Natural course, survivorship and therapy. *Am J Nephrol* 1:206–218, 1981.
122. Khauli RB, Steinmuller DR, Novick AC, Buszta C, Goormastic M, Nakamoto S, Vidt DG, Magnusson M, Paganini E, Schreiber MJ: A critical look at survival of diabetics with end stage renal disease. *Transplantation* 41(5):598–602, 1986.
123. Parfrey PS, Hutchinson TA, Harvey C, Guttmann RD: Transplantation versus dialysis in diabetic patients with renal failure. *Am J Kidney Dis* 5(2):112–116, 1985.
124. Nielsen VK: The peripheral nerve function in chronic renal failure VII. Recovery after renal transplantation. Clinical aspects. *Acta Med Scand* 195:163, 1976.
125. Friedman EA, Cohen C, Lowder G, Laungani GB, Butt KMH: Cytopathy does not preclude successful kidney transplantation in diabetics. *Kidney Int* 29:429, 1986.
126. Gonzalez–Carillo M, Bewick M, Rudge C, Parsons V, Watkins P, Maloney A: Vascular complications in diabetic patients with renal transplantation. *Transplant Proc* 14(1);33, 1982.
127. Peters C, Sutherland DER, Simmons RL, Fryd DS, Najarian JS: Patient and graft survival in amputated versus nonamputated diabetic primary renal allograft recipients. *Transplantation* 32(6);498–503, 1981.
128. Rimmer JM, Sussman M, Foster R, Gennari FJ: Renal transplantation in diabetes mellitus. Influence of preexisting vascular disease on outcome. *Nephron* 42:304–310, 1986.
129. Mitchell JC: End stage renal failure in juvenile diabetes mellitus: A 5-year follow-up of treatment. *Mayo Clin Proc* 52:281–288, 1977.
130. Rao KV: The influence of pre-existing vascular disease on the outcome of renal transplantation in diabetic patients. *Nephron* 48:74–75, 1988.
131. Weinrauch LA, D'Elia JA, Healy RW, et al.: Asymptomatic coronary artery disease: Angiography in diabetic patients before renal transplantation. *Ann Intern Med* 88:346–348, 1978.
132. Braun WE, Phillips DF, Vidt DG, Novick AC, Nakamoto S, Popowniak Kl, Paganini E, Magnusson M, Pohl M, Steinmuller DR, Protiva D, Buszta C: Coronary artery disease in 100 diabetics with end stage renal failure. *Transplant Proc* 16(3):603–607, 1984.
133. Feduska NJ, Vincenti F, Amend W, Iwaki I, Opel ZG, Terasaki P, Duca R, Hopper S, Salvatierra O: An alternative to cadaver kidney transplants for patients with insulin dependent diabetes mellitus. *Transplantation* 32(6):517–521, 1981.
134. Berloco P, Alfani D, Famulari A, Monari C, Trovati A, Poli L, Pritagostini R, Renna, Molajoni E, Cinti P, Marciani A, Cortesini R: Utilization of living donor organs for clinical transplantation. *Transplant Proc* 17(Suppl 2):13–17, 1983.
135. Sabbaga E, Ianhez LE, Chocair PR, Azevedo LS, Saturi PS, de Gors GM: Kidney transplants from living nonrelated donors. An analysis of 87 cases including 20 cases with specific blood transfusions from the donor. *Transplant Proc* 17:1741–1745, 1985.
136. Reding R, Squifflet JP, Pirson Y, Jamart J, Latinni D, Alexandre GPF: Unrelated living donor kidney transplantation: Experience with 16 cases. *Transplant Proc* 18:1087–1089, 1986.
137. Bowen PA, House MA, Bairas D, Kuremsarri K, Dennis AJ, Witherington R, Humphries AL: Successful renal transplantation using distantly related or unrelated living donors with donor-specific blood transfusion. *Transplantation* 39:450–453, 1985.
138. Morrow CE, Schwartz JS, Sutherland DER, Simmons RL, Ferguson RM, Kjellstrand CM, Najarian JS: Predictive value of thallium stress testing for coronary and cardiovascular events in uremic diabetic patients before renal transplantation. *Am J Surg* 146:331–335, 1983.
139. Philipson JD, Carpenter BJ, Itzkoff J, Hakala TR, Rosenthal JT, Taylor RJ, Puschett JB: Evaluation of cardiovascular risk for renal transplantation in diabetic patients. *Am J Med* 81:630–634, 1986.
140. Beutler E: The sickle cell diseases and related disorders. In: WJ Williams, E Beutler, AJ Erslew, MA Lichtman, eds, *Hematology*, 4th ed. McGraw-Hill, New York: pp 613–644, 1990.
141. Vaamonde CA, Oster JR, Strauss J: The kidney in sickle cell disease. In: WN Suki, G Eknoyan, eds, *The Kidney in Systemic Disease*, 2nd ed. Wiley Medical, New York: pp 159–196, 1981.
142. Thomas AN, Pattison C, Sergeant GR: Causes of death in sickle cell disease in Jamaica. *Br Med J* 285:633–635, 1982.
143. Chatterjee SN: National study in natural history of renal allografts in sickle cell disease or trait: A second report. *Transplant Proc* 19(2) (Suppl 2):33–35, 1987.
144. Chatterjee SN, Lundberg GD, Berne TV: Sickle cell trait: Possible contributory cause of renal allograft failure. *Urology* 11(3):266–269, 1978.
145. Spector D, Zachary JB, Sterioff S, Millan J: Painful crisis following renal transplantation in sickle cell anemia. *Am J Med* 64:835–839, 1978.
146. Miner DJ, Jorkasky DK, Perloff LJ, Grossman RA, Tomaszewski JE: Recurrent sickle cell nephropathy in a transplanted kidney. *Am J Kidney Dis* 10(4):306–313, 1987.
147. Gonzalez–Carillo M, Rudge CJ, Params V, Bewick M, White JM: Renal transplantation in sickle cell disease. *Clin Nephrol* 18(4):209–210, 1982.
148. Suki WN; Polycystic kidney disease. *Kidney Int* 22:571–580, 1982.
149. Mendez R, Mendez RG, Payne JE, Berne TV: Renal transplantation in adult patients with end stage polycystic kidney disease. *Urology* 5(1):26–28, 1975.
150. Salvatierra O, Wolfson M, Cochrum K, Ammend W, Belzer FO: End stage polycystic kidney disease: Management by renal transplantation and selective use of preliminary nephrectomy. *J Urol* 115:5–7, 1976.
151. DeBono DP, Evans DB: The management of polycystic kidney diesase with special reference to dialysis and transplantation. *Q J Med* (New Series) 66:353–363, 1977.
152. SanFilippo FP, Vaughn WK, Peters TF, Bollinger RR, Spees EK: Transplantation for polycystic kidney disease. *Transplantation* 36(1):54–59, 1983.
153. Valeri A, Hardy M, Stern L, Cohen D, Appel G: Outcome of transplantation in patients with polycystic kidney disease. *Kidney Int* 29:437, 1986.
154. Williams G, Mitcheson HD, Castro JE: Transplantation for polycystic kidney disease. *Urology* 12(6):628–630, 1978.
155. Wallenius M, Kuhlback B, Brotherus JW: Renal transplantation in polycystic kidney disease. *Scand J Urol Nephrol* 12:75–77, 1978.
156. Pechan W, Novick AC, Braun WE, Nakamoto S, Popowniak K, Steinmuller D: Management of end stage polycsytic kidney disease with renal transplantation. *J Urol* 125:622–624, 1981.
157. Lytton B: Surgery of the kidney. In: PC Walsh, RF Gitter, AD Perlmutter, TA Steney, eds, *Campbell's Urology*, 5th ed. Saunders, Philadelphia: pp 2430–2444, 1986.

158. Glassock RJ, Cohen AH, Adler SG, Word HJ: Secondary glomerular diseases. In: Brenner, Rector, eds, *The Kidney*, 3rd ed. pp 1056–1059, 1986.
159. McCoy RC, Johnson HK, Stone WJ, Wilson CB: Absence of nephritogenic GBM antigen(s) in some patients with hereditary nephritis. *Kidney Int* 21:642–652. 1982.
160. Brenner FP, Brynger H, Chantler C, Doncherwolche RA, Hathway RA, Jacobs C, Selwood NH, Wing AJ: Combined report on regular dialysis and transplantation in Europe. *Proc Eur Dial Transpl Assoc* 16:4–69, 1979.
161. Milliner DS, Pierdes AM, Holley KE: Renal transplantation in Alport's syndrome. Anti-glomerular basement membrane glomerulonephritis in the allograft. *Mayo Clin Proc* 57:35–43, 1982.
162. Querin S, Noel L-H, Grunfeld J-P, Droz D, Makieu P, Berger J, Kreis H: Linear glomerular IgG fixation in renal allografts: Incidence and significance in Alport's syndrome. *Clin Nephrol* 25(3):134–140, 1986.
163. Mathew TH, Mathews DC, Hobbs JB, Kincaid-Smith P: Glomerular lesion after renal transplantation. *Am J Med* 59:1177–190, 1975.
164. Williams HE, Smith LH: Primary hyperoxaluria. In: Stanbury JP, Wyngaardin JB, Frederickson DS, eds, *The Metabolic Basis of Inherited Disease*. McGraw Hill, New York, 1972.
165. Yendt ER, Cohanim M: Response to a physiologic dose of pyridoxine in type I primary hyperoxaluria. *N Engl J Med* 312(15):953–957, 1985.
166. Deodhar SD, Tung KSK, Zuhlke V, Nakamoto S: Renal homotransplantation in a patient with primary familial oxalosis. *Arch Pathol* 87:118–124, 1969.
167. Klauwers J, Wolf PL, Cohn R: Failure of renal transplantation in primary oxalosis. *JAMA* 209:551, 1969.
168. Saxon A, Busch GJ, Merrill JP: Franco V, Wilson RE: Renal transplantation in primary hyperoxaluria. *Arch Intern Med* 133:464–467, 1974.
169. Koch B, Irvine AH, Barr JR, Poxnanski WJ: Thru kidney transplantation in a patient with primary hereditary hyperoxaluria. *Can Med Assoc J* 106:1323–1331, 1972.
170. Morgan JM, Hartley MW, Miller AC, Diethelm AG: Successful renal transplantation in the hyperoxaluria. *Arch Surg* 109:430–433, 1974.
171. Toussaint C, Goffin Y, Potuliege P, Dupuis F, Dupont E, Toussaint D, Kinnaert P, van Gurtruyden J, Vereerstraeten P: Kidney transplantation in primary oxalosis. *Clin Nephrol* 5(5):239–244, 1976.
172. Leuman EP, Wegman W, Largiarder F: Prolonged survival after renal transplantation in primary hyperoxaluria of childhood. *Clin Nephrol* 9(1):29–34, 1978.
173. Scheinman JI, Najarian JS, Mauer SM: Successful strategies for renal transplantation in primary oxalosis. *Kidney Int* 25:804–811, 1984.
174. Halverstadt DB, Wenzl JE: Primary hyperoxaluria and renal transplantation. *J Urol* 111:398–402, 1974.
175. O'Regan P, Constable AR, Koekes AM, Kasidas GP, Rose GA: Successful renal transplantation in primary hyperoxaluria. *Postgrad Med J* 56:288–293, 1980.
176. Bohannon LL, Norman DJ, Barry J, Bennett WM: Cadaveric renal transplantation in a patient with primary hyperoxaluria. *Transplantation* 36(1):114–115, 1983.
177. David DS, Cheigh JS, Stenzel KH, Rubin AL: Successful renal transplantation in a patient with primary hyperoxaluria. *Transplant Proc* 15(4):2168–2171, 1983.
178. Whelchel JD, Alison DV, Luke RG, Curtis J, Diethelm AG: Successful renal transplantation in hyperoxaluria. *Transplantation* 35(2):161–164, 1983.
179. Adams ND, Carrera GF, Johnson RP, Latorracci R, Lemann J: Calcium-oxalate-crystal-induced bone disease. *Am J Kidney Dis* 1(5):294–299, 1982.
180. Blackburn WE, McRoberts JW, Bhathena D, Vazquez M, Luke RG, Severe vascular complications in oxalosis after bilateral nephrectomy. *Ann Intern Med* 82:44–46, 1975.
181. Veerenterghem Y, Vandamme B, Lerut T, Michielson P: Severe vascular complications in oxalosis after successful cadaveric kidney transplantation. *Transplantation* 38:93–95, 1984.
182. Watts RWE, Calne RY, Williams R, Mansell MA, Veall N, Purkiss P, Rolles K: Primary hyperoxaluria (type I): Attempted treatment by combined hepatic and renal transplantation. *Q J Med* 57:697–702, 1985.
183. Watts RWA, Rolles K, Morgan SH, William R, Calne RY, Danpure CJ, Mansell MA, Purkiss P: Successful treatment of primary hyperoxaluria type I by combined hepatic and renal transplantation. *Lancet* 2:474–485, 1987.
184. Schneider JA, Schulman JD: Cystinosis. In: JB Stanbury, JB Wyngaarden, DS Fredrickson, JL Goldstein, MS Brown, eds, *The Metabolic Basis of Inherited Disease*. McGraw-Hill. New York, pp 1844–1866, 1983.
185. Broyer M, Donderwolcke RA, Brunner FP, Brynger H, Jacobs C, Kramer P, Selwood NH, Wing AJ, Blake PH: Combined report on regular dialysis and transplantation of children in Europe, 1980. *Proc Eur Dial Transpl Assoc* 18:60–87, 1981.
186. Langlois RP, O'Regan S, Pelleteier M, Robitaille P: Kidney transplantation in uremic children with cystinosis. *Nephron* 28:273–275, 1981.
187. Gahl WA, Schneider JA, Thoene JG, Chesney R: Course of nephropathic cystinosis after age 10 years. *J Pediatr* 109:605–608, 1986.
188. Lawson RK, Talwalkar YB, Hodges CV: Renal transplantation in cystinosis. *J Urol* 113:552–555, 1975.
189. Malekzadeh MH, Pennisi AJ, Phillips L, Ettenger RD, Uittenbogaart CH, Fine RN: Growth and endocrine function in children with cystonosis following renal transplantation. *Trans Am Soc Artif Intern Org* 24:278–281, 1978.
190. West JC, Goodman SI, Seproter GP, Bloustein PA, Hambridge KM, Weil R: Pediatric kidney transplantation for cystonosis. *J Pediatr Surg* 12(5):651–655, 1977.
191. Malekzadeh MH, Neustein HB, Schneider JA, Pennisi AJ, Ettenger RB, Uittenbogaart CH, Kogut MD, Fine RN: Cadaver renal transplantation in children with cystinosis. *Am J Med* 63:525–533, 1977.
192. Mahoney CP, Striker GE, Hickman RO, Manning GB, Marchioro TL: Renal transplantation for childhood cystinosis. *N Engl Med* 283(8):397–402, 1970.
193. Mahoney CP, Striker GE, Fetherman GH, Hickman RO, Schneider JA, Marchioro TL: Renal transplantation in childhood cystinosis. Effects of the metabolic disease and renal allografts on each other. *Birth defects. Original article series* 9(2):140–141, 1973.
194. Broyer M, Gagnadoux UF, Bearton D, Parcal B, Lowifle J: Transplantation in children: Technical aspects, drug therapy and problems related to primary renal disease. *Proc Eur Dial Transpl Assoc* 18:313–321, 1981.
195. Desnick RJ, Sweeley CC: Fabry's disease: Galactosidase deficiency. In: JB Stanbury, JB Wyngaarden, DS Fredickson, JL Goldstein, MS Brown, eds. *The Metabolic Basis of Inherited Disease*, 5th ed. McGraw Hill, New York, pp 906–944, 1983.
196. Philippart M, Franklin SS, Gordon A: Reversal of an inborn

sphingolipidosis (Fabry's disease) by kidney transplantation. *Ann Intern Med* 77:195–200, 1972.
197. Philippart M: Fabry disease: Kidney Transplantation on an enzyme replacement therapy, *Birth Defects* 9(2):81–87, 1973.
198. Desnick RJ, Allen KY, Simmons RL, Woods JE, Anderson CF, Najarian JS, Krivit W: Fabry disease: Correction of the enzymatic deficiency by renal transplantation. *Birth Defects*. 9(2):88–96, 1973.
199. Venden Bergh FAJTM, Rietra PJGM, Kolh-Vegter AJ, Bosch E, Tager JM: Therapeutic implications of renal transplantation in a patient with Fabry's disease. *Acta Med Scand* 200:249–256, 1976.
200. Maizel SE, Simmons RL, Kjellstrand C, Fryd DS: Ten year experience in renal transplantation for Fabry's disease. *Transplant Proc* 13(1):57–59, 1981.
201. Donati D, Novari OR, Gastaedi L: Natural history and treatment of uremia secondary to Fabry's disease: An European experience. *Nephron* 46:353–359, 1987.
202. Kramer W, Thorman J, Mueller K, Frenzel H: Progressive cardiac involvement by Fabry's disease despite successful renal allo-transplantation. *Int J Cardiol* 7:72–75, 1985.

CHAPTER 60

Complications of Renal Transplantation

JOHN A. MURIE & PETER J. MORRIS

INTRODUCTION

Although complications following renal transplantation are now less than in previous years, they are nevertheless still responsible for appreciable morbidity and even mortality in the transplant recipient. Such complications are diverse in nature, ranging from technical problems related to the surgery to more widespread effects related to immunosuppression and/or poor renal function.

TECHNICAL

Vascular

Transplant renal artery thrombosis as a primary event is, fortunately, a rare complication in experienced units, for it will almost certainly result in loss of the transplanted kidney, even if recognized early and treated appropriately. In Oxford it has occurred after 0.3% of transplant operations, and it is generally due to technical error producing twisting or kinking of the renal artery when the kidney is placed in its extraperitoneal pouch. It should be suspected in any patient who suddenly becomes anuric within 48 hours of surgery, and, although rapid confirmation of arterial occlusion may be obtained by isotope renography, the problem is of such urgency that it may be more appropriate to return the patient immediately to the operating room for exploration. If the blood supply cannot be reconstituted within 90 minutes, warm ischemia will almost certainly cause irreversible damage to the graft. In the later weeks after transplantation, renal artery thrombosis may occur as a secondary event after arteriolar thrombosis in an acutely rejecting kidney.

Renal artery stenosis, on the other hand, is not uncommon. This has been recognized after 1.3% of transplant operations in Oxford, but it should be noted that when routine angiography is carried out in patients with hypertension after transplantation, a much higher incidence is found (1). When it occurs in the early months after transplantation, it generally affects the anastomotic site itself and is due to a technical defect. More often it presents one or more years after transplantation with poorly controlled hypertension and deterioration in graft function (1–3). Such stenoses typically lie distal to the site of anastomosis (Figure 1), and although they occur quite frequently they are not usually of functional significance (1). While the lesion may be demonstrated angiographically, it may be difficult to establish that it is the cause of hypertension and/or renal dysfunction, as both these factors may be due to vascular changes associated with chronic rejection. A renal biopsy may be helpful if it excludes chronic rejection and renal-vein renin studies may be of value in determining the functional significance of a radiologic stenosis.

Once the diagnosis is clear, if hypertension is difficult to control, and especially if renal function is compromised, an attempt to correct the stenosis should be made. Operative correction is difficult and should only be undertaken by those experienced in both transplant and vascular surgery. Twenty operations have been performed by one author (PJM) to correct a functional transplant renal artery stenosis, the technical aspects of which have been described elsewhere (4). In only one case was reconstruction not possible and a nephrectomy was performed. Eighteen out of 19 (95%) of the remaining procedures resulted in an improvement in hypertension. Excluding the nephrectomy and one patient who had good preoperative renal function, 16 out of 18 (89%) operations resulted in a significant improvement in renal function. While operative intervention has met with considerable success in Oxford, this has not been true of percutaneous transluminal angioplasty (PTA). Although this latter technique has been successful in treating atheromatous stenosis in the native renal artery (5), its use in the treatment of transplant renal artery stenosis has been attended by mixed results (2, 6). Complications such as renal artery thrombosis and graft loss have been reported, and the inferior results in the transplant recipient may be due to a pathologic process different from atheroma causing the lesion. Although PTA has never resulted in graft loss in Oxford and has occasionally been successful in dilating the stenosis, the majority of attempts have failed due to inability to negotiate the balloon catheter into the stenosis itself.

Secondary hemorrhage is an uncommon but life-threatening complication after transplantation and is due

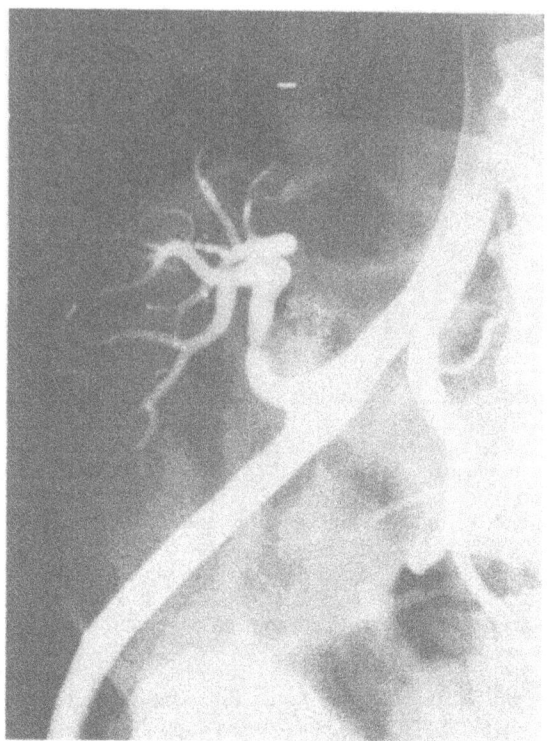

Figure 1. Angiogram showing transplant renal artery stenosis distal to the site of arterial anastomosis (renal artery end-to-side to external iliac artery).

to infection at the anastomosis. The source of sepsis may be contamination from the graft itself, but in any event the infection is usually introduced at the time of operation. It is fortunate that prophylactic antibiotics have reduced the incidence of this problem, since it inevitably requires graft nephrectomy and occasionally also the ligation of the external iliac artery if this has been used for renal revascularization. Surprisingly such a ligation does not always require the insertion of a vascular graft (7), but if arterial reconstruction is deemed necessary it should always be delayed if possible because of the associated infection.

Thrombosis of the renal vein may be seen in grafts removed after irrreversible rejection has occurred, but as a primary acute event it is most unusual. However, there is a suggestion that primary renal vein thrombosis may be occurring more frequently in the first week after transplantation in patients receiving cyclosporin (8). Renal vein thrombosis may be due to technical factors such as kinking or twisting of the vein (9) or to venous compression caused by swelling of the kidney durig an episode of rejection, acute tubular necrosis, or ureteric obstruction (10). Renal vein thrombosis at some later period after transplantation is probably more common than is realized. Here it may occur secondary to thrombosis of the common iliac vein (11) or occasionally as a primary event. Despite all these possibilities, only 0.6% of transplants in Oxford have been affected by this complication. The diagnosis may be suspected on clinical grounds after the onset of sudden pain and graft swelling. Hematuria and proteinuria may be observed, and isotope renography shows a failure of perfusion of the graft. Definitive diagnosis requires direct or pertrochanteric venography (12), but immediate surgical exploration may be more appropriate, although thrombectomy resulting in graft salvage is excessively rare. With or without surgical exploration, anticogulation is the only long-term treatment available.

Urologic

The two principal urologic complications after transplantation are ureteric obstruction and urine leakage (13, 14). Together they have complicated 7% of transplant operations in Oxford, obstruction being slightly more common than leakage. When obstruction occurs early in the post-transplant period, it is generally due to technical reasons at the site of implantation of the ureter into the bladder or twisting of the ureter. Oliguria or anuria in the immediate post-transplant period should make one suspect such problems. The diagnosis is confirmed by ultrasonography in the first instance (15, 16), followed by antegrade pyelography to define the exact site of obstruction. Early surgical revision is required. Ureteric obstruction by hematoma after a percutaneous needle biopsy is occasionally encountered, but this usually resolves spontaneously over a few days without active intervention. At times remote from the transplant operation, ureteric obstruction is often due to ureteric stricture formation, which is presumed to reflect ischemic damage to the ureter (2). Again, ultrasonography and an antegrade pyelogram or an intravenous urogram will confirm the diagnosis, which should always be considered when a gradual deterioration in renal function is seen, especially without evidence of significant chronic rejection. Ureteric strictures have been treated by ballon catheter dilatation, although formal surgical reconstruction is usually necessary.

Urine leakage usually occurs from the lower end of the ureter due to ischemia of this structure, perhaps as a result of skeletonization of the ureter at donor nephrectomy (2). Leakage from the cystotomy made at the time of ureteric implantation is relatively uncommon nowadays. Urine leakage is often not evident until at least 1 week after transplantation, and often several weeks pass before the diagnosis becomes obvious. Oliguria is noted in association with fever, local tenderness, and swelling. Ultrasonography followed by antegrade pyelography or intravenous urography allows a definitive diagnosis (17), for which surgery should be undertaken as soon as possible, as a delay will undoubtedly result in infection, making the inevitable surgery more difficult and hazardous.

There has been a marked reduction in the incidence of urologic complications, both obstruction and leakage, in recent years in the Oxford Transplant Unit. While the

Table 1. Urologic complications and immunosuppressive regimens for 600 consecutive transplant operations in Oxford

Regimen	Period of usage	Number of grafts	Number of primary complications (%)
High-dose pred + aza	1975–1979	171	16 (15.2)
Low-dose pred + aza	1978–1985	194	10 (5.2)
CyA*	1980–1985	102	5 (4.9)
CyA + pred	1983–1985	38	1 (1.1)
CyA + aza + pred	1985–1986	95	1 (1.1)
Total	1975–1986	600	43 (7.2)

Pred = prednisolone; aza = azathioprine; CyA = cyclosporin A.
* With conversion to aza + pred at 3 months post-transplantation.

surgical technique has remained constant, the immunosuppression protocols have changed significantly. From 1975 to 1979 when high-dose steroids (initially 100 mg prednisolone/day) were used, the rate of urologic complication was 15%. In later years, although a variety of protocols have been used, the steroid dose has been significantly lower (initially 20–30 mg/day) and primary urologic complications now affect only about 2% of transplants (Table 1).

Lymphatic

While lymph drainage in the first few days after transplantation is often evident if a suction drain has been inserted, this is rarely a problem. The major complication associated with the lymphatics is lymphocele formation, which usually occurs in the first 3 months after transplantation and presents as a large cystic mass in the vicinity of the kidney. A lymphocele always arises from the host lymphatics and is caused by a failure to ligate those lymphatics divided during exposure of the iliac vessels (18). Presenting features are due to the pressure of the lymphocele on the surrounding structures. Pressure on the ureter may reduce renal function, pressure on the iliac vein may cause swelling of the kidney, and strangury and diarrhea may occur due to pressure on the baldder and rectum, respectively (Figure 2). Ultrasonography allows definitive diagnosis, and the initial management is aspiration under ultrasonographic control. After two or three aspirations, the lymphocele often does not recur, but if continuing problems are met then marsupialization into the peritoneal cavity is performed (2, 18).

Wound

Prevention of contamination during donor nephrectomy, careful aseptic technique during transplantation, and the use of prophylactic antibiotics should ensure that the incidence of wound infection after the transplant operation is no more than 3%. This is a serious complication, since deep sepsis may involve the vascular anastomoses and cause secondary hemorrhage (see Vascular section). When wound infection occurs, adequate drainage must be provided immediately and appropriate antibiotic therapy should be introduced.

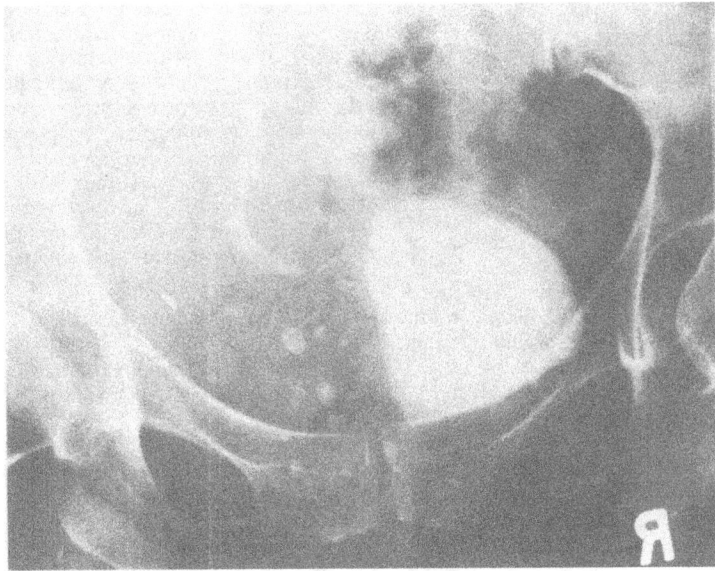

Figure 2. Urogram showing bladder filling defect due to post-transplantation lymphocele.

INFECTION

Incidence

Although the last decade has seen a decrease in the incidence of serious infections after transplantation, this complication remains a significant hazard for the transplant recipient, especially in the early months after surgery (19). The fall in incidence is primarily due to a general reduction in immunosuppressive therapy and, in particular, to modern low-dose steroid regimens (20–22). The reduction in morbidity and mortality from infection is also in some part due to fewer rejection episodes requiring immunosuppressive treatment due to the recognition of the transfusion effect and to HLA matching. A greater awareness of the hazard of infection and more aggressive diagnosis and treatment have also made a significant contribution. While postoperative bacterial chest infection and bacteriuria are not uncommon in transplant recipients, these rarely pose significant problems, unlike infections due to a variety of pathogens that may be encountered rather late in the post-transplant period.

After transplantation the most common presentation of an infection is fever. Although this may have a relatively trivial origin, such as gastroenteritis or influenza, thorough investigation is always required, and, depending on the clinical features, this may involve chest radiography; ultrasonography of the transplant wound area; cultures from the mouth and access sites; cultures of sputum, urine, blood, and stool; viral antibody titers; and even lumbar puncture. If the diagnosis remains elusive the possibility of cytomegalovirus (CMV) infection, in particular, or tuberculosis or fungal infection should be excluded by intensive investigation. Antibiotics should be withheld until an organism is identified if this is feasible, but on occasion empirical therapy is justified, especially in the neutropenic patient.

Pulmonary infection

This is a major cause of morbidity and mortality after renal transplantation. The diagnosis of fever in association with a pulmonary infiltrate on a chest radiograph may be difficult to ascertain and it is first necessary to exclude pulmonary edema, infarction, or hemorrhage as a cause of the radiologic appearance (23). It is worthy of note that in the first few weeks after transplantation, chest infections are usually due to those bacteria commonly encountered as pulmonary pathogens after any form of surgery. Opportunistic infections, on the other hand, such as those due to CMV, pneumocystis, legionella, nocardia, and fungi, occur after the first postoperative month and such organisms are encountered especially in the first year after transplantation (19, 24), with a declining incidence in later years, especially in those with good renal function on minimal immunosuppression. Pneumococcal pneumonia, however, may occur at any time and may run an aggressive course, leading to death, unless diagnosed and treated early.

The radiologic appearance may assist diagnosis. Rapidly progressive changes tend to be associated with bacterial infections, whereas a less rapid progression may indicate a viral or fungal causation. Consolidation is more commonly a feature of bacterial infection, whereas interstitial shadowing is compatible with viral or pneumocystis infection. Nodular infiltrates are associated with infection due to streptococcus, nocardia, tuberculosis, or fungi. While radiography is of undoubted importance in the management of the transplant patient with pulmonary infection, definitive diagnosis can only be made after identification of the responsible pathogen, and an aggressive approach to the acquisition of suitable specimens for bacteriologic study is needed. Although it is generally wise to withhold antibiotics until the pathogen has been identified, the condition of individual patients may make this unrealistic. Empirical treatment of suspected bacterial pneumonia must cover staphylococci, pneumococci, hemophilus, legionella, and gram-negative organisms, and a satisfactory antibiotic choice is flucloxacillin plus erthromycin in conjunction with an aminoglycoside. Suspected pneumocystis infection will often respond to high-dose cotrimoxazole, and in practice all four of the above drugs tend to be administered. If a definitive diagnosis is not reached or if empirical treatment is started without a response within 24 hours, bronchoscopy with bronchial alveolar lavage or open-lung biopsy is indicated (19).

CYTOMEGALOVIRUS PNEUMONIA

This does not occur in the first month after transplantation. A fever associated with changes on a chest radiograph, occurring between 1 and 4 months after transplantation in a patient who was seronegative at the time of operation and who received a kidney from a seropositive donor should be regarded as due to CMV infection when all other causes of fever and pulmonary infiltrate have been excluded. A leukopenia may develop in association with this infection, requiring a reduction in immunosuppression. Azathioprine, in particular, may have to be discontinued. Hyperimmune globulin and alpha-interferon have been claimed to have some benefit in CMV infection (25), but there is no generally accepted specific treatment for CMV pneumonia. CMV is discussed further in the section on viral infections.

PNEUMOCYSTIS CARINII PNEUMONIA

This is a relatively common pneumonia in transplant recipients who present with a fever, often associated with some dyspnea, but with few other physical signs. Radiography shows diffuse pulmonary shadowing with a linear distribution, and high-dose cotrimoxazole is the treatment of choice (Figure 3). This infection may now be occurring more frequently with the use of cyclosporin, and prophylactic cotrimoxazole has been given with benefit in Oxford and elsewhere over the first few months after transplantation.

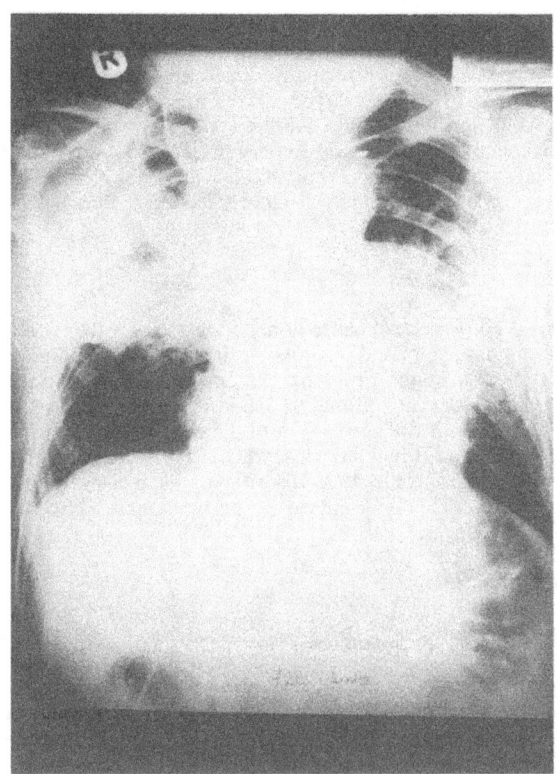

Figure 3. Pulmonary shadowing on a chest radiograph due to *Pneumocystis carinii* pneumonia in a transplant recipient.

PULMONARY TUBERCULOSIS

While the incidence of tuberculosis varies according to the region, it is undoubtedly more common in transplant recipients than in the general population. Symptoms are often nonspecific and the site of infection may be outside of the lungs. Established cases are treated with rifampicin and isoniazid, but both drugs are metabolized in the liver and rifampicin, in particular, is a potent inducer of hepatic enzymes. Such enzyme induction renders cyclosporin an unwise choice for immunosuppression, and this drug is better replaced by azathioprine if rifampicin is the chosen treatment. Mycobacterial infection is discussed further in the section on bacterial infections.

LEGIONELLA PNEUMONIA

The recent increase in the incidence of legionella pneumonia is probably due to an increasing awareness and identification of the organism, which proliferates in stagnant water and is often spread via airconditioning systems and showers (26). In the early stages, the chest radiograph shows irregular, nodular shadows, which may progress rapidly to lobar ro diffuse consolidation. Identification of the organism usually requires direct immunofluorescent staining, and it may be cultured from sputum or biopsy samples on specialized media. The drug of choice is high-dose erythromycin.

Urinary tract infection

A bacteriuria nearly always occurs in the first few weeks after transplantation because of the presence of an indwelling catheter for some days after the operation. Such a bacteriuria generally clears on removal of the catheter, especially in the presence of a good urine output. If it does not clear within a few days of catheter removal, or if a frank urinary tract infection is evident, active treatment with an appropriate antibiotic is warranted, as the continuing presence of bacteria in the urinary tract is a potential cause of septicemia in the immunosuppressed patient.

Wound infection

This serious complication has been discussed earlier. In cases of deep infection, diagnosis may be aided by ultrasonography or computerized tomography, but treatment should be prompt and consists of adequate drainage and appropriate antibiotic therapy.

Septicemia

This is not uncommon and is usually due to gram-negative organisms from the urinary tract. *Staphylococcus*, *Listeria*, and *Candida* may also cause septicemia. While awaiting the results of blood cultures, broad-spectrum antibiotic treatment should be started, and an aggressive search for the focus of infection should be made. The treatment of such a focus depends on its nature and site.

Viral infections

CYTOMEGALOVIRUS (CMV)

This is the most important of the viral infections encountered in transplant recipients and takes two forms (19, 25,

Table 2. Incidence of cytomegalovirus infection in 306 consecutive cadaver renal transplant recipients in Oxford with respect to CMV antibody status of donor and recipient (18).

	Recipient CMV +		Recipient CMV −	
	Donor CMV +	Donor CMV −	Donor CMV +	Donor CMV −
No. patients	84	98	60	64
No. infected	52 (62%)	52 (53%)	38 (63%)	0
	Reactivation		Primary infection	

27). The first is a primary infection and gives rise to more concern than the second, which is a secondary or reactivated infection. Primary infection occurs in patients who are seronegative at the time of transplantation and who receive a kidney from a seropositive donor (Table 2). Transmission of infection with the kidney is far commoner than transmission by blood transfusion (25), which has never been noted in the Oxford Transplant Unit.

Primary CMV infection often presents as a fever in the second or third month after transplantation and may be associated with neutropenia. Atypical lymphocytes may be seen on the blood film. Leukopenia will require a reduction in immunosuppression, especially if azathioprine has been used, and this drug in particular may need to be discontinued, putting the kidney at some risk of rejection. Primary CMV infection may cause penumonia and, less commonly, hepatitis, arthralgia, splenomegaly, myalgia, and gastrointestinal ulceration. Renal function may deteriorate during the early stages of infection and a glomerulopathy may occur (28). The infection is self-limiting within a period of 3 weeks, but great care is required to exclude other causes of fever in these patients until the diagnosis is firmly established by the appearance of CMV-specific IgM or IgG in the primary infection or by a rise in titer in secondary infections. No effective antiviral treatment exists for CMV infection, and management is, therefore, expectant. High-titer CMV immunoglobulin preparations may hold some hope for the future, but no data are available from controlled trials. Prophylactic alpha-interferon may decrease the incidence and severity of a primary infection, but again controlled data are missing (29).

Primary infection can be prevented by avoiding transplantation of a kidney from a seropositive donor into a seronegative recipient (Table 2), and this should be considered among the selection criteria for the donor and recipient. Nevertheless, other overriding considerations exist, which often mean that this ideal protocol cannot be followed. Vaccination against CMV prior to transplantation is being evaluated, but although a high proportion of patients seroconvert, it is not yet clear whether the incidence or severity of subsequent CMV infection is reduced. However, in Oxford our experience suggests that both the incidence and severity of CMV infection is indeed significantly decreased by prior vaccination.

HERPES SIMPLEX VIRUS (HSV)

Latent HSV infection may commonly be reactivated in immunosuppressed patients, especially in the early weeks after transplantation or in association with later complications. Local lesions are painted with 35% idoxuridine in dimethylsulphoxide or treated with acyclovir cream. If the local infection is severe, however, or if systemic infection has occurred, acyclovir chemotherapy should be started immediately, as widespread infection may occasionally cause death. The results of treatment with acyclovir for HSV infection are generally good and side effects are minimal.

VARICELLA ZOSTER

This is again a frequently encountered problem occurring at any stage after transplantation, and acyclovir is the treatment of choice. Patients who are seronegative for varicella antibody should avoid contact with children with chickenpox. Prophylactic hyperimmune globulin should be given after accidental contact, as chickenpox, although rare, can be an extremely virulent infection in a transplant recipient.

EPSTEIN-BARR VIRUS (EBV)

This is an occasional cause of a glandular fever-like illness in immunosuppressed patients. Although such an illness is not itself a major problem, patients taking cyclosporin may be especially prone to EBV infection because of suppression of the generation of T-cytotoxic cells against EBV-infected B lymphocytes, which in turn may cause an acute lymphoproliferative disorder or even a polyclonal lymphoma. This is discussed in the upcoming section on primary cancer.

HEPATITIS B VIRUS

Transplantation in patients who are carriers of the hepatitis B antigen is a relatively common problem in many countries. Graft survival in hepatitis B antigen carriers is rather better than in noncarriers, reflecting some innate immune defect, in addition to the effect of immunosuppressive drugs. There is great concern in carrier patients, however, about the progression of liver disease, which may accompany immunosuppression, even leading to liver failure (30–32). It may be that such patients are more appropriately treated by dialysis rather than transplantation, but if transplantation is chosen, then a case can be made for selecting only those patients who have a normal liver biopsy. In countries where hepatitis B is relatively common within the renal failure population, all new patients and all staff should be vaccinated.

HEPATITIS NON-A, NON-B VIRUS

This is increasing in incidence and occurs especially after blood transfusion. Like hepatitis B, it may be associated with progressive disease leading to hepatic failure (32).

OTHER VIRAL INFECTIONS

Many viruses commonly cause infections in the transplant patient. Fortunately most of these are a nuisance rather than a potential threat to life. They include parainfluenza, influenza A, influenza B, polyoma, and papilloma viruses.

Bacterial infections

Bacterial infections are common after transplantation and many have already been described in this section. Some rather less common bacteria also have to be remembered, which may affect the transplant recipient even many years after the operation.

LISTERIA MONOCYTOGENES

This may cause infection at any time after transplantation but usually after increased or excessive immunosuppression. It is the single commonest cause of meningoencephalitis in transplant recipients, and as soon as cerebrospinal fluid and blood cultures have been obtained, any patient with this condition should be given ampicillin as the drug of choice.

CLOSTRIDIUM DIFFICILE

Pseudomembranous colitis (PMC) is due to infection of the colon by *Clostridium difficile* and, although it typically occurs in patients who have been exposed to broad spectrum antibiotics, it may pose special problems in units where the organism has become endemic. This is likely in any unit with a large continuous ambulatory peritoneal dialysis program with its inevitable antibiotic-treated recurrent peritonitis. The drug of choice in PMC is oral vancomycin, but *Clostridium difficile* is highly infectious and appropriate steps must be take to avoid spread within the transplant unit (33).

NOCARDIA

This organism usually causes a respiratory illness with unproductive cough and malaise associated with a fever. Chest radiographs show a nodular pulmonary infiltrate. Spread to the brain, skin, and joints may result in local abscess formation. Sulphonamide is the drug of choice and this must be given for at least 2 months. Some have suggested that treatment continue for 1 year.

MYCOBACTERIUM TUBERCULOSIS

Although not very common, possible infection with this organism should be considered if an unusual infective process is encountered, especially in transplant recipients with a past history of active tuberculosis. In transplant patients extrapulmonary tuberculosis occurs just as often as pulmonary tuberculosis. It there is a past history of tuberculosis and doubt exists about the adequacy of previous treatment, prophylactic antituberculous chemotherapy should be given for the first 12 months after transplantation.

Fungal infection

While not particularly common in the transplant recipient, the possibility of fungal infection should be considered when fever and pneumonia occur in the presence of increased or excessive immunosuppression.

CANDIDA

This is the commonest fungal infection after transplantation and is often associated with debility from other complications, including other infections. Its most severe local manifestation is esophageal candidiasis, which should respond to local nystatin, but the rare septicemia will require treatment with amphotericin B.

ASPERGILLUS

This may cause pneumonia and disseminate to many sites including the brain, skin, kidney, and alimentary tract. It is treated with amphotericin B.

COCCIDIOIDES

This is rare in Europe but common in certain parts of North America. Lesions occur in the lungs, liver, brain, and spleen, and may be due to primary infection or reactivation of latent infection. Again amphotericin B is the treatment of choice.

CRYPTOCOCCUS

This is a rare cause of penumonitis and meningitis in immunosuppressed patients. Amphotericin B is again the treatment of choice.

HISTOPLASMA

Histoplasma may be a primary infection or the result of reactivation of a latent infection. Fever, skin lesions, and pneumonitis are seen and again amphotericin B is the treatment of choice.

Protozoal and helminthic infections

Pneumocystis carinii is by far the commonest of these organisms encountered in the transplant patient. However, infections due to *Giardia*, *Schistosoma*, *Toxoplasma*, *Leishmania*, and *Strongyloides* may be encountered. Many of these organisms have marked geographic limits and knowledge of these is helpful in diagnosis.

CARDIOVASCULAR COMPLICATIONS

Cardiovascular disease is a major cause of death in the general population, and this is even more pronounced in transplant recipients. No less than a quarter of deaths after renal transplantation in North America and Europe are due to cardiovascular complications (34). Much of the risk is associated with the underlying cause of renal failure, and patients whose renal impairment is due to hypertensive disease or diabetes mellitus fare particularly badly in this respect. Correction of risk factors, such as hypertension, obesity, and hyperlipidemia, is of major importance in the transplant patient, and although no direct evidence exists that smoking is a risk factor in the transplant population, its role in the normal population is well established, and it would seem unlikely that it does not similarly have a deleterious effect after transplantation. Strenuous effects should be made to persuade potential transplant recipients to stop smoking. The tendency to transplant increasing numbers of elderly and diabetic patients, combined with the longer graft survival that can now be achieved, will ensure that cardiovascular complications will become even more prominent in the future. The emphasis should be on prevention by correction of risk factors.

Hypertension

Although uremia itself may be associated with hypertension, elevated blood pressure also remains a major problem in those with functioning allografts. Despite improvements in renal function after operation, there must be new causes for hypertension, a problem that affects well over half of recipients of kidneys between 6 months and 3 years after surgery (35). Hypertension is also recognized as the commonest complication in long-term survivors after transplantation, affecting about half or these patients (36). The causes of such hypertension may include rejection, the influence of disease in the native kidneys, transplant renal artery stenosis, and immunosuppressive drugs, in particular, cyclosporin.

Hypertension is more common in recipients of cadaver grafts than in recipients of kidneys from living, related donors, which suggests that rejection is a significant factor in the high incidence of hypertension after transplantation (37). Chronic rejection, in particular, has a direct relationship with hypertension (36), and acute rejection too is often accompanied by elevation of blood pressure. This may involve the renin-angiotensin system in the allograft but reports are conflicting (38–40).

Some patients have poorly controlled hypertension attributable to disease of the native kidneys and may benefit from bilateral nephrectomy (41, 42). This is a major operation, however, and if the kidneys are small an alternative approach is bilateral renal embolization. This is a minor procedure with little morbidity and has been used with some success in the Oxford transplant unit (43).

The problem of transplant renal artery stenosis has been discussed earlier and, although the Oxford incidence is low, others have reported an incidence as high as 16% (44). Variation in the criteria for recognition accounts for some of the variation in incidence, but it must be appreciated that the association of renal artery stenosis and hypertension is not always causal. When other causes of hypertension have been excluded, percutaneous transluminal agioplasty is a useful initial approach, for while the results in Oxford have been poor, the technique has never resulted in graft loss and other units have reported good results. Reconstructive surgery can then be reserved for those in whom angioplasty fails.

Steroid immunosuppressive therapy contributes to hypertension (45), although modern low-dose steroid protocols are less hazardous in this respect (21). It is now apparent that the incidence of hypertension in patients treated with cyclosporin, with or without steroids, is probably greater than that seen in patients treated with prednisolone and azathioprine.

Lipid abnormalities

It is well known that uremic patients commonly have Type IV hyperlipidemia with marked hypertriglyceridemia (46). Cholesterol levels in the uremic patient tend to be normal or below normal. After transplantation, although the Type IV abnormality may persist, patients may also develop Type IIa or Type IIb hyperlipidemia with cholesterol as well as triglyceride elevation (47). An inverse relationship exists between very low-density lipoprotein (VLDL) and high-density lipoprotein (HDL) cholesterol. In patients receiving azathioprine and prednisolone, VLDL cholesterol may be raised after transplantation while HDL cholesterol is low, a feature known to predispose individuals to ischemic heart disease (48). In those receiving cyclosporin, cholesterol levels are high, this being entirely due to an increase in VLDL cholesterol (49). While HDL can be measured as a risk factor, it is unknown if raising its concentration by diet or drugs will reduce the risk of atheroma. Nevertheless, it would seem sensible to correct hyperlipidemia by restricting calorie, carbohydrate, and fat intake.

Deep venous thrombosis

This complication has occurred in 8% of transplant recipients in Oxford, the incidence increasing with age (50). Although it has been suggested that thromboembolic events in general occur with increased frequency in patients receiving cyclosporin (51), others have not found such as association (52, 53). Deep venous thrombosis exhibits two peaks in incidence, the first at the expected time about 1 week after the transplant operation and the second larger peak at about 4 months. It is noteworthy that a functioning allograft will largely correct the anemia and hemostatic defect associated with chronic renal failure by 4 months. The 4-month peak in incidence, and indeed all thrombosis distant to the time of the transplant operation itself, is usually associated with some complication requiring prolonged bed rest or further surgery (50). Thus, prophylaxis for thrombosis should be mandatory in patients with such complications. Our policy has been to investigate any significant leg swelling by venography or, if pulmonary symptoms suggest embolism, to carry out a ventilation/perfusion isotope scan of the lungs, whether or not such symptoms are accompanied by lower limb swelling. Treatment is immediate anticoagulation with heparin followed by oral warfarin for at least 4 months, as pulmonary embolism is responsible for about 4% of deaths in transplant recipients (4).

CANCER

Primary cancer

The incidence of cancer in transplant patients ranges from 1.6% in Europe to 24% in Australia (54, 55). Much of the difference is accounted for by the very high incidence of skin cancers in Australia. Transplant recipients also have a significantly increased risk of developing malignant lymphoma, but even if lymphoma and skin cancer are excluded, the transplant population still has a greater incidence of nearly all forms of cancer compared with the normal population. Increased susceptibility to neoplasia is due to several factors alone or in combination, which include depression of immune surveillance, increased susceptibility to oncogenic virus infection, chronic antigenic stimulation in the presence of immunosuppression, and a direct neoplastic action of immunosuppressive agents themselves (55).

Skin cancer is the commonest cancer encountered in transplant recipients, even in areas not known for a high incidence of such neoplasia in the general population. Squamous cell carcinoma is the commonest type and it may be very aggressive in the immunosuppressed patient, leading to death from metastatic disease. Bowen's disease, malignant melanoma, and basal cell carcinoma are also not infrequent in transplant recipients. Patients who develop skin cancers continued to do so even after treatment of specific lesions. In some cases, immunosuppression has to be discountinued and the kidney abandoned in order to save life. When immunosuppression is withdrawn new skin cancers do not occur. Because of the high incidence of this disease in warm climates, a serious attempt must be made at prevention. Transplant recipients should be advised on suitable clothing while in the sun and barrier creams should be used.

Malignant (non-Hodgkin) lymphomas occur 50–100 times more frequently in the transplant population than in the general population and account for nearly one third of all cancers in transplant recipients (54, 55). Nowadays these lymphomas are often described as lymphoproliferative disease, of which two types are recognized and for which differing treatments are appropriate (56). The first type is due to infection by the Epstein-Barr virus and presents as an infectious mononucleosislike illness within 1 year of transplantation. The fever and general lymphadenopathy often progress rapidly to a fatal conclusion, although withdrawal of immunosuppression will lead to regression in some patients. More recently, treatment with acyclovir without discontinuing immunosuppressive therapy has met with some success. The second type of lymphoproliferative disease presents as a local solid tumor, usually confined to the central nervous system. This disease responds to conventional therapy for non-Hodgkin's lymphoma, but it is often more aggressive than that seen in the general population, with short remissions and an eventually fatal outcome. In this type of disease neither discontinuing immunosuppression nor acyclovir appear to have any beneficial effect. The clinician should be aware that these two types of disease tend to merge, both in their presentation and in their histologic cytogenetic classification, which shows a spectrum ranging from polymorphic diffuse B-cell hyperplasia through a polymorphic B-cell lymphoma to a monomorphic B-cell lymphoma.

The behavior, and thus the treatment, of other cancers varies according to the cell type and site. Usually the treatment is not significantly different from that of the disease when it occurs in the general population. It is appropriate for the transplant recipient to adopt those prophylactic measures available to the general population, and in particular the increased incidence of cervical cancer in female transplant patients suggests that an annual cervical smear is a wise precaution.

Transferred cancer

Cancer has occasionally been transferred accidentally in the transplanted kidney from a cadaver donor with undetected neoplasia. If metastatic disease is present in the allograft this will soon appear in the recipient. Rapid spread tends to occur in the immunosuppressed patient, and treatment is withdrawal of immunosuppression and graft nephrectomy followed by a return to dialysis. This will occasionally lead to the regression of disease.

GASTROINTESTINAL COMPLICATIONS

Perforation or hemorrhage from a peptic ulcer is associated with a high mortality in the transplant patient, and many units screen potential recipients for peptic ulcer disease. In previous years in Oxford, patients with active ulceration have been treated surgically prior to transplantation, but more recently surgery has been restricted to those who fail to respond to histamine-receptor blockers or who have recurrent ulceration. All patients with a past history of peptic ulcer disease without evidence of active ulceration at the time of transplantation receive prophylactic ranitidine during the first few months after transplantation. If perforation or hemorrhage occur, these complications are treated promptly and aggressively by surgery.

Diverticular disease is no more common in transplant recipients than in the general population, but the problems of hemorrhage or sepsis, should they occur, pose an especially grave risk to the transplant recipient. Some consider the presence of diverticular disease in a potential recipient to be an indication for colectomy, but this is performed in Oxford prior to transplantation only in the most severe cases. Should a complication of diverticulosis occur after transplantation, it must be treated aggressively, and abscess formation or sepsis is an indication for early surgery.

The problems of gastrointestinal infection have been discussed previously. Pseudomembranous colitis may occur especially in units where *Clostridium difficile* is endemic. A necrotizing enterocolitis is also seen occasionally, which may result in gangrene of the colon and even the small bowel. When this occurs it is uniformly fatal and, although the cause is unknown, it may be associated with cytomegalovirus infection. Solitary ulcers may also occur in the bowel, notably in the cecum. These may bleed or perforate and require urgent surgery.

BONE COMPLICATIONS

Most bone complications after transplantation are due to steroid therapy. Avascular necrosis may affect many joints, including the wrists, elbows, knees, ankles, and shoulders, but it is most commonly seen in the hips, where it tends to occur bilaterally. This complication tends to occur between 1 and 3 years after transplantation and pain is the common presenting feature. Although the incidence of avascular necrosis has been as high as 15% in transplant recipients, with modern low-dose steroid immunosuppressive regimens this incidence has dropped dramatically. Eventually patients with avascular necrosis will require surgery. Replacement of the hip joint is well tolerated in transplant recipients and should be considered early to improve rehabilitation. Osteoporosis is the other principal steroid-related bone complication, although with low-dose steroid protocols this too has declined in incidence. Nevertheless, even low doses of steroid are likely to produce a significant degree of osteoporosis in postmenopausal women.

GROWTH IN CHILDREN

Retardation of growth in children with end-stage renal failure is well known, and although the rate of growth improves after transplantation, some reduction in eventual stature is likely. Growth rate is related both to the age of the child and to renal function, but it is the use of steroids in immunosuppressive regimens that causes most retardation after successful transplantation. While the use of alternate-day steroids improves the situation to some extent, a limitation of potential stature is still probable (57). When cyclosporin is used as the main immunosuppressive agent, on the other hand, especially if used without steroids, a normal growth rate is possible and there is evidence that catch-up growth may also occur (58, 59).

CATARACTS

Posterior lenticular cataracts occur in up to 10% of transplant recipients, and this is yet another complication associated with high-dose steroid therapy. While most cataracts remain small and cause little disability, some are large and require ophthalmic surgery to the lens.

SPECIFIC COMPLICATIONS OF DRUG THERAPY

Many of these complications have already been mentioned, especially in the case of steroid therapy. It would be inappropriate, however, to end this chapter without listing several important complications that are related to specific drugs. Azathioprine may cause bone marrow depression, hepatic dysfunction, and hair loss. Cyclosporin may cause nephrotoxicity, hepatic dysfunction, gingival hypertorphy, hypertrichosis, neurasthesia, and fluid retention. The more severe of these complications, when they occur, may require a reduction in the dosage or even withdrawal of the appropriate drug.

REFERENCES

1. Morris PJ, Yadav R, Kincaid-Smith P, Anderson J, Hare WSC, Johnson N, Johnson W, Marshall VC: Renal artery stenosis in renal transplantation. *Med J Aust* 1:1255–1257, 1971.
2. Belzer FO, Glass N, Sollinger H: Technical complications after renal transplantation. In: PJ Morris, ed, *Kidney Transplantation: Principles and Practice*, 2nd ed. Grune and Stratton, New York, pp 407–426, 1984.
3. Tilney NL, Rocha A, Strom TB, Kirkman RL: Renal artery stenosis in transplant patients. *Ann Surg* 199:454–460, 1984.
4. Morris PJ, Murie JA: Vascular complications after renal transplantation. In: RM Greenhalgh, CW Jamieson, AN Nicolaides, eds, *Vacular Surgery: Issues in Current Practice*. Grune Aand Stratton, New York, pp 255–265, 1986.
5. Gruntzig A, Velter W, Meier B, Kuhlmann U, Lutoff U, Siegenthaler W: Treatment of renovascular hypertension with percutaneous transluminal dilatation of renal artery stenosis. *Lancet* 1:801–802, 1978.
6. Grossman RA, Dafoe DC, Shoenfeld RB, Ring EJ, McLean GK, Oleaga JA, Freiman DB, Naji A, Perloff LJ, Barker CF: Percutaneous transluminal angioplasty treatment of renal transplant artery stenosis. *Transplantation* 34:339–343, 1982.
7. Chiverton SG, Muric JA, Allen RD, Morris PJ: Renal transplant nephrectomy: A ten year experience. *Surg Gynecol Obstet* 164:324–328, 1987.
8. Merion RM, Calne RY: Allograft renal vein trombosis. *Transplant Proc* 17:1746–1750, 1985.
9. D'Apuzzo V, Bretscher D, Oetliker O, Nachbur B: Renal vein thrombosis in kidney allografts. *Lancet* 2:975–976, 1973.
10. Sorensen BL, Hald T, Nissen HM: Silent iliac compression syndrome as a cause of renal vein thrombosis after transplantation. *Scand J Urol Nephrol* 6 (Suppl 15):75–77, 1972.
11. Arruda JAL, Gutierrez LF, Jonasson O, Pillay VKG, Kurtzman NA: Renal vein thrombosis in kidney allografts. *Lancet* 2:585–586, 1973.
12. Smellie WAB, Vinik M, Freed TA, Hume DM: Pertrochanteric venography in the study of human renal transplant recipients. *Surg Gynecol Obstet* 126:777–780, 1968.
13. Mundy AR, Podesta ML, Bewick M, Rudje CJ, Ellis FG: The urological complications of 1000 renal transplants. *Br J Urol* 53:397–402, 1981.
14. Loughlin KR, Tilney NL, Richie JP: Urologic complications in 718 renal transplant patients. *Surgery* 95:297–302, 1984.
15. Koehler PR, Kanemofo HH, Maxwell JC: Ultrasonic "B" scanning in the diagnosis of complications in renal transplant patients. *Radiology* 119:661–664, 1976.
16. Morley P, Barnett E, Bell P: Ultrasound in the diagnosis of fluid collections following renal transplantation. *Clin Radiol* 26:199–207, 1975.
17. Petrek J, Tilney NL, Smith EH, Williams JS, Vineyard GC: Ultrasound in renal transplantation. *Ann Surg* 185:441–447, 1975.
18. Griffiths AB, Fletcher EW, Mooris PJ: Lymphocele after renal transplantation. *Aust NZ J Surg* 49:626–628, 1979.
19. Winnearls CG, Lane DJ, Kurtz J: Infectious complications after renal transplantation. In: PJ Morris, ed, *Kidney Transplantation: Principles and Practice*, 2nd ed. Grune & Stratton,

New York, pp 427–467, 1984.
20. Morris PJ, Oliver DO, Bishop M, Cullen P, Fellows G, French M, Ledingham JG, Smith JC, Ting A, Williams K: Renal transplantation — A new unit's experience. *Lancet* 1:525–527, 1978.
21. Morris PJ, Chan L, French ME, Ting A: Low dose oral prednisolone in renal transplantation. *Lancet* 1:525–527, 1982.
22. Tilney NL, Strom TB, Vineyard GC, Merrill JP: Factors contibuting to the declining mortality rate in renal transplantation. *N Engl J Med* 299:1321–1325, 1978.
23. Fanta CH, Pennington JE: Pulmonary infections in the transplant patient. In: PJ Morris, NL Tilney, eds, *Progress in Transplantation II*. Churchill Livingstone, Edinburgh p 207, 1985.
24. Rubin RH, Wolfson JS, Cosimi AB, Tolkoff-Rubin NE: Infections in the renal transplant recipient. *Am J Med* 70:405–411, 1981.
25. Rubin RH: The problem of cytomegalovirus infection in transplantation. In: PJ Morris, NL Tilney, eds, *Progress in Transplantation II*. Churchill Livingstone, Edinburgh, pp 89–114, 1984.
26. Tobin JO'H Beare J, Dunnill MS, Fisher-Hoch S, French M, Mitchell RG, Morris PJ, Meurs MF: Legionnaire's disease in a transplant unit: Isolation of the causative agent from shower baths. *Lancet* 2:118–121, 1980.
27. Rubin RH, Tolkoff-Rubin NE, Oliver D, Rota TR, Hamilton J, Betts RF, Pass RF, Hillis W, Szuness W, Farrell ML, Hirsch MS: Multicentre seroepidemiologic study of the impact of cyctomegalovirus infection on renal transplantation. *Transplantation* 40:243–249, 1985.
28. Richardson WP, Colvin RB, Cheeseman H, Tolkoff-Rubin NE, Herrin JT, Cosimi AB, Collins AB, Hirsch MS, McCluskey RT, Russell PS, Rubin RH: Glomerulopathy associated with cytomegalovirus uremia in renal allografts. *N Engl J Med* 305:57–63, 1981.
29. Hirsch MS, Schooley RT, Cosimi AB, Russell PS, Delmonico FL, Tolkoff-Rubin NE, Herrin JT, Cantell K, Farrell ML, Rota TR, Rubin RH: Effects of interferon-alpha on cytomegalovirus reactivation syndromes in renal recipients. *N Engl J Med* 308:1489–1493, 1983.
30. Pirison Y, Alexandre GP, van Ypersele de Strihou C: Long-term effects of HBs antigenemia on patient survival after renal transplantation. *N Engl J Med* 296:194–196, 1977.
31. Parfrey PS, Forbes RDC, Hutchinson TA, Beaudoin JG, Dauphine WD, Hollomby DJ, Guttmann RD: The clinical and pathological cause of hepatitis B liver disease in renal transplant recipients. *Transplantation* 37:461–466, 1984.
32. La Quaglia MP, Tolkoff-Rubin NE, Dienstag JL, Cosimi AB, Herrin JT, Kelly M, Rubbin RH: Impact of hepatitis on renal transplantation. *Transplantation* 32:504–507, 1981.
33. Ritchie DB, Jennings LC, Lynn KL, Baily RR, Cook HB: Clostridium difficile-associated colitis: Cross-infection in predisposed patients with renal failure. *NZ Med J* 95:265, 1982.
34. Raine AEG, Ledingham JGG: Cardiovascular complications after renal transplantation. In: PJ Morris, ed, *Kidney Transplantation: Principles and Practice*, 2nd ed, Grune and Stratton, New York, pp 469–489, 11984.
35. Bachy C, Alexandre GPJ, de Strihou CY: Hypertension after renal transplantion. *Br Med J* 2:1287–1289, 1976.
36. Kirhman RL, Strom TB, Weir MR, Tilney NL: Late mortality and morbidity in recipients of long-term renal allografts. *Transplantion* 34:347–351, 1982.
37. Jacquot C, Idatte JM, Bedrossian J, Weiss Y, Safar M, Bariety J: Long-term blood pressure changes in renal homotransplantation. *Arch Intern Med* 138:233–236, 1978.
38. Bennett WM, McDonald WJ, Lawson RK, Potter GA: Post-transplant hypertension: Studies of cortical blood flow and the renal pressor system. *Kidney Int* 6:99–108, 1974.
39. Curtis JJ, Luke RG, Whelchel JD, Diethelm AG, Jones P, Dustan HP: Inhibition of angiotensin converting enzyme in renal transplant recipients with hypertension. *N Engl J Med* 308:377–381, 1983.
40. Linas SL, Miller PD, McDonald KM, Stables DP, Katz F, Weil R, Schrier RW: Role of the renin-angiotensin system in post-transplantation hypertension in patients with multiple kidneys. *N Engl J Med* 298:1440–1444, 1978.
41. Curtis JJ, Lucas BA, Kotchen TA, Luke RG: Surgical therapy for persistent hypertension after renal transplantation. *Transplantation* 31:125–128, 1981.
42. Curtis JJ, Luke RG, Diethelm AG, Whelchel JD, Jones P: Benefits of removal of native kidneys in hypertension after renal transplantation. *Lancet* 2:729–745, 1985.
43. Thompson JF, Flectcher EWL, Wood RFM, Chalmers DHK, Taylor HM, Benjamin IS, Morris PJ: Control of hypertension after renal transplantation by embolisation of host kidneys. *Lancet* 2:424–427, 1984.
44. Faenza A, Spolaore R, Poggioli G, Selleri S, Roversi R, Gozzetti G, Renal artery stenosis after renal transplantation. *Kidney Int* 23 (Suppl 14):S54, 1983.
45. Popovtzer MM, Pinnggera W, Katz FH, Corman JL, Robinette J, Lanois B, Halgrimson CG, Starzl TE: Variations in arterial blood pressure after kidney transplantation. *Circulation* 47:1297–1305, 1973.
46. Bagdade JD, Porte D, Bierman EL: Hypertriglyceridemia. A metabolic consequence of chronic renal failure. *N Engl J Med* 279:181–185, 1968.
47. Curtis JJ, Galla JH, Woodford SY, Lucas BA, Luke RG: Effect of alternate day prednisolone on plasma lipids, in renal transplant recipients. *Kidney Int* 22:42–47, 1982.
48. Kindler J, Sieberth HG, Hahn R, Glockner WM, Vlaho M, Pelzer R: Does atherosclerosis caused by dialysis limit this treatment? *Proc Eur Dial Transpl Assoc* 19:168–174, 1982.
49. Raine AEG, Carter RD, Chapman JR, Mann JI, Morris PJ: Hypercholesterolemia after renal transplantation associated with cyclosporin immunosuppression. *Transplant Proc*, in press.
50. Allen RD, Michie CA, Murie JA, Morris PJ: Deep venous thrombosis after renal transplantation. *Surg Gynecol Obstet* 164:137–142, 1987.
51. Vanrenterghem Y, Roels L, Lerut T, Gruwez J, Michielsen P, Gresele P, Deckmyn H, Colucci M, Arnout J, Vermylen J: Thromboembolic complications and haemostatic changes in cyclosporin-treated cadaveric kidney allograft recipients. *Lancet* 1:999–1002, 1985.
52. Allen RD, Michie CA, Morris PJ, Chapman JR: Venous thrombosis and cyclosporin. *Lancet* 2:1004, 1985.
53. Choudhury N, Neild GH, Brown Z, Cameron JS, Venkatesward RK: Thromboembolic complications in cyclosporin-treated kidney allograft recipients. *Lancet* 2:606–607, 1985.
54. Penn I: The incidence of malignancies in transplant recipients. *Transplant Proc* 7:323–326, 1975.
55. Sheil AGR: Cancer in dialysis and transplant patients. In: PJ Morris, ed, *Kidney Transplantation: Principles and Practice*, 2nd ed., Grune and Stratton, New York, pp 491–507, 1984.
56. Hanto DW, Simmons RL: Lymphoproliferative disease in immunosuppressed patients. In: PJ Morris, NL Tilney, eds, *Progress in Transplantation*, Vol 1. Churchill Livingstone, New York, pp 186–208, 1984.
57. Fine RN: Renal transplantation in children. In: PJ Morris,

ed, *Kidney Transplantation: Principles and Practice*, 2nd ed., Grune and Stratton, New York, pp 509–546, 1984.
58. Klare B, Walter JV, Hahn H, Emmrich P, Land W: Cyclosporin in renal transplantation in children. *Lancet* 2:692, 1984.
59. Fletcher SM, Conley SB, van Buren CT, Rose G, Kerman R, Kahan BD: Impact of cyclosporin on renal function and growth in pediatric renal transplant recipients. *Transplant Proc* 17:1284–1288, 1985.

CHAPTER 61

The Catheter

GRANNUM R. SANT & EDWIN M. MEARES, JR

INTRODUCTION

Catheter drainage of the urinary tract is a common medical practice. It is widely used to manage urinary tract obstruction, to facilitate surgical repair of the genitourinary tract, to monitor urinary output in hospitalized patients, manage incontinence, and to provide access to the upper urinary tract, i.e., kidneys and ureters.

Indwelling urethral catheters are an important cause of hospital-acquired (nosocomial) infections. Indeed, Beeson (1) in 1958 challenged the conventional practice of catheterization with his landmark editorial: "The case against the catheter." He emphasized the morbidity of bladder catheterization and stressed, "at times the catheter is indispensable for therapy... the decision to use this instrument should be made with the knowledge that it involves the risk of producing a serious disease which is often difficult to treat." This editorial led to an unfounded fear of the catheter by many clinicians, with some feeling compelled to withhold its use at all costs. Nevertheless, a redefinition of indications for urinary tract catheterization and a flurry of research aimed at reducing the morbidity associated with the indwelling urethral catheter ensued. The pathogenesis of catheter-related urinary tract infection(UTI) is now better understood, and alternative methods of urinary drainage and bladder management have replaced the indwelling urethral catheter in many clinical situations.

Catheterization is necessary in the management of various conditions in which its beneficial use far outweighs the potential complications. To minimize associated morbidity and mortality, however, clinicians must use urethral catheters judiciously and remove inlying catheters at the earliest opportunity. Alternative drainage methods include intermittent catheterization, external "condom" catheter drainage, percutaneous nephrostomy tubes, and ureteral stents (2–4). The widespread use of these techniques, unfortunately, has also produced both infectious and noninfectious complications. Indications for catheterization of the urinary tract always should be sound, techniques for catheter placement must be safe and aseptic, and every effort should be made to prevent infection during the period of drainage. Most importantly, the patient must be left with a sterile urinary tract after catheter removal.

TYPES OF URINARY CATHETERS

Urinary catheters are made in various shapes and sizes (Table 1). Catheter diameter is measured on the French (F) scale; this can be converted to millimeters by dividing by three. Indwelling urethral catheters have inflation bags or balloons to prevent dislodgement. The catheter tip may vary: coude tip to bypass urethral or bladder-neck strictures, mushroom (de Pezzer), or winged tip (Malecot) to provide drainage of urine and blood. The three-way Foley balloon catheter has a third lumen that permits continuous or intermittent bladder irrigation. This is useful to prevent postoperative clot retention and to administer continuous bladder irrigation with alum to control bleeding secondary to chemical, e.g., cyclophosphamide, or radiation cystitis. Indwelling catheters are made of soft latex rubber, silicone, or silastic, and feature a balloon (Foley) or phalanges (Malecot and de Pezzer) to prevent dislodgement. Catheters used to pass a urethral stricture or postprostatectomy bladder neck contracture usually are fashioned from woven silk, gum elastic, or plastic, and may have a distal curvature (coude) to facilitate passage. A small plastic or polyethylene catheter is suitable for intermittent urethral catheterization.

Catheters for percutaneous suprapubic cystostomy are usually polyethylene or silastic (8F–14F in diameter). Subsequently, if a larger catheter is required, the suprapubic tract usually can be dilated to facilitate insertion. When a suprapubic catheter is inserted during an open surgical procedure, a large Foley, Malecot, or de Pezzer catheter is used.

Most ureteral catheters (3F–8F in diameter) are made of soft polyethylene or silicone. Catheters fashioned to remain for prolonged periods within the ureter have phalanges on the shaft, terminal "pigtails," or J hooks (3,5).

Catheters designed for percutaneous nephrostomy are seldom larger than 14F in diameter and are usually made of polyethylene. They are anchored by suture attachment to the skin. Some also have a terminal pigtail that coils

Table 1. Common types of urinary tract catheters

Urethral
    Simple (straight)
    Retention (Foley, balloon)
    Coude tip (curved tip)
    Three-way (Foley, balloon)
Suprapubic
    Mushroom (dePezzer)
    Winged tip (Malecot)
    Percutaneous (Stamey, Cystocath)
Nephrostomy
    Open insertion (dePezzer, Malecot, Foley)
    Percutaneous insertion (angiocatheters, polyethylene tubes)
Ureteral stents
    External (standard ureteral catheters)
    Internal (double-J catheters)
External condom type

within the collecting system. During surgical procedures, large Foley, Malecot, or de Pezzer catheters are used for nephrostomy drainage; alternatively, soft polyethylene tubes may be used to minimize trauma to the renal pelvis and kidney.

INDICATIONS FOR URINARY CATHETERIZATION

Urinary retention

Acute urinary retention is the sudden inability of the patient to voluntarily empty the distended bladder. Predisposing factors include prostatic hypertrophy, bladder neck contracture, neuropathic bladders, trauma, gross hematuria with obstructing clots, and acute prostatitis. Postoperative retention can occur following inguinal, perirectal, or pelvic surgical procedures.

Acute bladder overdistention should be relieved promptly. One should first attempt to transurethrally pass a well-lubricated Foley balloon catheter (size 18F–22F). Small catheters (12F–14F) lack body and tend to coil at the level of the external urethral sphincter or the bladder neck in men. Obstruction to easy passage of a standard Foley catheter should lead instead to an attempt to pass a well-lubricated coude-tip catheter. The curved tip facilitates passage beyond the external sphincter and over the median prostatic lobe into the bladder. If urethral scars or other abnormalities prevent atraumatic catheterization, one should consult a clinician trained in the use of filiforms and followers. As an alternative, the bladder can be drained by suprapubic needle aspiration or by insertion of a suprapubic cystostomy tube using local anesthesia. The inexperienced person should never attempt to pass a catheter per urethram into the bladder by means of a catheter guide, lest severe urethral or prostatic trauma results. Percutaneous drainage minimizes urethral trauma, avoids dissemination of urethral bacteria into the blood stream, and allows subsequent radiographic or endoscopic evaluation of urethral and prostatic anatomy.

In patients with acute urinary retention associated with progressive "prostatism," the catheter should generally remain indwelling until corrective surgery is done. This allows decompression of the overdistended detrusor and facilitates early restoration of effective postoperative voiding. Postoperative urinary retention is usually managed by intermittent or short-term urethral catheterization. Restoration of normal voiding can be enhanced by administration of alpha-adrenergic blockers for a few days, e.g., prazosin, 1 mg, orally twice daily (6). This relaxes the smooth muscle of the bladder neck and prostate, and promotes bladder emptying. Intermittent urethral catheterization is preferred for the initial management of retention in acute spinal-cord injury patients (7). Techniques of intermittent catheterization are discussed elsewhere in this chapter.

Urinary incontinence

Leakage of urine can occur as a result of incompetence of the bladder outlet ("stress"), uninhibited detrusor contractions ("urge"), urinary fistulas (total), or, paradoxically, in urinary retention ("overflow"). Catheterization is used in the diagnosis of incontinence to measure postvoid residual urine, to introduce radiographic contrast for delineation of fistulas, and to study detrusor-sphincter function by means of cystometrography (CMG) and voiding cystourethrography (VCUG).

Cure of female stress incontinence is achieved by means of various operative prodecures designed to resuspend the bladder neck. Complete sphincteric dysfunction, e.g., neuropathic, postsurgical, and radiation injury, may produce severe incontinence that is difficult to correct surgically. In females, the only treatment alternatives may be an indwelling urethral catheter, surgical closure of the bladder neck plus suprapubic cystostomy, creation of a vesicostomy, or proximal urinary diversion, e.g., ileal conduit. Many clinicians argue that an indwelling catheter should not be used in the incontinent female patient for nursing and patient convenience alone (1). However, the avoidance of catheterization can result in decubitus ulcers, cellulitis, and bacteremia — morbidity exceeding that normally produced by an indwelling catheter. Two other management alternatives are available for incontinent males: penile clamps and condom catheters. Penile clamps, e.g., Cunningham clamps, are tolerated poorly and cause urethral fistulas or diverticula. Likewise, condom catheters can cause urethral obstruction and abrasions of the penile skin; furthermore, they predispose to urinary tract infection (8). The complications of condom catheter drainage will be discussed later. Uninhibited bladder contractions causing mild incontinence can be treated with anticholinergic drugs, e.g., propantheline bromide. However, total detrusor paralysis with retention is required to control severe incontinence caused by uninhibited bladder contractions. In such cases, intermittent bladder catheterization plus large doses of anticholinergics are needed to establish continence and effective bladder drainage. If bladder paralysis is not achieved or drug side effects become intolerable, supravesical urinary diversion may be required.

Patients with demyelinating diseases of the central nervous system, e.g., multiple sclerosis, or traumatic injuries involving the cervical or thoracic spinal cord, often present a special problem: They are incontinent but may empty their bladders incompletely due to bladder-external sphincter dyssynergia (9). Hydroureteronephrosis often develops because high intravesical pressure is produced by the simultaneous occurrence of uninhibited detrusor and external urethral sphincter contraction. Effective therapy in males usually requires external sphincterotomy, which results in low intravesical pressure and total urinary incontinence. Bladder drainage is then achieved using an external condom catheter system.

Urinary fistulas

Fistulas may occur at any point along the urinary tract. Usually, the diagnosis is suspected clinically and is confirmed by introducing radiographic contrast into the appropriate area by catheterization, i.e., retrograde urethrography, cystography, or retrograde ureteropyelography.

When recognized early, fistulas often close spontaneously following temporary urinary diversion above the level of the fistula. Initial treatment of renal pelvic or ureteral fistulas consists of percutaneous or open nephrostomy drainage or the use of a ureteral catheter to divert urine. Vesical fistulas can be managed with an indwelling catheter or by suprapubic drainage utilizing a Malecot or de Pezzer catheter. Urine can also be diverted supravesically by means of ureteral catheters or percutaneous nephrostomy tubes. Spontaneous closure of chronic or large vesical fistulas is unusual, however, and they usually require surgical repair, chronic indwelling catheter drainage, or permanent proximal urinary diversion. Urethral fistulas can be treated by an indwelling urethral catheter or the use of a suprapubic catheter.

Hydroureteronephrosis

Distention of the collecting system proximal to a pelviureteric, ureteric, or subvesical obstruction can be temporarily managed by placement of a catheter proximal to or through the obstruction. Surgical correction of the obstructing lesion is then performed as the patient's condition and disease state permit; otherwise, palliative catheter drainage or permanent proximal diversion is needed.

The percutaneous insertion of a drainage tube into the renal pelvis was introduced by Goodwin (10). Apart from providing urinary drainage, these tubes are used to define obstructive lesions by antegrade urography, to obtain urine for culture, to measure renal function, and to assess the hydrodynamic significance of the obstruction (2, 11, 12). Nevertheless, nephrostomy is an external drainage system that is seldom ideal for long-term "curative" or even "palliative" management.

Traditional ureteral catheters used for temporary urinary diversion must exit the urethra and be anchored to an indwelling urethral catheter; otherwise, migration (upward or downward) or dislodgment occurs. Predisposition of the patient to ascending renal infection is an obvious disadvantage. Internal ureteral catheters designed to prevent migration are now widely used for temporary relief of upper tract obstruction and as an adjunct to ureteroscopy and extracorporeal shock-wave lithotripsy (ESWL) (13, 14). Both percutaneous nephrostomy and internal ureteral stents are also useful in the management of symptomatic renal obstruction due to stones occurring in pregnant women. Indeed, these forms of temporary urinary diversion often allow a delay in definitive surgical correction of the obstructing lesion until after delivery (15). Stents and nephrostomy tube drainage are discussed in a subsequent section of this chapter.

Trauma and hematuria

Urethral catheterization is used in cases of trauma to monitor the urinary output of patients who are in shock. When a male patient suffers a pelvic fracture, the integrity of the urethra must be assessed before urethral catheterization is attempted. Once a normal urethra is visualized by means of retrograde urethrography, a Foley balloon catheter can be passed transurethrally and a cystogram done to assess bladder integrity. If the urethrogram shows urethral disruption, urethral catheterization is contraindicated. Instead, the bladder should be drained by means of a suprapubic catheter introduced percutaneously or at open cystostomy.

Transurethral catheterization with a large Foley catheter (22F or 24F) is indicated for patients with gross hematuria. The large lumen permits irrigation of clots from the bladder and the subsequent passage of fresh clots. The indwelling catheter allows egress of urine, monitoring of the hemorrhage, collapse of the bladder wall with concomitant contraction of bleeding vessels, and tamponade of prostatic or urethral bleeding.

Urinary infection

Voided urine specimens in women are often contaminated by periurethral bacterial flora; therefore, collection of a urine sample by "in-and-out" catheterization may be necessary for accurate diagnosis of UTI. Suprapubic needle bladder aspiration remains the least morbid and most accurate method of obtaining a urine sample for culture (16). To localize the site of infection (upper versus lower tract), the clinician can pass ureteral catheters via a cystoscope up each ureter to the renal pelvis following copious bladder irrigation. This allows procurement of differential renal and bladder cultures. A less accurate but less invasive procedure for upper tract localization of infection is the bladder washout technique of Fairley, which utilizes urethral catheterization only (17). Percutaneous aspiration of the renal pelvis for culture may prove necessary when ureteral catheterization is difficult or impossible, e.g., after ureteroneocystostomy or cutaneous ureteroileostomy.

When an obstructed urinary tract becomes infected, prompt drainage is required. Bladder outlet obstruction should be relieved by bladder catheterization; supravesical obstruction may necessitate the insertion of ureteral catheters or nephrostomy tubes (percutaneous or open). Intermittent urethral catheterization is an excellent adjunct in the therapy of cystitis associated with chronic urinary retention or indwelling catheters (4, 18).

Miscellaneous

Urethral catheterization is indicated for instillation of radiographic contrast for cystourethrography, intravesical chemotherapy for bladder carcinoma and interstitial cystitis, and for dissolution of certain calculi. Similarly, ureteral and nephrostomy catheters are used to deliver these agents to the renal pelvis and ureter in selected patients (19).

The recent introduction of percutaneous and extracorporeal shock-wave lithotripsy techniques have led to increased use of indwelling ureteral catheters and percutaneous nephrostomy tubes (20). These applications are dealt with later in this chapter.

INDWELLING URETHRAL CATHETERS

Incidence of infection

Of all patients hospitalized in the USA, about 5% develop nosocomial infections, 40% of which arise from the urinary tract (21, 22). Catheters and instrumentation account for about 80% of genitourinary tract hospital-acquired infections. An estimated 7–16% of all hospitalized patients undergo catheterization, and, of these, 1–3% develop bacteremia, with a mortality rate of about 10% (21). Risk factors for the development of nosocomial UTIs are shown in Table 2. The inlying Foley catheter is used for short-term drainage, e.g., after prostatic surgery, or for long-term drainage, e.g., patients with neuropathic bladders or incontinence. Most of the severe catheter-associated infections tend to occur in patients with catheters left in situ for prolonged periods (23). The National Nosocomial Infections Study (NNIS) (22) and the Study of the Efficiency of Nosocomial Infection Control (SENIC Project (24) show that urethral catheterization most often precedes the development of hospital-acquired urinary tract infection.

The rate of infection associated with in-and-out catheterization in hospitalized patients, mostly women, is about 6%, compared to less than 1% in outpatients (21, 25). This infection rate in hospitalized patients has remained unchanged throughout the past three decades. Single in-and-out catheterization is used to relieve temporary obstruction, to obtain urine from patients unable to provide a clean-catch specimen, to measure residual urine, and to allow radiographic or urodynamic study of the lower urinary tract. The risk of infection with single catheterization is increased in the elderly, the debilitated, the diabetic, the pregnant woman prior to delivery or postpartum, and the patient who carries significant postvoid residual urine (26). Brumfitt and associates (27) noted that women who are catheterized during labor are two to five times more susceptible to infection compared to their noncatheterized counterparts.

In contrast to in-and-out catheterization, the incidence of infection associated with indwelling urethral catheters in hospitalized patients has diminished during the past 30 years, mainly as a result of closed systems of urinary drainage (28). About 95% of patients develop significant bacteriuria within 96 hours of "open" urinary catheter drainage (29, 30). In contrast, with "closed" catheter drainage, the appearance of bacteriuria is usually delayed until the eighth day of catheterization, and only 50% of patients still catheterized at 14 days are infected (31). The SENIC Project documented a linear relationship between the duration of closed system catheterization and the incidence of UTI (24). Closed catheter drainage is clearly effective in reducing bacteriuria.

Diagnosis

Kass defined UTI as more than 100,000 bacteria per milliliter of urine in a single quantitative culture, regardless of symptoms or pyuria (29). Many still use these criteria to define catheter-related UTI; however, others accept lower colony counts (10,000/ml or 1000/ml) as significant levels of bacteriuria in catheterized patients (32, 33).

Urine samples for culture are best obtained from catheterized patients by needle aspiration of the catheter. The catheter is cleansed with alcohol or idophor solution at its junction with the collecting tube. It is then punctured with a 21-gauge (or smaller) needle connected to a syringe and urine is aspirated (34). The accuracy of this technique was confirmed by Bergqvist et al. (35), who found that cultures taken from the distal end of the catheter reliably agreed with those obtained by catheter puncture and percutaneous bladder aspiration. In general, disruption of a "closed" system to obtain a urine sample should not be done because the system may become contaminated. Per-

Table 2. Risk factors for nosocomial UTIs

Female sex
Prolonged catheterization
Advanced age
Debilitating disease
Immunosuppressive therapy
Granulocytopenia
Malnutrition
Alcoholism
Prolonged hospitalization

cutaneous suprapubic bladder aspiration is indicated only when a satisfactory sample cannot be obtained by needle aspiration of the catheter.

PATHOGENESIS OF CATHETER-RELATED INFECTION

Urethral catheterization can inoculate the bladder with bacteria from the perineum, the urethral meatus, or the urethra itself (26, 34). Thorough cleansing of the perineum and periurethral areas usually eradicates resident bacteria from these sites, but only temporarily. The distal third of the male urethra sometimes is colonized with coliforms or *Pseudomonas*; the female urethra, however, often is colonized by potentially pathogenic bacteria from the vagina and introitus (36–38). During catheterization, these urethral bacteria can be displaced into the bladder and cause infection. The normal urethra usually contains small numbers of bacteria, and only about 1% of healthy, nonhospitalized patients subjected to a single catheterization develop bacteriuria (21, 39). The rate of infection, however, is significantly higher in patients prone to urethral and meatal bacterial colonization, i.e., female, elderly, bedridden, and debilitated patients (26, 34). Fecal perineal contamination in incontinent patients also markedly enhances the risk of catheter-associated infection (23).

Other sources of catheter contamination include inadequate sterilization of instruments, catheters, antiseptic solutions, and even the hands of personnel (40, 41). A relationship exists between the extent of professional training of the person who inserts the urethral catheter and the subsequent incidence of bacteriuria. Women catheterized by licensed practical nurses develop about twice the incidence of bacteriuria during the first 48 hours after catheterization as do women who are catheterized by registered nurses or physicians (42).

Because the incidence of urethral bacterial colonization exceeds the rate of infection following in-and-out catheterization, intrinsic defense mechanisms must be operative at the bladder level. Provided the bladder empties completely and the vesical antibacterial factors are intact, infection seldom occurs (43). An active bacterial antiadherence mechanism apparently resides in the mucopolysaccharide glycosaminoglycan (GAG) layer of the bladder mucosa. A deficiency of this layer is thought to make the bladder more susceptible than normal to infection. Indwelling catheters may adversely affect this protective layer and cause increased bacterial adherence, colonization, and infection (44).

Bacteria causing infections while a catheter is inlying enter the bladder by two routes: around the catheter or via the lumen. The major pathway of infection in patients with indwelling catheters is the extraluminal migration of bacteria in the periurethral space (38, 42, 45). About 70% of catheter-associated nosocomial urinary tract infections are preceeded by colonization of the urinary meatus (38, 46). Pericatheter colonization is probably enhanced by the

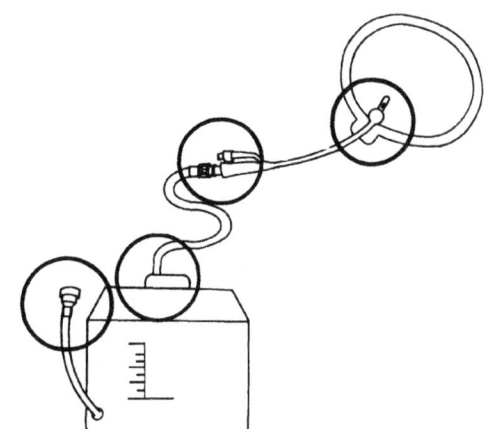

Figure 1. Entry points (circled areas) for bacteria to contaminate the urinary catheter drainage system.

accumulation of urethral secretions that normally are cleared by spontaneous voiding.

Bacteria can also enter the catheter drainage bag or tubing, and ascend within the catheter lumen against the direction of urine flow (47). Infection of bladder urine by this route generally occurs within 12–24 hours after the drainage bag becomes infected (30, 31). Sites of entry of bacteria into a collecting system include the junctions between the catheter and drainage tube, the drainage tube and collecting bag, and the drainage spigot of the collecting bag (42, 47–49) (Figure 1). Elimination of an open junction between the drainage tube and collecting bag markedly reduces infection associated with an indwelling urethral catheter (50). Disruption of the junction between the catheter and drainage tube done for irrigation or infusion of antimicrobics results in increased rates of bacteriuria, even in a closed drainage system (42, 51). Geographical grouping of high-risk catheterized patients, e.g., immunosuppressed, debilitated, those receiving antimicrobics, and those in intensive care units, may lead to bacteriuria caused by multidrug-resistant organisms owing to passive carriage on the hands of attendants (41). Indeed, epidemics of nosocomial catheter-associated bacteriuria have been traced to the transfer of pathogens on the contaminated hands of medical attendants from one drainage bag spigot to another. To prevent this iatrogenic form of infection, medical attendants must carefully wash their hands between attending each patient.

Bacterial isolates in catheter-associated UTIs are usually those organisms found in the gastrointestinal tract of the host. Strains of *Escherichia coli*, species of *Klebsiella* and *Enterobacter*, and enterococci constitute about 50% of isolates found in patients who have not received antibiotics (52). *Staphylococcus epidermidis*, non-group D streptococci, and yeast account for one third of the isolates, especially in patients receiving antibiotics (23, 52). Organisms such as *Pseudomonas* and *Serratia* cause infections late during hospitalization, particularly in patients receiving broad-spectrum antibiotics, bladder irrigations, antineoplastic agents, or immunosuppressive drugs (51–53).

SEQUELAE AND COMPLICATIONS

Although "closed" urinary catheter drainage and other preventive measures reduce the rate of catheter-related UTI, infected patients experience significant morbidity. At least 70% of symptomatic nosocomial bacteriuria cases are probably catheter related (21, 24). While most patients experience cystitis, some develop prostatitis, epididymitis, or pyelonephritis. A special risk exists if infection occurs with urea-splitting bacteria such as *Proteus* species — the rapid formation of "infected" struvite and apatite stones may occur.

Gram-negative bacteremia is the main threat to patients with indwelling catheters. The SENIC Project found that patients with catheters are 5.8 times more susceptible to bacteremia than noncatheterized patients (24). The risk of bacteremia increases with the duration of catheterization and reaches 10% by 37 days (24, 54). Sixty-five percent of bacteremias in the SENIC Project occurred in patients with urinary catheters. Patients who develop bacteremia as a consequence of urinary catheters have a mortality of about 10% (21, 53, 54). In the male patient, acute bacterial prostatitis, prostatic abscess, and epididymitis may develop as a consequence of urethral catheterization.

The noninfectious complications of chronic indwelling urethral catheterization include bladder calculi, contracted bladders, vesicoureteral reflux, urethral incompetence, urethral stricture, urethral fistula, and bladder carcinoma. The incidence of bladder carcinoma is higher than usual in catheterized patients, probably related to chronic inflammation and squamous metaplasia of the epithelium. The highest risk of bladder cancer is in patients managed with indwelling Foley catheters for more than 10 years (55). Chronic catheter use can also cause polypoid cystitis and nephrogenic adenoma. The latter is a nonmalignant metaplastic transformation of the bladder epithelium (56). Polypoid cystitis is a benign reactive but reversible catheter-associated lesion (57). Proper fixation of an indwelling catheter to the lower abdomen reduces the risk of urethral stricture. Such strictures have been reported to occur in many patients having open-heart surgery, probably as a result of mucosal ischemia (58). Catheter encrustation is common on indwelling catheters left in situ for more than 7–10 days. Calcium, magnesium, phosphorus, and urea nitrogen make up about 40% of the dry weight of the encrusted material. Encrustation can be retarded by bladder irrigation with 10% hemiacidrin solution (Renacidin®) or the oral administration of acetohydroxamic acid (Lithostat®). Both agents prevent precipitation of struvite and apatite salts, and thereby impede the formation of bladder calculi (59). Nonlatex catheters, e.g., silicone, are thought to cause less urethritis, catheter encrustation, and stone formation than latex catheters (59, 60).

Occasionally, the Foley balloon may not deflate and catheter removal is impossible (61). The balloon can be ruptured with mineral oil or ether injection. Care must then be taken to ensure that no fragments of the latex balloon remain in the bladder; this may predispose to infection and stone formation. The usual reason the balloon fails to deflate is mechanical collapse of the catheter material in the channel leading to the balloon. This may be overcome by insertion of a fine catheter stylet, such as one from a CVP manometer, to clear the channel (62). After prostatic surgery, a 30-ml balloon catheter is used to prevent slippage of the balloon into the prostatic fossa; however, this large balloon can cause troublesome postoperative bladder spasms that must be managed by the use of anticholinergic agents.

Bladder distension resulting from obstruction to catheter drainage in a quadriplegic patient can lead to autonomic dysreflexia. This occurs in patients with "high" spinal cord injury (above T7) and is manifested by hypertension, severe headache, sweating and piloerection above the level of the lesion, facial flushing, and bradycardia (63). Autonomic dysreflexia can be life threatening and must be treated promptly. The cause of the dysreflexia is uninhibited sympathetic discharge triggered by the bladder distension. The bradycardia is a result of reflex baroreceptor activation in the carotid sinus and aortic arch. Treatment consists of prompt decompression of the bladder and the use of an alphasympatholytic agent, e.g., phentolamine mesylate (63, 64). Chronic, mild dysreflexia may be treated pharmacologically with oral agents, e.g., prazosin 1 mg orally twice daily. Other devastating morbidities can occur as a consequence of urinary tract catheterization, such as bladder gangrene and perforation (65, 66).

PREVENTION AND MANAGEMENT OF CATHETER-ASSOCIATED BACTERIURIA

Indications for catheterization

Catheterization of the urinary tract should be limited to situations where the benefits outweigh the potential risks and complications. The best prophylaxis against catheter-related bacteriuria is avoidance of catheterization. When catheterization is required, in-and-out or intermittent catheterization is preferable to indwelling catheterization.

Aseptic catheterization

Catheter insertion should be performed under aseptic conditions by experienced, trained personnel after thorough cleansing of the meatus and perineum with an antiseptic solution. These solutions should be tested periodically to rule out bacterial contamination. The use of aseptic technique in the handling of the collecting apparatus, especially when the catheter-drainage tubing junction is assembled or when this seal is broken for irrigation, is important.

Closed urinary drainage system

Closed drainage systems reduce the frequency of catheter-associated bacteriuria. These systems feature a conventional two-way catheter attached aseptically to a sterile closed drainage bag or bottle. In 1928, Dukes (67) first described the potential benefits of such a system. However, four decades passed before closed drainage became popular, after studies showed closed systems reduce the rate of catheter-associated infection from more than 80% to 15–30% (42, 68). The incidence of bacteriuria rises sharply, however, when the integrity of the closed system is broken by disconnection of the drainage tube from the catheter for any reason. The system should never be disrupted merely to obtain a urine sample. Instead, one should aspirate urine aseptically from the catheter lumen by means of a syringe and needle. The bag should remain below the level of the patient and never be inverted; the drainage spigot must not be contaminated (69). The entry points for bacteria to contaminate the urinary drainage system are illustrated in Figure 1. These include a) the urethral meatus and around the catheter, b) the junction between the catheter and collection tube, c) the connection of the drainage tubing to the collection bag and reflux from the bag to the tubing, and d) the mouth of the bag drainage spigot.

Prophylaxis of extraluminal bacterial migration

Extraluminal migration of pathogens causes up to 70% of catheter-associated bacteriuria (38, 46). Improved catheters and catheter-care techniques have been designed, and urethral meatal cleansing and asepsis have been recommended, to reduce the incidence of infection caused by this route. However, trials of daily cleansing regimens show neither once-daily cleansing with green soap and water nor twice-daily applications of povidone-iodine solution and ointment are more beneficial than no meatal care in preventing bacteriuria during closed urinary drainage (70). The rates of bacteriuria actually are higher in the treated groups than in the untreated groups, particularly among elderly women with positive meatal cultures. Thus, the antiseptic benefits from meatal care in women may be negated by the adverse effect of urethral manipulation, which may enhance entry of bacteria into the bladder, whether or not the woman is catheterized (71). On the other hand, crusting occurs frequently at the catheter-meatal interface in men, and cleansing is a comfort measure that causes little adverse effect.

Conventional urethral catheters are made of latex. No significant differences in the rate of bacteriuria have been noted among latex and sialastic, polyvinylchloride, or hydro-polymer-coated latex indwelling catheters (72, 73). Moreover, catheters impregnated with antibiotics do not reduce infection rates, probably because the antibacterial activity is short lived (74). Hydrophilic polymer coating of latex catheters does reduce the precipitation of magnesium ammonium phosphate; however, whether this effect potentiates antibiotic therapy of established catheter-related bacteriuria remains unclear (75).

Antibacterial therapy — Prophylaxis and cure

Bacteria gain access to the bladder, drainage tubing, and drainage receptacle despite all efforts at prevention. Antibacterial therapy can be directed at prophylaxis or at cure of established infection.

Bladder irrigation with antimicrobial solutions — e.g., 0.25% acetic acid, neomycin-polmyxin solution — lower the incidence of catheter-associated UTI, but only temporarily. Irrigation can be intermittent or continuous via a three-way Foley catheter. However, constant bladder irrigation is expensive, requires extra nursing time, and can cause discomfort and gross hematuria (76). Systemic absorption may also occur in postoperative patients who have open vascular channels in the bladder or prostatic capsule. Superinfection with resistant bacteria or yeast often develops after extended periods of irrigation. The addition of bacitracin to neomycin/polymyxin can reduce the chance of superinfection with gram-positive cocci (77); however, bladder irrigations have a limited usefulness in the management of indwelling catheters.

Antiseptic solutions placed in drainage bags of closed systems are said to inhibit ascending bladder infections from the bag urine (30, 31, 48). In this regard, the addition of oxycyanide, formalin, chlorhexidine, hydrogen peroxide (3%), and povidone-iodine have all been recommended to reduce catheter-associated bacteriuria (48, 67, 78). However, other studies suggest that the periodic instillation of disinfectants into drainage bags is ineffective in reducing the rate of bacteriuria (79, 80). The matter appears to require additional study.

Experience with systemic antibiotics and urinary antiseptics has been disappointing in patients with indwelling catheters. Not only is the rate of infection seldom reduced, but antibiotic-resistant organisms may emerge (32, 76, 81). The use of antimicrobics combined with strictly closed urinary drainage of short duration can keep the urinary tract sterile or delay in the onset of infection (82–84). The system should be cultured at least weekly, and contaminated systems should be replaced promptly.

Prior to catheter removal, a urine culture should be obtained, and appropriate antibacterial therapy should be instituted to ensure a sterile urinary tract after removal. If the urine is sterile at the time of catheter removal, antibacterial therapy usually is not necessary. An exception is the high-risk patient who suffers from debilitating disease (76, 85). Use of a sulfonamide or nitrofurantoin will often suffice, although some advocate use of trimethoprim-sulfamethoxazole.

Miscellaneous factors

Catheter-care teams may play a role in minimizing catheter-associated bacteriuria and its sequelae (84, 86). Undoubtedly, the education of personnel regarding the importance of hand washing, the use of aseptic technique in catheter handling and care of the drainage bag, the avoidance of unnecessary disruption of a closed drainage system, and the wisdom of physical separation of catheterized patients, as well as of their urine-measuring equipment, will reduce the rate of infection (41, 49). Some argue that availability of a catheter-care team may increase the tendency of physicians to manage their patients with catheterization. Thus, although such a team may reduce the rate of infection, the number of patients catheterized may increase, leading to a greater absolute number of patients with catheter-related infection.

GUIDELINES FOR CATHETER MANAGEMENT

1. Indications for catheterization must be sound.
2. Aseptic intermittent catheterization is preferred to indwelling catheterization whenever possible.
3. Closed drainage is recommended. If contamination occurs, the bag and drainage system should be changed.
4. Urethral catheters should be inserted aseptically. The catheter should be secured to minimize movement.
5. Irrigation of the catheter is best avoided; however, aseptic technique must be used when irrigation is required. In selected patients, continuous irrigation of the bladder with neomycin-polymyxin-bacitracin via a three-way Foley catheter may be used in combination with a closed system.
6. The use of prophylactic systemic antibiotics is not routinely indicated. Symptomatic infections occurring in catheterized patients require therapy based upon urine culture and sensitivity testing.
7. Urine samples should be obtained by aseptic catheter aspiration once weekly for bacteriologic monitoring. Asymptomatic bacteriuria should not be treated until just before the catheter is removed. Exceptions include symptomatic infections or infections caused by urease-producing bacteria.
8. Catheterized patients with bacteriuria should be isolated from catheterized patients who are noninfected. This minimizes cross-contamination.
9. Prior to removal of the catheter, patients with positive urine cultures should be started on pathogen-specific antimicrobial therapy. Cultures should be repeated at 1 week and 1 month following therapy to assure a sterile urinary tract.
10. At the time of insertion or removal of the catheter, patients with bacteriuria (especially due to enterococcus) who have heart murmurs, valvular heart disease, or prosthetic devices should receive prophylactic antimicrobial therapy to prevent bacterial endocarditis or infection of the prosthesis. Prophylactic therapy against bacteremia related to catheter insertion or removal is recommended for all patients who have significant bacteriuria. Generally, therapy should begin about 1 hour before catheter removal or insertion and continue for 24 hours. We recommend gentamicin or tobramycin 1.5 mg/kg IM q 8 h 3 and ampicillin 1 g parenterally q 6 h 4.
11. Members of the hospital staff must be educated regarding all aspects of this system; urinary drainage, catheterization, and asepsis.

INTERMITTENT CATHETERIZATION

Intermittent catheterization is the method of choice for bladder drainage in acute spinal cord injury patients. Sterile intermittent catheterization was introduced by Guttmann to control urinary infection, rehabilitate bladders, and render patients catheter free (87).

The technique of intermittent catheterization requires trained personnel or a well-motivated patient with manual dexterity. Intermittent catheterization may not be practical in a quadriplegic patient who is unable to self-catheterize. The usual catheterization regime requires q 6 h catheterization. The volumes drained and the state of continence between catheterization are monitored, and every effort is made to limit the volumes to 400-600 ml (4, 7). Larger volumes require more frequent catheterization. Incontinence should be evaluated urodynamically to pinpoint the cause, e.g., hyperreflexia or bladder neck incompetence, and to direct pharmacologic therapy. Anticholinergics are used to paralyze the detrusor muscle, and alphasympathomimetics, e.g., ephedrine and phenyl propanolamine, are used to increase bladder neck competence.

The advantages of intermittent catheterization over indwelling Foley catheters include less bacteriuria and infection, increased patient comfort, and less interference with the patient's social and sexual life. Intermittent catheterization is used frequently in spinal cord injury patients, in patients with neurogenic bladder dysfunction, and in the short-term management of urinary retention (18, 88, 89).

Sterile versus clean intermittent catheterization

Guttmann used "sterile" intermittent catheterization because urethral or suprapubic drainage in spinal cord injury patients carries a high risk of infection, sepsis, and renal failure. The effectiveness of this management in paraplegics and quadriplegics was quickly apparent, and most patients were discharged from the hospital with sterile urine (87). Bacteriuria occurs in about 50% of patients on intermittent catheterization, but its significance is not fully known. Some clinicians recommend oral proplylaxis with nitrofurantoin or vitamin C plus methenamine mandelate or bladder instillations with a neomycin-polymyxin solution as methods to reduce this bacteriuria (7, 90, 91). Asymptomatic bacteriuria is, however, usually left untreated in patients who regularly empty their bladders by means of intermittent catheterization (92). Symptomatic patients should be appropriately cultured and treated with antimicrobics. Urethritis and epididymoorchitis often occur early in the course of intermittent catheterization; therefore, oral antibiotics are routinely prescribed for all patients during the first few weeks of the program (93).

Lapides et al. (18) believe that infection occurs secondary to decreased bladder resistance and vascularity resulting from bladder overdistension. Prevention of overdistension by frequent catheterization therefore allows the natural bladder defenses to overcome any bacteria introduced into the bladder during clean catheterization. Intermittent clean catheterization is now frequently used in adults and children to manage retention, detrusor areflexia, and bladder dysfunction. Clean catheterization more often leads to asymptomatic bacteriuria than sterile intermittent catheterization; however, each is a safe and effective method of bladder drainage that allows preservation of the patient's self-esteem, avoids the use of external collecting devices, and minimizes the occurrence of clinically significant infection and urosepsis. Sterile intermittent catheterization is recommended for hospitalized patients to avoid the risk of nosocomial UTIs. Nonhospitalized patients can be adequately managed with clean catheterization.

Correct methods must be carefully taught to patients performing intermittent, clean self-intermittent catheterization. Motivation and a good understanding of the external genitalia and urethral anatomy are prerequisites. The catheter size (8F–16 F) varies with the age of the patient; rubber, plastic, or metal catheters are used. In clean intermittent catheterization, soap and water are used to cleanse the catheter and external genitalia. Only water-soluble lubricants, e.g., K-Y jelly, are recommended. The catheter is boiled in hot water for about 5 minutes daily and then is stored in a clean, dry container between catheterizations.

In addition to bacteriuria and incontinence, there are other complications of intermittent catheterization (93). Mechanical problems secondary to adductor spasms, obesity, hypospadiac external urethral openings, and edema can make catheter insertion difficult. Whole catheters or tips of catheters can be "lost" inside the bladder and make cystoscopic removal necessary. Bladder calculi, usually calcium phosphate, can result from the introduction of oil-based lubricants or pubic hair into the bladder. These stones may be asymptomatic and only discovered on routine x-ray films, or they may cause recurrent infection, bladder spasms, or sudden interruption of urinary drainage via the catheter. Usually these stones are managed by endoscopic removal or lithotripsy.

NEPHROSTOMY TUBES

The technique of nonsurgical catheter placement within the renal pelvis (percutaneous nephrostomy) was first used by Goodwin to drain a hydronephrotic renal pelvis (10). This technique is now frequently used in treating various renal conditions: hydronephrosis, percutaneous endourological manipulations, postoperative urinary drainage, percutaneous stone dissolution, determination of renal function, and assessment of the degree of upper tract obstruction (the Whitaker pressure-perfusion test) (2, 11, 12).

Nephrostomy tubes are inserted via "open" or percutaneous routes. Large-diameter (18F–22F) Malecot or de Pezzer catheters can be placed in the renal pelvis during surgery, e.g., pyelolithotomy or anatrophic nephrolithotomy, to allow urinary drainage and to permit postoperative access for radiographic study or chemolysis of residual stone fragments (19). Small-diameter nephrostomy tubes (8F–14F) are inserted percutaneously using local anaesthesia, and an angiographic guide wire is controlled by fluoroscopy, ultrasound, or computed tomography (2). The nephrostomy "tract" obtained by the percutaneous approach can be dilated using fascial or balloon dilators (24F–32F), which affords easy access into the renal pelvis for percutaneous endourological procedures, e.g., stone removal or ultrasonic lithotripsy (94, 95). After endourological procedures, the nephrostomy tube is left in situ for 24–72 hours to monitor bleeding, to prevent urinary extravasation, and to provide urinary drainage. Percutaneous nephrostomy tube placement is now a routine hospital procedure performed under radiographic control and local anesthesia in most institutions.

Percutaneous nephrostomy tube placement and percutaneous stone removal (percutaneous nephrolithotomy) are associated with various complications, the most significant of which is bleeding (95). Transient venous bleeding, which occurs during tube placement, is usually self-limiting. Percutaneous stone manipulation (removal or lithotripsy) and tract dilatation can cause more troublesome parenchymal bleeding. This bleeding, mainly venous, generally is controlled by the tamponade effect of the rigid nephroscope sheath used for stone manipulation. Following manipulation, a large nephrostomy tube is left in the renal pelvis for drainage and a diuretic is given parenterally to assist in clot prevention (96, 97).

The most significant complication of percutaneous stone removal is sudden hemorrhage from a segmental branch of the renal artery, a pseudoaneurysm, or an arteriovanous fistula (98). Significant arterial bleeding, immediate or delayed, occurs in less than 1% of patients (96). Acute hemorrhage is manifested by gross hematuria or bleeding through or around the nephrostomy tube, either continuously or intermittently. Blood transfusions are given as needed, and an effort is made to control the bleeding using a Foley balloon or angiographic balloon to tamponade the nephrostomy tract. Persistent bleeding is managed by renal angiography with selective embolization of the bleeding vessel. This usually stops the bleeding and makes surgical exploration unnecessary. If angiographic embolization is unsuccessful, surgical exploration, often resulting in partial or total nephrectomy, is necessary.

Other important complications of percutaneous endourology are extravasation and sepsis. Rents in the renal pelvis occurring during tube placement or manipulation can lead to extravasation of fluid into the retroperitoneal space. Absorption of this fluid leads to fluid overload, to hyponatremia, and, if glycine is used, to hyperammonemia. Strict monitoring of fluid ingress and egress during percutaneous stone surgery is necessary (97). Prophylactic antibiotics are usually administered to reduce the chance of urosepsis.

Most problems with nephrostomy tubes are mechanical (99). The tube may become dislodged or urinary drainage may be blocked by sediment or clots. Dislodgement is prevented by anchoring the tube to the skin with a nonabsorbabale silk or nylon suture. Self-retaining nephrostomy tubes — e.g., Cope, Foley, Circle — reduce the chance of migration or dislodgement. If a tube is dislodged completely, the tract can usually be renegotiated using a guide wire and a new tube inserted under fluoroscopic control. Tube blockage is reduced by frequent gentle irrigation with normal saline solution, the use of a large-diameter tube, and by frequent tube changes. A high fluid intake with a brisk diuresis is also helpful (99). Skin care at the catheter entry site consists of cleansing with antiseptics and frequent sterile dressing changes.

Percutaneous chemolysis is a useful adjunct for dissolving struvite renal calculi. Chemolysis, occasionally performed as a primary procedure in selected poor-risk patients, generally is used to remove residual stone fragments after open renal surgery, extracorporeal shockwave lithotripsy, or percuttaneous lithotripsy. A 10% hemiacidrin solution (Renacidin®) is useful for dissolving triple phosphate calculi, whereas alkalinating agents, e.g., bicarbonate and Tham-E, dissolve uric acid calculi (19). Sepsis is always a potential complication of percutaneous irrigation, especially when infected struvite calculi are present. Marked elevations in renal pelvic pressure (> 30 cm H_2O are contraindicated and are best avoided by the use of a three-way irrigation system incorporating a manometer. This prevents backflow of urine and fluid into the vascular system and reduces the risk of bacteremia. Hemiacidrin solution contains magnesium; its excessive absorption can lead to hypermagnesemia with resultant neuromuscular paralysis. For this reason, serum magnesium levels should be monitored daily. Urine cultures are obtained frequently, and appropriate pathogen-specific antimicrobial drugs are administered during percutaneous irrigation (19).

Nephrostomy tubes left in situ for more than a few days cause bacteriuria. The responsible organisms often are common gram-positive skin bacteria (staphylococci and streptococci) that enter through or alongside the nephrostomy tube (100). Appropriate antimicrobial agents are used to treat symptomatic infections or are used at the time of tube removal. Antibiotic prophylaxis or treatment of asymptomatic infections require careful consideration because infection with more resistant pathogens may develop.

URETERAL STENTS

Stents are used for urinary drainage and to provide proper alignment of the ureter following surgical procedures. The recent introduction of ureteroscopic procedures, percutaneous endourology, and extracorporeal shock-wave lithotripsy (ESWL) has led to a marked increase in the use of ureteral stents (14, 20, 101). The stents are used to prevent obstruction by stone fragments (steinstrasse) following ESWL lithotripsy, to push ureteral stones back into the renal pelvis and thus allow ESWL treatment, and to "stent" the ureter following ureteroscopic manipulation and ureteral dilatation. Stents are also employed to relieve obstructive uropathy, e.g., metastatic retroperitoneal disease or benign retroperitoneal fibrosis; to manage ureteral fistulas; and to prevent leaks from ureteral surgery. The widespread use of stents has reduced the need for open surgery in many urologic conditions (102).

Ureteral stents may be external or internal. The distal end of external ureteral stents traverse the urethra and are usually tied externally to an indwelling catheter using silk ligatures. Stent migration (upward or downward) potential, the threat of ascending upper tract infection, and patient discomfort make external stents unsuitable for long-term use.

Internal or "indwelling" ureteral stents have the advantage of not requiring a Foley catheter for external fixation. The double-J ureteral catheter is the most widely used internal stent. J configurations at the upper and lower ends prevent migration, and its silicone composition affords flexibility and tissue biocompatibility. The softness of the silicone ensues patient comfort, although ureteral placement over a guide wire may prove difficult. Other materials used in the manufacture of stents include polyethylene, polyurethane, and C-flex (a copolymer of silicone). The use of the Gibbons ureteral stent (5), a flanged polyethylene catheter, has been supplanted by the newer double-J stents (3, 102).

Ureteral stents are inserted in various ways. Endoscopic retrograde insertion via the cystoscope or the ureteroscope is the most common technique. Stents are usually inserted over a guide wire under fluoroscopic control. Attention to stent position, size (usually 3F–8F diameter), and length (20–30 cm) is important. Improper stent selection can lead to traumatic bleeding from the renal pelvis or bladder, trigonal irritation, and poor urinary drainage. Stents can also be inserted percutaneously in an antegrade approach or by open operative placement (102).

Indwelling ureteral stents can result in vesicoureteral reflux, microscopic hematuria, pyuria, encrustation, and irritative bladder symptoms. Urosepsis is uncommon unless the stent becomes occluded. Unless very high intravesical pressures are generated, reflux occurs in only about 50% of patients. Bladder irritation (frequency, urgency, pain) generally indicates that the stent is too long and its distal end rests on the trigone or at the bladder neck. If these symptoms persist, the stent should be replaced with a shorter one. Pyuria is common in patients with indwelling stents; it usually represents a reaction to the stent's foreign material, not infection. Urine cultures should be obtained at least monthly in patients with indwelling stents; appropriate antibiotics should be prescribed as indicated. Encrustation of ureteral stents occurs commonly, especially in patients with bacteriuria or histories of urolithiasis (103, 104). Catheter encrustation can lead to struvite stone formation, which may necessitate treatment with percutaneous renal pelvic irrigation or open surgical removal. Long-term antimicriboal suppression, frequent abdominal x-ray studies, and short periods of internal stenting are recommended to reduce the occurrence of catheter encrustation and stone formation (104).

Upward migration of ureteral stents can cause obstruction, sepsis, or stone formation. Displaced stents generally can be retrieved from "below" using the ureteroscope or from "above" by a percutaneous approvach. Nondisplaced internal stents usually are removed or replaced via the cystoscope. Internal stents can be removed without cystoscopy if, during placement, a nonabsorbable suture is tied to the bladder end of the stent, is exteriorized through the urethra, and is taped to the penis or abdomen. A gentle tug on the suture usually suffices to remove the stent without urethral manipulation or cystoscopy (105). This method is used in children and in patients requiring short-term stents following shock-wave lithotripsy or ureteroscopic stone removal. Breakage can occur due to stent damage at the time of insertion or overzealous use of force during endoscopic removal (106). Stents used for long-term drainage must be changed frequently, especially in elderly, debilitated patients who tend to forget about their stents, become dehydrated, and thus promote catheter encrustation and stone formation. Patients with ureteral stents must be monitored carefully and evaluated promptly if fever, flank pain, gross hematuria, azotemia, or infection develop.

EXTERNAL "CONDOM" CATHETER DRAINAGE

"Condom" catheters are external collecting devices used in managing incontinent male patients who are able to empty their bladders: patients with central nervous system disease, e.g., cerebrovascular accidents; postprostatectomy incontinence; and detrusor hyperreflexia, e.g., quadriplegia or multiple sclerosis (107). Patients with hyperreflexia and associated detrusor-external sphincter dyssynergia are unsuitable for condom catheter drainage unless external sphincterotomy is performed. Condom drainage is not suitable for female patients.

Various types of condom catheters are commercially available. They can also be constructed makeshift using a condom or a finger cot. The condom part of the catheter is fixed to the penile shaft using tincture of benzoin, tape, and a surgical adhesive to provide a skin bond. Patients with short penile shafts have difficulty in keeping the condom on the penis, but this can be corrected by insertion of a penile prosthesis to provide increased length and rigidity.

Incontinent patients managed with condom catheters have a high rate of bacteriuria, particularly with *Proteus* and *Pseudomonas* species (8, 108, 109). Bacteria from the penis, perineum, and scrotum colonize the condom part of the collecting device, and this bacterial reservoir leads to ascending bacterial infection. Urine cultures are unreliable with the condom in place; instead, the condom device should be removed, the penis cleaned, and a midstream or catheterized specimen obtained.

In addition to problems with bacteriuria, a poorly fitted condom device can cause penile skin maceration, skin breakdown, skin necrosis, urethrocutaneous fistulas, and obstruction to urinary flow. These problems can be avoided by careful application of the catheter, prevention of kinking of the tubings, and frequent patient monitoring. The latter is particularly important in patients with neuropathic bladders who have absent or reduced penile sensation. Skin breakdown and pressure necrosis may go undetected in these patients because they lack pain sensation (110). Patients with condom catheters who are plagued by recurrent, symptomatic infections should be switched to another form of bladder drainage.

SUPRAPUBIC CATHETERS

The recognition that indwelling urethral catheters lead to many problems has resulted in an increased use of the suprapubic catheter for bladder drainage (111, 112). Suprapubic catheters are well tolerated, require less nursing care than indwelling urethral catheters, avoid ascending pericatheter urethral infection, and generally prevent prostatitis and epididymitis.

Suprapubic catheters can be inserted percutaneously or directly in the bladder during open surgical procedures. For the latter procedure, wide-bore catheters of the de Pezzer or Malecot variety are used. The recent development of various percutaneous suprapubic catheters, e.g., Stamey suprapubic catheter and sialistic Cysto-cath, allows percutaneous insertion under local anesthesia. This is a simple bedside procedure that is well tolerated by the patient. The patient should have a full bladder before the tube is inserted; otherwise, the bowel may be damaged. If the bladder is not palpable, a spinal needle (#20) should first be inserted percutaneously into the bladder, urine aspirated, and the bladder distended via the needle with sterile saline. Patients who have undergone previous lower abdominal or pelvic surgery may have bowel or peritoneum attached to the bladder, which often makes them better candidates for open suprapubic cystostomy than for percutaneous cystostomy.

Percutaneous suprapubic catheters are used for bladder drainage in various situations (113). They are preferred to indwelling urethral catheters in men who develop acute urinary retention associated with acute bacterial prostatitis. The suprapubic tube is also used following antiincontinence surgery, e.g., Stamey urethropexy or Burch colposuspension, to minimize infection and to measure residual urine during postoperative voiding trials.

The suprapubic catheter is well tolerated, and its short-term use produces few complications. Bladder irritability can develop if the catheter tip abuts the bladder trigone. This is managed by adjustment of catheter position or use of an oral anticholinergic, e.g., oxybutynin chloride or propantheline bromide. Bacteriuria may occur via the spread of skin bacteria alongside the tube into the bladder; however, bacteriuria rates are less with suprapubic tubes than with indwelling urethral catheters.

The long-term use of suprapubic tubes, especially in debilitated and elderly patient, results in a chronic foreign body reaction, with the risk of chronic cystitis, bladder contracture, bladder stones, and possible malignant transformation of the bladder epithelium.

REFERENCES

1. Beeson PB: The case against the catheter (editorial). *Am J Med* 24:1-3, 1958.
2. Fowler JE Jr, Meares EM Jr, Goldin RA: Percutaneous nephrostomy: Techniques, indications and results. *Urology* 6:428-434, 1975.
3. Finney RP: Experience with new double J ureteral catheter stents. *J Urol* 120:678-681, 1978.
4. Perkash I: Intermittent catheterization: The urologist's point of view. *J Urol* 111:356-360, 1974.
5. Gibbons RP, Correa RJ Jr, Cummings KB, Mason JT: Experience with indwelling ureteral stent catheter. *J Urol* 115:22-26, 1976.
6. Leventhal A, Pfau A: Pharmacologic management of postoperative overdistention of the bladder. *Surg Gynecol Obstet* 146:347-348, 1978.
7. Anderson RU: Non-sterile intermittent catheterization with antibiotic prophylaxis in the acute spinal cord injured male patient. *J Urol* 124:392-394, 1980.
8. Hirsh DD, Fainstein V, Musher DM: Do condom catheter collecting systems cause urinary tract infection? *JAMA* 242:340-341, 1979.
9. Fam BA, Rossier AB, Blunt K, Gabilondo FB, Sarkarati M, Sethi J, Yalla SV: Experience in the urologic management of 120 early spinal cord injury patients. *J Urol* 119:485-487, 1978.
10. Goodwin WE, Casey WC, Woolf W: Percutaneous trocar (needle) nephrostomy in hydronephrosis. *JAMA* 157:891-894, 1955.
11. Pfister RC, Newhouse JH: Interventional percutaneous pyeloureteral techniques. II. Percutaneous nephrostomy and other procedures. *Radiol Clin N Am* 17:351-362, 1979.
12. Whitaker RH: Methods of assessing obstruction in dilated ureters. *Br J Urol* 45:15-23, 1973.
13. Huffman JL, Bagley DH, Lyon ES: Extending cystoscopic techniques into the ureter and renal pelvis — experience with ureteroscopy and pyeloscopy. *JAMA* 250:2002-2005, 1983.
14. Campbell RJ, Griffith DP: Exchange ureteral stent insertion using pullout suture after extracorporeal shock wave lithotripsy. *Urology* 29:653-655, 1987.
15. Cass AS, Smith CS, Gleich P: Management of urinary calculi in pregnancy. *Urology* 28:370-372, 1986.
16. Stamey TA, Pfau A: Urinary infections: A selective review and some observations. *Calif Med* 113:16-35, 1970.
17. Fairley KF, Bond AG, Brown RB, Habersberger P: Simple test to determine the site of urinary tract infection. *Lancet* 2:427-428, 1967.
18. Lapides J, Diokno AC, Gould FR, Lowe BS: Further observations of self-catheterization. *J Urol* 116:169-171, 1976.
19. Sant GR, Blaivas JG, Meares EM Jr: Hemiacidrin irrigation in the management of struvite calculi: Longterm results. *J Urol* 1048-1050, 1983.
20. Dretler SP: Management of "steinstrasse." *Endourology* 1:1-2, 1986.
21. Meares EM Jr: Nosocomial urinary tract infections. *Infect Surg* 5:278-280, 1986.
22. Allen JR, Hightower AW, Martin SM, Dixon RE: Secular trends in nosocomial infections: 1970-1979. *Am J Med* 70:389-392, 1981.
23. Sant GR: Urinary tract infections in the elderly. *Semin Urol* 5:126-153, 1987.
24. Haley RW, Hooton TM, Culver DH, Stanley RC, Emori TG, Hardison CD, Quade D, Shachtman RH, Schaberg DR, Shah BV, Schatz GD: Nosocomial infections in U.S. hospitals, 1975-1976. Estimated frequency by selected characteristics of patients. *Am J Med* 70:947-959, 1981.
25. Marple CD: The frequency and character of urinary tract infections in an unselected group of women. *Ann Intern Med* 14:2220-2239, 1941.
26. Turck M, Goffe B, Petersdorf RG: The urethral catheter and urinary tract infection. *J Urol* 88:834-837, 1962.
27. Brumfitt W, Davies BI, Rosser E: Urethral catheter as a cause of urinary-tract infection in pregnancy and puerperium. *Lancet* 2:1059-1062, 1961.
28. Finkelberg R, Kunin CM: Clinical evaluation of closed urinary drainage systems. *JAMA* 207:1657-1662, 1969.
29. Kass EH: Asymptomatic infections of the urinary tract. *Trans Assoc Am Physicians* 69:56-63, 1956.
30. Kunin CM, McCormack RC: Prevention of catheter-induced urinary tract infections by sterile closed drainage. *N Engl J Med* 274:1155-1161, 1966.
31. Martin CM, Bookrajian EN: Bacteriuria prevention after indwelling urinary catheterization. A controlled study. *Arch Intern Med* 110:703-711, 1962.
32. Warren JW, Platt R, Thomas RJ, Rosner B, Kass EH: Antibiotic irrigation and catheter-associated urinary tract infections. *N Engl J Med* 299:570-573, 1978.
33. Stark R, Maki D: Bacteriuria in the catheterized patient. What quantitative level of bacteriuria is relevant. *N Engl J Med* 311:560-564, 1984.
34. Turck M, Stamm W: Nosocomial infection of the urinary tract. *Am J Med* 70:651-654, 1981.
35. Bergqvist D, Brönnestam R, Hedelin H, Stahl A: The relevance of urinary sampling methods in patients with indwelling foley catheters. *Br J Urol* 52:92-95, 1980.
36. Helmholtz HF: Determination of the bacterial content of the urethra. A new method, with results of a study of 82 men. *J Urol* 64:158-162, 1950.
37. Cox CE: The urethra and its relationship to urinary tract infection: The flora of the normal female urethra. *South Med J* 59:621-626, 1966.
38. Garibaldi RA, Burke JP, Britt MR, Miller WA, Smith CB: Meatal colonization and catheter-associated bacteriuria. *N Engl J Med* 303:316-318, 1980.
39. Guze LB, Beeson PB: Observations on the reliability and safety of bladder catheterization for bacteriologic study of the urine. *N Engl J Med* 255:474-475, 1956.
40. Hardy PG, Ederer GM, Matsen JM: Contamination of commercially packaged urinary catheter kits with pseudomonad EO-1. *N Engl J Med* 282:33-35, 1970.
41. Maki DG, Hennekens CH, Bennett JV: Prevention of catheter-associated urinary tract infection. An additional measure. *JAMA* 221:1270-1271, 1972.
42. Garibaldi RA, Burke JP, Dickman ML, Smith CB: Factors predisposing to bacteriuria during indwelling urethral catheterization. *N Engl J Med* 291:215-219, 1974.
43. Cox CE, Hinman F Jr: Experiments with induced bacteriuria, vesical emptying and bacterial growth on the mechan-

ism of bladder defense to infection. *J Urol* 86:739–748, 1961.
44. Daifuku R, Stamm WE: Bacterial adherence to bladder urothelial cells in catheter-associated urinary tract infection. *N Engl J Med* 314:1208–1213, 1986.
45. Kass EH, Schneiderman LJ: Entry of bacteria into the urinary tract of patients with inlying catheters. *N Engl J Med* 256:556–557, 1957.
46. Bultitude MI, Eykyn S: The relationship between the urethral flora and urinary infection in the catheterized male. *Br J Urol* 45:678–683, 1975.
47. Weyrauch HM, Bassett BJ: Ascending infection in an artificial urinary tract. *Stanford Med Bull* 9:25–29, 1951.
48. Maizels M, Schaeffer AJ: Decreased incidence of bacteriuria associated with periodic instillations of hydrogen peroxide into the urethral catheter drainage bag. *J Urol* 123:841–845, 1980.
49. Rutala WA, Kennedy VA, Loflin HB, Sarrubbi FA: Serratia marcescens nosocomial infections of the urinary tract associated with urine measuring containers and urinometers. *Am J Med* 70:659–663, 1981.
50. Gillespie WA, Lennon GG, Linton KB, Slade N: Prevention of catheter infection of urine in female patients. *Br Med J* 2:12–16, 1962.
51. Schaberg DR, Weinstein RA, Stamm WE: Epidemics of nosocomial urinary tract infection caused by multiple resistant gram-negative bacilli: Epidemiology and control. *J Infect Dis* 133:363–366, 1976.
52. McCormack RC: Nosocomial urinary tract infections. In: EW Hook, GL Mandell, JM Gwaltney Jr, MA Sande, eds, *Current Concepts of Infectious Diseases*. John Wiley & Sons, New York, pp 233–240, 1977.
53. Krieger JN, Kaiser DI, Wenzel RP: Nosocomial urinary tract infections. Secular trends, treatment and economics in a university hospital. *J Urol* 130:102–106, 1983.
54. McCabe WR, Jackson GG: Gram-negative bacteremia. I. Etiology and ecology. *Arch Intern Med* 110:847–855, 1962.
55. Locke JR, Hill DE, Walzer Y: Incidence of squamous cell carcinoma in patients with long-term catheter drainage. *J Urol* 131:1034–1035, 1985.
56. Ritchey ML, Novicki DE, Schultenover SJ: Nephrogenic adenoma of bladder: A report of 8 cases. *J Urol* 131:537–539, 1984.
57. Ekelund P, Johansson S: Polypoid cystitis: A catheter-associated lesion of the human bladder. *Acta Path Microb Scand* 87A:179, 1979.
58. Elhilali MM, Hassouna M, Abdel-Hakim A, Teijeira J: Urethral stricture following cardiovascular surgery: Role of urethral ischemia. *J Urol* 135:275–277, 1986.
59. Burns JR, Gauthier JF: Prevention of urinary catheter encrustations by acetohydroxamic acid. *J Urol* 132:455–456, 1984.
60. Nacey JN, Delahunt D, Tulloch AGS: The assessment of catheter-induced urethritis using an experimental dog model. *J Urol* 134:623–625, 1985.
61. Kelly TWJ, Griffiths GL: Ballon problems with Foley catheters. *Lancet* 2:1310, 1983.
62. Kleeman FJ: Technique for removal of Foley catheter when balloon does not deflate. *Urology* 21:416, 1983.
63. McGuire EJ, Wagner FM, Weiss RM: Treatment of autonomic dysreflexia with phenoxybenzamine. *J Urol* 115:53, 1976.
64. Texter JH Jr, Reece RW, Hranowsky N: Pentolinium in the management of autonomic hyperreflexia. *J Urol* 116:350–351, 1976.
65. Busse K, Altwein JE: Catheter-induced bladder gangrene. *J Urol* 112:461–462, 1974.
66. Freed JS, Krespi Y: Urologic catheter — unusual complication. *N Y State J Med* 79:1892–1893, 1979.
67. Dukes C: Urinary infections after excision of the rectum: Their cause and prevention. *Proc R Soc Med* 22:259–270, 1928.
68. Miller A, Linton KB, Gillispie WA, Slade N, Mitchell JP: Catheter drainage and infection in acute retention of urine. *Lancet* 1:310–312, 1960.
69. Buddington WT, Graves RC: Management of catheter drainage. *J Urol* 62:387–393, 1949.
70. Burke JP, Garibaldi RA, Britt MR, Jacobson JA, Conti M, Alling DW: Prevention of catheter-associated urinary tract infections. Efficacy of daily meatal care regimen. *Am J Med* 70:655–658, 1981.
71. Bran JL, Levison ME, Kaye D: Entrance of bacteria into the female urinary bladder. *N Engl J Med* 286:626–629, 1972.
72. Tidd MJ, Gow JG, Pennington JH, Shelton J, Scott MR: Comparison of hydrophilic polymer-coated latex, untreated latex and PVC indwelling balloon catheters in the prevention of urinary infection. *Br J Urol* 48:285–291, 1976.
73. Monson T, Kunin CM: Evaluation of a polymer-coated indwelling catheter in prevention of infection. *J Urol* 111:220–222, 1974.
74. Butler HK, Kunin CM: Evaluation of polymyxin catheter lubricant and impregnated catheters. *J Urol* 100:560–566, 1968.
75. Miller JM: The effect of hydron on latex urinary catheters. *J Urol* 113:530, 1975.
76. Andriole VT: Hospital acquired urinary infections and the indwelling catheter. *Urol Clin N Am* 451–469, 1975.
77. Fincke BG, Friedland G: Prevention and management of infection in the catheterized patient. *Urol Clin N Am* 3:313–321, 1976.
78. Webb JK, Blandy JP: Closed urinary drainage into plastic bags containing antiseptic *Br J Urol* 40:585–588, 1968.
79. Thompson RL, Haley CE, Searcy MA, Guenthner SM, Kaiser DL, Gröschel DHM, Gillenwater JY, Wenzel RP: Catheter-associated bacteriuria: Failure to reduce attack rates using periodic instillations of a disinfectant into urinary drainage systems. *JAMA* 251:747–751, 1984.
80. Kunin CM: The drainage bag additive saga. *Infect Control* 6:261–262, 1985.
81. Brocklehurst JC, Brocklehurst S: The management of indwelling catheters. *Br J Urol* 50:102–105, 1978.
82. Britt MR, Garibaldi RA, Miller WA, Hebertson RM, Burke JP: Antimicrobial prophylaxis for catheter-associated bacteriuria. *Antimicrob Agents Chemother* 11:240–243, 1977.
83. Turck M, Petersdorf RG: The role of antibiotics in the prevention of urinary tract infections. *J Chronic Dis* 15:683–689, 1962.
84. Shapito SR, Santamarina A, Harrison JH: Cather-associated urinary tract infections: Incidence and a new approach to prevention. *J Urol* 112:659–663, 1974.
85. Chodak GW, Plaut ME: Systemic antibiotics for prophylaxis in urologic surgery: A critical review. *J Urol* 121:695–699, 1979.
86. Stamm WE: Guidelines for prevention of catheter-associated urinary tract infection. *Ann Intern Med* 82:386–390, 1975.
87. Guttmann L: Initial treatment of traumatic paraplegia. *Proc R Soc Med* 47:1103, 1954.

88. Firlit CF, Canning JR, Lloyd FA, Cross RR, Brewer RJ Jr: Experience with intermittent catheterization in chronic spinal cord injury patients. *J Urol* 114:234–236, 1975.
89. Kyker J, Gregory JG, Shah J, Schoenberg HW: Comparison of intermittent catheterization and supravesical diversion in children with meningomyelocele. *J Urol* 118:90–91, 1977.
90. Anderson RU: Prophylaxis of bacteriuria during intermittent catheterization of the acute neurogenic bladder. *J Urol* 123:364–366, 1980.
91. Orikasa S, Koyanagi T, Motomura M, Kudo T, Tozashi M, Tsuju I: Experience with non-sterile, intermittent self-catheterization. *J Urol* 115:141–143, 1976.
92. Hinman F Jr: Intermittent catheterization and vesical defenses. *J Urol* 117:57–60, 1977.
93. Klauber GT, Sant GR: Complications of intermittent catheterization. *Urol Clin N Am* 10:557–562, 1983.
94. White EC, Smith AD: Percutaneous stone extraction from 200 patients. *J Urol* 132:437–438, 1984.
95. Segura JW: Endourology. *J Urol* 132:1079–1084, 1984.
96. Segura JW: Percutaneous endourology: Vascular complications. *World J Urol* 3:24–26, 1985.
97. Rudy DC, Woodside JR, Borden TA, Ball WS: Adult respiratory distress syndrome complicating percutaneous nephrolithotomy. *Urology* 23:376–377, 1984.
98. Kalash SS, Young JD Jr: Serious complications associated with percutaneous nephrolithotomy. *Urology* 29:290–293, 1987.
99. Roven SJ, Rosen RJ: Percutaneous nephrostomy and maintenance of nephrostomy drainage. *Urology* 23 (Special Issue, Part 1):25–28, 1984.
100. Sant GR, Hawes R, Meares EM Jr: "Bacteriuria" in patients with nephrostomy tubes — implications for antibiotic use in endourology. *J Urol* 135 (Supplement):255A, 1986.
101. El-Kappany H, Gaballah MA, Ghoneim MA: Rigid ureteroscopy for the treatment of ureteric calculi. Experience in 120 cases. *Br J Urol* 58:491–503, 1986.
102. Smith AD: Percutaneous ureteral surgery and stenting. *Urology* 23:37–42, 1984.
103. Spirnak JP, Resnick MI: Stone formation as a complication of indwelling ureteral stents: A report of 5 cases. *J Urol* 134:349–351, 1985.
104. Schulze KA, Wettlaufer JN, Oldani G: Encrustation and stone formation: Complication of indwelling ureteral stents. *Urology* 25:616–619, 1985.
105. Siegel A, Altadonna V, Ellis D, Hulbert W, Elder J, Duckett J: Simplified method of indwelling ureteral stent removal. *Urology* 28:429, 1986.
106. Sasagawa I, Nakada T, Akiya T, Umeda K, Sakamoto M, Katayama T: Use of indwelling double-curved ureteral stents and problems after stenting. *Eur Urol* 13:176–179, 1987.
107. Nanninga JB, Rosen J: Problems associated with the use of external urinary collectors in the male paraplegic. *Paraplegia* 13:56–58, 1975.
108. Johnson ET: The condom catheter: Urinary tract infection and other complications. *South Med J* 76:579–582, 1983.
109. Fierer J, Ekstrom M: An outbreak of *Providencia stuartii* urinary tract infections — Patients with condom catheters are a reservoir of the bacteria. *JAMA* 245:1553–1555, 1981.
110. Steinhardt G, McRoberts W: Total distal penile necrosis caused by condom catheter. *JAMA* 244:11–12, 1980.
111. Bruschchini H, Tanagho EA: Cystostomy drainage: Its efficacy in preventing residual urine and infection. *J Urol* 118:391–393, 1977.
112. Hodgkinson CP, Hodari AA: Trocar suprapubic cystostomy for post-operative bladder drainage in the female. *Gynecol* 96:773–783, 1966.
113. Peatfield RC, Burt AA: Smith PH: Suprapubic catheterization after spinal cord injury: A follow-up report. *Paraplegia* 21:220–226, 1983.

CHAPTER 62

Nonsurgical Management of Vesicourethral Dysfunction

J. KEITH LIGHT

INTRODUCTION

The conservative or nonsurgical treatment of voiding dysfunction has improved significantly, due predominantly to an improved understanding of the basic neurophysiologic mechanisms regulating the function of the bladder and urethra. Although still far from satisfactory, further research will undoubtedly open new avenues of treatment.

A basic understanding of the anatomy and physiology of the lower urinary tract is important when applying the principles of pharmacologic manipulation.

APPLIED NEUROPHYSIOLOGY

The lower urinary tract is innervated by both the autonomic and somatic nervous systems. The function of urine storage and expulsion is controlled by a complex set of reflex mechanisms involving both the central and peripheral circuits.

Autonomic nervous system

Both the parasympathetic and sympathetic components of the autonomic nervous system play a role in the lower urinary tract.

PARASYMPATHETIC NERVOUS SYSTEM

The parasympathetic nervous system via the pelvic nerve originates in the intermediolateral nuclei of the sacral spinal segments S2–S4. Both human and animal experiments suggest that S3 is the main segment affecting detrusor function (1, 2). Stimulation of the pelvic nerve results in a sustained detrusor contraction. Acetylcholine is the main neurotransmitter. Cholinergic receptor sites are found throughout the bladder and posterior urethra, being most common in the bladder body. Most are muscarinic in nature, i.e., atropine characteristically exhibits a complete blocking action at these sites. In most animals species, part of the bladder contraction elicited by electrical stimulation of the pelvic nerve is resistant to atropine. The finding of this atropine resistance in both the experimental animal and humans led researchers to believe that acetylcholine was not the sole transmitter and therefore the search for additional transmitters ensued (3, 4). The concept of nonadrenergic, noncholinergic transmitters and nerves arose, and led to the discovery that several other chemicals and nerves were indeed present in the lower urinary tract. These include vasoactive intestinal polypeptide, substance P, enkephalins, and the presence of p nerves, purinergic according to Burnstock and peptidergic according to Baumgarten (5, 6). Adenosine triphosphate was proposed as the nonadrenergic, noncholinergic neurotransmitter. Current opinion, however, holds that the noncholinergic excitatory component in the normal human bladder is very small (7). Available data, however, does not exclude the possibility that the atropine resistance component of bladder contraction may be important in abnormal detrusor behavior, e.g., instability. This may explain why anticholinergic drugs fail to inhibit involuntary detrusor contractions in some patients. The precise role that the other chemicals play in influencing the function of the lower urinary tract remains to be clarified. These neuropeptides, however, have been demonstrated in nerves in the bladder wall and may act by modulating the effect of the autonomic nervous system on the intrinsic ganglia within the bladder wall.

SYMPATHETIC NERVOUS SYSTEM

The superior hypogastric plexus (presacral nerve) is thought in humans to arise from the intermediolateral cell nuclei of T10–L2. The fibers cross the pelvic brim and continue as the inferior hypogastric plexus to reach the bladder. Sympathetic fibers join with parasympathetic fibers at this level to form the pelvic plexus. The pelvic plexus, which lies immediately adjacent to the bladder wall, thus receives both sympathetic and parasympathetic fibers, allowing modulation of one system by the other (8). Postganglionic fibers then spread out to supply the entire lower urinary tract. The neurotransmitter is norepinephrine and consequently adrenergic receptors are found throughout the bladder, posterior urethra, prostate, and seminal vesicles. Important sex differences occur in the distribution of these adrenergic nerves. They appear to be present in the male bladder neck, but morphologic studies have failed to demonstrate a significant number of catecholamine-containing nerve fibers in the female bladder neck and urethra. Pharmacologic studies, however, have demonstrated sympathetic-induced responses of smooth muscle in the female urethra. The adrenergic receptors are divided into alpha and beta, depending on whether stimulation results in contraction or relaxation, respectively, of the smooth muscle. Alpha receptors are further subdivided into $alpha_1$ and $alpha_2$. The term *alpha$_1$* refers to the postjunctional alpha receptor that mediates smooth muscle contraction. *Alpha$_2$* includes a group of presynaptic receptors that are responsible for a negative feedback mechanism inhibiting release of norepinephrine in response to postganglionic neural stimulation. The $alpha_1$ receptor type is thought to predominate in humans.

Although beta receptors are also present in the bladder, the density varies from investigator to investigator. The functional importance of these receptors in the human remains to be settled. Certainly from the clinical veiwpoint, beta blockade in humans does not result in significant changes.

Alpha receptors predominate in the bladder base and urethra, while beta receptors, although sparse, predominate in the bladder body. The sympathetic nervous system thus has the potential to enhance urine storage by relaxing the bladder body through stimulation of beta receptors, contracting the bladder outlet through stimulation of alpha receptors and by inhibition of nerve transmission along the pelvic nerve at the level of the pelvic ganglia. The precise role that the sympathetic nervous system plays in regulating bladder function in the normal person is, however, unclear at present. Once again, it may be in the abnormal situation that the sympathetic nervous system becomes important. Significant morphologic and histochemical changes have been described in bladder strips obtained from patients with damage to the parasympathetic nervous system, i.e., decentralized bladders. Phenylephedrine, an alpha-receptor stimulant, resulted in contraction of these bladder muscle strips, whereas there was little effect on normal bladder muscle (9). Similarly, in bladder outflow obstruction, noradrenaline caused contraction of muscle strips instead of the expected relaxation (10). These studies suggest that there may be an increased alpha adrenoceptor activity in response to denervation or obstruction.

Calcium has an important role in the excitation-contraction coupling of smooth muscle. The dependence of bladder muscle contractility of the inflow of exogenous calcium or release of endogenous calcium and the ability to interfere with this process is an additional potential for the mediation of bladder relaxation.

Somatic nervous system

The pudendal nerve arises from the anterior horn cells of the sacral segments S2–S4. This is the motor nerve to the pelvic floor muscles, including the periurethral muscle and striated muscle component of the distal sphinceteric mechanism. Whether the somatic fibers reach the sphincter muscle directly through the pudendal nerve or as vegetative fibers running with the pelvic nerves is still in dispute (11, 12).

APPLIED ANATOMY

Bladder

The bladder consists of intertwining bundles of smooth muscle. Discrete layers of smooth muscle are absent. Each muscle cell is in close apposition to the adjacent cells, except at certain junctional regions. This is termed a *region of close approach*, where intercellular distances of 10–20 nm occur, and it is through these junctional regions that the spread of an electrical stimulus from cell to cell is thought to occur.

The bladder neck smooth muscle differs histologically and pharmacologically from the detrusor proper. In males, the smooth muscle forms a complete circular collar, perhaps justifying the term *proximal internal urethral sphincter* (13). This collar arrangement is absent in the female (13). As mentioned previously, the male bladder neck has a rich noradrenergic but sparse cholinergic nerve supply. The female bladder, in contrast, has relatively few noradrenergic nerves.

Urethra

The part of the male urethra contributing to continence extends from the bladder neck to and including the membranous urethra. Extension of the smooth muscle from the bladder neck occurs down to the membranous urethra. At this level a layer of circularly orientated striated muscle fibers is found. This is termed the *striated component* of the distal urethral sphincter (13). The fibers differ, however, from those of the classic periurethral striated muscle, as they are smaller, are predominantly slow twitch, and are devoid of a muscle spindle (13). These characteristics allow for the sustained contraction that is so necessary for sphincteric function. The distal sphincteric mechanism is therefore composed of both smooth and striated muscle. The classic periurethral muscle plays no part in continence and is responsible for the volitional interruption of the urinary stream.

TREATMENT OF VOIDING DYSFUNCTION

There are a multitude of reasons why voiding does not occur in the smooth coordinated fashion that it is supposed to. A simplified functional approach divides these reasons into two main categories, failure of storage and failure to empty. Frequently these two problems coexist. It should be remembered that a normal voiding cycle depends on the presence of a stable bladder and a competent sphincteric mechanism. Urodynamic evaluation is often essential in determining which of the two problems occur so that rational treatment can be planned.

Failure of bladder storage

Any illness resulting in uninhibited detrusor contractions may cause urinary incontinence. Examples are multiple sclerosis, suprasacral spinal cord injuries, and stroke. Therapy is therefore aimed predominantly at controlling or ablating the detrusor contraction. A decrease in outlet resistance from any cause will likewise lead to urinary incontinence.

INHIBITION OF BLADDER CONTRACTILITY

Anticholinergic agents

As the main excitatory neurotransmitter for detrusor muscle contractility is acetylcholine, atropine and its cogeners will depress uninhibited contractions of any etiology. Atropine sulfate itself, however, is rarely used, although the tablet form is available.

Propantheline (Pro-Banthine®). This is a quaternary ammonium compound that is thought to competitively inhibit cholinergic transmission in the detrusor muscle and pelvic ganglia (14). In patients with detrusor hyperreflexia, the volume to the first contraction will generally increase, the force of the contraction will decrease, thus increasing the functional bladder capacity with a proportionate decrease in symptoms. Only the tablet form is now available in the United States. The usual adult dose is 15–30 mg every 4–6 hours per 24 hours. As with all the antimuscarinic agents, troublesome side effects may occur, which can interfere with patient compliance. These include inhibition of salivary secretion (dry mouth), blockade of the iris sphincter muscle (pupillary dilatation) and ciliary muscle (blurred vision), tachycardia, drowsiness, and constipation. The latter may require laxatives in patients with a neuropathic etiology for the voiding dysfunction. Antimuscarinic agents are contraindicated in patients with glaucoma and should be used with caution if significant outflow obstruction is present, as urinary retention may result.

Methantheline (Banthine®). This is also a quaternary ammonium compound and has a higher ratio of ganglionic blocking to antimuscarinic activity than propantheline. At the clinical level, however, there does not appear to be any significant difference between the two drugs. Methantheline has similar effects on the lower urinary tract. The usual dose is 50–100 mg every 4–6 hours per 24 hours. The side effects and contraindications are similar to propantheline.

Emepronium (Ceteprin®). This is a synthetic C_{10} quaternary ammonium base with anticholinergic properties. It has enjoyed more popularity and success in Europe than in the United States. The drug is currently unavailable in the United States. The standard adult does is 100–200 mg every 6 hours. Esophageal erosions have been reported if insufficient fluids are taken with each administration of the drug.

Antispasmodics

Agents that fall into this category are thought to act directly on the smooth muscle at a site distal to the cholinergic receptor mechanism. The agents also possess some antimuscarinic and local anesthetic properties. There are still some questions as to whether, in fact, the clinical effect is not simply due to their atropinelike effect. Because of the experimental evidence suggesting a different mode of action, however, these agents may be used in conjunction with true anticholinergic agents.

Oxybutynin chloride (Ditropan®). Oxybutynin is a tertiary amine with anticholinergic and musculotropic relaxant activity. The clinical effect is to suppress detrusor contractility. The recommended adult dose is 5 mg, three to four times per 24 hours. The side effects are similar to propantheline. Hyperthermia may occur secondary to interference with sudomotor responses, and peduncular hallucinosis has ben reported.

Flavoxate hydrochloride (Urispas®). Although reported to exhibit a direct inhibitory reaction on smooth muscle, in addition to anticholinergic properties, this drug appears clinically to be of limited value if used in situations where other agents have failed to control detrusor contractility (15). The adult dose is 100–300 mg, three to four times per 24 hours. The reported side effects are rare.

Alpha-adrenergic antagonists

The basis for using this class of drugs is the change in alpha-receptor density that occurs following outflow obstruction and damage to the nerve supply. The detrusor instability often present coincident with benign prostatic hypertrophy may improve following administration of these agents (10). With neurologic lesions above the conus medullaris resulting in detrusor hyerreflexia, however, these agents are of little clinical benefit in controlling detrusor contractility.

Alpha-adrenergic antagonists have, however, been reported to improve the tonus limb where decreased compliance has been observed on cystometrogram (16). This finding occurs most commonly in patients with meningomyelocele. Experimental studies in primates with decentralized bladders indicated a separate response to alpha-adrenergic blockade and anticholinergic agents (16). There is thus experimental evidence to try a combination of alpha antagonists and anticholinergics in patients with this type of bladder. Acquired neurologic lesions, e.g., cauda equina lesions, however, rarely show decreased compliance on cystometry.

Prazosin (Minipress®). This drug is now widely used in the United States following withdrawal of phenoxybenzamine because of possible mutagenic effects. Prazosin is thought to act by blocking the postsynaptic alpha adrenoceptors, i.e., alpha$_1$ receptors. The usual adult dose is 3–6 mg daily in divided doses. Higher doses, which are commonly used to control hypertension, are rarely required to achieve an effect on the bladder. Side effects include dizziness and syncope due to postural hypotension.

Calcium antagonists

The rationale for the use of this group of drugs has already been described. Both the initial experimental and clinical reports, however, have been disappointing (17, 18). Because of this, monotherapy with calcium antagonists was expanded to include the addition of an anticholinergic drug. Success has been encouraging using this combination, at least in the experimental animal (19). Terodiline, which has both anticholinergic and calcium-channel blocking effects, has been used with success in humans (20). The precise role that this class of drugs will play in controlling detrusor contractility remains to be clarified.

INCREASING OUTFLOW RESISTANCE

The human urethra contains both cholinergic and adrenergic innervation with both muscarinic and adrenergic receptors. It has been clearly shown that adrenoceptor-stimulating and -blocking drugs are far more important in regulating intraurethral pressure than cholinergic drugs. The predominant adrenoreceptor in humans is the alpha$_1$ subtype.

Alpha-adrenergic agonist

Ephedrine. This drug acts by releasing peripheral noradrenaline but also stimulates beta receptors. The oral adult dose is 25–50 mg, four times per 24 hours. Tachyphylaxis may develop. Pseudoephedrine (Sudafed®) has similar indications. The adult dose is 30–60 mg, four times per 24 hours.

The side effects include anxiety, insomnia, headache, and palpitations. The drug should be used with caution in patients with hypertension, hyperthyroidism, and cardiovascular disease. Urinary retention may be precipitated in the presence of outflow obstruction.

Phenylpropanolamine hydrochloride. This has the same properties as ephedrine while causing less central stimulation. The average adult dose is 50 mg, three times per 24 hours. The side effects are the same as ephedrine.

Imipramine and the lower urinary tract

Imipramine hydrochloride, a tricyclic antidepressant, exerts at least three pharmacologic effects on the lower urinary tract, facilitating urinary storage (21). The first is a central and peripheral anticholinergic action at some sites, the second is to block the active reuptake of norepinephrine by the presynaptic nerve, and third is a strong direct inhibitory effect on the bladder smooth muscle. The net clinical result is decreased bladder contactility and an increase in outflow resistance (21). This drug is also used commonly in nocturnal enuresis. In elderly patients, therapy is commenced with a single nighttime dose of 25 mg and is gradually increased until side effects appear or the dose reaches 150 mg (21). The usual adult dose is 25 mg, four times a day, for detrusor instability. The side effects include weakness, fatigue, tremor, mania, sedation, and postural hypotension. The drug is contraindicated when used in conjunction with monoamine oxidase inhibitors, as coma and seizures can be precipitated.

Failure of bladder emptying

Inadequate bladder emptying with large postvoid residuals may be secondary to abnormal detrusor contractility such as contractions of short duration or poor force, or an increase in outlet resistance. Therapy is therefore aimed at improving the detrusor contraction or decreasing the outlet resistance.

INCREASING INTRAVESICAL PRESSURE

Acetylcholine, the primary neurotransmitter in humans, cannot be used therapeutically because of actions at the central and ganglionic level and because of rapid hydrolysis by acetylcholinesterase.

Parasympathomimetic drugs

Bethanechol chloride (Urecholine®). This drug is cholinesterase resistant and cause in vivo contraction of bladder muscle. The clinical effectiveness in improving bladder emptying in the majority of patients with both neuropathic and non-neuropathic disease, however, has been disappointing (22, 23).

Bethanechol chloride does produce an increase in tension in the bladder muscle but fails to stimulate or facilitate a coordinated sustained detrusor contraction. The drug may be given subcutaneously in doses of 5 mg for postoperative urinary retention and repeated every 6 hours. The usual oral adult dose is 25–100 mg, four times per 24 hours. The side effects include nausea, vomiting, diarrhea, intestinal cramps, sweating, and salivation. Contraindications to the use of this drug are asthma, peptic ulcer, bowel obstruction, cardiac arrhythmia, and bladder outflow obstruction.

DECREASING OUTFLOW RESISTANCE

The spincteric mechanism in males, both proximal and distal, and the prostate contain an abundance of adrenergic nerves with alpha adrenoceptors (24, 25). The most common cause for organic obstruction in males is benign prostatic hypertrophy. Obstruction from an enlarged prostate may be secondary to either a mechanical effect or a functional effect. The former is produced by the physical presence of the tissue itself, while the latter is mediated through stimulation of the abundant alpha adrenoreceptors, resulting in increased tone of the prostatic smooth muscle. Although the mechanical component may gradually increase, fluctuation of symptoms does not occur. The functional or dynamic component, however, can vary quite rapidly according to the degree of sympathetic stimulation. Not infrequently a patient with relatively mild prostatic obstruction will develop sudden acute urinary retention due to associated factors such as chilling, nervous tension, or bladder overdistention. This is often transient and the use of an alpha-blocking agent may abort or relieve the retention. Alpha blockers are also useful in cases with bladder neck obstruction or "dyskinesia." This condition usually occurs in young males who complain of poor voiding. Urodynamic assessment reveals poor opening of the bladder neck associated with a normal detrusor contraction and relaxation of the striated periurethral muscle. Prazosin (Minipress®) has been found to be effective in reducing the obstructive symptoms of benign prostatic hypertrophy (26).

There is no class of pharmacologic agents that will selectively relax the striated muscle of the pelvic floor. The condition of detrusor-sphincter dyssynergia, where reflex contraction of the pelvic floor muscles occurs simultaneously with a bladder contraction, occurs exclusively in neuropathic voiding dysfunction and results in variable degrees of incomplete bladder emptying. Although skeletal muscle relaxants used to treat muscle spasticity have been tried, the clinical effectiveness of these agents is lacking.

INTERMITTENT CATHETERIZATION

Sterile intermittent catheterization was introduced in 1954 in the treatment of patients with spinal cord injury. The clean or nonsterile technique was described in 1972 (27). Since then, this technique has gained wide acceptance by virtue of its simplicity and effectiveness. To be truly effective, it must ensure social continence between catheterizations. This requires a bladder of adequate functional capacity that is capable of storing urine at low pressures. This is often not the case with neuropathic bladders, and pharmacology may be necessary to achieve this.

In addition, it is preferable to have the patients catheterize themselves, which for various reasons may not be possible. Intermittent catheterization as a definitive means of bladder drainage is usually performed every 4–6 hours. Care is taken to limit the volume drained to 300–500 cc per catheterization. This may necessitate limiting fluid intake or adjusting the catheterization interval. Bacteriuria is common in this population group but does not appear to have any long-term deleterious effects (28).

Intermittent catheterization may be used to ensure bladder drainage in voiding dysfunction of diverse etiology.

REFERENCES

1. Brindley GS, Polkey CE, Rushton DN: Sacral anterior root stimulators for bladder control in paraplegic and quadriplegic patients. *J Neurol Neurosurg Psychiatry* 45:952, 1983.
2. Juenemann K-P, Lue TF, Schmidt RA, Tanagho EA: The clinical significance of sacral and pudendal nerve anatomy. *J Urol* 139:74–80, 1988.
3. Ambache N, Zar MA: Noncholinergic transmission by postganglionic motor neurones in the mammalian bladder. *J Physiol* (London) 210:761, 1970.
4. Cowan WD, Daniel EE: Human female bladder and its noncholinergic contractile function. *Can J Physiol Pharmacol* 61:1236, 1983.
5. Burnstock G: Purinergic nerves. *Pharmacol Rev* 24:509, 1972.
6. Baumgarten HG, Holstein AF, Owman CH: Auerbach's plexus of mammals of man: Electron microscopic identification of three different types of neuronal processes in mesenteric ganglia of the large intestine from rhesus monkey, guinea-pigs and man. *Zeitschrift Zellforschung Mikroskopische Anatomie* 106:376, 1970.
7. Sjogren C, Andersson K-E, Husted S, Mattiasson A, Moller–Madsen B: Atropine resistance of transmurally stimulated isolated human bladder muscle. *J Urol* 128:1368, 1982.
8. DeGroot WC, Booth AM, Kriev J: Interaction between sacral parasympathetic and lumbar sympathetic inputs to pelvic ganglia. In: CM Brooks, K Koizani, A Sato, eds, *Integrative Functions of the Autonomic Nervous System*. University of Tokyo Press, Tokyo, pp 234–247, 19
9. Sundin T, Dahlstrom A, Norlen L, Svedmyr N: The sympathetic innervation and adrenoreceptor function of the human urinary tract in the normal state and after parasympathetic denervation. *Invest Urol* 14:322–328, 1977.
10. Perlberg S, Caine M: Adrenergic response of bladder muscle in prostatic obstruction. *Urology* 20:524–527, 1982.
11. Vodusek DB, Light JK: The motor nerve supply of the external urethral sphincter muscles: An electrophysiologic study. *Neurourol Urodynamics* 2:193–200, 1983.
12. Gosling JA: The structure of the bladder and urethra in relation to function. *Urol Clin North Am* 6:31–38, 1979.
13. Gosling JA, Dixon JS, Critchley HOD, Thompson SA: A comparative study of the human external sphincter and periurethral levator ani muscles. *Br J Urol* 53:35–41, 1981.
14. Benson GS, Sarshik Sa, Raezer D, Wein AJ: Bladder muscle contractility. Comparative effects of and mechanisms of actions of atropine, propantheline, flavoxate, and imipramine. *Urology* 9:31–35, 1977.
15. Briggs RS, Castleden CM, Asher MJ: The effect of flavoxate on uninhibited detrusor contractions and urinary incontinence in the elderly. *J Urol* 123:665–666, 1980.
16. McGuire EJ, Savastano JA: Effect of alpha-adrenergic blockade and anticholinergic agents on the decentralized primate bladder. *Neurourol Urodynamics* 4:139–142, 1985.
17. Forman A, Andersson K-E, Hendriksson L, Rud T, Ulmsten U: Effect of nifedripine on the smooth muscle of the human urinary tract. *Acta Pharmacol Toxicol* 43:111–118, 1978.
18. Leval KU, Lutzeyer W: Spontaneous phasic activity of the detrusor: A cause of uninhibited contractions in unstable bladder. *Urologia Int* 35:182–187, 1980.
19. Andersson K-E, Fovaeus M, Morgan E, McLorie G: Comparative effects of five different calcium channel blockers on the atropine-resistant contraction in electrically stimulated rabbit urinary bladder. *Neurourol Urodynamics* 5:579–586, 1986.

20. Peters D, et al.: Terodiline in the treatment of urinary frequency and motor urge incontinence. A controlled multicentre trial. *Scand J Urol Nephrol* (Suppl) 87:21–33, 1984.
21. Castleden CM, George CF, Renwick AG, Asher MJ: Imipramine — a possible alternative to current therapy for urinary incontinence in the elderly. *J Urol* 125:318–320, 1981.
22. Wein A, Malloy TR, Shofer F, Raezer DM: The effects of bethanechol chloride on urodynamic parameters in normal women and in women with significant residual urine volumes. *J Urol* 124:397–399, 1980.
23. Light JK, Scott FB: Bethanechol chloride and the traumatic cord bladder. *J Urol* 128:85–87, 1982.
24. Caine M, Raz S, Zeigler M: Adrenergic and cholinergic receptors in the human prostate, prostatic capsule and bladder neck. *Br J Urol* 47:193–202, 1975.
25. Ek A, Alm P, Andersson K-E, Persson CG: Adrenergic and cholinergic nerves of human urethra and urinary bladder. A histochemical study. *Acta Physiol Scand* 99:345–352, 1977.
26. Hedlund H, Andersson K-E, Ek A: Effects of prazosin in patients with benign prostatic obstruction. *J Urol* 130:275–278, 1983.
27. Lapides J, Diokno AC, Silber SJ, Lowe BS: Clean, intermittent self-catheterization in the treatment of urinary tract disease. *J Urol* 107:458–461, 1972.
28. Kass EJ, Koff SA, Diokno AC, Lapides J: The significance of bacilluria in children on long-term intermittent catheterization. *J Urol* 126:223–225, 1981.

Index

Abdominal aortic aneurysm surgery, 286–287
Acebutolol, dialysis for removal, 642
Acetaminophen, intoxication, 639, 643, 644
Acetate, dialysate composition, 801, 803–804, 842, 843
Acetazolamide, 29–30, 34, 37–38, 470, 624
    Bicarbonate reabsorption, 161, 163
    Hyperkalemia, 62, 63, 64
    Hyperkalemic periodic paralysis, 51
    Hyperphosphatemia, 133
    Hypokalemic periodic paralysis, 78
    Metabolic acidosis, 186, 188
    Metabolic alkalosis, 172
    Respiratory alkalosis, 229–230
Acetic acidosis, 239
Acetone, dialysis for removal, 643
Acetophenetidin, dialysis for removal, 643
Acetosalicylate, 179
Acetozolamide, uric acid stones, 154
N-Acetyl-beta-D-glucosaminidase, 613
N-Acetylprocainamide, 642, 644
Acetylsalicylic acid, 504–505, 643, 644, 645
Acid-base balance disorders, 258–260
Acid-base disorders, mixed, 233–242
Acid-base template, 235–237
Acidemia, acute renal failure, 297
Acid excretion, 164–166, 170–171, 208–209, 226, 238
Acipimox, dialysis for removal, 642
Acquired cystic disease, 543, 560–561
Acquired factor X deficiency, 463
Acquired ideopathic nephrotic syndrome with glomerulosclerosis, 216
Acquired immune deficiency syndrome (AIDS), 297, 326
Acroleine, 454
Acromegaly, 52
ACTH, 254, 263, 269, 307–308, 577
Active cytomegalic inclusion disease, 726
Acute appendicitis, 499
Acute fatty liver of pregnancy (AFLP), 504, 505
Acute glomerulonephritis syndrome, 305–312, 516, 547
Acute gouty arthritis, 472, 473
Acute hyperkalemia, 47
Acute hypokalemia, 47
Acute hyponatremia, 3–7
Acute interstitial nephritis, 288, 621, 626
Acute leukemia, 458, 469
Acute lobar nephronia, 369
Acute lymphoblastic leukemia, 132
Acute myocardial infarction, 65, 73, 79, 80, 116
Acute nephritis, 305, 307, 309, 343–344, 464
    Henoch-Schonlein nephritis, 419
Acute nonlymphocytic leukemia, amyloidosis, 461
Acute obstructive disease, 242
Acute pancreatitis, 101
Acute pericardial tamponade, 701
Acute peritoneal dialysis, hypokalemia, 81
Acute post-streptococcal glomerulonephritis, 287
Acute pyelonephritis, 287, 349–350, 352–355, 358–359, 498–500
    Pregnancy, 503–504
    Simple cysts, 564
Acute radiation nephritis, 628
Acute renal failure (ARF), 285–298, 391
    Amyloidosis, 463
    Azotemia, 285–289
    Cardiac failure, 285
    Chronic hyperuricemic nephropathy, 472
    Complications, 297
    Continuous arteriovenous hemodialysis (CAVHD), 296
    Continuous arteriovenous hemofiltration (CAVH), 295–296, 844
    Electroencephalogram, 720
    Etiologies, 285–287
    Hypercalcemia, 96
    Hyperkalemia, 298
    Hypocalcemia, 502
    Hypovolemia, 285
    IgA nephropathy, 344
    Intrinsic, 288
    Laboratory assessment and diagnosis, 288–289
    Metabolic acidosis, 502
    Mortality, 293–296, 298
    Multiple myeloma, 456–457
    Nephrotic syndrome, 320
    Nondialytic management, 292–298
    Nutritional management, 292–297
    Pathophysiology, 289–291
    Peritoneal dialysis, 296–297, 739–744
    Pregnancy, 500–506
    Renal ischemia, 615
    Slow continuous ultrafiltration (SCUF), 296
    Toxic nephropathies, 618–626

Treatment, 38
Ultrafiltration rate (UFR), 295, 296
Uric acid nephropathy, 469, 470
Acute renal vasculitis, 615
Acute tubular necrosis, 133, 187, 188, 286, 291–292
  Liver, hepatic dysfunction, 487
  Multiple myeloma, 458
  Nephrotic syndrome, 320
  Pregnancy, 505
Acute tumor lysis syndrome, 52, 132, 133
Acute uric acid nephropathy, 469–472
Acyclovir, 629, 643, 951
Addison's disease, 217, 254, 260, 270, 278–279
  Hyperkalemia, 53, 62
  Hypocalcemia, 256
  Hypoparathyroidism, 101
  Similarity of reflux nephropathy, 373
Adenoma, 80, 93
Adenosine diphosphate (ADP), 19–22, 99, 249–250, 815
Adenosine monophosphate (AMP), 101, 102, 128, 144, 146
Adenosine triphosphate (ATP), 63, 111, 121, 127–129, 194
ADPKD, see Autosomal dominant polycystic kidney disease
Adrenergic inhibitors, hypertension, 427
Adrenogenital syndromes, 170
Adriamycin, 455, 456, 626, 644
Adults
  Polycyctic kidney disease, 472
  Respiratory distress syndrome (ARDS), 186, 228–229, 499
  Sporadic hypophosphatemic osteomalacia, 584
Advanced liver disease, 80
Albumin, 37, 40, 116, 229, 248–249
Albuterol, 62, 63
Alcohol abuse, hyponatremia, 9
Alcoholic acidosis, 240
Alcoholic ketoacidosis, 126, 128, 187, 239
Alcoholic liver cirrhosis, 343, 344
Alcoholic liver disease, 479, 485, 487
Alcoholic patients, 727
  Acid-base disorders, 239–240
  Burns response, 281
  Hypomagnesemia, 272, 273
  Hypophosphatemia, 126, 128, 129, 273–274

Papillary necrosis, 359
Alcoholic withdrawal, 126, 239, 274
Alcohols, dialysis for removal, 642
Aldactone, 254
Aldosterone, 31, 32, 36, 40, 254
  Bicarbonate reabsorption, 162–163
  Cirrhosis sodium retention, 479
  Hypokalemia, 70–73, 78, 79
  Hypomagnesemia, 113, 115
  Metabolic alkalosis, 167–168, 169
  Potassium homeostasis, 46, 47, 49–51, 53–55
  Regulation of ammoniagenesis, 165, 166, 167
  Renal tubular acidosis, 583
  Surgery effect on, 263, 264
  Type 4 renal tubular acidosis, 216–217
Aldosteronism, 170, 253
Alkalemia, 59, 240, 242, 260
Alkali therapy
  Alcoholic acidosis, 240
  Cardiac arrest patients with acid-base disorders, 237–238
  Glycol nephrotoxicity, 620
  Medullary sponge kidney, 559
  Renal tubular acidosis, 214–215, 218
  Respiratory acidosis, 226
  Sepsis, 239
Alkyl phosphate, 643
Allantoin, 471
Allergic angiitis, 413
Allergic hepatitis, 471
Allograft rejection, see also Immunosuppression, 887–898
  Acute, 896–897
  Adjunctive use of antilymphocyte serum, 891
  Antilymphocyte and antithymocyte globulins, 897
  Antilymphocyte serum (ALS), 888–889
  Azathioprine, 888–891, 893, 894, 896
  Corticosteroids, 887–892, 894, 896–897
  Cyclosporin, 888, 891–896
  Methylprednisolone, 890, 891, 897
  Monoclonal antibodies, 889, 897
  Total lymph node irradiation (TLI), 889
Allopurinol, 133, 615, 292,

655–656, 891
Acute interstitial nephritis as result, 626
Chronic hyperuricemia nephropathy, 472–473
Hyperuricosuria, 148, 149, 154
Medullary sponge kidney, 559
Multiple myeloma, 454
Uric acid nephropathy, 471
Almitrene, 225
Alopecia, 101
Alpha-adrenergic blocking agents, 51, 52, 65, 512
Alpha- and beta-receptor antagonists, 511
Alpha blockers, hypertension, 427
Alpha ketoisocarproate, 295
Alpha methyldopa, 663
Alpha-receptor antagonists, 511
Alport's syndrome, 340, 517, 587, 659, 724
  GBM antigens, 338
  Renal transplantation, 870, 932–933
Aluminum bone disease, 727, 737
Aluminum gels, 134
Aluminum intoxication, 646, 717, 733–734, 737, 800
  Continuous ambulatory peritoneal dialysis, 762
  Dialysis dementia, 726–727
  Dialysis for removal, 642
  Dose-dependent tubular degeneration, 620
  Hemoperfusion for removal, 644
Alveolar gas equation, 223–224
Alzheimer's disease, 727
Amanita phalloides, 848
Amanitin, 643, 644
Amantadine, dialysis for removal, 643
Amikacin, 353, 354, 356, 622–623, 642
Amiloride, 29, 31, 32, 35, 320
  Hyperkalemia, 46, 52, 56
  Hypertension, 427
  Hypokalemia, 78, 79, 80, 81
  Hypomagnesemia, 115, 118
  Liver, hepatic dysfunction, 479
  Metabolic acidosis, 189
  Metabolic alkalosis, 161, 164
  Noninflammatory vascular diseases, 426
Amino acids, 2, 293–294
Aminoacidurias, 581–582
Aminoglycosides, 21, 70, 257–258, 281, 456, 548, 759
  Acute pyelonephritis, 499
  Acute renal failure, 287, 292, 298

Burn victims, 281
Hypocalcemia, 257–258
Infective endocarditis, 707, 708
Nephrotoxicity, 273, 622–623
Respiratory acidosis, 224
Urinary tract infections, 353, 356, 358
Aminohydroxypropylidene diphosphonate (ADP), 454
Aminophylline, 225, 642, 644
P-Aminosalicylate, acute interstitial nephritis, 626
Amitryptiline, 642, 644
Ammonia, 4, 164–165
Ammoniagenesis, 165
Ammonium acid urate stones, 139
Ammonium chloride, 229–230
Amobarbitol, 642, 644
Amoxapine, 624
Amoxicillin, 70, 353, 356, 626, 642
Amphetamines, 615, 624, 626, 642
Amphotericin, acute renal failure, 287
Amphotericin B, 21, 70, 115–116, 287, 629–630
Hypocalcemia, 257, 258
Nephropathy, 624
Peritonitis, 765
Ampicillin, 70, 497, 548, 636, 949
Acute interstitial nephritis as result, 626
Acute pyelonephritis, 499
Dialysis for removal, 642
Hemoperfusion for removal, 644
Infective endocarditis, 707
Urinary tract infections, 353, 354, 356, 358
Amyloid involvement of the collecting duct, 21
Amyloidosis, 38, 215, 397, 460–463
AA type, 459–463
AL type, 453, 456, 458, 459–463
End-stage renal disease and transplantation, 870
Pregnancy, 461
Renal transplantation, 912–913, 922–923
Renal vein thrombosis, 435
Amyloid tumors in bones, 826
Amyotrophic lateral sclerosis, 225
Anaesthesis, 667, 669–672
Analgesic nephropathy, end-stage renal disease and transplantation, 870
Analgesics, 287, 359, 627, 643, 644
Anaphylatoxins, 817–823, 827, 829–832, 847
Anaplastic carcinoma, 469
Androgen, 170, 604, 607–608, 737

Anemia, 183, 228, 697, 733–738, 891
Acute glomerulonephritis syndrome, 307
Anaesthesia, 669
Autosomal dominant polycystic kidney disease, 547
Chronic peritoneal dialysis, 747
Chronic renal failure, 703
Goodpasture's syndrome, 335, 339
Hemolytic, 358, 433
Pregnancy, 502, 521–522
Uremia, 664–665
Aneurysms, 780, 782, 784, 785
Angiographic dyes, polyuria, 19, 22, 23
Angiokeratoma corporis diffusum, 935
Angiotensin, renal ischemia as result, 614
Angiotensin II, 17
Angiotensin-converting enzyme (ACE) inhibitor, 79–80, 429–430, 433, 537–538, 663
Hyperkalemia causing, 270
Aniline, dialysis for removal, 642
Ankylosing spondylitis, 225
Anorexia nervosa, 67, 127, 189, 269
Anoxia, 8
Antacids, 125–129, 241, 477, 727, 804
Acute renal failure, 297, 298
Genitourinary tuberculosis, 391
Hypophosphatemia, 274
Multiple myeloma, 454
Phosphate-binding, 711–712, 714, 717, 727, 912
Antibiotics, 621–624, 626, 742
Acute glomerulonephritis syndrome, 307, 310, 311, 312
Acute interstitial nephritis as result, 626
Acute pyelonephritis, 499
Acute renal failure, 292, 298, 501, 502–503
Asymptomatic bacteriuria, 497–498
Autosomal dominant polycystic kidney disease, 547, 548, 556
Burns, 281, 282
Graft fistulas, 780–782
Hypokalemia, 70, 80, 81
Infective endocarditis, 706–708
Magnesurias, 586
Multiple myeloma, 454, 458

Peritonitis, 742, 764–766, 787–788
Pregnancy, 520
Pulmonary infections, 946
Sepsis, 239
Systemic lupus erythematosus, 395
Urinary tract infections, 351–356, 358, 660
Vasculitis, 418, 420
Anticholinergics, 672, 956–957
Anticoagulants, 625, 629, 661, 847–848
Epidural spinal hematoma, 726
Pregnancy, 513, 517
Antidepressants, 268, 642, 644
Antidiuretic hormone (ADH), 5, 264, 277, 280, 573
Surgical patients, 267, 269
Anti-glomerular basement membrane (GBM) antibody disease, 333–340, 870–872
Anti-GBM/ABM antibody disease, 333, 334–335
Antihistamines, 390, 799, 830
Antilymphocyte and antithymocyte globulins, allograft rejection, 897
Anti-lymphocyte serum (ALS), 888–889, 894–895
Antimicrobials/anticancer drugs, dialysis for removal, 642, 644
Antimony, 620
Antiplatelet agents, 445–446, 463, 506, 508, 518
Antipsychotics, 268
Antipyrine, acute interstitial nephritis as result, 626
Antirheumatics, dialysis for removal, 643, 644
Antithrombin III (AT-III), 322, 505
Antithymocyte globulin, diabetes mellitus, 533
Anuria, 140, 288
Anxiety, 721, 722
Aprobarbital, dialysis for removal, 642
Arginine hydrochloride (HCL), 51, 52, 270
Arginine vasopressin (AVP), 3, 4, 10, 264
Arrhythmias, 33, 36, 57, 100, 512
Acute renal failure, 298
Dialysis disequilibrium syndrome, 728
Hypokalemia, 66, 72–73, 76, 79–81, 270

Metabolic acidosis, 182
Metabolic alkalosis, 172
Pericarditis, 698, 700, 702
Peritoneal dialysis, 743
Renal transplantation, 935
Respiratory alkalosis, 229
Arsenic, 619, 642
Arteriolar nephrosclerosis, 870, 871
Arteriolar vasodilators, 511
Arteriosclerosis, shunt use, 779
Arteriosclerotic vascular disease, burn response, 281
Arthritis, amyloidosis, 461
Ascorbic acid, 151, 152, 686–687
Asphyxia, 257
Aspiration, 237
Aspirin, 327, 379–380, 420, 615, 815
   Hypercalcemia, 96, 98
   Preeclampsia, 513–514
   Pregnancy, 517
   Uremia, 845
Asthma, 65, 74, 225, 250, 260
Asymptomatic bacteriuria, 349–351, 357–358, 962, 963
Atenolol, 427, 511, 629, 642, 663
Atheroembolic disease, 435
Atherosclerotic heart disease (ASHD), 472, 536, 665, 697, 702
   Hypertension, 397
Atracurium, 672
Autoimmune hemolytic anemia, 132
Autonomic dysreflexia, 960
Autonomic neuropathy, 723–724
Autosomal dominant polycystic kidney disease (ADPKD), 543–554
   Aneurysms of cerebral and abdominal vessels, 549
   Basic fluid and electrolyte management, 544
   Characteristics, 544
   Counseling, 553–554
   Dialysis, 552–553
   Dietary management, 544
   Gastrointestinal problems, 550–551
   Hematuria, 546–547
   Hemorrhage, 546–547
   Hypertension, 544, 546, 549, 551, 553, 556
   Infection, 547–548
   Lifestyle, 546
   Neoplastic changes, 548
   Nephrolithiasis, 549–550
   Pain, 546
   Physical activity, 546
   Pregnancy, 551
   Prevention, 553–554
   Prognosis, 551–552
   Rovsing procedure, 546, 552, 553
   Transplantation, 552–553, 554
Autosomal recessive parathyroid hyperplasia, 256
Avascular necrosis, 952
AVP, see Arginine vasopressin
Azathioprine, 626, 643
   Allograft rejection, 888–891, 893, 894, 896
   Diabetes mellitus (IDDM), 539
   Familial Mediterranean fever, 923
   Goodpasture's syndrome, 339
   Renal transplantation, 446, 447, 877, 928–930, 952
   Systemic lupus erythematosus, 399–403, 924
   Transplant patients and pregnancy, 523, 524
   Uric acid nephropathy, 471
   Vasculitis, 415–418
Azlocillin, dialysis for removal, 642
Azotemia, 53, 79, 150–151
   Acute glomerulonephritis syndrome, 305, 308, 309
   Acute renal failure, 285–289
   Autosomal dominant polycystic kidney disease, 544
   Clinical disorders associated with, 286
   Diabetes mellitus (IDDM), 538, 539
   Diabetic ketoacidosis, 195
   Edematous states, 27, 31–32, 35, 38, 40
   Hypercalcemia, 96
   Hypertension, 432
   Management, 292
   Metabolic alkalosis, 172
   Nephrotic syndrome, 320, 321, 325, 328
   Polyuria, 21
   Pregnancy, 503, 518
   Renal ischemia, 614
   Scleroderma, 433
   Systemic lupus erythematosus, 398
   Urinary tract infections, 359
   Vasculitis, 420
Aztreonam, dialysis for removal, 642

Bacitracin, 624, 642
Backleak hypothesis, 290
Bacteremia, 238
Bacterial endocarditis, 310–312
Bacterial infections, renal transplantations, 948–949
Bacterial peritonitis, 479
Balkan nephropathy, 359, 597
Barbital, 642, 644
Barbiturates, 624, 642, 644, 645
Barium, 66, 269, 270, 619–620
Bartholin and Skene gland infection, 353
Bartter's syndrome, 64, 170, 253, 260, 269
   Hypomagnesemia, 115–116
   Inherited renal tubular disorders, 582, 586, 588–589
   Potassium metabolism disorders, 67, 70, 72–73, 75, 78–79
Basal cell carcinoma, 951
Bazzato double-bag system, 766
BCNU (carmustine), multiple myeloma, 455, 456
Bed rest, acute glomerulonephritis syndrome, 308
Behcet's syndrome, 355
Bence Jones (BJ) cast nephropathy (myeloma kidney), 453, 458
Benign familial hematuria syndrome, 517
Benoxaprofen, 626
Benzathine penicillin G, 308
Benzodiazepines, 241, 671, 724, 727
Benzolamide, 29, 161
Benzothiadiazide diuretics, acute glomerulonephritis, 309
Benzothiadiazine, 37
Berger's disease, 305, 325, 343, 870
Beryllium, 628
Beta-adrenergic receptor blockers, 98–99, 270, 379, 428, 663–664
   Hypertension, 427, 429
   Potassium metabolism disorders, 50–52, 55, 65–66, 73–74, 80
   Secondary hyperparathyroidism, 717
   Toxic nephropathies, 616, 629
Beta-adrenoceptor blocking agents, 512
Beta blockers, see Beta-adrenergic receptor blockers
Beta-cap system, 766
Betadine, 281
Beta-receptor antagonists, 511
Bicarbonate, 171
   Dialysate composition, 801, 804, 842, 843, 844

Excessive loads and metabolic alkalosis, 171
Fanconi syndrome, 459
Hypokalemia, 66–67, 69, 71, 77, 81
Uric acid nephropathy, 470
Uric acid stones, 154
Bicarbonate reabsorption
Diabetic ketoacidosis, 202–203
Edematous states, 27, 30, 37
Metabolic alkalosis, 160–163, 167–168
Bicarbonaturia, 57, 209, 267
Renal tubular acidosis, 212, 214, 216
Biguanides, 186
Bilateral adrenal hyperplasia, 169–170
Bilateral cervical cordotomy, 225
Bilateral diaphragmatic paralysis, 225
Bilateral hyperplasia, 80
Bilateral renal artery stenosis, 379, 429
Bilateral renovascular disease, 870
Bilateral ureteric occlusion, 286
Biliary tract disease, 484
Bismuth, 617, 619, 626
Bladder cancer, 600–603
Blood transfusions, 874–875
Blood urea nitrogen (BUN), 10, 35–36, 61, 197
Acute renal failure, 288, 292, 293, 294
Diabetes mellitus (IDDM), 534
Hemodialysis and nutritional management, 681–682
Nephrotic syndrome, 323
Peritoneal dialysis, 739
Urinary tract infections, 352
Volume depletion after surgery, 265
Body fluid composition disorders, 249–252
Bohr effect, 172
Bolus cyclophosphamide, 399, 403
Borates, dialysis for removal, 642
Boric acid, dialysis for removal, 642
Botulism, 224
Bowen's disease, 951
Brain
Adaptive response to altered plasma tonicity, 2
Death, 879, 880
Tumors, 250
Branched-chain amino acids (BCAAs), 294, 295
Breast carcinoma, invasive, 469

Bredinin, dialysis for removal, 643
Bretylium, dialysis for removal, 642
Bromide, dialysis for removal, 642
Bronchiectasis, 225
Bronchopneumonia, 402
Bulbar poliomyelitis, 225
Bulimarexia, 67
Bumetanide, 29–32, 36–38, 427–428, 470, 471
BUN, see Blood urea nitrogen
Burkitt's lymphoma, 132, 469
Burnet's syndrome, see Milk alkali syndrome
Burning foot syndrome, 722
Burns, 260–261, 267, 274, 281, 286
Burn shock, 277–280
Butabarbital, 642, 644

Cadaver donors, see also Donor selection in renal transplantation, 867–881
Allograft rejection, 892
Blood transfusions with renal transplantations, 874, 875
Diabetes mellitus (IDDM), 539
Graft survival, 928–932
Hypertension in recipients, 914, 950
Patient survival and pregnancy prospects, 523
Sickle-cell anemia, 578
Systemic lupus erythematosus, 923, 924
Tubular dysfunction, 905
Cadmium, 628, 629–630
Caffeine, hypokalemia, 66
Calcidiol, 91, 94–95, 99–101, 103–104
Calcifediol (25-OH vitamin D) deficiency, 271
Calciferol, 103
Calcitonin, 91, 95–100, 127, 272
Calcitriol, 91–95, 97, 99–101, 103–104, 271
Calcium
Balance disorders, 255–258
Dialysate composition, 801, 802–803, 842
Disordered metabolism, 215
Electrolyte disorders in surgical patient, 271–272
Hypocalcemia and hypercalcemia, 91–104
Metabolism and cell ischemia mechanism, 291
Metabolism in uremia, 664
Calcium-channel blockers, 36, 511, 625
Amyloidosis, 463
Diabetes mellitus (IDDM), 538
Hypertension, 428, 429
Calcium phosphate stones, medullary sponge kidney, 558, 559
Calcium salts, 58–59
Calcium stones, 139–153, 189, 911
Calculi, 359, 911
Camphor, dialysis for removal, 643
Cancer, 93, 678
Bladder, 600–603
Kidney, 593–597
Prostatic, 603–608
Renal pelvis and ureteral, 597–600
Renal transplantation, 950–951
Capreomycin, 70, 115–116, 624
Captopril, 79, 252–254, 616, 663–664
Acute interstitial nephritis as result, 626
Dialysis for removal, 642
Hypertension, 427, 430, 431, 511
Potassium metabolism disorders, 52, 54–55
Renal ischemia as result, 614
Renal transplantation, 914
Carbamazepine, 23, 625, 642
Carbenicillin, 70, 115–116, 626, 642
Carbenicillin indanyl, 356
Carbenoxolone, 70, 170
Carbon dioxide retention, 223–226
Carbon monoxide poisoning, 639, 643
Carbon tetrachloride, 643, 644
Carbromal, 642, 644
Carcinoma of the parathyroid glands, hypercalcemia, 93
Carcinomatosis, 358
Cardiac arrest, acid-base disorder, 233, 237–239, 267, 285
Cardiac complications, amyloidosis, 463
Cardiopulmonary bypass, 263
Cardiovascular complications, uremia and dialysis, 697–708
Infective endocarditis, 697, 704–708
Left ventricular dysfunction, 701–704
Pericarditis, 697–701, 702, 705
Cardiovascular disease, hyperuricemia, 473
Cardiovascular drugs, dialysis for removal, 644

Carmustine, hemoperfusion for removal, 644
Carnitine deficiency, 724
Carpal tunnel syndrome, 463, 729, 785, 786, 826
Catabolism, 661
Cataracts, 952
Catheters, 955–966, see also Urinary tract catheterization
   Associated bacteriuria, prevention and management of, 960–962
   "Condom," 965
   In-and-out, 958
   Indwelling urethral, 958
   Latex vs. nonlatex, 960
   Nephrostomy tubes, 963–964
   Related infection pathogenesis, 959–960
   Sterile vs. clean, 963–964
   Suprapubic, 965–966
   Types of, 955–956
CCNU, 626
Cefaclor, dialysis for removal, 642
Cefadroxil, 642, 859
Cefamandole, 356, 642
Cefezolin, dialysis for removal, 642
Cefixime, dialysis for removal, 642
Cefmenoxime, dialysis for removal, 642
Cefonicid, 642, 859
Cefoperazone, dialysis for removal, 642
Ceforanide, dialysis for removal, 642
Cefotaxime, dialysis for removal, 642
Cefotetan, dialysis for removal, 642
Cefotiam, dialysis for removal, 642
Cefoxitin, dialysis for removal, 642
Cefroxadine, dialysis for removal, 642
Cefsulodin, dialysis for removal, 642
Ceftazidime, dialysis for removal, 642
Ceftriaxone, dialysis for removal, 642
Cefuroxime, dialysis for removal, 642
Cell ischemia, 290–291
Cellophane (dialyzer membrane), 813, 820, 821
Cellulitis, 27
Cellulose acetate (dialyzer membrane), 813–814, 819–820, 823–824, 826, 828
   Comparison to cuprophan dialyzer, 831–832
   Phagocytic mobility decrease, 847
Central diabetes insipidus, 20–23
Central nervous system
   Acute hyponatremia, 5
   Hypernatremia, 269
   Hyponatremia, 3, 8, 267
Central pontine myelinolysis (CPM), 3, 8, 9
Cephacetrile, dialysis for removal, 642
Cephalexin, 70, 356, 377, 642
Cephaloridine, 642, 708
Cephalosporins, 354, 356, 358
   Acute interstitial nephritis as result, 626
   Acute pyelonephritis, 499
   Acute renal failure, 503
   Asymptomatic bacteriuria, 497
   Autosomal dominant polycystic kidney disease, 548
   Infective endocarditis, 707, 708
   Nephrotoxicity, 623
   Urinary tract infection, 660
Cephalothin, 623, 642, 764
Cephapirin, 548, 642
Cephradine, dialysis for removal, 642
Cerebral edema, 199, 204, 250
Cerebral hemorrhage, 726
Cerebral hyporia, 172
Cerebrovascular disease, acute renal failure, 296
Chagas' disease, 338
Chelation therapy, 258, 618–619, 620, 628, 646
Chemicals, removal of, 642–643, 644
Chemiluminescence, 824
Chemolysis, 964
Chemotherapy
   Bladder cancer, 602–603
   Genitourinary tuberculosis, 388–392
   Light chain deposition disease, 459
   Multiple myeloma, 457
Chicken pox, 948
Chlofibrate, 268
Chloral hydrate, 642, 644
Chlorambucil, 324–325, 328, 400, 418, 458
Chloramines, 800
Chloramphenicol, 548, 643, 644
Chlordane, hemoperfusion for removal, 644
Chlordiazepoxide, dialysis for removal, 642
Chloride, 642
   Dialysate composition, 801, 804
"Chloride shunt" syndrome, 46, 55, 64
Chlormethiazole, 515
Chloroquine, 66, 99, 643, 644
Chlorothiazide, 30
Chlorpromazine, 4, 644
Chlorpropamide, 22–23, 268, 642
Chlorthalidone, 30, 32, 37, 71, 549
   Hypertension, 427
   Hypocalcemia, 103
Cholecalciferol, 713
Cholestatic hepatocellular disease, 737
Cholestyramine, 152
Chromic acid, dialysis for removal, 642
Chromium, 620
Chronic anemia, 134
Chronic atrophic pyelonephritis, 363, 367, 376, 378
Chronic bacteriuria, 355–356
Chronic bronchitis, 225
Chronic glomerulonephritis, 374
   Pregnancy, 516–517
Chronic hypercapnia, 171
Chronic hyperchloremia, 55
Chronic hyperuricemic nephropathy, 472–473
Chronic hypokalemia, polyuria, 21–22
Chronic hyponatremia, 5–8
Chronic interstitial nephritis, 626–628
Chronic lead intoxication, 472
Chronic obstructive airway disease, 225
Chronic obstructive pulmonary disease (COPD), 226, 227, 242
Chronic peritoneal dialysis, 744–750
Chronic phosphate depletion, 166
Chronic pulmonary disease, metabolic alkalosis, 172
Chronic pyelonephritis, 217, 497, 874
   End-stage renal disease and transplantation, 870
   Pregnancy, 506
   Reflux nephropathy, 363, 367, 368
   Urinary tract infections, 349, 352, 357–360
Chronic radiation nephritis, 628
Chronic renal failure, 93, 101–102, 654–655, 720

Catabolism, 661
Components requiring management, 659
Congestive heart failure, 660–661
Dehydration, 659–660
Dietary intervention, 649–653
Extrarenal buffering, 166
Forms leading to renal transplantation, 870
Gout, 472
Hemofiltration, 843
Hypercalcemia, 98
Hyperkalemia, 53, 54
Hyperoxaluria, 152
Hyperphosphatemia, 132
Hypocalcemia, 104
Magnesium reabsorption, 115
Multiple myeloma, 457–458
Nutritional management, 675–688
Sequential ultrafiltration and dialysis, 843
Treatment, 38
Uncontrolled hypertension, 661
Urinary tract infection, 660
Urinary tract obstruction, 660
Chronic tubulointerstitial nephritis, 217, 352
Churg-Strauss syndrome, 333, 413
Cilastin, dialysis for removal, 642
Cimetidine, 98–99, 297, 626, 642, 717
  Hemoperfusion for removal, 644
  Renal ischemia as result, 614
Cimino Brescia fistula, 841
Ciprofloxacin, 548, 643
Cirrhosis of the liver, 17, 28, 32, 40, 249, 477–483, 485–488, 490
  Acid excretion, 165
  Acute hyponatremia, 7
  Acute renal failure, 292
  Burn response, 281
  Hyponatremia, 267, 268
  Renal transplantation, 870
  Septicemia, 358
  Spironolactone, 78
  With ascites, 5, 126
Cisplatin, 70–71, 80, 81, 115–116, 287
  Bladder cancer, 602
  Renal pelvis and ureteral cancer, 600
Cisplatinum nephropathy, 21, 100, 298, 619
  Hypocalcemia, 257, 258
  Hypomagnesemia, 273
Citrate, 100, 257, 258, 297, 459

Clavulinic acid, dialysis for removal, 642
Clindamycin, 548, 643, 644
Clinical stones disease, 154
Clofibrate therapy, 23, 626, 666, 685, 768
Clofibric acid, 321
Clonazepam, 666
Clonidine, 427, 428, 430, 511, 549
Clorox, 281
Clostridia antitoxin, acute renal failure, 502
Cloxacillin, 642, 707
Clycosurias, 582
Codeine, 352, 624
Colchicine, 643, 644, 922, 923
  Acute gouty arthritis, 473
  Amyloidosis, 462, 462, 463
  Hypocalcemia, 100
  Nephrogenic diabetes insipidus, 21
  Nephrotic syndrome, 913
Colistin, dialysis for removal, 642
Colonic ischemia, 60
Concentration product ratio (CPR), 144, 145, 147, 155
Congenital adrenal hyperplasia, 217, 269
Congenital chloride-losing diarrhea, 170, 171
Congenital disorders, end-stage renal disease and transplantation, 870
Congenital heart block, 215, 398
Congenital (meningomyelocele), end-stage renal disease and transplantation, 870
Congenital renal disease, 268
Congestive heart failure, 5, 17, 27–28, 32–34
  Acute glomerulonephritis syndrome, 307
  Acute hyponatremia, 7
  Acute renal failure, 292, 296
  Amyloidosis, 460, 461, 463
  Anaesthesia, 669
  Azotemia, 286
  Body fluid composition disorder, 249
  Chronic renal failure, 660–661
  Hypercalcemia, 98
  Hyperkalemia, 59, 63, 270
  Hypocalcemia, 100
  Hypomagnesemia, 115
  Hyponatremia, 268
  Liver, hepatic dysfunction, 480
  Metabolic acidosis, 187
  Metabolic alkalosis, 172
  Renal ischemia, 615

Respiratory acidosis, 226
Treatment, 34–36
Volume overload after surgery, 265
Conjunctivitis, 390
Continuous ambulatory peritoneal dialysis (CAPD), 539, 540, 724, 741, 755–769
  Aluminum bone disease, 717
  Compared to continuous cyclic peritoneal dialysis, 746
  Detoxification therapy, 737
  Dialyzability of specific drugs removed by 24 hours treatment, 860–862
  Increased intraabdominal pressure, 766–767
  Nutritional management, 683–687
  Pericarditis, 755
  Peritoneal sclerosis, 749
  Pregnancy, 522
  Ultrafiltration, 760–762, 767
Continuous arteriovenous hemodialysis (CAVHD), 133, 296, 482
Continuous arteriovenous hemofiltration (CAVH), 295–296, 482–483
  technique, 841, 844, 848
Continuous cyclic peritoneal dialysis (CCPD), 745–747, 749, 766
Continuous equilibration peritoneal dialysis (CEPD), 741–742
Continuous positive airway pressure (CPAP), 225–226
Contraction alkalosis (diuretic administration), 170
Contrast media nephrotoxicity, 661
Convertase, 327
Converting-enzyme inhibitors, 427, 511
Coomb's test, 511
Copper, 619, 642, 727, 800, 833
Cordis-Hakim ascites valve, 481
Coronary artery disease, 296, 873
Corticosteroids
  Acute glomerulonephritis syndrome, 307, 308
  Allograft rejection role, 887–892, 894, 896–897
  Catheter-related complications of peritoneal dialysis, 748
  Diabetes mellitus (IDDM), 539, 541
  First-use syndrome, 830
  Hemolytic uremic syndrome,

445, 504–505
Hypercalcemia, 99
Hypomagnesemia, 113
Infective endocarditis, 705
Obstructive uropathy, 629
Pericarditis, 700, 701
Pregnancy, 520
Respiratory acidosis, 226
Sulfonamide nephrotoxicity, 624
Systemic lupus erythematosus, 395, 399, 400, 402–404
Trimethadione hypersensitivity, 616
Vasculitis, 414–418, 420
Cortisol, 54, 70, 193, 196
Cortisone, 96, 272, 308
Co-trimoxazole, 372, 624
Cotrimoxazole lincomycin, 626
Coumadin, 327
Cox Proportional Hazard statistical technique, 540
Creatinine, 35, 36, 40, 391
  Acute renal failure, 293
  Autosomal dominant polycystic kidney disease, 552
  Dietary intervention effect, 649–653
  Goodpasture's syndrome, 339
  Hypocalcemia, 103
  Nephrotic syndrome, 323, 328
  Nondietary intervention, 654
  Reflux nephropathy, 374
  Urinary tract infections, 352
  Volume depletion after surgery, 265
Creutzfeldt-Jakob disease, 727
Crohn's disease, 115, 355
Crush syndrome, 132
Cryoglobulinemias, 463–464
Cryoprecipitate, 297
Cuprophan (dialyzer membrane), 813–824, 826–832, 845–847
Cushing's syndrome, 70, 93, 132, 269, 890
  Calcium stones formed, 141, 153
  Cyclosporin therapy, 896
Cyclobarbital, dialysis for removal, 642
Cyclophosphamide, 615, 643
  Cryoglobulinemias, 464
  Goodpasture's syndrome, 339
  IgA nephropathy, 345, 346
  Light chain deposition disease, 459
  Multiple myeloma, 454, 455, 456
  Nephrotic syndrome, 324–328
  Reflux nephropathy, 372
  Sickle hemoglobinemia, 577
  Systemic lupus erythematosus, 399–405
  Urinary tract infections, 355
  Vasculitis, 415–418, 420
  Waldenström's macroglobulinemia, 458
  Wegener's granulomatosis, 417, 925
Cycloserine, 388, 390, 643
Cyclosporin, 270, 287, 327, 487, 895–896
  Allograft rejection, 888, 891–896
  Diabetes mellitus (IDDM), 533, 534, 539, 541
  Familial Mediterranean fever, 923
  Magnesium deficiency cause, 115–116
  Potassium metabolism disorders, 52, 55
  Renal transplantation, 874–876, 880–881, 928, 930, 944
  Renal transplantation complications, 952
  Systemic lupus erythematosus, 400, 402, 405, 924
Cyclosporine A, 54, 418, 625–626
  Hemolytic uremic syndrome and transplantations, 446, 447
  Renal transplantation, 907, 909
  Transplant patients and pregnancy, 523, 524
Cystic disorders, see Renal cystic disorders
Cystic fibrosis, 79, 225, 250
Cystine depletion therapy, 934
Cystine stones, 139, 140, 141, 155
Cystinosis, 215, 216
Cystinuria, 155, 581, 582, 870
Cystitis, 498–499, 960
Cytomegalic inclusion disease, 730
Cytomegalovirus (CMV), 947–948
  Pneumonia, 946
Cytosine-arabinoside, 68, 70, 626

Danazol, 346, 399
Dantrolene, 52, 62, 63
Dapsone, hemoperfusion for removal, 644
Dazoxiben, preeclampsia, 514
DDAVP, 22, 297, 577
Deep venous thrombosis, renal transplantation, 950
Defective mononuclear phagocytosis, 396
Deferoxamine, 717, 727, 737
Dehydration, 245–249, 251, 659–660, 743
Delirium tremens, 269

Demeclocycline, 7, 250, 485, 624, 630
  Nephrogenic diabetes insipidus, 21
  Polyuria, 18, 21
Demeton sulfoxide, 643, 644
De-novo crescentic glomerulonephritis, 933
"De-novo" glomerular disease, 871
De-novo hypercholesterolemia, 768
Denver shunt, 481
Deoxycorticosterone acetate (DOCA), 55, 167, 170, 254
Depression, 721, 722
Desoxycorticosterone (DOC), 169, 170
Dexamethasone, 170, 358, 455
Dextroamphetamine, 629
Dextropropoxyphene, nephrogenic diabetes insipidus, 21
Diabetes
  Ketacidosis, 47, 126–129, 132, 193–204, 259–260
    Acid-base disorders, 237
    Classification, 184
    Hypokalemia, 65, 69–70, 252
    Hypomagnesemia, 273
    Hypophosphatemia, 274
    Magnesurias, 586
    Metabolic acidosis, 179, 181, 182, 183, 187
  Nephropathy, 270, 429, 533–541, 870
  Pregnancy, 516, 518
  Renal transplantation, 871
  Uremia, 666–667
Diabetes insipidus (DI), 18–22, 248, 264
  Hypernatremia, 12
  Hyponatremia, 268
  Nephrogenic, 7, 21–22, 630
  Renal losses, 247
Diabetes mellitus, 79, 199
  Acute renal failure, 287
  Anaesthesia, 670
  Beta-adrenergic receptor blockers, 428
  Chronic hyperuricemic nephropathy, 472
  Hyperkalemia, 254, 665
  Hypernatremia, 11, 51, 54
  Hypocalcemia, 101
  Hypophosphatemia, 126
  Hyporeninemic hypoaldosteronism (HRHA), 909
  Insulin-dependent (IDDM or Type I), 533–541

Iodide nephrotoxicity, 621
Metabolic acidosis, 189
Nephrotic syndrome, 319, 323
Non-insulin-dependent (NIDDM or Type II), 533–536, 538, 541
Renal losses, 247
Renal transplantation, 928–930
Renal tubular acidosis, 217
Renal vein thrombosis, 435
Urinary tract infections, 352–353, 358–359
Water volume disorders, 248
Diagoxin, hemoperfusion for removal, 644
Dialysance, 791, 794
Dialysate, production and composition, 800–805, 813, 842
Dialysis
  Access surgery, 775–788
  Acute renal failure, 485, 501, 504
  Adequacy, 729
  Autosomal dominant polycystic kidney disease, 552–553, 554
  Biocompatibility, 846–847
  Brain infections, 726
  Cardiovascular complications, 697–708
  Composition of dialysate, 716
  Degenerative brain disorders, 726–728
  Diabetes mellitus (IDDM), 538–539
  Dietary intervention, 652
  Drug elimination technique, 641–646
  Drugs used in, see also Drugs, uremia and dialysis, 853–865
  Embolic disease, 435
  Equilibration, 739
  Fluid and electrolyte disturbances, 725
  Hypercalcemia, 98
  Hyperkalemia and renal failure, 255
  Hyperosmolality, 11
  Hyperphosphatemia, 274
  Hypertension, 430
  Liver, hepatic dysfunction, 485–486, 488
  Membrane biocompatibility, 813–833
    Beta$_2$ microglobulin, 826
    Clinical effects, 826–833
    Clotting factors, 816
    Complement, 817–821
    Compositions of membranes, 813–814
    Erythrocytes, 814–815
    Febrile reactions, 832
    First-use syndrome (FUS), 828–831
    Interleukin-1, 825–826, 832
    Kallikrein and kinin, 816–817
    Leaching and spallation of materials, 832–833
    Leukocytes, 821–824
    Other sequelae, 832
    Platelets, 815–816
    Pyrexial reactions, 832
  Meninges infections, 726
  Metabolic acidosis, 187, 189
  Multiple myeloma, 457, 458
  Number of patients in U.S., 877
  Pericarditis, 700
  Psychological preparation and social adjustment, 666, 721–722
  Respiratory acidosis, 228
  Reverse osmosis proportioning systems, 744–745
  Single-needle, 844–845, 848–849
  Syndromes secondary to hemorrhage, 725–726
  Therapy options for uremic diabetic, 539
  Ultrafiltration, 791–795, 798, 801–803, 828, 843
  Underdialysis, 729
  Uremia, 667
  Uremic neuropathy, 724
Dialysis dementia, 719, 726–728
Dialysis encephalopathy, 712, 726–728
Dialysis equilibrium syndrome, 719–721, 726, 728, 743, 802
Dialysis therapy, 36, 38
Dialyzers, 791–800
  Coil, 793, 794, 814
  Complement activation, 799
  Fluid removal, 792–793
  High risk permeability membrane, 795–798, 805
  Hollow-fiber, 793–798, 814, 828–830
  Hypersensitivity, 828–831
  Large surface area, 795–798
  Plate, 793–794, 814, 828–830
  Residual blood volume, 798
  Reuse of, 799–800, 814, 820–821, 828, 831–832
    Hemodialysis, 846
  Solute removal, 791–792
  Thrombogenicity, 798
Diazepam, 354, 515, 624, 642, 644
Dialysis disequilibrium syndrome, 728
  Hypertension and pregnancy, 510
Diazoxide, 78, 309, 379, 642
  Hypertension, 429, 430, 514, 515
  Scleroderma, 433
Dibekacin, 623, 642
Dicarboxylic aminoaciduria, 581, 582
Dichloroacetate, 185, 186
Dichloromethylene diphosphonate (Cl$_2$ MDP), 99
Dichlorphenamide, 30, 78
Dietary sodium intake, 5
DI-2-ethylplexyl phthalate (DEHP), 833, 848
Diet therapy, calcium stones, 145–146
Diffuse proliferative glomerulonephritis, 396–397, 401, 403–405
Diffuse proximal polymyopathy, 724
Diflunisal, 615
DiGeorge syndrome, 258
Digitalis, 34–35, 51–52, 58, 61
  Acute glomerulonephritis syndrome, 307
  Acute renal failure, 298
  Hypercalcemia, 96
  Hyperkalemia, 63–64
  Hypocalcemia, 257, 258, 271–272
  Hypokalemia, 64, 72, 75, 80, 270
  Intoxication, 58, 270, 848
  Metabolic acidosis, 183
  Metabolic alkalosis, 172
  Serum magnesium concentration checks, 116
  Supraventricular arrhythmias, 704
Digitoxin, 644
Digotoxin, 503, 644
Digoxin, 35, 292, 642, 644–646, 661
  Amyloidosis, 463
  Half-life, 856–858
  Hypokalemia, 81
Dihydroergotamine, 629
Dihydrotachysterol, 103, 583, 713
1,25-Dihydroxycholecalciferol, 655
1,25-Dihydroxyvitamin D$_3$, 121, 126, 127, 713–717
Diltiazem, hypertension, 428
Dimercaprol (BAL), 618, 619
Dimethoate, 643, 644
Dimethylcystine, cystinuria, 581
Dimethylsulfoxide (DMSO),

amyloidosis, 461–462
Dinitro-o-cresol, dialysis for removal, 642
Diphenhydramine, hemoperfusion for removal, 644
Diphenylhydantoin, 287, 642
Diphenylhydramine, dialysis for removal, 642
Diphosphonates, hypercalcemia, 97, 272
Diplopia, 724
Dipyramidole, preeclampsia, 514
Dipyridamole, 327, 345, 346, 815
   Goodpasture's syndrome, 339
   Hemolytic uraenine syndrome, 504–505
   Reflux nephropathy, 372, 379, 380
Diquat, 643, 644
Disopyramide, hemoperfusion for removal, 644
Disseminated intravascular coagulation (DIC), 502, 503, 505
Distal renal tubular acidosis, 189, 210–215, 253, 270
   Inherited renal tubular disorders, 582–583, 587
   Renal transplantation, 912
   Tubular dysfunction, 906–907
Diuretics, 3, 18, 253
   Acid-base disorders, 242
   Acute interstitial nephritis as result, 626
   Acute renal failure, 292
   Amyloidosis, 462, 463
   Antihypertensive drugs in pregnancy, 511
   Autosomal dominant polycystic kidney disease, 549
   Bartter syndrome, 589
   Diabetes mellitus (IDDM), 538
   Discontinuation and hypokalemia, 269
   Edematous states, 27, 28–34
   Hypercalcemia, 98, 99
   Hyperkalemia, 61
   Hypertension, 427
   Hyperuricemia, 473
   Hypervolemia, 248
   Hypocalcemia, 258
   Hypokalemia, 71, 73–75, 77, 80
   Hypomagnesemia, 115
   Hyponatremia, 6, 267
   Hypophosphatemia, 126, 129
   Hyporeninemic hypoaldosteronism, 583–584
   Infantile recessive polycystic kidney disease, 556
Liver, hepatic dysfunction, 479–483
Metabolic acidosis, 183
Metabolic alkalosis, 170
Potassium-sparing, 78, 80
Preeclampsia during pregnancy, 512, 513
Respiratory acidosis, 226, 229
Uremia and hypertension, 663–664
Diverticulitis, 355, 873–874
Diverticulosis, 766, 951
Dobutamine, 36, 292
Donor
   Selection in renal transplantation, 867–881
   ABO groups, 880
   Age limits, 869
   Beating-heart donor, 875
   Blood transfusions, 874–875
   Cadaver donors, 878–880
   Disease causing death of donor, 877
   General health assessment, 867–868
   High-risk recipients, 869–870
   HLA-A, B and C loci, 880–881
   HLA-D or DR antigens, 880
   Immunological factors, 875–878
   Living related donor (LRD), 875–877
   Living unrelated donors, 877–879
   Metastatic malignancy, 869
   Nonimmunological factors, 868–870
   Pretransplant evaluation of recipient, 871–872, 878–879
   Psychological assessment, 877
   Renal studies, 870–871
   Tuberculosis, 869–870
   Viral infections, 881
L-Dopa, 71
Dopamine, 36, 721, 880
Doxorubicin, 455, 456, 626, 644
Doxycycline, 624
Droperidol, 671
Drugs
   Dosage with uremia, 666
   Intoxication, 233, 639–646
      Acid-base disorders, 239–241
      Diagnosis, 639–640
      Dialysis in treatment of, 641–646
      Exchange blood transfusion in treatment of, 645
      Future trends in therapy, 645–646
      Hemodialysis in treatment of, 641, 643–646
      Hemoperfusion in treatment of, 641–646
      Plasmapheresis in treatment of, 645
      "Scandinavian method," 639
      Techniques for enhancing drug removal, 640–645
      Treatment, 640
   Nephrotoxicity, 661
   Removable by dialysis, 642–643
   Rmovable by hemoperfusion, 644
   Uremia and dialysis, 853–865
      Absorption, 853, 856
      Active metabolites, 859, 863
      Analgesics, 859, 860, 863
      Anesthetics, 860, 863
      Antacids, 862
      Antianginal agents, 862
      Antianxiety agents, sedatives and hypnotics, 860
      Antiarrhythmics, 862, 863, 864
      Antibiotics, 858–859
      Anticholinergics, 860, 863
      Anticoagulants, 860, 863
      Anticonvulsants, 860, 863
      Antidepressants, 860
      Antifibrinolytics, 860, 863
      Antifungals, 861, 864
      Antihelmintics, 862, 863
      Antihypertensives, 862, 863, 864
      Antihistamines, 860, 863
      Antiinflammatory agents, 860, 863
      Antimalarials, 861
      Antimaniacals, 860
      Antimetabolites, 862, 863
      Antimicrobial agents/ antibacterials, 860–861, 863–864
      Antineoplastics, 862, 863
      Antiparasitics, 862, 863
      Antiplatelet agents, 860, 863
      Antipsychotics, 860
      Antispasticity agents, 863
      Antituberculous agents, 862, 864
      Antiulcer agents, 862
      Antiviral agents, 862, 864
      Blood-lipid lowering agents, 863, 864
      Bronchodilators, 862
      Cardiac inotropes, 862, 863, 864

Cardiovascular agents, 862, 863, 864
Cholinergics, 860, 863
Cyclosporine, 862
Dextran 40, 864
Diuretics, 863
Drug-dialysis interactions, 858–859
EDTA, 864
Half-life, 856–858
Hypoglycemic agents, 863
Hypouricemic agents, 862, 863, 864
Kidney failure and drug pharmokinetics, 853–856
Loading dose, 853–856
Renal clearance, 856–858
Steroids, 862
Duodenal atresia, 217
Dysarthria, 719–720
Dysproteinemias, 453–464
Amyloidosis (AA type), 459–463
Amyloidosis (AL type), 453, 456, 458, 459–463
Cryoglobulinemias, 463–464
Defined, 453
Multiple myeloma, 453–458
Waldenstrom's macroglobulinemia, 453, 458–459

ECF, see Extracellular fluid
Eclampsia, 39, 119, 514, 515
Ectopic pregnancy, 523
Edematous states, 27–40
Acute glomerulonephritis, 36–37
Acute renal failure (ARF), 38
Azotemia, 27
Bed rest, 28
Chronic renal failure, 33, 38
Cirrhosis, ascites, and hepatorenal syndrome, 39–40
Combination therapy, 33–34
Congestive heart failure, 27, 28, 32–36, 38
Diet therapy, 27–28, 33
Diuretics, 27–34
Hypoalbuminemia, 27
Hyponatremia, 29
Hypovolemia, 27
Idiopathic edema, 39
Nephrotic syndrome, 28, 32, 33, 37–38
Potassium-sparing agents, 32
Pregnancy toxemia, 39
Premenstrual syndrome, 39

Treatment of specific clinical conditions, 34–40
Effective plasma volume, 478
Effective renal plasma flow (ERPF), pregnancy, 495
EHDP (Didronel R), 99
Ehler-Danlos syndrome, 556
Eicosapentaenoic acid, 399
Eighth cranial nerve damage, 96
Electrolytes, 2, 32
Abnormalities in perioperative period, 267–274
Acute renal failure, 294
Anaesthesia, 670
Diabetic ketoacidosis, 194–198
Disorders in children, 245–261
Disorders in surgical patients, 263–274
Embolic disease, 433–435
Emphysema, 225
Enalapril, 52, 54–55, 427, 537, 663–664
Enalaprilat, 429
Encephalitis, 225, 268
Encephalopathy, 134, 479, 480
Endocrine therapy, 604, 607–608
Endotoxemia, 228
End-stage renal disease (ESRD), 363, 533
Causes, 870–871
Chronic peritoneal dialysis, 744
Degenerative brain disorders, 727
Drug pharmokinetics, 854–855
Infective endocarditis, 704–708
Kidney transplantation, 867–881
Pericarditis, 699, 700
End-stage restrictive lung disease, 225
Enflurane, 671
Englebreth-Holm-Swarm tumor, 338
Enteric hyperoxaluria, 141
Enterococcal endocarditis, 311
Enterocolitis, 951
Epanutin, 515
Epidemic pyodermarelated nephritis, 310
Epididymitis, 960, 965
Epididymoorchitis, 962
Epidural anesthesia in labor, 516
Epidural spinal hematoma, 726
Epinephrine, 46, 50, 193, 194, 225
Hyperkalemia, 49, 63
Hypersensitivity during hemodialysis, 799
Hypokalemia, 65, 73
Renal ischemia as result, 614
Epsilonaminocaproic acid, 577, 629

Epstein-Barr virus (EBV), 463, 948, 951
Equilibration dialysis, 739
Ergocalciferol, 103, 713
Ergot, renal ischemia as result, 614
Ergotamine, 629
Erythrocytes, 814–815
Erythrocytosis, renal transplantation, 915
Erythromycin, 377, 626, 643, 946, 947
Urinary tract infections, 353
Erythropoiesis, 734–736
Esophageal candidiasis, 949
Essential hypertension, end-stage renal disease and transplantation, 870
Estrogen, 113, 170
Ethacrynic acid, 29–32, 96, 170, 309, 427
Ethadione, 616
Ethambutol, 388–391, 643
Ethanol, 185, 186, 624, 642
Ethchlorvynol, 642, 644, 645
Ethiamate, dialysis for removal, 642
Ethionamide, genitourinary tuberculosis, 388
Ethosuximide, dialysis for removal, 642
Ethylene glycol, 186, 187, 620, 629, 642
Ethylene oxide (ETO), 644, 829, 830, 847–848
Ethyl-phosphorothioic acid (WR 2721, S-2-3-aminopropylamine), 99
Eucalyptus oil, dialysis for removal, 643
Euvolemia, 266, 267–269
Exchange blood transfusion, 645
Exercise hyperemia, 51
Extracellular fluid (ECF), 1, 2
Diabetic ketoacidosis, 195, 196, 197, 203
Hyponatremia, 8
Metabolic acidosis, 183, 184, 186
Potassium pool, 46
Thermal burns, 280, 281, 282
Volume depletion, 5, 7, 287
Volume expansion with hypercalcemia, 95–96

Fabry's disease, 870, 935
Familial hematuria syndrome, 517
Familial hypoclicuric hypercalcemia (FHH), 93

Familial hypokalemic or hyperkalemic periodic paralysis, 225
Familial Mediterranean fever (FMF), 460, 462, 463, 912–913, 922–923
Familial pseudohyperkalemia, 48
Fanconi syndrome, 216, 459, 557, 582, 586–588
  Cadmium intoxication, 628
  Renal tubular functional abnormalities, 629
  Streptozoticin, 625
  Tubular dysfunction, 907
Fat embolism, 258
Fenoprofen, 615, 617, 626
Fenoterol, hypokalemia, 65
Fibrinolytic agents, renal vein thrombosis, 436
First-use syndrome, 799, 828–831, 832, 847
Flail chest, 224
Floxacillin, dialysis for removal, 642
Fludrocortisone, 62, 63, 189, 210
Fluid disorders
  In children, 245–261
  In surgical patients, 263–274
Fluid therapy, 670
Fluoride intoxication, 52, 270
Fluoroacetamide, hemoperfusion for removal, 644
5-Fluorocytosine, dialysis for removal, 643
5-Fluorouracil, dialysis for removal, 643
Fluoxide, dialysis for removal, 642
Focal glomerulosclerosis, 38, 321, 326–327
  Pregnancy, 506
Focal proliferative glomerulonephritis, 396
Focal sclerosis, recurrence on posttransplant biopsies, 871, 872
Focal segmental sclerosis, 326–327, 870, 871
Folic acid, 642, 687, 738
Forced diuresis, 641
Forearm veins, preservation of, 666
Fosfomycin, dialysis for removal, 642
Fructose, 186, 215, 216
Fungal brain abscesses, 729
Fungal infections, 949
Furadantin, autosomal dominant polycystic kidney disease, 550

Furosemide
  Acute interstitial nephritis as result, 626
  Acute glomerulonephritis syndrome, 309
  Acute renal failure, 291
  Diabetes mellitus (IDDM), 538
  Diuretic therapy, 27, 29–38, 40
  Heavy metal intoxication, 619
  Hypercalcemia, 95, 96, 256
  Hyperkalemia, 61–64, 254
  Hypertension, 427, 428, 512, 514
  Hypervolemia, 248, 249
  Hypocalcemia, 100, 257
  Hypokalemia, 71, 78
  Hyponatremia, 7, 8
  Metabolic acidosis, 189
  Metabolic alkalosis, 170
  Nephrotic syndrome, 320
  Nephrotoxicity, 625
  Renal tubular acidosis, 210, 211, 217
  Ultrafiltration rate effect, 760
  Uric acid nephropathy, 470, 471

Galactosemia, 215, 216, 587
Gallamine, 642, 671–672
Gallbladder disease, 873
Gamma-aminobutyric acid (GABA), 721
Gamma globulin therapy, hemolytic uremic syndrome, 446
Gases, dialysis for removal, 643, 644
Gastric alkalosis, 168–169, 240
Gastroenteritis, hypernatremia, 12
Gemfibrozil, 321
Generalized lymphadenopathy, 390
Generalized prostaglandin deficiency, pregnancy, 513
Genioglossus nerve stimulation, 225–226
Genitourinary tuberculosis, 354, 387–393
Gentamicin, 115–116, 622, 623, 642, 644
  Acute renal failure, 503
  Autosomal dominant polycystic kidney disease, 548
  Infective endocarditis, 707, 708
  Urinary tract infections, 353, 354, 356, 660
Gibbs-Donnan effect, 295
"Giving-up-given-up" syndrome, 539
Glafenine, acute interstitial nephritis as result, 626
Glomerular cystic disease, 555
Glomerular disease, renal transplantation, 870, 871
Glomerular filtration rate (GFR), 28, 32, 34–38, 40
  Acute glomerulonephritis syndrome, 305, 306, 309
  Acute renal failure, 288–291
  Aminoglycoside nephrotoxicity, 622
  Anesthesia effect on, 263
  Bicarbonate reabsorption, 160, 161, 168
  Diabetes mellitus (IDDM), 534, 535, 536
  Differences between children and adults, 245–246, 247
  Hypercalcemia, 93
  Hyperkalemia, 45, 53–55, 62, 64
  Hypermagnesemia, 118
  Hypokalemia, 78
  Hypoosmolar states, 3
  IgA nephropathy, 345
  Metabolic acidosis, 177
  Metabolic alkalosis, 167
  Nephrotic syndrome, 317
  Pregnancy, 495, 496
  Reflux nephropathy, 379
  Renal failure, 241
  Renal ischemia, 615
  Renal sodium handling, 478
  Renal tubular acidosis, 214–217
  Urinary tract infections, 352
Glomerular hematuria, 343
Glomerular sclerosis, 310, 538
Glomerulonephritis, 287, 339, 343–345, 490–491, 872
  Plasma separation, 848
  Rapidly progressive, ESRD and transplantation, 870
  Urinary tract infections, 351
  Vasculitic kidney disease, 413, 415–418
Glomerulopathies, 323–328
Glomerulosclerosis, 79, 344, 397
Glucagon, 113, 193, 196, 198
Glucocorticoids, 267, 268
  Hemolytic uremic syndrome, 446
  Hypercalcemia, 94, 97–98
  Hyperkalemia, 51, 52, 62
  Hyperphosphatemia, 132
  Hypokalemia, 67, 70, 71
  Hypophosphatemia, 127
  Nephrotic syndrome, 324
  Respiratory acidosis, 229
Glucocorticosteroids, hypercalcemia, 99
Glucose, 19

Acute renal failure, 293–294, 298
Alcoholic acidosis, 240
Burn shock, 280
Clycosurias, 582
Diabetic ketoacidosis, 193, 194–195, 198, 200
Dialysate composition, 801, 804–805
Hyperkalemia, 52, 59
Hypernatremia, 11–12
Hyperosmolar states, 10
Hyperphosphatemia, 133
Hypokalemia, 77
Hypophosphatemia, 127
Lactic acidosis, 184
Metabolic alkalosis, 162, 171
Water volume disorders, 248
Glucosurias, 582
Glutamine, cystinuria, 582
Glutethimide, 642, 644, 645
Glycerol, 2, 19
Glycine, 4, 267, 268
Glycinuria, 582
Glycogen storage disease, 215, 587
Glycol nephrotoxicity, 620
Glycosuria, 126, 195
Glycyrrhizic acid, 170
Glycyrrhizinic acid, 70, 71
Gold, acute interstitial nephritis as result, 626
Gold nephrosis, 616, 617
Goodpasture's syndrome, 287, 333–340, 616, 848
Renal transplantation, 926
Gordon's syndrome, 55, 61, 64
Gore-Tex straight tube graft, 782–785
Gossypol, 70–71
Gout, 140, 472–473, 557, 655, 666
Graft occlusion, 783–784
Gram-negative bacteremia, 238, 286–287
Grand-mal seizure-induced lactic acidosis, 228
Granulomatosous diseases (sarcoid), 97, 255, 272
Gray syndrome in newborns, 358
Growth
Renal transplantation, 952
Renal tubular acidosis, 214–215, 216, 218
Retardation, 189
Guillain-Barre-Strohl syndrome, 305
Guillain-Barre syndrome, 128, 225
Guanabenz, 427, 428
Guanfacine, 427, 428

Hageman factor (factor XII), 816–817
Halogenated hydrocarbons, 620–621
Haloperidol, 4, 722
Hard water syndrome, 725, 800
Hartnup's disease, 581, 582
Hashimoto's disease, 93
Hashimoto's thyroiditis, 101
HbSC disease, 56
HbSS disease, 56
Head trauma, 250
Heavy metals, 617, 618
HELLP (Hemolysis, Elevated Liver enzymes, Low Platelets) syndrome, pregnancy, 504
Hemangiopericytomas, 169–170
Hematologic abnormalities, 733–738
Hematuria, 139, 328
  Acute glomerulonephritis syndrome, 308, 309, 311
  Bladder cancer, 601
  Cancer of renal pelvis and ureter, 597–598
  Sickle hemoglobinemia, 574, 577
Hemodiafiltration, 841, 843, 844, 848
Hemodialysis-associated hepatitis, 488–489
Hemofiltration, 646, 841, 843–844, 848
Hemolysis, 52, 270, 288, 733–734
Hemodialysis, 98, 623, 734–736, 798–799, 846–847
  Access surgery, 775–786
  Acquired cystic disease as result, 560
  Acute glomerulonephritis syndrome, 310
  Acute renal failure, 293, 295–297, 501, 506, 508
  Amyloidosis, 463, 913
  Asymptomatic bacteriuria, 497
  Autosomal dominant polycystic kidney disease, 552
  Carpal tunnel syndrome, 729
  Chronic renal failure, 848
  Diabetes mellitus (IDDM), 536, 538, 539, 540
  Dialysis disequilibrium syndrome, 719, 720, 721, 726, 728
  Dialyzability of specific drugs removed by one session, 860–862
  Drug elimination technique, 641, 643–646
  First-use syndrome, 799
  Heavy metal nephrotoxicity, 618–619
  Hypercalcemia, 272
  Hyperkalemia, 60–61, 255
  Hypermagnesemia, 118–119, 273
  Hyperphosphatemia, 133
  Hypervolemia, 248
  Hypocalcemia, 257
  Hypoxemia, 669
  IgA nephropathy, 346
  Infantile recessive polycystic kidney disease, 556
  Infective endocarditis, 704
  Iodide nephrotoxicity, 621
  Iron deficiency prone, 688
  Lead intoxication, 628
  Leukopenia induced by, 821–822
  Liver, hepatic dysfunction, 482, 486–489
  Management during pregnancy, 521–522
  Metabolic acidosis, 184, 186–188
  Metabolic alkalosis, 172, 173
  Multiple myeloma, 456–458
  Neuromuscular symptoms, 666
  Nutritional management, 680–683, 685
  Respiratory acidosis, 226
  Sickle-cell anemia, 577
  Solute clearance, 756
  Technique, 841–842
  Uric acid nephropathy, 471
  Water treatment, 800–805
Hemolytic-uremic syndrome (HUS), 287, 443–449, 500
  Acute renal failure, 286
  Clinical features, 443, 444
  End-stage renal disease and transplantation, 870
  Laboratory features, 444–445
  Pathogenesis, 443–444
  Plasma exchange (PE) therapy, 445–446
  Plasma infusion (PI) therapy, 445–446
  Pregnancy, 446, 504–505
  Renal transplantation, 446, 447, 926–927
  Treatment, 445–446
Hemoperfusion, 641–646, 841, 844, 848
Hemophan (dialyzer membrane), 814, 819, 820
Hemosiderosis, 665
Hemothorax, 224
Henderson-Hasselbalch equation, 163

Henoch-Schonlein purpura, 305, 333, 343, 344, 418–421
Henoch Schonlein purpura, renal transplantation, 870, 925
Heparin, 52–54, 270, 338, 758, 765
  Acute renal failure, 296–297, 503
  Anti-clotting for hemodialysis, 815
  Autosomal dominant polycystic kidney disease, 552
  For anticoagulation during dialysis, 779, 782, 798, 826, 847–848
  Hemodialysis and potassium homeostasis disorders, 909
  Hemolytic uremic syndrome, 445, 504–505
  Intraperitoneal, 741
  Liver, hepatic dysfunction, 482
  Pericarditis, 699, 700
  Reflux nephropathy, 379, 380, 381
  Renal vein thrombosis, 436
  Subdural hematoma, 726
Hepatitis, 297
Hepatitis B virus, 463, 488–491, 665, 872, 948
  Blood transfusions, 875
  Renal transplantation, 870, 879
  Surface antigen, 413
Hepatitis non-A, non-B virus, 948
Hepatorenal syndrome, 40, 479
Herbicides, dialysis for removal, 643–644
Hereditary cystinosis, renal transplantation, 934–935
Hereditary diseases, end-stage renal disease and transplantation, 870
Hereditary fructose intolerance, 587
Hereditary hyperoxaluria, renal transplantation, 933–934
Hereditary hypophosphatemic rickets with hypercalcuria, 584–585
Hereditary nephritis, pregnancy, 517
Heroin, 616, 624, 642
Herpes simplex virus, 355, 948
Hexabarbital, hemoperfusion for removal, 644
Heymann nephritis, 328
Histidnuria, 582
Hodgkin's disease, 334, 399
Human immunodeficiency virus (HIV), renal transplantation, 879, 881
Humoral hypercalcemia of malignancy (HHM), 92, 93
"Hungry bones" syndrome, 102, 104, 258, 271, 273
Huntington's disease, 554
Hydralazine, 36, 39, 292, 309, 404
  Autosomal dominant polycystic kidney disease, 549
  Hypertension, 427, 428–430, 511–512
    Pregnancy, 514, 515
  Improving myocardial performance, 704
  Scleroderma, 433
  Toxic nephropathies, 616, 629
Hydrochloric acid, 172–173, 229
Hydrochlorothiazide, 30, 32, 34–39, 71, 79
  Autosomal dominant polycystic kidney disease, 549
  Hypertension, 427
  Hypervolemia, 248
  Renal tubular acidosis, 216, 583
Hydrocortisone, 95, 256, 279
Hydrogen ion excretion, 246
Hydronephrosis, 21, 140
Hydroureter, polyuria, 21
Hydroureteronephrosis, 957–958
β-Hydroxybutyric acidosis, 239
25-Hydroxycholecalciferol, 320–321
1-α-Hydroxy cholecalciferol, 103, 104
11-Hydroxylase deficiency, 170
17-Hydroxylase deficiency, syndromes, 70
21-Hydroxylase deficiency, 54, 217
17-β-Hydroxylase deficiency, 170
1,25-$(OH)_2$ vitamin D_3 therapy, 586, 588, 664
25-Hydroxyvitamin D_3, 713
1α Hydroxyvitamin D_3, 713
Hyperacetemia, 803
Hyperaldosteronism, 32–33, 39, 53, 169, 273
  Metabolic alkalosis, 167, 169
Hyperalimentation, 125–127, 130, 273, 282, 869
  Acute renal failure, 293, 294–295
  Hypophosphatemia, 130, 274
Hyperammonemia, pregnancy, 504
Hyperbicarbonatemia, 236, 241, 260
Hyperbilirubinemia, 358, 504
Hypercalcemia, 79, 91–100, 255–256, 272, 625
  Acute renal failure, 288, 296, 298
  Bicarbonate reabsorption, 162, 163
  Calcium in dialysate composition, 803
  Calcium stones, 140, 150
  Diagnosis, 94–95
  Disequilibrium, 92, 95, 98, 99
  Drugs for management, 292
  Hereditary hypophosphatemic rickets, 585
  Hungry bones syndrome, 104
  Hyperphosphatemia, 132
  Hypervitaminosis-D, 99
  Hypokalemia, 96
  Hypomagnesemia, 273
  Malignant, 99
  Medullary carcinoma, 93
  Metabolic alkalosis, 166, 171
  Milk alkali syndrome, 99
  Multiple endocrine neoplasia (MEN) syndromes, 93
  Multiple myeloma, 93, 453–454, 456–458
  Polyuria, 19, 21, 22, 23
  Primary hyperparathyroidism, 98–99
  Renal insufficiency, 662
  Renal osteodystrophy, 713–717
  Renal transplantation, 910–911, 912
  Renal tubular acidosis, 215
  Signs and symptoms, 94, 95, 255
  T-cell lymphoma, 93
  Therapy, 95–100
  Thyrotoxicosis, 99
  Uremia, 664
Hypercalcemic hypocalciuria, 255
Hypercalciuria, 79, 94–95, 100, 583
  Hypocalcemia, 103
  Hypophosphatemia, 124
  Inherited trait, 142–143
  Nephrolithiasis, 140–147, 149–150, 153
  Renal tubular acidosis, 212, 215
Hypercapnia, 171, 223–227, 264
  Acid-base disorders, 234–237, 239, 241, 242
Hypercarbia, 128, 226, 229
Hyperchloremia, 171, 211
Hyperchloremic acidosis, 54, 95, 197
Hyperchloremic metabolic acidosis, 57, 64, 150
Hypercholesterolemia, nephrotic syndrome, 321
Hypercortisolism, 132
Hypercystinuria, 582
Hyperfiltration, 536–537, 576
Hypergammaglobulinemia, 164, 395

Index 989

Hyperglycemia, 2, 33, 249, 270, 743–744
  Acute glomerulonephritis syndrome, 309
  Burn response, 281, 282
  Diabetes mellitus (IDDM), 536–537, 538
  Diabetic ketoacidosis, 194–195, 198–201
  Hyperkalemia, 59–60, 270
  Hypernatremia, 11–12
  Peritoneal dialysis, 750
  Polyuria, 24
  Potassium uptake, 50, 51
  Pregnancy, 514
  Pseudohyponatremia, 267, 268
  Renal transplantation, 909
Hyper-hypomagnesemia, 258
Hypericarbonatremia, 239
Hyperinsulinemia, 65, 768
Hyperkalemia, 31–33, 37–38, 46–57, 63–64, 762
  Acute glomerulonephritis syndrome, 305, 308, 309, 310
  Acute renal failure, 293, 294, 296, 298
  Anaesthesia, 670, 671
  Autosomal dominant polycystic kidney disease, 556
  Blood transfusions, 67
  Burns, 261
  Causes, 50, 54, 254, 270
  Clinical approach, 48–49
  Clinical consequences, 56–57
  Congestive heart failure, 59, 63
  Diabetic ketoacidosis, 198, 201, 203, 204
  Diagnostic procedures, 49
  Dialysis patients, 725
  Diet therapy, 57
  Diuretics, 61
  Drug-induced, 52, 64
  Hematologic abnormalities, 736
  Hyperphosphatemia, 132–133
  Hypertension, 429
  Hyponatremia, 59
  Hypophosphatemia, 131
  Hypovolemia, 59
  Management, 57–64
  Medullary cystic disease, 558
  Metabolic acidosis, 180, 189
  Metabolic alkalosis, 162–165
  Perioperative surgical patient, 270–271
  Peritoneal dialysis required, 739–740
  Pigment nephropathy, 625
  Pneumonitis, 60
  Potassium metabolism disorders, 253–255
  Psychological noncompliance as cause, 721
  Redistribution, 270
  Renal ischemia, 614
  Renal transplantation, 908, 909
  Renal tubular acidosis, 207, 208, 216, 217
  Respiratory acidosis, 228
  Sickle hemoglobulinemia, 575, 576–577
  Therapy, 57–64
  Triamterene, 78
  Uremia, 665
  Urinary tract infections, 352
  Volume depletion after surgery, 265
Hyperkalemic periodic paralysis, 51, 63
Hyperkalemic renal tubular acidosis, 583
Hyperketonemia, 196
Hyperlipidemia, 249, 268, 321–322
  Dialysis patients, 768, 842
  Renal transplantation, 950
  Uremia, 665–666
Hypermagnesemia, 93, 95, 112, 118–119, 260
  Acute renal failure, 298
  Anaesthesia, 670
  Causes, 118–119
  Clinical manifestations, 119, 273
  Continuous ambulatory peritoneal dialysis, 762
  Dialysis composition, 725, 804
  Perioperative period surgical patient, 273
  Therapy guidelines, 119
Hypernatremia, 2, 7, 10–12, 250–252
  Acute renal failure, 297
  Diabetes insipidus, 12
  Diabetes mellitus, 11
  Dialysis patients, 725
  Limiting factor for hypertonic saline solution administration, 266
  Metabolic acidosis, 183, 251
  Perioperative period surgical patient, 267–269
  Peritoneal dialysis recommended, 740
  Polyuria, 21, 23, 24
  Signs and symptoms, 11, 12
Hyperosmolality, 10–12, 21, 23–24, 59, 266
  Acute peritoneal dialysis, 743–744
  Diabetic ketoacidosis, 194
  Treatment of, 1–12
Hyperosmolar nonketotic coma, 282
Hyperoxaluria, 140, 151–153, 870
Hyperparathyroid bone disease, 715
Hyperparathyroidism, 118, 166, 171, 255, 256
  Hypercalcemia, 272
  Hyperphosphatemia, 132
  Hypophosphatemia, 127
  Medullary cystic disease, 558
  Nephrotic syndrome, 318, 321
  Primary, 92–95, 97–99, 141–144, 149–151, 153
  Renal transplantation, 910–912
  Secondary, 215
Hyperphosphatemia, 102, 103, 131–134, 258, 271
  Acute metabolic acidosis, 132
  Acute renal failure, 298
  Acute respiratory acidosis, 132
  Causes, 131–132
  Hypophosphatemia, 131
  Perioperative period surgical patient, 274
  Rhabdomyolysis, 131
  Renal osteodystrophy, 711–714, 717
  Renal tubular acidosis, 216
  Sickle hemoglobinemia, 575
  Treatment, 133–134
  Tumor lysis syndrome, 131, 470
  Uremia, 664
Hyperplasia, hypercalcemia, 93
Hyperpotassemia, 802
Hyperproteinemia, 267, 268
Hyperreninemia, scleroderma, 433
Hypersensitivity angiitis, 333
Hypersensitivity reactions, polyarteritis, 413
Hypersplenism, 553, 555, 556, 874
Hypertension, 64, 165, 425–430, 516, 654
  Acid-base disorders, 237
  Acute glomerulonephritis syndrome, 306, 307, 309–310, 311
  Acute renal failure, 286
  Anaesthesia, 669
  Atherosclerotic cardiovascular disease, 697
  Autosomal dominant polycystic kidney disease, 544, 546, 549, 551, 553, 556
  Cardinal features of crisis, 429
  Chronic hyperuricemic nephropathy, 472

Chronic renal failure, 661
Continuous ambulatory peritoneal dialysis, 761
Cryoglobulinemias, 464
Diabetes mellitus (IDDM), 536–539, 541
Dietary intervention, 651–652
Edematous states, 27, 33, 38, 39
Embolic disease, 434, 435
Hypercalcemia, 94
Hyperkalemia, 55, 63, 255
Hyperuricemia, 473
Hypokalemia, 65, 70, 73, 80
Hypomagnesemia, 115
IgA nephropathy, 345
Malignant, 287
Metabolic alkalosis, 169, 170
Multicystic kidney disease, 560
Nephrotic syndrome, 320
Nondietary intervention, 653–655
Pharmacokinetics of drugs used in treatment, 427–428
Polyarteritis, 414
Pregnancy, 507–516, 518–526
Primary hyperparathyroidism, 150, 151
Radiation nephritis, 628
Reflux nephropathy, 367–368, 370, 371, 378–379, 381
Renal transplantation, 913–915, 943, 950
Renal tubular acidosis, 217
Renal vein thrombosis, 435
Renovascular, 430
Scleroderma, 433
Sickle-cell anemia, 575
Systemic lupus erythematosus, 397, 404
Uremia, 663–664
Venous, 780
Hypertensive encephalopathy, 305–306, 308–309, 429–430, 720, 726
Hyperthyroidism, 94, 112–113, 150, 255, 512
Hypertriglyceridemia, 267, 685–686, 746, 750
Acetate in dialysate composition, 803
Continuous ambulatory peritoneal dialysis, 763, 768
Renal transplantation, 950
Hypertrophic obstructive cardiomyopathy, 512
Hyperuricemia, 33, 79, 132–133, 217, 557
Acute renal failure, 288
Acute uric acid nephropathy, 469, 470
Asymptomatic, 473
Compared to gout, 655–656
Multiple myeloma, 454, 457
Nephropathies, 469–473
Pregnancy, 504
Sickle hemoglobulinemia, 575
Uremia, 666
Hyperuricosuria, 141, 144, 146–149, 153, 469
Diet therapy, 148–149
Treatment, 154
Hyperventilation, 124–128, 181, 182, 228, 238
Hyperviscosity syndrome, 458, 459, 848
Hypervitaminosis A, 687
Hypervitaminosis-D, 150, 153, 255–256, 629–630, 662
Hypercalcemia, 92–95, 97, 99, 104, 272
Renal transplantation, 910
Hypervolemia, 217, 248–249, 252, 320
Hypoalbuminemia, 27, 91–92, 188, 309, 317–322
Amyloidosis, 463
Diabetes mellitus, 535
Hypocalcemia, 271
Uremia, 678
Hypoaldosteronism, 54, 217, 254
Hypobicarbonatemia, 203–235–237
Hypocalcemia, 91, 96, 100–104, 203, 256–258
Acute renal failure, 257, 298, 502
Causes, 100, 101, 257
Clinical manifestations, 100–101
Diagnosis, 101–102
Disorders which may require therapy, 102–104
Hungry bones syndrome, 102, 104
Hyperparathyroidism, 101, 102
Hyperphosphatemia, 133–134, 258
Hypervitaminosis-D, 104
Hypophosphatemia, 131
Magnesurias, 586
Neonatals, 525
Nephrotic syndrome, 103, 318, 320–321
Perioperative period surgical patient, 271
Potassium metabolism disorders, 56, 58–59, 70
Renal tubular acidosis, 215
Signs and symptoms, 100, 101–102
Therapy, 102–104, 271–272
Uric acid nephropathy, 470
Vitamin D deficiency, 101–104
Hypocalciuria, 94, 101, 216, 318
Hypocapnia, acid-base disorders, 235–240, 242
Hypochloremia, 77, 167, 266
Hypocitraturia, 212, 215
Hypocomplementemia, 311, 312, 327, 435
Goodpasture's syndrome, 335
Pregnancy, 504
Renal transplantation, 924
Hypogammaglobulinemia, nephrotic syndrome, 318, 322
Hypoglycemia, 23, 200, 240, 428
Dialysis patients, 725, 805
Hyperkalemia, 60
Neonatals, 525
Hypokalemia, see also Potassium depletion, 28, 30, 32–35, 40, 64–81
Barium poisoning, 78
Bartter's syndrome, 67, 70, 72–73, 75, 78–79
Bicarbonate reabsorption, 162, 163
Causes in children, 252
Clinical approach, 48–49
Clinical consequences, 71
Diabetic ketoacidosis, 203, 204
Diagnosis, 49, 68–69
Drug-induced, 66, 70–71
Eating disorders, 80
Fanconi syndrome, 586
Hypercalcemia, 96
Hypercalciuria, 145
Hypervolemia, 248
Hyponatremia, 267
Hypophosphatemia, 127
Limiting factor for hypertonic saline solution administration, 266
Liver, hepatic dysfunction, 479, 480
Management, 74–78
Management of specific conditions, 78–81
Metabolic acidosis, 182, 187, 189
Metabolic alkalosis, 165, 167, 169, 170, 172
Nephrotic syndrome, 80, 320
Oral rehydration, 251
Oral replacement therapy, 76
Polyuria, 19, 21–22, 23
Potassium balance disorder, 252–253
Potassium total body intake, 47

Pregnancy, 512
Renal transplantation, 908
Renal tubular acidosis, 212, 213, 215
Respiratory acidosis, 229
Salicylate intoxication, 240
Surgical patient, 265, 269–270
Therapy, 74–78
Water volume disorders, 248
Hypokalemic myopathy, 225
Hypokalemic periodic paralysis, 65–66, 70, 72, 76–78
Hypomagnesemia, 96, 113, 258, 260
   Acute renal failure, 294, 298
   Bartter's syndrome, 115–116
   Causes, 115, 273
   Clinical manifestations, 273
   Diagnosis, 116–117
   Dialysis patients, 725
   Hypocalcemia, 102, 271
   Hypophosphatemia, 127
   Magnesurias, 586
   Metabolic alkalosis, 172
   Perioperative period surgical patients, 272–273
   Potassium metabolism disorders, 56, 70, 79–80
   Symptomatology, 116
   Therapy guidelines, 117–118
Hyponatremia, 1–12, 23–24, 36, 53, 56
   Acute renal failure, 293
   Body fluid composition disorder, 249–250
   Burns, 281
   Diabetic ketoacidosis, 199, 204
   Dialysis patients, 725
   Diuretic-induced, 6
   Hyperkalemia, 59
   Liver, hepatic dysfunction, 479, 486
   Pregnancy, 512
   Renal tubular acidosis, 217
   Resulting from diuretic therapy, 33
   Surgical patients, 6–7, 267–268
   Symptomatic, 6, 8–9, 29
   Therapy, 6–10, 29, 38
Hypoosmolality, 2–3, 21, 23
   Treatment of, 1–12
Hypoparathyroidism, 94, 102–103, 271
   Hyperphosphatemia, 132
   Hypocalcemia, 101–102
   Metabolic alkalosis, 171
Hypophosphatemia, see also Phosphorus depletion, 93, 104, 123–131, 272
   Acute renal failure, 294
   Alcoholic patient, 126, 128
   Causes, 123–124, 126, 128
   Clinical conditions, 127–128
   Clinical manifestations, 274
   Diabetic ketoacidosis (DKA), 126–127
   Hyperalimentation, 125, 130, 274
   Hypercalcemia, 272
   Hypercalciuria, 582
   Hyperphosphatemia, 134
   Incidence, 123
   Nutritional recovery syndrome, 127
   Perioperative period surgical patients, 273–274
   Primary hyperparathyroidism, 150
   Renal transplantation, 127, 910, 912
   Renal tubular acidosis, 908
   Respiratory alkalosis, 124–125, 127
   Respiratory muscle, 130
   Severe thermal burns, 127
   Side effects and complications of treatment, 131
   Treatment, 128
Hypophosphatemic bone disease, 582
Hypophosphatemic nonrachitic bone disease, 584–585
Hypoproteinemia, 306, 320, 420
Hyporeninemia, metabolic alkalosis, 169
Hyporeninemic hypoaldosteronism (HRHA) syndrome, 61, 62, 583–584, 909
Hyporeninism, 64, 254
Hyposthenuria, 21, 573, 576
Hypotension, 17, 96, 204
Hypothermia, 282, 740
Hypothyroidism, 93, 112–113, 118, 258, 267–268
   Hyperphosphatemia, 132
   Nephrotic syndrome, 318, 320
Hypouricemia, 186
Hypoventilation, 171, 224–230, 271
Hypovitaminosis D, nephrotic syndrome, 318
Hypovolemia, 27, 204, 247–248, 259, 261
   Acute renal failure, 285, 287
   Amyloidosis, 462
   Hyperkalemia, 59
   Liver, hepatic dysfunction, 483, 485
   Polyuria, 17, 18, 23, 24
   Pregnancy, 516
Hypoxanthine, 291, 292
Hypoxanthineguanine phosphoribosyl transferase (HGPRT) deficiency, 469
Hypoxemia, 183, 224–229, 241
   Dialysis related, 799, 803, 821–823, 826–828
Hypoxia, 8, 72, 128, 190, 264
Hytakerol, 103

Ibuprofen, 253, 615
   Acute interstitial nephritis as result, 626
   Cirrhosis, 479
Idiogenic osmoles, 2
Idiopathic bilateral diaphragmatic paralysis, 226
Idiopathic hypercalciuria, 141
Idiopathic hypoparathyroidism, 258
Idiopathic mesangiocapillary glomerulonephritis, 305
Idiopathic pulmonary hemosiderosis, 338
Ifosfamide, multiple myeloma, 454
IgA nephropathy (Berger's), see also Berger's nephropathy, 343–345
   End-stage renal disease and transplantation, 870
   Recurrence on posttransplant biopsies, 871
Ileostomy, 153–154, 179
Iminoglycinuria, 581
Imipinem, dialysis for removal, 642
Imipramine, 642, 644
Immunosuppression, see also specific topics, 887–898
   "Conventional" side effects, 891
   Maintenance with cyclosporin, 891–896
   Total lymph node irradiation (TLI), 896
   Urologic complications, 944–945
Immunotherapeutic (BCG) agents, bladder cancer, 602
Indomethacin, 23, 79, 253, 615–616
   Acute interstitial nephritis as result, 626
   Bartter syndrome, 589
   Cirrhosis, 479
   Diabetes mellitus, 535
   Hypercalcemia, 96, 98
   IgA nephropathy, 345
   Membrane biocompatibility, 828
   Pericarditis, 700

992 Index

Infantile recessive polycystic kidney disease (IRPKD), 543, 554–557
Infection stones, end-stage renal disease and transplantation, 870
Infections, end-stage renal disease and transplantation, 870
Infectious mononucleosis, 270
Infective endocarditis, 697, 704–708
Inflammatory bowel disease, 154
Inflammatory ileocolitis, 153
Influenza A virus, 948
Influenza B virus, 948
Inherited renal tubular disorders, 581–589
Inorganics, dialysis for removal, 642, 644
Insecticides, dialysis for removal, 643, 644
Insulin
 Aneurysms and autosomal dominant polycystic kidney disease, 549
 Bicarbonate reabsorption, 162
 Burn patient hyperosmolar nonketonic coma, 282
 Deficiency, 194–199
 Hyperkalemia, 59–60
 Hyperphosphatemia, 133
 Hypocalcemia, 257, 258
 Hypokalemia, 65, 66, 72, 73, 77
 Hypophosphatemia, 125, 126
 Physiology, 194
 Potassium homeostasis, 46, 50
 Serum magnesium concentration, 113
 Therapy for diabetic ketoacidosis, 203–204
Interaction reaction, 226–227
Interleukin-1 (IL-1), 825–826, 832, 887–888
Interleukin-2 (IL-2), 887–888
Intermittent peritoneal dialysis (IPD), 741, 745, 749, 755
 Solute clearance, 756
Interstitial disease, 79
 End-stage renal disease and transplantation, 870
Interstitial nephritis, 70, 217, 260, 343, 624
 Urinary tract infections, 359
Interstitial renal disease, metabolic acidosis, 180
Intestinal bypass, 154
Intestinal obstruction, 267
Intracellular fluid (ICF), potassium balance, 46

Intracranial hemorrhage, 11
 Hypernatremia, 12
Iodide, 615, 642
Iodide nephrotoxicity, 621
Iodinated radiographic contrast media, 621
Iron, 688
 Deficiency, 733, 737
 Dialysis for removal, 642
 Hemoperfusion for removal, 644
 Intoxication, 620, 646, 800
Ischemic heart disease, 321
Ischemic venipuncture, 270
Isocarboxazid, dialysis for removal, 642
Isoflurane, 671
Isoniazid, 186, 616
 Dialysis for removal, 643
 Genitourinary tuberculosis, 387–392
 Hemoperfusion for removal, 644
Isopropanol, dialysis for removal, 643
Isopropyl myristate, 833
Isoproterenol, 194
Italian Y connector, 766

Juvenile diabetes (IDDM), 533, 534
Juxtaglomerular apparatus hyperplasia, 169

Kaliuresis, 32, 35, 46, 71
 Hyperkalemia, 51
Kanamycin, 622, 623
 Dialysis for removal, 642
 Urinary tract infections, 353, 354
Kayexalate, 60, 62, 167, 189, 908
 Acute renal failure, 296, 298
Kayexalate R, 255
Ketamine, 671
Ketanserin, 515
Ketoacidosis, diabetic, see Diabetes, ketoacidosis
Ketoacids, 679–680
Ketoconazole, 53, 100
Ketonemia, 200
Ketonuria, 126
Ketoprofen, acute interstitial nephritis as result, 626
Kidney
 Cancer, 593–597
 Transplantation, see also specific topics
  Amyloidosis, 463, 912–913
  Autosomal dominant polycystic kidney disease,

552–554
  Bacterial infections, 948–949
  Bone complications, 952
  Cancer, 950–951
  Cardiovascular complications, 949–951
  Cataracts, 952
  Complications, 729–730
  Diabetes mellitus (IDDM), 539–541, 928–930
  Distal renal tubular acidosis, 912
  Divalent ion metabolism disorders, 910–911
  Donor and recipient selection, see also Donor selection, 867–881
  Drug therapy complications, 953
  Erythrocytosis, 915
  Familial Mediterranean fever, 912–913
  Fungal infections, 949
  Gastrointestinal complications, 951
  Goodpasture's syndrome, 340
  Growth in children, 952
  Hemolytic uremic syndrome, 446, 447
  Hypercalcemia, 910–912
  Hyperglycemia, 909
  Hyperkalemia, 908, 909
  Hyperparathyroidism, 911–912
  Hypertension, 913–915
  Hypokalemia, 908
  Hypophosphatemia, 274, 910, 912
  IgA nephropathy, 346
  Infections, 946–949
  Inherited and metabolic diseases, 930–935
  Light chain deposition disease, 459
  Liver, hepatic dysfunction, 487
  Lymphatic complications, 945
  Metabolic dysfunction, 905–915
  Nephrocalcinosis, 911–912
  Nephrolithiasis, 911–912
  Neuromuscular symptoms, 666
  Number of patients per year in U.S., 877, 878
  Obstructive uropathy, 910
  Patient reaction to, 721
  Pregnancy, 522–526, 927
  Pretransplant evaluation of

recipient, 871–873
Pretransplant surgical preparation, 873–874
Protozoal and helminthic infections, 949
Psychological preparation and social adjustment, 666, 667
Pulmonary infection, 946–947
Recipient selection, see also Recipient selection, 867–881
Renal artery stenosis, 914, 915
Renal function preservation, 672
Renin-angiotensin system, 913, 914
Rheumatologic disorders, 923–926
Sickle-cell anemia, 577–578
Systemic diseases, 921–923
Thrombotic microangiopathic disorders, 926–928
Tubular dysfunction, 905–915
Urinary dilution and concentration, 910
Urinary tract infection, 912
Urologic complications, 944–945
Vascular complications, 943–944
Vitamin-D intoxication, 910
Wound infections, 945
Kidneys-ureters-bladder (KUB) x-ray, acute renal failure, 287
Kimmelstiel-Wilson's disease, 667
Kock continent pouch technique, 603
Korsakoff psychosis, 725
Kussmaul respirations, 200
Kyphoscoliosis, 225

Labetalol
 Autosomal dominant polycystic kidney disease, 549
 Hypertension, 429, 430, 511, 512
Laceration of internal organs, 742
Lactic acidosis, 182–187, 190–191, 203, 259
 Acid-base disorders, 237–239, 241, 242
 Acute renal failure, 296
 Classification, 185
D-Lactic acidosis, 188
Laennec's cirrhosis, 477
Laminin, 338
Laxatives, 627, 804
 Acute renal failure, 298

Lead, 627–628, 642
Left ventricular dysfunction, 701–704
Legionella pneumonia, 947
Leigh's syndrome, 215, 587
Lesch-Nyhan syndrome, 153, 154
Leucine, 295
Leukemia, 70
 Hypercalcemia, 97
Leukocytosis, 270
Leukopenia, 821–823, 828, 846–847, 891
 Wegener's granulomatosis, 925
Leuprolide, 608
Le Veen peritoneal venous shunt (P-V), 7, 40, 481, 482
Levodopa, 722, 724
Licorice, 70
 Metabolic alkalosis, 170
Liddle's syndrome, 70, 170
Lidocaine, dialysis for removal, 642
Light chain deposition disease (LCDD), 453, 456, 458, 459
 Chemotherapy, 459
Light-chain disease, 921–922
Light chain nephropathies, 459
Lignac-Fanconi disease, 587
Lipiduria, 321
Lipoid nephrosis, 345
Listeria meningitis, 925
Lithium, 7, 250, 628, 630
 Dialysis for removal, 642
 Hypercalcemia, 272
 Hyperkalemia, 51, 52
 Nephrogenic diabetes insipidus, 21, 23
 Polyuria, 18, 21
Liver, hepatic dysfunction, see also Cirrhosis of the liver, 477–491
 Acute azotemia, 477, 479, 483–488, 491
 Acute intrinsic renal failure (ATN), 483–488
 Ascites, 477–483, 485, 487
 Edema, 477–483, 486
 Glomerular changes, 490–491
 Hemodialysis-associated hepatitis, 488–489
 Hepatorenal syndrome (HRS), 483–488
 Overflow theory of ascites formation, 478
 Renal sodium handling, 477–479
Lowe's syndrome, 215, 587
Lung disease, 226
Lung malignancies, 169, 250
Lupus glomerulonephritis, 400–405

Lupus nephritis, see also Systemic lupus erythematosus, 319, 395–405, 420
 Acute renal failure, 292
 Dietary management, 399
 Drug-induced, 616
 Histologic assessment, 397
 Mortality, 398
 Renal transplantation, 924
 Therapy, 403–404
Lupus nephropathy, 270
 Pregnancy, 506, 508
Lymphoblastic lymphoma, 132
Lymphoid granulomatosis, 333
Lymphoma, 97, 272, 729
Lymphoproliferative disease, 951
Lysolecthin, 321
Lysozymuria, 70

Macrodantin, reflux nephropathy, 377
Magnesium, 111–115
 Deficiency, see also Hypomagnesemia
  Hypophosphatemia, 126
 Dialysate composition, 801, 804
 Dialysis for removal, 642
 Electrolyte disorders in surgical patients, 272–273
 Excess, see Hypermagnesemia
 Hypercalcemia, 93, 102
 Hypokalemia, 69, 70, 73, 80
 Metabolism disorders, 260
 Renal stone disease, 118
Magnesium loading test (MLT), 117
Magnesium sulfate, 39, 515
Magnesurias, 582, 586
Magnetic resonance imaging (MRI), brainstem lesions in TURP patients, 4
Malabsorption, solute ingestion decrease, 3
Malabsorption syndromes, 257
Malignancy, renal tubular acidosis, 215
Malignant hyperthermia syndrome (MHS), 62, 63
Malignant hypertension, end-stage renal disease and transplantation, 870
Malignant melanoma, 951
Malnutrition, 127, 128, 224
 Diabetics, 667, 681
 Predisposing factor for catheter-related complications, 748, 749

Solute ingestion decrease, 3
Wernicke's encephalopathy, 725
Mandelamine, autosomal dominant polycystic kidney disease, 550
Mannitol, 267, 268
  Acute renal failure, 291
  Burns therapy (electrical burns), 281
  Burn treatment, 261
  Dialysis for removal, 642
  Heavy metal intoxication, 619
  Hyperosmolar states, 10
  Hypokalemia, 77
  Induction of hyperosmolar states, 2
  Irrigating fluid for TURP patients, 4
  Nephrocalcinosis, 629
  Nephrotoxicity, 625
  Polyuria, 19, 22, 23
  Uric acid nephropathy, 470, 471
MAO inhibitors, dialysis for removal, 642
Maple-syrup urine disease, 259
Mean whole-body response equations, 234
Meatal stenosis, 353
Mecillinam, dialysis for removal, 642
Meclofenamate, 615
Meconium aspiration, 260
Medica meatosum, 150
Medullary carcinoma, hypercalcemia, 93
Medullary cystic disease, 215, 268, 472, 543, 557–560
  End-stage renal disease and transplantation, 870
  Hereditary disorder associated with Fanconi syndrome, 587
  Juvenile nephronophthisis-medullary cystic disease (JN-MCD complex), 557–558
  Medullary sponge kidney, 543, 558–560
  Polyuria, 21
Medullary sponge kidney (MSK), 93, 140–141, 149–150, 543, 558–560
Mefanamic acid, 615, 626
Melphalan
  Amyloidosis, 461
  Light chain deposition disease, 459
  Multiple myeloma, 454, 455, 456
Membrane biocompatibility, 813–833

Membranoproliferative glomerulonephritis (MPGN), 327, 396, 435
  End-stage renal disease and transplantation, 870
  Pregnancy, 506, 517
  Recurrence on posttransplant biopsies, 871
  Sickle hemoglobinemia, 575–576
Membranous glomerulonephritis, 396, 397
Membranous nephropathy, 327–328
  End-stage renal disease and transplantation, 870
Meningitis, 250, 268, 949
Meningoencephalitis, 730, 949
Meperidine, 859
  Urinary tract infections, 352
Meprobamate, 642, 644
2-Mercaptoethane-sodium sulfonate (mesna), 454
2-Mercapto-propionylglycine (α-MPG), 581–582
Mercaptopurine, 907
6-Mercaptopurine, 400, 418
Mercury, 617, 618–619, 642
Mesangial glomerulonephritis, 396
Mesangial proliferative glomerulonephritis, 325–326, 345
Mesantoin, 616
Metabolic acidosis, 30, 31, 38, 177–191, 258–260
  Acid-base disorders, 233–234, 236–242
  Acid excretion, 165
  Acute renal failure, 188, 189, 502
  Aldosterone deficiency, 163
  Alkali therapy, 179, 182, 188, 189
  Autosomal dominant polycystic kidney disease, 544
  Bicarbonate therapy, 182–183, 184, 190–191
  Burn injuries, 277
  Classification, 184–185
  Diabetic ketoacidosis, 198, 200
  Diagnosis, 177–179
  Ethylene glycol intoxication, 187–188
  Gastrointestinal tract organic acid load, 188
  Hyperkalemia, 180, 187, 189
  Hypernatremia, 251
  Interstitial renal disease, 180
  Methanol intoxication, 186–187
  Renal failure, 183
  Renal tubular acidosis, 207–209, 211, 214, 215
  Respiratory acid-base disorders, 226–228
  Respiratory acidosis, 181, 182
  Respiratory alkalosis, 186
  Sickle hemoglobinemia, 575–577
  Therapy, 178–189
  Uremia, 665
Metabolic alkalosis, 32, 159–173, 259, 260
  Acid-base disorders, 234–237, 239–242
  Acid excretion, see also Acid excretion, 164–165
  Acute renal failure, 289, 297
  Aldosterone, 162–163, 165–169
  Bartter's syndrome, 170–171
  Congenital chloride-losing diarrhea, 170, 171
  Contraction, 170
  Effects, 172
  Excessive bicarbonate loads, 171
  Extracellular volume contraction, 163, 167–168
  Extrarenal buffering, 166
  Gastric alkalosis, 168–169
  Generation of, 166–167
  Hypercalcemia, 171
  Hypoparathyroidism, 171
  Maintenance of, 167–168
  Mineralcorticoid excess, 169
  Pathophysiologic states associated with, 168–172
  Postfasting, 171
  Posthypercapnic, 171, 172
  Potassium metabolism disorders, 162
  Reabsorption of bicarbonate, see also Bicarbonate reabsorption, 160–163
  Renal secretion of hydrogen, 159–166
  Respiratory acidosis, 229–230
  Respiratory alkalosis, 229
  Respiratory compensation, 171–172
  Therapy, 172–173
Metabolic dysfunction, 905–915
Metachromatic leukodystrophy, 216
Metallotoxins, 627–628
Metals
  Acute interstitial nephritis as result, 626
  Dialysis for removal, 642, 644
Metastatic breast adenocarcinoma, 132
Metastatic medulloblastoma, 132
Metastatic small-cell bronchogenic

carcinoma, 132
Metchromatic leukodystrophy, 215
Methadone, 624
Methanol, 183, 186–187, 643
  Lactic acidosis, 186
Methaqualone, 642, 644, 645
Methazolamide, 30
Methemoglobulinemia, 281
Methenamine mandelate, urinary tract infections, 356
Methicillin, 626
  Acute interstitial nephritis as result, 626
  Infective endocarditis, 707
Methohexital, 671
Methotrexate, 418, 643, 644
Methoxyflurane, 630
  Nephrogenic diabetes insipidus, 21
Methsuximide, 642, 644
Methyldopa, 270, 379, 629
  Autosomal dominant polycystic kidney disease, 549
  Dialysis for removal, 642
  Hypertension, 427, 428, 430, 511–512, 514–515
  Hypertension and pregnancy, 510–511
Methylguanidine, uremia, 845
Methylmercury complex, dialysis for removal, 643
Methylparathion, hemoperfusion for removal, 644
Methylprednisolone, 358, 403, 404
  Allograft rejection, 890, 891, 897
  Cryoglobulinemias, 464
  Dialysis for removal, 642
  Goodpasture's syndrome, 339
  Nephrotic syndrome, 325, 328
  Vasculitis, 420
Methylprylon, 642, 644
Methylsalicylate, 643, 644
Methylsergide, 629
Metocurine, 672
Metolazone
  Autosomal dominant polycystic kidney disease, 549
  Diabetes mellitus (IDDM), 538
  Diuretic therapy, 29–34, 36, 39, 40
  Hypertension, 427, 428
Metoprolol
  Autosomal dominant polycystic kidney disease, 549
  Dialysis for removal, 642
  Hypertension, 427, 511
Metronidazole
  Acute renal failure, 503
  Autosomal dominant polycystic

kidney disease, 548
Dialysis for removal, 643
Mevinolin, 321
Mezlocillin, dialysis for removal, 642
Microalbuminuria, diabetes mellitus, 534–536
Microangiopathic hemolytic anemia (MAHA), 444, 446, 448
Microscopic polyarteritis, 413, 414
Milk-alkali (Burnet's) syndrome, 99, 133, 167, 629
  Hypercalcemia, 92, 94, 255, 272
Mineral acidosis, 270
Mineral metabolism, 655
Mineralocorticoids
  Deficiency, 249, 269
  Excess and volume overload after surgery, 265
  Excess associated with metabolic alkalosis, 169–170
  Hyperkalemia, 51–52, 54–55, 62, 64, 254
  Hyperkalemia with uremia, 665
  Hypokalemia, 67, 70, 71
  Post-operative period, 263
  Potassium wasting, 253
Mineralocorticosteroids, renal tubular acidosis, 217
Minimal change disease (MCD), 324–326
Minimal-changed nephrotic syndrome, 517
Minoxidil, 310, 379
  Autosomal dominant polycystic kidney disease, 549
  Hypertension, 427, 429, 430, 511
  Renal transplantation, 914
  Scleroderma, 433
Minute ventilation (VE), 223
Mithramycin
  Hypercalcemia, 95–99, 272
  Hypocalcemia, 100
  Multiple myeloma, 453–454
Mithromycin, 625
Mitochondrial myopathy, 225
Mitomycin C, 626
Mixed essential cryoglobulinemia, 305, 333
Monoclonal antibodies, 889, 895
  Allograft rejection, 897
Monoclonal gammopathy of undetermined significance (MGUS), 459
Morphine, 140, 183
Moxalactam, 356, 642
Mucocutaneous candidiasis, 101
Mucomycosis, 727

Multicystic kidney, 543, 560
Multiple endocrine neoplasia (MEN) syndromes, hypercalcemia, 93
Multiple myeloma, 55, 150, 215, 453–458
  Chemotherapy, 454–457
  Cryoglobulinemias, 463
  End-stage renal failure, 453
  Hypercalcemia, 93, 97, 453–454, 456–458
  Hyperuricemia, 454, 457
  Iodide nephrotoxicity, 621
  Renal failure, 454–458
Multiple sclerosis, 225
Muscle crush injuries, acute renal failure, 285
Muscle relaxation, 671–672
Muscular dystrophy, 225
Myasthenia gravis crisis, 52, 224, 225
Mycobacterium tuberculosis, 949
Myeloma, 21, 922
Myocardial infarction, 204
  Acid-base disorders, 237
  Acute renal failure, 296
  Azotemia, 286
Myocardial ischemia, 72
Myocarditis
  Acute glomerulonephritis syndrome, 307
  Pericarditis, 699, 702
Myoglobinuria, 72, 281
  Acute renal failure, 291
Myopathy, 134
Myotonia, 51
Myxedema coma, 224

Nadolol, 379, 642
  Hypertension, 427, 428
Nafcillin, 70
  Acute interstitial nephritis as result, 626
  Dialysis for removal, 642
  Infective endocarditis, 707
Nafoxidine, systemic lupus erythematosus, 399
Na-K-ATPase, 49, 50, 53
  Hyperkalemia, 63
  Hypokalemia, 66
  Magnesium as cofactor, 116
  Sickle hemoglobinemia, 577
Na-K-ATPase pump, 1, 46
Naloxone, 225
Naproxen, 615
Narcotics overdoses, 241
Neomycin, 281, 623, 642
Neonatals, uric acid nephropathy,

469–470
Neostigmine, 225
Nephrocalcinosis, see also Calcium stones, 93–94, 103, 139–140, 153, 628–629
   Chronic renal tubular acidosis, 908
   Distal renal tubular acidosis, 189
   Hypercalcemia, 272
   Management, 140–141
   Medullary sponge kidney, 149
   Renal transplantation, 911–912
   Renal tubular acidosis, 207, 212–216, 218
Nephrogenic adenoma, 960
Nephrogenic diabetes insipidus
   Drugs causing, 21
   Lithium, 23
   Polyuria, 21–22
   Treatment, 23
Nephrolithiasis, see also Calcium stones, 93, 141, 146, 212
   Accelerated, 142
   Autosomal dominant polycystic kidney disease, 549–550, 553
   Chronic renal tubular acidosis, 908
   Distal renal tubular acidosis, 583
   End-stage renal disease and transplantation, 870
   Hypercalcemia, 272
   Medullary sponge kidney, 558, 559
   Renal transplantation, 911–912
Nephrosclerosis, 217
Nephrotic syndrome, 5, 28, 32–33, 215, 317–328
   Acute glomerulonephritis syndrome, 311, 312
   Acute renal failure, 292, 508
   Amyloidosis, 460–463, 913
   Antiinflammatory agents, 617–618
   Autosomal dominant polycystic kidney disease, 547
   Causes, 319
   Classification of glomerulopathies, 323–328
   Cryoglobulinemias, 464
   Defined, 317
   Diabetes mellitus, 534, 535
   Dietary restriction as therapy, 651, 652
   Etiology, 319
   Fanconi syndrome, 588
   Focal and segmental glomerulosclerosis, 326–327
   General management, 319–323
   Glomerulosclerosis, 616
   Goodpasture's syndrome, 335, 338
   Heavy metals as cause, 617
   Henoch-Schonlein nephritis, 419, 420
   Hepatitis B virus, 491
   Hyperlipidemia, 321–322
   Hypocalcemia with vitamin D deficiency, 91, 103
   Hypokalemia, 80
   Hypoproteinemia, 320
   Infectious complications, 322–323
   Initial clinical evaluation, 323
   Membranoproliferative glomerulonephritis (MPGN), 327
   Membranous nephropathy, 327–328
   Mercury-induced, 617
   Mesangial proliferative glomerulonephritis, 325–326
   Minimal change disease (MCD), 324–326
   Multiple myeloma, 318
   Nephrotoxic antecedents, 616
   Pathologic classification, 319
   Pathophysiology, 317–319
   Pregnancy, 508, 520
   Proteinuria, 371–373, 379–380
   Renal vein thrombosis, 435, 436
   Sickle-cell anemia, 575–577
   Systemic lupus erythematosus, 397, 398, 404
   Therapy, 37–38
   Thrombotic complications, 322
   Treatment of specific glomerulopathies causing, 323–328
   Waldenström's macroglobulinemia, 458
Neproxen, 626
Netilmicin, 622–623
Netilmicin, dialysis for removal, 642
Neurogenic bladder, end-stage renal disease and transplantation, 870
Neuroleptanalgesia (NLA), 671
Neurologic syndromes, 719–730
Neuromuscular symptoms, symptomatic therapy, 666
Neuropathy, 722–724
Neutrophils, 821–824, 847
New dialyzer syndrome, 828, 830
Nicotinamide, 581
Nicotine, effect on water clearance, 4
Nifedipine, 36
   Autosomal dominant polycystic kidney disease, 549
   Hypertension, 429, 428, 430, 511
   Hypertension and pregnancy, 514–515
Nitrates, 800
Nitrites, 800
Nitrofurantoin, 616
   Asymptomatic bacteriuria, 497
   Dialysis for removal, 643
   Reflux nephropathy, 377
   Urinary tract infections, 354, 356, 358
Nitrogen mustard, 400, 418
Nitroprusside, 511
   Hypertension except during pregnancy, 429, 514, 515
Nitrostigmine, hemoperfusion for removal, 644
Nocturnal myoclonus, 722
Nocturnal peritoneal dialysis (NPD), 747
Nodular and diffuse intercapillary glomerulosclerosis, 540
Nonbarbiturate anticonvulsants, dialysis for removal, 642
Nonbarbiturate hypnotics, dialysis for removal, 642, 644
Nonbarbiturate sedatives, dialysis for removal, 642, 644
Nonbarbiturate tranquilizers, dialysis for removal, 642, 644
Noncompliance, 721
Non-Hodgkin's lymphomas, 951
   Uric acid nephropathy, 469
Noninflammatory vascular diseases, 425–436
   Accelerated hypertension, 429–430
   Essential hypertension, 425–429
   Malignant hypertension, 429–430
   Renal embolization/embolic disease, 433–435
   Renal vein thrombosis (RVI), 435–436
   Renovascular hypertension, 430–432
   Scleroderma, 432–433
Nonketotic hyperosmolar coma, dialysis patients, 725
Nonsteroidal antiinflammatory agents, acute interstitial nephritis as result, 626
Nonsteroidal antiinflammatory drugs (NSAIDS), 268, 404

Norepinephrine, 193, 194
  Acute renal failure, 290
  Renal ischemia as result, 614
Norfloxacin, 356
Normocalcemia, 98
  Hypercalciuria, 142
Normocalciuria, 144
Normokalemia, 48, 73–75, 240
Normovolemia, 288
Nutritional management, see also specific topics, 675–688
  Amino acid metabolism, 678–680, 682, 684
  Chronic renal failure, progression of, 684–685
  Continuous ambulatory peritoneal dialysis, 686, 687, 763
  Hemodialysis patients, 680–683, 685
  Lipid-lowering regimens, 685–686
  Low-protein diets, 679–680
  Peritoneal dialysis, 683–686
  Protein metabolism, 678–680
  Septic autocannibalism, 675
  Trace elements, 687–688
  Uremia, 675–678
  Vitamins, 686–687
Nutritional recovery syndrome, 127
  Hypophosphatemia, 274
Nystagmus, 724

Oasthouse syndrome, 582
Obesity hypoventilation syndrome, 225, 226
Obstructive lung disease, 236
Obstructive nephropathy, 247, 270
Obstructive sleep apnea, 225, 226
Obstructive uropathy, 216, 217, 629
Oleander tea, 51, 52
Oliguria, 40, 54–55, 131
Ondine curse, 225
Opiates, 671
Oral contraceptive steroid therapy, 391
Oral rehydration therapy, 251–252
Oreopoulos-Zellerman connector, 766
Organic brain syndrome, 721, 722
Organic heart disease, 79–80
  Hypokalemia, 75
Organophosphates, 643, 644
Ornidazole, dialysis for removal, 643
Orthopnea, 248

Osmotic diuresis, 126, 127, 129
Osteitis fibrosa, 104, 272, 586, 715–716
  Chronic peritoneal dialysis, 750
Osteitis fibrosis, 272
Osteitis fibrosis cystica, 318
Osteodystropy, 216
Osteomalacia, 94, 97, 102–104, 134, 318
  Adult sporadic, 584, 585–586
  Aluminum intoxication, 727
  Chronic peritoneal dialysis, 750
  Hypophosphatemic, 584–585
  Inherited renal tubular disorders, 582, 586
  Phosphate depletion role, 712
  Renal osteodystrophy, 713–715
  Vitamin D for prevention, 459
Osteopenia, 189, 214
Osteopetrosis, 215, 216
Osteoporosis, 103, 586, 952
Ouabain, dialysis for removal, 642
Ovarian dysgenesis, 101
Oxacillin
  Acute interstitial nephritis as result, 626
  Infective endocarditis, 707
Oxipurinol, 471
Oxprenolol, peritoneal sclerosis, 749
Oxygen, metabolic acidosis, 183
Oxytocin, 268
  Antidiuretic potency, 4
  Hyponatremia, 3, 9

Paget's disease, 97, 132, 150, 153
Paget's syndrome, 141
Pancreatic cholera syndrome, 94
Pancreatitis, 93, 258, 267, 271
  Acute renal failure, 285
  Hypomagnesemia, 272
  Thrombotic thrombocytopenic purpura, 448
Pancuronium, 672
Pancytopenia, 874
Papaverine, to reduce vessel spasm, 779
Papillary necrosis, 140, 286, 287, 359
Papilloma virus, 948
Parainfluenza virus, 948
Paraldehyde, dialysis for removal, 642
Paramethadione, 616
Paraproteinemias, 921–923
Paraquat, 643, 644

Plasma drug extraction ratios, 645
Parathion, hemoperfusion for removal, 644
Parathyroid adenoma, 98
Parathyroidectomy, 271, 716–717, 733, 737, 873
  Hypercalcemia and renal transplantation, 910–911, 912
  Psychological function related, 722
Parathyroid hormone (PTH)
  Bicarbonate reabsorption, 162, 163
  Calcium deficiency, 91–104
  Erythropoiesis, 734
  Hypercalcemia, 255, 256, 258
  Hypercalciuria, 142–144, 146
  Hyperphosphatemia, 132, 133
  Hypocalcemia, 256, 258, 271
  Hypophosphatemia, 127
  Magnesium deficiency, 112, 115, 118
  Metabolic alkalosis, 162, 163, 166, 171
  Neuropathy, 723
  Primary hyperparathyroidism, 150
  Psychological function, 722
  Renal transplantation, 912
  Uremic encephalopathy, 720–721
  Vitamin-D compounds and renal osteodystrophy, 713–717
Parenchymal renal disease, 432
  Peritoneal dialysis, 740
  Pregnancy, 507
Pargyline, dialysis for removal, 642
Parkinson's disease, 71
Paromomycin, 623
Paroxysmal nocturnal dyspnea, 248
Patch-graft angioplasty, 783, 784
Pelvic cancer (female), 286
Penicillamine, 616–617
D-Penicillamine, 155, 333
  Amyloidosis, 461
  Cystinuria, 581–582
  Pregnancy, 519
  Wilson's disease, 587
Penicillin, 45–46, 70–71, 190, 615
  Acute glomerulonephritis syndrome, 307, 308
  Acute interstitial nephritis as result, 626
  Acute renal failure, 287
  Dialysis for removal, 642
  Dietary sodium restriction, 662
  Hyperkalemia, 53

Hypersensitivity, 626
Struvite stones, 156
Uremic encephalopathy, 720
Urinary tract infection, 660
Penicillin G, infective endocarditis, 707
Pentagastrin, 183, 188
Pentamadine, 624
Pentobarbital, 642, 644
Peptic ulcer disease, 125, 297, 873, 951
Percutaneous catheters, 775–776
Percutaneous transluminal angioplasty (PTA), 943
Periarteritis, pregnancy, 508
Periarteritis nodosa, 435
   Pregnancy, 516, 518
   Renal vein thrombosis, 435
Pericarditis, 697–701, 702, 705
   Continuous ambulatory peritoneal dialysis, 755
   Symptomatic, 700–701
Perinatal asphyxia, 250
Perinephric abscess, 358–359
Periodic paralysis, 269, 270
Periorbital edema, 251
Peripheral vascular disease, 428
Peritoneal dialysis, 98, 173, 739–750
   Access surgery, 786–788
   Acquired cystic disease as result, 560
   Acute glomerulonephritis syndrome, 310
   Acute renal failure, 296–297, 501, 506, 739–744
   Amyloidosis, 463
   Autosomal dominant polycystic kidney disease, 552
   Chronic, 744–750
   Continuous ambulatory (CAPD), see Continuous ambulatory peritoneal dialysis
   Continuous cyclic (CCPD), see Continuous cyclic peritoneal dialysis
   Continuous equilibration, see Continuous equilibration peritoneal dialysis
   Cyclers, 745
   Diabetes mellitus (IDDM), 539
   Drug elimination techniques, 641, 644
   Hyperkalemia, 60–61, 255
   Hypermagnesemia, 273
   Hypernatremia, 251
   Hyperphosphatemia, 133
   Hypervolemia, 248
   Intermittent (IPD), 741, 745, 749, 755
   Intraabdominal pressure (IAP), 749–750
   Left ventricular dysfunction, 703
   Liver, hepatic dysfunction, 486
   Medical complications, 750
   Metabolic acidosis, 184, 186, 187, 188
   Multiple myeloma, 456–457
   Nocturnal (NPD), 747
   Peritoneal sclerosis, 749
   Sickle-cell anemia, 577
   Solute clearance, 756
   Solutions, 741
   Tidal (TPD), 747
   Ultrafiltration failure syndrome, 749
   Uric acid nephropathy, 471
Peritoneal sclerosis, 749, 767
   Continuous ambulatory peritoneal dialysis, 760, 762, 768
Peritonevenous shunts (Le-Veen) (PVS), 7, 40, 481, 482, 486–487
Peritonitis, 267, 683–684, 742, 744–748, 750
   Continuous ambulatory peritoneal dialysis, 755, 756, 763–766
   Diagnosis, 764
   Peritoneal dialysis, 787
   Prevention of, 766
   Treatment, 764–766
Permanent urinary diversion, pregnancy, 516, 519
Pernicious anemia, 67, 101, 269
Phagocytosis, 823, 824
   Uremia, 845
Phalloidin, hemoperfusion for removal, 644
Phenacetin, 597
Phenazone, acute interstitial nephritis as result, 626
Phenazopyridine, 625
Phenazopyridine hydrochloride, urinary tract infections, 351
Phencyclidine, hemoperfusion for removal, 644
Phenelzine, dialysis for removal, 642
Pheninedione, 616, 626
   Acute interstitial nephritis as result, 626
Phenobarbital
   Acute interstitial nephritis as result, 626
   Dialysis for removal, 642
   Hemoperfusion for removal, 644
   Hypocalcemia, 256
   Serum concentrations for dialysis or hemoperfusion, 645
Phenolphthalein, 69
Phenols, hemoperfusion for removal, 644
Phenothiazines, 515
   Hypertension, 510
Phenylbutazone, 615
   Acute interstitial nephritis as result, 626
   Acute renal failure, 287
   Hemoperfusion for removal, 644
Phenytoin, 63, 616
   Acute interstitial nephritis as result, 626
   Hypocalcemia, 257
   IgA nephropathy, 346
Pheochromocytoma, 94
Phlebotomy, 183
Phosphate, 121
   Binders, 134
   Binding antacids, 125–126
   Deficiency
      Hereditary hypophosphatemic rickets, see also Hypophosphatemia, 585
   Depletion
      Acid excretion, 165
      Bicarbonate reabsorption, 162, 163
      Diabetic ketoacidosis, 198, 202
   Dialysis for removal, 642
   Homeostasis, 121–123
   Hypercalcemia, 95–99
   Hypophosphatemia, see Hypophosphatemia
   Restriction for management of disorders, 655
   Retention control and hyperphosphatemia, 711
   Routine replacement therapy, 129
Phosphaturia, 127, 216, 582, 584–586
Phosphorus, 121–134
   Compounds, 121
   Deficiency, see also Hypophosphatemia, 123, 127–129
   Depletion
      Intracellular, 131
      Respiratory alkalosis, 124–125
   Electrolyte disorders in surgical patients, 273–274
   Excess, see Hyperphosphatemia
   Homeostasis, 121–123

Hypercalcemia, 99
Hypocalcemia, 103
Metabolism in uremia, 664
Preparations commonly
   available, 130
Phosphorus deficiency syndrome,
   128
Phosphorus depletion syndrome,
   128
Pigmenturia, 287
Pindolol, 629, 663
   Hypertension, 427
Piperacillin, dialysis for removal,
   642
Piroxicam, 615
Plants, dialysis for removal,
   643–644
Plasma bicarbonate, 182, 223,
   225–227
   Acid-base disorders, 233–242
Plasma osmolarity, 1–2, 5–6, 9
   Hypernatremia, 10, 12
   Polyuria, 22
Plasmapheresis, 848
   Drug elimination technique, 645
   Glomerulonephritis, 616
   Hemolytic uremic syndrome, 446
   Mitomycin C nephrotoxicity, 626
   Multiple myeloma, 457
   Pregnancy, 518
   Thrombotic thrombocytopenic
      purpura, 449
Plasma separation, 841, 844, 848
Platelets, 815–816
Platinum, 619
Pneumococcal pneumonia, 946
Pneumocystis carinii pneumonia,
   946, 947
Pneumonia, 250, 260, 499, 949
Pneumonitis, 238, 949
   Hyperkalemia, 60
Pneumothorax, 224, 225, 237
Pneumovax, 398
Podophyllin, hemoperfusion for
   removal, 644
Polyacrylonitrile (PAN) (dialyzer
   membrane), 814, 819,
   822–824, 826–827, 832, 847
Polyamide, 814
Polyarteritis nodosa (classic
   polyarteritis), 287, 333,
   413–416, 425
   End-stage renal disease and
      transplantation, 416, 870
   Renal transplantation, 925–926
Polycarbonate (dialyzer
   membrane), 814, 826
Polychlorinate biphenyls,
   hemoperfusion for removal,
   644
Polycystic kidney disease, 21, 726
   End-stage renal disease and
      transplantation, 870
   Pregnancy, 516, 519
   Renal transplantation, 931–932
Polydipsia, 5, 7, 127
   Polyuria, 19, 21, 22
   Primary neurogenic, 22
   Psychogenic, 17, 20, 22, 23
   Renal tubular acidosis, 211
Polyethylene, 833
Polymethylmethacrylate (PMMA),
   814, 819, 823, 826, 827
Polymorphonuclear leukocytes
   (PMN), 333, 334
Polymyositis, 225
Polymyxin, acute interstitial
   nephritis as result, 626
Polymyxin B, 70
Polymyxin nephropathy, 623–624
Polyoma virus, 948
Polypoid cystitis, 960
Polysulfone (dialyzer membrane),
   814, 819, 823, 824, 826
Polyurethane, 833, 848
Polyuria, 7, 17–24, 127
   Amyloid involvement of the
      collecting duct, 21
   Angiographic dyes, 19
   Azotemia, 21
   Carbamazepine, 23
   Chlorpropamide, 22–23
   Classification of syndromes,
      18–19
   Clofibrate, 23
   DDAVP, 22
   Demeclocycline, 18, 21
   Diabetes insipidus, 18–22
   Diagnosis, 18–20
   Electrolytes, 24
   Glucose, 19
   Glycerol, 19
   Hypercalcemia, 19, 21–23
   Hyperglycemia, 24
   Hypernatremia, 21, 23, 24
   Hypoglycemia, 23
   Hypokalemia, 19, 21–22, 23, 252
   Hyponatremia, 23, 24
   Hyposthenuria, 21
   Hypotension, 17
   Hypovolemia, 18, 23, 24
   Indomethacin, 23
   Lithium, 18, 21
   Mannitol, 19, 22, 23
   Medullary cystic disease, 21
   Myeloma, 21
   Polycystic disease, 21
   Polydipsia, 19, 21, 22
   Renal tubular acidosis, 211, 213
   Serum sodium concentration,
      23–24
   Sickle-cell anemia, 21
   Sjogren's syndrome, 21
   Sulfonylureas, 23
   Therapeutic approaches, 22–23
   Tolbutamide, 22–23
   Treatment, 22–24
Polyuric syndromes, 17–24
Polyvinylchloride (PVC), 833, 848
Positive end-expiratory pressure
   (PEEP), 229
Posterior urethral valves,
   end-stage renal disease and
   transplantation, 870
Postfasting metabolic alkalosis, 171
Posthypercapnic alkalosis, 170
Posthypercapnic metabolic
   alkalosis, 171, 172
Postparathyroidectomy, 270
Post partum HUS (PHUS), 446
Postpartum renal failure (PPRF),
   renal transplantation,
   927–928
Post renal transplantation, 215
Post-streptococcal
   glomerulonephritis, 326,
   338
Potassium
   Balance disorders, 252–255
   Depletion, 50–57
      Alcoholic acidosis, 240
      Burn injuries, 277
      Diabetic ketoacidosis, 198,
         202
      Eating disorders, 67, 80
      External removal, 60–61
      Gastric alkalosis, 168–169
      Hyperaldosteronism, 68–71,
         74, 80–81
      Hypercatabolism, 53
      Hypoaldosteronism, 51,
         53–56, 59, 62, 64
      Hypokalemia, 64–81
      Management, 62–64
      Metabolic acidosis, 49–50,
         53–56, 69–71, 74, 77–78
      Metabolic alkalosis, 46, 53,
         60, 68–74, 77
      Renal tubal defects, 55–56
   Dialysis composition, 801, 802
   Dietary restriction, 61–62
   Electrolyte disorders in surgical
      patients, 269–271
   Formulations, 77–78
   Homeostasis, 45–48
      Disorders following kidney
         transplant, 908–910

Factors influencing potassium excretion, 45
Factors modifying potassium excretion, 46
Physiologic effects, 47–48
Hypertension, 429
Hypoosmolar and hyperosmolar states, 1, 2
Metabolic acidosis, 181–182
Metabolic alkalosis, 164–165, 170
Metabolism disorders, see Hyperkalemia; Hypokalemia; Potassium, depletion
Myopathy, 724
Renal tubular acidosis, 212, 214, 215
Supplements, 28, 32–38
Total body intake, 47, 52
Type 4 renal tubular acidosis and retention of, 216, 217
Potassium dichromate, dialysis for removal, 443, 642
Povidine-iodine, 787, 788
Practolol, dialysis for removal, 642
Prazosin, 36, 310, 379, 704
Autosomal dominant polycystic kidney disease, 549
Hypertension, 427, 429, 430
Scleroderma, 433
Prednisone, 95, 98, 615
Allograft rejection, 890–892, 894, 896, 897
Amyloidosis, 461, 463
Cryoglobulinemias, 464
Diabetes mellitus (IDDM), 539
Genitourinary tuberculosis, 390, 392
Glomerulonephritis, 517
Goodpasture's syndrome, 339
Hypercalcemia, 99, 256
IgA nephropathy, 345
Light chain deposition disease, 459
Multiple myeloma, 453–456
Nephrotic syndrome, 324, 326–327, 328
Pericarditis, 700
Preeclampsia, 662
Renal transplantation, 875, 876, 877
Systemic lupus erythematosus, 400–404
Transplant patients and pregnancy, 523
Vasculitis, 416–418, 420
Waldenstrom's macroglobulinemia, 458
Preeclampsia/eclampsia, 39
Pregnancy, 503–504, 507–518, 520, 524, 526
Hypertensive renal disease, 662
Pregnancy, 495–526
Acute cystitis, 498–499
Acute fatty liver of pregnancy (AFLP), 497, 504, 505
Acute glomerulonephritis, 516
Acute pyelonephritis, 498, 499–500
Acute renal failure, 287, 500–506
Acute symptomatic urinary tract infection, 498–500
Acute tubular necrosis, 503, 505
Amyloidosis, 461
Anatomical changes in kidney, 495
Anticoagulants, 513, 517
Asymptomatic bacteriuria, 496–498
Autosomal dominant polycystic kidney disease, 551
Azotemia, 503
Blood pressure regulation, 496
Blood transfusion, 516
Chronic glomerulonephritis, 516–517
Chronic hemodialysis, 521–522
Chronic pyelonephritis, 497, 506
Continuous ambulatory peritoneal dialysis (CAPD), 522
Cortical necrosis, 500–503, 505
Diabetic nephropathy, 516, 518
Disseminated intravascular coagulation (DIC), 502, 503, 505
Eclampsia, 508–510, 514
Ectopic, 523
End-stage renal failure, 505
Epidural anesthesia, 516
Functional changes in kidney, 495–496
General management plan, 507–511
HELLP syndrome, 504
Hemolytic uraenine syndrome (HUS), 504–505
Hemolytic uremic syndrome, 446, 500
Hereditary nephritis, 517
Hypertension, 508–516, 518–526
Hyperuricemia, 504
Hypovolemia, 516
Idiopathic postpartum renal failure, 504–505
Impact on renal function, 506–507
Magnesium sulphate, 515
Management important considerations, 505–506
Membranoproliferative glomerulonephritis, 517
Nephrotic syndrome, 520
Nontraumatic rupture of the urinary tract, 500
Offspring complications, 525–526
Overdistention syndrome, 500
Parenchymal renal disease, 507
D-Penicillamine, 519
Periarteritis nodosa, 516, 518
Permanent urinary diversion, 516, 519
Polycystic kidney disease, 516, 519
Preeclampsia, 508–510, 512–517, 520, 524, 526
Prostaglandin therapy, 513–514
Proteinuria, 520, 523
Pyelonephritis, 495, 516
Pyelonephrotis (tubulointerstitial disease), 518
Radiotherapy, 519, 520
Reflux nephropathy, 370–371, 379, 381, 516, 518–519
Renal hemodynamics, 495
Renal insufficiency, 662
Reye's syndrome, 504
Scleroderma, 516, 518
Sedation, 515
Sepsis, 502
Septic abortion, 502
Solitary kidney, 519–520
Systemic lupus erythematosus (SLE), 398, 399, 404–405, 516–518
Systemic sclerosis (SS), 518
Thrombotic thrombocytopenic purpura, 446
Transplant recipients, 522–526, 927, 928
Urinary tract infections, 357–358, 496–498
Urinary tract infection and sickle hemoglobinemia, 574
Urolithiasis, 516, 519
Volume expansion therapy, 513
Volume homeostasis, 495–496
Premature coronary heart disease, 321
Primaquin, 625
Primary hypophosphatemic rickets on X-linked

hypophosphatemic rickets, 585–586
Primidone, 616, 642
Probenecid, 31, 616, 618, 619, 625
   Chronic hyperuricemic nephropathy, 472
Procainamide, 404, 616, 859
   Dialysis for removal, 642
   Hemoperfusion for removal, 644
Progesterone, 225
Progressive systemic sclerosis (PSS), see also Scleroderma, 333
   Renal transplantation, 924–925
Promazine, hemoperfusion for removal, 644
Propoxyphene, 624
D-Propoxyphene, 643, 644
Propranolol, 51, 79, 309, 616, 717
   Acute interstitial nephritis as result, 626
   Autosomal dominant polycystic kidney disease, 549
   Dialysis for removal, 642
   Hypercalcemia, 94
   Hypertension, 427, 428, 430, 511
   Hypoglycemia, 725
   Peritoneal sclerosis, 749
   Scleroderma, 433
Propylthiouracil, 615–616
Prostacyclin, 297, 848
   Hemolytic uraenine syndrome, 505
   Hemolytic uremic syndrome, 445
Prostaglandins
   Acute renal failure, 291
   Bartter syndrome, 588–589
   Cirrhosis, 479
   Hypercalcemia, 97
   Hypokalemia, 72, 79
   Polyuria, 18, 21–23
   Synthesis, 31
   Systemic lupus erythematosus, 399
   Therapy during pregnancy, 513–514
Prostaglandin synthesis, 55
Prostaglandin synthetase inhibitors, 98
Prostate, transurethral resection of (TURP), 4, 9, 874
Prostatic abscess, urinary tract infections, 960
Prostatic cancer, 286, 603–608
Prostatitis, 349, 355, 356, 965
   Urinary tract infection, 960
Protein, dietary restriction, 649–654, 662–663; see also Proteinuria
Proteinuria, 36–37, 39, 317–322, 324–326, 343–346
   Acute glomerulonephritis syndrome, 308–311
   Amyloidosis, 462
   Bence Jones, 453, 454, 456, 458, 459
   Diabetes mellitus (IDDM), 534–537, 539–540
   Diet restriction effect, 649–654
   Dysproteinemias, 460, 461, 464
   Embolic disease, 434
   Hepatitis B virus, 490
   Multiple myeloma, Bence Jones, 453, 454, 456
   Nephrotic syndrome, 327, 328
   Penicillamine toxicity, 617
   Pregnancy, 506, 507, 518, 520, 523
   Reflux nephropathy, 364, 370–373, 378–381
   Renal vein thrombosis, 435
   Scleroderma, 432–433
   Sickle-cell anemia, 575, 576
   Simple cysts in children, 562
   Systemic lupus erythematosus, 397, 405
   Thrombotic thrombocytopenic purpura, 448
   Toxic nephropathies, 616–623
   Tubular, 318
   Waldenström's macroglobulinemia, 458
Prothrombin, 398
Protozoal and helminthic infections, 949
Protryptyline, 225
Proximal renal tubular acidosis (RTA), 188, 215–216, 253, 583
Prune-belly syndrome, 724
   End-stage renal disease and transplantation, 870
Pseudohypoaldosteronism, 55–56, 217, 254–255, 582–583
Pseudohyponatremia, 2, 267
Pseudohypoparathyroidism
   Hyperphosphatemia, 132
   Hypocalcemia, 101, 102–103
   Treatment, 102–103
Pseudomembranous colitis (PMC), 949, 951
Pseudonephrotic syndrome, 318
Psoriasis, amyloidosis as complication, 461
Psychiatric disorders, 719–730
Psychogenic polydipsia, 17
   Hyponatremia, 4

Psychological complications, 721–722
Psychosis, 267
   Water clearance affected by drug treatments, 4
Pulmonary capillary wedge pressure (PCWP), 228, 229
Pulmonary edema, 183, 227, 228, 237, 248
   Acute glomerulonephritis syndrome, 305, 308
   Burn response, 281
   Sedative overdose, 241
Pulmonary fibrosis, 228
Pulmonary tuberculosis, 947
Puromycin, aminonucleoside of, 616, 618
Pyelonephritis
   Autosomal dominant polycystic kidney disease, 547
   Bladder cancer surgery complication, 603
   Interstitial nephritis, 627
   Pregnancy, 516
   Systemic lupus erythematosus, 924
   Urinary tract infection, 960
Pyelonephritis (tubulointerstitial disease), pregnancy, 518
Pyloric stenosis, 260
Pyoderma, 307
Pyrazinamide
   Genitourinary tuberculosis, 388–391
   Hyperuricemic nephropathies, 469
Pyridoxine (B_6), 152, 391, 686
   Magnesium, 113
Pyruvate carboxylase deficiency, 215

Quadriparesis, 66, 77
Quinalbital, 642, 644
Quinethazone, 30
Quinidine, 642, 644, 666
Quinine, 615, 643
Quinolones, 625

Radiation nephropathy, 628
Radiation nephrotoxicity, 629
Radiographic contrast dyes, hyperosmolar states, 10
Radiotherapy
   Bladder cancer, 602
   Pregnancy, 519, 520
   Prostatic cancer, 607
Radium implant of cervix, 355

Ranitidine, 297, 643
Raynaud's phenomenon, 432, 433, 463, 924
Recipient selection in renal transplantation, 867–881
Recombinant alpha interferon, 455
Recombinant human erythropoietin (rhEPO), 665
Reflux nephropathy, 363–381
  Assessment, 381
  Defined, 363
  End-stage renal failure, 366, 370, 374, 375, 381
  Growth, 375–376, 380–381
  Hypertension, 367–368, 370, 371, 378, 381
  Infection, 376–378
  Management during pregnancy, 381
  Pregnancy, 370, 371, 379, 381, 516, 518–519
  Prevention of, 375–376
  Prognostic factors, 381
  Proteinuria, 364, 370–373, 378–381
  Reflux of urine, 368–369
  Renal insufficiency, 373–375
  Surgical management, 380–381
  Therapeutic approaches, 376–381
  Voiding disorders, 369–371
Refractory bactremic shock, 238
Regional analgesia, 672
Reiter's syndrome, 355
Rejection, see Allograft rejection
Renal adenocarcinoma, acquired cystic disease, 561
Renal agenesis, end-stage renal disease and transplantation, 870
Renal amyloidosis, 55
Renal artery stenosis, 252, 431
  Renal transplantation, 914, 915, 943–944, 950
  Unilateral, 169, 170
Renal bone disease, 804, 911
Renal calculi, 359, 911
Renal calculus disease, 359
Renal colic, 139, 140, 155
Renal cystic disorders, see also specific topics, 543–564
  Acquired cystic disease, 543, 560–561
  Autosomal dominant polycystic kidney disease, 543–554
  Infantile recessive polycystic kidney disease, 543, 554–557

Medullary cystic disease, 543, 557–560
Medullary sponge kidney, 543, 558–560
Multicystic kidney, 543, 560
Nephronophthisis, 543, 557–558
Simple cysts, 543, 561–564
Renal dysplasia, 248
  End-stage renal disease and transplantation, 870
Renal failure, see also Acute renal failure; Chronic renal failure; Renal insufficiency, 260
  Acid-base disorders, 233, 241
  Autosomal dominant polycystic kidney disease, 551
  Hepatitis B, 491
  Hypercalcemia, 272
  Hyperuricemic nephropathies, 469, 470
  Hypocalcemia, 257, 271
  Hyponatremia, 267, 268
  Pregnancy complications, 662
  Uric acid nephropathy, 472
Renal failure index, 288–289
Renal hamartomas, 169
Renal insufficiency, see also Renal failure, 649–656, 659–667
  Dietary intervention, 649–653
  Nondietary intervention, 653–656
Renal ischemia, 286, 614–615
Renal malignancy, end-stage renal disease and transplantation, 870
Renal osteodystrophy, 711–717, 750
  Aluminum bone disease, 717
  Dialysis, 716
  Hypercalcemia, 713–717
  Hyperphosphatemia, 711–714, 717
  Hypocalcemia, 712–713, 716–717
  Parathyroidectomy, 716–717
  Vitamin D sterols, 713–715
Renal parenchymal disease, 654
  Hypertension, 425–426
Renal parenchymal hematuria, 343
Renal pelvis, cancer, 597–600
Renal stone disease, 118
Renal transplantation, see Kidney, transplantation
Renal tubular acidosis (RTA), 23, 180, 207–218, 253, 582–584
  Acidification, 208–210, 213
  Alkali therapy, 214
  Calcium stones, 141, 152–153

Classification of types, 207–208
Clinical manifestations, 207–208
Diagnosis, 208–210
Fanconi syndrome, 216
Medullary sponge kidney, 558–559
Metabolic acidosis, 260
Nephrocalcinosis, 207, 212–215
Plasma bicarbonate, 207, 209
Potassium, 212, 215
Potassium metabolism disorder, 66–67, 70, 75, 77, 81
Proximal, see Proximal renal tubular acidosis
Sickle hemoglobinemia, 574
Tubular dysfunction, 905–908
Type I, see also Distal renal tubular acidosis, 210–215, 253, 582–583
Type II, 215–216, 253, 583, 586
Type IV, 216–218, 583, 906, 907
Renal tubular functional abnormalities, 629–630
Renal vein thrombosis (RVT), 215, 217, 322, 435–436, 661
  Amyloidosis, 461, 463
Renin-angiotensin system, renal transplantation, 913, 914
Renin antagonists, diabetes mellitus (IDDM), 538
Renovascular disease, 425
Reserpine, hypertension, 427, 430
Respiratory acid-base disorders, 223–230
  Metabolic acidosis, 226–228
  Respiratory acidosis, 223–228
  Respiratory alkalosis, 223–228–229
Respiratory acidosis, 128, 223–228, 259, 260
  Acid-base disorders, 233–237, 242
  Barbiturate-associated, 241
  Metabolic alkalosis, 229–230
Respiratory alkalosis, 223, 228–229, 259, 260
  Acid-base disorders, 234–236, 238–242
  Burns, 277, 281
  Hypocalcemia, 271
  Hypophosphatemia, 274
  Metabolic alkalosis, 229
Respiratory distress syndrome (RDS), 227
Respiratory failure, acid-base disorders, 242
Restless leg syndrome, 722, 724
Reticulum cell sarcoma, 729
Retrograde menstruation, 748

Retroperitoneal fibrosis, 286, 629
Reye's syndrome, 504
Rhabdomyolysis, 51–52, 58–59, 63, 132–133, 254
    Acute renal failure, 288, 291, 298
    Hyperkalemia, 270
    Hyperphosphatemia, 131
    Hypocalcemia, 101, 271
    Hypokalemia, 72
    Pigment nephropathy, 624–625
    Sickle hemoglobinemia, 576
Rheumatoid arthritis, 678
Rhodiascit machine, 480–483
Ribavirin, systemic lupus erythematosus, 399
Rickets, 94, 102–103, 256–258, 586, 713
    Adult sporadic hypophosphatemic, 582
    Oncogenous or tumoral, 582, 584
    Oncogenous with phosphaturia, 584, 585
    Renal tubular acidosis, 207, 214, 216
    X-linked hypophosphatemic, 582, 584–585
Rifampicin
    Acute renal failure, 391
    Genitourinary tuberculosis, 387–392
Rifampin, 70, 626
    Infective endocarditis, 707
Right-sided bacterial endocarditis, 311
Rocaltrol, 103
Rosearmycin, reflux nephropathy, 377–378

Salbutamol, 63
Salicylates, 186
    Acid-base disorders, 240
    Serum concentrates for dialysis or hemoperfusions, 645
Salicylic acid, 643, 644
Saline, hypercalcemia, 96
Salmon calcitonin, 256
    Multiple myeloma, 454
Sanarelli-Schwartman reaction, 505
Saralasin, 431, 914
Sarcoidosis, 92–95, 97, 99
    Calcium stones, 141, 150, 153
    Renal vein thrombosis, 435
Schistosomiasis, 874
    End-stage renal disease and transplantation, 870
Schizophrenia
    Acute hyponatremia, 4
    Water clearance affected by drug treatments, 4
Schonlein-Henoch purpura, 287
Scleroderma, 225, 425
    Acute renal failure, 286
    End-stage renal disease and transplantation, 870
    Pregnancy, 508, 516, 518
    Renal crisis, 432–433
    Renal transplantation, 924–925
Sclerosing peritonitis, 760, 762, 768
Secobarbital, 642, 644
Sedative overdose, 241
Selenium, 688
Sepsis, 183, 257–258
    Acute renal failure, 285, 296–297
    Anaesthesia, 670
    Burns, 281–282
    Gram-negative, 242
    Hypophosphatemia, 274
    Liver, hepatic dysfunction, 483
    Mixed acid-base disorders, 233, 238–239
    Multiple myeloma, 457, 458
    Pregnancy, 501, 502, 503
    Renal transplantation, 951
    Urinary tract infections, 356, 360
Septic autocannibalism, 675
Septicemia, 287, 358, 402, 525
    Renal transplantation complication, 947, 949
Sequential ultrafiltration and hemodialysis, 843, 848
Serotonin, 511, 515, 721
Serum albumin, 320
Serum bicarbonate, 165, 245
    Renal tubular acidosis, 216, 218
Serum calcium, hyperphosphatemia, 132–133
Serum chloride, diabetic ketoacidosis, 195
Serum ferritin, 664, 688, 737
Serum magnesium, 113–115, 116–117
    Hypophosphatemia, 130
Serum osmolarity, 11
Serum phosphorus, 126, 128, 130
Serum potassium, 59, 245, 253, 255
    Diabetic ketoacidosis, 202
    Hypokalemia, 64–67, 69, 71, 73–77, 79–80
    Hypophosphatemia, 127
    Metabolic acidosis, 260
Serum sickness, 287
Serum sodium, diabetic ketoacidosis, 195
Severe interstitial cystitis, 874
Shock lung syndrome, 844
Short bowel syndrome, 271
Shunts, 776–778
SIADH, see Syndrome of inappropriate ADH secretion (SIADH)
Sickle-cell anemia, see also Sickle hemoglobinemia, 56, 254, 287, 359, 573–578
    End-stage renal failure, 576, 577
    Polyuria, 21
    Renal transplantation, 908, 930–931
    Renal vein thrombosis, 435
Sickle cell nephropathy, 260
Sickle hemoglobinemia, see also Sickle-cell anemia, 573–578
Sickle-thalassemia, 574
Silicone, 832–833, 848
Silvadene, 281
Silver intoxication, 620
Silver nitrates, burns, 281
Simple cysts, 543, 561–564
Sisomicin, 623, 642
Sjogren's sydnrome, 21, 215, 463, 906
Skin breakdown, 27
Skin cancer, 951
Slow continuous ultrafiltration (SCUF), 296, 482
Small bowel bypass, 153
Smoking
    Bladder cancer, 600
    Lung cancer, 600
Snake bite, dialysis for removal, 643
Sodium
    Depletion, continuous ambulatory peritoneal dialysis, 762
    Dialysate composition, 801–802, 842
    Dialysis for removal, 642
    Dietary restriction, 662
    Edematous states, 27–29, 31
    Hypoosmolar and hyperosmolar states, 1, 2
    Hyporeninemic hypoaldosteronism, 583
    Perioperative period abnormalities, 267–269
    Potassium excretion, 45
    Pseudohypoaldosteronism, 583
Sodium bicarbonate, 10, 133
Sodium chlorate, dialysis for removal, 643
Sodium chloride, 7
    Edematous states, 27, 35

Reabsorption in polyuria
    syndromes, 18
Sodium citrate, dialysis for
    removal, 642
Sodium EDTA, hypercalcemia,
    272
Sodium nitroprusside,
    hypertension except during
    pregnancy, 430, 515
Sodium penicillin, 70
Sodium polystryene sulfonate, 60,
    62
Sodium sulfate, 55
Soft-tissue calcification, 804
Solvents, dialysis for removal,
    643–644
Sorbent hemoperfusion, 641–646
Sorbitol, 60, 186, 703
    Acute renal failure, 298
    Irrigating fluid for TURP
        patients, 4
Sotalol, dialysis for removal, 642
Spina bifida, 375
Spironolactone, 27, 29, 31–32, 35,
    39–40, 253
    Acute glomerulonephritis
        syndrome, 309
    Hyperkalemia, 52, 56
    Hypertension, 427
    Hypokalemia, 78
    Hypomagnesemia, 115, 118
    Liver, hepatic dysfunction, 479
    Metabolic alkalosis, 172
    Noninflammatory vascular
        diseases, 426
Spitzer-Weinstein syndrome, 254
Squamous cell carcinoma, 831
Steal syndrome, 785, 786
Stenosis
    Solitary kidney, 169
    Unilateral renal artery, 169
Stephen Johnson syndrome, 390
Steroids
    Acute renal failure, 502
    Embolic disease, 435
    Genitourinary tuberculosis, 390,
        392
    Gold nephrosis, 617
    Hypersensitivity during
        hemodialysis, 799
    IgA nephropathy, 345, 346
    Liver, hepatic dysfunction, 491
    Pregnancy, 517
    Psychotic episodes after
        transplantation, 721
    Sickle hemoglobinemia, 577
    Systemic lupus erythematosus,
        400
Streptococcal pharyngitis, 307, 308

Streptokinase, 322, 661
    Hemolytic uremic syndrome,
        445, 504–505
    Thrombosis, 783
Streptomycin, 622, 623
    Dialysis for removal, 642
    Genitourinary tuberculosis,
        387–391
    Infective endocarditis, 707
    Urinary tract infections, 353
Streptozotocin, 186, 537–539, 625
Strontium, dialysis for removal,
    642
Struvite stones, 139, 140, 155–156,
    359
    Dissolution of, 964
Subacute bacterial endocarditis,
    287
Subdural hematoma, 726
Succinocholine, 270
Succinylcholine, 52, 63, 270, 671
Sulfadiazine, 281
Sulfa drugs, acute renal failure, 292
Sulfamethoxazole, autosomal
    dominant polycystic kidney
    disease, 548
Sulfamylon, 281
Sulfinpyrazone
    Acute interstitial nephritis as
        result, 626
    Chronic hyperuricemic
        nephropathy, 472
    Goodpasture's syndrome, 339
Sulfisoxazole, 353, 356
Sulfonamides, 32, 626
    Acute interstitial nephritis as
        result, 626
    Acute renal failure, 287
    Acute renal vasculitis as result,
        615
    Asymptomatic bacteriuria, 497
    Dialysis for removal, 643
    Nephrotoxicity, 624, 628–629
    Reflux nephropathy, 377
    Urinary tract infections, 354,
        356, 358
Sulfonylureas, polyuria, 23
Sulindac, 615
Sulphate, 45–46
Suprofen, 469
    Renal ischemia as result, 615
Surgery
    Abdominal aortic aneurysm,
        286–287
    Acquired cystic disease, 561
    Acute renal failure, 502
    Amyloidosis, 463
    Anesthesia effect, 263
    Autosomal dominant polycystic

        kidney disease, 546, 547
    Bladder cancer, 602, 603
    Carpal tunnel syndrome, 729
    Cerebral hemorrhage, 726
    Consequences of, 263–264
    Diabetes mellitus (IDDM),
        539–541
    Dialysis access, 775–788
    Electrolyte abnormalities in
        perioperative period,
        267–274
    Fluid management in
        postoperative period, 266,
        267
    Genitourinary tuberculosis,
        391–393
    Hemolytic uremic syndrome,
        446
    Infective endocarditis, 708
    Intraoperative fluid
        management, 265–267
    Multicystic kidney, 560
    Obstructive uropathy in
        pregnancy, 505
    Prostatic cancer, 604–607
    Reconstructive, genitourinary
        tuberculosis, 392–393
    Reflux nephropathy, 377,
        380–381
    Renal cell carcinoma, 596
    Renal failure patients, 669–672
    Renal pelvic or ureteral
        carcinoma, 599
    Renal vein thrombosis, 436
    Simple cysts, 562
    Splenectomy, 874
    Thrombotic thrombocytopenic
        purpura, 449
    Volume disorders, 264–265
Surgical nephrectomy, end-stage
    renal disease and
    transplantation, 870
Surgical patient, fluid and
    electrolyte disorders,
    263–274
Swan Neck catheters, 756–758
Symptomatic bacteriuria, 349–350,
    351
Syndrome of hyporeninemic
    hypoaldosteronism (SHH),
    54, 55, 62–63
Syndrome of inappropriate ADH
    secretion (SIADH), 5, 7,
    23, 250, 268
    Hypomagnesemia, 273
    Treatment, 18
Synpharyngitic hematuria, 344
Systemic acidosis, acute renal
    failure, 298

Systemic diseases, end-stage renal
  disease and transplantation,
  870
Systemic lupus erythematosus
    (SLE), see also Lupus
    nephritis, 56, 287, 305, 333,
    395–405
  Atherosclerosis, 397
  Clinical features, 395
  Corticosteroid therapy, 395,
    399, 400
  Cytoxic drugs, 400–405
  Dietary management, 399
  Drug-induced, 616
  End-stage renal disease and
    transplantation, 870
  Fetal morbidity and mortality,
    398, 404–405
  Fluid and electrolyte disorder in
    children, 260
  Hypertension, 397, 404
  IgA nephropathy, 343–344
  Immunization, 397–398
  Infection, 397–398
  Maternal morbidity and
    mortality, 398
  Mortality, 395, 398
  Murine models of autoimmunity,
    398–400
  Nephritis-related complications,
    395–398
  Nephrotic syndrome, 319, 323,
    397
  Plasmapheresis, 402–403, 405
  Pregnancy, 398, 399, 404–405,
    516–518
  Proteinuria, 397, 405
  Renal insufficiency, 395–397
  Renal ischemia, 615
  Renal transplantation, 872, 908,
    923–924
  Renal tubular necrosis, 906
  Renal vein thrombosis, 435
  Serologic features, 395
  Therapy, 398–405
  Total lymphoid irradiation, 402
  Ultraviolet-light, 404
Systemic sclerosis (SS), pregnancy,
  518
Systemic vasculitis, 305

Tachyphylaxis, 38
Tachypnea, 247
  Hypernatremia, 11
Takayasu's arteritis, 413
Tamm-Horsfall proteinuria, 621
T-cell lymphoma, hypercalcemia,
  93

Tea-and-toast diet, 269
Temocillin, dialysis for removal,
  642
Tenckhoff peritoneal catheter,
  744, 748, 756, 787, 930
Terbutaline, 63
Testosterone, systemic lupus
  erythematosus, 399
Tetanus, 224
Tetany, 59, 96, 100, 133, 716
  Hypocalcemia, 256
  Hypokalemia, 252
  Neonatal, 260
  Uremic encephalopathy, 720
  Uric acid nephropathy, 470
Tetracyclines, 250, 356, 358, 615
  Acute renal failure, 287
  Asymptomatic bacteriuria, 497
  Dialysis for removal, 643
  Nephrotoxicity, 624
  Pregnancy, 504
  Reflux nephropathy, 377
Thalassemia, 101
Theophylline
  Dialysis for removal, 642
  Hemoperfusion for removal, 644
  Hypokalemia, 65, 66
  Plasma drug extraction ratios,
    645
  Serum concentrations for dialysis
    or hemoperfusion, 645
Therapeutic hyperthermia,
  hypophosphatemia, 274
Thermal burns, fluid and
  electrolyte disorders,
  277–282
Thiamine (B_1), 725
  Lactic acidosis, 184
  Magnesium, 113
Thiazides, 615
  Acute interstitial nephritis as
    result, 626
  Chronic hyponatremia, 6
  Diabetes mellitus (IDDM), 538
  Diuretic therapy, 27, 29–30,
    32–35, 38–40
  Hypercalcemia, 92, 94–96, 99,
    272
  Hypercalciuria, 144–146
  Hyperkalemia, 62–63
  Hyperkalemic periodic paralysis,
    51
  Hypertension, 427, 428
  Hyperuricosuria, 148, 149
  Hypocalcemia, 103
  Hypokalemia, 64, 71, 73, 77
  Hypomagnesemia, 115, 118
  Hyponatremia in surgical
    patient, 267

Medullary sponge kidney, 559
  Metabolic alkalosis, 170
  Noninflammatory vascular
    diseases, 426
  Preeclampsia, 512
  Reflux nephropathy, 379
  Renal tubular acidosis, 217
Thilopental, 671
Thiols, dialysis for removal, 643
Thiopental, hemoperfusion for
  removal, 644
Thiotexene, water clearance in
  hyponatremic psychotics, 4
Threshold for bicarbonate
  excretion, 188
Thrombocytopenia, 296, 815, 891
  Hypercalcemia, 98
Thrombocytopenic purpura, 848
Thrombocytosis, 270
Thrombosis, 10
  Dialysis access surgery, 778–780,
    782, 783, 785
  Membrane biocompatibility, 826
  Renal transplantation, 950
Thrombotic thrombocytopenic
    purpura (TTP), 443–449
  Acute renal failure, 286
  Clinical features, 443, 444,
    446–448
  Pathogenesis, 444, 448
  Pathology, 448
  Pregnancy, 446, 504
  Renal transplantation, 927
  Therapy, 448–449
Thromboxanes, 286, 297
Thromboxane synthetase
  inhibitors, 379, 380
Thyrocalcitonin, 166
Thyroidectomy, 271
Thyroparathyroidectomized
  (TPTX) animals, 166
Thyrotoxicosis, 78, 93, 99, 132
  Hypercalcemia, 272
Thyrotoxis, 848
Thyroxine, 623
Ticarcillin, 70
  Autosomal dominant polycystic
    kidney disease, 548
  Dialysis for removal, 642
Ticrynafen, 469
Tidal peritoneal dialysis (TPD),
  747
Timolol, hypertension, 427
Tin, dialysis for removal, 642
Tinidazole, dialysis for removal,
  643
Tissue hypoxia, 228, 237, 238
Tissue necrosis, 270
Titratable acid, 208

1006 Index

Tobramycin, 622–623
  Autosomal dominant polycystic kidney disease, 548
  Dialysis for removal, 642
  Infective endocarditis, 707
  Peritonitis, 764, 765
  Urinary tract infections, 353, 354, 356
Tocainide, dialysis for removal, 642
Tolbutamide, 616
  Polyuria, 22–23
Tolmetin, 615
  Acute interstitial nephritis as result, 626
Toluene, 620–621, 629–630
  Dialysis for removal, 643
  Hypokalemia, 66
Tonsillectomies, 345
Total lymph node irradiation (TLI), 896
  Allograft rejection, 889
Toxic nephropathy, see also specific topics, 613–631
  Acute interstitial nephritis, 626
  Acute renal failure, 618–626
  Acute renal vasculitis, 615
  Chronic interstitial nephritis, 626–628
  Diagnosis, 613
  End-stage renal disease and transplantation, 870
  Glomerulonephritis, 616–618
  Lesions, 614–630
  Nephrocalcinosis, 628–629
  Obstructive uropathy, 629
  Prevention, 630–631
  Renal ischemia, 614–615
  Renal tubular functional abnormalities, 629–630
  Renal vulnerability to toxins, 613, 614
  Syndromes, 614–630
  Treatment, 613–614
Toxic shock syndrome, 258
Toxoplasmosis, 730
Trace elements, 687–688, 727
Tracheal stenosis, 225
Transplantation, see Kidney, transplantation
Transurethral resection of the prostate (TURP), 9, 874
  Factor in acute hyponatremia, 4
Tranylcypromine, dialysis for removal, 642
Trauma, end-stage renal disease and transplantation, 870
Triameterene, acute glomerulonephritis syndrome, 309

Triampterine stones, 139
Triamterene, 27, 29, 31, 32, 35
  Hyperkalemia, 52, 56
  Hypertension, 427
  Hypokalemia, 78, 79
  Hypomagnesemia, 115, 118
  Noninflammatory vascular diseases, 426
Trichlomethiazide, hypertension, 427
Trichloroethanol hemoperfusion for removal, 644
Trichloroethylene, dialysis for removal, 643
Tricyclics, 642, 644
Trimethadione, 616
Trimethapan camsulate, hypertension, 430
Trimethoprim, 355, 356
  Autosomal dominant polycystic kidney disease, 548
  Reflux nephropathy, 377
Trimethoprim sulphamethoxazole, 891
  Reflux nephropathy, 376, 380
  Urinary tract infections, 353–356, 358
Tuberculosis, 140, 250, 874
  End-stage renal disease and transplantation, 870
  Renal transplantation, 869–870
  Simple cysts, 564
Tuberculous peritonitis, 764
Tubocurarine, 672
Tubular disorders, inherited, 581–589
Tubular dysfunction, 905–915
Tubular reabsorption of phosphorus (TRP), 95
Tubulointerstitial disease, 268, 270
Tumor lysis syndrome, 101, 153, 270, 470
  Hyperphosphatemia, 131
Tumors, 921
Tyrosinemia, 216, 587
Tyrosinosis, 215

Ultraviolet germicidal system, 766
Unilateral neonatal renal disease, 217
Unilateral sixth nerve palsy, 724
Untyped glycogen storage disease, 587
Uranium intoxication, 619
Urea nitrogen appearance (UNA), 676–677
  Continuous ambulatory peritoneal dialysis, 768

Uremia
  Acute glomerulonephritis syndrome, 305, 308, 310, 311, 312
  Anaesthesia, 667
  Anemia, 664–665
  Autonomic dysfunction, 723–724
  Calcium metabolism, 664
  Cardiovascular complications, 697–708
  Carnitine deficiency, 724
  Catabolism, 661
  Congestive heart failure, 660–661
  Conservative management, 662–667
  Contrast media nephrotoxicity, 661
  Detoxification therapy, 734–737
  Diabetics, 666–667
  Dietary protein restriction, 662–663
  Dietary sodium restriction, 662
  Drug dosage, 666
  Drug nephrotoxicity, 661
  Drugs used in, see also Drugs in uremia and dialysis, 853–865
  Fluid intake, 662
  Forearm veins, preservation of, 666
  Formation of idiogenic osmoles, 2
  Hypercalcemia, 662
  Hyperkalemia, 665
  Hyperlipidemia, 665–666
  Hypertension, 661, 663–664
  Hyperuricemia, 666
  Hypoalbuminemia, 678
  Metabolic acidosis, 665
  Neuropathy, 722–724
  Nutritional management, see also specific topics, 675–688
  Phosphorus metabolism, 664
  Pregnancy, 662
  Psychological complications, 721–722
  Psychological preparation, 666
  Psychological testing, 721–722
  Renal vein thrombosis, 661
  Social adjustment, 666
  Symptomatic therapy of neuromuscular symptoms, 666
  Toxic removal, 844–846
  Urinary tract infection, 660
  Urinary tract obstruction, 660
Uremic acidosis, 241

Uremic encephalopathy, 719–721
Uremic pericarditis, 669
Uremic polyneuropathy, 724
Ureter, carcinoma, 597–600
Ureterolithotomy, 140
Ureteropelvic junction obstruction, end-stage renal disease and transplantation, 870
Ureterosigmoid anastomosis, 216
Urethral carbuncle, 353
Urethral stricture disease, 874
Urethral syndrome, 354–355
Urethritis, 962
Uric acid nephrolithiasis, 473
Uric acid metabolism disorders, 655–656
Uric acid nephropathy, 469–472
Uric acid stones, 139–141, 147, 148, 153–155
  Autosomal dominant polycystic kidney disease, 548–550
  Dissolution of, 964
  Treatment, 154
Uricase, 471
Urinary fistulas, 957
Urinary incontinence, 956–957, 959, 963, 965
Urinary osmolarity, 10
Urinary retention, 956
Urinary tract catheterization, 955–966
  Antibacterial therapy, 961
  Aseptic, 960–961
  Closed urinary drainage system, 961
  External "condom" catheter drainage, 965
  Guidelines for management, 962
  Indications for, 956–957, 960
  Intermittent, 962–963
  Intermittent for vesicourethral dysfunction, 973
  Nephrostomy tubes, 963–964
  Prophylaxis of extraluminal bacterial migration, 960–961
  Sterile, 962–963
  Trauma and hematuria, 957
  Ureteral stents, 964–965
Urinary tract infections (UTI), 349–360, 496–498
  Acute pyelonephritis, 349, 350, 352–355, 358, 359
  Antibacterial therapy, 377
  Antibiotic therapy, 351–356, 358
  Asymptomatic bacteriuria, 349–351, 357–358
  Autosomal dominant polycystic kidney disease, 551, 556
  Calculi, 359
  Catheterization, 957–959
  Catheter-related, 955
  Chronic bacteriuria, 355–356
  Chronic pyelonephritis, 349, 352, 357–360
  Clinical patterns, 353–356
  Complications, 358–359
  Diabetes mellitus, 352, 353, 358–359
  Diagnosis, 350–351
  Diagnosis via catheterization, 958–959
  Fluid intake, 352
  Indwelling catheters, 356
  Multicystic kidney, 560
  Organisms responsible for, 349–351, 355
  Pain, 351–352
  Papillary necrosis, 359
  Perinephric abscess, 358–359
  Perirenal abscess, 352
  Pregnancy, 357–358
  Prevention of, 356–359
  Prophylactic therapy, 354, 359
  Prostatitis, 349, 355, 356
  Recurrent, 354
  Reflux nephropathy, 381
  Renal function alterations, 352–353
  Renal growth related, 375–376
  Renal transplantation, 912, 947
  Septicemia, 358
  Sequelae and complications, 960
  Sickle hemoglobinemia, 574
  Simple cysts, 564
  Symptomatic bacteriuria, 349–350, 351
  Urethral syndrome, 354–355
  Urinary pH alterations, 353, 354
  Vesicoureteral reflux (VUR), 356–357
  Volume depletion, 352
Urinary tract obstruction, 660
Urine ammonium, 178, 189–190
Urine calcium, 146
Urine magnesium, 152
Urine osmolal gap, 190
Urine osmolality, polyuria, 19–22
Urine osmolarity, 5, 7
  Hypernatremia, 10
Urokinase, 322, 661
Urolithiasis, pregnancy, 516, 519
Urosepsis, 963, 964, 965

Vaccines, hepatitis B infection, 488
VAD, 455
Vaginitis, 353, 358
Valium, 354
  Hypertension and pregnancy, 510
Valproic acid, dialysis for removal, 642
Vancomycin, 624, 757
  Dialysis for removal, 642
  Infective endocarditis, 707, 708
  Peritonitis, 764
  Urinary tract infections, 354
Varicella zoster virus, 948
Vascular access for extracorporeal therapy, 841–848
Vasculitis, 333, 335
  Acute renal failure, 286
  Atheroembolic disease, 435
  Cytotoxic drug therapy, 414–415, 416, 420
  Drug-related, 287
  End-stage renal failure, 417
  Methylprednisolone pulse therapy, 416, 420
  Nephrotic syndrome, 323
  Neuropathy, 723
  Plasma exchange therapy, 415, 418, 420
  Renal transplantation, 924–926
  Systemic, 288, 413–421, 463
  Systemic lupus erythematosus, 397
  Uric acid nephropathy, 471
Vasodilators, 7, 36, 429–430, 664
  Diabetes mellitus (IDDM), 538
  Hypertension, 427, 428
  Liver, hepatic dysfunction, 485
Vasopressin (ADH), 246
  Polyuria, 17–18
Vasopressinoic acid, chronic hyponatremia, 7
VBAP, 455
Vecuronium, 672
Ventilation, 190
  Alveolar, 223, 224, 228
  Acid-base disorders, 240
  Metabolic acidosis, 183
Ventilator therapy, 237
Verapamil, 63
  Autosomal dominant polycystic kidney disease, 549
  Hypertension, 428
Verotoxin-producing *E. coli* (VTEC), 443
Very low density lipoproteins (VLDL), 321
Vesicoureteral reflux (VUR), 363–381
  End-stage renal disease and transplantation, 870

Factors influencing segmental scar formation, 365
Functional deterioration, 372
Gender preference, 375
Presence in women, 381
Surgical correction, 377, 380–381
Treatment, 376
Urinary tract infections, 356–357
Voiding disorders, 369–371
Vesicourethral dysfunction, nonsurgical management, 969–972
　Alpha-adrenergic agonists, 972
　Alpha-adrenergic antagonists, 971–972
　Anticholinergic agents, 971
　Antispasmodics, 971
　Applied anatomy, 970
　Applied neurophysiology, 969–970
　Bladder training methods, 971–972
　Calcium antagonists, 972
　Emptying disorders, 972
　Intermittent catheterization, 973
　Parasympathomimetic drugs, 972
　Storage disorders, 972–973
　Treatment protocol, 970–972
Vinalbital, hemoperfusion for removal, 644
Vinblastine, nephrogenic diabetes insipidus, 21
Vincristine
　Multiple myeloma, 455, 456
　Thrombotic thrombocytopenic purpura, 449

Viomycin, 70, 624
Viral hepatitis, blood transfusions, 875
Viral infections, renal transplantation, 947–948
Vitamin A, 94, 255, 256, 687
Vitamin C, 724
Vitamin D
　Bicarbonate reabsorption, 163
　Deficiency, 258
　　Mineral metabolism disorders and chronic renal failure, 655
　　Renal tubular acidosis, 215, 216
　Extrarenal buffering, 166
　Fanconi syndrome, 459
　Intoxication, see Hypervitaminosis-D
　Magnesium metabolism, 113
　$1,25-(OH)_2$ vitamin D_3, 103, 142, 144
　　Intestinal calcium absorption, 802, 803
　1-alpha vitamin D_3, 103
Vitamin E, 687
Vitamins, 686–687
Vitiligo, 101
VMBCP, 455
VMCP, 455
Volume depletion syndrome (ECF), 281
Von Hippel-Landau syndrome, 593
Von Willebrand factor, 297
Von Willebrand's disease, 577

Waldenström's macroglobulinemia, 453, 458–459
　Cryoglobulinemias, 463
Warfarin, 327
　Embolic disease as complication, 435
　IgA nephropathy, 345, 346
　Mesangial proliferative glomerulonephritis, 345
　Reflux nephropathy, 372, 379, 380
Water balance, factors altering, 4
Water intoxication, 22, 23
Water treatment, for dialysis, 800–805
Water volume disorders, 246–249
Wegener's granulomatosis, 333, 413, 415, 416–418
　Renal transplantation, 924
Wernicke's encephalopathy, 725
Wiederheilm calculations, colloid osmotic pressure, 266
Williams syndrome, 255, 256
Wilm's tumors, 169, 520
Wilson's disease, 215, 587
Wound infections, 947

Xanthine stones, 139
Xylitol, 186

Y connectors, 766

Zinc, 687–688, 724
　Dialysis for removal, 642
Zomepirac, 615, 626

GPSR Compliance

The European Union's (EU) General Product Safety Regulation (GPSR) is a set of rules that requires consumer products to be safe and our obligations to ensure this.

If you have any concerns about our products, you can contact us on

ProductSafety@springernature.com

In case Publisher is established outside the EU, the EU authorized representative is:

Springer Nature Customer Service Center GmbH
Europaplatz 3
69115 Heidelberg, Germany

www.ingramcontent.com/pod-product-compliance
Lightning Source LLC
Chambersburg PA
CBHW082027260426
43749CB00057B/329